Be the Best
MyMAKit

Use the registration code below to gain access to this online study companion. This a a single source for all your student resources that support the textbook. By following the registration instructions below you will link to a wealth of opportunities to further your understanding of your course material. Use this website in conjunction with your textbook for a multidimensional learning experience. Enjoy!

STEP 1: Register

All you need to get started is a valid email address and the access code below. To register, simply:

1. Go to **www.mymakit.com**.
2. Click "**Students**" under "**First-time users.**"
3. Find the appropriate book cover. Cover must match the textbook edition being used for your class.
4. Click "**Register**" beside your book cover.
5. Read the **License Agreement** and **Private Policy**. If you accept, click "**I Accept.**"
6. Leave "**No**" selected under "**Do you have a Pearson account?**"
7. Using a coin scratch off the silver coating below to reveal your access code. Do not use a knife or other sharp object, which can damage the code.
8. Enter your access code in lowercase or uppercase, without the dashes.
9. Follow the on-screen instructions to complete registration.

During registration, you will establish a personal login name and password to use for logging into the Website. You will also be sent a registration confirmation email that contains your login name and password. Be sure to save this email.

Your Access Code is:

Note: If there is no silver foil covering the access code, it may already have been redeemed, and therefore may no longer be valid. In that case, you can purchase access online using a major credit card. To do so, go to www.mynursingkit.com. click "Students" under "First Time Users," find the cover of your textbook, then click "Buy Access," and follow the on-screen instructions.

STEP 2: Log in

1. Go to **www.mymakit.com** and click "**Students**" under "**Returning Users.**"
2. Find the appropriate book cover. Click on "**Login**" next to your book cover.
3. Enter the login name and password that you created during registration. If unsure of this information, refer to your registration confirmation email.
4. Click "**Login**."

Instructors

For premium-level access that includes testing and lecture support materials, please go to **www.mymakit.com** and click Request Access under the Instructors bar. You may also click on the Instructor Registration and Student Handout documents for additional information. For further assistance contact your local Pearson representative or call 800-852-4508

Got technical questions?

Customer Technical Support: To obtain support, please visit us online anytime at http://247pearsoned.custhelp.com where you can search our knowledgebase for common solutions, view product alerts, and review all options for additional assistance.

SITE REQUIREMENTS

For the latest updates on Site Requirements, go to www.mymakit.com. Click "**Students**" under "**Returning Users**". Pick your book and click "**Login**". Click on "**Need help**" at bottom of page for site requirements and other frequently asked questions.

Important: Please read the Subscription and End-User License agreement, accessible from the book website's login page, before using the *mymakit* website. By using the website, you indicate that you have read, understood, and accepted the terms of this agreement.

BRIEF CONTENTS

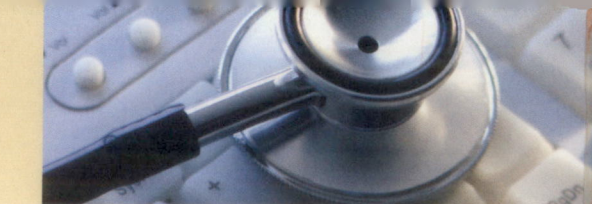

Unit I   **Introduction to the Medical Assisting Profession** 1

Chapter 1   The Medical Assistant Profession and the History of Healthcare 2

Chapter 2   Medical Assisting Today 19

Chapter 3   Professionalism in the Workplace 32

Chapter 4   Medical Law and Ethics 39

Chapter 5   Interpersonal Communication Skills 67

Chapter 6   Patient-Centered Care and Education 88

Chapter 7   Considerations of Extended Life 103

Unit II   **Administrative Responsibilities of the Medical Assistant** 115

Chapter 8   Written Communication 116

Chapter 9   Telephone Procedures 139

Chapter 10   Front Desk Reception 157

Chapter 11   Patient Scheduling 173

Unit III   **Managing Health Information in the Medical Office** 189

Chapter 12   Medical Records Management 190

Chapter 13   Electronic Medical Records 210

Chapter 14   Computers in the Medical Office 222

Unit IV   **Managing the Medical Office** 235

Chapter 15   Equipment, Maintenance, and Supply Inventory 236

Chapter 16   Office Policies and Procedures 248

Unit V   **Understanding Health Insurance: Billing and Coding Procedures** 259

Chapter 17   Insurance Billing and Authorizations 260

Chapter 18   ICD-9-CM Coding 321

Chapter 19   Procedural Coding 341

Unit VI   **Accounts Payable and Banking Procedures** 369

Chapter 20   Billing, Collections, and Credit 370

Unit VII   **Managing the Medical Office: Banking Procedures and Human Resources Management** 391

Chapter 21   Payroll, Accounts Payable, and Banking Procedures 392

Chapter 22   Managing the Medical Office 411

Unit VIII   **The Clinical Environment** 429

Chapter 23   The Clinical Environment and Safety in the Medical Office 430

Chapter 24   The Clinical Visit: Office Preparation and the Patient Encounter 444

Chapter 25   Medical Asepsis 458

Chapter 26   Surgical Asepsis 477

Chapter 27   Pharmacology and Medication Administration 502

Chapter 28   Vital Signs 540

Chapter 29   Minor Surgery 570

Unit IX   **Diagnostic Testing in the Medical Office** 595

Chapter 30   Diagnostic Procedures 596

Chapter 31   Microscopes and Microbiology 612

Chapter 32   Hematology and Chemistry 635

Unit X   **Medical Specialties and Testing** 673

Chapter 33   Urology and Nephrology 674

Chapter 34   Medical Imaging 711

Chapter 35   Cardiology and Cardiac Testing 729

Chapter 36   Pulmonology and Pulmonary Testing 769

Chapter 37   EENT 793

Chapter 38   Immunology and Allergies 823

Chapter 39   Dermatology 835

Chapter 40   Endocrinology 855

Chapter 41   Emergency Care 867

Chapter 42   Gastroenterology and Nutrition 914

Chapter 43   Orthopedics and Physical Therapy 949

Chapter 44   Obstetrics and Gynecology 983

Chapter 45   Pediatrics 1010

Chapter 46   Neurology 1036

Chapter 47   Mental Health 1054

Chapter 48   Oncology 1074

Chapter 49   Geriatrics 1086

Unit XI   **Nontraditional Medicine** 1097

Chapter 50   Alternative Medicine 1098

Unit XII   **Career Strategies** 1111

Chapter 51   Competing in the Job Market 1112

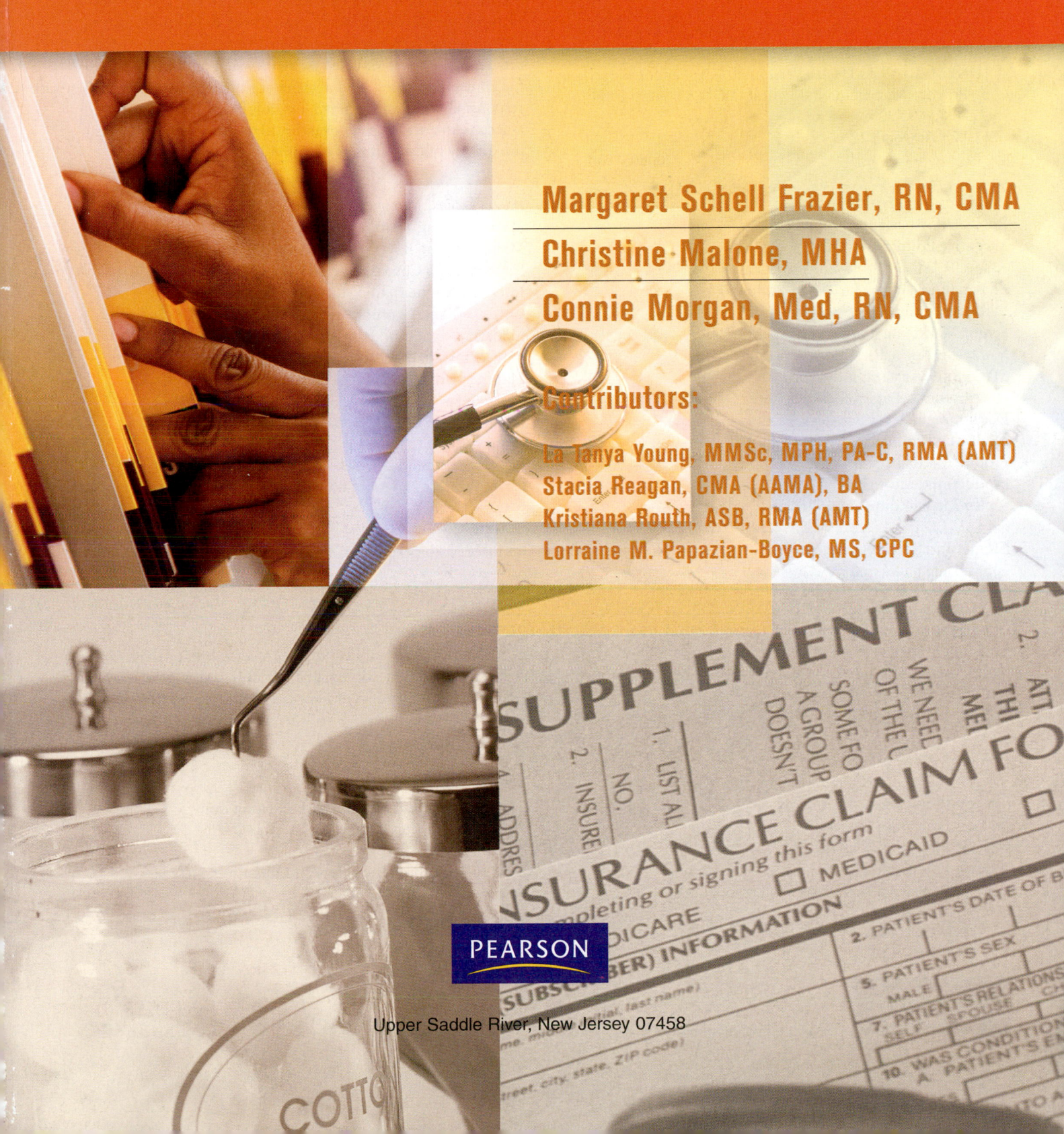

MEDICAL ASSISTING
Foundations and Practices

Margaret Schell Frazier, RN, CMA

Christine Malone, MHA

Connie Morgan, Med, RN, CMA

Contributors:

La Tanya Young, MMSc, MPH, PA-C, RMA (AMT)
Stacia Reagan, CMA (AAMA), BA
Kristiana Routh, ASB, RMA (AMT)
Lorraine M. Papazian-Boyce, MS, CPC

PEARSON

Upper Saddle River, New Jersey 07458

Library of Congress Cataloging-in-Publication Data

Frazier, Margaret Schell.
    Medical assisting : foundations and practices / Margaret
Schell Frazier, Christine Malone, Connie Morgan.
        p. ; cm.
    Includes bibliographical references and index.
    ISBN-13: 978-0-13-515058-0
    ISBN-10: 0-13-515058-2
    1. Medical assistants—Textbooks.   I. Malone, Christine.
    II. Morgan, Connie.   III. Title.
    [DNLM: 1. Allied Health Personnel.   2. Patient Care.
    3. Practice Management, Medical. W 21.5 F848m 2009]
    R728.8.F693 2009
    610.73'7069—dc22
                                            2008051933

Notice: The authors and the publisher of this volume have taken care that the information and technical recommendations contained herein are based on research and expert consultation, and are accurate and compatible with the standards generally accepted at the time of publication. Nevertheless, as new information becomes available, changes in clinical and technical practices become necessary. The reader is advised to carefully consult manufacturers' instructions and information material for all supplies and equipment before use, and to consult with a healthcare professional as necessary. This advice is especially important when using new supplies or equipment for clinical purposes. The authors and publisher disclaim all responsibility for any liability, loss, injury, or damage incurred as a consequence, directly or indirectly, of the use and application of any of the contents of this volume.

Publisher: Julie Levin Alexander
Publisher's Assistant: Regina Bruno
Executive Editor: Joan Gill
Associate Editor: Bronwen Glowacki
Editorial Assistant: Mary Ellen Ruitenberg
Director of Marketing: Karen Allman
Senior Marketing Manager: Harper Coles
Marketing Specialist: Michael Sirinides
Marketing Assistant: Judy Noh
Development: Triple SSS Press Media Development
Developmental Editor: Alexis Ferraro
Managing Production Editor: Patrick Walsh
Production Liaison: Julie Li
Production Editor: Karen Berry
Senior Media Editor: Amy Peltier

Media Project Manager: Rachel Collett
Manufacturing Manager: Ilene Sanford
Manufacturing Buyer: Pat Brown
Senior Design Coordinator: Maria Guglielmo
Interior Designer: Janice Bielawa
Cover Designer: Anthony Gemmellaro
Manager, Rights and Permissions: Zina Arabia
Manager, Visual Research: Beth Brenzel
Manager, Cover Visual Research and Permissions:
    Karen Sanatar
Image Permission Coordinator: Ang'john Ferreri
Composition: Laserwords
Printing and Binding: Webcrafters, Inc.
Cover Printer: Phoenix Color Corporation

Credits and acknowledgments borrowed from other sources and reproduced, with permission, in this textbook appear on the appropriate pages in text.

Pearson Education Ltd., London
Pearson Education Singapore, Pte. Ltd
Pearson Education, Canada, Inc.
Pearson Education—Japan
Pearson Education Australia PTY, Limited

Pearson Education North Asia Ltd, Hong Kong
Pearson Educación de Mexico, S.A. de C.V.
Pearson Education Malaysia, Pte. Ltd
Pearson Education, Inc., Upper Saddle River, New Jersey

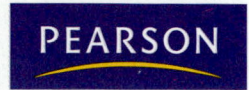

Prentice Hall
is an imprint of

www.pearsonhighered.com

10 9 8 7 6 5 4 3 2 1
ISBN-13: 978-0-13-515058-0
ISBN-10:   0-13-515058-2

To Dave, you are my strength, love and joy.

    I can never express the depth of my gratitude to you, my partner in life. Your patience, your encouragement, and your love carried me through the many toils and turmoil of writing this book. We also shared good times as we gathered information for the project. Without you at my side, I would have given up many times.

    To our grandchildren, you were so tolerant of the time I spent at the computer, at the libraries, and in general working on this project when I could have been spending time with you.

    To Dan Schell, my "little brother," and his wife Kathy. Thank you for all your help through the past and future years. You both are great.

Thanks.

Love, blessings and peace to all.

—Margie

To my Ian, whose life was a constant battle to improve the healthcare system for those who would come after him.

—Christine Malone

To my husband and children, you sacrificed family time and provided love and support for me to continue on this book.

    To my students and fellow educators, you are my lifelong inspiration to high standards for learning and teaching.

    To Margie, you are my loving, dedicated friend through all times and my encouragement for tenacity and endurance.

—Connie Morgan

CONTENTS

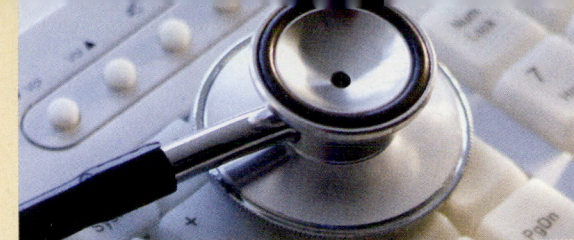

List of Procedures   xxvii
Preface   xxxiii
About the Authors   xxxv
Acknowledgments   xxxvii

Unit I   Introduction to the Medical Assisting Profession   1

Chapter 1   The Medical Assistant Profession and the History of Healthcare   2

Introduction   3
The Medical Assistant's Role in Healthcare   3
The History of Medicine   3
   Early Healing Practices   3
   Healing Based on the Supernatural   4
   Early Egyptian Medicine   4
   Early Chinese Medicine   4
   Early Native American Medicine   4
   Hippocrates and Early Contributors   4
The Beginning of Hand Washing in Healthcare   7
   Antisepsis Use in Healthcare   7
   The Medical Value of X-Rays   7
Important Organizations in Medical History   7
   The History of American Hospitals   8
   The History of the American Medical Association   8
   The Start of the American Red Cross   9
Important Women in Healthcare   9
   The Work of Marie Curie   9
   The Role of Florence Nightingale   9
   The Contributions of the Blackwell Sisters   10
The World Health Organization   10
Ethics and Patient Rights   10
   The American Hospital Association's Patient Bill of Rights (1973)   10
Professionalism   10
   Communication and Medical Terminology   12
   Physical Requirements   12
   Character   12
   Scope of Practice for Medical Assistants   12
Job Opportunities   13
Medical Assistant Educational Programs   13
Educational Requirements of Medical Assisting   13

Certification Examination   15
Multiple Medical-Assisting Statuses   15

Chapter 2   Medical Assisting Today   19

Introduction   20
The Medical Assistant's Role in Healthcare Today   20
The History of the Medical Assisting Profession   20
The Requirements of Other Allied Health Associations   21
   The American Medical Technologists (AMT)   21
   The American Academy of Professional Coders (AAPC)   22
   The American Health Information Management Association (AHIMA)   22
   The Association for Healthcare Documentation Integrity   22
Choosing Medical Assisting as a Career   22
   Understanding Medical-Assisting Responsibilities   22
   Identifying Positive Medical-Assisting Qualities   23
   Understanding the Medical Assistant's Role Outside the Office   25
Managing Time Effectively in the Medical Office   25
Procedure 2-1   Adapt to Change   25
Healthcare Team Members   26
   Physician   26
   Physician's Assistant   26
   Nurse Practitioner   26
   Nurse   26
   Pharmacist   26
   Other Healthcare Team Members   27
Medical Practice Specializations   28

Chapter 3   Professionalism in the Workplace   32

Introduction   33
The Medical Assistant's Role in Professionalism   33
What Is Professionalism?   33
   Characteristics of Professional Behavior   34
     Competence   34
     Honesty   34
     Compassion   34
     Respect for Others   35
     Responsibility   35
     Professional Demeanor   35
     Loyalty   35
     Attitude   35

Working Together as a Team 35
Prioritizing Tasks 36

Barriers to Professionalism 36
Bringing Personal Problems into the Workplace 36
Taking Care of Personal Business While at Work 36
Inappropriate Discussions in Front of Patients 36
Procrastination of Duties 36

Chapter 4   Medical Law and Ethics 39

Introduction 41

The Medical Assistant's Role in Medical Law and Ethics 42

The Sources of Law 42
Administrative Law 42
Comparing Public and Private Law 42
Criminal Law 42
Felonies 42
Misdemeanors 42
Civil Law 42
Tort Law 42

Understanding and Classifying Consent 43

Medical Malpractice 44
The Doctrine of *Respondeat Superior* 45
Types of Malpractice Insurance Policies 45

Procedure 4-1 ***Prepare an Informed Consent for Treatment Form*** 46
Proving Medical Malpractice 46
Medical Malpractice Awards 47
Preventing Medical Malpractice Claims 47
Defending Against Medical Malpractice Claims 47
The Statute of Limitations 48
Using Assumption of Risk as a Defense 48
Contributory and Comparative Negligence 48
Immunity from Negligence Suits 48
Res Judicata and *Res Ipsa* Locuitur 48
The Standard of Care 48

Tort Reform 48
Capping the Money Awarded to Injured Patients 48
Repeat Offender Providers 50

The Physician's Public Duties and Consequences 50
Reporting Vaccine Injuries 51
Reporting Cases of Abuse 51
Revoking Medical Licenses 52

The Physician-Patient Relationship 52
The Role of the Patient 52
The Role of the Physician 52

Contracts in Healthcare 52
Implied Contracts 52
Expressed Contracts 52
Terminating Contracts 53

The Good Samaritan Act 53

Maintaining Patient Confidentiality Through Proper Records Handling 53
Releasing Medical Records 53

Procedure 4-2 ***Obtain Authorization for the Release of Patient Medical Records*** 56
Accommodating Subpoenas of Medical Records 56
Disclosing Minors' Medical Information 56
Guarding Superprotected Medical Information 56

Procedure 4-3 ***Respond to a Request for Copies of a Patient's Medical Record*** 57
Faxing Medical Records 57
Disclosing Medical Records Improperly 57

The Health Insurance Portability and Accountability Act (HIPAA) 57
Title II of HIPAA 58
HIPAA and Computer Privacy 59
The HIPAA Privacy Officer 59
HIPAA Records Violations 59
The HIPAA Business Associate Agreement 59
Penalties for HIPAA Violations 60

Advance Directives 60

Employment Law and Healthcare 60
The Americans with Disabilities Act and Healthcare Employment 60
The ADA's Requirements 60

The Conscience Clause 62

The Patients' Bill of Rights 62

The Clinical Laboratory Improvement Amendments Act (CLIA) and Ambulatory Care 62

The Joint Commission on the Accreditation of Healthcare Organizations (JCAHO) and Ambulatory Care 62

Medical Ethics 62
Ethical Considerations 62
Ethical Model 63
Raising Ethical Issues in Healthcare 64

Bioethics 64

Chapter 5   Interpersonal Communication Skills 67

Introduction 69

The Medical Assistant's Role in Communication 69

Verbal Communication 69

Nonverbal Communication 70
Personal Space 70
Writing as a Means of Communication 71
Symbolic Language 71
Sign Language 71
Braille 71
Reading and Using Body Language 71

Eye Contact 73
Facial Expressions 73
Gestures 73
Posture 73
Therapeutic Touch 74
Demonstrating Active Listening 74
Interviewing the Patient 74
Employing Interviewing Techniques 74

Procedure 5-1 **Use Effective Listening Skills in Patient Interviews** 75
Identifying Factors That Hinder Communication 75
Communicating in Special Circumstances 75
Communicating with Physically Challenged Patients 75
Communicating with Hearing-Impaired Patients 76
Communicating with Sight-Impaired Patients 76
Communicating with Patients with Speech Impairments 76
Communicating with Patients via Interpreters 76

Procedure 5-2 **Communicate with a Hearing-Impaired Patient** 77
Communicating with Culturally Diverse Patients 77

Procedure 5-3 **Communicate with a Sight-Impaired Patient** 77

Procedure 5-4 **Communicate with a Patient via Interpreter** 78
Communicating with Mentally Ill Patients 78
Communicating with Angry or Distressed Patients 78
Communicating with Emotionally Challenged Patients 79
Communicating with Young Patients 79
Communicating with Geriatric Patients 79
Communicating with Grieving Patients 79
Maintaining Professional Patient Communication 80

Procedure 5-5 **Identify Community Resources** 81
Keeping a Professional Distance 81
Communicating with Coworkers 81
Communicating with Other Facilities 82
Developmental Stages of the Life Cycle and Their Impact on Communication 82

Procedure 5-6 **Prepare a Patient's Specialist Referral** 82
Maslow's Hierarchy of Human Needs 84
Defense Mechanisms 84

Chapter 6 **Patient-Centered Care and Education** 88

Introduction 90
The Medical Assistant's Role in Patient Education 90
Wellness 90
A Holistic Approach to Health Care 91
The Mind–Body Connection 91

Pain 91
Types of Pain 91
Physical Pain 91
Psychological Pain 91
Phantom Pain 92
Pain Assessment 92
Pain Management 93
Patient Teaching 94
Educating the Patient 94
Patient Miscommunication 95
Determining the Time Needed for Patient Education 95
Establishing a Proper Learning Environment 95
Teaching Resources 95
Patient Skills and Abilities 95
Culture and Patient Education 95
The Impact of Finances on Patient Education 96
Teaching Patients About Preventive Medicine 96
Preventing Medication Errors 96
Dieting and Weight-Loss Information 96
Information on Exercise 96
Stress Reduction 97
Smoking and Substance Abuse 97
Using the Internet for Education 98

Procedure 6-1 **Use the Internet to Find Patient Education Materials** 99

Chapter 7 **Considerations of Extended Life** 103

Introduction 104
The Medical Assistant's Role in Extended Life Care 105
Organ and Tissue Donations 105
Organ and Tissue Harvesting 105
Donation Issues and Concerns 105
Transplant Costs 107
Organ and Tissue Donation Rules and Regulations 107
Uniform Anatomical Gift Act 107
Hospitals 107
Advance Medical Directives 108
Durable Power of Attorney for Healthcare 108
Living Wills 108
Life-Prolonging Declarations 110
Hospice 111

Unit II **Administrative Responsibilities of the Medical Assistant** 115

Chapter 8 **Written Communication** 116
Introduction 118
The Medical Assistant's Role in Written Communications 118

Writing to Patients and Other Healthcare Professionals 118
    The Role of Spell-Checking 118
    Proper Spelling, Grammar, and Punctuation Use 118
    Sentence Structure 119
    Numbers in Correspondence 119
    Rules for Medical-Term Plurals 120

Components of the Business Letter 120
    Styles of Business Letters 123

Using Fonts in Typed Communication 123

Sending Letters to Patients 123

Proofreading 123

Working with Accepted Abbreviations 124

Creating Memos for the Office 126

Procedure 8-1   *Compose a Business Letter* 128

Mailing Written Communication 128

Procedure 8-2   *Prepare a Document for Photocopying* 128
    Window Envelopes 129

Procedure 8-3   *Send a Letter to a Patient About a Missed Appointment* 130
    Running and Resetting Postage Meters 130

Procedure 8-4   *Proofread Written Documents* 130
    Classifying Mail, Size Requirements, and Postage 131
    Buying Postage Online 133
    Using Multiline Optical Character Readers 133

Procedure 8-5   *Fold Documents for Window Envelopes* 133
    "ZIP + 4" Codes 134
    USPS-Approved Abbreviations in Addresses 134
    Restricted Materials 134
    Other Delivery Options 134

Using E-Mail to Communicate 135

Managing Mail and Correspondence 135
    Annotation 135

Procedure 8-6   *Open and Sort Mail* 136

Procedure 8-7   *Annotate Written Correspondence* 136

Chapter 9   Telephone Procedures 139

Introduction 141

The Medical Assistant's Role in Telephone Communications 141

Telephone System Features 141
    Making Calls with Hands-Free Devices 141
    Dialing Numbers Automatically 141
    Redialing Last Numbers Called 141
    Making Conference Calls 141
    Conversing via Speaker Telephone 142
    Call Forwarding 142

    Recording Telephone Calls 142
    Direct Telephone Lines 142
    Automatic Routing Units 142
    Placing Callers on Hold 142
    Other Special Features 143
    Using an Answering Service 143
    Using the Voicemail Feature 143

Patient Telephone Use 144

Answering the Telephone 144
    Screening Telephone Calls 144
    Directing Patient Calls to Physicians 144

Procedure 9-1   *Answer the Telephone in a Professional Manner* 145
    Prioritizing Telephone Calls 145
    Telephone Triage 146
    Taking Emergency Telephone Calls 146
    Being Professional on the Telephone 147
    Communicating with Hard-to-Understand Callers 148
    Handling Difficult Callers 148
    Receiving Calls from Emotional Patients 149
    Documenting Calls from Patients 149
    Taking Telephone Messages 149

Calling in Prescriptions and Refill Requests 149

Calling Patients 149

Procedure 9-2   *Take a Telephone Message* 151
    Leaving Messages 151
    Calling Other Healthcare Facilities 151

Using a Telephone Directory 152

Procedure 9-3   *Call a Pharmacy with Prescription Orders* 152
    Using an Online Directory 153
    Using a Rolodex System 153

Long Distance or Toll-Free Calls 153

Patient Confidentiality 153

Personal Telephone Calls 154

Telecommunication Relay Services 154

Chapter 10   Front Desk Reception 157

Introduction 158

The Medical Assistant's Role in Front Desk Reception 159

Characteristics of the Front Desk Receptionist 159

Opening the Office 159

Preparing Patient Files 159

HIPAA Compliance 159

Procedure 10-1   *Open the Office* 160

Greeting and Registering Patients 163
    Using Sign-in Sheets 163

Procedure 10-2   *Greet and Register Patients* 164
    Administering Patient Paperwork 164

Notifying Patients of Delays 165

Collecting Payments at the Front Desk 165

Escorting Patients 165

Managing Difficult Patients in the Reception Area 165

Procedure 10-3   *Collect Payments at the Front Desk* 167

Keeping Only Appropriate Patients in the Reception Area 167

Maintaining the Reception Room 167
    Providing Adequate Seating and Decoration 167
    Choosing Reading Material for the Reception Room 168
    Managing Children in the Reception Room 168
    Accommodating Patients with Disabilities 169
    Serving Patients with Service Animals 169

Caring for Patients as They Leave the Office 169

Closing the Office 169

Procedure 10-4   *Close the Office* 170

Chapter 11   Patient Scheduling   173

Introduction 175

The Medical Assistant's Role in Patient Scheduling 175

Scheduling New Patient Appointments 175
    New and Established Patients 176
    Allowing Appointments Adequate Time 177
    Creating an Appointment Matrix 177
    Balancing Patient and Office Needs in Scheduling 177
    Paper and Electronic Scheduling 177

Procedure 11-1   *Establish an Appointment Matrix* 178

Procedure 11-2   *Schedule New Patient* 179

Methods of Appointment Scheduling 179
    Cluster Scheduling 179
    Double Booking 179
    Fixed Appointment Scheduling 179
    Scheduling with Open Hours 179
    Wave Scheduling 179
        Modified Wave Scheduling 180
    Leaving Slack or Buffer Time 180
    Conducting Triage and Appointment Scheduling 180
    Using Appointment Reminder Systems 180

Procedure 11-3   *Schedule an Established Patient Appointment* 180

Correcting the Appointment Schedule 181

Documenting No-Show Appointments 181

Following Up on No-Show Appointments 181

Procedure 11-4   *Use Patient Reminder Cards* 181

Managing the Physician's Professional Schedule 183

Scheduling Hospital Services and Admissions 183

Procedure 11-5   *Reschedule a Missed Patient Appointment* 183

Procedure 11-6   *Manage the Physician's Professional Schedule and Travel* 184

Procedure 11-7   *Schedule a Hospital Procedure* 184

Procedure 11-8   *Schedule an Inpatient Admission* 185

    Specialty Referral Appointments 185

Arranging for Language Interpreters 185

Arranging Transportation for Patients 186

Achieving Efficiency in Scheduling 186

Unit III   Managing Health Information in the Medical Office   189

Chapter 12   Medical Records Management   190

Introduction 192

The Medical Assistant's Role in Medical Records Management 192

Information Contained in the Medical Record 192

The Purpose of the Medical Record 193

Signing Off on Medical Records 193

Procedure 12-1   *Prepare and Maintain the Medical Record* 195

Forms of Charting 196
    The Narrative Style 196
    Charting with SOAP 196
    Problem-Oriented Medical Record Charting 197
    Inserting Flow Charts in Medical Records 198
    Progress Notes 198

Using Abbreviations in Charting 199

Charting Patient Communication 199

Filing Systems 199
    Alphabetic Filing 199

Procedure 12-2   *Chart Patient Telephone Calls* 200

    Shingling Items for Medical Records 200
    Numeric Filing 200

Procedure 12-3   *File Documents Using the Alphabetic Filing System* 200

Procedure 12-4   *File Manually Using a Subject Filing System* 201

Procedure 12-5   *File Documents in Patient Medical Records* 202

File Storage Systems 202

Procedure 12-6   *Use the Numeric System to File Medical Records* 202

Active, Inactive, and Closed Patient Files 203

Converting Paper Records to Electronic Storage 203

Retaining Medical Records 204

Correcting Medical Records 204

Adding to Medical Records 205

Charting Conflicting Orders 205

"Owning" the Medical Record 205

Documenting Prescription Refill Requests 205

Procedure 12-7   *Correct Errors in the Patient Medical Record* 206

Releasing Medical Records 206

Releasing Information Whena Medical Practice Closes 207

Conducting Research with Medical Records 207

Chapter 13   Electronic Medical Records 210

Introduction 211

The Medical Assistant's Role in Using Electronic Medical Records 212

Electronic Medical Records Are Easily Accessible 212

How Does Paper Charting Differ from Electronic Charting? 212

Making the Conversion from Paper to Electronic Medical Records 213

   Training 213

Electronic Health Records and HIPAA Compliance 214

   Backing Up Computers and Electronic Medical Records 215

Using Personal Digital Assistants with Electronic Medical Records 216

Other Benefits of Electronic Medical Records 216

   Electronic Signatures 216

   Avoiding Medical Mistakes 216

   Saving Time 217

   Health Maintenance 218

   Using Electronic Medical Records with Diagnostic Equipment 218

   Marketing Purposes 218

   Communicating Between Staff Members 218

   Putting Medical Records Online 218

Procedure 13-1   *Correct an Electronic Medical Record* 219

Making Corrections in the Electronic Medical Record 219

Chapter 14   Computers in the Medical Office 222

Introduction 223

The Medical Assistant's Role in Computer Use in the Medical Office 224

Components of the Computer System 224

   Computer Hardware 224

     The Keyboard 224

     The Monitor 224

     The Computer Hard Drive 225

     Types of Computer Drives 225

     Computer Memory 225

     The Printer 225

   Surge Protection 226

   Backing Up Computer Systems 226

Computer Peripherals 226

   Scanners 226

   Digital Cameras 226

   Bar-Code Readers 226

   Electronic Sign-in Sheets 226

Maintaining Computer Equipment 227

Computer Software 227

Procedure 14-1   *Use Computer Software to Maintain Office Systems* 228

   Training Staff on Medical Software 228

   Types of Software Packages 228

Computer Security 228

   Computer Viruses 229

Internet Search Engines 229

Procedure 14-2   *Use an Internet Search Engine* 229

   Finding Appropriate Web Resources 230

Buying Medications Online 230

Procedure 14-3   *Verify Preferred Provider Status on an Insurance Company Web Site* 230

Allowing Personal Computer Use in the Office 231

Personal Digital Assistants 231

Computer Ergonomics 231

Unit IV   Managing the Medical Office 235

Chapter 15   Equipment, Maintenance, and Supply Inventory 236

Introduction 237

The Medical Assistant's Role in Equipment Maintenance and Supply Inventory 237

Working with Medical Office Equipment 238

   Training Employees to Use Medical Office Equipment 238

   Keeping a Maintenance Log for Medical Office Equipment 238

Replacing or Buying Medical Office Equipment 239

Weighing Equipment Leasing Against Buying 239

Using Fax Machines in the Medical Office 239

Procedure 15-1 *Take Inventory of Administrative and Clinical Equipment for Maintenance and Other Purposes* 239

Using Copy Machines in Healthcare Facilities 240

Adding Healthcare Data with Machines 240

Procedure 15-2 *Perform Routine Maintenance of a Computer Printer* 240

Medical Transcription 241

Finding Outside Transcription Services 241

Procedure 15-3 *Fax a Document* 241

Logging Medical Office Supplies 242

Inventorying Supplies 242

Checking for the Next Day's Supplies 243

Storing Supplies Upon Arrival 243

Procedure 15-4 *Prepare a Purchase Order* 243

Handling Drug Samples 244

Stocking Clerical Supplies 244

Tracking Supplies with Computer Software 244

Procedure 15-5 *Receive a Supply Shipment* 244

Chapter 16 Office Policies and Procedures 248

Introduction 249

The Medical Assistant's Role in Office Policies and Procedures 250

Creating Patient Information Pamphlets 250

Creating a Personnel Manual 250

Procedure 16-1 *Create an Office Brochure* 251

Creating Policies and Procedures for the Medical Office 251

Writing a Mission Statement 251

Preparing an Organisational Chart 251

Outlining Clinical Procedures 252

Procedure 16-2 *Create a Clinical Procedure for the Procedure Manual* 253

Outlining Administrative Procedures 253

Documenting Infection Control Procedures 253

Creating Quality Improvement and Risk Management Procedures 254

Writing Other Office Policies 254

Procedure 16-3 *Create an Administrative Procedure for the Procedure Manual* 254

Unit V Understanding Health Insurance: Billing and Coding Procedures 259

Chapter 17 Insurance Billing and Authorizations 260

Introduction 264

The Medical Assistant's Role in Insurance Claim Processing 264

The History of Health Insurance 265

Health Insurance Today 265

Health Insurance Terminology 265

Members and Their Families 266

Premiums 266

Fee Schedules and Approved Amounts 266

Deductibles 266

Copayments and Coinsurance 267

Stop Loss and Lifetime Maximum 267

Procedure 17-1 *Calculate Deductible, Coinsurance, and Allowable Amounts* 268

Waiting Period, Exclusions, and Pre-Existing Conditions 268

Private Health Insurance 269

Sources of Coverage 269

Group Insurance 269

Self-Insured Plan 269

COBRA Coverage 270

Individual Health Insurance Policies 270

Types of Plans 271

Fee-for-Service Plans 271

Managed Care Plans 271

Preferred Provider Organization (PPO) 271

Health Maintenance Organizations 272

Exclusive Provider Organizations 273

Point-of-Service (POS) Options 273

Consumer-Directed Healthcare Plans 273

Blue Cross/Blue Shield Plans 274

Other Related Benefits 274

Health Savings Accounts 274

Medical Savings Accounts 274

Flexible Spending Accounts 274

Third-Party Liability 275

Types of Coverage 276

Hospital 276

Medical 276

Surgical 276
Outpatient 276
Major Medical 276
Home Health Care 276
Catastrophic Health Insurance 276
Specialized Policies 276
Ancillary Coverage 276
   Prescription Drug Coverage 276
   Vision 277
   Dental 277
   Alternative Care 277

Government Insurance 278
Medicare Coverage 278
   The National Provider Identifier (NPI) 278
Medicare Part A 279
Medicare Part B 279
Medicare Part C: Advantage Plan 282
Medicare Part D 282
Medigap Plans 282
Medicare and Other Health Insurance (OHI) 282
Providers Participating in Medicare 282
Medicaid 283
   Covered Medicaid Services 284
State Children's Health Insurance Program
(SCHIP) 284
TRICARE 284
CHAMPVA 285

Worker's Compensation Insurance 285

Disability Insurance 286
Types of Disability Insurance 286
Definition of Disability 286
SSDI and SSI 286
The Medical Assistant's Role with Disability
Insurance 286

Reimbursement Methods 287

Processing Claims 287
Patient Registration 287
Verification of Benefits 289

Procedure 17-2   **Verify a Patient's Insurance
     Eligibility** 289
Determining Coordination of Benefits 290
Preparing Referrals, Authorizations, and
Precertifications 290
Documenting Insurance Company Calls 291

Health Insurance Claim Forms 291
The CMS-1500 Claim Form 291
Optical Character Recognition 291
Filing Timelines 300
Billing Insurance Companies Electronically 300

Procedure 17-3   **Obtain a Managed Care
     Referral** 303

Procedure 17-4   **Obtain Authorization from an
     Insurance Company for a
     Procedure** 303
Working with Fee Schedules 304
Charge-Based Fee Structure 304
Resource-Based Fee Structures 304
Medicare's Resource-Based Relative Value Scale 304
Posting Payments 305
Information on an EOB 305
Tracing Claims 307
Reconciling Payments and Rejections 307

Procedure 17-5   **Abstract Data to Complete a
     Paper CMS-1500 Claim Form** 308
Procedure 17-6   **Complete a computerized
     Insurance Claim Form** 314
Sending Supporting Documentation 314
Procedure 17-7   **Handle a Denied Insurance
     Claim** 315

The Office of the Insurance Commissioner 315
Projecting Health Insurance Costs in the Future 316

Chapter 18 ICD-9-CM Coding 321

Introduction 322
The Medical Assistant's Role in Diagnostic Coding 323
The History of Diagnostic Coding 323
Coding with the *ICD-9-CM* Book 324
The Volumes of ICD-9-CM 324
Volume II 324
Volume I 325
Supplementary Code Listings 325
ICD-9-CM Appendices 326
Volume III 326

Determining the Correct Diagnosis Code 326
Coding for Special Situations 331
Secondary Diagnoses 331

Procedure 18-1   **Perform Diagnostic Coding** 332
Combination Coding 332
Multiple Coding 332
Signs and Symptoms 332
Hypertension 332
Neoplasms 333
V codes 333
E codes 335
Poisonings and Adverse Effects 335
Coding for Fractures 336
Coding Burns 336
   Using the Rule of Nines in Coding Burns 336
Late Effects 337
Obstetrics 337

Diabetes 338

Inpatient Services 338

Pursuing Professional Certification 338

Chapter 19   Procedural Coding   341

Introduction 342

The Medical Assistant's Role in Procedural Coding 344

The History of Procedural Coding 344

Coding with the CPT-4 Manual 344

Fraud and Abuse 344

Organization of the CPT Manual 345

Tabular Index 345

Appendices 346

Alphabetical Index 346

Conventions and Symbols 346

Determining the Correct Procedure Code 346

Using CPT Modifiers* 353

Coding for Evaluation and Management Services 355

Coding for Special Situations* 359

Coding for Anesthesia 359

Procedure 19-1   Code for a Procedure   360

Coding for Surgery 360

Coding for Radiology 362

Coding for Pathology and Laboratory 363

Coding for Medicine 363

Unlisted Procedure Codes 364

The Health Care Common Procedure Coding System (HCPCS) 364

Ensuring Proper Reimbursement 365

Unit VI   Accounts Payable and Banking Procedures   369

Chapter 20   Billing, Collections, and Credit   370

Introduction 372

The Medical Assistant's Role in Billing, Collections, and Credit 372

Identifying Payment Basics 373

Manual Billing Systems 373

Computerized Billing Systems 373

Procedure 20-1   Post an Entry on a Day Sheet   374

Fee Schedules 374

Procedure 20-2   Prepare an Accounts Receivable Trial Balance   374

Participating Provider Agreements 375

Credit and Collections 375

Procedure 20-3   Explain Professional Fees to a Patient   376

Verifying Patient Identification 377

Managing Accounts Receivables 377

Collection in Managed Care 378

Forgiving Deductibles or Copayments 378

Procedure 20-4   Call a Patient Regarding an Overdue Account   378

Patients Who File for Bankruptcy 379

Professional Courtesy 379

Patient Billing Statements 379

Dismissing Patients Due to Nonpayment 380

Charging Interest on Medical Accounts 381

Addressing Checks That Fail to Clear 381

Procedure 20-5   Send a Patient Billing Statement   382

Contacting Nonpaying Patients 382

Sending Patients Collection Letters 382

Uncollectible Accounts 383

Collecting from Estates 384

Procedure 20-6   Post a Nonsufficient Funds Check   385

Overpaying on Accounts 385

Procedure 20-7   Post an Adjustment to a Patient Account   385

Procedure 20-8   Post a Collection Agency Payment   386

Procedure 20-9   Process a Patient Refund   386

Procedure 20-10   Process an Insurance Company Overpayment   387

Collections Through Small Claims Court 387

Unit VII   Managing the Medical Office: Banking Procedures and Human Resources Management   391

Chapter 21   Payroll, Accounts Payable, and Banking Procedures   392

Introduction 394

The Medical Assistant's Role in Payroll, Accounts Payable, and Banking Procedures 394

Processing Payroll 394

The History of Payroll 394

Present-Day Employment Issues 395
Payroll Processing 395
Creating New Employee Records 395
Updating Employee Records 395
The W-4 Form 397
Recording Employees' Work Hours 399
Calculating Payroll 399

Procedure 21-1 **Create a New Employee Record** 400

Employees Paid on an Hourly Basis 400
Salaried Employees 400
Computing Payroll Deductions 400
The Circular E 400
Other Deductions 400
Using Software to Calculate Payroll 401
Garnishing Wages 401

Accounts Payable 401
The Checkbook Register 402
Ordering and Receiving Supplies 404
Preparing a Deposit Slip 404

Procedure 21-2 **Calculate an Employee's Payroll** 405

Endorsement Stamps 405

Accessing Bank Accounts via the Internet 405

Procedure 21-3 **Write Checks to Pay Bills** 406

Petty Cash 406

Reconciling Bank Statements 406

Procedure 21-4 **Pay an Office Supply Invoice** 407
Procedure 21-5 **Complete a Deposit Slip** 407
Procedure 21-6 **Account for Petty Cash** 408
Procedure 21-7 **Reconcile a Bank Statement** 408

Chapter 22 **Managing the Medical Office** 411

Introduction 412

The Medical Assistant's Role in Managing the Medical Office 413

Characteristics of the Medical Office Manager 413

Responsibilities of the Office Manager 413

Leadership Styles 413

Conducting Effective Staff Meetings 414
Creating Staff Meeting Agendas 414
Staff Meeting Minutes 414

Staffing the Medical Office 415
Writing Job Descriptions 415
Creating Job Advertisements 415

Procedure 22-1 **Direct a Staff Meeting** 415
Recruiting and Interviewing Candidates 416
Avoiding Illegal Interview Questions 417

Procedure 22-2 **Write a Job Description** 417
Calling for Employment References 418
Hiring New Staff 418

Procedure 22-3 **Conduct an Interview** 419
Training New Staff 419
Supervising Staff 419

Overcoming Scheduling Issues 419

Procedure 22-4 **Call Employee References** 420

Performance Evaluations 420

Disciplining and Terminating Staff 420

Procedure 22-5 **Perform an Employee Evaluation** 421

Sexual Harrassment in the Medical Office 421

Procedure 22-6 **Discipline an Employee** 423

Employment Resources 423

Providing Employee References 423

Procedure 22-7 **Terminate an Employee** 423

Improving Quality and Managing Risk in the Medical Office 424
Creating a Quality Improvement Program 424
Working to Ensure Patient Safety 424
Reporting Office Incidents 425

Unit VIII **The Clinical Environment** 429

Chapter 23 **The Clinical Environment and Safety in the Medical Office** 430

Introduction 432

The Medical Assistant's Role in Office Safety 432

Personal Safety Measures 432
Body Mechanics 432

General Office Safety 432

Emergency Plans 434
Fire and Electrical Safety 434
Disasters 434
Workplace Violence 435
Workplace Security 435
Incident Reports 435

OSHA Bloodborne Pathogen Standards 436

Procedure 23-1 **File a Medical Incident Report** 436
Patient Safety 437

Exposure Control Plan 437
Standard Precautions and Infection Control Practices 437
Engineering and Work Practice Controls 437
Personal Protective Equipment 438

Procedure 23-2   Develop an Exposure Control Plan 439

Housekeeping and Laundry Decontamination 439
Hepatitis B Vaccinations 439
Hazard Communication Program 439
Training and Record Keeping 440
Exposure, Postexposure Evaluation, and Followup 441

Chapter 24   The Clinical Visit: Office Preparation and the Patient Encounter 444

Introduction 445
The Medical Assistant's Role in the Clinical Visit 446
The Standard Medical Office 446
Preparing and Maintaining Examination and Treatment Areas 447
Triage 447
Critically Ill or Severely Injured Patients 447
Consent 448
Charting the Medical History and Clinical Visit 449
Patient History 449
Personal History 449
Past Medical or Health History 449
Family Medical History 449
Chief Complaint 450
Present Illness 450
Assessment of Body Systems 450
Completing a Patient History Form 451
Charting a Clinical Visit 451

Procedure 24-1   Complete a Patient History Form 452

Charting Procedures 453
Documenting a Clinical Visit 453

Procedure 24-2   Document a Clinical Visit and Procedure 454

Chapter 25   Medical Asepsis 458

Introduction 459
The Medical Assistant's Role in Infection Control 460
The Cycle of Infection 460
Natural Defenses Against Infection 462
The Integumentary System 462
The Immune System 463
General Health 463
Other Natural Defenses 463
Asepsis and Infection Control 464
Occupational Safety and Health Administration (OSHA) 464
Centers for Disease Control and Prevention (CDC) 464

Infection Control Precautions 464
Personal Protective Equipment (PPE) 465
Hepatitis 465
Acquired Immunodeficiency Syndrome (AIDS) 467
Caring for the Patient with HIV/AIDS 469

Procedure 25-1   Perform Correct Handwashing 470

Latex Allergy 471

Procedure 25-2   Demonstrate Nonsterile Gloving 472

Education for the Patient or Health Professional 473

Chapter 26   Surgical Asepsis 477

Introduction 478
The Medical Assistant's Role in Surgical Asepsis 479
Surgical Asepsis 479
Sanitization, Disinfection, and Sterilization 479
Sanitization 479

Procedure 26-1   Demonstrate the Performance of Sanitization 480

Disinfection 481
Sodium Hypochlorite 482
Phenolics 482
Alcohol 482
Glutaraldehyde 482
Hydrogen Peroxide 482

Procedure 26-2   Demonstrate Disinfection Procedures 483

Sterilization 483
Autoclave Sterilization 483
Other Methods of Sterilization 484
Wrapping Instruments and Preparing Sterile Trays 485
Preparing the Surgical Field 485

Procedure 26-3   Demonstrate How to Wrap Surgical Instruments and Prepare Sterile Trays for Autoclave Sterilization 487

Procedure 26-4   Demonstrate Correct Procedure for Loading and Operating an Autoclave 488

Procedure 26-5   Demonstrate Correct Procedure for Pouring Sterile Solution onto a Sterile Field 489

Procedure 26-6   Demonstrate Correct Procedure for Opening a Sterile Surgical Pack to Create a Sterile Field 490

Procedure 26-7   Demonstrate the Correct Procedure for Using Transfer Forceps 492

Procedure 26-8   Demonstrate a Sterile Scrub (Surgical Hand Washing) 493

Alcohol-Based Hand Rubs 494

Procedure 26-9 Demonstrate How to Glove While Wearing Sterile Gown 496

Procedure 26-10 Demonstrate Sterile Gloving and Removal 497

Chapter 27 Pharmacology and Medication Administration 502

Introduction 504

The Medical Assistant's Role in Administering and Dispensing Drugs 504

Basic Pharmacology 505
    The General Effects of Drugs 506
    The Basic Functions of Drugs 506
    Prescription Versus Over-the-Counter Drugs 506
    Drug Nomenclature 506
    Drug Reference Sources 507
    Drug Classifications 507
    Controlled Substances 509

Medication Measurement and Conversion 512
    Dosage Calculation 512
        Metric and Household Systems of Measurement 514
        Calculating Pediatric Dosages by Body Weight 515

Safety Guidelines for Administering Medications 516

The Prescription 517

Procedure 27-1 Demonstrate Safety Measures to Prepare, Administer, and Document Medication 519
    Safeguarding Prescription Pads 519

Procedure 27-2 Demonstrate the Preparation of a Prescription for the Physician's Signature 520

Forms and Routes of Medication Administration 520
    Parenteral Administration 522
    Ampules and Vials 524

Procedure 27-3 Demonstrate Withdrawing Medication from an Ampule 525
    Intravenous Therapy 526

Procedure 27-4 Demonstrate Withdrawing Medication from a Vial 527

Procedure 27-5 Demonstrate the Reconstitution of a Powdered Drug for Injection Administration 529

Procedure 27-6 Demonstrate the Administration of Medication during Infusion Therapy 529

Procedure 27-7 Demonstrate the Preparation and Administration of Oral Medication 530

Procedure 27-8 Demonstrate the Administration of a Subcutaneous Injection 532

Procedure 27-9 Demonstrate the Administration of an Intramuscular Injection to Adults and Children 534

Procedure 27-10 Demonstrate the Administration of a Z-Track Injection 535

Chapter 28 Vital Signs 540

Introduction 541

The Medical Assistant's Role in the Initial Clinical Visit 542

Vital Signs Measurement 542
    Temperature 542
        Taking the Temperature 542
        Thermometers 544
    Pulse 544

Procedure 28-1 Obtain an Oral Temperature with an Electronic Digital Thermometer 544

Procedure 28-2 Obtain an Axillary Temperature with an Electronic Digital Thermometer 546

Procedure 28-3 Obtain a Rectal Temperature with an Electronic Digital Thermometer 547

Procedure 28-4 Obtain an Aural Temperature with a Tympanic Thermometer 548

Procedure 28-5 Obtain a Dermal Temperature with a Disposable Thermometer 549
    Respirations 550

Procedure 28-6 Perform a Radial Pulse Count 551

Procedure 28-7 Perform an Apical Pulse Count 552
    Blood Pressure 553

Procedure 28-8 Perform a Respiration Count 554
    Korotkoff Sounds 555
    Errors in Blood Pressure Readings 557

Weight and Height 557
    Weight 557

Procedure 28-9 Perform a Blood Pressure Measurement 557
    Height 559

Procedure 28-10 Obtain Weight and Height Measurements 559

Visual Acuity 561

Hearing Assessment 561

Preparing the Patient for a Physical Examination 561

Gowning   561
Draping   561
Positioning the Patient   561

Procedure 28-11   Demonstrate Patient Positions Used in a Medical Examination   563

Assessment Methods Used in an Examination   564
Assisting the Physician During the Examination   565
Recurrent Clinical Visits   566

Procedure 28-12   Prepare the Patient for Medical Examination and Assist the Physician   566

Chapter 29   Minor Surgery   570

Introduction   571

The Medical Assistant's Role in Office Surgery   572

Surgeries Performed in the Medical Office   572

Implied and Informed Consent   573

Preoperative Care and Patient Preparation   573
Setting Up the Room   574
Instruments   574
Clamping and Grasping   574
Cutting   575
Dilating, Probing, and Visualizing   576
Positioning and Draping   576

Procedure 29-1   Prepare the Skin for Surgical Procedure   577

Anesthesia   578
Local Anesthesia   579

Assisting During Minor Surgery   579

Procedure 29-2   Set Up a Sterile Tray and Assist the Physician with Minor Surgical Procedures   580

Sutures and Suture Removal   582
Suturing   583

Recovery/Postoperative Care   584

Procedure 29-3   Assist the Physician with Suturing   584

Procedure 29-4   Assist the Physician with Suture or Staple Removal   586

Patient Teaching and Dismissal   588
Wound Healing   588
Dressings and Bandages   589

Procedure 29-5   Change a Sterile Dressing   589

Unit IX   Diagnostic Testing in the Medical Office   595

Chapter 30   Diagnostic Procedures   596

Introduction   597

The Medical Assistant's Role in Diagnostic Testing   597

Clinical Laboratory Improvement Amendments (CLIA)   598
Waived Tests   598
PPMP Tests   598
Moderate-Complexity Tests   599
High-Complexity Tests   599
Quality Control and Quality Assurance   599

Procedure 30-1   Check the Accuracy of Glucometer Results Using Quality Control Methods   600

Regulations and Laboratory Safety   602
Joint Commission on the Accreditation of Healthcare Organizations   602
Safe Medical Devices Act   602

Hospital Laboratory Setting   602

The Physician Office Laboratory   603
POL Equipment   603
Centrifuge   603
Microscope   603
Electronic Equipment   604

Ordering Diagnostic Tests   604
The Physician's Order   604
In-House Ordering   605
Precertification   606
Precertification by Telephone   606
Scheduling with Outside Agencies   606
Screening and Follow Up of Test Results   606

Procedure 30-2   Screen and Follow Up Test Results   608

Chapter 31   Microscopes and Microbiology   612

Introduction   614

The Medical Assistant's Role in Specimen Collection   614

Microscopes   614
Types of Microscopes   614
Structure and Parts of a Microscope   614
Oculars   614
Objectives   615
Oil Immersion Objective   616
Arm and Focus Control   616
Light Source   616
Stage   616
Substage   616
Using the Microscope   616

Procedure 31-1   Demonstrate Correct Use of the Microscope   616

Microscope Maintenance   617

Microbiology   618

Scientific Nomenclature and Morphology 618
Normal Flora 618
Pathogens 619
  Bacteria 619
  Fungi 620
  Parasites 620
  Viruses 621

Preparing Specimens for Microscopic Examination 621
Preparing a Specimen Smear 621
Performing a Gram Stain 621
Preparing Wet Mounts 621
  Saline 621
  Potassium Hydroxide 621

Procedure 31-2 Prepare a Specimen Smear for Microbiological Examination 622

Procedure 31-3 Prepare a Gram Stain 623
  India Ink 624

Specimen Collection, Storage, and Transport 624
Collection of Stool Specimens 624
  Fecal Culture Testing for Ova, Parasites, and Other Infectious Organisms 624
  Fecal Occult Blood Testing 625
Culture and Sensitivity Testing 625

Procedure 31-4 Instruct a Patient in the Collection of a Fecal Specimen for Occult Blood or Culture Testing and Develop the Fecal Occult Blood Test 626

Procedure 31-5 Perform a Wound or Throat Culture Collection Using Sterile Swabs 628

Procedure 31-6 Perform Rapid Group A Strep Testing 630
  Performing a Wound or Throat Culture 630
Urine Cultures 631
  Storage and Transport of Urine Specimens 631

Chapter 32 Hematology and Chemistry 635

Introduction 637
The Medical Assistant's Role in Hematology and Chemistry 637
The Anatomy and Physiology of Blood 638
Plasma 638
Blood Cells 638
  Red Blood Cells 638
  White Blood Cells 638
  Platelets 639
Blood Cell Formation 639
Immunohematology 640

Blood Collection Equipment and Procedures 642
Tourniquets 642
Blood Collection Tubes 642
Order of Draw 642
Venipuncture 643
  Evacuated Tube 643
  Needle and Syringe 644
  Winged Infusion (Butterfly) 644
  Patient Reactions to Venipuncture 644

Procedure 32-1 Perform a Butterfly Draw Using a Hand Vein 645
Venipuncture Sites 646
Using the Evacuation System 646
  Verifying the Orders 646
  Obtaining Supplies 647
  Identifying the Patient 647
  Verifying Patient Preparation 648
  Proper Patient Care 648

Procedure 32-2 Perform a Venipuncture 648

Procedure 32-3 Demonstrate a Venipuncture Using the Syringe Method 650
  Capillary Puncture Collection 653
  Performing a Capillary Puncture 653

Procedure 32-4 Perform a Capillary Puncture 654
  Transporting Specimens 656

Performing Basic Laboratory Testing 656
Basics of Hematology Testing 657
Manual Tests 657
  Performing a WBC and Platelet Count with a Unopette Vial and Hematocytometer 657
  White Blood Cell Differential 657

Procedure 32-5 Perform a WBC and Platelet Count with a Unopette Vial and Hemacytometer 658

Procedure 32-6 Prepare a Blood Smear for a Differentiated Cell Count 659

Procedure 32-7 Prepare a Smear Stained with Wright's Stain 661
  Preparing a Blood Smear 662
  Manual Hematocrit 662
  Erythrocyte Sedimentation Rate 662

Procedure 32-8 Perform a Microhematocrit by Capillary Tube 662

Procedure 32-9 Perform a Hemoglobin Test Using a Hemoglobulinometer 664

Procedure 32-10 Perform an ESR Using the Westergren Method 664

Blood Chemistry Testing 665
Automated Chemistry Analyzers 665
  Measuring Blood Glucose 665

Procedure 32-11 **Measure Blood Glucose Using Accu-Chek™ Glucometer** 666

Procedure 32-12 **Perform a Blood Cholesterol Measurement Using the ProAct Testing Device** 667

Measuring Blood Cholesterol 668

Blood Typing and Grouping 669

Immunology Testing 669

Procedure 32-13 **Perform a Test for Infectious Mononucleosis** 669

Unit X   Medical Specialties and Testing 673

Chapter 33   Urology and Nephrology 674

Introduction 676

The Medical Assistant's Role in Urology and Nephrology 676

The Anatomy and Physiology of the Urinary System 677

Kidney Function 677

Nephrons 677

Urine Formation 678

Urinary System Infections 679

Renal Diseases 680

Dialysis 682

Neurogenic Bladder and Urinary Incontinence 683

Obstructive Conditions 683

Diagnostic Procedures 685

Urinalysis 685

Urinalysis Specimen Collection 685

Urine Containers 686

General Specimen Handling 687

Clean-Catch Urine Specimen Collection 687

Procedure 33-1 **Demonstrate Patient Instruction for a Clean-Catch Urine Specimen** 687

24-Hour Specimen Collection 688

Procedure 33-2 **Demonstrate Patient Instruction for Collection of 24-Hour Urine Specimen** 688

Specimen Collection by Catheterization 689

Physical Urinalysis 689

Procedure 33-3 **Perform Catheterization of a Female Patient** 690

Procedure 33-4 **Perform Catheterization of a Male Patient** 691

Appearance 693

Odor 694

Specific Gravity 694

Procedure 33-5 **Measure Urine Specific Gravity with a Refractometer** 694

Urinalysis with Chemical Test Strips 695

pH 696

Specific Gravity 696

Protein 696

Glucose 696

Ketones 697

Bilirubin and Urobilinogen 697

Blood 697

Leukocytes 697

Nitrite 697

Sediment Examination 698

Procedure 33-6 **Perform Urinalysis Using Chemical Test Strips** 698

Crystals 699

Procedure 33-7 **Perform a Multidrug Screen Urine Test Using the Instant-View Multi-Drug Screen Test** 701

The Male Reproductive System 701

Anatomy and Physiology 702

Penis 702

Scrotum 702

Internal Structures 703

Procedure 33-8 **Demonstrate Patient Instruction for Testicular Self-Examination** 703

Diseases and Disorders of the Male Reproductive System 704

Diseases and Disorders of the Prostate 704

Male Reproductive Disorders 704

Sexually Transmitted Diseases 706

Chapter 34   Medical Imaging 711

Introduction 712

The Medical Assistant's Role in Medical Imaging 712

Radiology 713

X-rays 713

Radiographs and Contrast Studies 713

Procedure 34-1 **Perform the General Procedure for an X-ray Examination** 714

Mammography 715

Angiography 715

Arthrography 716

Cholecystography 716

Fluoroscopy 717

Computed Tomography 717

Magnetic Resonance Imaging 717

Sonography 718

Nuclear Medicine 719

Equipment 719

Portable or Fluoroscopic Equipment 720

Safety Precautions and Patient Protection 720
   Radiation Shields 721
Limited-Scope Radiography 722
Scheduling Radiographs 722
Assisting with an X-ray 722
   Patient Preparation and Instructions 722
Preparation of the X-ray Room 722
   Terminology and Landmarks for Positioning 722
   Preparing a Patient for a Mammogram 722
   Preparing the Patient for Abdominal Contrast Studies 724
Filing and Loaning Radiographic Records 725
Procedure 34-2 **File and Loan Radiographic Records** 726

Chapter 35 Cardiology and Cardiac Testing 729

Introduction 732
The Medical Assistant's Role in Cardiology 732
Anatomy and Physiologyof the Heart 732
   Heart Conduction 733
Diseases and Disorders of the Heart 735
   Coronary Artery Disease 735
   Angina 735
   Myocardial Infarction 735
      Post-Myocardial Infarction 735
   Sudden Cardiac Arrest 735
   Hypertension/Hypertensive Heart Disease 736
   Congestive Heart Failure 736
   Pulmonary Edema 736
   Cardiomyopathy 737
   Arrhythmias 737
      Arrhythmias Resulting from Impulse Formation or Origin 737
      Arrhythmias Resulting from Conduction Disturbances 737
      Arrythmias Classified According to Consistency of Point of Origin 737
      Arrhythmias Classified According to Prognosis 737
      Treatment 738
   Infective Heart Disorders 738
      Endocarditis 738
      Myocarditis 739
      Pericarditis 739
      Rheumatic Fever and Rheumatic Heart Disease 739
   Valvular Disorders 739
   Vascular Disorders 740
      Phlebitis 740
      Thrombophlebitis 742
      Embolisms, Deep-Vein Thrombosis, and Thromboembolism 742

Arteriosclerosis and Atherosclerosis 742
Aneurysms 744
Raynaud's Disease 744
Buerger's Disease (Thromboangiitis Obliterans) 744
Diagnostic Tests 744
   Electrocardiogram 744
      Interpreting Waveforms on the ECG Tracing 746
      Artifacts 747
   Holter Monitor 749
Procedure 35-1 **Perform an Electrocardiogram** 750
Procedure 35-2 **Demonstrate the Application of a Holter Monitor** 753
   Stress Testing 755
   Echocardiogram 755
      Patient Preparation and Instructions 756
   Thallium Scan 756
   MUGA Scan 756
   Blood Studies 756
Identifying Arrhythmias/Dysrhythmias 756

Chapter 36 Pulmonology and Pulmonary Testing 769

Introduction 771
The Medical Assistant's Role in Pulmonology 771
The Anatomy and Physiology of the Pulmonary System 771
   The Upper Airway 771
   The Lower Airways 771
   Pulmonary Physiology 772
      The Mechanics of Gas Exchange 773
Diseases and Disorders of the Pulmonary System 773
   Lower Respiratory Obstructive Diseases 773
   Infectious and Inflammatory Conditions 775
   Malignancies 775
   Mechanical Insults 775
Pulmonary Assessment and Diagnosis 777
   Pulmonary Function and Other Common Diagnostic Testing 777
Procedure 36-1 **Demonstrate Performance of Spirometry** 780
      ABGs and Pulse Oximetry 781
      Peak Flow Testing 782
Procedure 36-2 **Demonstrate Performance of Measuring Oxygen Saturation Using a Pulse Oximeter** 782
      Mantoux Test 783
Procedure 36-3 **Demonstrate Performance of Peak Flow Testing** 784
Procedure 36-4 **Demonstrate Performance of the Mantoux Test by Intradermal Injection** 784
Inhalers and Nebulizers 786

Procedure 36-5 **Demonstrate Patient Instruction in the Use of an Inhaler** 787

Procedure 36-6 **Demonstrate Patient Instruction in the Use of a Nebulizer** 788

Oxygen Therapy 789
    Common Oxygen Therapy Equipment 790

Chapter 37 EENT 793

Introduction 795

The Medical Assistant's Role in an EENT Practice 795

The Anatomy and Physiology of the Eye 795
    Disorders and Diseases of the Eye 797
    Diagnostic Procedures 798
        Visual Acuity 798
        Color Blindness 801
    Eye Treatments 802

Procedure 37-1 **Measure Distance Visual Acuity with a Snellen Chart** 803

Procedure 37-2 **Perform the Ishihara Color Vision Test** 804

Procedure 37-3 **Perform Eye Irrigation** 804

Procedure 37-4 **Perform Instillation of Eye Medication** 806

The Anatomy and Physiology of the Ear 807
    Diseases and Disorders of the Ear 807
    Diagnostic Procedures 808
        Simple Audiometry 808
    Ear Treatments 808

Procedure 37-5 **Perform Simple Audiometry** 811

Procedure 37-6 **Perform Ear Irrigation** 812

Procedure 37-7 **Perform Instillation of Ear Medication** 813

The Anatomy and Physiology of the Nose 814
    Diseases and Disorders of the Nose and Nasal Passages 814
    Diagnosis and Treatment 815

The Anatomy and Physiology of the Throat 815

Procedure 37-8 **Assist with the Nasal Examination and Obtain Nasopharyngeal Specimen** 817

    Diseases of the Mouth and Throat 818
    Diagnosis and Treatment 818

Chapter 38 Immunology and Allergies 823

Introduction 824

The Medical Assistant's Role in Immunology and Allergy 824

The Anatomy and Physiology of the Immune System 825

Diseases and Disorders of the Immune System 827

Immunodeficiency Diseases 827
    HIV/AIDS Transmission Prevention Strategies 828
Autoimmune Diseases 828
Hypersensitivity and Allergic Reactions 831
    Diagnostic Procedures and Treatments 832

Chapter 39 Dermatology 835

Introduction 836

The Medical Assistant's Role in Dermatology 836

The Anatomy and Physiology of the Skin 837

Diseases and Disorders of the Skin 839
    Dermatitis 839
    Infectious Skin Disorders 841
    Fungal Skin Conditions 842
    Parasitic Skin Conditions 842
    Pigmentation Disorders 845
    Benign Neoplasms 845
    Cancerous Skin Disorders 846

Miscellaneous Integumentary Conditions 851

Cosmetic Treatment for Skin Conditions 852

Chapter 40 Endocrinology 855

Introduction 856

The Medical Assistant's Role in the Endocrinology Office 856

Anatomy and Physiology of the Endocrine System 857
    The Endocrine Glands 857

Endocrine Disorders 860
    Pituitary Gland Disorders 860
    Thyroid Gland Disorders 861
    Parathyroid Disorders 861
    Disorders of the Pancreas 861
    Adrenal Gland Disorders 863

Chapter 41 Emergency Care 867

Introduction 869

The Medical Assistant's Role in Emergencies 869

Emergency Resources 870
    EMS 870
    Good Samaritan Laws 870

Medical Office Preparedness 870
    Emergency Equipment and Supplies 870
        Crash Cart and Emergency Medical Box 870

Emergency Intervention 871
    Emergency Assessment 871
    OSHA Guidelines 873
    CPR, AED, and Obstructed Airway 874
        Airway 874

Breathing 876

Circulation 876

Defibrillation 876

Heimlich Maneuver 876

Procedure 41-1 **Perform Adult Rescue Breathing and One-Rescuer CPR** 878

Procedure 41-2 **Use an Automated External Defibrillator (AED)** 879

Chest Pain 881

Procedure 41-3 **Respond to an Adult with an Obstructed Airway** 882

Administering Nitroglycerin 883

Respiratory Distress 884

Shortness of Breath (SOB) 884

Hyperventilation 884

Procedure 41-4 **Administer Oxygen** 885

Chronic Obstructive Pulmonary Disease (COPD) 886

Pulmonary Edema 886

Shock and Anaphylactic Shock 886

Anaphylactic Shock 887

Assisting Patients in Shock 887

Bleeding 887

Pressure Points 888

Application of Direct Pressure 888

Internal Bleeding 888

Procedure 41-5 **Responding to a Patient Who Has Fainted** 888

Epistaxis 889

Open Wounds 889

Procedure 41-6 **Demonstrate the Application of a Pressure Bandage** 890

Abrasions 891

Avulsions and Amputations 891

Lacerations and Incisions 891

Puncture Wounds 892

Impaled Objects 892

Soft-Tissue Injuries 892

Traumatic Injury Emergencies 892

Procedure 41-7 **Demonstrate the Application of Triangular, Figure 8, and Tubular Bandages** 893

Pressure Bandages 895

Thermal Injuries: Integumentary and Systemic 895

Integumentary Insults: Burns 895

Frostbite 897

Heat Exhaustion 898

Hyperthermia 898

Hypothermia 898

Musculoskeletal Injuries 898

Fractures 899

Procedure 41-8 **Demonstrate the Application of a Splint** 900

Splint Application 901

Sprains, Strains, and Dislocations 901

Allergic Reactions 901

Neurological Emergencies 902

Decreased Level of Consciousness 902

Seizures 903

Cerebrovascular Accidents and Transient Ischemic Attacks 903

Head Injuries 904

Other Medical Emergencies 904

Acute Abdominal Pain 904

Diabetic Coma or Insulin Shock 905

Poisoning and Overdose 905

Poison Control Centers 906

Foreign Bodies in the Eye, Ear, and Nose 906

Psychosocial Emergencies 907

Domestic Violence 907

Sexual Abuse and Rape 907

Depression 907

Suicide 907

Rage 907

Alcohol Intoxication 907

Psychotic Behavior 907

Emergency Preparedness 908

Earthquakes 908

Fire 908

Floods 909

Hurricanes 909

Terrorism 909

Explosions 909

Biological Threats 909

Nuclear Blast 909

Mock-Environmental Exposures 909

Procedure 41-9 **Develop an Environmental Exposure Plan** 910

Chapter 42 Gastroenterology and Nutrition 914

Introduction 915

The Medical Assistant's Role in the Gastroenterology Office 916

The Anatomy and Physiology of the Gastrointestinal System 917

The Upper Gastrointestinal Tract (UGI) 917

Mouth 917

Teeth 918

Pharynx 919

Esophagus 919

Stomach 920

Duodenum 920

Lower Gastrointestinal Tract (LGI) 920

The Functions of the Gastrointestinal System 921

Diseases and Disorders of the GI Tract 922

Nutrition 927

The Food Guide Pyramid/MyPyramid Food Guidance System 931

How to Read a Food Label 932

Nutrition and Health 933

Factors That May Affect Caloric Intake 933

Obesity 934

The Effects of Alcohol on Nutrition 934

The Effects of Aging on Nutritional Status 935

Diseases and Disorders Involving Nutrition 935

Food Allergies and Food Intolerances 935

Diagnosis and Treatment of GI Disorders 936

Diagnostic Procedures 937

Colonoscopy 938

Procedure 42-1 **Assist with a Colon Endoscopic/Colonoscopy Exam** 939

Sigmoidoscopy 940

Rectal Suppositories 940

Patient Instruction in Nutrition 940

Procedure 42-2 **Assist with a Sigmoidoscopy** 942

Procedure 42-3 **Insert a Rectal Suppository** 944

Therapeutic Diets 944

Chapter 43 Orthopedics and Physical Therapy 949

Introduction 951

The Medical Assistant's Role in the Orthopedic Office 951

The Anatomy and Physiology of the Musculoskeletal System 952

Bones 952

Joints 954

Muscles 956

The Contraction of Muscle Cells 957

Common Musculoskeletal Diseases and Disorders 958

Neoplasia 961

Traumatic Musculoskeletal Conditions 961

Fractures 961

Other Traumatic Conditions 961

Amputation 962

Diagnostic Procedures 963

Treatment of Musculoskeletal Conditions in the Orthopedic Office 963

Splints and Braces 963

Casts 964

Cast Application 964

Procedure 43-1 **Assist with Fiberglass Cast Application** 965

Cast Removal 966

Physical Therapy Modalities 966

Procedure 43-2 **Assist with Cast Removal** 967

Thermodynamics 968

Ultrasonography 969

Assistive Aids for Ambulation 969

Crutches 969

Procedure 43-3 **Assist the Patient with Cold Application/Cold Compress** 970

Procedure 43-4 **Assist the Patient with Hot Moist Application/Hot Compress** 970

Procedure 43-5 **Assist with Therapeutic Ultrasonography** 971

Procedure 43-6 **Demonstrate Measuring for Axillary Crutches** 972

Canes 975

Walkers 975

Procedure 43-7 **Assist a Patient with Crutch Walking** 976

Procedure 43-8 **Assist a Patient in Using a Cane** 977

Prostheses 977

Procedure 43-9 **Assist a Patient in Using a Walker** 978

Body Mechanics 978

Procedure 43-10 **Assist a Patient in a Wheelchair to and from an Exam Table** 979

Chapter 44 Obstetrics and Gynecology 983

Introduction 985

The Medical Assistant's Role in the OB/GYN Office 985

The Anatomy and Physiology of the Female Reproductive System 985

Anatomy and Physiology of the Female Breast 987

The Menstrual Cycle 987

Menstrual Disorders 988

Contraception 988

Infertility 991

Pregnancy and the Birth Process 991

Delivery 992

Obstetrical History 992

Complications of Pregnancy 994

Procedure 44-1 **Assist with a Prenatal Exam** 994

Breastfeeding 996

Gynecological Diseases and Disorders 996

Assessing Vaginal Bleeding 996

Sexually Transmitted Diseases 998

Breast Disorders and Conditions 998

Procedure 44-2 **Instruct the Patient in Breast Self-Examination** 1000

Routine Assessment 1001

Diagnostic Procedures 1001

Procedure 44-3   *Assist the Physician in the Performance of a Pelvic Examination and Pap Test* 1001

Procedure 44-4   *Perform a Urine Pregnancy Test* 1004

Treatment Modalities 1004
   Cryosurgery 1005

Procedure 44-5   *Assist with Cryosurgery* 1005
   Psychological Considerations 1006

Chapter 45   Pediatrics 1010

Introduction 1011

The Medical Assistant's Role in Pediatrics 1012

Physical, Developmental, and Emotional Growth of a Child 1012
   Monitoring Growth Development 1012

Routine Visits (Well-Baby Checks) 1018
   Measuring Growth 1018

Procedure 45-1   *Perform and Record Measurements of Height or Length, Weight, and Head and Chest Circumference* 1018

Procedure 45-2   *Perform and Record Pediatric Vital Signs and Vision Screening* 1020
   Immunizations 1021

Procedure 45-3   *Perform Documentation of Immunizations, Both Stored and Administered* 1024
   Storing Vaccines 1025

Common Pediatric Diseases and Conditions 1025
   Common Contagious Diseases of Childhood 1025
   Congenital Neurological Disorders/Neural Tube Defects 1025
   Congenital Heart Conditions 1028
   Blood Disorders 1028
   Other Conditions 1029

Diagnostic Procedures 1029
   Positioning and Securing the Child for Examination and Treatment 1030
   Pediatric Urine Collection 1031

Procedure 45-4   *Perform Urine Collection with a Pediatric Urine Collection Bag* 1032

Chapter 46   Neurology 1036

Introduction 1038

The Medical Assistant's Role in Neurology and Neurosurgery 1038

The Anatomy and Physiology of the Nervous System 1038

The Central Nervous System 1039
The Peripheral Nervous System 1039
The Neuron 1040
Functions of the Nervous System 1041

Assessing the Neurological System 1041

Procedure 46-1   *Assist in a Neurological Exam* 1042
   The Glasgow Coma Scale 1043
   Lumbar Punctures 1043
   Electroencephalography 1043

Procedure 46-2   *Assist with a Lumbar Puncture* 1044

Procedure 46-3   *Prepare a Patient for an Electroencephalogram* 1045

Disorders and Diseases of the Central Nervous System 1045
   Cerebrovascular Accidents 1045
   Transient Ischemic Attack 1046
   Epilepsy 1046
   Amyotrophic Lateral Sclerosis 1047
   Parkinson's Disease 1047
   Multiple Sclerosis 1047
   Headache 1047
   Infectious Conditions of the Central Nervous System 1048
      Encephalitis 1048
      Meningitis 1048
      Brain Abscess 1048
   Brain Tumors 1049
   Head Trauma 1049
      Concussions and Contusions 1049
   Spinal Cord Injuries 1050
   Disk Disorders 1050

Diseases of the Peripheral Nervous System 1050
   Bell's Palsy 1050
   Trigeminal Neuralgia 1050
   Shingles (Herpes Zoster) 1051

Chapter 47   Mental Health 1054

Introduction 1055

The Medical Assistant's Role in the Mental Health Field 1056

The Anatomy and Physiology of Cognitive Functioning 1057

Mental Wellness 1058

General Mental Disorders 1058
   Schizophrenia 1058
   Mood Disorders 1059
      Major Depressive Disorder 1059
      Postpartum Depression 1062
      Seasonal Affective Disorder 1062
      Bipolar Disorder 1063
   Personality Disorders 1063

Anxiety Disorders   1063
   Generalized Anxiety Disorder and Panic Disorder   1064
   Phobic Disorder   1064
   Obsessive-Compulsive Disorder   1064
   Posttraumatic Stress Disorder   1064
Somatoform Disorders   1064
   Somatization Disorder   1064
   Conversion Disorder   1064
   Hypochondriasis   1065
   Factitious Disorders   1065
Gender Identity Disorder   1065
Mental Retardation   1066
Dementia   1066
   Alzheimer's Disease   1066
   Vascular Dementia   1066
   Dementia due to Head Trauma   1067
Mental Disorders Occurring During Childhood   1067
Substance-Related Disorders   1068
Assessment and Diagnosis   1070
Standard Treatments for Mental Disorders   1070

Chapter 48   Oncology   1074

Introduction   1075
The Medical Assistant's Role in the Oncology Practice   1076
The Classification and Physiology of Cancers   1076
Diagnostic Procedures   1077
   Routine Diagnostic Screening   1078
   Tumor Markers   1078
   Staging and Grading Malignant Tumors   1078
Cancer Treatment   1079
   Chemotherapy   1079
   Radiation   1080
   Surgery   1080
   Hormone Therapy and Immunotherapy   1081
   Side Effects of Cancer Treatment   1082
   Recent Developments in Cancer Treatment   1082
Hospice and Emotional Support   1082
The Cancer Prevention Lifestyle   1083

Chapter 49   Geriatrics   1086

Introduction   1087
The Medical Assistant's Role in the Geriatric Office   1088
The Aging Process   1088
   Physical Aspects of Aging   1088
   Social and Psychological Aspects of Aging   1089
   Nutritional Aspects of Aging   1090
   Economic Aspects of Aging   1090
***Procedure 49-1*   Role-Play Sensorimotor Changes
   of the Elderly**   1091
Cultural Views of Aging   1092
Promoting Health Among the Elderly   1093

Unit XI   Nontraditional Medicine   1097

Chapter 50   Alternative Medicine   1098

Introduction   1099
The Medical Assistant's Role in Alternative Medicine   1100
Complementary and Alternative Medical Systems   1100
Alternative Medicine   1100
   Ayurveda   1100
   Homeopathy   1100
   Naturopathy   1101
   Acupuncture   1101
Mind–Body Interventions   1101
   Biofeedback   1101
Integrative Medicine   1101
Biologically Based Therapies   1101
   Aromatherapy   1102
   Herbal Medicine   1102
Manipulative and Body-Based Methods   1102
   Hydrotherapy   1102
   Acupressure   1102
   Chiropractic   1103
   Craniosacral Therapy   1103
   Exercise   1103
   Reflexology   1103
   Massage   1104
      Lymphatic Massage   1104
      Sports Massage   1104
      Swedish Massage   1104
Energy Therapies   1105

Unit XII   Career Strategies   1111

Chapter 51   Competing in the Job Market   1112

Introduction   1113
The Medical Assistant's Role in Competing in the Job Market   1113
The Externship Experience   1114
   Understanding the Externship Site's Responsibilities   1114
   Outlining the Student's Responsibilities   1114
   The Responsibilities of the Medical Assisting Program   1114
Writing an Effective Resume   1114
Preparing a Cover Letter   1116
Identifying Places to Look for Employment   1116
***Procedure 51-1*   Write an Effective Resume**   1116
Completing Employment Applications   1117

Procedure 51-2   *Compose a Cover Letter* 1117

The Successful Interview 1120
    Preparing for the Interview 1120
    Dressing for the Interview 1120
    Presenting the Right Image 1121
    Following Up After the Interview 1121
Changing Jobs 1121

Procedure 51-3   *Follow Up with an Employer After an Interview* 1122

Appendix A: Correlation of Text to the General, Clinical, and Administrative Skills of the CMA (AAMA) 1125

Appendix B: Registered Medical Assistant (RMA) Medical Assisting Task List 1129

Appendix C: How to Become a Successful Student 1131

Appendix D: Preparing for the CMA (AAMA) and RMA (AMT) Certification Exams 1133

Appendix E: Translation of English–Spanish Phrases 1137

Appendix F: Normal Blood Values/Disease Conditions Evaluated for Abnormal Values 1139

Appendix G: Common Medical Abbreviations 1145

Appendix H: Medical Terminology Word Parts 1147

Appendix I: Answers to Chapter Case Study Critical Thinking Questions and In-Practice Scenarios 1159

Appendix J: Introduction to Medisoft Advanced (version 12) and Medisoft Simulation 1177

Glossary 1213
References 1239
Index 1241

LIST OF PROCEDURES

Chapter 2 **Medical Assisting Today** 19

Procedure 2-1 Adapt to Change 25

Chapter 4 **Medical Law and Ethics** 39

Procedure 4-1 Prepare an Informed Consent for Treatment Form 46

Procedure 4-2 Obtain Authorization for the Release of Patient Medical Records 56

Procedure 4-3 Respond to a Request for Copies of a Patient's Medical Record 57

Chapter 5 **Interpersonal Communication Skills** 67

Procedure 5-1 Use Effective Listening Skills in Patient Interviews 75

Procedure 5-2 Communicate with a Hearing-Impaired Patient 77

Procedure 5-3 Communicate with a Sight-Impaired Patient 77

Procedure 5-4 Communicate with a Patient via Interpreter 78

Procedure 5-5 Identify Community Resources 81

Procedure 5-6 Prepare a Patient's Specialist Referral 82

Chapter 6 **Patient-Centered Care and Education** 88

Procedure 6-1 Use the Internet to Find Patient Education Materials 99

Chapter 8 **Written Communication** 116

Procedure 8-1 Compose a Business Letter 128

Procedure 8-2 Prepare a Document for Photocopying 128

Procedure 8-3 Send a Letter to a Patient About a Missed Appointment 130

Procedure 8-4 Proofread Written Documents 130

Procedure 8-5 Fold Documents for Window Envelopes 133

Procedure 8-6 Open and Sort Mail 136

Procedure 8-7 Annotate Written Correspondence 136

Chapter 9 **Telephone Procedures** 139

Procedure 9-1 Answer the Telephone in a Professional Manner 145

Procedure 9-2 Take a Telephone Message 151

Procedure 9-3 Call a Pharmacy with Prescription Orders 152

Chapter 10 **Front Desk Reception** 157

Procedure 10-1 Open the Office 160

Procedure 10-2 Greet and Register Patients 164

Procedure 10-3 Collect Payments at the Front Desk 167

Procedure 10-4 Close the Office 170

Chapter 11 **Patient Scheduling** 173

Procedure 11-1 Establish an Appointment Matrix 178

Procedure 11-2 Schedule New Patient 179

Procedure 11-3 Schedule an Established Patient Appointment 180

Procedure 11-4 Use Patient Reminder Cards 181

Procedure 11-5 Reschedule a Missed Patient Appointment 183

Procedure 11-6 Manage the Physician's Professional Schedule and Travel 184

Procedure 11-7 Schedule a Hospital Procedure 184

Procedure 11-8 Schedule an Inpatient Admission 185

Chapter 12 **Medical Records Management** 190

Procedure 12-1 Prepare and Maintain the Medical Record 195

Procedure 12-2 Chart Patient Telephone Calls 200

Procedure 12-3 File Documents Using the Alphabetic Filing System 200

Procedure 12-4 File Manually Using a Subject Filing System 201

Procedure 12-5 File Documents in Patient Medical Records 202

Procedure 12-6   *Use the Numeric System to File Medical Records* 202

Procedure 12-7   *Correct Errors in the Patient Medical Record* 206

Chapter 13   Electronic Medical Records 210

Procedure 13-1   *Correct an Electronic Medical Record* 219

Chapter 14   Computers in the Medical Office 222

Procedure 14-1   *Use Computer Software to Maintain Office Systems* 228

Procedure 14-2   *Use an Internet Search Engine* 229

Procedure 14-3   *Verify Preferred Provider Status on an Insurance Company Web Site* 230

Chapter 15   Equipment, Maintenance, and Supply Inventory 236

Procedure 15-1   *Take Inventory of Administrative and Clinical Equipment for Maintenance and Other Purposes* 239

Procedure 15-2   *Perform Routine Maintenance of a Computer Printer* 240

Procedure 15-3   *Fax a Document* 241

Procedure 15-4   *Prepare a Purchase Order* 243

Procedure 15-5   *Receive a Supply Shipment* 244

Chapter 16   Office Policies and Procedures 248

Procedure 16-1   *Create an Office Brochure* 251

Procedure 16-2   *Create a Clinical Procedure for the Procedure Manual* 253

Procedure 16-3   *Create an Administrative Procedure for the Procedure Manual* 254

Chapter 17   Insurance Billing and Authorizations 260

Procedure 17-1   *Calculate Deductible, Coinsurance, and Allowable Amounts* 268

Procedure 17-2   *Verify a Patient's Insurance Eligibility* 289

Procedure 17-3   *Obtain a Managed Care Referral* 303

Procedure 17-4   *Obtain Authorization from an Insurance Company for a Procedure* 303

Procedure 17-5   *Abstract Data to Complete a Paper CMS-1500 Claim Form* 308

Procedure 17-6   *Complete a computerized Insurance Claim Form* 314

Procedure 17-7   *Handle a Denied Insurance Claim* 315

Chapter 18   ICD-9-CM Coding 321

Procedure 18-1   *Perform Diagnostic Coding* 332

Chapter 19   Procedural Coding 341

Procedure 19-1   *Code for a Procedure* 360

Chapter 20   Billing, Collections, and Credit 370

Procedure 20-1   *Post an Entry on a Day Sheet* 374

Procedure 20-2   *Prepare an Accounts Receivable Trial Balance* 374

Procedure 20-3   *Explain Professional Fees to a Patient* 376

Procedure 20-4   *Call a Patient Regarding an Overdue Account* 378

Procedure 20-5   *Send a Patient Billing Statement* 382

Procedure 20-6   *Post a Nonsufficient Funds Check* 385

Procedure 20-7   *Post an Adjustment to a Patient Account* 385

Procedure 20-8   *Post a Collection Agency Payment* 386

Procedure 20-9   *Process a Patient Refund* 386

Procedure 20-10   *Process an Insurance Company Overpayment* 387

Chapter 21   Payroll, Accounts Payable, and Banking Procedures 392

Procedure 21-1   *Create a New Employee Record* 400

Procedure 21-2   *Calculate an Employee's Payroll* 405

Procedure 21-3   *Write Checks to Pay Bills* 406

Procedure 21-4 **Pay an Office Supply Invoice** 407

Procedure 21-5 **Complete a Deposit Slip** 407

Procedure 21-6 **Account for Petty Cash** 408

Procedure 21-7 **Reconcile a Bank Statement** 408

Chapter 22 Managing the Medical Office 411

Procedure 22-1 **Direct a Staff Meeting** 415

Procedure 22-2 **Write a Job Description** 417

Procedure 22-3 **Conduct an Interview** 419

Procedure 22-4 **Call Employee References** 420

Procedure 22-5 **Perform an Employee Evaluation** 421

Procedure 22-6 **Discipline an Employee** 423

Procedure 22-7 **Terminate an Employee** 423

Chapter 23 The Clinical Environment and Safety in the Medical Office 430

Procedure 23-1 **File a Medical Incident Report** 436

Procedure 23-2 **Develop an Exposure Control Plan** 439

Chapter 24 The Clinical Visit: Office Preparation and the Patient Encounter 444

Procedure 24-1 **Complete a Patient History Form** 452

Procedure 24-2 **Document a Clinical Visit and Procedure** 454

Chapter 25 Medical Asepsis 458

Procedure 25-1 **Perform Correct Handwashing** 470

Procedure 25-2 **Demonstrate Nonsterile Gloving** 472

Chapter 26 Surgical Asepsis 477

Procedure 26-1 **Demonstrate the Performance of Sanitization** 480

Procedure 26-2 **Demonstrate Disinfection Procedures** 483

Procedure 26-3 **Demonstrate How to Wrap Surgical Instruments and Prepare Sterile Trays for Autoclave Sterilization** 487

Procedure 26-4 **Demonstrate Correct Procedure for Loading and Operating an Autoclave** 488

Procedure 26-5 **Demonstrate Correct Procedure for Pouring Sterile Solution onto a Sterile Field** 489

Procedure 26-6 **Demonstrate Correct Procedure for Opening a Sterile Surgical Pack to Create a Sterile Field** 490

Procedure 26-7 **Demonstrate the Correct Procedure for Using Transfer Forceps** 492

Procedure 26-8 **Demonstrate a Sterile Scrub (Surgical Hand Washing)** 493

Procedure 26-9 **Demonstrate How to Glove While Wearing a Sterile Gown** 496

Procedure 26-10 **Demonstrate Sterile Gloving and Removal** 497

Chapter 27 Pharmacology and Medication Administration 502

Procedure 27-1 **Demonstrate Safety Measures to Prepare, Administer, and Document Medication** 519

Procedure 27-2 **Demonstrate the Preparation of a Prescription for the Physician's Signature** 520

Procedure 27-3 **Demonstrate Withdrawing Medication from an Ampule** 525

Procedure 27-4 **Demonstrate Withdrawing Medication from a Vial** 527

Procedure 27-5 **Demonstrate the Reconstitution of a Powdered Drug for Injection Administration** 529

Procedure 27-6 **Demonstrate the Administration of Medication during Infusion Therapy** 529

Procedure 27-7 **Demonstrate the Preparation and Administration of Oral Medication** 530

Procedure 27-8 Demonstrate the Administration of a Subcutaneous Injection 532

Procedure 27-9 Demonstrate the Administration of an Intramuscular Injection to Adults and Children 534

Procedure 27-10 Demonstrate the Administration of a Z-Track Injection 535

Chapter 28 Vital Signs 540

Procedure 28-1 Obtain an Oral Temperature with an Electronic Digital Thermometer 544

Procedure 28-2 Obtain an Axillary Temperature with an Electronic Digital Thermometer 546

Procedure 28-3 Obtain a Rectal Temperature with an Electronic Digital Thermometer 547

Procedure 28-4 Obtain an Aural Temperature with a Tympanic Thermometer 548

Procedure 28-5 Obtain a Dermal Temperature with a Disposable Thermometer 549

Procedure 28-6 Perform a Radial Pulse Count 551

Procedure 28-7 Perform an Apical Pulse Count 552

Procedure 28-8 Perform a Respiration Count 554

Procedure 28-9 Perform a Blood Pressure Measurement 557

Procedure 28-10 Obtain Weight and Height Measurements 559

Procedure 28-11 Demonstrate Patient Positions Used in a Medical Examination 563

Procedure 28-12 Prepare the Patient for Medical Examination and Assist the Physician 566

Chapter 29 Minor Surgery 570

Procedure 29-1 Prepare the Skin for Surgical Procedure 577

Procedure 29-2 Set Up a Sterile Tray and Assist the Physician with Minor Surgical Procedures 580

Procedure 29-3 Assist the Physician with Suturing 584

Procedure 29-4 Assist the Physician with Suture or Staple Removal 586

Procedure 29-5 Change a Sterile Dressing 589

Chapter 30 Diagnostic Procedures 596

Procedure 30-1 Check the Accuracy of Glucometer Results Using Quality Control Methods 600

Procedure 30-2 Screen and Follow Up Test Results 608

Chapter 31 Microscopes and Microbiology 612

Procedure 31-1 Demonstrate Correct Use of the Microscope 616

Procedure 31-2 Prepare a Specimen Smear for Microbiological Examination 622

Procedure 31-3 Prepare a Gram Stain 623

Procedure 31-4 Instruct a Patient in the Collection of a Fecal Specimen for Occult Blood or Culture Testing and Develop the Fecal Occult Blood Test 626

Procedure 31-5 Perform a Wound or Throat Culture Collection Using Sterile Swabs 628

Procedure 31-6 Perform Rapid Group A Strep Testing 630

Chapter 32 Hematology and Chemistry 635

Procedure 32-1 Perform a Butterfly Draw Using a Hand Vein 645

Procedure 32-2 Perform a Venipuncture 648

Procedure 32-3 Demonstrate a Venipuncture Using the Syringe Method 650

Procedure 32-4 Perform a Capillary Puncture 654

Procedure 32-5 Perform a WBC and Platelet Count with a Unopette Vial and Hemacytometer 658

Procedure 32-6 Prepare a Blood Smear for a Differentiated Cell Count 659

Procedure 32-7 Prepare a Smear Stained with Wright's Stain 661

Procedure 32-8 Perform a Microhematocrit by Capillary Tube 662

Procedure 32-9 Perform a Hemoglobin Test Using a Hemoglobulinometer 664

Procedure 32-10 **Perform an ESR Using the Westergren Method** 664

Procedure 32-11 **Measure Blood Glucose Using Accu-Chek™ Glucometer** 666

Procedure 32-12 **Perform a Blood Cholesterol Measurement Using the ProAct Testing Device** 667

Procedure 32-13 **Perform a Test for Infectious Mononucleosis** 669

Chapter 33   Urology and Nephrology   674

Procedure 33-1 **Demonstrate Patient Instruction for a Clean-Catch Urine Specimen** 687

Procedure 33-2 **Demonstrate Patient Instruction for Collection of 24-Hour Urine Specimen** 688

Procedure 33-3 **Perform Catheterization of a Female Patient** 690

Procedure 33-4 **Perform Catheterization of a Male Patient** 691

Procedure 33-5 **Measure Urine Specific Gravity with a Refractometer** 694

Procedure 33-6 **Perform Urinalysis Using Chemical Test Strips** 698

Procedure 33-7 **Perform a Multidrug Screen Urine Test Using the Instant-View Multi-Drug Screen Test** 701

Procedure 33-8 **Demonstrate Patient Instruction for Testicular Self-Examination** 703

Chapter 34   Medical Imaging   711

Procedure 34-1 **Perform the General Procedure for an X-ray Examination** 714

Procedure 34-2 **File and Loan Radiographic Records** 726

Chapter 35   Cardiology and Cardiac Testing   729

Procedure 35-1 **Perform an Electrocardiogram** 750

Procedure 35-2 **Demonstrate the Application of a Holter Monitor** 753

Chapter 36   Pulmonology and Pulmonary Testing   769

Procedure 36-1 **Demonstrate Performance of Spirometry** 780

Procedure 36-2 **Demonstrate Performance of Measuring Oxygen Saturation Using a Pulse Oximeter** 782

Procedure 36-3 **Demonstrate Performance of Peak Flow Testing** 784

Procedure 36-4 **Demonstrate Performance of the Mantoux Test by Intradermal Injection** 784

Procedure 36-5 **Demonstrate Patient Instruction in the Use of an Inhaler** 787

Procedure 36-6 **Demonstrate Patient Instruction in the Use of a Nebulizer** 788

Chapter 37   EENT   793

Procedure 37-1 **Measure Distance Visual Acuity with a Snellen Chart** 803

Procedure 37-2 **Perform the Ishihara Color Vision Test** 804

Procedure 37-3 **Perform Eye Irrigation** 804

Procedure 37-4 **Perform Instillation of Eye Medication** 806

Procedure 37-5 **Perform Simple Audiometry** 811

Procedure 37-6 **Perform Ear Irrigation** 812

Procedure 37-7 **Perform Instillation of Ear Medication** 813

Procedure 37-8 **Assist with the Nasal Examination and Obtain Nasopharyngeal Specimen** 817

Chapter 41   Emergency Care   867

Procedure 41-1 **Perform Adult Rescue Breathing and One-Rescuer CPR** 878

Procedure 41-2 **Use an Automated External Defibrillator (AED)** 879

Procedure 41-3 **Respond to an Adult with an Obstructed Airway** 882

Procedure 41-4 **Administer Oxygen** 885

Procedure 41-5 **Responding to a Patient Who Has Fainted** 888

Procedure 41-6 **Demonstrate the Application of a Pressure Bandage** 890

Procedure 41-7 **Demonstrate the Application of Triangular, Figure 8, and Tubular Bandages** 893

Procedure 41-8 **Demonstrate the Application of a Splint** 900

Procedure 41-9 **Develop an Environmental Exposure Plan** 910

Chapter 42 Gastroenterology and Nutrition 914

Procedure 42-1 Assist with a Colon Endoscopic/Colonoscopy Exam 939

Procedure 42-2 Assist with a Sigmoidoscopy 942

Procedure 42-3 Insert a Rectal Suppository 944

Chapter 43 Orthopedics and Physical Therapy 949

Procedure 43-1 Assist with Fiberglass Cast Application 965

Procedure 43-2 Assist with Cast Removal 967

Procedure 43-3 Assist the Patient with Cold Application/Cold Compress 970

Procedure 43-4 Assist the Patient with Hot Moist Application/Hot Compress 970

Procedure 43-5 Assist with Therapeutic Ultrasonography 971

Procedure 43-6 Demonstrate Measuring for Axillary Crutches 972

Procedure 43-7 Assist a Patient with Crutch Walking 976

Procedure 43-8 Assist a Patient in Using a Cane 977

Procedure 43-9 Assist a Patient in Using a Walker 978

Procedure 43-10 Assist a Patient in a Wheelchair to and from an Exam Table 979

Chapter 44 Obstetrics and Gynecology 983

Procedure 44-1 Assist with a Prenatal Exam 994

Procedure 44-2 Instruct the Patient in Breast Self-Examination 1000

Procedure 44-3 Assist the Physician in the Performance of a Pelvic Examination and Pap Test 1001

Procedure 44-4 Perform a Urine Pregnancy Test 1004

Procedure 44-5 Assist with Cryosurgery 1005

Chapter 45 Pediatrics 1010

Procedure 45-1 Perform and Record Measurements of Height or Length, Weight, and Head and Chest Circumference 1018

Procedure 45-2 Perform and Record Pediatric Vital Signs and Vision Screening 1020

Procedure 45-3 Perform Documentation of Immunizations, Both Stored and Administered 1024

Procedure 45-4 Perform Urine Collection with a Pediatric Urine Collection Bag 1032

Chapter 46 Neurology 1036

Procedure 46-1 Assist in a Neurological Exam 1042

Procedure 46-2 Assist with a Lumbar Puncture 1044

Procedure 46-3 Prepare a Patient for an Electroencephalogram 1045

Chapter 49 Geriatrics 1086

Procedure 49-1 Role-Play Sensorimotor Changes of the Elderly 1091

Chapter 51 Competing in the Job Market 1112

Procedure 51-1 Write an Effective Resume 1116

Procedure 51-2 Compose a Cover Letter 1117

Procedure 51-3 Follow Up with an Employer After an Interview 1122

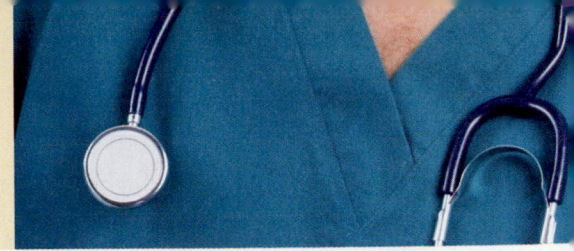

PREFACE

According to the U.S. Department of Labor statistics, medical assisting is one of the top ten fastest growing professions in the United States. This has been the trend for several years.

The increased employment opportunities for medical assistants in medical offices are in part a result of the nursing shortage. It is important to remember that nurses are trained to care for patients in the hospital, in bed. Many nurses now have specialized training in advanced care and are compensated according to their skills and time on the job. Medical assistants are trained in the care of ambulatory patients. Although working in the physician's office is the primary goal for employment, other options are available. Graduates find employment in clinics, pharmaceutical companies, insurance companies, medical laboratories, and in walk-in emergency and ambulatory care settings. Graduates should sit for the exams to become RMAs or CMAs, as the trend now is to hire credentialed assistants.

The Development of This Text

This unique text meets the highest standards outlined by CAAHEP and ABHES and provides all of the tools needed for student success. This comprehensive text can be used by both ABHES- and CAAHEP-accredited schools or those applying for accreditation to meet both content and competency requirements in the administrative and clinical areas.

This book presents a fresh approach to teaching medical assisting and includes the latest information on emergency preparedness, the electronic health record (an entire chapter is devoted to this important topic), and medical law and ethics. Our clinical chapters use a body systems approach. In this unique format, we include instruction of required clinical content and competencies in the body systems to which they apply. A discussion of anatomy and physiology is included in each of the body systems chapters and is an important tool for instructors who are unable to gauge the amount of anatomy and physiology a student has learned prior to the course or the level of the A&P course taken prior to enrollment. This, along with the medical terminology, can be used to reinforce the material in the rest of the chapter.

The material in this text is divided into twelve units. Unit 1 is an introduction to the medical assisting profession; Unit 2 delves into the administrative responsibilities of the medical assistant; Unit 3 focuses on managing health information in the medical office; Unit 4 highlights the area of managing the medical office; Unit 5 outlines understanding health insurance and billing and coding procedures; Unit 6 targets accounts payable and banking procedures; Unit 7 explores managing the medical office in the area of human resource management; Unit 8 considers the clinical environment; Unit 9 evaluates diagnostic testing in the medical office; Unit 10 focuses on medical specialties and testing; Unit 11 examines nontraditional medicine; and Unit 12 considers career strategies for the medical assistant.

Unique Features of This Text

- **CAAHEP and ABHES Entry-Level Standards:** Each chapter opens with a list of the CAAHEP and ABHES entry-level standards that are covered in the chapter. In addition, **Competency Skills Performance** boxes outline the procedures covered in each chapter.
- **Key terminology and abbreviations:** Terms and their definitions appear at the beginning of each chapter as well as in the narrative and comprehensive glossary. Phonetic pronunciations for difficult medical terminology are given in the comprehensive glossary.
- **MedMedia:** This link to the supplementary material available on the student CD describes the assets available to accompany each chapter (audio glossary, tips, legal and ethical scenarios, On the Job scenarios, HIPAA quizzes, multiple choice quizzes, and games)
- **Learning Objectives:** Specific learning objectives appear at the beginning of each chapter, stating what will be achieved upon successful completion of the chapter.
- **Case Studies with Critical Thinking Questions:** A thought-provoking case study is presented at the beginning of each chapter, with critical thinking questions interspersed throughout the chapter. Students must rely on the content in the text and their own critical thinking skills to answer the questions.
- **The Medical Assistant's Role:** Each chapter begins with a description of the medical assistant's specific role as it pertains to the content presented in the chapter.
- **HIPAA Compliance:** These feature boxes highlight the need-to-know law.
- **In Practice:** These real-life scenarios require students to pause and apply the knowledge presented in the chapter to answer critical thinking questions.
- **Keys to Success:** These are brief, helpful tips for professional success.
- **Concept Link:** This icon denotes reference to concepts presented in earlier or later chapters.
- **Competency Skills Performance:** Every procedure in the text includes the following main components to ensure student mastery of competencies: **Theory and Rationale; Materials; Competency** (includes **Task, Conditions,** and **Standard**), **Patient Education,** and **Charting Example.** Check-offs appear in the accompanying student workbook.
- **Anatomy and Physiology:** A discussion of anatomy and physiology is included in each of the body systems chapters, and is a great tool for instructors who need to gauge any student weakness in this area up front. Since instructors may not know the amount of A&P a student has learned prior to the course or the level of the A&P course taken previously, this, along with the medical terminology, should be used to reinforce the material in the rest of the chapter.

- **Informational Charts and Tables:** These appear throughout the text and summarize pertinent information for the reader. They provide students with visuals and comparisons to reinforce the lesson. In the specialty chapters they provide a quick reference for the disorders described in the chapter. Most tables include signs and symptoms, causes, diagnosis, and treatment. Students should refer to these tables for information not included in the text.
- **Color Photos and Illustrations:** These support the textual material presented and reinforce key concepts.
- **Chapter Summary:** The chapter summary is an excellent review of the chapter content and is often used for certification exams.

- **Chapter Review Questions:** End-of-chapter questions are provided in multiple-choice, true/false, short answer, and research format, and help reinforce learning. The review questions measure the students' understanding of the material presented in the chapter. These tools are available for use by the student or by the instructor as an outcomes assessment.
- **Externship Application:** This unique feature places the student in an externship site with a simulated situation the student may encounter.
- **Resource Guide:** This listing provides additional information (organization contact information, Web sites, etc.) related to chapter content.

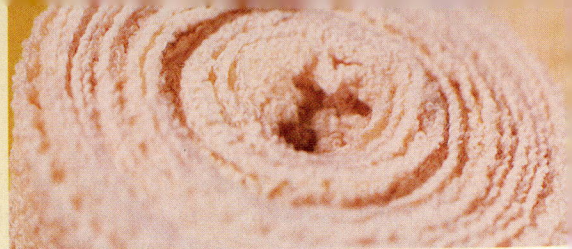

Margaret Schell Frazier, RN, CMA, B.S., studied nursing at Parkview Methodist School of Nursing, completing an ADN at Purdue University, then a B.S. in Health Sciences at St Francis University. She continued her formal education at Indiana State University, taking courses in technical education.

Margaret spent 13 years as an educator in the health careers field, specializing in medical assistant education. In addition to teaching mainly in medical assisting programs, she was assigned to curriculum development in pharmacology technology, physical therapy assistant, phlebotomy, massage therapy, EKG technician, and medical dictation. She also worked twice on the state-wide medical assisting curriculum review committee.

As an RN, she spent over 23 years at an intercity hospital working in maternal child health, including eight years in labor and delivery. She then transferred to the emergency department where she worked for over 15 years. This experience also afforded an opportunity to work in the ambulatory care center on weekends while teaching medical assisting classes. She also worked in the office of an ENT practitioner and in addition to office duties served as a private surgical scrub.

Margaret has been a member of AAMA since 1988 and a CMA during that time. She has served the organization at all three levels: local, state, and national. Her work has been published twice in the national professional journal, and she has published other books. She has presented at several national meetings in continuing education seminars. She is recognized by schools around the country as an expert in curriculum development and implementation.

Retirement from nursing and the teaching arena was not a retirement from the medical field. Margaret is president and consultant of M and M Consulting and still works in both areas of a physician's office, administrative and clinical. She spends many hours at her computer writing books and in her flower shop, Margie's Rose, where she relaxes while arranging flowers.

As early as she can remember, Margie (as she is known to her friends, students, and colleagues) has been interested in the medical field. She would read anything she could about medicine and still does. Her childhood neighbor was a physician, and he encouraged her, as did her father, to keep learning about medicine and to do her best in that field.

Margaret was married in 1957. She and her husband have four children, seven grandchildren, and one great-grandchild. They live on a small farm in rural northeast Indiana.

Christine Malone, BS, MHA, studied management practice and theory at Henry Cogswell College, receiving her B.S. in Professional Management. She continued her education at the University of Washington, obtaining her Master's Degree in Health Administration. Christine is currently working toward her Ph.D. in Business Administration with a Health Care focus.

Christine has over 20 years' experience in the healthcare field having spent time working as a dental assistant, a medical receptionist, an X-ray technician, medical clinic director, and as a consultant to healthcare providers, focusing on strategic management, efficient office flow, and human resource management. Since 2004, Christine has been teaching within the Health Professions Department at Everett Community College in Washington State. There she teaches Medical Office Management, Computer Applications in the Medical Office, Medical Practice Finances, Intercultural Communications in Healthcare, and Medical Law and Ethics. In 2006 Christine researched and developed a certificate program in Healthcare Risk Management. This series of three courses is offered via distance learning and provides the student who successfully completes the three courses a Certificate in Healthcare Risk Management.

Christine was elected to the Snohomish County Charter Review Commission, a 1-year position from 2005–2006. She is the co-chair of the Young Careerists Group within the Business and Professional Women's Association of Greater Everett, a member of the American College of Healthcare Executives (ACHE), a member of the Washington State Healthcare Executive Forum (WSHEF), a member of the American Society for Healthcare Risk Management (ASHRM), a member of the American College of Medical Practice Executives (ACMPE), and is active in healthcare politics on both a local and national level. Christine has been the guest speaker at various events on healthcare issues and in continuing education meetings across Washington State and has received her certification in vocational teaching, lean leader training in health care, as well as pediatric palliative care training.

Christine and her husband have five children and live in a 100-year-old home in Everett, Washington. In 1999, their third child, Ian, was injured due to medical negligence during his birth. Ian lived four and a half years before succumbing to his injuries in 2004. This was the genesis of Christine's work toward improving patient safety in healthcare. Her input has been sought by legislative committees, editorial boards, and many policy makers. A nationally recognized healthcare reform advocate, Christine has appeared on the *Today Show*, *NBC Nightly News*, *ABC Nightly News*, the CBC's *The National*, in *The New York Times*, *The Los Angeles Times*, and on *Salon.com*.

Connie Morgan, Med, RN, CMA, graduated from Indiana Wesleyan University in 1978 with a BS in Nursing and received RN licensure the same year. She was certified as a medical assistant in 1993 and remains current in skill level and certification. She went on to earn a master's degree in Education in 1995. Connie became "hooked" on teaching when she started assisting nursing students during their clinical rotation. In the years since, she has taught nursing students at St. Joseph's Diploma School of Nursing in Fort Wayne, Indiana, as well as the public; the general and clinical staff at Munising Memorial Hospital in Munising, Michigan; and medical assistant and practical nursing students at Ivy Tech Community College in Kokomo, Logansport, and Wabash, Indiana.

Connie has worked in a variety of clinical areas, including nursing homes and surgical, oncology, orthopedic, urology, obstetric, pediatric, intensive care, and ambulatory care settings as a nurse, and as a medical assistant in insurance, pediatric, and podiatry settings. In addition, she has worked to promote the medical assistant profession by maintaining membership in the American Association of Medical Assistants since 1993, serving as a CRB/CAAHEP surveyor since 1996, and editing articles for the magazine *Certified Medical Assistant* for the past few years. She continues to teach in the medical assistant program at Ivy Tech Community College.

ACKNOWLEDGMENTS

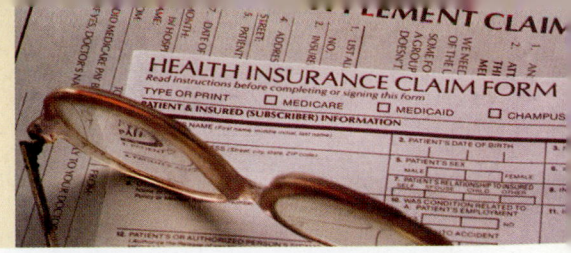

Many individuals played important roles in the concept, development, and final production of this unique, comprehensive medical assisting text. We would be remiss if we did not formally thank these wonderful people.

Our deepest gratitude goes to Julie Alexander, Publisher, for her confidence in the project and for her many astute observations and insightful comments at the very first "meeting of the minds." Her continued support as the project unfolded and continued is most appreciated. Joan Gill, our present executive editor, thanks. You have shown patience and have given us direction as the book approached completion. We would have never made it to the end without you.

Alexis Breen Ferraro, developmental editor, a big thanks for your constant pushing for material. Without that, we probably would have never made any deadlines. You had a very difficult job and brought everything together. Michel Heron, your photography is exceptional as usual, thanks for the fine job. Cindy Abel, thank you for providing your technical expertise and the direction necessary for the photos shot for the required illustrations.

A special thank you to Elizabeth Tinsley, who rewrote so much of the clinical content, and to Stacia Reagan, the book would not have been finished without you. You stepped in when we needed help and were most gracious about helping. Thank you to La Tanya Young for her insight and careful revision of the clinical chapters in preparation of this comprehensive text. There are many more individuals at Pearson we need to thank; however, it is impossible to remember all the names and titles. For anyone involved, a great big thank you. We thank the experts in their area who acted as contributing authors, James Thompson, Ph.D. MT (ASCP), and Christine E. Hollander, CMA (AAMA).

To others who have provided guidance and answers to so many questions, medical, technical, or otherwise, thank you. Dean Dauscher, MD, and Carolyn Dauscher, RN, you both were most kind and were always available to answer any medical question asked. Others who provided answers to medical questions or to technical questions about office forms, policies, or procedures include Carolyn Steinbacher, ORT; John Csisco, MD; Kimberly Weaver, RN, ADN; Mischelle Musser, RN, ADN; Jodie Inskeep, RN, AND; David Schlueter, MD; Eugenia Flucher, BSN, EdD; Bradley Boyd, MD; Mark Reecer, MD; and Jeffery Hudson, MD. Ronald Buskirk, St Joseph and Dupont Hospitals, you were readily available to answer technical questions about hospitals and compliance. Your help with providing forms was invaluable. Thank you.

Christine would like to extend a warm thank you to the staff of the Ka'anapali Beach Hotel in Maui, where much of the original draft was written. In addition, she'd like to thank her husband, Dylan, and children, Corey, Mallory, Molly, and Riley, for their patience while this project was completed.

Christine would also like to extend a special thank you to her students who have encouraged her throughout the process of writing this book., and to her colleagues at Everett Community College: Beth Adolphsen, CMA (AAMA); Karla Pouillon, RN, MEd; Julie Reiman, CMA (AAMA); and Francie Mooney, CMA (AAMA)—You have not only welcomed me into your midst, you have been immensely helpful in showing me the wonderful world of educating such a valuable member of the healthcare team: the medical assistant.

Reviewers

The authors and publisher wish to thank the following reviewers, all of whom provided valuable feedback and helped to shape the final text:

Cindy Abel, BS, CMA (AAMA), Pbt (ASCP)
Medical Assisting Program Chair/Assistant Professor
Ivy Tech Community College
Colorado Springs, CO

Kaye Acton, CMA (AAMA)
Department Head, Medical Assisting
Alamance Community College

Michaelann M. Allen, M.A. Ed., C.M.A. (AAMA)
Medical Assisting Program Coordinator/Instructor
North Seattle Community College
Seattle, WA

Kristen Anderson, R.N./B.S.N.
MA Instructor
Southwest Wisconsin Technical College
Fennimore, WI

Vanessa Armor
Instructor, Medical Assisting
Ivy Tech Community College of Indiana
Gary, IN
Warren, MI

Jennifer L. Barr, M.T., M.Ed., C.M.A. (AAMA)
Chairperson, Medical Assistant Technology
Sinclair Community College
Dayton, OH

Deborah J. Bedford, CMA (AAMA)
Program Coordinator/Instructor
North Seattle Community College

Tricia Berry, MATL, OTR/L
Director of Clinical Placement
School of Health Sciences
Kaplan University, FL

Kay E. Biggs, B.S., C.M.A. (AAMA)
Coordinator, Advisor Medical Assisting Technology
Columbus State Community College
Gahanna, OH

Sue Boulden, BSN, CMA (AAMA)
Mount Hood Community College

Janie Bowen
Alamance Community College

Jeannie Bower, B.S.
Instructor, Allied Health Department
Central Pennsylvania College
Camp Hill, PA

Rachel Bradshaw, AS, AA, AAS, CMA
 (AAMA)
Instructor, Medical Assisting
Western Piedmont Community
 College, NC

Charles Brown
Director of Career Services, MA
 Instructor
MedVance Institute
Eau Claire, WI

Mindy Brown, RMA (AMT)
Instructor, Medical Assisting
Pima Medical Institute, CO
Mooresville, NC

Susan Buboltz, RN, MS, CMA (AAMA)
Instructor and Co-director, Medical
 Assistant Program
Madison Area Technical College
Columbus, OH

Ginger Burleson, RN, CMA (AAMA)
Director, Medical Assistant Program
Northeast State Technical Community
 College

Kimberly Cannon
Guilford Technical Community College

Ellen Chiafolo
Medical Assisting Program Director
Keiser University, FL
Eugene, OR

Lisa L. Cook
MA Education Program Chair
Bryman College
Boca Raton, FL

Theresa Errante-Parrino, CMA (AAMA),
 EMT-P
Indian River Community College

Lorraine R. Fedorchak-Kraker, CMA-AC
Glen Oaks Community College

Janette Gallegos, RMA
Medical Assistant Instructor
Keiser College

Rebecca Gibson-Lee, M.S.T.E., C.M.A.
 (AAMA), A.S.P.T.
Professor/Program Director Medical
 Assisting Technology
The University of Akron
Akron, OH

Robyn Gohsman, A.A.S., R.M.A. (AMT),
 C.M.A.S.
Medical Assisting Program Director
Medical Careers Institute
Newport News, VA
Seattle, WA

Lisa M. Graese, C.M.T.
Instructor
Spokane Community College
Spokane, WA

Carol Hinricher
Program Director, Medical Information
 Technology
University of Montana College of
 Technology

Dolly R. Horton, C.M.A. (AAMA), B.S.,
 M.Ed.
Medical Assisting Coordinator
Mayland Community College
Spruce Pine, NC

DeAnn Knox, RN, BSN
Medical Assisting Instructor
Ivy Tech Community College, IN

Ann Kunze, BA, CMA (AAMA)
Instructor
Medical Careers Institute

Mary Marks, FNP-C, MSN, Pbt (ASCP)
Program Coordinator
Mitchell Community College
Norwalk, CT

Valerie Matson, BS, CLT
Adjunct Professor and Medical
 Technologist
Broome Community College
Newport News, VA

Nikki A. Marhefka
Medical Assisting Program Director
Central Pennsylvania College
Summerdale, PA

Deborah H. McCloskey, M.Ed., MT
 (AMT), CLS (NCA), CLT (HHS)
Program Director, Medical Assistant
 Program
Bluntville, TN

Natalie McBride
ICM School of Business and Medical
 Careers

DeLeesa Meashintubby
Medical Office Assistant/Health Records
 Technology Program Coordinator
Lane Community College

Aimee Michaelis
Lead Instructor
Pima Medical Institute, CO
Augusta, GA

Karen Minchella, PhD, CMA (AAMA)
Consultant/Faculty
Baker College
Macomb Community College
Fort Pierce, FL

Kinasha Myrick, CMA (AAMA), CAHI,
 BBA, MA
Medical Assisting/Billing and Coding
 Program Director
South Suburban College
Western School of Health and Business

Lisa Nagle, B.S.Ed., M.C.A.
Program Director, Medical Assisting
Augusta Technical College
Augusta, GA

Brigitte Niedzwiecki, RN, MSN
Medical Assistant Program Director
Chippewa Valley Technical College, WI

Mary S. Nichols, A.S., RMA (AMT)
Medical Assistant Program Manager
High-Tech Institute, CA

Deborah Odgaard
Medical Assistant Program
Des Moines Area Community College

Donna Patterson
Curriculum Manager
Corinthian Colleges, Inc., CA
Duquesne, PA

Lauren Perlstein, RN, MSN
Associate Professor, Medical Assistant
 Coordinator
Norwalk Community College
Gresham, OR

Stacia Reagan, CMA (AAMA), BA
Program Director
Spokane Community College, WA
Stuart, FL

Tiffany Rosta, CMA (AAMA)
Medical Assistant Instructor
ICM School of Business and Medical
    Careers
Pittsburgh, PA

Kristiana Routh, ASB, RMA (AMT)
Allied Health Consulting Services, PA

Sulea Rucker, C.M.A. (AAMA)
Division Manager
San Joaquin Valley College
Modesto, CA

Janet Sesser, RMA, CMA (AAMA), BSed
    Admin.
Corporate Director of Education
High-Tech Institute, Inc.
Phoenix, AZ

Lisa Schostek, BA, RMA (AMT), CPC,
    CAHI
Adjunct Faculty, Science and Health
    Division
Lakeland Community College

Lynn Slack, BS, CMA (AAMA)
Medical Programs Director
Kaplan Career Institute–ICM Campus, PA
Madison, WI

Judith D. Symons
McCann School of Business
Minersville, PA
Kalamazzo, MI

Jill M. Tarabula, MLS, CMA (AAMA)
Instructor
Bryant & Stratton College, NY

Cynthia J. Watkins, R.N., M.S.N.
Medical Assisting Program Director
Lorain County Community College
Lorain, OH

Kari Williams
Program Director, Medical Office
    Technology
Front Range Community College

Nancy S. Wright, RN BS CNOR
Instructor, School of Health Sciences
Virginia College
Port Orchard, WA

La Tanya Young, MMSc, MPH, PA-C,
    RMA (AMT)
Program Director, Assistant Professor
Clayton State University, GA
Lafayette, IN

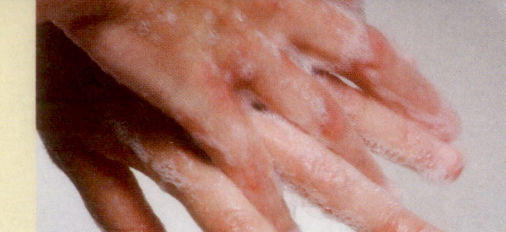

THE LEARNING PACKAGE

The Student Package

- Textbook

- Interactive CD ROM with exercises, learning games, skills review, medical office simulation for real-life application, skills videos, simulations, animations, resources, and audio glossary.

- Student Workbook that contains Chapter Outlines; Chapter Reviews; Learning Activities; Terminology Review; Critical Thinking Questions; Chapter Review Test, with Multiple Choice questions and additional True/False and Short Answer Questions; and Competency Check-Off Skill Sheets.

- CourseSmart eTextbook available for online purchase.

- MyMAKit is your key to student success. Use the code printed on the inside cover of this book to gain access to www. MyMAKit.com—the single source for all the resources that support this textbook!

The Instructional Package

- Instructor's Resource Guide with lesson plans, teaching tips, concepts for lecture, PowerPoint outline, suggestions for classroom activities, answers to all textbook and workbook questions; and sample syllabus.

- CD ROM with Test Gen and over 2,000 test questions, PowerPoint lecture slides, and Classroom Management software.

- Transition Guides to help make text implementation easy.

- MyMAKit is your key to instructor success. Ask your sales representative how you can gain access to this single source for all the instructor resources that support this textbook!

Chapter Opener Features

Case Study

Thought-provoking case studies provide scenarios that help students understand how the material presented in the chapter relates to the medical assisting profession.

Objectives

Each chapter opens with a list of learning objectives, which can be used to identify the material and skills the student show know upon successful completion of the chapter.

MedMedia

This link to the accompanying CD ROM and Companion Website provides a description of the many interactive resources available to supplement the content in each chapter.

Critical Thinking Questions

Critical thinking questions are interspersed within the body of the chapter, and students must rely on the content in the text and their own critical thinking skills to answer the questions.

CHAPTER **6**

Patient-Centered Care and Education

Case Study

Marina successfully passed her RMA exam and was excited to start her career as a medical assistant. After applying to several positions, she obtained employment with Dr. Gerard, a doctor of naturopathic medicine. Marina enjoys her work and loves teaching her patients about different approaches to a healthy lifestyle and effective stress and pain management.

After a particularly long, stressful morning, Marina takes her assigned break outside in the building's patio area. One of Marina's patients passes by and stops to say hello. His expression changes from one of happy recognition to one of confusion as Marina quickly extinguishes the cigarette she has been smoking. Suddenly feeling like a teenager caught by her parents doing something wrong, Marina forces a nervous smile as she greets her patient.

Objectives

After completing this chapter, you should be able to:

- Define and spell the key terminology in this chapter.
- Define the medical assistant's role in patient education.
- Define wellness.
- Discuss the holistic approach to healthcare.
- Explain the mind–body connection.
- Describe the types of pain, including physical, psychological, and phantom pain.
- Explain how pain is assessed.
- Describe different methods of pain management.
- Describe the factors the medical assistant must consider when facilitating an education program for patients.
- Describe how the medical assistant establishes a proper learning environment.
- Describe the types of information the medical assistant might provide the patient, including preventing medication errors, dieting and weight loss, exercise, stress reduction, smoking cessation, and substance abuse.
- Discuss the various teaching resources available in the medical office.

Med**Media**

http://www.MyMAKit.com

Additional interactive resources and activities for this chapter can be found on http://www.MyMAKit.com. For a video, tips, audio glossary, legal and ethical scenarios, on-the-job scenarios, quizzes, and games related to the content of this chapter, please access the accompanying CD-ROM in this book.

Video: *When English Is Not the Language*
Legal and Ethical Scenario: *Patient-Centered Care and Education*
On the Job Scenario: *Patient-Centered Care and Education*
Tips
Multiple Choice Quiz
Audio Glossary
HIPAA Quiz
Games: Spelling Bee, Crossword, and Strikeout

? Critical Thinking Question 6-1

In the case study, why do you think the patient looked confused when he noticed that Marina was smoking? Why do you think Marina felt guilty or uneasy about being seen by her patient while smoking? How would you feel if the person teaching you healthy habits and encouraging you did not follow his or her own advice?

Medical Assisting Standards

This boxed feature identifies the CAAHEP and ABHES Entry-Level Standards for the medical assistant that are discussed in each chapter. The CAAHEP standards are identified according to learning domain (cognitive, psychomotor, or affective).

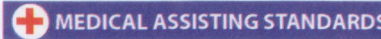

MEDICAL ASSISTING STANDARDS	
CAAHEP ENTRY-LEVEL STANDARDS	**ABHES ENTRY-LEVEL COMPETENCIES**
■ Perform within scope of practice (psychomotor) ■ Apply ethical behaviors, including honesty/integrity in performance of medical assisting practice (affective) ■ Discuss infection control procedures (cognitive) ■ Differentiate between medical and surgical asepsis used in ambulatory care settings, identifying when each is appropriate (cognitive) ■ Perform handwashing (psychomotor) ■ Prepare items for autoclaving (psychomotor) ■ Perform sterilization procedures (psychomotor) ■ Apply critical thinking skills in performing patient assessment and care (affective) ■ Assist physician with patient care (psychomotor)	■ Prepare patients for procedures. ■ Apply principles of aseptic techniques and infection control. ■ Prepare and maintain examination and treatment areas. ■ Prepare patient for and assist physician with routine and specialty examinations and treatments and minor office surgeries. ■ Use quality control. ■ Collect and process specimens. ■ Wrap items for autoclaving. ■ Perform sterilization techniques. ■ Dispose of biohazardous materials. ■ Practice Standard Precautions. ■ Operate and maintain facilities and equipment safely.

Medical Terminology and Abbreviations

Key Terminology

decontamination—use of physical means or chemical agents to remove, inactivate, or destroy pathogens on a surface or object to the point where they are no longer capable of transmitting infectious disease, thereby rendering the surface or object safe for handling, use, or disposal.

pathogen—disease-causing microorganism

Abbreviations

ADA—Americans with Disabilities Act

AIDS—acquired immunodeficiency syndrome

HBV—Hepatitis B virus

HIV—human immunodeficiency virus

MSDS—material safety data sheet

OSHA—Occupational Safety and Health Administration

The Medical Terminology and Abbreviations sections appear at the beginning of each chapter. The terms are listed in alphabetical order, a definition is provided, and the terminology appears in boldface on first introduction in the text. All terms are defined in the comprehensive glossary that appears at the back of the book, and phonetic pronunciations for difficult medical terminology are also provided.

Analyzing a Medical Term

You can often decipher the meaning of a medical term by breaking it down into its separate parts. Consider the following examples:

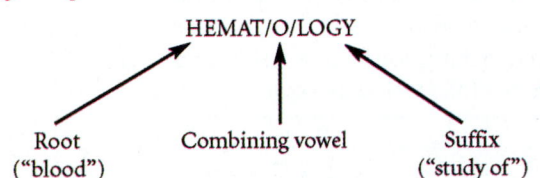

The text also features a separate appendix of Medical Terminology Word Parts, designed to help students analyze medical terms; understand word parts and word part guidelines; and define basic medical terms and terms used to describe major body systems, body direction, and diseases and disease conditions.

Additional Features

The Medical Assistant's Role

Each chapter begins with a description of the medical assistant's specific role as it pertains to the content presented in the chapter.

The Medical Assistant's Role in Office Safety

Medical assistants need to be aware of and trained in general and medical safety procedures. It is essential that MAS report any unsafe conditions to the proper person(s) immediately and follow all office safety rules. Following general and medical safety procedures will lower the potential for harm to employees and the public, and it will keep liability for injuries resulting from unsafe practices to a minimum.

Competency Skills Performance/ Procedures

This unique text meets the highest standards outlined by CAAHEP and ABHES, and provides all of the tools needed for student success. This comprehensive text can be used by both ABHES-and CAAHEP-accredited schools or those applying for accreditation to meet both content and competency requirements in the administrative and clinical areas.

A list of competencies appears at the beginning of each chapter in which procedures are presented. For each competency, Theory and Rationale are discussed, Required Materials are listed, and the procedure is presented in the proper format with the Conditions, Task, and Standards noted.

PROCEDURE 26-2 Demonstrate Disinfection Procedures

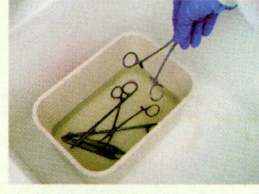

Theory and Rationale

All instruments to be sterilized must first undergo sanitization, then disinfection. When performed correctly, sanitization removes all organic materials and prepares instruments for effective disinfection. All organic material must be completely removed for the disinfectant to reach all areas of the article or instrument. Instruments must be dried thoroughly before they are placed in the disinfectant, as any water may dilute the chemical disinfectant.

Before proceeding with the disinfection of contaminated articles, the MA should read the MSDS for the disinfectant and look for general information regarding potential hazards, how to clean accidental spills, and which PPE to wear. Disposable gloves serve as a protective barrier against potentially infectious materials or contaminated instruments such as blood or body tissue. Additional utility gloves protect the skin from the irritating chemicals used for disinfection. Before moving the basin containing the contaminated instruments to another room, the MA should cover it with a cotton towel.

Materials

- Contaminated articles
- MSDS
- Disposable gloves
- Utility gloves
- Chemical disinfectant
- Soaking container
- Paper towels
- Cotton towel

Competency

(**Conditions**) With the necessary supplies, (**Task**) you will be able to perform the steps of disinfection (**Standards**) correctly and safely.

1. Review the MSDS, noting potential hazards, how to clean accidental spills, and whether PPE should be worn.
2. Apply disposable gloves to place the contaminated items into the basin. Then apply an additional layer of utility gloves.
3. Complete the sanitizing steps in Procedure 26-1. Remember to cover the basin of contaminated instruments with a cloth towel when you move them to the cleaning area.
4. Check the expiration date of the disinfectant and follow the manufacturer's directions for mixing and use (Figure 26-5 ◆).
5. With gloves on, completely immerse the contaminated articles in the container of disinfectant (Figure 26-6 ◆). Cover the container and soak the instruments for the length of time recommended by the manufacturer.
6. Remove and rinse each instrument thoroughly. Dry the instruments with paper towels.
7. Place the disinfected instruments on muslin or into sterilizing packets for the autoclave.

Figure 26-5 ◆ Follow the manufacturer's directions for mixing and use of the disinfectant.

Figure 26-6 ◆ Completely immerse the contaminated articles in the container of disinfectant.

✓ COMPETENCY SKILLS PERFORMANCE

1. Demonstrate the performance of sanitization.
2. Demonstrate disinfection procedures.
3. Demonstrate how to wrap surgical instruments and prepare sterile trays for autoclave sterilization.
4. Demonstrate the correct procedure for loading and operating an autoclave.
5. Demonstrate the correct procedure for pouring sterile solution onto a sterile field.
6. Demonstrate the correct procedure for opening a sterile surgical pack to create a sterile field.
7. Demonstrate the correct procedure for using transfer forceps.
8. Demonstrate a sterile scrub (surgical hand washing).
9. Demonstrate how to glove while wearing a sterile gown.
10. Demonstrate sterile gloving and removal.

Keys to Success

Helpful tips for career success are interspersed throughout the text to highlight the importance of professionalism.

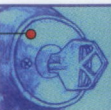

Keys to Success
OBTAINING INFORMED CONSENT

The physician is responsible for obtaining informed consent. For the consent to be truly "informed," however, patients must have the opportunity to ask the physician any and all questions. This task should never be delegated to the medical assistant. Instead, it is appropriate for the medical assistant to witness the patient's signature on the consent form.

A Consent to Release of Information form is signed by a patient before the care provider can apply for third-party reimbursement (Figure 24-3 ◆). Forms to release information should include the following:

- Name of the medical facility or practice that will be releasing the information
- Name of the individual who is to receive the information
- Patient's full name, specific information to be released
- Purpose of releasing the information

Special procedures and surgical procedures require informed consent. See Chapter 4, Medical Law and Ethics, for a more detailed discussion of informed consent. See Figure 4-4 for a sample of an informed consent form.

Concept Link

This visual link is a tool for providing concepts presented in earlier or later chapters.

In Practice

These real-life scenarios require students to pause and apply the knowledge presented in the chapter to answer critical thinking questions.

In Practice

The small physician's office where Jenny works as a front-desk medical assistant is on the first floor of a building where cars are parked outside the door. When Marion Wilson arrives for her appointment, she approaches the front desk and tells Jenny that she is going to leave her 2-year-old son sleeping in his car seat because Jenny can see the car from her desk. How should Jenny respond to Marion? What are some appropriate suggestions?

HIPAA Compliance

All discussions held within patient hearing range must be HIPAA-compliant. This means the medical assistant must never disclose patient confidential information when other patients can overhear.

HIPAA Compliance

These feature boxes highlight the need-to-know law.

Anatomy and Physiology

Our clinical chapters use a body systems approach. In this unique format, we include instruction of required clinical content and competencies in the body systems to which they apply. The discussion of A&P is a great tool for instructors who need to gauge any student weakness in this area up front. Since instructors may not know the amount of A&P a student has learned prior to the course—or the level of the A&P course taken previously—this along with the medical terminology should be used to reinforce the material in the rest of the chapter.

Anatomy and Physiology of the Endocrine System

There are two control systems in the body: the nervous system and the endocrine system.

- The nervous system, including the autonomic system, exerts control over body functions in a way similar to an electrical system. Impulses travel through the nerves at an extremely rapid speed and elicit an immediate response.
- The endocrine system is slightly slower in its elicited response, which is chemically mediated by **hormones.** The endocrine system is composed of **endocrine glands** that secrete and release hormones directly into the bloodstream (Figure 40-1 ◆). These glands include the pituitary gland, thyroid gland, parathyroid gland, pancreas, adrenal glands, gonads (testicles and ovaries), pineal gland, and thymus gland. (Refer to ∞ Chapter 33, Urology and Nephrology, and ∞ Chapter 44, Obstetrics and Gynecology, for a discussion of the sex hormones.)

Endocrine disorders are the result of too much or too little of a particular hormone being stimulated or released. Therefore, most endocrine disorders are referred to as either the hyper- or hypoactivity of the gland.

Hormones are chemical substances that influence and control body functions such as growth and development, sexual maturity, and metabolism. Hormones send messages to other glands and target organs (Figure 40-2 ◆). Regulation of this system is accomplished by a positive–negative feedback process. Negative feedback originates when blood hormone levels are elevated and a message is sent slowing or stopping of the gland's activity, thereby ceasing or reducing the production of the hormone. In this manner, blood levels of various hormones control the secretion of other hormones and their resulting blood levels.

The Endocrine Glands

The *pituitary gland* is a minute structure located in the midbrain, in the middle of the skull (Figure 40-3 ◆). It consists of two lobes, the anterior lobe and the posterior lobe. This gland

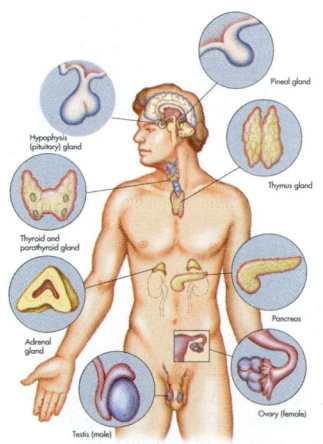

Figure 40-1 ◆ Endocrine glands scattered throughout the body.

Electronic Medical Records

An entire chapter of this text is devoted to the important topic of electronic health records.

 ## The Medical Assistant's Role in Using Electronic Medical Records

Electronic medical records will be a part of the medical assistant's job in any facility. Although the type of software used will vary from one office to the next, the basic premise is similar. The medical assistant will need to be comfortable using computers as well as be able to maneuver his or her way around the electronic medical record.

Electronic Medical Records Are Easily Accessible

Electronic medical records are simply the portions of patients' medical records that are kept on a computer's hard drive or a medical office's computer network rather than on paper. While physicians must retrieve paper files from separate and often large rooms, electronic records are easily accessible on a computer. In large offices where patients may see several different providers, electronic medical records allow physicians easily to locate patients' laboratory results, consultations, X-rays, and examination findings from other providers.

Using electronic health records (**EHRs**), medical offices are able to access any one patient's file from more than one networked computer in the office. For example, the billing office might have the patient's medical record open on a computer screen while it is accessing information needed for coding a specific procedure. At the same time, the physician might have the same patient's file open on a separate computer screen while she inputs treatment notes.

Charting patient information, such as telephone calls, is easily done within the electronic medical record. Typically, the software will contain a section for adding information, such as telephone calls or personal conversations that are related to the patient's medical care.

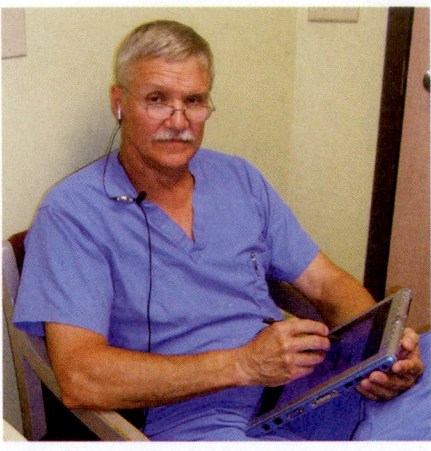

Figure 13-1 ◆ A physician uses a TabletPC to enter patient data while in the examination room.

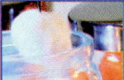 ## PROCEDURE 41-9 Develop an Environmental Exposure Plan

Theory and Rationale
Medical assistants are playing an increasing role in emergency preparedness. Emergencies include not only medical emergencies, but also natural disasters and man-made disasters. The most important rule to follow is to always be prepared for any situation that may arise. By adequate preparedness we not only help ourselves and our patients, but also the community that surrounds us.

Materials
- pen
- paper
- computer
- copy machine
- various emergency supplies
- waterproof containers

Competency
(**Condition**) With the necessary materials, you will be able to (**Task**) develop an environmental exposure plan (**Standards**) with correct items in the time designated by the instructor.

1. Create an emergency kit that can be used by your office in the event of an environmental emergency. Supplies may include:
   - flashlights
   - batteries
   - bottles of water
   - nonperishable food
   - bandages
   - alcohol and hydrogen peroxide
   - blankets
   - vinyl or latex gloves
   - tweezers, scissors
   - medication—ibuprofen, acetimetophen, antihistamines, antibiotic ointment, tetanus vaccines, etc.
   - self-powered radio
2. Enclose the kit in a waterproof container.
3. Place the kit in a safe area, such as a medicine closet or storage closet.
4. Create evacuation plans and make sure that every room in the medical office shows a detailed exit route.
5. Create a delineation chart that outlines responsibilities of office staff members in the event of an emergency.
6. Create a list of "safety zones" that can be used in the event of an emergency. For instance:
   - a safety zone in the event of a tornado
   - an outdoor safety zone in the event of a fire
   - a safety zone in the event of a flood
7. Make photocopies of the safety zone list, evacuation plan, and delineation chart for everyone in the office. Laminate and hang copies in the employee break room.
8. Train all office staff on the environmental exposure plan within ten days of hire.

Emergency Preparedness

This text includes the latest information on emergency preparedness and the medical assistant's role in protective practices.

Law and Ethics

Medical assistants face many situations that involve ethics and the law; therefore, a comprehensive chapter is provided to highlight the need-to-know law and present scenarios that may have a legal and ethical impact on patients. Informational tables and charts summarize key concepts.

The Sources of Law

U.S. law arises from varying sources. Court decisions establish **traditional law**. **Common law** comes from the English legal system. All U.S. states follow common law except Louisiana, which uses a system based on French law.

Courts set **precedents** when they decide cases. *Roe v. Wade*, for example, caused all states to revamp their legal approaches to abortion. Similarly, *Brown v. Board of Education* forced states to address the issue of segregation. **Segregation** is an example of how courts can overrule decisions and set new precedents. Years ago, court decisions deemed segregation a legal practice. Subsequent court decisions ruled segregation illegal, however, and thereby reversed the legal precedents.

Statutes are laws created by federal, state, or local legislators. Statutes are upheld by law enforcement, and cases may end up in local, state, or federal court systems. Medicare, Medicaid, and the Food and Drug Administration (**FDA**) are all agencies that create healthcare-related statutes.

Administrative Law

Administrative law, also called **regulatory law**, is passed by governmental agencies such as the Internal Revenue Service (**IRS**). Administrative law addresses issues of taxation, public transportation, manufacturing, the environment, and public broadcasting.

Comparing Public and Private Law

The United States' judicial system has two main branches of law: (1) public and (2) private. **Public law** focuses on issues between the government and citizens, such as criminal law, **constitutional law**, administrative law, and **international law**. Private or **civil law** focuses on issues between two or more citizens.

Criminal Law

Criminal law, also called penal law, focuses on the public's safety and welfare, addressing people who commit crimes or other illegal offenses. Classified by severity as felonies or misdemeanors, criminal law varies from one state to another. While all states have laws against such serious crimes as rape or murder, the laws for less serious crimes like theft or drug use may vary from one jurisdiction to another.

Felonies

Felonies are considered serious crimes, whereas misdemeanors are considered less serious offenses. States have varying definitions for each. Table 4-1 lists general felony categories. Some states, like New Jersey, classify felonies in four degrees. Other states place felonies in "classes," like Class A or Class 1. In cases like these, Class 1 is the most serious while Class 6 is the least.

Misdemeanors

Like felony classifications, misdemeanor classifications vary from state to state. Misdemeanors include such crimes as petty theft, prostitution, simple **assault,** and disorderly conduct. Because they are considered lesser crimes than felonies, misdemeanors are generally punished with lesser sentences.

Civil Law

The medical profession is primarily concerned with civil law, because it deals with issues relating to **contract law, commercial law,** and tort law. Contract and commercial laws address the rights and obligations one has to another, such as the doctor-patient relationship. Tort law deals with the injuries one has suffered at the hands of another, such as cases of medical malpractice.

Tort Law

Tort law deals with situations in which someone has been injured by another's actions or inactions. Torts are one of two types: unintentional or intentional. An **unintentional tort** occurs when a mistake is made. The vast majority of medical malpractice cases fall into this category, because unintentional torts usually involve negligence. **Negligence** is defined as an act that a reasonable health care provider would not have done or the omission of an act that a reasonable health care provider would have done. In contrast, an **intentional tort** occurs when someone purposefully does something that injures someone else. Table 4-2 defines intentional torts and gives healthcare examples.

? —Critical Thinking Question 4-1 —
How does the case study outlined at the beginning of this chapter illustrate one of the torts in Table 4-2? Please specify the tort.

TABLE 4-1 FELONY CATEGORIES

Felony Degree	Action of Person Being Charged
First	Committed the crime
Second	Was at the scene of the crime and assisted in the crime
Third	Assisted in the crime before the crime occurred
Fourth	Assisted the person who committed the crime after the fact

TABLE 35-1 RISK FACTORS IN HYPERTENSION

Nonmodifiable Risk Factors	Modifiable Risk Factors
Family history of hypertensive disease	Chronic stress
Being of African American descent	Obesity
Older age	Diet high in salt and fat
Diabetes	Oral contraceptives
Kidney disease	Sedentary lifestyle
	Smoking

Informational Charts and Tables

These appear throughout the text and summarize pertinent information for the reader. They provide students with visuals and comparisons to reinforce the lesson. In the specialty chapters they provide a quick reference for the disorders described in the chapter. Most tables include signs and symptoms, causes, diagnosis, and treatment.

Color Photos and Illustrations

Color photos and illustrations appear throughout the book to support the textual material presented and reinforce key concepts.

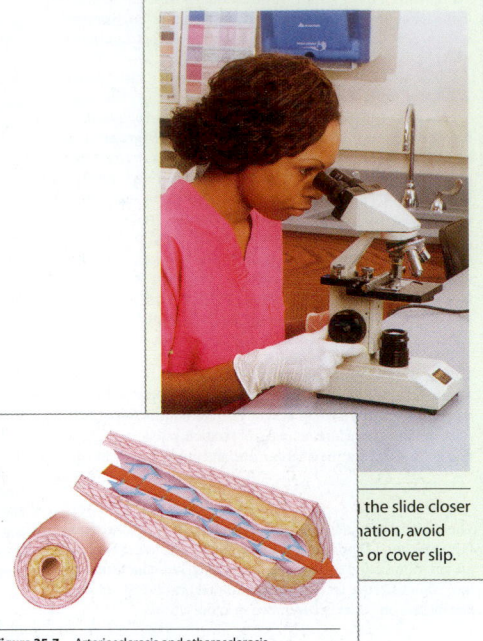

Figure 35-7   Arteriosclerosis and atherosclerosis.

... the slide closer ... nation, avoid ... e or cover slip.

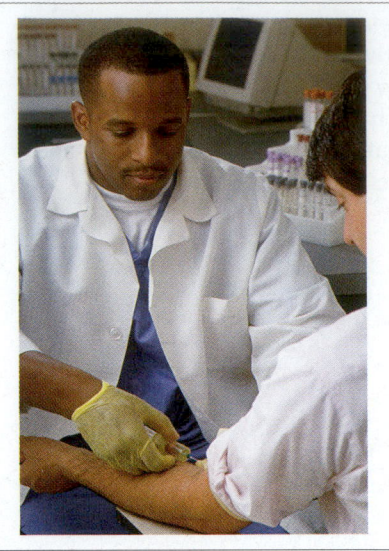

Figure 4-3 ◆ This patient has given implied consent to have her blood drawn.

Chapter Summary

Each chapter summary is an excellent review of the chapter content.

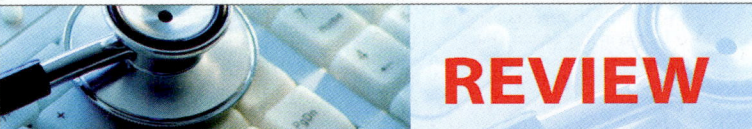

REVIEW

Chapter Summary

- The CPT coding book is designed to standardize the coding process by requiring healthcare providers to choose a procedure code based on the explicit description.
- Accurate CPT coding involves a number of steps, including determining correct codes via chart notes.
- Modifiers are an integral part of procedural coding, serving to add detail to procedure codes. By using modifiers, the coder is able to further identify any special circumstances that surround that particular service for that patient.
- The Health Care Common Procedure Coding System (HCPCS) provides codes for reporting nonphysician services, supplies, or durable medical equipment (DME), and certain physician services for medicare and medicaid.
- In all forms of coding, accurate documentation and reimbursement are tightly linked. Insurers will often request copies of patient healthcare records in order to determine the necessity of care rendered. Having accurate records of the services provided is helpful in timely and accurate payment of claims.
- Coding and billing fraud impose severe penalties. It includes falsifying medical records, billing for services not performed, and intentionally charging incorrect patients. Providers who are caught intentionally submitting fraudulent claims may be arrested and charged with crimes. In addition, they risk the loss of their licenses, practices, and preferred provider status.
- Bundling of services is the process of charging one procedure code for a group of charges that typically are performed at the same time. For bundled procedures, coders may not unbundle the charges, or charge for each procedure individually. This would be unbundling and insurance carriers consider this practice to be fraudulent.

Chapter Review Questions

End-of-chapter questions are provided in multiple-choice, true/false, short answer, and research format, and help reinforce learning. The review questions measure the students' understanding of the material presented in the chapter. These tools are available for use by the student or by the instructor as an outcome assessment.

Chapter Review

Multiple Choice

1. What is the proper way to address an elderly patient?
   a. Mrs. _____
   b. By first name
   c. "Honey" or "Sweetie"
   d. None of the above

2. The opinion that all people living in homeless shelters are likely to have lice is an example of
   a. stereotyping.
   b. discriminating.
   c. alienating.
   d. grieving.

3. Which of the following is *not* an example of keeping a professional distance?
   a. Giving a patient transportation options to the clinic
   b. Offering to pay a patient's copayment
   c. Reviewing a patient's billing charges with the patient
   d. None of the above

4. A common defense mechanism for a patient who has just received a serious diagnosis is
   a. denial.
   b. identification.
   c. conversion.
   d. compensation.

True/False

T F 1. Body language is far less important than verbal communication.

T F 2. Empathy and sympathy are really the same thing.

T F 3. When working with a hearing-impaired patient, the medical assistant should speak directly to the interpreter.

T F 4. When working with child patients, it is best to communicate directly with the parent during the visit rather than the child.

T F 5. Addressing the physician as "Dr." in front of patients gives patients the impression that the doctor is an authority figure who should be respected.

T F 6. Part of developing a good patient relationship includes sharing personal problems with the patients.

T F 7. Defense mechanisms protect a person's self-esteem and effectively deal with conflict.

T F 8. Patients will often share more information with the medical assistant that they will with the physician.

T F 9. It is best to use proper medical terminology when speaking with patients to demonstrate intelligence.

T F 10. A clinic's office policy dictates whether to allow service animals to accompany their owners to treatment rooms.

Short Answer

1. What is a good communication technique to use with angry patients?

2. Name the five stages of grief.

3. List six common defense mechanisms.

4. What is the difference between an open-ended question and a close-ended question?

5. When might it be appropriate to use therapeutic touch with a patient?

6. Describe the method you would use to communicate effectively with a hearing-impaired patient.

Research

1. Does the Americans with Disabilities Act (ADA) require that Braille be printed on public buildings to indicate bathrooms, elevators, etc.?

2. In your local area, are sign-language classes available to the public?

3. In your local area, what are the resources for patients who speak English as a second language?

4. If a non-English-speaking patient comes to your office alone, what local agency can you contact for an interpreter?

5. Search the Internet for books to read about communication skills. Which ones sound as if they might be helpful to the medical assistant?

6. What are the local resources for hearing-impaired people in your area?

7. What are the local resources for sight-impaired people in your area?

Externship Application Experience

This feature places the student in an externship site with a simulated situation the student may encounter. Critical thinking questions appear at the end of each brief scenario, and students must rely on the knowledge acquired in the chapter and their own critical thinking skills to answer each question.

Externship Application Experience

When Mrs. Rundholz calls to make an appointment for a complete physical examination, she says she can make the appointment but will not have child care for her 2-year-old and 6-month-old children. She asks if she can bring her children to her hour-long appointment. How should the medical assistant respond to Mrs. Rundholz? What are some appropriate suggestions?

Resource Guide

This listing provides additional information (organization contact information, websites, etc.) related to chapter content.

Resource Guide

American Association of Medical Assistants
20 N. Wacker Dr., Suite 1575
Chicago, IL 60606
Phone: (312) 899-1500
Fax: (312) 899-1259
www.aama-ntl.org/

Bioethics.com
http://bioethicsnews.com

Health Care Providers Service Organization
159 E. County Line Road
Hatboro, PA 19040-1218
Phone: (800) 982-9491
Fax: (800) 739-8818
www.hpso.com

Public Citizen
1600 20th St. NW
Washington, DC. 20009
Phone: (202) 588-1000
www.citizen.org

Sorry Works
P.O. Box 531
Glen Carbon, IL 62034
Phone: (618) 559-8168
www.sorryworks.net/

MedMedia

Reminds students to visit and explore the Student CD to supplement chapter content.

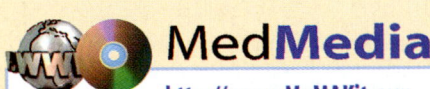

Med**Media**

http://www.MyMAKit.com

More on this chapter, including interactive resources, can be found on the Student CD-ROM accompanying this textbook and on http://www.MyMAKit.com.

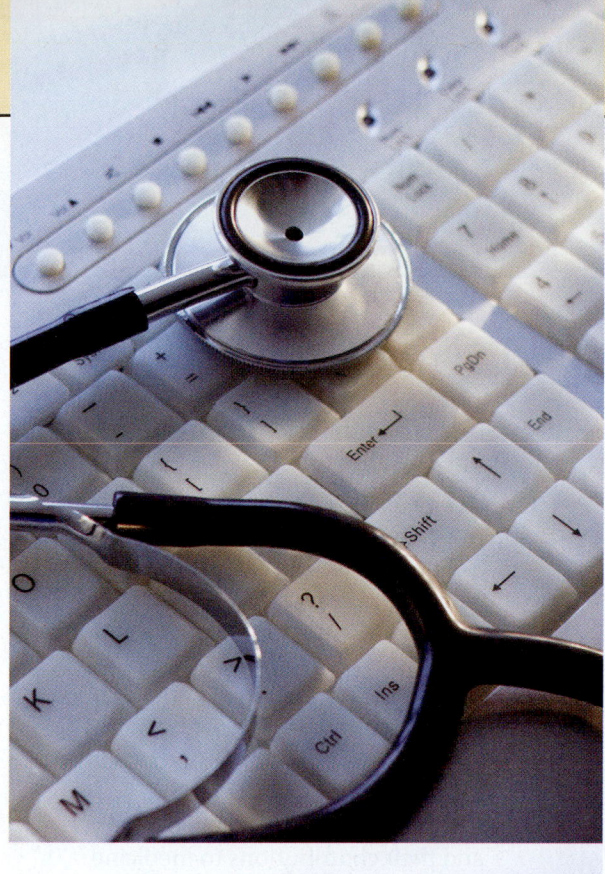

UNIT I

Introduction to the Medical Assisting Profession

Chapter 1   **The Medical Assistant Profession and the History of Healthcare**

Chapter 2   **Medical Assisting Today**

Chapter 3   **Professionalism in the Workplace**

Chapter 4   **Medical Law and Ethics**

Chapter 5   **Interpersonal Communication Skills**

Chapter 6   **Patient-Centered Care and Education**

Chapter 7   **Considerations of Extended Life**

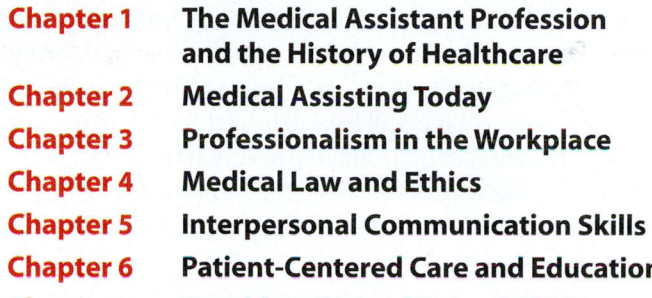

My name is Terri O'Connell, and I became a Certified Medical Assistant in June 2005. I have a BA in Communications and had worked for over fifteen years in the advertising profession as a businessperson before taking time off to raise a family. I became really interested in the Allied Health profession after taking a Medical Terminology course.

A medical assistant performs a combination of both clinical and administrative skills. In the final months of our training, the clinical experiences we had in various offices and facilities led me to take a first job at a busy pediatric practice. I knew I would have two patients in a pediatric office, the child and the parent. Sometimes either one of them could be difficult to work with. I had to learn how to keep the flow in the office moving, as the provider needed to be kept busy at all times. This entails finding the chief complaint of the patient quickly and making decisions as to what data the provider might need in order to make the final assessment and diagnosis.

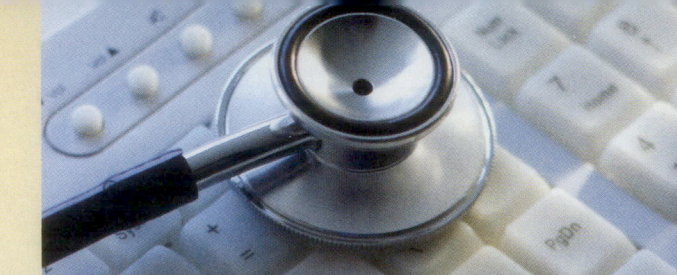

CHAPTER 1

The Medical Assistant Profession and the History of Healthcare

Case Study

Janet has been working with Dr. Fletcher for many years as a medical assistant and really enjoys her chosen profession. Next week the office will be celebrating Janet's thirty-year anniversary as a medical assistant, and everyone is excited about the celebration.

During Tuesday's staff meeting the office manager, Annette, announced that she will be updating files and implementing some employee certification changes that Dr. Fletcher learned about at a recent seminar. The biggest change will be that all medical assistants will have to be certified by taking and passing the AAMA certification exam within the next twelve months.

Janet is worried. She confides to a friend and coworker, Lucy, that she isn't really sure what Annette was talking about when she mentioned the AAMA certification exam. Lucy explains that she took the exam shortly after graduation last year and that is why her name pin bears the title "CMA (AAMA)."

Janet confesses that she has never taken a certification exam because she went to work right out of high school and got her first job in healthcare by being "grandfathered" in. When Janet started working thirty years ago, it was legal to train staff on the job, without certificates from accredited schools.

"You introduce yourself to patients as 'Dr. Fletcher's nurse,' so you must have gone to an RN program," Lucy says.

Janet looks offended. "No, I didn't. We're in the nursing profession, so I let my patients call me 'Nurse.' It's no big deal."

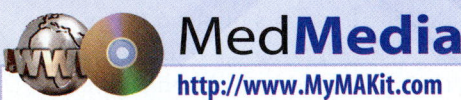

MedMedia

http://www.MyMAKit.com

Additional interactive resources and activities for this chapter can be found on http://www.MyMAKit.com. For a video, tips, audio glossary, legal and ethical scenarios, job scenarios, quizzes, and games related to the content of this chapter, please access the accompanying CD-ROM in this book.

Audio Glossary
Video
Legal and Ethical Scenario: *The Medical Assistant Profession and Healthcare*
On the Job Scenario: *The Medical Assistant Profession and Healthcare*
Tips
HIPAA Quiz
Multiple Choice Quiz
Games: Crossword, Strikeout, and Spelling Bee

Objectives

After completing this chapter, you should be able to:

- Define and spell the key terminology in this chapter.
- Define the medical assistant's role in the healthcare profession.
- Discuss the history of medicine and the purpose of the Hippocratic Oath.
- Discuss the beginning of hand washing in healthcare.
- Describe important organizations in medical history.
- Discuss important women in healthcare and their contributions to medicine.
- Describe the World Health Organization.
- Explain the American Medical Association's *Principles of Medical Ethics*.
- Describe the purpose of the American Hospital Association's *Patient Bill of Rights*.
- Identify the professional requirements of a medical assistant.
- Define the scope of practice of a medical assistant.
- Discuss the various opportunities for employment for medical assistants.
- Discuss the credentials of the American Association of Medical Assistants (AAMA) and American Medical Technologists (AMT).
- Identify medical assistant educational programs and list the educational requirements for medical assistants.

✚ MEDICAL ASSISTING STANDARDS

CAAHEP ENTRY-LEVEL STANDARDS	ABHES ENTRY-LEVEL COMPETENCIES
■ Perform within scope of practice (psychomotor) ■ Apply ethical behaviors, including honesty/integrity in performance of medical assisting practice (affective) ■ Summarize the Patient Bill of Rights (cognitive) ■ Use medical terminology, pronouncing medical terms correctly to communicate information, patient history, date and observations (psychomotor)	■ Project a positive attitude. ■ Maintain confidentiality at all times. ■ Be a "team player." ■ Be cognizant of ethical boundaries. ■ Exhibit initiative. ■ Adapt to change. ■ Evidence a responsible attitude. ■ Be courteous and diplomatic. ■ Conduct work within scope of education, training, and ability.

Introduction

Medical assisting is a fairly new profession in the healthcare delivery system, receiving professional recognition in 1955. Advances in medical science, a nursing shortage, and changes in the reimbursement system have made formal training and certification necessary for anyone wishing to work as a medical assistant in a medical office or clinic.

The Medical Assistant's Role in Healthcare

The medical assistant (MA) is vital to the healthcare field. In order to help fill the need for trained professionals, the medical assistant must have knowledge about the medical assisting profession and the evolution of medical science along with the practical skills to work in a fast-paced setting. Becoming an MA is stepping into a future filled with both challenges and an unlimited potential for growth.

The History of Medicine

Ancient treatments for illness and disease were practiced and passed down orally through the generations. Folk remedies evolved as certain plants were discovered to be harmful and others found to improve health. Early efforts to understand the origins of diseases and illnesses were largely based on belief in the supernatural.

Early Healing Practices

Early medicines were developed largely from plants and animals. Many plant remedies are still used today for heart conditions, **indigestion**, bleeding, and urinary tract infections. For example, garlic has recently been approved in Europe for treating cardiovascular conditions such as high cholesterol. Numerous other plant remedies are used around the world (Figure 1-1 ◆).

- Ginger treats conditions such as nausea, motion sickness, and lack of appetite.
- Licorice is used to soothe inflamed mucous membranes.
- The foxglove plant (*Digitalis lanata*) is the basis for digitalis preparations such as digoxin that are prescribed to slow and strengthen the heartbeat.
- Green tea is an antioxidant.
- Peppermint treats indigestion.
- Chamomile soothes the nerves.

Key Terminology *(continued)*

technical education programs—
program designed to give students skills
without higher education; also called vocational program (see following)

vocational programs—program designed
to give students skills without higher education; also called technical educational program (see preceding)

Abbreviations

AAMA—American Association of Medical
Assistants

ABHES—Accrediting Bureau of Health
Education Schools

AHA—American Hospital Association

AMA—American Medical Association

AMT—American Medical Technologists

CAAHEP—Commission on Accreditation
of Allied Health Education Programs

CMA—Certified Medical Assistant

EKG—electrocardiograph

HIPAA—Health Insurance Portability and
Accountability Act

JAMA—Journal of the American Medical
Association

NCCA—National Commission for Certifying
Agents

RMA—Registered Medical Assistant

WHO—World Health Organization

Animals are another source of treatments and cures.

- Leeches are used to treat wounds that require the draining of blood, such as reconstructive surgery for grafted
  tissue.
- Snake venom is commonly used to produce antivenin,
  the treatment for poisonous snakebites.

The use of nonpoisonous snakes by early Greek physicians is the origin of the caduceus symbol (Figure 1-2 ◆). Snakes
were thought to have regenerative powers, in part because they
regularly sloughed, or shed, their skin.

Healing Based on the Supernatural

Diseases were often believed to be of supernatural origin, caused
by evil spirits and angry gods. Treating these diseases was the
responsibility of sorcerers and shamans and often consisted of
torturing the patient to make the body unfit for demons to live
in. *Trepanning,* or boring a hole into the patient's skull, was
done to release evil spirits. Other, less painful treatments to
ward off demons included dancing, the use of talismans, or
magical charms, incantations, and magic (Figure 1-3 ◆).

Early Egyptian Medicine

As far back as 3000 B.C., there is evidence that the Egyptians
provided medical care for such conditions as tuberculosis and
pneumonia. Other records suggest that they were performing
surgery, as well. Fossils from this era indicate that an Egyptian
patient underwent brain surgery and survived. The patient's
skull bones had healed long before the patient died.

A practitioner named Imhotep, who lived from 2667
to 2648 B.C.E., is credited as founding Egyptian medicine in
the Third Dynasty (Figure 1-4 ◆). He authored some of the
original material on which the world's earliest known medical document, the *Edwin Smith Papyrus,* is based. Written
around 1600 B.C.E., the *Papyrus* details the known cures,
examination findings, and prognoses of the time and is
thought to be a compilation of multiple authors.

Early Chinese Medicine

Classical Chinese medicine has been traced as far back as 2700
B.C.E. Much of it reflects the culture's beliefs that everything,
including humans, is interconnected and that optimal health
comes from living harmoniously in the world. Classical Chinese practitioners believed the five methods in Figure 1-5 ◆
helped patients achieve good health. The Chinese also developed a list of the medical uses for many plants and herbs.

In the 1960s, the Chinese government commissioned ten
Western physicians to add scientific theory to classical Chinese
medicine. The result, called traditional Chinese medicine, is
taught in Chinese medical schools today.

Early Native American Medicine

Native Americans are among the earliest and most effective
medical practitioners. Native American healers, whose practices date as far back as 40,000 years in the United States,
believed they must always honor the patient's wishes and
never force treatment. Although medical treatments varied
among the Native American tribes, suicide was considered
one of the highest forms of bravery. The elderly and sick of
many tribes traditionally committed suicide during periods
of famine.

When treatment was an option, both the Navaho and the
Cherokee used herbs and such comfort measures as natural pain
relievers. Patients who recovered were often thought to have
supernatural powers. Because tribes lacked written language at
the time, early Native American healers used oral means to pass
their medical knowledge to younger tribe members.

Hippocrates and Early Contributors

Hippocrates (460 B.C.E.–377 B.C.E.), known as the Father of Medicine, practiced and taught medicine on the island of Kos, Greece.
He believed that disease was caused not by supernatural forces
but by natural causes. He believed the four elements of earth, air,
fire, and water were represented by the four humors (body
fluids): blood, phlegm, black bile, and yellow bile. Good health

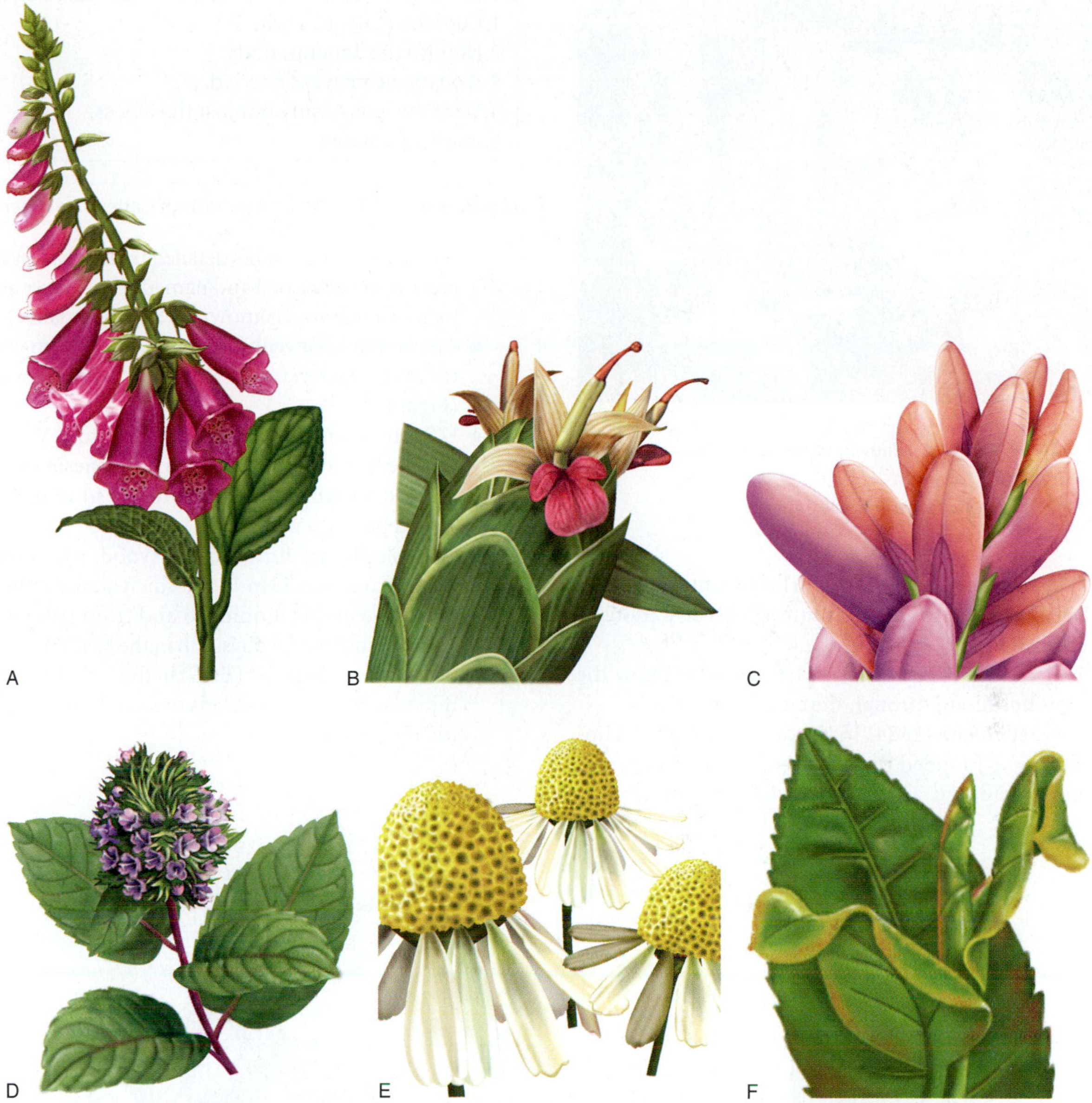

A

B

C

D

E

F

Figure 1-1 ◆ Numerous plant remedies are used around the world, such as (A) foxglove, (B) ginger, (C) licorice, (D) peppermint, (E) chamomile, and (F) green tea.

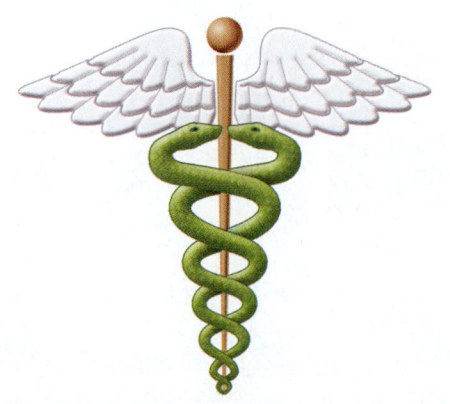

Figure 1-2 ◆ Caduceus symbol.

depended on keeping the humors balanced within the body. This belief was the basis for many theories of disease until the late 1800s.

Hippocrates taught a philosophy of wellness based on diet, exercise, moderation, rest, and positive outlook. His descriptions of disease identified symptoms and included a **prognosis**. The time-honored medical rule "First, do no harm" is attributed to Hippocrates.

Other early contributors to the medical field were the following:

- Galen (30–200 C.E.), who based his ideas about anatomy and physiology on his work with animal **cadavers**, a forerunner of later postmortem examinations. He also discovered that arteries carried blood instead of air and developed a technique for taking the pulse, a diagnostic tool used to this day.

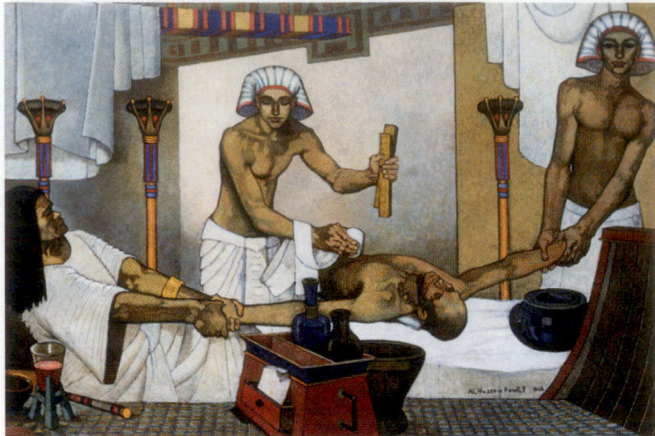

Figure 1-3 ◆ Diseases, often believed to be of supernatural origin, were treated by talismans.
Brian Warling/International Museum of Surgical Science

- Andreas Vesalius (1514–1564), who became known as the Father of Modern Anatomy through his dissections of the human body (Figure 1-6 ◆).
- William Harvey (1578–1657), who discovered how the heart pumps blood through the circulatory system.
- Thomas Sydenham (1624–1689), called the English Hippocrates, who founded the science of **epidemiology**. He is also considered an early **practitioner** of clinical

1. Cure the patient's spirit.
2. Nourish the patient's body.
3. Give medications as needed.
4. Treat the entire body, not just the illness.
5. Use acupuncture.

Figure 1-5 ◆ Early Chinese methods of patient treatment.

medicine because of his detailed patient observations and records. He described and named scarlet fever and Sydenham's chorea (once known as St. Vitus' dance).
- Antoni van Leeuwenhoek (1632–1723), who was the first to study bacteria and protozoa using a microscope (Figure 1-7 ◆).
- U.S. physician and pharmacist Crawford W. Long, who was the first to employ modern **anesthesia** in 1842 when he used an **ether**-based anesthesia to remove a tumor from a patient's neck.
- Scottish physician Alexander Wood, who invented the hypodermic needle in 1853, which allowed physicians to inject and extract liquids to and from patients' bodies.
- Willem Einthoven, a physician in the Netherlands, invented the electrocardiograph (**EKG**) in the early 1900's, an invention that enabled physicians to record the electrical activity of a patient's heart.

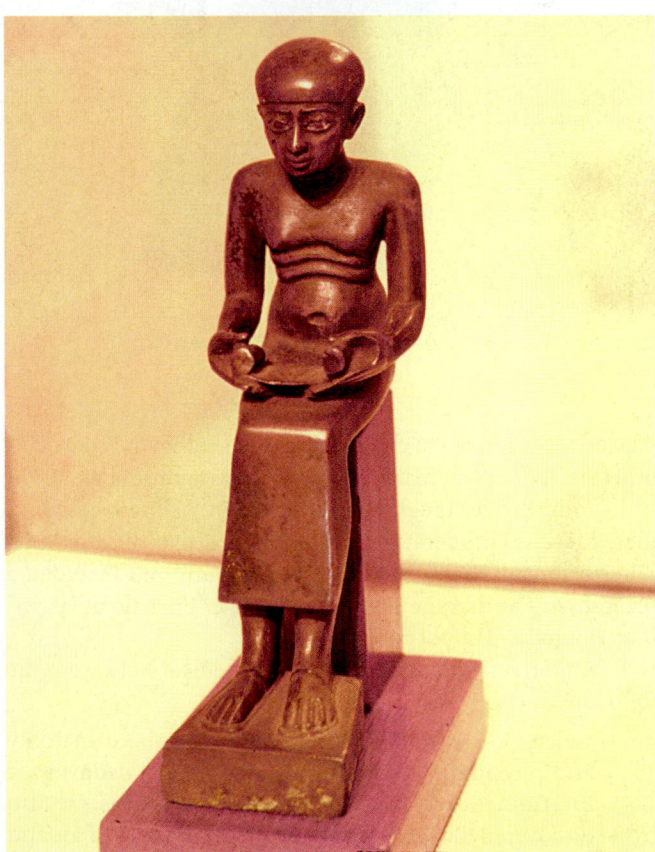

Figure 1-4 ◆ Imhotep (332–30 B.C.E.).

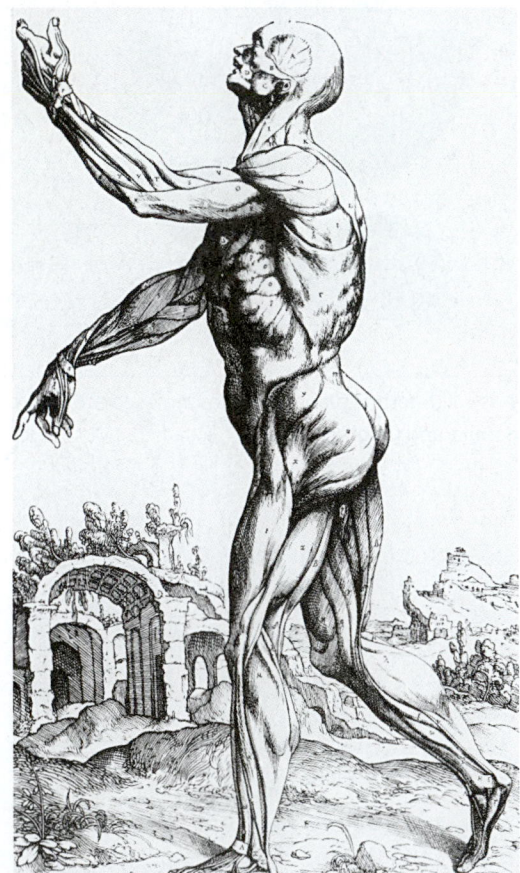

Figure 1-6 ◆ Andreas Vesalius (1514–1564), "Plate 25 from 'De Humani Corporis Fabrica,' Book II."

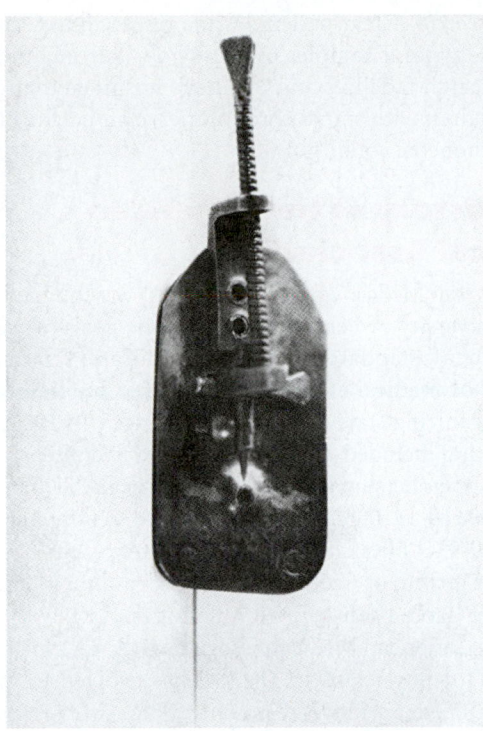

Figure 1-7 ◆ Anton Van Leeuwenhoek's prototype microscope.

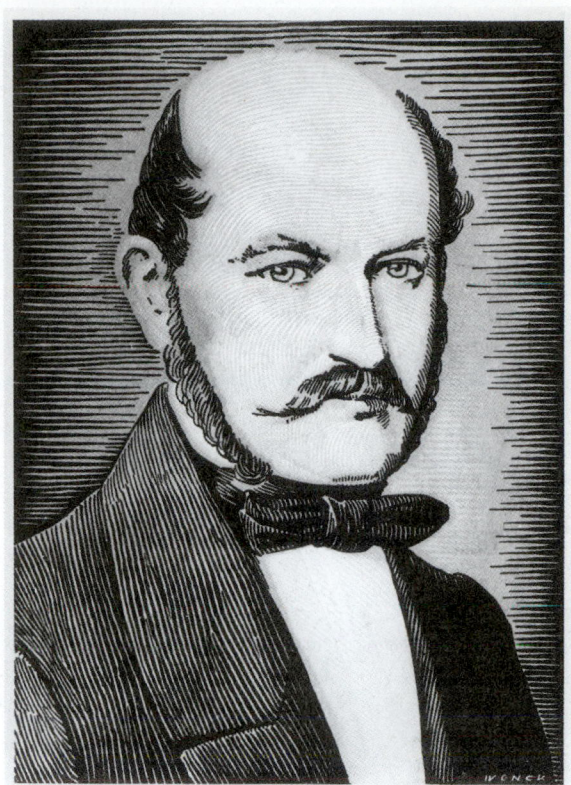

Figure 1-8 ◆ Ignaz Semmelweiss (1818–1865).

The Beginning of Hand Washing in Healthcare

In 1847, Hungarian physician Ignaz Semmelweiss (Figure 1-8 ◆) noticed a dramatic difference in the death rate of new mothers from childbed fever when the women delivered their babies at home with the help of midwives rather than in hospitals with surgeons. Childbed fever was a condition caused by a severe vaginal or uterine infection. Women who delivered at home were far more likely to survive. Because he suspected poor hospital hygiene as the cause, Dr. Semmelweiss began an experiment that required physicians to wash their hands before treating women in childbirth. At the time, physicians failed to wash their hands between patients, often attending to women in childbirth after working with recently deceased patients. The data from Semmelweiss's experiment showed that hand washing markedly reduced the death rate of women who delivered in hospitals.

Antisepsis Use in Healthcare

Despite his landmark discovery, Semmelweiss received little respect from his colleagues. As a result, hand washing between patients only began to enjoy widespread use in hospitals after British surgeon Joseph Lister discovered in 1867 that an **antiseptic** on wounds helped prevent infection. Lister based his study of **antisepsis** on the discoveries of French biologist Louis Pasteur.

While Pasteur is best known for inventing **pasteurization** in 1862, a process that uses heat to destroy bacteria, he also worked to prevent anthrax transmission and discovered the vaccine for rabies in 1885. Pasteur's pasteurization findings led to the use of heat in surgical-instrument sterilization. For all his work, Pasteur earned the title "Father of Preventive Medicine."

The Medical Value of X-Rays

Wilhem Roentgen revolutionized medical diagnosis in 1895 when he discovered X-rays while experimenting with vacuum tubes. His first X-ray image was of his wife's hand (Figure 1-9 ◆). Roentgen called the radiation rays he used "X" to indicate that they were unknown, but many of his colleagues called them Roentgen rays, a name that is still used in many languages today. In 1901, Roentgen received a Nobel Prize in physics for his discovery.

In Practice

Dawn Martinson, CMA (AAMA) is about to take an X-ray of Mrs. Boyan's hand. Mrs. Boyan asks Dawn if she knows how long X-rays have been used in healthcare. What can Dawn tell Mrs. Boyan about the discovery of this important medical discovery?

Other important figures in the history of medicine will be discussed in later chapters.

Important Organizations in Medical History

Throughout the years, a number of entities have formed to advance varying facets of the medical profession.

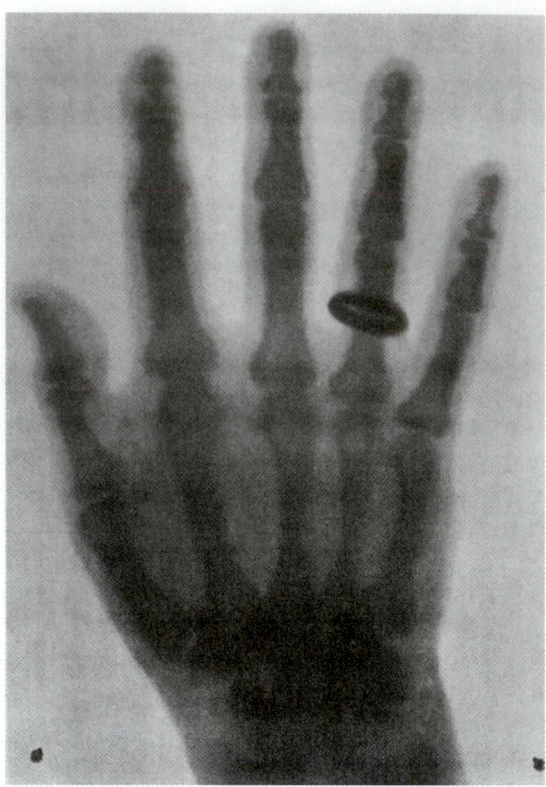

Figure 1-9 ◆ X-ray image of Roentgen's wife's hand, January 1896.

The History of American Hospitals

Early American hospitals bore little resemblance to the hospitals of today, in large part because people preferred to receive medical care in their own homes in the country's early days.

Benjamin Franklin built the first American hospital in Philadelphia in 1751. By 1910, that hospital and others like it had begun to run like today's scientific institutions. They used antiseptics, focused on cleanliness, and relieved pain with medications. In 1921, National Hospital Day was first celebrated on May 12, the birthday of famous nurse Florence Nightingale (see the following section on important female figures in medicine). The holiday continues to be recognized during the week of Nightingale's birth every year.

According to the American Hospital Association (**AHA**), by 2005 the United States had 5,756 hospitals with staffed beds totaling near 1 million. Hospitals today fall into the four following categories:

1. *General or community*—Range from ten beds to several hundred. Hospitals in this category, found in nearly every U.S. community, account for nearly 5,000 of the hospitals documented by the AHA in 2005.
2. *Teaching*—Found near university medical schools and have medical students, interns, and residents treating patients under the supervision of licensed physicians. In general, these facilities offer the same services as general hospitals (see preceding).
3. *Specialty*—Offer care to a certain patient type (e.g., children, burn victims, psychiatric patients, or patients undergoing drug or alcohol rehabilitation).

4. *Research*—Treat patients while researching certain disease types. Examples of these hospitals include cancer research facilities and Shriner's hospitals that care for children with spinal cord injuries, cleft palate, burns, or orthopedic conditions.

The History of the American Medical Association

The American Medical Association (**AMA**) was founded in 1847 at the University of Pennsylvania with the goals of "scientific advancement, standards for medical education, launching a program of medical ethics, and improved public health." It began organizing state and local associations in 1901, and its first meeting included 250 delegates from twenty-eight states. Physician membership in the group went from 8,000 in 1900 to over 70,000 by 1910. At that point, the AMA counted fully half of licensed U.S. physicians among its membership.

The growth of AMA marked the beginning of "organized medicine." Table 1-1 lists AMA milestones.

The American Medical Association (AMA) wrote a code of ethics for physicians in 1847. It has evolved to meet the changing needs of medical practice. The AMA *Principles of Medical Ethics* cover:

- Integrity
- Individual responsibility to society and community

TABLE 1-1 AMA MILESTONES

Year	Event
1847	The organization is founded.
1848	Makes dangers of "secretive remedies" the focus.
1858	Establishes Committee of Ethics.
1873	Sets up AMA Judicial Council.
1883	Launches *Journal of the American Medical Association* (**JAMA**).
1884	Supports experimentation on animals.
1897	Incorporates the organization.
1898	Starts Committee on Scientific Research to provide medical-research grants.
1899	Sets up Committee on National Legislation to represent group's interests in U.S. government.
1905	Launches Council on Pharmacy and Chemistry to set drug-manufacturing and advertising standards.
1912	Establishes Federation of State Medical Boards to deem group's rating of medical schools authoritative.
1948	Hires public relations firm to defeat government-run universal health care coverage.
1960	States that a blood alcohol level of 0.1% should be evidence of alcohol intoxication.
1970	Encourages the Federal Aviation Administration (FAA) to require all airlines to separate nonsmokers and smokers.
1974	Gives recommendations to ensure adequate protection of individuals used in human medical experimentation.
1982	Urges each state medical society to support laws to raise the legal drinking age to 21.
1988	Creates the Office of HIV/AIDS.
1995	Starts a campaign for liability reform.
2000	Supports Patients' Bill of Rights legislation in Congress.

Source: American Medical Association: www.ama-assn.org.

- Respect for human dignity
- Lifelong study
- Professional autonomy, or self-rule

Medical assistants should understand the *Principles of Medical Ethics* as explained by the AMA's Council on Ethical and Judicial Affairs. For example, the *Principles* state: "The term 'ethical' is used in opinions of the Council on Ethical and Judicial Affairs to refer to matters involving (1) moral principles or practices and (2) matters of social policy involving issues of morality in the practice of medicine. The term 'unethical' is used to refer to professional conduct which fails to conform to these moral standards or policies."

The American Association of Medical Assistants (**AAMA**) also has a Code of Ethics that sets guidelines for medical assistants in the practice of the profession. All medical assistants should be familiar with its contents.

The ten Standards of Practice for all individuals certified by the AMT are related to professionalism, ethics, standards of competence, and patient safety and welfare. Standard VI states, "The AMT professional shall respect the law and will pledge to avoid dishonest, unethical, or illegal practices."

The Start of the American Red Cross

In 1881, a nurse named Clara Barton formed the **American Red Cross**, now one of the largest humanitarian organizations in the world (Figure 1-10 ◆). During her life, Barton was the most

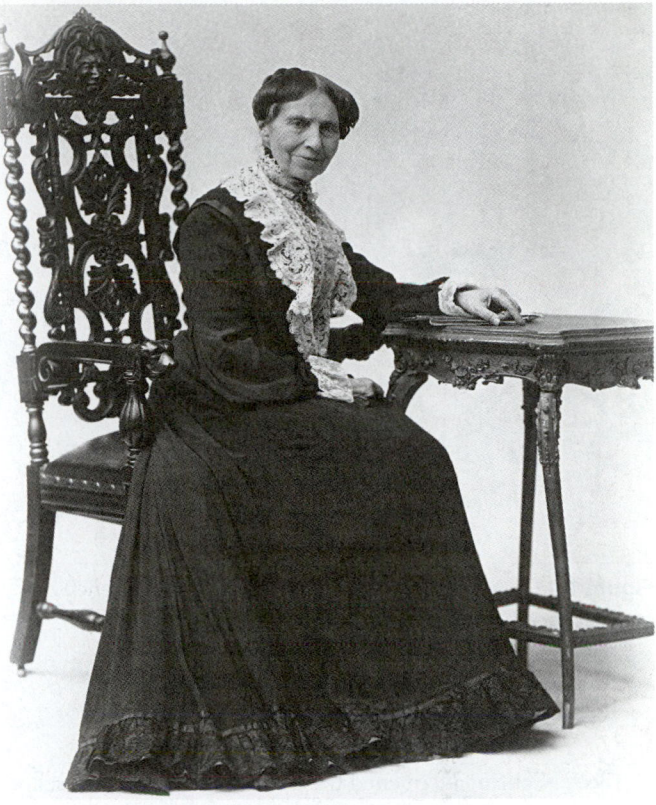

Figure 1-10 ◆ Clara Barton, founder of the American Red Cross.

decorated U.S. woman. She received the Iron Cross, the Cross of Imperial Russia, and the International Red Cross Medal. In 1904, at age 83, Barton founded the National First Aid Society.

Important Women in Healthcare

Women like Clara Barton have featured prominently in medical history throughout the years.

The Work of Marie Curie

One of the first notable women in health care was Marie Curie (Figure 1-11 ◆). This Polish woman became the first female instructor at the Sorbonne in France, and, in 1903, she became the first woman in France to complete her doctorate. Curie was the first person to win two Nobel Prizes in two different fields, and to this day she remains the only woman to have done so. Curie's work with radium eventually caused her death from radiation poisoning in 1934.

The Role of Florence Nightingale

Florence Nightingale is known as the founder of nursing. She was born in Florence, Italy, in 1820. At the time, nursing had a poor reputation. Nurses followed armies around, providing care and cooking meals. Nightingale helped advance the care of the poor, advocating improved medical care and commitment to the nursing profession. In 1860, she opened a nursing school in England. That school, the Nightingale School of Nursing, is still training nurses today.

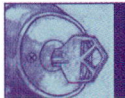

Keys to Success
AAMA CODE OF ETHICS

The Code of Ethics of AAMA shall set forth principles of ethical and moral conduct as they relate to the medical profession and the particular practice of medical assisting.

Members of AAMA dedicated to the conscientious pursuit of their profession, and thus desiring to merit the high regard of the entire medical profession and the respect of the general public which they serve, do pledge themselves to strive always to:

1. render service with full respect for the dignity of humanity;
2. respect confidential information obtained through employment unless legally authorized or required by responsible performance of duty to divulge such information;
3. uphold the honor and high principles of the profession and accept its disciplines;
4. seek to continually improve the knowledge and skills of medical assistants for the benefit of patients and professional colleagues;
5. participate in additional service activities aimed toward improving the health and well-being of the community.

Reprinted with permission of AAMA.

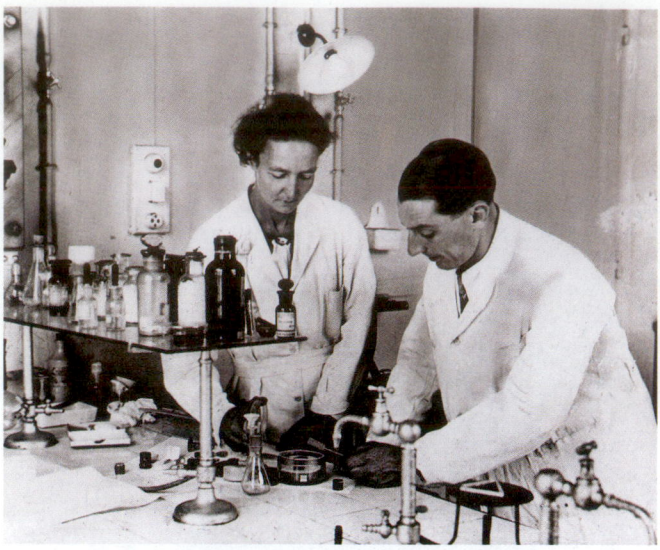

Figure 1-11 ◆ Marie Curie (1867–1934). Polish-born French physicist and her husband at work in the laboratory.

The Contributions of the Blackwell Sisters

In 1869, Nightingale opened the first women's medical school with Elizabeth Blackwell, the first woman to practice medicine in the United States with a degree (Figure 1-12 ◆). Given prejudices against women at the time, Blackwell herself had to apply to several medical schools before she was finally accepted by Geneva College in New York. She graduated at the top of her class. Although she was originally barred from practice in most hospitals because of her gender, Blackwell founded her own hospital in 1857, the New York Infirmary for Indigent Women and Children.

Blackwell's sister, Emily, was the third woman to earn a medical degree in the United States. The sisters worked together at the New York Infirmary for Indigent Women and Children for over forty years. In 1868, they founded the Women's Medical College in New York. By 1899, the college had graduated nearly 400 women doctors.

In 1970, 8 percent of all U.S. physicians were women. By 1980, that number had exceeded 12 percent. As of 2004, the number of female physicians in the United States was nearly 27 percent.

The World Health Organization

In 1945, when diplomats met to form the United Nations, one of the items discussed was the setting up of a global health organization. The World Health Organization (**WHO**) was launched on April 17, 1948, a date celebrated today as World Health Day. The WHO is responsible for providing leadership on many global health issues. Some of the stated goals of the WHO are to shape the health research agenda, set the norms and standards for health issues worldwide, articulate evidence-based policy options, provide technical support to countries and to monitor and assess health trends around the globe.

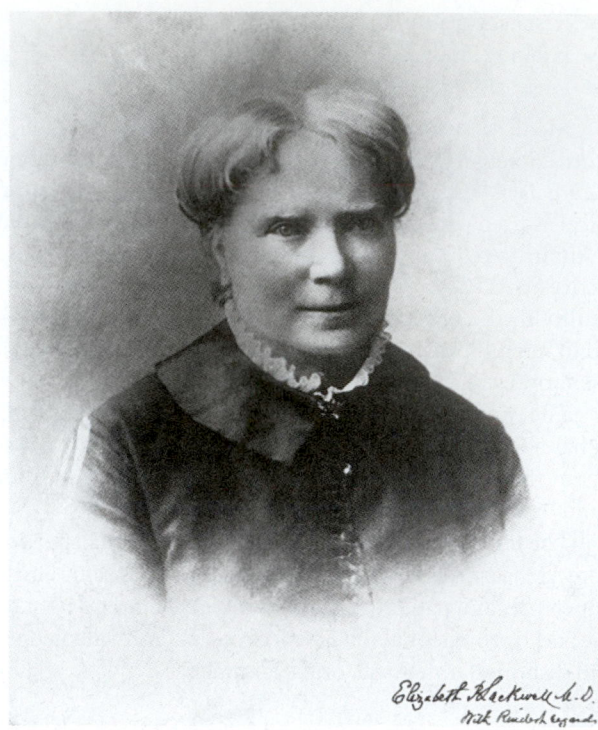

Figure 1-12 ◆ First female physician in the United States, Elizabeth Blackwell.

Ethics and Patient Rights

Ethics has been a part of medical practice since ancient times. In early Babylon, the Hammurabi Code set forth penalties for medical errors. The Hippocratic Oath followed (see Figures 1-13 ◆ and 1-14 ◆). For close to twenty-five centuries, the oath has guided physicians on issues of confidentiality, training practices, nondiscrimination, honesty, integrity, healing, morality, euthanasia, and abortion. It established medicine as an art of healing, not harming. The oath serves as the basis for medical ethics today.

The American Hospital Association's Patient Bill of Rights (1973)

As patients have become more involved in their own care, the focus has shifted from physicians telling patients what to do to physicians involving patients in decisions about their care. Patients today want to know more about the treatments their physicians recommends and any alternative treatments, including the benefits and risks of each. In 1992, hospitals were encouraged to adapt the revised bill to their facilities and communities. (∞ Chapter 4, Medical Law and Ethics, presents a more detailed discussion of this topic.)

Professionalism

As the average age of healthcare workers and the general population rises, the need for trained healthcare providers also rises. The training of nursing and allied healthcare professionals has not kept pace with the growing demand for healthcare services. The recognition of medical assistants as multiskilled health

I swear by Apollo the physician, and Aesculapius, and Health, and All-heal, and all the gods and goddesses, that, according to my ability and judgment, I will keep this Oath and this stipulation—to reckon him who taught me this Art equally dear to me as my parents, to share my substance with him, and relieve his necessities if required; to look upon his offspring in the same footing as my own brothers, and to teach them this art, if they shall wish to learn it, without fee or stipulation; and that by precept, lecture, and every other mode of instruction, I will impart a knowledge of the Art to my own sons, and those of my teachers, and to disciples bound by a stipulation and oath according to the law of medicine, but to none others. I will follow that system of regimen which, according to my ability and judgment, I consider for the benefit of my patients, and abstain from whatever is deleterious and mischievous. I will give no deadly medicine to anyone if asked, nor suggest any such counsel; and in like manner I will not give to a woman a pessary to produce abortion. With purity and with holiness I will pass my life and practice my Art. I will not cut persons laboring under the stone, but will leave this to be done by men who are practitioners of this work. Into whatever houses I enter, I will go into them for the benefit of the sick, and will abstain from every voluntary act of mischief and corruption; and, further from the seduction of females or males, of freemen and slaves. Whatever, in connection with my professional practice or not, in connection with it, I see or hear, in the life of men, which ought not to be spoken of abroad, I will not divulge, as reckoning that all such should be kept secret. While I continue to keep this Oath unviolated, may it be granted to me to enjoy life and the practice of the art, respected by all men, in all times! But should I trespass and violate this Oath, may the reverse be my lot!

—*Translated by Francis Adams*

From Edelstein, Lugwig. The Hippocratic Oath:Text, Translation and Interpretation. © 1996 Harold Cherniss. Reprinted with permission of The Johns Hopkins University Press.

Figure 1-13 ◆ Hippocratic Oath (classical version).

I swear to fulfill, to the best of my ability and judgment, this covenant:

I will respect the hard-won scientific gains of those physicians in whose steps I walk, and gladly share such knowledge as is mine with those who are to follow.

I will apply, for the benefit of the sick, all measures which are required, avoiding those twin traps of overtreatment and therapeutic nihilism.

I will remember that there is art to medicine as well as science, and that warmth, sympathy, and understanding may outweigh the surgeon's knife or the chemist's drug.

I will not be ashamed to say "I know not," nor will I fail to call in my colleagues when the skills of another are needed for a patient's recovery.

I will respect the privacy of my patients, for their problems are not disclosed to me that the world may know. Most especially must I tread with care in matters of life and death. If it is given me to save a life, all thanks. But it may also be within my power to take a life; this awesome responsibility must be faced with great humbleness and awareness of my own frailty. Above all, I must not play at God.

I will remember that I do not treat a fever chart, a cancerous growth, but a sick human being, whose illness may affect the person's family and economic stability. My responsibility includes these related problems, if I am to care adequately for the sick.

I will prevent disease whenever I can, for prevention is preferable to cure.

I will remember that I remain a member of society, with special obligations to all my fellow human beings, those sound of mind and body as well as the infirm.

If I do not violate this oath, may I enjoy life and art, respected while I live and remembered with affection thereafter. May I always act so as to preserve the finest traditions of my calling and may I long experience the joy of healing those who seek my help.

—*Written in 1964 by Louis Lasagna*
Academic Dean of the School of Medicine at Tufts University

Figure 1-14 ◆ Hippocratic Oath (modern version used in many medical schools today).

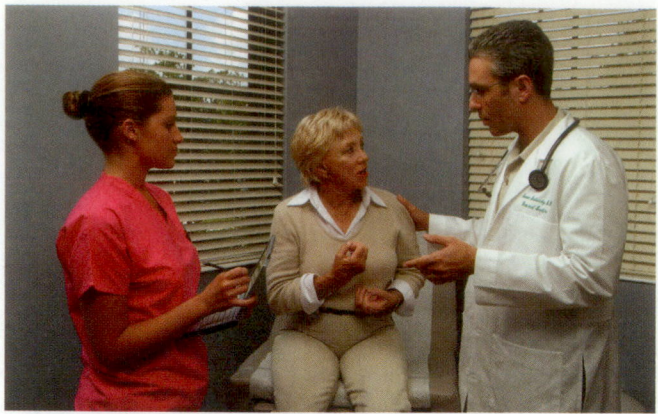

Figure 1-15 ◆ The recognition of medical assistants as multiskilled health professionals has expanded employment opportunities in the field.

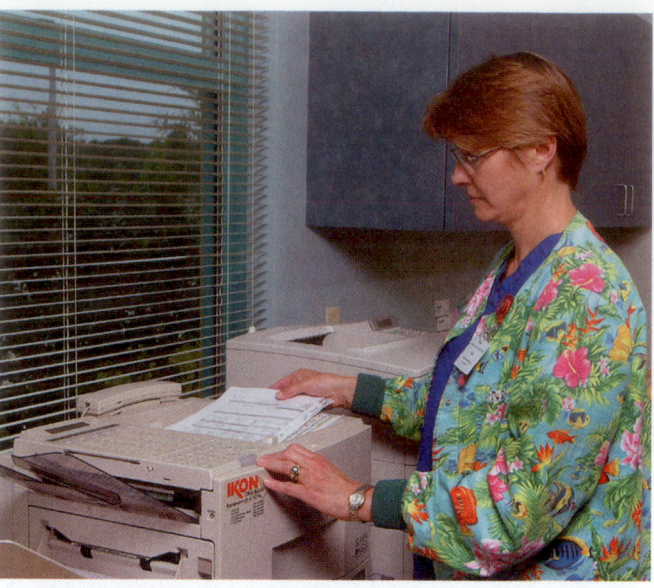

Figure 1-16 ◆ The medical assistant must have the dexterity to operate a variety of equipment.

professionals has expanded employment opportunities in the field (Figure 1-15 ◆).

Communication and Medical Terminology

Medical terminology is a basic language the MA will need to learn in order to speak with other health professionals, such as physicians and nurses. It comprises terms that are formed from roots, prefixes, suffixes, and combining forms. Learning medical terminology is the key to gaining medical knowledge and skills.

Another aspect of communication involves patients. When patients are ill or injured, they may be nervous or scared. It will be the MA's duty to calm them as much as possible so that they do not overreact physically or emotionally to physical examination or treatment. Therapeutic touch and an assuring manner help to defuse a patient's fear or anxiety. (∞ Chapter 5, Interpersonal Communication Skills, presents a more detailed discussion of this topic.)

Physical Requirements

Flexibility and strength are required for both clinical and administrative tasks. The medical assistant must be strong enough to perform various duties and have the dexterity to operate a variety of equipment (Figure 1-16 ◆). For example, the MA may need to transfer patients to exam tables or to wheelchairs. He or she may have to reach for supplies from higher storage shelves. Color vision must function normally to allow the MA to accurately describe the appearance of physical signs and symptoms. The medical assistant must be able to hear the telephone, voices, and patient sounds, especially when patients are distressed, and to listen to a patient's heartbeat with a stethoscope.

Character

Medical assistants must possess certain personality traits, including **empathy** for the patient as a whole person. The characteristics that are essential for working effectively with other medical team members and caring for patients are discussed in detail in ∞ Chapter 3, Professionalism in the Workplace.

Scope of Practice for Medical Assistants

The American Association of Medical Assistants defines medical assisting as an allied health profession whose practitioners function as members of the healthcare delivery team and perform administrative and clinical procedures. The medical assistant performs delegated clinical and administrative duties within the supervising physician's scope of practice consistent with the medical assistant's education, training, and experience. Such duties do not constitute the practice of medicine. Physician supervision shall be active and continuous but shall not be construed as necessarily requiring the physical presence of the supervising physician at the time and place that services are rendered.

It is not possible to devise a specific list of skills that covers all areas of performance for medical assistants. The AAMA defines and supports the medical assisting profession in its documents: *Occupational Analysis of the CMA (AAMA)*, the *Content Outline* of the CMA (AAMA) examination, the *Standards* and *Guidelines for Medical Assisting Educational Programs,* and *Advanced Practice of Medical Assisting*. To protect the public welfare and the right of the medical assistant to practice, and to provide a basis for legislation with the documents mentioned above, the AAMA has developed the *Scope of Practice for Medical Assistants.*

The MA is considered a dependent professional because performance is the result of assigned tasks within a job description and state law. Duties will often overlap those of licensed healthcare professionals.

It is the responsibility of the MA to know the laws concerning a medical assistant's scope of practice in the state in which he or she works. It is the responsibility of the employing agency to supply a job description that falls within legal regulations. It is the joint responsibility of the MA and the supervisor to monitor performance levels and provide training or supervision as necessary.

Patient Education

It is important for patients to understand the knowledge, skills, and scope of practice of all healthcare professionals, including the medical assistant. When patients incorrectly identify the medical assistant as a nurse, they should be politely corrected so they understand the medical assistant's role. For example, the medical assistant might say, "I am Dr. Smith's medical assistant. I have different skills from a nurse, and we perform different duties in the physician's office."

Job Opportunities

Medical assisting can be a chance for someone to step up in life. Medical assistants perform outpatient and inpatient services in many work settings, including medical offices, ambulatory clinics, hospitals, extended-care facilities, government agencies, rehabilitation facilities, and free-standing clinics. Jobs in a hospital or physician's office may include admissions, reception, billing, insurance, EKG, medical records, phlebotomy (with additional training), treatment/procedure, and emergency (registration or assistant). With further education and training, the MA may also find work as a pharmacy technician, for example (depending on state regulations), or an assistant to other professionals such as dentists and physical therapists.

The job outlook for medical assistants is promising. Job opportunities are expected to expand rapidly because of the rising numbers of elderly in the United States and because of advances in technology. With the likely growth in clinics and group practices, outpatient settings will continue to have the most openings. The strength of your training in administrative and clinical tasks will allow you a greater variety of job choices that meet your goals and interests.

Getting a job as a medical assistant may require previous experience in the field. In addition to an externship, which is an on-the-job learning experience, the MA can gain experience in an office setting by volunteering at a community clinic. Other volunteer possibilities include health screening clinics or fairs, well-baby clinics, senior citizen centers, and hospitals. Check with the college placement service to see what the community offers.

Medical assistants must have a proper resume when looking for a job. Most schools teach resume writing and also provide a chance to role-play a job interview. If you have access to the Internet, you may be able to get online help or advice on writing a resume. ∞ Chapter 51, Competing in the Job Market, provides detailed information on writing an effective resume.

Medical Assistant Educational Programs

In 1934, Dr. M. Mandl established the first school for training medical assistants. No longer just the physician's general helper, the medical assistant is now considered a multiskilled healthcare professional. Training today combines formal and clinical education along with an externship.

There are two options for credentials. One is the Certified Medical Assistant (**CMA**) (AAMA) credential through the American Association of Medical Assistants (AAMA). The second option is the Registered Medical Assistant (**RMA**) credential through the American Medical Technologists (**AMT**). In 2001, AAMA and AMT reached an agreement on a model state law that recognizes the scope of medical assisting. They also established minimum qualifications for practicing as an MA.

AMT was founded in 1939. AAMA, founded in 1955, develops the necessary structures to protect the MA's rights to practice. Both groups certify and represent medical assistants. AMT also represents and administers allied health certification examinations for medical laboratory technicians, medical technologists, phlebotomists, laboratory technicians, medical administrative assistants, allied health instructors, laboratory consultants, and dental assistants. AMT is accredited by the National Commission for Certifying Agencies (**NCCA**).

Along with the Committee for Accreditation of Allied Health Education Programs (**CAAHEP**), AAMA has established standards for accreditation (official approval) of medical assisting programs throughout the nation. The *Standards for an Accredited Educational Program for the Medical Assistant* may be viewed on the Internet at the CAAHEP site.

AMT is a member of the National Commission for Certifying Agents (NCCA), the accreditation arm of the National Organization for Competency Assurance (NOCA). NOCA sets standards for credentialing organizations in allied health fields.

The Accrediting Bureau of Health Education Schools (**ABHES**) is another accrediting agency. The U.S. Department of Education has granted recognition to ABHES as a specialized accreditor for training institutions with a healthcare educational focus. The evaluation standards of an ABHES-accredited program may be found on the Internet at www.abhes.org, in Chapter VI of the Accreditation Manual.

Educational Requirements of Medical Assisting

Vocational programs, **technical educational programs**, and **community colleges** all offer medical-assisting education. Programs take from six months to two years to complete. Many two-year programs award **associate degrees** as well as medical assisting certificates.

Accredited medical-assisting programs must teach in all areas of the AAMA Occupational Analysis, which lists medical-assisting skills for graduation, including **administrative**, **clinical**, and general ones (Figure 1-17 ◆). The AAMA composes the Occupational Analysis by randomly and periodically surveying medical assistants nationwide to determine their job duties.

Since 1998, applicants for the Certification Examination for Medical Assistants have been required to complete accredited medical assisting programs that include classes in clinical and administrative competencies (Table 1-2) and end with a required **externship** of a minimum number of hours. See ∞ Appendix C for tips on becoming a successful student.

Externships involve working as a medical assistant under a physician's supervision. Externships can run anywhere from 60

General, Clinical, and Administrative Skills* of the CMA (AAMA)

General Skills

◆ Communication
- Recognize and respect cultural diversity
- Adapt communications to individual's understanding
- Employ professional telephone and interpersonal techniques
- Recognize and respond effectively to verbal, nonverbal, and written communications
- Utilize and apply medical terminology appropriately
- Receive, organize, prioritize, store, and maintain transmittable information utilizing electronic technology
- Serve as "communication liaison" between the physician and patient
- Serve as patient advocate professional and health coach in a team approach in health care
- Identify basics of office emergency preparedness

◆ Legal Concepts
- Perform within legal (including federal and state statutes, regulations, opinions, and rulings) and ethical boundaries
- Document patient communication and clinical treatments accurately and appropriately
- Maintain medical records
- Follow employer's established policies dealing with the health care contract
- Comply with established risk management and safety procedures
- Recognize professional credentialing criteria
- Identify and respond to issues of confidentiality

◆ Instruction
- Function as a health care advocate to meet individual's needs
- Educate individuals in office policies and procedures
- Educate the patient within the scope of practice and as directed by supervising physician in health maintenance, disease prevention, and compliance with patient's treatment plan
- Identify community resources for health maintenance and disease prevention to meet individual patient needs

◆ Operational Functions
- Perform inventory of supplies and equipment
- Perform routine maintenance of administrative and clinical equipment
- Apply computer and other electronic equipment techniques to support office operations
- Perform methods of quality control
- Maintain current list of community resources, including those for emergency preparedness and other patient care needs
- Collaborate with local community resources for emergency preparedness
- Educate patients in their responsibilities relating to third-party reimbursements

Clinical Skills

◆ Fundamental Principles
- Identify the roles and responsibilities of the medical assistant in the clinical setting
- Identify the roles and responsibilities of other team members in the medical office
- Apply principles of aseptic technique and infection control
- Practice Standard Precautions, including handwashing and disposal of biohazardous materials
- Perform sterilization techniques
- Comply with quality assurance practices

◆ Diagnostic Procedures
- Collect and process specimens
- Perform CLIA-waived tests
- Perform electrocardiography and respiratory testing
- Perform phlebotomy, including venipuncture and capillary puncture
- Utilize knowledge of principles of radiology

◆ Patient Care
- Perform initial-response screening following protocols approved by supervising physician
- Obtain, evaluate, and record patient history employing critical thinking skills
- Obtain vital signs
- Prepare and maintain examination and treatment areas
- Prepare patient for examinations, procedures and treatments
- Assist with examinations, procedures, and treatments
- Maintain examination/treatment rooms, including inventory of supplies and equipment
- Prepare and administer oral and parenteral (excluding IV) medications and immunizations (as directed by supervising physician and as permitted by state law)
- Utilize knowledge of principles of IV therapy
- Maintain medication and immunization records
- Screen and follow up test results
- Recognize and respond to emergencies

Administrative Skills

◆ Administrative Procedures
- Schedule, coordinate, and monitor appointments
- Schedule inpatient/outpatient admissions and procedures
- Apply third-party and managed care policies, procedures, and guidelines
- Establish, organize, and maintain patient medical record
- File medical records appropriately

◆ Practice Finances
- Perform procedural and diagnostic coding for reimbursement
- Perform billing and collection procedures
- Perform administrative functions, including bookkeeping and financial procedures
- Prepare submittable ("clean") insurance forms

Figure 1-17 ◆ General, Clinical, and Administrative Skills* of the CMA (AAMA)

*All skills require decision making based on critical thinking concepts.

Reprinted by permission of the American Association of Medical Assistants (AAMA).

TABLE 1-2 SAMPLE ACCREDITED MEDICAL-ASSISTING CLASSES

Medical terminology	Medical law and ethics	Clinical surgical skills
Phlebotomy skills	Introduction to pharmacology	Clinical ambulatory skills
Intercultural communications	Administrative and office management skills	Medical billing and coding
Medical practice finances	Computer applications in the medical office	Anatomy and physiology
Medication administration	Disease and pathology	Cardiopulmonary resuscitation (CPR) and first aid skills
Clinical laboratory skills	Patient relations	Externship

to 240 hours, but many medical-assisting programs require externships of more than 240 hours. While externships are unpaid, students earn credits toward their medical assisting certificates.

HIPAA Compliance

All accredited medical-assisting programs include training on Health Insurance Portability and Accountability Act (**HIPAA**) regulations. HIPAA is critical for all healthcare professionals, because it provides a roadmap to avoiding patient-safety errors and malpractice lawsuits through vigilance to patient privacy. ∞ Chapter 4 details HIPAA and its implications for the medical assistant.

Certification Examination

To qualify for the CMA (AAMA) examination, the MA must meet the standards required by AAMA. The current standards require graduation from one of the following:

- A CAAHEP-accredited program, including externship, by January 31, June 30, or October 31 before the June, October, or late January test dates each year.
- An ABHES-accredited program completed by the deadline date.

As of January 5, 2009, the CMA (AAMA) Certification Examination began to be offered via computer-based testing. Candidates are able to select locations and flexible testing times at conveniently located computer-based testing centers throughout the United States. A pencil and paper examination will no longer be offered. The exam fee for the computer-based test is $125 for CAAHEP and ABHES graduating students, recent CAAHEP and ABHES graduates, and AAMA members. The exam fee is $250 for nonrecent CAAHEP and ABHES graduates and nonmembers. Exam fees are nonrefundable. After taking the computer-based exam, preliminary immediate pass/fail results will be provided. Official scores will be mailed within five to six weeks directly to candidates.

To keep your CMA (AAMA) status, you must recertify by testing on a five-year cycle or by fulfilling continuing education requirements.

To qualify for the RMA (AMT) examination, you must meet the standards set by AMT. The current standards require graduation from one of the following:

- A medical assistant program accredited by ABHES or CAAHEP.
- A medical assistant program accredited by a regional accrediting commission or a national accrediting organization approved by the U.S. Department of Education; the program must include 720 clock hours of medical assisting training and a clinical externship.
- A formal medical services training program of the U.S. Armed Forces.

Another way to qualify is to be employed in the medical assistant profession for at least five years, with no more than two as an instructor in a postsecondary medical assisting program. Upon passing the test, you obtain RMA (AMT) status.

AMT now has a Certification Continuation Program (CCP). AMT members are required to document activities supporting continuation of AMT certification every three years. Only newly certified members and reinstated members of AMT (after January 1, 2006) are required to attest to continuous employment while obtaining continuing education every three years. The goal is to promote, encourage, and reward practitioners who attempt to maintain the competencies required at initial certification throughout their careers.

Both AAMA and AMT offer networking possibilities at different levels within the organization and professional information through various publications. They also recognize the role of medical assistants during National Medical Assistant's Week, held yearly in October.

Multiple Medical-Assisting Statuses

Medical assistants who are certified by both the AAMA and the AMT can use both CMA (AAMA) and RMA (AMT) credentials. Both CMAs and RMAs are encouraged to join their local, state, and federal professional organizations. Although these organizations require fees to join, they help medical assistants maintain the skills needed in today's competitive job market through such benefits as:

- Educational presentations that offer CEUs
- Access to information on upcoming legislation related to the profession
- Subscription to professional journals
- Group insurance plans
- Professional malpractice insurance policies
- Networking opportunities

 **Critical Thinking Question 1-1**

Can Janet apply to take the AAMA exam at one of the three times offered this year? Why or why not? If not, explain what steps she might have to take to become eligible.

REVIEW

Chapter Summary

■ The early medical treatment of illness and disease consisted of folk remedies and sorcery. Knowledge of effective treatments was based on trial-and-error experiments with a wide range of plant and animal products. Some traditional treatments derived from plants, such as digoxin, are now manufactured in synthetic form.

■ Hippocrates is known as the Father of Medicine. In addition to teaching about health, he created the Hippocratic Oath, which sets ethical and professional guidelines for physicians. He also taught that disease had natural, rather than supernatural, causes.

■ In 1847 the AMA wrote a code of ethics for physicians. The code stressed professional and community responsibilities and promoted respect for human dignity, lifelong professional learning, and independence. The *Patient Bill of Rights* was developed by the AHA in 1973 to ensure effective care and satisfaction.

■ In 1847, Hungarian physician Ignaz Semmelweis began an experiment that required physicians to wash their hands before treating women in childbirth. The data from this experiment showed that hand washing markedly reduced the death rate of women who delivered in hospitals.

■ Throughout the years, a number of organizations have formed to advance varying facets of the medical profession. These include The American Hospital Association, the American Medical Association (AMA), and the American Red Cross.

■ Many women have featured prominently in medical history throughout the years. Marie Curie was one of the first notable women in healthcare, and to this day she remains the only woman to have won Nobel Prizes in two different fields. Florence Nightingale is known as the founder of nursing, and she helped advance the care of the poor, advocating improved medical care and commitment to the nursing profession. Elizabeth Blackwell was the first woman with a degree to practice medicine in the United States. Her sister, Emily, was the third woman to earn a medical degree in the United States. The Blackwell sisters worked together at the New York Infirmary for Indigent Women and Children for over forty years and in 1868 founded the Women's Medical College in New York.

■ Launched in 1948, the World Health Organization (WHO) is responsible for providing leadership on many global health issues.

■ As the medical field grew, requiring more highly trained people, the nursing profession developed to handle patient care. Economic changes in healthcare and a shortage of nurses have shaped the need for the trained multiskilled health professionals known as medical assistants.

■ A medical assistant needs solid communication, administrative, and clinical skills to project a professional image in the physician's office. Following ethical principles, including tolerance toward all persons, empathy, and maintaining patient confidentiality, is as important on the job as integrity, dependability, a sense of humor, and common sense. Good personal hygiene and certain physical capabilities are also necessary to perform the clinical aspects of patient care.

■ Jobs for medical assistants may be found in healthcare settings such as ambulatory care, physicians' offices, nursing homes, and hospitals.

■ It is the medical assistant's responsibility to maintain active membership in a professional organization. The AAMA and the AMT are two professional organizations for medical assistants, and their certification tests are nationally recognized. CMA (AAMA) recertification through continuing education is required to keep CMA credentials. RMA (AMT) recertification encourages voluntary continuing education for previously registered AMT members and a Certification Continuation Program for members joining after January 1, 2006.

■ The scope of medical-assisting practice is expected to continue to grow and change.

Chapter Review

Multiple Choice

1. Which of the following is an early medicine that is still used in medical treatment?
   a. cocoa
   b. ephedra
   c. foxglove
   d. geraniums

2. Trepanning was done to
   a. relieve pressure on the brain.
   b. release evil spirits.
   c. drain fluid after a head injury.
   d. allow good spirits to enter the head.

3. Who first used the term *prognosis*?
   a. Hammurabi
   b. Galen
   c. William Harvey
   d. Hippocrates

4. Which of the following is covered in the AMA's *Principles of Medical Ethics*?
   a. lifelong study
   b. humor
   c. personal hygiene
   d. personal gain

Chapter Review (continued)

5. On-the-job professionalism involves
   a. picking up and driving patients.
   b. scolding patients if they arrive late for an appointment.
   c. avoiding contact with patients.
   d. courtesy and patience with patients.

6. To become an MA, you should
   a. pass a recognized national certification test.
   b. apply for a license within your state.
   c. meet with local regulatory officials.
   d. take an oath before starting your job.

7. Experience in the field when you are still a student is called a(n)
   a. internship.
   b. externship.
   c. apprenticeship.
   d. clerkship.

8. In 2001, the AAMA and AMT established
   a. a working agreement to merge both organizations.
   b. a joint certification test for MAs.
   c. joint guidelines for the teaching of medical assisting.
   d. minimum qualification requirements to practice as an MA.

9. To maintain your CMA, you must continue your education or retest in
   a. six years.
   b. four years.
   c. five years.
   d. ten years.

True/False

T F 1. Medical assisting is a fairly new profession in the healthcare delivery system and did not receive professional recognition until the 1960s.

T F 2. Marie Curie is known as the founder of nursing.

T F 3. Physical flexibility and strength are not required if you plan to work only in the administrative section of the medical office.

T F 4. Nurses traditionally carried out both clinical and administrative duties in the physician's office.

T F 5. Scottish physician Alexander Wood invented the hypodermic needle.

Short Answer

1. What is the term for the written confirmation that an individual has met specific standards for the safe practice of a profession or service?

2. What is the granting of written permission to practice a profession called?

3. Explain how hand washing in healthcare began.

Research

1. What is the contact number for your local AAMA? Does it hold monthly meetings?

2. What is the process for applying to become a member of your local AAMA chapter?

3. Where would you research the specific laws that pertain to medical assistants working in your state?

4. Research the benefits and requirements of becoming a certified medical assistant.

Externship Application Experience

The medical assistant is performing her externship in a busy cardiology clinic. Toward the end of the externship, the clinic manager asks the medical assistant student if she has a resume she could leave with the clinic manager. The medical assistant has never prepared a professional resume. How should she proceed?

Resource Guide

Commission on Accreditation of Allied Health Education Programs (CAAHEP)

35 E Wacker Dr., Suite 1970
Chicago, IL 60601
1-312-553-9355
www.CAAHEP.org

American Association of Medical Assistants (AAMA)

20 N. Wacker Dr., Suite 1575
Chicago, IL 60606
1-800-228-2262
www.aama-ntl.org

Accrediting Bureau of Health Education Schools (ABHES)

7777 Leesburg Pike, Suite 314 N.
Falls Church, VA 22043
(703) 917-9503
www.abhes.org

American Medical Technologists

710 Higgins Road
Park Ridge, IL 60068
847.823.5169
www.amt1.com

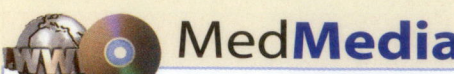

MedMedia

http://www.MyMAKit.com

More on this chapter, including interactive resources, can be found on the Student CD-ROM accompanying this textbook and on http://www.MyMAKit.com.

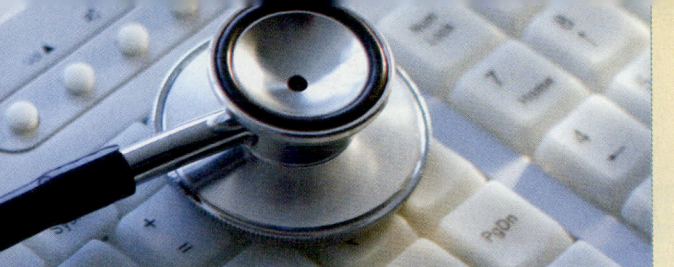

CHAPTER 2

Medical Assisting Today

Objectives

After completing this chapter, you should be able to:

- Define and spell the key terminology in this chapter.
- Define the role of the medical assistant in healthcare today.
- Describe the history of medical assisting.
- List the professional associations that certify other allied health professionals.
- List the qualities of a good medical assistant.
- List techniques for improving time-management skills.
- Define the jobs of other members of the healthcare team and their education requirements.

Case Study

Karla Wilkins and Carrie Smith, a medical assistant, were friends in high school. By the time the two unexpectedly meet at the local grocery store, they have not been in touch for several months. Carrie tells Karla about becoming certified as a medical assistant and includes such details as course load and topics. Looking confused, Karla responds, "If medical assistants don't *have* to be certified, why waste the time going to school? Why not just find a job and learn on the job?"

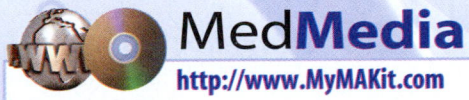

Med**Media**

http://www.MyMAKit.com

Additional interactive resources and activities for this chapter can be found on http://www.MyMAKit.com. For a video, tips, audio glossary, legal and ethical scenarios, on-the-job scenarios, quizzes, and games related to the content of this chapter, please access the accompanying CD-ROM in this book.

Video
Legal and Ethical Scenario: *Medical Assisting Today*
On the Job Scenario: *Medical Assisting Today*
Tips
Multiple Choice Quiz
Audio Glossary
HIPAA Quiz
Games: Spelling Bee, Crossword, and Strikeout

Key Terminology

accredited—endorsed by a reputable overseeing agency

administrative skills—clerical-type jobs (e.g., typing, filing)

advocate—one who defends or acts on behalf of another

American Association of Medical Assistants (AAMA)—national, professional association for medical assistants

American Medical Technologists (AMT)—national, professional association for medical technologists

body language—nonverbal means of communication (e.g., gestures, expressions)

clinical skills—abilities gained through hands-on patient care

rapport—trust and affection between parties

recertification—process of certificate renewal

Abbreviations

AAMA—American Association for Medical Assistants

AAPC—American Academy of Professional Coders

AHDI—Association for Healthcare Documentation Integrity

AHIMA—American Health Information Management Association

AMA—American Medical Association

AMT—American Medical Technologists

CAM—complementary alternative medicine

CLC—certified laboratory consultant

CMA—certified medical assistant

CMAS—certified medical administrative specialist

CMT—certified medical transcriptionist

COLT—certified office laboratory technician

CPC—certified professional coder

FDA—Federal Drug Administration

HIPAA—Health Insurance Portability and Accountability Act

HMO—health maintenance organization

LPN—licensed practical nurse

LVN—licensed vocational nurse

MLT—medical laboratory technician

MT—medical technologist

✚ MEDICAL ASSISTING STANDARDS

CAAHEP ENTRY-LEVEL STANDARDS	ABHES ENTRY-LEVEL COMPETENCIES
■ Perform within scope of practice (psychomotor) ■ Apply ethical behaviors, including honesty/integrity in performance of medical assisting practice (affective) ■ Apply active listening skills (affective) ■ Recognize the role of patient advocacy in the practice of medical assisting (cognitive) ■ Advocate on behalf of patients (psychomotor)	■ Adapt to change ■ Evidence a responsible attitude ■ Allied health professions and credentialing ■ Maintain licenses and accreditation

✔ COMPETENCY SKILLS PERFORMANCE

1. Adapt to change.

Introduction

With dramatic changes in healthcare over the past decade, including shorter hospital stays and managed care, physicians must rely on allied health personnel like medical assistants to help care for patients. With technology advancing and patient safety increasingly a focal point, many physicians today insist on hiring medical assistants who have been formally trained in accredited medical assisting programs. Part of this training includes complete knowledge of the medical assistant's role in patient care.

The Medical Assistant's Role in Healthcare Today

The medical assistant's role in healthcare is expanding. Medical assistants are working not only in ambulatory care settings, but also in unconventional locations such as insurance companies, hospitals, and skilled nursing facilities. As our population ages, the role of the medical assistant will likely grow further, as more patients enter the healthcare system.

The History of the Medical Assisting Profession

Traditionally, physicians hired nurses to work in their offices. With a shortage of nurses, physicians began to seek other qualified staff who could fulfill administrative and clinical duties. As a result, the demand for formally trained medical assistants began to rise.

When medical assisting began in the early 1950s, the Kansas Medical Assistants Society formed a professional organization for those in the field. A year later, the organization voted to rename itself the **American Association of Medical Assistants (AAMA)**. At the time, medical assistants lacked formal education; physicians trained most of their assistants on the job, and the AAMA held educational sessions designed to increase the professionalism of medical assisting. Since 1957, the AAMA has kept its national headquarters in Chicago, IL.

Abbreviations *(continued)*

TABLE 2-1 HISTORY OF THE AAMA

Year	Event
1961	Establishes certifying board.
1962	Offers sample exam.
1963	Holds first exams.
1977	Engages National Board of Medical Examiners as a test consultant.
1978	Gives exam in January and June at nationwide centers.
1980	Allows medical assistants to recertify via continuing education or exam.
1998	Requires exam candidates to complete medical assisting programs accredited by the Commission on Accreditation of Allied Health Education Programs (CAAHEP).
1999	Makes graduates of medical assisting programs accredited by the Accrediting Bureau of Health Education Schools eligible for the exam.
2002	Places certified medical assistant pin in space aboard a NASA shuttle.
2003	Renders recertification mandatory for certified medical assisting credential; adds October exam.
2005	Makes healthcare provider–level cardiopulmonary resuscitation mandatory to maintaining medical assisting certification.
2007	(AAMA) added to credential.
2009	Computerized testing offered.

Source: American Association for Medical Assistants: www.aama-ntl.org.

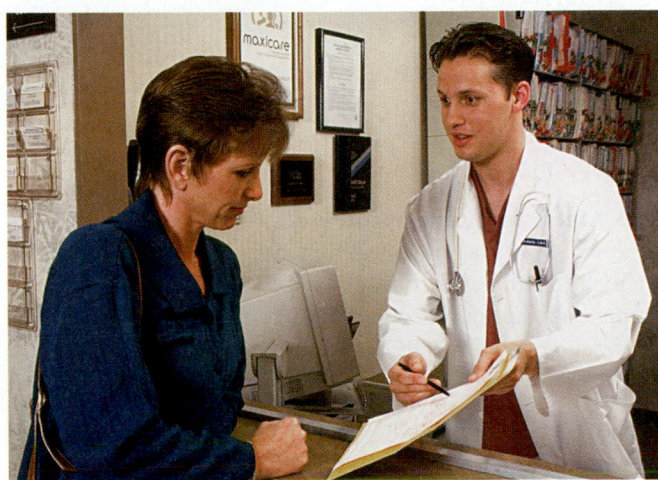

Figure 2-1 ◆ A medical assistant goes over paperwork with a patient.

The first AAMA president was Maxine Williams. Williams was a strong advocate for medical assisting. In 1959, she donated $200 of her own money to begin a fund to help needy students pursue their goal of becoming medical assistants. This fund, which still exists today, is called the Maxine Williams Scholarship Fund.

In 1978, the U.S. Department of Education followed suit of the **AMA** and recognized medical assisting as a profession. In 1991, the AAMA approved the current definition of medical assisting as, ". . . an allied health profession whose practitioners function as members of the health care delivery team and perform administrative and clinical procedures" (AAMA, 2007). Table 2-1 lists other AAMA milestones.

Today, medical assistants of both sexes are well trained, valuable members of the healthcare team (Figure 2-1 ◆).

? Critical Thinking Question 2-1

Referring to the case study at the beginning of the chapter, what evidence supports the argument that medical assistants should have a standardized base of knowledge?

The Requirements of Other Allied Health Associations

Healthcare is a very diverse community of professionals who work together as a team to care for patients. Allied health professionals have industry-specific associations; some have certification or registration exams. Postname initials indicate a professional's certification or registration status.

The American Medical Technologists (AMT)

In addition to the RMA certification discussed previously, the **American Medical Technologists** (**AMT**) (Figure 2-2 ◆) offers certification or registration as medical technologist (**MT**), medical laboratory technician (**MLT**), certified office laboratory technician (**COLT**), certified laboratory consultant (**CLC**), certified medical administrative specialist (**CMAS**), and registered phlebotomy technician (**RPT**).

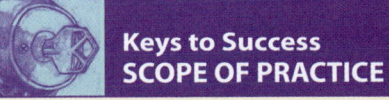

Keys to Success
SCOPE OF PRACTICE

Each state's Health Department outlines the exact scope of practice for medical assisting in that state.

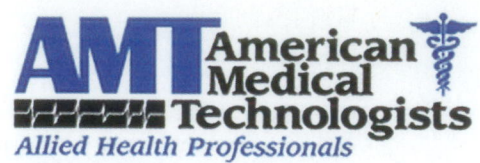

Figure 2-2 ◆ Logo for the American Medical Technologists Association (AMT).

Reprinted by permission.

The American Academy of Professional Coders (AAPC)

The American Academy of Professional Coders (**AAPC**) (Figure 2-3 ◆) is an organization for professionals focusing on medical billing and coding. The AAPC offers a voluntary credentialing program with examinations that confer certified professional coder (**CPC**) status.

The American Health Information Management Association (AHIMA)

The American Health Information Management Association (**AHIMA**) is a national organization of professionals who work in the field of medical records, coding, and health information management. This group was founded in 1928 to improve the quality of medical records. Currently, it is working to educate its membership on the changes required as healthcare records move toward becoming electronic.

The Association for Healthcare Documentation Integrity

In 1978, The Association for Healthcare Documentation Integrity (**AHDI**) was established as part of an effort to achieve recognition for the medical transcription profession. AHDI sets standards of education and practice for the medical transcription profession and offers a voluntary certification exam to individuals who wish to become Certified Medical Transcriptionists (CMTs). The **CMT** credential is awarded upon successfully passing the AHDI certification examination for medical transcriptionists (Figure 2-4 ◆).

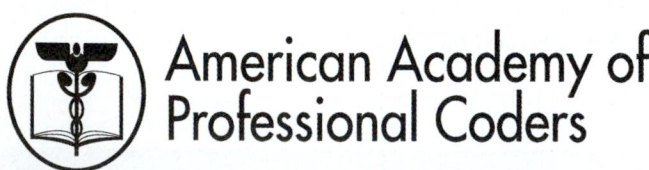

Figure 2-3 ◆ Logo for the American Academy of Professional Coders (AAPC).

Reprinted by permission.

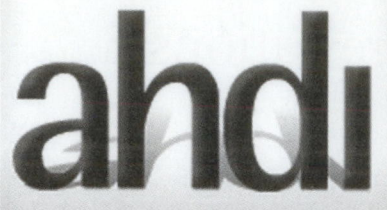

Figure 2-4 ◆ Logo for the Association for Healthcare Documentation Integrity.

Choosing Medical Assisting as a Career

Because medical assisting today is a career with multiple responsibilities, it requires a set of unique qualities.

Understanding Medical-Assisting Responsibilities

As mentioned in Chapter 1, the medical assistant helps the physician and the healthcare team provide patient care. To help keep patients safe, the medical assistant must practice good **clinical skills,** which include taking vital signs, collecting specimens, and administering medications and immunizations. Specific clinical duties for the medical assistant depend on the scope of practice in the state where the medical assistant is employed.

While patient care is part of medical assisting, the medical assistant's main responsibility is to be the patient's **advocate.** Because medical assistants will likely spend more time with patients than the physicians, medical assistants must develop a **rapport** with patients. Patients must be able to trust medical assistants, because those patients are more likely to share their personal information with assistants they trust. Patients may feel uncomfortable sharing their personal information with physicians, especially physicians they do not trust (Figure 2-5 ◆).

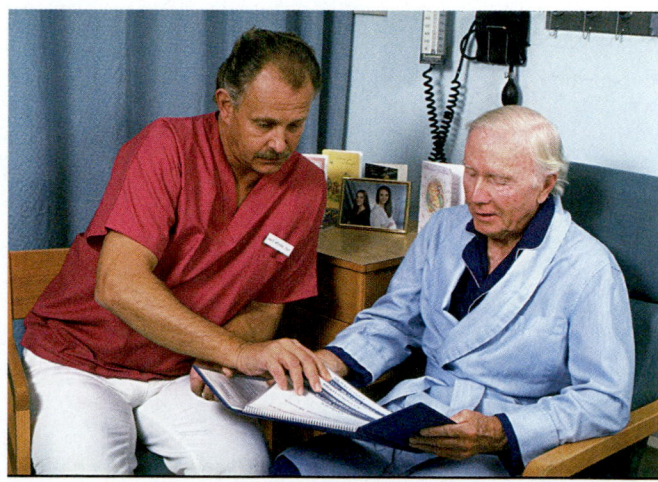

Figure 2-5 ◆ Medical assistants must develop a rapport with patients.

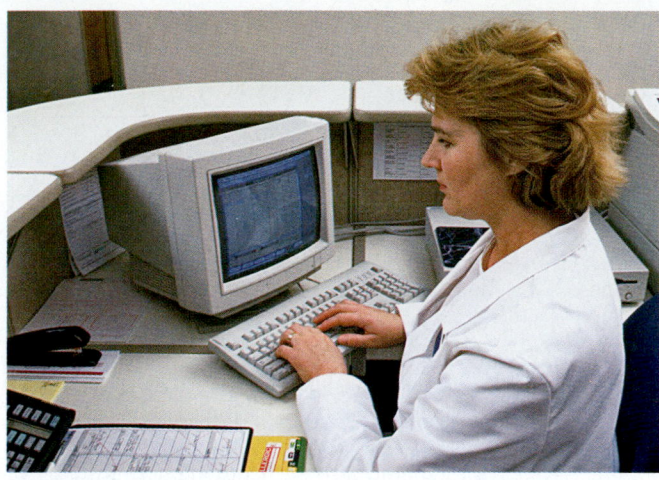

Figure 2-6 ◆ This medical assistant's responsibilities are weighted in the clerical arena.

In addition to clinical skills, medical assistants are responsible for performing **administrative skills**, such as appointment scheduling for physicians and insurance processing. The types of administrative duties medical assistants perform depend on the type and size of practice, as well as the assistants' preferences. Assistants may choose to apply for positions that have responsibilities weighted in the clerical or clinical arenas. In small clinics, medical assistants often perform both administrative and clinical functions. In large offices, job duties are often more specialized. Medical assistants in these offices may work in the clinical or administrative areas exclusively (Figure 2-6 ◆).

Identifying Positive Medical-Assisting Qualities

To be highly valued in today's competitive job market, medical assistants should have good clinical and administrative skills. The most sought-after assistants can perform varied duties in the medical office, applying their skills where those skills are needed most. To ensure they gain the proper skills, medical assistants should complete **accredited** programs. They should have a good understanding of medical terminology, and they should be well versed in the scope of their professional duties.

In addition to the proper background and training, good medical assistants have sound interpersonal skills. For a list of some desired qualities, see Table 2-2. Because many patients will stop seeing physicians when they feel uncomfortable with the office staff, patients should always feel welcome and cared for in the medical office. Good medical assistants remember patients' names, which helps make patients feel important and builds patient rapport.

In Practice

A new patient in town, Isaiah Rodriguez, arrives at the office needing a physician. According to Isaiah, his last physician had an unpleasant receptionist. Isaiah tells the medical assistant, "If I didn't like my doctor so much, I would have found another one." He adds that the person who answered his call for this appointment seemed like she was in a hurry. How should the medical assistant handle this situation? What can the medical assistant say to Isaiah? Should the medical assistant bring the situation to the doctor's attention? Why or why not?

TABLE 2-2 DESIRABLE MEDICAL ASSISTING QUALITIES

Quality	Explanation
Loyalty	■ Being faithful to one's employer, performing to the best of one's abilities, and arriving at work on time and ready to perform the job. Loyalty is staying with an employer through good days and bad.
Respect	■ Treating coworkers and patients with honor. Staff should demonstrate respect for physicians by using the title "Doctor" in front of patients, and doctors should show respect for their staff in return. Any corrective comments or disciplinary action should occur in private.
Dependability	■ Completing tasks on time and to the best of one's abilities. Dependability is arriving at work on time and staying to the end of the assigned shift. Late arrivals and frequent cancellations disrupt the whole office. Emergencies do happen, but dependable employees can generally be counted on to arrive and work when scheduled.
Courtesy	■ Extending kind words and compassion to patients and coworkers. Professional words and actions demonstrate courtesy.
Initiative	■ Taking action without being asked. A person with initiative knows what needs to be done and does it.
Flexibility	■ Willingness to exceed the job description whenever needed by changing one's schedule, if needed, or replacing someone who cannot work. Flexibility is the willingness to work late when the physician is running late and patients are still in the office. This is the ultimate sign of teamwork.
Credibility	■ Trustworthiness. Credibility is the feeling employers have toward employees when those employees have demonstrated that they are open and honest in their communications and actions.
Confidentiality	■ Ability to keep patient information private, to avoid sharing that information with inappropriate parties, like coworkers or neighbors.
Attitude	■ Overall approach. Positive attitudes foster positive work environments, while poor attitudes cultivate poor ones.

Effective medical assistants communicate well with patients as well as with other members of the healthcare team. Medical assistants should have empathy for others, and they should be comfortable in their role as patient advocates. In a country as diverse as the United States, good medical assistants know the prevailing cultural customs in their areas and can keep their personal beliefs separate from patient care. Good medical assistants also maintain patient confidentiality, disclosing personal patient information only when directed to do so by a patient or a court order.

Living and working in the same community can pose special challenges for healthcare staff who work with private patient information. Medical assistants know confidential patient information and are obligated by the Health Insurance Portability and Accountability Act (**HIPAA**), as well as ethical considerations, to keep that information private. In small communities, patients may ask about other patients outside the office. Medical assistants should never breach patient privacy, whatever the setting.

HIPAA Compliance

The Health Insurance Portability and Accountability Act (HIPAA) requires that medical assistants carefully guard patient confidentiality. Medical assistants should never release patient information without a patient's written authorization or a court order.

Like ethical behavior, a professional image is a critical part of medical assisting. Medical assistants are often patients' first contact with the office, and their behavior and appearance directly reflect the office and the physicians. Demonstrating professionalism means avoiding eating, drinking, and chewing gum while working or in patient view and maintaining a professional attitude. Part of maintaining a professional attitude includes remaining calm and polite and preventing patients from sensing any stress or irritation. Good medical assistants keep their personal feelings to themselves, never indicating disagreement with patients' healthcare or lifestyle choices. **Body language**, like facial expressions, may indicate disapproval. Table 2-3 provides examples of body language in different cultures.

Good medical assistants give the same level of professional care to all patients, even those who are rude and unpleasant. Good assistants also use proper grammar when communicating with patients, and that means avoiding slang terms or phrases. Patients who speak English as a second language may be unfamiliar with these terms and misinterpret their meanings.

TABLE 2-3	BODY LANGUAGE IN DIFFERENT CULTURES
Culture	**Examples**
Asian-Pacific	■ An open mouth, as when yawning, is considered rude. ■ Smiling can mean happiness, anger, confusion, or sadness. ■ Pointing with fingers is considered rude.
Chinese	■ Being physically intimidating, especially with an older person, is considered very rude. ■ Pointing is appropriate with an open hand, not just one finger.
Japanese	■ Bowing is a traditional greeting. ■ Staring is considered rude. ■ Standing with the hands in pockets is considered rude. ■ The "OK" symbol, the thumb and forefinger joined in a circle, may be interpreted as the signal for money.
Korean	■ Prolonged direct eye contact is considered rude. ■ Entering a room without knocking is considered rude. ■ Spitting and burping in public is acceptable.
Filipino	■ Hugging upon first meeting is acceptable. ■ Greetings include raised eyebrows. ■ Staring is considered rude.
Arabic	■ Failing to face a person while speaking is considered rude. ■ Men stand when women enter a room. ■ Men may shake hands with women only when the women offer their hands. ■ Only the right hand is used for eating.
Hispanic	■ Pointing with the index finger has a sexual meaning. ■ Standing closely together is appropriate.

Good personal hygiene, like professional behavior, is part of a professional image. Medical assistants should practice good personal hygiene for their body and their clothing. For example, American Medical Association (AMA) studies have shown that artificial nails may harbor bacteria, which is difficult to remove with hand washing. As a result, artificial nails should not be worn on the job. Medical assistants should also avoid wearing excessive or obtrusive jewelry, because hands will be washed and gloves donned several times a day. Body piercings, except for posts in the ear lobes, should not be visible, and tattoos and other body art should be covered during office hours. Hair should be clean and pulled back, and scented lotions and perfumes should be minimized out of respect for patients with allergies.

Uniforms, including shoes, should be clean and in good repair (Figure 2-7 ◆). The medical assistant's nametag should be in plain view and clearly identify the name and role of the medical assistant. Policies for dress, jewelry, hairstyles, piercings, and tattoos will vary from office to office, so medical assistants should review these policies when they are hired.

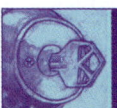

Keys to Success
PATIENT CONFIDENTIALITY

The job of protecting patient confidentiality extends beyond the work day. Never discuss patients by name outside the office, even when with coworkers. Always imagine that the patients, or people who know them, can hear the conversation. Imagine how breaching patient confidentiality would affect you and the physician.

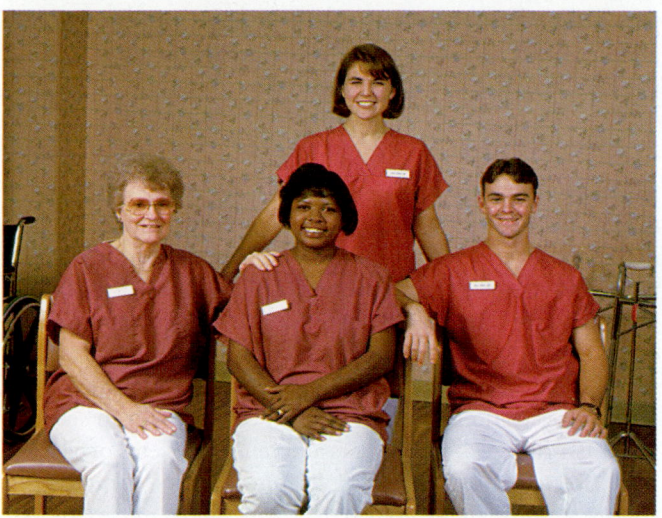

Figure 2-7 ◆ The medical assistant must maintain a professional image.

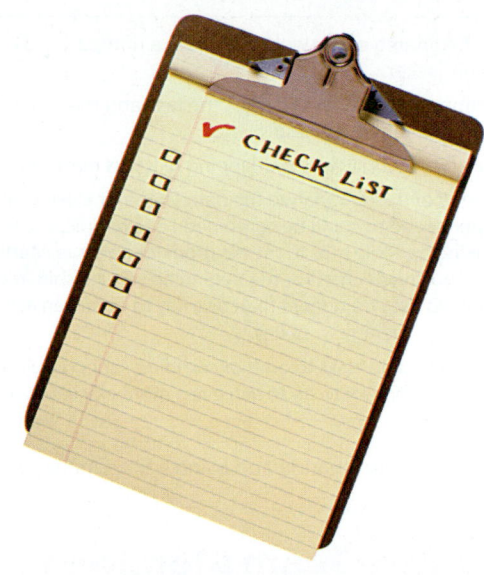

Figure 2-8 ◆ Using a checklist is a good way to stay organized.

Understanding the Medical Assistant's Role Outside the Office

In some ways, healthcare workers are held to a higher standard than those in many other fields. The medical assistant's professional image is expected to extend beyond the medical office, and the rules of patient confidentiality apply in all environments. When medical assistants work in the communities where they live, they are likely to see patients outside the clinical setting. Medical assistants must remember that they represent the medical office at all times, not just during business hours.

Managing Time Effectively in the Medical Office

In a busy healthcare setting, demands on the medical assistant's time can seem overwhelming. Depending on the office, one medical assistant may support several physicians. Especially in these situations, it is important for medical assistants to track their job duties and to know who to consult when their priorities conflict.

Good organization is key to medical-office time management. A time-management outline, which prioritizes projects, is one way for medical assistants to manage their time effectively. Writing down tasks is a good habit to develop. On paper, it is easier to divide big projects into smaller tasks or to organize tasks into a workable schedule. List items according to their due dates, and then categorize those items depending on how long they will take to complete. To stay on top of tasks, at the end of each day make a "to-do" list for the following day (Figure 2-8 ◆). Crossing items off the list as they are completed gives a sense of accomplishment and helps to ensure all items are completed.

If these techniques fail to help the medical assistant manage time effectively, try keeping a journal of each activity and the time it takes. Figure 2-9 ◆ lists the steps involved in creating and using such a time-management journal.

It is important for medical assistants to collaborate with their supervisors on time-management initiatives. Office managers and physicians should strive to keep their employees happy and efficient, and medical assistants who raise concerns about their use of time show that they are responsible members of the healthcare team.

PROCEDURE 2-1 Adapt to Change

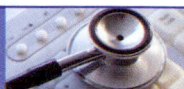

Theory and Rationale
Because physicians, supervisors, or office managers will often ask medical assistants to start a new task, it is crucial for medical assistants to adapt efficiently and effectively to changing priorities.

Materials
■ Notepad
■ Pen

Competency
(**Conditions**) With the necessary materials, you will be able to (**Task**) adapt to change when given a new task (**Standards**) within the time limit set by the instructor.

1. Listen closely as a new task is requested.
2. Ask questions to clarify the request, if needed.
3. Take notes about the task, if needed.
4. Begin working on the new task while maintaining a positive and professional attitude.

1. At the beginning of the work day, place a notepad and pen in the clinic jacket.

2. Each time you perform a task, list the task and the exact time it took from beginning to end.

3. Note any conflicts, such as overlapping requests from supervisors.

4. At the end of the day, analyze the data. Determine if any tasks were unneeded or could be combined. For example, you might be making multiple trips to the file room for patients' charts instead of pulling all charts at the beginning of each shift. You might need data from more than one day to obtain an accurate picture of an average work day.

5. When you find no tasks to omit or combine, schedule a meeting with your supervisor to try to achieve a more efficient workflow.

Figure 2-9 ◆ Steps to creating and using a time-management journal.

Healthcare Team Members

To be an effective member of a healthcare team, the medical assistant should understand the role of every other team member in patient-centered general care. Understanding the interaction of various roles adds to the quality of patient care and the efficiency of the physician's office.

Physician

Physicians provide the diagnosis and direction for patient treatment. Their training is long and rigorous, requiring a bachelor's degree, completion of medical school, licensure examination, and residency. Some physicians choose to specialize in a specific body system or treatment. For example, a physician who specializes in gastroenterology treats the gastrointestinal system, and a physician who specializes in gerontology deals with aging patients.

A physician must follow ethical practices. A physician's license may be suspended—the physician is temporarily barred from practicing—until the case is reviewed, or the license may be revoked—taken back by the government—if the misconduct is serious.

Health maintenance organizations (**HMOs**), managed care, and preferred providers have created another title for physicians: primary care physician (**PCP**), also called the *gatekeeper*. The PCP replaces what used to be referred to as the general practitioner (GP) or family physician. The PCP takes on the primary responsibility for patient care, makes referrals for additional treatment as necessary, and acquires precertification for care and procedures.

Medical assistant training should allow you to work with most physicians at the entry level. With additional on-the-job training the MA may be able to help a physician in specific settings. Be aware of the MAs responsibility to the physician(s) with whom the MA works. The physician is held as the *respondent superior* in court—if you make a patient error, both the MA and the physician are held responsible, or the physician employer is liable for his or her employee's actions.

Physician's Assistant

A physician's assistant (**PA**) provides patient care under the supervision of a physician. Training requirements and duties vary from state to state. Duties generally include taking the patient's medical history, performing physical examinations and diagnostic procedures, providing followup care, teaching patients, and, in some states, writing prescriptions.

Nurse Practitioner

Nurse practitioners (**NPs**) provide services similar to those of the PA. The main differences between these two professions are that the NP is also a trained nurse, and NPs require more training than PAs. Most NPs have advanced nursing degrees and many are able to open their own clinical practices, depending on the laws in their states. NPs are also allowed to prescribe medications and have Drug Enforcement Administration (**DEA**) registration numbers in most states. NPs can serve as patients' primary care providers and can see patients of all ages.

To be licensed as NPs, applicants must first complete the education and training needed to be a registered nurse (**RN**). In most states, NPs are also required to have a master's degree in nursing. Once applicants have secured their RN degree, they must complete an advanced nursing education program. Many of these programs specialize in a field like family practice, adult health, acute care, or women's health. NPs must be licensed by the states in which they practice.

Nurse

A licensed practical or vocation nurse (**LPN**, **LVN**) usually completes one year of training. A registered nurse (**RN**) can graduate from a two-year (associate), three-year (diploma), or four-year (baccalaureate) program. An RN receives more training in assessment and clinical skills, and as a result has greater responsibilities than an LPN or LVN.

Pharmacist

Pharmacists play an important role in patient care. They distribute the drugs prescribed by healthcare providers and educate patients about the medications they are taking. Some pharmacists work for pharmacies, while others own them. Many large healthcare facilities have pharmacies on their premises, which can be convenient for patients. Some pharmacists work for drug manufacturers researching new medications.

Pharmacists who work in community or retail pharmacies often counsel patients and answer questions about medications, both prescriptions and over-the-counter (OTC) medications, including possible side effects or drug interactions. Pharmacists may also advise patients about the use of durable medical equipment (DME), diet, exercise, or stress management.

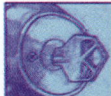

Keys to Success
YOUR TITLE

Medical assistants must *never* intentionally represent themselves as nurses. If a patient calls you "Nurse," carefully tell him or her your correct title. The best way to prevent misunderstandings is to wear a name pin with "CMA" or "RMA" following your name. *Never* refer to yourself as "the nurse".

Other Healthcare Team Members

Other members of the medical and dental healthcare team are described below.

- Blood bank technologist—tests blood to ensure donor-recipient compatibility.
- Certified nursing assistant (CNA)—helps nursing staff by providing bedside patient care in nursing home and extended care facilities, such as bed baths, feeding, walking, and vital signs.
- Clinical dietitian—coordinates patient's diet and medications.
- Dental assistant—works chairside with the dentist by preparing patients for treatment, taking dental X-rays, and making dental impressions.
- Dental hygienist—cleans patient's teeth, discusses findings with the dentist, and teaches dental health to the patient; in some states, may perform more advanced procedures with training.
- Electrocardiograph technologist—takes EKGs to provide a patient record of cardiac electrical activity.
- Electroencephalograph technologist—takes EEGs to provide a patient record of brain activity.
- Emergency medical technician (EMT)—from basic to paramedic levels, provides emergency stabilizing care at the scene of injury or trauma, then transports the patient to the nearest medical center. Three levels of EMT are basic, advanced or intermediate, and paramedic (Figure 2-10 ◆).
- Medical laboratory technologist—tests clinical specimens such as blood, urine, and other body specimens; also manages the department.
- Medical records technician—files patients' charts, ensures that stored records are kept confidential, and follows procedures for release of chart information to patients, courts of law, and insurance companies.
- Medical secretary—does a variety of administrative duties as directed based on the needs of the office, the professional staff, and the office manager.
- Medical transcriptionist—transfers physician/surgeon data from audio recordings to hard copies for the patient chart.
- Nuclear medicine technologist—responsible for dispensing radioactive substances before X-rays are performed.
- Occupational or physical therapy assistant—helps therapists by working with patients on specific activities.
- Occupational therapist (OT)—works with individuals who have conditions that are physically, emotionally, or developmentally disabling; helps patients to function at work and with daily living.
- Office manager—directs the activities of the administrative and clinical staff, such as physicians, nurses, and lab and respiratory technicians.
- Pharmacist—highly trained in dispensing of medications; fills prescriptions and provides patient education; mixes prescription pharmaceutical preparations as directed by the physician.
- Pharmacy technician—helps the pharmacist with routine tasks such as counting pills and labeling and helps the patient with healthcare items.

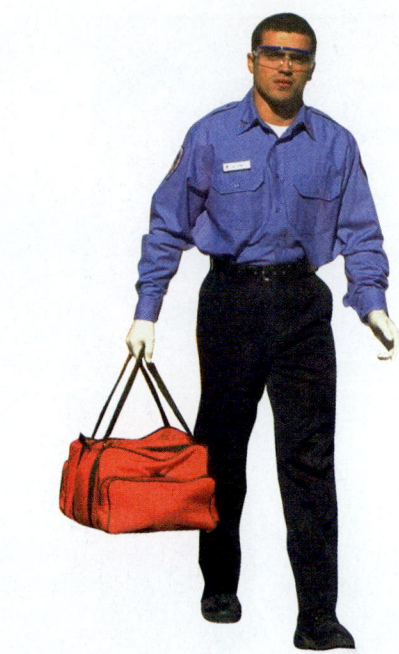

Figure 2-10 ◆ Emergency medical technician (EMT).

- Phlebotomist—specializes in taking blood specimens for laboratory analysis.
- Physical therapist (PT)—restores function, improves mobility, eases pain, and works to reestablish a patient in the workplace and community after an injury or illness (Figure 2-11 ◆).
- Respiratory therapist (also called respiratory care practitioner)—evaluates, treats, cares for, and educates patients with respiratory diseases.
- Social worker—connects patients with special needs to agencies that may help them; needs may be financial or may be the result of acute or long-term physical or mental illness.
- Ultrasound technologist—takes fetal and cardiac ultrasounds and others (Figure 2-12 ◆).

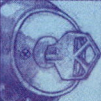

Keys to Success
LICENSING AND CERTIFICATION

Certification is written confirmation that an individual has met specified standards for the safe practice of a profession or service. Certified Medical Assistant (**CMA**) and Registered Medical Assistant (**RMA**) certificates are recognized nationally. Medical assistants and other health care professionals should complete an educational program and pass a national exam for voluntary certification.

Licensure is the granting of written permission to practice a profession. Physicians and nurses in all 50 states and the District of Columbia are required to have licenses. These licenses are recognized only in the state that grants them, although a license can be held in more than one state if the nurse or physician meets the requirements set by each state. State statutes (Practice Acts) define the scope of practice for these professionals.

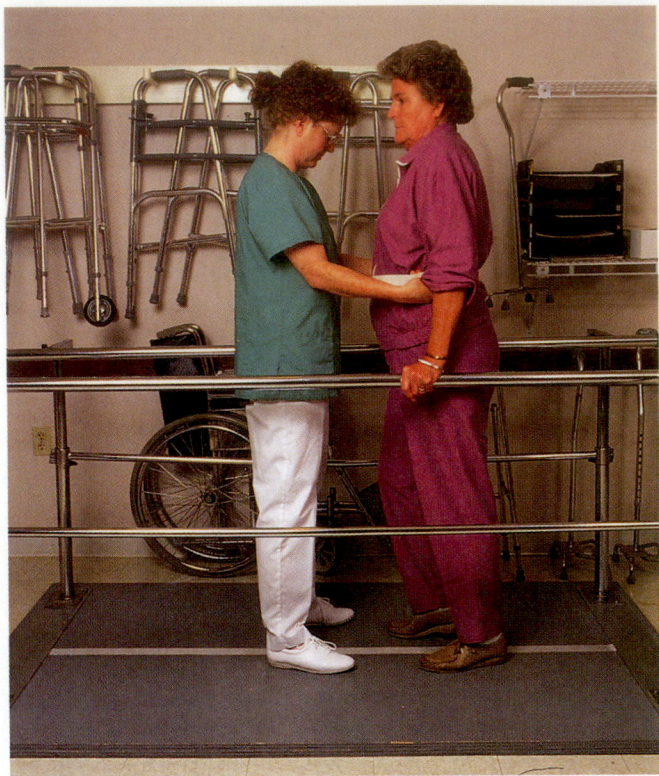

Figure 2-11 ◆ Physical therapist.

This list does not include every healthcare team member. As the medical field changes, so do job descriptions and training.

Medical Practice Specializations

Medical and surgical specialties today are varied. Table 2-4 lists several common medical specialties and the services they provide and Table 2-5 outlines several common surgical specialties.

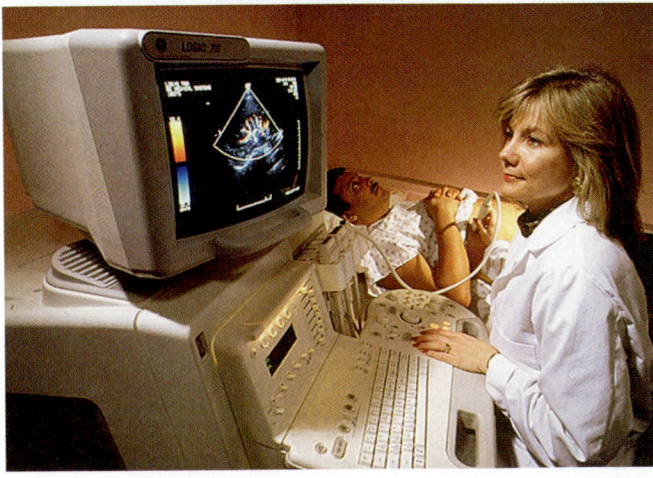

Figure 2-12 ◆ Ultrasound technologist.
Browne Harris / The Stock Market

TABLE 2-4 COMMON MEDICAL SPECIALTIES

Specialty Type	Service(s) Provided
Allergist	Diagnoses and treats allergic conditions
Cardiologist	Diagnoses and treats heart and cardiovascular system conditions
Dermatologist	Diagnoses and treats skin disorders
Emergency physician	Treats patients with emergent needs, such as in emergency rooms
Endocrinologist	Diagnoses and treats hormone-related disorders
Family practitioner	Acts as a primary care physician for patients of all ages, treating varied illnesses and performing routine screenings (e.g., physical examinations)
Gastroenterologist	Diagnoses and treats disorders related to the stomach and intestines
General practitioner	Same as the family practice physician (see preceding), except may not accept child patients
Gerontologist	Diagnoses and treats conditions of the elderly population
Gynecologist	Diagnoses and treats conditions related to the female reproductive system
Hematologist	Diagnoses and treats conditions associated with blood disorders
Infertility practitioner	Diagnoses and treats disorders related to infertility problems and helps achieve pregnancy via medical means
Intensive care physician	Treats patients in the hospital intensive care unit
Internist	Focuses on the prevention and treatment of adult diseases
Neonatologist	Diagnoses and treats newborns
Nephrologist	Diagnoses and treats conditions associated with the kidneys
Neurologist	Diagnoses and treats conditions associated with the nervous system
Obstetrician	Treats pregnant women through the postpartum period
Oncologist	Diagnoses and treats patients with cancerous conditions
Ophthalmologist	Diagnoses and treats eye conditions
Orthopedist	Diagnoses and treats conditions associated with the musculoskeletal system
Otolaryngologist	Diagnoses and treats conditions associated with the ears, nose, and throat
Pediatrician	Treats children
Podiatrist	Diagnoses and treats feet conditions
Proctologist	Diagnoses and treats conditions associated with the colon, rectum, and anus
Psychiatrist	Diagnoses and treats mental disorders
Pulmonologist	Diagnoses and treats conditions associated with the respiratory system
Radiologist	Interprets radiographs (X-rays) and other imaging studies (e.g., ultrasounds or mammograms)
Rheumatologist	Diagnoses and treats conditions associated with arthritis or other joint disorders
Urologist	Diagnoses and treats conditions associated with the urinary system

TABLE 2-5 COMMON SURGICAL SPECIALTIES

Surgical Specialty Type	Description
Cardiothoracic	Treats chest diseases and heart and lung conditions
Cosmetic	Repairs or reconstructs body parts, either due to accidents or disease or as elective surgery
General	Treats varied surgical cases
Maxillofacial	Repairs face and mouth disorders
Neurological	Repairs disorders of the neurologic system
Orthopedic	Repairs conditions of the musculoskeletal system
Vascular	Repairs conditions of the blood vessels

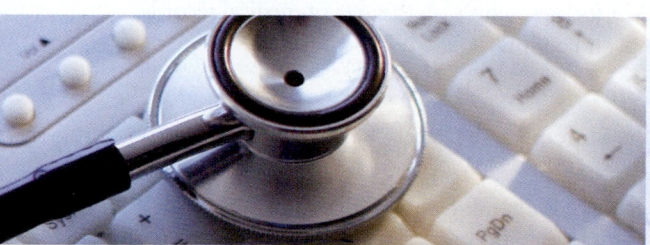

REVIEW

Chapter Summary

- Medical assistants perform varied tasks, both clinical and administrative, and keep the medical office running smoothly. The scope of medical assisting is expected to expand and to continue offering varied challenges and responsibilities.
- Traditionally, physicians hired nurses to work in their offices. Due to a shortage of nurses, physicians began to seek other qualified staff who could fulfill administrative and clinical duties, and therefore the demand for formally trained medical assistants began to rise.
- In the early 1950s, the Kansas Medical Assistants Society formed a professional organization for those in the field. One year later, the organization renamed itself the American Association of Medical Assistants (AAMA).
- In 1978, the U.S. Department of Education followed the AMA and recognized medical assisting as a profession.
- Healthcare is a very diverse community of professionals who work together as a team to care for patients. Allied health professionals have industry-specific associations, including the American Medical Technologists (AMT), the American Academy of Professional Coders (AAPC), the American Health Information Management Association (AHIMA), and the Association for Healthcare Documentation Integrity (AHDI).
- Effective medical assistants today have sound clinical and administrative skills, good interpersonal skills, and a professional image that extends outside the office.
- Organization and the proper tools are key to efficient time management in the medical office.
- To perform specialized treatments, you may need additional training specific to the physician's office. It is also very important to understand the roles of other healthcare team members to work successfully on a team.
- In order to be an effective member of a healthcare team, the medical assistant should understand the role of every other team member in patient-centered general care.

Chapter Review

Multiple Choice

1. Which of the following AAMA milestones happened first?
   a. The AAMA allows medical assistants to recertify via continuing education or exam.
   b. The AAMA places certified medical assistant pin in space aboard a NASA shuttle.
   c. The AAMA gives exam in January and June at nationwide centers.
   d. The AAMA makes healthcare provider-level CPR mandatory to maintaining medical assisting certification.

2. The AAPC offers a voluntary credentialing program for what category of health care professional?
   a. Medical Laboratory Technician
   b. Certified Medical Transcriptionist
   c. Certified Office Laboratory Technician
   d. Certified Professional Coder

Chapter Review (continued)

3. A medical assistant who has developed trust and affection between the patient and the medical assistant has shown which of the following?
   a. rapport
   b. advocate
   c. initiative
   d. courtesy

4. _____ is being faithful to one's employer, performing to the best of one's abilities, and arriving at work on time and ready to perform the job.
   a. Respect
   b. Loyalty
   c. Dependability
   d. Flexibility

5. The first president of the AAMA was
   a. Elizabeth Blackwell.
   b. Maxine Williams.
   c. Clara Barton.
   d. none of the above.

6. In what year did the U.S. Department of Education recognize medical assisting as a profession?
   a. 1958
   b. 1968
   c. 1978
   d. 1988

7. The AMT offers certification or registration to which of the following groups of professionals?
   a. CMAs
   b. CMAS
   c. CPCs
   d. All of the above

True/False

T F 1. Credibility is the feeling employers have toward employees when those employees have demonstrated that they are open and honest in their communications and actions.

T F 2. Medical assistants should never release patient information without a patient's written authorization or a court order.

T F 3. A person from the Chinese culture may find that staring is considered rude.

T F 4. A good medical assistant is able to keep his or her personal feelings private.

T F 5. A nurse practitioner typically has a master's degree in nursing.

T F 6. A dental assistant is a person who cleans a patient's teeth.

T F 7. AHIMA focuses mainly on the area of medical records, billing, and coding.

Short Answer

1. Explain the difference between a nurse and a nurse practitioner.
2. Explain what a blood bank technologist's duties include.
3. Describe the difference between a dental assistant and a dental hygienist.
4. Describe how certification differs from licensure.
5. Explain the pharmacist's role in patient care.
6. Explain how a social worker might be involved in a patient's care.

Research

1. Where does your local medical assisting association meet?
2. How would you go about becoming a member of your local medical assisting chapter?
3. What is the scope of practice of a medical assistant in your state?

Externship Application Experience

A patient at the externship site asks the medical assistant to differentiate between a nurse and a medical assistant. How should the medical assistant respond?

Resource Guide

American Academy of Professional Coders
2480 South 3850 West, Suite B
Salt Lake City, UT 84120
Phone: 800-626-2633
Fax: 801-236-2258
email:info@taapc.com, www.aapc.com

American Association of Medical Assistants
20 N. Wacker Dr., Ste. 1575
Chicago, IL 60606
Phone: (312) 899-1500
Fax: (312) 899-1259
www.aama-ntl.org

Association of Healthcare Documentation Integrity
4230 Kiernan Avenue
Suite 130
Modesto, CA 95356
Phone: (800) 982-2182
Fax: (209) 527-9633
email: ahdi@ahdionline.org

American Health Information Management Association
233 N. Michigan Avenue, 21st Floor
Chicago, IL 60601-5800
Phone: (312) 233-1100
Fax: (312) 233-1090
email: info@tahima.org, www.ahima.org

American Medical Technologists
10700 West Higgins Road, Suite 150
Rosemont, IL 60018
Phone: (800) 275-1268
Fax: (847) 823-0458
www.amt1.com

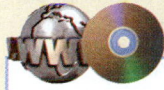 Med**Media**

http://www.MyMAKit.com

More on this chapter, including interactive resources, can be found on the Student CD-ROM accompanying this textbook and on http://www.MyMAKit.com.

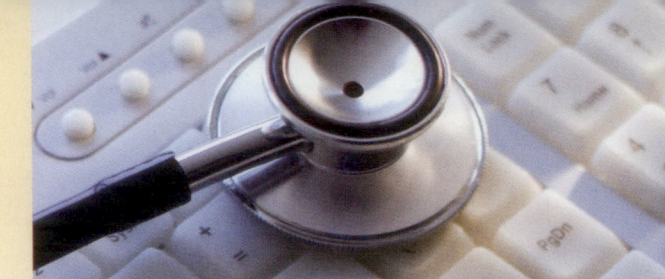

CHAPTER 3

Professionalism in the Workplace

Case Study

Jamie Kim has recently graduated from a medical assisting program. She has been interviewing at several clinics but has not been offered a position as a medical assistant yet. When Jamie discusses her frustration with her roommate, the roommate says, "Maybe you aren't portraying a professional image to the employers you are meeting."

Objectives

After completing this chapter, you should be able to:

- Define and spell the key terminology in this chapter.
- Define the medical assistant's role in the professional workplace.
- Explain the meaning of the word *professionalism* as it applies to working in a healthcare setting.
- Describe various positive traits the medical assistant should have in order to maintain a professional image.
- Describe various negative traits the medical assistant should avoid in order to maintain a professional image.

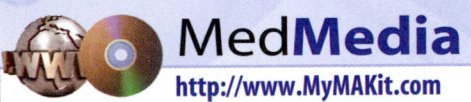

Med**Media**

http://www.MyMAKit.com

Additional interactive resources and activities for this chapter can be found on http://www.MyMAKit.com. For a video, tips, audio glossary, legal and ethical scenarios, on-the-job scenarios, quizzes, and games related to the content of this chapter, please access the accompanying CD-ROM in this book.

Video: *Patient Care*
Legal and Ethical Scenario: *Professionalism in the Workplace*
On the Job Scenario: *Professionalism in the Workplace*
Tips
Multiple Choice Quiz
Audio Glossary
HIPAA Quiz
Games: Spelling Bee, Crossword, and Strikeout

✚ MEDICAL ASSISTING STANDARDS

CAAHEP ENTRY-LEVEL STANDARDS	ABHES ENTRY-LEVEL COMPETENCIES
<ul><li>Perform within scope of practice (psychomotor)</li><li>Apply ethical behaviors, including honesty/integrity in performance of medical assisting practice (affective)</li><li>Apply active listening skills (affective)</li><li>Identify styles and types of verbal communication (cognitive)</li><li>Identify nonverbal communication (cognitive)</li><li>Demonstrate awareness of how an individual's personal appearance affects anticipated responses (affective)</li><li>Identify time management principles (cognitive)</li><li>Implement time management principles to maintain effective office function (affective)</li><li>Advocate on behalf of patients (psychomotor)</li><li>Recognize the role of patient advocacy in the practice of medical assisting (cognitive)</li></ul>	<ul><li>Adapt to change</li><li>Maintain confidentiality at all times</li><li>Project a positive attitude</li><li>Evidence a responsible attitude</li><li>Conduct work within scope of education, training, and ability</li><li>Instruct patients with special needs</li><li>Be courteous and diplomatic</li><li>Serve as a liaison between the physician and others</li><li>Orient patients to office policies and procedures</li><li>Adapt what is said to the recipient's level of comprehension</li><li>Adaptation for individualized needs</li><li>Exercise efficient time management</li><li>Receive, organize, prioritize, and transmit information expediently</li></ul>

Key Terminology

compassion—using empathy to sense others' concerns or feelings.

competence—the ability to perform one's job up to standard.

professionalism—acting in a businesslike manner in the workplace.

respect—treating others with dignity.

responsibility—taking ownership of one's actions.

Introduction

Professionalism in the healthcare setting is a must for the medical assistant as well as for all members of the healthcare team. A person who is acting in a professional manner is considered to be someone who has a high degree of self-control. This means the professional medical assistant is one who treats all patients and coworkers with a high level of respect.

The Medical Assistant's Role in Professionalism

As a medical assistant, you will have multiple encounters with patients every day. Each patient encounter has the potential to cause that patient's experience in your facility to be a positive or a negative one. Acting in a professional manner is one way to be the best advocate for your patient. As a medical assistant, you show professionalism by using complete sentences and correct spelling in your communications in the office and by not making rude or personal comments regarding a patient.

What Is Professionalism?

Professionalism is acting in a businesslike manner in the workplace. It is keeping calm, even in the most stressful of situations. The professional medical assistant is one who does not respond in anger when patients or coworkers are rude. Professionalism is both appearance and attitude, and it is something most patients will notice—especially if the medical assistant seems to fall short in this area (Figure 3-1 ◆).

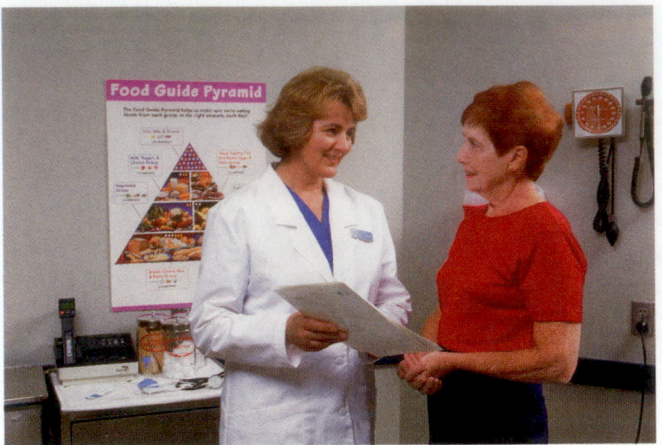

Figure 3-1 ◆ By remaining calm, the medical assistant helps the patient to remain calm as well.

Characteristics of Professional Behavior

There are many characteristics that embody the term *professional behavior*. While not all medical assistants will possess the same personality characteristics, there are some professional characteristics that should be present in all successful medical assistants.

Professionalism is portrayed to others by the medical assistant's manner of dress. Medical assistants should always dress in a manner that is acceptable for their place of employment. While many medical offices require medical assistants to wear scrubs when working in the clinical setting, administrative medical assistants may be asked to wear professional business attire. As mentioned in ∞ Chapter 2, the medical assistant's image must be professional at all times. This includes the cleanliness of the uniform, shoes, hair, and fingernails.

Competence

The medical assistant should have mastered the basic knowledge and skills associated with the profession of medical assisting. This **competence** will be obvious not only to coworkers, but also to the patients the medical assistant works with. Part of being competent is the motivation to continue learning. This is done by asking questions of the physician when needed and by attending classes or seminars in order to further advance the skills learned in the medical assisting training program.

? **Critical Thinking Question 3-1**
How can Jamie let a potential employer know her level of competence?

Honesty

The medical assistant must be honest when dealing with patients as well as coworkers. This includes reporting any actions or events that occur in the office that create an opportunity for a patient or employee injury. Honest behavior in the medical facility is recording data in the patient's chart only if it has been observed or verified. When dealing with patients, the medical assistant must honestly answer questions. This means admitting to the patient when the answer is unknown to the medical assistant. Of course, the medical assistant must only answer questions that are within the medical assisting scope of practice and should always refer the patient to the physician for questions that are beyond the medical assistant's scope of practice.

Compassion

Compassion is using empathy to sense others' concerns or feelings. The compassionate medical assistant is one who appreciates the experience the patient is enduring, including any pain or fears involved, and responds to that patient in a humane, healing manner. Compassionate behavior is also exhibited when the medical assistant shows empathy to coworkers who may be undergoing a challenging event or time in their lives (Figure 3-2 ◆).

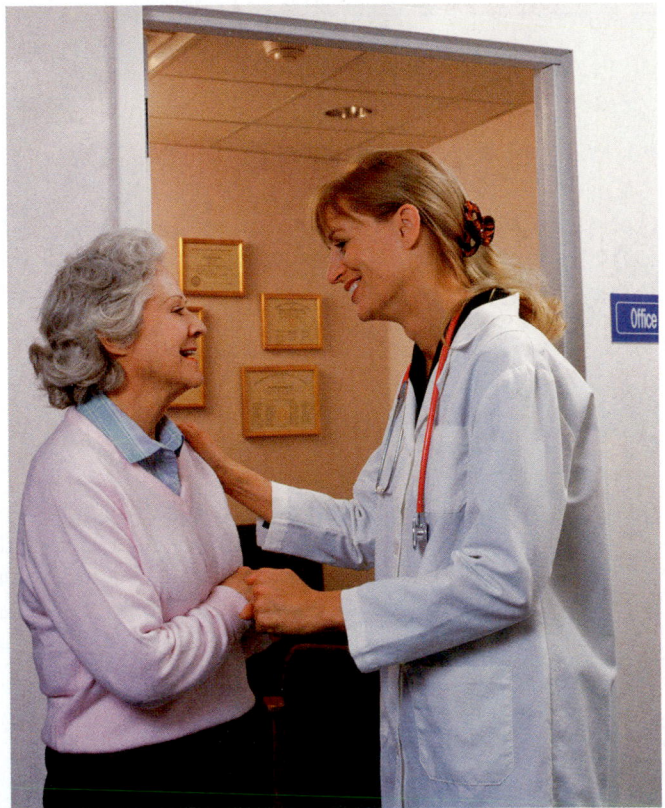

Figure 3-2 ◆ The medical assistant acts as the patient's advocate by showing compassion for the patient.

In Practice

Sylvia Gomez, RMA (AMT), has just roomed Mr. Paquette, a seventy-year-old patient. When Sylvia asks Mr. Paquette how he is feeling today, the man puts his head down and begins to cry. Sylvia asks him what is wrong and Mr. Paquette answers, "My wife passed away over the weekend." How might Sylvia proceed with the visit?

Respect for Others

The medical assistant shows **respect** to the patients she is working with by treating each patient as a valued person. Every patient must be treated with the same level of respect, allowing each patient to preserve his or her dignity, especially during times when the patient is feeling vulnerable. Since many patients will come from different social or cultural groups, the medical assistant who takes the time to learn something about each of those groups conveys to the patient that she respects their differences.

Respect is also shown to patients by the medical assistant who pays strict attention to patient confidentiality. This is also important when dealing with coworkers. The medical assistant must be sensitive to the needs, feelings, and wishes of coworkers, as well as in keeping confidences shared private.

Responsibility

The medical assistant must accept **responsibility** for his own actions. This includes being punctual for his shift and taking care of all aspects of his job while working. The medical assistant who exhibits this trait is one who does not attempt to place blame on others. Instead, the responsible medical assistant looks for ways to improve the functions within the medical office and learns from any mistakes made.

Critical Thinking Question 3-2

How can Jamie let the potential employer know that she will be a responsible employee?

Professional Demeanor

Professional demeanor is acting in a thoughtful way. The medical assistant shows a professional demeanor by acting in a way that shows respect for others as well as for herself. The medical assistant also exhibits a professional demeanor by maintaining a clean, neat appearance and dress that is accepted as appropriate for the clinical setting. In most clinical settings, proper attire is clean scrubs with clean shoes. Hair should be clean and pulled back and fingernails should be cut to the appropriate length and be painted only with a light, or clear, shade of polish.

Loyalty

The medical assistant shows loyalty to her employer by doing her best job in all aspects while working. This includes attitude as well. The medical assistant must strive to only comment on the positive nature of the physicians and the clinic. This gives the patient the picture of a facility that is run by professionals who respect and value one another. When the medical assistant complains about the facility, the available equipment, or the physician, the patient is given the impression that this is not the best clinic for one to seek care.

Attitude

The medical assistant's attitude will set the tone of the patient's visit in the medical office. Just as not making negative comments about the physician or the facility shows loyalty to the employer, the medical assistant's attitude toward those he works with will be apparent to the patient as well. The medical assistant must be able to keep calm, even when dealing with patients who are upset (Figure 3-3 ◆).

Working Together as a Team

All members of the healthcare staff must be able to work together as a team. Teamwork is vital to the success of the medical clinic in that all members must work together to provide the best quality of care to the patient. Part of good teamwork is the willingness to fill in for coworkers, if needed.

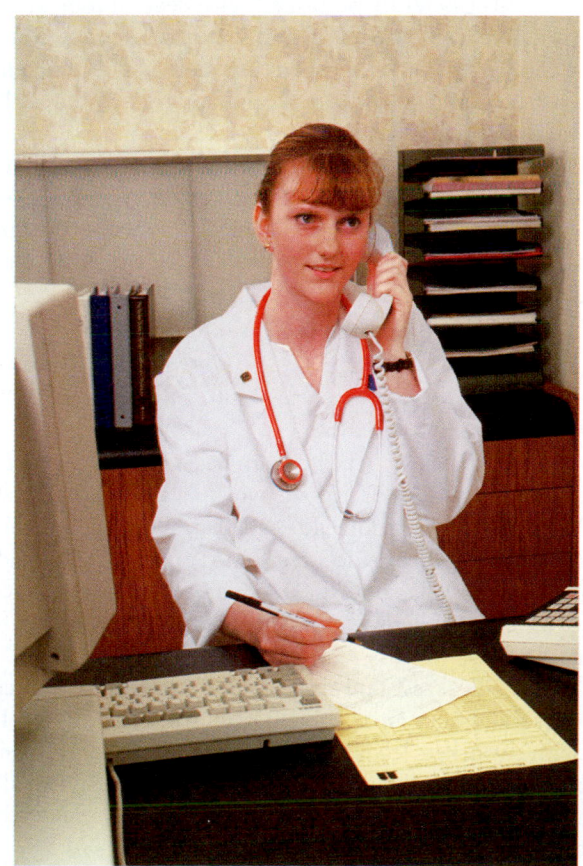

Figure 3-3 ◆ By maintaining a positive attitude on the telephone as well as in person, the medical assistant helps to make the patient's visit to the medical office a positive one.

Prioritizing Tasks

Because the medical office is a busy environment and the medical assistant will typically need to multitask in order to accomplish all of the tasks assigned on any given day, good time management is key to the efficient flow in the medical office.

In order to manage time effectively, the medical assistant must learn how to properly prioritize tasks throughout the day. Although it is not uncommon for the medical assistant to have only one task assigned at a time, it is more common for the medical assistant to have multiple tasks to complete in a specified time frame. Prioritizing is best done by determining which of the assigned tasks is needed sooner than the others. If all tasks are determined to be needed at the same level of importance, the medical assistant should perform the task that requires the least amount of time first. By handling tasks in this order, the medical assistant will be able to complete the smaller tasks first, leaving more time available to devote to the more time-consuming tasks.

Barriers to Professionalism

The medical office is often a very busy place. The medical assistant will frequently be tasked with several jobs at the same time. Because of this, sometimes remaining professional can be more difficult than others for the medical assistant. Some of the barriers to professionalism are avoidable. By avoiding these barriers in the first place, the medical assistant is better positioned to remain professional at all times while working.

When the patient observes the medical assistant performing in an unprofessional way, the patient is given a negative impression of the medical office and all who work there.

Bringing Personal Problems into the Workplace

Every member of the healthcare team has personal issues and conflicts that exist outside of the workplace. Finding a balance between work and home life can be challenging for many people, including the medical assistant. A good rule to abide by is to leave one's personal life outside of the medical office, in the same way bringing work problems home should be avoided.

The medical assistant should not burden his coworkers with personal issues and problems. Sharing personal problems with coworkers leads to gossip in the workplace. Gossip is detrimental to workplace morale in that it undermines the integrity of the person who retells the confidences shared by others.

If the medical assistant has a personal problem that needs to be dealt with, he should request time off from the clinic manager or physician in order to solve the problem.

? ─Critical Thinking Question 3-3 ─
What are some examples of personal issues that are not mentioned in the above section that Jamie should not bring up while working?

Taking Care of Personal Business While at Work

When the medical assistant uses work hours to take care of personal business, she is not exhibiting professionalism. The medical assistant should not entertain personal visitors while working. It is also inappropriate to discuss personal matters with patients or to engage in activities such as personal telephone calls, checking personal email while at work, or using the office computers for personal use during work hours.

Inappropriate Discussions in Front of Patients

The patients in the medical office will listen to what they hear the medical staff discussing. Unless the medical assistant is in an area of the office entirely out of the hearing range of patients, discussions between staff members should always be professional. Discussions should never be about issues that do not pertain to the medical office. For example, the patient should not overhear discussions about a television program the medical assistant recently viewed, or anything of a personal or gossiping nature. Of course, any discussion about other patients should not be overheard by other patients in order to avoid breaches in confidentiality (Figure 3-4 ◆).

HIPAA Compliance

All discussions held within patient hearing range must be HIPAA-compliant. This means the medical assistant must never disclose patient confidential information when other patients can overhear.

Procrastination of Duties

When given a task to perform, the medical assistant should strive to perform that task in the expected amount of time. Putting off tasks until the last minute leads to sloppy performance or poor work. The medical assistant exhibits professional behavior by performing requested or required tasks in the expected amount of time. This gives the employer the impression that the medical assistant can be counted upon to perform up to expectations. When the medical assistant realizes a task cannot be performed in the expected amount of time, he should go to the office manager or physician and explain the difficulty.

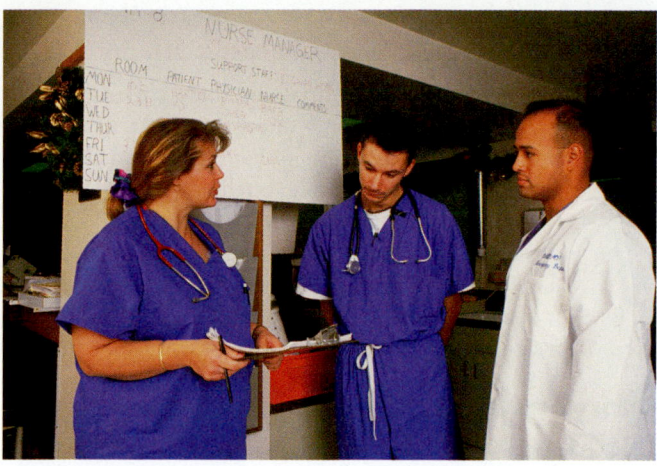

Figure 3-4 ◆ Every discussion within patient hearing range must be professional in nature.

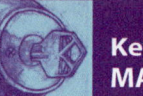

Keys to Success
MAINTAINING A PROFESSIONAL IMAGE

- **Leave personal problems at home.** As much as possible, avoid bringing personal problems to work. When personal problems become overwhelming, consider taking a day or two off to address them.
- **Avoid office gossip.** Refuse to gossip and spread rumors, because doing so is unproductive and can be harmful. Even when true, office information should be kept confidential. Consider how you would feel if you were the subject of the material.
- **Conduct no personal business during work hours.** Personal business takes time from the employer. Respect your employer's time, and conduct personal business, like telephone calls, during breaks or before or after work. Remember that patients may overhear your conversations, so always act professionally and courteously. When you must make a personal call during business hours, do so from a private room or outside the building.
- **Stay out of office politics.** Avoid office politics, because they are particularly destructive. Do not take credit for coworkers' accomplishments or blame others for your mistakes.
- **Do not procrastinate.** Practice prioritization rather than procrastination. Rank activities so you can complete them in an acceptable time frame. When a project seems too big to handle, try breaking it into smaller pieces or seeking help.

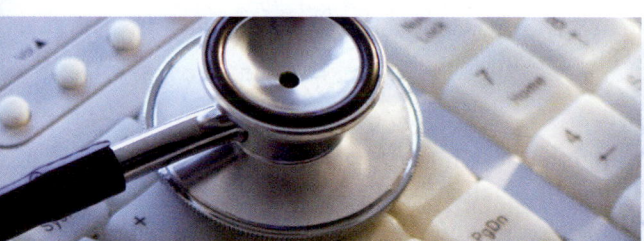

REVIEW

Chapter Summary

- The medical assistant plays a key role in maintaining the professional appearance in the medical office. Professionalism is acting in a businesslike manner in the workplace.
- By maintaining professionalism in the workplace, the medical assistant acts as an advocate for the patient.
- There are several qualities the medical assistant should exhibit in order to maintain a professional demeanor. These qualities include competence, honesty, compassion, respect for others,

responsibility, and loyalty. The attitude of the medical assistant, as well as the ability to prioritize tasks and work together as a team, also helps to project a professional appearance.
- Negative qualities will deter from the professionalism of the medical assistant. The medical assistant should leave personal problems at home, avoid office gossip, conduct no personal business during work hours, avoid office politics, and avoid procrastination.

Chapter Review

Multiple Choice

1. Which of the following would be an inappropriate discussion in front of a patient?
   a. The subject of an argument the medical assistant had with her spouse the prior evening
   b. The results of the patient's laboratory findings
   c. The need for a followup appointment with the physician
   d. All of the above

2. Why is maintaining a professional image important in the medical office?
   a. Patients may discontinue care with the physician if they feel the office staff are unprofessional
   b. Medical assistants may lose their job if their employer feels they are not providing a professional image
   c. Staff morale may decline if assistants are not maintaining a professional nature
   d. All of the above

3. Which of the following traits is exhibited when the medical assistant fills in for a coworker when needed?
   a. Time management
   b. Working together as a team
   c. Attitude
   d. Compassion

4. Which of the following is exhibited when the medical assistant comforts a patient who has recently lost her spouse?
   a. Time management
   b. Working together as a team
   c. Attitude
   d. Compassion

5. Which of the following is exhibited when the medical assistant only says positive things about the physician he works for?
   a. Time management
   b. Working together as a team
   c. Attitude
   d. Compassion

True/False

T F 1. The medical assistant has a minor role in portraying the professional nature of the clinic to the patient.

T F 2. The medical assistant may discuss a patient's confidential information with another patient.

T F 3. If the medical assistant is having a "bad day," the patient should not be able to tell.

T F 4. Every member of the healthcare team should say only positive things about one another in front of the patients.

T F 5. It is appropriate for the medical assistant to discuss his personal problems with the patient.

Short Answer

1. What are some examples of professional behavior the medical assistant should exhibit in the medical office?

2. What are some examples of negative behaviors that should not be exhibited in the medical office?

3. How might you respond to a coworker who begins to tell you about a personal problem?

4. How might you respond to a coworker who attempts to share gossip about another coworker with you?

5. What are examples of how the medical assistant can exhibit honesty in the medical office?

6. What are some examples of how the medical assistant can exhibit responsibility in the medical office?

7. What are some examples of how the medical assistant can exhibit respect for others in the medical office?

8. Describe a situation where a medical assistant will need to show compassion to the patient.

9. Describe a situation where a medical assistant will need to show compassion to a coworker.

10. Describe some ways you could show professionalism in an interview with a potential employer.

Research

1. Perform an Internet search of the word *professionalism*. What definitions do you find?

2. Describe an incident in your life where you were treated with professionalism.

Externship Application Experience

T.J. Perkins is performing his externship for a medical assisting program in a cardiology office. T.J. has been asked to room Mrs. Rutledge, a 80-year-old patient. As he walks Mrs. Rutledge down the hall, she asks T.J., "Tell me about yourself. Are you married? Do you have any children?" How should T.J. respond to Mrs. Rutledge and still maintain a professional demeanor with this patient?

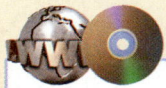 Med**Media**

http://www.MyMAKit.com

More on this chapter, including interactive resources, can be found on the Student CD-ROM accompanying this textbook and on http://www.MyMAKit.com.

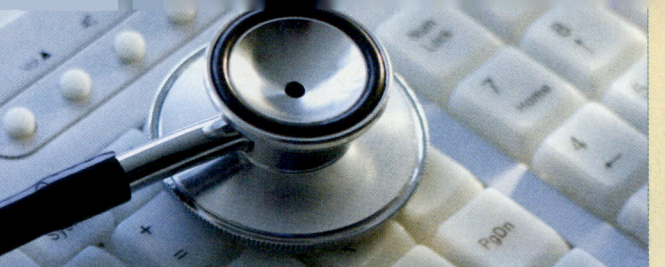

Objectives

After completing this chapter, you should be able to:

- Define and spell the key terminology in this chapter.
- Define the medical assistant's role as it pertains to medical law and ethics.
- Classify varied laws as they apply to healthcare.
- Describe malpractice, defenses to malpractice, and the different types of malpractice insurance policies.
- Outline the physician's public duties.
- Compare the duties of the physician and the patient in the physician-patient relationship.
- List ways in which medical assistants can help maintain patient confidentiality.
- Describe the history of the Health Insurance Portability and Accountability Act (HIPAA) and how it affects healthcare clinics.
- Define the conscience clause and how it applies to healthcare professionals.
- Discuss the patients' bill of rights.
- Describe JCAHO and how it impacts healthcare professionals.
- Explain why each healthcare profession has a code of ethics.
- Identify the monitoring agencies that address ambulatory healthcare.
- Explain the Blanchard and Peale ethical model.
- Discuss bioethics.

Medical Law and Ethics

Case Study

Victoria Mason is a medical assistant in Dr. Kozlowski's office. Victoria takes a telephone call from a man named Bart. He tells Victoria that one of his employees is a patient of Dr. Kozlowski's and asks her to tell him when his employee was last in the office and what treatment she received.

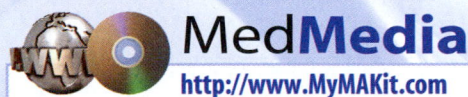

MedMedia

http://www.MyMAKit.com

Additional interactive resources and activities for this chapter can be found on http://www.MyMAKit.com. For a video, tips, audio glossary, legal and ethical scenarios, on-the-job scenarios, quizzes, and games related to the content of this chapter, please access the accompanying CD-ROM in this book.

Video: *Protecting Patient Privacy*
Legal and Ethical Scenario: *Medical Law and Ethics*
On the Job Scenario: *Medical Law and Ethics*
Tips
Multiple Choice Quiz
Audio Glossary
HIPAA Quiz
Games: Spelling Bee, Crossword, and Strikeout

Key Terminology

administrative law—legislation passed by governmental agencies

advance directives—directions for medical staff to follow in the event patients cannot speak for themselves

appeal—request for review of a denied service or claim, in an attempt to see the insurance company's denial reversed or overturned

assault—threat of touching or doing harm to another without their consent

assumption of risk—defense to medical malpractice in which the physician must prove the patient was fully informed of a procedure's risks

battery—act of touching or abusing another person without the person's consent

bioethics—issues surrounding life-and-death situations in health care (e.g., cloning, artificial insemination, abortion)

civil law—legislation that governs actions between two or more citizens

commercial law—legislation that relates to businesses

common law—legislation that stems from the English legal system; also called *traditional law*

comparative negligence—defense to medical malpractice in which the physician proves the patient was partly responsible for the patient's injury

conscience clauses—statements that allow health care workers to refuse to perform job tasks based on religious or personal objections

constitutional law—legislation that is based on the U.S. Constitution

contract law—legislation that relates to contracts

contributory negligence—defense to medical malpractice in which the physician proves an injury would not have occurred if not for the patient's actions

criminal law—legislation that relates to crimes

damages—money a patient is awarded for damages or injuries the patient sustained

defamation of character—act of saying negative things about a person that harm the person in some way

discovery rule—legislation that states the statute of limitations begins when an injury was discovered or should have been discovered

 MEDICAL ASSISTING STANDARDS

CAAHEP ENTRY-LEVEL STANDARDS	ABHES ENTRY-LEVEL COMPETENCIES
■ Perform within scope of practice (psychomotor)	■ Adapt to change
■ Apply ethical behaviors, including honesty/integrity in performance of medical assisting practice (affective)	■ Project a positive attitude
■ Explore issue of confidentiality as it applies to the medical assistant (cognitive)	■ Be cognizant of ethical boundaries
■ Respond to issues of confidentiality (psychomotor)	■ Evidence a responsible attitude
■ Demonstrate sensitivity to patient rights (affective)	■ Conduct work within scope of education, training, and ability
■ Apply local, state and federal health care legislation and regulation appropriate to the medical assisting practice setting (psychomotor)	■ Professional components
■ Recognize the importance of local, state and federal legislation and regulations in the practice setting (affective)	■ Maintain licenses and accreditation
■ Discuss legal scope of practice for medical assistants (cognitive)	■ Maintain liability coverage
■ Compare and contrast physician and medical assistant roles in terms of standard of care (cognitive)	■ Monitor legislation related to current healthcare issues and practices
■ Respond to issues of confidentiality (psychomotor)	■ Follow established policy in initiating or terminating medical treatment
■ Practice within the standard of care for a medical assistant (psychomotor)	
■ Perform within scope of practice for a medical assistant (psychomotor)	
■ Document accurately within the patient record (psychomotor)	
■ Demonstrate awareness of the consequences of not working within the legal scope of practice (affective)	
■ Demonstrate sensitivity to patient rights (affective)	

 COMPETENCY SKILLS PERFORMANCE

1. Prepare an informed consent for treatment form.
2. Obtain authorization for the release of patient medical records.
3. Respond to a request for copies of a patient's medical record.

Key Terminology *(continued)*

duress—act of coercing someone into an act

expert witness—person in a lawsuit who is considered an expert in a given field

expressed consent—agreement, either verbally or in writing, from the patient before a procedure is performed

expressed contract—agreement to a contract, either verbally or in writing

four Ds of negligence—elements patients must prove in malpractice (i.e., duty, dereliction of duty, direct cause, and damages)

fraud—deceitful act done to conceal the truth

Good Samaritan act—law that protects a person performing life-saving care to a stranger outside the medical setting

Health Insurance Portability and Accountability Act (HIPAA)—legislation that addresses patient privacy

implied consent—agreement through actions only

implied contract—agreement to a contract through actions only

informed consent—process in which a physician reviews with a patient the risks associated with a procedure, the risks of nontreatment, and accepted treatment alternatives

intentional tort—act of purposefully harming another

international law—legislation that relates to two or more countries

invasion of privacy—act of providing another person's information without that person's permission

malfeasance—state of performing an incorrect treatment

malpractice insurance policy—insurance to cover actions that have hurt a patient

misfeasance—state of performing a procedure incorrectly

negligence—action or inaction that injures another

nonfeasance—state of delaying or failing to perform a treatment

Patient Care Partnership—A list from the American Hospital Association (AHA) of patients' expectations, rights, and responsibilities while under care in the hospital setting

portability—state of being able to move an insurance policy from one employer to another

precedent—legal decision that sets the standard for subsequent, similar cases

public law—legislation that relates to citizens

regulatory law—legislation that relates to government regulations

res judicata—Latin phrase for "the thing has been decided"

respondeat superior—Latin phrase for "let the master answer"

segregation—act of keeping two parties apart due to such differences as race or gender

settled—state in which an offer of money is extended and accepted to drop a lawsuit

standard of care—care a reasonable provider with the same skills would provide in the same circumstances

statute of limitations—period after an injury happens within which a patient may file a malpractice lawsuit

tort of outrage—to intentionally inflict emotional upset on another

tort law—legislation that relates to one party injuring another

traditional law—also known as *common law*

undue influence—to persuade someone to do something they do not want to do

unintentional tort—to harm another person accidentally

Abbreviations

AAMA—American Association of Medical Assistants

ADA—Americans with Disabilities Act

AHIMA—American Health Information Management Association

AIDS—acquired immune deficiency syndrome

AMA—American Medical Association

CLIA—Clinical Laboratory Improvement Amendments Act

CMA—certified medical assistant

CMS—Centers for Medical and Medicaid Services

CPR—cardiopulmonary resuscitation

CPT—Current Procedural Terminology

DNR—do not resuscitate

EIN—employer identification number

FDA—Food and Drug Administration

HIPAA—Health Insurance Portability and Accountability Act

HIV—human immunodeficiency virus

IRS—Internal Revenue Service

JCAHO—Joint Commission on the Accreditation of Healthcare Organizations

MSA—medical savings account

STD—sexually transmitted disease

Introduction

Medical assistants face many situations that involve ethics and law. Ethics deals with issues of right and wrong, whereas the law serves to uphold what society feels is right and wrong. Ethical issues often take more thought than legal ones, because people have differing ideas about what is right. The law, in contrast, tends to allow little room for opinion. Each state has unique laws governing healthcare and the medical-assisting profession. It is crucial for medical assistants to know the laws of their states and to uphold those laws at all times. That adherence to law, paired with a clear understanding of what society and the medical-assisting profession spell out with regard to ethics, can help the medical assistant build a solid career.

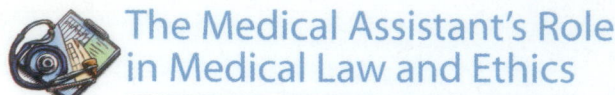

The Medical Assistant's Role in Medical Law and Ethics

Medical assistants are involved in many activities that have a legal and ethical impact on patients. Knowledge of state laws, as well as current ethical considerations prevailing within the AAMA, can make a positive difference in the lives of patients.

The Sources of Law

U.S. law arises from varying sources. Court decisions establish **traditional law**. **Common law** comes from the English legal system. All U.S. states follow common law except Louisiana, which uses a system based on French law.

Courts set **precedents** when they decide cases. *Roe v. Wade,* for example, caused all states to revamp their legal approaches to abortion. Similarly, *Brown* v. *Board of Education* forced states to address the issue of segregation. **Segregation** is an example of how courts can overrule decisions and set new precedents. Years ago, court decisions deemed segregation a legal practice. Subsequent court decisions ruled segregation illegal, however, and thereby reversed the legal precedents.

Statutes are laws created by federal, state, or local legislators. Statutes are upheld by law enforcement, and cases may end up in local, state, or federal court systems. Medicare, Medicaid, and the Food and Drug Administration (**FDA**) are all agencies that create healthcare-related statutes.

Administrative Law

Administrative law, also called **regulatory law**, is passed by governmental agencies such as the Internal Revenue Service (**IRS**). Administrative law addresses issues of taxation, public transportation, manufacturing, the environment, and public broadcasting.

Comparing Public and Private Law

The United States' judicial system has two main branches of law: (1) public and (2) private. **Public law** focuses on issues between the government and citizens, such as criminal law, **constitutional law**, administrative law, and **international law**. Private or **civil law** focuses on issues between two or more citizens.

Criminal Law

Criminal law, also called penal law, focuses on the public's safety and welfare, addressing people who commit crimes or other illegal offenses. Classified by severity as felonies or misdemeanors, criminal law varies from one state to another. While all states have laws against such serious crimes as rape or murder, the laws for less serious crimes like theft or drug use may vary from one jurisdiction to another.

Felonies

Felonies are considered serious crimes, whereas misdemeanors are considered less serious offenses. States have varying definitions for each. Table 4-1 lists general felony categories. Some states, like New Jersey, classify felonies in four degrees. Other states place felonies in "classes," like Class A or Class 1. In cases like these, Class 1 is the most serious while Class 6 is the least.

Misdemeanors

Like felony classifications, misdemeanor classifications vary from state to state. Misdemeanors include such crimes as petty theft, prostitution, simple **assault,** and disorderly conduct. Because they are considered lesser crimes than felonies, misdemeanors are generally punished with lesser sentences.

Civil Law

The medical profession is primarily concerned with civil law, because it deals with issues relating to **contract law, commercial law**, and tort law. Contract and commercial laws address the rights and obligations one has to another, such as the doctor-patient relationship. Tort law deals with the injuries one has suffered at the hands of another, such as cases of medical malpractice.

Tort Law

Tort law deals with situations in which someone has been injured by another's actions or inactions. Torts are one of two types: unintentional or intentional. An **unintentional tort** occurs when a mistake is made. The vast majority of medical malpractice cases fall into this category, because unintentional torts usually involve negligence. **Negligence** is defined as an act that a reasonable health care provider would not have done or the omission of an act that a reasonable health care provider would have done. In contrast, an **intentional tort** occurs when someone purposefully does something that injures someone else. Table 4-2 defines intentional torts and gives healthcare examples.

?—Critical Thinking Question 4-1—

How does the case study outlined at the beginning of this chapter illustrate one of the torts in Table 4-2? Please specify the tort.

TABLE 4-1 FELONY CATEGORIES	
Felony Degree	**Action of Person Being Charged**
First	Committed the crime
Second	Was at the scene of the crime and assisted in the crime
Third	Assisted in the crime before the crime occurred
Fourth	Assisted the person who committed the crime after the fact

TABLE 4-2 INTENTIONAL TORTS

Assault	Unauthorized attempt or threat to touch another person. *Example:* Telling a patient her temperature will be taken whether she wants it or not after she refuses to allow it.
Battery	Actual physical touching of another person without the person's consent; includes physical abuse. *Example:* Taking a patient's temperature against the patient's will.
Defamation of character	Making or publishing false or malicious statements about another person's character or reputation. *Example:* Telling patients they should not see the cardiologist across the street because that cardiologist has a drinking problem.
Duress	Act of coercing someone into an act. *Example:* Telling patients they must have a tetanus vaccine or they will develop a life-threatening infection. The patients feel they have no choice but to comply, even though they do not want the vaccine.
Fraud	Deceitful act made to conceal the truth. *Example:* Falsifying a patient's medical record to conceal a medical mistake.
Invasion of privacy	Releasing private information about another person without the person's consent. *Example:* Releasing a patient's medical records without the patient's consent or a court order.
Tort of outrage	Intentionally inflicting emotional distress on another person. *Example:* The physician yells at a patient for failing to follow instructions.
Undue influence	Intentionally persuading people to do things they do not want to do. *Example:* Convincing single mothers that they should give their children up for adoption when they clearly do not want to.

Understanding and Classifying Consent

Before patients are accepted for care in a medical office, they must give their consent to be examined and/or treated by the physician or healthcare provider and sign a consent form. Figure 4-1 ◆ lists the information that must be included on a consent form.

Only certain parties are legally able to sign consent forms (Figure 4-2 ◆). Consent forms must be written in the languages patients speak. Most facilities that treat patients from other cultures have consent forms in multiple languages.

Healthcare has two types of consent: (1) implied and (2) expressed. **Implied consent** is given when patients indicate through action only that they agree to submit. When patients

- ■ Name of the procedure to be performed
- ■ Name of the physician who will perform the procedure
- ■ Name of the person administering the anesthesia (if applicable)
- ■ Any potential risks to the patient from the procedure
- ■ Any risks to the patient if the procedure is *not* elected
- ■ Any accepted alternative treatments and their risks
- ■ Any exclusions the patient has requested
- ■ A statement indicating that all the patient's questions have been answered
- ■ The patient's and witnesses' signatures and the date signed

Figure 4-1 ◆ Necessary consent form information.

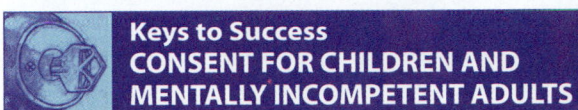

Keys to Success
CONSENT FOR CHILDREN AND MENTALLY INCOMPETENT ADULTS

Children or people who are mentally incompetent or temporarily incapacitated cannot legally give consent, just as they cannot legally enter into contracts. The parents or guardians of these patients must give consent for these patients.

are told they need to give blood samples and roll up their sleeves while saying nothing, they give implied consent (Figure 4-3 ◆).

Expressed consent occurs when patients agree either verbally or in writing to consent to a procedure. In healthcare, any invasive procedure should be done only after a patient has signed a consent form. This helps prove the patient knew the risks involved and agreed to them before the service.

- ■ Any mentally competent adult over age 18
- ■ The parent or legal guardian of a child, mentally incompetent adult, or temporarily incapacitated adult
- ■ Emancipated minors, defined as under age 18 but:
  - • Are married or self-supporting and responsible for their debts
  - • Have received a court order declaring them emancipated
- ■ A minor who is:
  - • In the armed services
  - • Being seen for treatment for sexually transmitted diseases
  - • Pregnant
  - • Being seen for information regarding birth control or abortion
  - • Being seen for treatment regarding drug or alcohol abuse

Figure 4-2 ◆ Parties who can sign a consent form.

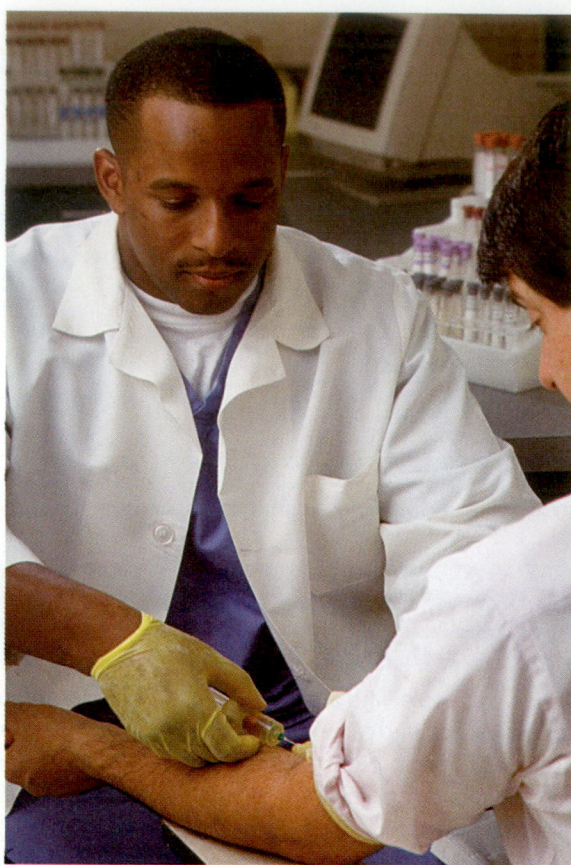

Figure 4-3 ◆ This patient has given implied consent to have his blood drawn.

Whether consent is implied or expressed, it must always be informed, meaning patients must be told the benefits and risks of any procedure, the risks of not having the procedure, and any accepted alternative treatments to the procedure (see Figure 4-4 ◆). Patients must also be clearly informed of any pain associated with the procedure or recovery and if they will require any assistance after the procedure.

Under the Doctrine of Informed Consent, all of the following must be explained to the patient in clear, easy-to-understand language before a procedure or surgery is performed:

■ The patient's diagnosis, if it is known
■ The purpose, advantages, and risks of the proposed treatment

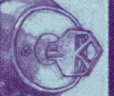

Keys to Success
SIGNING CONSENT FORMS

Patients must never be coerced or threatened into signing consent forms. Consent must be gained voluntarily and only after the patient has been fully informed of the procedure. Patients who fail to completely understand procedures, have any unanswered questions, or cannot read consent forms should never sign those forms.

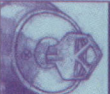

Keys to Success
OBTAINING INFORMED CONSENT

The physician is responsible for obtaining informed consent. For the consent to be truly "informed," however, patients must have the opportunity to ask the physician any and all questions. This task should never be delegated to the medical assistant. Instead, it is appropriate for the medical assistant to witness the patient's signature on the consent form.

■ Alternatives available to the patient, along with their risks and benefits
■ Potential treatment outcomes
■ Potential outcomes if there is no treatment

Procedures in an office or outpatient facility that may require special consent forms include, but are not limited to:

■ Administration of blood and blood products
■ Invasive diagnostic procedures, including lumbar punctures, cystoscopies, biopsies, and endoscopies
■ Chemotherapy
■ Cardiac or pulmonary stress testing

Patients may refuse treatment for any reason, including religious and personal beliefs. For example, a patient with end-stage cancer may refuse chemotherapy because the side effects may decrease the quality of life. A Jehovah's Witness may refuse blood products on religious grounds. When patients refuse treatment, they or their parents or guardians must sign a refusal-of-consent form. This form must indicate that the patient was given information on the risks and benefits of having the procedure or not.

Medical Malpractice

Doctors are sued for varied reasons. Some are sued for making serious errors, such as giving the wrong medications, performing the wrong surgeries, or failing to properly diagnose or treat patients. Other doctors, although few, commit Medicare or insurance fraud, or falsify patient records to conceal errors.

Malpractice is one of three types:

■ **Malfeasance** is performing an incorrect treatment, such as operating on the wrong patient.
■ **Misfeasance** is performing a treatment incorrectly, such as operating on a patient's arm and accidentally severing a nerve, leaving the patient without the use of the arm.

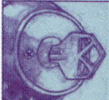

Keys to Success
WHEN PATIENTS REFUSE TREATMENT

Physicians have the right to refuse to perform elective surgery on patients who refuse to receive blood if needed.

MEMORIAL HEALTH

COMPLETE ORIGINAL IN INK FOR HOSPITAL CHART
PATIENT MUST BE AWAKE, ALERT AND ORIENTED WHEN SIGNING

DATE: _____ TIME: _____ □ AM □ PM

I AUTHORIZE THE PERFORMANCE UPON _____
OF THE FOLLOWING OPERATION (state nature and extent): _____
_____
_____

TO BE PERFORMED UNDER THE DIRECTION OF DR. _____

1. I HAVE BEEN ADVISED THAT THERE IS A FAVORABLE LIKELIHOOD OF SUCCESS, BUT I UNDERSTAND THAT A COMPLETELY SUCCESSFUL OUTCOME MAY NOT BE ACHIEVABLE, AND THERE ARE NO GUARANTEES REGARDING THE OUTCOME. I ALSO UNDERSTAND THAT CERTAIN ADVERSE EVENTS COULD OCCUR AS A RESULT OF THE PERFORMANCE OF THE PROCEDURE OR TREATMENT, INCLUDING PAIN, INFECTION, LACERATION OR PUNCTURE OF INTERNAL ORGANS, BLEEDING, NERVE DAMAGE OR EVEN IN RARE CASES, DEATH. I UNDERSTAND THAT HOSPITALIZATION OR OTHER INSTITUTIONAL CARE, HOME CARE OR CARE BY HEALTH PROFESSIONALS MAY BE NEEDED FOLLOWING THE PROCEDURE OR TREATMENT, RELATED TO FULL RECOVERY, RECUPERATION OR CONVALESCENCE. I UNDERSTAND THE ALTERNATIVES TO THIS PROCEDURE, INCLUDING MY RIGHT TO REFUSE TO CONSENT TO IT, AND I NEVERTHELESS HAVE DECIDED TO CONSENT TO PERFORMANCE OF THE PROCEDURE OR TREATMENT.

2. I CONSENT TO THE PERFORMANCE OF OPERATIONS AND PROCEDURES IN ADDITION TO OR DIFFERENT FROM THOSE NOW CONTEMPLATED, WHETHER OR NOT ARISING FROM PRESENTLY UNFORESEEN CONDITIONS WHICH THE ABOVE NAMED DOCTOR OR HIS/HER ASSOCIATES OR ASSISTANTS MAY CONSIDER NECESSARY OR ADVISABLE IN THE COURSE OF THE OPERATION.

3. I CONSENT TO THE DISPOSAL BY HOSPITAL AUTHORITIES OF ANY TISSUES OR PARTS WHICH MAY BE REMOVED.

4. THE NATURE AND PURPOSE OF THE OPERATION/PROCEDURE, POSSIBLE ALTERNATIVE METHODS OF TREATMENT, THE RISK AND BENEFITS INVOLVED, AND THE COURSE OF RECUPERATION HAVE BEEN FULLY EXPLAINED TO ME. NO GUARANTEE OR ASSURANCE HAS BEEN GIVEN BY ANYONE AS TO THE RESULTS THAT MAY BE OBTAINED.

5. I UNDERSTAND AND AGREE WITH THE ABOVE INFORMATION. I HAVE NO QUESTIONS WHICH HAVE NOT BEEN ANSWERED TO MY FULL SATISFACTION. I UNDERSTAND THAT I HAVE THE RIGHT TO ASK FOR FURTHER INFORMATION BEFORE SIGNING THIS CONSENT.

I have crossed out any paragraph above which does not apply or to which I do not give consent.

PATIENT SIGNATURE: _____   WITNESS SIGNATURE: _____
(OR PARENT OR GUARDIAN IF PATIENT IS UNDER 18 YEARS OF AGE)   *(OF PATIENT, PARENT OR GUARDIAN SIGNATURE)*
PATIENT DATE OF BIRTH: _____   WITNESS SIGNATURE: _____
RELATIONSHIP: _____   □ **TELEPHONE CONSENT** *(2ND WITNESS NEEDED FOR TELEPHONE CONSENT)*

Figure 4-4 ◆ Sample of an informed consent form.

■ **Nonfeasance** is delaying or failing to perform treatment, such as telling a patient a tumor does not need to be removed and the patient later has a bad outcome due to the nonremoval of the tumor.

The Doctrine of *Respondeat Superior*

Staff in the medical office can cause the office to be sued. If the medical assistant makes an error, for example, the lawsuit will usually be filed against the doctor who employs the medical assistant. This is called the doctrine of ***respondeat superior***, which is Latin for, "Let the master answer." Under this doctrine, physicians are responsible for the actions of their healthcare employees (Figure 4-5 ◆). Medical assistants can still be named in malpractice lawsuits, however, so each should seriously consider carrying a **malpractice insurance policy**. Because medical assistants have a low risk of injuring patients, insurance rates are generally low. Policies are available through local or state medical-assisting associations.

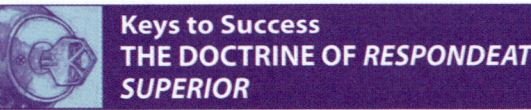

Keys to Success
THE DOCTRINE OF *RESPONDEAT SUPERIOR*

The doctrine of *respondeat superior* only covers employees performing within their scope of practice at the time of injury. In other words, a healthcare worker performing a duty outside the scope of practice in the worker's state is not covered by the physician's malpractice insurance policy.

Types of Malpractice Insurance Policies

Malpractice insurance policies are one of two types: (1) claims-made and (2) occurrence policies. Claims-made policies protect policyholders from malpractice claims only when the

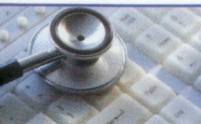

PROCEDURE 4-1 Prepare an Informed Consent for Treatment Form

Theory and Rationale

While the task of explaining the procedures, risks, and alternatives falls to the physician, the medical assistant is often the person who discusses the paperwork with the patient and obtains the patient's signature.

Materials

■ Informed consent for treatment form
■ Blue or black ink pen
■ Copy machine

Competency

(**Conditions**) With the necessary materials, you will be able to (**Task**) prepare an informed consent for treatment form (**Standards**) correctly within the time limit set by the instructor.

1. As the physician goes over the details of the upcoming procedure with the patient, fill in the informed consent form. The form must include:
   - The name of the procedure or treatment to be performed
   - The expected benefits of the procedure
   - Any possible risks of the procedure
   - Any accepted alternatives to the procedure and the risks or benefits associated with each
   - The fact that the patient may choose to forego the procedure and the possible risks or benefits associated with that choice

2. Be certain the form lists the patient's name, birth date, and the place the procedure is to be performed (in office, hospital, etc.).

3. Show the consent form to the physician for him or her to verify that all information is correct.

4. After the physician has left the room, go over the form with the patient. If the patient has further questions about the procedure, have the patient wait in the treatment room while you ask the physician to return to answer the questions. If the patient has no further questions about the procedure, have the patient sign the consent form.

5. Sign the consent form as a witness to the patient's signature.

6. Go over any specifics with the patient about the procedure day, such as any restrictions to eating or drinking on the day of the surgery, or where the patient should park the car.

7. Make a copy of the consent form for the patient. Place the original form in the patient's file.

---

insurance company insuring the policyholders at the time of the alleged malpractice is the same company at the time the claim is filed in court. Assume, for example, that on June 1,

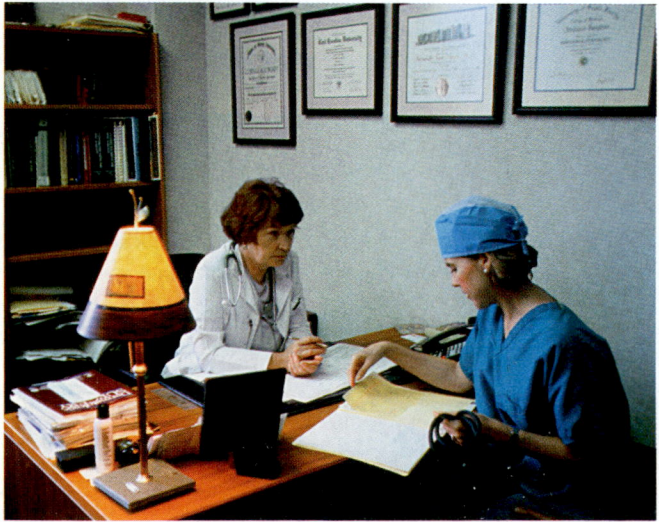

Figure 4-5 ◆ The physician and medical assistant work closely together to maintain safe care for their patients.

2009, Dr. Rasheem is covered under a claims-made policy provided by Allied Insurance when she performs an alleged malpractice event. If Dr. Rasheem is still covered by Allied Insurance when the claim is filed on December 10, 2009, she will be covered. If, however, she switches to a different insurance company before the filing date, Allied Insurance will not cover her. With her new plan, Dr. Rasheem could purchase a "tail" to cover her for the alleged malpractice incidence. A tail is a rider on the new policy that states the new company will cover any events for a certain period before the policy's purchase.

The second type of malpractice insurance policy, occurrence policies, cover policyholders regardless of when claims are filed provided the policies were in effect at the time of the alleged malpractice events. If Dr. Rasheem is covered by Unified Insurance under an occurrence-made policy on June 1, 2009, when an alleged malpractice event occurs, and then switches to a different company before the claim filing date of December 10, 2009, she would still be covered for the claim under her Unified Insurance policy.

Proving Medical Malpractice

The vast majority of medical malpractice lawsuits fail to make it to court. They are either **settled,** meaning the two sides

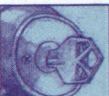

Keys to Success
INDIVIDUAL MALPRACTICE INSURANCE POLICIES FOR MEDICAL ASSISTANTS

Individual malpractice insurance policies for medical assistants are fairly inexpensive. For medical assistants working full time, rates are usually less than $100 per year for policies that cover up to $1 million per malpractice occurrence. For a quick online quote on malpractice insurance premiums, visit www.hpso.com.

agree on a financial award to the injured patient, or they are dismissed due to lack of proof. To prove medical malpractice, the patient must prove all of the following **four Ds of negligence:**

- *Duty*—Physicians have a duty to care for patients once they have taken those patients on. The patients must prove the physician breached this duty.
- *Dereliction of duty*—Physicians must meet **standard of care** guidelines for a health care provider with the same training, in the same location, under the same circumstances. The patients must prove the physician failed to perform to this standard.
- *Direct cause*—Patients must prove that the physicians' actions, or lack of action, directly caused the patients' injuries.
- *Damages*—Patients must prove they sustained **damages** due to the negligence.

Medical Malpractice Awards

Personal injury attorneys accept about one out of every twenty cases they review, but most cases are found in the physician's favor. Only one in ten cases accepted by an attorney results in an award or a settlement for the patient. When injured patients win cases, judges or juries may make one of the three following types of awards:

- *Nominal*—These are small awards or payments that are made when the negligence is proven but the damages are minimal.
- *Compensatory*—This is money that is awarded to the patient or the patient's family to compensate for the cost of medical care, the disability, mental suffering, any loss of income, and the loss of future income due to the injury.
- *Punitive*—Awards like these are made when judges or juries feel the healthcare providers should be punished for their actions. Courts may feel the providers were reckless or purposefully ignored signals that should have alerted them to the injuries. Punitive damages are typically high dollar amounts. Several states do not allow for punitive damages.

Preventing Medical Malpractice Claims

Patients file malpractice lawsuits for many reasons; lack of understanding is chief among them. Scientific advances in healthcare have allowed doctors to perform procedures that were considered too risky until recently. As procedures have become more complicated, patient risk has increased, and this has increased the likelihood of both poor outcomes and malpractice lawsuits, especially when the physician has failed to thoroughly explain the risks to patients. Physicians can help avoid lawsuits by completely explaining the risks of the procedures and obtaining the patients' **informed consent.** Informed consent should be written in detail and signed by both the patient and the healthcare provider (Figure 4-6 ◆).

Another means of lawsuit reduction has been gaining popularity recently, and that is if healthcare providers apologize to patients, those patients will be less likely to file malpractice claims. Many believe that patients sue because they are angry and only pursue legal recourse because they failed to receive acknowledgments of the errors and apologies. In research activities at the University of Michigan, healthcare providers were instructed to apologize to their patients when errors occurred. After one year, malpractice defense costs decreased from $3 million to $1 million. Today, twenty-nine states have laws that allow healthcare providers to apologize to patients after injuries without those apologies used as proof in lawsuits.

Defending Against Medical Malpractice Claims

Once a medical malpractice suit has been filed, the best defense is the medical record. Especially in the area of medical malpractice, an accurate and complete medical record is paramount. This record is the authoritative description of all care given a patient. It has all consent forms signed by the patient, as well as descriptions of the questions the patient asked and the answers the physician gave about needed care or treatment. For more on the medical record, see ∞ Chapter 12.

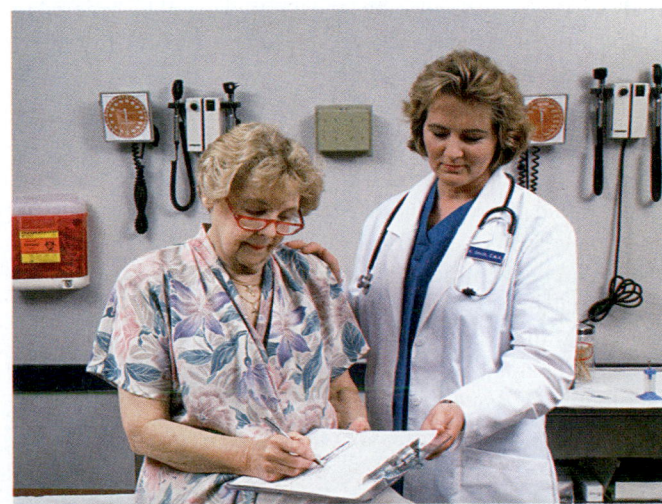

Figure 4-6 ◆ The medical assistant will frequently witness a patient's signature on a consent form.

The Statute of Limitations

Each state has a **statute of limitations** that sets the time within which an injured patient can file a malpractice lawsuit. Normally, this statute begins from the date of the injury. According to something called the **discovery rule,** some states allow the statute to begin when the injury was discovered or should have been discovered. This rule helps in cases in which the patient fails to discover the injury for several years after the injury has occurred. Other states allow the statute to begin when a minor child turns 18, allowing injured children to bring suits on their own behalf once they reach adulthood. Table 4-3 outlines the statute of limitations for each state.

Using Assumption of Risk as a Defense

Assumption of risk is a defense to medical malpractice physicians can use to prove they made the patients aware of the risks of their procedures. Under this defense, patients cannot sue the physicians when one of those risks occurs. This defense relies, however, on a detailed consent form signed by the patient.

Contributory and Comparative Negligence

The **contributory negligence** defense is one in which physicians may have been at fault for patients' injuries but can prove that the patient aggravated the injuries or in some way worsened them. For example, assume a physician sends a patient home with a sling instead of a cast and tells the patient to limit the motion of the arm to avoid aggravating the injury. If the patient then lifts groceries, worsening the fracture, that patient could be proven to have contributed to negligence.

Most states give patients no awards in contributory negligence cases. When awards are allowed, the court will normally assign a percentage of the award based on how responsible the patient was for the injury. For example, if the court finds the physician is 50 percent responsible for an injury and the patient is also 50 percent responsible, the physician will be ordered to pay 50 percent of the damages. These types of cases are typically called **comparative negligence**.

Immunity from Negligence Suits

The Feres doctrine was passed in response to a 1950 U.S. Supreme Court ruling regarding the Federal Tort Claims Act of 1946. The doctrine prevents members of the armed services from suing the U.S. federal government, its officials, or its facilities, unless an intentional tort was committed. Lawsuits resulting from a person acting within his or her scope of practice are examined on an individual basis with regard to the Federal Tort Claims Act, as exemplified in *Brown v. United States* and *Sherer v. United States.*

Res Judicata and *Res Ipsa Locuitur*

Res judicata is Latin for the phrase, "The thing has been decided." If patients lose their malpractice lawsuits, they cannot bring other suits against the physician for the same injuries.

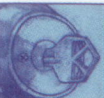

Keys to Success
PATIENT SAFETY

Every member of the healthcare team is responsible for patient safety. Any team member who witnesses something that seems wrong is compelled to speak with the physician about it out of the patient's hearing range. Team members who remain silent may be considered partly responsible for patients' injuries.

Once a case has been decided in a physician's favor, the case must be dropped. Conversely, when the court awards a patient damages, the physician can **appeal** the decision in the hope that the patient will settle for less than the awarded amount or the case will be found in the physician's favor.

Under the doctrine of *res ipsa locuitur,* the Latin phrase for, "The thing speaks for itself," physicians must prove what they did was correct. In all other malpractice cases, the patient must prove the physician's negligence. Cases of *res ipsa locuitur* are ones in which the malpractice is obvious. A wrong limb may have been amputated or an instrument left inside a patient.

The Standard of Care

The standard of care is a crucial tool for deciding most medical malpractice cases. The standard of care is the care a reasonably prudent person, in the same circumstances, with the same level of training, would perform. To determine if a healthcare provider has performed within the standard of care, one or both sides in the lawsuit will call on **expert witnesses**. An expert witness is a healthcare professional who is licensed or certified in the same specialty as the physician involved in the lawsuit. While expert witnesses must be licensed or certified, they need not be licensed or certified in the state where they are testifying.

Tort Reform

Some sources claim that the number of malpractice cases has risen over the past few years, causing an increase in medical malpractice insurance premiums, but those sources are mistaken. The medical malpractice insurance industry is cyclical, exhibiting the ups and downs of any other insurance industry. In fact, the number of malpractice cases that have awarded money to patients has decreased over the past decade and, once inflation is factored in, the amount of money awarded to patients has remained flat. Medical malpractice insurance carriers make most of their profits by investing premiums in the stock market. As the stock market ebbs and flows, so do the profits of insurance carriers.

Capping the Money Awarded to Injured Patients

About half the states in the United States have capped the awards that can be given to injured patients. These caps typically range from $250,000 to $1 million and fail to factor in the

TABLE 4-3 STATUTE OF LIMITATIONS IN EACH STATE

State	Statute of Limitations for Medical Malpractice
Alabama	2 years from the date of injury or 6 months from the date the injury was discovered to a maximum of 4 years from the date of injury.
Alaska	2 years from the date of injury.
Arizona	2 years from the date of injury.
Arkansas	2 years from the date of injury.
California	3 years from the date of injury or 1 year from the date the injury was discovered or should have been discovered. In the event a foreign object is found inside the plaintiff, the statute begins at the date the object was discovered or should have been discovered.
Colorado	2 years from the date of injury or date the injury was discovered or should have been discovered to a maximum of 3 years from the date of injury.
Connecticut	2 years from the date of injury or date the injury was discovered or should have been discovered to a maximum of 3 years from the date of injury.
Delaware	2 years from the date of injury or within 3 years if the injury was unknown and could not reasonably have been discovered.
Florida	2 years from the date of injury or date the injury was discovered or should have been discovered to a maximum of 4 years from the date of injury.
Georgia	2 years from the date of injury.
Hawaii	2 years from the date of injury or reasonable date of discovery. In the event an object is left inside a patient, a claim may be filed up to 1 year from the date of discovery. All claims must be filed within 6 years of the injury.
Idaho	2 years from the date of injury.
Illinois	2 years from the date of injury or up to 4 years if the injury could not reasonably have been discovered within 2 years.
Indiana	2 years from the date of injury.
Iowa	2 years from the date of injury or discovery of the injury. All claims must be filed within 6 years of the injury.
Kansas	2 years from the date of injury or up to 4 years if the injury could not reasonably have been discovered within 2 years.
Kentucky	1 year from the date of injury or up to 5 years if the injury could not reasonably have been discovered within 1 year.
Louisiana	3 years from the date of injury.
Maine	3 years from the date of injury.
Maryland	5 years from the date of injury or 3 years from the date the injury was discovered, whichever is greater.
Massachusetts	3 years from the date of injury or 3 years from the date of discovery. All claims must be filed within 7 years of the date of injury.
Michigan	2 years from the date of injury or 6 months from the date of discovery. All claims must be filed within 6 years of the date of injury.
Minnesota	4 years from the date of injury.
Mississippi	2 years from the date of injury or 2 years from the date of discovery. All claims must be filed within 7 years of the date of injury.
Missouri	2 years from the date of injury or date of discovery up to 10 years from the date of injury.
Montana	3 years from the date of injury or discovery up to 5 years from the date of injury.
Nebraska	2 years from the date of the injury or 1 year from the date the injury was discovered. All claims must be filed within 10 years of the date of injury.
Nevada	4 years from the date of injury.
New Hampshire	2 years from the date of the injury. In the event a foreign object is left inside a patient, the claim must be filed within 2 years of the discovery.
New Jersey	2 years from the date of the injury or 2 years from the date the injury was discovered or should have been discovered.
New Mexico	3 years from the date of injury.
New York	30 months from the date of injury. In the event a foreign object is left inside a patient, the claim must be filed within 1 year of the discovery.
North Carolina	3 years from the date of injury or the date the injury was discovered or should have been discovered. All claims must be filed within 10 years of the injury.
North Dakota	2 years from the date of injury or the date the injury was discovered or should have been discovered. All claims must be filed within 6 years of the injury.

continued

TABLE 4-3 STATUTE OF LIMITATIONS IN EACH STATE (CONTINUED)

State	Statute of Limitations for Medical Malpractice
Ohio	1 year from the date of injury. In the event a foreign object is left inside a patient, the claim must be filed within 1 year of the discovery.
Oklahoma	2 years from the date of injury.
Oregon	2 years from the date of injury or the date the injury was discovered or should have been discovered. All claims must be filed within 5 years of the injury.
Pennsylvania	2 years from the date of injury.
Rhode Island	3 years from the date of injury.
South Carolina	3 years from the date of injury or the date the injury was discovered or should have been discovered. In the event a foreign object is left inside a patient, the claim must be filed within 2 years of the discovery. All claims must be filed within 6 years of the date of injury.
South Dakota	2 years from the date of injury.
Tennessee	1 year from the date of injury.
Texas	2 years from the date of injury.
Utah	2 years from the date of injury or the date the injury was discovered or should have been discovered. In the event a foreign object is left inside a patient, the claim must be filed within 1 year of the discovery. All claims must be filed within 4 years of the date of injury.
Vermont	3 years from the date of injury or 2 years from the date the injury was discovered or should have been discovered. All claims must be filed within 7 years of the injury.
Virginia	2 years from the date of injury or the date the injury was discovered or should have been discovered. In the event a foreign object is left inside a patient, the claim must be filed within 1 year of the discovery. All claims must be filed within 10 years of the date of injury.
Washington, D.C.	3 years from the date of injury.
Washington	3 years from the date of injury or 1 year from the date the injury was discovered or should have been discovered. All claims must be filed within 8 years of the injury.
West Virginia	2 years from the date of injury or the date the injury was discovered or should have been discovered.
Wisconsin	3 years from the date of injury or 1 year from the date the injury was discovered or should have been discovered. All claims must be filed within 5 years of the injury.
Wyoming	2 years from the date of injury or the date the injury was discovered or should have been discovered.

Source: Expert Law.

severity of injuries, the number of physicians' prior malpractice cases, or if patients were injured due to physicians' reckless behavior.

Studies have shown that capping the money awarded to injured patients has not lowered medical malpractice premiums. Instead, premiums have continued to rise, even in states with caps. For example, a study performed by the Rand Corporation in 2004 found that caps on awards in the state of California resulted in payment of up to 30 percent less to injured patients than in states where no cap exists. In addition, this study found that patients who suffer the most severe injuries are typically compensated far less than patients with similar injuries in states without caps. Figure 4-7 ◆ outlines each state's record for providing safe care to patients.

There is a social cost of capping awards to injured patients, as well, and it is high. With too little money to cover their medical costs and expenses after an injury, patients often rely on their states' public healthcare systems (Medicaid), which means the taxpayers in those states pay for the injuries instead of the providers who are responsible for them.

Repeat Offender Providers

Studies in many states have shown that the vast majority of patient injuries arise from the same small handful of healthcare providers. Public Citizen, a nonprofit consumer rights group, performed a study in 1998 comparing the malpractice payouts in the United States to the number of doctors making payments. Their findings concluded that 5.9 percent of U.S. physicians were responsible for 57.8 percent of all medical malpractice payouts. In some states, like Kentucky, these providers are carefully disciplined to avoid injuring other patients. Other states, like Washington, have far worse records. In states like Washington, multiple offenders are likely to continue practicing and injuring patients. Figure 4-8 ◆ compares the number of healthcare providers in the United States who paid for a malpractice suit or settlement.

The Physician's Public Duties and Consequences

Physicians have certain responsibilities surrounding the reporting of certain events. Physicians who deliver babies must complete birth certificates, for example. Physicians who are the last to care for patients who have died are typically responsible for completing death certificates. All states list reporting requirements in the event of certain infectious or communicable diseases. Such lists can be obtained from state or local health departments and should be updated yearly.

State	Overall Grade	Access to Care	Quality and Patient Safety	Public Health and Injury Prevention	Medical Liability Environment
Alabama	D+	D+	C-	D+	D-
Alaska	C+	B+	D+	D	C
Arizona	D+	D+	C	C-	D-
Arkansas	D	D+	D	D	F
California	B	C	C+	A+	A+
Colorado	C	C+	D-	D+	B-
Conneticut	B	A-	A+	B	F
Delaware	C+	B-	A-	C+	D-
Dist. of Columbia	B	A+	A-	D+	F
Florida	C-	C-	B-	D-	D
Georgia	C+	D+	A	C	B-
Hawaii	C-	C+	D+	C+	D-
Idaho	D	D	D	D-	D
Illinois	C	B+	C	D+	D-
Indiana	D+	C-	D	C	D-
Iowa	C+	B-	A-	C	D
Kansas	C-	B-	F	D	D
Kentucky	C-	C	C	C	D-
Louisiana	C-	C-	B	D	D
Maine	B-	A	C+	C-	D
Maryland	B-	B+	B+	A+	F
Massachusetts	B	A	B	A-	D-
Michigan	B-	B+	B+	A	D-
Minnesota	C+	B+	C+	C	D-
Mississippi	C-	C	C+	D-	C-
Missouri	C+	B+	C-	D+	A-
Montana	C	C+	D-	F	A-
Nebraska	C-	C+	C-	D+	D+
Nevada	C-	D+	F	D-	A-
New Hampshire	C	B+	D-	C-	D-
New Jersey	C+	C+	A+	B+	F
New Mexico	D+	D+	C-	D+	D-
New York	C+	B-	B-	A+	D-
North Carolina	C-	C-	C	B+	F
North Dakota	C-	B-	D	D	D
Ohio	C+	A-	B-	D	D
Oklahoma	D+	C-	D-	C-	D-
Oregon	C-	C+	D	B+	D-
Pennsylvania	B-	A	A-	C-	F
Rhode Island	B-	A	B+	C-	F
South Carolina	B-	C	B+	D	B+
South Dakota	D+	C+	F	F	D
Tennessee	C-	C	C	D+	F
Texas	C	D+	D+	D	A+
Utah	D	D+	D-	D	D
Vermont	C	B+	C	C	F
Virginia	D+	C-	D+	C	F
Washington	D+	C	D	B-	D-
West Virginia	C+	C+	A	D	D
Wisconsin	C-	B-	D+	D+	D
Wyoming	D+	C+	D-	D-	F

Figure 4-7 ◆ Chart of information from the American College of Emergency Physicians regarding access to quality care in states with and without caps on malpractice awards.
Reprinted by permission of American College of Emergency Physicians®.

Reporting Vaccine Injuries

According to the 1986 National Childhood Vaccine Injury Act, vaccine injuries must be reported by physicians' offices to alert other physicians to possibly contaminated batches of vaccine. To report a vaccine injury, the medical assistant should obtain the patient's name and age, as well as the name and lot number of the vaccine. The call must be documented in the patient's file.

Reporting Cases of Abuse

Any incapacitated person, elderly person, or child who shows signs of suspected abuse or neglect must be protected. To that end,

Number of Payments Reported	Number of Doctors	Percent/Total Doctors in United States	Total Number of Payments	Total Amount of Payments	Percent of Total Number of Payments
All	147,378	17.6	219,272	$38,993,664,850	100
1	107,260	12.8	107,260	$18,131,973,750	48.9
2 or more	40,118	4.8	112,012	$20,861,691,100	51.1
3 or more	14,293	1.7	60,362	$11,084,300,850	27.5
4 or more	6,193	0.7	36,063	$6,481,629,350	16.5
5 or more	3,071	0.4	23,576	$4,073,749,100	10.8

Figure 4-8 ◆ Public Citizen study outlines the small number of physicians responsible for the vast number of malpractice payouts. *Reprinted with permission.*

physicians are required to report all cases of suspected child abuse to the proper authorities. After accidents, abuse is thought to be the second leading cause of death in children under age 5. When patients of any age sustain violent injuries, including injuries from gunshots or knives or criminal acts (like assault), attempted suicide, or rape, those injuries must be reported. The law protects healthcare workers from being sued for reporting suspected abuse.

Revoking Medical Licenses

Each state has its own medical practice acts. These acts list the duties and responsibilities of the physician and outline the actions that may be cause for disciplinary action, including suspension or revocation of the physician's license. In general, the more serious the action, the more serious the disciplinary action. For example, physicians who are convicted of felonies or proven to have abused patients may face license revocation.

The Physician-Patient Relationship

Both physicians and patients have responsibilities in their relationships.

The Role of the Patient

Patients are free to choose their physicians within the guidelines of their managed care plans. They can also choose whether they want to begin care or limit their care. Patients have the right to understand their treatment components, as well as side effects or benefits. All this information must be detailed for the patient before the procedure.

The Role of the Physician

Physicians have the right to refuse treatment to new patients, or even existing ones, unless those patients have life-threatening, emergent conditions. With proper notification, physicians can change their policies or their availabilities. When physicians are away from their practice for a period, like vacation, they must arrange for other physicians to cover their practice in the event of emergency. To simply close an office, with no emergency

referral, may be seen as abandonment of the patient and may result in a malpractice lawsuit.

Contracts in Healthcare

A contract is an agreement between two or more parties. All contracts must have the three following components:

1. An offer (the initiation of the contract)
2. Acceptance of the offer (both parties agree to the terms of the contract)
3. Some form of consideration (the exchange of fees for service)

Contracts can be verbal or written. In healthcare, a contract may be initiated when a patient calls the office to schedule an appointment. The offer is accepted when the medical assistant schedules the appointment. The patient is obligated to pay a fee for the service of seeing the physician, and the physician is obligated to treat the patient.

Physicians and patients operate using two types of contracts: (1) implied and (2) expressed.

Implied Contracts

Much like in implied consent discussed earlier, in an **implied contract**, nothing is written or spoken. Instead, patients imply through their actions alone that they agree to the contracts. For example, simply by arriving for care at the medical office patients imply that they will abide by the patient's portion of the doctor-patient contract and will pay for the services (Figure 4-9 ◆).

Expressed Contracts

Unlike implied contracts, **expressed contracts** have elements that are spoken or written. Expressed contracts occur when patients either verbally or in writing state that they will be responsible for their portion of contracts. For example, patients who sign payment agreements stating they will make payments of $100 per month for the next six months enter into an expressed contract. Figure 4-10 ◆ shows a sample expressed contract.

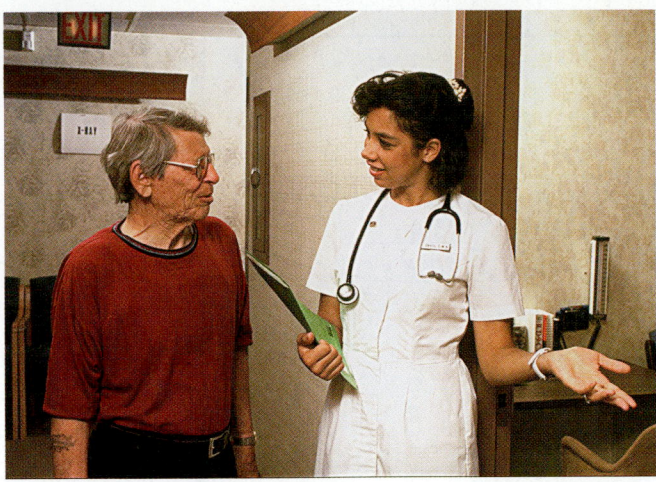

Figure 4-9 ◆ By arriving for care at the medical office, the patient implies that he or she will abide by the patient's portion of the doctor-patient contract and pay for services.

Terminating Contracts

The doctor-patient contract is typically resolved once the patient has completed the prescribed course of treatment outlined by the physician. While the patient may choose to end the doctor-patient relationship at any time, the physician must follow legal protocol to end the relationship.

Patients may choose to end their physician relationship for varied reasons, and they may or may not share those reasons with their provider. When patients do state reasons for ending their medical relationship, those reasons must be charted in the patients' charts. Physicians should send the patients letters acknowledging the termination and offer to refer the patients to other healthcare providers, if desired.

For their part, physicians may choose to terminate the doctor-patient relationship due to patients' noncompliance with treatment programs. They may also end patient relationships for personal reasons. Whatever the reason, physicians must follow legal protocol to avoid accusations of patient abandonment. This protocol includes sending a letter to a patient indicating the intent to terminate the relationship. This letter must include:

- A statement clearly indicating the intent to terminate the relationship
- The reason for the desire to terminate the relationship
- A statement that the patient's medical records will be available for transfer to another physician

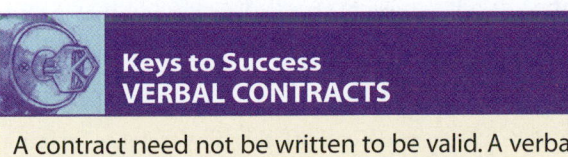

Keys to Success
VERBAL CONTRACTS

A contract need not be written to be valid. A verbal contract can be just as binding as a signed one.

- An offer to refer the patient to another physician
- A statement strongly encouraging the patient to seek care with another physician as needed

Figure 4-11 ◆ is a sample termination letter.

A termination-of-care letter must give the patient at least thirty days to find another physician. During that time, the present physician must continue to see the patient if the patient desires. Termination letters should be sent via certified mail with a signed return receipt requested. Copies of termination letters and signed receipts must be placed in patients' medical records.

The Good Samaritan Act

The **Good Samaritan act** protects healthcare workers from being sued when they render first aid in emergency situations outside the medical setting. If, for example, healthcare workers rendered cardiopulmonary resuscitation (**CPR**) at their local grocery store and the patient died or survived with poor outcomes, those healthcare workers would be protected. All states have Good Samaritan acts, although only Vermont requires those with CPR knowledge to stop and render first aid to victims.

Maintaining Patient Confidentiality Through Proper Records Handling

Because medical assistants are patient advocates, they must keep patients' best interests, notably patient confidentiality, at the forefront of their work. Medical assistants must never reveal patient information without a patient's signed consent or a court order. As a result, when patients' family members call the office, medical assistants can tell them nothing about the patients. Similarly, medical assistants are forbidden from releasing information to insurance companies, even bills for services, without patients' consent.

? — Critical Thinking Question 4-2 —
Referring back to the case study at the beginning of this chapter, assume that Victoria revealed information about Dr. Kozlowski's patient to the patient's employer. What is the potential impact on Victoria?

Releasing Medical Records

Requests for patients' medical records are common. Patients may need to see specialists, obtain second opinions, or seek care at different facilities. Any request for copies of patients' medical records must be accompanied by the patients' signed authorization. The medical assistant must be certain the authorization is directed to the correct facility and that it contains a date for when the signature was made. In addition to verifying the authorization,

September 4, 2010

I, __*Walter Backous*__ , agree to make payments of $100 per month to Morton Family Practice. My payment will be made by the ___15th___ of each month and will begin on the ___*15th of September, 2008*___ .

_____   _____
Parent or Guardian's Signature   Date

_____   _____
Witness's Signature   Date

Figure 4-10 ◆ Sample expressed contract agreement.

the medical assistant must also be completely clear about the nature of the request. Patients may authorize the release of their entire records, or they may authorize the release of information for one date of service only. Some physicians require their staff to alert them of any requests for records. In these offices, the medical assistant pulls the patient's file, attaches the request for copies, and gives the file to the physician for review.

Before sending any copies of medical records, however, the medical assistant must review the file to ensure that it is complete and that it contains only information about that patient. Some facilities provide counseling services that include patients and their family members. For these records, the medical assistant must obliterate any non–patient-specific information before sending copies.

In rare cases, medical offices may release original patient records. These requests are most often received via subpoena for court cases in which the judge or attorneys wish to see original material. When original medical records are

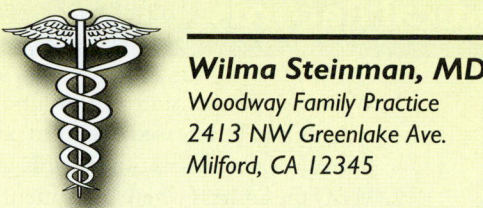

Wilma Steinman, MD
Woodway Family Practice
2413 NW Greenlake Ave.
Milford, CA 12345

August 25, 2010

Gloria Sanchez
891 NW Wallingford Ave.
Milford, CA 12345

Dear Ms. Sanchez:

Because you have missed your last four follow-up appointments to monitor your condition, I will no longer be able to provide you medical services. I believe your condition requires attention and strongly encourage you to seek care with a physician. When you have chosen a new physician, please advise this office by requesting, in writing, the transfer of your medical records.

If you wish, I would be happy to give you a referral. I will be available to treat you for no longer than 30 days from the receipt of this letter.

Sincerely,

Wilma Steinman, M.D.

Wilma Steinman, M.D.

Figure 4-11 ◆ Sample termination-of-care letter.

required, the medical assistant should make a complete copy of every item in the chart, and keep the copies in the office, recorded in a log, as proof of the contents at the time of release.

Occasionally, patients will ask to rescind the authorization to release information previously given. When this occurs, the patient will need to sign a separate form that states that previously given authorization is now rescinded. Many legal documents used for obtaining medical records have a disclosure included that states the amount of time the authorization is to be valid. For example, a form may say, "This authorization is valid for 90 days from the date of the signature." In the event one of these forms is used, the patient will not need to sign a separate form in order to rescind the authorization, unless the patient wishes to withdraw his or her authorization before the ninety-day time period.

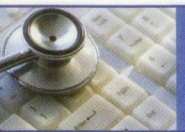

PROCEDURE 4-2 Obtain Authorization for the Release of Patient Medical Records

Theory and Rationale

The release of patient medical records requires strict attention to detail and relevant laws. The **Health Insurance Portability and Accountability Act (HIPAA)** requires healthcare providers to obtain patients' consent to release those patients' health information. The ability to properly obtain authorization for the release of patient medical records is vital to the medical assistant.

Materials

- Release-of-records authorization form
- Blue or black ink pen
- Copy machine

Competency

(Conditions) With the necessary materials, you will be able to **(Task)** obtain an authorization to release information from a patient **(Standards)** correctly within the time limit set by the instructor.

1. When the patient states all or a portion of the patient's records is to be released to a third party, ask the patient to sign and date a release-of-records form.
2. Verify the address where the patient would like the copies of the record sent.
3. Verify the records the patient would like released. If the patient requests specific release dates, ask the patient to write those dates on the release-of-records form.
4. Verify if the patient would like superprotected information (**HIV/AIDS**, mental health, drug or alcohol rehabilitation information, sexually transmitted disease information, or information about family planning), and ask the patient to check the appropriate box on the authorization form to allow the release of that information.
5. Identify which information in the medical record must be copied.
6. Copy the appropriate documents from the medical record.
7. Send the copies to the requested location.

Accommodating Subpoenas of Medical Records

Occasionally, medical offices may receive a subpoena for patients' medical records. Subpoenas may arise from lawsuits due to injury, such as from a car accident. A judge must sign a subpoena, which authorizes the physician to release the information without the patient's signature. Medical facilities are not required to notify the patient of the subpoena, but many will as a courtesy. HIPAA requires medical facilities to keep records of all patient-record disclosures, however, and to make those records available to patients upon request.

Critical Thinking Question 4-3

In the case study at the beginning of the chapter, imagine the patient's employer obtained a subpoena for her medical information. How would the medical assistant determine which information to release? What is the proper procedure?

Disclosing Minors' Medical Information

In most states, children under 18 may receive certain types of medical treatment without their parents' consent. Such treatments are limited to those for family planning (i.e., birth control

or abortion), sexually transmitted diseases (**STDs**), mental health, human immunodeficiency virus (HIV), acquired immune deficiency syndrome (AIDS), or alcohol or drug rehabilitation. Because laws for releasing minors' information vary from state to state, medical assistants must be very clear about the laws in the states where they practice.

Minors may receive copies of only those documents their parents cannot see. For example, minors could request and receive copies of their STD treatments, but they could not receive copies of the vaccines they received. Parents, in contrast, could receive copies of their children's vaccination record, but not their STD treatments.

Guarding Superprotected Medical Information

A few areas of medical information are considered "superprotected." While the definition varies from state to state, superprotected information is usually any material pertaining to family planning; STDs; mental illness; HIV or AIDS treatment, diagnosis, or testing; and alcohol or drug rehabilitation. Superprotected information normally requires a separate authorization before it can be released to a third party. In other words, if the medical assistant were to receive a request for copies of a patient's file, she would be unable to release superprotected information without a specific request from the patient.

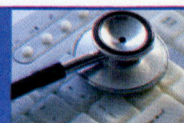

PROCEDURE 4-3 Respond to a Request for Copies of a Patient's Medical Record

Theory and Rationale

Releasing personal patient information without the patient's consent or a court order violates HIPAA. In fact, improperly copying documents in a patient's medical record could subject the physician to a lawsuit. Therefore, knowing how to properly respond to a request for copies of the patient's medical record is imperative for the medical assistant.

Materials

- Release-of-records authorization form
- Blue or black ink pen
- Copy machine

Competency

(**Conditions**) With the necessary materials, you will be able to (**Task**) respond to a request for copies of a patient's medical record (**Standards**) correctly within the time limit set by the instructor.

1. Verify that the release-of-records form has been signed and dated by the patient or the patient's legal representative.
2. Carefully review the release form for any specific date or information requests.
3. Check if the patient has authorized release of superprotected information (HIV/AIDS, mental health, drug or alcohol rehabilitation information, sexually transmitted disease information, or information about family planning).
4. Verify that you have the correct patient file.
5. Locate the documents to be copied.
6. Review the documents to be copied to verify that they carry the correct patient name and contain the information requested in the authorization to release information and only that information.
7. Copy the appropriate documents.
8. Send the copies to the requesting agency.
9. File the release-of-records request in the patient's medical record with a notation of the documents that were copied and sent.

Faxing Medical Records

Medical records should be faxed only when no other method of data transfer is available, because the risk of unintended recipients is too high. The American Health Information Management Association (**AHIMA**) recommends fax use for confidential patient information only when sending copies via postal service or messenger does not suffice. Medical offices should use a HIPAA-compliant fax cover sheet such as the one in Figure 4-12 ◆ any time they fax patient information.

Disclosing Medical Records Improperly

Disclosing confidential patient information without proper authorization or subpoena is cause for a lawsuit. Patients who feel they have been harmed by improper disclosure may sue a medical office for defamation of character, invasion of privacy, or breach of confidentiality. When information is disclosed improperly, the office is responsible for reporting the event to HIPAA.

The Health Insurance Portability and Accountability Act (HIPAA)

The Health Insurance Portability and Accountability Act (HIPAA) of 1996 was enacted to reform healthcare mainly by:

1. Improving **portability** and continuity in group and individual insurance
2. Combatting waste, fraud, and abuse in health insurance and healthcare delivery
3. Promoting the use of medical savings accounts (**MSAs**)
4. Improving access to long-term care services and coverage
5. Simplifying health insurance administration
6. Providing a means of paying for reforms and related initiatives

HIPAA is divided into the seven following titles:

Title I	Health Care Access, Portability, and Renewability
Title II	Preventing Health Care Fraud and Abuse; Administrative Simplification; Medical Liability Reform
Title III	Tax-Related Health Provisions
Title IV	Application and Enforcement of Group Health Plan Requirements
Title V	Revenue Offsets
Title XI	General Provisions, Peer Review, Administrative Simplification
Title XXVII	Assuring Portability, Availability, and Renewability of Health Insurance Coverage

HIPAA titles are nonsequential because some portions of the original legislation failed to pass.

Anne Wager, MD

Quan Lee, MD
8282 Arlington Way
Arlington, WA 12345
360-555-4545

Facsimile transmittal

To: _____ Fax number: _____

From: _____ Date: _____

Re: _____ No. of pages, including cover sheet: _____

___ Urgent ___ For Review ___ Please Comment ___ Please Reply

Comments:

CONFIDENTIAL INFORMATION

The information in this facsimile message and any accompanying documents is confidential. This information is intended for use only by the individual or entity named above. If you are not the intended recipient of this information, you are hereby notified that any disclosure, copying, or distribution of this information is strictly prohibited. Please notify the sender immediately by telephone. Thank you.

Figure 4-12 ◆ Sample HIPAA-compliant fax cover sheet.

Title II of HIPAA

Title II of HIPAA, which relates to healthcare providers, has three main goals, which are to:

- Prevent fraud and abuse in healthcare delivery and payment
- Improve Medicare and other programs through an efficient and effective standard
- Establish standards and requirements for all electronic transmission of certain health information

Title II dictated that, by July 2002, all healthcare providers begin using employer identification numbers (**EINs**) whenever they transmitted patient data electronically. The second portion of Title II imposed a privacy rule that addressed the:

- Rights individuals should have for their private health information
- Procedures that should be established for patients to exercise their rights to private health information

■ Uses and disclosures of private patient health information that should be authorized or required

This rule required all providers of healthcare or healthcare products to notify patients in writing how the patients' private health information would be handled and under what circumstances it would be released. The deadline for compliance was April 2003.

The third portion of Title II addresses the issue of electronically transmitting private health information. HIPAA mandated security measures to standardize electronic claim formats and eliminate outdated forms. The Security Ruling in Title II outlines the security measures that must be in place for healthcare providers to submit patient health information electronically.

HIPAA and Computer Privacy

HIPAA requires password protection for all computers used in healthcare. All employees who must access the computers must have their own passwords and log off when leaving their desks. In addition, computers must face away from patient areas of the clinic. Figure 4-13 ◆ outlines other computer-related requirements in the ambulatory setting.

The HIPAA Privacy Officer

While every member of the medical office should be well versed in HIPAA, every office must designate one person as the HIPAA privacy officer. The privacy officer is responsible for overseeing all aspects of the office's HIPAA compliance and helping patients who may question or file complaints about suspected violations.

Critical Thinking Question 4-4

Assume that the patient was fired after the medical office gave her employer her private health information without her permission. How should she go about filing a complaint with HIPAA?

HIPAA Records Violations

Patients who believe medical offices have inappropriately disclosed medical information may contact HIPAA authorities directly. Every medical office must have the complaint forms on file and help patients filing the proper paperwork. Normally, HIPAA will only issue fines or written warnings when violations were intentional or offices have logged a number of violations.

HIPAA Compliance

Patients can give anyone verbal access to their medical information by notifying the medical office in writing. Such information becomes part of the patients' permanent medical records. For example, if Julius Reiman gives written permission for his wife, Ruth, to have knowledge of his care, the physician can talk to Ruth about Julius's care or condition.

To be HIPAA compliant, the medical office must keep its computer systems secure. Knowing the proper procedure for keeping private patient information from being inappropriately viewed is an important function of the administrative medical assistant.

1. Before stepping away from an office computer for a moment or for the evening, be certain the computer is logged out so no one can obtain private patient information without logging in with a password.
2. Look around the desk area to be certain nothing in sight has private information viewable.
3. Cover or remove any files or papers that may contain patient information and may be viewable to patients.
4. When returning to the workstation, log back into the computer system using a personal password.
5. Ensure that your password is changed periodically and that it is not written anywhere near the computer station.

Figure 4-13 ◆ HIPAA compliancy for computers in the ambulatory setting.

The HIPAA Business Associate Agreement

HIPAA legislation stipulates that only those persons in the office who must have access to private patient information should have access. The office cleaners may work for the physician, but they do not need access to any private patient information.

Employees of medical offices are covered under HIPAA and are required to keep confidential information from leaving the office. Anyone who is not an employee of the medical office but may come into contact with private patient information must sign a HIPAA Business Associate Agreement. Such people include:

■ Copy-machine repairperson
■ Computer software support technician
■ Medical assistant externing in the clinic

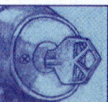

Keys to Success
WHAT IS AN EMPLOYEE?

Employees are people who work for wages and have payroll taxes taken out of their checks. People who work for the office but have no payroll taxes taken from their checks are not employees. These people must sign a HIPAA Business Associate Agreement if they might come into contact with patient private health information.

■ Medical assistant performing a shadow project
■ Consultants
■ Professional staff (e.g., accountants or lawyers)
■ Cleaning staff
■ Transcriptionists

Penalties for HIPAA Violations

The fines for HIPAA violations range from $100 to $25,000. Criminal penalties may also apply if it is determined that an individual knowingly obtained or disclosed personal health information without the proper authority. The most severe penalties under HIPAA legislation apply to anyone who commits an offense with the intent to sell, transfer, or use another person's health information. Figure 4-14 ◆ outlines the penalties for HIPAA violations.

Advance Directives

Today, many patients use **advance directives** to outline their wishes should they be unable to speak for themselves. Advance directives consist of living wills, orders outlining patients' desire to not be resuscitated, and durable power of attorney for healthcare. Any "Do Not Resuscitate" (**DNR**) order must be written and signed by the patient's doctor. A copy should rest in the patient's file. Concealing or altering an advance directive is a misdemeanor. Creating an advanced directive falsely is a felony.

General penalty for the failure to comply with requirements and standards:

■ Not more than $100 for each violation up to a $25,000 for all violations of an identical requirement during a calendar year.

Wrongful disclosure of protected health information:

■ A person who knowingly and in violation of HIPAA regulations:
  - Uses or causes to be used a unique health identifier
  - Obtains private health information relating to an individual
  - Discloses individually identifiable health information to another person

Shall be punished by:
  - A fine of not more than $50,000, imprisoned for not more than 1 year, or both
  - If the offense is committed under false pretenses, be fined not more that $100,000, imprisoned for not more than 5 years, or both
  - If the offense is done with the intent to sell, transfer, or use private health information for commercial purposes or to cause harm, be fined not more than $250,000, imprisoned not more than 10 years, or both

---

Figure 4-14 ◆ Penalties for HIPAA violations.

Living wills, which are legal in every state, state patients' desires should those patients become incapacitated. Instructions address patients' desire for life-support procedures.

Patients may sometimes give durable power of attorney to other people. The power of attorney names people who can speak or act for the patients in the event the patients cannot speak for themselves. Power-of-attorney documents normally address patients' desires for life support, but authorized parties may do such things as sign contracts or access bank accounts. A more detailed discussion of advance directives appears in ∞ Chapter 7, Considerations of Extended Life.

Employment Law and Healthcare

Title VII of the Civil Rights Act of 1964 was passed to protect employees from discrimination in the workplace. Under this act, employers cannot refuse to hire, refuse to equally compensate, or fire an employee based on race, color, sex, religion, or national origin.

During an interview, candidates cannot be asked questions that would reveal their age, marital status, religion, height, weight, or arrest record unless the information somehow relates to the job for which they are interviewing. For example, candidates who must reach objects on a shelf during the day can be polled about height to ensure they have the proper reach. Arrests are a forbidden topic, because mistakes can be made in the criminal justice system. Employers can, however, ask about convictions, as well as drug use. Drug screening before employment is also legal.

The Americans with Disabilities Act and Healthcare Employment

The Americans with Disabilities Act (**ADA**) prohibits employers from refusing to hire people with disabilities unless those disabilities prevent the people from performing the job. Employers would be justified in turning down wheelchair candidates for ditch-digging jobs, for example. A written, complete job description that includes any physical duties that are required helps candidates know if they can meet the requirements (Figure 4-15 ◆).

The ADA applies only to employers with fifteen or more employees, and a disability is defined as any condition that causes a person's major life activities to be limited. The act covers those who are HIV infected or have AIDS, cancer, a history of mental illness, and alcoholism.

The ADA's Requirements

The ADA requires employers to provide their employees basic accommodations, such as extra-wide parking spaces close to the door, accessible bathrooms, break rooms, and work-area accommodations. If an employer has fifteen or more employees and one of those employees suddenly becomes disabled, the employer must provide accommodations so the employee can continue to work. However, the employer has two years to provide the accommodations, and the accommodations must be reasonable.

Job Title: Certified Medical Assistant
Department: Pediatrics
Reports To: Clinical Manager

SUMMARY:

Under general supervision, is responsible for the physical care of patients through tasks of routine difficulty; responsible for maintaining the clinical area of the clinic.

ESSENTIAL DUTIES AND RESPONSIBILITIES:

Includes the following. Other duties may be assigned. Assists physicians with surgical procedures. Takes and records patients' blood pressure, temperature, pulse, respiration and weight. Makes routine entries into patients' charts. Shares responsibilities for use of equipment and supplies. Administers specified medication, by injection, orally or topically, and notes time and amount on patients' charts. Sterilizes equipment and supplies. Makes suggestions to improve work methods, trains new employees, makes routine entries into logs, records supplies and materials used. Completes requisitions for supplies and forwards to supervisor for approval.

QUALIFICATIONS:

To perform this job successfully, an individual must be able to perform each essential duty satisfactorily. The requirements listed below are representative of the knowledge, skill, and/or ability required. Reasonable accommodations may be made to enable individuals with disabilities to perform the essential functions.

EDUCATION:

Successful completion of an accredited medical assisting program.

LANGUAGE SKILLS:

Ability to read and comprehend simple instructions, short correspondence, and memos. Ability to write simple correspondence. Ability to effectively present information in one-on-one and small group situations to patients and other employees of the organization.

MATHEMATICAL SKILLS:

Ability to add and subtract two digit numbers and to multiply and divide with 10's and 100's. Ability to perform these operations using units of American money and weight measurement, volume and distance.

REASONING ABILITY:

Ability to apply common sense understanding to carry out instructions furnished in written, oral, or diagram form.

CERTIFICATES, LICENSES, REGISTRATIONS:

Must have certification of completion of CMA or RMA certification examination.

PHYSICAL DEMANDS:

The physical demands described here are representative of those that must be met by an employee to successfully perform the essential functions of this job. Reasonable accommodations may be made to enable individuals with disabilities to perform the essential functions. While performing the duties of this job, the employee is regularly required to stand; walk; use hands to finger, handle, or feel; reach with hands and arms; and talk or hear. The employee is occasionally required to sit; climb or balance; and stoop, kneel, crouch, or crawl. The employee must regularly lift and/or move up to 50 pounds. Specific vision abilities required by this job include close vision, distance vision, color vision, peripheral vision, depth perception, and ability to adjust focus.

The employee must have the ability to work overtime hours.

WORK ENVIRONMENT:

The work environment characteristics described here are representative of those an employee encounters while performing the essential functions of this job. Reasonable accommodations may be made to enable individuals with disabilities to perform the essential functions. While performing the duties of this job, the employee is occasionally exposed to outside weather conditions. The noise level in the work environment is usually moderate.

Figure 4-15 ◆ Sample detailed job description.

The Conscience Clause

A **conscience clause**, adopted in many states, outlines a healthcare worker's ability to refuse to participate in actions or care for reasons of religion or conscience. Usually, this clause is used when healthcare workers do not wish to be involved in abortion procedures, although it has recently been used when pharmacists do not wish to dispense certain pregnancy-preventing medications. When medical assistants have religious or conscientious objections to any actions or procedures in the office, they should familiarize themselves with the laws in their state and should fully inform their employer.

The Patients' Bill of Rights

As discussed in ∞ Chapter 1, The American Hospital Association (AHA) first adopted a Patients' Bill of Rights in 1972 and modified it in 1992. The AHA revamped this document in 2003, renaming the new version the **Patient Care Partnership**. This agreement is provided to all patients upon entering the inpatient hospital setting. The Patient Care Partnership outlines patients' expectations, rights, and responsibilities while in the hospital setting. Expectations are listed in areas such as the quality of care the patient can expect to receive, and a clean and safe environment should be provided to all patients.

Patients should expect to be involved in their care while in the hospital and should be involved in discussing their condition with the medical providers. These discussions should include the patient's treatment plan. Patients are directed to provide their healthcare team with all information relating to their treatment, including past illnesses and allergic reactions. Within the Patient Care Partnership, patients are told they should expect protection of their privacy while in the hospital setting, to be properly prepared for discharge when the time comes, and to be provided with help in filing insurance claims, if needed. The Patient Care Partnership can be viewed on the American Hospital Association website: http://www.aha.org.

In March 1997, President Bill Clinton appointed a committee to study the quality of healthcare in the United States. As part of its work, the committee issued a list of Consumer Bill of Rights and Responsibilities, which contained the Patients' Bill of Rights in Figure 4-16 ◆.

Many states have enacted their own patients' bills of rights. Contents vary, but most include patients' rights for obtaining care, completing the **appeal** process, and handling abuses by insurance carriers.

The Clinical Laboratory Improvement Amendments Act (CLIA) and Ambulatory Care

The Centers for Medicare and Medicaid Services (**CMS**) regulate all laboratory testing performed on humans in the United States, with the exception of testing done for medical research. CMS achieves this regulation via the Clinical Laboratory Improvement Amendments Act (**CLIA**) of 1988. These rules apply to any lab that is performing any work with specimens, including ambulatory care settings, and are in place to ensure safe, accurate laboratory testing. CLIA regulations are based on the complexity of the test method. The more complicated the test, the more stringent the requirements. Every facility that performs laboratory testing must establish a quality assurance program that includes quality control, personnel policies, patient test management, and proficiency testing. Facilities are inspected every two years to ensure compliance with federal CLIA regulations.

The Joint Commission on the Accreditation of Healthcare Organizations (JCAHO) and Ambulatory Care

The Joint Commission on the Accreditation of Healthcare Organizations (**JCAHO**), often simply called the Joint Commission, is a private organization that sets standards for healthcare administration and patient safety. Hospitals that receive federal funding, such as Medicare and Medicaid, are required to be JCAHO certified, while private hospitals and doctors' offices are not. Many facilities, including clinics that are not required to be JCAHO certified, still seek this accreditation, because it is a sign of excellence in patient safety.

Medical Ethics

Medical ethics are what govern the behavior of healthcare professionals. Each professional association has its own code of ethics that details the actions that are considered ethical by that profession. The American Association of Medical Assistants (**AAMA**) has a code of ethics that addresses five areas the medical assistant must strive for. Those areas are to:

1. Render services with respect for human dignity
2. Respect patient confidentiality, except when the law requires information
3. Uphold the honor and high principles set forth by the AAMA
4. Continually improve knowledge and skills for the benefit of patients and the healthcare team
5. Participate in community services that promote the good health and welfare of the general public

Since 1999, the AAMA has had a policy of sanctioning medical assistants who violate its disciplinary standards. Under this policy, called the AAMA's Disciplinary Standards and Procedures for CMAs, sanctions range from being denied eligibility to sit for the certification examination to permanent revocation of the certified medical assistant (**CMA**) credential.

Ethical Considerations

All medical assistants can expect to face legal and ethical situations that may require them to act to protect the patient

I. Information Disclosure You have the right to receive accurate and easily understood information about your health plan, health care professionals, and health care facilities. If you speak another language, have a physical or mental disability, or just do not understand something, assistance will be provided so you can make informed health care decisions.

II. Choice of Providers and Plans You have the right to a choice of health care providers that is sufficient to provide you with access to appropriate high-quality health care.

III. Access to Emergency Services If you have severe pain, an injury, or a sudden illness that convinces you that your health is in serious jeopardy, you have the right to receive screening and stabilization emergency services whenever and wherever needed, without prior authorization or financial penalty.

IV. Participation in Treatment Decisions You have the right to know all your treatment options and to participate in decisions about your care. Parents, guardians, family members, or other individuals that you designate can represent you if you cannot make your own decisions.

V. Respect and Nondiscrimination You have a right to considerate, respectful, and nondiscriminatory care from your doctors, health plan representatives, and other health care providers.

VI. Confidentiality of Health Information You have the right to talk in confidence with health care providers and to have your health care information protected. You also have the right to review and copy your own medical record and request that your physician amend your record if it is not accurate, relevant, or complete.

VII. Complaints and Appeals You have the right to a fair, fast, and objective review of any complaint you have against your health plan, doctors, hospitals, or other health care personnel. This includes complaints about waiting times, operating hours, the conduct of health care personnel, and the adequacy of health care facilities.

Figure 4-16 ◆ Patients' Bill of Rights.

yet remain within the bounds of law and the scope of practice. Sometimes, physicians may ask medical assistants to perform duties outside the scope of practice. Because this is illegal, the medical assistant should be comfortable declining to accept the task. To do so could cause patient injury and a lawsuit against both the medical assistant and the physician.

Similarly, most medical assistants will witness the physician or other members of the healthcare team perform procedures outside of the scope of practice for the medical assistant. In some practices, physicians may train medical assistants to perform some of these tasks. Because there are variations, medical assistants must be fully versed in their states' scopes of practice. Some procedures, like the application of a cast, may seem easy to perform after being shown by the physician, but if it is outside the scope of medical-assisting practice, it may be illegal to perform even with the physician's supervision.

Ethical Model

An unethical physician may ask the medical assistant to break the law. Medical assistants are legally bound by law and scope of practice to treat patients lawfully and ethically and to document correctly in patients' charts. If medical assistants wonder whether actions cross ethical or legal boundaries, they should consider the following questions based on the Blanchard and Peale Ethical Model:

1. Is the action legal?
2. Is the action ethical?
3. How will the action make me feel?
4. How would I feel if the action, and my involvement, was published in the local newspaper? If I had to explain my actions to my child/spouse/parent?

If the medical assistant is uncomfortable with any of the answers to these four questions, the action likely crosses an ethical or legal boundary, and the medical assistant should decline to participate. Any local Association of Medical Assistants chapter is a good place to call when in doubt about an action. Bad actions can hinder future employment. Prospective employers must believe new staff are ethical and will practice within their legal scopes of practice. Medical assistants who are associated with a medical practice or a physician who is practicing unethically or illegally will unfortunately gain that same reputation.

In Practice

Jan has been working as an administrative medical assistant for Dr. Borse for seven years. Dr. Borse frequently asks Jan to add charges to a patient account for services he did not perform.

Jan is paid well and feels she is harming no patients by complying with the doctor's requests. Dr. Borse says he only submits the false claims to make up for the money he loses by treating Medicare and Medicaid patients. One day, Dr. Borse is arrested for insurance fraud. He eventually serves two years in prison and loses his license to practice medicine. Jan has a very hard time getting a new job. Dr. Borse's story has been in all the local papers, and employers do not want to work with unethical staff.

How could Jan have changed the course of events? What advice would have helped Jan while she was working with Dr. Borse?

Raising Ethical Issues in Healthcare

The American Medical Association (**AMA**) has outlined several areas surrounding ethics in the management of patient care. A few appear in Figure 4-17 ◆ .

Other ethical standpoints by the AMA include areas surrounding finances in the healthcare setting. These include:

- Patient care should not be dictated by the patient's ability to pay. In other words, a physician should not order expensive tests for a patient who can pay and skip tests for one who cannot.
- Physicians can charge for missed appointments only when they notify the patients ahead of time.
- Patients must be able to receive copies of their medical record, regardless of any amounts owed the office. The

- With regard to organ transplantation, physicians must not consider age in the decision of who gets the organ. Priority must be given to the patient who has the strongest chance of obtaining long-term benefit; a person's individual worth to society must not be considered.
- With regard to clinical research, physicians must fully inform any patient involved in research and must give those patients the highest level of respect and care. The goal of any research program must be to obtain some type of scientific data.
- With regard to obstetrics, physicians must perform abortions within the boundaries of state and federal laws. If physicians do not wish to perform abortions, they must refer patients to physicians who will perform the procedure. If a patient undergoes genetic testing, the physician must give the results to both parents.

Figure 4-17 ◆ AMA ethical viewpoints.

physician cannot hold the medical record hostage for payment of the bill.

- Physicians can charge interest on medical bills in accordance with state law if they notify patients ahead of time.
- Fees for service must be reasonable and fair and must be based on Current Procedural Terminology (**CPT**) code guidelines regarding the nature of the care involved.

Bioethics

As medical technology advances, the issue of **bioethics** will continue to expand current thought, as well as some individuals' comfort zones. Bioethics addresses areas that affect human life. Examples are cloning, the use of embryonic stem cells, in-vitro fertilization, and abortion. Within bioethics, what is right for one person may not be right for another. The goal is to make decisions on a case-by-case basis, taking into consideration the individuals who are involved.

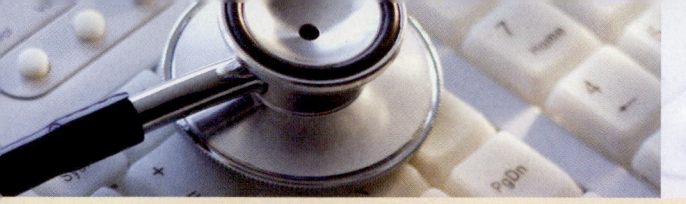

REVIEW

Chapter Summary

- U.S. laws arise from varying sources to achieve varying legal purposes.
- Malpractice is a serious, wide-ranging issue in healthcare that the medical assistant can address both individually and as a member of the healthcare team.
- Physicians have a number of public duties to perform to ensure patient safety and confidentiality are upheld.
- Medical assistants play a crucial role in patient confidentiality procedures.
- The Health Insurance Portability and Accountability Act (HIPAA) is in place to help steer the proper direction of contemporary healthcare.

- The various federal and state organizations driving current healthcare practices demand compliance from all members of the medical staff.
- Healthcare professionals must be vigilant about all relevant legislation, including the conscience clause, patients' bill of rights, and codes of ethics.
- Medical ethics govern the behavior of healthcare professionals. Each professional association has its own code of ethics that details the actions that are considered ethical by that profession

Chapter Review

Multiple Choice

1. *Res judicata* is Latin for
   a. The physician is responsible.
   b. The thing speaks for itself.
   c. Let the master answer.
   d. None of the above.

2. _____ is the unauthorized attempt or threat to touch another person.
   a. Assault
   b. Battery
   c. Duress
   d. Invasion of privacy

3. _____ is releasing private information about another person without the person's consent.
   a. Assault
   b. Battery
   c. Duress
   d. Invasion of privacy

4. _____ is the actual physical touching of another person without the person's consent; it includes physical abuse.
   a. Assault
   b. Battery
   c. Duress
   d. Invasion of privacy

5. _____ is the act of coercing someone into an act.
   a. Assault
   b. Battery
   c. Duress
   d. Invasion of privacy

True/False

T F 1. In most states, children under age 18 may receive medical attention for a sexually transmitted disease without parental consent.

T F 2. Patients win most medical malpractice cases.

T F 3. Patients may refuse treatment for any reason.

T F 4. Hospitals that receive federal funding, such as Medicare and Medicaid, are required to be JCAHO certified.

T F 5. The statute of limitations for medical malpractice cases is the same in every state.

T F 6. Classes of felony crimes are the same in every state.

T F 7. The physician must report any vaccine injuries.

Short Answer

1. What are the four steps in an ethical model, and how do they apply to an everyday situation, such as talking about a patient with coworkers outside the medical office?

2. What is the Good Samaritan Act?

3. What are the four Ds of negligence?

4. Differentiate implied consent from expressed consent.

5. Explain what is meant by *informed consent.*

6. Define the conscience clause and explain how it pertains to healthcare professionals.

7. Describe the steps the physician must take to legally terminate the physician-patient relationship.

8. Explain the function of the HIPAA Privacy Officer in the medical office.

Chapter Review (continued)

Research

1. Are there caps on the medical malpractice awards allowed in your state? If so, what are they?

2. Search the Internet for a medical malpractice case. What were the specifics of the case?

3. Search the Internet for a medical ethics case. What were the specifics of the case?

Externship Application Experience

Joe Rutigliano is a patient of Dr. Mallory's. As Joe is leaving the office after his appointment, he overhears Dr. Mallory and her medical assistant discussing his treatment plan in the hallway. He believes other patients also overhear their conversation, and he is upset. What should the medical assistant do?

Resource Guide

American Association of Medical Assistants
20 N. Wacker Dr., Suite 1575
Chicago, IL 60606
Phone: (312) 899-1500
Fax: (312) 899-1259
www.aama-ntl.org/

Bioethics.com
http://bioethicsnews.com

Health Care Providers Service Organization
159 E. County Line Road
Hatboro, PA 19040-1218
Phone: (800) 982-9491
Fax: (800) 739-8818
www.hpso.com

Public Citizen
1600 20th St. NW
Washington, DC 20009
Phone: (202) 588-1000
www.citizen.org

Sorry Works
P.O. Box 531
Glen Carbon, IL 62034
Phone: (618) 559-8168
www.sorryworks.net/

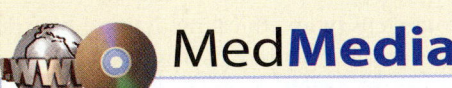

Med**Media**

http://www.MyMAKit.com

More on this chapter, including interactive resources, can be found on the Student CD-ROM accompanying this textbook and on http://www.MyMAKit.com.

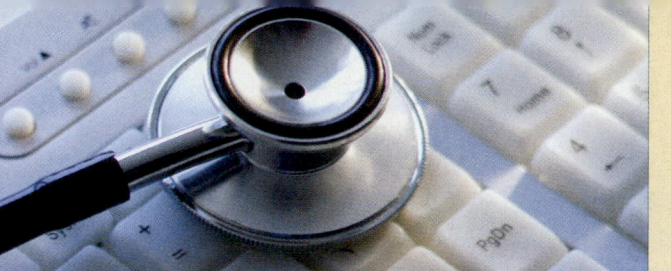

Objectives

After completing this chapter, you should be able to:

- Define and spell the key terminology in this chapter.
- Define the medical assistant's role in communicating with patients.
- Describe both verbal and nonverbal communication and how each can be used most effectively.
- List various listening skills.
- Identify how to communicate with patients in special circumstances.
- Explain how to communicate effectively with members of the healthcare team.
- Describe the developmental stages of the life cycle and Maslow's hierarchy of human needs.
- Discuss barriers to communication.

Interpersonal Communication Skills

Case Study

Katerina Bolshoy is a Russian patient who speaks broken English. The medical assistant, who does not speak Katerina's language, must schedule several appointments for Katerina, as well as explain insurance coverage to her.

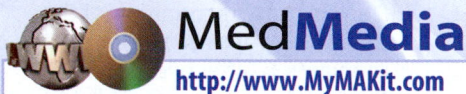

MedMedia
http://www.MyMAKit.com

Additional interactive resources and activities for this chapter can be found on http://www.MyMAKit.com. For a video, tips, audio glossary, legal and ethical scenarios, on-the-job scenarios, quizzes, and games related to the content of this chapter, please access the accompanying CD-ROM in this book.

Video: *Housekeeping 101; The Angry Patient; When English Is Not the Language*
Legal and Ethical Scenario: *Interpersonal Communication Skills*
On the Job Scenario: *Interpersonal Communication Skills*
Tips
Multiple Choice Quiz
Audio Glossary
HIPAA Quiz
Games: Spelling Bee, Crossword, and Strikeout

Key Terminology

anxiety—fear of the unknown; a feeling of fear or worry about the future

body language—set of nonverbal means of communication (e.g., facial expressions)

close-ended question—question that can be answered with "yes" or "no"

discriminating—acting against a person's interest due to a perceived difference in race, gender, economic, or other status

examples—illustrations of concepts or ideas

feedback—information that is reflected in an interpersonal exchange

hearing impaired—unable to hear or having a diminished sense of hearing

open-ended question—question that requires more than a "yes" or "no" answer

personal space—area around a person deemed the "comfort zone"

professional distance—professional relationship

reflecting—process of repeating information that is communicated

speech impaired—unable to speak or having a diminished ability to speak

stereotyping—process of shaping an opinion based solely on something like race, gender, or economic status

sympathy—pity

vocally impaired—unable to speak

Abbreviations

ASL—American Sign Language

✚ MEDICAL ASSISTING STANDARDS

CAAHEP ENTRY-LEVEL STANDARDS	ABHES ENTRY-LEVEL COMPETENCIES
■ Perform within scope of practice (psychomotor) ■ Apply ethical behaviors, including honesty/integrity in performance of medical assisting practice (affective) ■ Apply active listening skills (affective) ■ Identify styles and types of verbal communication (cognitive) ■ Identify nonverbal communication (cognitive) ■ Identify resources and adaptations that are required based on individual needs (cognitive) ■ Recognize the elements of oral communication using a sender-receiver processes (cognitive) ■ Recognize communication barriers (cognitive) ■ Identify techniques of overcoming communication barriers (cognitive) ■ Instruct patients according to their needs to promote health maintenance and disease prevention (psychomotor) ■ Demonstrate empathy in communicating with patients, family and staff (affective) ■ Use appropriate body language and other nonverbal skills in communicating with patients, family and staff (psychomotor) ■ Use reflection, restatement and clarification techniques to obtain a patient history (psychomotor) ■ Report relevant information to others succinctly and accurately (psychomotor) ■ Develop and maintain a current list of community resources related to patients' healthcare needs (psychomotor) ■ Demonstrate recognition of the patient's level of understanding in communication (affective) ■ Demonstrate respect for individual diversity, incorporating awareness of one's own biases in areas including gender, race, religion, age, and economic status (affective) ■ Differentiate between adaptive and non-adaptive coping mechanisms (cognitive) ■ Analyze communications in providing appropriate responses/feedback (affective) ■ Demonstrate awareness of the territorial boundaries of the person with whom communicating (affective) ■ Use language/verbal skills that enable patients' understanding (affective) ■ Demonstrate respect for diversity in approaching patients and families (affective)	■ Adapt to change ■ Maintain confidentiality at all times ■ Project a positive attitude ■ Be cognizant of ethical boundaries ■ Evidence a responsible attitude ■ Conduct work within scope of education, training, and ability ■ Adaptation for individualized needs ■ Instruct patients with special needs ■ Teach patients methods of health promotion and disease prevention ■ Locate resources and information for patients and employers ■ Instruct patients with special needs ■ Professional components ■ Monitor legislation related to current healthcare issues and practices ■ Orient patients to office policies and procedures ■ Adapt what is said to the recipient's level of comprehension ■ Use proper telephone techniques ■ Follow established policy in initiating or terminating medical treatment ■ Be courteous and diplomatic ■ Serve as a liaison between the physician and others ■ Exercise efficient time management ■ Receive, organize, prioritize, and transmit information expediently

✔ COMPETENCY SKILLS PERFORMANCE

1. Use effective listening skills in patient interviews.
2. Communicate with a hearing-impaired patient.
3. Communicate with a sight-impaired patient.
4. Communicate with patients via interpreters.
5. Prepare a patient's specialist referral.
6. Identify community resources.

Introduction

Communication is the process of sharing ideas between two or more people; it is sending and receiving messages verbally and nonverbally. Communication skills are vital for anyone working in healthcare, including the medical assistant. The medical assistant must share information accurately with patients, physicians, and coworkers and respond appropriately. The medical assistant must have a positive attitude and present information pleasantly.

The Medical Assistant's Role in Communication

How and why the medical assistant sends messages is important to the way in which they communicate to patients and staff in the medical office. Medical assistants will use more professional language, including medical terminology, than when conversing with friends. With patients, the medical assistant will use a warm, professional approach combined with empathy for the patient's situation.

Written office communication must also be professional. Charting is an essential form of communication in the medical office. Medical charts are legal documents that must be accurate and legible.

Verbal Communication

Communication takes different forms. Verbal communication uses spoken words. Professional medical assistants adopt polite tones of voice, avoid slang, and use proper grammar. Figure 5-1 ◆ outlines the Five Cs of better communication.

Communication must be geared to patients' ability to understand, which often means using basic terms rather than medical terminology. This applies even when patients are also healthcare professionals. Such patients may work in different fields and lack knowledge in the procedures they are undergoing.

Some patients may be embarrassed to admit a lack of understanding, and that can be dangerous. Patients who fail to understand may fail to follow medical directions. **Feedback,** which involves questioning patients to ensure comprehension, is the best way to avoid this situation. Medical assistants must

❑ **Content**—Address all areas of interest and fully answer all questions.

❑ **Conciseness**—Get to the point; say what needs to be said in as few words as possible.

❑ **Clarity**—Choose words that accurately and precisely convey meaning.

❑ **Coherence**—Create a logical, easy-to-follow train of thought.

❑ **Check**—Ask for feedback or clarification to ensure comprehension.

Figure 5-1 ◆ The five Cs of better communication.

ensure that patients understand what is being said. When communication barriers like language or disabilities limit patient comprehension, medical assistants must arrange for interpreters or family members to help facilitate the patient exchange.

Part of medical assisting is communicating carefully to ensure patients never feel demeaned. Sometimes, communication can be unintentionally offensive. Tone of voice, facial expression, and projection are all critical. Medical assistants who project the image that something is important inspire patients to do the same.

? — Critical Thinking Question 5-1 —

How can the medical assistant enhance communication with non-native English speakers like Katerina?

Nonverbal Communication

Some communication is verbal, while other communication is nonverbal. Nonverbal communication includes writing, using body language, and therapeutic touch. Nonverbal communication is sending a message without words. A smile and a touch are examples of nonverbal communication. Body language shows emotion and feeling. Learning to use and being able to read nonverbal communication are vital to working in a medical office. A patient's facial expressions, gestures, posture, and positioning provide clues to his or her mental state and health.

Personal Space

Personal space is the area immediately surrounding a person (Figures 5-2 ◆ through 5-5 ◆). It is a comfort zone. In U.S. culture, standing too close to someone sends a message of intrusiveness, while standing too far away sends a message of disinterest, rudeness, or lack of commitment to the conversation. Personal space varies with different cultures. In Arab countries, people converse at a distance that would be considered intimate in the United States, and backing away is considered an impolite gesture. As a medical assistant, it is important to be knowledgeable about personal space issues and respect patients' boundaries.

To understand the U.S. concept of personal space, ask yourself the following questions:

1. How do I feel when I am in a crowded elevator?
2. How would I feel at the library if I saw another student who had books and papers spread out on a table and all the other tables were in use?
3. How do I feel when a person whom I do not know enters my personal space?
4. How do I feel when a healthcare provider leans across me to reach for an item?

Often a person backs away when someone enters his or her personal space. This is an immediate cue for that person to stop or back away slightly. Some procedures will require the MA to be in a patient's personal space. Usually, the patient is aware of this, but make sure you ease the discomfort as much

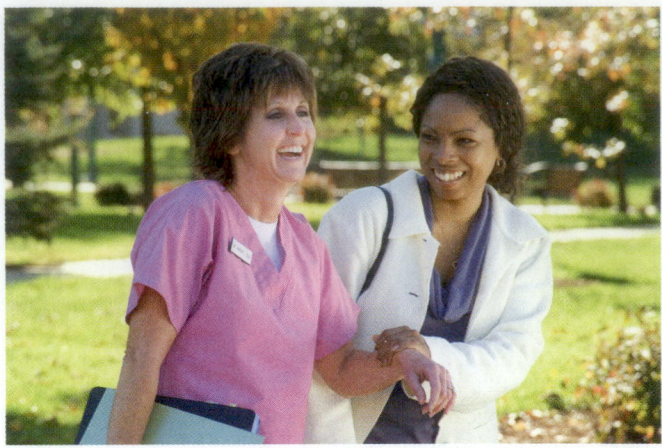

Figure 5-2 ◆ Intimate distance: shows affection, provides comfort and protection.

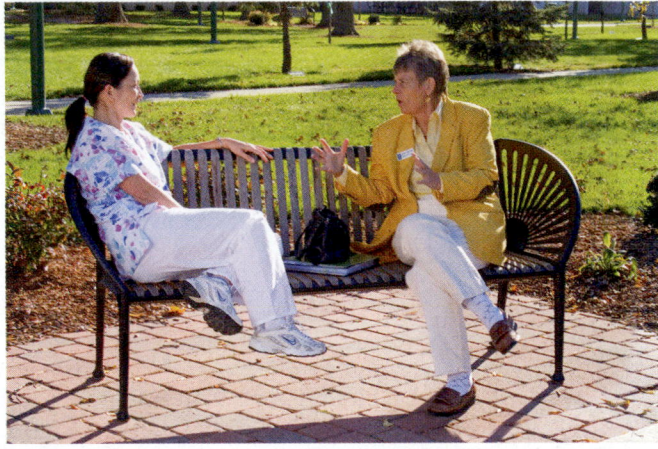

Figure 5-3 ◆ Personal distance: Most communication takes place at this distance.

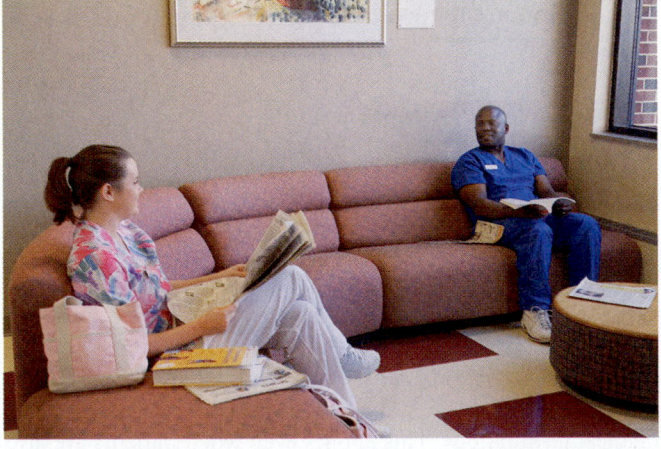

Figure 5-4 ◆ Social distance: less personal; used in social and business encounters.

as possible. Before invading the patient's personal space or touching the patient, say, "I need to take your pulse, so I am going to hold your wrist for approximately one minute. Is that

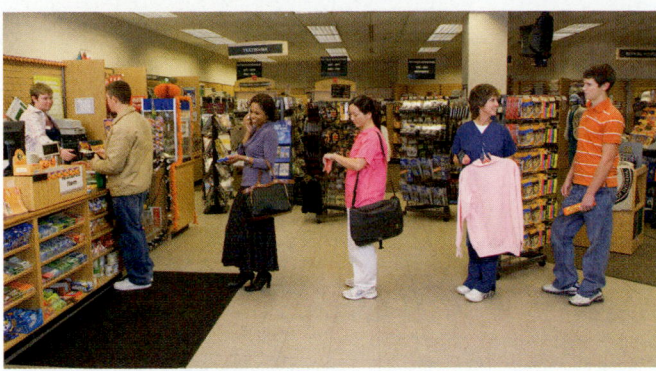

Figure 5-5 ◆ Public distance: least personal; observed in lectures, church, and impersonal social encounters.

OK?" It is important for the patient to give implied or verbal consent prior to any type of touching.

Writing as a Means of Communication

Written communication is one form of nonverbal communication that is crucial to both medical documentation and patient education. Medical assistants should use patients' charts both to capture patient information and to document that patients have understood the information given them.

In healthcare, patients typically receive written instructions after verbal instructions. Figure 5-6 ◆ provides a sample of written instructions. ∞ Chapter 8 goes into written communication in detail.

? — Critical Thinking Question 5-2 —
What is the value of written communication for patients like Katerina, who speak English as a second language? What characteristics would make that written communication most effective?

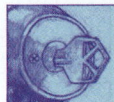

Keys to Success
PERSONAL SPACE MEASUREMENTS TYPICAL IN THE UNITED STATES

Intimate distance	0–18"	Shows affection, provides comfort and protection.
Personal distance	18"–4'	Most communication takes place at this distance.
Social distance	4'–12'	Less personal, used in social and business encounters.
Public distance	greater than 12'	Least personal, observed in lectures, church, and impersonal social encounters.

Keys to Success
ENGLISH AS A SECOND LANGUAGE

Remember that patients may not use English as their primary language. As a result, they may fail to understand phrases or slang common in English.

Symbolic Language

Symbolic language refers to an alternative way of communicating. Sign language is the most common form of symbolic language. Braille is the written form of language for people who are blind. It uses symbolic tactile (touch) images.

Sign Language

Sign language is used by a person who has total hearing loss or is unable to speak. Those who are unable to hear or who have a diminished sense of hearing are **hearing impaired,** sometimes called deaf; those who are unable to speak are called **vocally impaired.** The term *dumb* to denote inability to speak is less respectful. American Sign Language (**ASL**) is a complex language in its own right, with specific grammar rules and signs for words, using hand movements. Hand signs can also represent the letters of the alphabet, but communicating by spelling out words is considered "baby talk" and does not ensure informed consent (Figure 5-7 ◆). ASL is considered a formal communication method, where hand gestures, movements, and facial expressions enhance the meaning of signs.

When communicating with persons with hearing impairment, it is important to face them at all times, including when an interpreter is used. Many are able to read lips to some degree. Speak to the person in a normal tone of voice. Some patients can hear minimal sounds. It is also helpful to learn basic phrases in sign language, such as "please" or "thank you." Written communication can also be effective. Some patients are able to speak and be understood, while others make sounds that represent certain words. Listen carefully. Remember also the legal requirement to provide an interpreter.

Braille

Braille is a system of writing for the blind. Raised dots in certain patterns on paper represent letters of the alphabet. A blind person touches these dots with the fingertips to read words and numbers (Figure 5-8 ◆). (In ∞ Chapter 37, EENT, office procedures for blind patients are discussed.) Remember that it is not necessary to talk loudly to a person who is visually challenged; he or she is *not* hard of hearing.

Reading and Using Body Language

Research has shown that nonverbal communication sends primary messages more often than spoken words, and **body language** is an important part of nonverbal communication. Facial expressions, gestures, and eye movements can say more

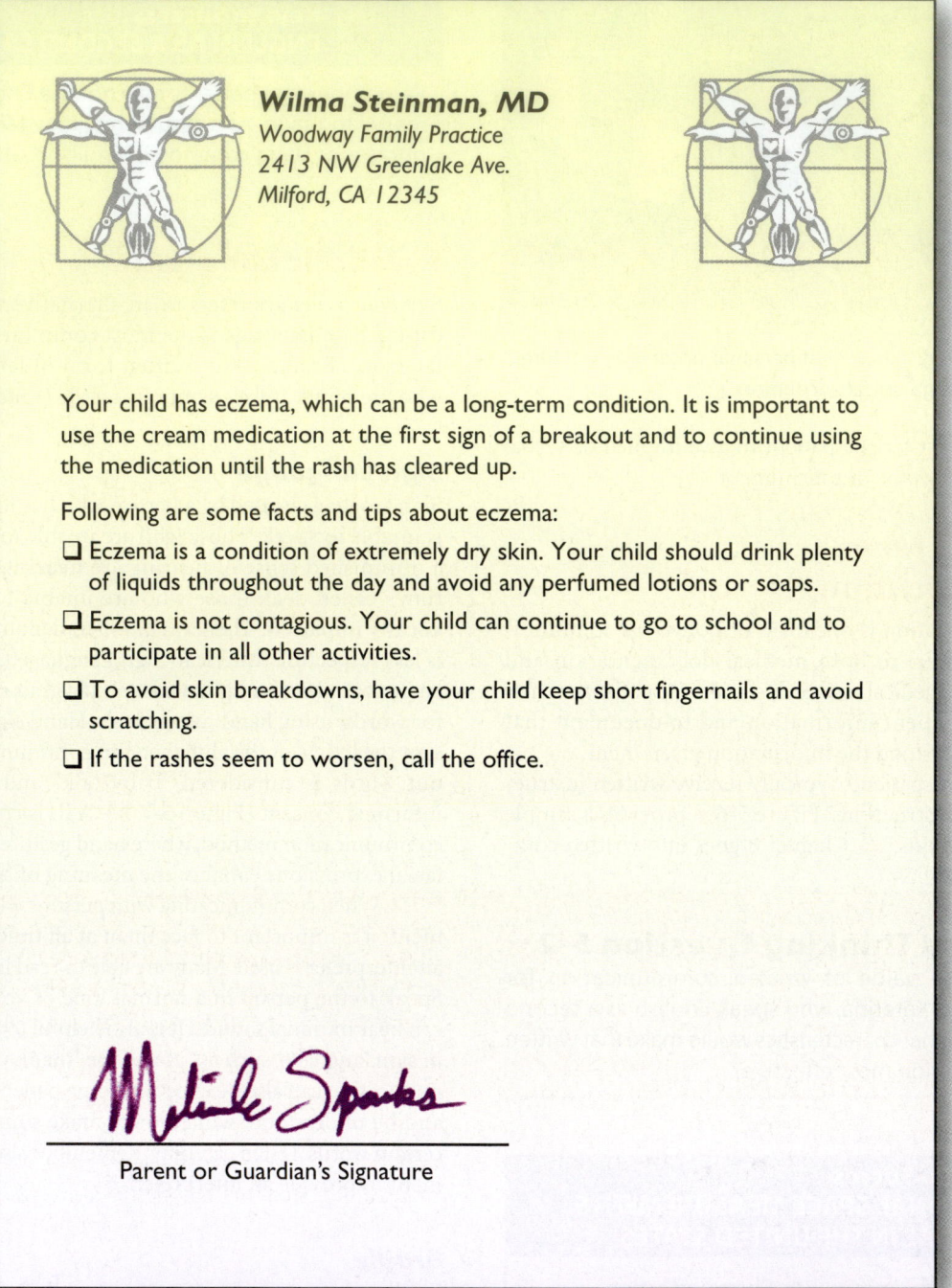

Wilma Steinman, MD
Woodway Family Practice
2413 NW Greenlake Ave.
Milford, CA 12345

Your child has eczema, which can be a long-term condition. It is important to use the cream medication at the first sign of a breakout and to continue using the medication until the rash has cleared up.

Following are some facts and tips about eczema:

❏ Eczema is a condition of extremely dry skin. Your child should drink plenty of liquids throughout the day and avoid any perfumed lotions or soaps.

❏ Eczema is not contagious. Your child can continue to go to school and to participate in all other activities.

❏ To avoid skin breakdowns, have your child keep short fingernails and avoid scratching.

❏ If the rashes seem to worsen, call the office.

_____
Parent or Guardian's Signature

Figure 5-6 ◆ Sample written instructions.

than words. For example, a shrug of the shoulders can be interpreted as a lack of interest.

Body language can help clarify verbal communication. A patient may, for example, claim to feel no pain but grimace when touched. The real message, then, is that the patient needs attention. Medical assistants should use nonverbal communication to ensure patient exchanges are effective and accurate. When patients say one thing but do another, medical assistants

should ask appropriate questions to ensure that patients provide accurate information.

Patients will read medical assistants' body language as well, so it is important for medical assistants to use neutral stances, even when patients are difficult. Medical assistants should always be professional and nonjudgmental, whatever the patient communication. Patients need to trust their medical assistants and should feel comfortable sharing personal information (Figure 5-9 ◆).

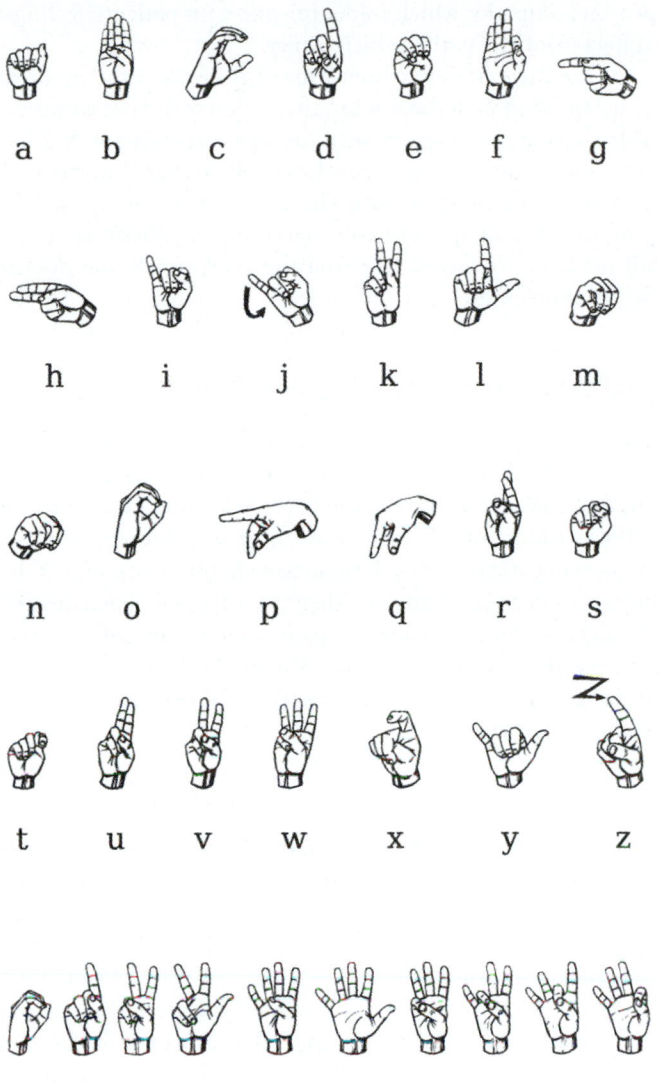

Figure 5-7 ◆ The American sign language alphabet.

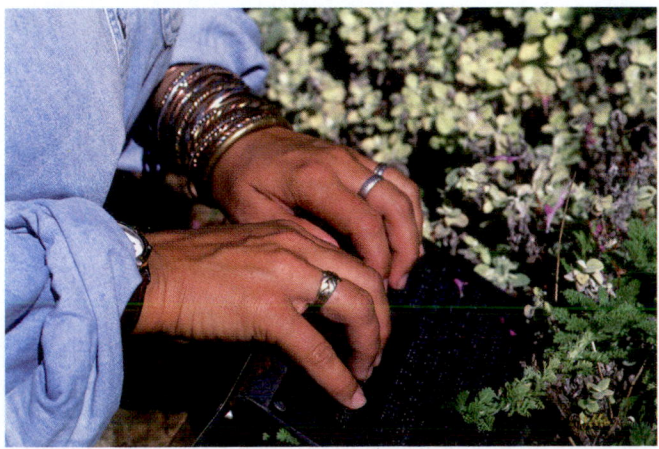

Figure 5-8 ◆ Braille is a system of writing for the blind.

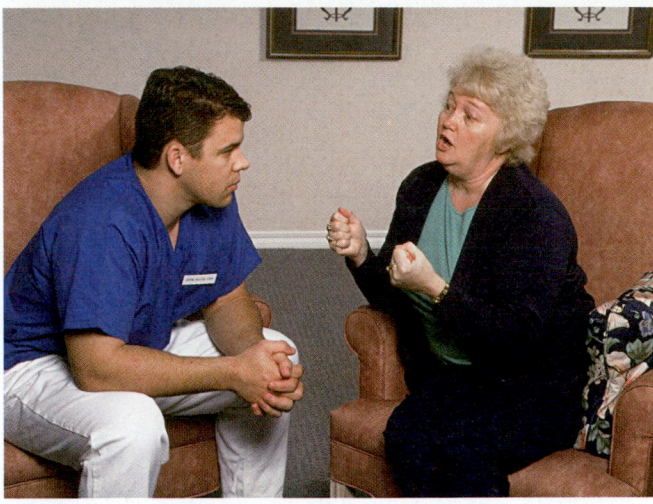

Figure 5-9 ◆ This patient's body language reflects her anger. The medical assistant must remain calm and show the patient with his body language that he is listening and he cares.

Eye Contact

Making eye contact shows you are listening to what the patient has to say or, as you are talking, if the patient understands what you are saying. The eyes express a range of emotions, including anger, love, and fear. Normal eye contact during conversation is not staring. Staring, a prolonged wide-eyed gaze, is a form of nonverbal communication. It can make a patient uncomfortable and can be interpreted as threatening.

Facial Expressions

Happiness, sadness, surprise, fear, anger, and disgust are basic facial expressions common to all cultures. Other, more subtle expressions are harder to read. For example, a raised eyebrow can mean that the patient is either questioning what you are saying or does not believe you.

Gestures

Gestures are movements that a person makes when he or she is talking. The hand may be used to indicate where the pain is located and if the pain is spreading to another area. Some people use gestures more than others, often to emphasize a point.

Posture

Posture involves body positioning and movement. A person who is listening carefully to what you are saying may lean toward you. Abruptly standing can indicate the conversation is over.

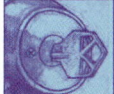
Keys to Success
BODY LANGUAGE AND CULTURE

Different cultures have different body-language norms. Some cultures consider direct eye contact a sign of disrespect, for example. As patient advocates, medical assistants must know the norms of their patients' cultures and observe those norms as signs of respect for patients' needs.

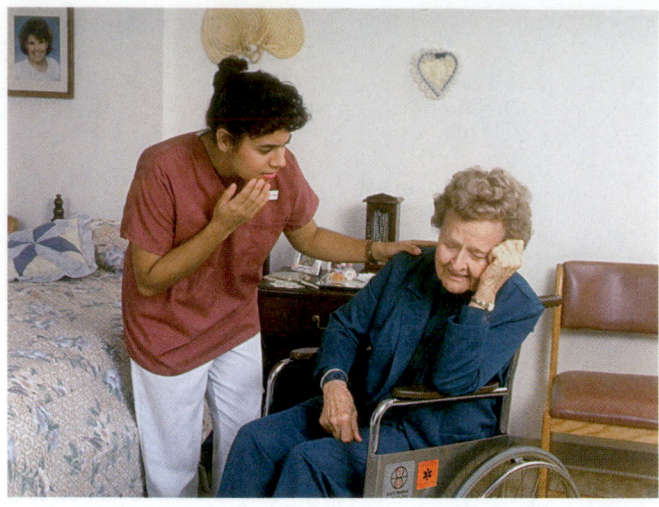

Figure 5-10 ◆ A medical assistant comforts a patient in distress.

Keep in mind that your body language is a reflection of how you are relating to others. A gentle nod of your head can be read as understanding. Keep it positive and open. Avoid folding your arms over your chest, as this is a closed position. It separates you from the patient. *Never* point a finger at anyone or gesture improperly. Even if someone is annoying, remain professional.

Therapeutic Touch

Nonverbal communication includes the use of touch. Touch can be very helpful to some patients. For example, touching a patient's arm during a time of sadness can relay a sense of kindness that most patients will appreciate. A patient in a good deal of emotional pain may appreciate a hand on the arm or shoulder (Figure 5-10 ◆).

Some patients prefer no touch. All people have a comfort zone called **personal space.** In general, personal space varies by culture. People from some cultures desire closeness, while others do not. Medical assistants can determine patients' personal spaces by observing how those patients react to differing levels of interaction. If, for example, the medical assistant reaches out to touch the patient's arm and the patient pulls away, the patient is likely uncomfortable and the medical assistant should withdraw the hand.

Demonstrating Active Listening

Medical assistants should always focus on patients' body language and spoken words. Active listening is the process of giving full attention during an exchange and minimizing interruptions. In the medical office, interruptions like telephone calls tell patients that they are less important than the callers.

Active listening is more listening than talking. This means the medical assistant should listen without interruption while the patient speaks, and then give the patient feedback so she feels understood. This is especially important when the patient is angry or upset. When medical assistants try to hurry conversations or fail to show empathy for patients, situations may

worsen. Empathy, which is identification for patients' feelings, differs from **sympathy,** which is pity.

Because patients spend more time with the medical assistant than with the doctor, they often feel more comfortable sharing information with the medical assistant. Studies have shown that patients grow less likely to share information as a person's authority rises. Therefore, the medical assistant should share any patient concerns with the physician, chart all medically relevant information, and notify the doctor when appropriate.

Interviewing the Patient

Medical assistants are often asked to obtain information from patients in the office. Medical assistants should always remain professional and organized and begin any patient conversation with introductions. With a working pen to document information in patient charts, the assistant should then conduct the interview in a private room. When the interview concludes, the medical assistant should let the patient know who will be entering the room next and when. When the medical assistant expects the physician or other provider to be delayed, the patient should be informed.

Employing Interviewing Techniques

Medical assistants may use different communication styles when interviewing patients. Some are more appropriate than others depending on the patient and the situation. **Open-ended questions** are appropriate when more than a "yes" or "no" response is needed. An example is, "Mrs. Dow, would you please describe your symptoms?" **Close-ended questions,** in contrast, can be answered with "yes" or "no." An example of this type of question is, "Mrs. Dow, have you had anything to eat or drink since midnight last night?"

Reflecting is another interviewing technique. This is the practice of repeating the patient's statement so the patient knows she has been understood. This technique allows the medical assistant to clarify parts of conversations. For example, a medical assistant might say, "Mrs. Dow, you said that for two weeks you have been having pain in your right shoulder and arm, and that the pain has been running down to your right hand. Is that right?"

Asking for **examples** is a technique that may help the medical assistant better understand the patient. In this case, a medical assistant may say, "With '1' being no pain, and '10' being extreme pain, can you tell me how you would rate the pain level you are having, Mrs. Dow?"

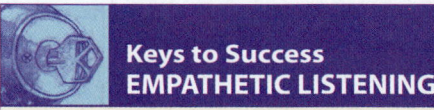

Keys to Success
EMPATHETIC LISTENING

Part of empathetic listening is making direct eye contact with the patient, nodding, and keeping an interested facial expression.

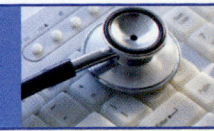

PROCEDURE 5-1 Use Effective Listening Skills in Patient Interviews

Theory and Rationale

Effective listening skills are vital for the medical assistant. By listening carefully to the patient and documenting appropriately, the medical assistant performs a valued function for the physician. Watching for the patient's nonverbal communication and paraphrasing the patient's statements verifies comprehension.

Materials
- Patient history form
- Pen

Competency

(**Conditions**) With the necessary materials, you will be able to (**Task**) use effective listening skills in interviewing the patient (**Standards**) correctly within the time limit set by the instructor.

1. Smile and introduce yourself to the patient.
2. Identify the patient by verifying the patient's birth date.
3. Verify that you have the correct patient chart.
4. Maintain a professional persona.
5. Maintain eye contact with the patient.
6. Ask the patient open-ended questions.
7. Do not interrupt the patient.
8. Paraphrase the patient's statements to verify comprehension.
9. Watch for the patient's nonverbal communication.
10. Summarize the patient's statements and conclude the interview.
11. Document appropriate information in the patient's file.

Allowing for periods of silence in conversations gives patients time to collect their thoughts or to think of answers. When patients fail to answer questions right away, the medical assistant should allow some time before asking more questions.

Another communication tool to use when speaking with patients is the indirect question. An indirect question is considered polite, especially when speaking with strangers. A sample direct question is, "Where is your son?" An indirect question is, "I was wondering if you know where your son is?" Figure 5-11 ◆ lists some common indirect phrases.

Critical Thinking Question 5-3

How does the reflecting conversation technique help ensure that medical assistants understand the concerns of patients like Katerina? What sort of questions would support this technique?

Identifying Factors That Hinder Communication

Various factors can impede communication. Culture is one, because messages can be perceived differently. Medical assis-

tants will encounter patients who think differently than they do, but assistants must treat all patients with dignity and respect. **Stereotyping** is prejudging patients based solely on gender, ethnic background, or other identifying factors. **Discriminating** is taking some sort of action against a person based solely on a stereotype. Whatever the medical assistant's personal feelings about a patient, he or she must always remain professional.

Communicating in Special Circumstances

Patients who are young, hearing impaired, sight impaired, mentally unable to understand, or sedated present special communication challenges. In all cases, medical assistants must always include the patients and their interpreters or guardians in conversations. Patients should always feel part of the process.

Communicating with Physically Challenged Patients

Patients experiencing physical challenges usually require assistance with activities. It is best to ask the patient for direction before assisting. For example, a wheelchair is helpful when movement to another area of the office is required. Ask the patient if

---

> Do you know . . . ?
>
> I was wondering. . . .
>
> Can you tell me . . . ?
>
> Do you happen to know . . . ?
>
> I'd like to know. . . .
>
> Have you any idea . . . ?

Figure 5-11 ◆ Common phrases used for asking indirect questions.

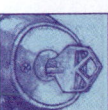

Keys to Success
SEEING-EYE DOGS

To ensure patient safety and honor the Americans with Disabilities Act (ADA), patients with service animals like seeing-eye dogs must be allowed to keep the animals with them at all times. These animals are working; however, so medical assistants should not pet or play with them unless invited to do so by the patient.

he or she would like a wheelchair. If the patient agrees, proceed. If the patient declines, take your time walking the patient to the area. (Refer to ∞ Chapter 43, Orthopedics and Physical Therapy, for additional information on patients with physical challenges.)

Communicating with Hearing-Impaired Patients

Communicating with **hearing-impaired** patients presents some special challenges. Many hearing-impaired people can read lips. When this is the case, medical assistants must speak slowly, facing the patient in a well-lighted room. The medical assistant can touch patients' arms to get their attention, and then begin the conversation (Figure 5-12 ◆).

When hearing-impaired patients have an interpreter, the conversation is still with the patient, not the interpreter. Medical assistants should face their patients and speak with them directly.

Communicating with Sight-Impaired Patients

Patients with sight impairments present communication challenges as well as raise special considerations about medical facilities. Medical assistants must escort patients who cannot see well to treatment rooms or the restroom, being careful to alert the patients to any steps, ramps, or slopes. Once in the treatment room, the medical assistant should place the patient's hand on the chair or table where the patient should sit (Figure 5-13 ◆). The medical assistant should then familiarize the patient with the room's layout and important features, such as the sink and door.

Sight-impaired patients often bring service animals to the medical office. These animals must stay with the patients throughout the visit, including when the patients use the restroom or visit the lab or radiology facilities.

Communicating with Patients with Speech Impairments

For the medical assistant, patients with **speech impairments** may be difficult to understand. When communication is difficult, the medical assistant should ask patients to repeat themselves. If medical assistants cannot understand patients

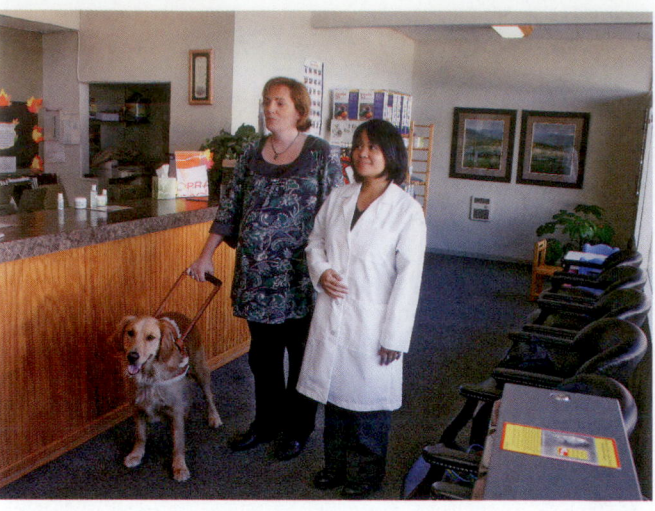

Figure 5-13 ◆ The medical assistant will need to assist the sight-impaired patient while in the office.

upon repetition, those medical assistants should ask the patients to write down what they are saying. At no time should the medical assistant act frustrated or hurried. Part of patient advocacy is being certain to correctly relate patient information to the physician.

Communicating with Patients via Interpreters

Patients who cannot communicate due to language barriers should be accompanied to the medical office by interpreters (Figure 5-14 ◆). The office may arrange interpreters, or the patient may bring a friend or family member to serve the role. The most important issues are that patients can understand the information being communicated to them and that healthcare professionals clearly understand what the patients are communicating. In communities with a high proportion of patients who speak languages other than English, the medical office will likely seek medical professionals who speak the

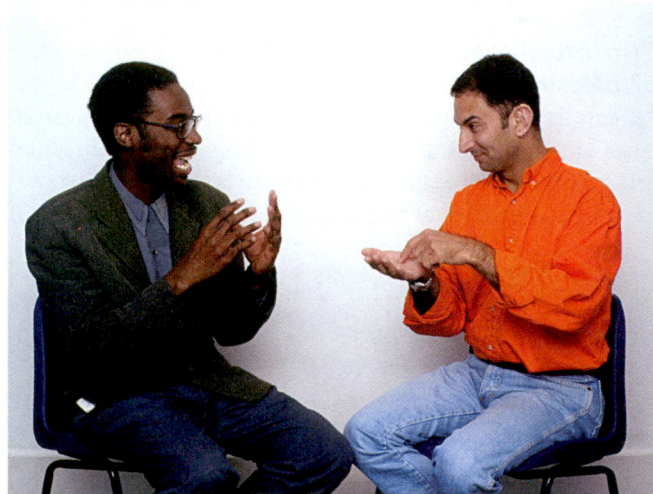

Figure 5-12 ◆ Hearing-impaired patients will often bring an interpreter.

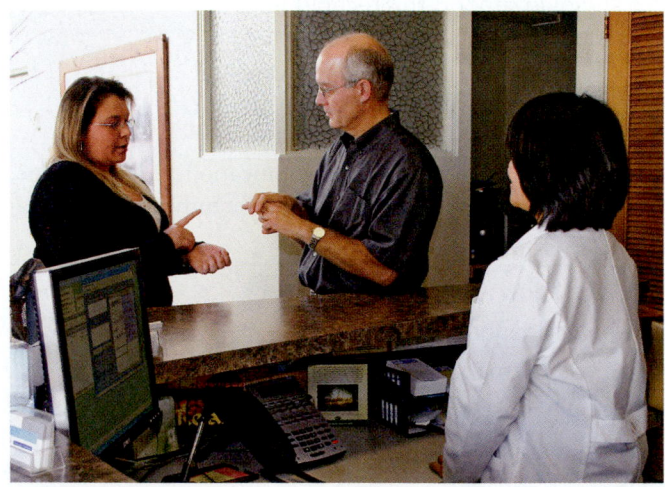

Figure 5-14 ◆ Interpreters should accompany those patients who cannot communicate due to language barriers.

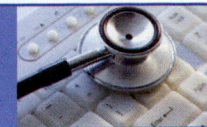

PROCEDURE 5-2   Communicate with a Hearing-Impaired Patient

Theory and Rationale

Communicating with hearing-impaired patients is a skill needed in any medical facility. Knowing how to get the patient's attention and how to communicate professionally and accurately is an important skill to master.

Materials

- Patient's file
- Blue or black pen

Competency

(**Conditions**) With the necessary materials, you will be able to (**Task**) communicate with a hearing-impaired patient (**Standards**) correctly within the time limit set by the instructor.

1. Alert the patient that you are ready to take him to the examination room by entering the reception area, touching the patient's arm to get his attention, and motioning to follow.
2. If the patient has an interpreter, also have the interpreter enter the examination room.
3. When speaking, look directly at the patient and speak slowly.
4. When the patient can read lips, verify understanding through patient questioning. When comprehension is lacking, write instructions for the patient.
5. When asking a patient to change into a gown, ask the patient to flip a switch or crack the door open when ready. People with hearing impairments cannot hear a knock to announce the physician's arrival.
6. At the end of the patient's visit, chart all communications, including verification of the patient's understanding.

community's prevalent language, in which case interpreters may be unneeded. The names and contact information of interpreters who accompany patients should be clearly noted in the patients' files so the interpreters can be contacted for comment or clarification.

Communicating with Culturally Diverse Patients

It is not possible for a medical office to hire a multilingual staff to communicate with patients from all ethnic and cultural backgrounds. But the medical assistant should try to

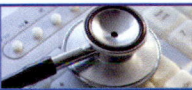

PROCEDURE 5-3   Communicate with a Sight-Impaired Patient

Theory and Rationale

Communicating with sight-impaired patients is a skill needed in any medical facility. The medical assistant may be called on to gather information from sight-impaired patients to facilitate paperwork completion in the office.

Materials

- Patient's file
- Blue or black pen

Competency

(**Conditions**) With the necessary materials, you will be able to (**Task**) communicate with a sight-impaired patient (**Standards**) correctly within the time limit set by the instructor.

1. Alert the patient that you are ready to visit the examination room by entering the reception area, touching the patient's arm, and offering your arm for the patient to hold.

2. Ensure any service animal accompanies the patient to the examination room.
3. Alert the patient to any steps, doorways, ramps, or slopes along the way.
4. Take the patient to a private area, outside of other patients' views or hearing ranges.
5. Place the patient's hand on the chair or table where sitting is desired.
6. Arrange for any service animal to sit directly next to the patient.
7. Ask the patient the questions on the history form, and write down the answers. Ensure the patient's responses are clearly understood.
8. At the end of the patient's visit, chart all communications, including how the patient's understanding was verified.
9. Sign and date the patient history form and note that the history form was completed for the patient due to sight impairment.

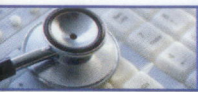

PROCEDURE 5-4 Communicate with a Patient via Interpreter

Theory and Rationale

Communicating with a patient via an interpreter is something the medical assistant may need to do both over the telephone when scheduling an appointment and when the patient arrives in the office for a visit. It is imperative that patients understand the information being communicated to them and that healthcare professionals understand what patients are communicating.

Materials

- Patient's file
- Pen

Competency

(**Conditions**) With the necessary materials, you will be able to (**Task**) communicate with a patient via an interpreter

(**Standards**) correctly within the time limit set by the instructor.

1. When the patient arrives in the office with an interpreter, obtain the name of the interpreter and verify the spelling.
2. Obtain the interpreter's contact information for the patient's medical record. If the interpreter has a business card, attach it to the patient's file.
3. Communicate with the patient directly; do not speak directly to the interpreter.
4. When any of the interpreter's comments are unclear, ask for clarification.
5. Document all essential parts of the interview in the patient's chart.

---

identify and be familiar with patients' backgrounds. Showing respect for different customs is essential. When working with a patient who speaks English as a second language; the MA must be patient and try to understand to the best of his ability and ask for assistance when necessary. Again, remember that providing an interpreter when necessary is a legal requirement.

Communicating with Mentally Ill Patients

Most patients who are mentally incompetent visit the medical office with their legal guardians. The medical assistant should speak with such patients first and then their guardians. Some patients have a mental illness and are mentally incompetent to speak for themselves. In these situations, the medical assistant must be certain the patient understands any instructions. Some effective techniques are to repeat patients' statements, ask patients to repeat what they have been told, or demonstrate the skills the patients have been shown.

Communicating with Angry or Distressed Patients

To avoid angering or distressing patients, the medical assistant should try to avoid the emotions' triggers. For example, the medical assistant can help avoid anger over a bill by reviewing the bill with the patient. The medical assistant should always explain things up front and give the patient written information on any relevant office policies.

When patients become angry or distressed, the medical assistant must always remain calm and professional (Figure 5-15 ◆). Typically, the best response to an angry patient is, "I'm sorry you're upset. Let's see if we can work this out." Most patients calm when the medical assistant responds calmly and demonstrates a sincere desire to help.

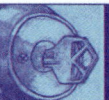

Keys to Success
THE INFLUENCE OF CULTURE AND AGE

The following are examples of different approaches to the same situation—a patient has just been diagnosed with insulin-dependent diabetes.

- You are teaching a seven-year-old boy how to give himself insulin injections. It is natural for the child to be worried. He may not listen well or remember instructions. One way to handle the situation is to find out more about the child's home situation, then instruct one or both parents in giving the insulin injection along with the child. The child will feel more secure when his parents are involved. It also satisfies the child's emotional needs, paving the way for easier learning. A parent or responsible caretaker should be present in the room during the teaching experience.

- A woman with a hearing impairment who is on Medicare and social security thinks she is going to die because she has no money for insulin and syringes. Explain that you will help her contact the appropriate agencies to help pay for the medications. Stress that she should contact you if she needs any other help. By relieving her concerns about money, you now have a patient ready to learn.

- A Chicano man learns he will have to take insulin for the rest of his life. He tells you, "I might as well die!" After talking with the man, you learn he is afraid he will no longer be able to work. Assure him that working should not be a problem. Tell him that learning how to take care of himself will help him continue taking care of his family.

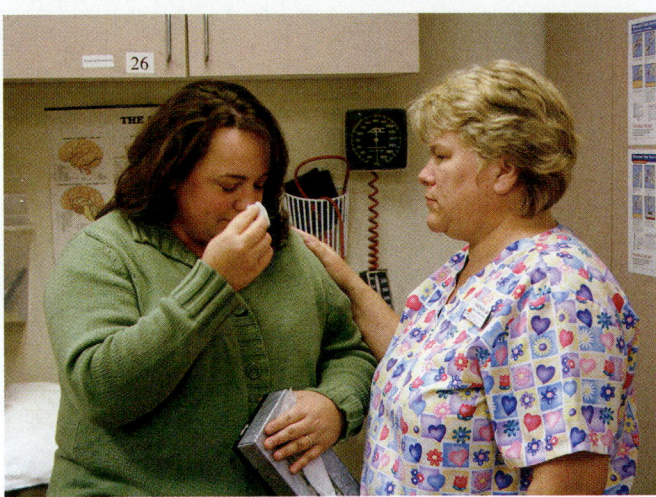

Figure 5-15 ◆ With an emotional patient, the medical assistant must remain calm.

Communicating with Emotionally Challenged Patients

A patient with emotional challenges may either acknowledge or deny those challenges. The medical assistant may be able to detect an emotional problem by observing actions and behavior. While anxiety is common in patients experiencing pain or waiting for the results of diagnostic tests, anger is not generally a normal response. Being kind and understanding will help ease a patient's anxiety or anger. In particular, medical assistants should speak in quiet, even tones. (Refer to ∞ Chapter 47, Mental Health, for a more thorough discussion of patients with emotional challenges.)

Communicating with Young Patients

When communicating with young patients, it is important that the medical assistant use words and questions the patients will understand. When the patients cannot articulate their feelings, the medical assistant can have them draw pictures. When talking to a young patient, the medical assistant should sit down in order to be at eye level with the patient. Before beginning any procedure on a young patient, even a simple one, the medical assistant should explain the procedure and show the equipment that will be used (Figure 5-16 ◆).

Young patients may at times be subjected to undesirable procedures. Vaccinations and blood draws, for example, may be uncomfortable and may require the patient to remain still for a few moments. For these types of procedures, parents may be helpful in or out of the room. Medical assistants should use their best judgment about parent presence and reassure the patient as much as possible. When the procedure concludes, the medical assistant should always praise the patient for being brave or "grown up." To help the patients view the medical office in a positive light, the office may reward young patients with a small prize, like a sticker.

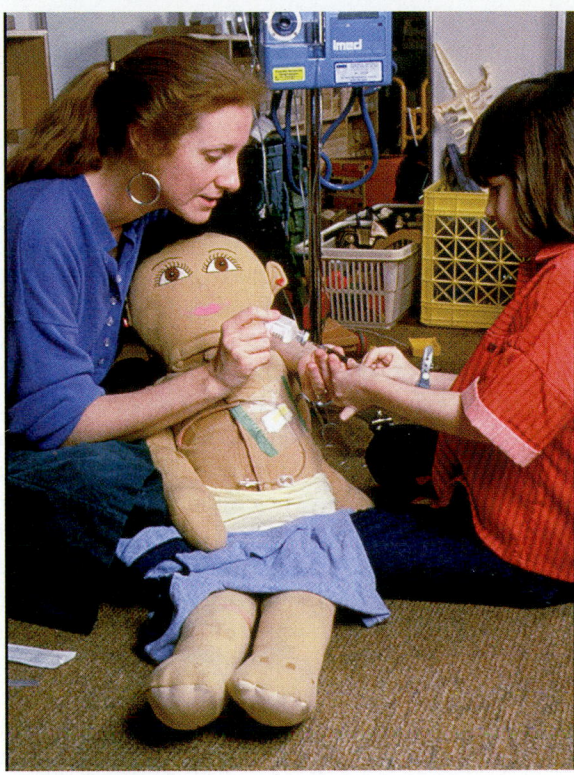

Figure 5-16 ◆ Often children will be more relaxed if the medical assistant demonstrates the procedure on a doll first.

Communicating with Geriatric Patients

In many geriatric patients, sight, hearing, and mobility may be compromised. Mental capacity may be diminished. Assisting with insurance forms, explaining how to take medications, providing information on outside agencies for assistance, and encouraging proper diet and social activities are some of the ways the medical assistant can help a geriatric patient. (Refer to ∞ Chapter 49, Geriatrics, for additional information on the elderly.)

Communicating with Grieving Patients

Communicating with grieving patients can be uniquely challenging. First, medical assistants must remember that the patients may be grieving for unique reasons: the loss of a loved one, a job, or a relationship. Patients may also grieve the diagnoses of chronic or terminal illnesses. Second, medical assistants must remember that people feel grief in individual ways.

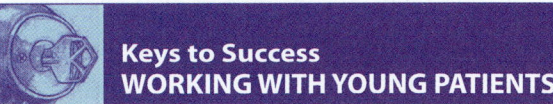

Keys to Success
WORKING WITH YOUNG PATIENTS

Treat young patients with respect. Do not lie to them. Misinformation about pain, for example, can instill long-standing distrust in healthcare professionals. Be honest and demonstrate on stuffed animals or dolls first so the patients can understand the plan and prepare.

Therefore, medical assistants should never belittle someone for feeling grief. Every person is entitled to grieve and for whatever reason. People feel what they feel. Medical assistants are not entitled to judge why.

Dr. Elisabeth Kübler-Ross was a pioneer in the field of working with dying or grieving patients. She advocated hospice care and wrote several books about the dying process. Kübler-Ross developed a list of the five stages of grief, noting that not every person experiences the stages in the same way, in the same order, or for the same period (Table 5-1).

It is important to remember that there is no "right" way to grieve. Medical assistants should listen to grieving patients and allow those patients time to express themselves. As appropriate, medical assistants should touch patients reassuringly on the arm or shoulder. Because there is no right thing to say, medical assistants should focus on offering support and empathy. Medical assistants can also offer information as needed. With physicians' permission, medical assistants can refer patients to a number of community and national resources that are available through hospice or other support groups (Table 5-2).

Maintaining Professional Patient Communication

The most effective medical assistants form positive relationships with their patients through mutual respect and professionalism. Medical assistants must be role models and earn their

TABLE 5-2 NATIONAL RESOURCES

Organization	Focus Area(s)
American Cancer Society www.cancer.org	Patients, families, friends and survivors of cancer
American Diabetes Association www.diabetes.org	Diabetes and related nutrition and recipes, prevention, and research
American Lung Association www.lungusa.org	Hayfever, asthma, lung cancer, and other respiratory illnesses
National Domestic Violence Hotline www.ndvh.org	Domestic violence, including a toll-free number to call 24 hours per day, 365 days per year
International Child Abuse Network www.yesican.org	Twenty-four-hour chat groups on child abuse, incest, and parenting; Web site is in English and Spanish
American Heart Association www.americanheart.org	Heart attack/stroke warning signs, high blood pressure, and healthy lifestyles; Web site is in English and Spanish
Centers for Disease Control HIV/AIDS www.cdc.gov/hiv/	Information on HIV/AIDS transmission, current research, and Internet links to testing centers or support groups

TABLE 5-1 KÜBLER-ROSS'S FIVE STAGES OF GRIEF

Stage	Description
Denial	Patients refuse to believe what is happening or has happened to them. This stage lasts until the patients accept the deaths or diagnoses.
Anger	Patients become angry, perhaps with the people who have died or the physicians who have given them the diagnoses. Patients may also become angry with God.
Bargaining	Patients try to make promises in return for the people who have died or new, nonterminal diagnoses (e.g., "I'll spend 20 hours a week doing volunteer work if God will bring back George").
Depression	Deep sadness over the loss sets in. Patients should seek help via counseling and/or medications, if needed.
Acceptance	Patients accept the deaths or diagnoses and begin to move on.

Reprinted with permission of Scribner, an imprint of Simon & Schuster Adult Publishing Group, from On Death and Dying *by Dr. Elisabeth Kübler-Ross. Copyright © 1969 by Elisabeth Kübler-Ross; copyright renewed © 1997 by Elisabeth Kübler-Ross. All rights reserved.*

patients' trust and admiration. In short, medical assistants are professionals and must always act like ones. Medical assistants' bad days should always be hidden from patients, and any personal problems or coworker difficulties should be continually concealed.

Medical assistants must speak respectfully and appropriately to patients, as well as to anyone within the patients' ranges of hearing. In addition, medical assistants should always use proper forms of address when speaking with patients. Elderly patients, for example, may prefer to be called either "Mrs. Thompson" or "Margaret."

To ensure patient respect, medical assistants should not assume they can shorten anyone's name; it is rude to shorten a person's name without permission. It is acceptable with permission, however. Take a patient named Richard, for example. The medical assistant should ask the patient if he would like to be called Richard. If he indicates he prefers to be called Rick, then the medical assistant should make a note in his chart so that all members of the healthcare team can address him properly.

The medical assistant should never use pet names for patients, like "Honey" or "Sweetie." It could offend some patients. The medical assistant should also avoid referring to patients as their conditions, such as "Back pain is in Room 2." In the same vein, the medical assistant should maintain patient confidentiality by only calling out full patient names outside the hearing of other patients.

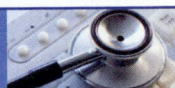

PROCEDURE 5-5 Identify Community Resources

Theory and Rationale

Medical assistants will frequently be asked to give patients referrals to community resources at the physician's request. Having this information in an easy and quick-to-locate format is one way to provide patients with excellent care.

Materials

- A computer with Internet access
- Written pamphlets and brochures
- Telephone directories

Competency

(**Conditions**) With the necessary materials, you will be able to (**Task**) identify community resources (**Standards**) correctly within the time limit set by the instructor.

1. Locate the name, address, telephone number, and Web site address for each of the following need categories in your community:
   a. Homeless services
   b. HIV/AIDS resources
   c. Disability services
   d. Domestic violence services
   e. Public assistance
   f. Housing authority/services
   g. Ombudsman services
   h. Foster care for children
   i. Foster care for adults
   j. Senior services
   k. Legal aid
   l. Rape victim services
   m. Crime victim services
   n. Culturally specific services (Native American, military, etc.)
   o. Medical assistant services (Medicaid, etc.)
2. Identify at least one to three resources for each need category.
3. Create a written document to give to patients.

HIPAA Compliance

To be Health Insurance Portability and Accountability Act (HIPAA)–compliant, the medical assistant should not call patients by their full names in the reception area. Instead, the assistant should use first or last name only. When two patients have the same first name, the last name is appropriate. For example, instead of "Jim," the medical assistant should call out "Mr. Costas."

Keeping a Professional Distance

It is important, both for the patient and the medical assistant, to keep a **professional distance,** but doing so can be difficult. Most healthcare professionals chose the field because they care about people and find it hard to remain detached when patients are hurting, dying, or in need. Medical assistants could become

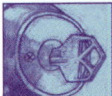

**Keys to Success
PROFESSIONAL COMMUNICATION WITH PATIENTS**

Medical assistants should conceal all personal stress from patients; voice and body language should mask any negative feelings. When medical assistants cannot keep their patient interactions free of personal stresses, they should consider asking their employer to find a temporary replacement.

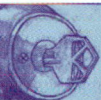

**Keys to Success
COMMUNITY RESOURCES**

Do not offer to drive patients to the store or to pay for prescriptions. Medical assistants serve patients best by finding them the appropriate community resources and making referrals with the doctor's permission.

very stressed if they became attached to every patient, and some patients may take advantage of medical assistants who are willing to go above and beyond the call of duty. Medical assistants need not abandon their concern for patients. They simply must keep a professional distance to maintain a professional image.

In addition to maintaining a professional distance, medical assistants must be very careful to avoid revealing personal details about themselves or the physician. It is acceptable for medical assistants to reveal an engagement when a patient notices an engagement ring, but the assistants should not tell the patient where they live or discuss personal relationships. Such details have no place in the patient–healthcare professional relationship.

Communicating with Coworkers

The medical assistant must maintain professional communication with coworkers and the doctors at all times while in the office. The medical assistant should minimize any nonwork conversations, remembering that patients may overhear them.

Just as in any work setting, the medical assistant may dislike some coworkers. Personal feelings aside, all members of the healthcare team should treat each other professionally and respectfully. Should medical assistants ever need to speak to a supervisor about coworkers, they should do so in a private setting. They should be professional, stating only facts, not opinions.

When communicating with the doctor in front of patients, the medical assistant must always address the doctor as "Dr." Even when the doctor is relaxed and informal, patients must have a level of respect for the doctor as an authority, and that image starts with the behavior of the other members of the healthcare team. Similarly, patients should never suspect that medical assistants are irritated with the physician.

All members of the healthcare team should be careful to use correct medical terminology and no slang when speaking with physicians and coworkers. The medical assistant should speak slowly, confidently, and always honestly. Jokes and non-work conversation have no place in the medical office when patients are present.

In Practice

Mark Minton, medical assistant, is completing paperwork in the reception area. Two of his coworkers, who are standing behind him at the front desk, begin a conversation about last night's episode of their favorite television show. Their conversation is loud enough to be heard in the reception area. What should Mark do?

Communicating with Other Facilities

Patient confidentiality is the most important factor when communicating with other facilities. When medical assistants schedule patients in another facility, they should give those facilities only the information they need to schedule the patients. This usually includes patient name and contact information, reason for referral, referring physician, and patient's insurance carrier. Any other information about the patient should come from the patient.

When making appointments for patients with other facilities, medical assistants must be out of hearing range of all other patients in the office. The assistants should have a telephone location for these types of calls, one that is not in the clinic hallway or at the front desk. Calling from the treatment room where the patient is waiting or from a private area is best.

Developmental Stages of the Life Cycle and Their Impact on Communication

Human development is a lifelong process. The individual faces certain tasks during each stage, builds on previous growth when entering each new stage, and gradually progresses to a higher

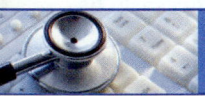

PROCEDURE 5-6 Prepare a Patient's Specialist Referral

Theory and Rationale
Medical assistants are often required to schedule patients to see specialists. This procedure must always be done in a private place and preferably with the patient present. Knowing the steps in this procedure, and how to communicate the necessary information to the patient, is part of being a patient's advocate in the medical office.

Materials
- Telephone
- Blue or black ink pen
- Patient's file
- Referral form to a specialist

Competency
(**Conditions**) With the necessary materials, you will be able to (**Task**) prepare a referral for a patient to see a specialist (**Standards**) correctly within the time limit set by the instructor.

1. Verify the patient file is correct.
2. Verify the referral form for the specialist is correct.

3. Verify the doctor's instructions (e.g., What does the doctor want the patient to be seen for? How soon does the patient need to be seen?).
4. Choose a private location, out of the hearing range of other patients.
5. If the pending referral is not an emergency and the patient is in the clinic, ask the patient for a convenient time or day to see the specialist.
6. Call the specialist's office and ask to speak to the person who handles the schedule.
7. Provide personal identification and the name of the referring doctor or clinic.
8. State the reason for the call.
9. Give patient information as requested by the specialist's office.
10. Set an appointment date and time. If the patient is in the clinic, verify the date and time.
11. Document the appointment's date and time on the referral form. If the patient is in the clinic, give the patient the referral form. Choose to mail the referral form when there is time before the appointment.
12. Document the call's results in the patient's chart.

level of development. The physical and emotional stages of the life cycle are often presented in psychology courses; understanding these stages helps in communication with all patients, regardless of age.

The stages of development are a complex subject that is presented more in depth during psychology courses. Depending on what theorist you subscribe to, you may believe that individuals will pass through life stages one at a time in chronological order without ever returning to the previous stage, they may skip stages and successfully navigate others in a random order, or they may pass unilaterally through stages and remain in one or more at any given time. It is important to understand that there is no "appropriate" method of development with people, because they will develop at an individual pace according to their own needs and environment.

An individual's ability to communicate and to interpret messages is greatly affected by his or her developmental stage. Jean Piaget, a Swiss philosopher and developmental theorist known for his theory of cognitive development as well as for his work studying children, conceived of physical and emotional stages of the life cycle (see Table 5-3). It is important to communicate with each person at his or her developmental level. As an example, an older female patient of 70-plus years might be beginning to prepare for the loss of her mate or for her own death. She may not hear or understand communication about medications, activity, or treatment because she is preoccupied with other concerns. A common mistake made by people who work with the elderly is to speak in babylike, patronizing tones. The usual response is one of annoyance or feeling insulted, and the elderly person may simply stop listening.

TABLE 5-3 APPROXIMATE PHYSICAL AND EMOTIONAL STAGES OF THE LIFE CYCLE, ACCORDING TO JEAN PIAGET

6 weeks	The baby begins to smile and develop facial expressions.
10 weeks	The baby begins to roll from prone to a supine position.
4 to 6 months	The baby raises its head and shoulders while lying in supine position.
6 to 8 months	The baby sits without support. Eye color may change.
8 to 12 months	The baby learns to crawl, stand, take steps, feed him- or herself, and develop autonomy.
1 year	The baby understands commands and simple conversation.
18 months	The toddler walks alone, feeds self, stacks objects, and is becoming more independent.
20 to 24 months	The toddler begins to learn bowel and bladder control and explores the environment.
3 to 4 years	The child talks in complete sentences.
4 to 5 years	The child dresses and undresses him- or herself.
5 to 6 years	The child's eye and body coordination improves. The child can skip and draw figures.
6 to 8 years	The child enters school, and physical skills improve.
8 to 13 years	The adolescent's rate of physical growth increases and adult sexual characteristics develop.
13 to 18 years	The teenager undergoes puberty and strives for independence.
18 to 20 years	The young adult becomes more independent, may continue his or her education, and/or may marry and have children.
20 to 30 years	The adult attempts to build a firm, safe foundation for the future. There may be a continuation of the educational process, marriage, and children.
30 to 40 years	The adult experiences more freedom, continuing to work and raise children.
40 to 50 years	The adult evaluates the first part of his or her life and continues working. The children may begin leaving the nest.
50 to 60 years	The adult experiences a sense of comfort, acceptance of life. Children continue leaving the home. The individual experiences freedom and success.
60 to 70 years	The adult looks forward to or begins retirement. Losing the mate and living alone become real possibilities. Less home committments mean greater sense of freedom to explore, travel, start a new hobby. Their rich fullfillment of life offers a great education they can pass on to younger generations.
70 plus years	The adult faces the facts of aging, may lose the mate and friends to illness and death, and begins to prepare for his or her own death. Less financial burdens bring the ability to fulfill wants and desires of traveling, gifts, vacations. More time can be spent enjoying family, friends and hobbies.

The last stage of life, old age, is often divided into three stages: early old age (55–65), old age (65–85), and very old age (85 and older). Adults in early old age become more aware of their own mortality, and significant lifestyle changes may occur. Some begin to acknowledge health problems, physical limitations, and a likely decline in earning power or working capacity in the years ahead.

Among the 65- to 85-year-old group, many have retired, are forced to live on lower incomes, and are experiencing progressively worse health problems. Living arrangements may change because of their financial situations or because they can no longer care for themselves. Some have lost partners, family members, and friends through death.

Most adults over age 85 have gone through all the experiences mentioned above. Many are in long-term-care facilities, many have severe memory problems, and many have no income. Others are in excellent health, are able to care for themselves, travel, and live life to the fullest.

The aging process affects different people in different ways. It is important not to stereotype the elderly—each person is unique in terms of genetic makeup, health status, financial status, and life experience.

In terms of personality and relationships, U.S. psychoanalyst Erik Erikson (1902–1994) believed that the development of trust, or lack of trust, in the first year of life is the foundation for the development of an individual's coping skills (Table 5-4). In each of the developmental stages described by Erikson, the positive resolution of any crisis is based on positive coping characteristics: trust, independence, initiative, competence, and integrity. Negative coping characteristics that contribute to negative resolution include mistrust, insecurity, and dependency, among others. An awareness of Erikson's life stages will help you better understand what patients experience as they grow and age and provides a foundation for more effective therapeutic communication with patients.

Maslow's Hierarchy of Human Needs

Communication may be influenced by people's needs. Abraham Maslow (1908–1970) was a U.S. psychologist who studied human motivation and developed what is known as Maslow's hierarchy of human needs (Figure 5-17 ◆). According to Maslow's principles, individuals fulfill their needs, partially or totally, at a basic level before moving toward higher levels of emotional satisfaction. For example, people must satisfy the most basic needs for food, shelter, and clothing before they can go on to fulfill their needs for family, employment, financial stability, or self-actualization.

Although the hierarchy is simplistic and cannot be applied to every situation, it does provide a perspective on communication problems in the medical setting. Health is not listed in Maslow's hierarchy, but it is a basic physiological need. Illness affects a person's emotional state. When an individual experiences chronic illness, recovery can take precedence over job stability, friendships, and self-actualization. During times of illness, some people worry about their job, family, and income over their own physiological needs. An individual who puts others' needs above his or her own health may sacrifice present needs for worsening health in the future.

TABLE 5-4 ERIK ERIKSON'S LIFE STAGES AND DEVELOPMENTAL TASKS	
1. Infancy	Develop trust.
2. Early childhood	Develop independence and self-direction.
3. Play age	Develop initiative.
4. School age	Develop competence.
5. Adolescence	Develop self-identity.
6. Early adulthood	Develop intimacy and love.
7. Middle adulthood	Develop concern for others and continue productivity.
8. Old age	Develop integrity.

Defense Mechanisms

Defense mechanisms are people's characteristic, usually unconscious ways of protecting themselves in stressful situations. Just as everyone has physical defenses that combat disease, everyone also has mental and emotional defenses to deal with stress and **anxiety.** These mechanisms may be engaged consciously or unconsciously, usually in combination with others. Table 5-5 lists some common defense mechanisms that may be encountered in patients. The medical assistant should also examine her own defense mechanisms as they arise in her interactions with patients and coworkers.

Defense mechanisms protect a person's self-esteem but do not effectively deal with conflict. It is important to recognize the coping style of the patient, patient's family, staff, and physicians. For example, one of the most common defense mechanisms is denial. A patient with a serious condition may refuse to believe what is happening. This refusal to accept reality is a factor in the patient's treatment and education.

An understanding of the psychological principles discussed in this chapter will improve your therapeutic communication skills and your interactions with patients.

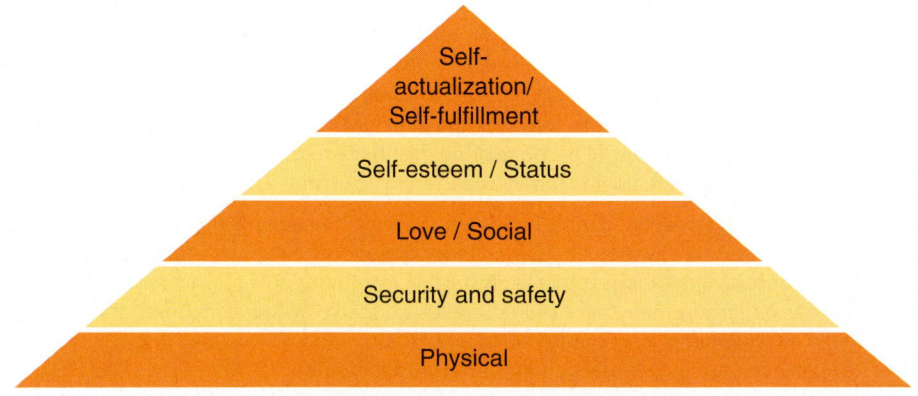

Figure 5-17 ◆ Maslow's hierarchy of needs.
Source: Maslow, Abraham H., Frager, Robert D. (ed.), and Fadiman, James (ed.). Motivation and personality, 3rd ed. © 1987. Reprinted by permission of Pearson Education, Inc. Upper Saddle River, NJ.

TABLE 5-5 COMMON DEFENSE MECHANISMS

Compensation	Trying to overcome some inability or inferiority. It helps to maintain one's self-respect and raise self-esteem.
Conversion	Changing an emotional problem into a physical symptom or other method of release that eases tension and anxiety related to conflict.
Denial	Avoiding or escaping the unpleasant or distasteful realities of living by ignoring or refusing to admit their existence.
Displacement	Transferring into another situation an emotion that was felt in a past situation where its expression would have been socially unacceptable.
Identification	Unconsciously imitating the mannerisms, behavior, and feelings of another person.
Overcompensation	Repressing unconscious attitudes and wishes and replacing them with conscious attitudes and behavior that are the opposite of the unconscious ones. Often referred to as *reaction formation*.
Projection	Blaming someone else for one's own failures or for specific events.
Rationalization	Explaining, excusing, or defending ideas, actions, and feelings. It helps to "save face" in embarrassing and anxiety-producing situations.
Regression	Escaping frustration and conflict anxiety by returning to methods used at an earlier stage of life.
Repression	Unconsciously storing unpleasant, unacceptable thoughts, desires, and impulses in the mind. The repressed information does not enter conscious awareness and may not be remembered unless there is an emotional trigger. Repression is sometimes termed *selective forgetting*.
Substitution	Accepting something in place of a desired object or need when the original cannot be obtained. The substitution helps to achieve at least some fulfillment.
Suppression	Storing away or forgetting unpleasant, emotionally painful experiences. This is a conscious forcing of unpleasant, anxiety-producing experiences into the unconscious mind.

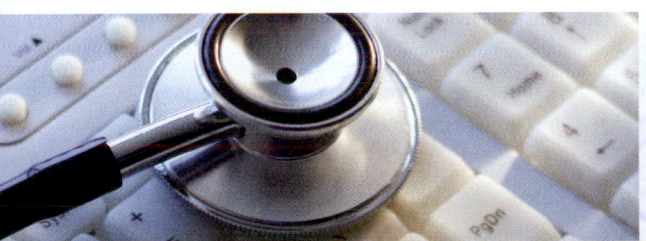

REVIEW

Chapter Summary

- Good communication skills are vital to anyone who works in healthcare, but especially for the medical assistant, who must demonstrate superior verbal and nonverbal communication.
- Listening is a crucial component of communication in healthcare.
- The medical assistant must identify barriers to communication and work to overcome them using the appropriate tools and techniques.
- Patient populations, including those with special needs and/or disabilities, dictate the ways in which the medical assistant should interact with them.
- Just as they do with patients, medical assistants must communicate properly, professionally, and respectfully with the other members of the healthcare team.

- According to Maslow's hierarchy of needs, individuals fulfill their needs at a basic level before moving toward higher levels of emotional satisfaction.
- A patient's age and cultural background can affect how the patient views healthcare. Careful listening and observing help with patient teaching.
- Defense mechanisms are the various ways people cope with life situations. Denial is a common defense mechanism shown by patients, especially those diagnosed with a serious illness.
- Elisabeth Kübler-Ross identified five emotional stages of grieving: denial, anger, bargaining, depression, and acceptance. Grieving applies to terminally ill patients as well as to patients who have experienced other kinds of losses.

Chapter Review

Multiple Choice

1. What is the proper way to address an elderly patient?
   a. Mrs. _____
   b. By first name
   c. "Honey" or "Sweetie"
   d. None of the above

2. The opinion that all people living in homeless shelters are likely to have lice is an example of
   a. stereotyping.
   b. discriminating.
   c. alienating.
   d. grieving.

3. Which of the following is *not* an example of keeping a professional distance?
   a. Giving a patient transportation options to the clinic
   b. Offering to pay a patient's copayment
   c. Reviewing a patient's billing charges with the patient
   d. None of the above

4. A common defense mechanism for a patient who has just received a serious diagnosis is
   a. denial.
   b. identification.
   c. conversion.
   d. compensation.

True/False

T F 1. Body language is far less important than verbal communication.

T F 2. Empathy and sympathy are really the same thing.

T F 3. When working with a hearing-impaired patient, the medical assistant should speak directly to the interpreter.

T F 4. When working with child patients, it is best to communicate directly with the parent during the visit rather than the child.

T F 5. Addressing the physician as "Dr." in front of patients gives patients the impression that the doctor is an authority figure who should be respected.

T F 6. Part of developing a good patient relationship includes sharing personal problems with the patients.

T F 7. Defense mechanisms protect a person's self-esteem and effectively deal with conflict.

T F 8. Patients will often share more information with the medical assistant that they will with the physician.

T F 9. It is best to use proper medical terminology when speaking with patients to demonstrate intelligence.

T F 10. A clinic's office policy dictates whether to allow service animals to accompany their owners to treatment rooms.

Short Answer

1. What is a good communication technique to use with angry patients?

2. Name the five stages of grief.

3. List six common defense mechanisms.

4. What is the difference between an open-ended question and a close-ended question?

5. When might it be appropriate to use therapeutic touch with a patient?

6. Describe the method you would use to communicate effectively with a hearing-impaired patient.

Research

1. Does the Americans with Disabilities Act (ADA) require that Braille be printed on public buildings to indicate bathrooms, elevators, etc.?

2. In your local area, are sign-language classes available to the public?

3. In your local area, what are the resources for patients who speak English as a second language?

4. If a non-English-speaking patient comes to your office alone, what local agency can you contact for an interpreter?

5. Search the Internet for books to read about communication skills. Which ones sound as if they might be helpful to the medical assistant?

6. What are the local resources for hearing-impaired people in your area?

7. What are the local resources for sight-impaired people in your area?

Externship Application Experience

Dr. Roberts wants Beth Parcher, a sight-impaired patient, to be scheduled for a series of physical therapy appointments and has asked the medical assistant to schedule the appointments. How will the medical assistant ensure Beth completely understands what Dr. Roberts wants her to do? How will the assistant ensure Beth is clear about the appointments scheduled for her?

Resource Guide

American Lung Association
61 Broadway, 6th Floor
New York, NY 10006
1-800-LUNGUSA
www.lungusa.org

American Diabetes Association
ATTN: National Call Center
1701 North Beauregard Street
Alexandria, VA 22311
1-800-DIABETES
www.diabetes.org

American Hospice Foundation
2120 L Street NW, Suite 200
Washington, DC 20037
1-800-347-1413
www.americanhospice.org

American Heart Association National Center
7272 Greenville Avenue
Dallas, TX 75231
1-800-AHA-USA-1
www.americanheart.org

Alzheimer's Association
225 N. Michigan Ave, Floor 17
Chicago, IL 60601
(312) 335-5886
www.alz.org

American Parkinson Disease Association Inc.
135 Parkinson Avenue
Staten Island, NY 10305
1-800-223-2732
www.apdaparkinson.org

The ALS Association
27001 Agoura Road, Suite 150
Calabasas Hills, CA 91301
(818) 880-9007
www.alsa.org

Online Communication Skills Test
http://discoveryhealth.queendom.com/
Seven Challenges: A guide to cooperative communication skills
http://www.newconversations.net/

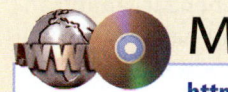

Med**Media**

http://www.MyMAKit.com

More on this chapter, including interactive resources, can be found on the Student CD-ROM accompanying this textbook and on http://www.MyMAKit.com.

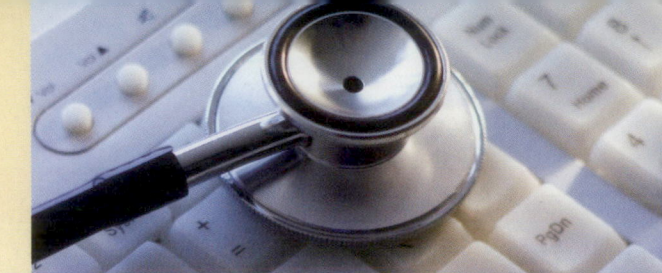

CHAPTER 6

Patient-Centered Care and Education

Case Study

Marina successfully passed her RMA exam and was excited to start her career as a medical assistant. After applying to several positions, she obtained employment with Dr. Gerard, a doctor of naturopathic medicine. Marina enjoys her work and loves teaching her patients about different approaches to a healthy lifestyle and effective stress and pain management.

After a particularly long, stressful morning, Marina takes her assigned break outside in the building's patio area. One of Marina's patients passes by and stops to say hello. His expression changes from one of happy recognition to one of confusion as Marina quickly extinguishes the cigarette she has been smoking. Suddenly feeling like a teenager caught by her parents doing something wrong, Marina forces a nervous smile as she greets her patient.

Objectives

After completing this chapter, you should be able to:

- Define and spell the key terminology in this chapter.
- Define the medical assistant's role in patient education.
- Define wellness.
- Discuss the holistic approach to healthcare.
- Explain the mind–body connection.
- Describe the types of pain, including physical, psychological, and phantom pain.
- Explain how pain is assessed.
- Describe different methods of pain management.
- Describe the factors the medical assistant must consider when facilitating an education program for patients.
- Describe how the medical assistant establishes a proper learning environment.
- Describe the types of information the medical assistant might provide the patient, including preventing medication errors, dieting and weight loss, exercise, stress reduction, smoking cessation, and substance abuse.
- Discuss the various teaching resources available in the medical office.

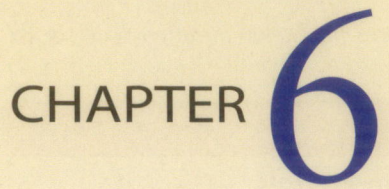

Med**Media**
http://www.MyMAKit.com

Additional interactive resources and activities for this chapter can be found on http://www.MyMAKit.com. For a video, tips, audio glossary, legal and ethical scenarios, on-the-job scenarios, quizzes, and games related to the content of this chapter, please access the accompanying CD-ROM in this book.

Video: *When English Is Not the Language*
Legal and Ethical Scenario: *Patient-Centered Care and Education*
On the Job Scenario: *Patient-Centered Care and Education*
Tips
Multiple Choice Quiz
Audio Glossary
HIPAA Quiz
Games: Spelling Bee, Crossword, and Strikeout

✚ MEDICAL ASSISTING STANDARDS

CAAHEP ENTRY-LEVEL STANDARDS	ABHES ENTRY-LEVEL COMPETENCIES
■ Perform within scope of practice (psychomotor) ■ Apply ethical behaviors, including honesty/integrity in performance of medical assisting practice (affective) ■ Explore issue of confidentiality as it applies to the medical assistant (cognitive) ■ Respond to issues of confidentiality (psychomotor) ■ Apply active listening skills (affective) ■ Identify styles and types of verbal communication (cognitive) ■ Identify nonverbal communication (cognitive) ■ Report relevant information to others succinctly and accurately (psychomotor) ■ Document patient education (psychomotor) ■ Document patient care (psychomotor) ■ Recognize the role of patient advocacy in the practice of medical assisting (cognitive) ■ Advocate on behalf of patients (psychomotor) ■ Practice within the standard of care for a medical assistant (psychomotor) ■ Demonstrate sensitivity to patient rights (affective) ■ Document accurately in the patient record (psychomotor) ■ Demonstrate empathy in communicating with patients, family and staff (affective) ■ Demonstrate recognition of patient's level of understanding in communications (affective) ■ Use internet to access information related to the medical office (psychomotor) ■ Instruct patients according to their needs to promote health maintenance and disease prevention (psychomotor) ■ Use language/verbal skills that enable patients' understanding (affective) ■ Demonstrate respect for diversity in approaching patients and families (affective)	■ Project a positive attitude ■ Maintain confidentiality at all times ■ Be a "team player" ■ Be cognizant of ethical boundaries ■ Exhibit initiative ■ Adapt to change ■ Evidence a responsible attitude ■ Be courteous and diplomatic ■ Conduct work within scope of education, training, and ability ■ Recognize and respond to verbal and nonverbal communication

Key Terminology

acute—sharp, severe, sudden; having a sudden onset and usually of short duration

afferent nerves—sensory nerves that carry impulses to the central nervous system

analgesic—pain reducing

assess—to evaluate

cerebral—pertaining to the cerebrum, the forepart of the brain

chronic—of long duration, often with slow progression

controlled substances—narcotics, stimulants, and certain sedatives

documenting—tracking the education process in the patient's medical record.

efferent nerves—motor nerves that carry impulses from the central nervous system to the peripheral nervous system

endorphins—proteins in the brain that have analgesic properties

evaluation—checking to see how well the patient has understood what has been taught

implementing—the actual teaching phase

planning—determining how to begin the task of teaching the patient

referred pain—pain that is felt in a different area from the injured or diseased part of the body

risk factor—factor that makes a person particularly vulnerable to certain diseases or disorders

Abbreviations

ACS—American Cancer Society

BMI—body mass index

JCAHO—Joint Commission on Accreditation of Healthcare Organizations

NIDA—National Institute on Drug Abuse

PSA—prostate-specific antigen

✔ COMPETENCY SKILLS PERFORMANCE

1. Use the Internet to find patient education materials

Introduction

Quality care involves focusing on the patient. Patient-centered care requires the medical assistant to be professional, communicate properly, understand the legal concepts, teach patients, and maintain the medical office.

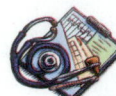

The Medical Assistant's Role in Patient Education

One of the many roles of the medical assistant involves teaching patients how to manage their pain and how to maintain wellness. The MA may also be involved in:

- Charting patients' pain levels
- Obtaining patient medical data
- Assisting patients with special needs

Wellness

Wellness is the ongoing process of practicing a healthy lifestyle. It depends on a balance between a person's physical and psychological states. Wellness is a personal matter, as each person is unique and has different needs. **Risk factors** are determined to assess the level or degree of wellness (Table 6-1). Then the individual takes action to reduce or eliminate these factors.

Critical Thinking Question 6-1

In the case study, why do you think the patient looked confused when he noticed that Marina was smoking? Why do you think Marina felt guilty or uneasy about being seen by her patient while smoking? How would you feel if the person teaching you healthy habits and encouraging you did not follow his or her own advice?

The average life span in the United States is 76 years. Smoking, abusing drugs and/or alcohol, diet, exercise, using seat belts, weight management, performing breast or testicular self-exams, prostate-specific antigen (**PSA**) screening, blood pressure screening, cholesterol screening, Pap smears, and safe sex are personal choices that can affect life span. Ignoring healthy lifestyle practices puts people at risk for developing chronic illnesses and/or debilitating (weakening) conditions.

People's lifestyles are based on their personal attitudes, experiences, and role models. For example, a child whose role model eats healthy foods, exercises, and does not smoke is more likely to practice the same healthy habits later in life. On the other hand, if the role model uses drugs, smokes, and is involved in criminal activity, the child is more likely to take up risky behavior. Positive experiences reinforce a healthier lifestyle. A person who starts exercising three times a week soon discovers that she has more energy for daily tasks. The energy is a positive outcome of exercising, which, in turn, motivates the person to continue.

Some risk factors cannot be changed, such as a genetic predisposition (tendency) toward developing a disease. Others, such as smoking, *can* be changed if the person has the desire to change them. Some healthy habits and attitudes are listed in Table 6-2.

TABLE 6-1 COMMON RISK FACTORS	
■ Smoking or tobacco product use ■ Poor physical fitness ■ High alcohol intake ■ Poor diet and nutrition ■ Disregarding auto safety measures ■ High stress level ■ Occupational health and environmental hazards ■ Drug abuse	■ Lack of immunizations ■ Poor dental care ■ High or very low blood pressure ■ Family history of cancer, heart attack, stroke, or diabetes ■ Unsafe sex ■ High or very low heart rate ■ Unhealthy body mass index (**BMI**) ■ Risk-taking behavior

TABLE 6-2 WELLNESS GUIDELINES	
■ Keep a positive attitude. ■ Cherish your values. ■ Exercise your mind, body, and spirit. ■ Control your stress. ■ Soothe your fears. ■ Think happy thoughts. ■ Stay active. ■ Challenge your mind. ■ Forgive and forget. ■ Avoid dangerous drugs. ■ Watch your sugar intake. ■ Walk briskly.	■ Enjoy the outdoors. ■ Maintain a healthy weight. ■ Eat a well-balanced diet. ■ Rinse fresh fruits and vegetables before eating. ■ Practice cleanliness. ■ Take medications as directed. ■ Stop smoking. ■ Lower your blood pressure and cholesterol. ■ Learn to breathe deeply.

A Holistic Approach to Health Care

Healthcare providers must understand the importance of the interaction between body and mind. A holistic approach to healthcare recognizes and addresses the complete care of the patient, including physical, social, psychological, spiritual, environmental, and economic elements. Holistic medicine facilitates healing and promotes wellness.

The patient should be involved in making decisions concerning the treatment or management of his or her general health. For example, stress is often a factor that contributes to illness or makes an illness worse. Part of holistic care consists of helping the patient learn how to control stress by using relaxation techniques, which contribute to overall healing.

The Mind–Body Connection

It has long been known that the human spirit and spirituality are driving forces in healing. Positive emotions such as joy, love, and happiness cause the brain to release endorphins. **Endorphins**, a group of proteins in the brain with **analgesic** properties, benefit physical functioning and boost immunity to disease. Negative feelings such as fear, anger, and grieving cause tightened muscles, faster heart and respiratory rates, and other heightened reactions.

Laughter, games, and relaxation activities have been used effectively in the treatment of chronic and terminal pain. Friendship, love, and spirituality give a sense of emotional security. The new area of pet therapy has been shown to be very beneficial for nursing home residents, hospital patients, and hospice patients.

Recognizing the connection between mental and emotional states and physical health is an important step in developing a healthier lifestyle. Finding ways to release or deal with negative emotions and replace them with positive, uplifting experiences is an excellent way to implement this step.

Pain

Pain is an unpleasant sensory and emotional experience. Each person responds differently to pain, depending on tolerance and pain threshold. Even when pain is seen as "imagined" by others, it can be very real to the person experiencing it. Factors that can affect how a person feels pain are cultural background and past experience. Anxiety, stress, and fear usually heighten the experience of pain.

In some cultures, people are taught not to show pain. Also, some patients may have a very high tolerance for pain, which means that some early warning signs may be ignored or undetected.

Pain is categorized as **acute** or **chronic**. Acute pain, such as surgical pain, usually lessens with treatment and time. Chronic pain, such as that of rheumatoid arthritis, lasts longer than a few weeks, often for a lifetime. It is the long-term effects of chronic pain on a patient's mental and physical state that are of the most concern. These effects include the following:

- Decreased activity or possibly inactivity
- Decreased sleep or poor quality of sleep
- Increased irritability and fatigue
- Chemical and/or medication dependency
- Mood swings
- Impaired ability to handle stress
- Lower self-esteem
- Anger
- Helplessness
- Sadness or depression

The treatment goal is to lessen the pain, keep it tolerable, and promote physical functioning.

Types of Pain

Physical Pain

Body pain is a signal of disease process or inflammation and serves as a protective mechanism. Pain causes a person to seek medical attention. For example, severe chest pain may be a heart attack, and severe abdominal pain could be internal bleeding. Without pain, there is no signal that something is wrong. Some patients have an impaired sense of pain. For example, a patient with diabetes may have reduced sensation in the feet. The patient may not be aware of a breakdown in tissues until it is so severe that the only treatment is amputation.

Pain intensity varies. Superficial pain is usually located on the body surface and does not penetrate deep into the tissue. Deep pain involves muscles, joints, and tendons. Visceral pain involves the internal organs and is usually the most severe.

Psychological Pain

Psychological pain can be either acute or chronic. Acute psychological pain may be described as terror, fear, despair, grief, rage, anger, helplessness, or hopelessness. If appropriate intervention does not take place to address and ease the pain, it often becomes chronic.

Chronic psychological pain may have a subtle onset. The person may not be aware of the symptoms he or she is experiencing. Diagnoses include anxiety disorders, posttraumatic

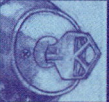

Keys to Success
HOW THE BODY RESPONDS TO PAIN

The nervous system carries electrical impulses to and from the brain (Figure 6-1 ◆). The brain interprets these signals and directs the body's response through chemical, hormonal, and muscular reactions. **Afferent nerves,** found in muscles, joints, organs, and skin, transmit impulses to the spinal cord and brain via the central nervous system. The brain sends signals through the **efferent nerves** to produce the appropriate body response. Afferent nerves send fast and slow signals for pain to the brain. This explains the occurrence of sharp, then throbbing pain after traumatic blunt injury. **Referred pain** confuses the brain because it is felt in a different area from where the pain originates.

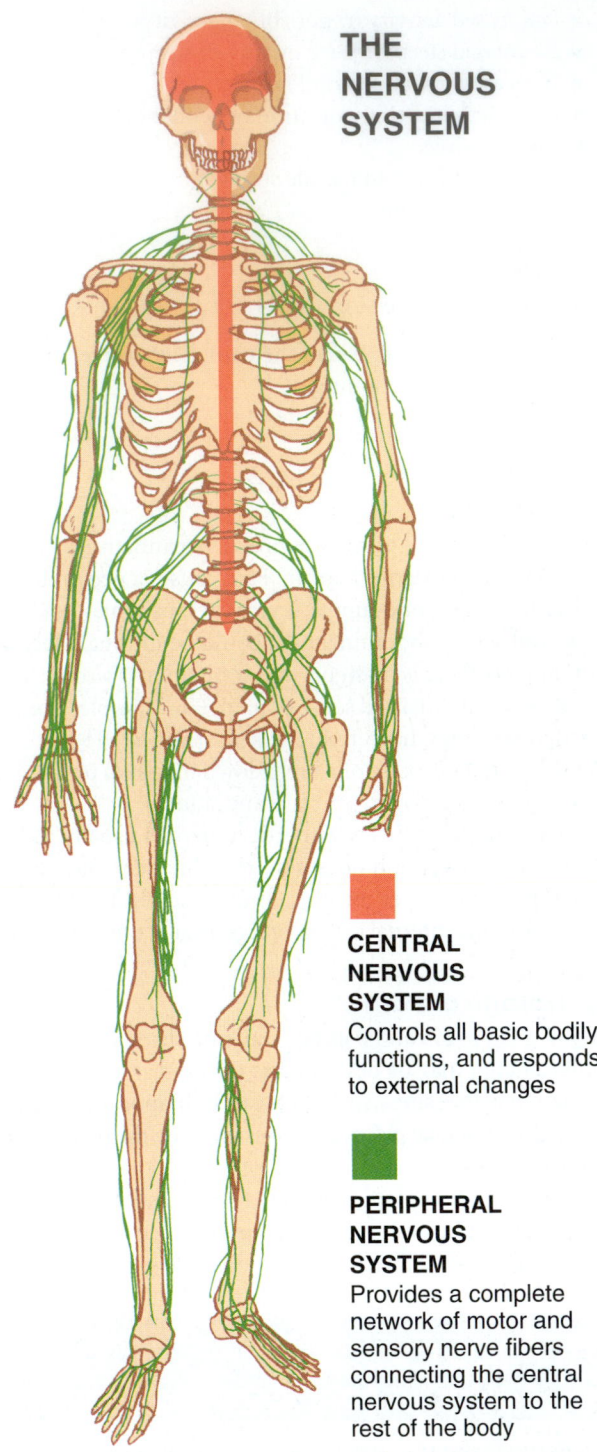

THE
NERVOUS
SYSTEM

■ CENTRAL
NERVOUS
SYSTEM
Controls all basic bodily
functions, and responds
to external changes

■ PERIPHERAL
NERVOUS
SYSTEM
Provides a complete
network of motor and
sensory nerve fibers
connecting the central
nervous system to the
rest of the body

Figure 6-1 ◆ The nervous system.

stress disorder, major depression, and other psychological disorders. (∞ Chapter 47, Mental Health, discusses psychological pain in greater detail.)

Phantom Pain

Phantom pain occurs after the amputation of a body part (Figure 6-2 ◆). The severed nerve endings feel as if they are still receiving stimuli from the amputated part, causing painful

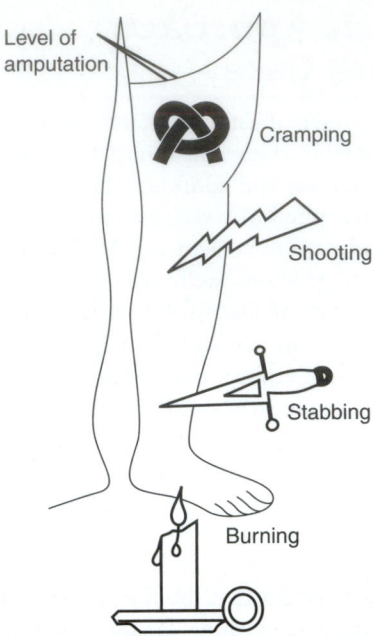

Level of
amputation

Cramping

Shooting

Stabbing

Burning

Figure 6-2 ◆ Phantom pain occurs after the amputation of a body part.

sensations as if the body part were still attached. The pain is usually severe but eases and disappears over time.

Pain Assessment

Part of the job of the MA may be to ask the patient to describe his or her pain (Table 6-3). It is best to use open-ended questions:

- When did the pain start?
- Where is the pain located?
- How frequently does the pain occur?
- Could you describe the pain for me?
- What actions or movements seem to lessen or increase the pain?

Three methods are commonly used to rate pain:

- Numerical or symbolic scale: The patient is asked to "grade" his or her pain on a scale of 0 (no pain) to 10 (the most severe pain) (Figure 6-3 ◆).
- Face scale: The patient is shown a series of faces ranging from a happy smiling face to a very unhappy face and

TABLE 6-3 COMMON WORDS USED TO DESCRIBE PAIN	
■ Stabbing	■ Intractable
■ Sharp	■ Unbearable
■ Cutting	■ Colicky
■ Tearing	■ Excruciating
■ Burning, stinging	■ Radiating
■ Dull	■ Penetrating
■ Intermittent	■ Aching
■ Continuous	■ Nagging, gnawing
■ Throbbing	■ Fleeting

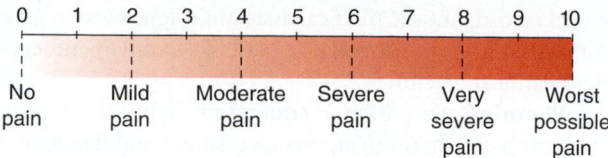

Figure 6-3 ◆ Numerical pain level chart with word modifiers.

points to the face that best illustrates his or her pain (Figure 6-4 ◆). The face scale works well with children and adults who have trouble using the number scale.

■ Full body picture (front and back): The patient marks the picture to indicate the areas where he or she feels pain, using different types of marks for different types of pain.

Pain Management

Pain management involves medication, comfort measures, alternative therapies, exercise, surgery, or a combination of methods. The choice of treatment depends on many factors including the severity or chronic nature of pain. Comfort measures include heat and cold therapy, elevation of the affected part, gentle massage, and other physical therapy. Surgery may involve severing the afferent nerve to stop the delivery of pain impulses to the brain. (∞ Chapter 43, Orthopedics and Physical Therapy, and Chapter 27, Pharmacology and Medication Administration, discuss pain management with physical therapy and medication.)

If these initial methods of pain control for patients with chronic pain are not effective, the physician may prescribe **controlled substances.** These medications are not prescribed over the phone or after office hours. The patient must be taught to strictly follow directions for dosage and use. The patient must keep scheduled appointments to obtain the next prescription.

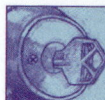

Keys to Success
GUIDELINES FOR PAIN ASSESSMENT AND MANAGEMENT

The Joint Commission on Accreditation of Health Care Organizations (**JCAHO**) has set guidelines for pain assessment and management. The guidelines became effective January 1, 2001, for hospitals and other healthcare facilities, including nursing homes, clinics, health maintenance organizations, and home health agencies. Agencies must comply with the regulations for pain assessment to remain fully accredited.

Pain assessment is now considered the fifth vital sign, to be charted along with temperature, pulse, respiration, and blood pressure. The patient evaluates the pain on a scale of 0 to 10. Happy and sad faces are used for children and those who cannot use the numerical scale. Pain relief is provided, and the patient is reassessed on a regular basis.

Additional medication is not supplied if the patient takes more than the prescribed dosage ahead of schedule. If the prescribing physician discovers the patient has obtained a controlled substance from another source, further pain management ceases. (Refer to ∞ Chapter 27, Pharmacology and Medication Administration, for additional information on controlled substances.)

A patient may choose to manage pain without medication because of potential side effects and drug dependence. Some examples of alternative therapy are relaxation exercises, herbal remedies, magnet therapy, biofeedback, acupuncture, acupressure, and chiropractic treatments. (Refer to ∞ Chapter 50, Alternative Medicine, for a more detailed discussion of alternative therapies.)

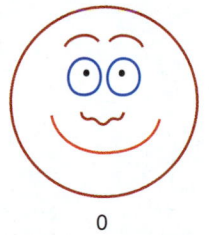 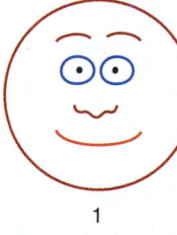 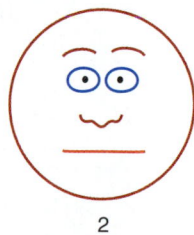 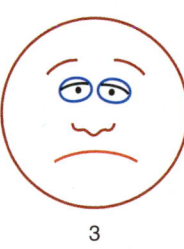 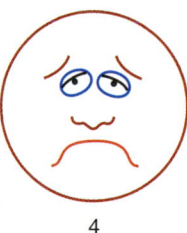 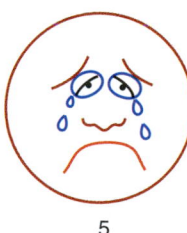

| 0 | 1 | 2 | 3 | 4 | 5 |

1. Explain to the child that each face is for a person who feels happy because he or she has no pain (hurt, or whatever word the child uses) or feels sad because he or she has some or a lot of pain.

2. Point to the appropriate face and state, "This face..." :

0—"is very happy because he (or she) doesn't hurt at all."
1—"hurts just a little bit."
2—"hurts a little more."
3—"hurts even more."
4—"hurts a whole lot."
5—"hurts as much as you can imagine, although you don't have to be crying to feel this bad."

3. Ask the child to choose the face that best describes how he or she feels. Be specific about which pain (e.g., "shot" or incision) and what time (e.g., Now? Earlier before lunch?)

Figure 6-4 ◆ The Wong/Baker FACES rating scale.

Source: From Hockenberry, M. J., Wilson, D., Winkelstein, M. L.: Wong's essentials of pediatric nursing, ed. 7, St. Louis, 2005, p. 1259. Used with permission. Copyright Mosby.

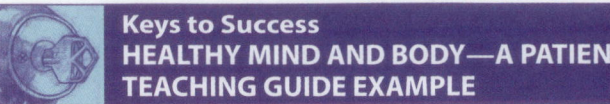

Keys to Success
HEALTHY MIND AND BODY—A PATIENT TEACHING GUIDE EXAMPLE

Take the time to keep healthy and prevent illness. If you already have a medical condition, make it a personal goal to stay as healthy as you can. Post the following reminders in a prominent place such as a refrigerator door or a bathroom mirror. Remember to focus on health even if you have a busy life.

- **Eat a healthy diet.** A balanced diet provides basic nutrients to boost immunity, keep the mind alert, and meet general body needs.
- **Exercise 30 minutes each day.** Regular exercise increases blood circulation, the movement of nutrients to the cells, muscle strength, and beneficial hormones. It also improves mental alertness and elevates the mood. Discuss an exercise plan with your physician before starting.
- **Get sufficient sleep.** While you rest, your body and mind are repairing, restoring, and refreshing.
- **Visit your physician for regular checkups and recommended screenings.** Come prepared with any questions you may have. If you are on medications, bring a list of drugs, dosages, and frequency of each. If you have a family pattern of medical conditions, tell the physician. Ask about periodic screening for those illnesses or diseases.

Patient Teaching

Patient teaching is vital for pain management. The medical office should make information and guidelines available to patients, such as:

- Discussion of the disease process that is causing the pain
- General information on treatments available for the disease
- Specific information relating to the individual patient
- Medication dosage and treatment frequency, explained in terms the patient can understand
- Changes in condition that should alert the patient to call the office immediately

Educating the Patient

Any patient education the medical assistant does in the office must be done under the direction of the physician. Part of patient education includes helping patients accept their conditions and providing positive reinforcement. To educate patients properly, the medical assistant must first **assess** the best way to teach them. For this step, the medical assistant will want to know how much pain patients are experiencing or if they are distressed. Patients cannot fully comprehend information when distracted by pain or anxiety.

After assessment, the medical assistant must gather the patient's information. Normally, this is found in the patient's

medical record, but the medical assistant might need to gather information from the doctor, the patient's family members, or other healthcare facilities.

Planning the patient's education includes taking the information gathered during the assessment and determining how to proceed in educating the patient. This step may include gathering pamphlets or printed information on the patient's condition or gathering equipment that will be used to demonstrate a new skill to the patient.

The **implementing** step is the actual teaching phase. During this step, it may be helpful for the medical assistant to demonstrate what he or she wants the patient to learn and then have the patient demonstrate the skill. For example, the medical assistant might show the patient how to use a pair of crutches and then ask the patient to demonstrate using the crutches. See Figure 6-5 ◆.

The next step in patient education is **documenting** what has been taught to the patient, the tools used in the teaching process, how well the patient demonstrated the skill, and any concerns the medical assistant may have, such as a patient's unwillingness to follow the doctor's instructions.

The **evaluation** step of patient education involves checking to see how well patients are using the information given to them. Some evaluation may need to be done over the phone if the doctor asks patients to call in to let the medical assistant know how they are doing. If the medical assistant discovers a patient is failing to comply with the doctor's instructions, either because she is unable or unwilling, the medical assistant will need to determine if there is a misunderstanding. If the patient is refusing to follow through, the

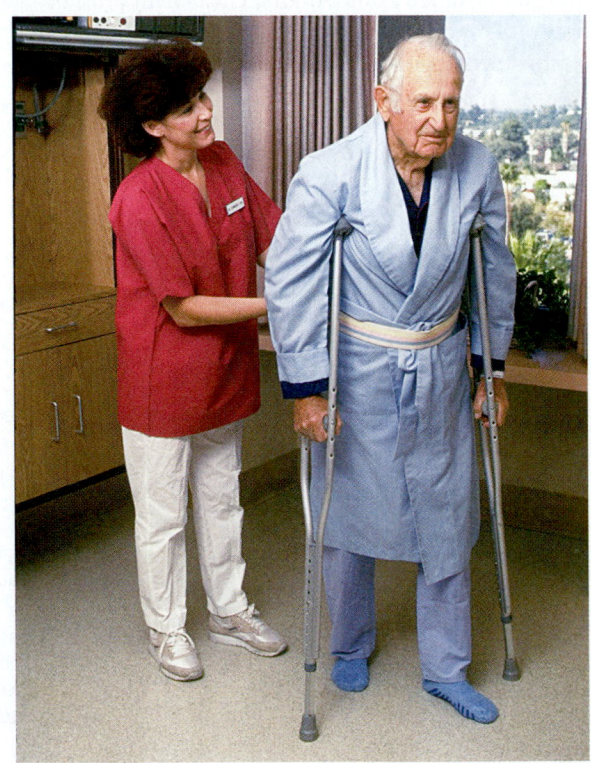

Figure 6-5 ◆ An MA assisting a man learning to use crutches.

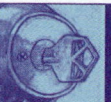

Keys to Success
PROPER CHARTING

The party who signs the patient's medical chart is assumed to have performed the tasks described. For example, if, after entering information on patient instruction, the medical assistant signs the chart, the assistant indicates that the assistant did the teaching. When that is not the case, notes must reflect the facts.

refusal must be charted and the doctor notified right away. Patients have the right to refuse treatment, but if they do so, their choices must be clearly documented.

Patient Miscommunication

Miscommunication can be disastrous, so medical assistants must be careful to be completely clear and watch for signs that patients may not understand instructions fully. Signs that the patient may not understand what has been said to them include a furrowed brow, a frown, and not making direct eye contact. Communicating with the patient cannot be hurried, so assistants will need to ensure they are comfortable with patients' levels of understanding before moving on.

HIPAA Compliance

All communication with the patient must be kept confidential. This means teaching episodes must take place in a private location, out of sight and hearing range of other patients or nonmedical staff.

Determining the Time Needed for Patient Education

Depending on the disease or illness, patient education can take several visits. Serious illnesses can be difficult to comprehend, and patients may need multiple visits to comprehend all the relevant information. When patients are willing to bring family members, those family members can be very helpful in patient-education initiatives. Often family members will recall information that the patient may have forgotten. Written instructions or information are also helpful, because they serve as reference materials outside the medical office.

Establishing a Proper Learning Environment

The teaching environment must be conducive to learning. It must be quiet and free from interruptions, and it should be well lighted. Hallways, the reception area, and any locations in view of other patients are inappropriate places for teaching. Patients must feel relaxed, comfortable, and able to ask questions.

Assume the medical assistant is teaching a patient how to use a piece of equipment. The equipment should be in the office,

and the medical assistant should be very familiar with the equipment's use and repair. The medical assistant should always provide written instructions on how to use any machinery.

Medical assistants must have solid knowledge of the skills they are trying to teach. When assistants are uncomfortable or less knowledgeable, they should request help before teaching patients. If patients ask a question and medical assistants do not know the answer, the assistants should admit they do not know and let the patients know they will find the answer and get back to them.

Teaching Resources

Teaching resources may be available for purchase, or the medical office can create its own. The medical assistant may use such teaching tools as audiocassettes, compact disks (CDs), food labels, videos, DVDs, or pamphlets in helping to demonstrate a new skill to a patient. Because people learn through seeing, hearing, and touch, and different patients may have different learning styles, the medical assistant may need to incorporate more than one teaching approach to educate the patient.

Patient Skills and Abilities

Before teaching patients new skills, the medical assistant must be aware of any of the patients' physical impairments. For example, assistants must know if patients cannot open a bottle of pills due to severe arthritis, especially when educating about medication use throughout the day. In cases like these, the medical assistants may need to improvise and devise other ways to help patients accomplish the doctor's directives. One way to help a patient such as this would be to contact the pharmacy to determine if the prescription can be filled in a bottle that does not contain a childproof cap.

Culture and Patient Education

Patients' cultures may prevent the medical assistant from teaching those patients certain skills. An example would be a patient from a culture where the custom is that a patient be taught by an assistant of the same gender as the patient. It is important for the medical assistant to know this and to come up with alternatives that are acceptable to both the physician and the patient. In the example of working with a patient who prefers an assistant of the same gender, the medical assistant must respect the patient's preference and ask a coworker of the same gender as the patient to assist that patient.

Cultural beliefs may have an impact on a patient's healthcare. For example, within the Asian culture, the family plays an important role. When working with a patient from this culture, it is important for the medical assistant to realize that the patient may refuse care if the family does not agree with or understand the need for care. Within this culture, it is also common to see many family members accompany the patient to the doctor's office.

No matter what culture the patient belongs to, the medical assistant should attempt to involve and educate the patient's family in the decision-making process, with the patient's permission. By having the patient's family involved, the likelihood of the patient's success in healthcare goals increases.

Religious beliefs may have an impact on a patient's healthcare as well. The Jehovah's Witness religion prohibits the use of blood products, for example. Many religions, such as the Catholic faith, restrict the use of birth control. The medical assistant and the provider should be aware of the patient's religious beliefs if those beliefs will cause a need for a different care plan.

The Impact of Finances on Patient Education

Financial difficulties may prevent patients from achieving desired educational goals. For example, patients may be unable to pay for appropriate shoes to begin a walking or exercise program. The patient may not have medical insurance that covers needed procedures or medications. The medical assistant must address any such restrictions before undertaking education. Rather than ask a patient about financial status, the medical assistant should simply ask the patient if he or she expects any problems following through with the physician's prescribed course of action. If the patient admits to a financial barrier, the medical assistant can then look for ways to assist the patient in finding resources or alternatives. Resources in the form of charities are available in many communities. With regard to medications, the physician may have samples in the office that may be given to the patient by the physician when the patient cannot afford to purchase needed drugs. In addition, some pharmaceutical manufacturers have free or reduced medication programs.

In Practice

Dr. Lopez has asked the medical assistant to schedule Sara Hardy for three followup visits, but Sara is not covered by insurance and states that she can afford just one visit. How should the medical assistant proceed?

Teaching Patients About Preventive Medicine

Studies have shown that if people practiced preventive medicine, they would greatly reduce the cost of healthcare in the United States. As discussed earlier in this chapter, preventive medicine, which includes mammograms or prostate exams, yearly physical exams, and scheduled immunizations for children, are personal choices that can affect life span. Medical assistants should promote health screenings to patients. They should keep educational literature available and ask patients about their last physical examinations to encourage screening appointments.

Preventing Medication Errors

Medication errors are far too common and are mostly preventable. Medical assistants can help prevent such errors by properly teaching patients about their medications. Patients do

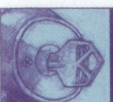

Keys to Success
PREVENTING CHILDHOOD INJURIES AND INJURIES IN THE ELDERLY

Preventable injuries are the leading cause of childhood death in the United States. Medical assistants working in family practices or pediatric offices should have educational materials on how to keep children safe and distribute them to new parents. Simple tips for preventing choking, drowning accidents, and fire hazards can help prevent tragedies.

Falls are common with the elderly, and they are preventable. Practices that treat elderly patients should distribute pamphlets detailing how to prevent falls. Such pamphlets should include details like removing throw rugs and ensuring steps are lined with slip-resistant material.

not always read the information the pharmacist gives them, and they sometimes fail to take time to consult with the pharmacist. Figure 6-6 ◆ is a sample medication-teaching tool that can be implemented in any medical office.

Dieting and Weight-Loss Information

Because patients will ask for information on dieting or weight loss, medical assistants should have information on hand to teach basic nutrition. This information should include copies of the new food guide (MyPyramid) and information on reading food labels (Figure 6-7 ◆). The MyPyramid food guide outlines the types of foods and food groups that are necessary for a balanced diet. Many people are unaware of the proper foods to eat to maintain a healthy lifestyle and giving this information to patients is one way to help them make healthy changes in their diet. However, the physician must authorize any information given to patients. A more detailed discussion of nutrition and how to read a food label can be found in ∞ Chapter 42, Gastroenterology and Nutrition.

Information on Exercise

Teaching patients about exercise is a common task. Medical assistants should have pamphlets on the benefits of exercise. Patients must be taught the importance of easing into exercise

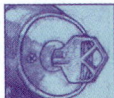

Keys to Success
IS THE INFORMATION PRACTICAL FOR THE PATIENT'S LIFESTYLE?

Be sure to think or ask about patients' lifestyles before teaching them about the medications they need to take. For example, does the patient work nights? If a prescription says to take a medication three times per day, does that mean the patient must rise in the middle of the night? Ensure patients understand how to administer medications and know the proper administration routes.

```
Name of
medication:_____

Dosage:_____

You will be taking this medication _____ times each
day.

This medication is being prescribed for the following
health condition:_____

Possible side effects of this medication include:
_____

If you experience any of the following signs or symp-
toms, please call the office right away:_____
_____
```

Figure 6-6 ◆ Sample medication teaching tool.

programs, how to stretch and warm up properly, and how to keep from injuring themselves. Patients over age 35 or with any underlying health conditions should seek the advice of their physician before beginning any new exercise program.

Stress Reduction

Most people are under various levels of stress every day. Sometimes, that stress gets too high to handle, and it impedes health. Having information on how to handle and reduce stress is one tool to help patients to maintain good health. Many physicians suggest their patients find a mechanism for reducing stress that works best for that patient's lifestyle. Some ideas for stress reduction are the following:

- Breathing exercises. Deep, slow breathing is believed to relax the muscles, oxygenate the blood, and calm the mind.
- Meditation. This technique goes a step further than deep breathing exercises. With meditation, the mind is literally focused on nothing—taking the stressful thoughts or situation out of mind for a period of time.
- Guided imagery. This technique is taught to women who take childbirth education classes. With this technique, the patient closes her eyes and focuses on a pleasant situation.
- Visualization. Taking guided imagery one step further, visualization is the technique of thinking of a task that needs to be done and thinking of doing it well. During a stressful situation, this technique might be used to visualize a resolution that is less stressful.
- Exercise. Many people find that exercise has the benefit of reducing stress.

- Sex. Although in stressful situations many people tend to have less sex, physicians recommend sex as a stress reliever.
- Music. Listening to relaxing music is a well-known mechanism for reducing stress levels.
- Yoga. This type of exercise incorporates breathing techniques and imagery, which can greatly reduce a person's stress level.

Smoking and Substance Abuse

Patients who smoke or abuse other substances will sometimes ask for help in stopping. Therefore, medical assistants should have information that has been approved by the physician on hand to give to patients to let them know what resources are available, both locally and nationally or on the Internet. The American Cancer Society (**ACS**) Web site (www.cancer.org) contains valuable resources for persons who wish to quit smoking. The ACS points out that tobacco addiction is both psychological and physical. For this reason, most persons who wish to quit smoking may need to try some combination of medicine, some method to change personal habits, and some level of emotional support. On the ACS website, patients or healthcare professionals can find links to information on the following:

- Using nicotine replacement therapy
- Various nicotine substitutes
- Choosing the right method to quit smoking
- Telephone support to help stop smoking
- Information on support groups
- Information about success rates

Anatomy of MyPyramid

One size doesn't fit all
USDA's new MyPyramid symbolizes a personalized approach to healthy eating and physical activity. The symbol has been designed to be simple. It has been developed to remind consumers to make healthy food choices and to be active every day. The different parts of the symbol are described below.

Activity
Activity is represented by the steps and the person climbing them, as a reminder of the importance of daily physical activity.

Moderation
Moderation is represented by the narrowing of each food group from bottom to top. The wider base stands for foods with little or no solid fats or added sugars. These should be selected more often. The narrower top area stands for foods containing more added sugars and solid fats. The more active you are, the more of these foods you can fit into your diet.

Personalization
Personalization is shown by the person on the steps, the slogan, and the URL. Find the kinds and amounts of food to eat each day at MyPyramid.gov.

Proportionality
Proportionality is shown by the different widths of the food group bands. The widths suggest how much food a person should choose from each group. The widths are just a general guide, not exact proportions. Check the website for how much is right for you.

Variety
Variety is symbolized by the 6 color bands representing the 5 food groups of the Pyramid and oils. This illustrates that foods from all groups are needed each day for good health.

Gradual Improvement
Gradual improvement is encouraged by the slogan. It suggests that individuals can benefit from taking small steps to improve their diet and lifestyle each day.

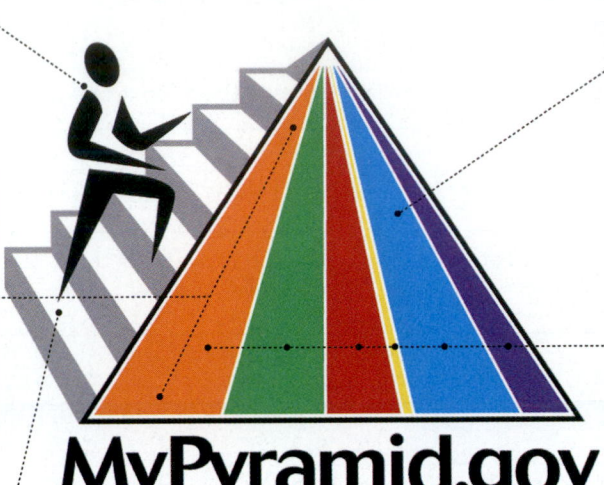

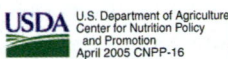

GRAINS   VEGETABLES   FRUITS   OILS   MILK   MEAT& BEANS

USDA U.S. Department of Agriculture Center for Nutrition Policy and Promotion April 2005 CNPP-16

USDA is an equal opportunity provider and employer.

Figure 6-7 ◆ MyPyramid food guide.

The National Institute on Drug Abuse (**NIDA**) maintains a Web site (www.nida.nih.gov) that contains a wealth of information on drug abuse and addiction. There the patient or healthcare professional will find information and resources for combating the abuse of these:

- Alcohol
- Club drugs
- Cocaine
- Heroin
- Inhalants
- LSD
- Marijuana
- Ectasy
- Methamphetamine
- PCP

- Prescription medications
- Tobacco
- Anabolic steroids

Using the Internet for Education

The Internet has patient education materials, but the medical assistant should use only reputable Web sites to gather information on conditions, medications, or illnesses (Table 6-4). Reputable Web sites are typically those that are associated with a university or college, the government, reputable news sources, such as CNN, and nonprofit organizations. Web sites that are maintained as "personal sites"—sites that are created and maintained by one person containing that person's beliefs—are not typically considered a reputable source for patient education materials. The physician should approve any material before the assistant gives it to patients.

TABLE 6-4 REPUTABLE WEB SITES FOR PATIENT EDUCATION

Web Site	Information
American Lung Association	Smoking cessation, asthma, hay fever, lung cancer (www.lungusa.org)
American Diabetes Associations	Nutrition and recipes, weight loss and exercise, diabetes prevention (www.diabetes.org)
Hospice	Guides for caregivers of and patients with terminal illnesses, talking to children about death, pain control, advance directives, finding a local hospice, healing after a loss (www.americanhospice.org)
American Heart Association	High blood pressure, controlling cholesterol levels, diet and nutrition (www.americanheart.org)
Alzheimer's Association	Living with Alzheimer's, guides for caregivers (www.alz.org)
American Parkinson Disease Association	Local support groups (www.apdaparkinson.org)
ALS Association	Local support groups, guides for caregivers (www.alsa.org)

PROCEDURE 6-1 Use the Internet to Find Patient Education Materials

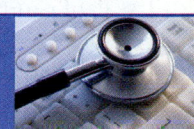

Theory and Rationale

Locating educational resources on the Internet is a fast way to find information. Often, the information can be printed and distributed to patients or incorporated into an educational piece created by the medical office.

Materials

- Computer and printer
- Patient chart
- Blue or black pen

Competency

(**Conditions**) With the necessary materials, you will be able to (**Task**) use the Internet to find patient education materials (**Standards**) correctly within the time limit set by the instructor.

1. Using the computer, locate reputable Web sites for desired materials.
2. Print copies of materials.
3. Show materials to the physician for approval.
4. Give/mail the materials to the patient.
5. Explain the materials to the patient as needed.
6. Place a copy of the materials in the patient's file.
7. Document how the materials were given to the patient and any verbal education provided with the materials.

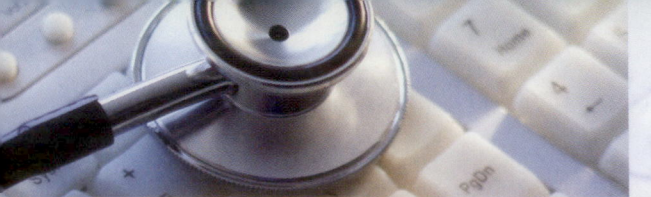

REVIEW

Chapter Summary

- Wellness is the ongoing process of practicing a healthy lifestyle.
- Holistic medicine addresses the whole patient and his or her needs. It involves the patient in making informed decisions about the course of treatment.
- Pain may be acute (short-term) or chronic (long-term). Chronic pain is the most serious and debilitating.
- Types of pain include physical, psychological, and phantom. Physical pain, as a symptom of disease process, inflammation, or trauma, serves as a protective mechanism by causing the person to seek medical attention. Psychological pain, while very real, is rarely caused by a pathological process but by a mental or emotional condition. Phantom pain occurs after the amputation of a body part. For a period of time the patient continues to feel pain as if the body part were still attached.
- Pain can be measured in three ways. The numerical scale ranges between 0 (no pain) and 10 (severe pain). The face scale is a series of faces ranging from happy to unhappy. On a picture of the body, front and back, the patient points to the location of pain.
- Pain is managed with medication, comfort measures, alternative therapies, exercise, surgery, or a combination of methods.
- An important part of an MA's job is patient teaching. The patient should understand the cause of the pain as well as how to manage it safely.
- The medical assistant is a key figure in educating the patient in the medical facility.
- Proper communication is critical to providing the patient with proper education.
- The medical assistant must verify with the physician the appropriateness of any educational materials that will be used to educate patients.
- Part of acting as the patient's advocate includes spending the appropriate amount of time assessing the patient's needs before, during, and after the education process.

Chapter Review

Multiple Choice

1. Which of the following is most likely a risk factor?
   a. Yoga
   b. Brisk walking
   c. Lower cholesterol
   d. High blood pressure

2. Positive emotions cause the brain to release proteins called
   a. endorphins.
   b. afferent neurons.
   c. efferent neurons.
   d. ganglia.

3. Phantom pain most likely occurs
   a. after strenuous exercise.
   b. before surgery.
   c. after an amputation.
   d. before resting.

4. Which of the following questions can you ask to assess a patient's pain?
   a. Are you sure you're in pain?
   b. Why didn't you come into the office sooner with this pain?
   c. How frequently does the pain occur?
   d. Do you really think the pain is serious?

5. Comfort measures for chronic pain include
   a. chiropractic treatments.
   b. heat and cold therapy.
   c. medications.
   d. surgery.

6. Controlled substances prescribed for chronic pain require the patient to
   a. schedule an appointment for the next prescription.
   b. call the office for a refill of the prescription.
   c. increase the dosage if the pain gets worse.
   d. seek alternative therapy.

7. Which of the following methods helps the patient to understand instructions?
   a. Speaking slowly and clearly
   b. Writing the instructions down
   c. Giving the patient time to ask questions
   d. All of the above

8. Which of the following healthcare members will the patient frequently share the most information with?
   a. The physician
   b. The medical assistant
   c. The nurse
   d. The receptionist

9. Which of the following are types of pain a patient may present with?
   a. Physical
   b. Psychological
   c. Phantom
   d. All of the above

Chapter Review (continued)

10. Which of the following resources might be valuable to your patient in the education process?
    a. Providing her with a local support group
    b. Providing her with educational pamphlets
    c. Providing her with links to online resources
    d. All of the above

True/False

T F   1. Pain is manifested only in physical complaints and does not affect mental ability.

T F   2. All types of stress have a negative impact on overall health.

T F   3. The Internet is a good source of information for educational materials you can provide to your patient.

T F   4. Your patient is on medications to control chronic pain. He had a particularly rough weekend and took an additional dose of medication. You may go ahead and refill the next prescription one day early to compensate for the change.

T F   5. All risk factors can be changed regardless of genetic predisposition.

T F   6. Challenging your mind frequently leads to additional stress and should be avoided in order to maintain a healthy lifestyle.

T F   7. It is important to use a reputable Web site when collecting patient education materials.

T F   8. Wellness is the ongoing process of practicing a healthy lifestyle.

T F   9. It is important for a patient to know how to manage pain safely and effectively.

T F 10. People's lifestyles are based on their personal attitudes, experiences, and role models.

Short Answer

1. Which motor nerves carry impulses from the central nervous system to the peripheral nervous system?

2. Sometimes severed nerve endings feel as if they are still receiving stimuli from the amputated part, causing painful sensations. What is this phenomenon called?

3. What kind of pain is felt in a different area from the injured or diseased part of the body?

4. What is the difference between acute and chronic pain?

5. What is the term for proteins in the brain that have analgesic properties?

Research

1. In your local area, what phone number(s) can patients call for assistance to stop smoking?

2. Where can patients find out about low-cost exercise programs in your community? Are any offered at the local YMCA or college?

3. In your local area, is there a pain management clinic for inpatient and outpatient treatment, or are patients treated by their primary care providers?

Externship Application Experience

Serena Milsom is a student medical assistant performing her externship in a pediatric practice. Serena is working with Marie, a 5-year-old child who is with her mother. Serena needs to teach Marie and her mother how to take care of the cast the doctor has applied to Marie's broken wrist. How should Serena go about accomplishing this task?

Resource Guide

ALS Association
27001 Agoura Road, Suite 150
Calabasas Hills, CA 91301
(818) 880-9007
www.alsa.org

Alzheimer's Association
225 N. Michigan Avenue, Floor 17
Chicago, IL 60601
(312) 335-5886
www.alz.org

American Diabetes Association
ATTN: National Call Center
1701 North Beauregard Street
Alexandria, VA 22311
1-800-DIABETES
www.diabetes.org

American Heart Association
7272 Greenville Avenue
Dallas, TX 75231
1-800-AHA-USA-1
www.americanheart.org

Resource Guide (continued)

American Holistic Health Association
P.O. Box 17400
Anaheim, CA 92817-7400
(714) 779-6152
www.ahha.org

American Lung Association
61 Broadway, 6th Floor
New York, NY 10006
1-800-LUNGUSA
www.lungusa.org

American Parkinson Disease Association
135 Parkinson Avenue
Staten Island, NY 10305
1-800-223-2732
www.apdaparkinson.org

Hospice
American Hospice Foundation
2120 L Street NW, Suite 200
Washington, DC 20037
1-800-347-1413
www.americanhospice.org

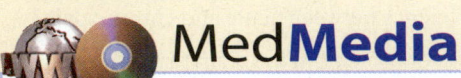

Med**Media**

http://www.MyMAKit.com

More on this chapter, including interactive resources, can be found on the Student CD-ROM accompanying this textbook and on http://www.MyMAKit.com.

Objectives

After completing this chapter, you should be able to:

- Define and spell the key terminology in this chapter.
- Define the medical assistant's role as it relates to extended life and terminal care.
- Discuss organ donation concepts, criteria, and resources for information.
- Discuss the selection of transplant recipients.
- Explain the uniform donor card and its importance.
- Summarize the Uniform Anatomical Gift Act.
- Explain how the 1987 amendments to the Social Security Act impact reimbursement for inpatient services.
- Discuss advance medical directives and the durable power of attorney in healthcare.
- Discuss living wills and life-prolonging declarations.
- Provide information regarding hospice.

Considerations of Extended Life

Case Study

One weekend, while home from college, Ori sat with his family watching a television special about organ transplants. Ori mentioned that when he renewed his driver's license, he had chosen to become an organ donor. Ori's younger sister said that she, too, wanted to be a donor as soon as she turned 18, because she felt it was important to help others, even in death.

Their mother, Katrina, said vehemently that she would not allow either of her children to be organ donors.

"Well, you can't stop me. I'm an adult now!" Ori shouted.

"Yes, I can, and I certainly will!" replied his mother. She went on to explain that if they got into an accident they would not be saved. It was her belief that rescue workers did not perform CPR or other life-saving measures on people who were known organ donors because it would be easier and less expensive for the hospital to just let them die and take the organs later.

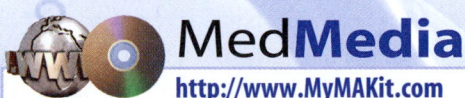

Med**Media**
http://www.MyMAKit.com

Additional interactive resources and activities for this chapter can be found on http://www.MyMAKit.com. For a video, audio glossary, legal and ethical scenarios, job scenarios, quizzes, tips, and games related to the content of this chapter, please access the accompanying CD-ROM in this book.

Video
Audio Glossary
Legal and Ethical Scenario: *Considerations of Extended Life*
On the Job Scenario: *Considerations of Extended Life*
Multiple Choice Quiz
Games: Crossword, Strikeout, and Spelling Bee
HIPAA
Tips

Key Terminology

cadaver—dead body

hospice—facility or program that provides care for the terminally ill in a home setting or hospice center

ischemic—pertaining to a decreased blood supply to tissue due to impaired circulation to the organ or part

organ—a group of tissues making up a structure that has a particular function in the body

palliative—relieving pain or discomfort

tissue—a group of cells that act together for a particular body function

Abbreviations

DNR—do not resuscitate

✚ MEDICAL ASSISTING STANDARDS

CAAHEP ENTRY-LEVEL STANDARDS	ABHES ENTRY-LEVEL COMPETENCIES
■ Perform within scope of practice (psychomotor) ■ Apply ethical behaviors, including honesty/integrity in performance of medical assisting practice (affective) ■ Apply active listening skills (affective) ■ Practice within the standard of care for a medical assistant (psychomotor) ■ Identify styles and types of verbal communication (cognitive) ■ Identify nonverbal communication (cognitive) ■ Explore issue of confidentiality as it applies to the medical assistant (cognitive) ■ Respond to issues of confidentiality (psychomotor) ■ Demonstrate sensitivity to patient rights (affective) ■ Document accurately in the patient record (psychomotor) ■ Demonstrate respect for individual diversity, incorporating awareness of one's own biases in areas including gender, race, religion, age, and economic status (affective) ■ Develop and maintain a current list of community resources related to patients' healthcare needs (psychomotor) ■ Apply local, state and federal health care legislation and regulation appropriate to the medical assisting practice setting (psychomotor) ■ Recognize the importance of local, state and federal legislation and regulations in the practice setting (affective)	■ Project a positive attitude. ■ Maintain confidentiality at all times. ■ Be a team player. ■ Be cognizant of ethical boundaries. ■ Exhibit initiative. ■ Adapt to change. ■ Evidence a responsible attitude. ■ Be courteous and diplomatic. ■ Conduct work within scope of education, training, and ability. ■ Be attentive, listen, and learn. ■ Be impartial and show empathy when dealing with patients. ■ Serve as a liaison between physician and others. ■ Use appropriate medical terminology. ■ Recognize and respond to verbal and nonverbal communication. ■ Adapt to individualized needs. ■ Instruct patients with special needs.

Introduction

New treatment technologies and techniques have significantly advanced medical care, particularly in the field of organ and tissue transplantation. Legal and educational strides in the area of organ donation have raised public awareness and interest.

While transplantation improves the quality of life, life-prolonging measures have raised quality-of-life questions. A living will allows a healthy person or a person with a terminal disease or catastrophic injury to state his or her wishes about prolonging life. A durable power of attorney for healthcare tells the physician and the family that if the patient is no longer mentally competent, the appointed person with power of attorney can make decisions regarding medical care in the patient's best interest. Hospice is an alternative to hospitalization for the terminal patient who wishes to die in comfort and with dignity.

The Medical Assistant's Role in Extended Life Care

The medical assistant must be aware of the rules regarding organ and tissue donations and transplants. Patients who need organ transplants or want to know about organ donation may ask the medical assistant for information. The MA may also be asked about medical directives, durable power of attorney for healthcare, living wills, and life-prolonging declarations. The MA will direct the patient and family to the proper sources of information, such as physicians, nurses, brochures, and Internet sites. Documenting the patient's questions and understanding the information provided is another responsibility.

Organ and Tissue Donations

Modern technology and scientific advances have made it possible to endow very ill people with the gift of life through other people's organs and tissues. It is now possible for one donor to provide organs and tissue for as many as fifty recipients. Table 7-1 lists organs and tissues that may be donated and transplanted.

Organ transplantation has been performed for over a century. Table 7-2 lists the highlights of this life-saving procedure's history.

Organ and Tissue Harvesting

Removal of organs or tissues is based on three factors:

1. Source of the donation—**cadaver** or live donor
2. Waiting period—cold **ischemic** (the body is in refrigeration in a morgue) or warm ischemic (the body is not refrigerated)
3. Removal order

Certain **tissues,** inner parts of the bone and ear, skin, corneas, connective tissue, and veins can be harvested (removed) from a donor who has been pronounced dead. Tissue compatibility must be determined before transplanting to reduce the chances of rejection by the recipient's body. The tissues may be removed some time after circulation and respiration have ceased. Warm ischemic time, however, cannot exceed four hours; cold ischemic time twelve hours. The cornea, for example, remains suitable for removal for transplantation when harvested within approximately six hours after the donor's heart has stopped beating.

One method of processing donated tissue is cryopreservation, in which tissues are frozen at a super cold temperature. The processor makes arrangements to transport the tissue to the tissue procurement organization. In some facilities the local medical examiner or coroner can release tissue for transplant when residual tissue can be returned for examination. An alternative is having a pathologist do a complete pathological tissue study.

Organs such as the heart, lungs, kidneys, liver, pancreas, stomach, and intestines must be harvested after the patient has been pronounced brain dead. The donor must have sustained brain death under circumstances in which respiration and circulation can be supported artificially, by means of ventilators and medications. The heart is removed first, then the other organs, as quickly as possible.

Live donors may donate certain tissues, bone marrow, stem cells, cord blood, kidneys, or a portion of the liver.

Donation Issues and Concerns

There is generally very little religious objection to organ or tissue donation. Most religions view donation as morally and ethically acceptable as long as it benefits individuals and society

TABLE 7-1 BODY PARTS THAT MAY BE DONATED

Tissues	Organs
Skin	Heart
Heart valves	Lungs
Bone	Liver
Corneas	Kidney
Islet cells	Pancreas
Bone marrow	Stomach
Stem cells	Small and large intestines
Cord blood	
Saphenous (leg) veins	
Tendons and ligaments	

TABLE 7-2 A SHORT HISTORY OF ORGAN TRANSPLANTATION

1905	First successful cornea transplant.
1933	First human-to-human kidney transplant (the kidney never functioned).
1954	First successful kidney transplant, identical twins.
1963	First successful lung transplant.
1967	First successful liver transplant.
1967	First heart transplant in South Africa.
1968	First successful heart transplant in the United States.
1968	Uniform Anatomical Gift Act passed.
1978	Uniform Brain Death Act passed, defining death as brain death.
1981	First successful heart/lung transplant.
1983	First anti-rejection drug approved for use.
1984	National Organ Transplant Act (NOTA) passed.
1986	Require Request Laws passed.
1989	First successful living-related liver transplant.
1990	First successful living-related lung transplant.
1991	First successful small intestine transplant.

and helps to ease the suffering of others. Jehovah's Witnesses, who do not believe in blood transfusions, do not object to organ and tissue transplants as long as all the blood has been removed before transplantation.

Obstacles to donation include distrust, fear of premature death, language differences, and family involvement. Some cultures may forbid organ donation because they believe the body should remain intact for burial.

? — Critical Thinking Question 7-1 —

How should Ori try to educate his mother about the process of organ donation?

In the United States, the sale and purchase of tissue and organs is prohibited. The donor's physician or the physician who pronounces the donor dead should not be involved in any part of the harvest procedure. The United Network for Organ Sharing (UNOS) is the agency that oversees tissue and organ harvest, preparation and testing of the tissue or organ, and storage and distribution of the tissue or organ. The cost of the harvest procedure is not passed on to the donor's family but is usually covered by the facility harvesting the tissue or organ or the regional organ procurement organization.

? — Critical Thinking Question 7-2 —

As you read in the case study, Ori's mother believes that hospitals save money if they let patients die and harvest organs later. Explain why the hospital cannot receive monetary compensation for organs. Also explain the difference between time frames in cold ischemic and warm ischemic donations.

When the organ or tissue comes from a live donor, it may go to a designated recipient. For example, if a mother is a match for a child who is experiencing kidney failure, she can donate her kidney to her child. The organ does not go into the general program.

In most states there is a statement on the front or the back of the driver's license that a person may sign declaring

Keys to Success
DONOR INFORMATION

Although there is no longer a specific age limit for donors, the recommended age is between birth and 75 years. The health and condition of the donor and of the organs and tissue at the time of death influence the suitability of the donation. Organs are harvested in such a way as to preserve the appearance of the body. Harvesting the heart may make the embalming procedure a little more difficult, but it can be done.

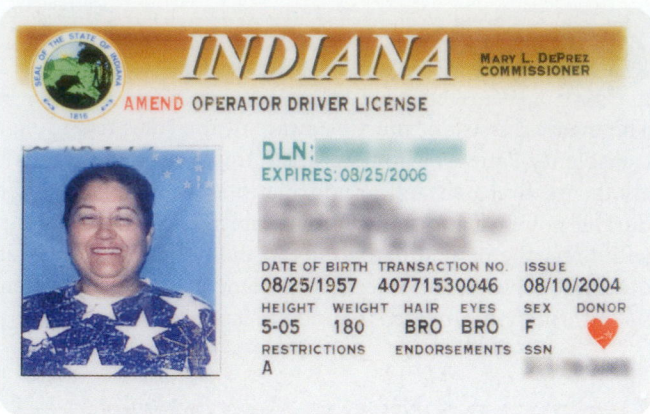

Figure 7-1 ◆ Individuals may declare their wish to be a tissue or organ donor on their driver's license.

his or her wish to be a tissue or organ donor at the time of death (Figure 7-1 ◆). The person may designate what tissue or organs may be harvested. This statement is only a statement of intent, however, and may be overridden by the next of kin in most states. Usually the next of kin makes the final decision.

Most states consider a signed universal donor card a legal document permitting the procurement of organs and tissue (Figure 7-2 ◆). However, some states require a signature on a universal donor card in addition to a signature on the back of a driver's license. Also, many institutions request permission from family members before procuring any organs. The decision

---

Organ Donor Card

I, _____, hereby make the following anatomical gift, if medically acceptable, to take effect upon my death.

_____Any organs or parts _____Entire body

Only the following specific organs or parts:

_____

Limitations or special wishes if any:

_____

(Signatures of donor and witnesses appear on reverse side.)

Front of card

Organ Donor Card (side two)

Signed by the donor and the following two witnesses in the presence of each other.

Donor Signature: _____

Date of Birth: _____ Date signed: _____

City and State: _____

Witness Signature: _____

Witness Signature: _____

This is a legal document under the Uniform Anatomical Gift Act or similar laws.

Back of card

Figure 7-2 ◆ Universal donor card.

is granted to a family member or guardian in the following order of priority:

1. Spouse
2. Adult son or daughter
3. Either parent
4. Adult sibling
5. Grandparent
6. Guardian

However, if the decedent, prior to the time of death, has indicated a refusal to make an organ donation, the institution or healthcare provider must honor that decision.

Sometimes a family member lower on the priority list may object to the donation. Most institutions abide by the wishes of the family and do not harvest any tissue or organs if all members are not in agreement.

 **— Critical Thinking Question 7-3 —**
Can Ori's mother disregard his signed intent to be an organ donor and refuse to allow the hospital to harvest organs upon his death?

Transplant Costs

Medical costs for transplants can include:

- Pretransplant evaluation and testing
- Hospital stay and surgical charges
- Followup care and testing
- Additional hospitalizations for complications or rejection
- Charges for anti-rejection drugs and other drug therapy
- Physicians' fees (including surgeons, radiologists, anesthesiologists, and pathologists)
- Procurement fees
- Rehabilitation, including physical, occupational, and vocational rehabilitation
- Insurance co-pays or deductibles

Out-of-pocket expenses include:

- Transportation to and from the transplant facility before, during, and after the transplant
- Food, lodging, and telephone charges for both the patient and the family
- Any childcare
- Lost wages for patient and family members

Patients must research the full cost(s) for a transplant procedure. Medicaid and many insurance policies do not cover transplants.

Organ and Tissue Donation Rules and Regulations

Many states have laws regarding the declared intent to donate body tissues or organs upon death. In the past, laws varied among the states and some states had no laws at all in this area. To address this inconsistency, the National Conference of Commissioners on Uniform State Laws approved the Uniform Anatomical Gift Act in 1968.

Uniform Anatomical Gift Act

As transplant methods advanced, the supply of donor organs and tissues was not meeting the demand. In 1987 the Uniform Anatomical Gift Act was updated with statutes to educate the public to the need for donated organs and tissues. Greater public awareness has since increased donations.

The Uniform Anatomical Gift Act includes the following rules:

- The donor must be at least 18 years old.
- The intent to donate must be made in writing.
- The donor may designate specific organs or tissue for transplantation, the entire body for research or transplantation, or any acceptable organs or tissues.
- The donor's valid statement takes precedence over other individuals' wishes except when an autopsy is required by law.
- If the donor has not acted during his or her lifetime, the survivors, in a specified order of priority, may act on the donor's behalf.
- If aware of the donor's wishes, the attending physician may dispose of the body under the act.
- The physician accepting the donor's organs in good faith is protected from lawsuits.
- The death of the donor may not be determined by any physician involved in the transplantation.
- The donor may revoke the intent to donate, or the gift may be refused by the recipient or by the healthcare provider (physician or facility).
- No financial arrangements can be made for donated organs.

Hospitals

A 1987 amendment to the Social Security Act requires written protocols, or sets of rules, from hospitals participating in Medicare or Medicaid that "assure that families of potential organ donors are made aware of the option of organ or tissue donation and their option to decline." Also, "No discussion or request is necessary if the medical record discloses a prior gift or a refusal to make a gift or if the gift would not be suitable according to accepted medical standards."

Hospitals generally ask certain routine questions during the admission procedure. They are now required to ask about organ donation in order to identify potential organ donors. With the consent of the attending physician, they are required to discuss organ donation with a person who answers in the negative.

When a patient agrees to donate, a request is made to see and document the organ donor card, driver's license, or other documentation of the intent to donate. Then it must be determined if there are any limitations (for example, a donor may wish to donate only his or her eyes or to donate for a single purpose, such as transplantation but not research). A copy is placed in the patient's medical record as evidence of a valid gift to be effective at death. This requirement is mandatory only during the admission process to hospitals.

Physicians are encouraged to ask their patients about donation. Hospitals are encouraged to ask patients who are scheduled for outpatient, emergency, or minor surgery, or any procedure that does not require being admitted to the hospital.

In 1998, the Organ Procurement and Transplant Network (OPTN) Final Rule was introduced by the Department of Health and Human Services. It requires that all hospitals performing transplants follow OPTN rules to receive Medicare or Medicaid reimbursement. Organ and tissue distribution was expanded from a local and regional system to a national system based on need. Also, three goals were established:

1. Minimum listing criteria establishing common guidelines for putting a patient on a waiting list.
2. Standard criteria for determining the medical status of a patient awaiting transplant, which allows a transplant center to release organs to patients with the most critical medical needs.
3. A reasonable collection policy permitting organs to be distributed over a larger geographic area, which has been made possible by newer methods of preserving organs for a longer period of time.

UNOS (United Network for Organ Sharing) established a national computer system for registering patients in need of transplants. Patient data entered into the system includes blood type, body size, medical urgency, length of time on the list, and tissue match. When a donor is identified, his or her data is entered to quickly find the closest matching candidate with the greatest need.

Tissue organizations process cardiovascular tissue, orthopedic tissue, and skin. The Food and Drug Administration (FDA) regulates tissue procurement, storage, and shipment.

Advance Medical Directives

Laws and guidelines for advance medical directives vary from state to state.

- *Advance medical directives* are signed legal documents in which an individual specifies his or her wishes concerning the provision of healthcare if he or she is ever in an incapacitated state.
- A *durable power of attorney for healthcare* tells the physician and the family that if the patient is no longer mentally competent, the appointed person with power of attorney can make decisions regarding medical care in the patient's best interests (Figure 7-3 ◆).

The patient should discuss these legal decisions with his or her family, the physician, and, if desired, with an attorney or clergy member. An attorney should be consulted to draft any documents and copies should be given to anyone who might be contacted in an emergency. The power of attorney can be revoked in writing.

Durable Power of Attorney for Healthcare

General guidelines for the appointment of a Durable Power of Attorney for Healthcare include the following (according to state law and requirements):

- The statement is voluntary, in writing, dated, and signed by the patient.
- If the patient is not capable of signing, another person may sign for the patient, in the patient's presence and at the patient's express direction.
- Two competent witnesses at least 18 years old, not related to the patient or responsible for the patient's healthcare, are usually required.
- The Power of Attorney must be notarized.
- Neither witness can sign on the patient's behalf.
- The person representing the patient must be at least 18 years old.
- The person representing the patient shall make decisions in the patient's best interest. The patient's family or physician cannot overrule the decisions without the court intervening.
- The appointment of this person becomes effective when the patient's physician certifies in writing that the patient is not able to consent.
- The appointment may be revoked by destroying the appointment document. Informing others in writing that the appointment is revoked will also revoke it. The final step in revoking the appointment is telling the physician. He or she must be aware of the revocation, or medical decisions will continue to be based on current knowledge of the durable power of attorney.

Living Wills

A living will is a document advising the physician of a person's wish to die naturally rather than be kept alive when death is inevitable (Figure 7-4 ◆). The living will may indicate treatments that should not be performed or treatments that should be terminated under clear circumstances. It can include a **DNR** order ("do not resuscitate"). Conditions of the declaration include certification in writing by the attending physician that:

- The patient has an incurable injury, disease, or illness.
- The patient's death will occur within a short time.
- Using life-prolonging procedures would serve only to artificially lengthen the dying process.

A provision in the will allows any medical procedure or medication necessary to provide comfort care and alleviate pain, even after other life-prolonging procedures have been withdrawn. Another possible provision addresses the wish to receive artificially supplied nutrition and hydration. If this provision is not included, the decision concerning nutrition and hydration will be made by the person with the power of attorney. States that do not honor living wills as legal documents recognize a person's right to decide to die naturally under the advance directive document.

POWER OF ATTORNEY FOR HEALTH CARE

(1) DESIGNATION OF AGENT: I designate the following individual as my agent to make health care decisions for me: _____
_____

(Name of individual you choose as agent)
_____

(address) (city) (state) (zip code)
_____

(home phone) (work phone)

OPTIONAL: If I revoke my agent's authority or if my agent is not willing, able, or reasonably available to make a health-care decision for me, I designate as my first alternate agent:
_____

(Name of individual you choose as first alternate agent)
_____

(address) (city) (state) (zip code)
_____

(home phone) (work phone)

OPTIONAL: If I revoke the authority of my agent and first alternate agent or if neither is willing, able, or reasonably available to make a health care decision for me, I designate as my second alternate agent:
_____

(Name of individual you choose as second alternate agent)
_____

(address) (city) (state) (zip code)
_____

(home phone) (work phone)

(2) AGENT'S AUTHORITY: My agent is authorized to make all health care decisions for me, including decisions to provide, withhold, or withdraw artificial nutrition and hydration, and all other forms of health care to keep me alive, **except** as I state here:

(3) WHEN AGENT'S AUTHORITY BECOMES EFFECTIVE: My agent's authority becomes effective when my primary physician determines that I am unable to make my own health care decisions unless I mark the following box. If I mark this box [ ], my agent's authority to make health care decisions for me takes effect immediately.

(4) AGENT'S OBLIGATION: My agent shall make health care decisions for me in accordance with this power of attorney for health care, any instructions I give below, and my other wishes to the extent known to my agent. To the extent my wishes are unknown, my agent shall make health care decisions for me in accordance with what my agent determines to be in my best interest. In determining my best interest, my agent shall consider my personal values to the extent known to my agent.

(5) AGENT'S POSTDEATH AUTHORITY: My agent is authorized to make anatomical gifts, authorize an autopsy, and direct disposition of my remains, except as I state here or elsewhere in this form:

INSTRUCTIONS FOR HEALTH CARE
Strike any wording you do not want.

(6) END-OF-LIFE DECISIONS: I direct that my health care providers and others involved in my care provide, withhold, or withdraw treatment in accordance with the choice I have marked below: **(Initial only one box)**
[ ] (a) **Choice NOT To Prolong Life**
I do not want my life to be prolonged if (1) I have an incurable and irreversible condition that will result in my death within a relatively short time, (2) I become unconscious and, to a reasonable degree of medical certainty, I will not regain consciousness, or (3) the likely risks and burdens of treatment would outweigh the expected benefits, **OR**
[ ] (b) **Choice To Prolong Life**
I want my life to be prolonged as long as possible within the limits of generally accepted health care standards.

(7) RELIEF FROM PAIN: Except as I state in the following space, I direct that treatment for alleviation of pain or discomfort should be provided at all times even if it hastens my death:

DONATION OF ORGANS AT DEATH
(8) Upon my death: (mark applicable box)
[ ] (a) I give any needed organs, tissues, or parts,
OR
[ ] (b) I give the following organs, tissues, or parts only: _____
[ ] (c) My gift is for the following purposes:
(strike any of the following you do not want)
(1) Transplant
(2) Therapy
(3) Research
(4) Education

(9) EFFECT OF COPY: A copy of this form has the same effect as the original.

(10) SIGNATURE: Sign and date the form here:

_____   _____
          (date)   (sign your name)

_____   _____
        (address)   (print your name)

_____   _____
          (city)   (state)

(11) WITNESSES: This advance health care directive will not be valid for making health care decisions unless it is either: (1) signed by two (2) qualified adult witnesses who are personally known to you and who are present when you sign or acknowledge your signature; or (2) acknowledged before a notary public.

Figure 7-3 ◆ Sample of power of attorney for healthcare.

Source: Ramont, Roberta Pavy, Niedrighaus, Dee Maldonado, Towle, Mary Ann, Comprehensive nursing care, © 2006, pp. 845, 900. Reprinted by permission of Pearson Education, Upper Saddle River, NJ.

LIVING WILL DECLARATION

Declaration made this _____ day of _____, 20_____ . I, _____ _____ being at least eighteen (18) years of age and of sound mind, willfully and voluntarily make known my desires that my dying shall not be artificially prolonged under the circumstances set forth below, and I declare:

If at any time my attending physician certifies in writing that: (1) I have an incurable injury, disease, or illness; (2) my death will occur within a short time; and (3) the use of life prolonging procedures would serve only to artificially prolong the dying process, I direct that such procedures be withheld or withdrawn, and that I be permitted to die naturally with only the performance or provision of any medical procedure or medication necessary to provide me with comfort care or to alleviate pain, and, if I have so indicated below, the provision of artificially supplied nutrition and hydration. (Indicate your choice by initialling or making your mark before signing this declaration):

_____ I wish to receive artificially supplied nutrition and hydration, even if the effort to sustain life is futile or excessively burdensome to me.

_____ I do not wish to receive artificially supplied nutrition and hydration, if the effort to sustain life is futile or excessively burdensome to me.

_____ I intentionally make no decision concerning artificially supplied nutrition and hydration, leaving the decision to my health care representative appointed under IC 16-36-1-7 or my attorney in fact with health care powers under IC 30-5-5.

In the absense of my ability to give directions regarding the use of life prolonging procedures, it is my intention that this declaration be honored by my family and physician as the final expression of my legal right to refuse medical or surgical treatment and accept the consequences of the refusal.

I understand the full import of this declaration.

I am a resident of

The declarant has been personally known to me, and I believe her to be of sound mind, I did not sign the declarant's signature above for or at the direction of the declarant. I am not a parent, spouse, or child of the declarant. I am not entitled to any part of the declarant's estate or directly financially responsible for the declarant's medical care. I am competent and at least eighteen (18) years of age.

_____
Witness Signature

_____
Printed Name

_____
Witness Signature

_____
Printed Name

_____
City and State of Residence

Date _____

_____
City and State of Residence

Date _____

Figure 7-4 ◆ Sample living will declaration.

Life-Prolonging Declarations

Some living wills include a "life-prolonging procedures" declaration, which states that the person wants healthcare providers to perform all possible life-prolonging medical treatments (Figure 7-5 ◆). As with other medical directives, the decision to sign this declaration should be made while the person is in good health and not under stress. The document must be signed, dated, and witnessed by two people over the age of 18 in advance of any hospitalization or admission to an inpatient facility. Furthermore, the decision should be discussed with family members, an attorney, and the physician. The patient's family and physician should be made aware of the declaration when it is completed. A copy should be placed in the patient's chart.

Life-Prolonging Procedures Declaration

Declaration made this _____ day of _____
(month, year). I, _____, being at least eighteen (18) years of age and of
sound mind, willfully and voluntarily make known my desire that if, at any time I have an incurable injury,
disease or illness determined to be a terminal condition, I request the use of life-prolonging procedures that
would extend my life. This includes appropriate nutrition and hydration, the administration of medication and
the performance of all other medical procedures necessary to extend my life, to provide comfort care or to
alleviate pain.

In the absence of my ability to give directions regarding the use of life-prolonging procedures, it is my
intention that this declaration be honored by my family and physician as the final expression of my legal
right to request medical or surgical treatment and accept the consequences of the request.

I understand the full import of this declaration.

Signed _____
City, Country, and State of Residence _____

_____

The declarant has been personally known to me, and I believe (him/her) to be of sound mind. I am
competent and at least eighteen (18) years of age.

Witness _____ Date _____
Witness _____ Date _____

Figure 7-5 ◆ Life-prolonging procedures declaration.
Source: Lutheran Health Network, Fort Wayne, Indiana. www.lutheranhealthnetwork.com

Hospice

During the nineteenth and early twentieth centuries, the terminally ill were cared for at home. With the advances in modern medicine and technology, many terminally ill patients are now cared for in hospitals, where multiple attempts are often made to extend their lives. These interventions often deny the patient the chance to die with dignity. Some patients are shocked or defibrillated, only to be kept alive in a vegetative state.

Hospice, an alternative to these interventions, originated in Europe. Hospice is a facility or program that provides care for the terminally ill in a home setting or hospice center. In 1974, the first hospice in the United States was established in New Haven, Connecticut. The objective is to improve the quality of the patient's last days by providing **palliative** care. No special interventions are used to prolong life. Pain medication is administered to keep the patient comfortable.

When the patient can no longer be cared for in the home setting, a long-term hospice center may be the next step. Family members care for the patient when they are able to do so. A team-oriented approach involves both family and professionals who offer emotional, social, and spiritual support to both the patient and the family along with bereavement counseling.

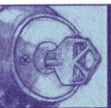

Keys to Success
PROVIDING INFORMATION

Medical assistants should acquire written information concerning tissue and organ donation, universal donor cards, living wills, advance medical directives, and durable power of attorney for health care. They should create an information file for the office to provide resource material for other staff and patients as needed.

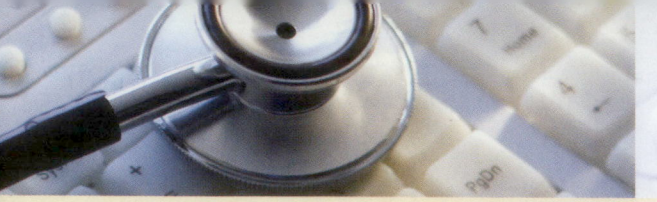

REVIEW

Chapter Summary

- Organ and tissue donation has become increasingly common with new breakthroughs in transplantation.
- An MA should be familiar with advanced medical directives, durable power of attorney for healthcare, living wills, and life-prolonging declarations in order to answer patients' questions. An MA should also understand how organs and tissues are harvested.
- Some organs and tissues are harvested after a patient has died. Others are harvested after the patient has been pronounced brain dead but respiration and circulation have been supported artificially. Living donors can donate certain organs and tissues.
- Patients should research transplant costs. They include medical costs, such as hospital stay and surgery, and out-of-pocket expenses, such as child care and lost wages.
- The Uniform Anatomical Gift Act governs organ donation.
- Hospitals must have written protocols concerning informing families of the option to donate and the option to decline.
- Organs and tissues are distributed via a national computer system. Donors and recipients are matched as closely as possible to avoid rejection of the tissue or organ. Distribution is also based on critical need.
- A durable power of attorney tells a physician and family that if the patient is no longer mentally competent, a person appointed by the patient has the power of attorney to make decisions for him or her.
- A living will is a document declaring a person's wish to die naturally.
- A life-prolonging declaration indicates that the person wants all possible medical treatment used to prolong his or her life.
- Hospice offers an alternative way for the terminally ill to die with dignity. The patient may be cared for at home or in a hospice center.

Chapter Review

Multiple Choice

1. Which of the following tissues can be transplanted?
   a. Pancreas
   b. Small intestine
   c. Large intestine
   d. Bone

2. Warm ischemic time cannot exceed
   a. 1 hour.
   b. 4 hours.
   c. 2 hours.
   d. 3 hours.

3. Cold ischemic time cannot exceed
   a. 4 hours.
   b. 8 hours.
   c. 10 hours.
   d. 12 hours.

4. Which of the following organs and tissues can be harvested after a donor has died and circulation and respiration have ceased?
   a. Pancreas
   b. Small intestine
   c. Corneas
   d. Kidney

5. Which of the following is true about a physician who pronounces the donor dead?
   a. The physician should not be involved in any part of the harvesting process.
   b. The physician should be involved in all parts of the harvesting process.
   c. The physician can oversee the harvesting by another physician.
   d. The physician cannot oversee harvesting but can oversee distribution.

6. A live donor understands that he or she
   a. cannot designate who receives the organ or tissue.
   b. can designate who receives the organ or tissue.
   c. is required to have a donor card.
   d. is responsible for all costs, including the patient's cost.

7. The updated version of the Uniform Anatomical Gift Act includes
   a. the ability to sue a physician who accepts the donor's organs in good faith.
   b. the provision that the donor may not revoke the donation.
   c. acceptable financial arrangements for donated organs.
   d. measures to raise awareness of the need for donated organs and tissue.

8. A durable power of attorney for healthcare allows
   a. a terminally ill patient to die naturally without life-prolonging medical procedures.
   b. a terminally ill patient to receive all possible life-prolonging medical treatments.
   c. an appointed person to make decisions for a patient who is no longer mentally capable.
   d. an appointed person to refuse any medication or treatment that eases the patient's pain.

Chapter Review (continued)

9. A living will allows
   a. a terminally ill patient to receive all possible life-prolonging medical treatments.
   b. a terminally ill patient to die naturally without life-prolonging medical procedures.
   c. an appointed person to make decisions for a patient who is no longer mentally capable.
   d. an appointed person to refuse any medication or treatment that eases the patient's pain.

10. Hospice is
    a. an alternative to hospital care.
    b. life-prolonging care.
    c. an alternative to home and family care.
    d. a transplantation care center.

True/False

T F   1. Hospitals must have written protocols about informing families of the option to donate organs and the option to decline.

T F   2. Due to advances in modern medicine and technology, many terminally ill patients are now cared for in hospitals, where multiple attempts are often made to extend their lives.

T F   3. If the decedent, prior to the time of death, indicated a refusal to make an organ donation, the institution or healthcare provider can choose not to honor that decision if the decedent had previously signed an organ donation card.

T F   4. The United Network for Organ Sharing (UNOS) is the agency that provides financing options for the family of the decedent making an organ donation.

T F   5. When a living will is signed advising the physician of a person's wish to die naturally rather than be kept alive when death is inevitable, the patient loses the right to receive any medication, including pain control.

Short Answer

1. What is a living will?

2. What is an alternative to hospitalization for the terminally ill patient who wishes to die in comfort and with dignity?

3. How many recipients can one donor provide organs and tissue for?

4. In which method of processing donated tissue are tissues frozen at a super cold temperature?

5. List the organs that must be harvested after the patient has been pronounced brain dead.

Research

1. Where do patients in your community go to have a living will drawn up? Must they use an attorney, or does someone offer this service free of charge?

2. Find the phone number and address of a local hospice your patients can utilize.

3. In your state, is the signed universal donor card a legal document permitting the procurement of organs and tissue? Does your state also require a signature on a universal donor card in addition to the signature on the back of the driver's license?

Externship Application Experience

A patient comes to the office to inquire about becoming a tissue and organ donor. She explains that her friend has been put on a waiting list for a heart and she wants information on how she and her family members can become donors upon their death. What would you, as the medical assistant, do in this situation?

Resource Guide

Hospice Foundation of America
1621 Connecticut Ave., NW, Suite 300
Washington, DC 20009
1-800-854-3402
www.hospicefoundation.org

International Association for Organ Donation
PO Box 545
Dearborn, MI 48121-0545
313-745-2235
www.iaod.org

United Network for Organ Sharing (UNOS)
PO Box 2484
Richmond, VA 23218
804-782-4800
www.unos.org

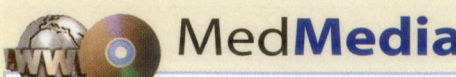

MedMedia

http://www.MyMAKit.com

More on this chapter, including interactive resources, can be found on the Student CD-ROM accompanying this textbook and on http://www.MyMAKit.com.

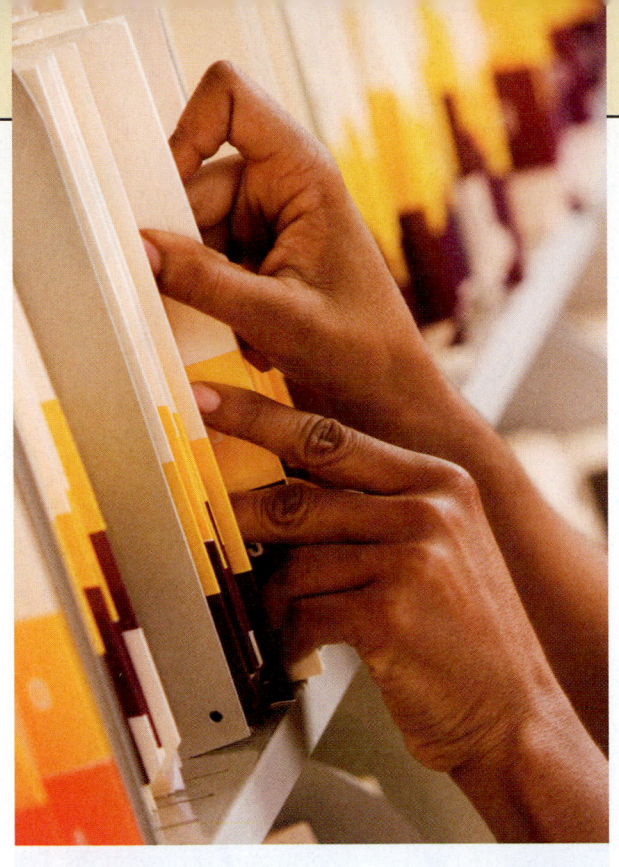

UNIT II

Administrative Responsibilities of the Medical Assistant

Chapter 8   **Written Communication**
Chapter 9   **Telephone Procedures**
Chapter 10 **Front Desk Reception**
Chapter 11 **Patient Scheduling**

My name is Kae Montgomery. When I first started working in a clinic during my externship, there was so much to learn. I had been taught all the basics in school, but now I had to apply this knowledge to the real world. One area I had to perfect was calling patients. On the electronic medical record (EMR) system we used, calling patients was referred to as phone notes. A patient would call in with a request, such as a referral or a prescription refill from the doctor. This would generate a phone note. Handling the phone notes was the easy part; calling the patient was sometimes tricky. We always called the home phone number, and since most people work, this would mean leaving a message on their answering machine. I had to be careful when leaving the message so that no specific details were given. I learned to leave just a general message such as "This is Kae calling from Dr. Yap's office. Your request is ready to be picked up."

If a spouse answered and I had no signed consent form for that person, I could not leave detailed information, even if he or she knew what the call was about. The spouse did not always understand why I could not leave a message since he or she was not aware of the fact that due to HIPAA privacy regulations, we were not allowed to share any of the patient's information with them, no matter what! One of the first things I learned in the EMR was where to look to find the patients' signed consent form.

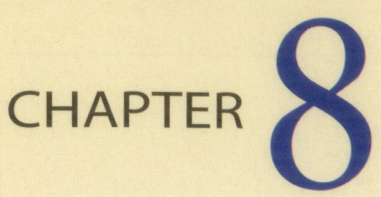

CHAPTER 8

Written Communication

Case Study

Dr. Calvin Jones brings the medical assistant a business card from the medical equipment salesperson he just had lunch with and asks the assistant to type a letter to the salesperson. In the letter, the physician would like to thank the salesperson for showing him a new electrocardiograph (**EKG**) machine and indicate that while he is uninterested in purchasing the machine now, the salesperson should call after the first of the year to assess the physician's willingness to purchase one at that time.

Objectives

After completing this chapter, you should be able to:

- Define and spell the key terminology in this chapter.
- Define the medical assistant's role in written communication in the medical office.
- Use correct grammar, spelling, and punctuation in all professional written communication.
- Discuss how to compose a patient letter.
- Detail the process of proofreading a business letter.
- List accepted healthcare abbreviations.
- Describe appropriate memo use in the medical office.
- Classify mail, including its size and postage requirements.
- Develop a policy for incoming and out-going e-mail to patients.
- Manage incoming mail and correspondence.

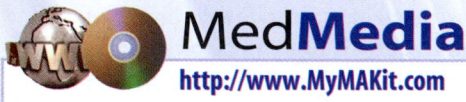

Med**Media**
http://www.MyMAKit.com

Additional interactive resources and activities for this chapter can be found on http://www.MyMAKit.com. For a video, tips, audio glossary, legal and ethical scenarios, on-the-job scenarios, quizzes, and games related to the content of this chapter, please access the accompanying CD-ROM in this book.

Video
Legal and Ethical Scenario: *Written Communication*
On the Job Scenario: *Written Communication*
Tips
Multiple Choice Quiz
Audio Glossary
HIPAA Quiz
Games: Spelling Bee, Crossword, and Strikeout

➕ MEDICAL ASSISTING STANDARDS

CAAHEP ENTRY-LEVEL STANDARDS	ABHES ENTRY-LEVEL COMPETENCIES
■ Perform within scope of practice (psychomotor)	■ Adapt to change
■ Apply ethical behaviors, including honesty/integrity in performance of medical assisting practice (affective)	■ Maintain confidentiality at all times
	■ Project a positive attitude
	■ Be cognizant of ethical boundaries
■ Identify nonverbal communication (cognitive)	■ Evidence a responsible attitude
■ Explore issue of confidentiality as it applies to the medical assistant (cognitive)	■ Conduct work within scope of education, training, and ability
	■ Be able to apply electronic technology
■ Respond to issues of confidentiality (psychomotor)	■ Apply computer concepts for office procedures
■ Practice within the standard of care for a medical assistant (psychomotor)	■ Be courteous and diplomatic
■ Recognize elements of fundamental writing skills (cognitive)	■ Serve as a liaison between the physician and others
■ Discuss applications of electronic technology in effective communication (cognitive)	■ Receive, organize, prioritize, and transmit information expediently
■ Organize technical information and summaries (cognitive)	■ Possess fundamental writing skills
■ Compose professional/business letters (psychomotor)	
■ Demonstrate sensitivity to the message being delivered (affective)	
■ Demonstrate awareness of the territorial boundaries of the person with whom communicating (affective)	
■ Analyze communications in providing appropriate responses/feedback (affective)	
■ Document accurately in the patient record (psychomotor)	

✓ COMPETENCY SKILLS PERFORMANCE

1. Compose a business letter.
2. Prepare a document for photocopying.
3. Send a letter to a patient about a missed appointment.
4. Proofread written documents.
5. Fold documents for window envelopes.
6. Open and sort mail.
7. Annotate written correspondence.

Key Terminology

annotation—process of reading a document and highlighting pertinent information

body—main portion of a business letter

closing—ending portion of a business letter

electronic mail—message sent electronically from one person to another; also called e-mail

font—style of type

letterhead—professional-quality stationery with a business' contact information (e.g., name, address, telephone and fax numbers)

logo—image that represents a business entity or brand

memo—interoffice note

postage meter—electronic scale used for weighing packages and printing postage labels

proofreading—process of reading and reviewing a document for errors

proofreader's marks—notations used when reading and reviewing a document for errors; see also *proofreading*

reference initials—in a professional letter, the all-capital initials of the author followed by the all-lowercase initials of the person who typed the letter (e.g., AJF/cmm)

salutation—greeting

spell-check—software that verifies word spellings

subject line—in a professional letter, the subject of the letter

thesaurus—resource for locating alternate words with similar meanings

Abbreviations

EKG—electrocardiograph

JCAHO—Joint Commission on the Accreditation of Healthcare Organizations

MLOCR—multiline optical character reader

OCR—optical character recognition

PDR—*Physician's Desk Reference*

UPS—United Parcel Service

USPS—United States Postal Service

Introduction

The ability to compose written documents is key for the administrative medical assistant. Physicians regularly ask medical assistants to type the letters they send to patients and other healthcare providers. Often, physicians will provide just basic facts and ask their medical assistants to compose letters with more detail. To perform these tasks well, the medical assistant must understand medical terminology as well as proper grammar, sentence structure, and punctuation.

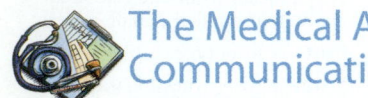

The Medical Assistant's Role in Written Communications

Medical assistants need to communicate in writing in many situations. The MA's communication style will need to differ depending upon the person he or she is writing to. For example, a letter written to a patient will use a different style than a professional letter to one physician from another.

Writing to Patients and Other Healthcare Professionals

Any written correspondence from the medical office reflects the physician and the office. Typographical, grammatical, and punctuation errors are not only confusing, they also reflect poorly on the medical office and may endanger the patient. Therefore, as a general rule, letters to patients and other healthcare professionals should be accurate, professional, and to the point. Each paragraph should address one topic and have no more than three to six sentences (Figure 8-1 ◆).

To compose and correct documents properly, every medical office should have a comprehensive medical dictionary, a **thesaurus** for acceptable alternate words, a desk dictionary, current coding books for procedure and diagnostic coding, and a *Physician's Desk Reference* (**PDR**) (Figures 8-2 ◆ through 8-4 ◆).

The Role of Spell-Checking

To help ensure written correspondence is error free, most computer software programs have built-in **spell-check** abilities, but medical assistants should not rely on such programs alone. Some words may pass spell checking because they are spelled correctly, but they may be used incorrectly. For example, the words "two," "to," and "too" all pass computerized spell checking, but each has a distinct meaning that is sometimes confused. An understanding of meaning is therefore important. Also, many spelling-verification programs lack the ability to check medical terms. As a result, medical assistants should keep medical dictionaries on hand for supplementary reference. While spell-check programs can be valuable tools, the medical assistant should take the time to read all documents for errors before giving those documents to physicians for final review and signing.

? — Critical Thinking Question 8-1—

Referring to the case study at the beginning of this chapter, how can the medical assistant help ensure the typed letter contains no errors?

Proper Spelling, Grammar, and Punctuation Use

Many words in the English language, especially medical words, are commonly misspelled. Table 8-1 gives some examples. When medical assistants are unsure of correct spellings, they should consult a comprehensive medical dictionary. Commonly used medical dictionaries include *Taber's Cyclopedic Medical Dictionary* and *Mosby's Medical Dictionary*.

Like accurate spelling, proper grammar is essential to a medical office's written correspondence. Poor grammar is unprofessional and reflects poorly on the physician and the office. Part of the medical assistant's role is to correct any grammar issues in physicians' drafts but retain the original intent of the content. Table 8-2 identifies common grammatical errors.

? — Critical Thinking Question 8-2 —

What are the possible ramifications for Dr. Jones if the medical assistant does not use accurate grammar, spelling, and punctuation?

Proper punctuation is another vital focus area in written documentation. Table 8-3 outlines the rules of use for common punctuation marks.

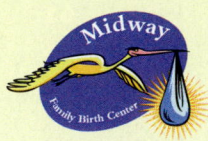

Jack Tsong, MD
Midway Family Birth Center
55 Long Island Way
Seattle, WA 12345

July 25, 2010

Suzanne Haufe
4728 California Ave E
Seattle, WA 12345

Dear Suzanne:

On behalf of my entire staff, I would like to welcome you to Midway Family Birth Center. Our goal is to provide our patients the highest quality service. If you ever feel we fall short, please bring it to my attention. I would consider it a personal favor.

It is an honor that you have placed your care in our hands. We look forward to working with you to meet your health goals.

Sincerely,

Jack Tsong, MD

Jack Tsong, MD
JKT/cmm

Figure 8-1 ◆ Sample patient letter.

Sentence Structure

In order to compose a proper sentence, certain components must be present. Every sentence must have a subject and a predicate in order to be a proper sentence. The subject is whom or what the sentence is about. The predicate is the word that says something about the subject. As an example, consider the sentence: "The patient arrived at 2:00 P.M." The subject is the word that the verb describes. In the example sentence, the verb "arrived" is describing the subject "patient." The predicate is what the subject did. In the example sentence, the predicate is "arrived at 2:00 P.M."

Numbers in Correspondence

In general, medical assistants should use words for quantities from one to ten in office correspondence but numbers for quantities over ten, like 24 or 876. When writing any unit of measurement, however, such as a medication dosage or weight or height, numbers always apply. For example, the medical assistant should type,

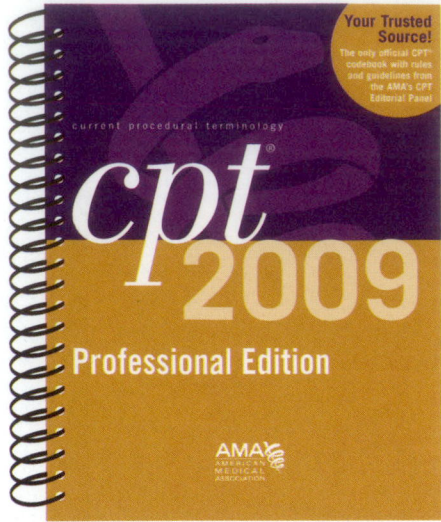

Figure 8-2 ◆ *Current Procedural Terminology (CPT) 2008 Professional Edition coding book.*
Reprinted by permission of the American Medical Association.

"The patient is taking 5 milligrams of the medication every hour." Numbers also always apply for the time of day, such as "1 P.M."

Rules for Medical-Term Plurals

The rules for creating plurals of medical terms can create confusion. Table 8-4 serves as a guide to the proper approaches.

Components of the Business Letter

All business letters, including those from medical offices, have the same basic components. First, each letter should appear on **letterhead.** Most medical offices have professionally printed

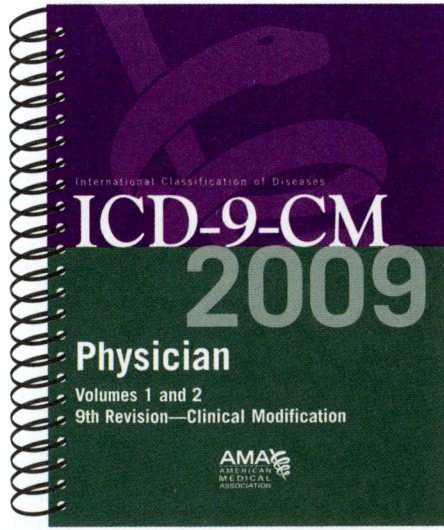

Figure 8-3 ◆ *International Classification of Diseases,* 9th Edition, Clinical Modification (ICD-9-CM) coding book.
Reprinted by permission of the American Medical Association.

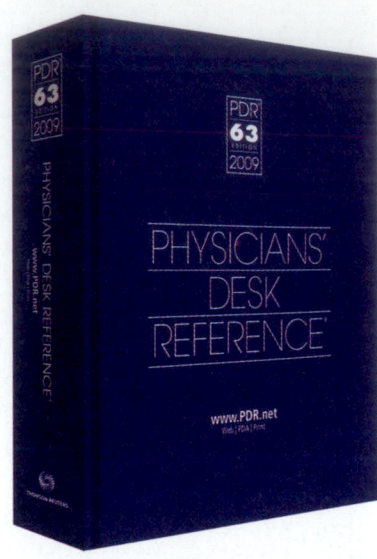

Figure 8-4 ◆ *Physician's Desk Reference (PDR).*

letterhead that carries the offices' names and addresses, telephone and fax numbers, e-mail addresses, and physicians' names (Figure 8-5 ◆). Letterhead may also contain a **logo,** some form of artwork that indicates the type of practice or other item of significance. For example, a pediatric office might have a logo that depicts children, while a chiropractic office might have a logo that includes a spine.

After letterhead, every piece of correspondence that is composed in the medical office must contain a nonabbreviated date, such as May 26, 2008, three lines down from the letterhead content at the top. Normally, a letter carries the date that the physician wrote or dictated it, not the date the medical assistant types it.

Three to six lines after the date comes the next component of the business letter: the inside address. The inside address appears against the left margin and includes the recipient's

TABLE 8-1 COMMONLY MISSPELLED WORDS		
acceptable	accidentally	accommodate
acquire	a lot	apparent
believe	calendar	category
cemetery	changeable	collectible
column	conscience	conscientious
conscious	discipline	embarrass
foreign	gauge	guarantee
harass	height	immediate
inoculate	judgment	leisure
liaison	maintenance	maneuver
miniature	minuscule	noticeable
occurrence	personnel	possession
privilege	publicly	questionnaire
receive	recommend	referred
relevant	schedule	threshold

TABLE 8-2 COMMON GRAMMATICAL ERRORS

Error	Example
Noun/verb mismatch	"The office feels this is a bad idea." (The office cannot feel, but people can.)
Adjective used as an adverb	"I did good on that exam." (The word *well* should replace *good*.)
Sentence that ends with a preposition	"This is something we need to work on." (A proper rewrite is, "This is something on which we need to work.")
Run-on sentence	"This lab is a dangerous place, patients should not be back here." (A semicolon should replace the comma.)
Misuse of words that sound alike but differ in spellings and meanings	"Their here, just two quiet." (The sentence should read, "They're here, just too quiet.")

TABLE 8-3 RULES OF USE FOR COMMON PUNCTUATION MARKS

Mark	Use(s)
Period (.)	Indicates the end of a sentence and separates the part of an abbreviation.
Comma (,)	Separates words, phrases, or two independent clauses and sets off elements that interrupt or add information in a sentence.
Semicolon (;)	Sets apart independent clauses and items in a list that contain commas.
Colon (:)	Follows a salutation in a business letter, precedes a list, separates independent clauses, helps express time.
Apostrophe (')	Indicates a missing letter from a contracted word and the possessive case of nouns.
Diagonal (/)	Separates the numbers in dates (e.g., 6/1/07) and fractions (e.g., 1/2) and sometimes indicates abbreviations (e.g., w/o).
Parentheses ( )	Set off part of a sentence that is not part of the main thought.
Quotation marks (" ")	Indicate a direct quote.
Ellipsis (. . .)	Shows that a thought trails off or represents missing material (e.g., "I was going to, but . . .").

name, title, company name, and address (Figure 8-6 ◆). Except for state name, the inside address includes no abbreviations. Table 8-5 lists the two-letter abbreviation for each state.

The **salutation** component of the business letter serves as the greeting. It typically appears two lines down from the inside address and carries the same name as the inside address. The salutations of formal letters should include the recipients' proper names and courtesy titles, such as "Dear Dr. Hagen." Table 8-6 provides guidelines for courtesy titles. For more informal correspondence, such as between two physicians who know each other well, salutations may use first names only, as in "Dear Shawn." When unsure of name spellings, medical assistants should ask for verification.

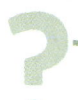

Critical Thinking Question 8-3

Which courtesy title is appropriate for a letter to a sales representative, and why?

The **subject line** is that part of the business letter that describes the letter's purpose. The subject line should appear two lines down from the salutation after the abbreviation "RE:"

TABLE 8-4 PLURALIZATION RULES FOR MEDICAL TERMS

Singular Form	Plural	Example
a	ae	bulla to bullae
ax	aces	thorax to thoraces
ex or ix	ices	appendix to appendices
on	a	ganglion to ganglia
um	a	ilium to illia
us	i	mellitus to melliti
y	ies	idiosyncrasy to idiosyncrasies
nx	nges	phalanx to phalanges

to indicate "regarding." A subject line might read, "RE: Sally Luder," for example. The subject line is the patient's name when the letter is about the patient (Figure 8-7 ◆).

The **body** is the main part of the business letter. It should start two lines down from the subject line, and each of its paragraphs should address only one issue, as mentioned earlier (see Figure 8-7).

The **closing** part of the letter typically appears two lines down from the ending portion of the body. The most common closing in a business letter is "Sincerely," but closing choice is at the physician's discretion. Four or five lines should be left between the closing and the physician's typed name to accommodate the physician's handwritten signature (see Figure 8-7).

Reference initials typically appear four to five lines down from the closing. Reference initials include the all-capital initials of the physician who wrote the letter, followed by the all-lowercase initials of the medical assistant who typed the letter (Figure 8-8 ◆).

Any information that may be enclosed with the letter should be indicated in the form of an enclosure notification two lines down from the reference initials. Such information can be indicated as "Enclosures" or "ENC.," followed by the number of items that are enclosed in parentheses. For example, a letter with two enclosures would have an enclosure notification that reads "Enclosures (2)" or "ENC. (2)." When there are no enclosures, this notation is omitted.

When the letter is to be copied to another party, the notation "c:" followed by that party's name should appear two lines down from the enclosure indication. For example, when Sally

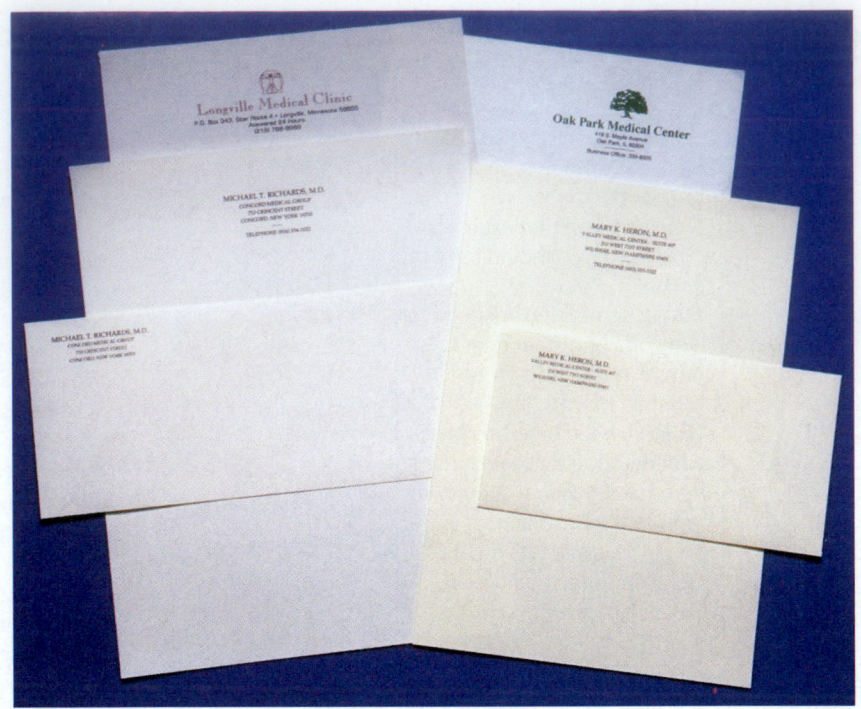

Figure 8-5 ◆ Sample physician letterhead stationery and envelopes.

Shawn D. Hagen, DC
19713 Scriber Lake Road
Lynnwood, WA 98036

Figure 8-6 ◆ Sample inside address.

TABLE 8-5 TWO-LETTER STATE ABBREVIATIONS

State	Abbreviation	State	Abbreviation
Alaska	AK	Kansas	KS
Alabama	AL	Kentucky	KY
Arkansas	AR	Louisiana	LA
Arizona	AZ	Massachusetts	MA
California	CA	Maryland	MD
Colorado	CO	Maine	ME
Connecticut	CT	Michigan	MI
Delaware	DE	Missouri	MO
Florida	FL	Mississippi	MS
Georgia	GA	Montana	MT
Hawaii	HI	North Carolina	NC
Iowa	IA	North Dakota	ND
Idaho	ID	Nebraska	NE
Illinois	IL	Oklahoma	OK
Indiana	IN	Oregon	OR

continued

TABLE 8-5 TWO-LETTER STATE ABBREVIATIONS   CONTINUED

State	Abbreviation	State	Abbreviation
Pennsylvania	PA	Virginia	VA
Rhode Island	RI	Vermont	VT
South Carolina	SC	Washington	WA
South Dakota	SD	Wisconsin	WI
Tennessee	TN	West Virginia	WV
Texas	TX	Wyoming	WY
Utah	UT		

Luder is to receive a copy of the letter, the copy notation would read, "c: Sally Luder."

Sometimes, business letters exceed one page. When they do, all subsequent pages must begin with the date of the letter, followed by the subject line. Pages after the first page require no letterhead, but they should appear on paper that matches the color and quality of the letterhead. Subsequent pages should be numbered.

In Practice

Dr. Mohammad asks Joanne Brennan, his new administrative medical assistant, to type a letter to a patient while he dictates. During dictation, Dr. Mohammad uses words unfamiliar to Joanne, so she guesses at how to spell some of the words, thinking that the patient probably won't notice.

What may happen if Joanne continues to guess at word spellings? Why is this issue important?

Styles of Business Letters

Medical offices use varied letter styles, including block, modified block, and modified block with indentations. Block and modified block are the most common styles, but the physician's preference dictates letter style. Figure 8-9 ◆ describes different styles and gives examples.

Using Fonts in Typed Communication

All word-processing software comes with a set of **fonts,** which are different styles of type. Professional letters should appear in 10-

TABLE 8-6 GUIDELINES FOR COURTESY TITLES

- ■ "Mr." is the appropriate title for males.
- ■ Professional titles like "MD" or "DO" replace the courtesy title. For example, "John Aye, MD," should replace "Mr. John Aye."
- ■ "Ms." is used when a woman's marital status is unknown, or when the woman prefers.
- ■ "Mrs." is used for a married woman.
- ■ "Miss" is used for a young girl or an unmarried woman who prefers it. When in doubt, use "Ms." rather than "Miss."
- ■ Two people at the same address should appear separately (e.g., "Mr. Joseph Paterniti and Ms. Beth Dorio").

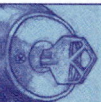

Keys to Success
SIGNING LETTERS FOR THE PHYSICIAN

Occasionally, physicians will be out of the office when letters must be mailed, so they may ask their medical assistants to send those letters without their signatures. The review process, however, should remain the same. The physicians should still read or otherwise review the letters and give their approvals before the letters are sent. Approved letters can be stamped with lines like, "Read but not signed due to time constraints." When offices lack preprinted stamps like this, the medical assistant can print the physician's name where the signature belongs and follow the printing with a personal signature to indicate that the assistant signed for the physician.

to 12-point formal fonts, like Times New Roman, Garamond, or Arial (Figure 8-10 ◆). While informal fonts may function for things like interoffice informational sheets, they are considered inappropriate for professional business letters.

Sending Letters to Patients

Medical offices send letters to patients for a number of reasons, including to communicate changes in office policy or procedure. Personalized letters serve to notify patients they need to see or who have missed appointments. Whatever the reasons they are sent, patient letters should be professional and accurate. Copies of all written patient correspondence should be filed in the patients' medical records.

Proofreading

As discussed earlier, while most word-processing software can check spelling and grammar, such programs are neither failsafe nor complete substitutes for manual error-checking processes. Because most documents today are composed electronically, medical assistants can proofread and correct those documents before printing. **Proofreading** is the process of checking written information for spelling or other errors. Sometimes, proofreading includes modifying a letter's style (e.g., line format) to make the letter more appealing on paper.

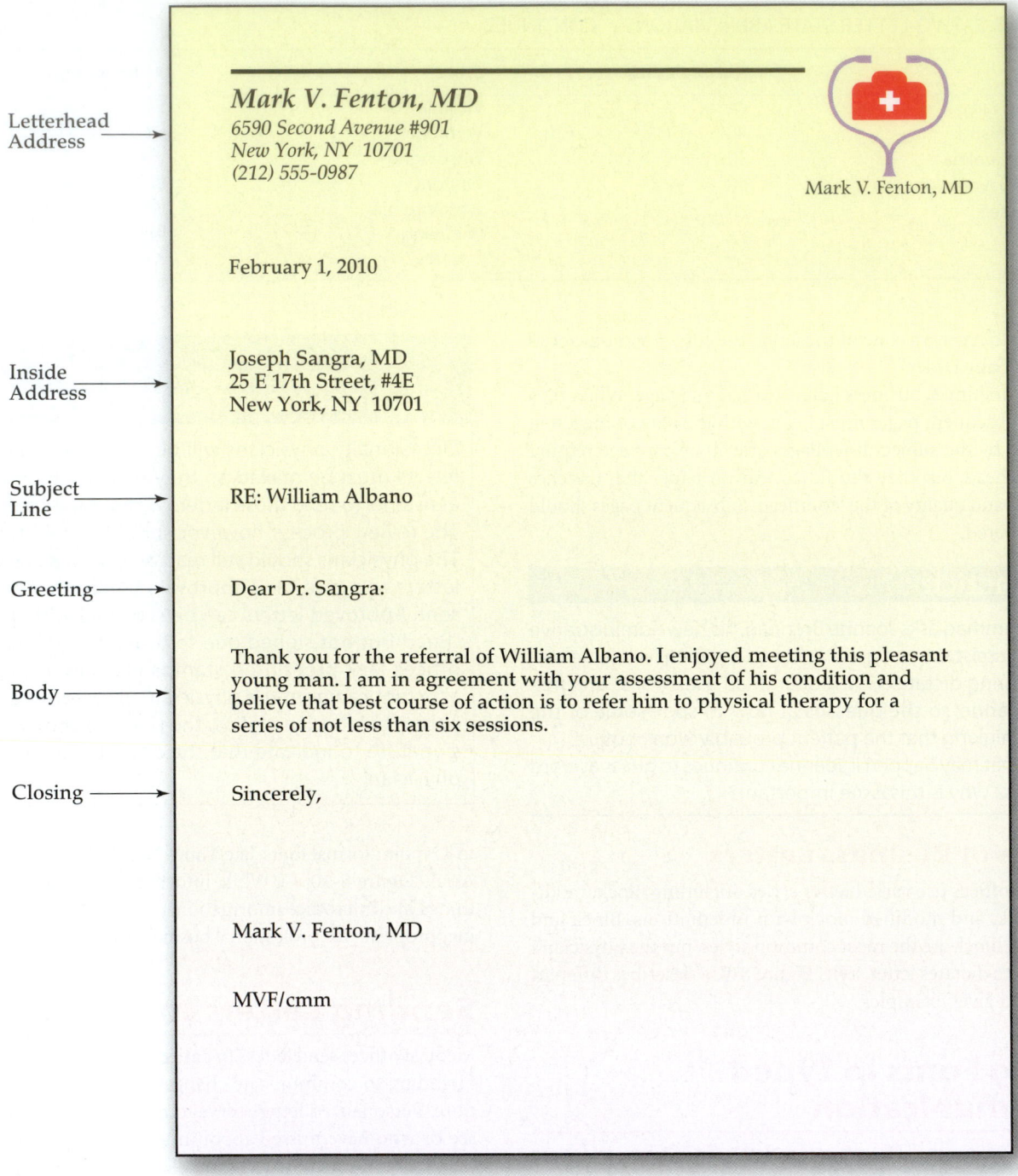

Letterhead Address →

Mark V. Fenton, MD
6590 Second Avenue #901
New York, NY 10701
(212) 555-0987

Mark V. Fenton, MD

February 1, 2010

Inside Address →

Joseph Sangra, MD
25 E 17th Street, #4E
New York, NY 10701

Subject Line →

RE: William Albano

Greeting →

Dear Dr. Sangra:

Body →

Thank you for the referral of William Albano. I enjoyed meeting this pleasant young man. I am in agreement with your assessment of his condition and believe that best course of action is to refer him to physical therapy for a series of not less than six sessions.

Closing →

Sincerely,

Mark V. Fenton, MD

MVF/cmm

Figure 8-7 ◆ Sample business letter.

Proofreading requires medical assistants to read documents slowly and check that the documents are clear and logically organized. To indicate needed changes, medical assistants place **proofreader's marks** on printed documents (Figure 8-11 ◆).

To catch all errors, medical assistants should read all letters at least twice. Documents should be printed only after they have been proofread. Once documents are printed, medical assistants should proofread them one last time to determine if format changes, like more or less space between lines, would make the documents more attractive.

Working with Accepted Abbreviations

Abbreviations are common in medical terminology. For all members of the healthcare team, however, it is essential to use only accepted abbreviations in office communication. The Joint Commission on the Accreditation of Healthcare Organizations (**JCAHO**) has identified the standard abbreviations its members are required to use, as well as avoid. Table 8-7 lists the latter. JCAHO prepared this list due to the growing concern that the

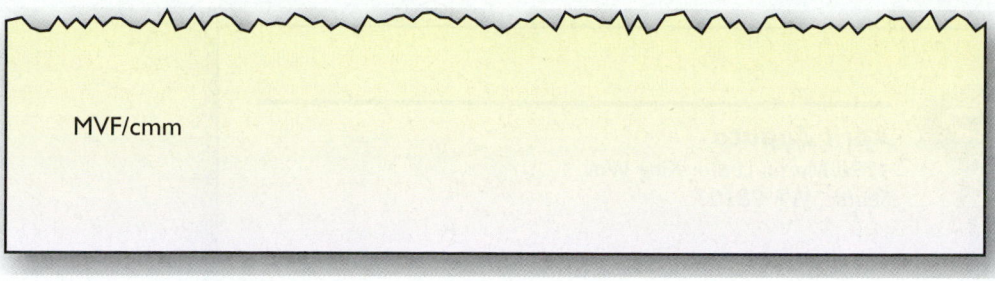

MVF/cmm

Figure 8-8 ◆ Sample reference initials.

April Zapata
4190 Martin Luther King Way
Seattle, WA 98107

June 2, 2010

April Zapata
4190 Martin Luther King Way
Seattle, WA 98107

RE: Lab results

Dear April:

Your lab results are in, and we have been trying to reach you to schedule an appointment to review them. Please call us at (206) 555-9000 to schedule an appointment at your earliest convenience.

Sincerely,

Martin Hurst, MD

MLH/idm

4 lines between date and inside address

3 lines between inside address and subject line

2 lines between subject line and salutation

2 lines between salutation and body of the letter

2 lines between the body and the closing

4 lines between the closing and the signature line

2 lines between the signature line and the identification line

A

Figure 8-9a ◆ Block style.

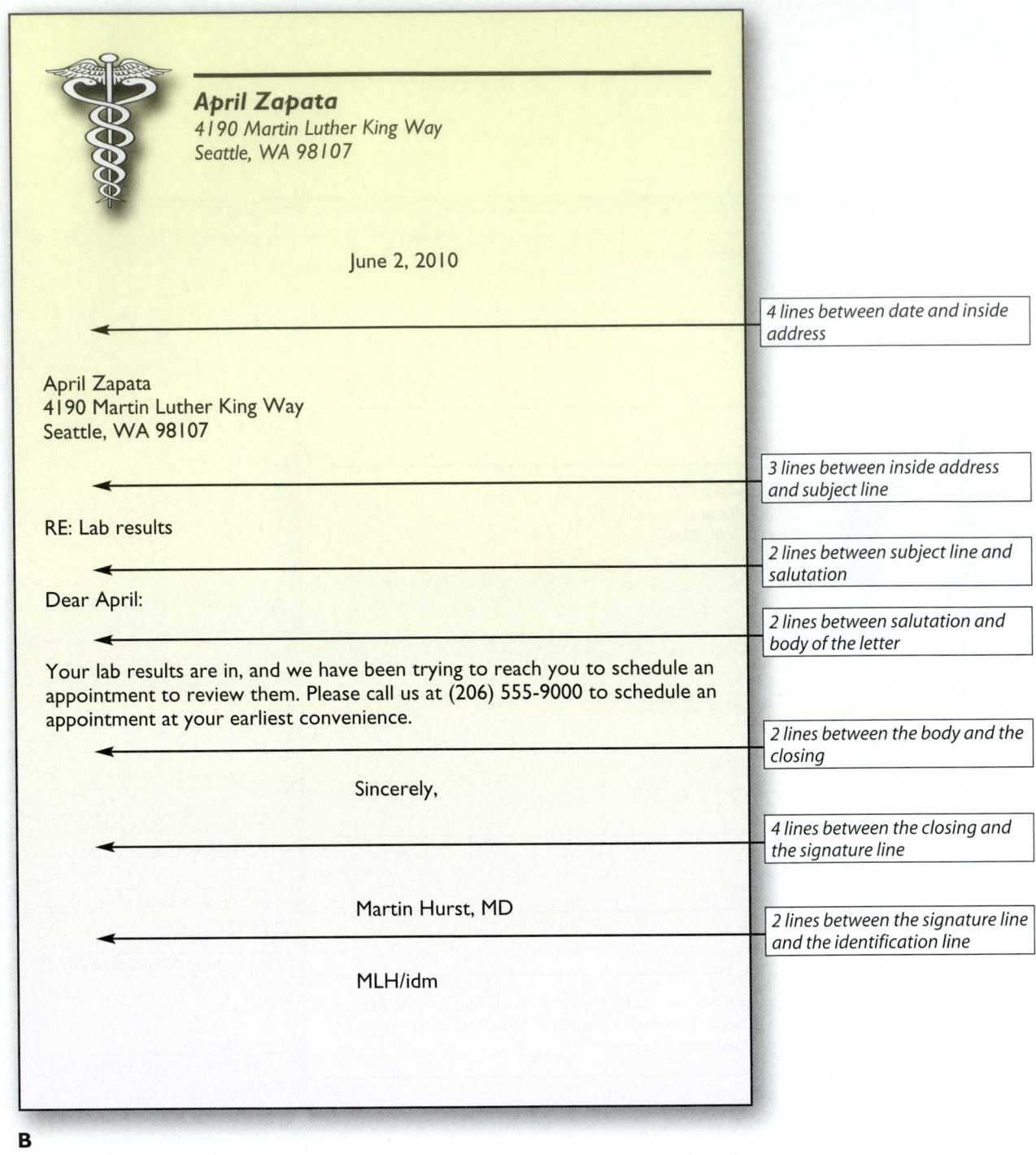

April Zapata
4190 Martin Luther King Way
Seattle, WA 98107

June 2, 2010

← *4 lines between date and inside address*

April Zapata
4190 Martin Luther King Way
Seattle, WA 98107

← *3 lines between inside address and subject line*

RE: Lab results

← *2 lines between subject line and salutation*

Dear April:

← *2 lines between salutation and body of the letter*

Your lab results are in, and we have been trying to reach you to schedule an appointment to review them. Please call us at (206) 555-9000 to schedule an appointment at your earliest convenience.

← *2 lines between the body and the closing*

Sincerely,

← *4 lines between the closing and the signature line*

Martin Hurst, MD

← *2 lines between the signature line and the identification line*

MLH/idm

B

Figure 8-9b ◆ Modified block style: date, closing, signature, and identification lines center; all other lines are flush left.

use of more than one abbreviation for the same medical term created a situation where confusion, misdiagnosis, or even injury to the patient could occur. In the medical office, lists like these help staff maintain consistent terminology and avoid confusion and errors. Medical assistants who are unclear about abbreviations should always err on the side of caution and spell out the corresponding words.

Creating Memos for the Office

A **memo** is a type of interoffice correspondence. Memos are a quick and efficient means of communication. They require no postage and are designed to have clear messages. Office managers might compose memos to communicate with their entire staff, or staff members may write memos to communicate with other staff.

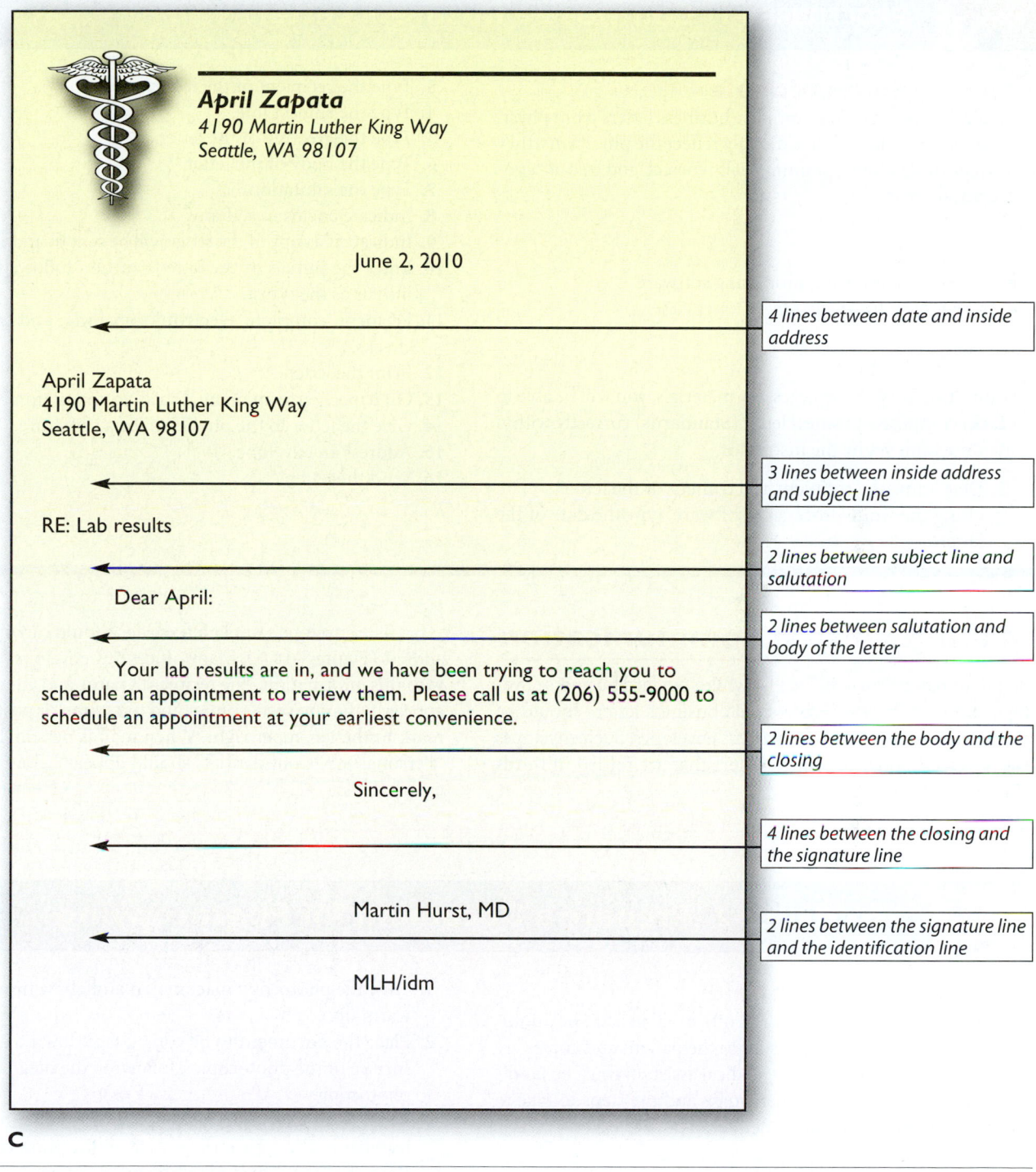

April Zapata
4190 Martin Luther King Way
Seattle, WA 98107

June 2, 2010

← *4 lines between date and inside address*

April Zapata
4190 Martin Luther King Way
Seattle, WA 98107

← *3 lines between inside address and subject line*

RE: Lab results

← *2 lines between subject line and salutation*

Dear April:

← *2 lines between salutation and body of the letter*

Your lab results are in, and we have been trying to reach you to schedule an appointment to review them. Please call us at (206) 555-9000 to schedule an appointment at your earliest convenience.

← *2 lines between the body and the closing*

Sincerely,

← *4 lines between the closing and the signature line*

Martin Hurst, MD

← *2 lines between the signature line and the identification line*

MLH/idm

C

Figure 8-9c ◆ Modified block with indentations. Resembles modified block style, except that each paragraph is indented five spaces.

Arial 10-point font	Arial 12-point font
Garamond 10-point font	Garamond 12-point font
Times New Roman 10-point font	Times New Roman 12-point font

Figure 8-10 ◆ Sample fonts.

Most memos begin with the word "MEMO" or "MEM-ORANDUM" at their tops. Below that, typically the date, recipient, and author appear (Figure 8-12 ◆). Many medical offices preprint memo paper, but some print memo paper on an as-needed basis.

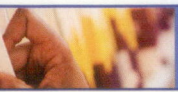

PROCEDURE 8-1   Compose a Business Letter

Theory and Rationale

Medical assistants often compose business letters from physicians. Because these letters directly reflect the physicians, they must be professional, grammatically correct, and free of typographical errors.

Materials

- Computer with word-processing software
- Information for the letter

Competency

(**Conditions**) With the necessary materials, you will be able to (**Task**) compose a business letter (**Standards**) correctly within the time limit set by the instructor.

1. Determine the recipient and content of the letter.
2. Using the word-processing software, type the date of the letter.
3. Type the recipient of the letter.
4. Type the subject line.
5. Type the greeting of the letter.
6. Type the body of the letter.
7. Type the salutation.
8. Indicate enclosures, if any.
9. Indicate if a copy of the letter will be sent to another party.
10. Enter the initials of the letter's author, followed by your initials as the typist.
11. Perform complete electronic spelling and grammar checks.
12. Print the letter.
13. On paper, perform manual spelling and grammar checks.
14. Give the letter to the physician for a signature.
15. Address an envelope.
16. Send the letter.

Mailing Written Communication

Standard paper size is 8½″ × 11″, while standard business envelope size is 4⅛″ × 9½″. Professional business letters should be mailed in business-sized or "Size 10" envelopes. Such envelopes easily accommodate business letters that are folded in thirds (Figure 8-13 ◆).

The envelope's upper left corner should carry the office's address (Figure 8-14 ◆). Many offices buy envelopes preprinted with this information. The recipient's name and address should appear in the envelope's center and the stamp or postage-meter mark in the far upper right. When mail is personal, the word "Personal" or "Confidential" should appear below the recipient's address.

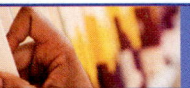

PROCEDURE 8-2   Prepare a Document for Photocopying

Theory and Rationale

Many documents in the medical office will need to be photocopied. Often, originals are sent to the patient and copies are kept in the patient's file. The medical assistant must be familiar with how the photocopier works and the steps to take to correctly copy needed documents.

Materials

- Photocopier
- Document to be copied
- Envelope
- Patient medical record

Competency

(**Conditions**) With the necessary materials, you will be able to (**Task**) prepare a document for photocopying (**Standards**) correctly within the time limit set by the instructor.

1. Turn the photocopy machine on and allow time for it to warm up.
2. Place the document to be copied face down on the glass surface of the photocopier, following the diagram on the photocopier.
3. Indicate the number of copies needed by entering the number in the appropriate place on the photocopier.
4. Press the "copy" button on the photocopier.
5. Once the copy has been made, remove the original.
6. Place the original document into an envelope to be mailed to the patient.
7. Place the photocopy of the document into the patient's file.

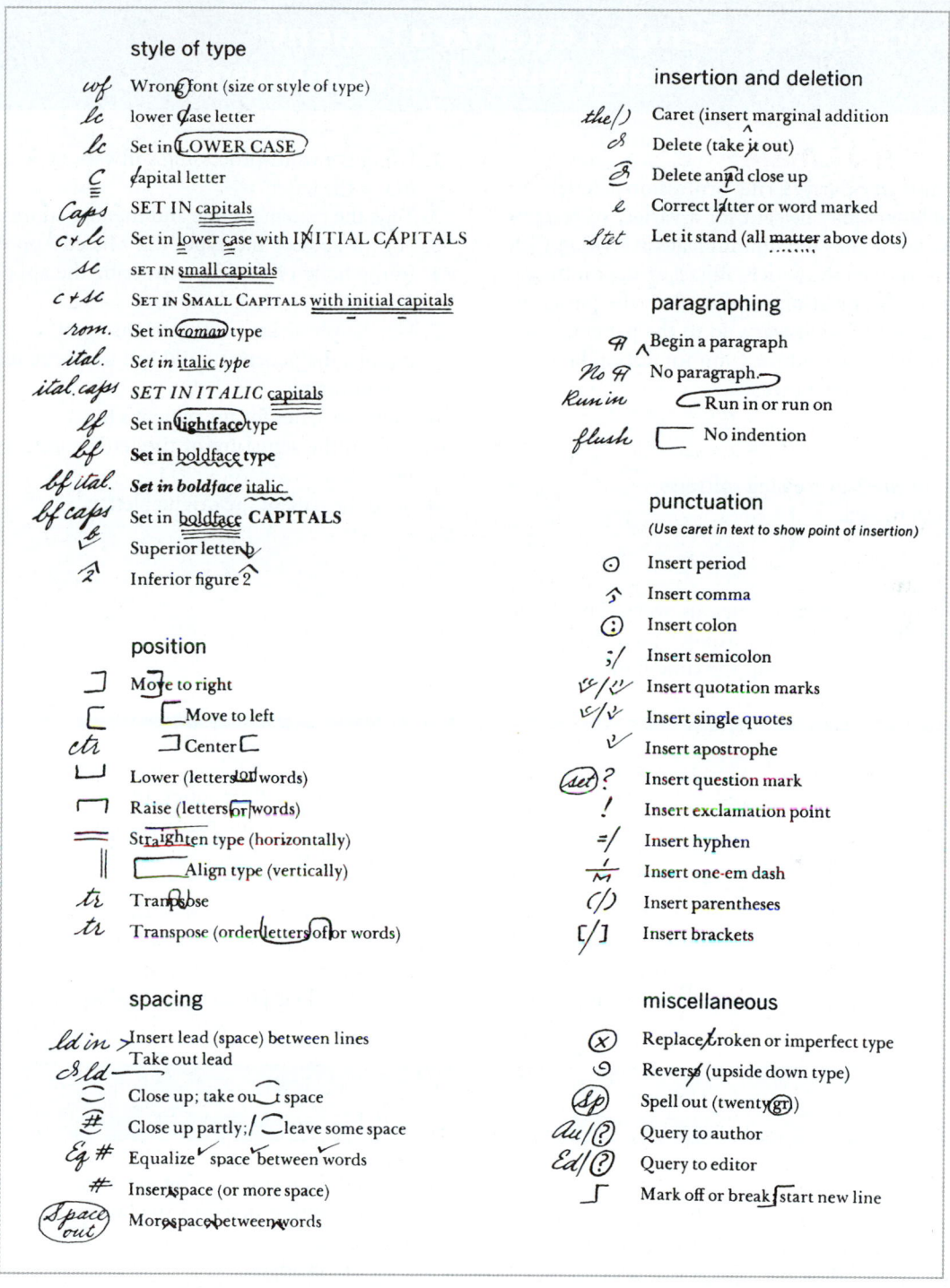

Figure 8-11 ◆ Proofreader's marks.

Some medical offices place their required registration forms on their Web site. By directing patients who have computers to access the Web site to download, print, and fill out the needed forms, the medical office saves the cost of printing the packets and mailing them to the patient ahead of time.

Window Envelopes

For certain types of mail, like insurance billing forms or patient billing statements, medical offices often use window envelopes.

Before such envelopes are sealed, however, medical assistants should ensure that addresses appear in the windows (Figure 8-15 ◆).

HIPAA Compliance

Regardless of size or type, for personal patient information medical offices must use security envelopes. Security envelopes have internal patterns that keep the contents of documents obscured. Figure 8-16 ◆ shows a security envelope.

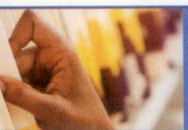

PROCEDURE 8-3   Send a Letter to a Patient About a Missed Appointment

Theory and Rationale

Medical assistants regularly write professional letters to patients. These letters may be sent for a variety of reasons when the physician wishes to communicate in writing with the patient, such as when the patient misses an appointment. Often, written communication is used when the physician desires written proof of what was said to the patient. Strict attention to detail helps avoid miscommunication between the patient and the medical office.

Materials

- Computer with word-processing software
- Patient medical record

Competency

(**Conditions**) With the necessary materials, you will be able to (**Task**) send a letter to a patient regarding a missed appointment (**Standards**) correctly within the time limit set by the instructor.

1. Using the word-processing software, type the date at the top of the letter.
2. Type the patient's name and mailing address.
3. For the subject line, type "RE: Missed Appointment."
4. In the body of the letter, describe the appointment that was missed, including its date.
5. Per the physician's instructions or office policy, list the reasons the patient should call to reschedule the missed appointment.
6. Copy the letter for the patient's file.
7. Obtain the signature of the letter's author (you or the physician).
8. Send the patient the original letter.

Running and Resetting Postage Meters

Many medical clinics have **postage meters**, which weigh mail pieces, determine correct postage and print postage on envelopes or labels (Figure 8-17 ◆). Basic models simply weigh pieces of mail and print postage, while advanced versions accept stacks of mail, insert documents into envelopes, seal envelopes, and affix proper postage. Postage meters are extremely useful to the medical office because they are generally user friendly and reduce wasted postage as well as time spent at the post office.

Most medical offices lease their postage meters from companies that supply the meters as well as corresponding supplies (e.g., ink cartridges, ribbons, labels). Once offices have arranged payment for their postage, medical assistants facilitate meter

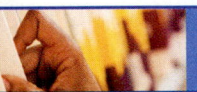

PROCEDURE 8-4   Proofread Written Documents

Theory and Rationale

Proofreading skills are imperative to the medical assistant, because the composition of written documents is a large part of medical assisting. Sending documents out without proofreading them may lead to confusion on the part of the recipient, or even to possible misdiagnosis or treatment of a patient.

Materials

- Computer document to be proofread
- Computer with word-processing software

Competency

(**Conditions**) With the necessary materials, you will be able to (**Task**) proofread a written document (**Standards**) correctly within the time limit set by the instructor.

1. Open the document using the word-processing software.
2. Use the word processor's spelling and grammar checking functions.
3. Save any changes.
4. Starting at the top, read the entire document to verify that all spelling, punctuation, and grammatical errors were corrected.
5. Save any changes.
6. Print the document.
7. Review the entire document to verify that all spelling, punctuation, and grammatical errors were corrected. If changes were made, reprint the document.
8. Give the document to the physician for signature.

TABLE 8-7 MEDICAL ABBREVIATIONS TO AVOID

Abbreviation	Potential Problem	Preferred Replacement(s)
U (unit)	Mistaken for "0" (zero), the number "4" (four), or "cc."	"unit"
IU (International Unit)	Mistaken for IV (intravenous) or the number 10 (ten).	"International Unit"
Q.D., QD, q.d., qd (daily); Q.O.D., QOD, q.o.d., qod (every other day)	Mistaken for each other. The period after the Q is mistaken for "I" and the "O" is mistaken for "I" (q.i.d. is four times a day dosing).	"daily" or "every other day"
Trailing zero (X.0 mg); Lack of leading zero (.X)	Decimal point is missed.	X mg or 0.X mg
MS	Can mean morphine sulfate or magnesium sulfate.	"morphine sulfate"
MS04 and MgS04	Confused for one another.	"magnesium sulfate"

Source: Joint Commission on the Accreditation of Healthcare Organizations.

use by calling the postage companies' customer service departments and providing their user identification numbers, office passwords, and meters' serial numbers and access codes.

Classifying Mail, Size Requirements, and Postage

The United States Postal Service (**USPS**) varies its services for mailing letters and packages according to urgency and value. A standard postage stamp facilitates first-class mail service, which is available for items weighing no more than 13 ounces. Mail that weighs over 13 ounces must be sent via Priority Mail or Parcel Post.

After Express Mail, which is the fastest USPS service (with a guaranteed next-day delivery seven days a week), Priority Mail is the U.S. government's fastest mail service. For most destinations in the United States, Priority Mail arrives within two to three days. However, Priority Mail items must weigh no more than 70 pounds, and packages cannot exceed a combined length, width, and depth of 108 inches. When senders use envelopes and packages provided by USPS that clearly state "Flat Rate," Priority Mail is available at a flat rate (Figure 8-18 ◆).

Media Mail, or Standard Mail, is strictly for printed or bound materials, such as books or magazines, sound recordings, videotapes, or CDs and DVDs. This service is more economical than the other services, but it tends to take longer, usually two to ten days. Advertising cannot be sent by Media Mail.

In addition to its base services, the USPS offers a variety of optional services for added costs. Certified mail, for example, provides a mailing receipt and a record of the mailing at

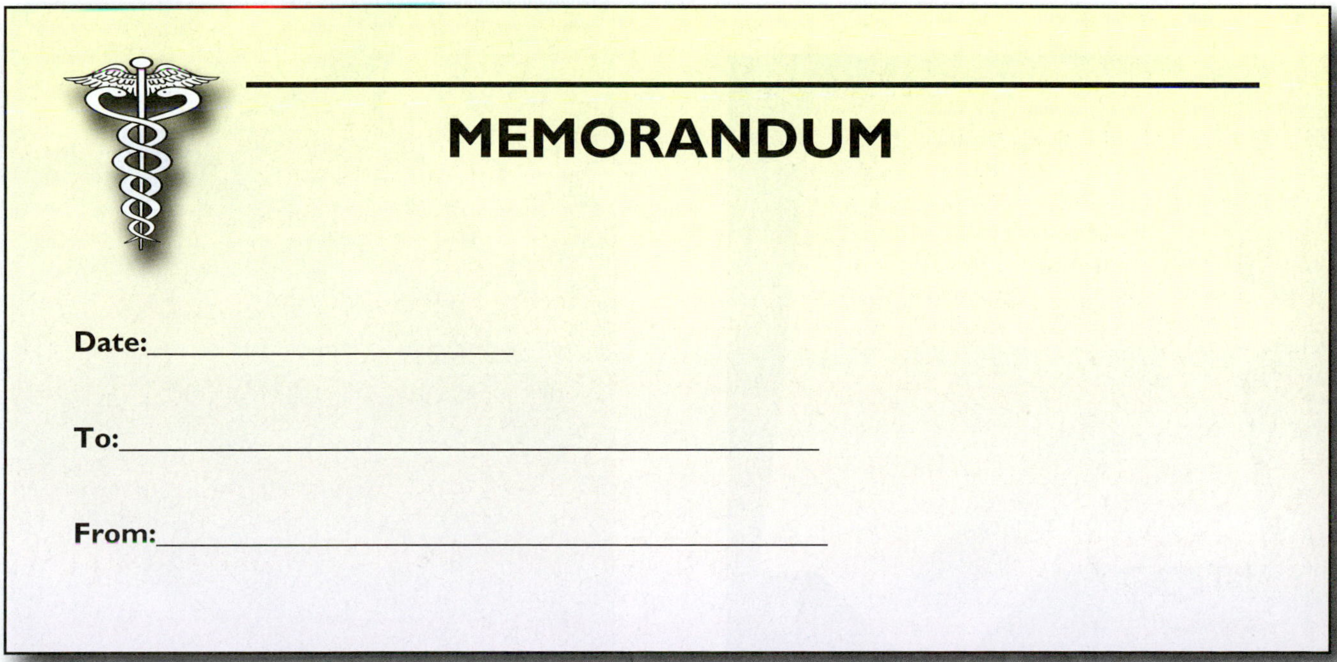

MEMORANDUM

Date:_____

To:_____

From:_____

Figure 8-12 ◆ Sample opening of an interoffice memo.

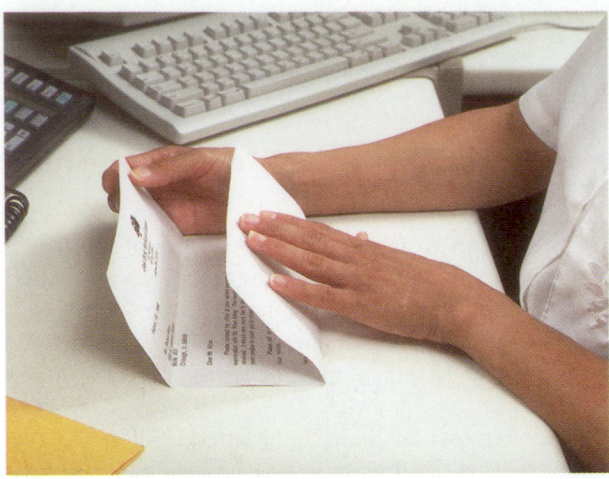

Figure 8-13 ◆ When folded into thirds, the letter will easily fit within the standard business envelope.

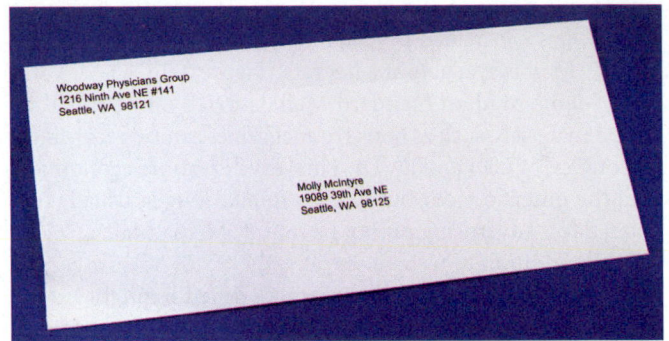

Figure 8-14 ◆ Example of a properly addressed business envelope.

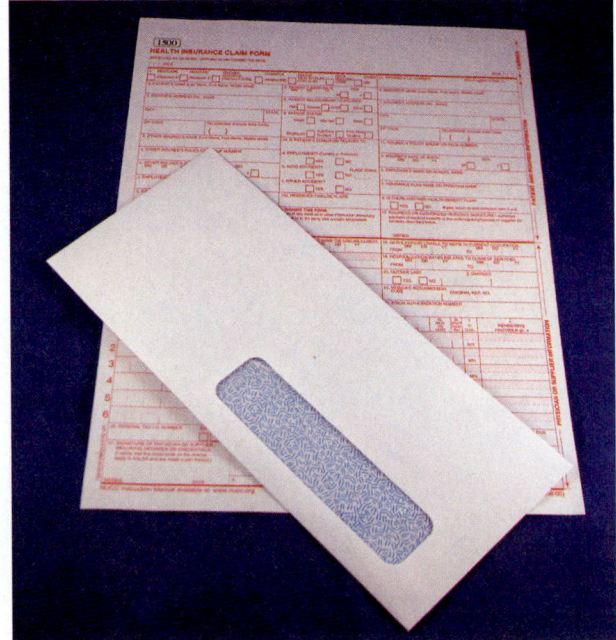

Figure 8-15 ◆ Photo of window envelope.

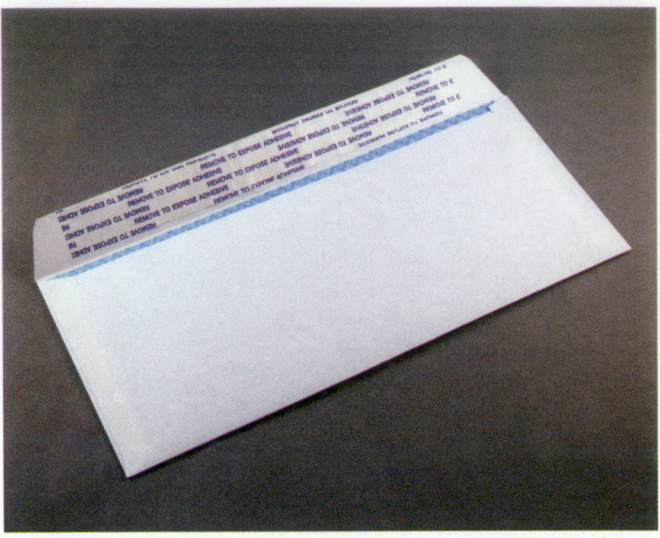

Figure 8-16 ◆ A security envelope.

the local post office, but it is available only for First-Class and Priority Mail packages and letters. Confirmation receipts are another, added service (Figure 8-19 ◆). Delivery confirmation allows senders and receivers to track pieces of mail or packages online. Registered mail, another option available for only First Class and Priority Mail, offers the ability to purchase insurance up to $25,000 for the value of the item. A return receipt can also be added to this service. Insurance can be purchased for

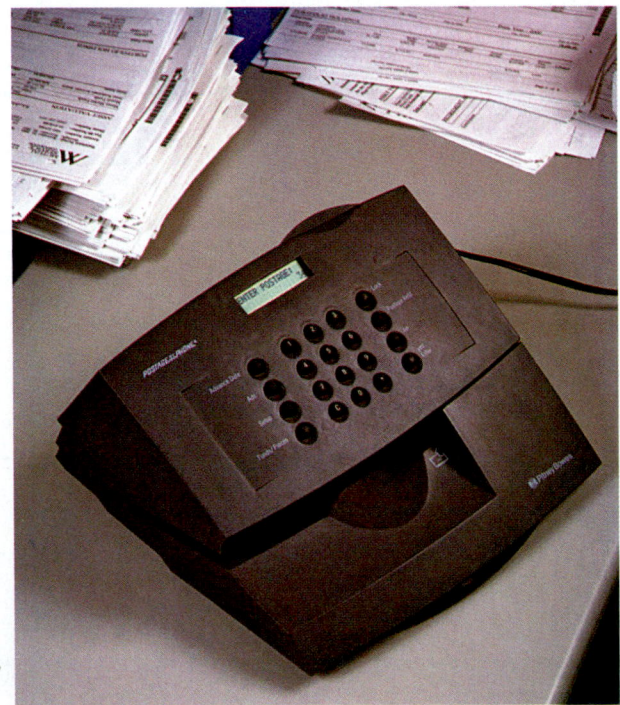

Figure 8-17 ◆ An electronic postage meter.

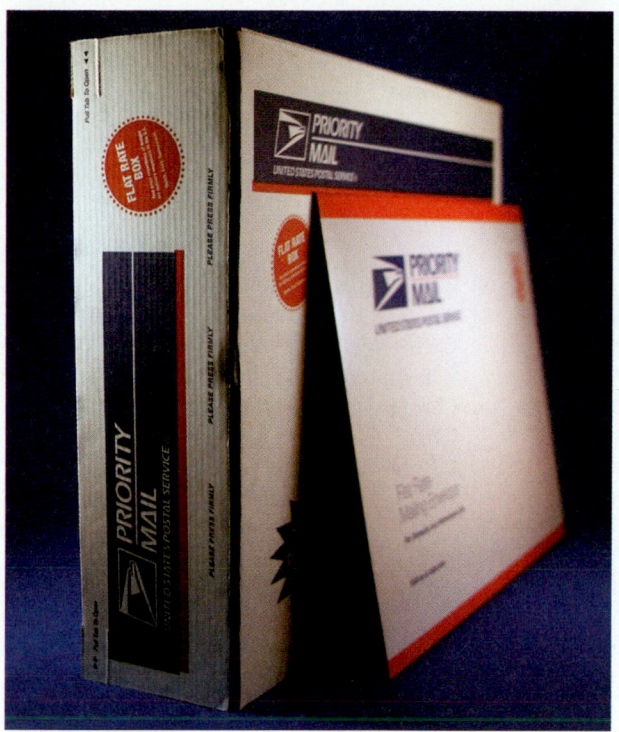

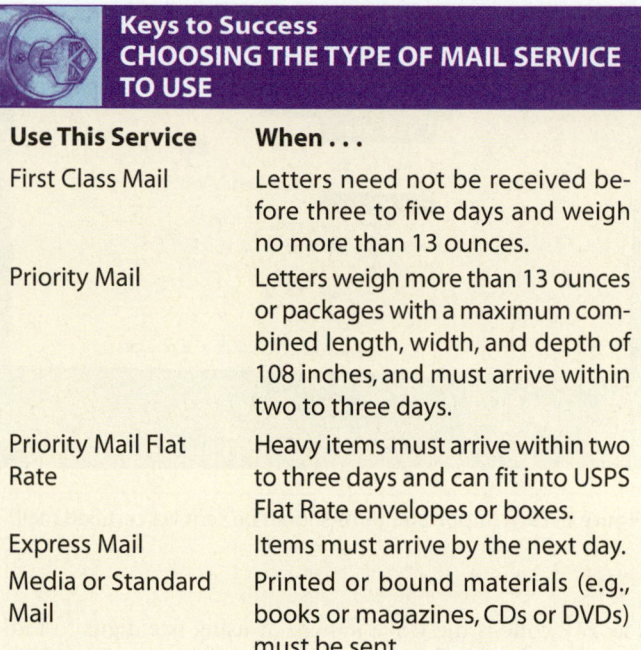

Figure 8-18 ◆ The USPS charges one flat rate to use its flat rate envelopes and boxes, regardless of where the item is being shipped within the United States or how much it weighs.

any item shipped via the USPS, but the cost of the insurance rises with the value of the item.

Buying Postage Online

The USPS now sells postage online to any consumer with a computer and a printer. This service is available for both domestic and international shipments and includes such options as insurance (up to a $500 value) and delivery confirmation.

Using Multiline Optical Character Readers

The USPS uses multiline optical character readers (**MLOCRs**), which use optical character recognition (**OCR**) to determine how to route mail through its systems. MLOCRs capture images of the fronts of pieces of mail, look up postal codes, print barcodes, and perform mail sorts.

MLOCRs cannot read all mail, however. Some handwriting is hard to read and addresses may sometimes appear in incorrect locations. This type of mail is either sent to another, more powerful computer for scanning or to a human operator.

PROCEDURE 8-5   Fold Documents for Window Envelopes

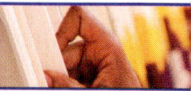

Theory and Rationale
When documents are folded properly before they are placed in window envelopes, post-office machinery can read addresses correctly and deliver mail in a timely manner.

Materials
- Document to be mailed
- Window envelope

Competency
(**Conditions**) With the necessary materials, you will be able to (**Task**) fold a document for use with a window envelope (**Standards**) correctly within the time limit set by the instructor.

1. Locate the mailing address on the document.
2. Compare the location of the mailing address to the location of the window on the envelope.
3. Fold the document such that the mailing address will be viewable through the envelope's window once the document has been inserted in the envelope.
4. Insert the document in the envelope.
5. Verify that the address is viewable through the window.
6. Seal the envelope.

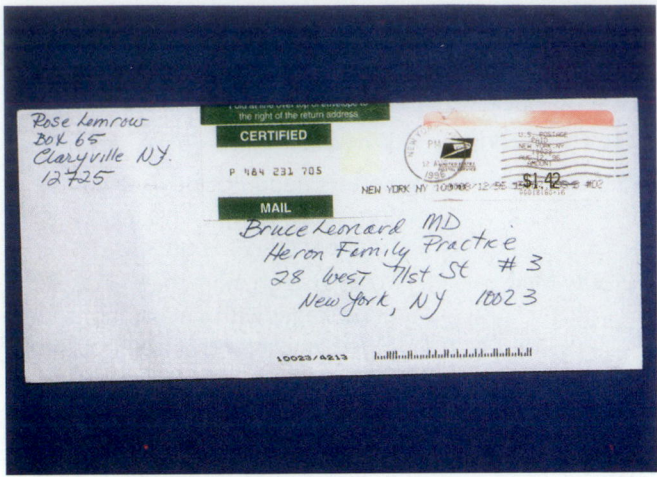

Figure 8-19 ◆ Important items should be sent via certified mail.

"ZIP + 4" Codes

The ZIP code is the USPS system of using five digits to indicate mail's intended destination. Since 1983, the USPS has been using "ZIP + 4" codes to expedite postal service by directing mail to more precise locations. These codes, which as their name suggests, extend traditional ZIP codes by four digits, appear on the USPS Web site at http://zip4.usps.com/zip4/welcome.jsp.

USPS-Approved Abbreviations in Addresses

Mail that follows USPS recommendations reaches its destination far more quickly than mail that does not. Some of these recommendations, approved abbreviations for mailing addresses, appear in Table 8-8.

Restricted Materials

The USPS will mail no item that is outwardly or of its own force dangerous or injurious to life, health, or property. Similarly, it will not transport most hazardous material. The following items are also subject to certain restrictions:

- Intoxicating liquors
- Firearms
- Knives or other sharp instruments
- Odor-producing chemicals
- Liquids and powders
- Controlled substances

When in doubt about the mailability of an item, the medical assistant should call or visit the USPS.

Other Delivery Options

Some services compete with the USPS by offering package tracking, insurance, and delivery services that include Federal Express, United Parcel Service (**UPS**), and DHL. Federal Express (FedEx) offers overnight courier, ground, heavy freight, and document copying services. FedEx services are

TABLE 8-8 USPS-APPROVED ABBREVIATIONS

For Streets and Towns

Alley	ALY	Hill	HL
Annex	ANX	Island	IS
Avenue	AVE	Junction	JCT
Boulevard	BLVD	Lake	LK
Bridge	BRG	Lane	LN
Brook	BRK	Manor	MNR
Bypass	BYP	Meadow	MDW
Canyon	CYN	Mountain	MTN
Cape	CPE	Orchard	ORCH
Causeway	CSWY	Parkway	PKWY
Center	CTR	Place	PL
Circle	CIR	Plaza	PLZ
Cliff	CLF	Point	PT
Club	CLB	Port	PRT
Common	CMN	Ridge	RDG
Corner	COR	River	RIV
Court	CRT	Road	RD
Cove	CV	Route	RTE
Creek	CRK	Shore	SHR
Crossing	XING	Spring	SPG
Drive	DR	Square	SQ
Estate	EST	Station	STA
Expressway	EXPY	Street	ST
Forest	FRST	Terrace	TER
Freeway	FWY	Throughway	TRWY
Garden	GDN	Trail	TRL
Gateway	GTWY	Tunnel	TUNL
Grove	GRV	Turnpike	TPKE
Harbor	HBR	Valley	VLY
Heights	HTS	View	VW
Highway	HWY	Village	VLG

For Secondary Unit Designators

Apartment	APT	Office	OFC
Basement	BSMT	Penthouse	PH
Building	BLDG	Room	RM
Department	DEPT	Space	SPC
Floor	FL	Suite	STE
Front	FRNT	Trailer	TRLR
Lobby	LBBY	Upper	UPPR
Lower	LOWR		

available both to home and business customers, and FedEx offers shipping services via Express, Ground, Freight, and International services. The United Parcel Service (UPS), much like FedEx, offers shipping services both within the United States and worldwide via various shipping speeds and methods. Both of these companies offer package pickup, which alleviates the need to take a package to a FedEx or UPS retail location. The Deutsche Post World Net (DHL) offers shipping services worldwide at a variety of shipping speeds. In 2003, DHL purchased Airborne Express—then the third largest private express delivery company in the United States.

Using E-Mail to Communicate

Electronic mail, or e-mail, is an electronic means of communication. Many medical offices use e-mail to communicate with patients. As a general rule, patients who give medical offices their e-mail addresses authorize those offices to send them e-mail. However, it is crucial that medical staff remember that e-mail is far from secure. For example, e-mail addresses can be misspelled, causing incorrect parties to receive messages. Also, employers have the right to view any e-mail their employees send on company systems. Because confidentiality is not guaranteed, all medical staff, including the medical assistant, should only use e-mail to send patients such nonconfidential information as appointment reminders.

Managing Mail and Correspondence

Administrative medical assistants are typically in charge of sorting and distributing the medical office's incoming mail (Figure 8-20 ◆). Because many such items, such as pathology reports or consultation letters, are time sensitive, assistants should sort and distribute incoming mail daily.

Many times, the person who sorts and distributes the mail is also asked to stamp the date the mail was received. Many offices also require the person sorting the mail to open each piece so recipients can easily access the contents. Items marked "personal" or "confidential" should be left unopened, however.

To avoid confusion, each office should have a mail sorting and distribution policy that includes a list of the items each staff member should receive. For example, the physician may receive all communications or reports regarding patients, any professional journals, and literature from professional organizations. The office manager, by contrast, may receive all bills, advertisements for services or supplies, and samples from drug or supply companies.

HIPAA Compliance

Because many of the items sent to the medical office contain private patient information, mail should never be left where other people can access it, even when unopened.

Annotation

To abbreviate their reviews of the information they receive, some physicians charge their administrative medical assistants with **annotation,** a process that involves reading, highlighting, and summarizing information. Medical assistants who annotate should clarify the information physicians consider pertinent before they undertake the task (Figure 8-21 ◆). Typically, the physician will ask the medical assistant to highlight the patient's name, any pertinent information about the patient, such as a diagnosis or treatment plan, and the name of the sender of the letter.

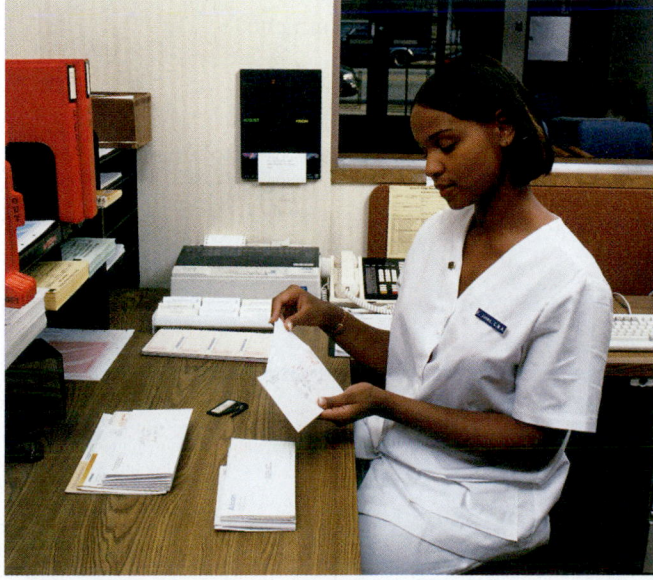

Figure 8-20 ◆ The medical assistant is commonly the person to open and sort the mail.

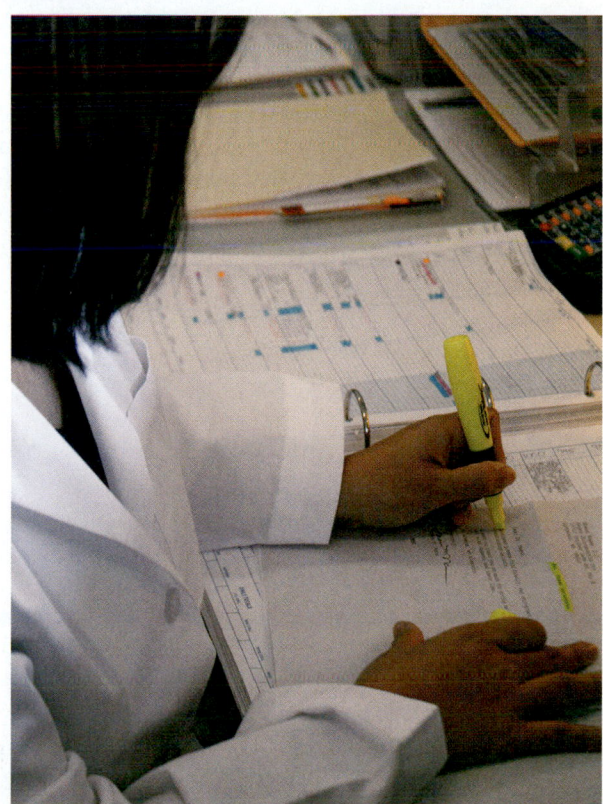

Figure 8-21 ◆ The medical assistant may be asked to open and annotate portions of the physician's incoming mail.

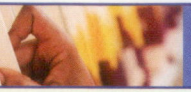

PROCEDURE 8-6 Open and Sort Mail

Theory and Rationale

The medical office receives various kinds of mail daily. Some mail contains important, private patient information, whereas other is considered "junk." The medical assistant will likely need to learn to sort mail properly.

Materials

- A stack of incoming mail, including payments from insurance companies and patients, advertisements, drug samples, magazines, professional journals, bills for office services, a letter to the physician marked "Personal and Confidential," and consultation reports from other physicians
- Date stamp
- Letter opener

Competency

(**Conditions**) With the necessary materials, you will be able to (**Task**) open and sort the office mail (**Standards**) correctly within the time limit set by the instructor.

1. Using a date stamp, stamp the date on each received item.
2. Sort the mail into the appropriate files according to the following:
   - Physician—correspondence from other physicians, hospitals, or laboratories, as well as any professional journals
   - Office manager—bills for office services, drug samples, advertisements for supplies or services
   - Receptionist—magazines
   - Billing office—payments from patients or insurance companies, correspondence from insurance companies
3. Open each piece of mail, except for the piece marked "Personal and Confidential."
4. Distribute the mail appropriately. Leave the mail piece marked "Personal and Confidential" on the physician's desk.

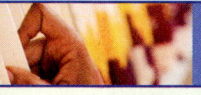

PROCEDURE 8-7 Annotate Written Correspondence

Theory and Rationale

In a busy medical office, the physician may want the medical assistant to scan and annotate medical reports to save time. Medical assistants who know what information to look for save time for the physician and can point out key pieces of information.

Material

- Written correspondence
- Highlighter pen
- Letter opener

Competency

(**Conditions**) With the necessary materials, you will be able to (**Task**) annotate a written correspondence (**Standards**) correctly within the time limit set by the instructor.

1. Open the envelope with the document to be annotated.
2. Read the document once in its entirety.
3. Using the highlighter pen, review the document again, highlighting such pertinent information as:
   - Patient's name
   - Findings of any examination or laboratory work
   - Dates for followup appointments
   - Diagnosis
4. Read the document a third time to ensure all pertinent information has been noted.
5. Place the annotated document on the physician's desk for review.

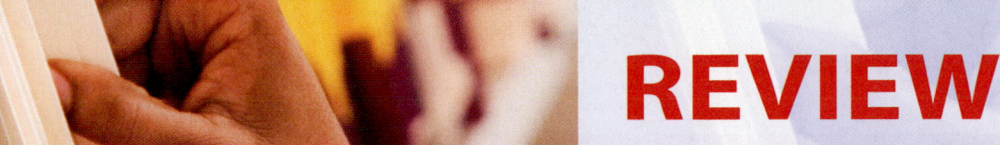

REVIEW

Chapter Summary

- Proper grammar, spelling, and punctuation are all paramount to a medical office's positive image.
- Medical assistants should follow a defined process when composing letters to patients and other members of the healthcare team.
- Medical assistants must be familiar with the use of a medical dictionary.
- The proofreading of business letters, which involves attention to detail as well as a solid understanding of English essentials, is a means by which the medical assistant can help support a positive professional image for the office.
- In all correspondence, medical assistants should use only abbreviations that are accepted in the healthcare industry.
- Memos are one vehicle healthcare staff can use to communicate with other team members.
- The U.S. mail system is governed by a set of rules and restrictions the medical assistant should be familiar with to function as part of the healthcare team.
- E-mail is governed by its own unique set of rules and policies.
- The medical assistant is responsible for managing incoming mail and correspondence according to office policy.
- The medical assistant may be called upon to annotate the physician's mail correspondence.

Chapter Review

Multiple Choice

1. Which of the following USPS mail types is appropriate for mailing a DVD?
   - a. Media
   - b. Priority
   - c. Express
   - d. Ground

2. Which of the following mail types is appropriate for sending a letter that must arrive the next day?
   - a. Media
   - b. Priority
   - c. Express
   - d. Ground

3. A piece of mail marked _____ should be left unopened and given directly to the intended recipient.
   - a. "Open Immediately"
   - b. "Personal"
   - c. "Important"
   - d. All of the above

4. Which of the following substances may be prohibited by the USPS for mailing?
   - a. Alcoholic beverages
   - b. Firearms
   - c. Flammable material
   - d. All of the above

5. In the medical office, it is appropriate to use a memo when the:
   - a. Office manager wishes to notify staff of a holiday party
   - b. Medical assistant must notify a patient of a missed appointment
   - c. Physician would like to contact a patient with test results
   - d. All of the above

True/False

T F 1. Any written correspondence in the medical office reflects on the physician and the office.

T F 2. As a general rule, numbers from one to ten should be written out when writing letters.

T F 3. The rules for making medical terms plural confuse the medical office.

T F 4. "Miss" is the appropriate title to use when addressing a woman of unknown marital status.

T F 5. The most common salutation in professional letters is "Yours Truly."

T F 6. E-mail is a secure way to send patients test results.

Short Answer

1. What is the purpose of the subject line in a professional letter?

2. What is a typical closing in a professional letter?

3. What are the reference initials for Mark S. Stevens, MD, who authors a letter, and medical assistant Sarah Ellen Parker, who types it?

4. Which three fonts appear most often in a business letter?

5. Explain the process of annotation.

6. Describe the function of spell-check software.

7. Give several examples of words in English that sound the same yet have different meanings.

8. What is a logo, and why is it used?

Research

1. What classes could you take at your local community college to help improve your written communication skills?

Chapter Review (continued)

2. Looking at the USPS Web site, how would you calculate postage to various locations throughout the United States? Outside the United States?

3. Review the Web sites for both FedEx and UPS. Compare their services. Does either offer a service the other does not?

Externship Application Experience

When Dr. Yi asks office manager Marnie Glaser, CMA, to open and distribute the day's mail, Marnie accidentally opens a piece to Dr. Yi marked "Personal." What is the proper way to handle this situation?

Resource Guide

United States Postal Service
Phone: (800) 275-8777
www.usps.com

Federal Express
www.fedex.com
Phone: 1-800-GO-FEDEX

United Parcel Service
www.ups.com
Phone: 1-800-PICK-UPS

DHL
www.dhl-usa.com
Phone: 1-800-CALL-DHL

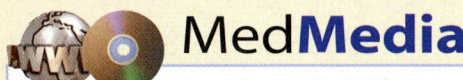

Med**Media**

http://www.MyMAKit.com

More on this chapter, including interactive resources, can be found on the Student CD-ROM accompanying this textbook and on http://www.MyMAKit.com.

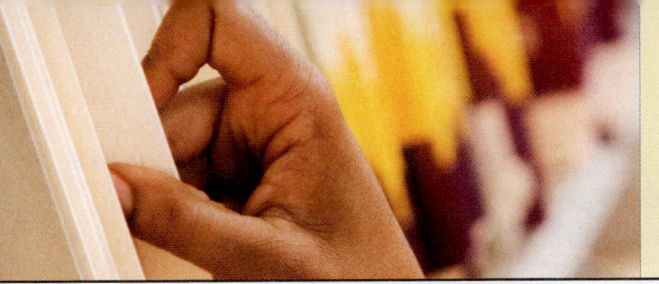

Objectives

After completing this chapter, you should be able to:

- Define and spell the key terminology in this chapter.
- Define the medical assistant's role as it pertains to telephone procedures.
- Describe the main features of telephone systems.
- Outline the benefits of an answering service.
- Explain how to perform telephone triage, including a list of the steps to take when triaging patients this way.
- Describe how to handle emergency calls and calls with difficult patients.
- Outline the procedure for taking a proper telephone message.
- Respond to telephone prescription requests.
- Describe the steps to take when calling patients via telephone.
- Use a telephone directory effectively.
- Discuss how the medical assistant can protect patient confidentiality when using the telephone.

Telephone Procedures

Case Study

Martha Hagen, one of the medical office's established patients, calls to notify the office that she is having chest pains. Martha is not sure if she should make an appointment to come into the office or if she should go to the emergency room.

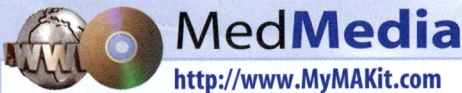

MedMedia
http://www.MyMAKit.com

Additional interactive resources and activities for this chapter can be found on http://www.MyMAKit.com. For videos, tips, audio glossary, legal and ethical scenarios, on-the-job scenarios, quizzes, and games related to the content of this chapter, please access the accompanying CD-ROM in this book.

Video: *Patient Reception, Telephone Procedures*
Legal and Ethical Scenario: *Telephone Procedures*
On the Job Scenario: *Telephone Procedures*
Tips
Multiple Choice Quiz
Audio Glossary
HIPAA Quiz
Games: Spelling Bee, Crossword, and Strikeout

Key Terminology

automatic dialer—telephone feature that dials numbers programmed into the system using codes; see also *speed dial*

automatic routing unit—telephone equipment that allows callers to self-select their call destinations via an automated, electronic prompt system

call forwarding—telephone feature that forwards incoming calls to other numbers

conference call—telephone feature that allows parties in different locations to participate in one call

direct telephone lines—telephone number that reaches a person directly rather than an operator or a receptionist

established patient—patient whom the medical office has seen previously

generic message—telephone answering message that fails to identify the receiver specifically

hands-free telephone device—headset or headphones with a speaker and microphone that allow users to participate in calls without picking up the telephone's receiver

hold feature—telephone feature that allows the user to place one call on hold and take another

last number redial—telephone feature that dials the last number dialed from that telephone

route—to direct telephone calls to other numbers

speaker phone—telephone feature that broadcasts the speaker's voice

speed dial—telephone feature that dials numbers programmed into the system using codes; see also *automatic dialer*

triage notebook—notebook the administrative medical assistant uses to properly handle calls from patients with potentially life-threatening conditions

triaging—process of prioritizing patients based on need

Abbreviations

ADA—Americans with Disabilities Act

HIPAA—Health Insurance Portability and Accountability Act

TTY—teletypewriter system

✚ MEDICAL ASSISTING STANDARDS

CAAHEP ENTRY-LEVEL STANDARDS	ABHES ENTRY-LEVEL COMPETENCIES
■ Perform within scope of practice (psychomotor)	■ Adapt to change
■ Apply ethical behaviors, including honesty/integrity in performance of medical assisting practice (affective)	■ Maintain confidentiality at all times
■ Apply active listening skills (affective)	■ Use appropriate guidelines when releasing records or information
■ Practice within the standard of care for a medical assistant (psychomotor)	■ Project a positive attitude
■ Identify styles and types of verbal communication (cognitive)	■ Be cognizant of ethical boundaries
■ Identify nonverbal communication (cognitive)	■ Evidence a responsible attitude
■ Explore issue of confidentiality as it applies to the medical assistant (cognitive)	■ Conduct work within scope of education, training, and ability
■ Respond to issues of confidentiality (psychomotor)	■ Professional components
■ Demonstrate sensitivity to patient rights (affective)	■ Monitor legislation related to current healthcare issues and practices
■ Demonstrate respect for individual diversity, incorporating awareness of one's own biases in areas including gender, race, religion, age, and economic status (affective)	■ Orient patients to office policies and procedures
■ Demonstrate sensitivity to the message being delivered (affective)	■ Adapt what is said to the recipient's level of comprehension
■ Demonstrate awareness of the territorial boundaries of the person with whom communicating (affective)	■ Adaptation for individualized needs
■ Analyze communications in providing appropriate responses/feedback (affective)	■ Instruct patients with special needs
■ Document accurately in the patient record (psychomotor)	■ Locate resources and information for patients and employers
■ Identify resources and adaptations that are required based on individual needs (cognitive)	■ Use proper telephone techniques
■ Discuss applications of electronic technology in effective communication (cognitive)	■ Be courteous and diplomatic
■ Explain general office policies (psychomotor)	■ Serve as a liaison between the physician and others
■ Report relevant information to others succinctly and accurately (psychomotor)	■ Exercise efficient time management
■ Demonstrate telephone techniques (psychomotor)	■ Receive, organize, prioritize, and transmit information expediently
■ Perform patient screening using established protocols (psychomotor)	

Introduction

Professional telephone skills are essential for the medical assistant. Often, the telephone is the first contact a patient has with the physician's office and can set the tone of the patient's relationship with the clinic. Allowing the telephone to ring too long before answering or placing a patient on hold for extended periods are two examples of poor telephone procedure. One disadvantage to using the telephone is that neither party can use nonverbal communication to determine the attitude or sincerity of the other party. For this reason, it is important for medical assistants to keep their voice pleasant, polite, and professional while on the telephone. Handling telephone calls courteously and efficiently is the best way to make a good first impression on callers.

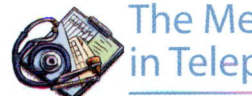
The Medical Assistant's Role in Telephone Communications

Since the telephone is often the patients' primary means of communicating with the medical office, the medical assistant must be capable of handling many kinds of calls. These calls range from those to schedule appointments to those of an emergency nature. The MA must be professional and able to remain calm, no matter what the demeanor of the caller.

Telephone System Features

Today's telephone systems are sophisticated, multifeature units that require training for new employees, including medical assistants.

Making Calls with Hands-Free Devices

For staff who answer telephone calls often throughout the day, **hands-free telephone devices** not only free the hands, they place little stress on the body. Wireless versions of these devices also allow medical assistants to conduct calls away from the telephone system, a feature that is particularly helpful when patient files must be pulled or assistants must move to different workstations (Figure 9-1 ◆). Assistants can wear wireless headsets all day throughout the office.

Dialing Numbers Automatically

Many telephone systems today have **automatic dialer** or **speed dial** functions that allow medical assistants to dial up to 100 programmed numbers with the push of a few buttons instead of dialing the whole number (Figure 9-2 ◆). Such features save medical assistants a great deal of time when contacting insurance companies, pharmacies, hospitals, laboratories, and physicians via the phone.

Redialing Last Numbers Called

The **last number redial** telephone feature, common today in home and office systems, dials the last number called from the phone with one button. Some systems offer a feature that will redial the last number called until there is an answer.

Making Conference Calls

The **conference call** feature allows two or more parties to speak on the same phone line at once. Conversation flows more easily and misunderstandings between parties diminish when all parties involved are on the line at the same time. In the medical office, the physician may use this feature to speak with a patient and another member of the healthcare team, such as the physical therapist.

As the parties to a conversation increase, however, so does the potential for confusion. Therefore, when conference calls have more than three parties, all parties should identify themselves before commenting.

broadcast the voice of another healthcare professional while a patient is in the office, for example. Medical professionals can work hands free, which means they can do things like write in patients' charts while taking part in the conversation. Whenever the speaker phone feature is used, however, it is important and courteous to advise speakers that they are being broadcast and to advise them of all other listeners in the room.

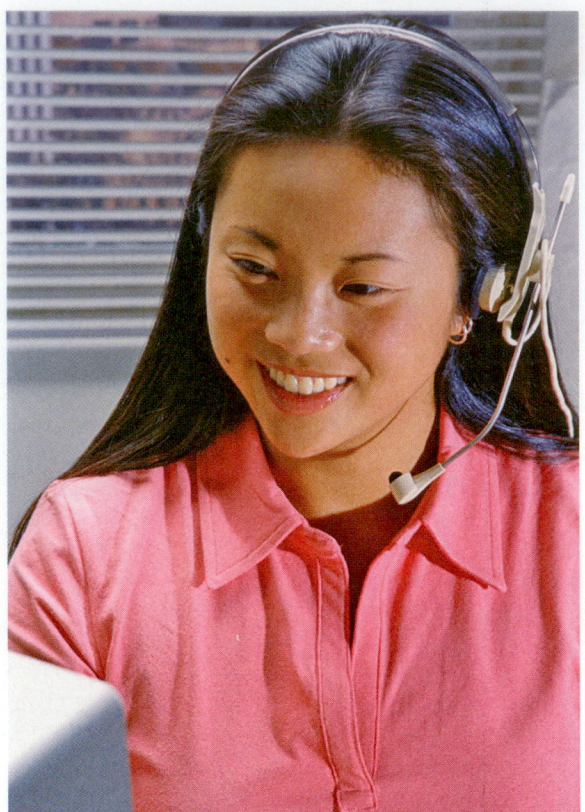

Figure 9-1 ◆ Using a hands-free headset makes the medical assistant's job easier.

Conversing via Speaker Telephone

The **speaker telephone** feature, which broadcasts the speaker's voice from the unit, helps when more than one party at the same location wishes to participate in a telephone conversation. In the medical office, the physician may use this feature to

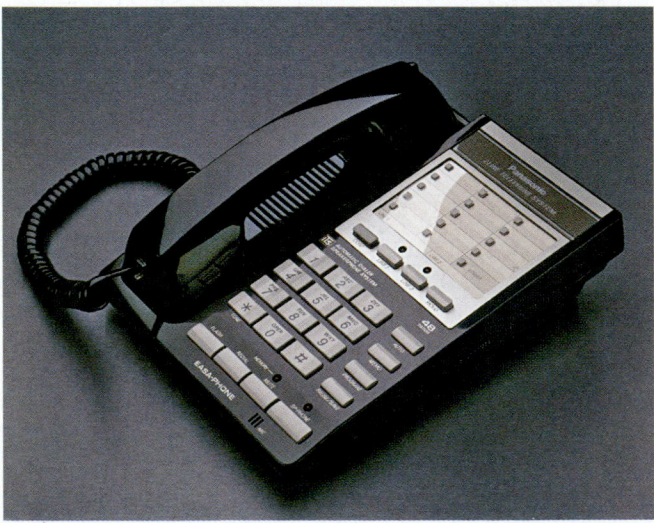

Figure 9-2 ◆ Most telephone systems in the medical facility have features such as speed dial.

HIPAA Compliance

Patient confidentiality is an important part of Health Insurance Portability and Accountability Act (**HIPAA**) compliancy. The speaker-phone feature must only be used to discuss confidential patient information when parties unauthorized to have the patient's information are unable to overhear the conversation.

Call Forwarding

Call forwarding automatically routes incoming calls to other telephone numbers. In the medical office, this feature is most commonly used after business hours to direct incoming calls to an answering service.

Recording Telephone Calls

The medical office, like other businesses, may wish to record incoming calls. Recorded calls support both quality-assurance efforts and training initiatives.

Direct Telephone Lines

Many medical offices use **direct telephone lines** that **route** to select members of the staff. Patients can call the billing department, for example, or staff in charge of appointment scheduling. While direct lines can eliminate the need for hold times, they require patients to have multiple telephone numbers for the office.

Automatic Routing Units

In many medical offices, callers can use **automatic routing units** to choose the parties they wish to reach by dialing the main line and choosing extensions. Automated instructions direct callers to the parties they wish to reach. While such systems can be beneficial, they can also have drawbacks. For example, such systems may impose long wait periods on callers or require multiple steps to reach desired extensions.

Placing Callers on Hold

The **hold feature** of telephone systems places callers on hold so users can complete other tasks. With this feature, staff can juggle multiple telephone lines or handle calls while assisting patients in person. Callers cannot see who is in the medical office when they call, however, so medical assistants must use the hold feature judiciously. Improper use can extend wait times and give the impression that the patient on hold is not important.

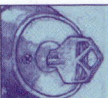

Recording telephone calls without the callers' consent is illegal. Medical offices that wish to record calls should do one of the following:

- Prerecord a message that plays before the medical assistant takes the line. Such a recording may say, "This call may be recorded to maintain quality customer service."
- Have the medical assistant advise callers that calls may be recorded.

Callers can choose to avoid participating in recorded calls. When they do, medical offices cannot record calls.

Medical assistants should verify that callers have only non-emergency issues before placing those callers on hold. In general, all members of the healthcare team should use the hold function in such a way that minimizes wait times and treats all patients equally.

Even the simplest telephone systems can play music or recorded information during hold times. The most rudimentary systems connect the telephone system to a radio, while more advanced units allow callers to choose the type of information they will hear. Many medical offices record or buy messages for this purpose. Such messages can be specific to the practice, such as messages about well-child checkups for pediatric offices, or informational, like those about seasonal allergies for allergists' offices. Some physicians use **generic messages**, and some will even record their own messages in their own voices. Messages like these add a personal touch that can both reassure patients and fortify their trust in the practice. However, only physicians with warm, pleasant-sounding, and clear voices should record messages like these. As mentioned earlier, the telephone is usually the patient's first contact with the medical office. Unpleasant-sounding physicians may unnerve new patients. Medical assistants with proper speaking voices can sometimes record such messages effectively.

Like the recorded information that is played during hold periods, hold music should be used with some stipulations. First, the music must be clear and generally pleasant. Callers are a captive audience who may become irritated by music that is broken by static or considered offensive. Religious music, for example, should be avoided, because it could offend followers of different faiths. So that they may better understand their callers' experiences, it is good practice for medical assistants periodically to call the offices where they work and assess the offices' recordings.

Critical Thinking Question 9-1

If the medical office uses an automated system where callers are greeted by a recording, how can the medical assistant best serve a patient who has a possible emergency?

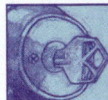

Never place a caller on hold without first asking for and receiving permission. When callers agree to hold, they should wait no more than 20 to 30 seconds before a member of the healthcare team checks in with an update. Long periods of hold time give the impression that patients are forgotten or unvalued when callers should instead feel that the medical office values them and their time.

Other Special Features

Large medical offices may have the funds to purchase special telephone features, such as programs that call patients with electronic appointment reminders or requests. "Automatic redial in reverse," which prevents long wait periods, is another such feature. With this feature, patients call the medical office and choose a number for the type of service they need, such as "1 to schedule an appointment." The patients then record their names, enter their telephone numbers, and hang up. When a medical assistant becomes available, the system automatically redials the patient and connects the call. Patients are free to go about other tasks, and office staff need not retrieve messages.

Using an Answering Service

When they are closed, perhaps during lunch or after conventional business hours, most medical offices use professional answering services to handle their calls. Such services forward calls to appropriate parties and thereby eliminate the need for the call forwarding feature mentioned earlier. Some telephone systems are designed to forward any calls not answered by the fourth ring to an answering service.

To ensure patients always receive high-quality customer service, medical offices should only use answering services experienced in healthcare. In addition, answering services should always have the contact information for the physicians on call. This way, the service can reach the physicians in the event of patient emergency. To retrieve any of the messages the service has taken, the medical office usually must call the service once the office reopens. Some answering services send messages via fax or e-mail.

Using the Voicemail Feature

Most medical offices use voicemail within their system. Often, voicemail is used at each employee's personal extension. When a patient calls the office after hours via the main office telephone line, the patient will typically reach an answering service. If the call comes through to an internal extension within the medical office, for example, the billing office, a voicemail may be reached after hours.

When using the voicemail feature, each employee should leave his or her name, department name, and information to let the caller know when to expect a return telephone call. An example might be: "This is Debra Meyers in the billing office at

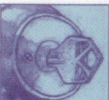

Martha Lake Family Practice. I am away from my phone right now. If you will leave me a message, including your name and telephone number, I will return your call within 24 hours."

Patient Telephone Use

Some medical offices provide telephones for patient use, often in the reception area or at the front desk, although growing cellular-phone use is eroding this practice. Offices that do provide patient phones will typically install a separate line that does not interfere with incoming calls, as well as restrict the phone to local calls only.

In Practice

Established patient Josie Welton often arrives early for her appointments. While she waits in the reception area, Josie uses the patient phone to make a call during which she details her healthcare problems and other personal information. The other patients in the reception area overhear the entire conversation. How should the medical assistant address this situation?

Answering the Telephone

Answering calls professionally is an art form that medical assistants should master, because telephone work is a large part of medical assisting. Before answering any calls, the medical assistant should obtain a pen and paper and prepare a cheerful yet professional greeting. Many assistants find practicing before a mirror, or even placing a "smile" symbol near the telephone, to be helpful when preparing for telephone work.

When medical assistants answer calls, they should speak clearly as they identify their office and themselves. Some offices identify themselves by physician names, while others use the names of their offices. Some offices even use original greetings, such as, "It's a great day at Mountain View Clinic. This is Sara."

As customer-service representatives are trained to do, medical assistants should answer calls within two to three rings. Any longer period gives a negative impression, perhaps that staffing in the office is inadequate or the office is overburdened.

Once the caller begins speaking, the medical assistant should try to match his or her rate of speech, although the assistant should always strive for a moderate pace.

As soon as the caller gives his or her name, the assistant should write the name down. Throughout patient calls, the medical assistant should refer to the caller by name, reinforcing that the caller is important. When the call is complete, the medical assistant should always say goodbye and allow the caller to hang up first. This reinforces the impression that the caller remains important and that the medical assistant is in no hurry to move on.

In terms of call content, medical assistants should be familiar enough with their office location to be able to give most callers directions, as well as such related information as parking fees and availability. In addition to office location, medical assistants should be familiar with the insurance plans their office participate in so they are armed to answer patient questions in that arena. Printed lists near the phone serve as good reference. Figure 9-3 ◆ identifies some behaviors to avoid while on the phone.

Screening Telephone Calls

As part of their telephone duties, medical assistants are charged with screening calls, which involves determining a call's purpose and whether that purpose is an emergency. To give assistants solid guidelines, every medical office should have a written policy for screening calls. ∞ Chapter 16 provides more information on creating office policies.

Directing Patient Calls to Physicians

Often, the calls medical assistants take are from parties who ask to speak with the physician directly. As a result, physicians should outline criteria for when they will accept patient calls (Figure 9-4 ◆). In addition to meeting physicians' needs and desires, such policies give medical assistants guidelines for

- Acting with no authority or out of the scope of training (e.g., reducing fees, agreeing to refill prescriptions without the physician's consent, making diagnoses).
- Arguing with callers. Medical assistants must remain professional and calm.
- Violating patient confidentiality. Medical assistants must never release any patient information without the patient's permission, including the fact that the patient patronizes the medical office.
- Answering telephone calls where other patients can hear them.
- Taking inaccurate or incomplete messages.
- Eating or drinking while using the telephone.
- Allowing callers to remain on hold for more than 30 seconds with no contact.

Figure 9-3 ◆ Improper telephone procedures.

PROCEDURE 9-1 Answer the Telephone in a Professional Manner

Theory and Rationale

One of the medical assistant's main duties, which is critical to the medical office, is to answer the office telephone. To complete this task, the assistant must have attention to detail, as well as the ability to multitask.

Materials

- Pen
- Paper
- Telephone

Competency

(**Conditions**) With the necessary materials, you will be able to (**Task**) answer the medical office telephone (**Standards**) correctly within the time limit set by the instructor.

1. Answer the telephone between the second and third rings.
2. State the office's name, followed by your name.
3. If the caller fails to provide a personal name, ask for it and write it down.
4. Determine the reason for the call.
5. If the caller is having a medical emergency, ask if someone can come to the phone to speak about it. If not, motion a coworker to dial for emergency services while keeping the patient on the line.
6. If the patient is calling to speak with another member of the healthcare team, transfer the call to that person if available.
7. When a requested party is unavailable, record a message. Include the name of the caller, the date and time of the call, the telephone number where the caller can be reached, the reason for the call, and the name of the person the caller wishes to reach.
8. When taking a message, inform the caller when the call will likely be returned.
9. Clarify information (e.g., appointment time) as appropriate.
10. Allow the caller to hang up before hanging up.
11. Route any message to the proper staff member.
12. Chart any healthcare-related information into the patient's chart as appropriate.

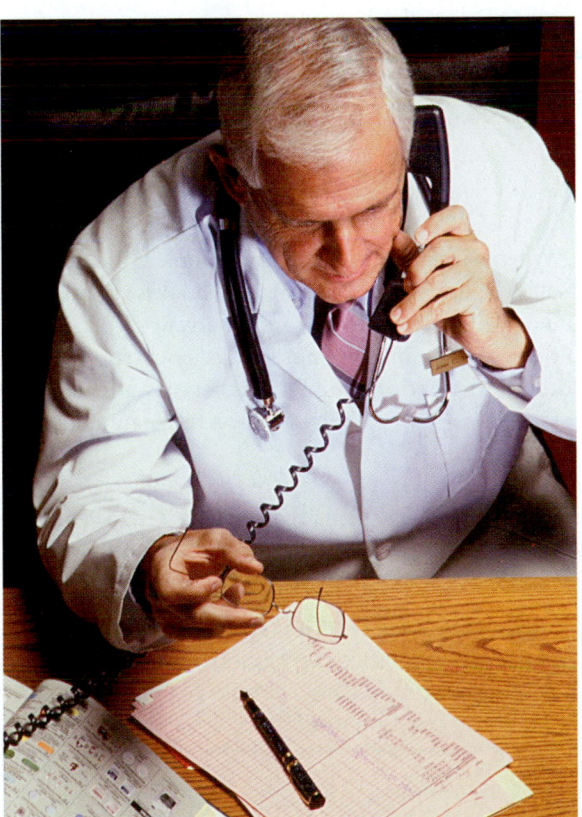

Figure 9-4 ◆ A physician takes a telephone call at his desk.

telephone use. Many physicians accept no telephone calls, even when not with patients.

When patients ask physicians to return their calls, the medical assistant should place the message with the patient's chart on the physician's desk. In offices with several physicians, typically only one physician will be "on call" after hours, a role the physicians serve on a rotating basis. Any physician who is on call after hours must have some way of being reached. Due to the nature of the occupation, physicians must be available at all times, whether by telephone or pager. In addition to being readily available to the medical assistant, such numbers must be readily available to the office's answering service. When physicians do accept calls, the medical assistant should gather a caller's name and reason for calling before transferring the call to the physician.

Prioritizing Telephone Calls

In general, it is most efficient to address short telephone calls before longer ones. Short calls include those that simply need to be routed to staff or that derive from **established patients** needing to make appointments. Long, time-consuming calls include those from new patients or patients with elaborate questions. Calls from angry or agitated patients take precedence above all others, however. Hold periods, even short ones, could worsen the situation. The sooner medical assistants provide for patient needs, the happier patients are. Figure 9-5 ◆ outlines some common call scenarios.

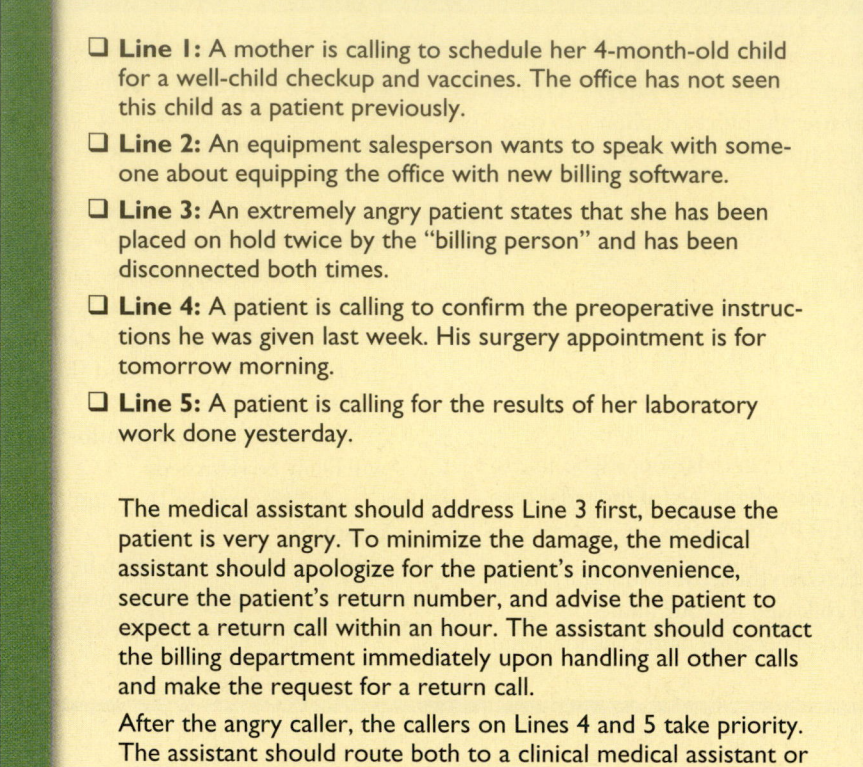

❑ **Line 1:** A mother is calling to schedule her 4-month-old child for a well-child checkup and vaccines. The office has not seen this child as a patient previously.

❑ **Line 2:** An equipment salesperson wants to speak with someone about equipping the office with new billing software.

❑ **Line 3:** An extremely angry patient states that she has been placed on hold twice by the "billing person" and has been disconnected both times.

❑ **Line 4:** A patient is calling to confirm the preoperative instructions he was given last week. His surgery appointment is for tomorrow morning.

❑ **Line 5:** A patient is calling for the results of her laboratory work done yesterday.

The medical assistant should address Line 3 first, because the patient is very angry. To minimize the damage, the medical assistant should apologize for the patient's inconvenience, secure the patient's return number, and advise the patient to expect a return call within an hour. The assistant should contact the billing department immediately upon handling all other calls and make the request for a return call.

After the angry caller, the callers on Lines 4 and 5 take priority. The assistant should route both to a clinical medical assistant or the nurse on staff. Line 2 is the next call in priority order. The medical assistant should route this call to the office manager, and then turn to the caller on Line 1. The Line 1 caller comes last in this situation, because a new-patient call takes the longest to resolve.

Figure 9-5 ◆ Prioritization of telephone calls.

Telephone Triage

The ability to **triage** patient telephone calls, or place them in priority order, is important not only for patient safety and well being, but also because it cultivates a positive office image. To triage calls properly, the medical assistant must know the types of complaints considered emergencies and, of those, which demand immediate attention. Calls from patients with potentially life-threatening emergencies must be handled before all other calls. Potentially life-threatening emergencies include, but are not limited to:

- Complaints of chest pain
- Complaints of heavy bleeding due to an injury
- Bleeding in a pregnant woman
- High fever in an infant or child
- Severe asthma attack
- Severe shortness of breath
- Possible poisoning or allergic reaction
- Obvious broken bone
- Sudden confusion, loss of consciousness, or change in mental status
- Mention of suicide or harm to themselves or others.

When triaging calls, a **triage notebook** at the front desk is invaluable (Figure 9-6 ◆). The triage notebook is typically a three-ring binder with sections for call and emergency types. Physicians should participate in these notebooks' construction so they can dictate the actions medical assistants and other staff must take. Figure 9-7 ◆ explains how a triage notebook might be used.

A more detailed discussion of triage and care of critically ill or severely injured patients is in ∞ Chapter 24, The Clinical Visit: Office Preparation and the Patient Encounter.

? — Critical Thinking Question 9-2 —
If the medical office mentioned in the case study lacks a triage notebook, how should the medical assistant go about creating one?

Taking Emergency Telephone Calls

When patients need immediate transport to the hospital, the medical assistant may be asked to call for emergency services.

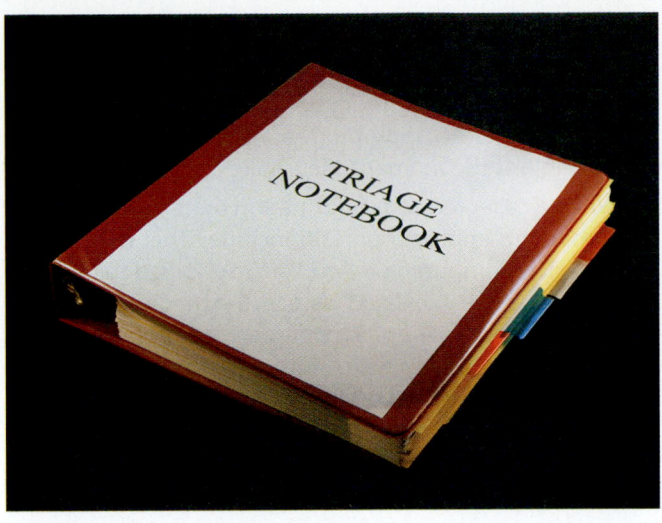

Figure 9-6 ◆ A triage notebook.

If the emergency has occurred in the medical office, the medical assistant will need to direct emergency services to the office to pick up the patient (Figure 9-8 ◆). The medical assistant should have the patient's name, age, and gender before making the call, as well as the problem type and type of care the physician is requesting. The medical assistant will need to be sure to give any specific directions, such as the office or suite number, and then advise the physician of the estimated time of arrival of the emergency services team.

Being Professional on the Telephone

When using the telephone, the medical assistant must be professional. Professionalism includes never chewing gum or eating while using the telephone and being careful to pronounce words, including names, correctly. Assistants should avoid using

---

Scenario: A patient calls the office complaining of chest pain.

Action:

❑ The medical assistant turns to the page in the triage notebook labeled "Chest Pain."

❑ The medical assistant asks the patient to describe the pain.

Situation 1: The patient states the pain is radiating down the arm.

Action:

❑ The medical assistant asks the patient to verify his or her present address. When the physician is in the office, the medical assistant asks a coworker to notify the physician of the emergency call. The physician will typically take the call when in the office.

❑ If the physician is not in the office, the medical assistant motions for a coworker to call for emergency services on another line.

❑ The medical assistant keeps the patient on the line while giving the second medical assistant the information to give to emergency medical service personnel.

❑ The medical assistant lets the patient know that emergency help is on the way and remains on the line with the patient until emergency services arrive.

❑ The medical assistant charts the entire situation in the patient's medical chart and gives the chart to the physician for review.

Situation 2: The patient indicates some pain in the chest and stomach that has persisted for the past week but remained at a steady intensity.

Action:

❑ The medical assistant schedules the patient to see the physician.

❑ The medical assistant confirms the time and date of the appointment with the patient.

Figure 9-7 ◆ Sample triage notebook use.

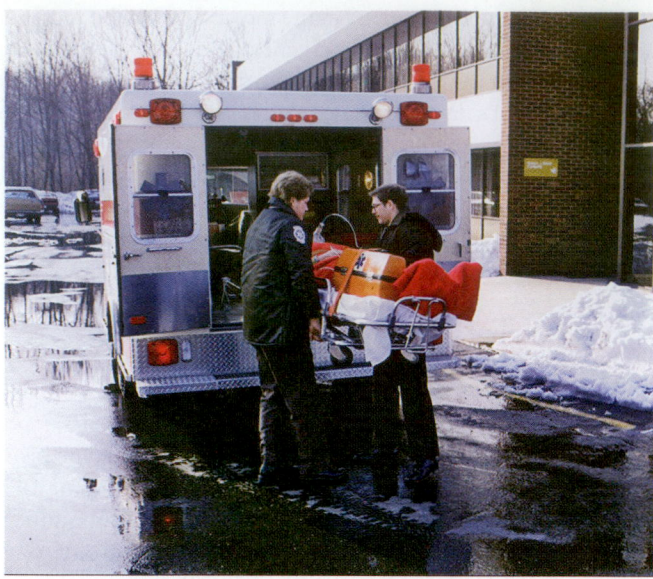

Figure 9-8 ◆ In the event of a medical emergency, an ambulance may be called to the medical office to transport the patient to the hospital.

unfamiliar words or slang, especially when speaking to people who use English as a second language. The medical assistant's voice should be calm and pleasant and its tone polite and warm. Callers should feel they have the medical assistant's complete attention.

In addition to using proper words and a soothing voice, medical assistants must be organized and prepared to answer the telephone properly. They should have a pen or pencil and paper ready before picking up the line. Never should assistants be rushed or anxious to end patient calls. When the time callers need exceeds the time medical assistants have, those assistants should take the callers' names and numbers and get permission to call them back.

Especially over the telephone, many people get into habits of using phrases or terminology that fail to work in healthcare. Figure 9-9 ◆ provides some examples with proposed improvements.

Communicating with Hard-to-Understand Callers

Part of acting like a professional includes listening to patients speak without interruption. When patients have speech impediments or English that is unclear, medical assistants may have to ask those patients to repeat themselves. When confusion persists, the medical assistant should try repeating what they heard to verify the patient's message was understood correctly.

Handling Difficult Callers

Occasionally, patients call the office while very upset. With calls like these, the most important thing the medical assistant can do is to remain calm and professional and avoid both attacking the patient personally and taking the patient's emotions personally. Medical assistants must always speak politely and courteously, whatever the callers' attitudes. While the medical assistant's job

- When a caller asks for a staff member who is not in the office, inappropriate phrases include, "He isn't in yet," "She's in the restroom right now," or "I don't know where she is." An appropriate substitution is, "He's unavailable at the moment. May I take a message?"

- When a caller requests information or help with something, improper phrases include, "That isn't my job," "The computer is down," or "You'll need to talk with someone in billing." Instead, the medical assistant should take the caller's name and number, commit to checking with another member of the healthcare team, and promise to call the patient with the desired information.

- When a new patient calls to schedule an appointment, the medical assistant should not say things like, "We don't accept that insurance," "We don't take patients with your condition," or "I've never heard of the doctor who referred you." Instead it is appropriate to say, "We are not preferred with your insurance plan, but let me find out who is and call you back," or "Our office doesn't specialize in conditions such as yours, but let me check with the doctor to see who she would refer you to and call you back." Another appropriate response is, "Will you please spell the referring doctor's last name, and do you have that office telephone number?" These statements are unlikely to offend the caller.

- The habit of asking patients, "How are you?" is an undesired one. Although common in American culture as a generic opener, some patients take the question literally and provide personal information. As has been discussed before, personal patient information must be guarded, especially at an office's busy front desk.

- Medical assistants should anticipate how terms may be interpreted. For example, the term "waiting room" implies an area where patients wait, but a more positive term is "reception room," because it means patients are received into the office.

Figure 9-9 ◆ Appropriate telephone phrases.

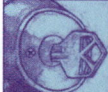

Keys to Success
EMERGENCY PHONE NUMBERS

Every medical office should keep a list of emergency telephone numbers near every office telephone. This list should include numbers for police nonemergency services, the sheriff's department, and poison control, among others.

is not to take verbal abuse, most angry callers will calm quickly when the medical assistant remains calm and polite. Any calls like this, however, must be documented in patients' files.

To resolve matters involving difficult callers, the medical assistant should apologize for whatever the patient is angry about and determine how to correct the situation. Any calls from patients that cannot be resolved must be brought to the physician's attention. The physician may choose to call the patient in the hope of finding resolution.

Receiving Calls from Emotional Patients

Emotional patients, such as those who are grieving or have been in accidents, will likely need more of the medical assistant's time. If the patient is emotional and calling to schedule an appointment, the medical assistant will need to determine if the patient needs to be seen right away. In a situation like this, the medical assistant should chart in the patient's medical record what happened during the telephone call and bring the situation to the physician's attention. It may be appropriate for the physician to call the patient back.

Documenting Calls from Patients

While not all patient calls must be documented in the patients' chart, any related to the patients' healthcare should be charted. Figure 9-10 ◆ outlines which calls should and should not be charted. Every medical office should have a policy about when and how to chart telephone calls, and medical assistants should be familiar with their offices' policies. In most offices, the administrative medical assistant makes the entry in the patient's chart and places the chart on the physician's desk for review or possible followup action.

Taking Telephone Messages

Taking a telephone message properly saves time for the member of the healthcare team who is returning the call. Most offices have message pads for this purpose (Figure 9-11 ◆). Such pads, which serve as reminders to the medical assistant, have spaces for all the information needed from patients.

Calling in Prescriptions and Refill Requests

Guidelines for prescription refills vary from one office to another. Generally, most offices require at least 24 hours' notice to refill prescriptions. Medical assistants should forward these calls, which may come from patients or pharmacists, to the clinical medical assistant or nurse. Alternatively, the medical assistant can check with the physician to see if the physician wishes to see the patient before allowing his or her refill. When office policy requires the medical assistant to check with the physician on all prescription refill requests but the physician is unavailable when the call comes in, the assistant must take the patient's name; the medication requested, including dosage; and the number where the patient or pharmacist can be reached. The medical assistant must then pull patient's file and place it, with the corresponding message, on the physician's desk (Figure 9-12 ◆).

Calling Patients

Before making telephone calls, medical assistants should have all materials and information at hand, including the patients' medical charts. Assistants who are calling patients to schedule

---

Calls That Typically Must Appear in Patients' Charts

- Patients who cancel appointments and fail to reschedule
- Patients who say they are in the hospital
- Relatives of patients who say the patient has died
- Patients who indicate they are not returning to the office for care
- Patients who contend they cannot afford to keep their appointments, fill their prescriptions, or see specialists

Calls That Typically Require No Charting

- Patients confirming appointment times
- Patients rescheduling appointments
- Patients complaining about their bills

Figure 9-10 ◆ Charting telephone calls in patient charts.

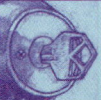

Keys to Success
TAKING A TELEPHONE MESSAGE

Obtain all the following information when taking telephone messages:

- Date and time of telephone call
- Name of person with whom the caller wishes to speak
- Name of the caller (verify the spelling when unsure)
- Telephone number, including area code, where the caller can be reached
- Nature or reason for the call
- Your name

Advise the caller when to expect a return call. If, for example, the caller is calling for Jane in the billing department but Jane is out, tell the caller when to expect a return call. This way, the caller can avoid wasting time waiting for the call. Also, be sure to route messages to appropriate parties in a timely manner.

Figure 9-11 ◆ Telephone message pads should be located near every office telephone in the administrative portion of the medical office.

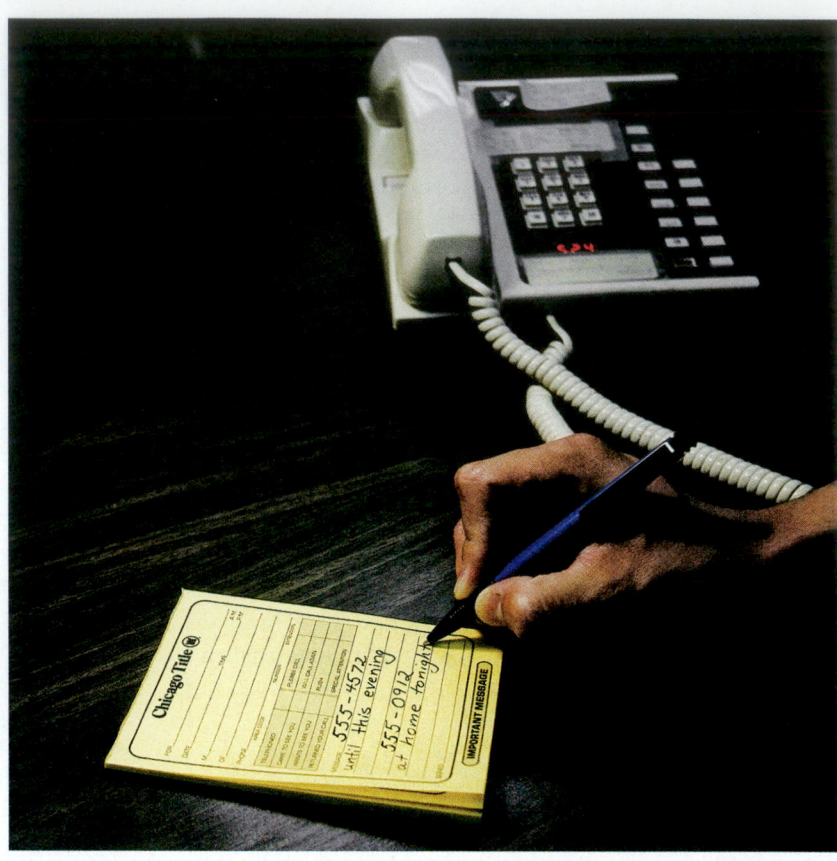

Figure 9-12 ◆ When prescription refill requests come into the office, the medical assistant should pull the patient's file and give both to the physician.

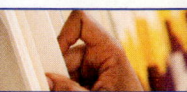

PROCEDURE 9-2 Take a Telephone Message

Theory and Rationale

Medical assistants often take telephone messages for other members of the healthcare team. In this task, accuracy is paramount. A simple numeric transposition, for example, can make a message useless.

Materials

- Pen
- Telephone message pad
- Telephone

Competency

(**Conditions**) With the necessary materials, you will be able to (**Task**) take a telephone message (**Standards**) correctly within the time limit set by the instructor.

1. Answer the telephone call by the second ring.
2. Once the caller identifies the desired party, reach for the message pad.
3. Ask for the caller's full name, verify the spelling, and document it on the pad.

4. Verify the name of the party the caller is trying to reach, and document it on the pad.
5. Ask for the reason for the call, and document it on the pad.
6. Ask for the caller's telephone number, including area code, and document it on the pad.
7. Repeat the telephone number to the caller to verify it was documented correctly.
8. Write the date and time of the call on the pad.
9. Write your name or initials on the pad.
10. Tell the caller when to expect a return call.
11. Bid goodbye to the caller, and allow the caller to hang up before hanging up.
12. Route the message to its intended recipient.

---

appointments should be well versed in the time each procedure takes, as well as any special patient instructions, such as not eating for 12 hours before a particular visit. Any patient calls that are medically relevant must be charted in the patients' charts.

Leaving Messages

To remain HIPAA compliant, medical assistants must maintain confidentiality at all times, including while on the telephone. When leaving messages, for example, assistants must remember that the people taking those messages, such as the patients' spouses or parents of minors seeking treatment for pregnancy, sexually transmitted diseases, mental illnesses, or drug and alcohol counseling, may lack the patients' permission to know the nature of the calls. ∞ Chapter 4 provides more information on the legalities of releasing information for minors.

When medical assistants must leave messages for patients, those assistants should leave their names, the physicians' names, and the appropriate telephone numbers. When an office's name self-identifies, such as "Marysville Oncology Specialists" or "Monroe Women's Care and Family Planning Clinic," the medical assistant should not leave the office's name, because doing so discloses some of the patient's confidential information. Instead, medical assistants should leave the names of physicians only, as in, "This is Christine calling

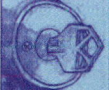

Keys to Success
LONG-DISTANCE CALLS

Factor in time zones before making long-distance calls (Figure 9-13 ◆). When calling California from New York, for example, the medical office must factor in a three-hour time difference.

from Dr. Wilson's office. I'm leaving a message for Jose. Please call me at 555-123-4567."

Calling Other Healthcare Facilities

Medical assistants often will be asked to call other healthcare facilities involved in the care of mutual patients, whether to schedule appointments with specialists or obtain information from patients' primary care providers. Whatever the reason for the call, the medical assistant will need to maintain patient confidentiality at all times. This means disclosing only absolutely necessary information to the other office staff when placing the call. If the medical assistant is scheduling a patient with a specialist, for example, that assistant will need to provide the patient's contact and insurance information. Other private patient information, like lifestyle habits and payment history, should remain

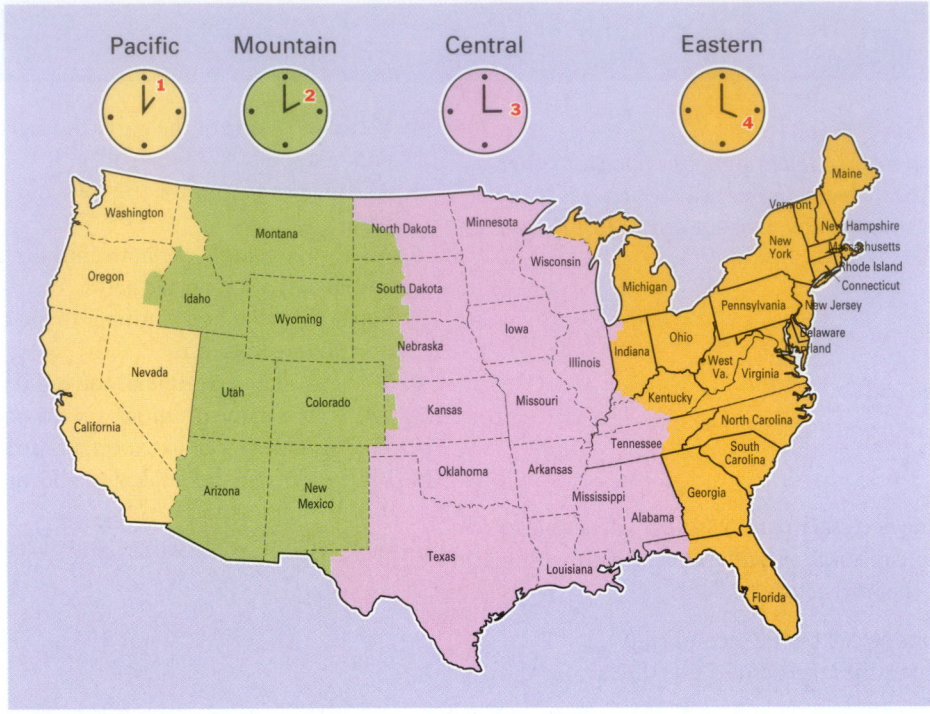

Figure 9-13 ◆ A time zone map.

undisclosed. Figure 9-14 ◆ provides tips on patient-related exchanges via telephone.

Using a Telephone Directory

In the past, a "telephone directory" usually meant a "telephone book," but today several different companies produce telephone books. The medical office may have one book for white pages and one for yellow pages, for example. When a medical office is in a large metropolitan area, it may have several books to cover its surrounding areas. Listings in the white pages are alphabetical by the person's name and alphabetical by business type in the yellow pages. Most telephone books create sublistings for business types, as well. For example, under the directory for physicians may be an alphabetical listing of physicians by type, such as pediatrician.

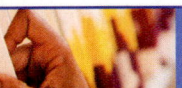

PROCEDURE 9-3 Call a Pharmacy with Prescription Orders

Theory and Rationale
As part of their duties in the medical office, medical assistants often call pharmacies with new or refill prescriptions. To complete this task properly and ensure patient safety, assistants must demonstrate strict attention to detail.

Materials
- Telephone
- Patient's chart
- Pen
- Prescription information
- Pharmacy telephone number

Competency
(Conditions) With the necessary materials, you will be able to **(Task)** call a pharmacy with a new or refill prescription order **(Standards)** correctly within the time limit set by the instructor.

1. Carefully read the prescription the physician has ordered.
2. Ask the physician any questions about the prescription if needed.
3. Call the pharmacy where the patient would like the prescription filled.
4. Give the pharmacist the patient's name, and verify the spelling.
5. Give the pharmacist the patient's birth date.
6. Give the pharmacist the medication's name, dosage, and directions per the physician. Alert the pharmacist to any drug allergies the patient has.
7. Ask the pharmacist to repeat the information for verification, and inform the pharmacist if the patient is en route to the pharmacy.
8. Note the prescription, including pharmacy name and telephone number, on the medication record in the patient's medical chart.

- If your physician is running behind on appointments or has been delayed getting to the office, call patients who will be impacted. Offer to reschedule when a delay is unacceptable.
- When the physician cannot do so, have the medical assistant make followup calls to patients after surgical procedures. When patients report anything unusual, transfer the call to the physician.
- Call new patients with all administrative information, such as parking and preferred manner of dress, medications and foods to avoid for certain tests and procedures.
- Advise patients of important policies (e.g., pay at the time services are rendered) before they visit the office.
- Remind all patients to bring necessary information to visits (e.g., insurance cards or lists of medications).
- Stagger staff lunch hours so a live person always answers the telephone.

Figure 9-14 ◆ Ways to show patient importance through telephone use.

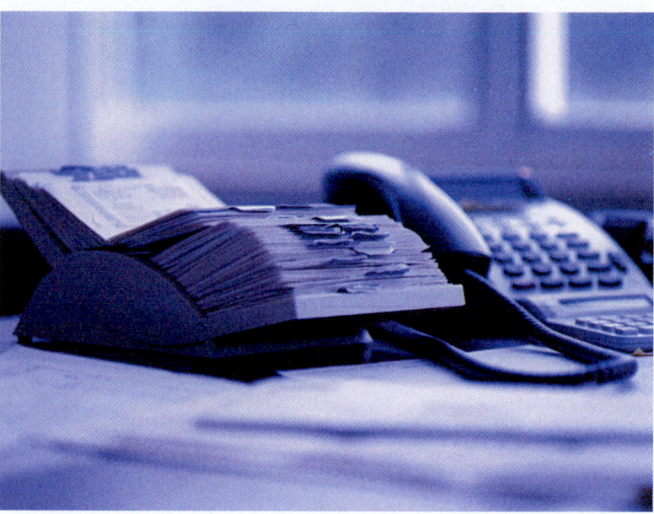

Figure 9-15 ◆ A Rolodex™ card system next to the telephone allows the medical assistant to quickly locate commonly called numbers.

Most telephone directories are color coded for ease of use. Many precede their white pages with business sections in different colors. Directories typically have listings for local ZIP codes at their beginnings and a government section that includes listings for federal, local, and state agencies. These pages are typically colored differently, sometimes blue.

Using an Online Directory

Many medical offices today use the Internet to look up telephone numbers. Many Web sites, including www.Yahoo.com, www.anywho.com, www.dexknows.com, www.yellowpages.com, www.superpages.com, and www.bigbook.com, search for both local and national telephone numbers for both personal and business information.

Using a Rolodex System

Every medical office should keep a directory of commonly called telephone numbers on the computer or in a Rolodex card file (Figure 9-15 ◆). Such tools make it easier to locate the number for the cardiac specialist the physician refers patients to, for example.

Long-Distance or Toll-Free Calls

The medical assistant may frequently make long-distance telephone calls on behalf of the medical office. Some offices require staff to log any long-distance telephone calls with the call's purpose,

as well as the name and number of the party being called. To comply with such requests, medical assistants should familiarize themselves with their offices' policies.

Most suppliers and businesses the medical office buys from will have toll-free telephone numbers, which typically begin with 1-800, 1-888, or 1-866, and impose no charges on callers.

Patient Confidentiality

Maintaining patient confidentiality is extremely important. Violations of patient privacy are serious offenses punishable by fines under HIPAA. Patients must know that their private information will be kept confidential. One of the best ways to do this is for the medical assistant to refrain from discussing any patient information within hearing distance of other patients. When patients hear office staff discussing other patients, they may assume that their private information is similarly discussed. Keeping conversations professional, and never resorting to gossip about other staff members or patients, is one way to reinforce to patients that the medical assistant is trustworthy and professional.

HIPAA Compliance

The medical office must treat all callers requesting patient information cautiously. Because callers' identities cannot be determined via telephone, the office should disclose no confidential information over the telephone. Instead, members of the healthcare team should advise callers to send any requests via fax or mail and to accompany those requests with a signed authorization from the patient or a court order.

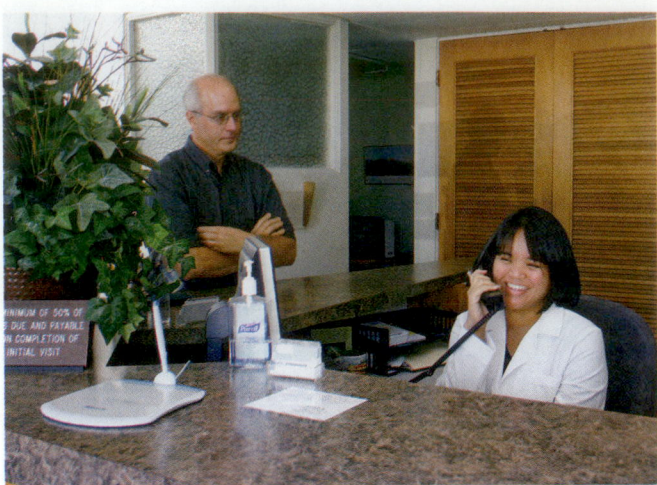

Figure 9-16 ◆ Making or receiving personal telephone calls is unprofessional. When medical assistants must make personal calls, they should do so on break and out of patients' hearing.

Personal Telephone Calls

Studies on businesses across America have found that the average employee spends 65 hours per year on personal calls while at work. Because personal calls are very expensive for employers, they are generally frowned on. Some employers feel that employees who spend time on personal telephone calls during work hours are stealing from them.

To avoid ill will, medical assistants should review and abide by their offices' policies for personal telephone use. Making or receiving personal telephone calls is unprofessional, and it ties up a business's telephone line (Figure 9-16 ◆). Most offices allow employees to receive only emergency telephone calls during work hours. When medical assistants must make personal calls, they should do so on break or during lunch and out of patients' hearing range.

- The caller types a message into a special telephone.
- The message transmits to the relay service.
- An operator calls the medical office.
- When the medical assistant answers, the operator self-identifies and identifies the caller.
- The operator mediates between the medical assistant and the caller, reading messages to the assistant and typing responses to the caller.
- When the call is complete, the medical assistant bids the patient goodbye, awaits the interpreter's response, and then hangs up.

Figure 9-17 ◆ Using a telecommunication relay service.

Telecommunication Relay Services

Patients who are hearing or speech impaired may use a telecommunication relay system to contact the medical office. The Americans with Disabilities Act (**ADA**) requires that telephone companies have telecommunication relay systems available 24 hours per day, 365 days per year. Figure 9-17 ◆ describes how a telecommunication relay system works.

A medical office with a large number of hearing-impaired patients, perhaps an audiology practice, may have a teletypewriter (**TTY**) system (Figure 9-18 ◆). TTY systems connect to the telephone, allowing both parties to the call to type their responses and thereby eliminate the need for a telecommunication relay service.

When using services like these, it is important to note that conversations be aimed at the caller, not the operator. The operator is charged with typing every spoken word, not serving as the call's recipient. In other words, the medical assistant should not say, "Tell Sharon the physician can see her at 10 A.M." Instead, the assistant should say, "Sharon, the physician can see you at 10 A.M. Will that time work?"

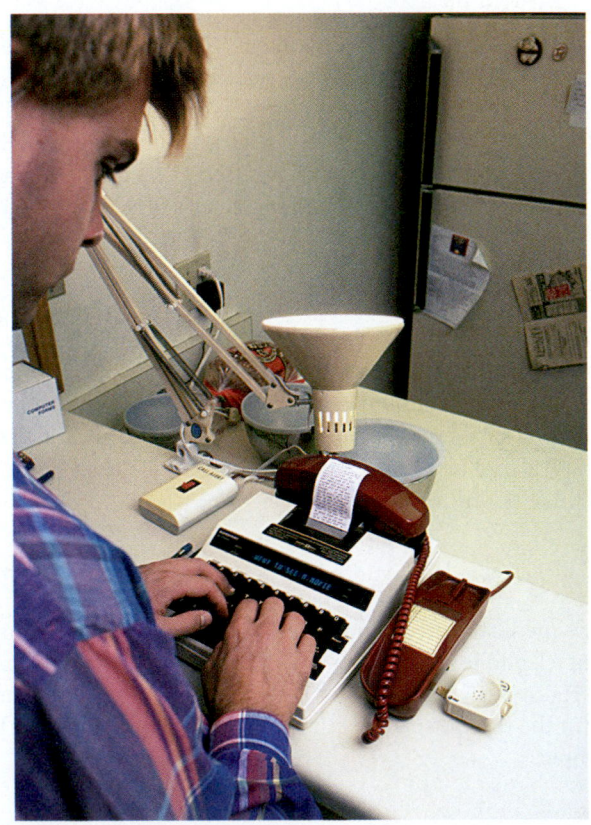

Figure 9-18 ◆ A patient using a teletypewriter (TTY) system.

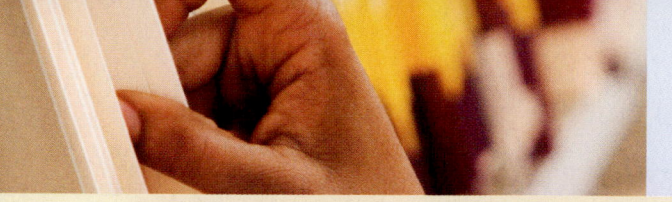

REVIEW

Chapter Summary

- Like the medical assistant, an answering service serves a crucial role in handling telephone calls efficiently and professionally.
- To triage the medical office's incoming calls properly, medical assistants need a distinct skill set, including a good understanding of any procedure's time requirements.
- Emergency calls dictate special telephone attention, as do callers who are angry or otherwise upset.
- When answering calls in the medical office, the medical assistant should follow all office policies for taking messages properly.
- Prescription requests must be made using proper, professional telephone procedure.
- When calling patients on medical offices' behalf, it is crucial that medical assistants remain calm and professional at all times.
- Telephone directories, both electronic and conventional hard-copy versions, are helpful tools in the office's search for telephone numbers.
- While conducting telephone procedures in the medical office, the medical assistant's most crucial task is to maintain patient confidentiality.

Chapter Review

Multiple Choice

1. Which of the following telephone features dials a number with the push of just one button?
   a. Last number redial
   b. Speed dialer
   c. Automatic dialer
   d. All of the above

2. Which of the following pieces of information need not be included when taking a message?
   a. Caller's name
   b. Call date
   c. Patient's insurance information
   d. Medical assistant's name

3. Which of the following is an appropriate way to handle an angry caller?
   a. Hang up the phone
   b. Remain calm
   c. Use the hold feature
   d. None of the above

4. Which of the following calls should be handled first?
   a. Patient calling for lab results
   b. Doctor's college roommate calling for the doctor
   c. Patient complaining of shortness of breath
   d. Patient confirming an appointment time

5. Which of the following is the best choice for patients on hold?
   a. Generic message thanking callers for holding
   b. Local news station with slight static
   c. Physician's gruff voice
   d. Any of the above

6. For a caller with a life-threatening emergency who needs emergency medical services, the medical assistant should
   a. ask the caller to hold while dialing emergency medical services on another line.
   b. ask the caller to hang up and immediately dial 9-1-1.
   c. ask the caller to hold while transferring the call to a clinical medical assistant.
   d. hang up on the caller and dial 9-1-1.

7. To find the telephone number for a medical supplier, the medical assistant could
   a. use an Internet directory.
   b. check a telephone book.
   c. search Rolodex card file.
   d. all of the above.

True/False

T F 1. Telephone triage is the ability to transfer calls to voicemail.

T F 2. When patients call to cancel their appointments but fail to reschedule, the calls should be charted in the patients' medical charts.

T F 3. When leaving messages for a patient, it is acceptable to tell the patient's spouse the purpose for the patient's visit.

T F 4. When calling other healthcare facilities to schedule appointments for patients, the medical assistant should disclose only needed patient information.

T F 5. Before answering the office telephone, medical assistants should know the insurance plans the office participates with.

Chapter Review (continued)

T F 6. Because medical terminology is unfamiliar to most patients, layman's terms are best when speaking with patients.

T F 7. Unidentified callers should be routed directly to the physician.

Short Answer

1. Why is it important to speak clearly on the telephone?

2. Explain why taking personal telephone calls during office hours is problematic.

3. Explain how a telephone relay system works.

4. What is the purpose of a telephone triage notebook?

5. Explain how a medical office can legally record patient telephone calls.

6. Differentiate between screening and prioritizing telephone calls.

Research

1. Look online for companies that sell multiline telephone systems. What kind of features do they offer?

2. What local companies can you find in your area that offer answering services to medical offices? What services do they offer?

3. Research companies that offer telephone translation services in your area. What languages do they offer translation for? How much does the service cost?

Externship Application Experience

When Sofie Pouillon calls the office, she says wants to cancel her upcoming appointment because she is very unhappy with the physician. What can the medical assistant say to this patient? What is the proper way to chart this call and notify the physician?

Resource Guide

Amateur Radio Research and Development Corporation
Telecommunications for the Deaf
Post Office Drawer 6148
McLean, VA 22106-6148
www.amrad.org

Online Yellow Pages
www.yellowpages.com

SkillPath Seminars
"The Secrets to Being a Front Desk Superstar" Seminar
P.O. Box 2768
Mission, KS 66201-2768
Phone: (800) 873-7545
Fax: (913) 362-4241
www.skillpath.com

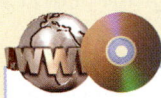

Med**Media**

http://www.MyMAKit.com

More on this chapter, including interactive resources, can be found on the Student CD-ROM accompanying this textbook and on http://www.MyMAKit.com.

Objectives

After completing this chapter, you should be able to:

- Define and spell the key terminology in this chapter.
- Define the medical assistant's role in front desk reception.
- Describe the steps to opening and closing the office efficiently.
- List the steps to prepare files for patient arrivals.
- Describe appropriate ways to greet and register both new and established patients.
- Identify means of maintaining patient confidentiality in all front-desk activities.
- Communicate with patients regarding scheduling delays and cancellations.
- Manage difficult patients effectively in the reception area.
- List the types of patients who should not be left in the reception room.
- Discuss how to maintain a safe and pleasant reception-room environment.
- Name appropriate reading materials for the reception room.
- Describe safe and effective ways to incorporate a children's area in the reception room.

Front Desk Reception

Case Study

When Marilyn Peterson enters the medical office for a new patient appointment, the medical assistant greets her and gives her paperwork to complete. In response, Marilyn frowns and says, "I don't want to fill all of that out. I'm only here to see the doctor about a sore throat. I don't have time for paperwork."

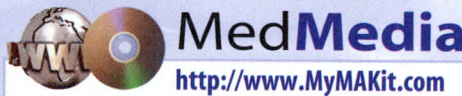

MedMedia
http://www.MyMAKit.com

Additional interactive resources and activities for this chapter can be found on http://www.MyMAKit.com. For a video on patient reception, tips, audio glossary, legal and ethical scenarios, on-the-job scenarios, quizzes, and games related to the content of this chapter, please access the accompanying CD-ROM in this book.

Video: *Patient Reception*
Legal and Ethical Scenario: *Front Desk Reception*
On the Job Scenario: *Front Desk Reception*
Tips
Multiple Choice Quiz
Audio Glossary
HIPAA Quiz
Games: Spelling Bee, Crossword, and Strikeout

Key Terminology

Americans with Disabilities Act (ADA)—federal law that outlines appropriate treatment or accommodations for patients or employees with disabilities

checklist—list of activities or steps to take to perform a task

copayment—a predetermined amount of money a patient must pay for each physician's visit

front desk—place in a medical office where the receptionist welcomes patients as they enter

hazard—something that is dangerous or possibly dangerous

HIPAA compliant—in line with federal patient confidentiality laws

office policy—agreed-upon standard for handling a situation or procedure in the office

reception area—waiting area for patients in the medical office

receptionist—medical staff member who greets patients, answers the telephone, and directs office flow

service animal—animal that has been trained to assist a person with a handicap

sign-in sheet—paper or electronic document on which patients sign their names upon entering the office

Abbreviations

ADA—Americans with Disabilities Act

HIPAA—Health Insurance Portability and Accountability Act

MEDICAL ASSISTING STANDARDS

CAAHEP ENTRY-LEVEL STANDARDS	ABHES ENTRY-LEVEL COMPETENCIES
■ Perform within scope of practice (psychomotor) ■ Apply ethical behaviors, including honesty/integrity in performance of medical assisting practice (affective) ■ Apply active listening skills (affective) ■ Practice within the standard of care for a medical assistant (psychomotor) ■ Identify styles and types of verbal communication (cognitive) ■ Identify nonverbal communication (cognitive) ■ Demonstrate sensitivity to patient rights (affective) ■ Analyze communications in providing appropriate responses/feedback (affective) ■ Document accurately in the patient record (psychomotor) ■ Identify resources and adaptations that are required based on individual needs (cognitive) ■ Explain general office policies (psychomotor) ■ Report relevant information to others succinctly and accurately (psychomotor) ■ Perform patient screening using established protocols (psychomotor) ■ Discuss applications of electronic technology in effective communication (cognitive)	■ Adapt to change ■ Maintain confidentiality at all times ■ Project a positive attitude ■ Show a responsible attitude ■ Conduct work within scope of education, training, and ability ■ Instruct patients with special needs ■ Be courteous and diplomatic ■ Serve as a liaison between the physician and others ■ Orient patients to office policies and procedures ■ Adapt what is said to the recipient's level of comprehension ■ Adaptation for individualized needs ■ Exercise efficient time management ■ Receive, organize, prioritize, and transmit information expediently

✓ COMPETENCY SKILLS PERFORMANCE

1. Open the office.
2. Greet and register patients.
3. Collect payments at the front desk.
4. Close the office.

Introduction

The adage "There is no second chance to make a good first impression" holds as true for the medical office as it does for any other business. In the medical office, the person who answers the telephone, often the medical assistant, plays a substantial role in patients' first impressions. Because poor impressions can prompt patients to seek care in other facilities, the medical assistant who is serving as **receptionist** at the **front desk** must treat all patients with a high level of customer service. That level of service should carry through from the telephone, into the **reception area** when patients arrive, and beyond into the clinical and treatment areas. The visual impressions made by the presentation of the reception area, in conjunction with the appearances and professional manners of the healthcare staff, greatly impact a patient's first impression of the office.

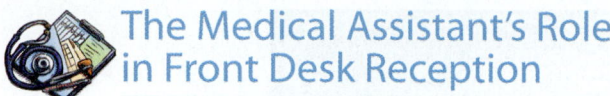

The Medical Assistant's Role in Front Desk Reception

The medical assistant's role at the front desk of the medical office is to greet all patients and visitors as they enter the office. The medical assistant must be aware of the various types of paperwork that may be required of patients as they arrive in the office. As the front desk receptionist, the MA should be aware of the office policy regarding the type of patients who may need to be taken back before others due to their condition or needs.

Characteristics of the Front Desk Receptionist

While people can learn the skills they need to be adequate front-desk receptionists, they must exhibit positive personality traits to excel at the job. When receptionists excel, they can positively impact the medical office's bottom line. Studies have shown that patients will continue to seek treatment with physicians they do not really like just because they feel well cared for by the rest of the healthcare team. Conversely, many patients will not return to the office when they feel a lack of caring about their needs on the part of the staff (Figure 10-1 ◆).

In short, front desk receptionists should really enjoy interacting with people. Successful front-desk receptionists remember patients' names. Remarkable receptionists remember the names of patients' children or spouses. Superior front-desk receptionists also remain calm, even with the rudest of patients or in the busiest of circumstances. Because receptionists can rarely start and finish their tasks without interruption, they must be open to constantly shifting their focus. The best front-desk receptionists are happy, kind people who genuinely care about patients and who have the utmost faith in the clinical staff and physicians on their healthcare teams.

?—Critical Thinking Question 10-1—

How can the medical assistant demonstrate caring and concern to Marilyn?

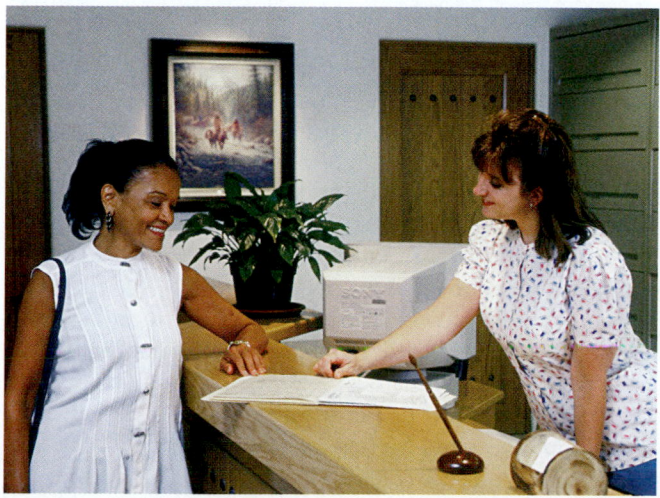

Figure 10-1 ◆ The front desk receptionist must be kind and professional with all patients.

Opening the Office

The task of opening and closing the medical office usually falls to the front-desk receptionist. A policy that outlines the steps to opening and closing the office helps train new staff and ensures that other, established staff can follow the proper procedures when serving in a cross-functional capacity. A printed **checklist** helps ensure that all staff follow all necessary steps.

While opening and closing procedures vary from office to office, most offices follow some basic steps. In general, staff should arrive at the office 30 or more minutes before patients are expected to arrive to ensure the facility is ready for business. Scrambling to find supplies or searching for files while patients are in the office is unprofessional and gives the impression that the healthcare team is unprepared.

Upon entering the office, the receptionist should turn on the lights and disarm the alarm system. Next, he should check the office answering system to identify patients who need visits that day or who have canceled their appointments. Calls should be handled in order of importance.

After making necessary calls, the front-desk receptionist should ensure that the reception room is ready to receive patients. This means making sure the room is tidy and free of litter. When the office provides coffee or water, the receptionist should ensure that related supplies are adequate.

Preparing Patient Files

Before the office closes for the night, staff should pull all patient files needed for the next morning. Any new patient files should be started, which means inserting all appropriate paperwork. Figure 10-2 ◆ depicts a new patient file folder with various paperwork the patient and healthcare professionals will fill out. The amount and type of paperwork contained within the patient file depends upon the type of practice and the policies regarding necessary forms in that particular facility.

Figure 10-3 ◆ is an example of a new patient history form. These forms may be purchased from a variety of medical office supply retailers, though many medical facilities create their own. Figure 10-4 ◆ shows an example of a HIPAA authorization agreement. This form is necessary in any medical setting where private patient information will be gathered and kept on file.

HIPAA Compliance

There are some patients who will refuse to sign the HIPAA authorization agreement form in the medical office. This is an infrequent event. When this happens, the medical assistant

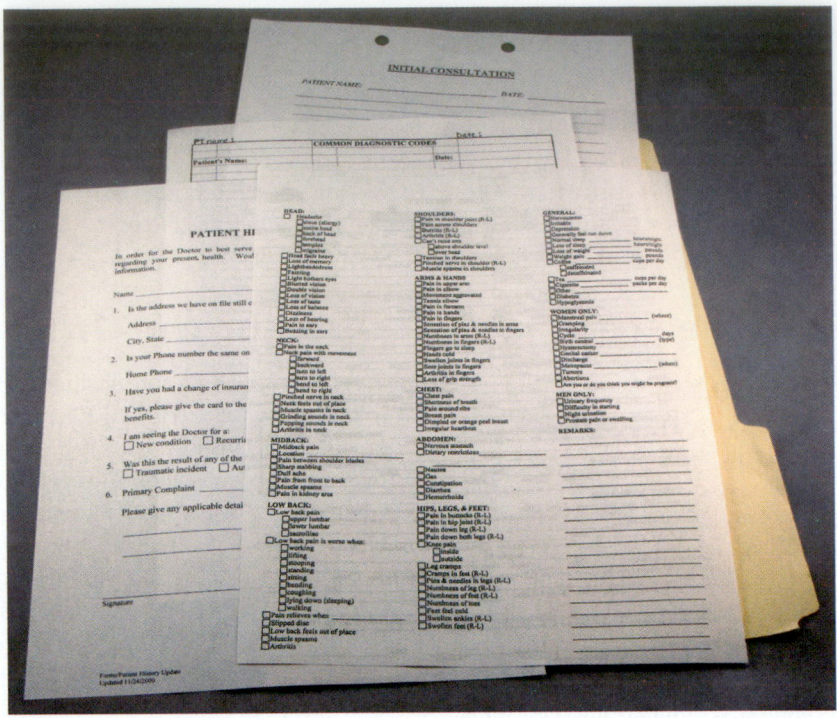

Figure 10-2 ◆ A new patient medical record with various forms.

should simply write "refused to sign" where the patient's signature is indicated, along with the date. The fact that the patient has refused to sign the form should be brought to the physician's attention and the form, with the medical assistant's notation, should be filed in the patient's medical record.

Before patients arrive, the receptionist must verify that all patient files have all necessary paperwork, such as laboratory results reports (outlining the findings of a patient's blood tests, urine tests, or analysis of secretions taken from the patient) and pathology reports (a report outlining the findings of any gross or microscopic tissue examination). When the billing office asks to see patients about their accounts, notes should be placed on the patients' files so those patients can be routed to the billing office before seeing the physician. To ensure patient confidentiality, all patient files must be kept out of sight of nonessential staff and other patients.

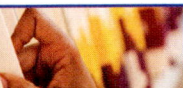

PROCEDURE 10-1   Open the Office

Theory and Rationale
When a medical office documents its standard opening procedures in a list, that list can help ensure that all members of the healthcare team have the tools to perform those procedures fully, accurately, and consistently.

Materials
■ Checklist of office opening procedures

Competency
(**Conditions**) With the necessary materials, you will be able to (**Task**) open the medical office (**Standards**) correctly within the time limit set by the instructor.

1. Arrive in the office at least 30 minutes before the first patient appointment.
2. Turn off the office alarm system.
3. Turn on all appropriate lights and equipment.
4. Retrieve messages from the office answering system, and return telephone calls as appropriate.
5. Verify that all patient charts needed for the morning were pulled the night before and that all needed information is attached to those charts.
6. Check the office for safety and cleanliness issues. For example, be sure all garbage cans are empty.
7. When the office is ready, unlock the door for patients to enter.

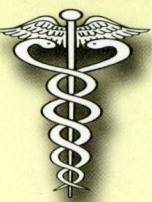

Victory Medical Center
4100 SW Highway 6
Victorville, WA 12345
(509) 555-9832

Patient Name: _____

                    Last Name   First Name   Middle Initial

Address: _____

                Street   City   State   Zip

Home Phone: _____ Work Phone: _____

Mobile Phone: _____ Birthdate: _____

Social Security Number: _____ Age: _____

Sex: _____ Marital Status: S M D W Children: _____

How do you prefer to be addressed? _____

Spouse's Name: _____

Primary Care Physician: _____ Phone No.: _____

Name of Person Responsible for Bill: _____

Relationship to Patient: _____ Phone No.: _____

Address of Person Responsible for Bill: _____

Patient's Employer: _____ Phone No.: _____

Occupation: _____

Spouse's Employer: _____ Phone No.: _____

Occupation: _____

INSURANCE INFORMATION

Primary Insurance: _____ Policy No.: _____

Name of Policyholder: _____ Birthdate: _____

SS#: _____ Relationship to Insured: _____

Secondary Insurance: _____ Policy No.: _____

Name of Policyholder: _____ Birthdate: _____

If Injured: Date: _____ Place: _____

Claim Number: _____ Nature or Cause of Injury: _____

Employer at Time of Injury: _____ Phone No.: _____

EMERGENCY INFORMATION

In case of emergency, local friend or relative to be notified (not living at same address)

Name: _____ Relationship to Patient: _____

Address: _____ Phone No.: _____

I hereby authorize the healthcare professionals in this clinic to diagnose and treat my condition. I clearly understand and agree that all services rendered me are charged directly to me and that I am personally responsible for payment. I agree that I am responsible for all bills incurred at this clinic. I hereby authorize assignment of my insurance rights and benefits directly to the provider for services rendered. I also authorize the healthcare professionals to discuss my care with other healthcare providers who I am currently treating with.

_____   _____

Patient's Signature   Date   Parent or Guardian Signature   Date

Figure 10-3 ◆ Sample new patient history form.

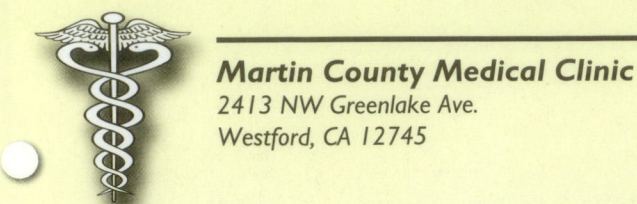

Martin County Medical Clinic
2413 NW Greenlake Ave.
Westford, CA 12745

AUTHORIZATION TO RELEASE INFORMATION

ACKNOWLEDGMENT OF RECEIPT of the Notice of Privacy Practices of the Martin County Medical Clinic (MCMC)

I acknowledge that I have received or been offered the Notice of Privacy Practices of the Martin County Medical Clinic. I understand that the Notice describes the uses and disclosures of my protected health information by the Covered Entities and informs me of my rights with respect to my protected health information.

_____

Name of Patient

_____

Patient Date of Birth

_____

Signature of Patient or Personal Representative

_____

Printed Name of Patient or Personal Representative

_____

Date

If Personal Representative, indicate relationship:

_____

Declinations

_____ The Individual declined to accept a copy of the Notice of Privacy Practices.

_____ The Individual received a copy of the Notice of Privacy Practices but declined to sign an Acknowledgment of Receipt.

_____

Signature of MCMC Healthcare Representative

_____

Name of MCMC HealthCare Representative

Figure 10-4 ◆ Sample HIPAA authorization form.

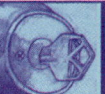

When patients' first visits are scheduled at least a week after those patients call to schedule, administrative medical assistants may mail those patients new patient history forms to complete before arriving at the office. This system has one potential drawback, however: Patients may forget to bring their paperwork to their first visit.

Critical Thinking Question 10-2

Thinking back to the case study at the beginning of the chapter, how can the medical assistant argue to the physician or office manager that sending new patient history forms before patients' first visits will in fact benefit the office?

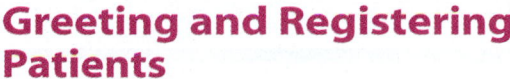

Greeting and Registering Patients

The front-desk receptionist is the host or hostess of the medical office. As such, the receptionist should welcome all patients upon arrival, even when busy with other tasks. If, for example, the receptionist is on the telephone when a patient arrives, the receptionist should look up and smile at the patient and hold up an index finger to indicate a slight delay in service (Figure 10-5 ◆).

Years ago, a window separated the receptionist's desk and the reception room to keep conversations behind the front desk private. Today, most medical offices have adopted a friendlier, more open system in the reception room (Figure 10-6 ◆). Now when medical assistants must have private conversations with patients, they must either lower their voices or move the patients to private areas of the office. In modern times, the window is seen as a barrier to effective customer service.

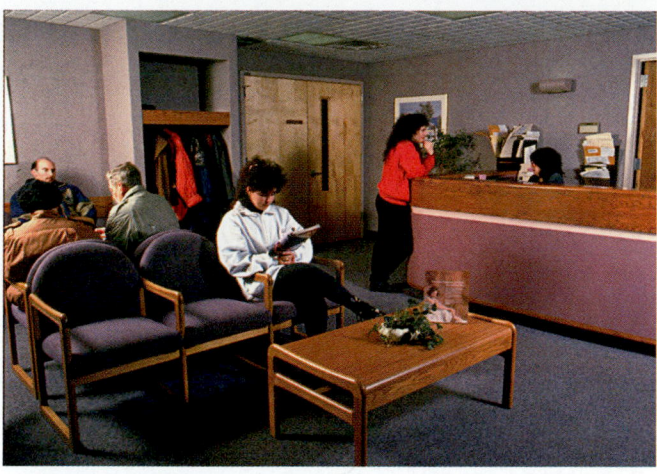

Figure 10-6 ◆ Many reception rooms in medical offices today have adopted a friendlier, more open system.

As part of greeting new patients, medical assistants should orient patients to the office with such information as the locations of the restroom and coat rack and where to find reading materials. When greeting established patients, assistants should confirm that all information on file (e.g., address, telephone number, and insurance carrier) remains the same as the last visit. When patients' insurance information has changed, the medical assistant should photocopy both sides of new insurance cards.

Patient confidentiality at the front desk is essential to the medical office. Whenever the medical assistant must discuss confidential health or financial information with a patient, all exchanges must occur out of the hearing range of other patients (Figure 10-7 ◆).

Using Sign-in Sheets

Some medical offices require patients to sign in upon arrival. Before the Health Insurance Portability and Accountability Act

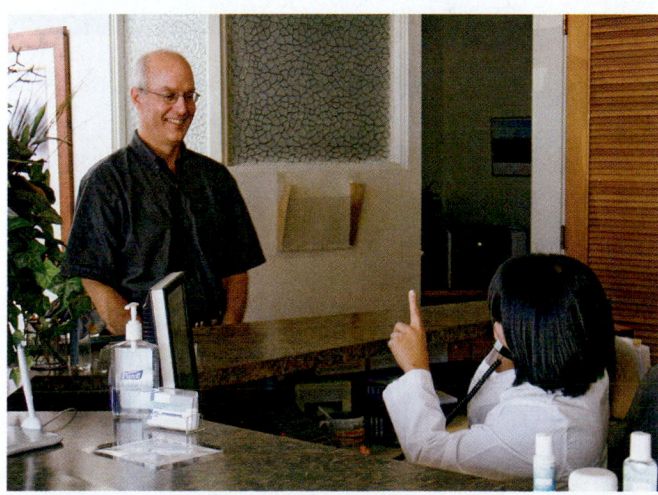

Figure 10-5 ◆ If the receptionist is on the telephone when a patient comes in, she should look up and make eye contact with the patient immediately.

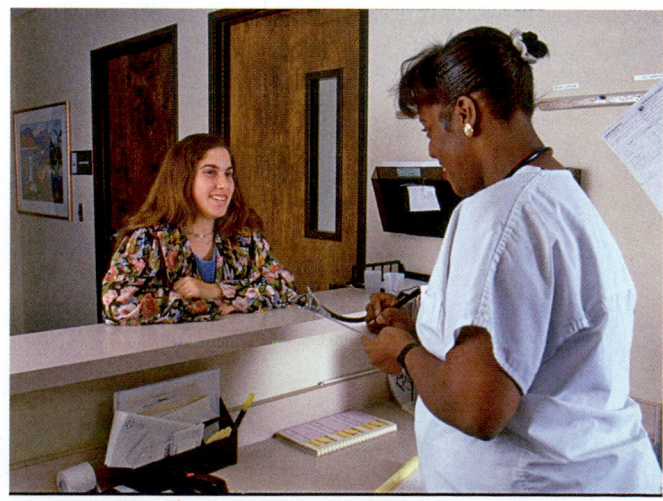

Figure 10-7 ◆ The receptionist must maintain patient confidentiality at the front desk by keeping her voice low.

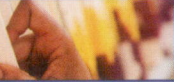

PROCEDURE 10-2 Greet and Register Patients

Theory and Rationale

As patients enter the medical office, each needs to be greeted by the medical assistant and then registered according to his or her needs.

Materials

- Patient history form
- Pen
- Clipboard

Competency

(**Conditions**) With the necessary materials, you will be able to (**Task**) greet and register patients (**Standards**) correctly within the time limit set by the instructor.

1. As the patient arrives at the front desk, look up and make eye contact right away. If you are on the telephone, make a motion to the patient with your index finger to indicate you will be with the patient in one moment. If you are not on the telephone, smile and ask the patient for his or her name.
2. Once you have obtained the patient's name, check the appointment schedule to verify the patient is there at the right time and to verify the type of appointment the patient is scheduled to have.
3. If the patient is new to the office, give him or her the appropriate new patient forms to fill out on a clipboard, along with a pen.
4. Ask the patient to take a seat in the reception area and provide the patient with an approximate amount of time he or she can expect to wait before being taken back to see the provider.
5. Alert the clinical medical assistant to the patient's arrival.

(**HIPAA**) was enacted, **sign-in sheets** were typically sheets of paper that patients signed when entering the office. Such sheets alerted the medical assistant to a patient's arrival and served as proof of the patient's visit. Today, any office sign-in sheets must be **HIPAA compliant**, which means that a patient's signature must be invisible to the next patient who signs the sheet. Offices often use separate sheets for physicians, although this is not a legal requirement.

HIPAA Compliance

Simply covering a sign-in sheet or blacking out patients' names after check-in fails to meet HIPAA standards, because signatures can still easily be viewed. Several other sign-in methods, however, are HIPAA compliant. One convenient method stores patient signatures electronically, much like department stores do (Figure 10-8 ◆). Another method keeps individual sign-in sheets in patients' files.

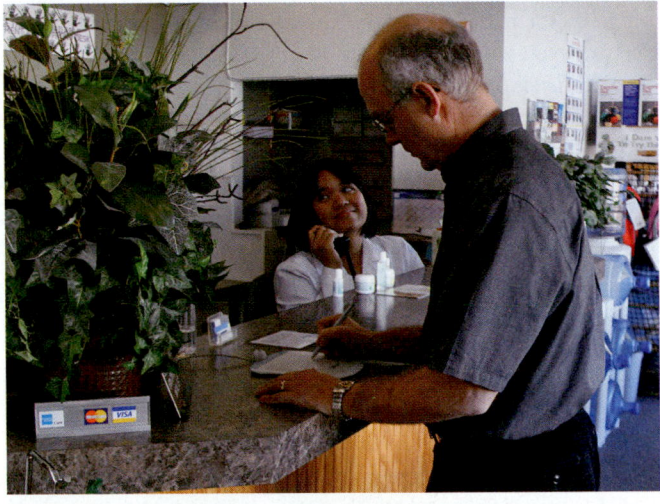

Figure 10-8 ◆ A patient signs an electronic sign-in sheet.

Administering Patient Paperwork

When patients arrive at the office, the medical assistant must give them any necessary forms to complete and identify any important landmarks, such as where signatures are needed. At this time, the assistant should also copy new patients' identification and insurance cards.

The patient registration form (Figure 10-3) is one of the medical office's most important forms, because it contains all information needed to bill for patient care. To ensure billing processes remain up to date, this form should be verified at every visit but no more than once every month. When working with patient paperwork, medical assistants must keep all information confidential. For example, assistants should only ask patients to verify their birth dates or addresses when other patients cannot overhear. Similarly, the reasons for patients' visits should only be disclosed when other patients cannot overhear.

Sometimes, patients will refuse to disclose certain information. Patients most commonly balk at providing their Social Security numbers and birth dates, often because they fear identity theft. When medical assistants encounter patients like these, they should gently remind the patients that all information in medical files is confidential and is only released with the patients' written consent or a court order. When these facts fail to persuade a patient, the medical assistant should note on the patient's chart the information that was refused and give the chart to the clinical staff. Ultimately, the physician must decide whether to accept the patient for treatment.

Keys to Success
HELPING THE PATIENT COMPLETE THE HISTORY FORM

Medical assistants must sometimes help patients complete their patient history forms. To maintain patient confidentiality, assistants should provide all such assistance out of the hearing range of other patients. Before asking any personal history questions, for example, medical assistants should escort patients to a private area away from the reception room. When medical assistants have completed patient forms for patients, they must sign those forms and note why the patients could not complete those forms themselves. Some patients cannot complete patient history forms due to disability, pain, illiteracy, or other factors. For these patients, medical assistants should enlist administrative support.

Notifying Patients of Delays

Once a patient has completed all necessary paperwork, the medical assistant must notify the clinical staff of that patient's arrival. Delays happen in the medical office regularly, often due to unforeseen circumstances with emergencies or competing priorities. When delays occur, it is important for the assistant to keep patients apprised. Such consideration demonstrates sound customer service, because it lets patients know that the medical assistant and the physician value patients' time.

Some offices use electronic signs at the front desk to broadcast physicians' schedules, but such signs are only as good as the staff updating them. Therefore, whenever electronic signs are used, the medical assistant must ensure they accurately depict wait times. Whatever system is used, when delays start to exceed 20 minutes, the medical assistant should try to reach patients before they arrive at the office and suggest that they visit the office later or even reschedule.

Collecting Payments at the Front Desk

Part of greeting patients at the front desk includes collecting patients' **copayments** as those patients register. Most offices have signs at their front desks that state, "Copayments are due at the time of service." Patient files should clearly list any copays

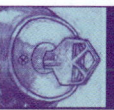

Keys to Success
OBTAINING BIRTH DATES FROM PATIENTS

Because insurance carriers use birth dates to help identify their members, they will not process claims when that information is missing. When patients refuse to disclose their birth dates, they may have to forego insurance coverage and self-fund their charges.

that are expected. For patients' convenience, the medical office should accept multiple forms of payment (e.g., cash, personal check, credit/debit card). To ensure payments are somehow procured, offices should have policies for addressing patients who cannot pay their copayments at the time of service. Some offices allow patients to mail their copayments or to discuss payment with the billing office.

To track fees, most offices use preprinted fee slips, also called encounter forms or superbills. Fee slips follow patients through the office. The physician and/or clinical medical assistant circles the services or procedures that were performed, as well as any diagnoses the physician assigns to the patient (Figure 10-9 ◆). While medical office supply companies sell standard fee slips, many medical offices customize fee slips to include the diagnoses and procedures they commonly use. Because procedural and diagnosis codes change every year, fee slips should be reviewed for accuracy annually and reprinted as needed.

Typically, the medical assistant who is working at the front desk when the patient arrives prepares the patient's fee slip for that date of service. The medical assistant attaches the slip to the patient's file and routes the file to the clinical medical assistant.

Escorting Patients

Almost always, a medical assistant or clinical medical assistant should escort patients to the examination room after verifying the patients' identities. To do this, the assistant should open the door to the reception area and call out a patient's first name. When more than one patient stands, the assistant should then call out the patient's last name. Once in the back office area, the assistant should confirm the patient's birth date using the patient's file.

Managing Difficult Patients in the Reception Area

As the hub of the reception area, the front desk is on display for the rest of the office. Occasionally, the front-desk receptionist must manage difficult patients in the reception area. Many difficulties can be avoided by keeping patients apprised of expected delay times. Medical assistants who remain calm and professional are best equipped to function in and defuse patient interactions.

When the medical assistant encounters a difficult patient in the reception area, the first goal is to remove the patient from the area. Patients who are out of the sight and hearing ranges of other patients tend to have less leverage. Once an angry patient is in another location, the medical assistant should work to address the patient's issue or find someone who can.

 Critical Thinking Question 10-3
How should the medical assistant respond to Marilyn? What is appropriate for facial expression and tone of voice?

WINDY CITY CLINIC
Beth Williams, M.D.
123 Michigan Avenue, Chicago, IL 60610
(312) 123-1234

UROLOGIC GYNECOLOGY
GENERAL GYNECOLOGY
OBSTETRICS

ID.# 20-1342846
No. 4815

PATIENT INFORMATION

PATIENT'S LAST NAME		FIRST		INITIAL	BIRTHDATE		SEX ☐ MALE ☐ FEMALE		TODAY'S DATE / /
ADDRESS	CITY		STATE	ZIP	RELATION TO SUBSCRIBER		REFERRING PHYSICIAN		
SUBSCRIBER or POLICY HOLDER					INSURANCE				
ADDRESS	CITY		STATE	ZIP	INSURANCE ID.#		COVERAGE CODE		GROUP

OTHER HEALTH COVERAGE?
☐ NO
☐ YES   IDENTIFY _____

DISABILITY RELATED TO:
☐ ACCIDENT ☐ PREGNANCY
☐ INDEPENDENT ☐ OTHER

DATE SYMPTOMS APPEARED, INCEPTION OF PREGNANCY, OR
ACCIDENT OCCURED: / /

ASSIGNMENT and RELEASE: *I hereby assign my insurance benefits to be paid directly to the undersigned physician. I am financially responsible for noncovered services. I also authorize the physician to release any information required to process this claim.*

SIGNATURE OF PATIENT (or Parent, if Minor) _____   DATE / /

✓	PROCEDURES	CPT-Mod	AMOUNT	✓	PROCEDURES	CPT-Mod	AMOUNT	✓	PROCEDURES	CPT-Mod	AMOUNT
	A. OFFICE VISITS			31	Post-Partum	59430		60	PG Test, Urine	86006	
1	New GYN, Limited	90010			**F. GYN PROCEDURES**			61	Antigen Test	86006	
2	New GYN, Intermediate	90015		32	Irrigation of Vagina	57150*		62	Cytopathology Smear	88155	
3	New GYN, Extensive	90017		33	Insert Pessary	57160*		63	Specimen Handling	99000	
4	New GYN, Comprehensive	90020		34	Pessary Supplies	99070			**I. MISCELLANEOUS**		
5	Return GYN, Minimal	90030		35	Colposcopy	57452		64	Surgical Tray	99070	
6	Return GYN, Brief	90040		36	Biopsy, Cervix	57500		65	Therapeutic Injection	90782	
7	Return GYN, Limited	90050		37	Biopsy, Vagina	57100		66	Injection, Kenalog	J1870	
8	Return GYN, Intermediate	90060		38	Biopsy, Vulva	56600		67	Injection, Xylocaine	J3480	
9	Return GYN, Extended	90070		39	Biopsy, Endometrium	58100		68	Injection, Estrogen	J2655	
10	Return GYN, Comprehensive	90080		40	Biopsy, Skin			69	Injection, Progesterone	J2675	
11	Return GYN, Post-Operative	99024			0.5 cm.	11420		70	Injection, Vitamin B12	P4320	
	B. CONSULTATION				0.6 to 1.0 cm.	11421		71	Special Reports	99080	
12	GYN Consultation, Limited	90600			1.1 to 2.0 cm.	11423					
13	GYN Consultation, Intermed.	90605		41	Cryotherapy, Cervix	57511					
14	GYN Consultation, Compreh.	90620		42	Destruct. Condyloma	56501					
15	GYN Consultation, Complex	90630		43	Diaphragm Fitting	57170					
16	Second Opinion Surgery	90653		44	Diaphragm Supplies	99070					
	C. TELEPHONE CONSULTATION			45	IUD Insertion	58300					
17	Telephone Consult., Simple	99013		46	IUD Supplies	99070					
18	Telephone Consult., Intermed.	99014		47	IUD Removal	58301					
19	Telephone Consult., Compreh.	99015			**G. UROLOGIC PROCEDURES**						
	D. SPECIAL SERVICES			48	Urethral Dilation	53660					
20	ER Service after Office Hrs.	99064		49	Urethral Dilation, Repeat	53661					
21	ER Service during Office Hrs.	99065		50	Bladder Instillation	51700					
22	Night Call before 10 pm	99050		51	Periurethral Injection	53665					
23	Night Call after 10 pm	99052		52	Simple Catheterization	53670					
24	Sunday or Holiday Service	99054		53	Manual Electric Stimulation	97118					
25	Office Non-Schedule	99058			**H. LAB**						
	E. OB CARE			54	Urine Analysis	81000					
26	Prenatal Dx, Consultation	90620		55	Urine Culture	87068					
27	Initial OB, NOrmal	59400		56	Hematocrit	85015					
28	Initial OB, High Risk	59400.22		57	Hemogram	85021					
29	Return OB, Normal	59420		58	Commercial-Lat.	87087			**TODAY'S TOTAL FEE**	$	
30	Return OB, High Risk	59420.22		59	Wet Mount	87210					

✓	DIAGNOSIS	CODE	✓	DIAGNOSIS	CODE	✓	DIAGNOSIS	CODE	✓	DIAGNOSIS	CODE
	Abortion:			Breasts	216.5		Galactorrhea	676.6		Pregnancy Postpartum	V24.2
	Threatened	640.0		Vulva	221.2		Hemorrhoids	455.0		Rectocele	618.0
	Incomplete	637.1		Breast Disorder (Mass)	611.72		Hypertension	401		Retention of Urine	788.2
	Habitual	646.3		Bronchitis	491		Incontinence of Urine	788.3		Stress Incontinence	625.6
	Abnormal Urination	788.6		Carcinoma In Situ:			Interstitial Cystitis	595.1		Urethral Stricture	598
	Abnormal PAP Smear	795.0		Cervix	233.1		Irritable Colon	564.1		Urethral Syndrome	597.81
	Adenomyosis	617.0		Uterus	233.2		Irregular Menstrual Cycle	626.4		Uterine Leiomyoma	218
	Adnexal MAss	625.8		Female Genital Organs	233.3		Malignant Neoplasm:			Uterine Prolapse:	
	Amenorrhera	626.0		Cervical Dysplasia	622.1		Cervix	180.9		Incomplete	618.2
	Anemia	285.9		Cervicitis	616.0		Uterus	182.0		Complete	618.3
	Arthritis	716.9		Contraceptive Management	V25.0		Ovary	183.0		Vaginal Discharge-Non Specific	623.5
	Artificial Menopause	627.4		Cystocele	618.0		Vagina	184.0		Vaginal Enterocele	618.6
	Asthma-Hayfever	493.0		Cystourethritis	595.0		Vulva	184.4		Vaginal Prolapse	618.0
	Atrophic Vaginitis	627.3		Diabetes Mellicus	250.0		Menopausal Syndrome	627.2		Vaginal Vault Prolapse Post	
	Bartholin Abscess	616.3		Thyroid Disorder	246.9		Menometrorrhagia	626.2		Hysterectomy	618.5
	Benign Neoplasm:			Dysmenorrhea	625.3		Oligomenorrhea	626.1		Vulvovaginitis:	
	Cervix	219.0		Dyspareunia	625.0		Obesity	278.0		Non Specific	616.1
	Uterus	219.1		Dysuria	788.1		Ovarian Cyst	620.2		Candida	112.1
	Ovary	220		Ectopic Pregnancy	617.0		Pelvic Inflammatory Disease	614.9		Trichomonas	131.01
	Vagina	221.1		Endometriosis	617.9		Pelvic Peritoneal Adhesions	614.6			
	Vulva	221.2		Enuresis-Unstable Bladder	788.3		Polycystic Ovaries	256.4			
	Benign Neoplasm of Skin:			Frequency of Urination	788.4		Postmenopausal Bleeding	627.1			
	Buttocks	216.5		Functional Disorder:			Post-Op Wound Infection	998.5			
	Abdomen	216.5		Bladder Instability	596.5		Pregnancy Prenatal	V22			

MISCELLANEOUS DIAGNOSIS

DOCTOR'S SIGNATURE _____

DATE _____ / /

SERVICES PERFORMED AT: ☐ Office ☐ Emergency Room
☐ **WINDY CITY CLINIC**
123 Michigan Avenue, Chicago, IL 60610
(312) 123-1234
☐ Hospital Calls at $_____ per Visit

ADMITTED _____ / /
DISCHARGED _____ / /

RETURN VISIT INFORMATION
15 • 30 • 45 • 60
___ DAYS ___ WEEKS ___ MONTHS ☐ WILL CALL
Procedure: _____

ACCEPT ASSIGNMENT
☐ YES
☐ NO

INSTRUCTIONS TO PATIENT FOR FILING INSURANCE CLAIMS

1. Complete patient information portion of this form.
2. Sign and date.
3. Mail this form directly to your insurance company with your own insurance company's form.
4. Patients with health care insurance please remember:
   A. Professional services are charged to the patient, and not to the insurance company.
   B. Insured patients are expected to take care of their fees as services are rendered.
   C. This office cannot accept responsibility for collecting your insurance claim or for negotiating a settlement on a disputed claim.
   D. You are responsible for payment of your account.

TODAY'S FEE	$
OLD BALANCE	$
ADJUSTMENTS	$
TOTAL DUE	$
AMOUNT RECEIVED TODAY	$
☐ CASH ☐ CHECK ☐ C.C.	
NEW BALANCE	$

Figure 10-9 ◆ Sample medical office fee slip.

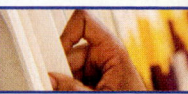

PROCEDURE 10-3   Collect Payments at the Front Desk

Theory and Rationale

Most medical insurance plans today require the patient to pay an out of pocket amount at the time of each visit. This payment, known as a copay, should be collected from the patient upon arrival in the medical office.

Materials

■ Pen
■ Cash receipt book
■ Credit card machine
■ Check endorsement stamp

Competency

(**Conditions**) With the necessary materials, you will be able to (**Task**) collect payments at the front desk (**Standards**) correctly within the time limit set by the instructor.

1. As the patient arrives at the front desk, check the computer or chart to verify the patient's copayment amount.
2. After registering the patient, let the patient know the amount of the expected payment.
3. Ask the patient if he or she would prefer to make the payment via cash, check, or credit card.
4. If the patient pays via cash, write a receipt from the cash receipt book.
5. If the patient pays via check, endorse the check with the bank endorsement stamp. Ask the patient if he or she would like a written receipt. If so, write a receipt from the cash receipt book.
6. If the patient pays via credit card, process the card on the credit card machine, have the patient sign the slip, and provide the patient with the correct portion as a receipt.

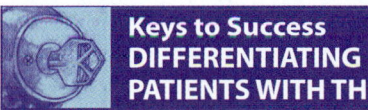

Keys to Success
DIFFERENTIATING BETWEEN TWO PATIENTS WITH THE SAME NAME

Because patients may sometimes have the same first and last names, medical assistants must verify files for all patients. Patient birth date is one way to differentiate files.

Keeping Only Appropriate Patients in the Reception Area

In general, patients visit their physicians when they are ill. Depending on the type of practice, medical assistants may help support patients with contagious diseases or life-threatening conditions. As a rule, any patients with contagious conditions should not be left in the reception room. This includes children suspected of having chicken pox and anyone with a high fever (Figure 10-10 ◆).

■ A patient who is bleeding
■ A patient who is visibly ill
■ A patient who has broken out in a contagious rash, such as chickenpox
■ A patient who states he or she feels about to vomit
■ A patient who is complaining of shortness of breath
■ A patient who is complaining of chest pain
■ A patient who states he is feeling very dizzy or light-headed

---

Figure 10-10 ◆ Examples of patients who should not be kept waiting in the reception area.

Any patient who is exhibiting signs of a condition that makes other patients in the reception room uncomfortable should also be moved. This includes patients who are coughing continuously, are bleeding or visibly ill, or have conditions that may cause other patients to stare. Moving these patients out of the reception room addresses those patients' comfort, as well as the comfort of the other patients. Any emergency patient must be brought back to see the physician right away.

Maintaining the Reception Room

The reception room should be quiet and peaceful. Patients who are waiting for appointments should be able to sit calmly, undisturbed by loud noises and other distractions. In addition to being quiet, the reception room must be kept clean and free of **hazards**. To attain this goal, medical assistants must check the reception room throughout the day to remove any garbage and retrieve any lost or forgotten items. To keep control of the room, the assistant must do things like ask children to be quiet and instruct patients to take food outside. Many offices play relaxing music in the reception area.

Providing Adequate Seating and Decoration

To ensure patient comfort, the reception room should have an adequate amount of comfortable, easy-to-clean furniture. Experts in medical office space planning believe medical offices should have enough seating to accommodate at least one hour's worth of patients per physician, as well as the friends or relatives who accompany those patients. The furniture should be at a level from which most patients can rise easily and without

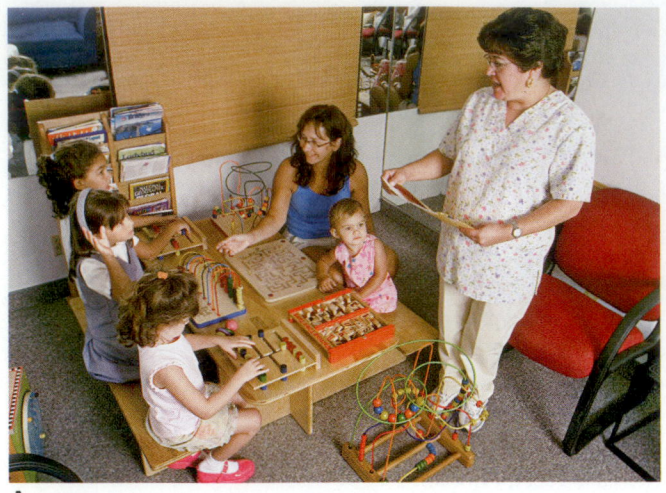
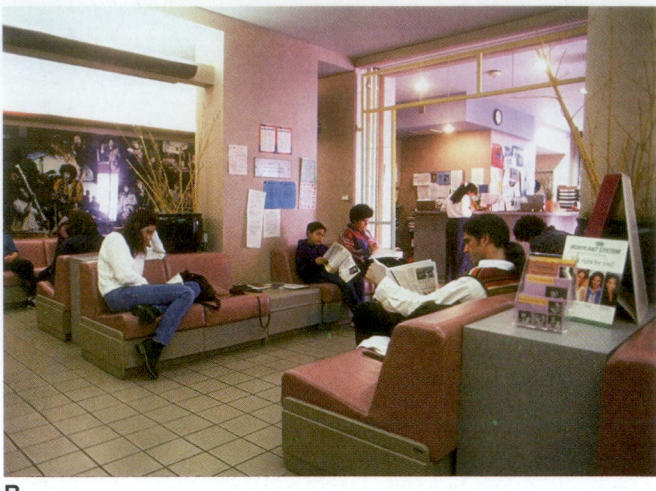

A   B

Figure 10-11 ◆ (a) A pediatric reception room will typically have child-size furniture and toys; (b) a family practice reception room will cater to patients of all ages.

assistance. Many offices have coat racks for patients' coats or umbrellas.

Practice type dictates the reception room's décor. A pediatric practice has a very different reception room than a women's healthcare practice, for example. A pediatric practice should have videos and toys, whereas a practice that caters to geriatric patients might have a fish tank or other soothing decorations (Figure 10-11 ◆).

Choosing Reading Material for the Reception Room

Like décor, reading material in the reception area is dictated by practice type. Reading material that is current and tailored to office clientele is a nice customer service touch. For example, a practice that specializes in prostate problems might have magazines about fishing, hunting, or sports activities, while a practice that specializes in women's breast surgery might have magazines about women's fashion (Figure 10-12 ◆).

Managing Children in the Reception Room

Pediatric offices or family practices often have reception areas geared toward children. In offices where children are not the primary patient population, reception areas may have small areas devoted to children. All child-geared areas should have toys and books and other items of interest to children. In all cases, child-geared reception areas and materials must be safe and clean. For example, any toys must be checked regularly to confirm they are safe and in good working order. Young children may place small items, including toys, in their mouths. Most states have laws that dictate how to clean toys for public settings. In Washington State, for example, the law dictates that toys must be cleaned with a 10 percent bleach solution after every use.

At no time, including when parents see physicians, should children be left unattended in the reception room. Medical assistants who allow children to be unattended give unspoken consent and assume responsibility for those children on behalf of the office. To ensure safety, children must remain with their parents throughout the parents' office visits. To be proactive, medical assistants might speak with parents before

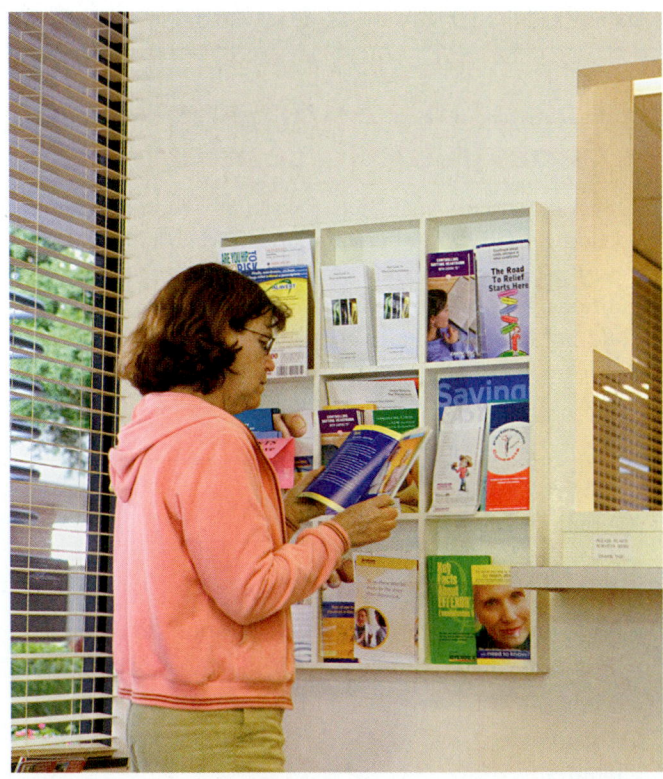

Figure 10-12 ◆ Having educational materials available to the patients in the reception area is very common.

scheduling those parents' next appointments. To underscore the message, an office might post a sign in the reception area that states, "Children May Not Be Left Unattended in the Reception Area."

In Practice

The small physician's office where Jenny works as a front-desk medical assistant is on the first floor of a building where cars are parked outside the door. When Marion Wilson arrives for her appointment, she approaches the front desk and tells Jenny that she is going to leave her 2-year-old son sleeping in his car seat because Jenny can see the car from her desk. How should Jenny respond to Marion? What are some appropriate suggestions?

Accommodating Patients with Disabilities

The **Americans with Disabilities Act (ADA)** stipulates that patients with disabilities must be able to access all public buildings, including medical facilities. Medical offices must therefore be able to accommodate people who are in wheelchairs or otherwise unable to use stairs. Ramps and elevators can render medical offices accessible.

Any entrance door must be at least 36 inches wide to accommodate a wheelchair. Any interior door, such as to a restroom or treatment room, must also be accessible by wheelchair. Any carpeting in the facility must be no more than 1/2 in. high, because wheelchair users find deeper carpeting difficult to navigate. In addition, all restrooms must be clearly marked and all doorknobs operational with a closed fist.

Serving Patients with Service Animals

Service animals, usually easily identifiable by their collars or harnesses, must accompany their owners throughout those owners' office visits. Service animals of all kinds assist their owners by doing such things as:

- Pulling wheelchairs
- Carrying or picking up items
- Alerting to hazards

While dogs serve as service animals most often, some patients enlist cats, monkeys, or even ferrets in this role (Figure 10-13 ◆).

Caring for Patients as They Leave the Office

In most medical offices, patients pass the reception desk as they exit. Offices are designed this way to ensure that patients complete any final activities, such as scheduling followup

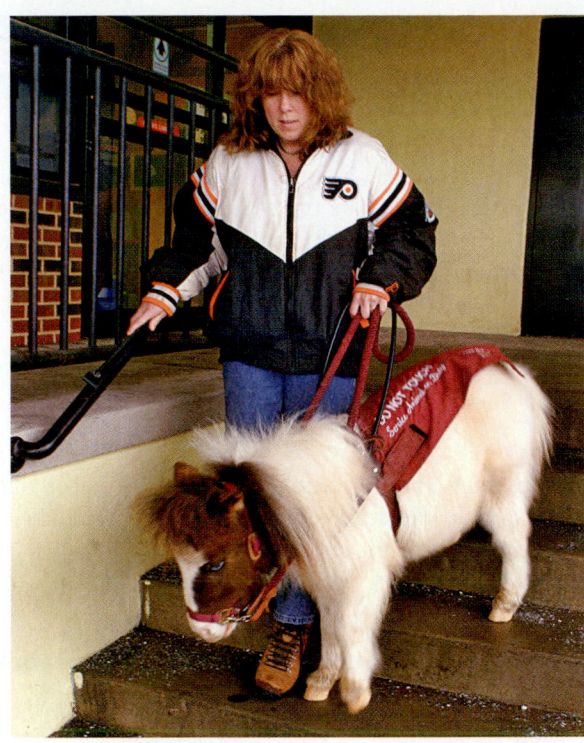

Figure 10-13 ◆ A woman is guided down a flight of stairs by her seeing eye miniature horse.

appointments. In some large offices, staff in the back office may schedule followup appointments. In small offices, the front-desk receptionist makes such appointments. In all cases, exiting patients should be instructed to give the receptionist their super bills or fee slips. On these forms, the physicians should have noted any followup appointments they would like scheduled. Only with this information in hand should the front-desk receptionist schedule the followup appointment. In some offices, the fee slip is kept with the patient's chart to go to billing, rather than carried to the front desk by the patient.

The receptionist should bid goodbye to all patients exiting the office, even those who need no followup. This small act not only reinforces that the office staff care about their patients, it promotes a friendly, warm environment.

Closing the Office

To ensure the medical office is closed consistently, properly, and comprehensively, offices should document their desired procedures in **office policies**. Any member of the healthcare team who is charged with closing the office should complete such tasks as pulling charts for patients scheduled for the following morning, transferring telephone lines to the office answering system, turning off all machinery and lights, locking the doors, and enabling the office alarm system.

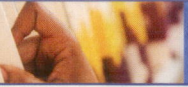

PROCEDURE 10-4 Close the Office

Theory and Rationale

Medical assistants are often tasked with closing the medical office. Just as it supports the office-opening procedure, a checklist helps ensure that medical staff complete this procedure correctly.

Materials

■ Checklist of office closing procedures

Competency

(**Conditions**) With the necessary materials, you will be able to (**Task**) close the medical office (**Standards**) correctly within the time limit set by the instructor.

1. Ensure all patients have exited the office. Check treatment rooms and restrooms.

2. Verify that all the day's patient files have been routed to the appropriate area (e.g., billing, physician, clinical medical assistant).
3. Pull all files for patients scheduled for the following morning.
4. Confirm that all information needed for the morning's patients (e.g., lab reports or consultations) is available.
5. Attach needed information to patient files.
6. Call to confirm any patient appointments made prior to three days ago.
7. Forward the telephones over to the answering system.
8. Turn off all appropriate equipment and lights.
9. Activate the alarm and lock the doors when leaving the building.

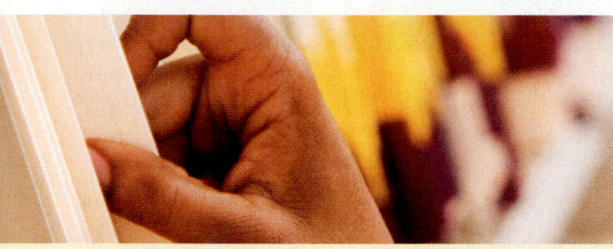

REVIEW

Chapter Summary

■ Office policies are invaluable tools for ensuring medical offices are closed and opened properly by all members of the healthcare team.
■ When patients arrive, office staff should be prepared with all necessary information and paperwork.
■ Both new and established patients deserve the highest level of customer service from the medical office.
■ It is paramount that the entire healthcare team safeguard patient confidentiality at the front desk and throughout the medical office.
■ When patients are difficult, medical assistants must strive to remain calm and diffuse the situation.

■ Medical assistants should ensure that the reception area is used only for patients who may be left alone and is always in a condition that is appropriate both for the patients and the overall image and goals of the office.
■ When patients have special needs, medical assistants should strive to provide them appropriate care.
■ It is particularly important that children and other unique populations receive the care and attention that is appropriate for their needs.

Chapter Review

Multiple Choice

1. Staff members should arrive in the office _____ minutes before the first patient appointment.
   a. 10
   b. 15
   c. 30
   d. 40

2. Which of the following patients should not be left alone in the reception room?
   a. Child with symptoms of chicken pox
   b. Adult with HIV
   c. Patient with eczema
   d. Patient with a sight impairment

Chapter Review (continued)

3. When a physician is running 30 minutes behind schedule, the medical assistant should
   a. notify patients of the delay as they enter the office.
   b. avoid eye contact with patients in the waiting area.
   c. ask a clinical medical assistant to notify the patients in the reception area.
   d. all of the above.

True/False

T F 1. Studies have shown that patients will stay with physicians they do not really like when they feel the rest of the staff care about their needs.

T F 2. A window between the reception room and the receptionist's desk is the best way to keep patients from overhearing the receptionist's conversations.

T F 3. Copayments should never be collected at the front desk.

T F 4. An electric sign that relays the physician's scheduling delays precludes staff from having to communicate those delays verbally.

T F 5. HIPAA prevents staff from calling patients' names in the reception room.

T F 6. When patients refuse to disclose all necessary information, medical assistants should ask them to leave.

T F 7. Patients who are bleeding visibly should not be left in the reception room.

T F 8. Reading materials in the reception room should be geared toward the type of patients receiving services.

T F 9. Educational materials that are specific to the type of practice make good reading materials for the reception room.

Short Answer

1. Describe how, while on the telephone, the front-desk receptionist should greet patients entering the office.

2. Explain how to render a sign-in sheet HIPAA compliant.

3. Why is it important to notify patients of any delays in the office?

4. What does it mean to escort a patient?

5. Why may patients become irritable in the reception room?

6. What is the best way to handle a loud, angry patient in the reception room?

7. Why is it important to regularly inspect children's toys in the reception room?

8. Why is it important to have a policy that states no children may be left unattended in the reception room?

Research

1. What classes could you take at your local community college that would help you to communicate better with patients at the front desk?

2. What are the laws in your state that pertain to how often toys in the office must be cleaned?

3. Interview someone who works in a medical office. Ask the person how the reception staff in his or her office deal with difficult patients.

Externship Application Experience

When Mrs. Rundholz calls to make an appointment for a complete physical examination, she says she can make the appointment but will not have child care for her 2-year-old and 6-month-old children. She asks if she can bring her children to her hour-long appointment. How should the medical assistant respond to Mrs. Rundholz? What are some appropriate suggestions?

Resource Guide

The Americans with Disabilities Act (ADA) Homepage
www.ada.gov

Microsoft Office Online
Work Essentials
http://office.microsoft.com/en-us/workessentials/

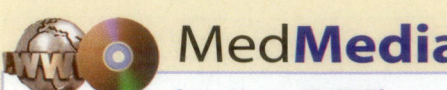

MedMedia

http://www.MyMAKit.com

More on this chapter, including interactive resources, can be found on the Student CD-ROM accompanying this textbook and on http://www.MyMAKit.com.

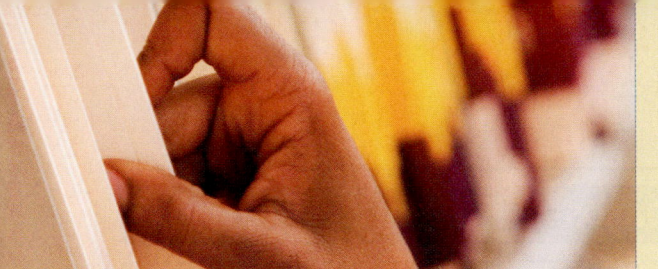

Objectives

After completing this chapter, you should be able to:

- Define and spell the key terminology in this chapter.
- Define the medical assistant's role in patient scheduling.
- Create guidelines for scheduling patient appointments.
- Differentiate between paper and electronic scheduling systems.
- Chart patient no-shows accurately.
- Follow up on patients who miss their appointments.
- Manage the physician's appointment calendar for professional travel.
- Schedule patients for hospital services and admissions.
- Arrange for language interpreters for non–English-speaking patients.
- Arrange for patient transportation.

Patient Scheduling

Case Study

When Glenn Jenson calls the office to set up an appointment, he says he has never been in to see the physician before. When the medical assistant asks him why he must see the physician, he responds, "I'd rather not go into that with you. I'll tell the doctor when I see her."

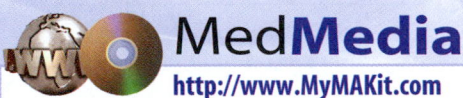

MedMedia

http://www.MyMAKit.com

Additional interactive resources and activities for this chapter can be found on http://www.MyMAKit.com. For a video, tips, audio glossary, legal and ethical scenarios, on-the-job scenarios, quizzes, and games related to the content of this chapter, please access the accompanying CD-ROM in this book.

Video: *Scheduling Patients*
Legal and Ethical Scenario: *Patient Scheduling*
On the Job Scenario: *Patient Scheduling*
Tips
Multiple Choice Quiz
Audio Glossary
HIPAA Quiz
Games: Spelling Bee, Crossword, and Strikeout

Key Terminology

buffer time—an appointment scheduling method of leaving certain times of day open to accommodate situations such as patients who call for same-day appointments or physicians who need to catch up on charting

cluster scheduling—scheduling method that groups patients with similar appointments around the same time of day

double booking—scheduling more than one patient for the same appointment time

established patient—patient whom the medical office has seen previously

fixed-appointment scheduling—scheduling system that assigns every patient a specific appointment time

matrix—process of blocking out times in the appointment schedule when the provider is unavailable or out of the office

modified wave scheduling—a scheduling system where two or three patients are scheduled at the beginning of each hour, followed by single patient appointments every 10 to 20 minutes for the rest of that hour

new patient—patient whom no provider of the same specialty in the office has seen for three or more years

new patient checklist—list of information new patients must provide when calling to schedule appointments

office brochure—pamphlet outlining an office's staff and services

open hours—scheduling method that allows patients to seek treatment without appointment times

preapprovals—the process of calling a patient's insurance carrier prior to a service in order to obtain preapproval or authorization for the service to be performed

slack time—an appointment scheduling method of leaving certain times of day open to accommodate situations such as when patients call for same-day appointments or physicians who need to catch up on charting

✚ MEDICAL ASSISTING STANDARDS

CAAHEP ENTRY-LEVEL STANDARDS

- Perform within scope of practice (psychomotor)
- Apply ethical behaviors, including honesty/integrity in performance of medical assisting practice (affective)
- Apply active listening skills (affective)
- Practice within the standard of care for a medical assistant (psychomotor)
- Demonstrate sensitivity to patient rights (affective)
- Analyze communications in providing appropriate responses/feedback (affective)
- Document accurately in the patient record (psychomotor)
- Explain general office policies (psychomotor)
- Demonstrate telephone techniques (psychomotor)
- Discuss pros and cons of various types of appointment management systems (cognitive)
- Manage appointment schedule using established priorities (psychomotor)
- Describe scheduling guidelines (cognitive)
- Schedule patient admissions and/or procedures (psychomotor)
- Recognize office policies and protocols for handling appointments (cognitive)
- Use office hardware and software to maintain office systems (psychomotor)
- Identify critical information required for scheduling patient admissions and or procedures (cognitive)

ABHES ENTRY-LEVEL COMPETENCIES

- Adapt to change
- Maintain confidentiality at all times
- Project a positive attitude
- Be cognizant of ethical boundaries
- Show a responsible attitude
- Orient patients to office policies and procedures
- Adapt what is said to the recipient's level of comprehension
- Instruct patients with special needs
- Manage physician's professional schedule and travel
- Use proper telephone technique
- Application of electronic technology
- Schedule and monitor appointments
- Apply computer concepts for office procedures
- Be courteous and diplomatic
- Serve as a liaison between the physician and others
- Exercise efficient time management

✓ COMPETENCY SKILLS PERFORMANCE

1. Establish an appointment matrix.
2. Schedule a new patient.
3. Schedule an established patient appointment.
4. Use patient reminder cards.
5. Reschedule a missed patient appointment.
6. Manage the physician's professional schedule and travel.
7. Schedule a hospital procedure.
8. Schedule an inpatient admission.

Key Terminology *(continued)*

triage notebook—notebook kept near the administrative medical assistant answering incoming telephone calls that

outlines questions and steps to follow in the event callers have potentially life-threatening conditions

wave scheduling—a scheduling system where patients are scheduled only during the first half of each hour.

Abbreviations

EKG—Electrocardiogram

Introduction

While the specifics of appointment scheduling vary from one medical office to another, the basic concepts remain the same. Patients may call to schedule their first visit or routine followup appointments. They may also call with medical emergencies. Medical assistants must know how to best handle each of these situations.

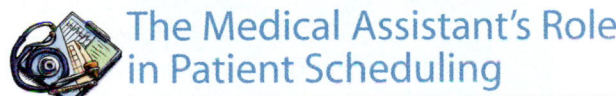

The Medical Assistant's Role in Patient Scheduling

Medical assistants are responsible for scheduling patients for a variety of appointments. Both new and established patients will need to be scheduled for appointments in the medical facility. The MA will also need to schedule patients for procedures in the outpatient and inpatient setting, as well as for laboratory or X-ray tests and procedures.

Scheduling New Patient Appointments

When a **new patient** calls the medical office to schedule an appointment, it is important to collect all needed information (Figure 11-1 ◆) while remaining professional, objective, and consistent. A patient's financial information should not command special attention from the medical assistant and should not be the first question the medical assistant asks of the caller. A **new patient checklist** (Figure 11-2 ◆) can help ensure that medical assistants ask appropriate questions, cover all bases, and gather information from all new patients consistently.

? —Critical Thinking Question 11-1-
If Glenn fails to state his reason for requesting a physician visit, how can the medical assistant determine the time to allot for the appointment?

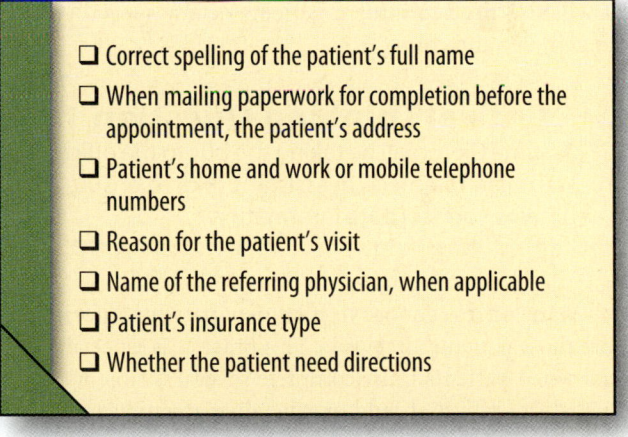

❑ Correct spelling of the patient's full name
❑ When mailing paperwork for completion before the appointment, the patient's address
❑ Patient's home and work or mobile telephone numbers
❑ Reason for the patient's visit
❑ Name of the referring physician, when applicable
❑ Patient's insurance type
❑ Whether the patient need directions

Figure 11-1 ◆ Information to gather from new patients over the telephone.

Because most healthcare providers are members of several managed care plans as preferred providers, it is important that medical assistants ask for patients' insurance information before scheduling appointments. When patients refuse to provide this information, assistants should let the patients know that this information is needed for patients to receive the highest benefits from their plans and that the patients may need to pay in full for their visits if the physician is not participating with their plans. When the medical office requires payment at the time of the visit, the medical assistant must also inform patients of this policy.

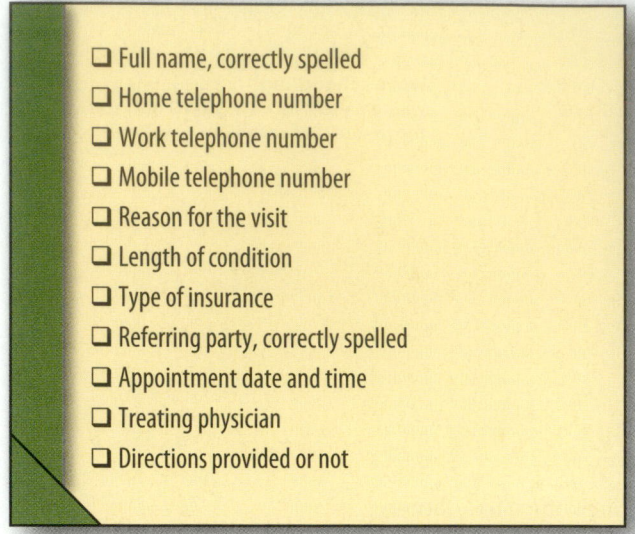

❑ Full name, correctly spelled
❑ Home telephone number
❑ Work telephone number
❑ Mobile telephone number
❑ Reason for the visit
❑ Length of condition
❑ Type of insurance
❑ Referring party, correctly spelled
❑ Appointment date and time
❑ Treating physician
❑ Directions provided or not

Figure 11-2 ◆ Sample new patient checklist.

?—Critical Thinking Question 11-2

How should the medical assistant respond if Glenn refuses to disclose his insurance information?

In addition to obtaining information, the medical assistant may need to provide the patient with information. Patients sometimes need directions to the office or information regarding bus routes that reach the office. Preprinted directions near the office telephone can serve as clear guides. The medical assistant will also need to inform patients of any special parking arrangements and costs.

?—Critical Thinking Question 11-3

Assume Glenn will be taking the bus to the office. What steps can the medical assistant take to ensure Glenn obtains correct route information?

Many offices choose to mail new patients information before those patients' first visits. This practice is especially beneficial when patients must complete several forms. As added information, offices should expand their mailings to include their **office brochure** and information about the physicians or office policies (Figure 11-3 ◆).

When medical assistants will be mailing forms to patients, they must advise the patients that they will be receiving the forms and should complete them before arriving for their first appointment. When offices do not send forms as a practice, assistants will need to ask patients to arrive early for their appointments so they can complete their paperwork before seeing the physician. The number of forms drives how much time patients will need for this task, but in general, 10 to 20 minutes will suffice. When other healthcare providers have referred new

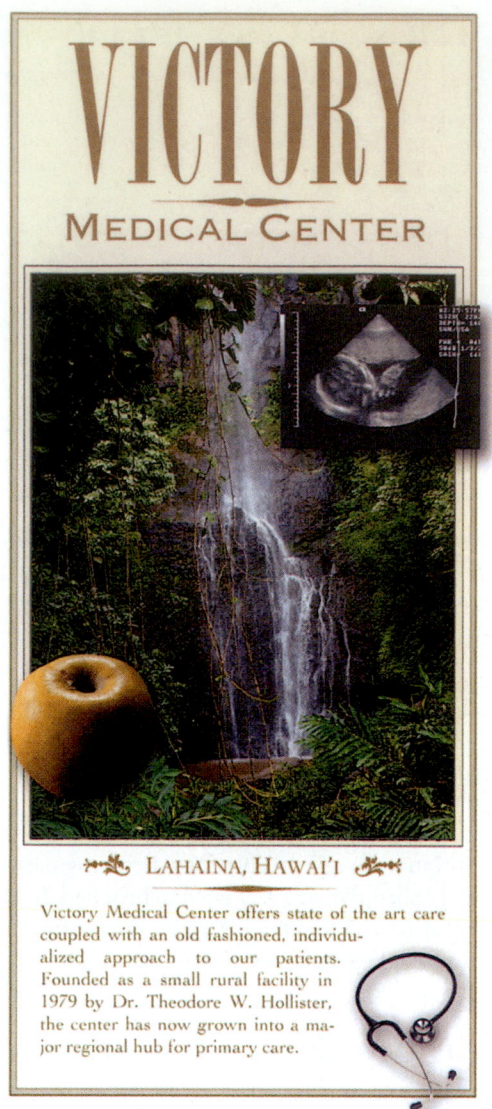

VICTORY
MEDICAL CENTER

❀✿ LAHAINA, HAWAI'I ❀✿

Victory Medical Center offers state of the art care coupled with an old fashioned, individualized approach to our patients. Founded as a small rural facility in 1979 by Dr. Theodore W. Hollister, the center has now grown into a major regional hub for primary care.

Figure 11-3 ◆ Sample medical office brochure.

patients to the office, medical assistants may want to ask those patients to bring their referral forms and any other relevant materials (e.g., X-rays or laboratory reports) to their visits. Sometimes, however, referring providers send such information separately.

New and Established Patients

Medical offices have varying policies on what constitutes "new" and "established" patients. In general, a new patient has not been seen in the medical office by any of the healthcare providers of the same specialty within the past three years. Conversely, an **established patient** has seen one of the healthcare providers of the same specialty in the medical office within the past three years. This rule especially applies when billing patients' health insurance plans. When patients have been seen in the medical office, even by practitioners different from the one they are seeing on their next visit, those patients are considered established by their insurance carriers.

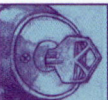

Keys to Success
ACCIDENTAL INJURY FILES

Keep patients' accidental injury files separate from those patients' general medical files. Then, when insurance companies request copies of patients' medical records due to the accidental injury, the copying task is far easier.

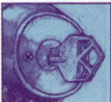

Keys to Success
CONSIDERING PATIENT REQUIREMENTS

Every office has a few patients who need extended appointment times due to disability or complex health issues. Staff should note these unique requirements on the patients' hard-copy or electronic records so that the medical assistant who is scheduling appointments can allot appropriate amounts of time.

Patients who have been involved in accidents, such as car or on-the-job injuries, may be considered "new" when seeking care for related injuries because they will likely need to provide accidental-injury information and undergo evaluations as if the office has never seen them before. Therefore, it is important for medical assistants to know their offices' policies for "new" and "established" patients and to follow those policies consistently.

Allowing Appointments Adequate Time

The time patient appointments require depends on the type of practice and the preferences of the healthcare providers. Table 11-1 lists general appointment types and times allowed. In typical offices, new patients are seen for longer periods than established ones. For example, a new patient appointment may be scheduled for 30 minutes, whereas an established patient appointment may extend only 10 or 15 minutes. Each medical office should document its policy for allotting appointment time and review it regularly to ensure it continues to be appropriate for patients and physicians.

Many physicians prefer to limit certain types of appointments in any given day. For example, a pediatrician may only want to see one or two sports physicals in a day. An OB/GYN physician may only want to see one or two new maternity patients in a day. Again, documented policies are beneficial, because they can clarify physicians' preferences and help the medical assistant schedule appointments properly. If, for example, the pediatrician will only allow two sports physicals a day, the office may schedule those appointments for 10 A.M. and 3 P.M. Once those appointments are filled, the medical assistant can easily see that the schedule will support no more sports physicals that day.

Creating an Appointment Matrix

The process of scheduling medical office appointments begins with an appointment **matrix.** An appointment matrix, which can be applied to both paper and computerized appointment schedules, depicts the appointment times available in the medical office. Medical assistants block out the times on the matrix when physicians are unavailable due to hospital rounds, vacations, or holidays. When appointment matrices are paired with appointment systems, medical assistants can also block times for certain pieces of equipment so equipment conflicts do not arise.

Depending on the type of practice or the specialties of the physicians, medical assistants use certain abbreviations in their matrix notations. Within an office, however, these abbreviations must be standard so that all members of the healthcare team can interpret the abbreviations accurately. For example, an office may use the abbreviation "NP" for a new patient.

Balancing Patient and Office Needs in Scheduling

When medical assistants schedule appointments, they must pay attention to patients' needs. For example, assistants should schedule patients who need fasting blood draws at the beginning of the day. Just as assistants should heed patient needs, they should factor in what is appropriate for the office. For example, if the office has only one electrocardiogram (**EKG**) machine, it would be inappropriate for the medical assistant to schedule two patients who need the machine at once. When only one staff member performs a certain procedure or test, the medical assistant must keep that person's availability in mind when scheduling appointments.

Paper and Electronic Scheduling

Today, most large medical offices use computer software to manage their patient appointments (Figure 11-4 ◆). Electronic appointment scheduling offers many advantages. With computerized systems, several staff members can access the appointment schedule at once and from different locations in the office. Some computerized systems allow staff and/or physicians to access the appointment schedule from outside the office.

Offices that use paper appointment books should choose books that support their number of physicians and patients. In multiphysician practices, appointment books might be color coded by provider (Figure 11-5 ◆).

TABLE 11-1 TIME ALLOTTED FOR PATIENT APPOINTMENTS

Appointment Type	Allotted Time (in Minutes)
New patient	30
Physical exam	60
Routine checkup	15
Well child checkup	15
Blood pressure check	5

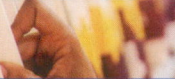

PROCEDURE 11-1 Establish an Appointment Matrix

Theory and Rationale

With an appointment matrix, the medical assistant is able to create time slots for the various appointment types in the medical office. Using this method, the medical assistant is better able to accurately schedule patients for the necessary amount of time and facilitate efficient flow in the office.

Materials

■ Pen
■ Appointment book

Competency

(**Conditions**) With the necessary materials, you will be able to (**Task**) establish an appointment matrix (**Standards**) correctly within the time limit set by the instructor.

1. Determine the amount of time the providers want patients to have for each appointment type.
2. Within the appointment book, block out the time when the providers will be out of the office (e.g., for lunch, other appointments, vacations, or conferences).
3. Highlight or create blocks of time in the appointment book for appointments the provider specifies as those she would like only a limited number of, such as physical exams.
4. Go over the created appointment matrix with the providers to determine where any adjustments need to be made.

Even in one-physician practices, different columns of the appointment book may be used for different procedures. For example, all new patients might be scheduled in the far left column and all followup appointments in the far right one. In some offices, appointment types are highlighted in different colors to indicate type of patient or procedure. For example, patients undergoing laboratory work might be highlighted in orange while patients having X-rays might be highlighted in blue. Each office devises a system that works for it.

HIPAA Compliance

The appointment book, whether hard copy or electronic, is considered a legal document. Paper appointment books, like all hard-copy medical records, must be kept in a safe location. Computerized appointment schedules must be protected just like any other item that contains private patient information. Computerized schedules are secured through secure computer systems and password use by all administrative staff. At the end of the day, any prints of the computerized system should be shredded to protect patient confidentiality.

Figure 11-4 ◆ Scheduling appointments on the computer saves time over using a manual scheduling system.

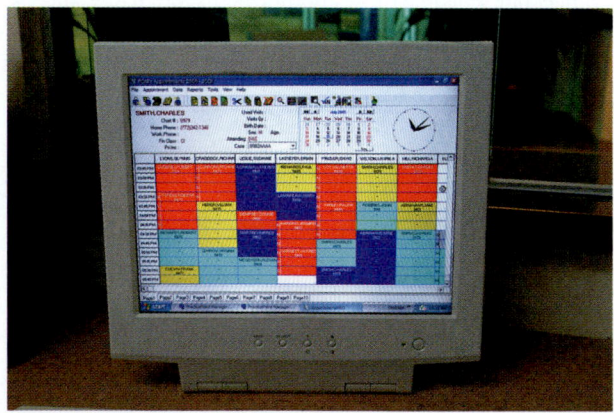

Figure 11-5 ◆ Using a color-coded scheme is easier in a multiphysician practice.

PROCEDURE 11-2 Schedule a New Patient

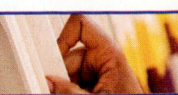

Theory and Rationale

Most patients who schedule appointments in the medical office do so over the telephone. The administrative medical assistant must know the information needed from each new patient and be able to answer any questions professionally.

Materials

- Telephone
- Blue or black pen
- Paper
- Appointment book

Competency

(**Conditions**) With the necessary materials, you will be able to (**Task**) schedule a new patient who calls the medical office (**Standards**) correctly within the time limit set by the instructor.

1. Using a professional, friendly voice, answer the telephone by the second ring.
2. State the office name followed by your name.
3. When the caller does not self-identify as a new patient, ask the caller if he or she has been in to the office previously.
4. Ask the patient to spell his or her first and last names.
5. Write the patient's full name on the checklist.
6. Ask the patient for work and home telephone numbers, and home address.
7. Ask the patient how he or she was referred to the office.
8. Ask the patient to identify the type of health insurance he or she will be using.
9. Confirm that your physician participates in the patient's health care plan.
10. If the physician does not participate in the patient's health care plan, advise the patient that he or she may fail to receive preferred benefits or may need to pay in full for their services.
11. Ask the patient to state the condition prompting the visit.
12. Ask the patient to define the length of the condition.
13. Offer the patient appointment times to see the physician.
14. Schedule the patient.
15. If mailing paperwork to the patient to complete before the appointment, direct the patient to complete the paperwork before the visit.
16. If the patient will need to complete the paperwork at the first visit, direct him or her to arrive 15 minutes before the appointment's scheduled start time.
17. Document the patient's information in the manual or electronic appointment schedule.
18. Ask the patient if directions to the office are needed.
19. Give the patient any needed parking information.
20. Confirm the appointment's date and time with the patient.
21. Allow the patient to hang up the telephone before hanging up yourself.

Methods of Appointment Scheduling

Ambulatory healthcare uses several different methods to schedule patient appointments. Practice type and physician preference determine which method is used.

Cluster Scheduling

Cluster scheduling is a system of booking several patients around the same block of time. This method is normally used when the patients all need the same type of service, such as laboratory work or consultations. By clustering similar appointments, the office can serve patients most efficiently.

Double Booking

Double booking is done when two or more patients are scheduled to see the same healthcare provider at once. This method serves when an emergency patient must be seen that day, or it may be used to accommodate patients who need added services while in the office. For example, if the medical office has two patients who are both going to need laboratory work, the

medical assistant might schedule both patients for the same appointment time. This option works, because the clinical medical assistant can perform laboratory work with one patient while the physician sees the other. This system uses the treatment rooms as well as the clinical staff's time effectively.

Fixed Appointment Scheduling

The most common method of scheduling patients is **fixed-appointment scheduling.** In this method, the office gives each patient a specific appointment time.

Scheduling with Open Hours

The **open hours** scheduling method works for patients who do not need specific appointment times. This system is used in walk-in clinics, laboratories, and X-ray facilities where patients are normally seen on a first-come, first-served basis.

Wave Scheduling

Medical clinics with large numbers of procedure rooms and clinical staff may use something called **wave scheduling.** In

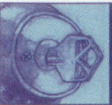

Keys to Success
CHRONICALLY LATE PATIENTS

When patients are habitually late for their appointments, the medical office should give those patients times that precede scheduled appointment times by 15 minutes. When a chronically late patient is scheduled for a 2:15 P.M. appointment, for example, the office should advise the patient to arrive at 2:00 P.M.

wave scheduling, patients are scheduled only for the first half of each hour. The first patient to arrive is seen first. If two or more patients arrive at once, the clinical medical assistant will need to triage the patients to make the decision on who to take first.

Modified Wave Scheduling

The **modified wave scheduling** method is a variation on the wave method just discussed. With modified wave scheduling, two or three patients are scheduled at the beginning of each hour, followed by single patient appointments every 10 to 20 minutes for the rest of that hour. Complicated cases are generally scheduled at the beginning of the hour, while minor cases are usually scheduled toward the end.

Leaving Slack or Buffer Time

Most medical offices that use scheduling systems for patient appointments leave certain times of day open to accommodate things like patients who call for same-day appointments or physicians who need to catch up on charting. Such open periods, called **slack** or **buffer time,** are generally 15- to 30-minute slots at the end of the morning and the end of the afternoon or evening.

Conducting Triage and Appointment Scheduling

Patients with medical emergencies will sometimes call their physicians' offices for assistance. When they do, administrative medical assistants should have clearly written protocols for handling the situations. A **triage notebook,** detailed in ∞ Chapter 9, outlines these protocols, as well as questions to ask patients who call with possible medical emergencies. Such a notebook, which should be clear, concise, and written under the physicians' direction, should be left near the telephone where patient calls are answered. ∞ See Chapter 10 for more information on the triage notebook.

Using Appointment Reminder Systems

Typically, patients are given appointment reminder cards as they leave the office (Figure 11-6 ◆). These reminder cards are normally the size of a business card and contain the date, day, and time of the patient's next appointment, as well as the office's name and telephone number.

Even with reminder cards, patients may forget their appointments. For this reason, many offices call patients the day before their appointment to remind them. Such calls must remain confidential. When leaving messages, staff should disclose no patient information. Instead, the assistant can leave a message like, "This is Jared calling from Dr. Barker's office to remind Kaneesha of her appointment tomorrow at 2 P.M. If you have any questions, please call me back at 201-555-6000."

For patients who schedule followup appointments a month or more in the future, many offices choose to send reminder cards. These cards can be postcards only when they contain no personal patient information such as the reason for the visit. If the name of the office discloses the reason for the

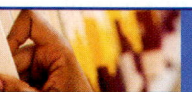

PROCEDURE 11-3 Schedule an Established Patient Appointment

Theory and Rationale

Patient scheduling, which constitutes a large portion of the medical assistant's job, is vital to proper time management in the medical office. Therefore, the assistant must be properly trained to perform this task.

Materials

- Appointment schedule
- Blue or black pen
- Patient's chart

Competency

(**Conditions**) With the necessary materials, you will be able to (**Task**) schedule a patient appointment (**Standards**) correctly within the time limit set by the instructor.

1. Locate the chart of the patient to be scheduled.
2. Determine the type of appointment that is needed.
3. Determine the patient's schedule.
4. Determine the physician's schedule.
5. Enter the patient in the appointment schedule.
6. Restate the appointment date and time to the patient. If the patient is in the office, provide a written reminder card. Remind the patient to bring any needed items to the appointment or to follow any procedures (e.g., fasting before the visit).

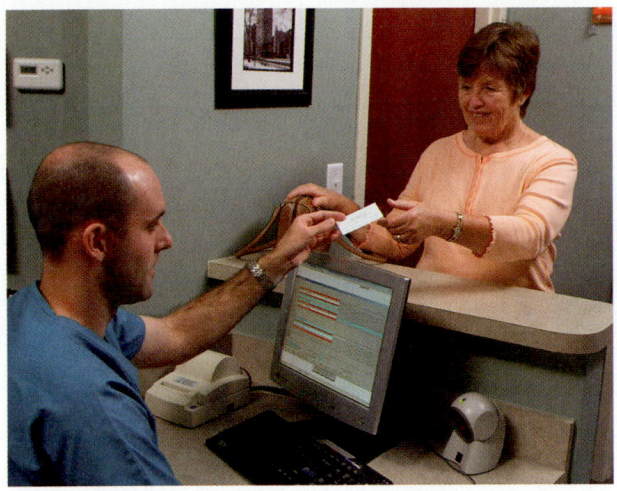

Figure 11-6 ◆ Typically, patients are given appointment reminder cards when they leave the office.

patient's visit, the office should not use postcard reminders. For example, if the office is called "Woodland Oncology Center," someone who sees a postcard with this name may assume the patient has cancer. Offices like these should either mail appointment reminders in envelopes or call patients with reminders. Some form of reminder card or call has been proven to reduce dramatically the number of no-show appointments.

Correcting the Appointment Schedule

White correction fluid, as with patients' medical records, is disallowed from the appointment book. When an appointment is changed in the appointment book, it should not be obliterated or erased or blacked out with a marker. Instead, the medical assistant should draw one line through the patient's name and note

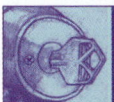

Keys to Success
AUTOMATED TELEPHONE REMINDER SYSTEMS

Many medical offices today use automated telephone reminder systems to remind patients of their upcoming appointments. These systems, typically paired with computerized appointment systems, automatically dial patients' contact telephone numbers and play recorded reminder messages.

why the patient failed to keep the appointment (Figure 11-7 ◆). Some medical offices use color-coded systems to indicate schedule changes. For example, a red "X" next to a patient's name might indicate an appointment cancellation. Electronic schedules accept notations, cancellations, and rescheduled or missed appointments.

Documenting No-Show Appointments

Patients who fail to arrive for their appointment and do not call to reschedule are considered "no-shows." The medical office must try to reach all no-shows. Typically, this is done via telephone 15 to 30 minutes after a patient's appointed time. When medical assistants reach such patients, they should try to reschedule the appointment. When they cannot reach patients, however, they should leave messages requesting return calls to reschedule. When assistants can neither reach patients nor leave messages, they may mail notes requesting rescheduling.

Following Up on No-Show Appointments

Missed patient appointments, for whatever reason, must be documented in the patients' medical records. Any steps the

---

PROCEDURE 11-4 Use Patient Reminder Cards

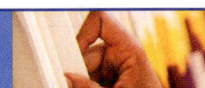

Theory and Rationale

Many patients, as they leave the medical office, will require a followup appointment. The medical assistant will need to schedule that appointment for the patient and provide the patient with a reminder card.

Materials

- Pen
- Appointment book
- Appointment reminder card

Competency

(**Conditions**) With the necessary materials, you will be able to (**Task**) use patient reminder cards (**Standards**) correctly within the time limit set by the instructor.

1. As the patient arrives at the reception desk, look at the fee slip to verify when the provider wants the patient to return for an appointment.
2. Ask the patient if there is a day or time that works best for his or her schedule for the appointment.
3. Check the appointment book to find an appointment time that fits with the patient's schedule.
4. After verifying that the appointment will work with the patient's schedule, write or type the appointment into the appointment schedule.
5. Write the patient's appointment on a reminder card and give the card to the patient.

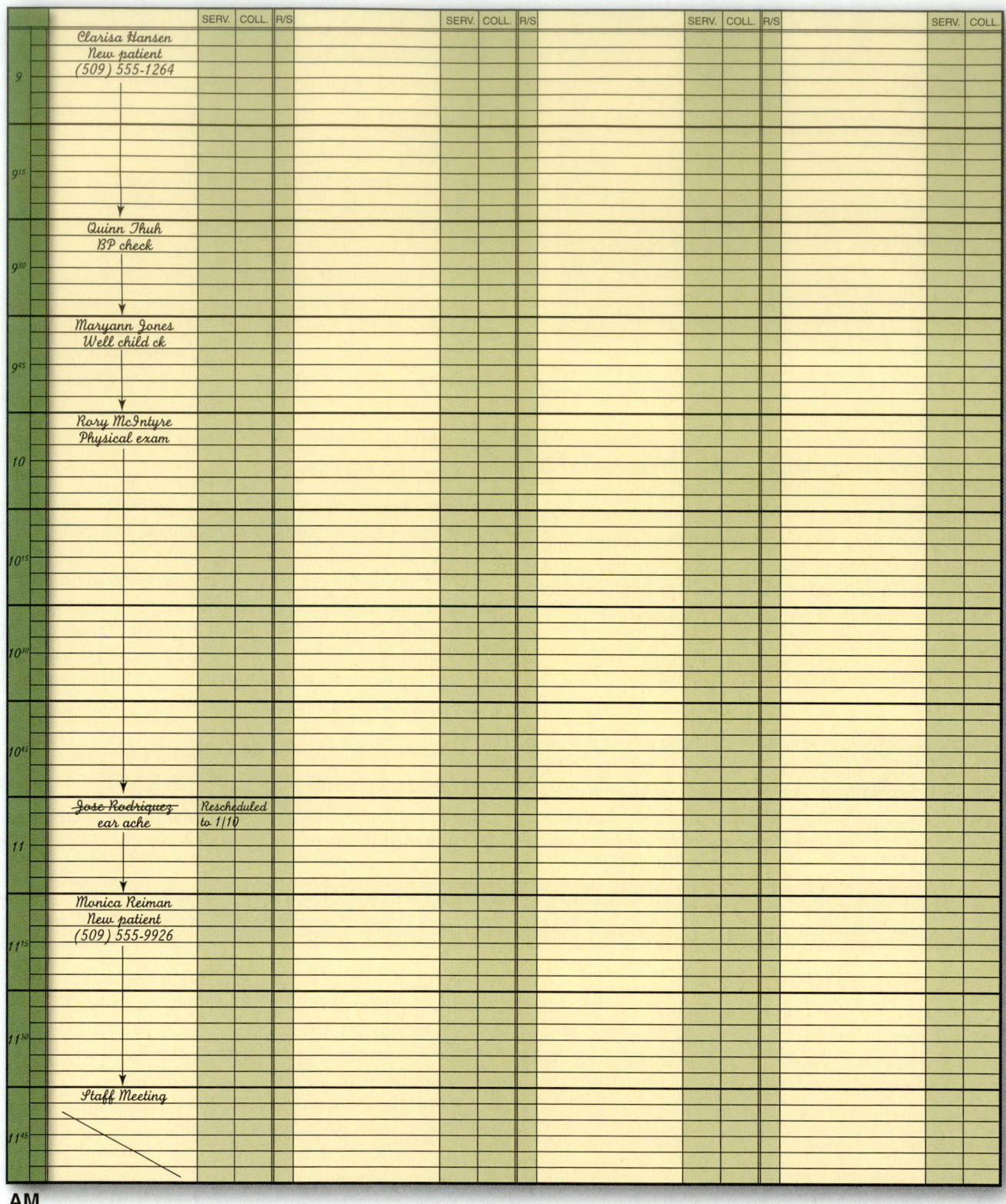

Figure 11-7 ◆ Sample appointment book indicating a patient who has changed an appointment.

medical office staff takes to try to reschedule those patients must be documented as well. When patients refuse to reschedule or remain unreachable, medical assistants must make notes in those patients' medical records and submit those records to the physician for review.

Well-documented patient medical records become particularly important when patients experience adverse outcomes due to missed appointments. Medical offices with clear, comprehensive patient records are better able to defend against malpractice suits. Some offices take the extra step of sending patients certified letters when they miss important followup appointments, such as postoperative appointments. Proof of the patients' receipt of such letters demonstrates the office took every step possible to encourage patients to obtain needed care.

In Practice

Dr. Brosnan performed a vasectomy on William Grissom and asked him, as he asks all patients who have undergone this procedure, to have a followup evaluation and laboratory work to determine the procedure's effectiveness. Mr. Grissom, however, failed to show for his followup appointment. Three months later, Dr. Brosnan received a notice that Mr. Grissom has filed a malpractice suit. According to the notice, Mr. Grissom is alleging that Dr. Brosnan was negligent because Mr. Grissom's wife is newly pregnant. How could Dr. Brosnan's office have protected itself against this situation?

Managing the Physician's Professional Schedule

Many physicians attend professional meetings outside the office. These range from lunches with colleagues to traveling to out-of-state seminars. In many medical offices, the administrative medical assistant manages the physician's professional schedule. At minimum, this task includes blocking out times in the appointment schedule when the physician is unavailable for patient appointments. The assistant may also be asked to book airline flights or hotel rooms, or to reserve seats at conferences.

To ensure accuracy and efficiency, medical assistants should clearly write all information on the physician's travel plans, including any confirmation numbers (Figure 11-8 ◆). A copy of all such information should remain in the office to keep the rest of the healthcare team apprised of the physician's schedule. The physician can retain any original documents. When the physician attends a seminar or conference that awards continuing-education credits, the medical assistant should track that information, as well.

Scheduling Hospital Services and Admissions

Many physicians care for or perform procedures on patients in hospital settings as well as in ambulatory clinics. For this reason, administrative medical assistants must be well versed in the procedures for scheduling patients for hospital services.

PROCEDURE 11-5 Reschedule a Missed Patient Appointment

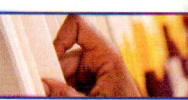

Theory and Rationale

The medical office must follow up on all missed patient appointments. The medical assistant must call the patient to attempt to reschedule the missed appointment and document notes in the medical record.

Materials

- Appointment schedule
- Pen
- Patient's chart

Competency

(**Conditions**) With the necessary materials, you will be able to (**Task**) reschedule a missed patient appointment (**Standards**) correctly within the time limit set by the instructor.

1. Fifteen minutes after the patient's appointment time, call the patient's home telephone number.
2. If the patient answers:
   - Point out the missed appointment time and ask for an appropriate time to reschedule.

- If the patient reschedules the appointment, document the new appointment in the appointment book as well as the patient's chart. Also chart that the patient missed the originally scheduled appointment.
- If the patient does not wish to reschedule, politely state that you will inform the physician. Chart the missed appointment and refusal to reschedule in the patient's chart, and give the chart to the physician.

3. If the patient fails to answer:
   - Leave a message on voice mail or with the person who answers. Be certain to disclose no confidential patient information. An appropriate message is, "This is Juan at Dr. Saunders's office. I'm calling for Mrs. Banfield. We had you scheduled for an appointment today at 9:00 A.M., and I'm calling to reschedule. Please call me back at 715-555-6789."
   - In the patient's chart, document the missed appointment and the message.

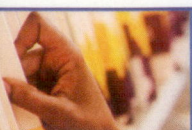

PROCEDURE 11-6 Manage the Physician's Professional Schedule and Travel

Theory and Rationale

Many physicians travel out of town for speaking engagements or seminars while gaining continuing-education credits for relicensure. The medical assistant will often be asked to coordinate the physician's schedule and make all necessary travel arrangements for these trips.

Materials

- A telephone
- A list of the physician's travel needs, including dates and times of the meeting or seminar, place of the seminar, and physician preference for airline and hotel arrangements.
- Paper and pen

Competency

(**Conditions**) With the necessary materials, you will be able to (**Task**) manage the physician's professional schedule and travel (**Standards**) correctly within the time limit set by the instructor.

1. Call the physician's preferred airline and book the appropriate flight.
2. Make a note of the date, time, airline, and flight number for the departure time and arrival time for both the outgoing flight and the return flight.
3. Call the physician's preferred hotel and book the appropriate room.
4. Make a note of the confirmation number for the hotel room.
5. Arrange for any necessary transportation to or from the hotel and airport.
6. Create a list of all arrangements made and give the list to the physician.
7. Give a copy of the list of arrangements to the office manager and to the receptionist.
8. Verify the receptionist has blocked out the dates the physician will be away, if applicable.

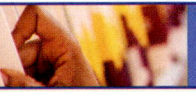

PROCEDURE 11-7 Schedule a Hospital Procedure

Theory and Rationale

When procedures cannot be performed in the medical office or patients would be better served in hospitals, physicians ask the medical assistant to schedule patients for hospital procedures.

Materials

- Patient's chart
- Hospital/surgery scheduling form
- Scheduling guidelines
- Calendar
- Telephone
- Notepad
- Pen

Competency

(**Conditions**) With the necessary materials, you will be able to (**Task**) schedule a patient for a hospital procedure (**Standards**) correctly within the time limit set by the instructor.

1. Obtain information from the physician or clinical medical assistant about the needed surgery or procedure and the desired hospital.
2. Call the patient's insurance carrier to obtain preauthorization for the procedure.

3. Document the preauthorization number in the patient's chart along with the name of the insurance company customer service representative spoken to.
4. If the patient is in the clinic, ask what date or time would be most convenient for the procedure. If the patient is not in the clinic, call the patient to determine scheduling needs.
5. Call the hospital to communicate the procedure the physician has planned, the amount of time needed for the procedure, and the date preferred for the procedure.
6. Provide the hospital staff the patient's information, including name, birth date, address, telephone number, insurance information, and preauthorization number. Also relay all pertinent health information, such as allergies or disabilities.
7. After agreeing on a date and time, give the information to the patient and enter it in the physician's appointment schedule.
8. Advise the patient that the hospital will likely call to provide instructions and verify the check-in date and time.
9. Schedule the patient for a postoperative appointment in the physician's office, if needed.
10. Chart all information in the patient's medical record, and give the chart to the physician for review.

PROCEDURE 11-8 Schedule an Inpatient Admission

Theory and Rationale

When patients require inpatient procedures or observations, physicians will ask medical assistants to schedule those patients for inpatient hospitalizations. Medical assistants who know the proper procedure help ensure that the scheduling process goes smoothly.

Materials

- Patient's chart
- Inpatient scheduling guidelines
- Calendar
- Telephone
- Notepad
- Pen

Competency

(**Conditions**) With the necessary materials, you will be able to (**Task**) schedule an inpatient admission (**Standards**) correctly within the time limit set by the instructor.

1. Call the patient's insurance carrier to obtain preauthorization for the procedure, the needed followup, and the allowable number of hospital days.
2. Document the preauthorization number in the patient's chart along with the name of the insurance company customer service representative spoken to.
3. Call the hospital admissions office with the patient's name, physician's name, and reason for admission.
4. Let the admissions office know when the physician would like the patient to be admitted.
5. Give the admissions office the patient's contact information, birth date, insurance information, and preauthorization number.
6. Instruct the patient when to arrive at the hospital and where to go once there.
7. Give the patient any specifics on what to bring (or not) to the hospital.
8. Chart all information in the patient's medical record, and give the chart to the physician for review.

- Leaving on United Airlines Flight #12 at 7:10 P.M. Thursday.
- Arriving in Chicago at 10:02 P.M.
- Reservations with Hertz car rental, Confirmation #1298745.
- Reservations at the Red Lion hotel, Confirmation #LEN987.
- Seminar starts in the Capital Boardroom at 9 A.M. Friday.
- Return on United Airlines Flight #81 at 9:10 A.M. Sunday.

Figure 11-8 ◆ Sample physician's travel schedule.

To facilitate the hospital scheduling process, the medical office should keep all hospital and related telephone numbers near the telephone or program them into speed dial. Most health insurance plans require physicians to obtain **preapprovals** for surgical procedures. Unless the procedure is an emergency, the medical assistant should call the patient's insurance carrier to obtain authorization for the procedure before scheduling the patient. Whenever possible, medical assistants should schedule patients for hospital services while those patients are in the office. With patients present, assistants are better able to coordinate patients' schedules.

Every office should have guidelines for scheduling patients for hospital services. Such guidelines should list the type of procedure, the physician, the time the physician needs, and any information that must be relayed to the patient, such as fasting presurgery. The medical office should also have preprinted informational forms from the hospital or outpatient facility that gives such specifics as directions to the facility and check-in procedures. Patients should receive such forms before they leave the office.

Specialty Referral Appointments

Many patients in the medical office will need to be scheduled for appointments with specialists. When this happens, the physician will notify the medical assistant of the patient's need for a specialty referral. The physician will also state the name of the specialist the patient is to be referred to, information regarding the condition for which the patient needs to be seen, and a time frame within which the appointment should be made.

Depending upon the policy in the medical clinic, the medical assistant may call to schedule the referral for the patient directly. In other offices, the medical assistant may supply the information about the referral to the patient and the patient makes the telephone call directly. Either way, the medical assistant must supply the patient with the needed information regarding the need for the additional appointment.

Arranging for Language Interpreters

Occasionally, the medical office will treat patients who are not fluent in English or who cannot communicate due to a disability. Typically, these patients visit the office with family members or friends who can translate for them. When patients cannot arrange for interpreters, the medical office must arrange interpreter services. Many states offer translation services for

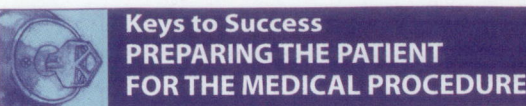

Keys to Success
PREPARING THE PATIENT
FOR THE MEDICAL PROCEDURE

Medical procedures make many patients nervous. Medical assistants can help make patients' experiences positive ones by letting them know exactly what to expect before, during, and after their procedures. Assistants should include any dietary or activity restrictions before or after procedures, specify how long the procedures are expected to take, and provide information on warning signs.

their Medicaid-covered patients. When translation services are needed, offices should keep interpreters' telephone numbers at the front desk. When using a translator, the medical assistant must document the name and contact information of the translator in the patient's chart.

To bring translation services in house, many medical offices, especially those in communities with large non–English-speaking populations, seek employees who are fluent in other languages. Members of the healthcare team who can translate for patients are valuable assets to the medical office.

Arranging Transportation for Patients

Many medical offices treat patients who cannot drive themselves to the office. Patients may have disabilities or offices may be in challenging locations. As a courtesy to patients, medical assistants should keep telephone lists of transportation services. Such lists should include taxicab services as well as local services for the elderly or disabled.

Achieving Efficiency in Scheduling

All medical offices at some point realize that their appointment scheduling procedures could be improved. Physicians may routinely exceed scheduled appointment times, or

extended delays may regularly irritate patients. When flaws like these become apparent, it is important for the healthcare team as a whole to re-evaluate how the office schedules appointments. Every member of the team should participate in improvement efforts, because scheduling affects every staff member (Figure 11-9 ◆).

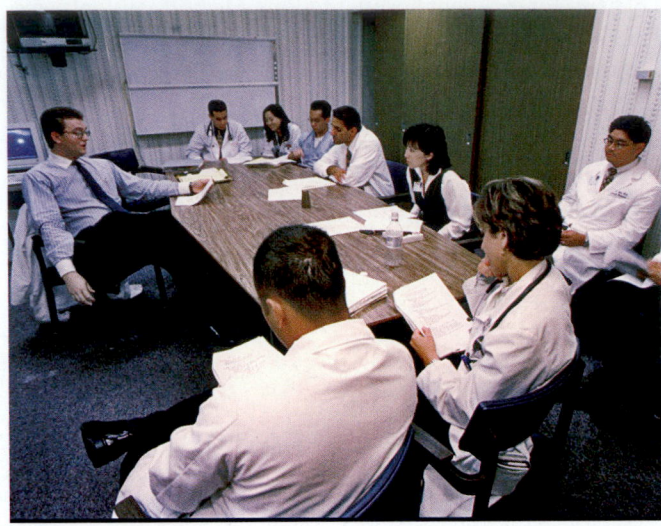

Figure 11-9 ◆ When scheduling flaws become apparent, each member of the healthcare team should participate in improvement efforts.

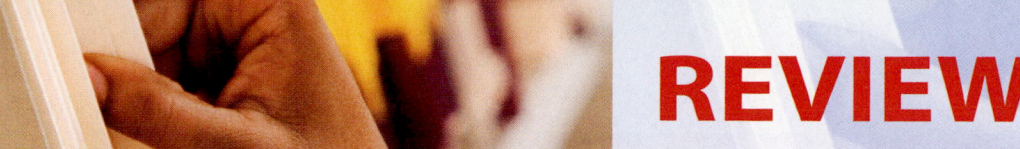

REVIEW

Chapter Summary

- Guidelines for scheduling patient appointments are invaluable tools for medical offices intent on providing effective, efficient patient service.
- Today, medical offices can choose between paper and electronic scheduling systems.
- Both paper and electronic scheduling systems accommodate patient no-shows, which always must be documented properly for legal and other purposes.
- Whenever patients miss their appointments, the medical assistant should follow up to attempt rescheduling.

- The physician's professional schedule, which includes travel, is part of a medical office's overall scheduling scheme.
- Like the physician's travel, the medical assistant must be able to accommodate patients' hospital appointments in the office's scheduling system.
- Effective medical assistants arrange appropriate transportation services or language interpreters for patients in need.

Chapter Review

Multiple Choice

1. At _____ minutes after a patient has missed an appointment, the medical assistant should call to reschedule.
    a. 5
    b. 10
    c. 15
    d. 60

2. A new patient is defined as someone who has
    a. not been seen in the medical office for more than one year.
    b. not been seen by any physician in the office for more than three years.
    c. been seen by another physician in the office within the last year but is now seeing a new provider in the office.
    d. all of the above.

3. A new patient checklist is worthwhile when scheduling new patient appointments to ensure the medical assistant
    a. gathers all necessary information from the new patient.
    b. provides directions to the office, if needed.
    c. gives information on parking arrangements.
    d. all of the above.

4. The medical office should ask new patients to arrive _____ minutes before their scheduled appointments to complete new patient paperwork.
    a. 5
    b. 15
    c. 25
    d. 35

5. Which of the following scheduling methods books several patients around the same time?
    a. Cluster booking
    b. Stream scheduling
    c. Set appointment time scheduling
    d. None of the above

True/False

T F 1. The time allowed for patient appointments remains constant from practitioner to practitioner.

T F 2. The appointment book is a legal document.

T F 3. Double booking is the process of allowing patients to arrive for appointments at their leisure.

T F 4. It is appropriate to tell chronically late patients that their appointments are 15 minutes before the times scheduled in the appointment book.

T F 5. It is unnecessary to chart a no-show appointment in a patient's chart.

T F 6. Medical offices that chart patients' missed appointments can avoid losing malpractice lawsuits.

T F 7. When scheduling patients for procedures, it is important to disclose everything to expect.

T F 8. Medical assistants do not arrange transportation services.

T F 9. A medical office's appointment scheduling system should be reviewed periodically to determine its efficiency.

Short Answer

1. What is one way to prepare the appointment schedule to allow appointments for patients who call and want same-day appointments?

2. Describe a triage notebook and its role in the medical office.

3. How can medical assistants help patients remember to keep their appointments?

4. What is meant by a "no-show" appointment?

5. What can medical assistants do when they find that patients are waiting long periods for their appointments?

6. Describe how an appointment matrix is used in the medical office.

Chapter Review (continued)

Research

1. Research online for companies that sell medical office appointment scheduling software. How do these companies compare to one another?

2. Interview someone who works in a medical office. Do the physicians in this office travel for out-of-town events related to their practice? If so, who in the office handles the scheduling arrangements?

3. What local resources are available in your area for arranging for medical language interpreters?

Externship Application Experience

When Shawn Guthmein calls to schedule a new patient appointment with Dr. Gootkind, he mentions that he will be bringing his service animal to his appointment because he is legally blind.

Because Shawn is a new patient, he will need to complete several forms once he is in the clinic. How can the medical assistant best assist this patient?

Resource Guide

MicroWiz Medical Appointment Scheduling Software
http://www.microwize.com/ohpro.htm

MedStar Medical Appointment Scheduling Software
http://www.medstarsystems.com

NewMedia Medicine Medical Appointment Scheduling Software
http://www.newmediamedicine.com/

ScheduleView Medical Appointment Software
http://www.scheduleview.com/

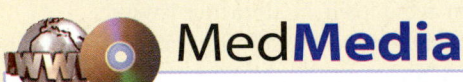 Med**Media**

http://www.MyMAKit.com

More on this chapter, including interactive resources, can be found on the Student CD-ROM accompanying this textbook and on http://www.MyMAKit.com.

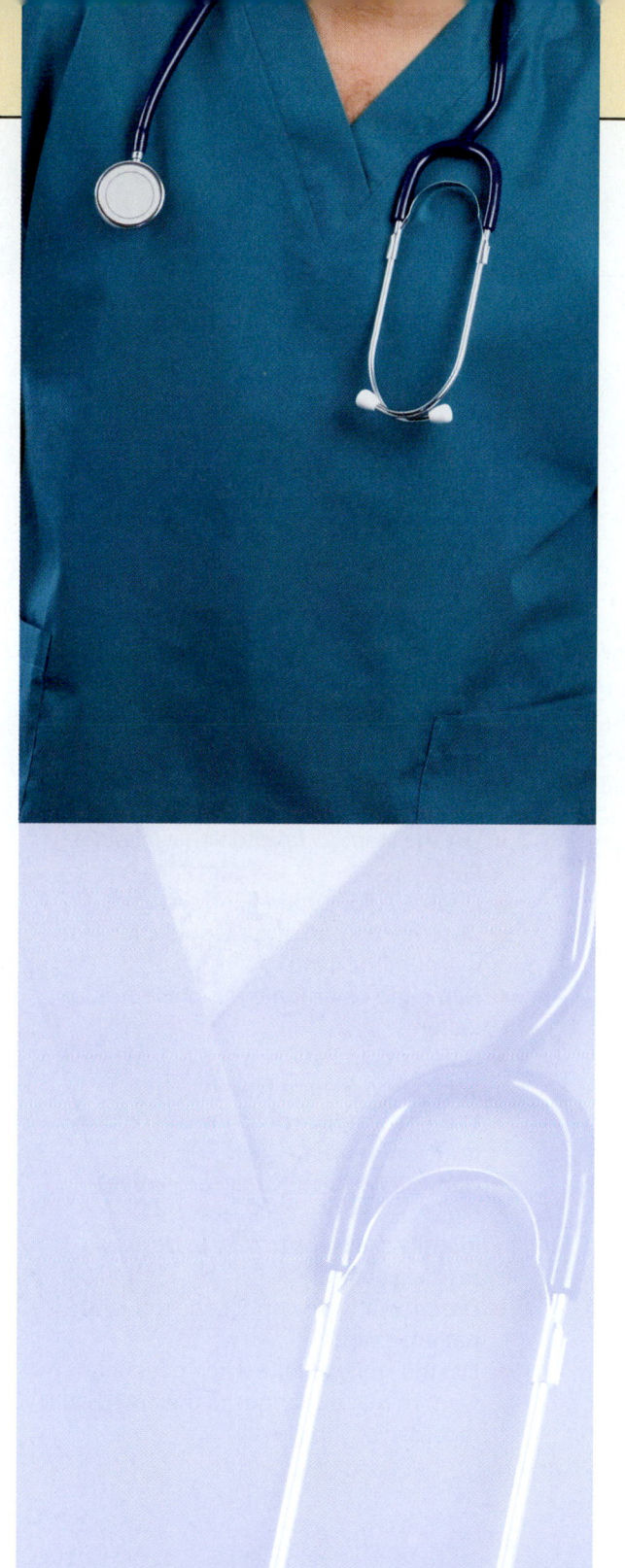

UNIT III

Managing Health Information in the Medical Office

Chapter 12   **Medical Records Management**
Chapter 13   **Electronic Medical Records**
Chapter 14   **Computers in the Medical Office**

My name is Sharon Martincak. I am a recent graduate of the medical assisting program at Everett Community College. I learned a lot about the importance of maintaining patient privacy in my training, and during my externship I realized how important that training was to my career as a medical assistant. Without this knowledge, I would be lost. I am responsible for a lot of information about each patient, and I am responsible for everything that is included in the patient's medical chart. I have to deal with patients' friends, relatives, and insurance companies, and I have to be aware of what I can disclose about the patient and what I cannot.

Every day I work with telephone messages, fax messages, and information that the patient entrusts to me. This information must be kept from anyone who is not supposed to have it. Medical assistants must be very careful in the way this information is used in order to protect both the patient and the physician. As a medical assistant, I am held liable for patient information and how it is used. I cannot stress enough the importance of knowing HIPAA privacy laws. This knowledge has made my job safer and easier.

CHAPTER 12

Medical Records Management

Case Study

When Melissa begins working for Dr. Kingsley, Caroline, one of the physician's longtime medical assistants, is charged with training her. One day, as Caroline pulls charts for patients scheduled for that afternoon, she points out a note on the outside of Robert Olson's chart that reads, "Problem." Caroline explains that the note alerts the medical assistants and the physician to patients who are "hard to work with." She says these patients complain, are late to their appointments, or are just generally unpleasant.

Objectives

After completing this chapter, you should be able to:

- Define and spell the key terminology in this chapter.
- Define the medical assistant's role in medical records management.
- List information contained in the medical record.
- Explain various charting styles.
- Discuss how to chart patient communication.
- Define cross-referencing and how it should be used.
- List the steps to take to find a missing file.
- Discuss color-coded filing systems.
- Describe why an office would choose to use numeric filing.
- Name the common types of file storage systems.
- Differentiate between active, inactive, and closed patient files.
- Distinguish electronic medical records from paper ones.
- Name ways to store inactive patient files.
- Identify the steps to take to destroy a medical record.
- Describe how to correct an error in a patient chart.
- List the steps to take when patients want to make changes to their medical records.

MedMedia

http://www.MyMAKit.com

Additional interactive resources and activities for this chapter can be found on http://www.MyMAKit.com. For videos, tips, audio glossary, legal and ethical scenarios, on-the-job scenarios, quizzes, and games related to the content of this chapter, please access the accompanying CD-ROM in this book.

Video: *Medical Records Management, Getting Along with Coworkers*
Legal and Ethical Scenario: *Medical Records Management*
On the Job Scenario: *Medical Records Management*
Tips
Multiple Choice Quiz
Audio Glossary
HIPAA Quiz
Games: Spelling Bee, Crossword, and Strikeout

✚ MEDICAL ASSISTING STANDARDS

CAAHEP ENTRY-LEVEL STANDARDS	ABHES ENTRY-LEVEL COMPETENCIES
■ Perform within scope of practice (psychomotor) ■ Apply ethical behaviors, including honesty/integrity in performance of medical assisting practice (affective) ■ Practice within the standard of care for a medical assistant (psychomotor) ■ Demonstrate sensitivity to patient rights (affective) ■ Document accurately in the patient record (psychomotor) ■ Explain general office policies (psychomotor) ■ Identify systems for organizing medical records (cognitive) ■ Describe various types of content maintained in the patient's medical record (cognitive) ■ Discuss pros and cons of various filing systems (cognitive) ■ Identify both equipment and supplies needed for filing medical records (cognitive) ■ Describe indexing rules (cognitive) ■ Discuss filing procedures (cognitive) ■ Identify types of records common to the healthcare setting (cognitive) ■ Organize a patient's medical record (psychomotor) ■ File medical records (psychomotor) ■ Maintain organization by filing (psychomotor) ■ Consider staff needs and limitations in establishment of a filing system (affective) ■ Demonstrate telephone techniques (psychomotor)	■ Maintain confidentiality at all times ■ Use appropriate guidelines when releasing records or information ■ Be cognizant of ethical boundaries ■ Evidence a responsible attitude ■ Application of electronic technology ■ Apply computer concepts for office procedures ■ Prepare and maintain medical records ■ File medical records ■ Perform medical transcriptions

✓ COMPETENCY SKILLS PERFORMANCE

1. Prepare and maintain the medical record.
2. Chart patient telephone calls.
3. File documents using the alphabetic filing system.
4. File manually using a subject filing system.
5. File documents in patient medical records.
6. Use the numeric system to file medical records.
7. Correct errors in the patient medical record.

Key Terminology

active patient files—files for patients who have appointments or who have been in to see the physician recently

advance directives—documents that outline patients' wishes regarding healthcare should those patients be unable to speak for themselves

chief complaint—main reason a patient seeks care

closed patient files—files for patients who will not be returning to the clinic

cross-referencing—method of tracking and finding patient files for patients with multiple last names

electronic medical records—medical records kept via computer; also called electronic health records

electronic signature—electronic version of a person's signature to be used in electronic medical records (see preceding entry)

financial information—data on payment record or ledger, health insurance identification numbers, and policy numbers

flow charts—graphs in patient medical records that track such things as weight gain or newborn growth

inactive patient files—files for patients who have not seen the physician for extended periods

indecipherable—unreadable

medical information—information on a patient's medical care and history

medical record—legal document consisting of medical information obtained from the patient via consultations, examinations, and tests

medical research program—research conducted to determine the effectiveness or harm of certain medications or medical treatments

narrative—type of medical charting in which the healthcare provider writes a narrative version of patient contact

nontherapeutic research—research programs that do not benefit the study's patients

obliterate—to make unreadable or unrecognizable

patient information—the information contained within the patient's medical record

personal information—information such as patient's name, birth

Key Terminology *(continued)*

date, gender, marital status, occupation, next of kin, and any other items collected for personal identification.

problem-oriented medical record (POMR) charting—type of medical record charting that focuses on patients' healthcare problems and addresses those problems at each visit

progress notes—notes in patients' medical charts outlining those patients' progress or complaints

purge—to remove closed or inactive patient medical records from the medical office

shingling—process of attaching small pieces of paper to standard-size sheets of paper so the small items are easy to locate in patients' charts

SOAP note charting—type of charting that considers the patient's subjective and objective findings, the provider's assessment of the patient's condition, and the prescribed plan of action for treatment

social information—information about a patient's social habits, such as tobacco, drug, or alcohol use

standard of care—legal term that describes the type of care a reasonable healthcare provider is expected to provide under the same situation

statute of limitations—period within which a patient must file a lawsuit after an injury

subpoena—court order demanding that a party appear in court or copies of the medical record be sent to a third party

Abbreviations

FDA—Food and Drug Administration

HIPAA—Health Insurance Portability and Accountability Act

POMR—problem-oriented medical record

SOAP—subjective, objective, assessment, and plan

Introduction

Medical records play an important role in healthcare delivery, so they must be accurate and complete. Healthcare providers rely on patients' medical records as accurate depictions of patients. With patients' consent, medical records are often sent between physicians and hospitals to give physicians complete pictures of patients' medical histories.

As legal documents, medical records are often the single most important tools healthcare providers can use to defend against medical malpractice lawsuits. Risk management and quality improvement programs rely on medical records to catch errors in patient care. Insurance companies often request copies of patient medical records to determine the appropriateness of billing codes and reimbursement levels. Medical records that are incomplete or **indecipherable** may cause problems in patient care.

The Medical Assistant's Role in Medical Records Management

The medical assistant works with patient medical records on a regular basis. Having a clear understanding of how to work with patient medical records is imperative to the medical assistant, since the office can be subject to civil litigation if patient privacy is breached. ∞ Chapter 13 provides a discussion of working with the electronic medical record.

Information Contained in the Medical Record

Medical records have four types of **patient information**: (1) **personal information,** (2) **financial information,** (3) **medical information,** and (4) **social information.** Personal information is the information patients supply when first seeing physicians for care. Such information includes a patient's name, birth date, gender, marital status, occupation, next of kin, and any other items collected for personal identification. Personal information may also include any comments the medical assistant might write in the patient's file regarding the patient's language or cultural background, if such information pertains to the patient's healthcare.

A patient's financial information includes a patient's ledger and insurance information, which includes policy and identification numbers and insurance-plan contact information, as well as any other information needed to bill the insurance company for the patient's care. In many medical offices, some portion of the patient's financial information is kept in a separate file from medical information. Financial information also includes copies of insurance company correspondence, and signed authorizations from the patient allowing the medical provider to release information to the insurance company.

Medical information includes the **chief complaint,** or the main reason a person seeks care; any family medical history; the patient's medical history; the results of examinations; the physical examination form; the prescribed course of treatment, including any medications or referrals; and the patient's diagnoses, progress notes, operative reports, radiology reports, laboratory reports, and any other reports or information that pertains to the patient's healthcare (Figure 12-1 ◆).

Social information is any personal information on the patient, such as race and ethnicity, hobbies, and regular sports participation. Social information also includes such lifestyle choices as smoking, alcohol consumption, drug use, and sexual habits.

In addition to personal, financial, medical, and social information, other documents are routinely part of the patient's medical record. These documents include the **HIPAA** understanding form, which indicates the patient has been notified of the office's privacy policies; the HIPAA release form (see ∞ Chapter 10), which authorizes the medical provider to discuss the patient's care with other parties; documents from hospitalizations; and any items the patient brings to the appointment, such as a list of current medications or copies of information from other medical providers' files.

The Purpose of the Medical Record

A patient's medical record documents a patient's treatment plan and goals in paper or electronic form. The medical record must contain a full account of all patient treatment, including what treatment was given and why it was given or if treatment was withheld and why.

In whatever form, medical records must be complete, accurate, organized, concise, timely, and factual. They should never contain opinions or judgments about patients. Whenever medical records are **subpoenaed** for trials, physicians may have to explain notations. A jury who thinks a physician is judgmental or unkind could hand down an unfavorable verdict. In addition, unprofessional notations may predispose other healthcare professionals to treat patients differently. The best way to keep medical charting professional is to always write as if the patient will be reading the comments. Anything the medical assistant would not say to the patient should remain out of the patient's medical record.

? —Critical Thinking Question 12-1—
Recall the case study at the beginning of this chapter. How would writing "Problem" on the patient's chart work against the physician's office?

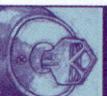

Keys to Success
THE FIVE Cs OF MEDICAL CHARTING

Medical charting must adhere to the following "Five Cs rule," which means patient charts must be

- **Concise**—Patient charts must be to the point and contain no entries that fail to relate to the patient's healthcare in some way.
- **Complete**—Medical records must be complete and objective. All pertinent information must be included while opinions and judgments are excluded.
- **Clear**—When handwritten, patient information should be printed, not written in cursive, and delivered in a clear, easy-to-read manner.
- **Correct**—Medical records must be error free. Errors are both improper additions and omissions. When errors are made, their creators must correct them as soon as possible.
- **Chronologic**—Medical records should be in chronologic order, with the latest entries on top.

Risk management departments use medical records to determine if the **standard of care** has been met. The standard of care states that a healthcare provider must use reasonable and necessary skill when caring for patients, the same care another provider with the same training would use in the same circumstances. The best defense against malpractice claims are well-kept, accurate medical records. Some civil cases have held healthcare providers liable for their failure to maintain proper records. ∞ Chapter 4 provides more detail on medical malpractice.

Some healthcare providers may review patient medical records as part of consultation visits or "second opinions." Others will review medical records when patients transfer to other offices.

When patients have completed **advance directives,** a copy of those documents should be placed in the patient's medical record.

Medical records are frequently used to determine reimbursement. The coding professionals who work in the medical office will often review the medical record in order to determine the proper code to use for billing purposes. This is another example of why proper documentation in the medical record is so important.

Signing Off on Medical Records

Any entry in a patient's medical record must have an identifying mark indicating the person who made the entry. Policies on this will vary from one medical office to the next, but the minimum should be no less than the initials and credentials of the person making the entry. Some medical offices require a complete signature along with credentials; others allow a first initial, last name, and credentials (Figure 12-2 ◆).

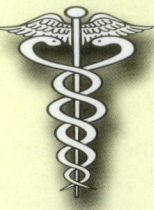

Maria Fernandez-Raul, MD
Woodway Family Practice
2413 NW Greenlake Ave.
Milford, CA 12345

OPERATION DATE: 8/11/08

PATIENT: ADAM PARCHER

SURGEON: MARIA FERNANDEZ-RAUL, MD

PREOPERATIVE DIAGNOSIS:

Congenital external nasal deformity.

POSTOPERATIVE DIAGNOSIS:

Congenital external nasal deformity.

PROCEDURE:

Aesthetic rhinoplasty

DESCRIPTION OF PROCEDURE:

The patient is a 33-year-old male who presented with concerns for nasal airway obstruction and discontent with the external appearance of his nose. Examination confirms the above-noted concerns with a widened nasal base, palpable and visible dorsal cartilage and nasal bones.

Correction of the external deformity by open rhinoplasty, lowering of the dorsum, lowering of the cartilaginous dorsum, narrowing of the nasal bones, resection and narrowing of the nasal tip, excision of caudal septum and nasal spine were discussed. The nature of the procedures and risks, including bleeding, hematoma, infection, poor wound healing, scarring, asymmetry, airway difficulties, palpable or visible nasal structures, and possible need for secondary procedures were all discussed. The patient understands and wishes to proceed as outlined.

FINDINGS:

The patient underwent open rhinoplasty through a columellar chevron incision. The nose was copiously infiltrated with 1% lidocaine with epinephrine prior to incision. The chevron incision was incised and carried to bilateral rim incisions. The nasal skin was then degloved using sharp dissecting scissors. This was opened over the nose up to the root of the nose to allow full exposure. The irregular nasal bones were initially smoothed with a rasp. Excision of the dorsal nasal bone was then carried out using a straight guarded osteotome. Approximately 1 mm thickness of bone was removed. After osteotomy was completed from a low to high position, infracture of the nasal bones was carried out. This provided good narrowing of the nasal base. A small piece of septal cartilage was crushed and flattened using the cartilage crusher and this was placed over the nasal dorsum. Hemostasis was assured. The skin was redraped and closure was carried out using interrupted 6-0 Prolene for the columellar and stab incisions. Interrupted 5-0 plain gut sutures were used to close the rim incisions and the septal transfixion incision. Xeroform packs were removed and nasal splints were placed. A second set of Xeroform packs was placed lateral to the nasal splints. The dorsum of the nose was taped and a dorsal thermoplast splint was also placed. The procedure was well tolerated. The posterior throat was suctioned and a throat pack that had been placed at the beginning of the procedure was removed. The patient was awakened and extubated and discharged to the recovery room in stable condition.

Maria Fernandez-Raul, MD

Figure 12-1 ◆ Sample operative report.

PROCEDURE 12-1 **Prepare and Maintain the Medical Record**

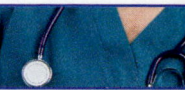

Theory and Rationale

Medical records contain information concerning the patient's medical history, including treatment records and previous outcomes, personal information, insurance information, and consent for treatment. Any signed releases of information or informed consent are also included, as well as a signed HIPAA form. Only information requested can be released to third parties after signed consent is obtained. To release more than requested and consented to is a breach of confidentiality. Offices have various forms and a variety of ways for compiling this information.

The patient registration form and health questionnaire may be completed by a new patient before or at the beginning of the first visit. This form includes current date, patient's name, address, and phone number, Social Security number, healthcare insurance information, occupation, marital status, and next of kin or emergency contact person.

It may be necessary for the medical assistant to assist the patient in completing these forms. For example, a patient who is illiterate or for whom English is a second language may have difficulty, as would an elderly patient with arthritic hands.

Medical records include the following.

Demographic information

- Patient name
- Address and telephone number
- Occupation
- Next-of-kin information

Administrative information

- Patient registration record (usually in patient's handwriting)
- Correspondence (from medical professionals, the patient, or other sources)
- Insurance coverage and copies of insurance cards
- Name of individual responsible for payment

Consent documents

- Consent for treatment
- Consent to release information
- Signed HIPAA form

Clinical information

- Patient's medical or health history
- Progress notes
- Current complaint or condition
- Physical examination and assessment findings
- Allergies
- Medical treatment plan or services received
- Current medications and medications prescribed, dispensed, or administered
- Immunization record
- Consultation reports
- Home healthcare reports
- Outcomes and response to care

Laboratory documents

- Chemistry reports
- Cytology reports
- Hematology reports
- Histology reports
- Microbiology reports
- Serology reports
- Urinalysis reports
- Miscellaneous laboratory reports

Diagnostic procedure reports

- Electrocardiogram and other cardiology testing reports
- Imaging and other radiology reports
- Respiratory therapy reports
- Miscellaneous diagnostic procedure reports

Hospital documents

- Admission notes
- Emergency room reports
- History and physical
- Operative reports
- Pathology reports
- Discharge summary report

Therapeutic service reports

- Nutritional therapy reports
- Occupational therapy reports
- Physical therapy reports
- Speech therapy reports
- Rehabilitation therapy reports

Materials

- File folder for chart
- Black or blue ink pen
- Allergy label or red pen for noting allergies
- Fasteners
- Chart dividers
- Double- or triple-hole punch
- Name and alphabetic, color-coded file labels
- Preprinted forms listed below (the practice or specialty of the medical office will determine if some or all of the forms will be used):
  - Administrative documents
  - Patient registration record (usually in patient's handwriting)
  - Correspondence (from medical professionals, the patient, or other sources)
  - Consent documents
  - Consent for treatment
  - Consent to release information
  - Clinical documents
  - Patient history

continued

PROCEDURE 12-1 **Prepare and Maintain the Medical Record** (continued)

Competency

(**Conditions**) Using the listed materials (**Task**), you will prepare and maintain record readiness for the medical office (**Standards**) according to established office policy within the time and to the degree of accuracy designated by the instructor.

1. Greet and identify the new patient.
2. Instruct the patient to complete a registration form if he or she has not mailed one in or brought a completed form to the appointment.
3. Upon completion of the registration form, clarify any information the patient left blank or illegible.
4. Enter the registration data into the computer.
5. Organize forms and dividers according to office requirements and place in the record. Some charts require that forms be double- or triple-hole punched.
6. Label the record and each form with the patient's name and record identification number.
7. Place the registration form in the record location as directed by office policy.
8. If necessary, add an allergy label to the record folder and to appropriate chart forms.
9. For each patient return visit, check and place additional forms in the record as necessary.

Patient Education

Discuss with the patient the importance of filling out the forms completely and legibly. Answer any questions about the forms that the patient may ask.

Initials only—*SPM, CMA (AAMA)*
Full signature—*Sara P. Mendoza, CMA (AAMA)*
Variation—*S. Mendoza, CMA (AAMA)*

Figure 12-2 ◆ Sample sign-off signatures.

Any time a medical record contains a signature with initials rather than the full name, the medical office must keep a permanent record of the signer. In Figure 12-2, for example, Sara Mendoza's full signature must be on file in the administrative office so that her initials "SPM" or partial name "S. Mendoza" can be easily mapped to Sara Mendoza.

An office that uses **electronic medical records** may use an **electronic signature.** In offices where medical notes are dictated

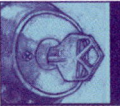

Keys to Success
DOCUMENTING THE PATIENT'S MEDICAL RECORD

There is a phrase in healthcare, "If it wasn't charted, it wasn't done," which means anything that is not documented in a patient's medical record did not happen as far as the law is concerned. Similarly, anything that is charted in a record did happen from a legal standpoint. Therefore, ensure medical records are comprehensive and accurate, because even the smallest omission or incorrect statement can cause a host of problems, including malpractice lawsuits, incorrect patient care, patient injury, and miscommunication between healthcare providers.

and printed for patient files, an electronic signature or rubber-stamp signature may replace handwritten signatures. Again, there must be a permanent record of the signer, as well as an original version of the signature on file.

Forms of Charting

Just as medical offices vary, so, too, do the methods of inserting information into medical records.

The Narrative Style

Narrative notes are simply written descriptions of patients' visits. As one of the oldest forms of medical charting, narratives are chronological. Findings of the visit appear with the doctor's instructions or prescriptions. Many physicians dictate their narrative notes about patient care, have their notes transcribed, and place the typewritten notes in the patients' files, although narratives can be manual or electronic. In some offices, physicians underline or outline certain terms in narrative notes to add emphasis (Figure 12-3 ◆).

Charting with SOAP

SOAP note charting is a method that tracks the subjective, objective, assessment, and plan (**SOAP**) for a patient's visit. Subjective findings include patient statements, including any information about the chief complaint. This section would include any quotes the patient may make about his condition ("My back feels as if I have a heavy weight on it") and any other information provided by the patient regarding the duration and intensity of the complaint.

Objective findings are observations by the medical assistant and the healthcare provider, examination findings, and patient vital signs. This section would include the results of any tests performed, such as orthopedic or neurological tests, as

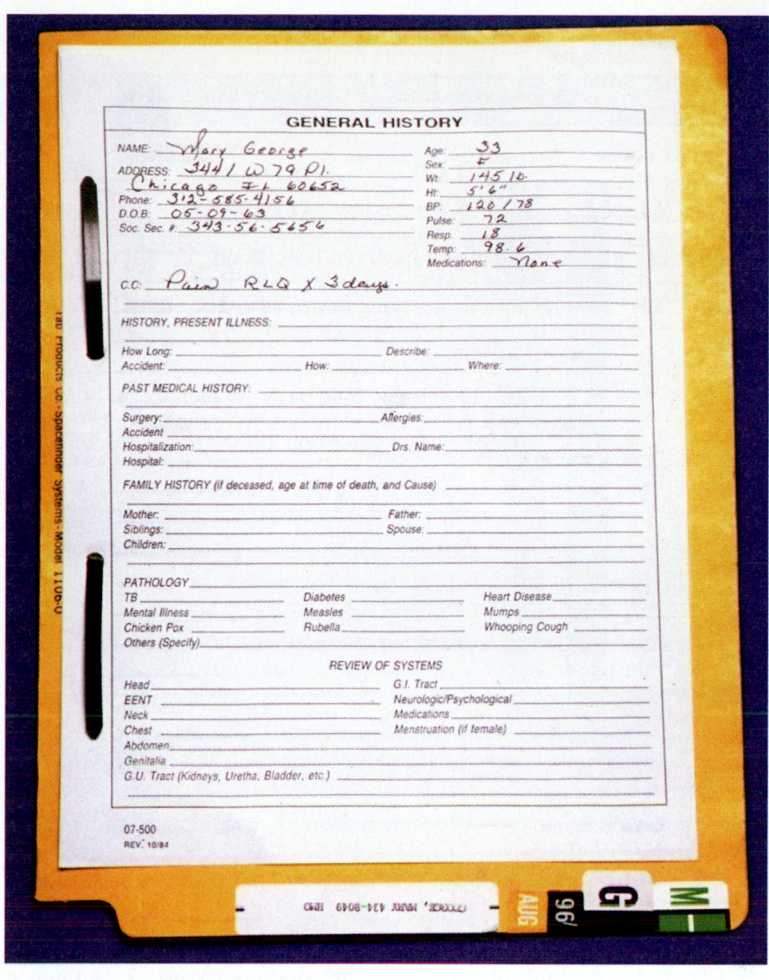

Figure 12-3 ◆ Sample handwritten chart documentation.

well as any visual examination findings made by the physician, such as rashes the patient is exhibiting or the fact that the patient winces when the physician touches a certain body part.

The assessment of the patient is the doctor's diagnosis, possible diagnosis, or the diagnosis that the physician wishes to rule out for that visit. In the event that the diagnosis is one the physician can make at the time of the visit, the assessment will

include that information. An example would be an assessment of "eczema" when the physician can clearly see this condition on the patient. If the physician must access certain test results before she can make a definitive diagnosis, the assessment might list "possible pneumonia" while the physician waits to see the patient's chest X-ray to make a definitive diagnosis.

The plan is the healthcare provider's prescribed plan of action, which includes any prescriptions, tests, instructions, or referrals to other providers or therapies. This section will include any information about both prescription and over-the-counter medications, herbal remedies, or diet plans the physician has recommended for the patient.

The SOAP method of charting is extremely popular and easy to use. By clearly identifying the four areas in the SOAP format, anyone reading the notes can easily locate information within the patient medical record notes (Figure 12-4 ◆).

Problem-Oriented Medical Record Charting

Problem-oriented medical record (POMR) charting tracks a patient's problems throughout medical care. Each problem is assigned a number, and that number is referenced when the patient comes in for care (Figure 12-5 ◆). Advocates for POMR

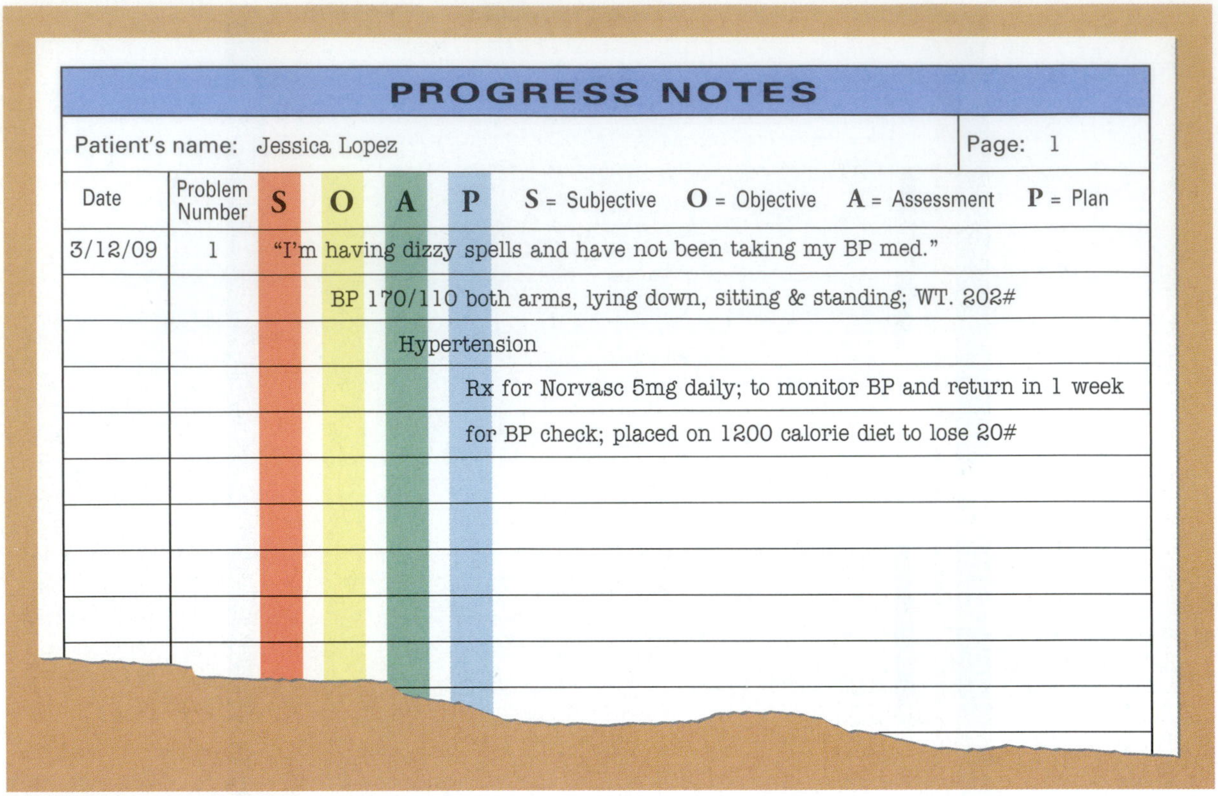

Figure 12-4 ◆ Sample SOAP note charting.

charting believe that charting according to patients' problems renders healthcare providers less likely to overlook previous problems. For example, assume Horatio Black arrives for an initial appointment with Dr. Stella Bartlett. When Horatio arrives, he mentions he has had trouble with back pain for the past year or so. He also states that he has been diagnosed as "borderline diabetic." The main reason for today's visit, however, is for Horatio to discuss problems with depression and sleeplessness.

Using the POMR method of charting, Dr Bartlett would assign a number to each of the problems Horatio mentioned. She might assign the main reason for the visit, depression and sleeplessness, the number 1, Horatio's back pain number 2, and possible diabetes number 3. Each of these problems would have its own page in the medical chart so Dr. Bartlett can easily reference the problems at each visit. Once a condition is resolved, a notation is made so the doctor need not reference the problem on subsequent visits. As new problems arise, new numbers are assigned, and new pages are allotted for tracking the problems.

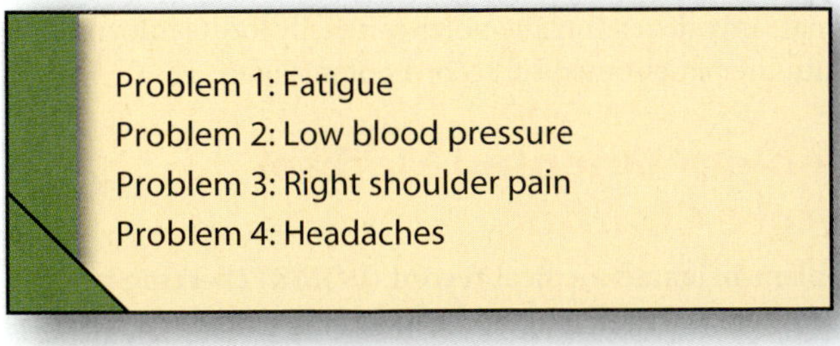

Inserting Flow Charts in Medical Records

Flow charts are visual tools that help track certain information in patients' medical records. Take the growth of children, for example. Each time the physician sees an infant, the clinical medical assistant will measure the child's weight, length, and head circumference and make notations on a flow chart that the physician can then use when discussing any concerns with the child's parent or guardian. An example of a growth chart is in ∞ Chapter 45, Pediatrics.

Progress Notes

Progress notes are daily chart notes made during patient visits to document patients' progress or status with certain conditions. Assume a patient arrives for an appointment complaining of fatigue. On the patient's subsequent visits, progress notes would outline the patient's current condition, any treatment recommendations, and outcomes. Depending on the office, progress notes may be made in SOAP, POMR, or narrative format. The notes may also be handwritten or electronic.

Problem 1: Fatigue
Problem 2: Low blood pressure
Problem 3: Right shoulder pain
Problem 4: Headaches

Figure 12-5 ◆ Sample POMR charting.

Using Abbreviations in Charting

Given that abbreviations can lead to confusion in healthcare, or even errors in patient care, medical assistants must be extremely careful when using abbreviations in patients' charts and ensure that the abbreviations are accepted by their facilities. Because different facilities may use different abbreviations for medical terms, when in doubt assistants should write out rather than abbreviate words. For example, one office may use the abbreviation "cx" to mean appointment cancellation. Another office may use the same abbreviation to indicate a cancer diagnosis.

Confusion among abbreviations can be avoided with a standard list of abbreviations between facilities. ∞ Chapter 8 lists abbreviations that are common in healthcare, as well as abbreviations that should never be used.

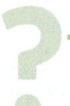

Critical Thinking Question 12-2

What are the potential implications of abbreviations for "problem" patients? How does this approach compare to full notes on patient charts, as described in the chapter-opening case study?

Charting Patient Communication

Communications with patients, outside of office visits, must be documented in patients' charts when it is medically relevant. Such communications include telephone calls or e-mails from patients that relate to those patients' medical care, missed or cancelled appointments, or pharmacy requests to refill prescriptions. It is important to accurately chart all such exchanges in patients' medical records. Each office should have a policy regarding the type of communication that requires charting, and all members of the healthcare team should closely follow that policy. Such chart notes help to safeguard the medical office from malpractice claims or misunderstandings.

While thoroughness is important, not all patient conversations merit charting. Medical assistants should use their best judgment to determine if conversations are medically relevant.

In Practice

Dylan McElvaney, RMA, (AMT) has taken a telephone call from Lynn Kinney, a patient in the office. Lynn states she is very unhappy with the office because she has been waiting for three days for her laboratory results to be conveyed to her. She says she won't be coming back to the office and will be calling to have copies of her medical file sent to another facility. What should Dylan say to Lynn? How should Dylan chart this telephone call in Lynn's medical record?

Filing Systems

Most medical offices use one of two types of filing systems: (1) alphabetic or (2) numeric. While alphabetic is far more common overall, numeric filing is more common in facilities where patient treatment records must be kept extremely confidential, such as in facilities specializing in mental health, HIV or AIDS treatment, or reproductive healthcare.

Alphabetic Filing

In alphabetic filing, patient information is filed alphabetically by last name. Some offices file according to the first two letters of the patient's last name; others use the patient's first and last name initials. Still others use a portion of the patient's last name and the first initial of the first name. Offices that use alphabetic filing place color-coded alphabetic stickers on the outside of patients' charts (Figure 12-6 ◆). Color coding helps misfiled charts stand out.

Patients with hyphenated last names can confuse filing practices in medical offices. When a patient's last name is Morris-Davidson, for example, some staff may file the patient's chart under the first part of the hyphenated name, Morris, while other staff may file according to the latter part, which is Davidson. To avoid confusion, medical offices should have clear policies for filing the charts of patients with hyphenated names and strictly follow those policies.

Unfortunately, even with clear policies, hyphenated names can still be confusing. A patient with the last name Morris-Davidson may go by Morris on some occasions yet use Morris-Davidson or even Davidson at others. **Cross-referencing** files with cards that direct staff to proper files can help address such variations. In the case of Morris-Davidson, for example, the patient's original medical record would be filed under the correct full name of Morris-Davidson and a blank patient file, labeled with the name's other combinations, would be filed under Morris and Davidson. Under this system, if the patient called and identified herself as "Mrs. Ann Davidson," the medical assistant would look in the "Davidson" file and find a blank file that said "Ann Morris-Davidson's file is under Morris-Davidson."

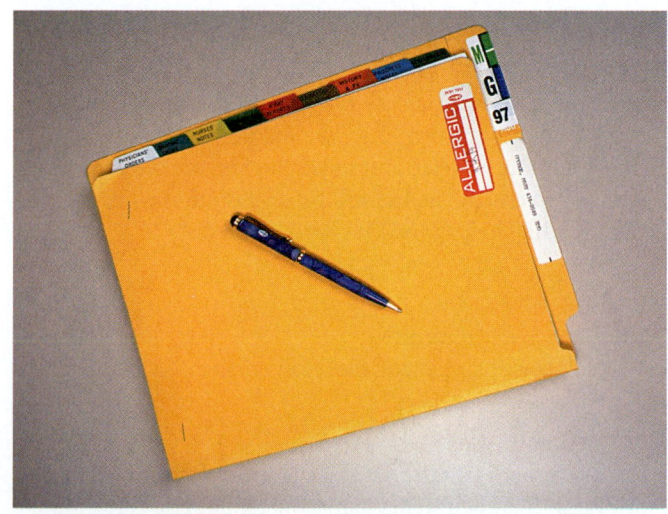

Figure 12-6 ◆ Using color-coded labels enables the medical assistant to quickly locate a misfiled chart.

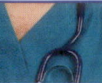

PROCEDURE 12-2 Chart Patient Telephone Calls

Theory and Rationale

Patient telephone calls are frequently noted in patients' medical records. Medical offices should have clear policies for charting patient calls, and medical assistants should understand their offices' policies. Clear chart notes help to safeguard the medical office from misunderstandings or malpractice claims.

Materials

■ Notepad and pen
■ Patient's chart

Competency

(**Conditions**) With the necessary materials, you will be able to (**Task**) chart a telephone call from a patient (**Standards**) correctly within the time limit set by the instructor.

1. While answering an incoming patient call, determine if the call is medically relevant to the patient's care in the office.

2. When the call is medically relevant to the patient's care, note the call's time and date, the patient's complete name and telephone number, and the nature of the message.
3. When the call ends, pull the patient's chart.
4. In the progress notes section of the patient's chart, note the current date and time.
5. Write the medically relevant portion of the call in the patient's medical record, using quotation marks to indicate any direct quotes from the patient.
6. Sign your name and credentials at the end of the chart entry.
7. When the call requires the physician's attention, leave the chart on the physician's desk. When the call does not require the physician's attention, file the chart.
8. After transferring all relevant information to the chart, shred any notes from the call that contain personal patient information.

Shingling Items for Medical Records

Many medical offices file such small items in patients' medical records as written telephone messages or half-size sheets containing patient progress notes. To keep these small items from being lost in the records, offices employ **shingling,** which is the process of simply taping the small items to an 8½″ × 11″ sheet of paper and then filing the paper in the patient's chart (Figure 12-7 ◆).

Numeric Filing

Some patient files, such as those in offices devoted to HIV or AIDS–related care, mental health, pregnancy or family planning, or alcohol and drug rehabilitation, may demand a higher level of security. Numeric filing is often used in these types of offices. Because the numeric system masks the identity of patients, it is difficult to retrieve filed information without the

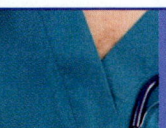

PROCEDURE 12-3 File Documents Using the Alphabetic Filing System

Theory and Rationale

Most medical facilities use the alphabetic method for filing patient medical record files. The medical assistant must pay close attention to detail and be certain files are filed accurately in order to ensure the file will be easily found when needed. Color coding helps misfiled charts stand out.

Materials

■ Patient medical records
■ Color-coded alphabetic file letter stickers

Competency

(**Conditions**) With the necessary materials, you will be able to (**Task**) file documents using the alphabetic filing system

(**Standards**) correctly within the time limit set by the instructor.

1. Using the color-coded alphabetic file letter stickers, apply stickers to each medical record using the patient's first two letters from the last name.
2. Arrange the medical records into alphabetical order by last name.
3. File the medical records accurately into the filing cabinet.

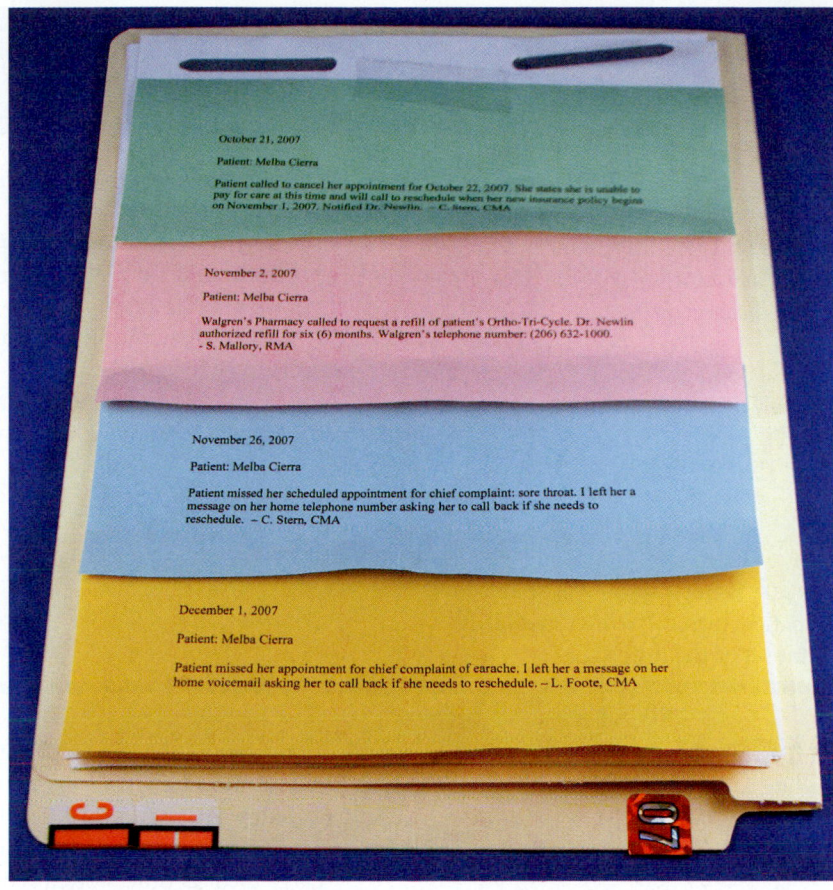

Figure 12-7 ◆ Sample shingled chart note.

PROCEDURE 12-4   File Manually Using a Subject Filing System

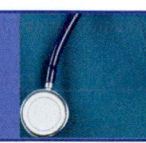

Theory and Rationale

Medical facilities will often keep documents relating to various diseases or illnesses on file in the office. These documents may be given to patients as part of the education process. Using a subject filing system for these documents allows the medical assistant and other staff to locate specific information.

Materials

- Documents to be filed by subject
- Alphabetic card file
- Index card listing subjects

Competency

(**Conditions**) With the necessary materials, you will be able to (**Task**) file manually using a subject filing system (**Standards**) correctly within the time limit set by the instructor.

1. Organize the documents by subject matter.
2. Match the subject of the document to the appropriate category on the index cards.
3. Underline the subject title on the document.
4. File the document under the appropriate category.
5. If the document fits into more than one category, create an index card as a cross-reference listing the name of the document and the category under which it is filed.

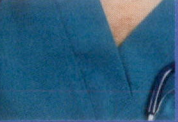

PROCEDURE 12-5 File Documents in Patient Medical Records

Theory and Rationale

A patient's medical record expands as new documents, test results, and consultations from other healthcare facilities are added to it. Often, the medical assistant is responsible for filing documents in patients' medical records.

Materials

- Patient medical record
- Documents to be filed
- Two-hole punch

Competency

(Conditions) With the necessary materials, you will be able to **(Task)** file documents into a patient medical record **(Standards)** correctly within the time limit set by the instructor.

1. Using the two-hole punch, punch holes in the top of each document to be filed.
2. Verify that the physician has viewed any report to be filed (e.g., laboratory or pathology report) by locating the physician's initials on the report.
3. Verify that the patient file matches the name on the documents to be filed.
4. Using the metal clips in the file, place the documents in the patient medical record with the most recent documents on top.
5. Fasten the metal clips.

---

proper codes. In offices that file with numeric systems, lists of patient names and corresponding codes must be kept in a secure location for the systems to work.

File Storage Systems

Most medical office filing systems consist of metal cabinets that hold paper patient charts in alphabetical order. Old-style filing cabinets were designed in a tower shape, with drawers that pulled out to reveal the files within. Other styles of freestanding filing cabinets have drawers that reveal the sides of files. These cabinets are useful for identifying files by their color-coded alphabetic or numeric tabs (Figure 12-8 ◆).

Large medical offices often require large file storage systems. These offices use filing systems that allow the entire filing cabinet to move to access files (Figure 12-9 ◆). These types of filing systems take up less space than stationary models and are ideal for large facilities that must accommodate large numbers of paper files.

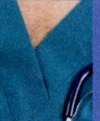

PROCEDURE 12-6 Use the Numeric System to File Medical Records

Theory and Rationale

Some medical facilities use the numeric method for filing patient medical record files. These facilities are typically ones where the patient medical information is considered of a highly sensitive nature. The medical assistant must pay close attention to detail and be certain files are filed accurately in order to ensure the file will be easily found when needed.

Materials

- Patient medical records
- Color-coded numeric file stickers

Competency

(Conditions) With the necessary materials, you will be able to **(Task)** use the numeric system to file medical records **(Standards)** correctly within the time limit set by the instructor.

1. Using the color-coded numeric file stickers, attach the first two numbers of the patient's medical record number to the patient's medical record.
2. After verifying that the patient's numeric identification number is accurately recorded on a master sheet kept away from the patient files, organize the records in numerical order.
3. File the medical records in numerical order into the medical records filing cabinet.

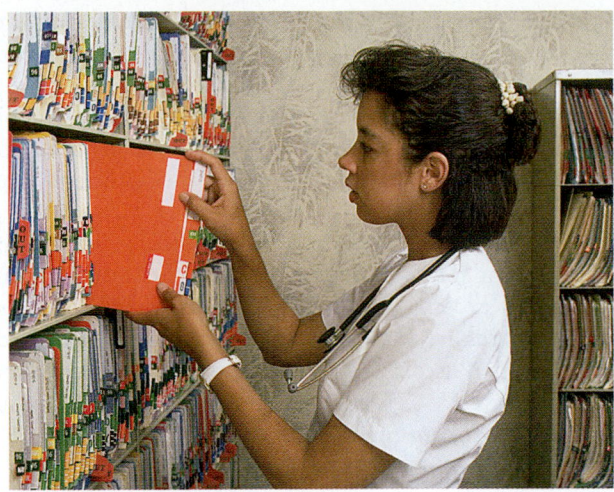

Figure 12-8 ◆ A medical office filing system.

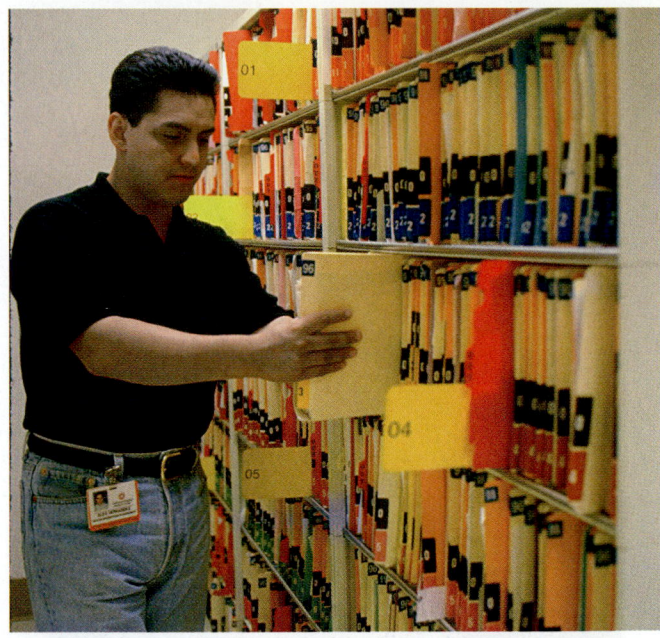

Figure 12-9 ◆ A space-saving filing system allows the user to move the entire cabinet to access files.

Active, Inactive, and Closed Patient Files

Paper medical charts take up a lot of space, especially in large offices or offices where physicians have been in practice for long periods. Keeping all patient charts in the same filing system can be overwhelming and increases the time it takes to find patients' files. For these reasons, many clinics **purge** inactive or closed patient files. This process entails moving medical files to other locations or perhaps scanning the documents in the files and then digitally storing the data on microfilm, microfiche, CD, DVD, or other electronic storage system. Once this process is done, the paper medical records can be destroyed. To purge properly, however, a clear policy on what constitutes a closed or inactive file must be written.

Most offices would agree that files for patients who actively have appointments or who have been in to see the physician recently are considered **active patient files. Inactive patient files** are normally those for patients who have not been in to see the physician for a period between two and five years,

depending on the type of practice, the number of files the practice must store, and the office policy. Removing inactive patient files leaves room for new patient files and makes it easier to find active patient files.

The term "closed" is normally reserved for the files of patients who have moved and will not be continuing to treat with the physician or facility. It is also used to describe files for patients who are deceased or files for patients who have stated they will be discontinuing treatment in that facility. **Closed patient files** are normally moved to other storage systems, leaving the space available for active patient files. Patient files fluctuate among active, inactive, and closed status. A file that is considered active today may be closed tomorrow if the patient contacts the office to report an out-of-state move. That same file may return to active status if the patient moves back and resumes care in the medical office.

Converting Paper Records to Electronic Storage

Paper records can be converted to an electronic format for long-term storage. When this happens, the paper records are typically no longer needed. Paper records that are no longer needed must be destroyed so their information cannot be related to patients. Typically, paper records are shredded after copying or scanning (Figure 12-10 ◆). All medical offices should have paper shredders to destroy confidential information. Shredding companies can complete large projects. Such companies will shred documents and provide certifying notices to the medical office.

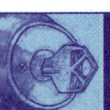

**Keys to Success
MISFILED MEDICAL INFORMATION**

When medical records are misplaced, look first under the patients' first names instead of their last. When the file for Krystle Shawger is not filed under "S" for "Shawger," for example, look under "K" for Krystle. If the file is not there, next determine when Krystle was last in the office. Identify the other patients who were in the office at the same time, and determine if Krystle's file was accidentally filed with one of those patient's files. Apply the same method to misfiled medical information. If, for example, Krystle's lab results are missing, check the files of patients who had lab work around the same time.

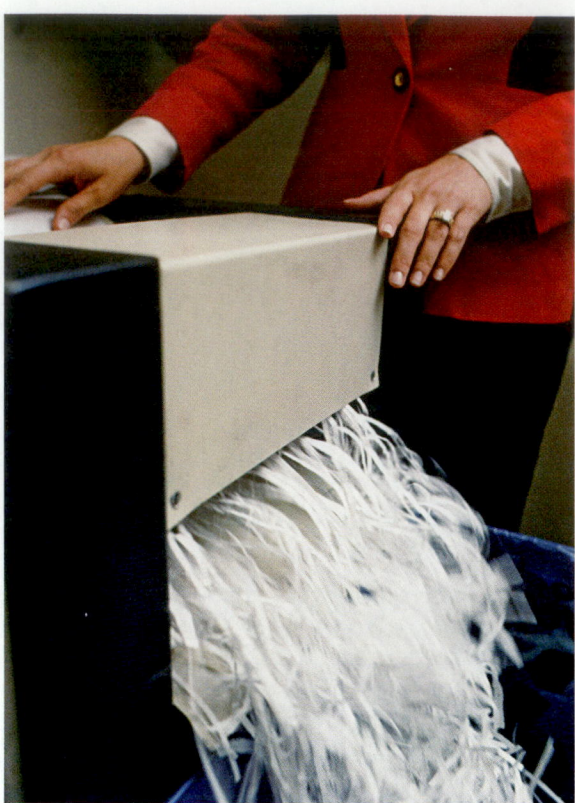

Figure 12-10 ◆ Using a paper shredder ensures patient confidentiality.

Retaining Medical Records

State and federal regulations dictate how long medical records must be kept. To comply with those regulations, medical assistants should know the statute of limitations in the state where they practice and help their offices keep medical records at least as long as those statutes require. Patients can bring malpractice lawsuits during the **statute of limitations,** which typically begins when the injury occurs. In many states, however, the discovery rule can greatly alter the statute of limitations. The discovery rule states that the statute of limitations starts on the day the injury was discovered or should have been discovered. Take a patient who has had surgery during which the surgeon leaves a surgical sponge in the surgical site. This patient

may fail to realize the medical error for some time. In states where the discovery rule applies, the statute of limitations would begin when the injury, the sponge in this case, is discovered, even if it is many years later. This rule can also apply to minors by beginning the statute of limitations on the day the minor child turns 18. ∞ Chapter 4 lists the statutes of limitations for each state.

Medicare guidelines state that medical records must be retained for at least five years. Because the statute of limitations may exceed five years in some states, and because medical records are an extremely important part of defending any claim of medical negligence, it is a good idea to keep medical records for as long as possible. Once an office is out of room for storing medical record files, records can be scanned and kept on CDs, DVDs, microfilm, or any other safe electronic format. In all forms, medical records must be stored in a secure environment, safe from any water or fire damage, and easily accessible by the healthcare team as needed.

HIPAA Compliance

HIPAA states that medical records must be kept confidential. A record can only be disclosed with a patient's consent or a court order. When it is determined appropriate to destroy a medical record, HIPAA dictates that the record must be shredded beyond recognition. It cannot be in a condition such that it can be put back together to reveal personal patient information.

Correcting Medical Records

Medical records must be corrected lawfully, or it may appear the medical office is trying to conceal an error in patient care. When errors do happen, they must be corrected as soon as possible. The correct way to address an error is to draw one line through the error, initial and date the correction, and write the correct information above or beside the inserted line (Figure 12-11 ◆).

When an error is an entire line or several lines in the patient chart, the entire portion of the entry that is in error should be struck with a line. When an entire entry is in error,

---

1/10/10 CMJ, CMA (AAMA) right

1/10/10 Patient complains of pain in her ~~left~~ hand, constant for the past 2 days.

C. Jones, CMA (AAMA)

Figure 12-11 ◆ Sample correction of a charting error.

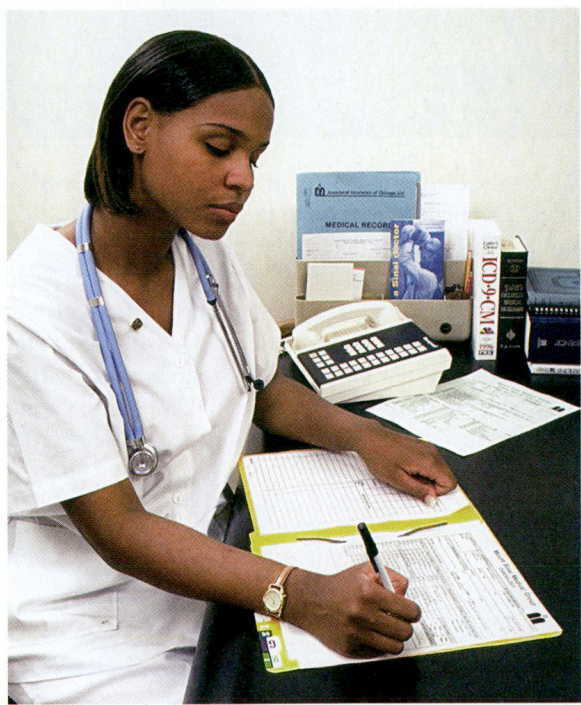

Figure 12-12 ◆ The medical assistant must chart accurately.

TABLE 12-1	ADDITIONS TO THE MEDICAL RECORD
Addition Type	**Example**
Late entry	Oct. 3, 2007 LATE ENTRY FOR Sept. 25, 2007: Patient stated she was unable to fill her prescription due to cost. *S. Nguyen,* CMA (AAMA)
Addendum	Oct. 2, 2007 ADDENDUM for Sept. 25, 2007: Ms. Manfredo stated she had been involved in an automobile accident on Sept. 24, 2007. She was seen in the emergency room of Brattleboro Community Hospital. Ms. Manfredo stated, "The pain in my right arm was so bad I could not put on my jacket." *S. Nguyen,* CMA (AAMA)

which can happen if the medical assistant accidentally charts in the wrong patient's chart, the assistant should draw a line through the entire entry, make a notation such as "wrong patient's chart," and include the date and the medical assistant's initials and credentials. Only the person who made the error should correct the medical chart (Figure 12-12 ◆).

Errors in medical charts should never be **obliterated,** scribbled out, or covered with correction fluid, because records with such effects are viewed as attempts to hide the truth or cover wrongdoing. One line through an incorrect entry leaves no doubt as to the information being corrected.

?— Critical Thinking Question 12-3

Imagine that the medical office has decided to discontinue notes like "Problem" on patient charts. How should the office go about removing such notes from patient files?

Adding to Medical Records

When an error in a medical chart is one of omission, information may be added to the medical record after the fact by beginning the entry with the date the addition is being added, followed by the words "Late Entry," the date of the visit the late entry pertains to, the notes that were originally omitted, and the signature of the person making the entry. When a correction exceeds the space where the error is, the medical assistant can insert an addendum to the medical record. This insertion should read "ADDENDUM to [date of the visit]" just before the entry. The use of all capitals is significant in such entries. Table 12-1 provides examples.

Charting Conflicting Orders

Every member of the healthcare team is obligated to take reasonable action to ensure patient safety. Medical assistants should follow no orders they feel may harm patients. Instead, they should consult the physicians out of patients' hearing range. When physicians insist that their orders be followed according to their instructions and they explain why the orders will not cause patient injury, the medical assistants should chart the events, including the fact that they questioned the doctor as to the accuracy of the orders. They should also include the physicians' responses.

"Owning" the Medical Record

Medical records belong to the physicians or facilities where they are created. The information inside, however, belongs to the patients. Patients have a right to access their medical records and to correct those records when they feel errors have been made. Patients should not, however, be left alone to peruse their chart. When patients request corrections to their medical records, the healthcare team must determine whether errors exist. If the physician agrees an error has been made, the correction should be made as described earlier in this chapter. If the physician feels the entry was not in error, the physician cannot be forced to treat the entry as an error. In this case, patients must be allowed to create their own version of the event, and copies of those written statements must be placed in the medical records (Figure 12-13 ◆). Such statements become permanent parts of the patients' medical records.

Documenting Prescription Refill Requests

Pharmacies call in prescription refill requests to the medical office. Each medical office should have a policy that requires at least 24 hours for refill requests so physicians have time to review patients' files.

When a pharmacy calls with a prescription request, the medical assistant must pull the patient's file and place the

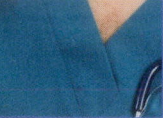

PROCEDURE 12-7 Correct Errors in the Patient Medical Record

Theory and Rationale

Medical assistants regularly make notations and entries in patients' medical records. When assistants make errors, they must follow legal protocol to correct those errors so it does not appear as though the medical office is trying to conceal errors in patient care.

Materials

- Patient medical record
- Blue or black ink pen

Competency

(**Conditions**) With the necessary materials, you will be able to (**Task**) correct an error in the patient medical record (**Standards**) correctly within the time limit set by the instructor.

1. Locate the error in the patient's medical record.
2. Draw a straight line through the error.
3. Initial and place the date above the line.
4. When the corrected entry will fit above the line, write the correction there. Include the date of the new entry and your initials. When the corrected entry will not fit above the line, add a new entry to the progress notes with the day's date and the word "ADDENDUM" in all capitals. Include the date of the addendum, enter the corrected entry, and initial the entry.

---

request and patient file on the physician's desk for review. If the physician feels the patient should be seen in the office before a prescription refill, the medical assistant should first call the pharmacy to notify it of the physician's request and then call the patient to schedule an appointment. If the physician authorizes the refill request, the medical assistant should call the pharmacy back with the appropriate information. All information about the refill request, authorized or not, must be charted in the patient's medical record. ∞ Chapter 9 lists the steps to calling in and charting prescription refills.

Releasing Medical Records

Requests for copies of the patient's medical record are common. These requests may come from insurance companies, other healthcare facilities, or from the patient. Any request for copies of the patient's medical record must be accompanied by a signed authorization from the patient or a court order.

Copies of the medical record cannot be released to anyone, including the patient's spouse, without the patient's consent. HIPAA legislation allows for the medical facility to obtain

---

November 1, 2008

Dr. Langko's medical assistant made a notation on March 15, 2008, of a telephone call I made. The notation claims I called to cancel my appointment and refused to reschedule. I do not believe this happened. I do not remember making that call and believe that the entry was made in error.

Signed,

Gloria Bowman

Figure 12-13 ◆ Sample addition to the medical record from the patient.

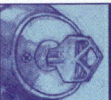

a signature from the patient allowing the medical office to discuss the patient's care with anyone listed on the list. Frequently, patients will use this form to indicate they wish to have their spouse or adult child be given access to the patient's medical record.

When copies of the chart are needed right away, some insurance companies or other entities may request the copies be faxed. It is important to note that faxing personal patient information should never be done unless it is absolutely necessary as use of the fax in this manner is not considered to be an appropriate way to safeguard patient confidential information.

Releasing Information When a Medical Practice Closes

When a medical practice closes and no other facility takes responsibility for the patient's medical records, notices must be sent to all patients with medical files at the facility. Such notices should give patients a reasonable timeline within which to contact the office to request file transfers. Regardless of whether transfer requests are made, the physician or the physician's estate will be responsible for the original files for the period outlined by the state's statute of limitations.

Conducting Research with Medical Records

When patients participate in **medical research programs,** their medical records must be kept indefinitely. If adverse effects arise, even in other generations, the medical office must be able to prove the physician had the patient's consent to participate in the research. Medical research involves patients taking experimental medication or patients involved in **nontherapeutic research.**

In nontherapeutic research, a pharmaceutical company develops a new drug to combat a certain disease or disorder. Before that company can market the drug, however, it must receive approval from the Food and Drug Administration (**FDA**). The FDA requires extensive testing before drugs are considered safe and effective enough to be released. Part of FDA testing usually includes a nontherapeutic research trial in which companies pay physicians to dispense the drug to healthy patients who do not have the disease or disorder the drug is targeting so as to identify any side effects. Patients in these types of research programs must be fully aware of the risks and must sign consent forms to that effect.

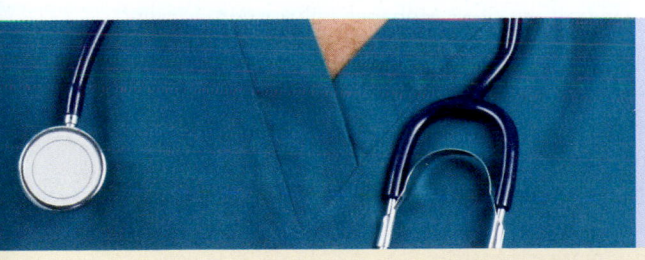

REVIEW

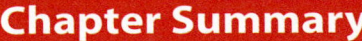

Chapter Summary

- Medical records are integral in the healthcare process, so it is crucial that they are complete, accurate, and effective.
- Medical offices should have systems in place to find missing files.
- Color-coded filing systems are one efficient way for offices to find patient information.
- Offices desiring a high level of security might choose a numeric filing system, as it masks patient identity.

- Depending on their size and intent, medical offices may choose varying file storage systems.
- Patient files fluctuate between active, inactive, and closed status as patients traverse the healthcare system.
- Medical offices should correct errors in a patient charts according to accepted protocol.

Chapter Review

Multiple Choice

1. Which of the following is NOT one of the four types of patient information contained in medical records?
   a. Personal information
   b. Social information
   c. Geographic information
   d. Financial information

2. Which of the following describes the patient's chief complaint?
   a. The main reason the patient is seeking care that day
   b. The most significant finding on the patient's exam
   c. The highest level diagnosis code assigned to the patient
   d. The most noticeable symptom the patient has

3. Which of the following describes a reason why a "late entry" might be made in a patient's chart?
   a. The medical assistant realizes he forgot to add a relevant fact into the patient's medical chart. He makes that entry the following day.
   b. The patient asks the medical assistant to make a correction in the medical record.
   c. The medical assistant realizes she has charted something in the wrong patient's file.
   d. The medical assistant doesn't chart in the patient's chart until the end of her shift.

4. Which of the following type of medical record keeping is the oldest form of medical charting?
   a. SOAP format
   b. POMR
   c. Narrative style
   d. None of the above

True/False

T F 1. Flow charts are used to note patients' progress relative to others in the population.

T F 2. Numeric filing systems are more secure than alphabetic filing systems.

T F 3. All medical facilities use the same medical abbreviations.

T F 4. Nontherapeutic studies do not benefit the patient/subject.

T F 5. Inactive patient files are typically those patients who have not been in to see the physician for a period of two to five years.

T F 6. Healthcare facilities in all states must keep patient medical records on file for the same period of time.

T F 7. The term "closed" patient files typically describes patients who have moved or will not be continuing treatment with the physician or facility.

Short Answer

1. What is the most common reason for a cross-referencing system in the medical office?

2. Medical records should be faxed only under what circumstances?

3. What does the acronym POMR stand for?

4. Describe how a prescription refill request should be handled.

5. What are the "Five Cs" of medical charting?

6. What does the acronym SOAP stand for?

7. What is another term for "electronic medical record (EMR)"?

8. Describe how a late entry should be charted in a patient's medical chart.

9. Outline the steps to take to locate a missing patient chart.

Research

1. Interview a person who works in a medical office. How does that office file patient files? Alphabetically or numerically? How are the files labeled? Are color-coded labels used?

2. Research online for local companies that offer shredding services. How much do they charge for their services? How do they guarantee confidentiality?

3. Look online for companies that sell filing systems to medical offices. What type of systems can you find? What type of system is more expensive?

Externship Application Experience

Sylvia Bissey, a patient of Dr. Borshack's for over twenty years, tells the medical assistant that she would like to get a copy of her husband's current lab results. The medical assistant explains that she will need a signed authorization from Mr. Bissey in order to release the information to his wife. Sylvia becomes upset and says, "I have *always* been given copies of his lab results in the past." How should the medical assistant respond to Sylvia?

Resource Guide

Health Insurance Portability and Accountability Act (HIPAA) Web site
http://www.hhs.gov/ocr/hipaa/

The Institute of Medicine
http://www.iom.edu

iHealth Record Web site
http://www.ihealthrecord.org/
This Web site allows users/consumers to house their medical records online.

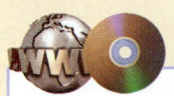

Med**Media**

http://www.MyMAKit.com

More on this chapter, including interactive resources, can be found on the Student CD-ROM accompanying this textbook and on http://www.MyMAKit.com

CHAPTER 13

Electronic Medical Records

Case Study

Walter Reardon is an 80-year-old patient in Dr. Rand's office. Dr. Rand has recently converted his patient files from paper medical records to electronic medical records. David is Dr. Rand's medical assistant. David escorts Mr. Reardon to the examination room and then begins to perform his initial assessment using the electronic medical record he accesses from the computer in the examination room. When he notices this, Mr. Reardon becomes upset, saying he doesn't trust computers and doesn't want his private medical information "out there for everyone to see."

Objectives

After completing this chapter, you should be able to:

- Define and spell the key terminology in this chapter.
- Define the medical assistant's role in using electronic medical records.
- Distinguish between the use of electronic medical records and paper medical records.
- Understand how to convert from paper to electronic medical records.
- Identify the steps to complete an electronic medical record.
- Describe the steps to correct a mistake in the electronic medical record.
- Identify the steps to take to properly destroy a paper medical record after it has been converted to electronic format.
- Understand HIPAA compliance with regard to the use of electronic medical records.
- Describe the use of personal digital assistants with electronic medical records.
- Know the benefits of using electronic medical records.

Med**Media**
http://www.MyMAKit.com

Additional interactive resources and activities for this chapter can be found on http://www.MyMAKit.com. For a video, tips, audio glossary, legal and ethical scenarios, on-the-job scenarios, quizzes, and games related to the content of this chapter, please access the accompanying CD-ROM in this book.

Video
Legal and Ethical Scenario: *Electronic Medical Records*
On the Job Scenario: *Electronic Medical Records*
Tips
Multiple Choice Quiz
Audio Glossary
HIPAA Quiz
Games: Spelling Bee, Crossword, and Strikeout

MEDICAL ASSISTING STANDARDS

CAAHEP ENTRY-LEVEL STANDARDS	ABHES ENTRY-LEVEL COMPETENCIES
■ Perform within scope of practice (psychomotor) ■ Apply ethical behaviors, including honesty/integrity in performance of medical assisting practice (affective) ■ Practice within the standard of care for a medical assistant (psychomotor) ■ Demonstrate sensitivity to patient rights (affective) ■ Document accurately in the patient record (psychomotor) ■ Discuss principles of using Electronic Medical Records (EMR) (cognitive) ■ Identify types of records common to the healthcare setting (cognitive) ■ Maintain organization by filing (psychomotor) ■ Organize a patient's medical record (psychomotor) ■ Execute data management using electronic healthcare records such as the EMR (psychomotor) ■ Use office hardware and software to maintain office systems (psychomotor) ■ Discuss applications of electronic technology in effective communication (cognitive)	■ Maintain confidentiality at all times ■ Use appropriate guidelines when releasing records or information ■ Be cognizant of ethical boundaries ■ Evidence a responsible attitude ■ Application of electronic technology ■ Apply computer concepts for office procedures ■ Prepare and maintain medical records

Key Terminology

electronic medical records—medical records kept via computer; also called electronic health records

electronic signature—electronic version of a person's signature to be used in electronic medical records (see preceding entry)

indecipherable—unreadable

Abbreviations

EHR—electronic health record
EMR—electronic medical record
HIPAA—Health Insurance Portability and Accountability Act

✓ COMPETENCY SKILLS PERFORMANCE

1. Correct an electronic medical record.

Introduction

Electronic medical records, sometimes called electronic health records, are part of healthcare's future. Although electronic medical records have been around since the Mayo Clinic began using them in the 1960s, the technology has been slow to move into ambulatory care. As today's healthcare providers strive to make healthcare safer and allow for efficient team communication, electronic records are playing a more prominent role.

In his 2004 State of the Union address, President George W. Bush stated, "By computerizing health records, we can avoid dangerous medical mistakes, reduce costs, and improve care." Shortly after this speech, President Bush outlined a plan to ensure that most Americans have electronic health records by 2014.

The Medical Assistant's Role in Using Electronic Medical Records

Electronic medical records will be a part of the medical assistant's job in any facility. Although the type of software used will vary from one office to the next, the basic premise is similar. The medical assistant will need to be comfortable using computers as well as be able to maneuver his or her way around the electronic medical record.

Electronic Medical Records Are Easily Accessible

Electronic medical records are simply the portions of patients' medical records that are kept on a computer's hard drive or a medical office's computer network rather than on paper. While physicians must retrieve paper files from separate and often large rooms, electronic records are easily accessible on a computer. In large offices where patients may see several different providers, electronic medical records allow physicians easily to locate patients' laboratory results, consultations, X-rays, and examination findings from other providers.

Using electronic health records (**EHRs**), medical offices are able to access any one patient's file from more than one networked computer in the office. For example, the billing office might have the patient's medical record open on a computer screen while it is accessing information needed for coding a specific procedure. At the same time, the physician might have the same patient's file open on a separate computer screen while she inputs treatment notes.

Charting patient information, such as telephone calls, is easily done within the electronic medical record. Typically, the software will contain a section for adding information, such as telephone calls or personal conversations that are related to the patient's medical care.

Many medical offices have computer terminals in each examination room, allowing the medical personnel to add information to the patient's electronic medical record, download test results, or research past medication records while the patient is in the room. In some offices, the physician or medical assistant uses a portable electronic tablet to enter patient data into the computer system (Figure 13-1 ◆).

How Does Paper Charting Differ from Electronic Charting?

With paper charting, the patient's chart is only available to one staff member at a time. The following example illustrates the steps an office using paper charting might take:

1. The patient telephones the medical office and schedules an appointment to see the physician. The receptionist writes down the information the patient gives her, such as the patient's name, address, telephone numbers, insurance information, and the patient's current complaint.
2. Sometime before the patient's appointment, the receptionist or the billing office may call the patient's insurance carrier to verify the patient's benefits.

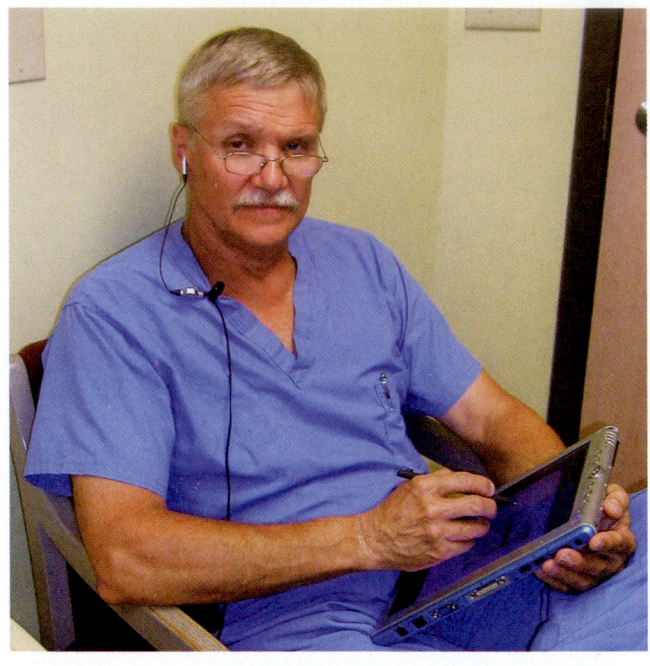

Figure 13-1 ◆ A physician uses a TabletPC to enter patient data while in the examination room.

3. The day before the patient's appointment, the receptionist may call the patient to remind him of his appointment for the next day.
4. The day before the patient's appointment, the receptionist will prepare the new patient's chart. This is typically done by gathering a paper file folder, color-coded labels to identify the patient's last name, and any other paper forms the patient and the medical staff will fill out on that first visit.
5. When the patient arrives for his visit, the receptionist will give the patient the necessary papers to fill out.
6. When the patient is taken back to the examination room, the clinical medical assistant will begin taking vital signs, such as blood pressure, pulse, and temperature, and begin noting this information by writing in the patient's paper medical chart.
7. When the physician sees the patient, she will review the information the patient has filled out along with the information the medical assistant has filled out and begin making notes of her own into the patient's paper chart. If the physician writes a prescription, she will make a note of this in the patient's chart, along with writing the actual prescription on a paper for the patient to take to the pharmacy.

In some offices, the physician does not make written notes in the patient's chart and instead dictates her findings into a tape recorder. Those notes will be transcribed by an assistant or a transcription service, then added to the patient's paper chart.

8. If the physician orders X-rays or laboratory tests, the patient's paper chart will be pulled once those reports are returned to the office in order for the physician to review the results along with the patient's chart (Figure 13-2 ◆). Figure 13-3 ◆ shows the workflow in a medical office using paper charts.

In contrast, here are the steps an office using electronic charting might take:

1. A patient calls the office to schedule a new appointment. The receptionist begins an electronic chart while she has the patient on the telephone, adding information about telephone numbers, insurance information, and symptoms into the software program.

2. Sometime before the patient's appointment, the software may be programmed to confirm electronically the patient's health insurance coverage.

3. The day before the patient's appointment, the software may be programmed to call and remind the patient of his appointment the next day. If not, it may send a reminder for office personnel to make this phone call.

4. When the patient arrives in the office, he may be escorted to an examination room, where a medical assistant will fill out the patient information form on the computer while the patient is present to answer any questions.

5. The medical assistant will then take the patient's vital signs, entering all gathered information into the electronic medical record as she goes.

6. When the physician comes into the room, he will review the patient's information in the electronic medical record and make his own notes there while interviewing and examining the patient. If a prescription is written, the physician will fill this information out in the electronic medical record, including faxing the prescription to the pharmacy the patient chooses. If any laboratory work or X-rays are ordered, the physician or medical assistant will fill this out within the electronic medical record. If the physician wishes to give the patient any educational materials, such as information on reducing cholesterol, this information may be quickly printed from within the computer system, including making a notation within the patient's electronic medical record that the information was given.

7. If laboratory work or X-rays were ordered, the physician will need only to review the patient's electronic medical record on the computer, which may be done from any computer terminal within the clinic (Figure 13-4 ◆). Figure 13-5 ◆ shows the workflow in a medical office using electronic medical records.

Making the Conversion from Paper to Electronic Medical Records

Although many healthcare providers and clinical support staff find that the process of changing from paper to electronic medical records format is time consuming, most would agree that once the **EMRs** have been implemented, using the computer rather than writing in the patient's chart by hand saves a great deal of time.

The conversion from paper to electronic medical record format is typically done over a period of time. Some clinics are able to use a scanner to scan documents from the patient's paper medical record to the electronic record. Other clinics may need to enter information from the paper chart to the electronic record manually. The process depends on the type of electronic medical record software being used and the preferences of the medical staff (Figure 13-6 ◆).

Once the information from the paper medical record has been transferred to the electronic medical record, the clinic staff may choose to destroy the paper record. This must be done by shredding the documents contained in the medical record. In some offices, the staff chooses to simply store the paper record in a secure location rather than destroy the file. When documents such as written reports or consultations from other facilities come into the office, these documents are typically added to the electronic medical record using a scanner. If the original document is no longer needed, it can be shredded in order to protect patient privacy.

Training

Any software company that sells electronic medical records software should supply the medical office with a certain amount of training for the staff to learn to use the equipment. This training should be attended by anyone within the office who will be using the software, including the physicians. In addition, a training manual should be supplied for use in training future staff

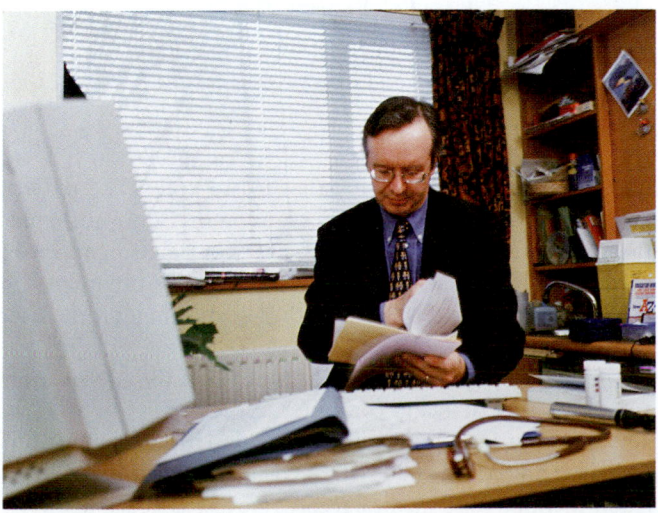

Figure 13-2 ◆ The physician will pull the patient's paper charts to review the results of tests alongside the patient's chart.

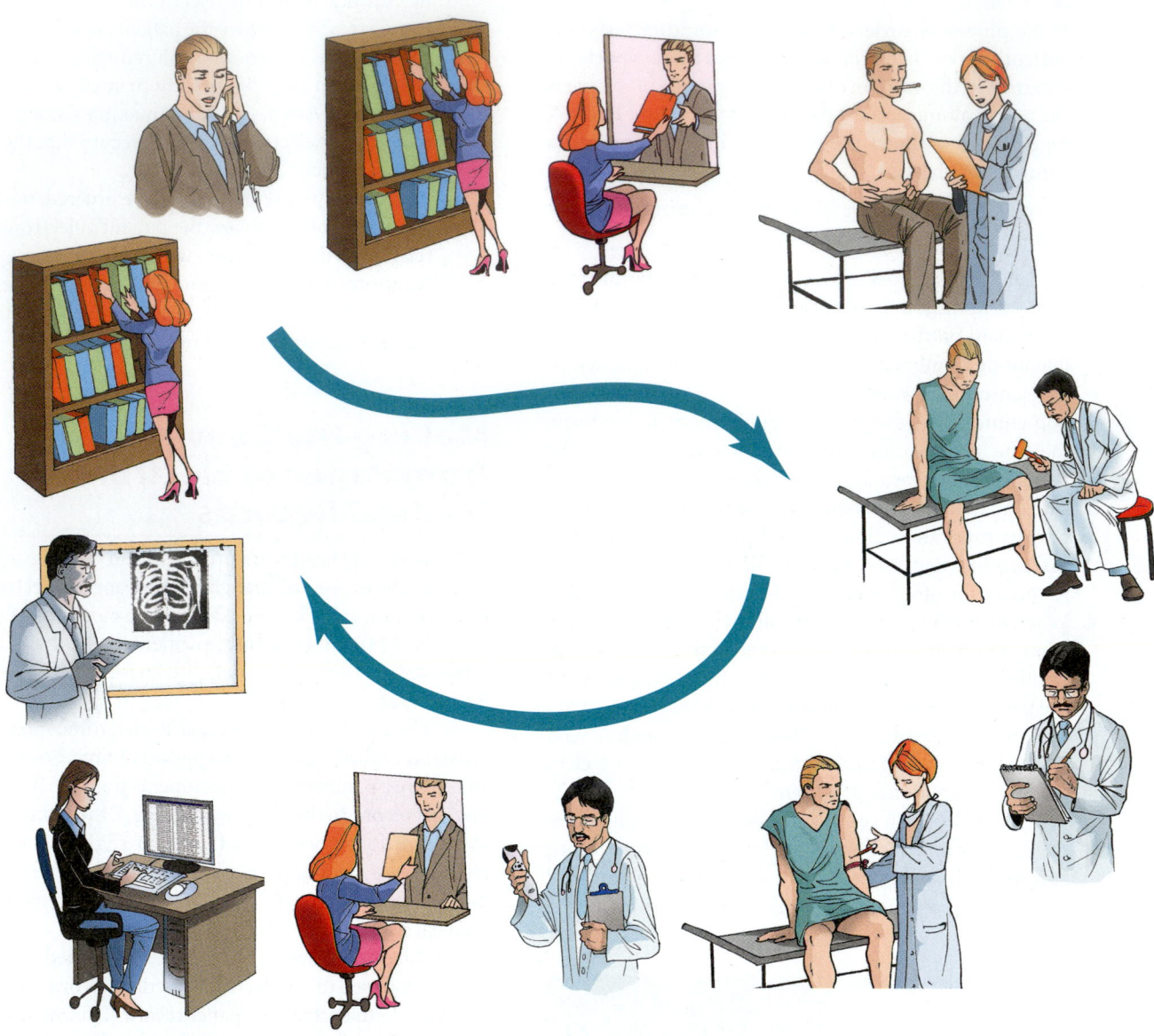

Figure 13-3 ◆ Workflow in a medical office using paper charts.

members. Software companies that sell electronic medical record software should also supply the office with contact information to reach a technical support person in the event a question or concern with the new software should arise within the medical clinic.

Electronic Health Records and HIPAA Compliance

Just as with paper medical records, electronic medical records must be kept private. In order to assure patient privacy and compliance with **HIPAA** legislation, all computer users must have their own password to access the patient medical records. With each person having login information, the software can track each entry or deletion and who made it. With paper records, it is not always obvious who last had a record and who made the latest changes if the user is not identified.

Each station must be logged off when the user is away from his or her desk and computer screens must not be viewable by other patients while private patient information is displayed on the screen. Given the regulations in HIPAA legislation, computerized medical records are just as safe, if not more so, than paper medical records with regard to possible improper disclosure of information.

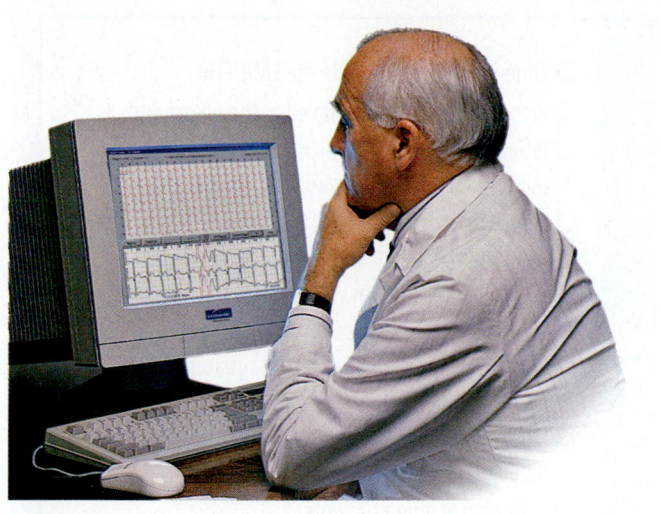

Figure 13-4 ◆ A physician uses a computer to access a patient's electronic medical record.

IQ mark™ Advanced Holter. Courtesy of Midmark Diagnostic Group.

Backing Up Computers and Electronic Medical Records

In order to remain in compliance with HIPAA regulations, medical offices must use data backup systems to safeguard the information contained on the office computer systems, including patient medical records. This is typically done on a daily basis and in most offices the computer backup system is set to work automatically. By having daily backup files, the medical office will not likely lose computer data, even if the entire computer system goes down.

?—Critical Thinking Question 13-1—

Recall the case study at the beginning of this chapter. What can you tell Mr. Reardon about the safety of his private patient information as it is contained within the electronic health record? How can you reassure him that his information isn't "out there"?

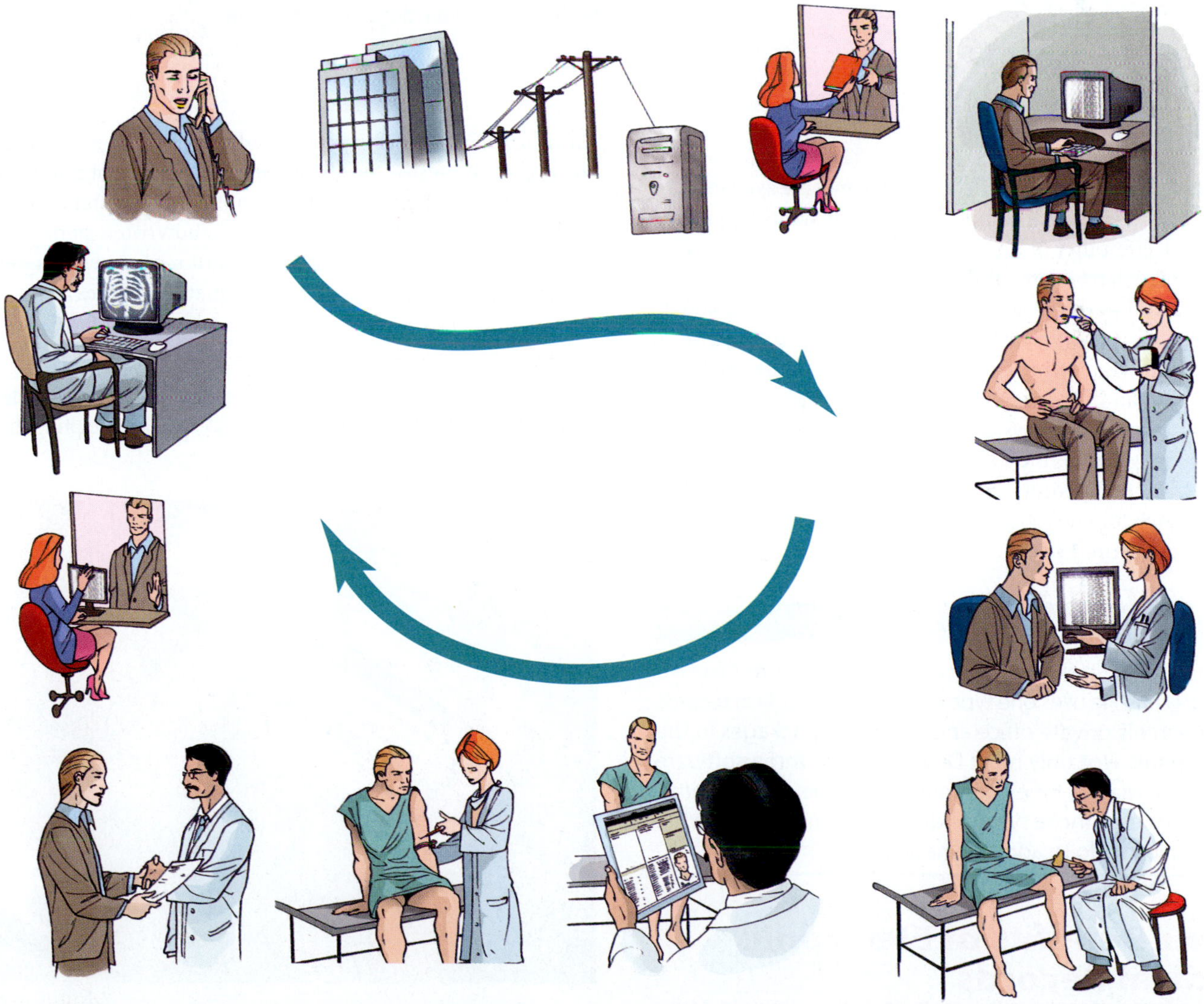

Figure 13-5 ◆ Workflow in a medical office using electronic medical records.

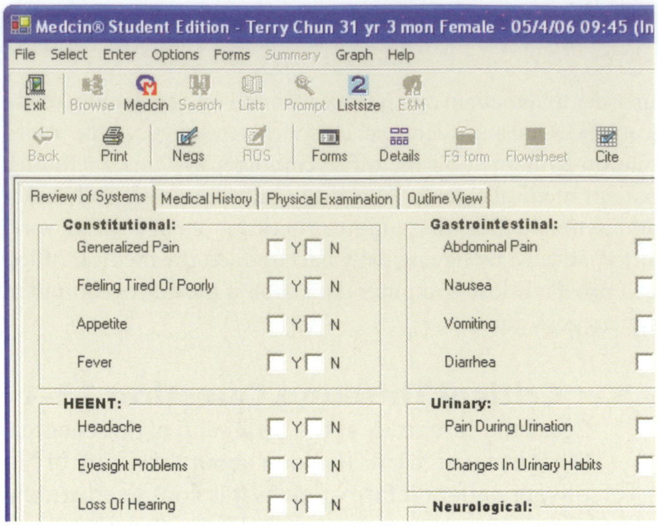

Figure 13-6 ◆ Some clinics are able to use a scanner to scan documents from the patient's paper medical record to the electronic medical record.

ImpactMD Document Scanner. Courtesy of Allscripts LLC.

❏ Time-stamp recordings in the EMR/EHR

❏ Prescriptions printed or faxed to the pharmacy

❏ Printed patient education information that directly relates to the patient's care

❏ Search for a certain type of condition or certain age or geographic location of a group of patients

❏ Digital photos or X-rays attached in the patient's EMR/EHR

❏ Electronically ordered lab results, imaging items, or medical tests

❏ Electronic graphs of lab results of height, weight, or blood pressure data

❏ Letters to or about patients

❏ Electronic data transmission to other healthcare providers

Figure 13-7 ◆ Functions of an EMR/EHR.

Using Personal Digital Assistants with Electronic Medical Records

Depending on the program, electronic records are available via keyboard connected to a computer system or stylus tapped on a notebook computer or on a personal digital assistant (PDA). These devices have many of the same functions as a full-size computer and have the added benefit of being small enough for physicians to carry with them from patient to patient. Most electronic medical records systems can be configured to work according to an office's specific needs. Figure 13-7 ◆ lists the functions many of these systems provide. One of the many benefits of such systems is the ability to access medical record information from many locations in the health care facility and to quickly search for and retrieve information in the patient's medical record (Figure 13-8 ◆).

In Practice

Dr. Jonas runs a private practice and makes rounds in two local hospitals. He uses one type of electronic medical records software in his private office and two other packages in the two hospitals. Not only must Dr. Jonas learn three software systems, he may at times be unable to move patient information between those systems due to incompatibility. What might Dr. Jonas do to address these issues?

Other Benefits of Electronic Medical Records

There are additional benefits to using electronic medical records, which are discussed in the following sections.

Electronic Signatures

An office that uses **electronic medical records** may use an **electronic signature.** In offices where medical notes are dictated and printed for patient files, an electronic signature or rubber-stamp signature may replace handwritten signatures. In these offices, there must be permanent record of the signer, as well as an original version of the signature on file.

Avoiding Medical Mistakes

Electronic medical records can be used to alert healthcare providers to possible medication reactions. This is especially helpful when

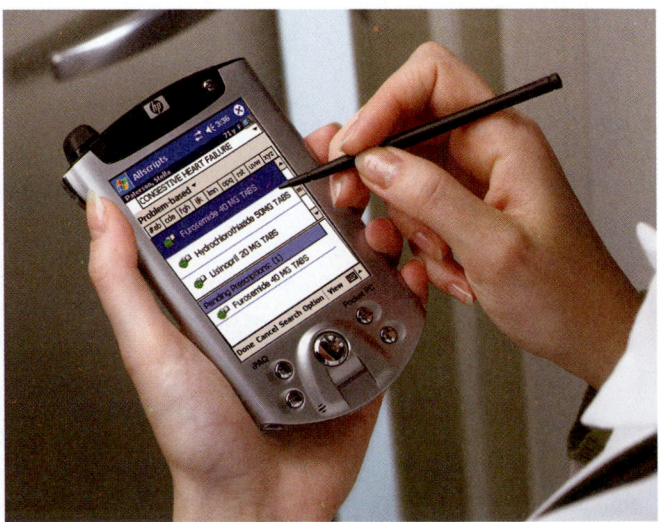

Figure 13-8 ◆ A handheld PDA.

Courtesy of Allscripts LLC.

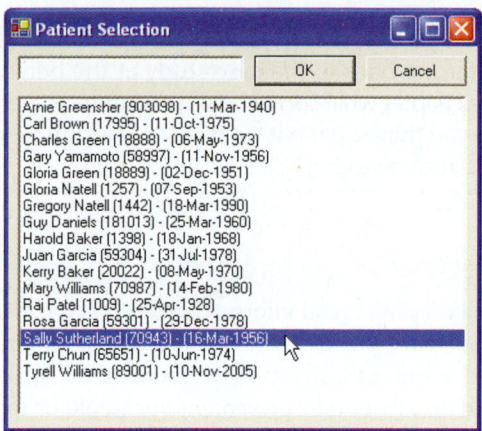

Figure 13-9 ◆ Selecting the right patient is easy with electronic medical records.
Courtesy of Medcin.

treating patients who are cotreating with several specialists. The EMR software will typically have a safeguard mechanism built in that alerts the prescribing physician to any contraindicated medications a particular patient may have (Figure 13-9 ◆).

One of the most convincing arguments for converting paper medical records to an electronic format is based on patient safety. In 1999, the Institute of Medicine published a report called "To Err Is Human: Building a Safer Health System." This report stated, "At least 44,000 people, and perhaps as many as 98,000 people, die in hospitals every year as a result of

medical errors that could have been prevented." One of the Institute's recommendations was to move to electronic medical records. Their conclusions suggested that some medical errors are caused by **indecipherable** handwriting, a problem that would be eliminated if providers made their entries electronically rather than in handwritten form.

Some states have enacted legislation to address the issue of illegible handwriting and medical errors. In March 2006, Washington State passed a law that requires all prescriptions written by physicians to be submitted electronically to pharmacists or to be printed rather than written in cursive.

?— Critical Thinking Question 13-2

Recall the case study at the beginning of this chapter. What might you say to Mr. Reardon to convince him the change from paper to electronic medical records is in his best interest?

Saving Time

The time saved by electronic medical records may be better invested in patient care. Many healthcare providers believe they spend a great deal of time charting, far more time than they spend on actual patient care. With the cost of healthcare rising, it makes sense to free up the healthcare provider's time while decreasing avoidable patient injuries (Figure 13-10 ◆).

Most electronic medical records programs have drop-down menus that allow the user to choose information or

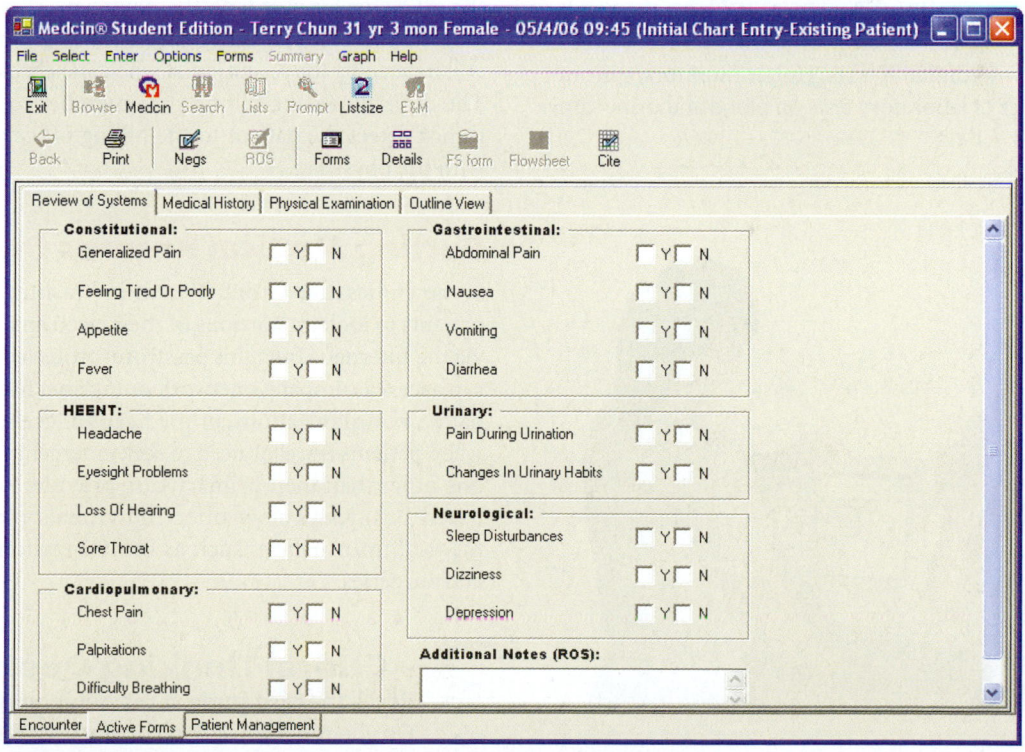

Figure 13-10 ◆ An intake screen in an electronic medical record.
Courtesy of Medcin.

symptoms from a preprogrammed list. For example, when the user inserts a diagnosis of "diabetes," the software may display a list of possible symptoms the patient may be having, such as excessive thirst or frequent urination. Many EMR programs also include lists of possible diagnoses for the physician to choose from based on the symptoms the patient lists. For example, if the patient complains of excessive thirst and frequent urination, the program may offer "diabetes" as a possible diagnosis for the physician to choose from.

Electronic medical records allow medical staff easily to transmit patient information to patients' health insurance companies when requested, rather than having to photocopy the paper records and send them via the postal service. It is just as important to follow HIPAA guidelines for releasing medical records electronically as it is for releasing photocopies of the patient's paper medical record.

Health Maintenance

Many medical offices send reminder cards or letters to patients regarding the need for upcoming services. These are typically used to remind patients of the need for a dental exam, a mammogram, a yearly physical, immunizations, or well-child checkups. Using electronic medical records, the administrative medical assistant can ask the software program to print these reminders.

Using Electronic Medical Records with Diagnostic Equipment

With electronic medical records software, the medical office is able to perform many tests in the office and have the results show immediately within the electronic medical record. This can also be done with digital X-rays, Holter monitors, spirometers, and a number of laboratory tests on blood and urine samples (Figure 13-11 ◆).

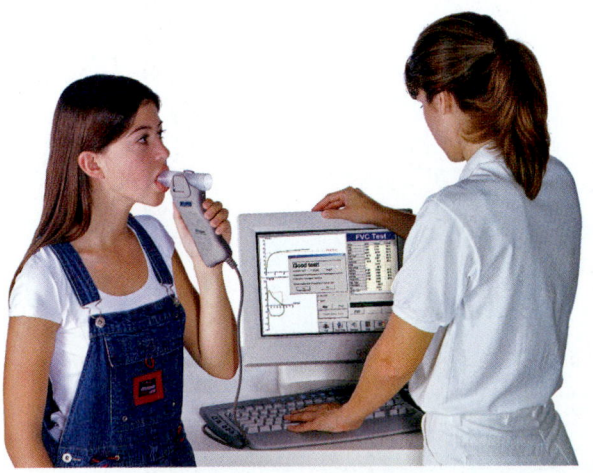

Figure 13-11 ◆ A medical assistant performs a spirometry test using electronic medical record software.
Courtesy of Midmark Diagnostic Group.

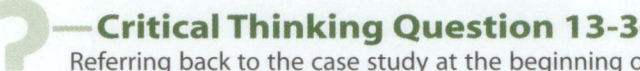

? Critical Thinking Question 13-3

Referring back to the case study at the beginning of the chapter, what sort of health maintenance reminders do you think a patient such as Mr. Reardon might benefit from receiving?

Marketing Purposes

Many medical clinics send informational flyers to patients on a regular basis. An example would be a flyer that is sent during flu season and describes the signs and symptoms of the flu along with prevention tips. Part of the prevention tips would be to encourage readers to come into the physician's office for a flu vaccine.

With electronic medical records, the administrative staff is also able to create a list of patients according to specific parameters. For example, if the office has recently welcomed a physician who specializes in allergies to the office, the administrative staff can create a list of patients who have been treated for allergies and use that list to send a letter to patients to let them know of the availability of the new physician.

Communicating Between Staff Members

There are times in the medical office when one member of the staff needs to communicate with another staff member about a particular patient. An example would be a patient who has an outstanding balance owing in the medical office. The billing staff member may need to see the patient when he comes into the office for his visit with the physician. Using the electronic medical record, the billing staff member can post an alert that will be seen by the receptionist when she checks the patient in. The alert allows the billing staff member to have the receptionist direct the patient to the billing office prior to his visit with the physician.

Putting Medical Records Online

Some clinics, like Group Health in Washington State, allow patients to look up portions of their electronic medical records via the Internet. Using this password-protected system, patients can access a company's network or intranet for their lab results, dates of immunizations, or medication levels, which can help when patients travel or need to seek emergency care with someone other than their primary care provider. Several Internet-based businesses now offer individuals online storage of medical information, such as immunizations, medications, and surgeries.

? Critical Thinking Question 13-4

Recall the case study at the beginning of this chapter. Do you think you could convince Mr. Reardon that having access to his medical records online might be helpful to him?

PROCEDURE 13-1   Correct an Electronic Medical Record

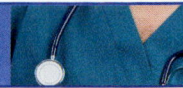

Theory and Rationale

As with a paper medical record, mistakes may be made within an electronic medical record. The medical assistant must be aware of how to make appropriate corrections to the electronic medical record in an accurate manner. The MA must correct the mistake as soon as possible, following legal protocol to correct those errors.

Materials

■ Computer with electronic patient medical record

Competency

(**Conditions**) With the necessary materials, you will be able to (**Task**) correct an electronic medical record (**Standards**) correctly within the time limit set by the instructor.

1. Identify the correct patient electronic medical record where the error was made.
2. Locate the error within the record.
3. Using the rules associated with the software you are using, make the appropriate correction within the medical record.
4. Sign off on the changes as necessary, according to the steps required within the software program.
5. Verify the change made is correct before closing the patient's electronic medical record.

Making Corrections in the Electronic Medical Record

Just as with paper medical records, medical staff entering data into the electronic medical record may make mistakes in their entries. When this happens, the mistake must be corrected as soon as possible. With electronic health records, the steps to take to make the correction will depend upon the software. Most often, the user will make the correction by crossing out the error and entering the correct information. The original entry will still be viewable, although it may show on a separate screen or it may show as having a line drawn through the entry (Figure 13-12 ◆).

> Patient complains of ~~right~~ left leg pain.

Figure 13-12 ◆ Mistakes in the electronic medical record must be corrected as soon as possible. Most often, the user will cross out the error and enter the correct information, as shown in this example.

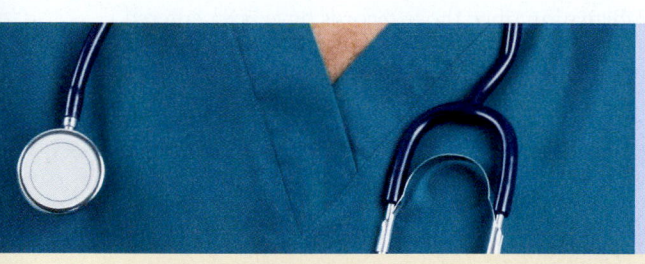

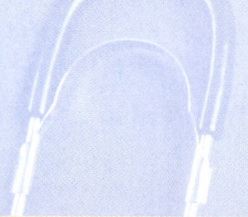

REVIEW

Chapter Summary

■ Electronic medical records are the portions of a patient's medical record that are kept on a computer's hard drive or a medical office's computer network rather than on paper.

■ Electronic medical records are gaining popularity over conventional paper files because they offer enhanced ease, efficiency, and accessibility.

■ With paper charting, the patient's chart is only available to one staff member at a time. Electronic medical records make the patient's chart available to many healthcare team members at the same time.

■ The conversion from paper to electronic medical record format is typically done over time. Once paper medical records are converted to electronic versions, those paper records must be appropriately destroyed.

■ Medical offices should correct errors in a patient chart according to accepted protocol.

Chapter Summary (continued)

■ By using electronic medical records, a medical office is able to perform tasks such as sending reminder post cards more easily than performing these same tasks with paper medical records.

■ Other benefits of electronic medical records include using electronic signatures, avoiding medical mistakes, saving time, and communicating between staff members.

Chapter Review

Multiple Choice

1. A PDA is often used in the medical office. What does PDA stand for?
   a. Professional desk assistant
   b. Personal digital assistant
   c. Progressive digital assistant
   d. None of the above

2. Which of the following is a reason the medical office would send postcard reminders to patients?
   a. Yearly physical examination
   b. Mammogram
   c. Immunizations
   d. All of the above

3. Using EMR, the medical staff will typically be able to do which of the following?
   a. Locate possible contraindications with prescribed medications
   b. Allow two or more staff members to access the same patient file at the same time
   c. Fax medical records to other medical offices
   d. All of the above

4. Which of the following is a reason a patient may want to access her own medical records online?
   a. View current medications
   b. View the date of a vaccination
   c. Read a current lab report
   d. All of the above

True/False

T F 1. Electronic medical records do not have to comply with HIPAA regulations.

T F 2. Electronic medical records are the same thing as electronic health records.

T F 3. Converting from paper to electronic medical records is a quick and easy process.

T F 4. Correcting charting errors in an electronic medical record is much the same as correcting an error in a paper chart.

T F 5. Electronic medical records allow one staff member to communicate with another staff member via electronic notes.

T F 6. Using PDAs, physicians can transfer data about their patients from one computer system to another.

Short Answer

1. Explain how the use of EMR can help to avoid medication prescription errors.

2. Why would it be important for all staff members, even those with extensive computer experience, to attend a training session for new electronic medical records software?

3. Explain how a medical office might enter a letter from an outside medical facility into a patient's electronic medical record.

4. How would a medical office use the information contained within their electronic medical records software for marketing purposes?

5. Who is quoted as saying "By computerizing health records, we can avoid dangerous medical mistakes, reduce costs, and improve care"?

6. Explain how an electronic signature is used.

7. What is a drop-down menu?

8. How would using electronic medical records save time over using paper medical records?

9. What was the first medical clinic to begin using electronic medical records?

10. Why should a medical office shred papers that contain patient information once those records have been entered into an electronic format?

Research

1. Interview a person who works in a medical office that is using electronic medical records. How does that person feel about working with electronic medical records as opposed to using paper records?

2. Research the various personal digital assistants (PDAs) that are available for medical personnel to purchase. What kind of features do they offer?

3. Search the Internet for companies that offer an electronic medical record. How do the services offered compare?

Externship Application Experience

Dr. Shelley Fredrich is a pediatrician working in a busy family practice clinic. When the office begins the conversion from paper to electronic medical records, Dr. Fredrich says she does not think she needs to attend the orientation and training session scheduled for the remainder of the staff. She believes that she is "computer-savvy" and that the training session will be a waste of her time. How could Dr. Fredrich be convinced to attend the training session?

Resource Guide

Epic (a computerized electronic health record system)
1979 Milky Way
Verona, WI 53593
Phone: (608) 271-9000
Fax: (608) 271-7237
http://www.epicsystems.com

Health Insurance Portability and Accountability Act (HIPAA) Web site
http://www.hhs.gov/ocr/hipaa/

The Institute of Medicine
http://www.iom.edu

Medical Records Institute
425 Boylston Street, 4th Floor
Boston, MA 02116-3315
Phone: (617) 964-3923
Fax: (617) 964-3926
http://www.medrecinst.com/

PowerMed (a computerized electronic health record system)
48 Free Street
Portland, Maine 04101
Phone: (207) 772-3920
Fax: (207) 772-3281
http://www.powermed.com/

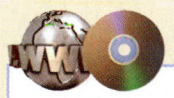 Med**Media**

http://www.MyMAKit.com

More on this chapter, including interactive resources, can be found on the Student CD-ROM accompanying this textbook and on http://www.MyMAKit.com.

CHAPTER 14

Computers in the Medical Office

Case Study

Dr. Crates has asked the medical assistant to research options for adding a new computer terminal to the office. The physician wants to ensure that the chosen system can run all the latest software in addition to the practice management and electronic health record software used in the office.

Objectives

After completing this chapter, you should be able to:

- Define and spell the key terminology in this chapter.
- Define the medical assistant's role in computer use in the medical office.
- Describe the functions and uses of computers in the medical office.
- List the steps to researching the purchase of a new computer system.
- Name the components of a computer system.
- Explain how properly to maintain computer equipment.
- Describe ways to secure office computers.
- Use the Internet to search for information.
- Create a policy for personal computer use in the office.
- Describe a personal digital assistant and how it works with computers.
- Explain the basic principles of computer ergonomics.

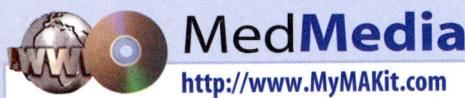

MedMedia

http://www.MyMAKit.com

Additional interactive resources and activities for this chapter can be found on http://www.MyMAKit.com. For a video, tips, audio glossary, legal and ethical scenarios, on-the-job scenarios, quizzes, and games related to the content of this chapter, please access the accompanying CD-ROM in this book.

Video
Legal and Ethical Scenario: *Computers in the Medical Office*
On the Job Scenario: *Computers in the Medical Office*
Tips
Multiple Choice Quiz
Audio Glossary
HIPAA Quiz
Games: Spelling Bee, Crossword, and Strikeout

MEDICAL ASSISTING STANDARDS

CAAHEP ENTRY-LEVEL STANDARDS	ABHES ENTRY-LEVEL COMPETENCIES
■ Perform within scope of practice (psychomotor) ■ Apply ethical behaviors, including honesty/integrity in performance of medical assisting practice (affective) ■ Discuss the importance of routine maintenance of office equipment (cognitive) ■ Perform routine maintenance of office equipment with documentation (psychomotor) ■ Recognize the importance of local, state and federal legislation and regulations in the practice setting (affective) ■ Use office hardware and software to maintain office systems (psychomotor) ■ Use Internet to access information related to the medical office (psychomotor) ■ Discuss applications of electronic technology in effective communication (cognitive) ■ Verify eligibility for managed care services (psychomotor) ■ Identify principles of body mechanics and ergonomics (cognitive)	■ Maintain confidentiality at all times ■ Use appropriate guidelines when releasing records or information ■ Be cognizant of ethical boundaries ■ Conduct work within scope of education, training, and ability ■ Monitor legislation related to current healthcare issues and practices ■ Application of electronic technology ■ Apply computer concepts for office procedures ■ Perform medical transcriptions ■ Exercise efficient time management ■ Receive, organize, prioritize, and transmit information expediently ■ Fundamental writing skills

✓ COMPETENCY SKILLS PERFORMANCE

1. Use computer software to maintain office systems.
2. Use an Internet search engine.
3. Verify preferred provider status on an insurance company Web site.

Introduction

Most medical offices use computer systems for some form of operations. From appointment scheduling to bookkeeping and electronic charting, computers have become integral to medical offices. To function most effectively, medical assistants should understand the components of the computer system, as well as how to maintain parts and update software. Computer systems and software programs advance quickly, so it is important to maintain skills and attend training classes as needed.

Key Terminology

bar-code scanners—devices that scan or view bar codes for transfer to attached computers

battery backup systems—systems that protect computers in the event of power surges or power outages

computer peripherals—devices that connect to computers to add function or use

computer viruses—programs written to disrupt computer function

electronic sign-in sheets—computer programs that display the names of those who sign in

ergonomic—designed for proper body posture

flash drives—small, external computer storage devices; see *thumb drives*

health-related calculators—computer programs that quantify health-related conditions (e.g., target body weight)

Internet search engines—Web sites that search the Internet for information based on set criteria

malware—computer programs that can destroy computer programs

medical management software—software medical offices use to perform day-to-day functions (e.g., billing, appointment scheduling)

personal digital assistants (PDAs)—small, portable devices that store and transmit data

scanners—devices that copy documents or pictures for transfer to computer systems

thumb drives—small, external computer storage devices; see *flash drives*

Abbreviations

AMA—American Medical Association
CD—compact disc
CDC—Centers for Disease Control
CPU—central processing unit
DPI—dots per square inch
DVD—digital versatile/video disc
FDA—Food and Drug Administration

HIPAA—Health Insurance Portability and Accountability Act
JAMA—*Journal of the American Medical Association*
JCAHO—Joint Commission for the Accreditation of Healthcare Organizations
PDA—personal digital assistant
PHI—patient health information

RAM—random access memory
ROM—read-only memory
URL—universal resource locator
USB—universal system bus
VIPPS—Verified Internet Pharmacy Practice Site

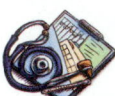

The Medical Assistant's Role in Computer Use in the Medical Office

Medical assistants use computers in the medical office for a variety of tasks. From the time the new patient begins care in the medical office, through each appointment, the computers are used for entering patient data, charging and coding for services, and keeping track of appointments.

Components of the Computer System

Computer systems have three main components:

1. **Hardware**—the equipment itself
2. **Software**—programs in the system
3. **Peripherals**—extras that can attach to or be installed in the hardware

Each computer component is intricately intertwined with the others. An office can have the most powerful hardware available yet be limited by software. Similarly, an office can have top-of-the-line software that fails to work due to old, outdated systems. Table 14-1 discusses main computer-system types.

Computer Hardware

Computer hardware consists of several parts. For example, firewalls, which allow or deny computer access, may sometimes be considered hardware, but they can be software as well. All computers have a central processing unit (**CPU**), which is the computer's

brain. The CPU enables the computer to process data and run software. All CPUs function in the same basic way but differ in speed and capabilities. Generally, the faster the CPU, the higher the computer's cost.

Virtually all computers have ports that serve as keyboard, monitor, mouse, printer, and speaker connections (Figure 14-1 ◆). Other ports may be used for such add-on items as scanners or backup drives.

? Critical Thinking Question 14-1

What must the medical assistant know about the medical office's computer needs? How does office need dictate computer choice?

The Keyboard

Computer keyboards may be standard or **ergonomic** (Figure 14-2 ◆). Ergonomic keyboards reduce typing stress by supporting the hands and wrists comfortably. Keyboards typically attach to computers via cords, but many offices now have wireless models that work from any spot within the computer's range, typically 15 to 30 feet.

The Monitor

Computer monitors come in various sizes and qualities. To conserve desk space, many offices opt for flat-screen models. Monitor display is based on the number of dots per square inch (**DPI**). The higher a monitor's DPI, the clearer its picture. Much like with the CPU just discussed, cost increases as DPI increases.

? Critical Thinking Question 14-2

What factors would justifiably influence the medical office to fund a flat-screen monitor?

TABLE 14-1	MAIN COMPUTER SYSTEM TYPES
Supercomputers	Introduced in the 1960s; have the fastest processing capacity of today's computers
Mainframe computers	Used for large-volume applications (e.g., government statistics)
Minicomputers	Multiuser computers that fall between mainframe computers and microcomputers in size and capabilities
Microcomputers	Generally small, ranging from desktop models to handheld versions; commonly used in healthcare facilities

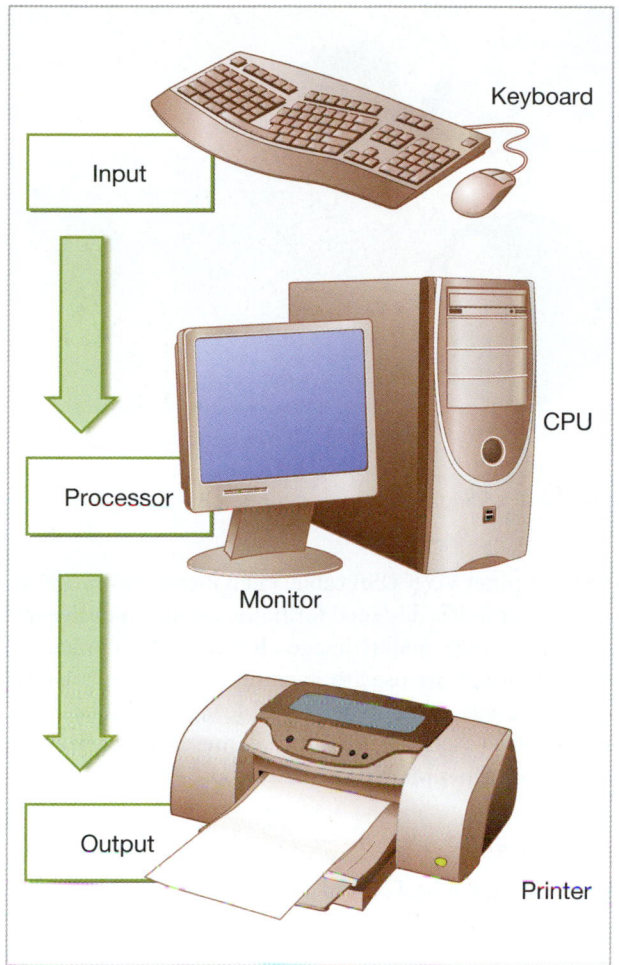

Figure 14-1 ◆ Components of a computer system.

The Computer Hard Drive

A computer's hard drive houses the computer's files and programs as a read/write device. The term read/write refers to the computer's ability to read data that is introduced from other sources and its ability to write (save) data to its own hard drive.

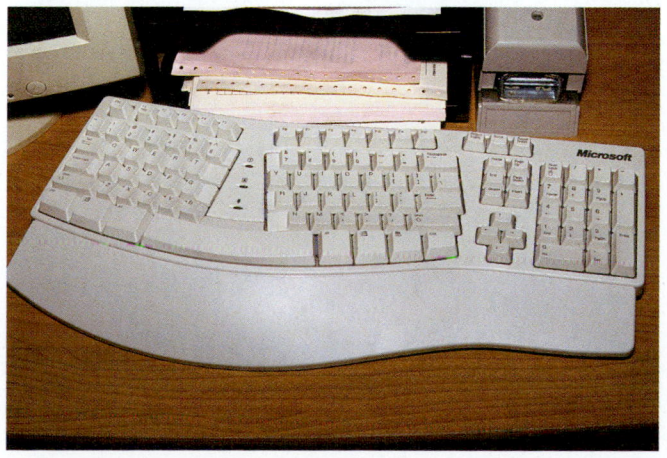

Figure 14-2 ◆ Ergonomic keyboard.

Because hard drives can fail, jeopardizing critical data, medical offices should back up their hard drives regularly. This is typically done with a backup system, such as using a separate computer to save data to, or using some form of external device designed to save the computer data. Again, the larger the hard drive, the more expensive the computer.

Types of Computer Drives

Computers have varied types of drives. Most systems come with compact disc (**CD**) drives that allow computers to access files and programs on CDs. CDs are plastic discs used to store data or programs. Digital versatile disc (**DVD**) drives, an option for most contemporary computers, provide access to files on DVDs. DVDs, like CDs, are plastic discs that are used to store data or programs. DVDs have the ability to hold approximately six times the amount of information than a CD can hold. Floppy drives, for their part, provide a route to information on floppy disks. Floppy discs are data storage devices composed of a thin flexible magnetic sheet enclosed in a square or rectangle plastic shell. As technology advances, floppy disks are becoming obsolete. Apple® computers, for example, no longer come with floppy disk drives.

Flash drives are small memory devices with no moving parts. These devices, sometimes called **thumb drives**, vary in size from 8 megabytes to 64 gigabytes and are used to store files for transport between computer systems. These drives are small enough to carry in a pocket; many attach to neck chains for convenience. Flash drives usually connect to computers via a universal system bus (**USB**) port. The USB port may be located on the back or side of the computer and consists of a plug-in for the USB device. Just as with other computer components, the greater the storage capability, the higher the price.

Like flash drives, Zip drives and Jaz drives store data. These devices are slightly larger than floppy drives and hold much more data. Because they are portable, Zip and Jaz drives can be used to transport data between computers. They are also commonly used for file backup.

Computer Memory

A computer's memory consists of read-only memory (**ROM**) and random access memory (**RAM**). ROM is a class of storage media that is not easily modified. It is used mainly to hold permanent data: programs that do not change or alter with use. RAM is a type of storage media that allows the data contained to be accessed in any order. The computer manufacturer writes permanent instructions on ROM chips, which are installed on the computer's motherboard. The amount of RAM, which varies according to users' needs, is also in chip form on the motherboard. Information stored in RAM erases when the computer shuts down or experiences a power failure. When a computer's RAM is insufficient, the computer typically runs more slowly.

The Printer

When a printer is attached to a computer, the user can print information housed on the computer. Printers come in varied types, sizes, and speeds. Some, called inkjet printers, use liquid ink, whereas laser printers use toner to print. Offices may sometimes need to order printer supplies from manufacturers. Other printer supplies may be found at office supply stores. Because the cost of printing supplies can vary greatly, offices should factor in these costs when selecting printers.

 **—Critical Thinking Question 14-3—**
What type of information can the medical assistant gather to give the physician an accurate idea of printer costs?

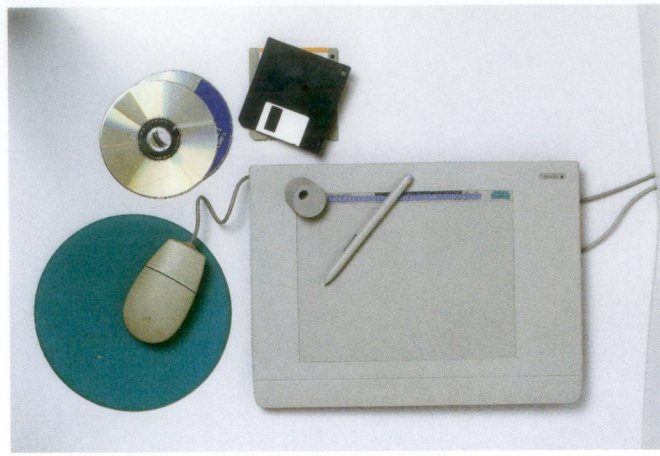

Figure 14-3 ◆ Various computer peripherals.

Surge Protection

Computers should be protected against damage caused by power outages or electrical surges. All computers in the medical office should be connected to an uninterruptible power supply or **battery backup systems.** All computer power supplies should also have surge protection to prevent voltage surges, which can be very damaging to computer components.

Backing Up Computer Systems

To avoid critical data loss, computers in the medical office should be backed up regularly. Offices can use the various tapes or drives discussed earlier in this chapter, or they can back up data from one computer system to another. Whatever backup system the medical office uses, the backup tape, drive, and computer should be housed in a location separate from the originating computer so fire, flood, or theft cannot threaten the data.

HIPAA Compliance

Health Insurance Portability and Accountability Act (**HIPAA**) regulations require medical offices to prevent unauthorized users from accessing office computers. Virus-detection and elimination software, firewall technology, and intrusion-detection tools all serve this purpose by keeping unauthorized users from violating office computers and patient information.

Computer Peripherals

Computer peripherals connect to computer systems to offer useful functions. Examples include scanners, digital cameras, bar-code readers, and electronic sign-in sheets (Figure 14-3 ◆).

Scanners

Scanners are similar to photocopiers in that they copy documents. Unlike photocopiers, however, scanners can transfer electronic versions of documents or images to computers.

Digital Cameras

Digital cameras take pictures without film. Images store electronically in the camera until the user downloads them to a computer. Typically, images are downloaded from the camera

to the computer via a USB cable. Digital cameras range from inexpensive models designed for home use to expensive models capable of high-quality images. In the medical office, these cameras typically are used to document patient injuries, such as a patient who presents with visible signs of abuse. Other medical offices might use these cameras to create office brochures or other marketing materials.

Bar-Code Readers

Many modern medical offices use bar coding to manage information. Some offices use bar codes to identify patient files or enter patient data in computers. Others use the technology to track inventory or supplies. **Bar-code scanners,** one type of reader, vary in size and type. Some models work via trigger, while others use what looks like an ink pen (Figure 14-4 ◆).

Electronic Sign-in Sheets

Electronic sign-in sheets, which work like the devices department stores use at checkout, arose because HIPAA deemed

Figure 14-4 ◆ Bar-code scanner.

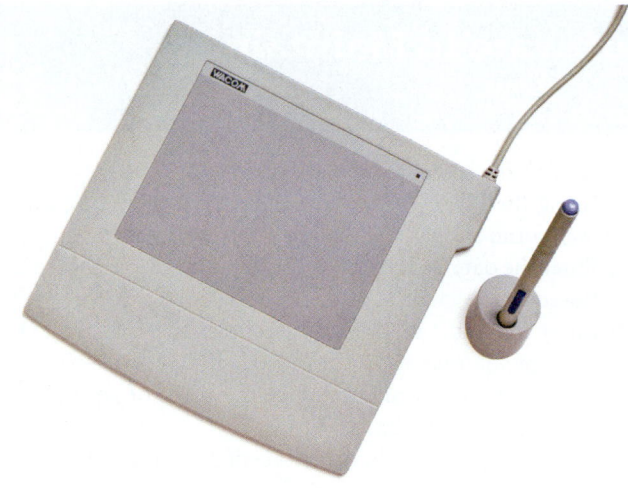

Figure 14-5 ◆ Electronic sign-in sheet.

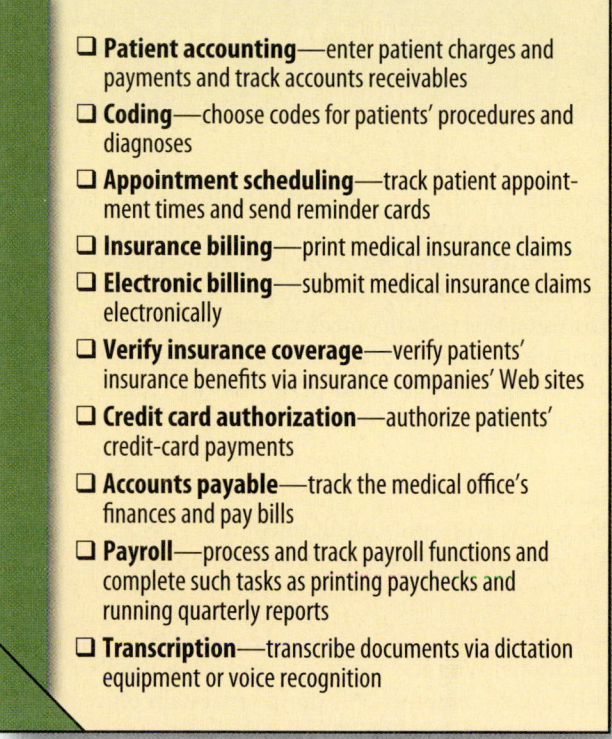

- ❑ **Patient accounting**—enter patient charges and payments and track accounts receivables
- ❑ **Coding**—choose codes for patients' procedures and diagnoses
- ❑ **Appointment scheduling**—track patient appointment times and send reminder cards
- ❑ **Insurance billing**—print medical insurance claims
- ❑ **Electronic billing**—submit medical insurance claims electronically
- ❑ **Verify insurance coverage**—verify patients' insurance benefits via insurance companies' Web sites
- ❑ **Credit card authorization**—authorize patients' credit-card payments
- ❑ **Accounts payable**—track the medical office's finances and pay bills
- ❑ **Payroll**—process and track payroll functions and complete such tasks as printing paychecks and running quarterly reports
- ❑ **Transcription**—transcribe documents via dictation equipment or voice recognition

Figure 14-6 ◆ Common features in medical management software.

paper sign-in sheets insufficient for safeguarding patient information. With **electronic sign-in sheets,** patients enter their names electronically on tablets or pads, and the sheets display the resulting signatures on receptionists' computer screens (Figure 14-5 ◆).

Maintaining Computer Equipment

Because computer equipment is expensive and fragile, the medical office should strive to maintain it. To start, office policies should disallow food and drink near computers. One liquid spill can irreversibly damage a computer or destroy a keyboard. In addition, computer systems, as well as CDs, DVDs, and other discs, should be kept in cool, dry places, out of direct sunlight and away from potentially damaging items. Discs should be handled carefully and cleaned only with static-free, soft cloths and appropriate chemicals. All parts of the computer, including the keyboard and mouse, should be dusted regularly. A trained professional should perform any maintenance.

Computer Software

Most medical offices use some form of **medical management software** that performs such functions as appointment scheduling, patient charting, electronic medical record management, bookkeeping, insurance billing, and task and prescription managing. An office's needs determine which software it uses. Demonstrations by the software salesperson can help medical offices ensure that they buy programs that are appropriate for their needs. Following the trend in other areas of technology, feature-rich management software tends to cost more than simple programs. Figure 14-6 ◆ identifies common features in medical management software. Figure 14-7 ◆ identifies medical software companies.

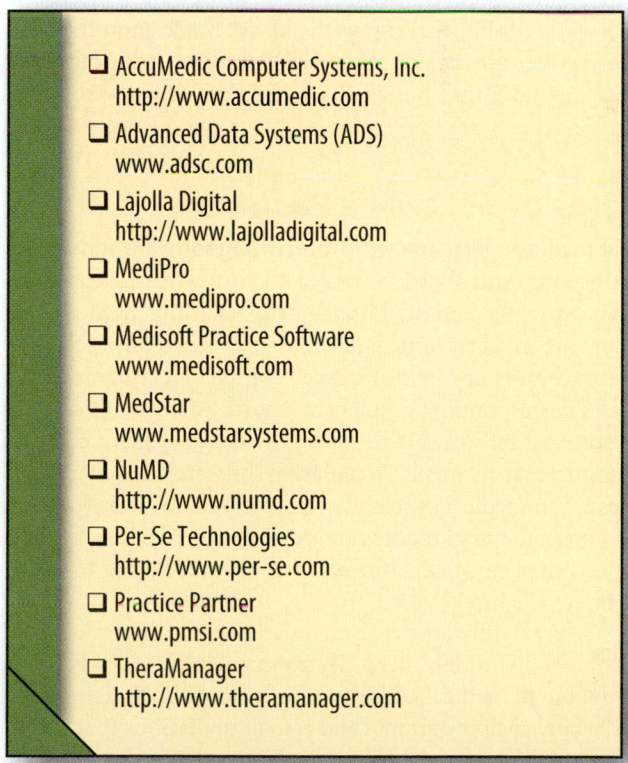

- ❑ AccuMedic Computer Systems, Inc. http://www.accumedic.com
- ❑ Advanced Data Systems (ADS) www.adsc.com
- ❑ Lajolla Digital http://www.lajolladigital.com
- ❑ MediPro www.medipro.com
- ❑ Medisoft Practice Software www.medisoft.com
- ❑ MedStar www.medstarsystems.com
- ❑ NuMD http://www.numd.com
- ❑ Per-Se Technologies http://www.per-se.com
- ❑ Practice Partner www.pmsi.com
- ❑ TheraManager http://www.theramanager.com

Figure 14-7 ◆ Medical software companies.

PROCEDURE 14-1 Use Computer Software to Maintain Office Systems

Theory and Rationale

The computer software used in the medical office is capable of performing a multitude of tasks. One such task is to maintain the office systems. An example of such a task would be to keep track of the equipment used in the medical office. By performing this task, the medical assistant can keep track of information pertaining to needed maintenance, such as the name of the company that performs the repairs, and the schedule for equipment maintenance.

Materials

- Computer with spreadsheet software
- List of equipment to enter into the computer

Competency

(**Conditions**) With the necessary materials, you will be able to (**Task**) utilize computer software to maintain office systems (**Standards**) correctly within the time limit set by the instructor.

1. Launch the spreadsheet software.
2. Using the list of equipment, enter each piece of equipment onto a separate line on the spreadsheet.
3. Enter the date each piece of equipment was purchased or leased by the medical office.
4. Enter the name of the manufacturer that supplied the piece of equipment.
5. Enter the type of maintenance the piece of equipment needs on a regular basis.
6. Enter information about the needed maintenance, such as the name of the company that performs the repairs, and the schedule for equipment maintenance.

Training Staff on Medical Software

Medical office management software should come with an onsite training option that includes telephone customer service support and manuals or demos for future training needs. All staff who will be working with the software should attend training. Because such training may incur costs, medical offices should explore that possibility before making any software purchases.

Types of Software Packages

Most medical offices use word-processing software, most commonly Microsoft Word.® Using such software, medical assistants can type patient letters, print mailing lists, format documents and brochures, and create charts and forms. Spreadsheet software like Microsoft Excel® completes calculations and creates corresponding graphs and charts. Medical offices may use spreadsheet software to track statistics on patient care and personnel management. Presentation software like PowerPoint® helps when medical offices plan educational meetings or seminars for patients. Not only can presenters create slides for projection, they can print those slides as note-taking tools for attendees (Figure 14-8 ◆).

Several software programs currently on the market, such as Microsoft Outlook®, keep electronic calendars, which can be invaluable to medical offices trying to coordinate staff schedules. Many such programs send e-mail invitations that recipients can add to their electronic calendars, as well as print in daily, weekly, or monthly slices.

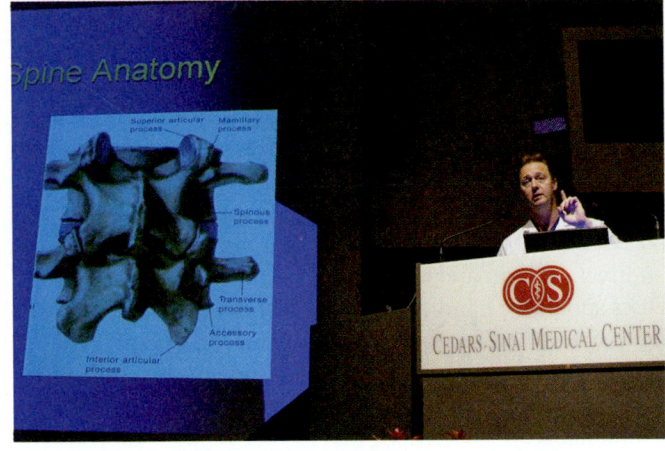

Figure 14-8 ◆ Physician giving a PowerPoint presentation.

Computer Security

To safeguard computer systems, staff members should be required to use alphanumeric passwords to access them. To thwart hackers, users should choose unobvious passwords, taking care to avoid initials, birth dates, and telephone numbers. Users should also be careful to avoid sharing their passwords and leaving their passwords in plain view. It is good practice for users to log off whenever leaving their computer workstations unattended. Figure 14-9 ◆ outlines HIPAA standards for safeguarding patient health information.

- ❑ Patient health information (**PHI**) must be backed up periodically.
- ❑ An audit trail must exist for backed-up data that leaves the medical facility.
- ❑ Access to backed-up data must be restricted to authorized parties.
- ❑ A backup plan and disaster recovery plan must be in place.
- ❑ Data must be a retrievable, exact copy.
- ❑ All computers must be password protected.

Figure 14-9 ◆ HIPAA standards for safeguarding patient health information.

Computer Viruses

Computer viruses are programs designed to perform mischievous functions. **Malware**, a twist on the computer virus, is designed to damage computer programs by infiltrating computers. Malware includes spyware, adware, Trojan horses, and worms. These programs can damage or corrupt hard drives, as well as infect other computers without users' knowledge. Because these types of programs exist, every computer in the medical office should have virus-protection software that is updated regularly. The two most commonly used antivirus software programs are made by McAfee and Norton.

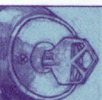

Keys to Success
USING THE COMPUTER FOR WORK-RELATED PURPOSES ONLY

Because the computer systems in a medical office belong to the physician or the office, they should only be used for private use when employers grant permission. Even with permission, staff should download no screen savers or other, similar files. Most computers get viruses and malware when users open malicious e-mails or visit certain Web sites. Therefore, to protect computers, medical assistants should open no attachments from unknown sources or Web sites.

Internet Search Engines

Internet search engines use key words and phrases to retrieve information from the Internet. Popular search engines are Yahoo, Google, Dog Pile, and Ask.com. Contemporary healthcare providers often search the Internet for medical information. Medical offices often need source material for patient brochures or presentations, and the Internet can be a valuable resource in this area.

In Practice

Dr. Victor is giving a presentation on a new procedure she is performing for scar-tissue removal. Dr. Victor has asked Jamie, her medical assistant, to use the Internet to find information on other, similar procedures for comparison. How should Jamie begin, and where? What key words would be appropriate for the search engine?

PROCEDURE 14-2   Use an Internet Search Engine

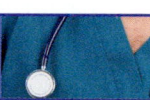

Theory and Rationale

The Internet has a vast amount of information the medical office can use to educate patients, research new technologies and equipment, and contact patients. Search engines can quickly locate desired information and resources.

Materials

■ A computer with Internet access

Competency

(**Conditions**) With the necessary materials, you will be able to (**Task**) use the computer to search for a topic via an Internet search engine (**Standards**) correctly within the time limit set by the instructor.

1. Turn on the computer.
2. Launch an Internet browser.
3. Visit the uniform resource locator (URL) of the search engine.
4. Enter the search keywords.
5. Visit retrieved Web sites to obtain the desired information.
6. To refine the search, enter more or different key words.

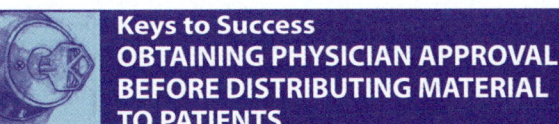

- ❑ American Medical Association (**AMA**) (www.ama-assn.org)
- ❑ Joint Commission for the Accreditation of Healthcare Organizations (**JCAHO**) (www.jcaho.org)
- ❑ Journal of the American Centers for Disease Control and Prevention (**CDC**) (www.cdc.gov)
- ❑ Lancet (www.lancet.org)
- ❑ Medical Association (**JAMA**) (www.jama.ama-assn.org)
- ❑ New England Journal of Medicine (www.nejm.org)

Figure 14-10 ◆ Medical Web sites.

Finding Appropriate Web Resources

When newly diagnosed with conditions or illnesses, patients often have many questions for their healthcare providers. Many such providers find it helpful to give patients lists of reputable Web sites for further information. When patients have long-term or chronic illnesses or conditions and may be seeking support groups, such lists can be especially beneficial.

Professional medical Web sites are the sites physicians visit when seeking up-to-date information on conditions, illnesses, or pharmaceuticals. Figure 14-10 ◆ lists some reputable examples.

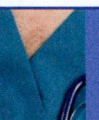

Keys to Success
OBTAINING PHYSICIAN APPROVAL BEFORE DISTRIBUTING MATERIAL TO PATIENTS

Before giving Web site information to patients, be sure to obtain the physician's permission. Give patients only information from reputable Web sites.

Many physicians subscribe to online journals that charge for access but offer the latest information on research, medications, and techniques. Seminars and conferences can be informative, but Web sites serve as ongoing resources as topics arise.

Many Web sites have **health-related calculators** that aid both patients and healthcare staff. Such calculators address such factors as basal metabolic rate, body mass index, pregnancy and due date, ovulation, target heart rate, children's adult height predictions, smoking costs, and seafood mercury intake.

Often, major health insurance carriers maintain their own comprehensive Web sites that allow subscribers and physicians alike to access a wide span of information. Some sites even give physicians access to patients' benefit information, although direct contact with the insurance companies is often still needed, especially when authorizations are required. Such sites are particularly helpful for offices wishing to verify that patients have active policies at the time of visit.

Buying Medications Online

Patients who lack prescription drug coverage may leverage the Internet as an economical way to obtain medications. Online medication purchase can be dangerous, however, so medical offices should encourage patients to use only sites certified by the Verified Internet Pharmacy Practice Site (**VIPPS**). VIPPS certification ensures that the National Association of Boards of Pharmacy has reviewed the online pharmacy for safety and compliance. Certified online pharmacies provide information on prescribed medications, including possible adverse reactions or side effects and any safety concerns.

Patient Education

Medical offices should advise patients never to purchase medications from Internet sites outside the United States. Direct patients to the U.S. Food and Drug Administration (**FDA**) (www.fda.gov) Web site for tips on buying medications online.

PROCEDURE 14-3 **Verify Preferred Provider Status on an Insurance Company Web Site**

Theory and Rationale

Insurance company names can change when companies merge. Medical assistants must keep abreast of the insurance plans their offices participate with. The ability to verify preferred provider status is a valuable function for both the physician and the patient.

Materials

- Computer with Internet connection
- Insurance company's URL
- Name of target physician

Competency

(**Conditions**) With the necessary materials, you will be able to (**Task**) verify a provider's preferred status on an insurance company Web site (**Standards**) within the time limit set by the instructor.

1. Using the computer, launch an Internet browser.
2. Enter the URL of the insurance company.
3. Navigate to the provider page or section.
4. In the search field, enter the provider's name and/or location.
5. Verify if the physician is preferred with the target insurance company.

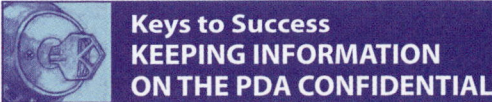

Keys to Success
KEEPING INFORMATION
ON THE PDA CONFIDENTIAL

When a physician's PDA contains private patient information, it must be kept inaccessible to unauthorized parties. Passwords protect PDAs just like computers.

Allowing Personal Computer Use in the Office

All medical offices should write policies for personal use of office computers and ensure that all members of the healthcare team follow those policies strictly. Patients who feel office computers are being used for personal reasons may develop negative impressions of the office. As a result, some offices forbid all personal computer use, while others allow personal use during breaks or the periods before and after shifts. Policies should reflect an office's approach. For example, personal computer use may be allowed, but not within sight of patients.

Personal Digital Assistants

Many physicians today use **personal digital assistants (PDAs)** to do things like quickly check medication dosages or research drug interactions. *Personal digital assistant* is a term used to describe any small, mobile hand-held device that provides computing and information storage retrieval capabilities for personal

or business use, often for keeping schedule calendars and address book information handy. Outside the medical office, PDAs can serve to record patients' hospital visits or the calls physicians take while on call (Figure 14-11 ◆).

Because PDAs can connect to computer systems, information can transfer between the two. For example, physicians can enter patient information into their PDA and then later download that information to their desktop computers. PDAs especially benefit physicians who wish to review patient charts outside the office. Rather than remove patient charts from the office, physicians can record the necessary information in their PDA.

Computer Ergonomics

Long-term computer use has prompted a number of recommendations that help address health concerns. For example, members of the healthcare team can avoid eye strain by frequently looking away from the computer screen. Antiglare screens are another option, as is placing the monitor at an angle to avoid glare. Carpal tunnel syndrome is associated with repeated use of the wrists, such as when typing on a keyboard. Many computer users find that the ergonomic keyboards mentioned earlier in this chapter alleviate this syndrome's symptoms. Keyboard wrist supports are also helpful.

Proper posture and equipment placement are crucial to avoiding computer-related injuries. Users should sit straight in chairs that support the lower back (Figure 14-12 ◆). Chairs should have armrests, but users should only use those features when not typing. Keyboards should be placed to allow a 90-degree angle at the elbows and close enough so users need not reach forward. Monitors should be at eye level, with a viewing angle of 5 to 30 degrees. Users should not have to twist to see their monitors. Users' feet should be flat on the floor, and legs should be uncrossed.

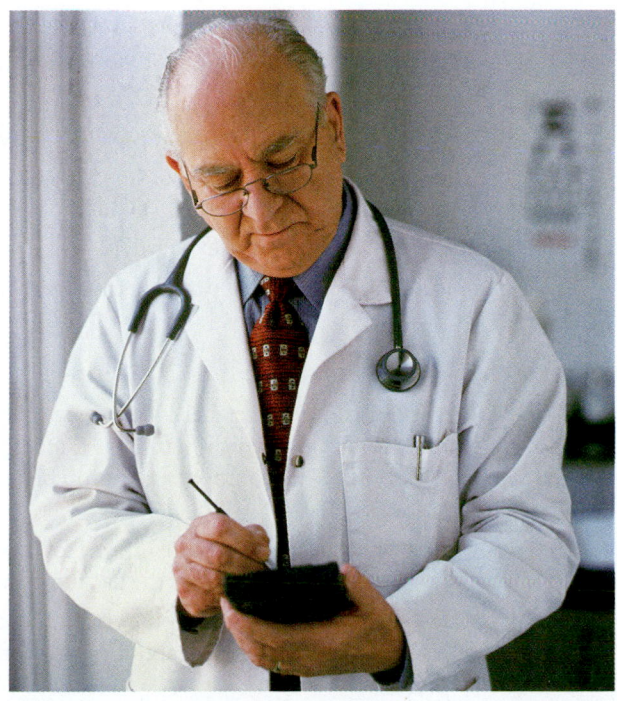

Figure 14-11 ◆ A physician using a personal digital assistant (PDA).

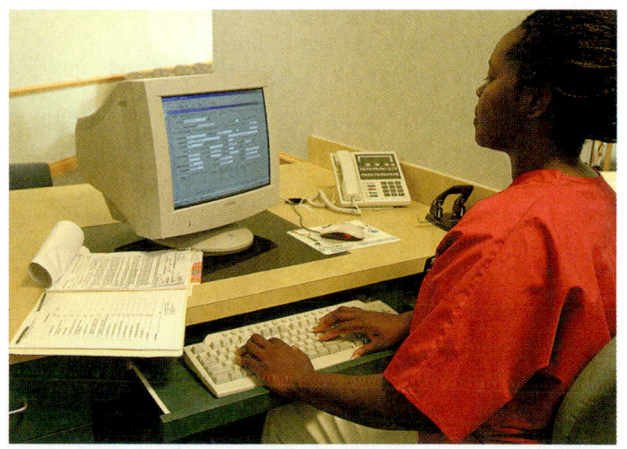

Figure 14-12 ◆ The medical assistant should have an ergonomically correct desk, chair, and keyboard.

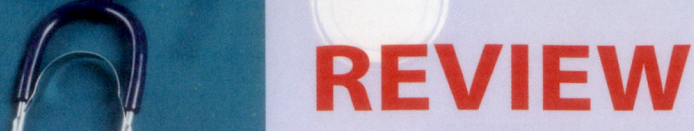

REVIEW

Chapter Summary

- Computers serve varied functions and uses in the medical office, all of which the medical assistant should be familiar with.
- The purchase of a new computer system entails careful, informed research to ensure that the needs of the medical office are met.
- The components of a computer system include hardware, software, and peripherals.
- Office staff can take steps to maintain computer equipment, but repairs should be left to professionals.

- Security is an important part of office computing, because it helps ensure the confidentiality of patient information.
- The Internet can serve as a resource for nearly infinite medical information.
- When using computers, medical offices should instate clear policies for the computers' use.
- Personal digital assistants can help bridge the computing gap when out of the office.
- Ergonomically designed computer equipment helps ensure that all members of the healthcare team work safely.

Chapter Review

Multiple Choice

1. Computer peripherals include
   a. printers.
   b. scanners.
   c. external hard drives.
   d. all of the above.

2. Another term for flash drive is _____ drive.
   a. star
   b. thumb
   c. media
   d. small

3. An electronic sign-in sheet is designed to
   a. maintain patient confidentiality.
   b. ensure HIPAA compliance.
   c. track patients in the office.
   d. all of the above.

4. A medical office may use a scanner to
   a. copy photos into a patient's chart.
   b. photocopy documents to give to patients.
   c. track insurance correspondence.
   d. maintain patient confidentiality.

5. Which brand of computer no longer comes with floppy disc drives?
   a. Apple
   b. Dell
   c. Hewlett-Packard
   d. All of the above

True/False

T F 1. The CPU is considered the computer's brain.
T F 2. Flat-panel monitors are often used when desk space is at a premium.
T F 3. Computer passwords should be easy to remember, such as birth date or addresses.
T F 4. Medical management software companies should provide onsite training of staff.
T F 5. A trained professional should perform any maintenance on office computers.
T F 6. Bar-code scanners are used in healthcare to track supplies, among other things.

Short Answer

1. What is PowerPoint software used for?
2. What is the importance of an external battery backup system?
3. What is a thumb drive used for?
4. What is the difference between a computer virus and malware?
5. What is the main danger in downloading files to an office computer?
6. Name Internet search engines for finding information online.
7. Name some functions of a health-related calculator.
8. What is an "ergonomically correct keyboard"?
9. Describe the functions of medical practice management software.

Research

1. Search the Internet for computer retailers. What type of system do you think would be a typical setup for a medical office computer station? What components do you believe would be included?
2. Interview a person who works in a medical office. How does that facility back up its data? How often is the backup done?
3. Research online for information on computer ergonomics. What kind of information did you find about posture and working at a computer?

Externship Application Experience

As Monica Friedenrich is training the medical assistant on the medical office's computer systems, she explains the HIPAA regulations for passwords, which includes a unique password for every staff member. Monica then directs the medical assistant to use her own password during training. Should the medical assistant comply? If the assistant chooses to comply, what issues could result?

Resource Guide

AltaVista Translation Services
www.altavista.com

CSGNetwork and Computer Support Group Health-Related Calculators
http://www.csgnetwork.com

Occupational Safety and Health Administration (OSHA) Web site
www.osha.gov

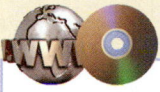

Med**Media**

http://www.MyMAKit.com

More on this chapter, including interactive resources, can be found on the Student CD-ROM accompanying this textbook and on http://www.MyMAKit.com.

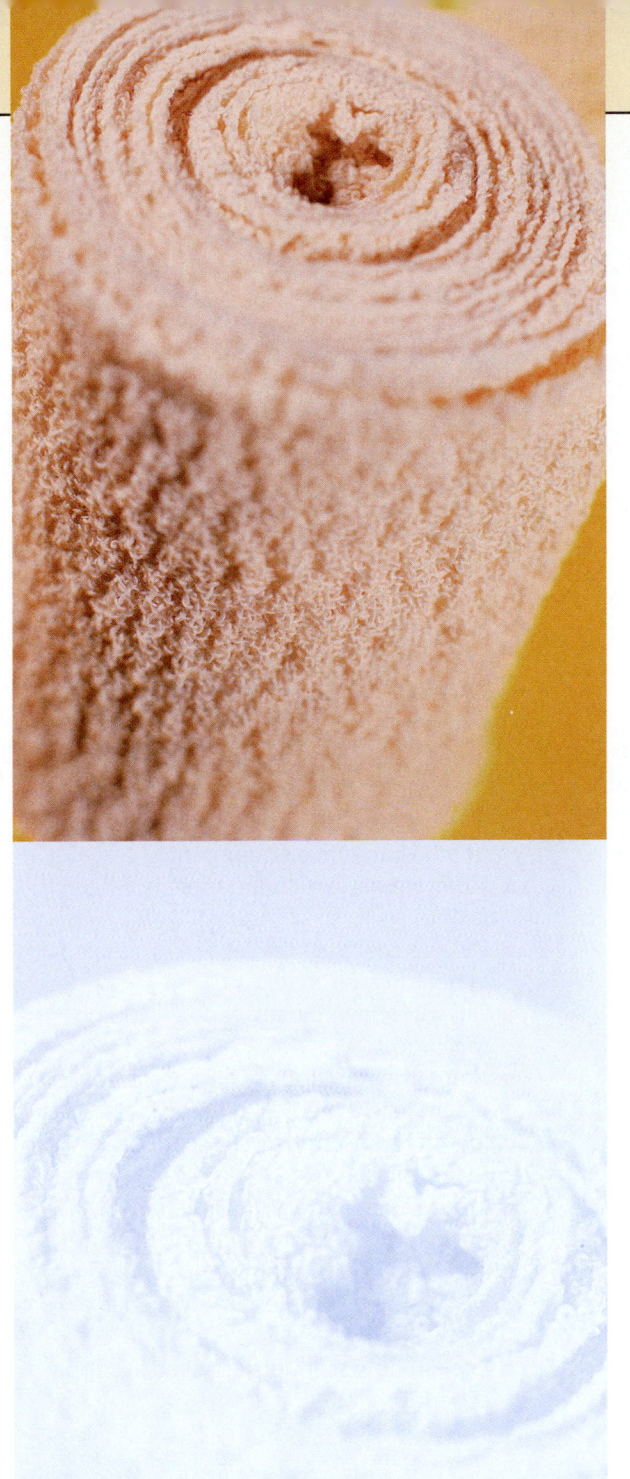

UNIT IV

Managing the Medical Office

Chapter 15   **Equipment, Maintenance, and Supply Inventory**

Chapter 16   **Office Policies and Procedures**

My name is Johnna Connell, and I'm a Certified Medical Assistant. I worked as a medical assistant for ten years before embarking on a teaching career.

One of the highlights of medical assisting is the diversity of the career. The training a medical assistant receives in both the clinical and administrative areas makes for a versatile employee. Some of my job duties included assessing patients; assisting the physician with exams; setting up and assisting with minor surgeries, X-rays, EKGs, PFS studies, and lab testing; preparing inventory of supplies; ordering supplies; purging files; and more.

Unlike other clinical employees, I could also flex and work in the front office. Even though my everyday duties involved the clinical areas, I also wanted to keep my administrative skills up to date. This administrative expertise became invaluable to my employers when the group decided to open a satellite office. I was given the job of setting up this office and working it singlehandedly several afternoons a week, including both administrative and clinical duties. It was a huge responsibility and challenge, but what a great feeling to know I could run an entire office alone!

One of my favorite parts of the job was getting to know the patients. I tried to treat each of them as I would want my own family members to be treated. Some of my patients did seem like dear friends after many years of assisting them. It was a joy to serve them. The desire to serve should be at the heart of every medical assistant.

Today, I have the challenge of serving medical assisting students— I teach medical assisting at the Winder campus of Lanier Technical College. I am so proud to promote such an exciting career.

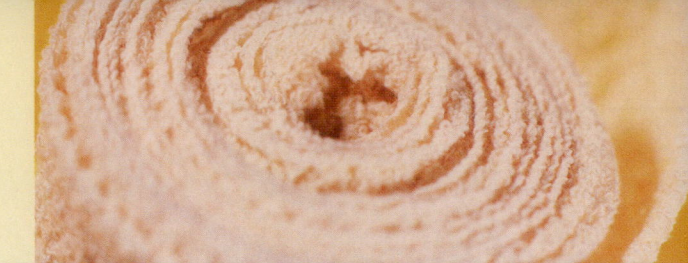

CHAPTER 15

Equipment, Maintenance, and Supply Inventory

Case Study

During a medical office's weekly staff meeting, several staff members voice their frustration over frequently running out of clerical supplies before new supplies are received. As the person in charge of inventory and supply ordering in the administrative office, the office manager asks the medical assistant to devise a system to address the situation.

Objectives

After completing this chapter, you should be able to:

- Define and spell the key terminology in this chapter.
- Define the medical assistant's role in equipment, maintenance, and supply inventory.
- Write an office equipment maintenance manual.
- Research the best options for purchasing supplies and equipment.
- Explain the pros and cons of leasing and purchasing office equipment.
- Maintain patient confidentiality while faxing.
- Discuss the functions of a photocopier in healthcare.
- Describe how to use a ten-key adding machine.
- Name the functions of a transcription machine in a medical office.
- Identify transcription services outside the medical office.
- Create an inventory control manual.
- Explain the steps involved in receiving and logging drug samples.
- Discuss how supplies are stocked in a medical office.
- Explain how scanners are used in supply ordering.

Med**Media**

http://www.MyMAKit.com

Additional interactive resources and activities for this chapter can be found on http://www.MyMAKit.com. For a video, tips, audio glossary, legal and ethical scenarios, on-the-job scenarios, quizzes, and games related to the content of this chapter, please access the accompanying CD-ROM in this book.

Video
Legal and Ethical Scenario: *Equipment, Maintenance, and Supply Inventory*
On the Job Scenario: *Equipment, Maintenance, and Supply Inventory*
Tips
Multiple Choice Quiz
Audio Glossary
HIPAA Quiz
Games: Spelling Bee, Crossword, and Strikeout

➕ MEDICAL ASSISTING STANDARDS

CAAHEP ENTRY-LEVEL STANDARDS	ABHES ENTRY-LEVEL COMPETENCIES
■ Perform within scope of practice (psychomotor) ■ Apply ethical behaviors, including honesty/integrity in performance of medical assisting practice (affective) ■ Discuss the importance of routine maintenance of office equipment (cognitive) ■ Perform routine maintenance of office equipment with documentation (psychomotor) ■ Perform an office inventory (psychomotor) ■ Use office hardware and software to maintain office systems (psychomotor)	■ Conduct work within scope of education, training, and ability ■ Dispose of controlled substances in compliance with government regulations ■ Application of electronic technology ■ Maintain records for accounting and banking purposes ■ Serve as a liaison between the physicians and others ■ Exercise efficient time management ■ Receive, organize, prioritize, and transmit information expediently ■ Maintain physical plant ■ Operate and maintain facilities and equipment safely ■ Inventory equipment and supplies ■ Evaluate and recommend equipment and supplies for practice

✔ COMPETENCY SKILLS PERFORMANCE

1. Take inventory of administrative and clinical equipment for maintenance and other purposes.
2. Perform routine maintenance of a computer printer.
3. Fax a document.
4. Prepare a purchase order
5. Receive a supply shipment.

Key Terminology

expiration date—date on which something loses full strength or validity

inventory—supplies on hand

maintained—kept in good working order

packing slip—list of supplies ordered and included in a shipment

scanner—piece of equipment that takes an exact image of a photo or document and transfers that image to a computer

transcribe—to type words as they are spoken

transcription machine—piece of equipment that allows the user to listen to and type taped words

user manual—document that describes how something (e.g., equipment) is used

warranty—period within which a piece of equipment is repaired without cost to the buyer

Abbreviations

EPA—Environmental Protection Agency

HIPAA—Health Insurance Portability and Accountability Act

OSHA—Occupational Safety and Health Administration

WHO—World Health Organization

Introduction

In medical offices that run smoothly, equipment is well **maintained** and supplies and **inventory** are effectively managed. While some large offices track their supplies and inventories electronically, others opt for manual processes. Medical assistants who are adept at equipment use in the medical office are both efficient at their jobs and competitive in the job market.

The Medical Assistant's Role in Equipment Maintenance and Supply Inventory

Medical assistants are responsible for maintaining many parts of the medical office. Depending on the size of the facility, the MA may be responsible for maintaining the equipment and keeping track of supplies and inventory.

Working with Medical Office Equipment

Every piece of equipment a medical office buys or leases comes with a **user manual**. A new piece of equipment typically also comes with a **warranty**, a guarantee from the vendor that certain defects or problems will be repaired for a predetermined period. Many companies sell extended warranties that cover equipment for longer periods. To track warranty periods and expedite repairs or replacement, the date a piece of equipment was leased or purchased should be written on the equipment's user manual. When possible, any receipts should be included. User manuals should be kept in a central location, like a file cabinet, so they can quickly and easily be found when needed.

Training Employees to Use Medical Office Equipment

Every employee who is asked to use a piece of office equipment must be trained on that equipment's proper use and care. Many suppliers train employees when equipment is purchased, but often just once, which means staff who have been trained must document their training if future employees are to be trained, as well.

Training manuals can be invaluable tools for documenting training content in the medical office. Manuals should devote one page to each piece of equipment. In addition to explaining how to use and maintain the equipment, each page should provide a place for employees to sign and date once properly trained (Figure 15-1 ◆). In addition to furthering training objectives, such manuals keep the medical office in compliance with Occupational Safety and Health Administration (**OSHA**) safety regulations. ∞ Chapter 23 details OSHA safety regulations in the medical office.

Training employees on the use of the photocopier.
Familiarize employees with:
❑ On/off switch
❑ Paper placement on glass
❑ Paper replacement
❑ Use of enlarge/reduce feature
❑ Toner replacement
❑ Location of telephone number for repairs
❑ Location of telephone number for supplies
Signature of Employee:
Signature of Trainer:
Date:

Figure 15-1 ◆ Sample office equipment training manual.

Keeping a Maintenance Log for Medical Office Equipment

For each piece of equipment that requires regular maintenance, the medical office should keep a log of the maintenance requirements, schedule, and responsible party. When equipment must be maintained by the manufacturer or another professional repair person, the log should include those parties' contact information. Anyone who performs maintenance should sign and date the maintenance log. A complete maintenance log helps the medical office prove that its equipment has been well maintained, which can in turn help expedite warranty work (Figure 15-2 ◆).

Office Equipment Maintenance Log				
Equipment name	**Maintenance to be performed**	**Maintenance schedule**	**Name of person performing the maintenance**	**Signature and date**
Photocopier	Clean spilled toner inside the machine	Once monthly	Louise Glaser, CMA	*L. Glaser, CMA (AAMA) 9/4/10*

Figure 15-2 ◆ Sample office equipment maintenance log.

Replacing or Buying Medical Office Equipment

When the time comes to replace or acquire equipment, the physician may ask the medical assistant to research options. For small, easy-to-transport pieces, assistants may ask sales representatives to bring samples to the office for review. Assistants may also research equipment online or visit stores where equipment is displayed. For high-dollar purchases, sales representatives should give medical assistants references of customers who are using the products. In turn, the assistants should take the time to call those references and poll them on customer service and ease of the equipment's use.

When calling other medical offices for equipment references, the medical assistant should be sure to talk to the staff members who actually use the equipment. Those staff will accurately depict how that equipment works.

Weighing Equipment Leasing Against Buying

Leasing and buying have distinct advantages when it comes to equipment. Leasing does not award ownership, but it typically requires no downpayment. In the event the equipment breaks or malfunctions, the manufacturer usually replaces or repairs it as part of the lease. Purchased equipment generally requires full funding up front or a downpayment and financed balance. Buying, however, confers ownership. Once the equipment is paid for, the owner need only cover the costs associated with maintenance or repairs. Physician's preference, price, and intended use all help drive the lease/buy decision.

Using Fax Machines in the Medical Office

Facsimile or fax machines are common pieces of medical office equipment that come in varied sizes and prices (Figure 15-3 ◆). Via telephone lines, fax machines make it possible to send and receive printed documents anywhere in the world where other fax machines are located. Simple, relatively inexpensive models simply fax documents from one location to another. Higher-end versions also serve as photocopiers and **scanners**.

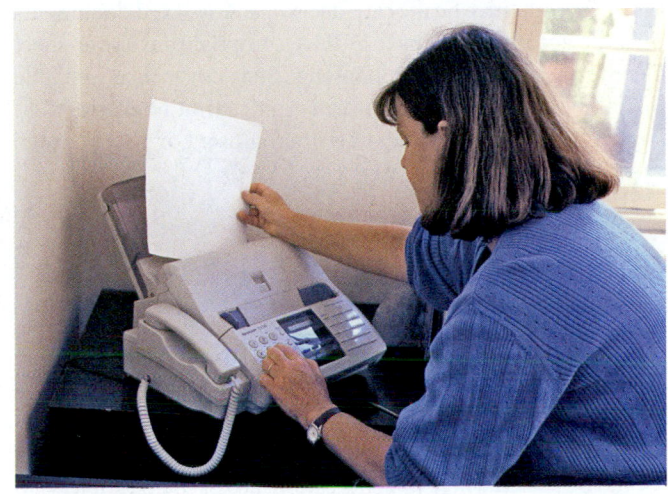

Figure 15-3 ◆ The fax machine in the medical office must be located outside of areas frequented by patients.

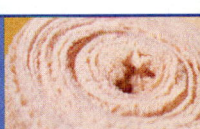

PROCEDURE 15-1 **Take Inventory of Administrative and Clinical Equipment for Maintenance and Other Purposes**

Theory and Rationale

An up-to-date list of a medical office's equipment helps determine the equipment's age in the event the equipment needs repair, or if fire, flood, or theft occurs.

Materials

- Paper
- Pen
- Computer with word-processing or spreadsheet software

Competency

(**Conditions**) With the necessary materials, you will be able to (**Task**) perform an inventory of equipment (**Standards**) correctly within the time limit set by the instructor.

1. Locate all administrative and clinical equipment in the medical office.

2. List each piece of equipment with manufacturer name, serial number, and date of purchase, when known.
3. Include information about the company maintaining the equipment.
4. Include information about the supplies needed to maintain the equipment, including where those supplies are purchased.
5. Using word-processing or spreadsheet software, create an inventory sheet of all equipment information.
6. Update the inventory sheet as needed when new equipment is purchased or older equipment is replaced.

To guard patient confidentiality, fax machines must be kept in areas of the office that are inaccessible to patients. Such machines should not reside on the counter at the front desk or in a hallway, for example. While medical offices commonly use fax machines to send and receive confidential patient information, the Health Insurance Portability and Accountability Act (HIPAA) dictates that fax machines only be used in the event other modes of transmission fail to suffice. Therefore, when medical offices must transmit information on patients' behalf, medical assistants should use conventional mail when there is time. Some medical offices use courier services in lieu of faxing, especially for such highly confidential information as HIV status or reproductive healthcare decisions. Any faxed documents must be accompanied by a HIPAA-compliant fax cover sheet like the one shown in ∞ Chapter 4. Such cover sheets include disclaimers that the faxed information cannot be disclosed to any party without the patient's written consent or a court order.

Using Copy Machines in Healthcare Facilities

Copy machines, like fax machines, come in all sizes and price levels. Medical offices should have high-quality copiers that are maintained and serviced regularly. Because medical offices tend to use their copiers heavily, unreliable machines can severely impede office functioning. Like fax machines, office copiers should be placed where patients cannot access them. Copiers are best placed behind the front desk or near the billing office, as staff in those areas use copiers the most. See ∞ Chapter 8 for a procedure on preparing a document for photocopying.

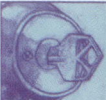

Keys to Success
EQUIPMENT MALFUNCTION

Medical office equipment may sometimes malfunction. When it does, report the malfunction to the office manager or physician immediately. Malfunctions in some equipment, especially clinical equipment, can injure patients or medical staff.

When researching copiers, medical offices should consider various factors. While price and warranty items are of obvious concern, the cost of supplies is also an important consideration. Some copiers require difficult-to-find or expensive parts.

Adding Healthcare Data with Machines

Upon hearing "adding machine," many people envision ten-key calculators. Such calculators are normally electronic, and most have tape for printing (Figure 15-4 ◆). Through consistent use, most administrative staff in the medical office become able to use ten-key calculators by touch. This skill is especially helpful when adding long columns of numbers, like those on pegboard day sheets, deposit slips, or patient ledgers. Medical staff also often use handheld calculators. These machines come in all shapes and sizes, typically run on battery power, and are convenient when ten-key systems are impractical. Some handheld calculators are small enough to fit in the pocket of a clinic jacket.

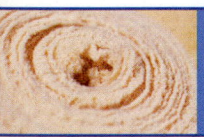

PROCEDURE 15-2 **Perform Routine Maintenance of a Computer Printer**

Theory and Rationale

While most equipment in the medical office requires trained technicians to provide maintenance, the medical assistant performs basic maintenance on many pieces, such as the computer printer.

Materials

- Paper
- Pen
- Computer printer
- Maintenance logbook

Competency

(**Conditions**) With the necessary materials, you will be able to (**Task**) perform routine maintenance of a computer printer (**Standards**) correctly within the time limit set by the instructor.

1. Review the maintenance logbook for the computer printer.
2. Following the manufacturer's directions, open the printer cover and remove the toner cartridge.
3. Using the manufacturer-provided cleaning tool, clean any dust and spilled toner from within the printer.
4. Replace the cleaning tool and the toner cartridge.
5. Close the printer cover.
6. In the maintenance logbook, enter information about the maintenance, including the date and your signature.

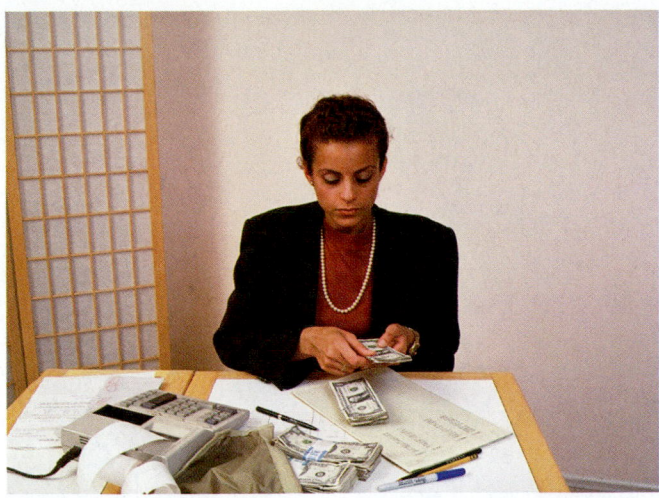

Figure 15-4 ◆ The medical assistant will use a ten-key calculator for tasks such as totaling the daily deposit.

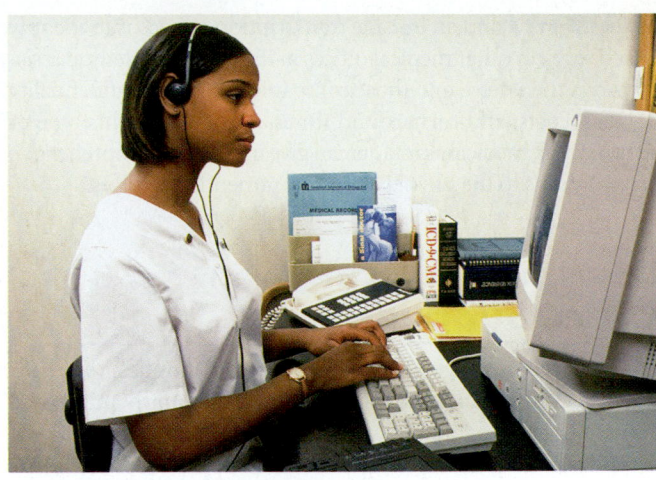

Figure 15-5 ◆ A medical assistant using a transcription machine.

Medical Transcription

In years past, **transcription machines** were common in medical offices (Figure 15-5 ◆). Physicians would dictate patient information into these tape recorder–devices and give the tapes to administrative staff, who would **transcribe** the spoken words to printed form. Staff would use headphones to hear the tapes and foot pedals to control the tapes. Volume and speed buttons would control those functions.

Physicians must be afforded the opportunity to review the transcripts of transcribed tapes before the tapes are erased. Physicians may verify wording or correct errors. Once physicians have approved transcriptions, the tapes can be erased and reused.

Finding Outside Transcription Services

Most medical offices today use outside transcription services. Such services typically require physicians to call a recorded telephone line to dictate their information. The corresponding printed documents arrive via fax, e-mail, or postal service.

For a number of reasons, thorough research is important when choosing outside transcription services. Many transcription services are based outside the United States, where patient privacy laws can vary and fail to meet U.S. **HIPAA** regulations. Research should reveal companies' reputations as well as prices and services. While the Internet can be a valuable research tool in this realm,

---

PROCEDURE 15-3 Fax a Document

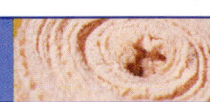

Theory and Rationale

Faxing documents from the medical office requires strict attention to HIPAA regulations for safeguarding private patient information.

Materials

■ Document to be faxed
■ HIPAA-compliant fax cover sheet
■ Pen
■ Fax machine

Competency

(**Conditions**) With the necessary materials, you will be able to (**Task**) fax a document using a fax machine (**Standards**) correctly within the time limit set by the instructor.

1. Complete the fax cover sheet with personal name, phone number, and clinic contact information.
2. Fill in the name and fax number of the fax recipient.
3. List the number of pages in the fax, including the cover sheet.
4. Properly orient the fax cover sheet and document to be faxed in the fax machine.
5. Dial the target fax number.
6. When the fax has fully transmitted, remove the documents and file them with the fax confirmation sheet in the patient's file.

the best way to find an outside transcription service is to identify which services other medical offices in the area use. Medical assistants can then delve into those companies' patient confidentiality policies, costs, and turnaround times. Armed with this type of information, medical assistants can give informed, comprehensive presentations to the physician on recommended services.

Logging Medical Office Supplies

To effectively manage office inventory and supplies, the medical office should create a master list of all regularly purchased items. This list should include all disposable supplies; separate lists should detail clinical and clerical supplies. All such lists should include the supply, the order or part number, the name of the company, and the typical quantity and frequency of ordering (Figure 15-6 ◆).

Inventorying Supplies

To ensure that the medical office remains at fully functioning status, one member of the healthcare team should regularly inventory all supplies to ensure they remain in stock (Figure 15-7 ◆). Out-of-stock items force offices to reschedule procedures or incur high next-day reordering expenses. Offices use supplies at different rates, and their reorder schedules should reflect those differences. Most offices inventory supplies weekly, while others adhere to monthly or daily schedules. Because medical assistants' vacation schedules and days off vary, the inventory task works best when shared by more than one staff member.

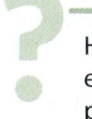
Critical Thinking Question 15-1

How does rotating the person in charge of inventory each week benefit the medical office's inventory process?

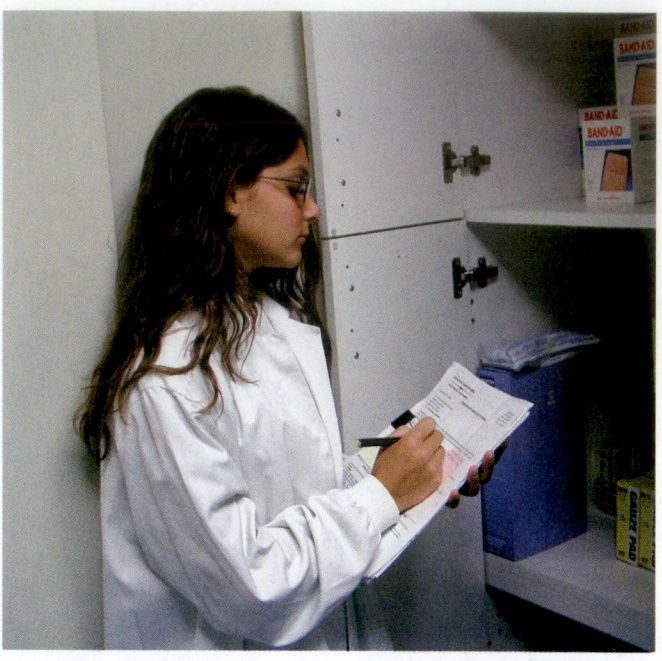

Figure 15-7 ◆ Medical supplies must be inventoried on a regular basis.

The key to effective supply management is to have enough supplies to efficiently run the office but not so much as to risk expiration or storage issues. Many of the supplies used in the clinical part of the office, such as laboratory collection containers or medications and vaccines, have expiration dates. Some supplies, especially medications, have expiration dates of no more than one year from the date of manufacture. A medical office might get a good price on gloves by ordering 500 boxes at once, for example, but if the staff will take two years to use those gloves and storage space is at a premium, the savings is not likely worth the inconvenience. Many offices devise systems to remind themselves when certain supplies must be ordered. If, for example, staff know to

Inventory Supply Log				
Supply	**Order or Part Number**	**Supplier**	**Number in Order**	**Frequency of Order**
Fee slips	N/A	Minuteman Press (425) 555–9000	5,000	Twice annually
Fax toner cartridges	HP6545	Office Depot (800) 345-3000	2	Once monthly

Figure 15-6 ◆ Sample inventory supply log.

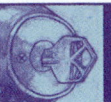

reorder gloves once only ten boxes are left in stock, a reorder reminder note can be attached to the tenth box of gloves.

Some medical offices use purchase orders for ordering supplies or equipment needed in the office. In some facilities, these purchase orders must be authorized by the office manager or the physician; in other facilities they are filled out by the person in charge of ordering supplies and sent directly by that person to the supplier.

In Practice

Before the medical assistant was hired, the medical office lacked a system for ordering supplies. Members of the healthcare team simply ordered supplies as they felt necessary. As a result, the office now has cupboards full of supplies that will expire in a month. As a new employee, the medical assistant is charged with devising a system for tracking office inventory. Where should the assistant start? What steps will help ensure all supplies are counted correctly?

Checking for the Next Day's Supplies

At the end of the workday, one member of the healthcare team should ensure that the office has enough supplies for all procedures scheduled the next day. Rescheduling due to supply deficiencies reflects poorly on the office as well as impedes efficient office operation. The medical office should develop a good relationship with other, nearby offices so that supplies can be borrowed in the event of unexpected shortages.

Storing Supplies Upon Arrival

When supplies arrive in the medical office, one staff member must locate the **packing slip** and check to ensure all supplies are included. Usually, this slip is sealed in a plastic envelope and attached to the outside of the box, or it may be in the box with the supplies. The packing slip lists the supplies that were ordered and the supplies in the shipment. This slip may also serve as an invoice. If so, it must be routed to the accounts payable office after the order is checked for completeness. When part of an order is missing or backordered, the medical assistant must

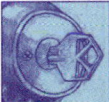

PROCEDURE 15-4   Prepare a Purchase Order

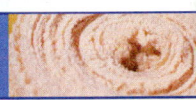

Theory and Rationale
The use of purchase orders is one way the medical office can accurately keep track of the supplies that are needed and used in the clinic, as well as how often these supplies are being ordered.

Materials
- List of needed supplies
- Purchase order form
- Pen
- Fax machine or telephone

Competency
(**Conditions**) With the necessary materials, you will be able to (**Task**) prepare a purchase order (**Standards**) correctly within the time limit set by the instructor.

1. Review the list of needed supplies, grouping them according to the vendor they will be ordered from.

2. Fill in the name and fax number of the company the supplies are to be ordered from.
3. List each supply individually on the purchase order, taking care to note the quantity needed and the part number associated with each item.
4. If the physician's signature is required, obtain his or her signature. If it is not required, sign and date the form with your own signature.
5. If the purchase order can be faxed to the supplier, fax the document and make a note of the date and time the fax went through.
6. If the purchase order cannot be faxed to the supplier, call the supplier and place the order over the telephone. Document the name of the person you spoke to and the date and time of the call.
7. File the purchase order in a folder for pending orders.

make a notation and keep the packing slip until the remaining supplies arrive in the office.

Except for clerical supplies, all newly arrived medical office supplies should be stored behind older inventory so older supplies are used first. Because many medical supplies have **expiration dates**, this procedure helps eliminate waste.

Handling Drug Samples

Many medical offices welcome the pharmaceutical representatives who supply them drug samples, which are normally small amounts of the drugs pharmaceutical companies sell. Usually, samples are name-brand, costly drugs new to the market. Companies give physicians drug samples in the hope those physicians will prescribe the drugs to their patients. Typically, physicians set aside short periods to meet with drug-company representatives. In most states, medical assistants may sign for the drug samples that sales representatives leave. Not all medical offices permit pharmaceutical representatives access to the physicians or other clinical staff.

In medical offices, drugs should be grouped according to type. Antibiotics should be kept together, for example, as should antidepressants or cough medicines. All medications, including drug samples, must be kept out of patient access areas. Medications, including drug samples, have expiration dates and must be discarded once those dates have passed. In some states, sample drugs must also be tracked. Medical offices should track samples even when the law does not require it. Tracking discourages staff from taking drugs and supplies for personal use.

Stocking Clerical Supplies

Clerical supplies are easier to stock than clinical supplies because most medical offices know how many envelopes, stamps, and forms they regularly use. In addition, clerical

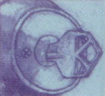

Keys to Success
DISCARDING MEDICATIONS

The Environmental Protection Agency (**EPA**) and World Health Organization (**WHO**) recommend discarding expired medications by wrapping those medications in plastic or sealing them in plastic bags before disposal. Flushing medications is not recommended because it exposes people, pets, and the environment to potential harm.

supplies do not expire and most such items, except for preprinted business cards or letterhead (Figure 15-8 ◆), are readily available at local supply stores. While an abundance of clerical supplies can present a storage problem, many suppliers offer volume discounts.

Tracking Supplies with Computer Software

Many medical offices today use barcode-equipped computer software to ensure that they have adequate supplies. When members of the healthcare team take items from the supply room, they use the software to scan those items' bar codes and note the departments using the supplies. When supplies drop below a preprogrammed level, the staff member in charge of ordering supplies is notified to order more of that supply. Software ordering systems are only as accurate as the staff members who use them, however. When supplies are scanned inaccurately, they cannot be tracked and supplies may not be adequately stocked.

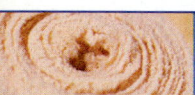

PROCEDURE 15-5 Receive a Supply Shipment

Theory and Rationale
Medical office supplies are ordered and received regularly. To ensure that all ordered supplies have been received, the medical assistant must carefully check the supplies' packing slip.

Materials
- Box of supplies
- Packing slip
- Supply inventory logbook
- Pen

Competency
(**Conditions**) With the necessary materials, you will be able to (**Task**) receive a supply shipment (**Standards**) correctly within the time limit set by the instructor.

1. Open the box of supplies and locate the packing slip.
2. Remove each item from the box, checking it on the packing slip.
3. On the packing slip, circle any missing supplies.
4. Put the supplies away, newer ones behind older ones.
5. Note in the supply log that the supplies have been received.
6. When any supplies on the packing slip are absent from the shipment, notify the supplier.
7. When any supplies on the packing slip are on back order, retain the slip until the backordered supplies arrive.
8. When the packing slip also serves as an invoice, route it to the accounts payable department.
9. Discard packing materials appropriately.

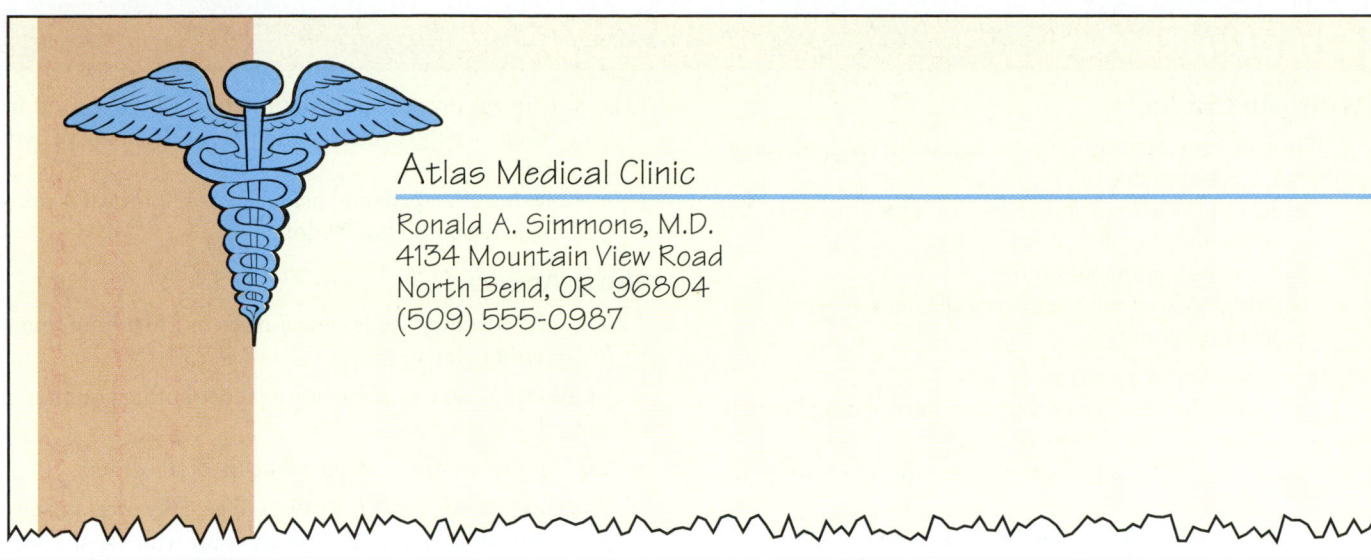

Atlas Medical Clinic

Ronald A. Simmons, M.D.
4134 Mountain View Road
North Bend, OR 96804
(509) 555-0987

Figure 15-8 ◆ Sample of medical office letterhead paper.

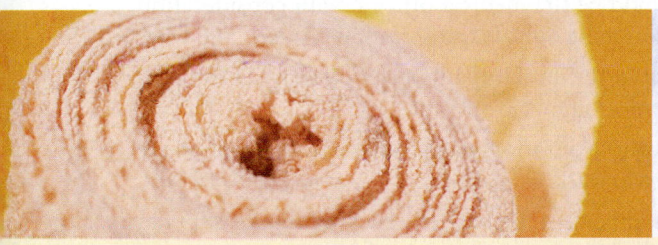

REVIEW

Chapter Summary

- For the medical office, an equipment maintenance manual serves to ensure all needed equipment is in working order and able to support business initiatives.
- At the physician's request, the medical assistant is often charged with researching the best options for buying supplies and equipment.
- Depending on factors like need, cost, and long-term objectives, medical offices may choose to lease or buy their business equipment.
- Fax machines are just one common piece of equipment that require all members of the healthcare team to remain vigilant to patient confidentiality.
- A photocopier in the medical office functions to provide copies of documents for patient and office use.
- Staff in the medical office often become adept at using ten-key calculators to manipulate numbers.
- Transcription machines, once predominant in healthcare, are still sometimes used today to convert spoken words to written ones.
- When researching transcription services outside the medical office, the medical assistant should be conscious of such factors as location and cost.
- An inventory control manual helps a medical office ensure that it is always fully equipped with needed supplies.
- Medical supplies may have expiration dates and should be ordered with the goal of using all supplies before they expire.
- Drug samples must be tracked and notice must be taken of any expiration dates on these samples.

Chapter Review

Multiple Choice

1. When investigating options for replacing medical equipment, it is acceptable to
   a. have a salesperson bring the equipment to the office to demonstrate it.
   b. view the equipment online.
   c. visit a local supplier and view the item in person.
   d. all of the above.

2. In the medical office, fax machines
   a. should be used to send patient information between offices because it saves postage.
   b. can be placed anywhere where most convenient for office staff.
   c. come in all sizes and prices.
   d. all of the above.

3. The best way to dispose of expired medications is to
   a. donate them to an agency that will use them outside the United States.
   b. give them to patients who might want them.
   c. sell them on eBay.
   d. wrap them in plastic and place them in the garbage.

4. It is important to keep a maintenance log for medical office equipment to
   a. prove the equipment has been maintained in the event warranty work is needed.
   b. ensure the equipment is being maintained so it will work properly.
   c. avoid having to purchase a replacement piece.
   d. all of the above.

5. When looking to purchase a new copy machine for the medical office, staff should consider the
   a. cost of supplies.
   b. features of the machine.
   c. availability of supplies.
   d. all of the above.

True/False

T F 1. It is always a good idea to call for references with any new supplier before making an expensive purchase.

T F 2. Many transcription services use employees in the United States.

T F 3. Clinical inventory in the medical office should be taken weekly, whatever the practice type or patient load.

T F 4. Taking office pens and paperclips for home use is stealing and should not be done.

Short Answer

1. Give one advantage to leasing a piece of office equipment instead of buying it.

2. Name one advantage to buying a piece of office equipment instead of leasing it.

3. Explain the use of a scanner in the medical office.

4. When calling other medical offices to get references for supply companies, why speak with the staff who use the supplies or equipment?

5. Explain why the medical office should keep an employee training manual for office equipment.

6. What should be the medical office's main consideration when researching outside transcription services, and why?

7. Why separate the inventory list of clerical supplies from the list for clinical supplies?

8. Explain why expiration dates on medical supplies are important to track.

9. Why is it important to check the packing slip for supplies shipment?

10. Why do pharmaceutical companies give medical offices free drug samples?

11. What clerical supplies are usually ordered with an office's name, address, and telephone number preprinted?

Research Questions

1. Interview a person who works in a medical office. How does that office keep track of the various supplies needed and used?

2. Research various office supply companies online for information about photocopiers. What type of machine do you think would be appropriate for a medical office?

3. Call a medical office supply company. How quickly are orders typically shipped? Are there discounts offered for higher quantity purchases?

Externship Application Experience

A package of medical office supplies arrives at the medical office. While checking off the supplies received on the packing slip, the medical assistant notices five items on the packing slip are not in the box. How should the medical assistant handle the situation?

Resource Guide

Child Family Health International (this agency takes donated, unused medical supplies)
995 Market Street, Suite 1104
San Francisco, CA 94103
Phone: (415) 957-9000 or (866) 345-4674
Fax: (415) 840-0486
www.cfhi.org

Par Inventory Management System (manufactures bar code scanning software for inventory control management)
Phone: (800) 272-7537
Fax: (440) 266-7400
www.parker.com

Visual Supply Pro (manufactures bar code scanning software for inventory control management)
2689 Danforth Terrace
Wellington, FL 33414
Phone: (561) 792-1477
Fax: (561) 792-1677
www.decisionsw.com

World Health Organization
Avenue Appia 20
CH - 1211 Geneva 27
Switzerland
Phone: +41 22 791 2111
Fax: +41 22 791 3111
www.who.org

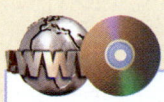

Med**Media**

http://www.MyMAKit.com

More on this chapter, including interactive resources, can be found on the Student CD-ROM accompanying this textbook and on http://www.MyMAKit.com.

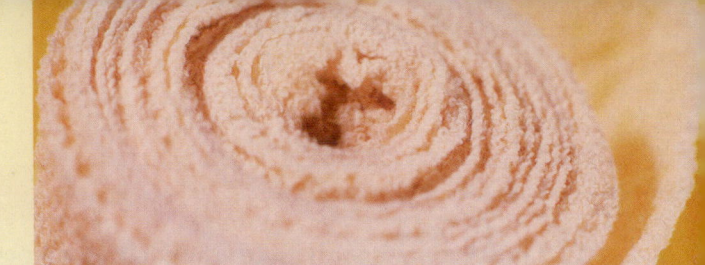

CHAPTER 16

Office Policies and Procedures

Case Study

Monte Taylor recently passed the medical assisting registration exam and has just obtained his first job as a registered medical assistant. Dr. Radcliff, an internist who shares her office space with several other physicians, has hired Monte. On Monte's first day, he asks the office manager if there is a manual that outlines office procedures. The office manager tells Monte that office staff have never taken the time to compose a procedures manual. She asks Monte if he would be willing to take on such a task.

Objectives

After completing this chapter, you should be able to:

- Define and spell the key terminology in this chapter.
- Define the medical assistants role in office policies and procedures.
- Create patient information pamphlets.
- Develop a personnel manual.
- Create a policies and procedures manual for the medical office.

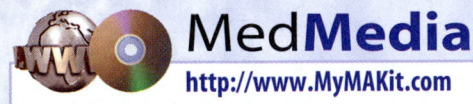

MedMedia
http://www.MyMAKit.com

Additional interactive resources and activities for this chapter can be found on http://www.MyMAKit.com. For a video, tips, audio glossary, legal and ethical scenarios, on-the-job scenarios, quizzes, and games related to the content of this chapter, please access the accompanying CD-ROM in this book.

Video: *Coping with Sales Calls*
Legal and Ethical Scenario: *Office Policies and Procedures*
On the Job Scenario: *Office Policies and Procedures*
Tips
Multiple Choice Quiz
Audio Glossary
HIPAA Quiz
Games: Spelling Bee, Crossword, and Strikeout

✚ MEDICAL ASSISTING STANDARDS

CAAHEP ENTRY-LEVEL STANDARDS	ABHES ENTRY-LEVEL COMPETENCIES
■ Perform within scope of practice (psychomotor) ■ Apply ethical behaviors, including honesty/integrity in performance of medical assisting practice (affective) ■ Practice within the standard of care for a medical assistant (psychomotor) ■ Explain general office policies (psychomotor) ■ Report relevant information to others succinctly and accurately (psychomotor) ■ Document accurately in the patient record (psychomotor) ■ Identify resources and adaptations that are required based on individual needs (cognitive) ■ Use office hardware and software to maintain office systems (psychomotor) ■ Report relevant information to others succinctly and accurately (psychomotor) ■ Explain general office policies (psychomotor) ■ Apply local, state and federal health care legislation and regulation appropriate to the medical assisting practice setting (psychomotor) ■ Recognize the importance of local, state and federal legislation and regulations in the practice setting (affective)	■ Maintain confidentiality at all times ■ Be cognizant of ethical boundaries ■ Conduct work within scope of education, training, and ability ■ Orient patients to office policies and procedures ■ Adapt what is said to the recipient's level of comprehension ■ Adaptation for individualized needs ■ Apply computer concepts for office procedures ■ Exercise efficient time management ■ Fundamental writing skills

✔ COMPETENCY SKILLS PERFORMANCE

1. Create an office brochure.
2. Create a clinical procedure for the procedure manual.
3. Create an administrative procedure for the procedure manual.

Introduction

Every business needs written policies and procedures to ensure that employees know how to perform their jobs correctly, and healthcare is no exception. Policies and procedures are perhaps even more important in the medical field than in others because they may contribute to patient safety and risk reduction. A **policy** is a statement of guidelines or rules on a given topic. A **procedure** describes how to perform a given task or project.

Key Terminology

brochure—document containing information about a topic

compulsory—required

mission statement—statement that describes the medical office's reason for existing

organizational chart—breakdown of the chain of command in a business

personnel manual—compilation of employment policies for an office; also called an employee handbook

policy—guidelines or rules for an issue

procedure—steps to perform a task or project

Abbreviations

HIPAA—Health Insurance Portability and Accountability Act

OSHA—Occupational Safety and Health Administration

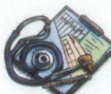

The Medical Assistant's Role in Office Policies and Procedures

Upon hire in a medical facility, the medical assistant should be given access to the clinic's policy and procedure manual. This manual will guide the MA as she learns the job and will continue to be a resource throughout employment in that facility. The medical assistant should be sure to point out any areas of the job where she feels a policy or procedure should be written if one does not already exist. Having an up-to-date policy and procedure manual makes the job of the medical assistant easier and helps to avoid miscommunication.

Creating Patient Information Pamphlets

Every member of the healthcare team is responsible for educating patients. Much of the information physicians ask that patients receive may be in written form. Many medical offices buy educational **brochures** to give to patients. These documents are available on a multitude of topics, including back pain, child immunizations, and menopause (Figure 16-1 ◆).

For physicians who want to provide more detailed information, brochures may be created with the help of in-house staff or a professional printing company. However the office chooses to create patient educational pamphlets, those pamphlets must be professional. All printed material must be accurate and free of typographical errors. Depending on the cultural makeup of an office's patients, brochures may be printed in various languages (Figure 16-2 ◆).

Creating a Personnel Manual

A **personnel manual,** also called an employee handbook, lists the rules and regulations that apply to all staff in the medical office (Figure 16-3 ◆). This manual also breaks down the office's benefits for health, life, and disability insurance, among others. Many offices give all new employees copies of their personnel manuals upon hire. Other offices keep single copies in central locations or in an electronic format accessible to all employees.

To create a personnel manual, the office manager and/or physician should list desired manual items. For ideas, a medical office might consult the personnel manuals of other offices. For all material, it is important to keep federal and state laws in mind to ensure all policies are within legal boundaries. Figure 16-4 ◆ lists items commonly found in personnel manuals.

? Critical Thinking Question 16-1
What type of policies and procedures should Monte start identifying for his office?

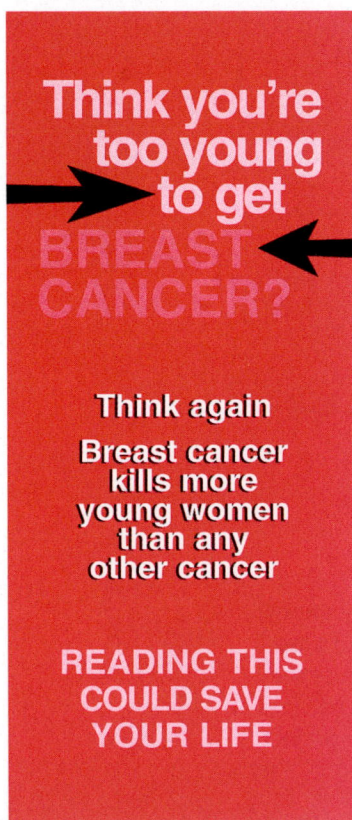

Figure 16-1 ◆ A patient education pamphlet on breast cancer.

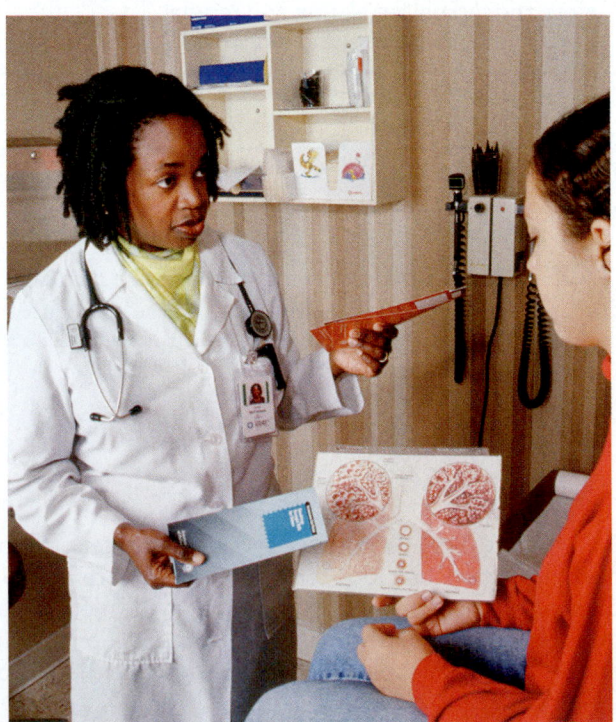

Figure 16-2 ◆ A medical assistant explains the dangers of smoking to a young patient.

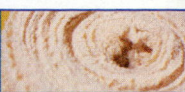

PROCEDURE 16-1 Create an Office Brochure

Theory and Rationale
Office brochures are a useful way to educate patients on the physician's specific types of treatment or therapy. All office brochures must be professional, accurate, and free of typographical errors.

Materials
- Computer with word-processing software
- List of information the physician would like in an office brochure

Competency
(**Conditions**) With the necessary materials, you will be able to (**Task**) create an office brochure (**Standards**) correctly within the time limit set by the instructor.

1. Gather information on the brochure's subject.
2. Launch the word-processing software.
3. Create a title for the brochure, such as "Living with Diabetes."
4. Add information to the brochure in an easy-to-read format. Use simple terms rather than medical terminology.
5. Add information regarding where the patient can look for further resources, such as Web sites.
6. Include the office's name, address, and telephone number.
7. Check for typographical and grammatical errors.
8. Print the brochure, and give it to the physician for review before making copies for patients.

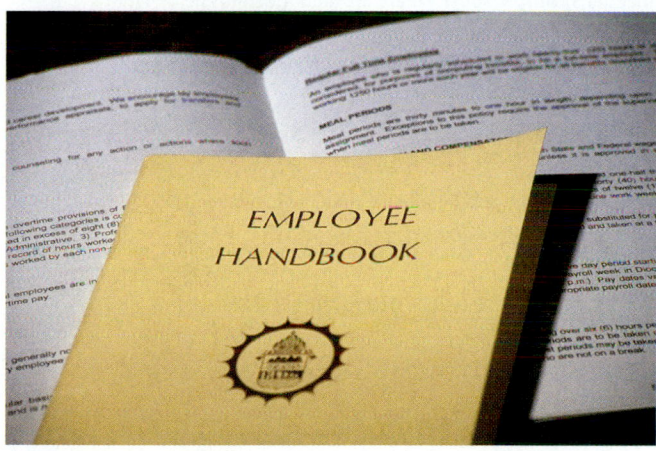

Figure 16-3 ◆ The employee handbook should be updated on a regular basis and made available to each new employee.

Creating Policies and Procedures for the Medical Office

The medical office's policy and procedures manual may contain both policies and procedures, or policies and procedures may be separated. Whatever the approach, each policy and procedure manual should contain the following items in separate sections:

- Mission statement
- Organizational chart
- Personnel policies
- Clinical procedures
- Administrative procedures

A table of contents should clearly direct readers to desired pages. Per Occupational Safety and Health Administration

(**OSHA**) and **HIPAA** regulations, infection control and quality improvement and risk management procedures must be kept in separate notebooks and reviewed and updated regularly.

Writing a Mission Statement
The policy and procedures manual for a medical office should begin with an office **mission statement** that is concise and communicated to all staff. For example, a mission statement might read, "To care for all patients in a compassionate and dignified manner, with a focus on patient safety and satisfaction." Many medical offices frame and hang their mission statements for patients to see.

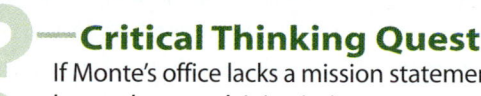

Critical Thinking Question 16-2
If Monte's office lacks a mission statement, how should he go about explaining its importance to the physician?

Preparing an Organizational Chart
In addition to the mission statement, all policy and procedure manuals should break down the offices' organizational structures

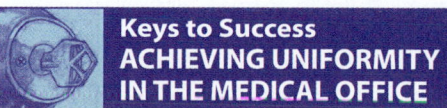

Keys to Success
ACHIEVING UNIFORMITY IN THE MEDICAL OFFICE

One of the most important reasons for having a medical office policy and procedure manual is to clarify rules and regulations and the physician's expectations for procedures. Strict adherence to policies as they are outlined achieves uniformity in the office and provides a fair method of treating staff.

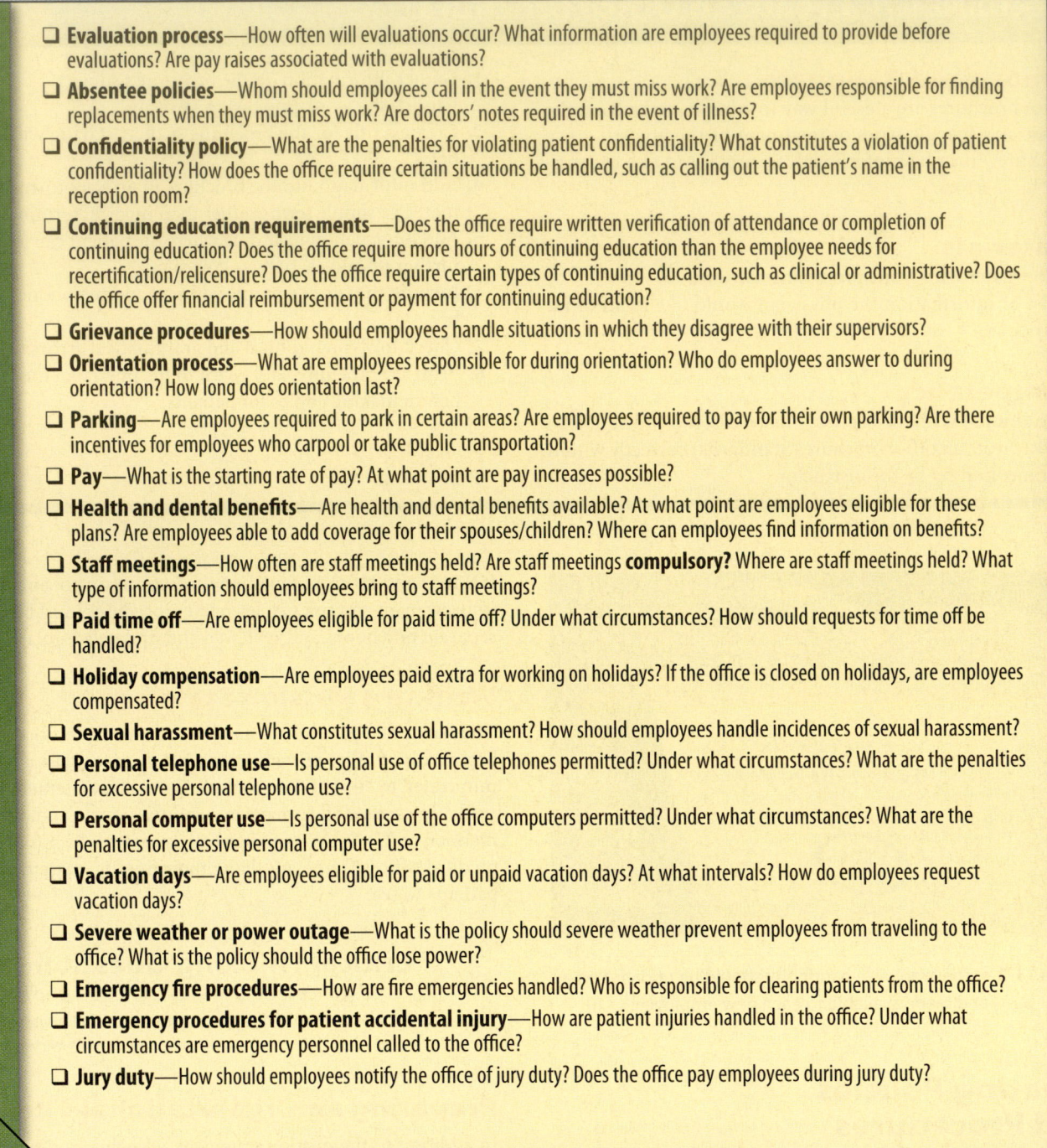

❑ **Evaluation process**—How often will evaluations occur? What information are employees required to provide before evaluations? Are pay raises associated with evaluations?

❑ **Absentee policies**—Whom should employees call in the event they must miss work? Are employees responsible for finding replacements when they must miss work? Are doctors' notes required in the event of illness?

❑ **Confidentiality policy**—What are the penalties for violating patient confidentiality? What constitutes a violation of patient confidentiality? How does the office require certain situations be handled, such as calling out the patient's name in the reception room?

❑ **Continuing education requirements**—Does the office require written verification of attendance or completion of continuing education? Does the office require more hours of continuing education than the employee needs for recertification/relicensure? Does the office require certain types of continuing education, such as clinical or administrative? Does the office offer financial reimbursement or payment for continuing education?

❑ **Grievance procedures**—How should employees handle situations in which they disagree with their supervisors?

❑ **Orientation process**—What are employees responsible for during orientation? Who do employees answer to during orientation? How long does orientation last?

❑ **Parking**—Are employees required to park in certain areas? Are employees required to pay for their own parking? Are there incentives for employees who carpool or take public transportation?

❑ **Pay**—What is the starting rate of pay? At what point are pay increases possible?

❑ **Health and dental benefits**—Are health and dental benefits available? At what point are employees eligible for these plans? Are employees able to add coverage for their spouses/children? Where can employees find information on benefits?

❑ **Staff meetings**—How often are staff meetings held? Are staff meetings **compulsory?** Where are staff meetings held? What type of information should employees bring to staff meetings?

❑ **Paid time off**—Are employees eligible for paid time off? Under what circumstances? How should requests for time off be handled?

❑ **Holiday compensation**—Are employees paid extra for working on holidays? If the office is closed on holidays, are employees compensated?

❑ **Sexual harassment**—What constitutes sexual harassment? How should employees handle incidences of sexual harassment?

❑ **Personal telephone use**—Is personal use of office telephones permitted? Under what circumstances? What are the penalties for excessive personal telephone use?

❑ **Personal computer use**—Is personal use of the office computers permitted? Under what circumstances? What are the penalties for excessive personal computer use?

❑ **Vacation days**—Are employees eligible for paid or unpaid vacation days? At what intervals? How do employees request vacation days?

❑ **Severe weather or power outage**—What is the policy should severe weather prevent employees from traveling to the office? What is the policy should the office lose power?

❑ **Emergency fire procedures**—How are fire emergencies handled? Who is responsible for clearing patients from the office?

❑ **Emergency procedures for patient accidental injury**—How are patient injuries handled in the office? Under what circumstances are emergency personnel called to the office?

❑ **Jury duty**—How should employees notify the office of jury duty? Does the office pay employees during jury duty?

Figure 16-4 ◆ Common personnel manual items.

in **organizational charts** (Figure 16-5 ◆). Organizational charts are maps to office hierarchies, from physicians to entry-level staff. Members of the healthcare team should be able to use these charts to identify their supervisors, as well as their supervisors' supervisors, all the way to the top of the chain of command. In addition to reporting structure, an organizational chart might explain how employees can contact varied healthcare staff.

Outlining Clinical Procedures

Any clinical procedure that requires patient intervention should be documented for employee reference. Procedures should clearly list appropriate steps, as well as information on patient education, documentation, and infection control. The type of clinical procedures found in a policies and procedures manual varies according to the type of medical practice and the physician's specialty.

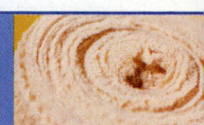

PROCEDURE 16-2 Create a Clinical Procedure for the Procedure Manual

Theory and Rationale

Just as with administrative, infection control, personnel, quality improvement, or risk management procedures, clinical procedures must be clear in order for medical assistants to perform them at the required standard.

Materials

- Computer with word processing software

Competency

(**Conditions**) With the necessary materials, you will be able to (**Task**) create a clinical procedure for an office procedure manual (**Standards**) correctly within the time limit set by the instructor.

1. Determine the type of clinical procedure for which you need to create a written description.
2. Gather the information on how this clinical procedure should be performed.
3. Title the procedure (e.g., "Collecting a Urine Sample").
4. Describe the policy's purpose (e.g., "Purpose: To describe the method for collecting a urine sample from a patient").
5. List each step in the procedure.
6. Print the procedure and give it to the office manager for approval.
7. Once approved, place the procedure in the clinical portion of the office procedure manual.

Outlining Administrative Procedures

Administrative procedures should be documented to include such topics as:

- Office opening and closing
- Inventory and supply ordering
- Appointment scheduling
- Patient accounting and bookkeeping
- Insurance processing
- Insurance benefit verification
- Patients' records release
- Medical records management
- Operation of administrative office machinery

Like clinical procedures, administrative procedures vary according to the type of medical practice, but the vast majority of administrative policies remain constant from office to office (Figure 16-6 ◆).

 ## Critical Thinking Question 16-3

How should Monte determine which policies should appear in his office's policy manual?

Documenting Infection Control Procedures

Infection control procedures should be written for all of a medical office's applicable procedures, including the following:

- Biohazardous waste disposal
- Employee needlestick injuries
- Employee exposure to infectious materials
- Employee education for infection control
- OSHA-required documentation
- Local, state, and federal reporting requirements for infectious agents

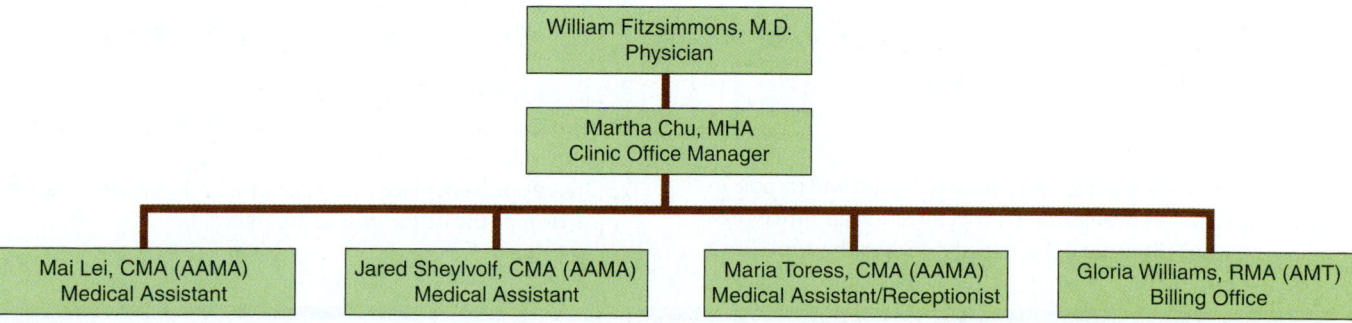

Fitzsimmons Family Practice Organization Chart

William Fitzsimmons, M.D.
Physician

Martha Chu, MHA
Clinic Office Manager

Mai Lei, CMA (AAMA)
Medical Assistant

Jared Sheylvolf, CMA (AAMA)
Medical Assistant

Maria Toress, CMA (AAMA)
Medical Assistant/Receptionist

Gloria Williams, RMA (AMT)
Billing Office

Figure 16-5 ◆ Sample organizational chart for a medical office.

Policy: Releasing Medical Records to a Patient

Purpose: To release medical records to the patient following legal guidelines.

❏ Verify the patient's identity by requesting photo identification.

❏ Obtain the patient's signature on the release of records form.

❏ Ensure the patient has dated the release form.

❏ Check to see if the patient has made any alterations to the release form, such as restricting the records release to a limited date.

❏ Check to see if the patient has checked the boxes allowing release of information regarding HIV/AIDS, reproductive health, mental health, or drug and alcohol rehabilitation.

❏ Pull the patient's medical record.

❏ Photocopy the appropriate parts of the medical record according to any limitations noted by the patient on the release form.

❏ Send copies of the records to the patient.

❏ Note in the patient's file when the records were released.

❏ File the original signed release form.

Figure 16-6 ◆ Sample administrative procedure.

As mandated by OSHA, infection control procedures must be part of the office's exposure control plan, which must be kept separate from other procedure manuals in the office and must be made available to an OSHA inspector if needed.

In Practice

Anka is a registered medical assistant working for Dr. Radliffe. While Anka is finishing a blood draw on a patient, she accidentally sticks herself with the contaminated needle. How will Anka know what to do now that this injury has happened?

Creating Quality Improvement and Risk Management Procedures

Quality improvement and risk management procedures are designed to reduce patient or staff injury in the medical office. These policies range from information on washing children's toys in the reception room to handling life-threatening patient events in the office. While quality improvement and risk management procedures policies vary according to office needs, the vast majority apply to all office types. According to HIPAA, quality improvement and risk management procedures must be kept in a separate notebook that is clearly marked and updated regularly.

Writing Other Office Policies

To ensure ongoing compliance and relevance, all medical office policies should be reviewed and updated regularly. Many large medical offices separate their policy manuals into clinical and

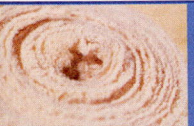

PROCEDURE 16-3   Create an Administrative Procedure for the Procedure Manual

Theory and Rationale
Medical offices need clearly written policies and procedures for all members of the healthcare team to understand how each task is performed.

Materials
■ Computer with word-processing software

Competency
(**Conditions**) With the necessary materials, you will be able to (**Task**) create an administrative procedure for an office procedure manual (**Standards**) correctly within the time limit set by the instructor.

1. Determine the type of procedure to be created.
2. Gather the information on how this administrative procedure is to be performed.
3. Title the procedure (e.g., "Policy: Sorting Incoming Mail").
4. Describe the policy's purpose (e.g., "Purpose: To describe the method of routing incoming mail to appropriate staff").
5. List each step in the procedure.
6. Print the procedure, and give it to the office manager for approval.
7. Once approved, place the procedure in the administrative portion of the office procedure manual.

administrative sections. Some offices further divide their manuals according to position or department. Table 16-1 identifies policies that may be found in medical office policy and procedure manuals.

TABLE 16-1 SAMPLE POLICIES AND PROCEDURES

Policy or Procedure	Purpose
Emergency Closure Policy	Outlines the steps to take in the event the office closes due to emergency
Building Lockup Policy	Describes the steps to take to lock the building at the end of the day
Publications and Distribution Policy	Outlines the policy with regard to allowing publications or pamphlets to be distributed to patients and staff
Smoking Policy	Describes the availability of smoking areas near the office
Personal Relationships Between Office Staff	Outlines the policy for personal relationships between coworkers
Personal Relationships Between Staff and Patients	Outlines the policy for personal relationships between office staff and patients
Termination Policy	Describes the policy for terminating employment
Disciplinary Policy	Describes the policy for disciplining of employees. Includes an outline of the offenses justifying discipline
Grievance Policy	Describes the process staff must follow to file grievances
Continuing Education	Outlines the requirements for continuing education
Malpractice Insurance	Describes the requirements for holding malpractice insurance
Reimbursement for Seminars	Outlines the policy for reimbursing staff who attend medical-related seminars
Computers for Personal Use Policy	Describes the policy for personal use of office computers
Petty Cash Funds	Describes the policy for using petty cash, including the type of expenses that qualify as petty cash and the amount to be kept as petty cash
Parking Policy	Outlines where employees may park, as well as reimbursement for parking expenses
Dress Code Policy	Describes the dress code for each office position
Opening Office Policy	Outlines the steps to take to open the office at the beginning of the day
Disclosure of Patient Information Policy	Describes the procedure for disclosing patient information, including the forms required and the Health Insurance Portability and Accountability Act (HIPAA regulations
Job Descriptions	Provides a job description for each office position
HIPAA Privacy Officer Duties	Outlines the duties of the HIPAA privacy officer in the medical office
Calling Patients from the Reception Room	Describes the procedure for calling patients from the reception room
Missed Patient Appointments	Describes the steps to take when patients miss their appointments. Includes proper charting technique
Termination of the Physician/Patient Relationship	Outlines the steps to legally terminate the physician/patient relationship
E-mail Policy	Describes the conditions under which the medical office may e-mail information to patients or other facilities
Obtaining Consent for a Procedure	Describes the consent forms used in the medical office and outlines the process of witnessing patient signatures
Prescription Refill Requests	Outlines the policy for taking telephone calls for prescription refills, including documentation in the patient's medical record
Jury Duty Policy	Describes the policy for employees called for jury duty
Sick Leave Policy	Describes the policy for employees who take sick leave
Personal Telephone Calls	Describes the policy for employees making and receiving personal telephone calls

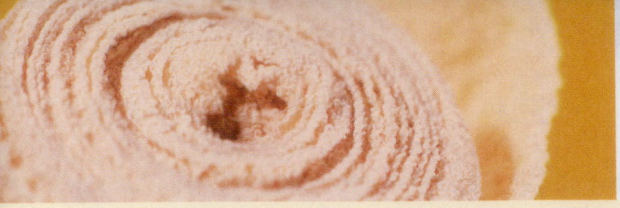

REVIEW

Chapter Summary

- Informational pamphlets are effective vehicles for educating patients.
- Office personnel manuals are needed to ensure all members of the healthcare team perform appropriately and to consistent standards.
- A policies and procedure manual in the medical office serves as written record of the legal, desired behavior of all health-care staff.

Chapter Review

Multiple Choice

1. Any _____ procedure that requires patient intervention should be documented for patient reference.
   a. clinical
   b. administrative
   c. infection control
   d. all of the above

2. Quality improvement and risk management procedures are designed to
   a. reduce patient injury.
   b. limit employee injury.
   c. avoid liability lawsuits.
   d. all of the above.

3. A procedure for filing insurance claims would be found under which policies section of the office procedure manual?
   a. Clinical
   b. Infection control
   c. Risk management
   d. Administrative

4. Once a policy and procedure manual has been written, it should be updated
   a. once a month.
   b. once a year.
   c. once every five years.
   d. as a policy or procedure changes.

5. The office mission statement should be shared with
   a. administrative staff.
   b. clinical staff.
   c. patients.
   d. all of the above.
   e. A and B.

True/False

T F 1. Only the office manager can compose a procedure for the office manual.

T F 2. An organizational chart outlines the chain of command in the office.

T F 3. By strictly following a policy and procedure manual, medical office management gives the impression that all staff members will be treated consistently.

T F 4. Office policies for quality improvement and risk management must be kept in a separate notebook.

T F 5. Compulsory means choosing to participate.

Short Answer

1. List the sections all policy and procedure manuals should include.

2. What is the purpose of an office mission statement?

3. Give five examples of an administrative policy.

4. Give five examples of a clinical policy.

5. Give five examples of a quality improvement or risk management policy.

6. Give five examples of an infection control policy.

7. Differentiate between a policy and a procedure.

8. Describe the steps to take to create an educational brochure.

9. Why might a medical office have separate policy and procedure manuals for its administrative and clinical areas?

10. Differentiate between a clinical policy and an administrative policy.

Research

1. Search online for policy and procedure manuals for medical facilities. Describe what each of these companies has in common with one another.

2. Call a local medical office. Ask the office manager if the office has a policy and procedure manual. How often is it updated? How are employees given access to the manual?

3. Search the Internet for companies that make office educational brochures. What type of information can you get ready-made pamphlets for?

Externship Application Experience

Manuel is unsure how to handle a patient who refuses to schedule a followup appointment. He asks two other members of the healthcare team to explain the office policy for proceeding and receives two vastly different responses. Should Manuel follow the advice of one staff member over the other? How can he know how this situation is supposed to be handled?

Resource Guide

Employee Manual (offers downloadable and customizable employee manuals)
www.theemployeemanual.com/

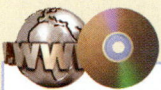

Med**Media**

http://www.MyMAKit.com

More on this chapter, including interactive resources, can be found on the Student CD-ROM accompanying this textbook and on http://www.MyMAKit.com.

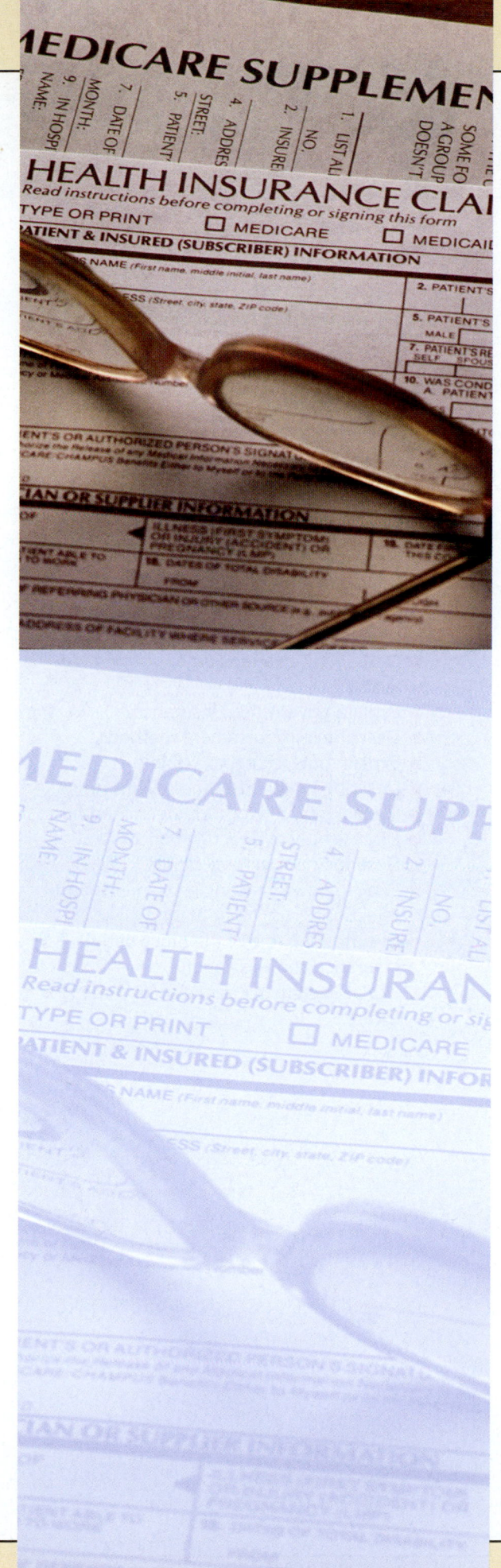

Understanding Health Insurance: Billing and Coding Procedures

Chapter 17   Insurance Billing and Authorizations
Chapter 18   ICD-9-CM Coding
Chapter 19   Procedural Coding

My name is Teresa Godyn. I have been working as a medical assistant for about a year. One of the things I have found when working in the medical field is that medical assistants have to remember that we are not just performing a task, but providing patients with a sense of comfort and well-being. We offer this by being conscientious about how we deliver pertinent information. Leaving phone messages plays a dominant role in patient communication when patients are out of the office. A patient may feel frustrated because a needed medication cannot be authorized through insurance, a diagnostic is not covered, or a specialist appointment may not be available in a timely fashion. The way the medical assistant handles this can dramatically change the way a patient views the quality of their healthcare.

Making sure the patient can hear a caring, empathetic tone is important. Though we only hear of their aches and pains, from time to time these can be all encompassing for your patient. I have found that truly listening to my patients shows them I care about them.

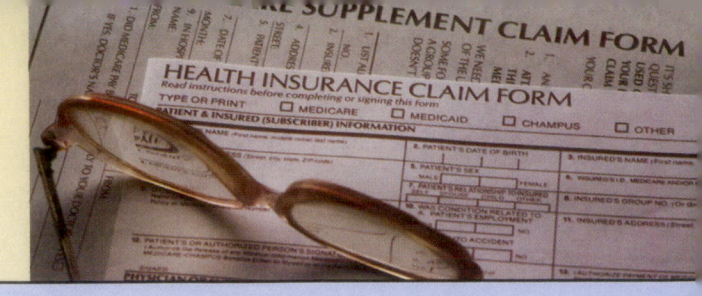

CHAPTER 17

Insurance Billing and Authorizations

Case Study

Martin Zamora is a patient at Woodway Health Care. Martin has recently gotten married and his new wife has health coverage through her employer. Martin says he believes his wife's coverage is better than what he has through his own employer, and he wants her policy billed for his care.

Objectives

After completing this chapter, you should be able to:

- Define and spell the key terminology in this chapter.
- Define the medical assistant's role in insurance claim processing.
- Describe the history of health insurance.
- Define health insurance terminology.
- Describe private health insurance and the various sources of coverage.
- Describe the types of managed care plans.
- Describe the various types of coverage available.
- Explain government insurance.
- Describe reimbursement methods.
- Explain how to prepare claims.
- Describe health insurance claims forms.
- Explain how to work with fee schedules.
- Discuss how to post payments.
- Describe how to trace claims.
- Explain how to reconcile payments and rejections.
- Describe the role of the office of the insurance commissioner.
- Explain health insurance costs in the future.

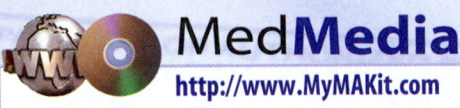

MedMedia
http://www.MyMAKit.com

Additional interactive resources and activities for this chapter can be found on http://www.MyMAKit.com. For a video on getting precertification, tips, audio glossary, legal and ethical scenarios, on-the-job scenarios, quizzes, and games related to the content of this chapter, please access the accompanying CD-ROM in this book.

Video: *Getting Precertification*
Legal and Ethical Scenario: *Insurance Billing and Authorizations*
On the Job Scenario: *Insurance Billing and Authorizations*
Tips
Multiple Choice Quiz
Audio Glossary
HIPAA Quiz
Games: Spelling Bee, Crossword, and Strikeout

MEDICAL ASSISTING STANDARDS

CAAHEP ENTRY-LEVEL STANDARDS	ABHES ENTRY-LEVEL COMPETENCIES
■ Perform within scope of practice (psychomotor) ■ Apply ethical behaviors, including honesty/integrity in performance of medical assisting practice (affective) ■ Explore issue of confidentiality as it applies to the medical assistant (cognitive) ■ Respond to issues of confidentiality (psychomotor) ■ Demonstrate sensitivity to patient rights (affective) ■ Identify types of insurance plans (cognitive) ■ Discuss referral process for patients in a managed care program (cognitive) ■ Apply both managed care policies and procedures (psychomotor) ■ Identify models of managed care (cognitive) ■ Discuss workers' compensation as it applies to patients (cognitive) ■ Apply third party guidelines (psychomotor) ■ Demonstrate assertive communication with managed care and/or insurance providers (affective) ■ Complete insurance claim forms (psychomotor) ■ Obtain precertification, including documentation (psychomotor) ■ Obtain preauthorization, including documentation (psychomotor) ■ Describe procedures for implementing both managed care and insurance plans (cognitive) ■ Demonstrate sensitivity in communicating with both providers and patients (affective) ■ Obtain precertification, including documentation (psychomotor) ■ Obtain preauthorization, including documentation (psychomotor) ■ Discuss how guidelines are used in processing an insurance claim (cognitive) ■ Compare processes for filing insurance claims both manually and electronically (cognitive) ■ Describe guidelines for third-party claims (cognitive) ■ Discuss types of physician fee schedules (cognitive) ■ Describe the concept of RBRVS (cognitive) ■ Define Diagnosis-Related Groups (DRGs) (cognitive) ■ Communicate in a language the patient can understand regarding managed care and insurance plans (affective)	■ Maintain confidentiality at all times ■ Use appropriate guidelines when releasing records or information ■ Be cognizant of ethical boundaries ■ Monitor legislation related to current healthcare issues and practices ■ Apply computer concepts for office procedures ■ Use manual and computerized bookkeeping systems ■ Serve as a liaison between physician and others ■ Perform billing and collection procedures ■ Exercise efficient time management ■ Receive, organize, prioritize, and transmit information expediently ■ Analyze and use current third-party guidelines for reimbursement ■ Perform billing and collection procedures ■ Complete insurance claim forms ■ Implement current procedural terminology and ICD-9 coding ■ Use physician fee schedule

Key Terminology

abstracting—the process of locating data in multiple source documents and accurately transferring it to a form

accept assignment—physician agrees to accept the amount approved by the insurance company as payment in full for a given service

advance beneficiary notice—a form patients sign agreeing to pay for covered Medicare services that may be denied due to medical necessity or frequency

allowed amount—the dollar amount for a service that an insurance company considers acceptable and uses to determine benefit payments; also called *approved amount*

ancillary coverage—insurance coverage for services provided by other than a physician or hospital, such as dental, vision, or chiropractic care

appeal—process of asking for a review of a denied service or claim

approved amount—see *allowed amount*

assignment of benefits—request made by a patient to allow the insurance carrier to pay the healthcare professional directly rather than issuing monies to the patient

balance billing—billing a patient for the dollar difference between the provider's charge and the insurance approved amount; usually not permitted for participating providers

beneficiary—person who is eligible to receive benefits/services under an insurance policy

birthday rule—according to this rule, the parent with the birthday earlier in the year is the primary carrier for the children; the parent with the later birthday is the secondary carrier

bundling—combining multiple services under a single all inclusive CPT code and one charge

capitation plans—healthcare plans in which providers are paid set fees per month per member patients

caretaker—person or entity responsible for determining when and if a patient needs specific types of healthcare; also called gatekeeper or primary care provider (PCP)

carve outs—services that are reimbursed in addition to the base rate for the patient

Key Terminology *(continued)*

catastrophic—large and usually unforeseen

categorically needy—Medicaid eligible patients who qualify for cash assistance as well as medical services

certificate of coverage—a letter from the insurance company that provides proof of type and timeframe of coverage when a patient terminates a health insurance policy

CHAMPVA—insurance plan administered by the Civilian Health and Medical Program of the Veterans Administration that covers dependents of veterans who have total and permanent service-connected disabilities

charge slip—document on which the physician indicates procedure and diagnosis codes; also called a routing slip or an encounter form

clean claim—insurance claim with no errors

coinsurance—percentage of medical charges patients are responsible for according to their insurance plan contracts

commercial insurance—see *private insurance*

consumer-directed healthcare plans—health insurance plans that place patients in charge of how their healthcare dollars are spent

conversion factor—a constant dollar value multiplied by the relative value unit to determine the price of individual services

coordination of benefits—the process of determining which insurance policy should be billed first, second, or third, when a patient is covered by multiple policies

copayment—set dollar fee per visit or service that patients are responsible for according to their insurance plan contracts

covered—services potentially eligible for reimbursement

deductible—monetary amount patients must pay to the provider for healthcare services before their health insurance benefits begin to pay

denied—a claim processed by an insurer and determined not eligible for payment

dependent—a family member or other individual who qualifies for coverage on the insured's policy; also called beneficiary. See also *insured; policyholder*

disability insurance—insurance that covers lost wages and certain other benefits due to a disability that prevents the individual from working

elective procedure—procedure that will benefit the patient but does not need to be scheduled immediately

eligibility—the process to determine if a patient is qualified to receive coverage/paid benefits according to the insurance policy guidelines

end stage renal disease—total or nearly complete failure of the kidneys

encounter form—document on which the physician indicates procedure and diagnosis codes; also called a routing slip or charge slip

exclusive provider organization—a managed care contract with a smaller network of providers under which the employer agrees to not use any other networks in return for favorable pricing

exclusions—procedures or services not covered under an insurance plan

explanation of benefits—a statement that accompanies payment from the insurance company that summarizes how the payment for each billed service was calculated and gives reasons for any items not paid

fee-for-service—process in which insurance companies pay providers fees for each service provided to covered patients

fee schedule—list of the approved fees insurance carriers agree to pay to participating providers who agree to contract with the carriers. Also refers to the standard set of fees the provider charges to all insurers

flexible spending account—account into which employees place pretax earnings for projected medical expenses; also called *healthcare reimbursement account*

form locators—the boxes to be completed on the CMS-1500 claim form

formulary—tiered list of drugs covered by an insurance company

gatekeeper—see *caretaker*

generic drugs—low-cost medications that duplicate their name-brand counterparts in active ingredient and effect

geographic adjustment factor—a numeric multiplier used by Medicare to adjust fees for the varying costs of practicing medicine in different areas of the country

group health insurance—a commercial insurance policy with rates based on a group of people, usually offered by an employer

health maintenance organization—a group of physicians or medical center that provides comprehensive service to members under a capitated payment plan; members' care is covered only when using these designated providers

health savings account—tax-free savings accounts used for medical expenses in conjunction with a high-deductible health plan

healthcare reimbursement account—see *flexible spending account*

hospice—facility or service for patients who are diagnosed with terminal illnesses and are expected to have six or fewer months to live

hospital services—patient care provided by a licensed acute care hospital

indemnity—see *fee-for-service*

individual health insurance—a commercial insurance policy with rates based on individual health criteria

individual practice association—HMOs that are the most decentralized and involve contracting with individual physicians to create a healthcare delivery system

inpatient—a person who is admitted to the hospital for a minimum of 24 hours

insured—person who holds or owns an insurance policy; same as the member or the policyholder

liability insurance—type of insurance that covers injuries that occur on, in, or because of the insured's property

lifetime maximum benefit—monetary amount allowed by an insurance carrier for a covered member's covered expenses over the member's lifetime

limiting charge—the maximum amount a Medicare non-PAR provider may bill the patient on an unassigned claim; 115% of the non-PAR fee schedule

long-term care—insurance that covers lost wages and certain other benefits due to a disability that prevents the individual from working, usually for more than one year

managed care—a system of healthcare delivery focused on reducing costs by transferring risk to the provider and may limit the type and frequency of care members may receive

Medicaid—a joint federal and state program that helps with medical costs for some people with low incomes and limited resources

medical necessity—criteria establishing when a service is appropriate

medically needy—Medicaid-eligible patients who are eligible for medical services, but not cash assistance

medical savings account—tax-free savings accounts for small employers and self employed; used for medical expenses in conjunction with a high-deductible health plan

Medicare—federal program that covers medical expenses for those aged 65 and over, those with end-stage renal disease, and those with long-term disabilities

member—the person who owns the insurance policy

negotiated fee schedule—a common reimbursement method in managed care whereby the MCO develops a list of fees for providers that they agree to accept in the participating provider contract; fees may be determined based on a percentage of the provider's usual fee or arrived at through negotiation

non-covered—services not eligible for reimbursement under any circumstance

non-participating provider—healthcare provider who has not contracted with a particular health insurance carrier

outliers—exceptional circumstances that cost far more or less than the average

outpatient—a person who receives medical care at a hospital or other medical facility but who is not admitted for more than 24 hours

participating provider—healthcare provider who has contracted with a particular health insurance carrier

past timely filing limits—time beyond which an insurance carrier will accept an insurance claim

payer number—unique identifying number assigned to each insurance carrier for the purpose of directing electronic claims

per case—*per case* payment method used for hospitals. Under this method, the hospital receives a pre-established amount per patient for the entire stay, based on the patients diagnosis, regardless of how long they are in or what services are provided

per diem—*per day* payment method whereby the facility is paid a flat amount per day the patient remains, regardless of what services are provided

physician services—patient care provided by a licensed physician

point of service—an insurance offering in which a patient has access to multiple plans, such as an HMO, PPO, and indemnity, and may choose to use any of them for any given service

policyholder—person who holds or owns an insurance policy; same as the member or the insured

preauthorization—approval for treatment or service obtained from an insurance company before the care is provided

precertification—see *preauthorization*

pre-existing condition—condition for which a patient received treatment in a certain period before beginning coverage with a new insurance plan

preferred provider—organization that contracts with independent providers to perform services for members at discounted rates

premium—dollar amount paid to the insurance company to have coverage in force; usually paid monthly; employers may pay part or all of the premium as an employee benefit

preventive care—healthcare designed to keep a person healthy

private insurance—insurance not provided by the government but by an independent not-for-profit or for-profit company; also called *commercial insurance*

rejected—a claim that is returned to the provider without processing due to a technical error

relative value unit—unit of measure assigned to medical services based on the resources required to provide it; includes work, practice expense, and liability insurance

resource-based relative value scale—the methodology Medicare uses to establish physician fees, based on the relative value unit, the geographic adjustment factor, and the conversion factor

respite care—temporary care provided by an outside party to relieve the usual caregiver

self-insurance—type of insurance where rather than purchasing a commercial insurance policy, an employer sets aside a large reserve fund to directly reimburse employees for medical expenses

skilled nursing facility—a licensed facility that primarily provides inpatient, skilled nursing care to patients who require medical, nursing, or rehabilitative services but does not provide the level of care or treatment available in a hospital

sliding fee scale—a provider's fee schedule that charges varying fees for a service based on a patient's financial ability to pay

staff model HMO—employs salaried physicians who treat members in facilities owned and operated by the HMO

stop loss—the maximum amount the patient must pay out-of-pocket for copayments and coinsurance

subscriber—person who holds or owns an insurance policy; same as the member or the insured

superbill—document on which the physician indicates procedure and diagnosis codes; also called a routing slip or an encounter form

third-party administrator—a company that processes paperwork for claims for a self-insured employer

TRICARE—health insurance administered by the U.S Department of Defense for active duty military personnel, retired service personnel, and their eligible dependents; formerly known as Civilian Health and Medical Program (CHAMPUS)

unbundling—billing multiple services with separate CPT codes and separate charges that should be combined under a single CPT code and one charge

usual, customary, and reasonable (UCR) fee—a fee determined by third-party payers to reimburse providers based on the provider's normal fee, the range of fees charged by providers of the same specialty in the same geographic area, and other factors to determine appropriate fees in unusual situations

waiting period—period after a new health insurance plan begins during which certain services are not covered

waiver—see *advance beneficiary notice*

worker's compensation—insurance coverage for job-related illness or injury provided by employers by law

Abbreviations

ABN—advance beneficiary notice

ADA—American Dental Association

CDHP—consumer-directed health plan

CF—conversion factor

CHAMPVA—Civilian Health and Medical Program of the Veterans Administration

CMS—Centers for Medicare and Medicaid Services

COB—coordination of benefits

COBRA—Consolidated Omnibus Budget Reconciliation Act

CPT—Current Procedural Terminology

CSRS—civil service

DEERS—defense enrollment eligibility reporting system

DME—durable medical equipment

EMC—electronic media claims

EOB—explanation of benefits

EPO—exclusive provider organization

ESRD—end stage renal disease

FERS—federal employee retirement system

FL—form locator

FSA—flexible spending account

GAF—geographic adjustment factor

HCFA—Health Care Financing Administration

HCRA—healthcare reimbursement account

HIPAA—Health Insurance Portability and Accountability Act

HMO—health maintenance organization

HSA—health savings account

ICD-9-CM—*International Classification of Diseases,* 9th ed., *Clinical Modification*

IRS—Internal Revenue Service

LC—limiting charge (Medicare)

MAC—Medicare administrative contractor

MCO—managed care organization

MSA—medical savings account

MSP—Medicare secondary payer

NON-PAR—non-participating physician (Medicare)

NPI—national provider identifier

PCP—primary care provider

PIP—personal injury protection

POS—point of service

PPO—preferred provider organization

RBRVS—resource-based relative value scale

RVU—relative value unit

SCHIP—State Children's Health Insurance Program

Abbreviations *(continued)*

SSDI—Social Security Disability Insurance
SSI—Supplemental Security Income
TEFRA—Tax Equity and Fiscal Responsibility Act

TPA—third-party administrator
TPL—third-party liability
UCR—usual, customary, and reasonable

UPIN—unique provider identification number

 COMPETENCY SKILLS PERFORMANCE

1. Calculate deductible, coinsurance, and allowable amounts.
2. Verify a patient's insurance eligibility.
3. Obtain a managed care referral.
4. Obtain authorization from an insurance company for a procedure.
5. Abstract data to complete a paper CMS-1500 form.
6. Complete a computerized insurance claim form.
7. Handle a denied insurance claim.

Introduction

Processing insurance claims accurately is vital to the success of any medical practice. Just as basic knowledge of medical terminology is the first step to medical assisting success, an understanding of basic insurance terminology is vital to those responsible for processing claims.

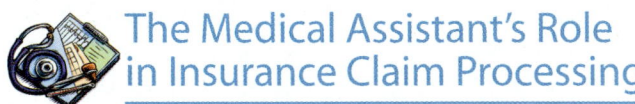

The Medical Assistant's Role in Insurance Claim Processing

Medical assistants must be able to answer patients' questions regarding how managed care works and how owed amounts are determined for any given procedure. Medical assistants must also be able to verify patients' insurance coverage and explain that coverage to the patients. In addition, MAs must know how to process health insurance claims accurately, follow up on past-due claims, and pursue accounts collection. Medical assistants must possess an understanding of how medical insurance is applied in various situations in order to be an advocate for patients. Since patients are not commonly aware of their insurance coverage, it is up to the medical assistant to check to see if authorizations are needed and to obtain them if necessary.

Developing skills in this area will enable the MA to be a patient advocate, helping patients obtain the benefits they are eligible for and helping them understand the reasons when a cost is not covered. Just as in other areas of medical assisting, the medical assistant's involvement in the insurance billing area will depend on the type of practice. In a large physician's office, there often is a separate department that handles most of the insurance matters. In a smaller office, the medical assistant may have more responsibilities in this area. Regardless of the type or size of office, in every situation the medical assistant is a vital team player in helping patients access their insurance benefits.

The History of Health Insurance

Health insurance in the United States began in the mid-1800s, when it was used to replace the income of people injured in accidents or ill from certain diseases. The first group policy giving comprehensive benefits was offered by Massachusetts Health Insurance of Boston in 1847. Insurance companies issued the first individual disability and illness policies around 1890. Hospital insurance coverage began in 1929, when a group of schoolteachers in Texas formed a contract with a local hospital to guarantee up to 21 days of hospital care for a premium of $6 per year. This plan became quite popular, and other groups of employers joined the plan, which eventually became known as the Blue Cross Plan.

During World War II, when wages were frozen, employers began offering their employees **group health insurance** as a benefit. Group health insurance plans cover entire groups of individuals, usually through employers or other large associations or defined groups. These early plans were designed to protect employees from the high costs of hospitalization and eventually evolved into the healthcare plans common today.

Employee benefit plans became popular in the 1940s and 1950s. The unions that represented large groups of workers bargained for better benefit packages, including tax-free, employer-sponsored health insurance.

During the 1950s and 1960s government programs began to cover healthcare costs. Social security coverage included disability benefits for the first time in 1954, and the government created the Medicare and Medicaid programs in 1965. By the end of 1995, individuals and companies paid for about one-half of the healthcare received in the United States, with the government paying for the other half.

The 1980s and 1990s saw a rapid rise in the cost of healthcare. During this time the majority of employer-sponsored group insurance plans moved to less expensive managed care plans. This move had been facilitated by the federal HMO Act of 1973, which allowed use of federal funds and policy to promote health maintenance organizations (HMOs), and the Tax Equity and Fiscal Responsibility Act (TEFRA) in 1982, which made it easier and more attractive for HMOs to contract with the Medicare program. By the mid-1990s, most Americans who had health insurance were enrolled in managed care plans.

Patient Education

Although most insurance plans began as safety mechanisms in the event of **catastrophic** health events, most plans today cover **preventive care**. Catastrophic health events are defined as chronic illnesses or serious injuries that require expensive, specialized, or long-term care. An example is a person diagnosed with cancer or a person who needs several surgeries after a serious accident. Preventive care is care a patient receives to stay well. Examples include well-child checks and yearly mammograms or physicals.

Health Insurance Today

Today, Americans obtain health insurance from a variety of sources. Medical assistants need to be knowledgeable about the rules and requirements of each. These will be discussed in detail later in the chapter.

About half of insured people in the United States have health insurance through a private or commercial insurance company. Usually this is through a **group health insurance** policy sponsored by an employer. Some employers **self-insure**, paying directly for employees' medical bills. Individuals who do not have employer-sponsored health insurance may purchase an **individual health insurance** policy. **Liability insurance**, such as automobile and homeowner insurance, provides for medical expenses related to certain accidents.

Most Americans who do not have private insurance receive health insurance benefits from the state or federal government. Government programs include **Medicare**, a federal program for persons over age 65, the disabled, and **end stage renal disease** (**ESRD**) patients; **Medicaid**, a federal/state program primarily for low-income people; **TRICARE**, for active duty and retired service personnel and their families; and **CHAMPVA** for veterans with service-related disabilities. **Workers' compensation** provides coverage for employees for job-related injuries or illnesses.

Despite the many options available for health insurance, it is estimated that 45 to 50 million people in the United State have no health insurance coverage. Often this is because individuals do not have or do not qualify for employer-based coverage, do not qualify for federal programs, or cannot afford individual policies. For these patients, many offices establish a **sliding fee scale** that charges fees based on a patient's financial ability to pay. Some cities also have free or low cost clinics established and run by volunteers or not-for-profit agencies.

In addition to determining the source of patients' insurance, medical assistants need to determine what type of coverage they have. Insurance may cover **hospital services, physician services,** preventive care, catastrophic care, **long-term care, ancillary** services such as prescription drugs, vision, dental, chiropractic, and special risks such as cancer. With each type of coverage and each source of coverage, medical assistants need to identify how patients' insurance relates to the specific services being provided in a specific situation. Research, attention to detail, careful communication, and patient advocacy are skills that successful medical assistants use in the insurance arena.

Health Insurance Terminology

Just as medical assistants need to understand medical terminology to provide physical care for patients, a knowledge of insurance terminology is critical to helping patients utilize their health insurance. In many situations, there are multiple terms that essentially have the same meanings. In other situations, terms that seem similar to the layperson have different and specific meanings in the world of health insurance. Patients are often unfamiliar with their insurance benefits and may not understand the terms they hear. Medical assistants who understand insurance terms can advocate for patients and communicate in ways that patients understand.

Members and Their Families

Health insurance, also called medical insurance, is a contract between an insurance carrier and the person who owns the insurance policy, known as the **member**, **subscriber**, **insured**, or **policyholder**. For those who receive insurance through their employers, the member is the employee. For those who buy individual policies, the member is the person who purchased the plan. For those covered by government policies, the term **beneficiary** is often used and refers to the individual who qualifies for the program.

Many commercial policies allow members to include family members on the plan. Family members are called **dependents** and may include a spouse, children, unmarried domestic partners, and stepchildren. Inclusion of family members is not automatic and it is possible for some, but not all, family members to be covered. The member must obtain forms from the employer or the insurance company to specifically designate dependents' coverage. The medical assistant will need to ask the patient, and possibly call the insurance company, to determine who is eligible for benefits. It is also important to know exactly how each dependent is legally related to the member.

Premiums

In order to obtain a commercial health insurance policy, the policyholder pays a **premium** to the insurance carrier. The premium is usually paid in monthly installments for the next month's coverage. In group coverage, the employer often pays the majority of the premium and employees authorize the remainder to be deducted from paychecks. If dependent coverage is selected, the premium is higher. Some government plans require a premium as well.

Fee Schedules and Approved Amounts

Providers establish a **fee schedule**, which lists their charge for each service they provide. This is normally organized by type of service and CPT code (see Figure 17-1 ◆). Providers may set their charges in any manner they desire; however, in most states they are required to charge the same fee to every patient and every insurance company. They cannot discuss their fees with other providers and use that information to set prices, a practice known as price fixing. The charge on the fee schedule is known as the providers usual charge.

Insurance companies are not required to pay providers' usual charges. Insurers can use any method they desire to establish a payment level. Often they calculate what they determine to be an average or customary price among providers of the same specialty and in the same geographic area. This is called the approved or **allowed amount**. When a provider's actual charge is less than the allowed amount, the insurer will pay the actual charge. Providers cannot increase their charge for a given

New Patient Examinations		
Office Visit, Level 1	99201	$ 55.00
Office Visit, Level 2	99202	$110.00
Office Visit, Level 3	99203	$154.00
Office Visit, Level 4	99204	$226.00
Office Visit, Level 5	99205	$299.00
Established Patient Examinations		
Office Visit, Level 1	99211	$ 45.00
Office Visit, Level 2	99212	$ 60.00
Office Visit, Level 3	99213	$ 80.00
Office Visit, Level 4	99214	$123.00
Office Visit, Level 5	99215	$199.00

Figure 17-1 ◆ Sample fee schedule.

service to selected insurance companies in order to receive higher payment. When providers' charges are more than the insurance allowable, the insurance pays the allowed amount. This method of determining insurance payments is called **usual, customary, and reasonable (UCR)**. When calculating benefits and amounts owed, the first step is to identify the allowed charge.

Deductibles

Few health insurance plans cover 100 percent of the care patients receive, so patients will experience several different kinds of out-of-pocket expenses. Before the insurance plan pays any benefits, patients may have a **deductible** to meet. The deductible is a monetary amount patients must pay to the provider for healthcare services before health insurance benefits begin to pay. Deductible amounts can be as low as $100 or as high as $10,000. Plans with low deductibles tend to have higher premiums than plans with high deductibles. Some government plans also have deductibles. When calculating benefits and amounts owed, the second step is to subtract the deductible from the allowed charge (see Figure 17-2 ◆).

In some policies, the deductible will not be required for all services. A preventive care visit may not require a deductible, whereas a sick visit will. This is to encourage patients to seek preventive care. When patients include family members on the policy, there is usually an individual deductible and a family deductible. The individual deductible is the maximum deductible that any given family member must pay; the family deductible is the maximum deductible for all family members combined.

For example, John Jacobs is the policyholder and carries his wife Jeanne and his two children Jana and James on the policy. The individual deductible is $100, and the family deductible is $300. Jeanne receives medical care for a cost of $150, she pays her deductible of $100, and insurance benefits will apply to the

Scenario 1: Martina Kahlo has health insurance through her employer's plan. She has a $100 yearly deductible, and then she is covered at 100 percent. Martina sees Dr. Jacobson for an office call that includes lab work. The cost of the office call is $128. How much does Martina owe for her visit?

$128 charge for medical services.

$100 for Martina's annual deductible.

Martina must pay her $100 deductible. The insurance company will pay the $28 balance.

Scenario 2: Jorge Garcia has an individual health insurance plan. He has a $1,000 yearly deductible, and then he is covered at 80 percent. Jorge sees Dr. Jacobson for an office call that includes lab work and two X-rays. The cost of the office call is $217. How much does Jorge owe for his visit?

$217 charge for medical services.

$1,000 for Jorge's annual deductible.

Insurance company will pay $0 because Jorge has not met his $1,000 annual deductible. Jorge must pay the $217 charge.

Figure 17-2 ◆ Calculating a patient's insurance deductible.

remaining $50. A short time later, Jana becomes ill and sees the doctor for a charge of $50. The entire $50 will be applied to her deductible and must be paid out of pocket. Now the family has accumulated $150 toward the family deductible. Next, John receives care for $200. He has not met his individual deductible, and the family deductible has not been met yet. He will pay $100 out of pocket for his individual deductible and insurance benefits will apply to the remaining $100 of his bill. $250 of the family deductible has now been met. Unfortunately, James becomes ill and sees the doctor for a $100 visit. Even though he has not met his individual deductible, only $50 is owed on the family deductible, so $50 is paid out of pocket for James, and insurance benefits apply to the remaining $50. Now that the $300 family deductible has been met, no family member will be required to pay a deductible for the remainder of the year, even if the individual deductible for that dependent has not been met. The family deductible presents a savings for families of more than three members.

Copayments and Coinsurance

After the deductible is met, most patients still have out-of-pocket expenses they are responsible for. **Copayments** are set dollar amounts that patients pay at the time of service, such as $10 or $20 per visit. **Coinsurance** is a set percentage of charges that patients pay. An 80/20 coinsurance plan means that the insurance company pays 80 percent of approved charges and the patient pays 20 percent. A 70/30 plan means that the insurance company pays 70% of approved charges and the patient pays 30%. Different types of visits or different types of providers

may have different copayment or coinsurance amounts. For example, preventive care may have no copayment or coinsurance while sick care does. A specialist visit may require a higher copayment or coinsurance than a primary care visit. The specific rules are set by the insurance company and clearly spelled out in the patient's policy. Most government programs require a copayment or coinsurance.

When calculating benefits and amounts owed, after the deductible is subtracted from the allowed amount, coinsurance is calculated by multiplying the remaining balance times the coinsurance percentage. Then, subtract the copayment or coinsurance amount from the remaining balance.

When providers have a **participating** or **preferred** provider contract with the insurance company, they agree to accept the insurance allowed amount as payment in full and cannot bill patients the difference between their actual charge and the allowed amount. However, when the provider is not participating or contracted with an insurance company, the patient is responsible for the entire balance not covered by insurance. This is called **balance billing**. The insurance company calculates deductibles, coinsurance, and copayments based on the allowed amounts, which may be less than the provider's actual charge. Figure 17-3 ◆ shows how copayments and coinsurance amounts are calculated.

Stop Loss and Lifetime Maximum

Many insurance policies have **stop loss** and **lifetime maximum** benefits clauses. A stop loss is the maximum amount the patient must pay out-of-pocket for copayments and coinsurance. After this amount is reached in a year, the insurance pays 100% of the remaining expenses. The stop loss amount starts over the next year. Lifetime maximum benefit is the maximum amount the insurance company will pay for individual members over the course of the patient's life. A common lifetime maximum benefit is $1 million, but it could be as low as $100,000 in a very inexpensive policy. Sometimes patients will select a low cost policy and not be aware of provisions such as the lifetime maximum. While

Scenario 1: Dr. Jones charges $75 for an office call. Mary Smith is insured with Premera Blue Cross Insurance and has a 20 percent coinsurance obligation. Dr. Jones is a preferred provider with Premera Blue Cross and has agreed to accept $64.25 as payment in full for his office call. Mary owes 20 percent of the $64.25 fee ($12.85).

Scenario 2: Dr. Barro charges $70 for an office call. Molly Manchero is insured with Regence Blue Shield Insurance and has a $10 copayment obligation. Dr. Barro is a preferred provider with Regence Blue Shield and has agreed to accept $62.50 as payment in full for his office call. Molly owes $10 of the $62.50 fee.

Figure 17-3 ◆ Calculating copayments and coinsurance.

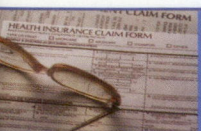

PROCEDURE 17-1 Calculate Deductible, Coinsurance, and Allowable Amounts

Theory and Rationale

The medical assistant will frequently explain to patients how their deductible, coinsurance, and allowable amounts are calculated. Attention to detail is very important as misquoted figures can be cause for patients to become dissatisfied with the medical staff.

Materials

- Pen
- Paper
- Insurance verification form
- Patient's insurance identification card

Competency

(**Conditions**) With the necessary materials, you will be able to (**Task**) calculate deductible, coinsurance, and allowable amounts (**Standards**) correctly within the time limit set by the instructor.

1. After the patient's insurance coverage has been verified, locate the information on the verification form regarding any deductible and coinsurance amount.
2. Inform the patient of the deductible amount that will need to be paid at the beginning of the calendar or fiscal year.
3. Explain to the patient that the amount charged for any particular procedure in the medical office will likely be reduced to a lower amount (called the allowed amount) when processed by the insurance carrier.
4. Imagine the patient has a $100 yearly deductible and a 10 percent copayment. The patient has had an examination, with a charge of $95.00, an X-ray with a charge of $75.00, and laboratory work with a charge of $102.00.
5. Imagine the insurance carrier in this situation allows $72.00 for the examination, $51.00 for the X-ray, and $80.00 for the laboratory work.
6. Calculate the patient's amount owing by adding the allowed figures to come to a total of allowed charges.
7. Subtract the $100.00 deductible from the total of the allowed charges.
8. Multiply the remaining allowed amount by 20 percent to determine the patient's coinsurance.
9. Add the $100.00 deductible to the 20 percent coinsurance amount to determine the amount the patient will need to pay out of pocket for the visit.
10. Explain the figures to the patient and collect the fees.

$1 million or even $100,000 may sound like a lot of money, medical expenses can accumulate very quickly with a serious illness such as cancer or an organ transplant.

Waiting Period, Exclusions, and Pre-Existing Conditions

In addition to out-of-pocket expenses, many health insurance plans have **waiting periods** and **exclusions** that limit what the insurance plan needs to pay in benefits. A waiting period is a set period of time that must pass before a member's **pre-existing condition** is covered. A pre-existing condition is any condition a patient was diagnosed with or treated for, including receiving prescription medications, before beginning coverage with a new insurance plan.

HIPAA Compliance

Although waiting periods for pre-existing condition coverage vary from one insurance plan to another, a pre-existing condition is covered without a waiting period when the patient has been insured the 24 months before joining the new plan. Therefore, if patients remain insured for 24 or more months, they can change jobs and retain pre-existing condition coverage without added waiting periods even when

they have chronic illnesses. Patients should obtain a **certificate of coverage** from the previous insurance plan. This letter documents the nature and length of coverage with the plan. Patients submit it to the new plan to establish proof of continuous coverage. If patients have had more than one insurance plan during the previous 24 months, certificates of coverage from each plan should be submitted. Even when patients have not been insured the 24 months before joining new insurance plans, Health Insurance Portability and Accountability Act (HIPAA) legislation restricts insurance companies from requiring patients to wait any longer than 12 months from the dates their new insurance coverage began.

Any uncovered services or diagnoses are called exclusions. Some plans exclude such things as routine eye exams and hearing tests. Others exclude any service related to an uncovered or excluded diagnosis. For instance, if a patient's insurance plan does not cover services related to a "hearing loss" diagnosis, that patient would have no coverage for hearing tests. If, however, that same patient presented with complaints of multiple ear infections, hearing tests with a diagnosis of "ear infection" may be covered.

Some insurance plans will not cover certain **elective procedures** considered medically unnecessary, such as some kinds of plastic surgery. Because the definition of "elective" varies between insurance plans, it is crucial that medical assistants verify eligibility for all procedures with patients' insurance carriers before providers perform services. It is also important to inform patients of all findings.

Private Health Insurance

An overview of the health insurance industry and a basic understanding of key insurance terms has been presented. Next is a discussion of private and commercial insurance.

A number of national commercial insurance carriers, including Blue Cross/Blue Shield, Aetna, and Cigna, offer health insurance coverage. Some national carriers offer both managed care and preferred provider policies; most offer policies that can be purchased secondary to Medicare. Policies through national commercial carriers might be purchased by employers for a group of employees or by individuals who lack health insurance through their places of employment. Coverage amounts and premiums vary according to policy type.

Sources of Coverage

The most common sources of private health insurance are group insurance through an employer or other organization, a self-insured plan through an employer or labor union, COBRA continuation of group coverage, and individual insurance.

Group Insurance

Group insurance is a policy offered to groups of people where the risk or cost of insurance is spread across everyone equally for a given level of coverage. It is usually the least expensive type of insurance because statistics show that a few people in a group will use a large amount of services, but many people in the group will use few if any services. Everyone pays the same rate for protection, so the high costs of a few members are shared equally by everyone in the group. The most common group is the employees of a company. However, various professional organizations also offer group coverage. Group insurance is the most common source of private insurance in the United States.

Employers initiate negotiations with an insurance company to cover their employees. Employers determine how large their financial budget is for employee health insurance premiums and how much they want employees to contribute toward the premium. The insurance company then presents a list of benefits available for that price. The more that can be paid in premiums, the more benefits will be available. Employers will select the insurance company and the benefit package that best meets the budget and the employees' anticipated needs.

It is common for an employer to allow employees to select among a variety of benefit packages from the chosen insurance company. The employer designates the amount the company will pay per month toward the premium, which is usually constant among all packages. Employees are able to select the package that best meets their needs for medical care and premium cost. Packages with high deductibles and copayments or coinsurance will cost less than packages with low deductibles and

out-of-pocket expenses. Employees may have the option to add dependents for an additional premium. Some employers pay part of the dependents' premiums and others require the employee to pay the full amount. Because most companies offer a variety of health insurance options for employees, two patients with the same employer and the same insurance company may have different benefits. Figure 17-4 ◆ gives such a sample scenario. To avoid giving out incorrect information, it is important for medical assistants to determine the specific benefits available to each patient. Often this information is available online through the insurer's secured Web site or by calling the insurance company.

Critical Thinking Question 17-1

How should the medical assistant explain to Martin that his wife will need to add him to her policy if she has not yet done so?

Employer-based coverage typically begins with the next calendar month following 30 days of employment, but this timeframe can vary. It is important to determine when coverage begins for a patient who has recently changed jobs. It is also important to determine when coverage ends for a patient leaving a job. Coverage may end the last day of employment, the end of the month, or the end of the following month.

Self-Insured Plan

For patients, health insurance through a self-insured plan is very similar to group insurance. In fact, employees may not even recognize the difference. An employer or labor union who self-insures does not purchase a policy through a commercial insurance company. Instead, it sets aside a large pool of money, or reserve, and uses that fund to reimburse employees for their healthcare expenses. Sometimes it will contract with a **third party administrator (TPA),** an outside company that processes the paperwork for claims, but any payments come from the employer's or labor union's funds, not an insurance company.

Two patients, Sara and George, present Premera Blue Cross insurance identification cards. ABC Marketing, a large employer that provides its employees an extensive insurance plan, employs Sara. Lone Star Plumbing, a small employer that has purchased a plan with minimal employee coverage, employs George. Although they present similar insurance cards, Sara and George have vastly different coverage.

Figure 17-4 ◆ Same insurance company, different benefits.

?— Critical Thinking Question 17-2-

Is it advisable to call the insurance carrier of Martin's wife to check on benefits and spousal eligibility? Why or why not?

COBRA Coverage

When employees have been covered under group insurance and leave employment, they may have the opportunity to continue the group coverage at their own expense. The premium is the same as that for the group, but because often the employer has been paying a large portion of the employees' premium, patients may be surprised at the cost of the premium. Nonetheless, the premium is usually less, and the benefits better, than an individual policy. This option allows employees to keep insurance in force until they obtain new insurance coverage.

The federal Consolidated Omnibus Reconciliation Act (**COBRA**) requires employers to extend health insurance coverage at group rates, usually for up to 18 months, to any employee who is laid off, quits, or is fired, except under certain circumstances (Figure 17-5 ◆).

COBRA coverage is available to employees who work for employers with twenty or more employees. Both full- and part-time employees are counted to determine whether a plan is subject to COBRA. A qualified beneficiary is typically an individual who was covered by the employer's group health insurance plan on the day before a qualifying event. This beneficiary can be the employee, the employee's spouse, and the retired employee's dependent children or any child born to or placed for adoption with a covered employee during the period of COBRA coverage.

In order to be qualified for COBRA coverage, the qualified beneficiary must have experienced a qualifying event. Qualifying events for employees include:

- The voluntary or involuntary termination of employment for reasons other than gross misconduct
- Reduction in the number of hours of employment resulting in the termination of health insurance coverage

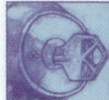

Keys to Success
PROVIDING COVERAGE INFORMATION TO PATIENTS

Most patients are only vaguely aware of their insurance plan coverage. Therefore, be sure to check with patients' insurance companies before providing patients expensive treatment and to relay coverage information to patients. Remember that insurance companies only give reviews of patients' benefits. They do not guarantee actual benefits when claims are received. Make sure patients understand that you are only relaying information from their insurance carriers. Direct any questions the patient may have about coverage to those carriers.

Qualifying events for spouses include:

- The covered employee's becoming entitled to Medicare coverage
- Divorce or legal separation of the covered employee
- Death of the covered employee

Qualifying events for dependent children include:

- Loss of dependent child status under the plan rules
- Voluntary or involuntary termination of the covered employee's employment for any reason other than gross misconduct
- Reduction in the hours worked by the covered employee resulting in the termination of health insurance coverage
- Covered employee's becoming entitled to Medicare
- Divorce or legal separation of the covered employee
- Death of the covered employee

In order to be eligible for COBRA coverage, a qualified beneficiary must notify the employer's plan administrator of a qualifying event within 60 days after divorce or legal separation or a child's ceasing to be a dependent under plan rules. Employers must notify the plan administrator of a qualifying event within 30 days after an employee's death, termination, reduced hours of employment, or entitlement to Medicare.

Individual Health Insurance Policies

Another type of insurance plan is the individual plan or policy, which individuals buy directly through insurance carriers. These plans are often the most expensive, because group rates are unavailable.

The benefits are often not as good as group policies, resulting in higher deductibles and other out-of-pocket expenses. The minimum level of benefit package for individual insurance policies is regulated by each state, and in some states, only a few companies offer individual policies due to restrictive requirements. Employees who have been on a COBRA plan can convert to an individual policy with the same insurance company when the COBRA benefits expire, but the group rates and benefits will no longer apply.

Congress passed COBRA health benefit provisions in 1986 to provide certain former employees, retirees, spouses, former spouses, and dependent children the right to temporarily continue health coverage at group rates. To be eligible for COBRA coverage, employees must have been enrolled in their employers' health plans when they worked and those health plans must continue to be in effect for active employees.

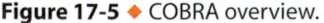

Figure 17-5 ◆ COBRA overview.

Types of Plans

Since the passage of the HMO ACT of 1973 and the Tax Equity and Fiscal Responsibility Act (**TEFRA**), the insurance industry has introduced health insurance plans that allow patients a variety of ways to access providers and share in the cost of care. These various plans also differ in how insurance companies pay providers.

Fee-for-Service Plans

Back in the 1980s, **fee-for-service**, also known as **indemnity**, plans were the norm. Rare today, and typically among the most expensive offerings, fee-for-service plans allow patients to seek care with any covered healthcare providers, for any covered services. Neither the list of physicians patients may see, nor the fee schedules are prearranged. These plans are private health insurance plans that reimburse healthcare providers on the basis of a fee for each health service provided to the covered person. Fee-for-service plans typically include a yearly deductible, after which the insurance company will pay at a certain coinsurance rate. Most commonly the coinsurance rate is 70/30 or 80/20 percent, with the insurance company paying the higher percentage and the member paying the lower.

Fee-for-service plans are among the most expensive because they do not contain managed care or cost-control measures. The type of person who generally opts for the fee-for-service plan is an individual with a serious medical condition who needs frequent treatment or those who can afford the plan and want to have complete freedom of choice to see the provider of their choice whenever they wish.

Managed Care Plans

Today, most patients are covered by **managed care**. Managed care plans control the costs associated with plan purchase by controlling the amounts they reimburse health care providers. Managed care organizations (**MCOs**) contract with healthcare providers to provide care for a certain group of patients. Those providers, called participating providers, sign a contract with the MCO that stipulates discounted reimbursement rates, billing guidelines, and other rules. A provider will usually have contracts with several different MCOs. The MCO then contracts with insurance companies to offer lower reimbursement rates through its network of participating providers. The MCO will list the provider's name in a directory given to patients. Patients will have lower out-of-pocket expenses if they use a participating provider.

Providers who do not contract with a specific MCO are called **nonparticipating providers**. Some MCOs cover patients who see nonparticipating providers, but usually at the patients' higher out-of-pocket expense. Other MCOs offer no coverage if the insured sees a nonparticipating provider. Therefore, it is important for medical assistants to let patients know whether providers participate with the patients' health plans. A provider may be participating with some patients' MCOs and nonparticipating with others. Most offices ask about healthcare coverage the first time patients call. When in doubt, assistants should ask patients for their insurance information and then call or research the insurance companies online.

Managed care plans are divided into four basic types: Health Maintenance Organizations (**HMOs**), Preferred Provider Organizations (**PPOs**), Exclusive Provider Organizations (**EPOs**), and Point of Service (**POS**) Plans.

Table 17-1 summarizes the various types of MCOs and their characteristics.

In Practice

Georgia Collins calls the medical office to schedule an appointment as a new patient. When the medical assistant asks her about her insurance coverage, she says she is unsure of her insurance company's name and cannot locate her insurance card. How should the medical assistant respond? Is insurance information needed before patients seek care? Why or why not? If Georgia becomes angry, how should the medical assistant react?

Preferred Provider Organization (PPO)

The preferred provider organization (PPO) contracts with physicians and facilities to perform services for PPO members at specified rates. These rates, or fees, are contractually adjusted so that the PPO member is charged less than nonmembers. The PPO gives subscribers a list of PPO member-providers from which subscribers can receive healthcare at PPO rates. If a patient chooses to receive treatment from a provider who is not in the PPO network, the patient has to pay any difference between the PPO's rate and the outside provider's rate. PPOs generally require preauthorization for major medical services.

Each physician in a practice may be a member of more than one PPO, and all the doctors in the practice may not necessarily belong to the same PPO. Some of the main features of PPOs include the following:

- PPOs are similar to HMOs in that they enter into contractual arrangements with healthcare providers (e.g., physicians, hospitals, and other healthcare professionals) and together form a provider network.
- Unlike an HMO, members don't have a PCP (gatekeeper) nor do they have to use an in-network provider for their care. However, PPOs offer members higher benefits as financial incentives to use network providers. The incentives may include lower deductibles, lower copayments, and higher reimbursements. For example, if the subscriber sees an in-network family physician for a routine visit, she may only have a small copayment or deductible. If she sees a non-network family physician for a routine visit, she may have to pay as much as 50% of the total bill.
- PPO members typically do not have to get a referral to see a specialist. However, there is a financial incentive to use a specialist who is a member of a PPO's provider network.

TABLE 17-1 VARIOUS TYPES OF MCOs AND THEIR CHARACTERISTICS

HMO	PPO	POS	EPO
■ State licensed ■ Most stringent guidelines ■ Limited network of providers ■ Members assigned to PCPs ■ Members must use network except in emergencies or pay a penalty ■ Usually there is a financial reward to providers for managing the cost of care	■ Limited network of providers but larger than HMO ■ Members may be assigned to PCPs but restrictions on accessing other physicians not as tight as in HMO ■ Financial penalty for accessing non-network providers less severe than in an HMO ■ Usually there is no reward to providers for managing the cost of care	■ Hybrid of HMO and PPO networks ■ Members may choose from a primary or secondary network ■ Primary network is HMO-like ■ Secondary network is often a PPO network ■ Out-of-pocket expenses are lower within the primary network and higher when using the secondary network ■ Members have more choices with less expense than with a PPO	■ Doesn't have an HMO license ■ Members are eligible for benefits only when they use network providers ■ Financial penalties for members leaving the network are similar to those of HMO ■ Priced lower than a PPO but higher than an HMO

IPA Model HMO	Staff Model HMO	Network Model HMO	Group Model HMO
■ An association formed by physicians with separately owned practices (solo or small group) ■ HMO may contract with physicians separately or through the IPA	■ HMO hires the physicians and pays them salaries ■ HMO owns the network ■ HMO owns the clinic sites and health centers	■ HMO uses two or more group practices or a group practice plus a combination of staff physicians and contracted independent physicians to form a network of providers ■ Allow members to choose their providers	■ HMO contracts with multi-specialty groups. ■ May be open-panel or closed-panel

Source: Vines, Deborah, Braceland, Ann, Rollins, Elizabeth, and Miller, Susan. Comprehensive Health Insurance: Billing, Coding, and Reimbursement. *©2008 Pearson Education, Upper Saddle River, NJ. Reprinted with permission.*

■ PPOs are less restrictive than HMOs in the choice of healthcare provider. However, they tend to require greater out-of-pocket payments from their members.*

Critical Thinking Question 17-3

Assume the medical assistant determined that Martin's wife's insurance plan was not one of the physician's preferred plans. What should the medical assistant say to Martin?

Health Maintenance Organizations

Health maintenance organizations (HMOs) are managed care plans that cover members only when those members seek care from a list of healthcare providers and suppliers who have contracted with the HMO. When members wish to seek care from providers not on the list, they must pay for the care. Most HMOs require patients to choose primary care providers (PCPs) who belong to the network of covered providers. The primary care provider serves as the **caretaker** or **gatekeeper**, the person who arranges any specialist services or hospitalizations.

*Source: Vines, Deborah, Braceland, Ann, Rollins, Elizabeth, and Miller, Susan. *Comprehensive Health Insurance: Billing, Coding, and Reimbursement.* © 2008, pp. 29–30. Reprinted by permission of Pearson Education Inc., Upper Saddle River: NJ.

The plans have various rules for copayment, coinsurance, and deductible amounts. The subscriber to an HMO plan is able to obtain healthcare on a regular basis with unlimited medical attention. Thus, HMOs encourage subscribers to take advantage of preventive healthcare services in an attempt to make healthcare coverage more cost efficient. HMOs do tend to cover more preventive procedures such as annual physicals, prostate cancer testing, and mammography.

■ A distinctive feature of an HMO is that the subscriber chooses a primary care physician. The PCP arranges, provides, coordinates, and authorizes all aspects of a member's healthcare. PCPs are usually family doctors, internal medicine doctors, general practitioners, or OB/GYNs.

■ An HMO enters into contractual arrangements with healthcare providers (e.g., physicians, hospitals, and other healthcare professionals) and together form a provider network.

■ Members are required to see only providers within this network if they are to have their healthcare paid for by the HMO. If the member receives care from a provider who isn't in the network, the HMO will not pay for care unless it was preauthorized by the HMO or deemed an emergency.

- Members can only see a specialist (e.g., cardiologist, dermatologist, rheumatologist) if they are referred and the PCP authorizes the service. The referral must be approved by the HMO. If the member sees a specialist without a referral, the HMO will not pay for the service.
- HMOs are the most restrictive type of health plan because of the restrictions the members have in selecting a healthcare provider. However, HMOs typically provide members with a greater range of health benefits for the lowest out-of-pocket expenses, such as either no or a very low copayment and deductible.

The four main types of HMOs, discussed next, vary in the way they link providers in order to create a healthcare delivery system.

Group Model HMO   A group model HMO is an organization that contracts with a multispecialty physicians' group to provide physician services to an enrolled group. Physicians are employees of the group practice and generally are limited to providing care only to the HMO's members.

Individual Practice Association HMO **Individual practice association (IPA)** HMOs are the most decentralized and involve contracting with individual physicians to create a healthcare delivery system. The HMO contracts with community hospitals and providers of services such as laboratories and diagnostics. Pharmacy services are provided through a contracted network of independent and chain community pharmacies and mail order service.

Network Model HMO   Network HMOs contract with more than one community-based multispecialty group to provide wider geographical coverage. The group practices under contract with one HMO vary from large to small, from primary care to multispecialty practice.

Staff Model HMO   The **staff model HMOs** employ salaried physicians who treat members in facilities owned and operated by the HMO. Most services, including diagnostic, laboratory, and pharmacy services, are provided on-site. A team of health professionals delivers the care.*

Exclusive Provider Organizations

Exclusive provider organizations (EPOs) are types of managed care plans that cover members who seek care from healthcare providers in a small network. In these plans, groups of healthcare procrm their own networks and then contract with employers to provide exclusive care to their employees. EPOs often have hospitals in their networks, and physicians contracted with these networks must perform their hospital services in the contracted hospitals.

An EPO is referred to as exclusive because employers agree not to contract with any other plan. Members are eligible for benefits only when they use the services of the network of providers with certain exceptions for emergency or out-of-area services. If a patient decides to seek care outside the network, generally he is not reimbursed for the cost of treatment. Technically, many HMOs can be considered EPOs except that EPOs are regulated under insurance statutes rather than federal and state HMO regulations. As a result, the EPO is priced lower than a PPO to the employer, but an EPO's premiums are usually more expensive than an HMO's premiums.

Point-of-Service (POS) Options

Because many patients do not wish to accept services from only their HMO providers, some HMO plans add a point-of-service option. Patients who choose this option do not have to use only the HMO's physicians. However, if they choose to see physicians outside the network, they must pay increased deductibles and coinsurance. This option makes the HMO more like a PPO, in terms of choices available to the patients.

- The reason it is called a *point-of-service* option is because members choose which option—HMO or PPO—they will use each time they seek healthcare.
- Like an HMO and a PPO, a POS plan has a contracted provider network.
- POS plans encourage, but do not require, members to choose a primary care physician. As in a traditional HMO, the PCP acts as a gatekeeper when making referrals. Members who choose not to use their PCPs for referrals (but still seek care from an in-network provider) still receive benefits but will pay higher copays and/or deductibles than members who use their PCPs.
- POS members also may opt to visit an out-of-network provider at their discretion. If that happens, the member's copayments, coinsurance, and deductibles will be substantially higher.[†]

A triple option plan is a type of POS that offers patients a choice between an HMO, a PPO, and a traditional indemnity plan. For example, they may choose to use the HMO or PPO, where their out-of-pocket costs are lower for routine checkups, but may have an out-of-network specialist they have seen for many years for a particular medical problem, and choose to pay a higher out-of-pocket cost to continue to see that specialist under the traditional indemnity plan. A POS offers patients the greatest amount of control over both their providers and their out-of-pocket costs.

Consumer-Directed Healthcare Plans

The newest type of insurance plan, which is becoming increasingly popular in response to rising healthcare costs, is the **consumer-directed healthcare plan (CDHP)**. These plans place

---

*Source: Vines, Deborah, Braceland, Ann, Rollins, Elizabeth, and Miller, Susan. *Comprehensive Health Insurance: Billing, Coding, and Reimbursement*. © 2008, pp. 28–29. Reprinted by permission of Pearson Education, Inc. Upper Saddle River, NJ.

[†]Source: Vines, Deborah, Braceland, Ann, Rollins, Elizabeth, and Miller, Susan. *Comprehensive Health Insurance: Billing, Coding, and Reimbursement*. © 2008, p. 30. Reprinted by permission of Pearson Education, Inc. Upper Saddle River, NJ.

consumers in charge of how their healthcare dollars are spent, rendering those consumers more likely to ask questions about, or research the need for, their health-related services. Just as with traditional employer-paid plans, employers who support consumer-directed healthcare plans retain a certain amount of money from employees' paychecks to fund healthcare premiums. Generally, a consumer-driven health plan includes a three-tier structure of payment for healthcare: a tax-exempt health savings account or medical savings account that an individual uses to pay for health expenses up to a certain amount, a high-deductible health insurance policy that pays for expenses over the deductible, and a gap between those two in which individuals pay any healthcare expenses out of their own pocket. These out-of-pocket expenses may be eligible for reimbursement through a flexible spending account. Accounts are administered by insurance companies, which process claims and issue payments. Employees receive lists of covered services, just as with traditional plans.

From the medical provider's point of view, consumer-directed healthcare plans work much the same as traditional health insurance plans in that the physician's office sends bills directly to healthcare plans and is reimbursed by healthcare plans. Patients pay any portion not covered by the healthcare plan.

Blue Cross/Blue Shield Plans

Patients may have Blue Cross (BC) and Blue Shield (BS) plans through group health coverage or individual insurance. According to the BCBS Association (BCBSA), nearly one-third of people in the United States are covered by some type of BCBS plan (www.bcbsa.com). BC began at Baylor University Hospital in Texas to provide teachers with prepaid hospitalization benefits. BS was begun in Palo Alto, California, in 1939 as a response to an AMA resolution encouraging physicians to cooperate with prepaid health plans. Historically, BC plans provided hospital service benefits and BS plans provided physician service benefits. Each BC and BS plan was an independent not-for-profit health plan, with one or more plans in most states across the country. The national associations merged in 1977 to form BCBSA, with 450 member plans. Today the national association is for-profit and many of the local plans have either gone for-profit or have been purchased by for-profit insurance companies.

Patients may have a BC plan, a BS plan, or a combination BCBS plan depending on the geographic area. It is important to remember that each BCBS plan is separate and unique in terms of benefits, cost sharing, and other requirements, just as private commercial insurance companies are unique from each other.

BCBS coverage includes fee-for-service traditional coverage, managed care plans, a federal employee program (FEP), Medicare supplemental plans, and healthcare anywhere plans. The type of coverage is indicated on the member ID card. Members with a PPO plan have cards that contain the letters "PPO" in the upper right-hand corner. FEP member cards display a logo of an outline of the USA map and the words "federal employee program" and "government-wide service benefit plan." The healthcare anywhere coverage, also called BlueCard, contains a logo of a suitcase. This coverage enables members traveling in the service area of another BCBS plan to utilize local preferred providers and receive benefits under their home plan. Most BCBS member ID numbers begin with three letters that are a code indicating the member's home plan. It is essential to include these letters when reporting the member ID number on a claim. Figure 17-6 ◆ shows a sample BCBS member ID card.

Each BCBS processes its own claims, so medical assistants need to verify the correct filing address. In the past, most local BCBS plans would forward claims to the correct home plan, but that practice has become less common in recent years as many plans have joined commercial for-profit companies.

Other Related Benefits

Legislation has created the opportunity for several types of tax-advantaged financial accounts in which patients can set aside some of their income to help cover healthcare expenses not paid by insurance. Employers are able to contribute to some of these funds. Patients submit their own expenses for reimbursement to these funds, so medical assistants are not directly involved in the billing. But, it is important to be aware of them in case patients have questions or need receipts or other documentation from the provider to submit to these plans.

Health Savings Accounts

Health savings accounts (HSAs) are personal savings accounts that can be used along with a high-deductible health plan to help pay for unreimbursed medical expenses. These accounts offer certain tax advantages to the individual in that the employee places pretax dollars into the savings accounts. Contributions to HSAs can be made by employers and/or individuals. Annual contributions are limited, as are out-of-pocket maximums, although persons aged 55 and over can make additional contributions. HSAs are portable from one job to another.

Medical Savings Accounts

The Health Insurance Portability and Accountability Act of 1996 (HIPAA) permits eligible individuals to establish a medical savings account (**MSA**). These accounts may be used to pay for medical expenses along with a high-deductible health insurance plan. In order to be eligible for a medical savings account an individual must be employed by a small employer that provides a high-deductible health insurance plan or be self-employed and covered by a high-deductible health insurance plan. Contributions may be made by the individual and/or the employer, but not both in the same year.

Flexible Spending Accounts

Flexible spending accounts (FSA) also called **healthcare reimbursement accounts (HCRA)** allow individuals to set aside a portion of their pretaxed wages to pay for certain out-of-pocket healthcare expenses. Money from flexible spending accounts can be used to pay for expenses not covered by health insurance, such as:

■ Deductibles and copays
■ Prescription drugs and medical supplies
■ Dental services, dentures, and orthodontics
■ Eyeglasses, contacts, solutions, and eye surgery

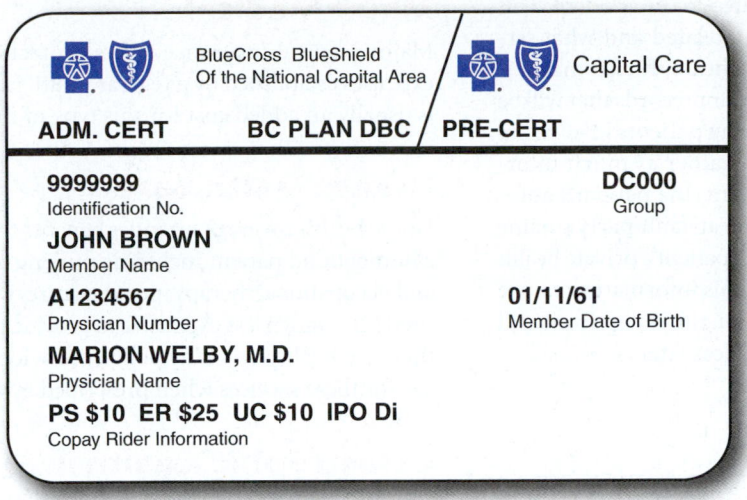

Figure 17-6 ◆ Sample BCBS member ID card.

- Chiropractic services
- Psychiatric care and psychologists' fees
- Smoking cessation programs

Money set aside in flexible spending accounts in any given year must be spent by a certain date, typically March 15th of the following year or the money is forfeited. Figure 17-7 ◆ explains how a flexible spending account works.

Third-Party Liability

When patients are involved in a non-work-related accident, there may be third-party liability (**TPL**) insurance that covers medical bills. Most businesses, homeowners, and vehicle owners have liability insurance to cover injuries that occur on their properties or in vehicle accidents. For example, when patients are injured in an automobile accident, the automobile owner's auto liability insurance typically covers the patients' medical expenses.

State laws vary regarding how automobile insurance is handled, but many states have no-fault coverage. Under no-fault coverage, the injured person's own auto insurance pays the medical bills, even if someone else was at fault. This is paid under the personal injury protection (**PIP**) of the injured person's policy. The injured person's auto insurance company then works with the at-fault party's company to recover the expenses. If the injured person does not have PIP coverage, or expenses exceed the limit, then the at-fault party's insurance is billed. If the injured party files a lawsuit against the at-fault party, then medical bills may be sent to the patient's attorney. In these cases, the provider may need to wait until the case is settled to receive payment, which can take several years. Providers should ask their own attorney to file a lien with the patient's attorney, which establishes the provider's legal right be paid upon settlement.

If payment from a TPL company is delayed more than a specified number of days, such as 45 or 60 days, some insurers will *pay and pursue*. This means they will accept claims for services related to the injuries, pay them, then pursue the TPL insurance for reimbursement. If the provider or patient receives payment or a settlement from the TPL, that party needs to reimburse the plan that originally paid the bills. When patients' bills exceed the amount covered by the TPL, private and government plans can be billed for the denied expenses.

Patients often are responsible for a deductible and sometimes copayments or coinsurance on a TPL policy. Insurers often have a maximum approved charge that they will pay. Usually balance billing is permitted because providers are not contracted with TPL insurers.

When injured patients are already established in the practice, a new medical record and a new financial account should

Chris Tamparo works for an employer that offers to put Chris's pretax earnings into a flex spending account for Chris' health care expenses. Chris has a health insurance plan through his employer that has a $500 deductible and then coverage for 80 percent of his care.

Chris visits his physician for an office call and lab work. The cost for the visit is $145. During the office call, Chris gets a prescription that costs $43. Chris's health insurance policy lacks a prescription drug benefit.

Cost of physician visit and lab work: $145

Cost of prescription medication: $ 43

Total $188

Chris has a $500 annual deductible, so his insurance plan will pay $0 of the physician visit. Because Chris lacks prescription drug coverage, his insurance plan will pay $0 of the prescription cost. Chris pays the full $188 and gives the receipts to his employer. The employer reimburses Chris $188 out of Chris' flex spending account.

Figure 17-7 ◆ Flexible spending or healthcare reimbursement accounts.

be created specifically for treatment related to the accident. This helps clarify what services are accident-related and what services are part of patients' ongoing healthcare. It also makes it easier to provide copies of accident-relevant records that will be required by the insurers. When registering patients involved in an accident, medical assistants should gather as much information as possible regarding the accident, the patient's automobile coverage if an auto accident, the at-fault party's name and insurance information, as well as the patient's private health insurance or Medicare coverage. While this information can be confusing to collect and organize, thoroughness up front will make it easier to bill and collect for services later.

Types of Coverage

Regardless of patients' source of coverage or the type of plans they have, many alternatives exist as to the type of coverage included in a plan. Type of coverage refers to the specific services covered under the plan. Each insurance policy is tailored to include the benefits most desired and most affordable for each group or individual. Understanding some of the most common alternatives for coverage types will enable medical assistants to clarify for patients what can be expected from their policies (Vines, p. 35).

Hospital

Hospital coverage provides protection against the costs of hospital care. It generally provides a room allowance (a stated amount per day for a semiprivate room) with a maximum number of days per year. Special provisions are made for operating room charges, X-rays, laboratory work, drugs, and other medically necessary items while the insured person is an **inpatient**. An inpatient is a person who is admitted to the hospital for a minimum of 24 hours.

Medical

Medical coverage provides benefits for **outpatient** medical care including physicians' fees for hospital visits and nonsurgical procedures. The term *medical* refers to physicians' costs. Special provisions are made for diagnostic services such as laboratory, X-ray, and pathology costs. An outpatient is a person who receives medical care at a hospital or other medical facility but who is not admitted for more than 24 hours.

Surgical

Surgical coverage provides protection for the cost of a physician's fee for surgery, whether it is performed in a hospital, in a doctor's office, or elsewhere, such as a surgical center. Charges for anesthesia generally are covered by surgical insurance.

Outpatient

Outpatient coverage usually provides protection for emergency department visits and other outpatient divisions in a hospital or medical facility such as X-ray, pathology, and psychological services.

Major Medical

Major medical insurance offers protection for large medical expenses established by a regular health insurance policy. There is usually an added cost for this type of insurance coverage.*

Home Health Care

Home health coverage provides benefits for services received by a homebound patient including nursing care; physical, speech, and occupational therapy; personal caregivers; and other related needs. It is much less expensive to provide these services at home than in a facility, so many policies provide high levels of coverage for these services when prescribed by a physician.

Catastrophic Health Insurance

Catastrophic insurance provides protection only for the most expensive medical needs and is only suitable for individuals with the financial means to handle routine illnesses and hospitalizations. It is among the least expensive forms of health insurance because deductibles are generally large and there may be caps on the amount the policy will pay.

Specialized Policies

Patients can also purchase separate specialized policies to provide protection for unique situations. Special risk insurance provides protection against specific illnesses, such as cancer, or against certain types of high-risk accidents that may be excluded from traditional policies, such as sky diving or mountain climbing.

Long-term care insurance covers custodial services such as assistance with personal and household chores either at home or in a facility. The degree of care is based on the condition and requirements of the patients. Long-term care insurance is best purchased many years before a person anticipates needing it, because the annual premium increases with age and health status decline. Many financial advisers recommend that people consider purchasing long-term care policies in their early 50s.

Ancillary Coverage

Ancillary coverage is insurance for services provided by other than a physician or hospital, such as prescription drugs, vision, dental and alternative care. These are often packaged in with the main policy, but are actually provided by other insurance companies and other MCOs. Usually, patients have separate deductibles and copayments/coinsurance for ancillary coverage. Out-of-pocket costs from these plans may not count toward the overall stop loss provision.

Prescription Drug Coverage

Most insurance plans today have some form of prescription drug coverage because prescription medications are often very expensive,

*Source: Vines, Deborah, Braceland, Ann, Rollins, Elizabeth, and Miller, Susan. *Comprehensive Health Insurance: Billing, Coding, and Reimbursement.* © 2008, p. 35. Reprinted by permission of Pearson Education, Inc., Upper Saddle River, NJ.

and name brands are often far more costly than their generic counterparts. On behalf of pharmaceutical companies, pharmaceutical representatives visit medical offices to showcase the latest drugs on the market. As a marketing tactic, representatives often leave free samples for physicians to dispense. Through free samples on a short-term basis, physicians can provide needed medications to patients with financial issues or insurance companies that do not offer coverage. Physicians may also use free samples as trials before writing prescriptions. Plans typically have a **formulary**, a list of drugs they will cover. Usually the formulary is subdivided into two or more tiers with each tier having a different level of coverage (Figure 17-8 ◆). For example, tier 1 may include most generic drugs and perhaps a few brand name drugs that have no generic equivalent. Patients might have a small copayment, perhaps only a few dollars, for tier 1 drugs. Tier 2 may include preferred brand name drugs, ones for which there is no generic equivalent. Patients would have a slightly higher copayment for these drugs. Tier 3 may include brand name drugs that have generic equivalents or similar brand name drugs at a lower cost. Patients would have the highest out-of-pocket expense for these drugs, perhaps as high as 50 percent coinsurance. There may be some drugs that are not on the formulary at all. Patients need to present evidence of medical necessity in order to receive coverage for nonformulary drugs. Medical assistants can advocate for patients if their plan will not cover a specific drug the provider prescribed. They can help identify potentially similar medications from the formulary or from a lower tier of the formulary that the provider could evaluate and consider prescribing an equally effective drug at a lower cost to the patient. This could create a financial savings to the patient while maintaining safe and high-quality care.

Most drug plans are administered separately from the main insurance plan. Patients usually have a separate deductible and different copayments or coinsurance amounts than their core health insurance plan. This can be confusing to patients who think they have met the medical deductible, only to find out they owe a drug deductible as well.

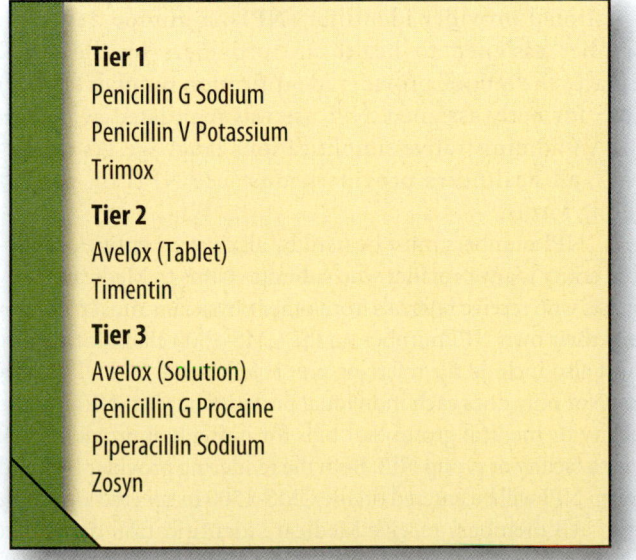

Tier 1
Penicillin G Sodium
Penicillin V Potassium
Trimox

Tier 2
Avelox (Tablet)
Timentin

Tier 3
Avelox (Solution)
Penicillin G Procaine
Piperacillin Sodium
Zosyn

Figure 17-8 ◆ Sample tiered drug formulary for antibiotics.

Some drug plans provide a mail order option for maintenance medications, which are medications patients take on a long-term basis to treat a chronic condition such as high cholesterol, arthritis, or heart conditions. The mail order plan may allow patients to order three months of medication for two copayments. This saves the patient four copayments per year for each medication ordered in this manner. In order to fill prescriptions in this manner, the mail order pharmacy will require that the prescription be written to dispense 90 days of medication at a time, with three refills for the remainder of the year. Medical assistants may need to make the prescriber aware of this requirement so the script can be written in the appropriate format.

Vision

Vision benefits include examinations and corrective hardware. Usually, patients can receive these services from an ophthalmologist or a licensed optometrist. An ophthalmologist is a medical doctor who specializes in examining, diagnosing, and treating eyes and eye diseases. An optometrist is an eye care professional who is a PCP for most vision and ocular healthcare concerns.

Examinations may be allowed annually or biannually. Contact lens wearers have a vision examination followed by a contact lens fitting/examination. If contact lenses are not medically necessary, the cost of the contact lens exam may not be covered.

Corrective hardware includes lenses, frames, and contact lenses. Hardware usually has a maximum dollar amount approved annually. Contact lenses needed after cataract surgery are usually covered under the patient's medical benefit, not the vision benefit.

Dental

Dental services are provided by a licensed dentist (DDS or DMD) or denturist, as well as a registered hygienist operating under a licensed dentist. Benefits may include diagnostic/preventive, basic, major, and orthodontia. Diagnostic/preventive services typically include examinations, cleaning, X-rays, space maintainers, and fluoride treatments. Basic may include amalgam fillings, simple and surgical extractions, endodontics, root canal, and treatment of periodontal disease. Major service covers crown, bridges, partials, and dentures. Orthodontia includes initial banding fees as well as monthly maintenance fees. Certain high-cost services such as dentures and orthodontia may require a significant waiting period before being eligible for coverage. Dental services directly related to medical conditions can often be billed to medical rather than dental insurance. An example of this would be tooth decay as a result of radiation therapy for a bone tumor in the jaw.

Alternative Care

Alternative care, also called complementary care, includes services such as chiropractic, massage therapy, and acupuncture. A chiropractor (DC) diagnoses and treats back problems by manually manipulating the bones in the spine to ease pain and restore mobility. "Chiropractors are . . . also trained to recommend therapeutic and rehabilitative exercises, as well as to provide nutritional, dietary and lifestyle counseling. Chiropractic care is used most often to treat neuromusculoskeletal complaints, including but not limited to back pain, neck pain, pain in the joints of the arms or legs, and headaches" (American Chiropractic Association). Depending on the state and the insurance company, chiropractic coverage may or may not require a referral from a medical doctor.

Massage therapy is "a profession in which the practitioner applies manual techniques, and may apply adjunctive therapies, with the intention of positively affecting the health and well-being of the client" (American Massage Therapy Association). Massage therapy improves functioning of the circulatory, lymphatic, muscular, skeletal, and nervous systems and may improve the rate at which the body recovers from injury and illness. It is often used in treating musculoskeletal conditions and injuries. Training and licensing requirements for massage therapists vary from state to state. Insurance coverage for services of a massage therapist usually requires a prescription from a chiropractor or medical doctor.

Acupuncture is part of traditional Chinese medicine. Acupuncture is the stimulation of specific points on the body by a variety of techniques, including the insertion of thin metal needles though the skin. It aims to restore and maintain health through the stimulation of specific points on the body. The service is provided by a licensed acupuncturist (LAc).

Some plans require a referral or authorization from the PCP in order for a patient to receive benefits for alternative care services. Medical assistants may need to facilitate such requests for referrals. Other plans will allow the patient to self-refer, meaning the patient receives these services without a referral or authorization. Typically, chiropractic, massage therapy, and acupuncture visits are limited in terms of how often the patient may receive them and the number of visits in a year. Anything above this cap may need a PCP referral or may not be covered at all. It is important for medical assistants to help patients understand how their policies are structured in this area.

Government Insurance

The U.S. government provides health insurance through a number of different programs for designated groups of people, such as the elderly, disabled, military personnel and retirees, and injured workers. Each of these programs has its own eligibility requirements and benefit structure. An overview of these programs follows.

Medicare Coverage

Medicare, established in 1965, is a federal program that provides health insurance for approximately 43 million Americans, including people aged 65 and older, patients who have been disabled for more than 24 months, and patients with end-stage renal disease (ESRD).

The program is administered by the Centers for Medicare and Medicaid Services (**CMS**) formerly known as the Health Care Financing Administration (**HCFA**). CMS contracts with private companies called Medicare administrative contractors (**MAC**) to educate and work with providers, process claims, and other functions.

One of CMS's obligations is to keep providers informed about proper Medicare billing. To this end, a vast array of information is available to providers free of charge on the CMS website www.cms.gov. A section called MedLearn provides free online training on many Medicare topics, free newsletters, articles, and other informative products.

The MACs also disseminate free billing information relevant to that particular region. Providers can sign up for e-mail alerts and announcements from the MAC to be sure they remain up to date. The MACs for each region are listed on the CMS website. Medical assistants involved in Medicare billing should learn how to access and use this vital information. Just as in many other areas of law, ignorance of Medicare rules is not an acceptable response.

Medicare claims should be submitted within 365 days of date of service. Those submitted later than this will be subject to a 10 percent penalty, unless the provider can prove that late submission was due to factors beyond its control, such as obtaining information from the MAC. The final submission deadline for claims to be considered at all is determined by a unique timetable based on the Medicare fiscal year. To simplify, services provided from January 1 through September 30 should be billed by the end of the next calendar year. Services provided between October 1 and December 31 have until the end of two calendar years to be billed. Figure 17-9 ◆ illustrates the schedule.

This means that providers have 13 to 27 months to bill for services, depending on the date the service was provided. This is longer than many private carriers allow and longer than many think they have. Medical assistants should not assume that a Medicare bill more than a year old is too old to submit, even though it will usually be penalized 10 percent. The MA should keep a chart like that in Figure 17-9 handy for quick reference to determine what deadlines exist.

The Medicare program has major component parts called Part A (hospital insurance), Part B (provider coverage), Part C (Medicare Advantage), and Part D (prescription drug).

The National Provider Identifier (NPI)

A national provider identifier (**NPI**), a unique, ten-digit number assigned to healthcare providers by the CMS, replaces the unique provider identification number (**UPIN**) CMS formerly assigned. NPI use was mandated as part of HIPAA administrative simplifications language. As of May 2007, all healthcare providers must use NPIs on patient billing forms.

NPI numbers must be used by all covered entities. A covered entity is any provider who submits claims to Medicare. Specialists who receive referrals from other physicians must place not only their own NPI number on the CMS-1500 claim form, they must also include the referring physician's name and NPI number. Not only does each individual provider have an NPI but the facility or medical group that bills for individual providers will have a facility or group NPI. Both the rendering provider NPI and group NPI will be entered on the CMS-1500 in specific locations.

All members receive Medicare identification cards that list their names, identification numbers, plans (Part A, Part B, or both), and effective dates (Figure 17-10◆).

Service provided (date)	Should be billed by (date)
10/1/07–9/30/08	12/31/09
10/1/08–9/30/09	12/31/10
10/1/09–9/30/10	12/31/11
10/1/10–9/30/11	12/31/12

Figure 17-9 ◆ Medicare submission deadlines.

Medicare Part A

Part A Medicare coverage is hospital insurance that covers most care for patients who have been hospitalized (for up to 90 days in a given period of time), patients in **skilled nursing facilities** (facilities for long-term care or other care facilities where patients must be monitored by nursing staff regularly) for given periods, patients who receive medical care at home, patients with life-limiting illnesses requiring **hospice** care (comfort care provided to patients who have 6 or fewer months to live), patients who require psychiatric treatment for given periods, and patients who require **respite** care (care provided in a skilled nursing facility on a short-term basis for patients normally treated at home). Citizens who receive Social Security benefits are automatically enrolled in Medicare Part A benefits with no premiums. There are deductibles and coinsurance for most services in Part A.

Medicare Part B

Part B Medicare coverage covers such services as physician care, therapy, and laboratory testing. Because Part B is voluntary, members must pay income-based premiums to enroll, which is a requirement as of January 1, 2007. In 2008, the standard monthly premium was $96.40, although this premium fluctuates depending upon the Medicare recipient's income level.

Patients also have out-of-pocket expenses under Part B. There is an annual deductible ($128 in 2008) that increases each year and 20 percent coinsurance on most services.

Physicians must choose if they will participate with Medicare. A participating provider, also called PAR, must accept the Medicare fee schedule (MFS) amounts as payment in full for its services. If the MFS is higher than the physician's normal fee for a service, the normal fee is the maximum amount that can be billed. The provider must bill Medicare for all services, even those known to not be covered by Medicare. They also **accept assignment** on all claims, which means they accept the MFS amounts and the payment is sent to the provider. Approximately 95 percent of all physicians are PARs.

For example, consider an office visit with a physician charge of $118 and an assumed rate of $100 on the MFS. The PAR physician receives $100 × 80% = $80 from Medicare and

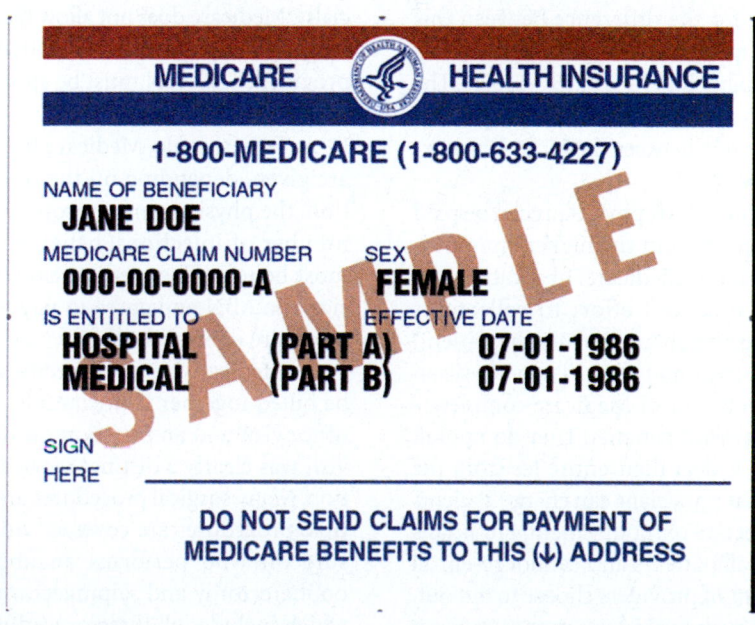

Figure 17-10 ◆ A Medicare ID card.

must collect $100 × 20% = $20 coinsurance from the patient. The Medicare payment is sent to the physician. The physician writes off the difference between the MFS and the normal charge: $118 – $100 = $18.

Nonparticipating physicians (non-PAR) also need to bill Medicare for all services, including those not covered. However, they can decide to accept assignment on a case-by-case basis. If they accept assignment, they agree to accept the non-PAR MFS as payment in full. The non-PAR MFS is 5 percent less than the PAR MFS, so non-PAR physicians are paid less than PAR physicians on assigned claims. Medicare sends the payment to the non-PAR physician on assigned claims. Approximately 5 percent of all providers are non-PAR.

For example, consider the example above for a non-PAR physician who accepts assignment. The office visit charge is $118. The non-PAR MFS is $100 × 95% = $95. The non-PAR physician receives $95 × 80% = $76 from Medicare and must collect $95 × 20% = $19 coinsurance from the patient. The Medicare payment is sent to the physician. The physician writes off the difference between the MFS and the normal charge: $118 – $95 = $23.

If non-PAR providers do not accept assignment, they must accept the **limiting charge (LC)** as payment in full. The LC amount is 15 percent higher than the non-PAR MFS. If the LC is higher than the physician's normal fee for a service, the normal fee is the maximum amount that can be billed. However, Medicare will reimburse 80 percent of the non-PAR MFS amount only. Patients pay 20 percent coinsurance of the non-PAR MFS and also pay the additional 15 percent difference that makes up the LC. Medicare sends payment to the patient on nonassigned claims, and providers must collect the full amount of the LC from the patient.

Consider the example above once more for a non-PAR physician who does not accept assignment. The office visit charge is $118. The non-PAR MFS is $100 × 95% = $95. Medicare sends its portion to the patient $95 × 80% = $76. The patient has out-of-pocket responsibility for the coinsurance: $95 × 20% = $19. The LC is $95 × 115% = $109.25, and the patient is also responsible for the difference between this and the Medicare approved charge: $109.25 – $95 = $14.25. Thus, the patient's total responsibility is $19 + $14.25 = $33.25. The total amount of $109.25 must be collected from the patient. The physician writes off the difference between the LC and the normal charge $118 – $109.25 = $8.75.

On nonassigned claims, non-PAR physicians can be paid at higher rates than PAR physicians, but the higher amount is the responsibility of the patient, not Medicare. In addition, the provider must devote more time and effort to collections because the entire amount must be obtained from the patient.

Physicians, dentists, podiatrists, and selected non-physician providers may also choose to opt out of Medicare completely and enter into private contracts with patients. They do not bill Medicare for any services and collect their entire fee from the patient. There is no limit on what physicians can charge. Patients bill Medicare themselves and receive reimbursement. Physicians who opt out must opt out for all patients and cannot re-enroll for two years. Less than 1 percent of providers choose to opt out. Some non-physician providers such as chiropractors cannot opt out and are required to bill Medicare for all patients.

One very important aspect to billing Medicare is a form called the **advance beneficiary notice (ABN)** or **waiver** (Figure 17-11 ◆). The ABN must be signed by patients before receiving covered services that may be denied payment by Medicare. If, during the encounter, physicians recommend services that may be denied, patients need to be informed and given the opportunity to accept or decline the service, knowing they will be obligated to pay if Medicare does deny it. If patients do not understand that Medicare could deny the service, they are not obligated to pay for and cannot be billed for it. Medical assistants are vital to facilitating this because they are the link between the medical care and the billing rules. Medical assistants need to review the ABN with the patient and obtain a signature before the service is provided. The ABN notifies patients that the service may not be paid by Medicare and patients agree to be responsible for payment. Medicare does not allow the ABN to be completed after the service is provided.

To understand when the ABN is needed, it is important to understand how Medicare classifies its services. **Non-covered** services are those that are not eligible for reimbursement under any circumstance and do require an ABN to be completed. **Covered** services are those potentially eligible for reimbursement; however, they are not automatically paid. Covered services must meet **medical necessity** and other criteria, such as frequency in order to be paid. Medical necessity refers to more than whether a physician believes the service is needed. Medicare medical necessity means services or supplies that are proper and needed for the diagnosis or treatment of the patient's medical condition are provided for the diagnosis, direct care, and treatment of the medical condition, meet the standards of good medical practice in the local area, and are not mainly for the convenience of the patient or provider. If they do not meet these criteria, services may be denied. It is providers' responsibility to become familiar with what covered services may be denied under what circumstances, based on their specialty. Medicare does not allow blanket ABNs, which is the practice of having all Medicare patients sign ABNs for any service provided. The ABN must be specific to the patient's particular circumstance.

For example, Medicare limits how often B-12 injections are given, depending on the diagnosis. In a particular situation, the physician may recommend more than the stipulated number of injections, believing the patient will receive the most benefit. The medical assistant would ask the patient to sign the ABN and agree to pay for the additional injection if Medicare denies payment.

Medicare has very specific rules about what services can be billed together. For example Medicare will not pay for an office visit and an injection on the same day, unless the office visit was clearly a distinct service, such as a physical examination. Many surgical procedures are **bundled**, meaning that multiple procedures are covered with one charge. For example, a surgeon who performs an abdominal hysterectomy with oopherectomy and salpingectomy must bill one charge only, which includes all three procedures. To bill this as three separate services would be called **unbundling**, which is considered

(A) **Notifier(s):**
(B) **Patient Name:** _____ *(C)* **Identification Number:** _____

ADVANCE BENEFICIARY NOTICE OF NONCOVERAGE (ABN)

NOTE: If Medicare doesn't pay for *(D)*_____ below, you may have to pay.

Medicare does not pay for everything, even some care that you or your health care provider have good reason to think you need. We expect Medicare may not pay for the *(D)*_____ below.

(D) _____	*(E)* Reason Medicare May Not Pay:	*(F)* Estimated Cost:

WHAT YOU NEED TO DO NOW:

- Read this notice, so you can make an informed decision about your care.
- Ask us any questions that you may have after you finish reading.
- Choose an option below about whether to receive the *(D)*_____listed above.
  Note: If you choose Option 1 or 2, we may help you to use any other insurance that you might have, but Medicare cannot require us to do this.

(G) OPTIONS: Check only one box. We cannot choose a box for you.
❑ **OPTION 1.** I want the *(D)*_____ listed above. You may ask to be paid now, but I also want Medicare billed for an official decision on payment, which is sent to me on a Medicare Summary Notice (MSN). I understand that if Medicare doesn't pay, I am responsible for payment, but **I can appeal to Medicare** by following the directions on the MSN. If Medicare does pay, you will refund any payments I made to you, less co-pays or deductibles.
❑ **OPTION 2.** I want the *(D)*_____ listed above, but do not bill Medicare. You may ask to be paid now as I am responsible for payment. **I cannot appeal if Medicare is not billed.**
❑ **OPTION 3.** I don't want the *(D)*_____listed above. I understand with this choice I am **not** responsible for payment, and **I cannot appeal to see if Medicare would pay.**

(H) **Additional Information:**

This notice gives our opinion, not an official Medicare decision. If you have other questions on this notice or Medicare billing, call **1-800-MEDICARE** (1-800-633-4227/**TTY:** 1-877-486-2048).

Signing below means that you have received and understand this notice. You also receive a copy.

(I) **Signature:**	*(J)* **Date:**

Form CMS-R-131 (03/08)   Form Approved OMB No. 0938-0566

Figure 17-11 ◆ Advance beneficiary notice (ABN) form.

fraud. This will be discussed further in Chapter 19, Procedural Coding.

Medicare Part C: Advantage Plan

Medicare Part C is managed care, known as Medicare Advantage plans. Formerly known as Medicare + Choice, these plans are offered by private insurance companies and replace Parts A, B, and D. The benefit to the patient is potentially more comprehensive care at the same or lower cost than Medicare. The disadvantage, as with any managed care plan, is that the choice of providers is limited. Patients keep their Medicare identification card and receive an additional card from the Advantage plan. Because patients may not understand the difference between the two cards, it is a good practice for medical assistants to ask patients if they belong to an Advantage plan or have another identification card. When billing, the Medicare Advantage plan is billed, not Medicare. When patients have secondary coverage, medical assistants bill the secondary plans after the Medicare Advantage plan has made a payment or decision.

Medicare Part D

As of January 2006, the newest Medicare coverage plan is Part D, the prescription drug plan. Members covered by Medicare may opt to purchase Part D coverage, which covers both name-brand and generic prescription drugs at participating pharmacies. The Part D plans are provided by private companies. Not all drugs are covered under every plan, so patients need to determine which plans cover their most common or most expensive medications. Medical assistants can assist patients by providing them with complete medication lists. The Medicare website for patients, www.medicare.gov, has a prescription drug plan finder tool to assist patients to evaluate their options. Medicare Part D has an annual deductible, copayments or coinsurance and a maximum benefit level, and a stop loss for patients who have out of pocket costs over a certain level. The deductible and stop loss levels are updated annually.

Medicare Part D enrollees have several mail-in pharmacy options from companies that typically offer low out-of-pocket expenses. Enrollees should view this option cautiously, however. It may be less than ideal for patients on short-term medications, like antibiotics, because delivery may take a week or more.

Medigap Plans

Medigap or Medicare Supplemental Plans are insurance plans offered by private companies to reimburse patients for the out-of-pocket expenses they incur with Medicare. CMS regulates what benefits can be offered by these plans and which companies can offer them. Not all Medigap plans cover the same expenses. The basic benefit is coverage of patients' coinsurance, but some also offer coverage of deductibles for Parts A and B, skilled nursing facility coinsurance, foreign travel, and other specific expenses. Medigap is billed after Medicare has determined its portion of the payment. Most Medigap plans have an agreement with CMS so that the MACs will electronically send the claims information to the Medigap carrier, relieving the provider of the need to directly bill the Medigap policy. Medical assistants should ask patients if they have a Medigap policy so that information can be included on the billing to Medicare.

Medicare and Other Health Insurance (OHI)

Patients may have other health insurance (OHI) in addition to Medicare. CMS requires providers to be very vigilant in determining when Medicare is obligated to pay first and when they are the secondary payer. These are known as Medicare secondary payer (MSP) rules. When Medicare is the secondary payer, it pays a lower portion of the bill than when they are primary. Medicare provides a detailed questionnaire on the CMS Web site, which medical assistants should review with patients to determine MSP. In general, Medicare is primary to Medicaid and secondary to most other insurance, including workers' compensation, liability, TRICARE, or when covered by a spouse's group health policy. Medicare is usually secondary when patients over age 65 are still working and covered by an employer's group heath plan. There are exceptions to this, which the MSP questionnaire will aid in determining.

Providers Participating in Medicare

Medicare must accredit any health care providers who wish to participate in its program in a process very similar to the application process of any managed care plan. Because most health insurance plans follow Medicare's lead when it comes to accreditation and fee schedules, it is crucial for medical assistants or office managers to stay up to date by consulting Medicare's published guidelines or Web site.

As of July 2005, Medicare requires all medical offices to file medical claims electronically, or via e-billing. Some clinics may be allowed to continue to bill claims on paper. Those clinics must have no more than ten full-time employees, or the equivalent of ten full-time employees, such as twenty part-time employees whose combined working hours total that of ten full-time employees.

Medicare prefers to use electronic funds transfer for payment to physicians and medical facilities. This is set up by filling out an Authorization Agreement for Electronic Funds Transfer form. This form is returned to Medicare along with a copy of a voided check or deposit ticket. After receipt of this

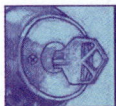

Keys to Success
EXPLAINING MEDICARE COVERAGE

The medical assistant should clearly explain to the Medicare-covered patient any services and costs that may not be paid by Medicare. Medicare requires services be listed on the waiver form that the patient must sign. Be sure to give a copy of the form to the patient and keep a copy in the patient's permanent file.

information, Medicare will begin directly depositing funds into the physician or facility's account within three weeks.

Medicare maintains a provider directory of participating providers nationwide. A search for a provider can be performed by state or specialty. This list contains the provider's name, specialty, education, residency, gender, foreign languages spoken by the physician, hospital affiliation, and practice location.

Medicare provides a variety of in-person as well as online workshops for providers to learn more about topics such as payment notices and reimbursements, the appeals process, using the Medicare Web site, and updates on changes that apply to physicians or medical facilities.

Medicaid

Medicaid coverage is a health benefit program for low-income patients. Like Medicare, Medicaid is run by CMS, although each state dictates the amount and type of services Medicaid covers. The federal government provides funds to every state, and every state adds its own funds to cover qualified enrollees. As of 2001, the last year for which Medicaid has compiled extensive data, more than 46 million persons received healthcare services through the Medicaid program. Because every state runs its own Medicaid program, identification cards or coupons differ (Figure 17-12 ◆).

Because Medicaid reimbursement is extremely low in most states, most healthcare providers cannot afford to treat a large number of Medicaid patients. The low reimbursement rate has caused many healthcare providers to stop accepting Medicaid patients altogether, or to stringently limit the number of patients. As a result, Medicaid-covered patients may wait longer for care or travel to find accepting providers.

If they wish to accept Medicaid patients, healthcare providers must apply to become Medicaid accredited in their state. As part of this process, which is very similar to any other managed care application process, Medicaid provides physicians fee schedules of covered expenses.

Medicaid programs offer coverage on a month-to-month basis in most states, which means that Medicaid may not cover a patient one month just because Medicaid covered the patient in a previous month. It is vital for medical assistants to know the Medicaid rules and regulations in their state as those rules and regulations apply to their practice types and to ask Medicaid patients for proof of coverage in the plan.

Low-income elderly or disabled patients often have both Medicare and Medicaid coverage. Medicare is always primary in these cases, and Medicaid is secondary. Often, Medicare's reimbursement rate is higher than what Medicaid will allow, resulting in no Medicaid payment. The CMS estimates that there are approximately 6.5 million persons receiving benefits from both Medicare and Medicaid. When physicians accept assignment from both Medicare and Medicaid, or participate in both programs, those physicians must accept what the two agencies together pay as payment in full for covered services. In these cases, billing patients for any portion of covered services is illegal. To do so can result in fines and/or removal from the Medicare and/or Medicaid programs as a participating provider.

It is important to note that Medicaid coverage is not simply based upon a person's income level. An individual in a particular state may be considered low income yet not qualify for Medicaid benefits within that state. Medicaid coverage is based upon a list of qualifications, including the person's age, whether the patient is pregnant, disabled, or blind, whether the person is a U.S. citizen or a lawfully admitted immigrant, as well as income level. Medicaid also includes special rules for persons who live in nursing homes or disabled children who live at home.

Medicaid-eligible patients may qualify under different sets of criteria for different programs. One major distinction is between the **categorically needy** (CN) and **medically needy** (MN). CN patients qualify for cash assistance as well as medical services. MN patients generally have a higher income than CN patients and are eligible for medical services but not cash assistance. In addition, they may be eligible for fewer medical

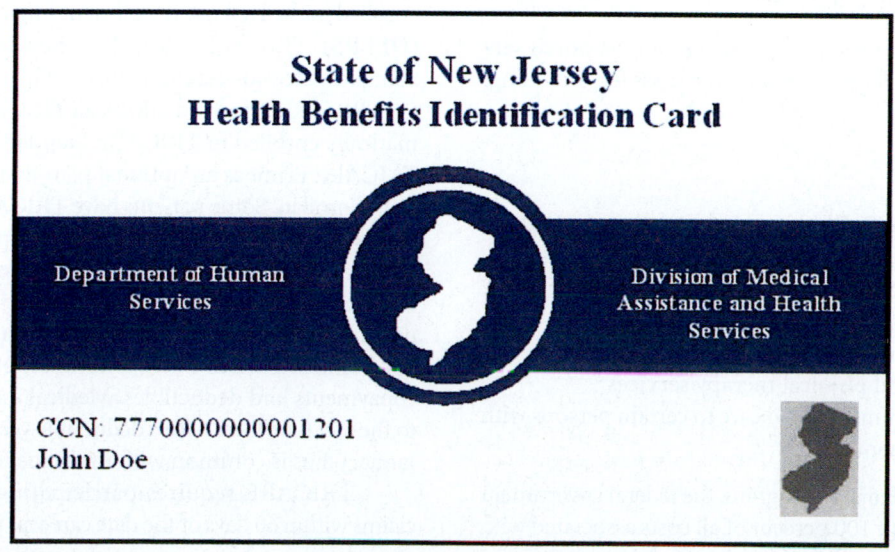

Figure 17-12 ◆ Medicaid coupon from New Jersey.

services than CN patients. Medical assistants need to verify which specific services and programs covered patients are eligible for. For example, some patients will be eligible for certain children's programs that cover a subset of specific services.

Medicaid is always the "payer of last resort," meaning that all other insurances should be billed before Medicaid. If the payment from the other insurance is higher than Medicaid's approved rate, Medicaid will pay nothing.

Medicaid has introduced cost-sharing in recent years, which means that some patients may be responsible for copayments, deductibles, or premiums based on income level, family size, and other factors. If working for Medicaid providers, medical assistants should become familiar with their state's Medicaid identification card and eligibility verification system, as these tools provide much information about patients' coverage, eligibility, and financial responsibility.

Covered Medicaid Services

Although each state determines who will be covered by Medicaid, what type of services will be covered, and the reimbursement provided for the covered services, the federal government requires certain basic services be provided in order for the state to qualify for federal funding. These services include:

- Inpatient hospital services
- Outpatient hospital services
- Prenatal care
- Vaccines for children
- Physician services
- Nursing facility services for persons aged 21 or older
- Family planning services and supplies
- Rural health clinic services
- Home healthcare for persons eligible for skilled-nursing services
- Laboratory and X-ray services
- Pediatric and family nurse practitioner services
- Nurse-midwife services
- Early and periodic screening, diagnostic, and treatment services for children under age 21

The federal government also lists certain optional services for which states will receive matching funds for providing. These include:

- Diagnostic services
- Clinic services
- Intermediate care facilities for the mentally retarded
- Prescribed drugs and prosthetic devices
- Optometrist services and eyeglasses
- Nursing facility services for children under age 21
- Transportation services
- Rehabilitation and physical therapy services
- Home and community-based care to certain persons with chronic impairments

Along with the Medicaid program, the federal government also reimburses states for 100 percent of all costs associated with providing healthcare in facilities of the Indian Health Service. This program is responsible for providing health services to native Americans and Alaskan natives. The federal government also provides financial assistance to the twelve states that provide the highest number of emergency services to undocumented aliens.

State Children's Health Insurance Program (SCHIP)

In 1997, as part of the Balanced Budget Act, Congress created the State Children's Health Insurance Program (**SCHIP**). This program was created to cover children who did not have another form of health insurance coverage. Similar to basic Medicaid, SCHIP was designed to function as a federal/state joint program. Children within families who earned too much income to qualify for Medicaid, but not enough income to purchase other health insurance, are to be covered by the SCHIP program.

Beginning in October 1997, the federal government provided $24 billion in funds over five years to help states expand healthcare coverage to the estimated 5 million uninsured children who fall into the category targeted by SCHIP. There are three options states can choose from in order to comply with the SCHIP program. These choices are the following:

1. Use the federal SCHIP funds to expand Medicaid eligibility to children who did not previously qualify
2. Design a separate children's health insurance fund that is entirely separate from Medicaid
3. Combine both the Medicaid and the separate children's health insurance fund

Every state had an approved SCHIP program in place by October 1999.

TRICARE

TRICARE, formerly called CHAMPUS, is a federal program that provides healthcare benefits to families of current and retired military personnel. The active duty service member is called a sponsor and eligible family members are called beneficiaries. To be eligible for TRICARE, sponsors and beneficiaries must be enrolled in the Defense Enrollment Eligibility Reporting System (**DEERS**). TRICARE offers three benefit types: (1) TRICARE Standard, a fee-for-service plan. (2) TRICARE Extra, a PPO; and (3) TRICARE Prime, an HMO; all TRICARE enrollees are automatically enrolled in TRICARE Standard and TRICARE Extra. TRICARE Prime is an optional plan that enrollees must specifically enroll in. Some patients have TRICARE for Life, a plan that acts as secondary insurance coverage for patients over age 65. For primary insurance, these patients have Medicare. TRICARE requires preauthorization for medical services, and patients must use in-network providers. Active duty families on TRICARE Standard and TRICARE Extra and most retirees will usually owe copayments and deductibles. Medical assistants should be alert to the fact that TRICARE's deductible year begins October 1, not January 1 as is common with many insurance plans.

TRICARE requires participating providers to submit claims within 60 days of the date care was provided. Non-network providers have up to one year from the date the care was provided to submit claims.

CHAMPVA

The Civilian Health and Medical Program of the Veterans Administration (CHAMPVA) is a federal program that covers the healthcare expenses of the families of veterans with total, permanent, service-related, covered disabilities and the spouses and dependent children of veterans who died in the line of duty. Patients with CHAMPVA coverage may use any civilian healthcare provider, without preauthorization.

If a patient has other coverage besides CHAMPVA, the other coverage should be billed first. By law, CHAMPVA is always the secondary payer, except to Medicaid, State Victims of Crime Compensation, and supplemental CHAMPVA policies. Once the primary insurance carrier has made payment, a CMS-1500 claim form is sent to CHAMPVA along with a copy of the primary carrier's explanation of benefits.

CHAMPVA requires preauthorization in the following areas only:

- Organ and bone marrow transplants
- Hospice care
- Dental care
- Durable medical equipment (**DME**) worth more than $300
- Most mental health or substance abuse services

Worker's Compensation Insurance

Worker's compensation insurance covers employees injured in the workplace or suffering from a workplace-related illness. Occupational injuries are those that occur during the course of employment, but they do not have to occur on company property or while performing work duties. Accidents that occur off-site, such as while driving on company business, at a remote work site, or during a paid break are covered. Occupational illnesses are conditions that arise from short- or long-term exposure to a workplace hazard or condition, such as dust, chemical allergens, radiation, repetitive motion, and loud noises. The challenge with occupational illnesses is identifying, diagnosing, and reporting them, as some—such as repetitive stress injuries (RSI), hearing loss, and various respiratory disorders—may take years to manifest themselves.

All employers must offer workers' compensation insurance, although laws vary from state to state. Insurance may be obtained from a state-managed fund, private insurers, or employer self-insurance. Some states do not allow private insurers to offer workers' compensation policies, so coverage must be obtained from the state or through self-insurance. Federal laws cover workers in Washington, DC, coal miners, federal employees, and maritime workers.

A workers' compensation claim is initiated by filing the First Report of Illness or Injury. State laws vary widely on the time frame required for filing and the responsible party. In some states, the employer may be required to file this report, and in other states the first provider who treats the injured worker is responsible. Medical assistants need to be familiar with how the filing process works in their state.

Benefits to the injured worker include coverage of the cost of medical care related to the illness or injury, wages for time lost from work due to illness or injury, death benefits for survivors when the accident is the cause of the worker's death, and rehabilitation or retraining benefits that enable the worker to return to work or learn a different line of work if necessary.

A non-disability (ND) claim means the worker was injured and treated by a physician, but no time was lost from work. In a ND claim, no lost wages are paid. Temporary disability (TD) means that the worker is able to return to previous or modified work at a later time; permanent disability (PD) means that no further improvement is expected and the worker is unable to return to work.

Healthcare providers must enroll with their states' worker compensation programs before accepting worker compensation cases. Providers receive identification numbers for billing purposes. Workers' compensation programs reimburse physicians based on an established schedule. If physician charges are higher than the reimbursement amount, patients cannot be balance billed. In some states, workers' compensation operates under a managed care model.

To ensure the program runs properly, healthcare providers must keep good records on worker's compensation cases. This includes verifying patients' injuries with employers and contacting insurance companies to obtain claim numbers and verify the date of injury on file. Medical assistants must know their state laws for worker's compensation coverage should patients need preauthorization before care.

Patients in worker's compensation cases should have new files created so the medical office can separate that documentation from patients' other records, and thereby keep reporting and claim filing accurate. Most states' labor departments provide free physician reporting forms and claim information for injured workers.

HIPAA Compliance

Medical providers often receive requests for copies of medical records for patients who have been injured on the job or elsewhere. To practice within HIPAA guidelines for information release, be sure to look closely to determine the exact information being requested. For example, a requesting

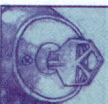

Keys to Success
MEDICAL CLAIMS FOR INJURIES

Any patient who has a medical claim for an injury, whether through workmen's compensation or other liability insurance, will have a claim number and a claims manager or department to handle the claim. At the beginning of the patient's care in the medical office, locate the name and phone number of the claims manager. Readily available contact information will allow the office easily to contact the claims manager in the event the physician orders tests or procedures that require preauthorization.

agency may ask for medical records pertaining to injury care only. A separate file for injury claims makes it easier to determine the information that is to be copied and sent. Also, be sure you have a signed release from the patient or a court order before releasing any information to a third party.

Disability Insurance

Disability insurance reimburses a patient for lost wages due to a non-work-related disability that prevents the individual from working. Benefits are based on a percentage of employees' wages, often 66 percent, because benefits are not subject to income tax. Lost wages due to a work-related disability are covered by worker's compensation insurance; lost wages due to a disability related to an automobile or other liability accident are covered by liability insurance.

With only a few exceptions, disability insurance does not pay for medical treatment; therefore, medical assistants will not often be billing a disability plan for medical services. However, medical assistants may need to assist patients who are applying for disability coverage or benefits by providing information from the medical record regarding the patient's past health history or current disability. Even though patients have disability insurance, they may not have medical coverage because they are not employed and cannot afford or are not eligible for individual health insurance policies.

Types of Disability Insurance

Disability insurance is offered by federal, state, and private sources. Federal disability policies include Social Security Disability Insurance (**SSDI**) for workers who are permanently disabled, but not from a job-related incident; Supplemental Security Income (**SSI**) for low-income disabled persons without a qualifying work history; Veteran's Disability Compensation for veterans whose injuries or diseases are the result of active duty service; Veteran's Disability Pension Benefits for wartime veterans with limited income and who are no longer able to work; Civil Service (**CSRS**) and Federal Employees Retirement System (**FERS**) disability for federal and civil service employees who become disabled. Veterans benefits include certain medical services, which medical assistants will submit bills for and for which the insurance payment must be accepted as payment in full. Five states (California, Hawaii, New Jersey, New York, and Rhode Island) and Puerto Rico provide disability insurance. State policies tend to provide short-term coverage that begins about a week after disability and extends from six to twelve months. Private policies may be obtained through employers or purchased individually. Usually, a waiting period is required after the disability begins before benefits are paid. A longer waiting period will result in a lower premium. An employer-sponsored policy will be terminated when employment ends. The advantage of an individual policy is that employees keep it when changing employers, and it can be renewed without regard to health or employment status.

Definition of Disability

No standard definition of a disability exists; rather, the conditions of a disability are defined by each individual plan. The Social Security definition of a disability is the strictest, and own-occupation disability offered by some private companies is the most liberal. Under the Social Security definition, patients are considered disabled if they cannot do work that they did before, they cannot adjust to other work because of their medical condition(s), and their disability has lasted or is expected to last for at least one year or to result in death. Social security pays no benefits for temporary or partial disability. This definition applies to both SSI and SSDI.

Own-occupation disability means that, because of sickness or injury, patients are not able to perform the substantial duties of their occupation that they were performing at the time of disability. Patients may be considered totally disabled even if they are at work in some other capacity so long as they are not able to work in their occupation. Of course, a private own-occupation disability policy will be more expensive to purchase than one with a more strict definition, similar to the one used by Social Security. Patients may be tempted to purchase the least expensive policy only to be disappointed when they find the definition of disability is so strict that it is difficult to meet eligibility requirements.

SSDI and SSI

To establish disability under SSDI or SSI, individuals complete the required forms, usually with the help of a social worker, and go through a determination process. Patients' personal physicians do not make a determination regarding whether a patient is disabled; this is determined by the insurance plan based on medical information in the patient's record. An appeals process is also available for patients who disagree with the determination of disability.

To be eligible for SSDI, workers must meet Social Security eligibility standards in terms of the number of quarters worked and the amount of wages earned per quarter. Eligible workers include disabled workers under the age of 65 and their families; individuals who become disabled before age 22 if a parent who is covered under Social Security retires, becomes disabled, or dies; certain disabled widows, widowers, or divorced spouses; and blind workers meeting specific vision criteria. After 24 months of disability payments, disabled individuals become eligible for Medicare, which will cover many of the medical expenses.

SSI was created for disabled individuals with low incomes not meeting the work and wage criteria for SSDI. Eligible persons include disabled individuals under the age of 65 with very limited income and resources, disabled children under the age of 18, and blind adults and children meeting specific vision criteria. Many SSI recipients also qualify for Medicaid and as such, some of their medical expenses may be covered.

The Medical Assistant's Role with Disability Insurance

Medical assistants should be familiar with the various ways physicians may be involved with the disability determination process, for both government and private insurers. Physicians may be treating disability applicants and need to provide medical records or testimony regarding patients' functioning. Information provided may include facts such as the date the disability occurred, a description of how the disability occurred, description of how the disability prevents the patient from working, examination and test results that document the extent of disability, and the level and timeframe of expected recovery. The wording of information provided by physicians can affect the determination, based on the disability definition being used by the insurer. Physicians may also work as paid consultative examiners who provide an outside medical or psychological examination of applicants. In this case, patients may come to the office who are disability applicants and not part of the physician's established patient base. Physicians also may be paid medical review officers who review claims from a medical perspective for the insurer. Part of the physician's regular schedule may be set aside for this activity.

Reimbursement Methods

Insurance companies reimburse providers using a variety of methods, so it is important for medical assistants to understand how this impacts the practice. The most traditional reimbursement method is a usual, customary and reasonable (UCR) fee schedule maintained by each insurance company. The insurer establishes an acceptable "customary" fee based on the range of what other providers of the same specialty in the same geographic area charge. The insurer will pay either this amount or the provider's normal fee ("usual"), whichever is less. In unusual circumstances, they will negotiate a specific "reasonable" for a given bill. The insurer is not required to publicize what its UCR fees are, but the practice learns by experience the amount each company approves.

A common reimbursement method in managed care is a **negotiated fee schedule**. The MCO develops of list of fees for providers that they agree to accept in the participating provider contract. Fees may be determined based on a percentage of the provider's usual fee (for example, 80%) or may be arrived at through negotiation.

Capitation is most often used by HMOs. Capitation means *per head*. Under a capitation plan, the insurer pays providers a flat amount per member per month, regardless of what services the patient uses. If they come in many times, or not at all, the provider receives the same payment. The objective of capitation is to put the responsibility and risk on the provider to manage the patient's care in a cost effective yet medically appropriate manner.

For inpatient care a **per diem** or *per day* payment method may be used. The facility is paid a flat amount per day the patient remains, regardless of what services are provided. This method places much of the cost management on the facility to provide the services that are medically appropriate, because they will not be paid more for unnecessary services. The risk is partially shared with the insurer, who pays more for a longer stay than a shorter one. However, there may be maximum number days that will be paid for any given condition.

Per case payment is also used for hospitals. Under this method, the hospital receives a pre-established amount per patient for the entire stay, based on the patient's diagnosis, regardless of how long they are in or what services are provided. When Medicare uses this form of reimbursement, it is called Diagnosis Related Groups (DRG), because patients with similar conditions and care requirements are classified or grouped together and all are eligible for the same amount of reimbursement.

In capitation, per diem and per case reimbursement methods it is not uncommon for additional payment to be made for **outliers**, or exceptional circumstances that cost far more or far less than the average. Most contracts also include **carve outs**, services that are reimbursed in addition to the base rate for the patient. The details of each MCO contract are different; there are no general rules. The medical assistant needs to become familiar with the details of each contract the provider has to be sure the billing and payment are appropriate.

Processing Claims

The first step to properly reimbursing insurance claims is obtaining accurate information. Many medical offices ask patients for their health insurance information over the phone, before their first visits. Other offices simply ask patients for their insurance type over the phone and then ask those patients to bring their insurance card to their visit.

Patient Registration

Each new patient in the medical office should complete a registration form (Figure 17-13 ◆) that is verified at each visit and updated annually. Before releasing private patient information to insurance carriers, medical assistants must obtain signed authorization from patients. To do otherwise is to violate HIPAA regulations for patient confidentiality. Insurance claim forms give patients' names, addresses, birth dates, diagnoses, and types of treatment, all highly protected patient information.

After obtaining pertinent patient information, medical assistants must identify the name and birth date of the insured. When the patient is the spouse or child of the insured, the medical assistant must ask the patient for the additional information. The assistant will need to know if the patient is covered by more than one plan. If so, the assistant will then have to determine which plan is primary and which is secondary.

Medical assistants must photocopy both sides of patients' insurance identification cards when patients arrive for their first visits (Figure 17-14a ◆). The front of cards typically carry the names and identification numbers of the insured or members. Each patient is uniquely identified by a member identification number assigned by the insurance company. Patients have a different number with each separate insurance plan they may have. HIPAA originally made provision for a unique patient identification number that would be the same for all insurance companies, but concerns about privacy and identity theft have put this on hold indefinitely.

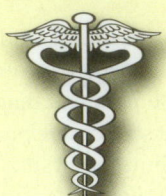

Victory Medical Center

4100 SW Highway 6
Victorville, WA 12345
(509) 555-9832

Patient Name: _____
        Last Name   First Name   Middle Initial

Address: _____
        Street   City   State   Zip

Home Phone: _____ Work Phone: _____

Mobile Phone: _____ Birthdate: _____

Social Security Number: _____ Age: _____

Sex: _____ Marital Status: S M D W Children: _____

How do you prefer to be addressed? _____

Spouse's Name: _____

Primary Care Physician: _____ Phone No: _____

Name of Person Responsible for Bill: _____

Relationship to Patient: _____ Phone No: _____

Address of Person Responsible for Bill: _____

Patient's Employer: _____ Phone No: _____

Occupation: _____

Spouse's Employer: _____ Phone No: _____

Occupation: _____

INSURANCE INFORMATION

Primary Insurance: _____ Policy No: _____ Group No: _____

Name of Policyholder: _____ Birthdate: _____

SS#: _____ Relationship to Insured: _____

Secondary Insurance: _____ Policy No: _____ Group No: _____

Name of Policyholder: _____ Birthdate: _____

If Injured: Date: _____ Place: _____

Claim Number: _____ Nature or Cause of Injury: _____

Employer at Time of Injury: _____ Phone No: _____

EMERGENCY INFORMATION

In case of emergency, local friend or relative to be notified (not living at same address)

Name: _____ Relationship to Patient: _____

Address: _____ Phone No: _____

I hereby authorize the healthcare professionals in this clinic to diagnose and treat my condition. I clearly understand and agree that all services rendered me are charged directly to me and that I am personally responsible for payment. I agree that I am responsible for all bills incurred at this clinic. I hereby authorize assignment of my insurance rights and benefits directly to the provider for services rendered. I also authorize the healthcare professionals to discuss my care with other healthcare providers who I am currently treating with.

_____   _____
Patient's Signature   Date   Parent or Guardian Signature   Date

Figure 17-13 ◆ Sample new patient registration form.

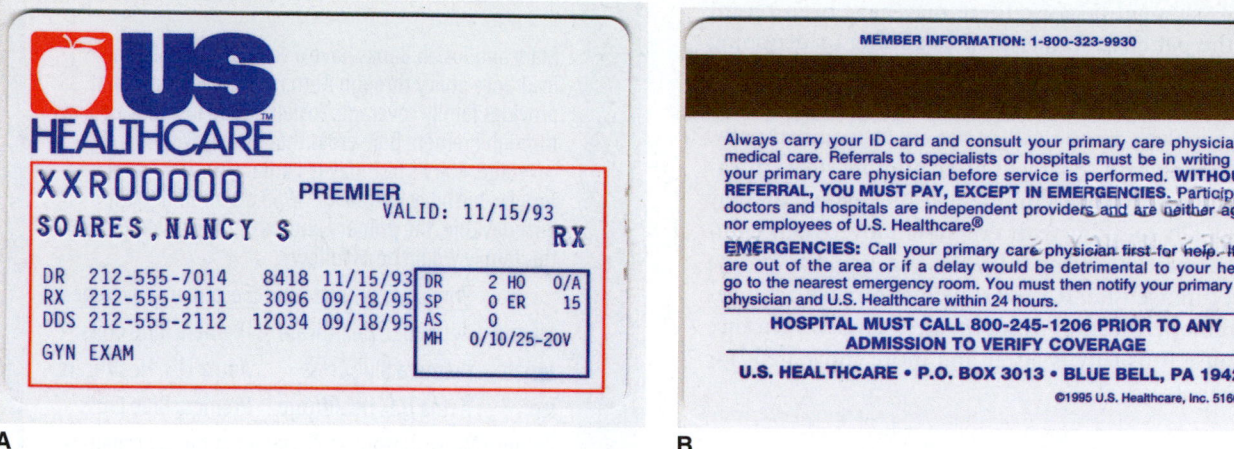

Figure 17-14 ◆ (a) The front of an insurance identification card; (b) the back of an insurance identification card.

In today's world of identity theft, most insurance plans no longer use Social Security numbers for identification. Instead, many identification numbers now have alphabetic prefixes followed by numbers. Some have alphabetic characters only. Plans may have their own group or plan numbers, as well. A **payer number**, a number that identifies an insurance company, allows medical offices to submit claims electronically. The back of the card typically has the claims mailing addresses (Figure 17-14b). Insurance telephone numbers appear on the front or back of cards. Typically, one number is for "customer or member service"

and another is for "providers." Medical assistants call the latter for information on patients' coverage or claims.

Verification of Benefits

After obtaining insurance information from patients, medical assistants should verify coverage with the insurance company. By doing this, medical assistants ensure they have the most current and accurate information possible. However, even verifying benefits with the insurance company is not a

---

PROCEDURE 17-2 Verify a Patient's Insurance Eligibility

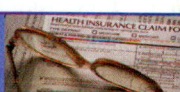

Theory and Rationale

Many patients who seek medical care are covered by some form of medical insurance. Verifying a patient's eligibility is an important part of the medical assistant's job. Verifying benefits with the insurance company ensures that the medical assistant has the most current and accurate information possible.

Materials

- Insurance identification card
- Patient's registration form
- Telephone
- Paper
- Pen

Competency

(**Conditions**) With the necessary materials, you will be able to (**Task**) verify a patient's insurance eligibility (**Standards**) correctly within the time limit set by the instructor.

1. Looking at the patient's registration form, locate the patient's birth date and the patient's relationship to the insured.

2. Looking at the patient's insurance identification card, locate the name of the insured, the insured's member identification number, and the telephone number of the insurance company.

3. Call the insurance company at the provider customer service telephone number listed on the insurance identification card.

4. When the customer service representative answers the call, write down the name of the customer service representative and the date and time of the call.

5. Verify spelling of policyholder's name and birth date.

6. Verify patient's name and birth date.

7. Verify coverage for type of service to be rendered, including frequency or number of visits.

8. Verify when preauthorization is needed.

9. Verify patient's financial responsibility for deductible, copayment, or coinsurance amounts.

10. Verify coordination of benefits rules if more than one policy covers the patient.

11. Verify provider's participating or non-partipating status.

12. Verify the address where insurance claims are to be mailed or the payer number needed for electronic billing.

guarantee of payment because there may have been recent changes in the patient's status, such as adding or dropping coverage, that have not been input into the computer system at the time of verification. The most common way to verify benefits is to make a phone call to the insurance company. Some companies have a separate phone number for verification. The process may be completely automated or may include personally speaking with a representative. Many companies also offer the option of verifying benefits online through a secure website. It is worthwhile to make arrangements for online verification with providers' largest insurance carriers because it usually is faster and more convenient for medical assistants.

Determining Coordination of Benefits

Patients may be covered by more than one insurance plan. Most often this is because spouses each have a group health plan and each has purchased coverage for the other. Also, both spouses may elect to cover their children under both policies. Insurance companies, in cooperation with state insurance commissioners, have established specific rules that determine which coverage is billed first, called primary, and which is billed second, called the secondary policy. This process is called **coordination of benefits (COB)**. Patients do not have the option of specifying which insurance should be primary or secondary.

When spouses or partners are covered by each other's policy, the patient's own policy is always primary for him or her, and the spouse's or partner's policy is secondary. Likewise, when spouses are patients, their own policy is primary. Medical assistants should not assume that spouses are covered by each other's policy because such coverage is entirely their choice, based on their insurance needs and costs associated with covering other family members. It is possible, for example, for the husband's insurance to cover himself and his wife, but the wife's insurance may cover only her. In this case, the husband would have only one insurance, his own. The wife would have two policies; hers would be primary and her husband's would be secondary.

When both parents carry coverage for the children, most health insurance plans decide which insurance plan is primary and which is secondary based on the **birthday rule** (Figure 17-15 ◆). According to this rule, the parent with the birthday earlier in the year is the primary carrier for the children; the parent with the later birthday is the secondary carrier for the children.

The birthday rule relies only on the month and day of the parents' birthday. The year is not used. The insurance commissioners of most states have agreed to use the birthday rule. If a state does not use the birthday rule, the COB rules of plan in the non-birthday rule state apply. Medical assistants need to ask about this when verifying benefits.

Complicated issues can arise with child patients covered by three companies, perhaps through both biological parents and one stepparent. In these cases, typically the custodial parent's

Mary and Josiah Banks have a son, Ian. Mary has an insurance policy through Aetna U.S. Health Care that provides family coverage. Josiah has an insurance policy through Premera Blue Cross that also provides family coverage. Mary's birthday is January 10, 1977, and Josiah's birthday is April 15, 1968. According to the birthday rule, the primary and secondary coverage for this family would be as follows:

	Primary Coverage	Secondary Coverage
Mary	Aetna U.S. Healthcare	Premera Blue Cross
Josiah	Premera Blue Cross	Aetna U.S. Healthcare
Ian	Aetna U.S. Healthcare	Premera Blue Cross

Because Mary's birthday falls earlier in the year than Josiah's, her policy is primary for her and Ian. Because Josiah's birthday falls later, his plan is secondary for Ian. Policyholders are primary on their own policies, so Josiah's primary carrier is his own policy through Premera Blue Cross.

Figure 17-15 ◆ Using the birthday rule.

plan is primary, the spouse of the custodial parent's plan is secondary, and the noncustodial parent's plan is tertiary. The easiest way to get patients' claims paid on time is to ask the insurance carriers to identify the order in which to bill.

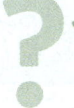

Critical Thinking Question 17-4

Using the birthday rule as a guide, what types of questions should the medical assistant ask Martin?

Preparing Referrals, Authorizations, and Precertifications

Before scheduling any nonemergency procedures or costly tests, medical assistants should call insurance carriers to both verify patients' eligibility for those services and to complete any needed **preauthorizations**. Preauthorization, sometimes called **precertification**, is the process of calling the patient's insurance carrier to obtain permission for patients to receive prescribed procedures. Depending on the insurance plan,

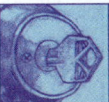

**Keys to Success
DOCUMENTING THE PATIENT FILE**

Any service billed by the medical office must be documented in the patient's file. Billing for services that have not been documented is considered fraud and is illegal. Therefore, it is crucial that all billed-for services and diagnoses are documented as patient complaints or services performed by members of the healthcare team.

some managed care companies require referrals from patients' primary care providers for specialized care. In these cases, medical assistants may need to call patients' primary care providers to coordinate the patients' referrals. Any time assistants receive preauthorization or precertification numbers for patients, they should include those numbers on the CMS-1500 insurance billing form as well as make note of them in the patient's file.

When patients require specialist care, managed care plans may require referrals from patients' **PCPs**. Medical assistants who work for PCPs may be asked to arrange those specialist referrals, which entails verifying that specialists are covered under patients' managed care plans. To accomplish this task, assistants can either phone insurance carriers' customer service departments or look online. Medical assistants in specialist offices must ensure that patients' PCPs have arranged referrals before those patients visit the specialists' offices.

Many HMOs penalize physicians who fail to obtain authorization before rendering service. Many times, insurance carriers will deny claims that were not properly preauthorized. In managed care, physicians are then restricted from billing patients for denied services. In effect, the physicians perform the procedures for free. With penalties this severe, it is imperative that healthcare providers verify the need for referrals, authorizations, or precertifications before providing service.

Documenting Insurance Company Calls

While comprehensive, in-depth knowledge of all insurance plans is unrealistic, administrative medical assistants should know where to find answers and information. Many insurance companies provide coverage information on line. Insurance companies' Web site addresses typically appear on patients' identification cards. These resources are recommended for general information, not procedure authorization. When assistants have questions about patients' insurance coverage, the provider customer service department of the patients' insurance carriers is the best place to call.

Medical assistants should document any calls made to an insurance carrier, including date and time, number used, party on the phone, and information obtained. Such data becomes part of patients' permanent financial record and can be referenced should there ever be a discrepancy between what the medical assistant was told by the insurance carrier and how the insurance carrier processed the claim.

Health Insurance Claim Forms

Before the 1990s, health insurance carriers required healthcare providers to use unique forms to bill for patient services. Patients were required to obtain these forms from their employers or insurance carriers. Healthcare providers would attach **superbills**, also called **charge slips** or **encounter forms**, which are preprinted lists of procedures and diagnosis codes commonly used in the office. Providers would circle the services they provided, along with the applicable diagnoses; attach the

superbill to the unique insurance claim form; and mail the form to the appropriate insurance carrier for reimbursement.

The CMS-1500 Claim Form

To help standardize the insurance billing industry, the former HCFA (now CMS), created a uniform billing form to be used by physicians and other professional providers. This form, now called the CMS-1500, is used today by all health insurance carriers, including Medicare, Medicaid, and workmen's compensation carriers, to complete paper billed claims (Figure 17-16 ◆). Dental claims are sent via the American Dental Association (**ADA**) standard form. The ADA form and the CMS-1500 are the only two insurance claim forms medical assistants use to submit paper claims today.

The boxes to be completed on the CMS-1500 form are referred to as **form locators** (FL). The form is divided into two major sections: Patient and Insured Information (FL 1–13) and Physician or Supplier Information (FL 14–33). The top right margin is the Carrier's Area and is used to print the insurance company's address on the form.

Specific guidelines exist for completing a CMS-1500 claim form. TRICARE, CHAMPVA, Medicare, Medicaid, and workers' compensation carriers have their own rules. Private insurance companies also have their own variations. Because guidelines vary at the state and local levels for completing the CMS-1500, the medical assistant should check with his local intermediaries or private carriers. For Blue Cross Blue Shield claims, the medial assistant should refer to the provider manual for his state's Blue Cross Blue Shield plans for guidelines for completing the CMS-1500 claim form.

When completing the form, medical assistants will be **abstracting** data, or using several source documents to find the required information. It is the medical assistants' responsibility to locate all needed data on established documents and accurately transfer it to the CMS-1500 form. The patient registration form provides information about the patient's and insured's name, address, birth date, and related data. The insurance card provides information on the insurance policy, identification and group numbers, mailing address for claims, as well as basic coverage and cost information. The clinic's encounter form will provide the date of service, services rendered, and treating provider. The encounter form may contain fees or the medical assistant may need to refer to the clinic's fee schedule for charges. The encounter form or patient registration form may contain the clinic's address, tax identification number, and NPI numbers, or the medical assistant may need to refer to other office records for this information. Table 17-2 provides general guidelines for completing the form and identifies the most common source documents needed for each form locator. Accuracy in identifying and transferring the data is paramount; a single transposition in a critical field such as name, identification number, birth date, or CPT code could cause the claim to be rejected. A few extra minutes spent proofreading data will prevent the need to rework claims later.

Optical Character Recognition

The CMS-1500 is printed in red ink so that it is recognizable by OCR scanners. Optical character recognition (OCR)

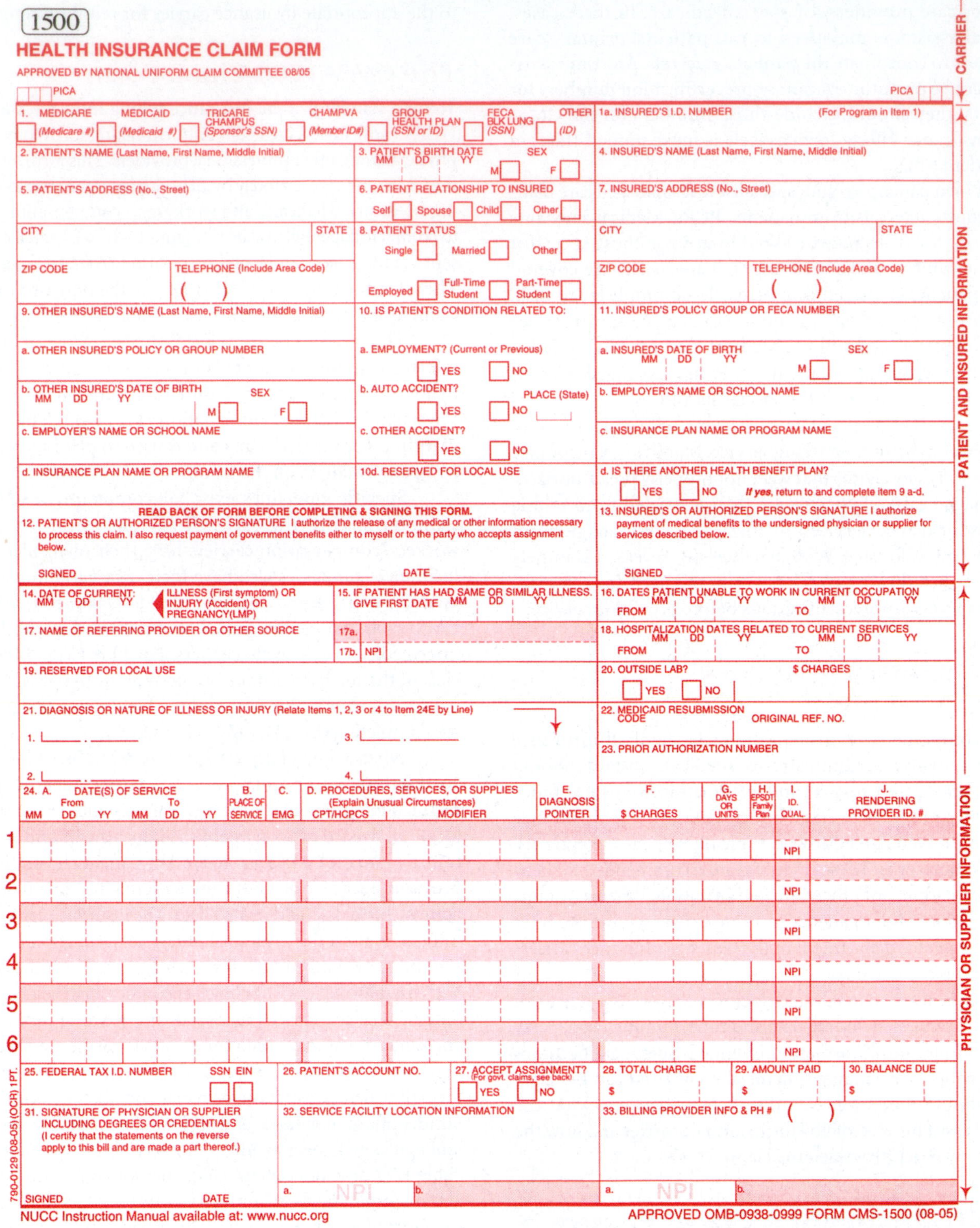

Figure 17-16 ◆ CMS-1500 claim form.

devices (scanners) are being used frequently across the nation for processing paper insurance claims because of their speed and efficiency.

A scanner can transfer printed or typed text and bar codes to the insurance company's computer memory. Scanners read at such a fast speed that they reduce the cost of data entry and decrease the processing time. More control is gained over data input by using OCR. It improves accuracy, thus reducing coding errors because the claim is entered exactly as coded by the medical assistant.

text continues on page 300

TABLE 17-2 INSTRUCTIONS FOR COMPLETING THE CMS-1500 CLAIM FORM

FL Number, Name, and Use (R = required; C = conditional depending on claim)	Source Document
Carrier area (top right-hand margin) Enter the insurance plan's mailing address for claims from this policy. Be sure to verify. Some insurance companies have different addresses and different PO boxes for different types of plans, such as group, individual, or government.	Insurance ID card
FL 1 – FL 13: PATIENT AND INSURED INFORMATION	
FL 1: Type of Insurance (R) FL 1 identifies what type of insurance the patient carries. The form lists five government plans: Medicare, Medicaid, TRICARE/CHAMPUS, CHAMPVA, and FECA/Black Lung. There are two other options: Group Health Plan and Other. These are utilized based on what type of plan the insured is enrolled in. BCBS is usually marked Other.	Insurance ID card
FL 1a: Insured's ID Number (R) FL 1a asks for the insured's insurance ID number as reflected on the insurance card. The insured could be the patient or it could be someone else such as spouse, mother, or father.	Insurance ID card
FL 2: Patient's Name (R) In FL 2, enter the name of the patient who received services. This information is input last name, first name, and middle name or initial. The spelling should match the insurance card exactly. If the name on the card is misspelled, then the name in the computer should be misspelled until the patient provides a new card with the correct spelling.	Patient registration form Encounter form
FL 3: Patient's Date of Birth/Sex (R) In FL 3, enter the patient's date of birth and sex/gender. The date of birth is entered using the eight-digit format: MMDDCCYY. Enter an X in the correct box for male or female. Do not try to guess the gender based on the patient's name.	Patient registration form Encounter form
FL 4: Insured's Name (R) FL 4 asks for the name of the person who is the insured. This may or may not be the patient. If the patient is the insured, the word "SAME" should be entered. The insured's name should be entered last name, first name, middle name or initial.	Insurance ID card
FL 5: Patient's Address (R) Enter the patient's home address and telephone number in FL 5. This information is taken from the patient information form when the patient registers in the office. The address should include the street name and number, city, state (two-letter abbreviation), and zip code. Do not use commas, periods, or other punctuation in the address. Do not use the # sign for apartment numbers. When entering a nine-digit zip code, include the hyphen. Do not use a hyphen or space as a separator within the telephone number.	Patient registration form
FL 6: Patient's Relationship to the Insured (R) Once FL 4 has been completed, in FL 6 enter an X in the correct box to indicate the patient's relationship to the insured. Options include Self, Spouse, Child, or Other. If the patient is the insured person, the "Self" entry is marked here. Only one box can be marked.	Patient registration form
FL 7: Insured's Address (R) In FL 7, enter the insured's address. If the insured person is not the patient (see FL 4), then this field should be completed. This information should include the street name and number, city, state (two-letter abbreviation), zip code, and phone number. If the patient is the insured, leave this FL blank.	Patient registration form

continued

TABLE 17-2 INSTRUCTIONS FOR COMPLETING THE CMS-1500 CLAIM FORM (CONTINUED)

FL Number, Name, and Use (R = required; C = conditional depending on claim)	Source Document
FL 8: Patient Status (R) Indicate the patient's status in FL 8: Single, Married, or Other. It also requires the patient's employment status: Employed, Full-Time Student, or Part-Time Student. Enter an X in the box for the patient's marital status and for the employment or student status. Only one box on each line can be marked. Divorced and widowed should be marked as Single. Full-Time Student indicates that the patient is registered as a full-time student as defined by the post-secondary school or university. Do not mark this box for students in elementary or high school. This information is important for determination of liability and coordination of benefits.	Patient registration form
FL 9: Other Insured's Name (C) If FL 11d is marked YES, complete FL 9 and 9a–d; otherwise, leave them blank. FL 9 indicates that there is a holder of another policy that may cover the patient. When there is additional group health coverage, enter the other insured's full last name, first name, and middle initial of the enrollee in another health plan if it is different from that shown in FL 2. If there is no secondary policy, FL 9 is left blank.	Insurance ID card
FL 9a: Other Insured's Policy or Group Number (C) Enter the policy number or group number of the secondary insurance policy in FL 9a. The number should be entered exactly as it appears on the insurance card.	Insurance ID card
FL 9b: Other Insured's Date of Birth/Sex (C) FL 9b requires the date of birth of the insured of the secondary policy. The date of birth should be entered in the eight-digit format: MMDDCCYY. Choose either male or female accordingly.	Insurance ID card Patient registration form
FL 9c: Employer's Name or School Name (C) Enter the name of the insured's employer or school in FL 9c.	Patient registration form Insurance ID card
FL 9d: Insurance Plan Name or Program Name (C) FL 9d asks for the name of the secondary insurance plan. This information is taken directly from the secondary insurance card. Enter the name exactly as it appears on the card.	Insurance ID card
FL 10a–c: Is Patient's Condition Related To? (R) FL 10 identifies whether the patient's visit was related to an employment accident, auto accident, or other accident. This FL is used when filing workers' compensation claims, auto accident claims, or claims for other types of injuries. If the patient's visit does not pertain to an accident of any kind, the default answer will be NO. Enter an X in the correct box. If this box is not marked, or marked incorrectly, the claim could be delayed.	Encounter form Medical record
FL 10d: Reserved for Local Use (C) Different insurance carriers for different reasons use FL 10d. One example of use would be a specific insurance carrier requiring the word "Attachment" to be placed here in the event that there are paper attachments with the claim. This box is completed with the Medicaid ID number on Medi-Medi claims.	
FL 11: Insured's Policy Group or FECA Number (C) If FL 4 is completed, then FL 11 should be completed. FL 11 identifies the insured's policy group number listed on the insurance card. This number should be entered exactly as it appears on the insurance card. A FECA number (nine-digit alphanumeric identifier) is listed here when employees of the federal government are filing workers' compensation claims.	Insurance ID card

TABLE 17-2 INSTRUCTIONS FOR COMPLETING THE CMS-1500 CLAIM FORM (CONTINUED)

FL Number, Name, and Use (R = required; C = conditional depending on claim)	Source Document
FL 11a: Insured's Date of Birth/Sex (C) In FL 11a, list the date of birth of the insured. The date of birth should be listed in the eight-digit format: MMDDCCYY. If the patient and the insured are the same person, this space can be left blank. Mark an X in either male or female accordingly. If gender is unknown, leave blank.	Insurance ID card Patient registration form
FL 11b: Employer's Name or School Name (C) In FL 11b, list the insured's place of employment or school that is attended, if a full-time university student as marked in FL 8. If the patient/insured is unemployed, leave blank.	Insurance ID card Patient registration form
FL 11c: Insurance Plan Name or Program Name (C) FL 11c identifies the insurance plan name. The information should be taken directly from the insurance card and spelled exactly as it appears on the card.	Insurance ID card
FL 11d: Is There Another Health Benefit Plan? (R) In FL 11d, indicate whether there is another health benefit plan. If there is another plan, YES is marked with an X and the information is entered into form locators 9a–d. If there is no additional insurance plan, NO is marked.	Patient registration form
FL 12: Patient's or Authorized Person's Signature (R) FL 12 is where the patient or guarantor signs, allowing the release of any medical information to the insurance company for billing purposes. This release is only valid for billing information. Any other request for records will require a formal release of information form to be signed by the patient or guarantor. This signature is good for one year from the date it is signed and should be updated annually. When submitting claims, the words "Signature on File" or "SOF" may be printed here in place of a signature. The actual patient signature will be on file in the patient's chart. If the patient signs the form, enter the date in the six-digit format (MM/DD/YY) or eight-digit format (MM/DD/CCYY). If "Signature on File" or "SOF" is entered, do not enter a date. If there is no signature on file, leave blank or enter "No Signature on File."	Patient registration form
FL 13: Insured's or Authorized Person's Signature (C) FL 13 is where the patient or insured signs, authorizing the insurance company to reimburse the physician or supplier directly. As just stated, the words "Signature on File" or "SOF" may be printed here in place of a written signature when filing claims. If the patient signs the form, enter the date in the six-digit format (MM/DD/YY) or eight-digit format (MM/DD/CCYY). If "Signature on File" or "SOF" is entered, do not enter a date. If there is no signature on file, leave blank or enter "No Signature on File." Not required for government claims such as Medicare, Medicaid, Workers Compensation.	Patient registration form
FL 14 – FL 33 PHYSICIAN OR SUPPLIER INFORMATION	
FL 14: Date of Current: Illness, Injury, Pregnancy (C) Indicate the first date of the current illness, injury, or pregnancy in FL 14. The date should be entered in the six-digit (MM/DD/YY) or eight-digit format (MM/DD/CCYY). For a pregnancy, the first day of the woman's last menstrual period (LMP) is used. If this information is not known, leave blank.	Encounter form Medical record
FL 15: If Patient Has Had Same or Similar Illness (C) In FL 15, enter the first date of treatment for the same or similar illness in the past. The date should be entered in the six-digit (MM/DD/YY) or eight-digit format (MM/DD/CCYY). If the information is not known, leave blank.	Encounter form Medical record

continued

TABLE 17-2 INSTRUCTIONS FOR COMPLETING THE CMS-1500 CLAIM FORM (CONTINUED)

FL Number, Name, and Use (R = required; C = conditional depending on claim)	Source Document
FL 16: Dates Patient Unable to Work in Current Occupation (C) In FL 16, list the dates the patient is unable to work due to his or her illness or injury. These dates will be required when filing workers' compensation or disability claims. The dates should be entered in the six-digit (MM/DD/YY) or eight-digit format (MM/DD/CCYY). If the information is not required, leave blank.	Encounter form Medical record
FL 17: Name of Referring Physician or Other Source (C) FL 17 requests the name of the physician referring the patient. Some insurance companies, such as health maintenance organizations (HMOs) or exclusive provider organizations (EPOs), require this information to be on a claim. The information entered should include the physician's last name, first name, and credentials. If multiple providers are involved, enter one provider using the following priority order: 1. Referring provider 2. Ordering provider 3. Supervising provider. If there is no referring physician, leave blank.	Encounter form Referral form
FL 17a: ID Number of Referring Physician (C) The insurance plan's ID number of the referring, ordering, or supervising provider is reported in FL 17a, if required by the plan. Since the implementation of the NPI, this field is rarely used.	Referral form
FL 17b: NPI Number (C) Enter the NPI number of the referring, ordering, or supervising provider in FL 17b.	Referral form
FL 19: Reserved for Local Use (C) FL 19 is used for miscellaneous information that may be required by the insurance policy.	
FL 20: Outside Lab (C) FL 20 is used only if lab tests appear in section 24. A YES answer indicates that an entity other than the entity billing for the service performed the purchased services. If YES is chosen, enter the purchased price under Charges and complete FL 32. If the lab tests were performed by the provider's office, mark NO. If no lab tests were ordered, leave this FL blank.	Encounter form Medical record
FL 21: Diagnosis or Nature of Illness or Injury (R) In FL 21, the ICD-9 codes for the diagnoses applied to this claim are entered. At least one code must be entered and up to four codes can be used on a claim. They are placed in order of precedence, line 1 being the primary diagnosis, and so forth. No diagnosis descriptions are used on a claim form. The ICD-9 codes should be checked for medical necessity to make sure they are used appropriately with the CPT codes used in FL 24D. Relate lines 1, 2, 3, and 4 to the lines of service in 24E by line number.	Encounter form Medical record
FL 22: Medicaid Resubmission Code (C) If required, FL 22 is where the Medicaid resubmission code used for Medicaid claims is entered. List the original reference number and the code for resubmitted claims.	Medicaid EOB Phone call to insurance company
FL 23: Prior Authorization Number (C) Some insurance plans, such as those of HMOs and PPOs, require a prior authorization number. If required, when preauthorization is obtained from an insurance company for services, the number assigned is input in FL 23. Also, HMO-required referral numbers are input in this form locator. If prior authorization is required and is omitted, the claim will be denied. If no prior authorization is required, leave blank.	Referral form

TABLE 17-2 INSTRUCTIONS FOR COMPLETING THE CMS-1500 CLAIM FORM (CONTINUED)	
FL Number, Name, and Use (R = required; C = conditional depending on claim)	**Source Document**
Section 24 The six service lines in Section 24 were divided horizontally to accommodate submission of supplemental information to support the billed service, such as anesthesia and drug information.	
FL 24A: Dates of Service (R) In FL 24A, enter the dates of service for the services provided. Depending on the insurance carrier, these columns are filled in using different formats. Some require both the To and From dates to be listed in six-digit format (MM/DD/YY). Some require just the From date to be listed or just the To date. If the same procedure was provided multiple times on a single date, the specific date is entered once and the number of procedures is listed in FL 24G.	Encounter form Medical record
FL 24B: Place of Service (R) Place of service in FL 24B is a mandatory field to be completed because it describes the place where the procedure or service was performed. This place could be many places, such as the physician's office, hospital, emergency department, skilled nursing facility, or even the patient's home. A code is used (see following list) to indicate the place of service. Note that the CMS has stated that the place of service must also be fully written out in FL 32. Consider this example: The patient was an inpatient (hospital) and the physician saw the patient in the hospital for an evaluation and management service. Therefore, the code 21 (see following list) would be entered in FL 24B and the name and address of the hospital entered in FL 32. Common place of service codes include the following: 11. Physician's office 20. Urgent care facility 21. Inpatient hospital 22. Outpatient hospital 23. Hospital emergency department 31. Skilled nursing facility	Encounter form Medical record
FL 24C: EMG (Emergency) (C) FL 24C is used only with Medicaid to indicate whether the service was provided on an emergency basis. This FL should be marked with a Y for YES or left blank for NO. The definition of an emergency can be defined differently by each payer.	Encounter form Medical record
FL 24D: Procedures, Services, or Supplies (R) In FL 24D, enter the CPT or HCPCS codes used to identify the procedures, services, or supplies provided. Modifiers are also listed in FL 24D. If more than three modifiers are used, list 99 here and enter the modifiers in FL 19.	Encounter form Medical record
FL 24E: Diagnosis Pointer (R) FL 24E indicates the line number (1, 2, 3, and 4) of the diagnosis code listed in FL 21 as it relates to each service or procedure. If more than one diagnosis is attached to a single procedure or service, list the primary diagnosis first. Leave a space between each number. It is critical to be sure that each CPT code has a corresponding diagnosis code to justify the need. Some insurances, such as Medicare, require only one diagnosis reference number per service.	Encounter form Medical record

continued

TABLE 17-2 INSTRUCTIONS FOR COMPLETING THE CMS-1500 CLAIM FORM (CONTINUED)

FL Number, Name, and Use (R = required; C = conditional depending on claim)	Source Document
FL 24F: Charges (R) FL 24F lists the charges that are assigned to each CPT or HCPCS code listed. The amount should be entered without a decimal point or dollar sign. If multiple units are entered in FL 24G, the charges should reflect the total charge for amount of the procedure times the number of units. It is not a per unit charge. The charge entered should be the provider's established fee schedule, not the discounted or contracted rate. Medicare claims should contain the Medicare fee schedule charge.	Encounter form Physician fee schedule
FL 24G: Days or Units (R) Enter the number of units per procedure or service provided to a patient in FL 24G. If multiple units are entered in 24G, the charges should reflect the amount of the procedure multiplied by the number of units. When required by payers to provide supplemental information such as the National Drug Code (NDC) units in addition to the HCPCS units, enter the applicable NDC units' qualifier and related units in the shaded line. The following qualifiers are to be used when reporting NDC units: F2 International Unit; ML Milliliter; GR Gram; UN Unit.	Encounter form Medical record
FL 24H: EPSDT Family Plan (C) FL 24H is used on Medicaid claims only to identify whether the patient is receiving her services through Medicaid's Early and Periodic Screening, Diagnosis, and Treatment (EPSDT) program. Enter "Y" for YES or "N" for NO or follow state-specific guidelines.	Insurance (Medicaid) ID card
FL 24I: ID Qualifier (C) If the insurance plan requires use of a plan specific provider ID number for the provider who delivered the service, enter the code for type of plan. Otherwise, leave blank.	Office records
FL 24J: Rendering Provider (R) The provider rendering the service is reported in FL 24J. Enter the NPI number in the unshaded area of the field. If the insurance plan also requires use of a plan specific provider ID number for the provider who delivered the service, enter the ID number in the shaded portion. Otherwise, leave the shaded portion blank.	Encounter form Medical record
FL 25: Federal Tax ID Number (R) List in FL 25 the physician's federal tax ID number or the employer identification number (EIN) of the billing entity. Do not enter hyphens with numbers. The appropriate box (SSN or EIN) should be marked with an X.	Encounter form Office records
FL 26: Patient's Account Number (C) In FL 26, enter the patient's account number assigned by the medical office. The computer system used in the office will generate the number, and it should be entered on the claim. This in turn will allow for the account number to appear on the Explanation of Benefits (EOB) form, which makes it easier to locate the correct patient to post insurance payments.	Encounter form Medical record
FL 27: Accept Assignment? (C) FL 27 is used with Medicare claims to indicate whether the physician accepts assignment on this claim. PAR physicians will always mark YES. Non-PAR physicians must select YES or NO on each claim.	Encounter form Office records
FL 28: Total Charge (R) FL 28 lists the total charges, added together from those listed in FL 24F. The charges should be checked for accuracy to ensure proper reimbursement. Do not use decimal points or dollar signs in this entry.	Calculator

TABLE 17-2   INSTRUCTIONS ON COMPLETING THE CMS-1500 CLAIM FORM (CONTINUED)

FL Number, Name, and Use (R = required; C = conditional depending on claim)	Source Document
FL 29: Amount Paid FL 29 indicates the amount paid by primary insurance on this claim. This amount is added after the primary EOB is received and payment is posted. A secondary claim is printed to be sent to the secondary insurance carrier along with a copy of the primary insurance carrier's EOB. Do not use decimal points or dollar signs in this entry. Do not enter any patient payments unless instructed to do so by the insurance plan. Some managed care plans require copayments to be reported here.	Encounter form
FL 30: Balance Due (C) FL 30 is used to record the difference between the amounts in FL 28 and 29. If FL 29 is blank, leave FL 30 blank also. This amount is the balance due for the claim being submitted. When a claim is submitted electronically, this locator or "balance due" does not appear. Do not use decimal points or dollar signs in this entry.	Calculator
FL 31: Signature of Physician or Supplier Including Degrees or Credentials (R) FL 31 identifies the name of the physician or supplier who has provided the services to the patient along with professional credentials (MD, PA-C, or NP). If a paper claim is submitted, the physician or supplier's name must be typed/printed. "Signature on File" or "SOF" is not acceptable in this FL. Enter a six-digit date (MM/DD/YY), eight-digit date (MM/DD/CCYY), or alphanumeric date. A signature stamp may be used instead of a written signature. The stamp must leave a clear, nonsmeared image on the claim.	Typed Signature stamp
FL 32: Name and Address of Facility Where Services Were Rendered (C) FL 32 identifies the name of the facility where services were provided. Enter the name, address, zip code, and NPI number. When more than one supplier is used, a separate CMS-1500 form should be used for each supplier.	Encounter form Medical record
FL 32a: NPI Number (C) Enter the NPI number of the service facility location in FL 32a.	Encounter form Office records
FL 32b: Other ID Number (C) If required by the insurance plan, enter the plan specific ID number here.	Encounter form Office records
FL 33: Billing Provider Information and Phone Number (R) Enter the provider's or supplier's billing name, address, zip code, and phone number in FL 33. The phone number is to be entered in the area to the right of the field title. Enter the name and address information in the following format: First line: Name Second line: Address Third line: City, state, and zip code	Encounter form Office records
FL 33a: NPI Number (R) Enter the NPI number of the billing provider in FL 33a.	Encounter form Office records
FL 33b: Other ID Number (C) If required by the insurance plan, enter the plan-specific ID number here.	Encounter form Office records

Source: Adapted from Vines, Deborah, Braceland, Ann, Rollins, Elizabeth, and Miller, Susan. Comprehensive Health Insurance: Billing, Coding, and Reimbursement. *© 2008, pp. 223–232.*

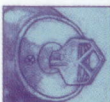

Keys to Success
PATIENT ACCOUNT NUMBERS

Including the medical office's patient account number on the CMS-1500 claim form helps identify when payment is made. Most insurance companies list offices' patient account numbers on the explanation of benefits, making patient accounts easier to find and payments easier to post in computer systems.

The CMS-1500 form was developed so insurance carriers could process claims efficiently by OCR. Keying a form for OCR scanning requires different techniques than preparing one for standard claims submission. Because the majority of insurance carriers accept the OCR format, it is suggested that it be routinely used. Successful OCR begins with the proper submission of claims data. Printed characters must conform to the preprogrammed specifications relative to character size and alignment on the CMS-1500 form. Only the current CMS-1500 form with red dropout ink is acceptable for OCR. These characteristics cannot be copied; therefore, original forms are necessary. OCR guidelines include the following:

- Use original approved forms only.
- Use all capital letters.
- Use a standard mono-spaced serif font (one that has little lines on the ends of the letters such as Courier).
- Do not use any punctuation such as . , / # -.
- Keep all text within the boundaries of the red box for each FL.
- Use eight digit dates for birthdates. Other dates can be either six or eight digits, but should be consistent.
- Do not erase, strike out, overtype, or white out. If you make a mistake, start over.
- Do not use highlighters or pen to make any extra markings on the form.
- Do not tape or staple anything to the form.*

Using diagnostic coding (**ICD-9-CM**) ∞ (Chapter 18) and procedural (CPT) coding ∞ (Chapter 19), medical assistants can file accurate CMS-1500 health insurance claim forms. Most medical offices have software that creates these forms, but medical assistants must input proper, comprehensive information to obtain accurate results. For example, assistants enter an insurance company's address in the blank portion in the upper right of the form. When preparing to send printed documents, assistants should fold the CMS-1500 such that address information shows through a window envelope (Figure 17-17 ◆).

*Source: Vines, Deborah, Braceland, Ann, Rollins, Elizabeth and Miller, Susan. *Comprehensive Health Insurance: Billing, Coding, and Reimbursement.* © 2008, p. 35. Reprinted by permission of Pearson Education, Inc. Upper Saddle River, NJ.

HIPAA Compliance

Once completed, CMS-1500 claim forms contain confidential patient information. As a result, these forms must be protected from view by anyone who is unauthorized to see patient information. Keep these forms in a secure area, never in a nonsecure area even when in envelopes. When errors are made on CMS-1500 claim forms and new ones must be printed, shred the forms with errors to protect patient privacy.

The CMS-1500 form accommodates only four diagnostic codes, which should appear in order of importance. The first code is always for the patient's chief complaint. Box 24E on the CMS-1500 form links each service on the form to the appropriate diagnosis code in box 21 (see Table 17-2). A completed form CMS-1500 is shown in Figure 17-18 ◆.

Filing Timelines

Most insurance carriers accept claims up to one year from the date of service, although some have much shorter timelines, such as 90 days. After filing timelines pass, claims are considered **past timely filing limits** and will likely be rejected. With most managed care plans, claims rejected due to timely filing limits cannot be billed to the patient. To avoid rejection, it is best to submit claims soon after service is rendered.

Billing Insurance Companies Electronically

Electronic claims, also called electronic media claims or **EMCs**, are submitted to the insurance carrier via a central processing unit (CPU), tape diskette, direct data entry, direct wire, telephone line via modem, or personal computer. Electronic claims are never printed on paper. When claims are sent electronically to the insurance carriers for processing, an electronic signature is used to verify that the information received is true and correct. Medicare requires electronic transmission of claims for providers with ten or more employees or facilities with twenty-five or more employees. Paper claims will not be processed for these submitters.

Electronic claims have a number of advantages:

- Administrative costs are lower because fewer personnel hours are needed to prepare forms, and supply and postage costs are lower.
- Fewer claims are rejected because technical errors are detected and corrected before the claim arrives at the payer.
- Processing is faster with fewer errors. An electronic claim is received by the payer in minutes. The payer does not have to perform data entry, so there is less opportunity for errors to be introduced. In addition, most claims can be automatically adjudicated by the computer, rather than being processed by a claims analyst.
- Errors can be corrected faster. If errors are found on claims by carriers or the claim is denied, the office is notified immediately and medical assistants can begin work on resolving the issue.

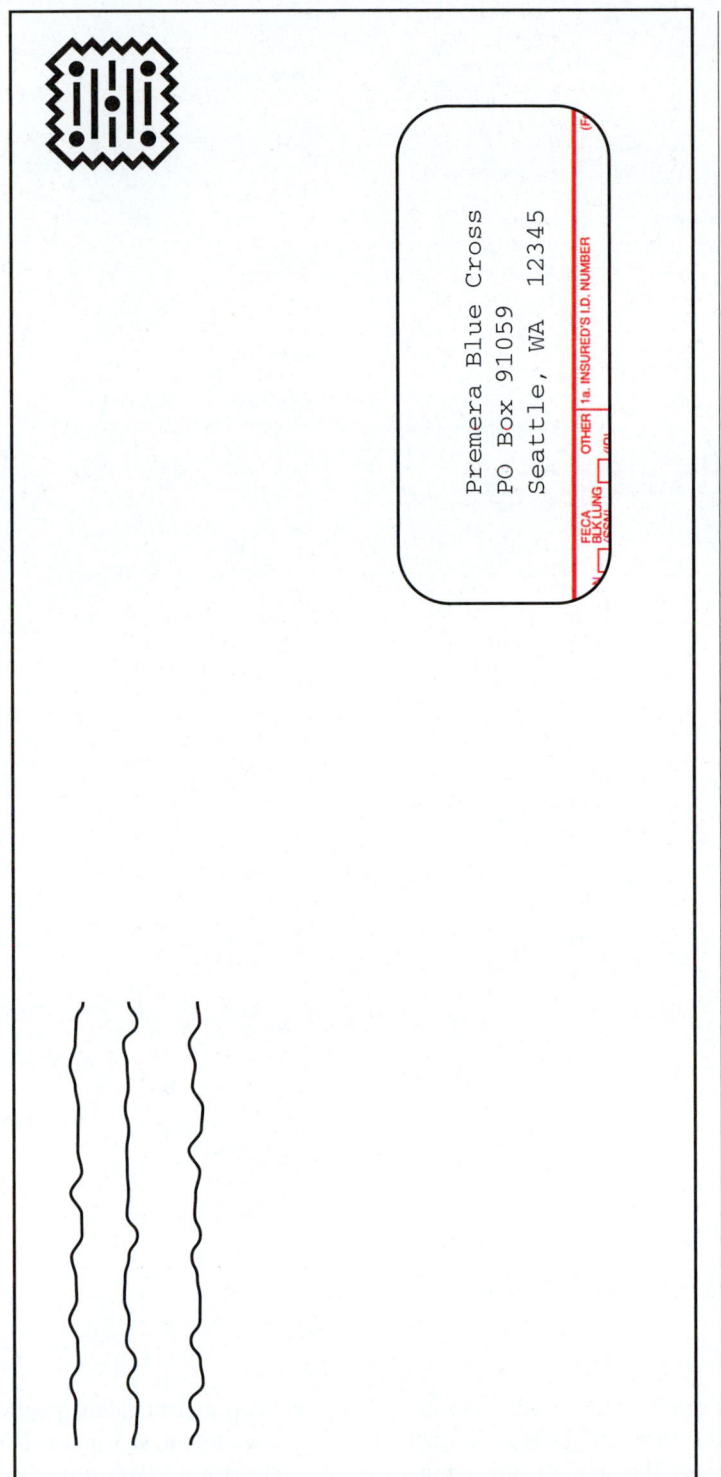

Figure 17-17 ◆ Fold the CMS-1500 such that address information shows through the window envelope.

301

(1500)

HEALTH INSURANCE CLAIM FORM
APPROVED BY NATIONAL UNIFORM CLAIM COMMITTEE 08/05

BLUE CROSS BLUE SHIELD
379 BLUE PLZ
CAPITAL CITY NY 12345

PICA   PICA

1. MEDICARE MEDICAID TRICARE CHAMPUS CHAMPVA GROUP HEALTH PLAN FECA BLK LUNG OTHER	1a. INSURED'S I.D. NUMBER (For Program in Item 1)
☐ (Medicare #) ☐ (Medicaid #) ☐ (Sponsor's SSN) ☐ (Member ID#) ☐ (SSN or ID) ☐ (SSN) ☒ (ID)	YYJ744258013

2. PATIENT'S NAME (Last Name, First Name, Middle Initial): ABNER AARON
3. PATIENT'S BIRTH DATE: 01 28 1976 SEX: M ☒ F ☐
4. INSURED'S NAME (Last Name, First Name, Middle Initial): ABNER MELISSA

5. PATIENT'S ADDRESS (No, Street): 98 N ROSEWOOD DR
6. PATIENT RELATIONSHIP TO INSURED: Self ☐ Spouse ☒ Child ☐ Other ☐
7. INSURED'S ADDRESS (No, Street): SAME

CITY: TOWNSHIP STATE: NY
8. PATIENT STATUS: Single ☐ Married ☒ Other ☐
CITY STATE

ZIP CODE: 12345 TELEPHONE: (555) 5558552
Employed ☒ Full-Time Student ☐ Part-Time Student ☐
ZIP CODE TELEPHONE ( )

9. OTHER INSURED'S NAME (Last Name, First Name, Middle Initial)
10. IS PATIENT'S CONDITION RELATED TO:
11. INSURED'S POLICY GROUP OR FECA NUMBER: 015386

a. OTHER INSURED'S POLICY OR GROUP NUMBER
a. EMPLOYMENT? (Current or Previous) ☐ YES ☒ NO
a. INSURED'S DATE OF BIRTH: 08 04 1974 SEX: M ☐ F ☒

b. OTHER INSURED'S DATE OF BIRTH SEX: M ☐ F ☐
b. AUTO ACCIDENT? PLACE (State) ☐ YES ☒ NO
b. EMPLOYER'S NAME OR SCHOOL NAME: PASTA USA

c. EMPLOYER'S NAME OR SCHOOL NAME
c. OTHER ACCIDENT? ☐ YES ☒ NO
c. INSURANCE PLAN NAME OR PROGRAM NAME: BLUE CROSS BLUE SHIELD

d. INSURANCE PLAN NAME OR PROGRAM NAME
10d. RESERVED FOR LOCAL USE
d. IS THERE ANOTHER HEALTH BENEFIT PLAN? ☐ YES ☒ NO *If yes, return to and complete item 9 a-d*

READ BACK OF FORM BEFORE COMPLETING & SIGNING THIS FORM.
12. PATIENT'S OR AUTHORIZED PERSON'S SIGNATURE I authorize the release of any medical or other information necessary to process this claim. I also request payment of government benefits either to myself or to the party who accepts assignment below.
SIGNED SOF DATE

13. INSURED'S OR AUTHORIZED PERSON'S SIGNATURE I authorize payment of medical benefits to the undersigned physician or supplier for services described below.
SIGNED SOF

14. DATE OF CURRENT ILLNESS (First symptom) OR INJURY (Accident) OR PREGNANCY (LMP)
15. IF PATIENT HAS HAD SAME OR SIMILAR ILLNESS, GIVE FIRST DATE
16. DATES PATIENT UNABLE TO WORK IN CURRENT OCCUPATION FROM TO

17. NAME OF REFERRING PHYSICIAN OR OTHER SOURCE
17a.
17b. NPI
18. HOSPITALIZATION DATES RELATED TO CURRENT SERVICES FROM TO

19. RESERVED FOR LOCAL USE
20. OUTSIDE LAB? ☐ YES ☒ NO $ CHARGES

21. DIAGNOSIS OR NATURE OF ILLNESS OR INJURY (Relate Items 1,2,3 or 4 to Item 24E by Line)
1. 300 01   3. V17 3
2. 305 1   4. V17 5

22. MEDICAID RESUBMISSION CODE ORIGINAL REF. NO.
23. PRIOR AUTHORIZATION NUMBER

24. A. DATE(S) OF SERVICE From MM DD YY To MM DD YY	B. PLACE OF SERVICE	C. EMG	D. PROCEDURES, SERVICES, OR SUPPLIES CPT/HCPCS MODIFIER	E. DIAGNOSIS POINTER	F. $ CHARGES	G. DAYS OR UNITS	H. EPSDT Family Plan	I. ID. QUAL	J. RENDERING PROVIDER ID. #
1	12 01 XX 12 01 XX	11		99203	1234	85 00	1		NPI	1234567890
2	12 01 XX 12 01 XX	11		85025	123	95 00	1		NPI	1234567890
3	12 01 XX 12 01 XX	11		93000	123	75 00	1		NPI	1234567890
4	12 01 XX 12 01 XX	11		80053	123	75 00	1		NPI	1234567890
5	12 01 XX 12 01 XX	11		36415	123	15 00	1		NPI	1234567890
6									NPI	

25. FEDERAL TAX ID. NUMBER SSN ☐ EIN ☒: 750246810
26. PATIENT'S ACCOUNT NO.: B2
27. ACCEPT ASSIGNMENT? ☐ YES ☐ NO
28. TOTAL CHARGE $ 345 00
29. AMOUNT PAID $
30. BALANCE DUE $

31. SIGNATURE OF PHYSICIAN OR SUPPLIER INCLUDING DEGREES OR CREDENTIALS (I certify that the statements on the reverse apply to this bill and are made a part thereof)
SIGNED PHIL WELLS MD DATE 12/01/XX

32. SERVICE FACILITY LOCATION INFORMATION
CAPITAL CITY MEDICAL
123 UNKNOWN BLVD
CAPITAL CITY NY 12345
a. 1513171216 b.

33. BILLING PROVIDER INFO & PH. # (555) 5551234
CAPITAL CITY MEDICAL
123 UNKNOWN BLVD
CAPITAL CITY NY 12345
a. 1513171216 b.

NUCC Instruction Manual available at: www.nucc.org
WCMS-1500CS
APPROVED OMB 0938-0999 FORM CMS-1500 (08/05)

Figure 17-18 ◆ A completed CMS-1500 claim form.

- Payment is faster. Payment can be transferred electronically to the provider's bank, eliminating delays in cash flow. These payments are referred to as electronic remittances. Medicare is required by law to process electronic claims in fourteen days, and is prohibited from processing paper claims for at least twenty-eight days after receipt.

Electronic claims also have disadvantages:

- Claims transmission can be disrupted occasionally due to power failures or computer hardware or software problems that might require claims to be resubmitted.

- Many patient billing programs cannot create an electronic attachment, so when a claim attachment is required, the electronic claim must be sent separately from mailed attachments, which sometimes causes problems for the payer in matching up the two. In some cases, the claim must instead be submitted on paper when it must be accompanied by a claim attachment.

Electronic claims, which are the leading method of claims submission by providers, are submitted through a clearinghouse, a billing service, or directly to the carrier. A physician

PROCEDURE 17-3   Obtain a Managed Care Referral

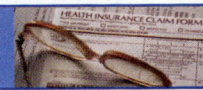

Theory and Rationale

Medical assistants in primary care or family practice physicians' offices are often required to obtain managed care referrals for patients who need to see specialists or other healthcare providers. Whenever needed, medical assistants in specialists' offices should ensure that managed care referrals are obtained for patients covered by managed care policies.

Materials

- Telephone
- Patient's medical chart
- Name and telephone number of patient's primary care provider

Competency

(**Conditions**) With the necessary materials, you will be able to (**Task**) obtain a managed care referral for a patient (**Standards**) correctly within the time limit set by the instructor.

1. Call the patient's primary care provider's office, and ask for the person in charge of referrals.
2. Give the referral assistant the patient's information, including name and birth date.
3. Inform the referral assistant of the need for a referral to the physician, including the reason for the patient's visit in the medical office.
4. Ask the referral assistant if any information from the patient's file is needed to process the referral.
5. Ask the referral assistant when to expect the referral. If needed, provide the office fax number for information transmittal.
6. Document in the patient's file the content of the telephone call.
7. Notify the physician and the patient of the content of the telephone call.

PROCEDURE 17-4   Obtain Authorization from an Insurance Company for a Procedure

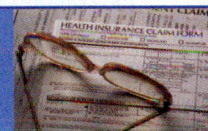

Theory and Rationale

Most insurance companies require preauthorization before physicians perform any nonemergency services. Without insurance carrier authorization, physicians may not be paid for their services.

Materials

- Patient insurance information (i.e., ID number, birth date of the insured, name and telephone number for provider customer service at the insurance company)
- Paper and pen
- Description of the procedure the doctor has prescribed, including Current Procedural Terminology (**CPT**) code
- Patient's diagnosis pertaining to the needed procedure
- Location where procedure is to be performed (e.g., office, outpatient surgery, inpatient hospitalization)
- Date by which the procedure must be performed

Competency

(**Conditions**) With the necessary materials, you will be able to (**Task**) obtain an authorization from an insurance carrier for a procedure (**Standards**) correctly within the time limit set by the instructor.

1. Write down the date and time of the call, the name of the insurance company, and the name of the insurance company representative on the phone.
2. Give the insurance company representative your name and your office's/physician's name.
3. Give the insurance company representative the name of the patient, the name of the insured, and the insured's ID number.
4. Let the representative know what the procedure is your doctor has prescribed for the patient and the date by which the procedure must be performed.
5. Provide the representative any other requested information (e.g., procedure code, diagnosis code, and place where the procedure is to be performed).
6. Write down the authorization number the representative provides.
7. Ask the representative if any supporting documentation (e.g., chart notes, operative report, laboratory report, or pathology report) will be needed with the CMS-1500 billing form. If so, write down the required documentation.
8. Keep all preceding information in the patient's file for reference in case the claim is not paid by the insurance carrier.

who plans to use electronic billing must contact all major insurers and carriers for a list of the vendors approved to handle electronic claims and must have a signed agreement with each. Each carrier has special electronic billing requirements and is knowledgeable about which systems meet its criteria and which are compatible in format. The field data that is requested by the carriers is almost identical to the information on the CMS-1500 claim form. Insurance carriers also provide information about how to submit an electronic bill for patients who have secondary coverage. Medicare provides the software and training for electronic submissions. Medicare, Medicaid, TRICARE, and many private insurance carriers allow providers to submit insurance claims directly to them with no "middle man." In this type of system, the medical practice must have special software or the physician must lease a terminal from the carrier to key in claims data. The data is transmitted via modem (dedicated telephone line) directly to the carrier's computer for processing.

If the physician is not sending the data directly to the carrier, a clearinghouse may be used. A clearinghouse is a company that receives claims from providers, puts them through a series of audits to check for errors, and then forwards them to the appropriate insurance carrier in the carrier's required data format. Clearinghouses may charge a flat fee per claim or charge a percentage of the claim's dollar value. It is very important for the physicians' practices to negotiate the best possible fee for using a clearinghouse's services.

The clearinghouse conducts an audit to determine if any data on the claim is incorrect or missing; such a claim is referred to as a dirty claim. The results of the audit are sent back to the provider from the clearinghouse in the form of an audit/edit report. The medical assistant will need to correct any claims with incorrect data (as indicated on the audit/edit report) and resubmit them to the clearinghouse. Dirty claims, those with errors, will not be transmitted to the carriers. When the claims are corrected and resubmitted to the clearinghouse, they are considered clean claims, which are then formatted and forwarded to the carrier. Each time the claim is returned there is an additional charge, so the medical assistant should ensure that clean claims are transmitted initially.*

Working with Fee Schedules

Providers have different methods in determining their fee structure (the amount charged for each procedure performed). As stated by the American Medical Association (AMA), "Physicians have the right to establish their fees at a level which they believe fairly reflects the costs of providing a service and the value of the professional judgment." Two main methods are used for determining fees: charged-based and resource based fee structures.

Charge-Based Fee Structure

Charge-based fees are the fees that many providers charge for similar services. To set their fees, providers begin with an analysis of their procedure codes. To determine if their fees are in range with other providers of the same specialty, they may research a nationwide fee database. This information can be purchased by the provider to ascertain how fees compare to national averages. The database is divided into categories to indicate fees that are 25, 50, 75, and 90 percent higher based on fees charged throughout the nation. A provider can decide if her usual fees should be on the high, low, or midpoint range.

Resource-Based Fee Structures

Resource-based fees are based on the following three factors:

1. How difficult it is for the provider to perform the procedure (work).
2. How much office overhead the procedure involves (practice expense).
3. The relative risk that the procedure presents to the patient and the provider (malpractice).

Third-party payers also establish the amount they will reimburse providers. Each payer will determine the usual, customary, and reasonable (UCR) fee it feels should be charged by the provider by determining the percentage of the published fee in the national database that it will pay.[†]

Medicare's Resource-Based Relative Value Scale

Medicare bases its payment system on the resource-based relative value scale (**RBRVS**), which assigns a unit of relative value for provider's services based on the amount Medicare believes those services actually cost to provide.

The RBRVS has three parts: (1) national relative value (**RVU**), (2) **geographic adjustment factor** (**GAF**), and (3) national uniform conversion factor (**CF**). The national relative value is based on the type of work a physician does, the cost of practicing (overhead), and the cost of the provider's medical malpractice insurance. For example, the relative value for a basic office visit is lower than the value of a surgical procedure. The second part of RBRVS, the geographic adjustment factor, considers the area of the country in which a physician practices, adjusting higher or lower based on that area's cost of living. The third and final RBRVS part, the national uniform conversion factor, is a dollar amount used to determine the payment amount for a service. Each year, Medicare adjusts this factor according to the cost-of-living index.

Before agreeing to participate with any plan, healthcare providers should carefully review the fee schedules the managed care companies provide. Once contracts are in place, physicians have little leverage to adjust fee schedules

---

*Source: Vines, Deborah, Braceland, Ann, Rollins, Elizabeth, and Miller, Susan. *Comprehensive Health Insurance: Billing, Coding, and Reimbursement.* © 2008, pp. 215–216. Reprinted by permission of Pearson Education, Inc. Upper Saddle River, NJ.

[†]Vines, Deborah, Braceland, Ann, Rollins, Elizabeth, and Miller, Susan. *Comprehensive Health Insurance: Billing, Coding, and Reimbursement.* © 2008, p. 419. Reprinted by permission of Pearson Education, Inc. Upper Saddle River, NJ.

and may find some, or all, fees are lower than they can afford to accept.

Posting Payments

Once an insurance carrier has processed a claim, a check is sent to the healthcare provider with an **explanation of benefits (EOB)** (Figure 17-19 ◆). With large insurance carriers, providers may receive one EOB and check as payment for several patients. The EOB lists the name of the patient, the name of the insured, the date of service, the amount billed, the amount allowed (should it be a managed care insurance carrier), the amount paid, and the amount the provider may bill the patient. Medical assistants must check EOBs to ensure all services that were billed are accurately listed and that service payment matches the amount in the insurance company contract.

An explanation will not always be accompanied by payment, but it will state the status of the claim. The claim may be pending waiting for additional information. A pending claim is one that is received but not processed by the carrier because additional information is needed or there is an error. For claims submitted electronically, the EOB is referred to as the Electronic Remittance Advice (ERA). The EOB lists the patient, dates of services, types of service, and the charges filed on the insurance claim form. The EOB also describes how the amount of the benefit payment was determined. If claim forms were filed for more than one patient with the same insurance carrier at the same time, the provider's EOB may include information on more than one patient.

The format and contents of each EOB vary based on the benefit plan and the services provided. No universal form for explaining benefits is available. It has been a point of debate that all providers are required to use the CMS-1500 and the UB-04 standardized forms, yet carriers can customize their EOBs in any way. Terminology is also different on various EOBs. For example, some EOBs show the "Allowed Amount or Charge" and some EOBs read "Deducted Amount." The medical assistant will eventually become accustomed to the carriers with whom the provider contracts, but should always review all EOBs carefully prior to entering data.

However, many terms and categories are common to all carriers. Insurance carriers often use codes on the EOB to refer to these terms or situations. These codes are called reason codes and remark codes. Usually, these codes are explained on the face or back of the EOB. If one line is read at a time, the descriptions and calculations for each patient are easily understood. An EOB statement has three sections that explain how a claim was processed:

1. Service Information. Identifies the provider (hospital or other facility, doctor, specialist, or clinic), dates of service, and charges from the provider.
2. Coverage Determination. Summarizes the total deductions, charges not covered by the plan, and the amount the patient may owe the provider.
3. Benefit Payment Information. Indicates who was paid, how much, and when.

Information on an EOB

The following information appears on an EOB:

1. Account name: company name
2. Date the EOB statement was finalized
3. Member's or insured's name and ID number
4. Patient's identification number as it appears on his or her ID card
5. Number assigned to the claim
6. Name of the person who received the service (the patient)
7. Provider's name
8. Service description column, which indicates:

   - Dates of the services provided (DOS)
   - Procedures performed (CPT codes)
   - Total charge for each procedure
   - The portion of the bill not covered by the plan
   - The contractual allowed amount
   - Patient's copay
   - Patient's deductible or noncovered procedures or amounts
   - Patient's coinsurance

9. Total payment to the provider
10. The total amount that is the patient's responsibility to the provider of services

After posting the payment to the specific date and procedure, an adjustment may be needed. An adjustment is a positive or negative change to a patient's account balance. Corrections, changes, and write-offs to patients' accounts are made by means of adjustments to the existing transactions. The medical assistant will also adjust a patient's bill as a result of any discounts given. If the provider is a PAR provider, the difference between the billed amount (the provider's UCR fee) and the allowed amount is adjusted from the amount the patient owes. Also note whether a balance is due from the patient, or whether a refund is due the patient or insurance carrier. For example, if a patient paid for a service in advance and was reimbursed by the carrier or if the patient or insurance carrier overpaid on an account, then a refund is due.*

In addition to sending EOBs to providers, insurance carriers send EOB copies to the insured. When providers contract with insurance carriers, they must accept the allowed amount of the claim as payment in full. Billing the patient for the difference between the billed amount and the allowed amount, a practice called **balance billing**, violates the healthcare provider's contract with the insurance carrier. Figure 17-20 ◆ shows how this works. If providers are not contracted with the carriers, they should balance bill.

When patients have set copayments, those copays should be collected at the time of service. When patients owe coinsurance or deductible amounts, medical assistants must bill patients once the insurance carriers send notification.

---

*Adapted from Vines, Deborah, Braceland, Ann, Rollins, Elizabeth, and Miller, Susan. *Comprehensive Health Insurance: Billing, Coding, and Reimbursement.* © 2008, pp. 433–434, 444–445.

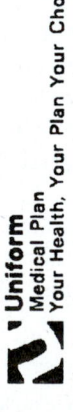

Uniform
Medical Plan
Your Health, Your Plan Your Choice

Explanation of Benefits
This is not a bill.
06/08/2007

Your UMP ID Number: W125370058
Subscriber Name: CHRIS R LONEMA
Patient Name CHRIS R LONEMA
Claim Number: K100925-0038

CHRIS R LONEMA
3160 GRAND AVE 12345
EVERETT   WA

Provider Information

CATHERINE N DORTON ARNP
7620 44TH ST NE   12345
MARYSVILLE   WA

If you have questions, contact us:

By Mail:
Uniform Medical Plan   98124-1578
PO Box 84578
Seattle, WA

By Phone/E-mail:
Local: 425-555-3000
Toll Free: 1-800-555-6004
E-mail: www.ump.hca.wa.gov

Provider Name:	Date(s) of Service	Service(s) Provided	Amount Charged	UMP Allowed	PPO Savings	Non-Cov'd Amount	Deductible	Copay	Co-Ins. %	UMP Paid	Patient's Responsibility	See Notes Section
CATHERINE N DORTON -ARNP	05 07 07 -05 07 07	87621 90 PATHOLOGY-PHYS CHGS	125.00	66.94	58.06				6.69	90	60.25	6.69	PPU
CATHERINE N DORTON -ARNP	05 07 07 -05 07 07	88142 90 PATHOLOGY-PHYS CHGS	72.00	28.31	43.69				2.83	90	25.48	2.83	PPU
		TOTALS	197.00	95.25	101.75	0.00	0.00		9.52		85.73	9.52	

Other Insurance Paid Amount   0.00
(*) See Notes Adjustment   0.00
UMP Final Paid Amount/Check   85.73   # 43984431

Total Payment to Enrollee: ********0.00

Total Payment to Provider: *******85.73

NOTES:

THANK YOU FOR USING A UNIFORM MEDICAL PLAN PARTICIPATING PROVIDER

PPU   THIS IS YOUR PLANS PARTICIPATING PROVIDERS CONTRACTUAL ALLOWANCE FOR THIS SERVICE. PROVIDER AGREES TO REDUCE THE FEE TO THE AMOUNT ALLOWED.

DEDUCTIBLE
YOU HAVE MET 200.00 OF YOUR 200.00 DEDUCTIBLE FOR 01/01/2007 - 12/31/2007

Figure 17-19 ◆ Explanation of benefits (EOB).

How Much Should the Patient Be Billed?

❑ Corey Johansen is insured with Medicare.

❑ His service with Dr. Anholm was billed at $100.00.

❑ Dr. Anholm is a participating provider with Medicare.

❑ Medicare allows $78.45 for this service.

❑ Medicare paid $62.76.

How much does Corey owe?

$100 for the service

$78.45 is allowed

Provider must write off the difference between the amount charged ($100.00) and the amount allowed ($78.45). This means the provider must write off $21.55.

Corey owes the difference between the allowed amount ($78.45) and the amount paid by Medicare ($62.76). Corey owes $15.69 for his service with Dr. Anholm.

Figure 17-20 ◆ Sample billing when provider is contracted with the insurance carrier.

Tracing Claims

Each state has its own guidelines that outline the timeframe within which an insurance carrier must pay or deny a claim. In Washington State, for example, that timeframe is 30 days. Any claims that have not been processed within that timeframe are subject to interest in the amount allowed by state law. As a general rule, any claim that has not been paid or denied within 45 days of submission on paper, or 20 days of submission electronically, may be considered past due and warrants a telephone call to the insurance carrier. Most medical office software can print a list of past due claims, making it easy to identify the claims that require further investigation.

When a claim is past due, the medical assistant should call the insurance carrier to follow up on or trace the claim. During this call, the medical assistant may be told that the insurance carrier does not have the claim on file. If this is the case, the medical assistant can request a fax number to send the claim to the customer service representative for processing personally. The medical assistant may also be told that there was an error on the claim. Sometimes, the medical assistant may be able to clarify the error over the phone; other times, the claim will need to be resubmitted. The medical assistant should always document any phone call made to an insurance carrier, noting the date and time of the call, the name of the person spoken to, and the results of the call.

Reconciling Payments and Rejections

Claims are sometimes denied or rejected, many times for errors the medical office made. Incorrect identification numbers, incorrect birthdates, missing diagnosis codes, and missing

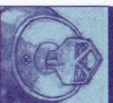

Keys to Success
QUICK REFERENCES FOR REASONS FOR DENIED CLAIMS

Reason claim was denied: Need supporting documentation

Tip for avoiding this denial: When calling for preauthorization of any procedure, ask the insurance company customer service representative if supporting documentation will be required. If so, copy the chart notes, operative report, laboratory report, or other documentation and send it in with the CMS-1500 billing form.

Reason claim was denied: Diagnosis code does not match procedure performed

Tip for avoiding this denial: Before sending the claim, look at the diagnosis codes the physician assigns to the patient in the *ICD-9* coding book to verify that the code matches the procedure.

Reason claim was denied: Patient is no longer eligible for coverage

Tip for avoiding this denial: Before scheduling any procedure, call to verify coverage with the insurance carrier.

Reason claim was denied: Missing information on the CMS-1500 claim form

Tip for avoiding this denial: Quickly scan all CMS-1500 claim forms prior to sending to determine any missing information or blank boxes.

Reason claim was denied: Past timely filing limits

Tip for avoiding this denial: Submit all insurance claim forms in a timely manner, usually within 30 days of the date of the procedure.

Reason claim was denied: Preauthorization was not obtained before performing the service

Tip for avoiding this denial: Before scheduling any procedure, call to verify coverage with the insurance carrier.

supporting documentation all delay payment of insurance claims. Attention to detail in the claim submission process saves time and effort in the end.

A **rejected** claim is one that never entered the carrier's system due to an incorrect identification number or similar technical problem. These are often returned to the provider during the EMC process. Rejected claims should be corrected and resubmitted as a new claim. A **denied** claim is one the carrier received and processed but did not pay due to benefits or coverage issues. The reason for denial is usually listed on the EOB. Be careful to differentiate between denials of total charges and disallowances. Disallowances represent partial payment on claims because they are above the maximum allowable fee. If the reason cannot be determined or the medical assistant or patient disagrees with the reason, a telephone call should be placed to the insurance company. Often denials can be handled on the phone. If a corrected claim needs to be resubmitted, the carrier should provide specific directions on how to do this. Denied claims that are resubmitted as new claims, rather than corrected claims, will usually be rejected due to a duplicate date of service.

text continues on page 314

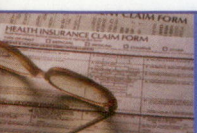

PROCEDURE 17-5 Abstract Data to Complete a Paper CMS-1500 Claim Form

Theory and Rationale

Even though few offices still complete CMS-1500 forms manually, and without the aid of a computer, some small offices do. Proper completion of a paper CMS-1500 claim acquaints medical assistants with the form locator fields and data requirements, all of which will be required when using a computer program. This procedure allows medical assistants to focus on how to abstract or locate required information from the source documents without learning a computer software program at the same time.

Materials

- Klaus Davies patient registration form (Figure 17-21 ◆)
- insurance ID card (Figure 17-22 ◆)
- encounter form (Figure 17-23 ◆)
- Capital City Medical fee schedule (Figure 17-24 ◆)
- Table 17-2: Instructions on Completing the CMS-1500 Claim Form
- blank CMS-1500 form (Photocopy Figure 17-16 or obtain from instructor)
- black ink pen
- calculator

Competency

(**Conditions**) With the necessary materials, you will be able to (**Task**) abstract data from the medical record to complete a CMS-1500 form (**Standards**) correctly within the time limit set by the instructor.

Refer to Table 17-2 to identify how each field is to be completed and where to find the information. Print all information neatly, in capital letters, with a pen. Erasing, crossouts, writeovers, and white-out may not be used. You may wish to fill in a draft form in pencil, then recopy it in ink when finished.

1. Enter the insurance company name and mailing address in the carrier area.
2. Check the correct box in FL 1.
3. Enter the insured's ID number in FL1a.
4. Enter the patient's name in FL 2.
5. Complete FL 3.
6. Complete FL 4.
7. Enter the patient's address and phone in FL 5. Note there are three lines of information to complete.
8. Complete FL 6.
9. Leave FL 7 blank.
10. Complete FL 8 for marital status and employment status.
11. Leave FL 9a to 9d blank.
12. Complete FL 10a, 10b, 10c.
13. Leave FL 10d blank.
14. Enter the groups number in FL 11.
15. Leave FL 11a blank.
16. Enter the employer in FL 11a.
17. Enter the insurance plan name in FL 11c.
18. Mark NO in Fl 11d.
19. Enter "SOF" in FL 12.
20. Enter "SOF" in FL 13.
21. Leave FL 14 to FL 19 blank.
22. Mark NO in FL 20.
23. Enter the first diagnosis code in FL 21, line 1.
24. Enter the second diagnosis code in FL 21, line 2.
25. Leave FL 22 to FL 23 blank.
26. In FL 24A, line one, enter the date of service in both the FROM and TO fields.
27. Enter the code number for place of service in FL 24B.
28. Leave FL 24C blank.
29. Enter the first CPT code in FL 24D.
30. In FL 24E enter "1 2" to designate that both diagnoses 1 and 2 relate to this service.
31. Look on the encounter form to find the description for CPT code 99231. Then look on the fee schedule to find the fee for this service and enter it in FL 24F.
32. Enter 1 for units in FL 24G.
33. Leave blank FL 24H and FL 24I.
34. Enter the physician's NPI number on the unshaded portion of 24J. You will find this on the encounter form.
35. Repeat these steps for lines 2 through 6. In FL 24E be certain you designate the correct diagnoses reference for each service, as some lines will be only "1" or only "2."
36. When all services are completed, enter the EIN in FL 25 and mark X in the appropriate box. You will find this on the patient registration form.
37. Enter the patient's account number in FL 26. You will find this on the patient registration form.
38. Leave FL 27 blank.
39. Add up the total charges in column 24F. Write the total in FL 28.
40. Leave FL 29 and FL 30 blank.
41. Enter the physicians signature, credentials and date in FL 31. Be certain to stay within the lines of the box.
42. Enter the name and address of the clinic in FL 32.
43. Enter the clinic's group NPI number in 32a. You will find this on the patient registration form.
44. Leave FL 32b blank.
45. In FL 33, enter the clinic's phone number in the top right corner.
46. Enter the clinic's name and address in the FL 33.
47. Enter the clinic's NPI number in FL 33a.
48. Leave FL 33b blank.
49. Proofread your work. Check all spelling and numbers against your source documents.
50. Check your claim against the sample CMS-1500 form in Figure 17-25 ◆.

PROCEDURE 17-5 **Abstract Data to Complete a Paper CMS-1500 Claim Form** (*continued*)

Capital City Medical—123 Unknown Boulevard, Capital City, NY 12345-2222 (555)555-1234 Phil Wells, MD, Mannie Mends, MD, Bette R. Soone, MD	Patient Information Form Tax ID: 75-0246810 Group NPI: 1513171216

Patient Information:

Name: (Last, First) Davies, Klaus   ☒ Male   ☐ Female   Birth Date: 10/24/1965

Address: 19 Willow Rd. Capital City, NY 12345   Phone: (555) 555-1276

Social Security Number: 631-03-4305   Full-Time Student: ☐ Yes   ☒ No

Marital Status: ☐ Single   ☒ Married   ☐ Divorced   ☐ Other

- -

Employment:

Employer: Organic Food Mart   Phone: ( ) (555) 555-5619

Address: 13 Mile Blvd, Township, NY 12345

Condition Related to: ☐ Auto Accident   ☐ Employment   ☐ Other Accident

Date of Accident: _____ State _____

Emergency Contact: _____ **Phone: ( )** _____

- -

Primary Insurance: Blue Cross Blue Shield PPO   Phone: ( ) _____

Address: 379 Blue Plaza, Capital City, NY 12345

Insurance Policyholder's Name: Same   ☐ M ☐ F DOB: _____

Address: _____

Phone: _____ Relationship to Insured: ☒ Self ☐ Spouse ☐ Child ☐ Other

Employer: _____   Phone: _____

Employer's Address: _____

Policy/ID No: YYZ8436489   Group No: 326463 Percent Covered: ____%, Copay Amt: $35.00

- -

Secondary Insurance: _____   Phone: ( ) _____

Address: _____

Insurance Policyholder's Name: _____   ☐ M ☐ F DOB: _____

Address: _____

Phone: _____ Relationship to Insured: ☐ Self ☐ Spouse ☐ Child ☐ Other

Employer: _____   Phone: ( ) _____

Employer's Address: _____

Policy/ID No: _____ Group No: _____ Percent Covered: ____%, Copay Amt: $_____

- -

Reason for Visit: Need my blood pressure and cholesterol checked today

Known Allergies: _____

Were you referred here? If so, by whom?: _____

Figure 17-21 ◆ Klaus Davies sample patient registration form.

(*continued*)

PROCEDURE 17-5 Abstract Data to Complete a Paper CMS-1500 Claim Form *(continued)*

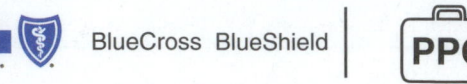

BlueCross BlueShield | PPO

Group Name **ORGANIC FOOD MART**

ID **YY28436489**   Group **32643**   BC Plan **252** BC Plan **353**

Subscriber/Dependents   M RX
01: KLAUS DAVIES   Y Y
02: SARA DAVIES   Y Y

Card Issue Date   10/09/XX

An independent License of the Blue Cross and Blue Shield Association

Provider: Please submit medical and/or vision claims to your local Blue Cross and/or Blue Shield plan in whose Service Area the Member received services. Submit all other claims to 379 BLUE PLZ CAPITAL CITY NY 12345

Member: To locate a preferred or participating Blue Provider outside your service area please call 1 (555) 810-BLUE (2583). For all other questions, please call 1-555-9978 This card is not an authorization for services or a guarantee of payment.

PPP Network   DED $300: COMP CARE $35 COPAY
                           IN-NTWK 20%/OUT-NTWK 40%

REGENCE RX BIN **09870**   PCN **246800**

OV $35   ER $100 $10 GEN
SP $50 $35 FORM
                         $50 NON-FORM

Figure 17-22 ◆ Klaus Davies sample insurance ID card.

PROCEDURE 17-5 Abstract Data to Complete a Paper CMS-1500 Claim Form (continued)

Patient Name Klaus Davies

Capital City Medical
123 Unknown Boulevard, Capital City, NY 12345-2222
Physician: Phil Wells, MD NPI 1234567890

Date of Service
10-26-20XX

New Patient		Other Invasive/Noninvasive			Laboratory		
Problem Focused	99201	Arthrocentesis/Aspiration/Injection			Amylase	82150	
Expanded Problem, Focused	99202	Small Joint		20600	B12	82607	
Detailed	99203	Interm Joint		20605	CBC & Diff	85025	X
Comprehensive	99204	Major Joint		20610	Comp Metabolic Panel	80053	
Comprehensive/High Complex	99205	**Other Invasive/Noninvasive**			Chlamydia Screen	87110	
Well Exam Infant (up to 12 mos.)	99381	Audiometry		92552	Cholesterol	82465	
Well Exam 1–4 yrs.	99382	Cast Application			Digoxin	80162	
Well Exam 5–11 yrs.	99383	Location Long Short			Electrolytes	80051	
Well Exam 12–17 yrs.	99384	Catheterization		51701	Ferritin	82728	
Well Exam 18–39 yrs.	99385	Circumcision		54150	Folate	82746	
Well Exam 40–64 yrs.	99386	Colposcopy		57452	GC Screen	87070	
		Colposcopy w/Biopsy		57454	Glucose	82947	
		Cryosurgery Premalignant Lesion			Glucose 1 HR	82950	
		Location (s):			Glycosylated HGB A1C	83036	
Established Patient		Cryosurgery Warts			HCT	85014	
Post-Op Follow Up Visit	99024	Location (s):			HDL	83718	
Minimum	99211	Curettement Lesion			Hep BSAG	87340	
Problem Focused	99212	Single		11055	Hepatitis panel, acute	80074	
Expanded Problem Focused	99213 X	2–4		11056	HGB	85018	
Detailed	99214	>4		11057	HIV	86703	
Comprehensive/High Complex	99215	Diaphragm Fitting		57170	Iron & TIBC	83550	
Well Exam Infant (up to 12 mos.)	99391	Ear Irrigation		69210	Kidney Profile	80069	
Well exam 1–4 yrs.	99392	ECG		93000	Lead	83655	
Well Exam 5–11 yrs.	99393	Endometrial Biopsy		58100	Liver Profile	80076	X
Well Exam 12–17 yrs.	99394	Exc. Lesion Malignant			Mono Test	86308	
Well Exam 18–39 yrs.	99395	Benign			Pap Smear	88155	
Well Exam 40–64 yrs.	99396	Location			Pregnancy Test	84703	
Obstetrics		Exc. Skin Tags (1–15)		11200	Obstetric Panel	80055	
Total OB Care	59400	Each Additional 10		11201	Pro Time	85610	
Injections		Fracture Treatment			PSA	84153	
Administration Sub. / IM	90772	Loc			RPR	86592	
Drug		w/Reduc	w/o Reduc		Sed. Rate	85651	
Dosage		I & D Abscess Single/Simple		10060	Stool Culture	87045	
Allergy	95115	Multiple or Comp		10061	Stool O & P	87177	
Cocci Skin Test	86490	I & D Pilonidal Cyst Simple		10080	Strep Screen	87880	
DPT	90701	Pilonidal Cyst Complex		10081	Theophylline	80198	
Hemophilus	90646	IV Therapy—To One Hour		90760	Thyroid Uptake	84479	
Influenza	90658	Each Additional Hour		90761	TSH	84443	
MMR	90707	Laceration Repair			Urinalysis	81000	
OPV	90712	Location Size Simp/Comp			Urine Culture	87088	
Pneumovax	90732	Laryngoscopy		31505	Drawing Fee	36415	X
TB Skin Test	86580	Oximetry		94760	Specimen Collection	99000	
TD	90718	Punch Biopsy			**Other:**		
Unlisted Immun	90749	Rhythm Strip		93040			
Tetanus Toxoid	90703	Treadmill		93015			
Vaccine/Toxoid Admin <8 Yr Old w/ Counseling	90465	Trigger Point or Tendon Sheath Inj.		20550			
Vaccine/Toxoid Administration for Adult	90471	Tympanometry		92567			

Diagnosis/ICD-9: **401.9, 272.0**

| | | | | | Lipid Panel | 80061 | X |

I acknowledge receipt of medical services and authorize the release of any medical information necessary to process this claim for healthcare payment only. I do authorize payment to the provider.

Patient Signature *Klaus Davies*

Total Estimated Charges: _____

Payment Amount: _____

Next Appointment: _____

Figure 17-23 ◆ Klaus Davies sample encounter form.

(continued)

PROCEDURE 17-5 **Abstract Data to Complete a Paper CMS-1500 Claim Form** (*continued*)

Capital City Medical
Fee Schedule

New Patient OV		Laceration Repair various codes	$60
Problem Focused 99201	$45	Punch Biopsy various codes	$80
Expanded Problem Focused 99202	$65	Nebulizer various codes	$45
Detailed 99203	$85	Cast Application various codes	$85
Comprehensive 99204	$105	Laryngoscopy 31505	$255
Comprehensive/High Complex 99205	$115	Audiometry 92552	$85
Well Exam infant (less than 1 year) 99381	$45	Tympanometry 92567	$85
Well Exam 1–4 yrs. 99382	$50	Ear Irrigation 69210	$25
Well Exam 5–11 yrs. 99383	$55	Diaphragm Fitting 57170	$30
Well Exam 12–17 yrs. 99384	$65	IV Therapy (up to one hour) 90760	$65
Well Exam 18–39 yrs. 99385	$85	Each additional hour 90761	$50
Well Exam 40–64 yrs. 99386	$105	Oximetry 94760	$10
Established Patient OV		ECG 93000	$75
Post Op Follow Up Visit 99024	$0	Holter Monitor various codes	$170
Minimum 99211	$35	Rhythm Strip 93040	$60
Problem Focused 99212	$45	Treadmill 93015	$375
Expanded Problem Focused 99213	$55	Cocci Skin Test 86490	$20
Detailed 99214	$65	X-ray, spine, chest, bone—any area various codes	$275
Comprehensive/High Complex 99215	$75	Avulsion Nail 11730	$200
Well exam infant (less than 1 year) 99391	$35	Laboratory	
Well Exam 1–4 yrs. 99392	$40	Amylase 82150	$40
Well Exam 5–11 yrs. 99393	$45	B12 82607	$30
Well Exam 12–17 yrs. 99394	$55	CBC & Diff 85025	$95
Well Exam 18–39 yrs. 99395	$65	Comp Metabolic Panel 80053	$75
Well Exam 40–64 yrs. 99396	$75	Chlamydia Screen 87110	$70
Obstetrics		Cholestrerol 82465	$75
Total OB Care 59400	$1700	Digoxin 80162	$40
Injections		Electrolytes 80051	$70
Administration 90772	$10	Estrogen, Total 82672	$50
Allergy 95115	$35	Ferritin 82728	$40
DPT 90701	$50	Folate 82746	$30
Drug various codes	$35	GC Screen 87070	$60
Influenza 90658	$25	Glucose 82947	$35
MMR 90707	$50	Glycosylated HGB A1C 83036	$45
OPV 90712	$40	HCT 85014	$30
Pneumovax 90732	$35	HDL 83718	$35
TB Skin Test 86580	$15	HGB 85018	$30
TD 90718	$40	Hep BSAG 83740	$40
Tetanus Toxoid 90703	$40	Hepatitis panel, acute 80074	$95
Vaccine/Toxoid Administration for Younger		HIV 86703	$100
Than 8 Years Old w/ counseling 90465	$10	Iron & TIBC 83550	$45
Vaccine/Toxoid Administration for Adult 90471	$10	Kidney Profile 80069	$95
Arthrocentesis/Aspiration/Injection		Lead 83665	$55
Small Joint 20600	$50	Lipase 83690	$40
Interm Joint 20605	$60	Lipid Panel 80061	$95
Major Joint 20610	$70	Liver Profile 80076	$95
Trigger Point/Tendon Sheath Inj. 20550	$90	Mono Test 86308	$30
Other Invasive/Noninvasive Procedures		Pap Smear 88155	$90
Catheterization 51701	$55	Pap Collection/Supervision 88142	$95
Circumcision 54150	$150	Pregnancy Test 84703	$90
Colposcopy 57452	$225	Obstetric Panel 80055	$85
Colposcopy w/Biopsy 57454	$250	Pro Time 85610	$50
Cryosurgery Premalignant Lesion various codes	$160	PSA 84153	$50
Endometrial Biopsy 58100	$190	RPR 86592	$55
Excision Lesion Malignant various codes	$145	Sed. Rate 85651	$50
Excision Lesion Benign various codes	$125	Stool Culture 87045	$80
Curettement Lesion		Stool O & P 87177	$105
Single 11055	$70	Strep Screen 87880	$35
2–4 11056	$80	Theophylline 80198	$40
>4 11057	$90	Thyroid Uptake 84479	$75
Excision Skin Tags (1–15) 11200	$55	TSH 84443	$50
Each Additional 10 11201	$30	Urinalysis 81000	$35
I & D Abscess Single/Simple 10060	$75	Urine Culture 87088	$80
Multiple/Complex 10061	$95	Drawing Fee 36415	$15
I & D Pilonidal Cyst Simple 10080	$105	Specimen Collection 99000	$10
I & D Pilonidal Cyst Complex 10081	$130		

Figure 17-24 ◆ Capital City Medical fee schedule.

PROCEDURE 17-5 Abstract Data to Complete a Paper CMS-1500 Claim Form (continued)

1500

HEALTH INSURANCE CLAIM FORM
APPROVED BY NATIONAL UNIFORM CLAIM COMMITTEE 08/05

BLUE CROSS BLUE SHIELD
379 BLUE PLZ
CAPITAL CITY NY 12345

☐☐ PICA | PICA ☐☐☐

1. MEDICARE MEDICAID TRICARE CHAMPVA GROUP FECA OTHER	1a. INSURED'S I.D. NUMBER (For Program in Item 1)
CHAMPUS	HEALTH PLAN BLK LUNG	

☐ (Medicare #) ☐ (Medicaid #) ☐ (Sponsor's SSN) ☐ (Member ID#) ☐ (SSN or ID) ☐ (SSN) ☒ (ID)

1a. INSURED'S I.D. NUMBER: YYZ8436489

2. PATIENT'S NAME (Last Name, First Name, Middle Initial)
DAVIES KLAUS

3. PATIENT'S BIRTH DATE MM 10 DD 22 YY 1965 **SEX** M ☒ F ☐

4. INSURED'S NAME (Last Name, First Name, Middle Initial)
SAME

5. PATIENT'S ADDRESS (No, Street)
19 WILLOW RD

6. PATIENT RELATIONSHIP TO INSURED
Self ☒ Spouse ☐ Child ☐ Other ☐

7. INSURED'S ADDRESS (No, Street)

CITY: CAPITAL CITY STATE: NY

8. PATIENT STATUS
Single ☐ Married ☒ Other ☐

CITY STATE

ZIP CODE: 12345 TELEPHONE (Include Area Code) (555) 5551276

Employed ☒ Full-Time Student ☐ Part-Time Student ☐

ZIP CODE TELEPHONE (Include Area Code) ( )

9. OTHER INSURED'S NAME (Last Name, First Name, Middle Initial)

10. IS PATIENT'S CONDITION RELATED TO:

11. INSURED'S POLICY GROUP OR FECA NUMBER
326463

a. OTHER INSURED'S POLICY OR GROUP NUMBER

a. EMPLOYMENT? (Current or Previous) ☐ YES ☒ NO

a. INSURED'S DATE OF BIRTH MM DD 04 YY **SEX** M ☐ F ☐

b. OTHER INSURED'S DATE OF BIRTH MM DD YY SEX M ☐ F ☐

b. AUTO ACCIDENT? PLACE (State) ☐ YES ☒ NO

b. EMPLOYER'S NAME OR SCHOOL NAME
ORGANIC FOOD MART

c. EMPLOYER'S NAME OR SCHOOL NAME

c. OTHER ACCIDENT? ☐ YES ☒ NO

c. INSURANCE PLAN NAME OR PROGRAM NAME
BLUE CROSS BLUE SHIELD PPO

d. INSURANCE PLAN NAME OR PROGRAM NAME

10d. RESERVED FOR LOCAL USE

d. IS THERE ANOTHER HEALTH BENEFIT PLAN?
☐ YES ☒ NO *If yes, return to and complete item 9 a-d*

READ BACK OF FORM BEFORE COMPLETING & SIGNING THIS FORM.

12. PATIENT'S OR AUTHORIZED PERSON'S SIGNATURE I authorize the release of any medical or other information necessary to process this claim. I also request payment of government benefits either to myself or to the party who accepts assignment below.

SIGNED SOF   DATE

13. INSURED'S OR AUTHORIZED PERSON'S SIGNATURE I authorize payment of medical benefits to the undersigned physician or supplier for services described below.

SIGNED SOF

14. DATE OF CURRENT MM DD YY ILLNESS (First symptom) OR INJURY (Accident) OR PREGNANCY (LMP)

15. IF PATIENT HAS HAD SAME OR SIMILAR ILLNESS, GIVE FIRST DATE MM DD YY

16. DATES PATIENT UNABLE TO WORK IN CURRENT OCCUPATION
FROM MM DD YY TO MM DD YY

17. NAME OF REFERRING PHYSICIAN OR OTHER SOURCE
17a.
17b. NPI

18. HOSPITALIZATION DATES RELATED TO CURRENT SERVICES
FROM MM DD YY TO MM DD YY

19. RESERVED FOR LOCAL USE

20. OUTSIDE LAB? ☐ YES ☒ NO $ CHARGES

21. DIAGNOSIS OR NATURE OF ILLNESS OR INJURY (Relate Items 1,2,3 or 4 to Item 24E by Line)
1. 401 09   3.
2. 272 0   4.

22. MEDICAID RESUBMISSION CODE ORIGINAL REF. NO.

23. PRIOR AUTHORIZATION NUMBER

24. A. DATE(S) OF SERVICE From			To			B. PLACE OF SERVICE	C. EMG	D. PROCEDURES, SERVICES, OR SUPPLIES (Explain Unusual Circumstances) CPT/HCPCS MODIFIER	E. DIAGNOSIS POINTER	F. $ CHARGES	G. DAYS OR UNITS	H. EPSDT Family Plan	I. ID. QUAL	J. RENDERING PROVIDER ID. #
MM	DD	YY	MM	DD	YY									
10	26	XX	10	26	XX	11		99213	12	55 00	1		NPI	1234567890
10	26	XX	10	26	XX	11		85025	1	95 00	1		NPI	1234567890
10	26	XX	10	26	XX	11		80061	2	95 00	1		NPI	1234567890
10	26	XX	10	26	XX	11		80076	2	95 00	1		NPI	1234567890
10	26	XX	10	26	XX	11		36415	12	15 00	1		NPI	1234567890
													NPI	

25. FEDERAL TAX ID. NUMBER SSN EIN
750246810 ☐ ☒

26. FEDERAL TAX ID. NUMBER
A8

27. ACCEPT ASSIGNMENT? (For govt. claims, see back) ☐ YES ☐ NO

28. TOTAL CHARGE $ 355 00

29. AMOUNT PAID $

30. BALANCE DUE $

31. SIGNATURE OF PHYSICIAN OR SUPPLIER INCLUDING DEGREES OR CREDENTIALS (I certify that the statements on the reverse apply to this bill and are made a part thereof)
PHIL WELLS MD 10/26/XX
SIGNED DATE

32. SERVICE FACILITY LOCATION INFORMATION
CAPITAL CITY MEDICAL
123 UNKNOWN BLVD
CAPITAL CITY NY 12345
a. 1513171216 b.

33. BILLING PROVIDER INFO & PH. # (555) 5551234
CAPITAL CITY MEDICAL
123 UNKNOWN BLVD
CAPITAL CITY NY 12345
a. 1513171216 b.

NUCC Instruction Manual available at: www.nucc.org
WCMS-1500CS

APPROVED OMB 0938-0999 FORM CMS-1500 (08/05)

Figure 17-25 ◆ Klaus Davies sample completed CMS-1500 form.

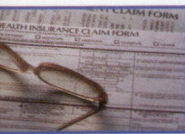

PROCEDURE 17-6 Complete a Computerized Insurance Claim Form

Theory and Rationale

Proper completion of the CMS-1500 insurance claim form is vital to prompt payment of claims in the medical office. So that forms print properly, medical assistants must accurately enter necessary patient data in the computer system.

Materials

- Computer with medical billing software
- Patient medical chart
- Fee slip for patient's visit

Competency

(**Conditions**) With the necessary materials, you will be able to (**Task**) complete an insurance claim form (**Standards**) correctly within the time limit set by the instructor.

1. Choose the patient's account ledger in the computer billing software.
2. Verify that the fee slip is for the patient with the account opened on the computer.
3. Enter the charges and coding as appropriate.
4. Complete the patient insurance information field.
5. Enter the patient's information, including address, telephone number, and birth date.
6. Enter the insured's information, including address, telephone number, and birth date.

7. Enter the patient's relationship to the insured.
8. Enter the insured's identification and group number.
9. Check the appropriate box to indicate the patient has authorized the release of information to the insurance company.
10. Check the appropriate box to indicate the patient has assigned the benefits (payment) to the provider.
11. Check the appropriate boxes to indicate if the visit was related to an accident.
12. If the visit was due to an accident, enter the accident's date.
13. Enter any information regarding a referring physician, if applicable.
14. Enter any information regarding the patient's need for hospitalization for these charges, if applicable.
15. Enter the treating provider's name, address, telephone number, national provider identification (NPI) number, and Internal Revenue Service (**IRS**) tax identification number.
16. Enter information regarding the facility where the services were performed if not performed in the provider's office.
17. Check the appropriate box to indicate the provider accepts assignment.
18. Print the patient's insurance claim form.
19. Review the form for accuracy and completeness.
20. Send the claim to the insurance company.

Submitting a formal appeal is very different from submitting a new claim because an appeal involves extra time and paperwork. Additional information and paperwork must be supplied, and detailed clinical information that may involve the physician might also be requested by the carrier. The appeals process involves a lot of administrative work by the medical assistant and other staff members. Because the appeals process is time consuming, it is often not done properly or consistently. Rather than appeal, some facilities take the "easy road" by submitting a statement to the patient and requiring the patient to deal with the carrier, instead of doing so themselves.

If the decision is made to go ahead with an appeal, the first step is to know and follow the appeals policy of the payer. For example, medical assistants must register the appeal in a timely manner, because there is often a cutoff date for doing so. Most practices learn about the appeals policies of the major plans they work with by referring to physician administrative manuals, contracts, and newsletters. Plan representatives may also be contacted to learn about specific policies. In general, an appeal includes writing a letter that clearly states why the provider believes the denial was not justified. It is best to be clear and factual rather than emotional, angry, or threatening when writing appeal letters. Attach the EOB and any additional supporting documentation

to the letter. Be aware that some plans are instituting paperless review procedures, which will decrease the time spent gathering and documenting detailed information.*

Assistants should also send a copy to the patients. Because healthcare coverage is an agreement between the patient and the insurance carrier, the patient often gets better results when requesting an appeal. For this reason, the medical assistant should always ask the patient to become involved in any appeal process.

Sending Supporting Documentation

Many insurance plans require supporting documentation, things like chart notes, surgical/operative reports, laboratory reports, pathology reports, before they will pay for certain, usually high-cost services, like surgeries (Figure 17-26 ◆). When calling insurance carriers to obtain preauthorization for services, medical assistants should ask customer service representatives if they need supporting documentation with the insurance claim forms. Sending proper documentation with

---

*Source: Adapted from Vines, Deborah, Braceland, Ann, Rollins, Elizabeth, and Miller, Susan. *Comprehensive Health Insurance: Billing, Coding, and Reimbursement.* © 2008, p. 473. Pearson Education, Inc. Upper Saddle River, NJ.

PROCEDURE 17-7 Handle a Denied Insurance Claim

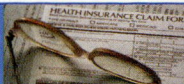

Theory and Rationale

Even after taking care to enter all information into the computer system management software program, insurance claims will occasionally be returned to the medical office. To determine the cause of the denial and the proper action to take, denied claims must be acted on in a timely fashion.

Materials

- Patient insurance information (i.e., ID number, birth date of the insured, name and provider customer service telephone number of insurance company)
- Paper and pen
- Copy of the explanation of benefits (EOB) received
- Description of the procedure the doctor has performed, including CPT code
- Patient's diagnosis pertaining to the procedure performed
- Location where procedure was performed (e.g., office, outpatient surgery, inpatient hospitalization)
- Date the procedure was performed
- Any documentation of the service having been preauthorized by the office

Competency

(**Conditions**) With the necessary materials, you will be able to (**Task**) handle a denied insurance claim (**Standards**) correctly within the time limit set by the instructor.

1. Organize all materials.
2. Call the insurance company's provider customer service phone number as listed on the patient's insurance identification card.
3. Write down the date and time of the telephone call, the number called, and the name of the customer service representative on the phone.
4. Self-identify to the customer service representative, and provide the patient's identification number and date of service.
5. If the service was preauthorized, give that information to the customer service representative.
6. Ask the customer service representative why the procedure was not paid as anticipated.
7. If there was an error in processing the service for payment, ask the customer service representative if any other information is needed to process the claim correctly. Ask the customer service representative when the office can expect payment for the procedure.
8. If the customer service representative says the claim was correctly processed, request the reason for the denial.
9. If the reason for the denial was lack of supporting documentation, ask the customer service representative if faxing the information is a solution. If the answer is yes, get the customer service representative's direct fax line and fax the needed documentation.
10. If the reason for the denial requires an appeal be filed, ask the customer service representative to explain the insurance company's process for appeals.
11. Write down any pertinent information, such as where to mail the appeal and what information the appeal should contain.
12. Call the patient with the findings and get the patient involved as needed.

---

the CMS-1500 billing form often avoids claims return and therefore delayed payment.

At other times, the insurance will ask for additional documentation while reviewing the claim. The request usually comes in the form of a letter. When replying to such requests, medical assistants should be certain to identify exactly what information is being requested and respond specifically. It is not necessary to send a voluminous amount of records when only one or two specific items are being requested.

With worker's compensation and TPL claims, carriers may request a progress report. A written progress report clearly describes the extent of the patient's recovery since the injury, what further treatment is needed, and the expected result. Include any test results such as X-rays, lab tests, or physical function tests, such as range of motion or lifting capacity, to document the patient's status. Medical assistants should respond to such requests immediately because no further payment will be made on the claim until the report is received. Medical assistants may have the responsibility of abstracting the pertinent information from the medical record, drafting the report, and presenting it to the provider for review and signature.

The Office of the Insurance Commissioner

Each state has an Office of the Insurance Commissioner, a valuable resource for both the medical office and the patient. When medical assistants or patients believe claims were incorrectly processed and appeal attempts have been fruitless, assistants may file formal written complaints with the state's insurance commissioner. It is important to involve patients in this process because they are the consumers the insurance commissioner is charged with protecting. Patients may be reluctant to appeal to the commissioner on their own initiative because they are unfamiliar with the process. One good approach is for medical assistants to write a letter on behalf of the patient and ask the patient to sign it. Sometimes, the threat of complaint alone can inspire insurance carriers to review denied claims.

OPERATION DATE: 10/7/08

SURGEON: GREGORY PROVENCE, MD

PREOPERATIVE DIAGNOSIS:

Right parotid mass.

POSTOPERATIVE DIAGNOSIS:

Same.

PROCEDURE:

Right deep lobe parotid resection, removal of right parotid tumor with facial nerve preservation and with facial nerve monitoring.

DESCRIPTION OF PROCEDURE:

The patient is a 54-year-old female who noted a growing mass in the right parotid area. Fine needle biopsy reported benign cells and CT scan confirmed a large bilobed cystic lesion. Risks, expectations, complications, procedure, and alternative treatment measures were discussed prior to consent.

FINDINGS:

A bilobed tumor extending medial to the facial nerve branches into the "turquoise" space superior to the thyroid process and most of the deep lobe parotid were absent. Facial nerve was preserved with the facial nerve monitoring.

General endotracheal anesthesia was given. 1% Xylocaine was used for facial skin infiltration. Incision was drawn with an ink pen and incision was carried along the preauricular crease around the "yellow" lobule to the upper neck along the skin crease. Incision carried through the platysmas and the sternomastoid muscle and the external ear canal. The posterior facial vein was identified and dissected laterally, lifting the gland away from the facial vein for the purpose of identifying the lower branch of the facial nerve. Superiorly, the facial branch was identified. It was then carefully preserved and as the parotid gland was lifted, the superficial lobe of the parotid gland was lifted laterally and anteriorly. The lower division of the facial nerve was found and medial to the nerve was the tumor. The tumor was then gently grasped with forceps and the lower division was carefully lifted and shifted superiorly as the tumor was shifted inferiorly for excision. Blunt and sharp dissection was made to free the nerve from surrounding tissue. The deep lobe of the parotid was generally absent because of the size of the mass. The mass was cynlindrical bilobed-shaped, and extending beyond the styloid process, placed superior to the styloid process into the "turquoise" space.

Finally the entire tumor was isolated and removed. Bleeding was controlled with bipolar cautery. An Avitene sheet was used for hemostasis. A 15 Blake drain was inserted, secured with 3-0 nylon. The skin incision was closed with 4-0 chromic and 5-0 nylon. Blood loss was about 25 cc. Dressing applied. Antiobiotic ointment was placed on the incision.

The patient was then extubated and sent to the recovery room in good condition. Postop facial nerve function was intact. She was given Keflex for prophylaxis and Lortab 7.5 mg for pain. She will be seen as needed and drain will be removed in the next 48 hours.

GREGORY PROVENCE, MD

Figure 17-26 ◆ Sample operative report.

Projecting Health Insurance Costs in the Future

With the cost of healthcare and health insurance coverage rising far beyond the rate of inflation in the United States, most experts would agree that the U.S. healthcare system will differ dramatically in the future. In the past, many employees were covered by health insurance plans that covered 100 percent of all healthcare expenses. These plans are few and far between today; the vast majority of employer-provided health insurance policies require patients to share in the cost of their healthcare in the form of deductibles, coinsurance, and copays.

One possibility for the future is for employers to offer employees vouchers for health insurance coverage. Employees could use these vouchers to purchase plans that suit their needs. In an attempt to find ways to cover the 47 million Americans currently without health insurance coverage, experts studying these types of plans believe all Americans could be offered tax incentives or rebates for purchasing health insurance coverage. Whatever the future may bring, the medical assistant should stay current on the legislation that affects healthcare and health insurance coverage, both locally and nationally.

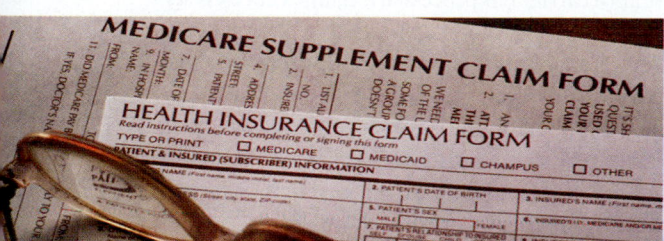
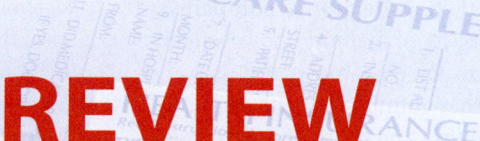

REVIEW

Chapter Summary

- Medical assistants play a central role in insurance claim processing and are responsible for accuracy and responsiveness as well as patient relations.

- Health insurance in the United States began in the mid-1800s. The first group policy giving comprehensive benefits was offered by Massachusetts Health Insurance of Boston in 1847. Insurance companies issued the first individual disability and illness policies around 1890. Hospital insurance coverage began in 1929. During World War II, when wages were frozen, employers began offering their employees group health insurance as a benefit. Employee benefit plans became popular in the 1940s and 1950s. During the 1950s and 1960s government programs began to cover healthcare costs. Social security coverage included disability benefits for the first time in 1954, and the government created the Medicare and Medicaid programs in 1965. By the end of 1995, individuals and companies paid for about one-half of the healthcare received in the United States, with the government paying for the other half. The 1980s and 1990s saw a rapid rise in the cost of healthcare. During this time, the majority of employer-sponsored group insurance plans moved to less expensive managed care plans.

- People in the United States obtain health insurance from a variety of sources. Medical assistants need to be knowledgeable about the rules and requirements of each. They must understand insurance terminology in order to help patients utilize their health insurance. Patients are often unfamiliar with their insurance benefits and may not understand the terms they hear. MAs who understand insurance terms can advocate for patients and communicate in ways that patients understand.

- A number of national commercial insurance carriers offer health insurance coverage. Examples include Blue Cross/Blue Shield, Aetna, and Cigna. Policies might be purchased by employers for a group of employees or by individuals who lack health insurance through their places of employment. Coverage amounts and premiums vary according to policy type.

- The most common sources of private health insurance are group insurance, self-insured plans, and individual insurance.

- The federal Consolidated Omnibus Reconciliation Act (COBRA) requires employers to extend health insurance coverage at group rates, usually for up to 18 months, to any employee who is laid off, quits, or is fired, except under certain circumstances.

- The HMO Act of 1973 and the Tax Equity and Fiscal Responsibility Act (TEFRA) introduced health insurance plans that allow patients a variety of ways to access providers and share in the cost of care. These various plans differ in how insurance companies pay providers.

- Managed care plans control the costs associated with plan purchase by controlling the amounts they reimburse healthcare providers. MCOs contract with healthcare providers to provide care for a certain group of patients. Managed care plans are divided into the following types: Health Maintenance Organizations (HMOs), Preferred Provider Organizations (PPOs), Exclusive Provider Organizations (EPOs), and Point of Service Plans (POS). These healthcare plans all support the insurance needs of patient populations, but in varying ways and at varying levels of cost and coverage.

- It is important for the medical assistant to be familiar with all aspects of the Medicare program, divided into Parts A, B, C, and D, because more and more patients will be covered by this type of insurance as the U.S. population ages.

- Medicare and Medicaid both provide vital services such as hospitalization, physician visits, and prescription drug coverage to substantial patient populations.

- Medigap or Medicare supplemental plans are insurance plans offered by private companies to reimburse patients for the out-of-pocket expenses they incur with Medicare.

- In 1997, The State Children's Health Insurance Program (SCHIP) was created to cover children who do not have another form of health insurance coverage. It is similar to

Chapter Summary (continued)

Medicaid in that SCHIP is designed to function as a federal/state joint program.

■ The TRICARE and CHAMPVA programs deliver insurance coverage to patients who are in the military or families of military members.

■ Worker's compensation is a program designed to provide employees who are injured on the job an insurance safety net.

■ It is important for medical assistants to understand how reimbursement affects the practice. Insurance companies reimburse providers using a variety of methods; however, the most traditional method is a usual, customary, and reasonable (UCR) fee schedule. Other reimbursement methods include a negotiated fee schedule, capitation, per-diem payment method, or per-case payments. When Medicare uses a per-case form of reimbursement, it is called Diagnosis Related Groups (DRG).

■ Healthcare claim preparation is an involved process that requires attention to detail, knowledge of healthcare regulations, and the ability to interface with a broad array of healthcare entities.

■ The CMS-1500 claim form is used by all health insurance carriers, including Medicare, Medicaid, and workmen's compensation carriers, to complete paper billed claims. The form is divided into two major sections and includes 33 form locators (boxes to be completed on the form).

■ Electronic claims are submitted to the insurance carrier via a central processing unit (CPU), tape diskette, direct data entry, direct wire, telephone line via modem, or personal computer. Medicare requires electronic transmission of claims for providers with ten or more employees or facilities with twenty-five or more employees.

■ Providers have different methods in determining their fee structure. Two main methods used for determining fees are charge-based and resource-based fee structures.

■ Once an insurance carrier has processed a claim, a check is sent to the healthcare provider with an Explanation of Benefits (EOB) statement. Medical assistants must check EOBs to ensure all services that were billed are accurately listed and that service payment matches the amount in the insurance company contract.

■ Medical assistants should call insurance carriers to follow up on or trace claims that are past due. Each state has its own guidelines that outline the timeframe within which an insurance carrier must pay or deny a claim.

■ Claims can be rejected or denied for errors made by the medical office. Attention to detail in the claim submission process saves time and effort in the end.

■ The Office of the Insurance Commissioner is a valuable resource for both the medical office and the patient. Assistants may file formal written complaints with the state's insurance commissioner.

■ Many experts believe that due to the rising cost of health care and health insurance coverage, the U.S. healthcare system will differ dramatically in the future. Today, the vast majority of employer-provided health insurance policies require patients to share in the cost of their healthcare in the form of deductibles, coinsurance, and copays.

Chapter Review

Multiple Choice

1. Typically, the most expensive health plans to buy are
   a. employer provided.
   b. individual.
   c. Medicare Part B.
   d. Medicare Part A.

2. With most insurance carriers, timely filing limits refer to submitting claims within _____ days from the date of service.
   a. 365
   b. 120
   c. 45
   d. 30

3. The best way to trace an overdue insurance claim is to
   a. send another copy of the original claim.
   b. send a bill to the patient.
   c. call the insurance company regarding the claim.
   d. call the state's Office of the Insurance Commissioner.

4. Which of the following might be eligible for COBRA benefits?
   a. Recently fired employee
   b. Recently laid off employee
   c. Employee who recently quit
   d. All of the above

5. Consumer-directed healthcare plans
   a. offer patients a wide variety of in-network physicians.
   b. cause patients to be more aware of healthcare costs.
   c. are offered by Medicare.
   d. are called "capitated plans."

6. Balance billing occurs when the physician
   a. bills the secondary insurance company after receiving payment from the primary insurance company.
   b. bills the primary insurance company.
   c. bills Medicare.
   d. bills the patient an amount that should be written off under the preferred provider contract.

Chapter Review (continued)

7. Using the birthday rule, the parent who is usually primary when billing for a child's services is the parent who
   a. has a birthday earlier in the year.
   b. has birthday later in the year.
   c. is older.
   d. is younger.

8. Many insurance plans exclude coverage for
   a. routine hearing tests.
   b. elective surgery.
   c. plastic surgery.
   d. all of the above.

9. HIPAA requires medical offices to give patients
   a. copies of the office's privacy practices.
   b. access to their medical records on request.
   c. accounts of any disclosures of their medical records on request.
   d. all of the above.

True/False

T F 1. Many managed care plans require the medical office to obtain preauthorization before rendering certain services to patients.

T F 2. When insurance companies deny payment for services, the only recourse is to bill the patient for the fee directly.

T F 3. Medicare fee schedules are the same wherever physicians practice.

T F 4. Medicaid is funded entirely by each state.

T F 5. Sending any information to an insurance company without the patient's permission violates HIPAA.

Short Answer

1. Explain the term *pre-existing condition* as it applies to healthcare.

2. Why is it a good idea to start a new file for an existing patient who has just recently been involved in a worker's compensation claim?

3. Which other terms mean the same as "subscriber" with regard to health insurance coverage?

4. What is another term for the Medicare advance beneficiary notice?

5. List two reasons a claim might be denied by an insurance company and suggest how to avoid those denials.

6. What does CMS stand for and what is its role?

Research

1. Interview a person who works in a medical office. How does that office handle insurance authorizations for patients with managed care?

2. Look at the Medicare Web site. Where is the office for providers in your state to call for help with claims processing or questions?

3. Look at your state's Medicaid Web site. What telephone number do providers in your state call in order to obtain authorization for procedures on a Medicaid-covered patient?

Externship Application Experience

Phyllis Allen is a patient of Dr. King's. The physician would like to have Phyllis scheduled for a biopsy procedure to be performed in the office. What information should the medical assistant gather before calling the insurance carrier? What information should the assistant write down during the telephone call?

Resource Guide

Centers for Medicare and Medicaid Services
7500 Security Boulevard
Baltimore, MD 21244
Phone: (877) 267-2323
www.cms.hhs.gov

U.S. Department of Defense Military Health System
Skyline 5, Suite 810
5111 Leesburg Pike
Falls Church, VA 22041-3206
www.tricare.org

U.S. Department of Health and Human Services
200 Independence Avenue, SW
Room 509F, HHH Building
Washington, DC 20201
Phone: (800) 368-1019
www.hhs.gov/ocr/hipaa

U.S. Department of Labor
Frances Perkins Building, 200 Constitution Ave., NW
Washington, DC 20210
Phone: (866) 4-USA-DOL
www.dol.gov

Med**Media**

http://www.MyMAKit.com.

More on this chapter, including interactive resources, can be found on the Student CD-ROM accompanying this textbook and on http://www.MyMAKit.com.

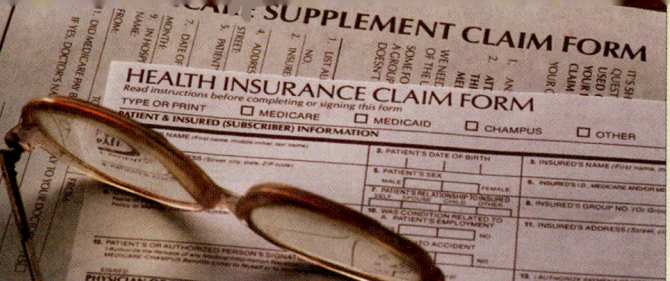

Objectives

After completing this chapter, you should be able to:

- Define and spell the key terminology in this chapter.
- Define the medical assistant's role in diagnostic coding.
- Explain the history of diagnostic coding.
- Describe the function and layout of the ICD-9 coding book.
- List the steps to correctly choose diagnosis codes.
- Explain how to code for various special situations.
- Describe how the medical assistant might pursue professional certification.

ICD-9-CM Coding

Case Study

Recently hired in the billing department of Dr. Johnson's medical office, Mary is asked to assign a diagnostic code to a patient's visit and bill for the charges. Unfortunately, Mary has a difficult time deciphering Dr. Johnson's handwriting. After deciding she cannot read the writing in the patient's chart, she says, "Well, it looks like the visit has something to do with the patient's ear, so I'll just code the visit as an earache."

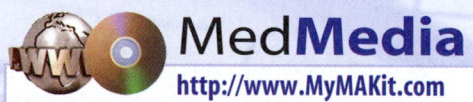

MedMedia
http://www.MyMAKit.com

Additional interactive resources and activities for this chapter can be found on http://www.MyMAKit.com. For a video, tips, audio glossary, legal and ethical scenarios, on-the-job scenarios, quizzes, and games related to the content of this chapter, please access the accompanying CD-ROM in this book.

Video: *Insurance Coding*
Legal and Ethical Scenario: *ICD-9-CM Coding*
On the Job Scenario: *ICD-9-CM Coding*
Tips
Multiple Choice Quiz
Audio Glossary
HIPAA Quiz
Games: Spelling Bee, Crossword, and Strikeout

Key Terminology

adverse reaction—unexpected or dangerous reaction to a drug

and—interpreted as *either/and/or* in a diagnostic code description

category—a three-digit code in *ICD-9-CM* tabular list

chapter—one of seventeen major sections of *ICD-9-CM* Volume I tabular list, organized by body system and etiology

chief complaint—statement in the patient's own words of the reason for seeking medical care

combination code—a single code that describes two or more conditions that frequently occur together

conventions—*ICD-9-CM* coding rules, abbreviations, symbols, or formatting intended to ensure consistency in coding

E codes—codes that indicate the cause of an illness or condition

etiology—cause of a disease or an illness

first-listed—the diagnosis that is chiefly responsible for the outpatient services provided; formerly called primary diagnosis

late effect—current condition that results from a previous, resolved condition

main term—words by which conditions and diseases are alphabetized in *ICD-9-CM* Volume II; may be name of condition, eponym, acronym, or synonym, but not an anatomical site

manifestation—outward or associated condition resulting from an underlying disease

M codes—identify neoplasm type and tumor behavior, used by tumor registries

morbidity—illness or injury

mortality—death

multiple coding—a diagnosis that requires more than one *ICD-9-CM* code to completely describe it; often indicated by a second code in slanted brackets

neoplasm—the medical term for an abnormal growth of new tissue, often referred to as a tumor

nonessential modifiers—words in parentheses after a main term in the *ICD-9-CM*, clarifying the main term, but need not be present in the medical record

not otherwise specified (NOS)—a general code used when details are not available in the medical record

---

MEDICAL ASSISTING STANDARDS

CAAHEP ENTRY-LEVEL STANDARDS	ABHES ENTRY-LEVEL COMPETENCIES
■ Perform within scope of practice (psychomotor) ■ Apply ethical behaviors, including honesty/integrity in performance of medical assisting practice (affective) ■ Explore issue of confidentiality as it applies to the medical assistant (cognitive) ■ Respond to issues of confidentiality (psychomotor) ■ Apply local, state and federal health care legislation and regulation appropriate to the medical assisting practice setting (psychomotor) ■ Recognize the importance of local, state and federal legislation and regulations in the practice setting (affective) ■ Document accurately in the patient record (psychomotor) ■ Use office hardware and software to maintain office systems (psychomotor) ■ Describe procedures for implementing both managed care and insurance plans (cognitive) ■ Work with physician to achieve the maximum reimbursement (affective) ■ Apply both managed care policies and procedures (psychomotor) ■ Apply third party guidelines (psychomotor) ■ Describe how to use the most current diagnostic coding classification system (cognitive) ■ Perform diagnostic coding (psychomotor)	■ Conduct work within scope of education, training, and ability ■ Monitor legislation related to current health care issues and practices ■ Apply managed care policies and procedures ■ Obtain managed care referrals and precertification ■ Exercise efficient time management ■ Analyze and use current third party guidelines for reimbursement ■ Perform diagnostic coding ■ Implement current procedural terminology and ICD-9 coding

---

✔ COMPETENCY SKILLS PERFORMANCE

1. Perform diagnostic coding.

Introduction

Diagnostic coding is the process of assigning a number to a description of the patient's condition, illness, or disease as it appears in the healthcare provider's listing in the patient's medical chart. Procedure codes, discussed in Chapter 19, describe services performed on patients; diagnostic codes outline the reasons services were needed. Diagnostic codes are used to group and identify diseases and illnesses and to track causes of **morbidity** and **mortality.** Diagnostic codes must be accurate, because they inform insurance companies of the severity of patients' conditions and therefore the need for services, procedures, or tests.

Key Terminology *(continued)*

principal diagnosis—the reason determined, after study, to be responsible for an inpatient stay

qualified—diagnosis statement accompanied by terms such as possible, probable, suspected, rule out (R/O), or working diagnosis indicating the physician has not determined the root cause

secondary diagnoses—conditions, diseases, or reasons for seeking care in addition to the first-listed diagnosis; they may or may not be related to the first-listed diagnosis

section—an organizational division of a chapter that groups together multiple categories

sequela—an abnormal condition resulting from a previous injury, condition, or disease

sign—a physical sign of a condition that can observed or measured by a physician

subcategory—a four-digit code in *ICD-9-CM* tabular list

subclassification—a five-digit code in *ICD-9-CM* tabular list

subterm—indented two spaces under the boldfaced main term in the *ICD-9-CM* and further describes the condition, in terms of etiology, co-existing conditions, anatomic site, episode, or similar descriptor

symptom—indication of a condition reported by the patient that the physician cannot observe or measure

tabular list—Volume I of *ICD-9-CM* that lists all diagnostic codes in numerical order

uncertain—see *qualified*

V codes—codes for visits' reasons, other than disease or illness

with—interpreted as *both, together with* in a diagnostic code description

Abbreviations

AAPC—American Academy of Professional Coders

AHIMA—American Health Information Management Association

APHA—American Public Health Association

CCS-P—Certified Coding Specialist-Physician based

CPC—Certified Professional Coder

DM—diabetes mellitus

ICD-9-CM—*International Classification of Diseases, 9th Rev., Clinical Modification*

TBSA—total body surface area, of burns

The Medical Assistant's Role in Diagnostic Coding

Because proper coding is vital to appropriate reimbursement, the medical assistant's role in diagnostic coding must be done with the utmost attention to detail. While it is the physician's role to assign diagnoses to the patient, the MA is responsible for applying the proper code to match the diagnosis the physician provides. Accurate diagnostic coding is the first step in obtaining reimbursement for services. Inaccurate diagnosis codes on bills can result in improper payment or nonpayment for services provided. While a large medical office may hire professional, certified coders, medical assistants are a vital link in communication between coders and physicians. Medical assistants are also responsible for maintaining medical records appropriately so they can be easily utilized by coders. Some medical assistants choose to pursue certification as professional coders.

The History of Diagnostic Coding

Diagnostic coding has existed for more than a century, beginning in 1893 with French physician Jacques Bertillon. Dr. Bertillon composed the Bertillon Classification of Causes of Death, which the American Public Health Association (**APHA**) adopted in 1898. At the time, the classification contained an alphabetic index and a tabular list and was quite small compared to coding references used today. The APHA recommended the classification be revised every ten years to ensure it was current.

In 1901, the APHA published a coding book called the *International Classification of Diseases (ICD), Volume I*. The *ICD-1* was used until 1910, when the second volume, *ICD-2*, was published. Volume updates continued to be published approximately every ten years until the *International Classification*

of Diseases, Volume 9, Clinical Modification (**ICD-9-CM**) was published in 1979.

ICD-10 was completed in 1999, and has replaced the *ICD-9-CM* in all major countries except the United States. An implementation date for the United States has not been established, but it is expected that there will be a transition period of at least two years. The *ICD-10* will provide a revised and expanded code structure that will incorporate updated terminology, make it easier to add codes, such as for new technologies, allow for greater specificity and consistency, and comply with code set standards outlined by HIPAA.

Table 18-1 compares the *ICD-9-CM* and *ICD-10* coding manuals. Once *ICD-10* is incorporated into common use, the *ICD-9-CM* will become obsolete, and physicians, clinics, and hospitals will have to change their electronic and manual coding systems to reflect the new coding structure.

TABLE 18-1 COMPARISON OF ICD-9 AND ICD-10

ICD-9-CM	ICD-10
Title: *International Classification of Diseases,* 9th Rev., *Clinical Modifications*	Title: *International Statistical Classification of Diseases and Related Health Problems*
Contains a chapter titled, "Diseases of the Nervous System and Sense Organs"	Divides the chapter into three chapters titled: "Diseases of the Nervous System" "Diseases of the Eye and Adnexa" "Diseases of the Ear and Mastoid Process"
Contains a chapter titled "Mental Disorders"	Renames this chapter "Mental and Behavioral Disorders"
Contains a supplement titled "V Codes"	"V Codes" becomes a chapter rather than a supplement
Contains a supplement titled "E Codes"	"E Codes" becomes a chapter rather than a supplement
Contains numeric codes that require four and five digits	Contains alpha numeric codes that require up to seven digits and letters
Contains two volumes for diagnosis coding	Contains three volumes for diagnosis coding

Coding with the *ICD-9-CM* Book

The *ICD-9-CM* book lists the codes to use for any diagnoses physicians give patients. The challenge is to find appropriate codes. Diagnostic codes describe the medical need of visits. If, for example, a patient presents in the office complaining of a headache and sore throat and the physician orders a throat culture, the medical assistant must ensure the claim form carries a diagnostic code that relates to a sore throat. If instead the medical assistant codes only for a headache, the office will not likely be paid for the throat culture.

Incorrect diagnostic coding may not only impede the office's ability to get paid by the insurance carrier, it may adversely affect the patient's ability to obtain health insurance coverage in the future. Assume the medical assistant incorrectly assigns a patient a diagnostic code for acute myocardial infarction when that patient was treated for chest pain due to heartburn. That patient might be incorrectly perceived as having heart disease and therefore experience insurance coverage issues, such as denial of coverage in the future.

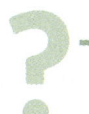

Critical Thinking Question 18-1

Referring to the case study at the beginning of the chapter, what is the potential harm in Mary's guessing at the patient's diagnostic code?

The *ICD-9-CM* lists over 10,000 diagnostic codes in three volumes. *ICD-9-CM* codes are updated annually and take effect October 1 of each year. Medical assistants should use the edition of the *ICD-9-CM* that was in effect on the date of service. For example, patients seen on September 30, 2009, would be coded using the 2009 coding manual, while those seen on October 1, 2009 would be coded using the 2010 coding manual. The transition date for diagnosis coding differs from the one used for procedural coding, January 1, which will be addressed in ∞ Chapter 19. *ICD-9-CM* updates are needed to amend current listings and reflect new diseases or illnesses. The World Health Organization (WHO) has updated ICD codes since 1948. Code changes are published by the National

Center for Health Statistics and the Centers for Medicare and Medicaid Services (CMS), in conjunction with the WHO.

The Volumes of ICD-9-CM

Each of the three *ICD-9-CM* volumes has a distinct purpose. Volume I is a tabular list of diseases, Volume II is an alphabetic index of diseases, and Volume III is a tabular list and alphabetic index of hospital procedures. Physicians use Volumes I and II of *ICD-9-CM;* hospitals use all three volumes.

In the physical organization of the manual, Volume II appears first, followed by Volume I, then Volume III. Many publishers print *ICD-9-CM* manuals for physicians' offices that contain only Volumes I and II, in order to save on cost. We will first provide an overview of each volume, in the order it appears in the book. Later in the chapter, detailed coding instructions will be presented. Each volume also uses a number of specialized rules, abbreviations, formatting, and symbols called **conventions**. These are also described at the beginning of the manual. A key to selected symbols usually appears at the bottom of each page. The conventions and symbols are specific to each volume.

Volume II

Volume II, which appears first in the coding manual, contains two sections.

- **Section 1: Alphabetic Index to Diseases**. This is the section of the *ICD-9-CM* that medical assistants need to utilize as the first step in coding. Conditions, diseases, and reasons for seeking medical care are listed alphabetically by **main term** and **subterms** that aid in locating the most appropriate code. After identifying potential codes in the index, they are verified in Volume I, the Tabular List. Final code selection should never be done based only on the index. Section 1 also contains two tables that contain cross-tabbed index entries for hypertension table and neoplasms. Detailed use of the index and tables will be described later.
- **Section 2: Alphabetic Index to External Causes of Adverse Effects of Drugs and Other Chemical Substances, Injuries and Poisonings.** When a condition is

caused by an accident or poisoning, there are supplemental codes used to describe the circumstances. The first part of this section is the Table of Drugs and Chemicals. This table contains an alphabetical list of drugs and other chemical substances, cross-tabbed with a list of causes, to identify poisonings and external causes of drug-related adverse effects, such as drug-induced attempted suicide or an adverse reaction to penicillin. This is followed by an alphabetic index used to locate the external cause of an injury, such as a fall or motor vehicle accident. Detailed use of this will be described later.

Volume I

After locating the diagnosis in the appropriate index in Volume II, it will be verified by referencing the tabular list in Volume I. Volume I is a numerically sequenced list of all diagnosis codes, divided into seventeen chapters based on cause, or **etiology**, of the disease or injury, as well as by location of the disease or injury on or in the body. Every chapter title describes the conditions within, followed by the range of three-digit codes within. Table 18-2 gives an overview of Volume I chapters.

In addition to a title, each Volume I chapter has a sub-title in large print followed by a range of three-digit codes in that category. Each three-digit code combination describes a general

> 3-digit code: 037 Tetanus
> 4-digit code: 245.0 Acute thyroiditis
> 5-digit code: 372.05 Acute atopic conjunctivitis

Figure 18-1 ◆ Sample three-, four-, and five-digit codes from the *ICD-9-CM* coding book.

disease; subsequent fourth and fifth digits add more specificity. Five-digit codes confer the highest level of definition. Volume I indicates the number of digits needed for coding: three, four, or five. Figure 18-1 ◆ shows sample three-, four-, and five- digit codes from the *ICD-9-CM* coding book.

Supplementary Code Listings

Following the seventeen chapters listing codes 000-999, there are two sections with supplemental codes. The first of these, Supplementary Classification of Factors Influencing Health Status and Contact with Health Services, are commonly referred to as V codes, because these codes begin with the letter "V" and range from V01 to V83 (Figure 18-2 ◆). These codes classify the reason for care, other than an active illness. V codes are located

TABLE 18-2   CONTENTS OF *ICD-9-CM* VOLUME I

Chapter Number	Chapter Name	Code Numbers Included
1	Infectious and Parasitic Diseases	001–139
2	Neoplasms	140–239
3	Endocrine, Nutritional, and Metabolic Diseases and Immunity Disorders	240–279
4	Diseases of the Blood and Blood-Forming Organs	280–289
5	Mental Disorders	290–319
6	Diseases of the Nervous System and Sense Organs	390–459
7	Diseases of the Circulatory System	390–459
8	Diseases of the Respiratory System	460–519
9	Diseases of the Digestive System	520–579
10	Diseases of the Genitourinary System	580–629
11	Complications of Pregnancy, Childbirth, and the Puerperium	630–677
12	Diseases of the Skin and Subcutaneous Tissue	680–709
13	Diseases of the Musculoskeletal System and Connective Tissue	710–739
14	Congenital Anomalies	740–759
15	Certain Conditions Originating in the Perinatal Period	760–799
16	Symptoms, Signs, and Ill-Defined Conditions	780–799
17	Injury and Poisoning	800–999
	Supplementary Classification of Factors Influencing Health Status and Contact with Health Services	V01–V83
	Supplementary Classification of External Causes of Injury and Poisoning	E800–E999
Appendix A	Morphology of Neoplasms	
Appendix C	Classification of Drugs by American Hospital Formulary Service	
Appendix D	Classification of Industrial Accidents	
Appendix E	List of three-digit categories	

V61.3 Problems with aged parents or in-laws

V21.0 Period of rapid growth in childhood

V65.44 HIV counseling

Figure 18-2 ◆ Sample V codes.

E836 Machinery accident in water transport

E878.3 Surgical operation with formation of external stoma

E904.0 Abandonment or neglect of infants and helpless persons

Figure 18-3 ◆ Sample E codes.

through the alphabetical index in Volume II, Section 1. The second supplementary classification in Volume I is the Supplementary Classification of External Causes of Injury and Poisoning, commonly called E codes, because each code begins with the letter "E" and range from E800-E899 (Figure 18-3 ◆). E codes classify causes of injury and poisoning. E codes are located through the index in Volume I, Section 2.

ICD-9-CM Appendices

Volume I of the *ICD-9-CM* book has four appendices. These appendices are used as a reference to the user in order to provide a clinical picture or further information about the patient's diagnosis. The appendices are used to further define the diagnosis, to classify new drugs, or to reference the type and cause of on-the-job injury the patient has sustained.

- **Appendix A: Morphology of Neoplasms**—This appendix provides "M" codes that indicate how neoplasms (tumors) have morphed to other body areas. M codes are not used for billing, they are used only by tumor registries.
- **Appendix B: Glossary of Mental Disorders**—Appendix B was officially deleted from the *ICD-9-CM* coding manual on October 1, 2004.
- **Appendix C: Classification of Drugs by American Hospital Formulary Service**—Each drug currently on the market appears here. This appendix is used to code any adverse effects of drugs on the patient.
- **Appendix D: Classification of Industrial Accidents**—This appendix describes on-the-job accidents. This list contains codes to describe accidents according to the type or place of accident. The following list shows the categories of on the job accidents and an example of a code found under each list.
- **Appendix E: List of Three-Digit Categories**—All three-digit categories in the *ICD-9-CM* book appear here.

Volume III

Because Volume III of *ICD-9-CM* is for inpatient procedure coding, medical assistants will only use it if working in hospital settings. Although medical assistants may be hired by hospital-owned physician practices, the majority of hospitals hire professional certified coders to code inpatient charts.

Volume III contains an Index to Procedures, followed by the Tabular List of Procedures. Hospital procedure codes are three or four digits long and range from 00.01 to 99.99

(Figure 18-4 ◆). Physicians use the CPT manual to code for procedures and services, which will be discussed in ∞ Chapter 19 .

Determining the Correct Diagnosis Code

Coding begins and ends with the patient's medical record. Medical assistants abstract information from the medical record in order to code for services and the reasons they were provided. Coding is to be done to the highest level of certainty, meaning that all relevant information in the chart should be coded, but missing information should not be assumed or coded. Only conditions, diseases, and symptoms documented in the medical record can be coded and billed. If the medical record is incomplete or inaccurate, it should be corrected or amended before attempting to code (Figure 18-5 ◆).

In Practice

Sharon is the medical assistant who completes billing work in the office. One day when she receives a patient file for billing, Sharon notices that the fee slip the physician completed indicates that he drained a cyst on the patient's wrist. When Sharon reviews the chart notes to assign a diagnosis code, she finds that the physician has written nothing in the chart about the cyst or the procedure. In situations like these, Sharon usually just "jots something" in the chart. What might be wrong with this scenario?

There are a number of documents within the medical record that may contain needed information. When coding for

00.02 Therapeutic ultrasound of the heart

53.61 Incisional hernia repair with prosthesis

87.43 X-ray of ribs, sternum, and clavicle

Figure 18-4 ◆ Sample hospital procedure codes.

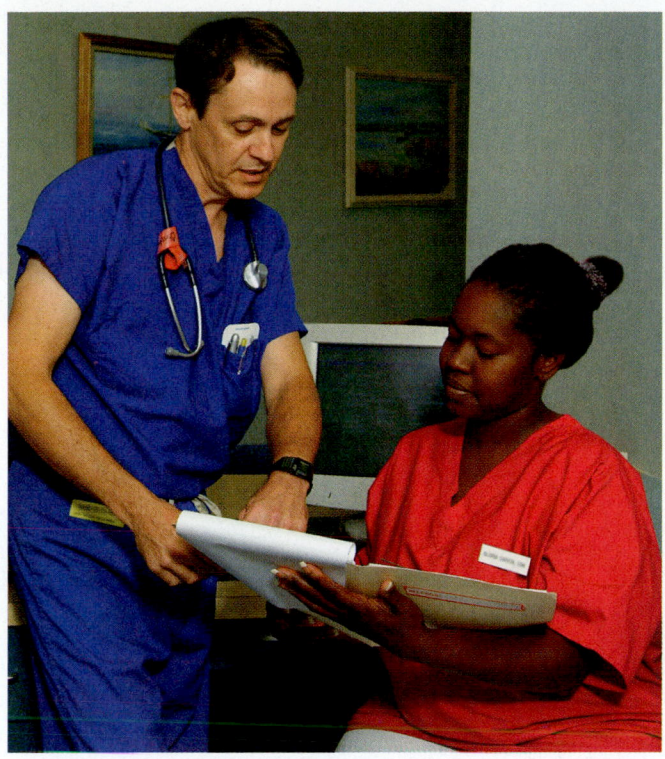

Figure 18-5 ◆ The medical assistant may need to consult the physician in order to obtain the correct code to use.

office-based or other outpatient services, medical assistants will refer to the patient registration form, the encounter form, visit notes, lab and radiology reports, and operative reports for outpatient procedures. When coding for services physicians provide to inpatients, medical assistants will refer to the admitting history and physical (H&P), daily progress notes, operative reports, lab and radiology reports, and the discharge summary.

It is important to keep in mind that when performing diagnosis coding in order to bill for services, the diagnosis must describe the reasons the specific service was provided and related medical conditions that may affect the specific service. Diagnosis codes should not repeat patients' entire problem list, which is a comprehensive list of all active conditions that often appears in the front of the medical record.

For example, assume a patient is seen for a sinus infection, and she also has chronic gastric reflux. An antibiotic is prescribed for the sinus infection and the physician inquires how the gastric reflux is doing, but does not actively treat it. Only the sinus infection would be coded.

In another example, assume a patient is seen for a burn on the hand, and he also has diabetes. The physician indicates that the diabetes may slow the healing process and requires more frequent followup visits due to the diabetes impact. Therefore, both the burn and the diabetes would be coded.

The following coding steps provide the practical details medical assistants need to patiently and accurately execute the process. The majority of this discussion will be oriented toward office-based coding. Inpatient coding guidelines have some variations and these will be highlighted at the end of the chapter.

1. **Identify the first-listed diagnosis as stated in the medical record.** Often the physician will indicate a diagnosis code on the encounter form, but it is wise to verify it against the medical record. Look for a definitive diagnostic statement by the physician for reason for the visit. The diagnosis may be indicated with the word *impression* or, in SOAP notes, it will be under *A (Assessment)*. This will be the **first-listed** or **primary diagnosis**, the reason chiefly responsible for the services provided.

Uncertain or **qualified** diagnoses are those accompanied by terms such as possible, probable, suspected, rule out (R/O), or working diagnosis, indicating the physician has not determined the root cause. For outpatient coding, do not use uncertain diagnoses. Instead, look for the patient's **signs** or **symptoms** that are part of the patient's **chief complaint**. The chief complaint is a statement in the patient's own words of the reason for the visit. Signs are indications of a condition that the physician can observe or measure, such as a rash. Symptoms are indications reported by the patient that the physician cannot observe or measure, such as a headache.

Additional conditions or complaints will become **secondary** diagnoses, which will be coded in the same way as the primary, but listed after them on the CMS-1500 billing form. Signs and symptoms that are routinely associated with the first-listed diagnosis are not coded as secondary diagnoses.

The following sample patient scenarios illustrate the difference between a definitive diagnosis and signs and symptoms. These same scenarios will be developed throughout each step in the coding process discussed.

Sample Patient Scenario
Selecting the First Listed Diagnosis

Scenario 1—A patient presents with difficulty breathing and fever. The physician takes a sputum culture and diagnoses acute pneumonia. The first-listed diagnosis is pneumonia, acute. Difficulty breathing and fever are commonly associated symptoms of pneumonia, so they would not be coded.

Scenario 2—A patient presents with difficulty breathing and fever. The physician orders a chest X-ray for "suspected pneumonia." The first-listed diagnosis would be difficulty breathing and the secondary diagnosis would be fever.

2. **Locate the main term in the alphabetic index, Volume II.** Identify the word(s) from the first-listed diagnosis to be looked up under the main term in the index (Figure 18-6 ◆). It may be the name of a *condition*, such as "Fracture"; a *disease*, such as "Pneumonia"; or *reason* for a visit, such as "Screening." The main term may also be located by *eponym* (a disease or condition named after an individual) such as "Colle's fracture"; an abbreviation or *acronym*, such as "AIDS"; a nontechnical *synonym* (a word similar in meaning) such as "broken" instead of fracture; and occasionally, an *adjective*, such as "twisted." Some main terms are rather generic with pages of subterms, such as "Disease," while others are quite specific with only a single code, such as "Duroziez's disease." It

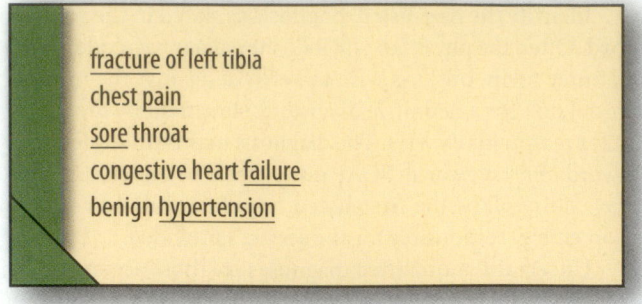

fracture of left tibia

chest pain

sore throat

congestive heart failure

benign hypertension

Figure 18-6 ◆ Examples of diagnostic statements with main term underlined.

is helpful to note that diagnoses usually cannot be located by looking up the anatomic site. The main term is always bold-faced with an initial capital letter. After locating the main term, the tentative code(s) will be verified in Volume I. Never code from the index. The steps for verifying codes will be described later.

Exercise
Getting Acquainted with the Alphabetical Index

Look at the first few pages of your *ICD-9-CM* Volume II index. Find examples of each the following types of main terms:

condition _____

disease _____

reason for visit _____

eponym _____

acronym _____

synonym _____

Sample Patient Scenario
Identifying the Main Term

Scenario 1—*Diagnosis*: Acute pneumonia. *Main term*: Pneumonia.

Scenario 2—*Diagnosis*: Difficulty breathing. Fever. Suspected pneumonia. *Main term*: Breathing, for the first-listed diagnosis. Fever would be the main term for a secondary diagnosis. "Suspected" pneumonia is a qualified or uncertain diagnosis and should not be coded.

3. **Review any modifiers, instructional notes, or subterms associated with the main term.** Subterms are indented two spaces under the boldfaced main term and further describe the condition, in terms of etiology, such as *Pneumonia, allergic;* coexisting conditions, such as *Pneumonia, with influenza;* anatomic site, such as *Pneumonia, interstitial;* episode, such as *Pneumonia, chronic* or similar descriptors. Subterms often have

additional layers of one or more of their own subterms, each of which are indented another two spaces.

Carry over lines are indented more than two spaces from the level of the preceding line. If the main term or subterm is too long to fit on one line, a carry over line is used. It is important to read carefully to distinguish between carry over lines and subterms.

Main terms may also have **nonessential modifiers**, words that appear in parentheses immediately after the main term. These words do not have to be present in the medical record in order to use the code, but if they are present, it confirms the user has located the appropriate code. For example, Pneumonia has many non-essential modifiers including *(acute), (Alpenstich), (benign),* and others.

Main terms or subterms may contain instructional notes, such as *see* or *see also,* which direct the user to other entries. For example, *Pneumonia, alveolar—see Pneumonia, other.* This instructs the user where to look for the code needed. Terms may also contain special formatting, such as slanted brackets, indicating that **multiple coding** may be required. For example, *Pneumonia, anthrax* is followed by the codes "022.0 *[484.5]* " The second code in slanted brackets is required in addition to the first code to completely describe the condition.

Exercise
Identifying Conventions in Volume II

Look up the main term Pneumonia in the alphabetical index and locate examples of the following:

nonessential modifier _____

subterms _____

subterms of a subterm _____

instructional note _____

multiple coding _____

The acronym NEC (not elsewhere classifiable) means that a more specific code is not available for a certain variation of a condition.

Sample Patient Scenario
Using Volume II Conventions

Scenario 1—*Main term*: Pneumonia. *Nonessential modifier*: (acute). *Subterm*: No further description is provided, so no subterms are required.

Scenario 2—*Main term*: Breathing. *Nonessential modifier*: None. *Subterm*: The word "difficulty" is not listed as a subterm, but the synonym "labored" appears and would be an appropriate choice.

4. **Identify the tentative code(s) associated with the most appropriate subterm(s).** When the appropriate subterms are

located, the tentative code(s) is printed immediately to the left. It is helpful to jot down the potential appropriate codes before verifying in the tabular list. Never use the index to make the final code selection.

Sample Patient Scenario
Selecting the Tentative Code(s)

Scenario 1—Pnemonia (acute) 486
Scenario 2—Breathing, labored 786.09

5. **Locate the tentative code(s) in the tabular list of Volume I.** Look for the tentative code number in the tabular list where codes are arranged in numerical order (Figure 18-7 ◆). Volume I is organized into seventeen **chapters** based on etiology or the body system. The chapter numbers do not correlate directly with the code numbers. Refer back to Table 18-2. Chapters are divided into **sections** with boldfaced or highlighted headings. Within the sections, the actual code numbers are tabulated in three levels: **category** (three-digit codes), **subcategeory** (four-digit codes), and **subclassification** (five-digit codes). It is helpful to learn the specific meanings of these designations, because the terms are used frequently in coding instructions.

6. **Interpret the Volume I conventions used with the category.** Before verifying and finalizing the code, the MA must first interpret the conventions presented with the code and its category. Volume I conventions include punctuation, instructional notes, and symbols and may appear on the same line with the code, above it, below it, or at the beginning of a subcategory, category, section, or chapter. Look carefully for any information that may be relevant to your tentative code selection, as the additional information may direct you when to use a different code or an additional code, depending on your original diagnostic statement.

In Volume I, the way in which punctuation is used has meaning (Figure 18-8 ◆). Medical assistants should become familiar with these meanings:

:   Colons are used after an incomplete phrase or term that requires one or more of the modifiers indented under it to make it assignable to a given category.
[ ] Square brackets are used to enclose synonyms, alternate wordings, or explanatory phrases.
( ) Parentheses are used to enclose optional or supplementary words that may be present or absent in a physician's statement of condition without affecting the code assignment.

Instructional notes are used to define terms, provide coding instructions, and provide fifth-digit information.

Use Additional Code or *Code Also* This instruction is placed in the tabular list in the categories where the coder may wish to add further information, by means of an additional code, to give a more complete picture of the diagnosis or procedure.

Code First Underlying Disease As Used for those codes not intended to be used as the first-listed diagnosis. These codes are for symptoms only (**manifestation**) and never for causes. The codes and their descriptions are in italic type, meaning that the code cannot be listed first, even if the diagnostic statement is written that way.

Includes Indicates separate terms, such as modifying adjectives, sites, conditions entered under a subdivision (such as a category), to further define or give examples of the content of the category.

Excludes Exclusion terms are enclosed in a box and are printed in italics to draw attention to their presence. The importance of this instructional term is its use as a guideline to direct the coder to the proper code assignment. In other words, all terms following the word Excludes: are to be coded elsewhere as indicated in each instance.

NOS (**not otherwise specified**) means unspecified. This acronym refers to a lack of sufficient detail in the diagnostic statement to be able to assign it to a more specific subdivision within the classification.

Level	Code	Description
Chapter	None	3. Endocrine, Nutritional and metabolic diseases, and immunity disorders (240–279)
Section	None	Diseases of other endocrine glands (250–259)
Category	250	Diabetes mellitus
Subcategory	250.0	Diabetes mellitus without mention of complication
Subclassification	250.00	Diabetes mellitus without mention of complication, type II, not stated as uncontrolled

Figure 18-7 ◆ Example of Volume I tabulation levels.

482.82 Escherichia coli [E. coli]
490 Bronchitis, not specific as acute or chronic
Bronchitis NOS:
    catarrhal
    with tracheitis NOS

Figure 18-8 ◆ Examples of punctuation conventions.

NEC (not elsewhere classified) is used to alert coders that some forms of the condition may be classified differently, but there is not a more specific code for their condition. In other words, the coder may have more specific information than what the codes provide for. An everyday example would be if a friend were to ask you, "What is your favorite color, red, yellow, blue, or other?" Perhaps your favorite color is purple, so you would respond "Other." You have a more specific response than what your friend provided. In coding, NOS and NEC should be used with caution, only as a last resort if no more appropriate code exists.

Symbols are used to alert the coder that something is different with the code.

▲ ►◄   upright or sideways triangles mean that there is a revision to the description of an existing code number

•   a round bullet means that the code number is new to this revision.

⬤   an octagon, or a number within a circle (❹ ❺), depending on the publisher, means that the code must be coded either to the fourth level or the fifth level of specificity.

✖   an "x" or ☐ empty box, depending on the publisher, indicates a nonspecific (NEC or NOS) code. These should be used only when absolutely necessary because doing so may delay payment on the claim.

Certain words also have special meaning in Volume I. For example, *and* is interpreted as *either/and/or* in a diagnostic code description; *with* is interpreted as *both, together with* in a diagnostic code description (Figure 18-9 ◆).

Sample Patient Scenario
Interpreting Volume I Conventions

Scenario 1—Tentative code 486 is designated as an "Unspecified Code." Review the documentation for any additional specific information. None appears. Because the index

directed us to this code for acute pneumonia, this choice is acceptable. Also note that the category contains an "excludes" statement that redirects the coder to more specific codes for specific types of pneumonia. None of these apply.

Scenario 2—Tentative code 786.09 is a subclassification. First locate the subcategory (786.0 Dyspnea and respiratory abnormalities) and category (786 Symptoms involving respiratory systems and other chest symptoms) headings for conventions. The only convention is a symbol indicating that five digits must be used. Going back to 786.09 we find some explanatory notes with synonyms and "excludes" notes. Read these. None apply to our patient. We also note that 786.09 is designated as an "Unspecified Code," but since we cannot code any more certainty based on the documentation, use of the code is acceptable.

7. **Select the code with the highest level of specificity.** There is no general rule regarding how many digits any given code will have. This is determined only after reading all the instructional notes and conventions available in the category. Assign a three-digit code if there are no four-digit codes in that category. Assign a four-digit code if there are no five-digit codes in the subcategory. Fourth- and fifth-digit codes may be found in one of several possible locations, depending on the number of options available. They may be located sequentially in the **tabular list**, at the beginning of the category, section, or chapter. Fifth digits may be found sequentially in the tabular list, or at the beginning of the subcategory, category, section, or chapter. Be certain to review these areas thoroughly to locate the correct fourth and fifth digits when required. It sometimes requires a little detective work and reviewing several pages of codes to locate the appropriate listing.

Sample Patient Scenario
Selecting the Code with the Highest Level of Specificity

Scenario 1—Pneumonia, organism unspecified, 486. This code matches the physician's diagnostic statement and there are no subcategories or subclassifications available. This is an example of a final code with only three digits.

Scenario 2—Dyspnea and respiratory abnormalities, other, 786.09. This is a five-digit subclassification so no additional digits are required. While there are other subclassifications in this category for more specific variations of the condition, none accurately describe this patient.

8. **Review the code for appropriate age, gender, and reimbursement edits.** The bottom of the page in the *ICD-9-CM* manual contains additional symbols that indicate codes that should be used only with specific age groups and genders, as well as those that may contain reimbursement alerts. The symbols used vary by publisher and are usually described in a key at the bottom of each page or two-page spread.

> 787.0 Nausia **and** vomiting → codes for both symptoms are included in this subcategory
>
> 787.01 Nausia **with** vomiting → patient with both symptoms
>
> 787.02 Nausea **alone** → patient presents with only nausea
>
> 787.03 Vomiting **alone** → patient presents with only vomiting

Figure 18-9 ◆ Example of usage of words "*and*" and "*with*."

Exercise
Identifying Volume I Conventions and Edits

The following is a sample entry from the *ICD-9-CM* manual. How many conventions and edits can you identify? Circle each one and write next to it the meaning of the punctuation, symbol, or instruction.

❹ **600 Hyperplasia of prostate**
  INCLUDES enlarged prostate
❺ **600.0 Hypertrophy (benign) of prostate**
  Benign prostatic hypertrophy
  Enlargement of prostate
  600.00 Hypertrophy (benign) of prostate without urinary obstruction and other lower urinary tract symptoms (LUTS) ♂ 𝔸
    Hypertrophy (benign) of prostate NOS
  600.01 Hypertrophy (benign) of prostate with urinary obstruction and other lower urinary tract symptoms (LUTS) ♂ 𝔸
    Hypertrophy (benign) of prostate with urinary retention
    Use additional code to identify symptoms:
    nocturia (788.43)
    straining on urination (888.65)
    urinary urgency (788.63)

♂ Male 𝔸 Adult (15+) years 𝕄 Maternity (12-55 yr) ℕ Newborn (0 yr)

Sample Patient Scenario
Reviewing the Code for Age, Gender, or Reimbursement Edits

Scenario 1—486 There are no age, gender, or reimbursement edits for this code.
Scenario 2—786.09 There no age, gender, or reimbursement edits for this code.

9. Verify the final code against the documentation. As a final check, with coding manual instructions fresh in your mind, refer back to the original documentation and verify that all conditions of the code agree with the medical record. If a discrepancy arises, work through the process again from the beginning.

Sample Patient Scenario
Verifying the Final Code Against Documentation

Scenario 1—Pneumonia, organism unspecified, 486. The final code matches the documentation.
Scenario 2—Dyspnea and respiratory abnormalities, other, 786.09
You would repeat this entire process to code for the other symptom, fever.

10. Assign the code. Write down the final code where indicated on your worksheet or documentation. Be certain to proofread the number as you wrote or keyboarded it to avoid transcription errors that are easy to make.

11. Repeat this process for any additional codes required by the medical record. Selecting a diagnosis code may seem like a long and tedious process at first. As medical assistants become familiar with the services and codes used by their medical office, coding becomes faster and easier, but accuracy and attention to detail is always paramount. Taking time and care to learn the fundamentals correctly will help create long-term success in the medical assistant's coding role.

— Critical Thinking Question 18-2 —
When Mary cannot decipher the physician's handwriting, what should she do?

HIPAA Compliance

Some physicians outsource their billing services. Because the information needed to process insurance claims is confidential, offices using outside billing services must sign a Business Associates Agreement which verifies that those services are **HIPAA** compliant and will keep patient information confidential.

Coding for Special Situations

As with any activity, there are always special situations that require additional information and knowledge. Diagnosis coding is the same. There are a number of conditions and circumstances that have unique tables, codes, and guidelines. An overview of these are provided in the remainder of the chapter.

Secondary Diagnoses

Patients may present with more than one complaint or condition that needs to be treated. Up to four diagnosis codes may be entered on the CMS-1500 form. As discussed earlier, the main reason for the visit is the first-listed diagnosis. Other conditions may be listed as secondary diagnoses, in the priority documented in the medical record. If two complaints are equal in

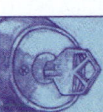

Keys to Success
MEDICAL BILLING SOFTWARE UPDATES

Medical billing software typically comes programmed with *ICD-9-CM* codes. To keep current and insert accurate diagnosis code information in insurance claims, it is crucial that such software be updated regularly. Claims with outdated or expired codes will likely experience delays or denials by insurance carriers.

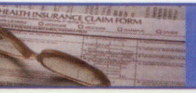

PROCEDURE 18-1 Perform Diagnostic Coding

Theory and Rationale

Proper diagnostic coding is key to proper reimbursement from insurance carriers. The medical assistant must know precisely where to look in the *ICD-9-CM* coding book in order to obtain proper codes, as well as which steps to take when unsure of the proper code.

Materials

- Patient's medical chart
- Current *ICD-9-CM* coding book
- Superbill with doctor's written diagnosis

Competency

(Conditions) With the necessary materials, you will be able to **(Task)** perform diagnostic coding **(Standards)** correctly within the time limit set by the instructor.

1. Locate the patient's diagnostic code(s) or description on the superbill or in the chart notes.
2. Verify that the diagnostic code(s) or description on the superbill also appear in the patient's chart in the form of a patient complaint (subjective finding) or a test finding (objective finding).
3. Using Volume II (the Alphabetic Index) of the *ICD-9-CM* coding book, find the diagnostic code(s).
4. Using Volume I (the Tabular Index), confirm that the written description matches the chart notes. If in doubt, check with the physician.
5. Read and defer to the conventions in the Tabular List.
6. Assign the code for each diagnosis, beginning with the appropriate first-listed diagnosis.

---

priority, either can be listed first. If signs and symptoms are common to the diagnosed condition, only the condition is coded, not the signs and symptoms.

EXAMPLE

The patient presents to the office with complaints of a sore throat. The physician finds upon examination that the patient has an abscess on his tonsil. In addition, the physician assigns diagnoses for this patient for ringing in the ears and sinus infection. The first-listed diagnosis is 475 peritonsillar abscess, followed by 388.31 subjective tinnitus, followed by 473.1 frontal sinusitis.

Combination Coding

Some conditions that frequently occur together may be described with a **combination code**. Careful reading of subterms in the index and category *includes* and *excludes* notes in the tabular list will guide the medical assistant as to when a combination code is available. Combination code descriptions frequently contain specific words that indicate more than one condition is covered, such as associated *with, due to, secondary to, without, with, complicated by, and following.* In Figure 18-9, code *787.1 Nausea with vomiting* is a combination code.

Multiple Coding

Multiple coding is when a condition requires two or more codes to fully describe it. In the index, multiple coding may be indicated by a second code in slanted brackets. In the tabular list, it is indicated by the instructional note *Code also (condition)* or *Code first (condition)* or *Use additional code.* Omission of the additional codes could result in denial or delay of payment.

In the earlier example of *600.01 Hypertrophy (benign) of prostate with urinary obstruction and other lower urinary tract*

symptoms (LUTS), there was an instructional note to *Use additional code to identify symptoms* followed by commonly paired conditions. This is an example of multiple coding.

Multiple codes are also used when an underlying condition (etiology) causes a second condition (manifestation.) For example, *Diabetes, type II, with renal manifestations* (250.40) requires a second code for the specific kidney disease, such as *Chronic kidney disease, stage III* (585.3).

Signs and Symptoms

When a definitive diagnosis is not yet available, the medical assistant may assign a sign or symptom diagnosis code. Assume, for example, the physician suspects pneumonia is the patient's diagnosis but will be unsure until an X-ray is taken and read. The medical assistant can assign diagnoses related to the patient's symptoms, such as wheezing, fever, cough, and shortness of breath. Signs, symptoms, and ill-defined conditions are found in the *ICD-9-CM* code book under codes 780.56 to 781.1.

EXAMPLE

780.6 fever, 786.07 wheezing, 786.2 cough, 785.05 shortness of breath.

Hypertension

Hypertension in medical terms refers to a condition of elevated blood pressure regardless of the cause. It has been called "the silent killer" because it usually does not cause symptoms for many years—often not until a vital organ has been damaged.

When blood pressure is checked, two values are recorded. The higher one occurs when the heart contracts (systole); the lower occurs when the heart relaxes between beats (diastole). Blood pressure is written as the systolic pressure followed by a

ICD-9-CM Index to Diseases Addenda (FY08) Effective October 1, 2007

Hypertension Table	Malignant	Benign	Unspecified
Hypertension, hypertensive (arterial) (arteriolar) (crisis) (degeneration) (disease) (essential) (fluctuating) (idiopathic) (intermittent) (labile) (low renin) (orthostatic) (paroxysmal) (primary) (systemic) (uncontrolled) (vascular)	401.0	401.1	401.9
cardiorenal (disease)	404.00	404.10	404.90
with			
heart failure	404.01	404.11	404.91
and chronic kidney disease	404.01	404.11	404.91
stage I through stage IV or unspecified	404.01	404.11	404.91
venous, chronic (asymptomatic) (idiopathic)	—	—	459.30

Figure 18-10 ◆ Conditions due to or associated with hypertension.

Source: International Classification of Diseases, Ninth Revision, Clinical Modification (2008). Reprinted from National Center for Health Statistics, http://www.cdc.gov/nchs/datawh/ftpserv/ftpicd9/ftpicd9.htm#guidlines.

slash and the diastolic pressure, for example, 120/80 mm Hg (millimeters of mercury). This reading would be referred to as "one twenty over eighty." Hypertension is defined in adults as 140 mm Hg systolic or 90 mm Hg diastolic on three separate readings recorded several weeks apart.

Figure 18-10 ◆ provides a complete listing of all conditions associated with hypertension. Four columns are shown:

- Condition (not titled as such in the excerpt)
- Malignant
- Benign
- Unspecified

The first column identifies the hypertensive condition, such as:

Accelerated
Cardiovascular disease
Renal involvement
Heart involvement

The last three columns identify the subcategories of the disease as malignant, benign, or unspecified. Do not select a code from the malignant or benign category unless the documentation indicates the specific type of hypertension. When the documentation does not indicate the type of hypertension, ask the physician to specify the type. If that alternative is not available, select "unspecified" (Vines, pp. 91–92).

EXAMPLE

Hypertension (arterial) (essential) (primary) (systemic) NOS to Category 401 with the appropriate fourth digit. Do not use either .0 (malignant) or .1 (benign) unless the medical record documentation supports it. Otherwise assign .9 (unspecified).*

*Vines, Deborah, Braceland, Ann, Rollins, Elizabeth, and Miller, Susan. *Comprehensive Health Insurance: Billing, Coding, and Reimbursement.* © 2008, p. 92. Reprinted by permission of Pearson Education. Upper Saddle River, NJ.

As with any other code, after the tentative code has been identified in the hypertension table, it should be verified in the tabular list.

Neoplasms

Neoplasm is the medical term for an abnormal growth of new tissue, often referred to as a tumor. Neoplasms can occur in any type of tissue anywhere in the body, and they can be either malignant or benign. Tumors that have cellular characteristics that cause it to invade adjacent healthy tissue or spread to distant sites are malignant, or life threatening. The spreading of malignant neoplasm is called metastasis. Tumors that do not have these characteristics are benign. The neoplasm table in Volume II provides the index to the behaviors and anatomic sites of neoplasms (Figure 18-11 ◆).

The neoplasm table lists the anatomical sites alphabetically. For each site there are six possible codes, depending on the type of neoplasm behavior. Malignant neoplasms will be identified as primary (site of origin), secondary (site of metastasis), or ca in situ (cells that have begun to change but have not yet invaded normal tissue). Malignant neoplasms are coded as primary unless the medical record indicates secondary (metastasis) or ca in situ (preinvasive carcinoma). Benign neoplasms will be stated as such in the medical record. "Uncertain behavior" refers to situations in which the pathologist clearly indicates that further study is needed before determining the benign or malignant behavior. "Unspecified" is used when the medical record does not contain adequate description of the neoplasm, such as a patient who has relocated and whose previous medical records are not yet available.

After determining the anatomic site and the type of behavior, select the code from the appropriate column, then verify it in the tabular list. For example, primary carcinoma of the anal canal, 154.2.

V codes

Not all patients who seek healthcare services have a specific disease or condition. They may receive services such as preventive

	Malignant					
	Primary	Secondary	Ca In situ	Benign	Uncertain Behavior	Unspecified
Neoplasm, neoplastic	199.1	199.1	234.9	229.9	238.9	239.9
abdomen, abdominal	195.2	198.89	234.8	229.8	238.8	239.8
cavity	195.2	198.89	234.8	229.8	238.8	239.8
organ	195.2	198.89	234.8	229.8	238.8	239.8
viscera	195.2	198.89	234.8	229.8	238.8	239.8
acoustic nerve	192.0	198.4	–	225.1	237.9	239.7
acromion (process)	170.4	198.5	–	213.4	238.0	239.2
adenoid (pharynx) (tissue)	147.1	198.89	230.0	210.7	235.1	239.0

Figure 18-11 ◆ Sample entries from neoplasm table.

care, therapy, followup, suture removal, or pregnancy supervision. They may have problems that require screening. They may carry certain risk factors or have a certain health status that may affect treatment and require coding. All of these are examples of situations that require V codes.

V codes can be used in many different ways. Depending on the encounter, the V code could be primary or supplemental. Usually, if the V code is primary, the reason for this encounter was not due to an injury or illness. That is, V codes are mainly used for encounters other than disease or injury such as annual checkups, physical exams, and immunizations. The V code would be the primary reason for the encounter since there is no chief complaint at these types of visits. These visits are also referred to as *well checkups*. There are three exceptions in which the V code is used as the primary code when there *is* a disease:

1. Chemotherapy
2. Radiation
3. Rehabilitation

EXAMPLE

HIV/AIDS—the code must distinguish between exposure and/or testing positive for the presence of the acquired immunodeficiency syndrome (AIDS) virus.

The question that must be asked is "Why is the patient here today?" Although the patient may have cancer for which he is receiving chemotherapy or radiation, the encounter today is not for the disease but for the treatment. In this case, the V code is primary and the disease is secondary.

V codes fall into one of three categories: problems, services, or factual.

1. **Problems**—V codes identify a problem that could affect a patient's overall health status but is not itself a current illness or injury. The V code in this example is supplemental.

EXAMPLE

Allergy to drug

2. **Services**—As mentioned, a V code can be used to describe circumstances other than an illness or injury that prompted the patient's visit. This is an exception to the rule for coding V codes. Although there is a disease, the V code is coded primary because it is the main reason for the encounter. The disease would be coded supplemental to the V code.

EXAMPLE

Chemotherapy
Radiation
Rehabilitation

3. **Factual**—V codes are used to describe certain facts that do not fall into the "problem" or "service" categories. For example, coding the type of birth, look under "Outcome of Delivery."

EXAMPLE

Single liveborn to indicate birth status.

V codes indicate a reason for an encounter—*they are not diagnosis codes.* A corresponding diagnosis code must accompany a V code to describe the reason the procedure was performed. Key words found in statements that may result in selection of a V code are shown in Figure 18-12 ◆.

EXAMPLE

A patient who has a family history of colon cancer presents with rectal bleeding (569.3).
   Alphabetic index: History (personal) of Family malignant neoplasm (of) colon
   Tabular List: V16.0
   Correct code: V16.0
   Correct code sequence: 569.3, V16.0

Admission for	Dialysis	Maladjustment
Aftercare (of)	Donor	Observation
Attention to	Examination	Problem (with)
Care (of)	Fitting of	Prophylactic
Carrier	Follow-up	Replacement (by) (of)
Checking/checkup	Health or healthy	Screening
Contact	History (of)	Transplant
Contraception	Maintenance	Vaccination
Counseling		

Figure 18-12 ◆ Key words in diagnostic statements that may result in selection of a V code.
Source: Vines, Deborah, Braceland, Ann, Rollins, Elizabeth, and Miller, Susan, *Comprehensive Health Insurance: Billing, Coding, and Reimbursements* © 2008 Pearson Education, Upper Saddle River, NJ. Reprinted with permission.

EXAMPLE

A patient presents to a healthcare facility for care after having unprotected sex with a partner who has tested positive for human immunodeficiency virus (HIV).

   Alphabetic index: Exposure to HIV
   Tabular list: V01.7, contact with or exposure to other viral diseases
   Correct code: V01.79*

V codes are indexed in the alphabetical index of Volume II. The V code tabular list appears in Volume I after category 999.

E codes

E codes are a supplementary classification that describes the external cause of illness or injury. They are never the first-listed diagnosis and are never used alone. They must be preceded by a diagnostic code from 001 to 999. For example, if a patient is being treated for a fractured ulna because he fell off a ladder, a code from category 813 would describe the fracture and E881.0 would describe the cause, fall from ladder.

In the event medical treatment is due to a drug overdose, whether accidental or due to attempted suicide, E codes are mandatory. Figure 18-13 ◆ lists other rules for E code use.

Some examples of when E codes would be used are as follows:

- A patient was involved in a motor vehicle accident.
- A patient was a pedestrian who was struck by a car while crossing the street.
- A patient fell off a ladder at home.
- A patient has accidentally ingested rat poison.
- A patient was injured as a result of a medical mistake, such as the physician operating on the wrong limb.
- A patient was bitten by a poisonous spider.
- A patient was knocked down at a sporting event.
- A patient was assaulted by another person.

*Source: Vines, Deborah, Braceland, Ann, Rollins, Elizabeth, and Miller, Susan. *Comprehensive Health Insurance: Billing, Coding, and Reimbursement.* © 2008, pp. 83–85.

E codes have a separate index in Volume II, which begins after the alphabetic index and after the table of drugs and chemicals. E codes also have a separate tabular list, which appears in Volume I after the V codes.

Poisonings and Adverse Effects

The Table of Drugs and Chemicals is a cross-tabulated index to poisoning and external causes of adverse effects of drugs and other chemical substances.

When coding for drugs or chemicals that have caused poisonings or **adverse reactions,** the medical assistant will need to determine the type of drug or chemical involved, if the event was accidental or purposeful, and whether the substance was prescribed by a health care provider. Table 18-3 outlines external causes, event descriptions, and ranges where codes can be found.

If the adverse reaction is due to therapeutic use of a drug, code the adverse reaction first, followed by the appropriate E code from the table. For example, rash due to adverse reaction to initial dose of penicillin, 693.0, E930.0. A poisoning code from column 1 is never used with a therapeutic use code from column 3.

Any situation other than therapeutic use will be coded with first, a poisoning code from column 1; second, a code for

Never use as primary diagnostic codes.

Use does affect reimbursement from insurance carriers.

Can hasten reimbursement by providing the insurance carrier information.

Child abuse codes have top priority.

After child abuse codes, cataclysmic events take priority.

After cataclysmic events and child abuse codes, transportation codes take priority.

Figure 18-13 ◆ Rules for E code use.

TABLE 18-3 DRUG AND CHEMICAL POISONING OR ADVERSE EFFECT CODE

External Cause	Code Description	Code Range
Poisoning	Assigned to a patient according to the classification of the drug or chemical in the poisoning	960–989
Accidental	Used for accidental overdose, wrong substance given or taken, drug taken accidentally, or accidental use of a drug or chemical during a medical procedure	E850–E869
Therapeutic use	Used for the external effect caused by a correct substance properly administered that caused an adverse or allergic reaction	E930–E952
Suicide attempt	Used to report attempted suicide via drugs or chemicals	E950–E952
Assault	Used to report a poisoning that was inflicted on another person with the intent to harm or kill	E961–E962
Unknown	Used when the medical record is unclear whether the poisoning was intentional or accidental	E980–E982

the adverse effect from 000 to 999; third, an E-code for the intent, from the columns *accident, suicide attempt, assault,* or *undetermined.* If more than one adverse effect is present, multiple codes may be used.

Coding for Fractures

When coding fractures, the medical assistant will need to know the type of fracture and whether that fracture is open or closed. The *ICD-9-CM* coding book contains codes to indicate fractures in the following categories:

- *Spiral*—Typically occurs due to twisting.
- *Fissure or hairline*—Usually imposes minimal trauma to the bone and tissues.
- *Comminuted*—Has more than two fragments of bone that have been broken off, are unstable, and include tissue damage.
- *Linear*—Runs the length of the bone.
- *Closed*—Keeps the skin intact.
- *Double*—Refers to multiple fractures of the same bone.
- *Simple*—Does not break the skin and has little tissue damage.
- *Greenstick*—Is bend-like fracture in which the bone is not broken through; mostly found in children.
- *Infected*—Is in an infected area.
- *Compound/Open*—Breaks the skin.
- *Depressed*—Is a skull fracture with the bone broken inward.
- *Oblique*—Presents as an oblique break in the bone; very rare.
- *Pathological*—Caused by disease.
- *Impact/Compression*—Refers to a situation in which the vertebral (spinal) column is compressed and then breaks under the pressure.
- *Complex*—Severely damages the tissue around the fracture site.
- *Stress*—Caused by repeated stress to the bone.
- *Impacted*—Diagnosed when bones are broken and the ends smash together.
- *Fragmented*—Occurs when trauma breaks many bones inside the patient.

Coding for fractures requires specific identification of the exact bone fractured and often, the location of the fracture on the bone. For example, Closed fracture of the humerus, upper end,

surgical neck 812.01. Fifth digits are required on most fracture codes and are often located at the beginning of the category or section rather than in the sequential tabular listing. Fractures of the skull, neck, and trunk include combination codes for associated conditions. For example, Fracture of base of the skull, closed with subarachnoid, subdural, and extradural hemorrhage, with moderate loss of consciousness 801.23. In this code, 801 category describes Fracture of base of skull. The fourth digit .2 describes closed with subarachnoid, subdural, and extradural hemorrhage. The fifth digit subclassfication 3, which appears at the beginning of the section Fracture of the skull (800-804), describes moderate [1–24 hours] loss of consciousness.

Coding Burns

When coding for burns (codes 940-948), the medical assistant must know the depth and extent of the burn, as well as the burn-causing agent. Burns are classified by depth as first degree (redness of the skin), second degree (blistering of the skin), and third degree (full thickness of skin involved). To code burns, first code the site(s) and degree of the burn, with the most severe first; second, code the percentage of total body surface area (TBSA) with third degree burns, based on the rule of nines; third, if the burn is infected, use code 958.3; finally, use an E code to describe the cause of the burn. With multiple burns, the first code should indicate the highest burn degree. If a patient has a first, second, or third degree burn in the same body area, the highest degree code is given to that burn. In other words, if a patient sees the physician for first and second degree burns of the right hand, the medical assistant will only code for the second degree burn since it is the highest degree of burn. If that same patient also has a first degree burn on the lower leg, the medical assistant would code for the second degree burn of the right hand and the first degree burn of the lower leg.

Using the Rule of Nines in Coding Burns

The medical assistant should assign codes from category 948 when coding burns according to the extent of the total body surface area (**TBSA**) involved, or when the site of the burn is not specified. Category 948 codes are based on the "rule of nines" in estimating the body surfaces involved. The head and neck are assigned 9%, each arm is assigned 9%, each leg is assigned 18%, the anterior and posterior trunk are each assigned 18%, and the genitalia are assigned 1%. Physicians may change these percentages when treating infants or children in order to accurately describe the amount of skin that has been burned, or when treating larger adults who may have more body surface area (Figure 18-14 ◆).

For example, assume a patient suffered third degree burns to the back and back of left arm, and second degree burns to the back of the right arm when she fell into a campfire. The third degree burn of back is coded as 942, burn of trunk, plus fourth digit .3 for third degree and fifth digit 4 for back, creating the code 942.34; third degree burn of left back upper arm and forearm is 943 upper extremities, fourth digit .3 for third degree, fifth digit 9 for multiple sites (upper arm and forearm), arriving at the code 943.39; the second degree burn of right back upper arm and forearm is similar, but uses a fourth digit of .2 for second degree burn, for a code of 943.29. To code for TBSA, first add up the percentage of each body area: 18% for the back and 9% for each arm totaling 36%. This gives a subcategory code of 948.3. The fifth digit describes the TBSA with third degree burns, which is 27% for the back and back of left arm, for a final code 948.32. To code for the cause of the burn, use E897, accident caused by controlled fire not in building or structure, including bonfire. Total coding for this patient is 942.34, 943.39, 943.29, 948.32, E897.

Late Effects

Late effects are conditions that arise from acute illnesses, old injuries, or previous conditions that have been resolved. There is no specific guideline for how much time must pass between the original event and its manifestation or **sequela** for it to be classified as a late effect. It is largely dependent on the physician's judgment, which should be documented in the medical record.

Key words that indicate a late effect include *due to (an old injury), late, following (previous condition)*. For example, a

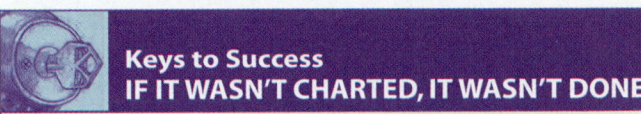

Keys to Success
IF IT WASN'T CHARTED, IT WASN'T DONE

The saying in the medical office, "If it wasn't charted, it wasn't done," holds true for coding. A provider can only charge for items noted in patients' charts.

malunion due to a previous fracture, hemiplegia following a stroke, or scarring due to a burn. First code the current condition or sequelae; second, assign a late effect code from categories 905 through 909; third, assign a late effects E code from category E929 late effects of accidental injury, if applicable. For example, Malunion of fracture of the humerus, 733.11, Late effect of fracture of upper extremities, 905.2.

Obstetrics

Obstetric coding is one of the more complex areas of coding because multiple codes are required for anything other than a normal delivery of a single liveborn infant. All visits for supervision of a pregnancy require a V code from the category V22 for a normal pregnancy or V23 for a high-risk pregnancy. These codes can be located in the index under *Pregnancy, supervision.* Carefully review the subcategories to ensure correct code selection. Complications of pregnancy are located in the index under *Pregnancy, complicated by* or *Pregnancy, management affected by.* Chapter 11 of the tabular list (630-677) contains the codes for complications of pregnancy, childbirth and the puerperium (six weeks after delivery). These codes are used only on the record of the mother. Most complications of pregnancy

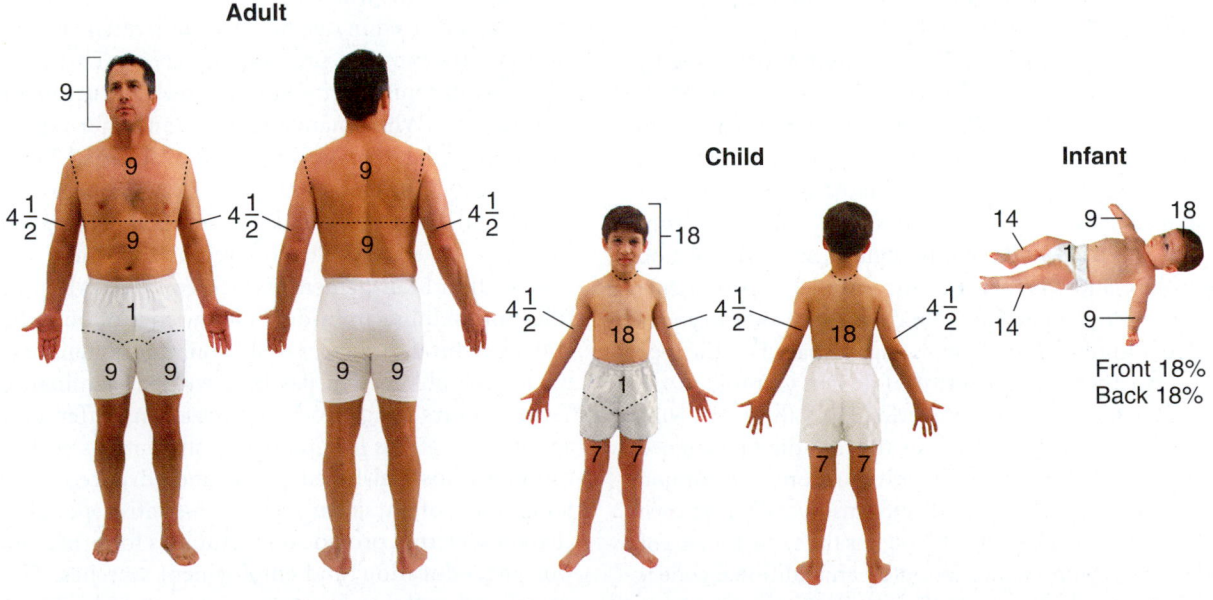

Note: Each arm totals 9% (front of arm $4\frac{1}{2}$ %, back of arm $4\frac{1}{2}$ %)

Figure 18-14 ◆ Rule of nines.

have a unique code from Chapter 11 that is to be used in place of, or in addition to, a code for the same condition in a non-pregnant person. For example, when pregnancy causes diabetes, called gestational diabetes, a code from the subcategory 648.8 is used, rather than a code from the diabetes category, 250. When a woman with pre-existing type I or type II diabetes becomes pregnant, a code from the subcategory 648.0 is used in addition to a secondary code from the category 250. For example, DM complicating pregnancy, 648.03, 250.00.

The birth itself will include codes for the delivery, any complications, and the outcome of delivery. A normal delivery is defined as a vaginal delivery needing minimal or no assistance, resulting in a single liveborn infant. In addition, the code V27.0 is required to indicate the outcome of delivery.

Multiple births, caesarean sections, and complicated deliveries require multiple codes that describe all the circumstances. In addition, codes from the range V27.1 to V27.9 are used to indicate the number of liveborn infants and stillborn fetuses. For example, delivery of twins by vaginal delivery with no antepartum or postpartum complication, both liveborn, 651.01, V27.2.

A separate medical record is opened for all liveborn infants. The record will have a code from the range V30-V39 that describes the location of birth and the existence of multiple liveborn or stillborn mates. Any other medical conditions of the infant are separately coded. For example, Twin, mate liveborn, V31.

Diabetes

Not only is diabetes mellitus (**DM**) a common condition, it causes and impacts many other conditions, so medical assistants will frequently encounter the need to code for it. Category 250 Diabetes Mellitus is the category used. It excludes gestational diabetes, neonatal DM, nonclinical diabetes, and hyperglycemia that has not been diagnosed as DM.

DM is always coded to the fifth digit and frequently involves combination coding as well as multiple coding. Medical assistants need to thoroughly review the medical record to abstract certain facts about patients' DM: whether it is type I, type II, or unspecified; whether it is stated as being uncontrolled; what complications exist. If no complications exist, subcategory 250.0 is used, and the fifth digit is assigned based on the type of DM and whether it is uncontrolled or not. Acute manifestations or complications are coded with subcategories 250.1 to 250.3, and the fifth digit is assigned based on the type of DM and whether it is uncontrolled or not. Chronic manifestations are coded with subcategories 250.4 through 250.9, based on body system affected. Again, the fifth digit is assigned based on the type of DM and whether it is uncontrolled or not. If more than one body system is affected, use a code from each body system, and be certain the fifth digit is the same for all. For each body system with manifestation(s), an additional code is required to specify the nature of the manifestation. The most common manifestations are listed in the instructional notes within each subcategory. Verify the manifestation code where it originally appears within the tabular list. If a type II diabetic

requires long-term insulin use, assign the additional code V58.67 to report this information.

For example, type II DM, with long-term insulin use and associated glaucoma. The first code is 250.50 for DM. The fourth digit ".5" indicates ophthalmic manifestations. The fifth digit "0" indicates type II, not stated as uncontrolled. The second code is 365.44 for Glaucoma associated with systemic disorders. Note that this is a different code in the tabular list category, 365 Glaucoma, than if the glaucoma had developed independent of DM. Finally, assign V58.67 to report long-term insulin use by a type II diabetic. The complete coding would be 250.50, 365.44, V58.67.

Inpatient Services

When coding for services provided by the physician in the inpatient setting, a few guidelines are different. The patient will be assigned an admitting diagnosis code, which describes the reason for the admission. After all tests and studies are completed and results reported, a **principal diagnosis** is assigned based on these results. The principal diagnosis must be assigned prior to final billing. Uncertain conditions, which are not coded in the outpatient setting, are coded "as though they exist" in the inpatient setting. Patients may have multiple diagnoses for co-existing conditions, so physicians should report only the diagnoses that pertain to their services. For example, if a patient has a fractured leg and is also diabetic, the orthopedic surgeon would report the fracture as the diagnosis while the endocrinologist would report the DM.

Pursuing Professional Certification

Medical assistants who enjoy the problem-solving and detective work involved in diagnostic coding often choose to pursue certification as a professional coder. This career path allows them to use their clinical knowledge to enhance their coding skills. While many organizations offer certifications, the most widely recognized are the Certified Professional Coder (**CPC**), offered by the American Academy of Professional Coders (**AAPC**), and the Certified Coding Specialist-Physician based (**CCS-P**), offered by the American Health Information Management Association (**AHIMA**). Both certifications require an in-depth knowledge of both diagnostic and procedural coding, as well as reimbursement basics. Certification is obtained by passing a written examination that is several hours long. Both organizations offer entry level apprentice options for graduating students, as well as certification for hospital-based coders and advanced certification for a variety of physician and administrative specialties. Local chapter meetings provide opportunities for professional networking, education, and employment searches. Their websites, listed at the end of the chapter, provide more detailed information and requirements.

Whether medical assistants decide to become certified professional coders or remain in a largely clinical role, diagnostic coding skills are important to their career. Some medical assistants may perform hands-on coding, while others review encounter forms or serve as an interpreter or communication link for other coders. Understanding how to abstract diagnostic information from the medical record and accurately translate it into codes that justify reimbursement will enable medical assistants to play a vital role in supporting both patients and their medical office.

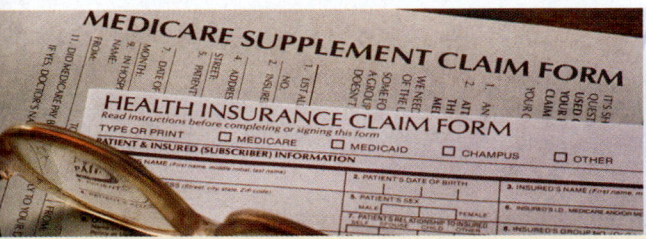
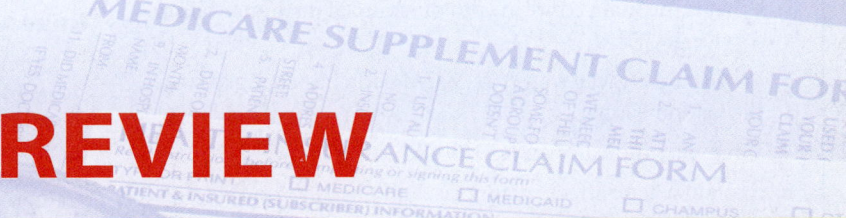

REVIEW

Chapter Summary

- The medical assistant's role in diagnostic coding must be done with the utmost attention to detail. The physician is responsible for assigning diagnoses to patients; however, the MA is responsible for applying the correct code to match the diagnosis the physician provides.

- Proper coding and health insurance reimbursement are tightly linked. If coded incorrectly, procedures may not be reimbursed at the proper level.

- Diagnostic coding has existed for more than a century. French physician Jacques Bertillon composed the Bertillon Classification of Causes of Death in 1893, which the American Public Health Association (APHA) adopted in 1898. In 1901, the APHA published a coding book called the *International Classification of Diseases (ICD), Volume I,* which was used until 1910, when the second volume was published. Volume updates continued to be published every ten years until the *ICD-9-CM* was published in 1979.

- *ICD-10* was completed in 1999 and has replaced *ICD-9-CM* in all major countries except the United States.

- Proper prioritization of diagnosis codes helps ensure both proper documentation and appropriate insurance reimbursement.

- To choose diagnosis codes correctly, medical assistants must follow a number of predefined steps.

- Coding for various special situations must be done accurately in order to properly describe the patients' condition to the insurance carrier.

- Medical assistants may choose to pursue certification as a professional coder. The most widely recognized organizations that offer certifications are the Certified Professional Coder (CPC) offered by the American Academy of Professional Coders (AAPC) and the Certified Coding Specialist-Physician based (CCS-P) offered by the American Health Information Management Association (AHIMA).

Chapter Review

Multiple Choice

1. To locate the proper diagnosis code, which volume of the *ICD-9-CM* coding book should be consulted first?
   a. I
   b. II
   c. III
   d. None of the above

2. The *ICD-9-CM* coding book has how many volumes?
   a. 1
   b. 2
   c. 3
   d. 4

3. *ICD-9-CM* codes are how many digits?
   a. 3
   b. 4
   c. 5
   d. All of the above

4. Which of the following volumes is the alphabetic index of the *ICD-9-CM* coding book?
   a. I
   b. II
   c. III
   d. None of the above

True/False

T F 1. Volume I is only used for hospital codes.

T F 2. Volume I indicates the number of digits required for coding.

T F 3. V codes indicate the reason for care, other than present illness.

T F 4. V codes cover HIV testing.

T F 5. E codes greatly affect reimbursement by insurance carriers.

T F 6. Diagnosis codes describe the need for medical care.

T F 7. Each visit a patient has with a healthcare provider can only have one diagnosis code.

Chapter Review (continued)

Short Answer

1. How do you determine the first-listed diagnosis given to a patient?

2. What is the main concern with outsourced insurance billing services?

3. What clue indicates an *ICD-9-CM* code has changed since the last revision?

4. What clue indicates an *ICD-9-CM* code is new?

5. Explain a "late effect" diagnosis, and give an example.

6. Why would a physician code a condition as suspected?

7. What does the saying, "If it wasn't charted, it wasn't done," mean?

8. When is the *ICD-10* coding book expected to be used in ambulatory care?

9. What is meant by the etiology of a disease?

Research

1. Interview a person who works in the billing office of a local medical office. How does that office handle the process of coding? Do the physicians assign the codes? What is the role of medical assistants in coding?

2. Look at the Medicare Web site. What are some of the rules Medicare applies regarding the use of diagnostic codes?

3. Look at your state's Medicaid Web site. What are some of the rules Medicaid applies regarding the use of diagnostic codes?

Externship Application Experience

Mabel Donchez, a patient of Dr. Bridges, is being seen today for an accidental overdose of a prescription medication Dr. Bridges prescribed. What part of the *ICD-9-CM* coding book would hold the proper code for this diagnosis?

Resource Guide

American Academy of Professional Coders
2480 South 3850 West, Suite B
Salt Lake City, UT 84120
Toll Free Phone: (800) 626-CODE (2633)
Phone: (801) 236-2200
Fax: (801) 236-2258
Email: info@aapc.com
www.aapc.com

American Health Information Management Association
233 N. Michigan Avenue, 21st Floor
Chicago, IL 60601-5800
Toll Free Phone: (800) 335-5535
Phone: (312) 233-1100
Fax: (312) 233-1090
Email: info@ahima.org
www.ahima.org

American Medical Association
515 N State Street
Chicago, IL 60610
Phone: (800) 621-8335
www.ama-assn.org/

Centers for Disease Control and Prevention
1600 Clifton Road
Atlanta, GA 30333
Phone: (800) 311-3435
www.cdc.gov

Flash Code (provides information on proper ICD-9-CM coding)
Phone: (800) 711-7873
www.icd9coding1.com

Ingenix
12125 Technology Drive
Eden Prairie, MN 55344
Phone: (888) 445-8745
Fax: (952) 833-7079
www.ingenix.com/

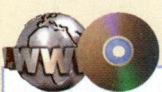 Med**Media**

http://www.MyMAKit.com

More on this chapter, including interactive resources, can be found on the Student CD-ROM accompanying this textbook and on http://www.MyMAKit.com.

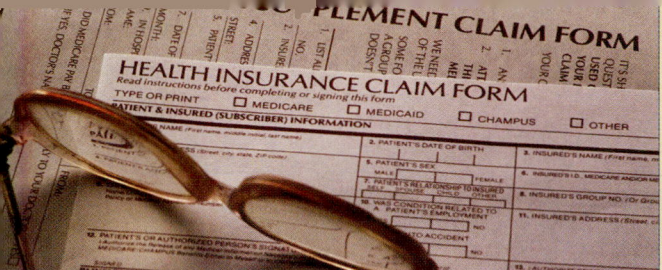

Objectives

After completing this chapter you should be able to:

- Define and spell the key terminology in this chapter.
- Define the medical assistant's role in procedural coding.
- Understand the history of procedural coding.
- Describe the purpose of the CPT-4® book.
- Identify fraudulent practices in coding and billing.
- Describe the layout of the CPT-4 book.
- List the steps to accurate CPT coding, including determining correct codes via chart notes.
- Discuss how modifiers are used in procedural coding.
- Describe how to code for evaluation and management services.
- Explain the use of the Health Care Common Procedure Coding System (HCPCS) and coding guides for specialized medical practices.
- Explain the relationship between accurate documentation and reimbursement.

Procedural Coding

Case Study

At Monday morning's staff meeting, Dr. Anderson mentions she is unhappy with the amount she is being reimbursed for her Medicare patients' office visits. To boost reimbursement, Dr. Anderson asks her medical assistant, Lydia, to use higher codes for those patients.

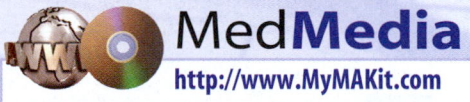

MedMedia
http://www.MyMAKit.com

Additional interactive resources and activities for this chapter can be found on http://www.MyMAKit.com. For a video, tips, audio glossary, legal and ethical scenarios, on-the-job scenarios, quizzes, and games related to the content of this chapter, please access the accompanying CD-ROM in this book.

Video: *Insurance Coding*
Legal and Ethical Scenario: *Procedural Coding*
On the Job Scenario: *Procedural Coding*
Tips
Multiple Choice Quiz
Audio Glossary
HIPAA Quiz
Games: Spelling Bee, Crossword, and Strikeout

Key Terminology

abuse—improper behavior and billing practices that result in financial gain but are not fraudulent

add-on code—a CPT code designated by the plus sign (+) that cannot be used alone; must be used together with another CPT code

alphabetical index—alphabetical listing of CPT codes by procedure name, condition, eponym, and acronym

audit—a review process that verifies that every detail of a CPT code is clearly documented in the medical record

bilateral—on both sides of the body

bundling—combining multiple services under a single, all-inclusive CPT code and one charge

category—a division of a subheading within the tabular index

Category I codes—CPT codes numbered 00100 to 99999 representing widely used services and procedures approved by the FDA

Category II codes—supplemental tracking codes that can be used for performance measurement; four numbers followed by the letter F, such as 1002F.

Category III codes—temporary codes for data collection and tracking the use of emerging technology, services, and procedures; four numbers followed by the letter T, such as 0162T.

common descriptor—the portion of a standalone code before the semicolon that is shared with the indented codes that follow

contributing factors—three secondary criteria, in addition to the key components, that may influence the selection of an E&M code; includes presenting problem, counseling/coordination of care, and physicians' face to face time with patients and families

coordination of care—a contributory factor in E&M coding that describes physicians' work in arranging care with other providers

counseling—a contributory factor in E&M coding that describes physicians' discussion with patients and family members regarding diagnosis, treatment options, instructions and followup

CPT-4 manual—procedural coding book used in all U.S. healthcare settings

downcode—to assign a code for a lower level of service than was

---

 MEDICAL ASSISTING STANDARDS

CAAHEP ENTRY-LEVEL STANDARDS	ABHES ENTRY-LEVEL COMPETENCIES
■ Perform within scope of practice (psychomotor) ■ Apply ethical behaviors, including honesty/integrity in performance of medical assisting practice (affective) ■ Explore issue of confidentiality as it applies to the medical assistant (cognitive) ■ Respond to issues of confidentiality (psychomotor) ■ Apply local, state, and federal health care legislation and regulation appropriate to the medical assisting practice setting (psychomotor) ■ Recognize the importance of local, state, and federal legislation and regulations in the practice setting (affective) ■ Document accurately in the patient record (psychomotor) ■ Describe procedures for implementing both managed care and insurance plans (cognitive) ■ Use office hardware and software to maintain office systems (psychomotor) ■ Work with physician to achieve the maximum reimbursement (affective) ■ Apply both managed care policies and procedures (psychomotor) ■ Apply third party guidelines (psychomotor) ■ Describe how to use the most current procedural coding system (cognitive) ■ Define upcoding and why it should be avoided (cognitive) ■ Describe how to use the most current HCPCS coding (cognitive)	■ Conduct work within scope of education, training, and ability ■ Monitor legislation related to current healthcare issues and practices ■ Apply managed care policies and procedures ■ Obtain managed care referrals and precertification ■ Receive, organize, prioritize, and transmit information expediently ■ Analyze and use current third-party guidelines for reimbursement ■ Use physician fee schedule ■ Implement current procedural terminology and ICD-9 coding

---

 COMPETENCY SKILLS PERFORMANCE

1. Code for a procedure.

Introduction

Procedural coding is the act of assigning a code to a patient's procedure or service. Since 1966, procedure codes have been **standardized**, which has rendered coding both more efficient and more accurate. Accuracy in procedural coding is essential, because incorrect or inadequate coding may lead to denial or delay of insurance claims.

Key Terminology *(continued)*

actually performed; done by some insurance companies to save money; done by some physicians to avoid fraud or abuse charges

established patient—patients who have seen the same provider, or another provider of the same specialty in the same practice, within the past three years

Evaluation and Management (E&M)—CPT codes used for billing physician services to evaluate and manage patient care, such as office visits

examination—a key component of E&M coding that describes the complexity of the physical assessment of the patient

face-to-face time—a contributory factor in E&M coding that measures the amount of time the provider spent in the presence of the patient and/or family, as opposed to time spent documenting the visit or arranging referrals

fraud—to intentionally bill for services that were never given, including billing for a service that has a higher reimbursement than the service produced

global period—refers to the number of days surrounding a surgical procedure during which all services relating to that procedure—preoperative, during the surgery, and postoperative—are considered part of the surgical package

global surgical concept—see *global period*

guidelines—specific instructions at the beginning of each section of the CPT manual that define terms and describe specific information about how to use codes in that section

Health Care Common Procedure Coding System (HCPCS)—process for coding procedures and services

history—a key component of E&M coding that describes the background, onset, and progression of the patient's current condition

indented code—a CPT code whose description is indented three spaces under another (standalone) code and whose definition includes the portion before the semicolon (;) in the standalone code; done to save space in the CPT manual

inpatient—patient who has been formally admitted to a facility with written admission orders from a physician

instructional notes—directions in the tabular index, which appear in parentheses before or after a code entry, to point the user to alternative codes for closely related procedures or to codes that must or must not be used together

key components—three primary determining criteria in selecting an E&M code; include history, examination, and medical decision making

Level I codes—same as CPT

Level II codes—HCPCS alphanumeric codes created by CMS to bill supplies, drugs, and certain services

Level III HCPCS codes—HCPCS alphanumeric codes created by regional Medicare carriers; being phased out under HIPAA

main term—words by which procedures and services are alphabetized in the CPT index; may be a procedure, service, anatomic site, condition, synonym, eponym, or abbreviation

medical decision making (MDM)—a key component of E&M coding that describes the complexity establishing a diagnosis and/or selecting a management option

modifier—two-digit alphanumeric codes appended to CPT or Level II codes to further describe circumstances

modifying term—descriptive words in the alphabetic index that appear indented under the main term to further describe the service or procedure

new patient—patients who have not seen the same provider, or another provider of the same specialty in the same practice, for more than three years

observation status—a designated type of care in which a patient is hospitalized for monitoring, but not formally admitted

outpatient—patient who has not been formally admitted to a facility, such as office visits, emergency department, and observation status

parent code—see standalone code

patient status—classification of patients as new or established

physical status modifier—two-digit alphanumeric codes (P1 to P6) appended to anesthesia codes that indicate the health status of the patient at the beginning of the procedure

postoperative period—the number of days following a procedure during which follow-up visits are bundled with the primary procedure and are not billed separately

presenting problem—a contributory factor in E&M coding that consists of a disease, condition, illness, injury, symptom, sign, finding complaint, or other reason for the encounter, as stated by the patient

procedural coding—process of assigning codes to healthcare services and procedures

procedures—services healthcare providers perform on patients

relative value unit (RVU)—unit of measure assigned to medical services based on the resources required to provide it; includes work, practice expense, and liability insurance

section—one of six major divisions of the CPT manual: evaluation and management; anesthesia; surgery; radiology; pathology and laboratory; medicine

semicolon (;)—a punctuation mark in a standalone code; the part of the definition before the semi-colon is used by the indented codes that follow

special instructions—directions within each section describing specific rules and definitions for use of codes within a particular category or subcategory

standalone code—a CPT code that contains a full description and is not dependent on another code for complete meaning

standardized—uniform practice

subcategory—a division of a category within the tabular index

subheading—a division of a subsection within the tabular index

subsection—subdivisions within a CPT section of the tabular index

tabular index—the numerical listing of all CPT codes, accompanied by guidelines and notes

unbundling—billing multiple services with separate CPT codes and separate charges that should be combined under a single CPT code and one charge

upcode—to code and bill for a higher level of service than was actually provided

usual, customary, and reasonable (UCR)—reimbursement method in which insurance companies compare provider's charges against their normal charge, other providers' charges, and unusual circumstances

Abbreviations

AMA—American Medical Association

ASA—American Society of Anesthesiologists

B*T*M—Basic unit, Time, Modifying circumstances; formula for anesthesia reimbursement

CMS—Centers for Medicare and Medicaid Services

CPT—Current Procedural Terminology

DME—durable medical equipment

E/EX—examination (component of E&M codes)

E&M—evaluation and management

FDA—Food and Drug Administration

H—history (component of E&M codes)

HCPCS—Health Care Common Procedure Coding System

MDM—medical decision making (component of E&M codes)

POS—place of service

RVU—relative value unit

UCR—usual, customary, and reasonable

The Medical Assistant's Role in Procedural Coding

Medical assistants are responsible for finding the proper procedure code that correlates with the procedure performed by the provider as documented in the medical record. If the provider has not provided enough information to determine the proper code, the MA may need to consult the physician to ascertain more precisely what was done. The physician should amend the documentation to clarify the details before a code is assigned. The medical assistant may also be responsible for communicating with insurance companies regarding why a certain code was assigned to a patient.

The History of Procedural Coding

Before the mid-1960s, healthcare providers used the **usual, customary, and reasonable (UCR)** system to determine fair charges for their services. The UCR system was designed by insurance carriers to determine what the usual, customary, and reasonable fee was for providers of healthcare services. In other words, insurance companies would look at billing records to see what providers in a certain geographic area charged for any given procedure code. The average of those charges was taken and then called the usual, customary, and reasonable charge for that service in that geographic area by that type of provider. Insurance companies would reimburse charges based on what they believed to be usual, customary, and reasonable. Most patients paid for their services, and when they had health insurance, they submitted their own reimbursement claims. There were no standard medical billing forms or procedure codes.

To standardize medical fees and increase the accuracy of the coding process, in 1992 the U.S. Congress developed a system that assigned a **relative value unit (RVU)** to every healthcare procedure or treatment. ∞ Chapter 17 details how RVUs are used to determine fee schedules.

Coding with the CPT-4 Manual

Today, the CPT-4 manual covers all procedures approved by the Federal Drug Administration (**FDA**). When it was first published in 1966, however, the book focused mainly on surgical procedures. Some codes covered radiology, laboratory, and pathology services. Although the book is updated annually, the last major revision, the fourth, occurred in 1977.

In an effort to establish industry standards, in the 1980s the U.S. Congress began requiring providers to use CPT codes for all services Medicare patients receive. The codes, which are five digits long, must now appear on the CMS-1500 insurance claim form. ∞ Chapter 17 explains how to complete the CMS-1500 insurance claim form.

Procedures and services performed by physicians are reported using codes from the *Current Procedural Terminology, Fourth Edition,* which is published by the American Medical Association (**AMA**). The purpose of CPT® is to provide uniform language that will accurately describe medical, surgical, and diagnostic services so that those involved with health management and reimbursement will have an effective means of communication.

CPT is a registered trademark of the American Medical Association.

As with diagnostic coding, the challenge is to find the most appropriate and accurate code. Patient encounters for what is commonly referred to as an "office visit," for example, may be reported with any of thirty-plus codes, depending on a number of circumstances surrounding the visit, but only one of these code choices is correct in any given situation. Likewise, more than fifty codes exist for a patient who receives sutures for a wound, depending on location, length and depth of the wound. Medical assistants need to be familiar with all the criteria for coding services offered by their office to be certain they select the most accurate code.

Fraud and Abuse

When uncertain of the best code, it may be tempting to **upcode**, that is to code for a higher level of service than what was actually provided in order to gain higher reimbursement, or **downcode**, to code for a lower level of service than what was actually provided in order to avoid potential **fraud** or **abuse**. Fraud is intentionally billing for services that were never given, which includes upcoding. Abuse is improper behavior and billing practices that result in financial gain but are not fraudulent. As in all areas of healthcare, "ignorance is no excuse." When medical assistants are unsure regarding a coding issue, they may consult with the physician, a colleague, or a professional organization.

Coding fraud in healthcare is a serious offense. It includes falsifying medical records, billing for services not performed, and intentionally charging incorrect patients. Coding fraud is not worth the risk. Providers caught intentionally submitting fraudulent claims may be arrested and charged with crimes. These providers risk the loss of their licenses, practices, and preferred provider status, as well as their reputations.

Some offices feel upcoding, using inappropriately high codes to boost reimbursement amounts, is justified given rising health care costs. Insurance carriers have actively been seeking out such fraudulent providers, however, and imposing stiff penalties such as deterrents. For providers like these, insurance companies often seek maximum penalties, even jail time.

Unlike upcoding, some coding practices are perfectly legitimate, but providers must be careful to make the distinction. For example, some laboratory codes, like lipid or electrolyte panels, are placed together or bundled because they are commonly ordered together. When physicians order only some tests in a panel, those tests should be billed individually. When doctors order entire panels, however, they cannot bill tests separately.

To do so would be to **unbundle** the codes, and that is insurance fraud.

Critical Thinking Question 19-1

How would Lydia describe upcoding to Dr. Anderson?

The CPT lists over 8,800 procedural codes. They are updated every year and take effect January 1. Medical assistants should use the edition of the CPT that was in effect on the date of service. For example, patients seen on December 31, 2009, would be coded using the 2009 coding manual while those seen on January 1, 2010 would be coded using the 2010 coding manual. The transition date for diagnosis coding differs from the one used for procedural coding, which is October 1. This is addressed in ∞ Chapter 18. CPT updates are needed to amend current listing and reflect new technologies and equipment. Code changes are published by the AMA in conjunction with CMS.

Organization of the CPT Manual

The organization of the 2008 CPT manual appears in Figure 19-1 ◆. The content and labeling of the many appendices sometimes change when the manual is updated.

While it may seem unusual to discuss the covers of a manual, the inside front and back covers contain helpful information for medical assistants. Inside the front cover is a list of commonly used symbols, **modifiers**, and place of service codes. These will be discussed in detail later. Inside the back cover are commonly used medical abbreviations. Following the covers is a section of introductory matter that presents the table of contents by page number, instructions for use of the codebook, and other valuable information, depending on the publisher. Possible inclusions are a review of medical terminology and anatomical plates.

Tabular Index

The **tabular index** is a numerical listing of all CPT codes, divided into **Category I**, **Category II**, and **Category III**. Category I codes, which comprise the bulk of the CPT, are numbered 00100 to 99999. They describe widely used services and procedures approved by the FDA and are organized into six **sections** (see Table 19-1). While most of the codes are in numeric order, the codes 99201 through 99499 appear in the first section: Evaluation and Management. This is done for ease of use, because these codes are the most frequently used and are used by all medical specialties. Other codes are used more selectively, based on the specific services provided by each office. The majority of this chapter will discuss Category I codes in detail.

Category II codes are supplemental tracking codes and can be used for performance measurement. The use of these codes is optional and should not be used to replace Category I codes. They are four numbers followed by the letter F, such as 1002F. Most medical assistants will likely not use these codes often.

CPT is a registered trademark of the American Medical Association.

Inside covers
Introductory matter
Tabular index
    Category I
    Category II
    Category III
Appendices
    A — Modifiers
    B — Summary of Additions, Deletions and Revisions
    C — Clinical Examples
    D — Summary of CPT Add-on Codes
    E — Summary of CPT Codes Exempt from Modifier 51
    F — Summary of CPT Codes Exempt from Modifier 63
    G — Summary of CPT Copes That Include Moderate (Conscious) Sedation
    H — Alphabetic Index of Performance Measures by Clinical Conditions or Topic
    I — Genetic Testing Code Modifiers
    J — Electrodiagnostic Medicine Listing of Sensory, Motor, and Mixed Nerves
    K — Product Pending FDA Approval
    L — Vascular Families
    M — Crosswalk to Deleted CPT Codes.
Alphabetical index

Figure 19-1 ◆ Organization of the CPT manual.
CPT only copyright 2008 American Medical Association. All rights reserved.

Category III codes are temporary codes for data collection and tracking the use of emerging technology, services, and procedures. The codes are four numbers followed by the letter T, such as 0162T. If a Category III code is available, medical assistants should use it in place of a Category I code. Category III technology and procedures may be in the FDA approval process. Services may be items that the AMA is considering adding to Category I. For example, online medical evaluation was a temporary code, 0074T, from 2005 to 2007; in 2008 it was assigned to Category I as 99444.

TABLE 19-1 SECTIONS OF THE CPT-4 CATEGORY I CODES	
Section	**Code Range(s)**
Evaluation and Management (E&M)	99201–99499
Anesthesiology	00100–01999
	99100–99140
Surgery	10021–69990
Radiology	70010–79999
Laboratory/Pathology	80048–89356
Medicine	90281–99199
	99500–99602

Appendices

The CPT manual has several appendices, which provide additional reference information.

Appendix A—Modifiers presents a complete description of all modifiers applicable to the current year codes. Modifiers are two-digit alphanumeric codes appended to CPT or **Level II codes** to further describe circumstances. An abbreviated list of commonly used modifiers appears inside the front cover, but medical assistants should develop the habit of referring to Appendix A until they are familiar with the details of how a specific modifier is to be used. Use of modifiers will be introduced later in the chapter.

Appendix B—Summary of Additions, Deletions, and Revisions is a valuable reference at the beginning of the year when the new CPT codes are released. Medical assistants can quickly cross-reference the CPT codes on encounter forms to Appendix B in order to determine what commonly used codes in their office might be affected by the annual revision.

Appendix C—Clinical Examples provides examples of E&M code scenarios for many medical specialties. These should not be used for coding, but for learning and understanding how various patient encounters might be coded. Every E&M code has at least one example.

Appendix D—Summary of CPT **Add-on Codes** lists the code numbers for those codes than cannot be used alone. Add-on codes are also designated with a + sign in the tabular index. Use of add-on codes will be described later.

Appendix E—Summary of CPT Codes Exempt from Modifier 51 is a summary, not exhaustive, list of code numbers that do not require modifier 51, multiple procedures. These are codes that are typically performed with another procedure but are not subject to reimbursement reductions that typically accompany multiple procedures performed at the same time. Since multiple procedures usually are billed with modifier 51, these codes do not require modifier 51. Modifier 51 exempt codes are also designated with a ⊘ sign in the tabular index. Use of modifier 51 will be described later.

Appendix F—Summary of CPT Codes Exempt from Modifier 63 lists code numbers that do not require modifier 63 procedure performed on infants less than 4 kg. Modifier 63 exempt codes are also designated with a parenthetical instruction in the tabular index.

Appendix G—Summary of CPT Codes That Include Moderate (Conscious) Sedation is a list of codes in which moderate sedation by the surgeon is an inherent part of the procedure. For these codes, sedation should not be billed separately. Moderate sedation codes are also designated with a ⊙ symbol in the tabular index.

Appendix H—Alphabetic Index of Performance Measures by Clinical Condition or Topic is a cross-reference between Category II codes and situations in which they might be used. Most medical assistants will likely not use this appendix often.

Appendix I—Genetic Testing Code Modifiers lists modifiers for reporting molecular laboratory procedures related to genetic testing. This enables providers to be more precise in coding without altering the test description. Only medical assistants working in the area of genetic testing will use these modifiers.

Appendix J—Electrodiagnostic Medicine Listing of Sensory, Motor, and Mixed Nerves is used in accurately coding nerve conduction studies with CPT codes 95900, 95903, and 95904. Only medical assistants who work in an office performing nerve conduction studies will use this appendix.

Appendix K—Product Pending FDA Approval lists CPT category I codes for vaccines expected to be approved FDA at some point after the CPT manual is published, often in July. This enables a code to be immediately available once approval is granted. These codes are also designated with a dagger symbol † in the tabular index.

Appendix L—Vascular Families depicts the structure of first-, second-, and third-order vascular branches. It aids medical assistants in coding for catheterization of the aorta.

Appendix M—Crosswalk to Deleted CPT Codes cross-references codes from the previous year that have been deleted with suggested replacement codes in the current year's manual. Medical assistants can quickly cross-reference the CPT codes on encounter forms that were deleted in the annual revision to Appendix M in order to determine what codes they can consider using instead.

Alphabetical Index

As in the *ICD-9-CM* manual, CPT coding begins with the **alphabetical index**. All procedures and services in the CPT manual are listed alphabetically by **main term** and **modifying terms** that aid in locating the most appropriate code or range of codes. After identifying potential codes in the index, they are verified in the tabular index. Final code selection should never be done based only on the alphabetical index. Detailed use of the index will be described later.

Conventions and Symbols

The CPT manual uses a number of formatting conventions and special symbols to provide information and to use space efficiently. Many of these are printed inside the front cover of the manual. They will be discussed in detail in the next section.

Determining the Correct Procedure Code

As with diagnostic coding, procedure coding also begins and ends with the patient's medical record. Medical assistants abstract information from the medical record in order to code

CPT is a registered trademark of the American Medical Association.

for services and the reasons they were provided. Coding is to be done to the highest level of certainty, meaning that all relevant information in the chart should be coded, but missing information should not be assumed or coded. Only procedures and services documented in the medical record can be coded and billed. If the medical record is incomplete or inaccurate, it should be corrected or amended before attempting to code.

There are a number of documents within the medical record that may contain needed information. When coding for office-based or other outpatient services, medical assistants will refer to the encounter form, visit notes, in-house lab and radiology reports, and operative reports for outpatient procedures. When coding for services physicians provide to inpatients, medical assistants will refer to the daily rounds sheet, which lists the patients seen in the hospital, daily progress notes, and operative reports.

It is important to keep in mind that when performing procedure coding, the MA must code and bill only for the services actually delivered on a specific date by a specific provider. Do not bill for services previously completed, performed by a different provider, or ordered to be completed in the future.

EXAMPLE

A patient, Henry, makes a followup visit to Dr. Jessop related to back pain. Dr. Jessop discusses Henry's progress and current condition, performs a physical examination, reviews X-rays taken by the hospital outpatient department, adjusts Henry's medication, provides therapeutic ultrasound, and orders a magnetic resonance imaging (MRI) study. The medical assistant, Heather, codes for the E&M visit and the therapeutic ultrasound, both of which Dr. Jessop performed today. The X-ray was not performed by Dr. Jessop; it was done previously at another location, so Heather doesn't code for the X-ray. Reviewing the X-ray and adjusting the medication are part of the medical decision making in the E&M visit, so there are not separate codes for these activities. The prescription itself is filled by the pharmacy, so she does not code for it. Heather also does not code for the MRI, which will be performed in the future at another location. If Dr. Jessop had a physical therapist on staff who provided the therapeutic ultrasound treatment, Heather would have still coded for it, but when she billed it, she would indicate on the CMS-1500 form (FL 24J) who actually performed that service.

The eleven coding steps described below provide the practical details medical assistants need to patiently and accurately execute the process of procedural coding.

1. Identify the primary and secondary services or procedures performed, as stated in the medical record. Often the physician will indicate procedure codes on the encounter form, but it is wise to verify them against the medical record. When abstracting from the medical record, be certain to not write in the record. Make a photocopy of the pertinent pages that can be annotated and highlighted or keep a separate paper for notes.

Look first for the chief complaint or reason for the visit. Services or procedures may be indicated in SOAP notes, under *O (Observation)*. Identify the primary procedure, or the main

CPT is a registered trademark of the American Medical Association.

service provided during the encounter. Often, this may simply be the E&M encounter, the history, examination, and recommendations. It is common for the E&M to be the only service provided. E&M coding will be discussed in detail later. It may be a treatment, such as an injection, or a minor surgical procedure, such as removal of a lesion or repair of a laceration.

Additional services documented in the medical record should be identified by the medical assistant as secondary procedures. Secondary procedures are coded in the same way as primary procedures and prioritized from highest cost to lowest cost on the CMS-1500 form. This is because many insurance companies pay the first procedure in full, but discount additional procedures performed at the same time. Generally, the E&M is identified first, with additional procedures to follow, but some insurers may request that all services be listed in descending cost order.

Finally, note the quantity of each procedure. For many procedures, such as E&M, the quantity will be one. For services such as removal of lesions, it is important to identify the type and number of lesions removed. For services based on time, such as therapeutic ultrasound, identify the number of minutes spent providing the service.

The following sample patient scenario illustrates how to identify procedures. The same scenario will be developed throughout each step in the coding process discussed. An example of coding for E&M services will be presented later.

Sample Patient Scenario
Selecting the Primary and Secondary Procedures

Patient presents with a lesion on the back. The physician prepares the area, administers local anesthetic, and removes a 0.7 cm benign lesion from the back. The site is closed with simple sutures.

The primary procedure is removal of a lesion on the back.

2. Locate the main term in the alphabetic index. The index of the CPT manual lists main terms used to locate procedure codes. The main term may be located in one of four ways.

1. It may be the name of the *procedure* or *service,* such as "Endoscopy" or "Splint."
2. It may the name of the *organ* or *anatomic* site, such as "Colon" or "Tibia."
3. It may be the name of a *condition,* such as "Fracture"; a *disease,* such as "Polyp" or "Fracture."
4. It may also be located by *eponym* (a disease or condition named after an individual) such as "Colle's fracture"; an abbreviation or *acronym,* such as "AIDS"; a nontechnical *synonym* (a word similar in meaning) such as "Removal" instead of "excision."

While in many ways these options are similar to those used in the *ICD-9-CM* index, the biggest difference is that in the CPT index, main terms include organs and anatomic sites, whereas in the *ICD-9-CM* anatomical site was not an option (Figure 19-2 ◆). Because there are so many choices of how to

Eponym/ Acronym	Procedure	Anatomic Site	Condition	Synonym
(Eponym) Colles fracture	Repair	Wrist	Fracture	
(Acronym) EKG	Electrocardiogram	Heart		Monitoring
	Excision	Eye	Cataract	Removal

Figure 19-2 ◆ Alternative methods for locating the CPT main term.

locate a main term, a good guideline is to search in this order: eponym or abbreviation; procedure or service; organ or anatomical site; disease or condition; synonym.

Some main terms are rather generic with pages of modifying terms, such as "Excision," while others are quite specific with only a single code, such as "Color Vision Examination." The main term is always boldfaced with each word beginning with a capital letter. After locating the main term, the tentative code(s) will be verified in Volume I. Never code from the index. The steps for verifying codes will be described later.

Exercise
Getting Acquainted with the Alphabetical Index

Look at the first few pages of your CPT alphabetical index. Find examples of each the following types of main terms:

eponym _____

acronym _____

procedure _____

organ _____

anatomic site _____

condition _____

Sample Patient Scenario
Identifying the Main Term

There is no acronym or eponym for removal of lesions. The first choice is to look under the procedure, Excision. When looking by organ system or anatomic site, the medical assistant remembers that lesions are located on the "skin," not on the back or other body area. In the CPT manual, entries for back procedures reference the internal musculoskeletal structure, not the skin itself. To locate by condition, the medical assistant would look under "Lesion."

3. Review any modifying terms or instructional notes associated with the main term. Main terms rarely provide the

CPT is a registered trademark of the American Medical Association.

exact code needed. Frequently, main terms function as major headings that have up to three series of modifying terms. Modifying terms are descriptive words in the alphabetic index that appear indented under the main term to further describe the service or procedure (modifying terms different than two-digit modifiers that are appended to Category I codes). When modifying terms appear, it is important to review the entire list, as they do affect the appropriate code selection.

The first series of modifying terms is aligned on the same margin as the main term, but in smaller, non-boldfaced type. The second and third levels of modifying terms are each indented several spaces beyond the previous level. They further describe the main term, in reference to anatomical site such as *Excision, kidney*; extent, such as *Excision, Clavicle, Partial*; procedure, such as *Electrocardiography, 24-Hour Monitoring*; or similar descriptors.

If the main term or modifying term is too long to fit on one line, a carry over line is used. Carry over lines are indented the same number of spaces as the beginning of the line. It is important to read carefully to distinguish between carry over lines and modifying terms.

Main terms and modifying terms contain instructional notes, such as *see* or *see also*, which direct the user to synonyms. For example, *Pneumonotomy—see Excision, Lung*. This instructs the user where to look for the code needed.

Codes may be listed singly, as a range, or as a nonsequential list. A range of codes is presented with a hyphen "-," such as *Bone Graft, Harvesting 20900-20902*. This indicates that all codes beginning with 20900 and ending with and including 20902 should be reviewed. Nonsequential codes are presented with a comma "," such as *Biopsy, Urethra 52204, 52354, 53200*. This indicates that three codes should be reviewed, but the intervening code numbers are probably not applicable.

Exercise
Identifying Conventions in the CPT Index

Look up the main term Blood in the alphabetical index and locate examples of the following:

Main term _____

Instructional note _____

First-level modifying term _____

Second-level modifying term _____

Third-level modifying term _____

Carry over line _____

Sample Patient Scenario
Using CPT Alphabetical Index Conventions

Main term: Excision
Instructional note: See Debridement; Destruction
First modifying term: Lesion
Second modifying term: Skin
Third modifying term: Benign.

There is not a modifying term for the location of the lesion. This will be identified once the tabular index is consulted.

4. Identify the tentative code(s) associated with the most appropriate modifying term(s). When the appropriate modifying terms are located, the tentative code(s) is printed immediately to the right. It is helpful to jot down the potential appropriate codes before verifying in the tabular list. Never use the index to make the final code selection. Even if only one code appears, it must be verified in the tabular index to be certain the code selection is accurate.

Sample Patient Scenario
Selecting the Tentative Code(s)

Excision
  Lesion
    Benign   Code range: 11400-11471

5. Locate the tentative code(s) in the tabular index. Look for the tentative code number in the tabular index where codes are arranged in numerical order. The tabular index contains six sections based on medical specialty. Chapters are divided into **subsections**, **subheadings**, **categories**, and **subcategories** based on anatomy, procedure, condition, or descriptor. The name of each of these divisions is printed with a specific typeface and text formatting, depending on the publisher. Not all of the divisions appear under every subsection; it depends on the amount of information in each specific subsection. All codes appear under the lowest division. It is helpful to learn the specific meanings of these designations, because the terms are used frequently in coding instructions (Figure 19-3 ◆).

CPT is a registered trademark of the American Medical Association.

6. Interpret the conventions used in the tabular index.[*] Even though you are now eager to verify and finalize your code, you first need to interpret the conventions presented with the code. The codes are presented as a five-digit number with no decimal point, and a description to the right. Tabular index conventions include formatting, punctuation, instructional notes, and symbols and may appear on the same line with the code, above it, below it, or at the beginning of a subcategory, category, subheading, subsection, or section. Look carefully for any information that may be relevant to your tentative code selection, as the additional information may direct you when to use a different code or an additional code, depending on the specific procedure performed.

In the tabular index, the most critical convention is the paired use of the **semicolon** (;) and indents. To conserve space and avoid having to repeat common terminology, some of the procedure descriptors in the tabular index are not printed in their entirety, but rather refer back to a common portion of the procedure descriptor listed in a preceding entry. The **standalone** or **parent code** is the one whose description is left-justified and begins with a capital letter. The shared portion of the code before the semicolon is the common descriptor, which is shared with indented codes. The portion after the semicolon is the unique descriptor that applies to only one code number. The **indented code** description is indented three spaces and begins with a small letter. It is only the unique descriptor for that code number. This unique descriptor must be combined with the unique descriptor from the standalone code in order to obtain a full description of the code. Within any series of indented codes, you *must* refer back to the standalone code within that series to determine the common descriptor of the indented code(s). Indented codes describe variations on the standalone code, such as alternative anatomic site, alternative procedure, or extent of services.

Figure 19-4 ◆ illustrates this formatting convention. The standalone code is 27134. The common part its of description is the words before the semicolon ("Revision of total hip arthroplasty"). This **common descriptor** should be considered part of each of the following indented codes in that series. For example, the full procedure descriptor represented by code 27137 is as follows:

27137 Revision of total hip arthroplasty, acetabular component only, with or without autograft or allograft

An indented code does not have to be billed together with the standalone code. They are considered two distinct procedures or services. The common descriptor is simply a space-saving convention in the printed book.

Instructional notes, which appear in parentheses, are used in the tabular index to point the user to alternative codes for closely related procedures or to codes that must or must not be used together (Figure 19-5 ◆).

---

[*]Adapted from Vines, Deborah, Braceland, Ann, Rollins, Elizabeth, and Miller, Susan. *Comprehensive Health Insurance: Billing, Coding, and Reimbursement*, pp. 133–135.

Level	Description					
Section	Anesthesia		Surgery			
Subsection	HEAD	NECK	CARDIOVASCULAR SYSTEM			
Subheading	*none*	*none*	<u>Heart and Pericardium</u>			<u>Arteries & Vessels</u>
Category	*none*	*none*	*Pericardium*	*Cardiac Valves*	*Arterial Grafting*	*multiple*
Subcategory	*none*	*none*	*none*	**Aortic** **Mitral** **Tricuspid** **Pulmonary**	*none*	*multiple*

Figure 19-3 ◆ Example of tabular index organization levels and formatting.

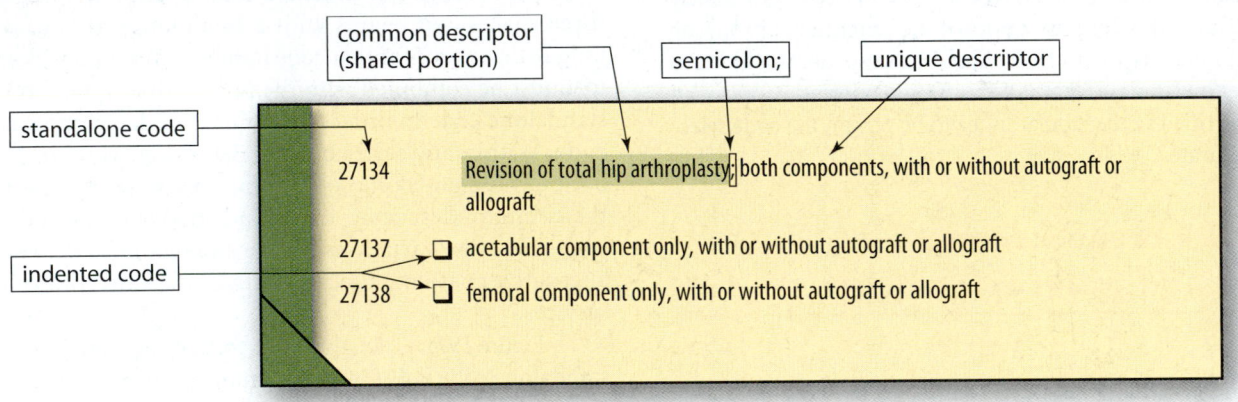

Figure 19-4 ◆ Example of standalone and indented codes.
CPT only copyright 2008 American Medical Association. All rights reserved.

Special instructions are directions within each section describing specific rules and definitions for use of codes within a particular category or subcategory. These also should be read and interpreted before assigning a code, even if it means going back to the top of the page or a previous page to find them. **Guidelines** are instructions that appear at the beginning of each of the six sections and apply to all codes in that section. Guidelines also list commonly used modifiers and provide subsection information.

Symbols are used in the tabular index to alert the user to certain circumstances that may affect use or interpretation of codes. There is a key at the bottom of each page. Medical assistants should become familiar with these meanings:

CPT is a registered trademark of the American Medical Association.

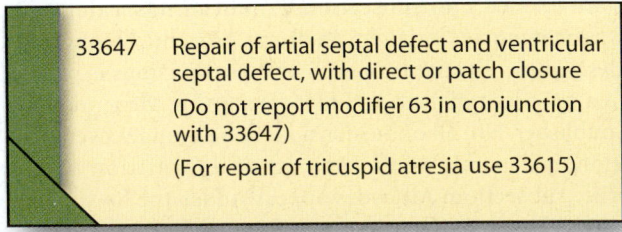

Figure 19-5 ◆ Example of instructional notes.
CPT only copyright 2008 American Medical Association. All rights reserved.

⊙   Moderate sedation is automatically included in the code description

◐   Modifier 51 exempt. When billing multiple procedures, a code with this symbol does not require using modifier 51.

+   Add-on code must be used in conjunction with another CPT code. Frequently, the accepted companion codes are provided in an instructional note.

✗   FDA approval pending. FDA approval of the vaccine described is expected to come during the current year.

( )   Parentheses are used to enclose synonyms, eponyms, or supplementary descriptors that may be present or absent in a physician's statement of condition without affecting the code assignment.

●   New code in this edition of the CPT manual

▲   Revised code – the code number is the same, but the descriptor has been updated

►◄   Contains new or revised text

New and revised code symbols are an important aid to medical assistants experienced in coding. They alert the user to the fact that a code they may be accustomed to using in a certain manner has been updated and may no longer be appropriate.

Exercise
Interpreting Special Instructions

Look up CPT code 11400 in the tabular index. Locate the special instructions under the subheading *Excision—Benign Lesions*. Read the instructions, then write down answers to the questions below:

1. Is anesthesia included? _____
2. Where should one look for codes for shave removal? _____
3. Where should one look for codes for electrosurgical and other methods of removal? _____
4. What is the definition of *excision?* _____
5. What is the margin? _____
6. What is included in the size of the excised lesion? _____
7. What type of closure is included? _____
8. Where should one look for codes for intermediate closures? _____
9. Where should one look for codes for complex closures? _____
10. Where should one look for codes for adjacent tissue transfer? _____
11. What part of the instructions contains new or revised information? _____

CPT is a registered trademark of the American Medical Association.

Sample Patient Scenario
Interpreting Tabular Index Conventions

The index directed us to Excision, Lesion, Benign 11400-11471. The task now is to look up this range of codes in the tabular index to select the one that best describes the procedure (0.7 cm lesion from the back, closed with simple sutures, benign.) First, read the special instructions at the beginning of the subheading *Excision – Benign Lesions* and complete the exercise on interpreting special instructions to help understand what is being said.

Scan all the codes in this range. The last six codes, 11450 to 11471, describe *Excision of skin and subcutaneous tissue for hidradenetis*, which is not appropriate for this case. You quickly see among codes 11400 to 11446 that there are many indented codes that appear to be the same. For example, 11401, 11421, 11441 all state *excised diameter 0.6 to 1.0 cm.*

To understand the differences between these codes, it is necessary to compare the common portion of the accompanying standalone codes, 11400, 11420, 11440. The first part of the common portion of the standalone codes is also the same *Excision, benign lesion including margins, except skin tag (unless listed elsewhere).* The last half line of the common portion that describes the body area is what varies among the standalone codes.

7. **Select the code with the highest level of specificity.** There is no universal rule that describes how many codes need to be reviewed before identifying the one with the highest specificity. Sometimes, the best code is the first one listed; other times, there may be a dozen or more codes to review, and additional ones to cross-reference. There also is no universal rule that describes how precise the correct code will be in its description. For example, many codes on the integumentary system include the size of the area treated, but the size is usually a range, such as 1.1 cm to 2.0 cm. If a treatment covers 1.5 cm exactly, there is not a more specific code or modifier to describe the exact size. The medical record often contains more detail than what is coded. Only by carefully interpreting the conventions associated with each code, category, and section can one be certain. As medical assistants become experienced in a particular office, they become very familiar with the most frequently used codes.

Sample Patient Scenario
Selecting the Code with the Highest Level of Specificity

First, select the standalone code that contains the description for this patient. The term *back* does not appear, but using knowledge of anatomy, you know that *trunk* includes the back. 11400, *trunk, arms, or legs* is the appropriate stand-alone code.

Now select the indented code that describes the diameter of 0.7 cm. Code 11401 is *excised diameter 0.6 to 1.0 cm,* so this is the best code.

8. Review the code for appropriate bundling, add on codes and quantity. Carefully review code descriptions, instructional notes, and special instructions one more time to be certain that the code selected is accurate. Pay special attention to **bundling** edits, frequently triggered by the words *includes* and *not separately reportable.* This indicates that multiple services are included in a single code. The words *report separately* or *use in conjunction with* indicate that additional codes should be used. For example, the special instructions for *33510 to 33516 Coronary artery bypass, vein only* include both bundling and multiple coding situations. For bundling, the instructions state *Procurement of the saphenous vein graft is included in the description of the work for 33510-33516 and should not be reported as a separate service or co-surgery.* However, an additional code is needed in other situations, *to report harvesting of an upper extremity vein, use 35500 in addition to the bypass procedure.*

CPT codes also differ regarding how the quantity of procedures is to be reported. This information is provided in the code description or special instructions. For example, to report removal of skin tags, a single code, 11200, describes *up to and including 15 lesions.* While the code is reported with a quantity of *1* on the CMS-1500 form, block 24G, it describes as many as 15 lesions. For shaving of epidermal or dermal lesions (11300-11313) each code describes a single lesion; multiple lesions of the same size and body area are reported by designating the number of lesions in block 24G on the CMS-1500 form. End stage renal disease services are reported with a single code for the entire month (90918-90921); the special instructions describe the scope of services included. Codes that include a time-based element also vary in how quantity is reported. For example, codes for certain physical therapy treatments (97032-97039) describe 15 minutes of treatment with a quantity of *1* on the CMS-1500 form, block 24G. Thirty minutes of treatment is reported with a quantity of *2* on the CMS-1500 form, block 24G.

Add-on codes should also be verified. Use of add-on codes may be limited to only a few codes that are listed in instructional notes. For example, when coding for discectomy of multiple disks, the code for each additional interspace is reported in addition to a specific primary procedure code. CPT add-on code 63078 should be used in conjunction with 60377.

Sample Patient Scenario
Reviewing the Bundling, Add-on Code, and Quantity Edits

The special instructions describe that local anesthesia and simple closure are included (bundled) with the codes in this subheading. No add-on codes apply. No additional coding is

required for these services. Only a single lesion was excised, so there are no quantity edits.

Note: If a second lesion in the same location and same size range is performed, the code is reported with a quantity of *2* on the CMS-1500 form, block 24G.

9. Determine if modifiers are required. Modifiers affect the complete description of a service and frequently have a significant impact on reimbursement and coding compliance. Use of modifiers may be described in the instructional notes, special instructions, or guidelines. It is usually dependent on the experience of the coder to determine if the situation calls for any modifiers. Detailed use of modifiers is discussed later in the chapter.

Sample Patient Scenario
Determining if Modifiers Are Required

No modifiers are required for this case. If more than one lesion had been excised, of a different size range or body area, modifier 51, multiple procedures, would be used on the subsequent procedures.

10. Verify the final code against the documentation. As a final check, with coding manual instructions fresh in your mind, refer back to the original documentation and verify that all conditions of the code agree with the medical record. If a discrepancy arises, work through the process again from the beginning.

Sample Patient Scenario
Verifying the Final Code Against Documentation

11401 Excision, benign lesion including margins, except skin tag, trunk arms or legs, excised diameter 0.6 cm to 1.0 cm accurately matches our description of excision of 0.7 cm lesion from the back, closed with simple sutures, benign.

11. Assign the code. Write down the final code where indicated on your worksheet or documentation. Be certain to proofread the number as you wrote or keyboarded it to avoid transcription errors that are easy to make.

Repeat this process for any additional codes required by the medical record.

Selecting a procedure code may seem like a long and tedious process at first. As medical assistants become familiar with the services and codes used by their medical office, coding becomes faster and easier, but accuracy and attention to detail is always paramount. Taking time and care to learn the fundamentals correctly will help create long-term success in your coding role.

Using CPT Modifiers*

Modifiers are two-digit suffixes used with CPT codes to report a service or procedure that has been modified by some specific circumstance without altering or modifying the basic definition or CPT code (Table 19-2). The proper use of modifiers can speed up claims processing and increase reimbursement, whereas the improper use of CPT modifiers may result in claim delays or denials. A complete list of modifiers can be found in the CPT book in Appendix A with their full definitions. Modifiers may be used for these reasons:

- To report only the professional component of a procedure or service
- To report a service mandated by a third-party payer
- To indicate that a procedure was performed bilaterally

*Adapted from Vines, Deborah, Braceland, Ann, Rollins, Elizabeth, and Miller, Susan. *Comprehensive Health Insurance: Billing, Coding, and Reimbursements,* pp. 135–140.

- To report multiple procedures performed at the same session by the same provider
- To report a portion of a service or procedure that was reduced or eliminated at the physician's discretion
- To report assistant surgeon services.

The most commonly used modifiers are discussed next.

22 Unusual Procedural Service—This modifier is used when the service provided is higher than that usually required for the listed procedure. A special report should be submitted with the claim. A special report is a report that details the reasons for a new, variable, or unlisted procedure or service; it explains the patient's condition and justifies the procedure's medical necessity. An unlisted procedure is a service or procedure that is not listed in the CPT codebook. Each section's guidelines have codes for unlisted procedures.

47 Anesthesia by Surgeon—Regional or general anesthesia provided by the surgeon may be reported by

TABLE 19-2 CPT MODIFIERS

Modifier	Use
21	Prolonged Evaluation and Management Services
22	Unusual Procedural Services
23	Unusual Anesthesia
24	Unrelated Evaluation and Management Service by the Same Physician during a **Postoperative** Period
25	Significant, Separately Identifiable Evaluation and Management Service by the Same Physician on the Same Day of the Procedure or Other Service
26	Professional Component
32	Mandated Services
47	Anesthesia by Surgeon
50	Bilateral Procedure
51	Multiple Procedures
52	Reduced Services
53	Discontinued Procedure
54	Surgical Care Only
55	Postoperative Management Only
56	Preoperative Management Only
57	Decision for Surgery
58	Staged or Related Procedure or Service by the Same Physician during the Postoperative Period
59	Distinct Procedural Service
62	Two Surgeons
63	Procedure Performed on Infants
66	Surgical Team
76	Repeat Procedure by Same Physicians
77	Repeat Procedure by Another Physician
78	Return to the Operating Room for a Related Procedure during the Postoperative Period
79	Unrelated Procedure or Service by the Same Physician during the Postoperative Period
80	Assistant Surgeon
81	Minimum Assistant Surgeon
82	Assistant Surgeon (when qualified resident surgeon is unavailable)
90	Reference (Outside) Laboratory
91	Repeat Clinical Diagnostic Laboratory Test
99	Multiple Modifiers

Source: CPT 2008. Copyright 2007 American Medical Association. All rights reserved.

CPT is a registered trademark of the American Medical Association.

adding modifier 47 to the basic service. This does not include local anesthesia.

50 Bilateral Procedure—Bilateral means pertaining to two sides. Unless otherwise identified in the descriptor, bilateral procedures that are performed at the same operative session should be identified by appending modifier 50 to the procedure.

51 Multiple Procedures—When multiple procedures are performed, other than evaluation and management (E/M) services, at the same session by the same provider, the primary procedure may be listed first. The additional procedures may be identified by appending modifier 51 to the additional procedure. Modifier 51 has four applications, namely, to identify:

- multiple medical procedures performed at the same session by the same provider.
- multiple, related operative procedures performed at the same session by the same provider.
- operative procedures performed in combination, at the same operative session, by the same provider, whether through the same or another incision or involving the same or different anatomy.
- a combination of medical and operative procedures performed at the same session by the same provider.

Many insurers reimburse a lesser amount for procedures using modifier 51, because there is a potential cost savings for the surgeon performing multiple procedures at one session, compared to performing only a single procedure. Modifier 51 should not be appended to designated add-on codes or those with the symbol ⊘, which means "exempt from modifier 51."

53 Discontinued Procedure—Under certain circumstances, the physician may elect to terminate a surgical or diagnostic procedure. Due to extenuating circumstances or those that threaten the well-being of the patient, it may be necessary to indicate that a surgical or diagnostic procedure was started but discontinued. This circumstance may be reported by adding the modifier 53 to the code reported by the physician for the discontinued procedure.

54 Surgical Care Only—When one physician performs a surgical procedure and another provides preoperative and/or postoperative management, surgical services may be identified by adding modifier 54 to the usual procedure number.

55 Postoperative Management Only—When one physician performed the postoperative management and another performed the surgical procedure, modifier 55 is appended to the usual procedure number.

56 Preoperative Management Only—When one physician performed the preoperative care and evaluation and another physician performed the surgical procedure, the preoperative component may be identified by adding modifier 56 to the usual procedure number. Modifier 53 is not used to report the elective cancellation of a procedure prior to the patient's

anesthesia induction or surgical preparation in the operating suite. This modifier is not used to report the treatment of a problem that requires a return to the operating room; see modifier 78 instead.

EXAMPLE FOR MODIFIERS 54, 55, AND 56

A physician may intend to perform all three components of a global service (preoperative management, surgical care, and postoperative management); however, after providing the preoperative management and performing the surgical procedure, he is unexpectedly called out of town. The surgeon in this case reports the surgical procedure with the modifiers 54 and 56 appended. The physician who performed the postoperative management reports the operative procedure code with modifier 55 appended. Reporting the postoperative management indicates that the physician performed all of the postoperative care.

58 Staged or Related Procedure by the Same Physician During the Postoperative Period—The physician may need to indicate that the performance of a procedure or service during the postoperative period was

1. planned prospectively at the time of the original procedure (staged).
2. more extensive than the original procedure.
3. for therapy following a diagnostic surgical procedure. This circumstance may be reported by appending modifier 58 to the staged or related procedure.

59 Distinct Procedural Service—Under certain circumstances, the physician may need to indicate that a procedure or service was distinct or independent from other services performed on the same day. Modifier 59 is used to identify procedures that are not normally reported together, but are appropriate under the circumstances.

62 Two Surgeons—When two surgeons work together as primary surgeons performing a distinct part of a procedure, each surgeon should report his or her distinct operative work by adding modifier 62 to the procedure and any associated add-on codes for that procedure as long as both surgeons continue to work together as primary surgeons.

78 Return to the Operating Room for a Related Procedure During the Postoperative Period—The physician may need to indicate that another procedure was performed during the postoperative period of the initial procedure. When this subsequent procedure is related to the first and requires the use of the operating room, it may be reported by adding modifier 78 to the related procedure. If the return is due to a complication, it is eligible for reimbursement, even though it occurs during the postoperative period.

79 Unrelated Procedure or Service by the Same Physician During the Postoperative Period—The physician may need to indicate that the performance of a procedure during the postoperative period was unrelated to the original procedure.

80 Assistant Surgeon—Surgical assistant services may be identified by adding modifier 80 to the usual procedure number.

Coding for Evaluation and Management Services

Evaluation and Management (E&M) codes describe patient encounters with a physician for the evaluation and management of a health problem. Although these codes begin with 99, they are located out of numerical sequence in the CPT manual, at the front of the manual, as the first section. E&M codes are selected based on the category of service, which may be the location or the type of service provided, depending on the category.

Normally, the physician marks the E&M code on the encounter form. Medical assistants need to ensure that documentation in the medical record is consistent with the codes checked off. It is also a good idea to **audit** bills on a regular basis. Auditing is a detailed process that verifies that every detail of the E&M code is clearly documented. E&M coding possesses some differences from the rest of CPT coding. The key steps for E&M coding are described next. Do not be tempted to rush through E&M coding by skipping or abbreviating any of these steps, because this could result in inaccurate coding and payment.

1. **Identify the category of service.** When coding for E&M services, it is important to select the category of service first, before trying to determine the specific code. Categories may describe the location of service, such as office visit or hospital inpatient visit, or the type of service, such as consultation, critical care, or preventive care. This can be confusing because not all services provided in the medical office, for example, are coded from the *Office Visit* category. They may be coded from *Consultation, Preventive Care,* or several other categories as well. It is important to be familiar with CPT definitions of these services, which are described in special instructions at the beginning of each subsection. Table 19-3 lists the most commonly used categories of E&M service with a brief description of each. To locate codes, look first in the alphabetical index, under the main term *Evaluation and Management,* then select the appropriate category.

2. **Identify the subcategory of service.** Most of the E&M categories are further subdivided based on patient status (new vs. established), location (office vs. inpatient), frequency (initial vs. subsequent), or other relevant characteristic. These criteria are defined in the section guidelines or subsection special instructions. Some of the commonly used terms are discussed in the section that follows.

Medical assistants will frequently need to determine **patient status**; that is, to distinguish between **new patients** and **established patients**, as this criterion is used for office visits and preventive care. A new patient is one who has not received any professional services from the physician, or another physician of the same specialty who belongs to the same group practice, within the past three years. An established patient is one who

TABLE 19-3 COMMONLY USED CATEGORIES OF E&M CODES

Office (and Other Outpatient) Services	99201–99215
Hospital Observation Services	99217–99220
Hospital (Inpatient) Services	99221–99239
Consultations (Office)	99241–99245
Consultations (Inpatient)	99251–99255
Emergency Department Services	99281–99288
Pediatric Critical Care Patient Transport	99289, +99290
Critical Care Services	99291, +99292
Inpatient Pediatric and Neonatal Critical Care	99293–99300
Nursing Facility Services	99304–99318
Rest Home, Custodial Care, Domiciliary	99324–99337
Oversight Services for Domiciliary, Rest Home or Home	99339–99340
Home Services	99341–99350

Source: CPT 2008, Copyright 2008 American Medical Association. All rights reserved.

has received professional services from the physician, or another physician of the same specialty who belongs to the same group practice, within the past three years (Figure 19-6 ◆).

Some codes are determined based on whether the patient is an **outpatient** or an **inpatient.** An inpatient is someone who has been formally admitted to a facility with written admission orders from a physician. All others are considered outpatients, even though they may occupy a hospital bed, for example, on **observation status** and emergency department patients. Observation status is a designated type of care in which a patient is hospitalized for monitoring, but not formally admitted.

3. **Review the reporting instructions for the selected category or subcategory.** Each category and subcategory within the E&M section contains definitions and instructions that describe key terms, how the codes are to be reported, and what may be bundled into the code description. Even though this can sometimes be lengthy, take time to read and understand what is being said. For example, when reporting critical care services, lengthy examples are provided of what comprises critical care, where it can be provided, and the age of the patient appropriate for the codes. In addition, a list of bundled CPT codes is provided, which cannot be reported separately.

4. **Determine the key components.** Within each subcategory, there are three to five levels of codes, in increasing order of complexity. It is necessary to determine the **key components** or other criteria used for code selection within each subcategory of E&M codes. Many codes are based on the extent of the history (H), the examination (E), and the medical decision making (MDM). Other codes are based on time or age. A summary of the three key components (H, E, MDM) follows. More detailed guidelines can be found in the CPT guidelines and reference texts.

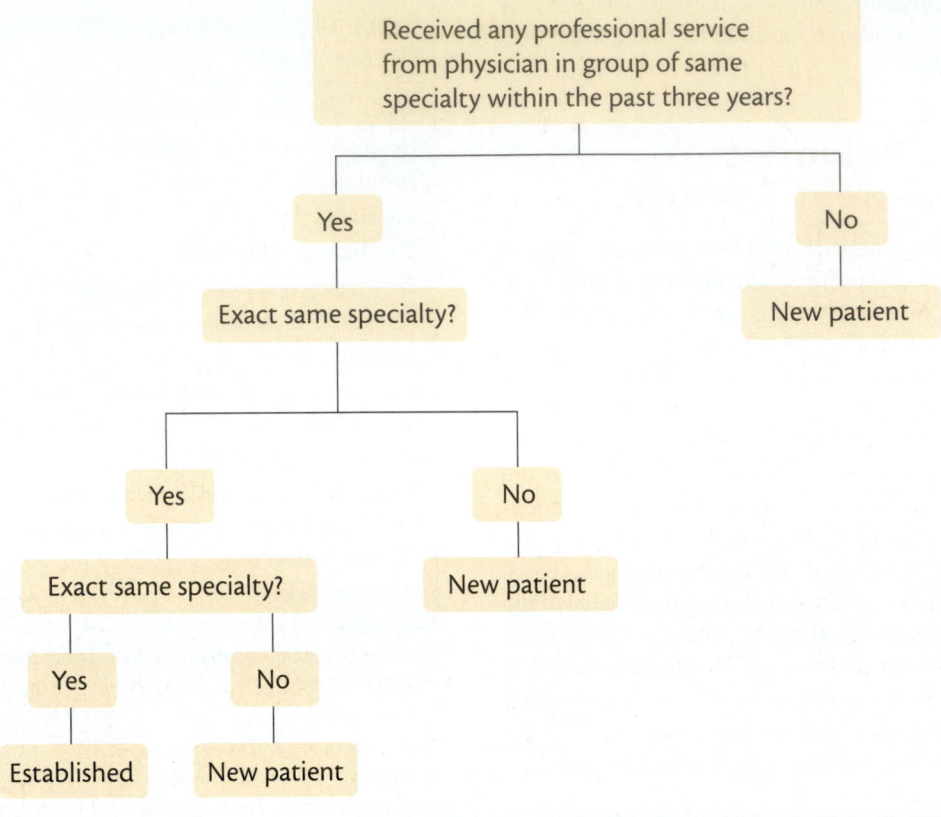

Figure 19-6 ◆ Decision tree for new versus established patients.
Source: CPT 2008, Professional Edition, p. 2. American Medical Association. Reprinted with permission.

a. History (H) To determine the proper level of **history** for the E&M code, the following descriptions are used:

   Problem focused—patient's problem is small; he has only one chief complaint and gives a brief history of his present illness or problem

   Expanded problem focused—patient's problem is mild to moderate; she has more than one chief complaint and/or a more extensive history of her present illness or problem.

   Detailed—patient's problem is moderate to severe and he has pertinent past, family and/or social history that is directly related to his current problem.

   Comprehensive—patient's problem is moderate to severe; she has a more extensive history and needs a complete review of all additional body systems.

b. Examination (E/Ex) To determine the proper level of **examination** for the E&M code, the following descriptions are used:

   Problem focused—A limited examination of the affected body area is done.

   Expanded problem focused—A limited examination of the affected body area is done along with other related organ systems.

   Detailed—An extended examination of the affected body area and other related organ systems is performed.

   Comprehensive—A general multisystem examination is performed.

For the purposes of determining a body area, the CPT-4 code book lists the following body areas to be recognized:

■ Head, including the face
■ Neck
■ Chest, including breasts and axilla
■ Abdomen
■ Genitalia, groin, buttocks
■ Back
■ Each extremity

For the purpose of definition of organ systems, the CPT-4 code book lists the following organ systems:

■ Eyes
■ Ears, nose, mouth, and throat
■ Cardiovascular
■ Respiratory
■ Gastrointestinal
■ Genitourinary
■ Musculoskeletal
■ Skin
■ Neurologic
■ Psychiatric
■ Hematologic/Lymphatic/Immunologic

c. Medical Decision Making (MDM) In order to determine the proper level of **medical decision making**

CPT is a registered trademark of the American Medical Association.

(MDM) for the E&M codes, the medical assistant should consider the following:

- The number of possible diagnoses the patient has
- The amount or complexity of the medical records the provider must go through to treat the patient
- The risk of significant complications as a result of this treatment.

There are four types of medical decision making recognized by the CPT-4. These are listed as: straightforward; low complexity; moderate complexity; and high complexity. Straightforward is listed as minimal diagnoses, minimal complexity, and minimal risk of complications. Low complexity is listed as limited diagnoses, limited complexity, and low risk of complications. Moderate complexity is listed as multiple diagnoses, moderate complexity, and moderate risk of complications. High complexity is listed as extensive diagnoses, extensive complexity, and high risk of complications.

The specific E&M code is selected based on how it meets the criteria of the key components. The criteria for each component are described in the code definition in the CPT manual. Some categories of E&M codes require that all three key components be at the level specified in the code description or a higher level in order to assign the code. Other categories require that only two of the key components be at the level specified in the code description or a higher level in order to assign the code. The number of components required is stated in the code description.

5. Identify the contributing factors. E&M codes that contain the three key components H, E, and MDM also have three **contributing factors**: counseling, coordination of care, and nature of the **presenting problem**. These factors rarely determine the code, but should be consistent with the code selected.

Counseling is defined as a discussion with the patient and/or a family concerning the patient's diagnosis, test results, impressions, prognosis, risks and benefits of treatment options, and instructions for management of the condition.

Coordination of care is the task of working with other providers or agencies to provide the patient with needed care, such as referral to home healthcare.

E&M codes take the following into consideration in determining the nature of the presenting problem:

- **Minimal**—The problem may not require the presence of the physician, but service is provided under the physician's supervision.
- **Self-limited or minor**—The problem runs a definite and prescribed course, is temporary, and is not likely to permanently alter the patient's health status.
- **Low severity**—The problem has a low risk of causing the patient's death without treatment and full recovery is expected.
- **Moderate severity**—The problem has a risk of death without treatment, there is an uncertain prognosis, or an increased likelihood the problem will cause permanent health problems for the patient.

CPT is a registered trademark of the American Medical Association.

- **High severity**—The problem has a high risk of causing the patient's death without treatment, or there may be a high probability of prolonged functional impairment to the patient as a result of this condition.

Finally, time is a consideration in E&M coding. Codes with the three key components also include an indication of the amount of time the physician typically spends **face-to-face** with the patient and/or family. While these E&M codes should never be selected based on time, there are unusual situations in which a code level can be increased. If the time spent in counseling and coordination of care is more than 50 percent of total visit time, time may be considered a controlling factor to qualify for a higher level E&M code. In order to do this, documentation needs to indicate the total amount of time spent with the patient and/or family, the amount of time spent in counseling and coordination of care, and a description of why the additional time was required.

6. Verify and assign the code. After verifying documentation against CPT guidelines, special instructions, and code descriptions, determine the appropriate code and write it on your coding worksheet or enter it into the computer system. Be certain to verify the accuracy of the code number, as transpositions easily occur.

7. Identify bundled and separately billable services. Certain services are included in the E&M code: discussions with patients and their families about the current problem; physical examination; reviewing test results, reports from other providers, and records of outside services; ordering tests and services; writing prescriptions; scheduling procedures; providing instructions and education to patients and their families. Certain codes, such as critical care, include a more specific list of bundled services. If a visit is related to postoperative followup, it should not be billed separately. If an office or emergency department encounter develops into another E&M service on the same date, such as inpatient admission, the first E&M is bundled into the hospital admission.

Identify as separately billable any other services provided in the office such as venipuncture, immunizations, EKGs, X-rays, and lab tests performed in the office and proceed with the coding of these services.

8. Identify modifiers.* Certain modifiers are used specifically for E&M coding. It is important to assign modifiers correctly to ensure appropriate reimbursement. Commonly used modifiers for E&M codes include the following:

21 *Prolonged Evaluation and Management Service.* Used when the service provided is greater than the highest level described for the code range.

24 *Unrelated Evaluation and Management Service by the Same Physician During a Postoperative Period.* Used when the E&M service is not related to the reason for surgery and is provided within the postoperative time period (global period) in the payer's reimbursement; for example, during a postoperative period for an appendectomy, patient sprains an ankle.

25 *Significant, Separately Identifiable Evaluation and Management Service by the Same Physician on the Same Day of the Procedure or Other Service.* Used when the physician provides an E&M service in addition to another E&M service or procedure on the same day; for example, during a preventive care visit, a heart problem is identified and the physician does a cardiac work up in addition to the preventive care visit. The cardiac workup is billed with an office visit E&M (99212-99215) with modifier 25 in addition to the code for preventive care.

32 *Mandated Services.* Used when the encounter is requested by the payer; for example, a second opinion required or independent medical examination in a liability case.

52 *Reduced Service.* Used when an E&M service is less extensive than the descriptor indicates.

57 *Decision for Surgery.* Used to indicate a decision for major surgery within 24 hours was made during the visit. The modifier indicates that this visit was more than the preoperative assessment that is included in the surgical code.

9. Identify place of service code for the CMS-1500. While not a direct component of CPT coding, medical assistants who are responsible for completing the CMS-1500 billing form need to assign a place of service (POS) code in block 24B that is consistent with the place of service defined in the CPT code (Table 19-4). These codes can also be found inside the front cover of many CPT manuals. For example, if using CPT code 99213 for a new patient office visit, the POS code on the CMS-1500 cannot be 21 inpatient hospital.

?—Critical Thinking Question 19-2—

What should Lydia tell Dr. Anderson about the relationship between appropriate codes and medical chart documentation?

In addition to leveraging documentation to code properly, medical assistants must remember that codes and the physician's time are sometimes indirectly related. Some patients simply take

TABLE 19-4 CURRENT PLACE OF SERVICE CODES TO BE USED IN BILLING FOR HEALTHCARE SERVICES

Place of Service Code	Place of Service Name	Place of Service Description
01	Pharmacy	A facility where drugs are sold, dispensed, or provided directly to patients
02	Unassigned	Not currently used
03	School	An educational facility
04	Homeless Shelter	A temporary housing facility
05	Indian Health Service Free-Standing Facility	A facility owned and operated by the Indian Health Service to provide services to American Indians and Alaskan Natives who do not require hospitalization
06	Indian Health Service Provider-Based Facility	A facility owned and operated by the Indian Health Service to provide services to American Indians and Alaskan Natives who are admitted as inpatients or outpatients
07	Tribal 638 Free-Standing Facility	A facility owned and operated by a federally recognized American Indian or Alaskan Native tribe to provide services to tribal members who do not require hospitalization
08	Tribal 638 Provider-Based Facility	A facility owned and operated by a federally recognized American Indian or Alaskan Native tribe to provide services to tribal members who are admitted as inpatients or outpatients
09	Prison-Correctional Facility	A prison or jail maintained by federal, state, or local authorities
10	Unassigned	Not currently used
11	Office	An ambulatory care clinic where the physician sees the patient
12	Home	The patient's private residence
13	Assisted Living Facility	A residential facility that provides on-site support 24 hours every day
14	Group Home	A residence with shared living areas where the patient receives supervision
15	Mobile Unit	A facility that moves from place to place to provide preventive, treatment or screening services
16–19	Unassigned	Not currently used
20	Urgent Care Facility	A location other than the hospital emergency room where patients are seen for unscheduled emergency care
21	Inpatient Hospital	A hospital facility where the patient is admitted for 24 hours or more
22	Outpatient Hospital	A portion of a hospital facility where the patient is seen for care as an outpatient

CPT is a registered trademark of the American Medical Association.

TABLE 19-4 CURRENT PLACE OF SERVICE CODES TO BE USED IN BILLING FOR HEALTHCARE SERVICES (CONTINUED)

Place of Service Code	Place of Service Name	Place of Service Description
23	Emergency Room—Hospital	The Emergency Room of a hospital
24	Ambulatory Surgical Center	A free-standing facility, other than the physician's office, where the patient is seen for surgical and diagnostic services on an ambulatory basis
25	Birthing Center	A facility, other than a hospital's maternity facility, which provides a setting for labor and delivery
26	Military Treatment Facility	A medical facility operated by a branch of the United States military
27–30	Unassigned	Not currently used
31	Skilled Nursing Facility	A facility that provides inpatient skilled nursing care but does not provide the level of care available in the hospital
32	Nursing Facility	A facility that provides care to patients who require care above the level of custodial care
33	Custodial Care Facility	A facility that provides supervision of patients who requires assistance that is not medically related
34	Hospice	A facility other than the patient's home where palliative care is given to terminally ill patients
35–40	Unassigned	Not currently used
41	Ambulance—Land	A land vehicle used for transporting the sick or injured
42	Ambulance—Air or Water	An air or water vehicle used for transporting the sick or injured
43–48	Unassigned	Not currently used
49	Independent Clinic	A location, other than a hospital, that is operated to provide medical services to outpatients only
50	Federally Qualified Health Center	A facility located in a medically underserved area that provides Medicare patients preventive medical care under the direction of a physician
51	Inpatient Psychiatric Facility	A facility that provides inpatient psychiatric services supervised by a physician
52	Psychiatric-Facility Partial Hospitalization	A facility that provides treatment for mental illnesses for patients who do not require full-time hospitalization
53	Community Mental Health Center	A facility that provides mental health benefits on an outpatient basis
54	Intermediate Care Facility/Mentally Retarded	A facility that provides custodial care to mentally retarded individuals
55	Residential Substance Abuse Treatment Facility	A facility that provides treatment for substance abuse
56	Psychiatric Residential Treatment Center	A facility that provides 24-hour psychiatric care
57	Nonresidential Substance Abuse Treatment Facility	A facility that provides treatment for substance abuse on an ambulatory basis
58–59	Unassigned	Not currently used
60	Mass Immunization Center	A facility where providers administer vaccines

Source: http://www.cms.gov/placeofservicecodes

more of the physician's time. When, however, patients require longer visits because they need translators or are severely disabled, codes that reflect extended visits are appropriate.

Coding for Special Situations*

Coding for Anesthesia

Anesthesia codes have their own section, which is located before the Surgery section. Basic anesthesia administration services are those services provided by or under the responsible supervision of a physician. These services include general and regional anesthesia, as well as supplementation of local anesthesia. Anesthesia is coded and reimbursed according to the formula **B*T*M**. B is basic unit, the relative value assigned by the American Society of Anesthesiologists (**ASA**). The relative value is a number that reflects how complicated a particular procedure is compared to others. T stands for time, reported as the minutes from when the anesthesiologist begins preparing the patient until the patient is no longer under the care of the anesthesiologist. Depending on the insurer, the minutes may be reported on the CMS-1500 form as total minutes, 15-minute units, or 30-minute units. M is the modifying unit, for the **physical status modifier**, which indicates the condition of the patient at the time anesthesia is administered (Table 19-5).

*Adapted from Vines, Deborah, Braceland, Ann, Rollins, Elizabeth, and Miller, Susan. *Comprehensive Health Insurance: Billing, Coding, and Reimbursement.* pp. 141–153. © Pearson Education. Upper Saddle River, NJ.

CPT is a registered trademark of the American Medical Association.

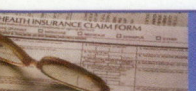

PROCEDURE 19-1 Code for a Procedure

Theory and Rationale

Proper procedure coding in the medical office facilitates timely payment of providers' claims. Therefore, medical assistants must be familiar with the steps involved in locating and assigning proper procedure codes.

Materials

- CPT-4 coding book
- Superbill/encounter form
- Patient's chart

Competency

(**Conditions**) With the necessary materials, you will be able to (**Task**) assign a procedure code (**Standards**) correctly within the time limit set by the instructor.

1. On the superbill, locate the procedure code the physician has circled.

2. Identify the primary and secondary services or procedures performed, as stated in the medical record.
3. Locate the main term in the alphabetic index.
4. Review any modifying terms or instructional notes associated with the main term.
5. Identify the tentative code(s) associated with the most appropriate modifying term(s).
6. Locate the tentative code(s) in the tabular index.
7. Interpret the conventions used in the tabular index.
8. Select the code with the highest level of specificity.
9. Review the code for appropriate bundling, add-on codes, and quantity.
10. Determine if modifiers are required.
11. Verify the final code against the documentation.
12. Assign the code.

In the case of difficult and/or extraordinary circumstances such as extreme youth or age (under 1 year of age or over 70 years) or other unusual risk factors, it may be appropriate to report one or more of the qualifying circumstances by using an add-on code listed in Figure 19-7 ◆ addition to the anesthesia services.

The index is researched for the procedure under the main term Anesthesia. The section's subsections are organized by body site. Under each subsection the codes are arranged by procedures. For example, under the heading "Neck," codes for procedures performed on various parts of the neck, the

esophagus, thyroid, larynx, trachea; lymphatic system; and the major vessels are listed.

Coding for Surgery

The Surgery section is the largest section in CPT. The subsections found in the Surgery section and how they are broken down into the body systems is shown in Figure 19-8 ◆.

The anatomic arrangement of each subsection is as follows:

- Head
- Neck (Soft Tissue) and Thorax

TABLE 19-5 P CODE MODIFIERS FOR ANESTHESIA BILLING

P Code	Patient Condition	Description
P1	Normal and healthy	Modifier indicates the patient is normal and healthy
P2	Mild systemic disease	Modifier indicates the patient has some form of mild systemic disease, such as hypertension
P3	Severe systemic disease	Modifier indicates the patient has a severe systemic disease that could affect the care of the patient. May be used for a patient who has congestive heart failure or uncontrolled diabetes.
P4	Severe systemic disease that threatens life	Modifier indicates the patient has a severe systemic disease that is a threat to life, such as a patient with a life-threatening blood clot
P5	Expected to die without the procedure	Modifier used for patients who are critically injured and require emergency surgery
P6	Brain-dead and being prepped to remove organs for transplant	Modifier used for a patient who is brain dead and being maintained on life support for organ removal

Source: CPT 2008. Copyright 2008 American Medical Association. All rights reserved.

CPT is a registered trademark of the American Medical Association.

+99100	Anesthesia for patient of extreme age; younger than 1 one year and older than 70
+99116	Anesthesia complicated by utilization of total body hypothermia
+99135	Anesthesia complicated by utilization of controlled hypotension
+99140	Anesthesia complicated by emergency conditions (specify) (list separately in addition to code for primary anesthesia procedure)

Figure 19-7 ◆ Qualifying circumstances for anesthesia.
CPT only copyright 2008 American Medical Association. All rights reserved.

- Back and Flank
- Spine (Vertebral Column)
- Abdomen
- Shoulder
- Humerus (Upper Arm) and Elbow
- Forearm and Wrist
- Hand and Fingers
- Pelvis and Hip Joint
- Femur (Thigh Region) and Knee Joint
- Leg (Tibia and Fibula) and Ankle Joint
- Foot and Toes
- Application of Casts and Strapping
- Endoscopy/Arthroscopy.

Within each heading there is also a consistent theme of procedures described, such as:

- Incision
- Excision
- Introduction or Removal
- Repair, Revision, and/or Reconstruction

Integumentary System	10021–19499
Musculoskeletal System	20000–29999
Respiratory System	30000–32999
Cardiovascular System	33010–39599
Digestive System	40490–49999
Urinary System	50010–53899
Male Genital System	54000–55980
Female Genital System	56405–58999
Maternity Care and Delivery	59000–59899
Endocrine System	60000–60699
Nervous System	61000–64999
Eye and Ocular Adnexa	65091–68899
Auditory System	69000–69979
Operating Microscope	69990

Figure 19-8 ◆ The subsections found in the Surgery section.
CPT only copyright 2008 American Medical Association. All rights reserved.

CPT is a registered trademark of the American Medical Association.

- Fracture and/or Dislocation
- Arthrodesis/Amputation

A surgical CPT code is a bundled code. As mentioned earlier, a *bundled code* is a single CPT code used to report a group of related procedures as in the surgical package. Unbundling occurs when separate procedures are reported that should have been included under a bundled code. This practice will result in denial of a claim.

A surgical package includes specific services in addition to the operation, including these:

- One related E/M encounter on the date immediately prior to or on the date of procedure, subsequent to the decision for surgery
- Preparing the patient for surgery including local infiltration, topical anesthesia
- Performing the operation, including normal additional procedures, such as debridement
- Immediate postoperative care, including dictating operative notes, talking with the family and other physicians
- Writing orders
- Evaluating the patient in the postanesthesia recovery area
- Typical postoperative followup.

The typical postoperative care includes follow up visits for normal uncomplicated care. Each third-party payer determines the number of days in which this followup care may take place. Therefore, it is important when certifying for surgery to ask the global period of the third-party payer. The **global period** refers to the number of days surrounding a surgical procedure during which all services relating to that procedure—preoperative, during the surgery, and **postoperative**—are considered part of the surgical package. This is also referred to as the **global surgical concept**. To determine global days, information from the insurance carrier or other payers may need to be obtained. Many publications and software packages on the market address global days for most carriers and unbundling.

Third-party payers have varying definitions of what constitutes a surgical package and varying policies about what is to be included in the surgical package. Because surgical package rules define what is or is not included in addition to the surgical procedure, the surgery also defines the services for which additional charges can or cannot be submitted.

Two types of services are not included in surgical package codes. These services are reported separately and reimbursed in addition to the surgical package fee:

- Complications, exacerbations, recurrence, or the presence of other diseases or injuries requiring additional services should be reported separately.
- Care for the condition for which a diagnostic surgical procedure was performed or of other coexisting conditions is not included and may be reported separately.

An area of great concern in medical billing is inaccurately billing separately for procedures considered incidental to the major procedure. Many CPT surgical narratives in the CPT book include "with or without" or other language to include or exclude incidental services. Numerous procedures are done in conjunction with other procedures, and often the CPT code subsection notes and guidelines will indicate that a particular code includes a variety of the supporting procedures.

The CPT book further states that followup care for complications, exacerbations, recurrence, and the presence of other diseases that require additional services is not included in the surgery package. General anesthesia for surgical procedures is not part of the surgical package, and the anesthesiologist bills general anesthesia services separately.

Supplies and materials provided by the physician (e.g., sterile trays/drugs) over and above those usually included with procedures rendered are listed separately.*

Wound repair is coded according to wound size and location. The *CPT-4* describes three types of wound repair: (1) simple, (2) intermediate, and (3) complex. Simple wound repairs involve closing partial or full-thickness wounds to the skin and subcutaneous tissues with no deep structure involvement. Intermediate repairs impact one or more deep layers of subcutaneous tissue and nonmuscle fascia, as well as the skin. Complex repairs are closures of layered wounds that require such added work as scar revision, debridement, or retention sutures.

To bill for wounds appropriately, healthcare providers must measure and record all repairs in centimeters. When more than one wound classification is repaired, the most complicated should be listed as the primary procedure and the less complicated should appear as secondary. When wound repair involves nerves, blood vessels, and/or tendons, medical assistants should locate codes from the proper surgery sections of the CPT-4 code book.

EXAMPLE

A patient presents to the medical office with a laceration on his scalp. The laceration measures 2 cm and is therefore coded with CPT code 13120—Repair, complex, scalp, arms and/or legs; 1.1 cm to 2.5 cm.

When providers complete multiple procedures on the same day, they must code those procedures separately and order them on the CMS-1500 claim form from major to minor. Major procedures are complex, "serious" surgeries, while minor procedures

are simpler ones. Assume, for example, a patient has a tonsillectomy, a chin wound repair, and a small mole removed from the nose all on the same day. For this patient, the medical assistant would place the most important surgery, the tonsillectomy, at the top of the claim form, and the least serious one, the small mole removal, at the bottom.

EXAMPLE

Coding for the above patient would be listed as follows: 42826—Tonsillectomy, primary or secondary; age 12 or over, followed by code 12011—Simple repair of superficial wound of face, ears, eyelids, lips and/or mucous membranes; 2.5 cm or less, followed by code 11400–Excision benign lesion including margins, trunk, arms, or legs; excised diameter 0.5 cm or less.

Coding for Radiology

The codes in the Radiology section are used to report radiological services performed by or supervised by a physician. Radiology codes may have two parts:

1. Results are the technical component of a service. Testing leads to results. The technical component is the part of the relative value associated with the procedure that reflects the test, technologist, the equipment, and processing including preinjection and postinjection services such as local anesthesia, placement of a needle or catheter, and injection of contrast material. The technical component of taking the x-ray would be reported with the procedure code and the modifier "-TC" attached to the procedure.
2. Results lead to interpretation. Reports are the work product of the interpretation of numerous test results. The professional component is the part of the relative value associated with a procedure that represents a physician's skill, time, and expertise used in performing it, as opposed to the technical component. The reading, interpretation, and the written report of the radiological examination by the physician would be the professional component and the modifier "-26" would be attached to the procedure.

These modifiers are to be used only when the physician's office states that only part of the radiological procedure was done; otherwise, the descriptor remains as stated with no modifier.*

Contrast material is commonly used for imaging enhancement. Contrast material improves visualization and evaluation of the body structure or organ studied. Some of the procedures listed in the Radiology section of the CPT book may be performed with or without the use of contrast material for imaging enhancement. The phrase "with contrast" used in the codes for procedures using contrast for imaging enhancement represents contrast material administered intravascularly, intra-articularly, or intrathecally. When contrast materials are only administered orally and/or rectally, the study does not qualify as "with contrast" and should be coded "without contrast."

*Source: Vines, Deborah, Braceland, Ann, Rollins, Elizabeth, and Miller, Susan. *Comprehensive Health Insurance: Billing, Coding, and Reimbursement.* © 2008, Pearson Education, Inc. Upper Saddle River, NJ. Reprinted with permission.

CPT is a registered trademark of the American Medical Association.

Coding for Pathology and Laboratory

The codes in the Pathology/Laboratory section cover services provided by physicians or by technicians under the supervision of a physician. A complete procedure includes:

- Ordering the test
- Taking and handling the sample
- Performing the actual test
- Analyzing and reporting on the test results.

The 8000 series codes are used to report the performance of specific laboratory tests only and do not include the collection of the specimen via venipuncture (or finger/heel/ear stick), arterial puncture, or other collection methodology (e.g., lumbar puncture). The collection of the specimen by venipuncture or by arterial puncture is not considered an integral part of the laboratory procedure(s) performed. Codes in the 36400-36425 series are used to report venipuncture for obtaining blood samples.

Organ or disease-oriented panels are reported with the codes from the 80048–80076 series. These panels were developed for coding purposes and should not be interpreted as clinical standards for testing. A *panel* is a group of tests ordered together to detect particular diseases or malfunctioning organs. When a panel is reported, all of the listed tests must have been performed with no substitution. If fewer tests are performed than those listed in the panel code (unbundling), then the individual code number(s) for each test should be listed rather than the panel code.

EXAMPLE

80051 Electrolyte Panel
This panel must include the following:

Carbon dioxide	(82374)
Chloride	(82435)
Potassium	(84132)
Sodium	(84295)

Procedures and services are listed in the index under the following types of main terms:

- Name of the test, such as urinalysis, drug test
- Procedure such as hormone assay
- Abbreviations such as CBC, RBS, TLC
- Panel of tests, under Blood Tests.

Some medical practices have laboratory equipment and perform their own testing. In office labs must be certified by the Clinical Laboratory Improvement Amendment (CLIA) of 1988, which awards three levels of certification. The lowest level for an in-office certified lab can perform dipstick urinalysis and

urine pregnancy. If the medical practice does not have a lab but obtains the specimen for the lab, the venipuncture code 36415 may be billed for obtaining the blood sample. As in every medical setting, the Occupational and Safety and Health Administration (OSHA) regulates safety.

Although Medicare does not allow physicians to bill for lab work they did not perform, other third-party payers do. When a medical practice has a contract with a lab (pays the lab for the work), it may bill for the tests reported. The modifier 90 is attached to the code for the lab test. On the CMS-1500, form locator 20 must say "yes" and the fee the medical practice pays the lab must be entered under "Charges." Also, form locator 32 must report the name and address of the lab.

Coding for Medicine

The Medicine section of the CPT book contains a variety of listings for reporting procedures and services provided by many different types of healthcare providers. In addition, many services and procedures provided by nonphysician practitioners can be found in the Medicine section. For example, codes in the physical medicine and rehabilitation subsection are often used to report the services and procedures provided by physical and occupational therapists. Audiologists and speech therapists find listings in the special otorhinolaryngologic services subsection that describes some of the technical procedures and services they provide.

Codes from the Medicine section may be used with codes from any other section. Add-on codes and separate procedure codes are included in the Medicine section.

Immunizations require two codes, one for administering the immunization and the other for the particular vaccine or toxoid that is given (Figure 19-9 ◆).

The descriptors for injections require two codes, one for administering the immunization and the other for the particular vaccine or toxoid that is given.

Cardiac catheterizations are the most commonly performed surgical procedure, with more than 1 million performed each year. Complete coding of cardiac catheterization requires at least three codes: a code for the catheterization procedure itself, a code for the injection procedure, and a code for the imaging supervision and interpretation. Each of these has a professional and a technical component. Unless the physician owns the laboratory, those codes are billed using modifier 2.6.*

*Source: Vines, Deborah, Braceland, Ann, Rollins, Elizabeth, and Miller, Susan. *Comprehensive Health Insurance: Billing, Coding, and Reimbursement.* © 2008 Pearson Education, Inc. Upper Saddle River, NJ. Reprinted with permission.

90471	Immunization administration
90710	Measles, mumps, rubella, and varicella vaccine (MMRV), live, for subcutaneous use

Figure 19-9 ◆ Coding for immunizations.

CPT is a registered trademark of the American Medical Association.

Unlisted Procedure Codes

When physicians perform procedures not in the coding book, medical assistants must use "unlisted procedure codes" and submit copies of procedure reports with claims. When procedure reports are not submitted, claims may be denied or delayed. To ensure timely, accurate processing, procedure reports should contain the following:

- Reason the procedure was needed
- Time the procedure took
- Complexity of patient's symptoms
- Patient's final diagnosis
- Examination findings pertinent to the procedure
- Diagnostic or therapeutic procedures that led to the procedure
- Any concurrent patient problems
- Any needed followup care

The Health Care Common Procedure Coding System (HCPCS)

The **Health Care Common Procedure Coding System (HCPCS),** called "Hick Picks" in the industry is a set of codes developed and maintained by CMS for the reporting of professional services, non-physician services, supplies, durable medical equipment (**DME**) and injectable drugs. Historically, HCPCS has had three levels.

CPT codes are Level I HCPCS codes for professional services.

Level II codes are alphanumeric codes that begin with a letter, followed by four numbers, for example, A4356. Typically, when professionals refer to "HCPCS codes," they are referring to Level II codes. Level II codes cover supplies, DME, drugs, non-physician providers, and certain physician services for Medicare and Medicaid. When CPT and HCPCS codes exist for the same service, use the CPT code. When procedure descriptions differ, HCPCS Level II codes have priority. They are required by Medicare and Medicaid. They have been mandated as a HIPAA uniform code set for all insurance carriers, but implementation is in progress. Be sure to check with private carriers to verify if they accept HCPCS Level II codes. Reimbursement for supplies and equipment is usually faster when HCPCS codes are used, because they are more specific than

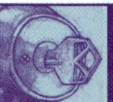

Keys to Success
BILLING FOR MEDICARE PATIENTS

For Medicare patients, avoid billing for injections on the same day as exams. Medicare will not pay visit codes and injections on the same visits. When offices accidentally bill for both, Medicare throws out the visit code and funds the injection only. As a result, the office receives the lesser of two fees.

CPT is a registered trademark of the American Medical Association.

using the generic CPT code for supplies, 99070. A list of the categories in Level II appears in Table 19-6. Level II codes are updated on a quarterly basis; the manual is published annually in October. Quarterly updates are available on the CMS Web site at www.cms.gov.

Level III HCPCS codes were developed by regional Medicare carriers, but are being phased out under HIPAA's administrative simplification provision, which requires uniform code sets.

The HCPCS Level II coding manual contains an alphabetical index and a tabular listing. As with the other coding manuals, use the alphabetical index first to locate the item or service, then refer to the tabular list to verify. Many DME manufacturers print a suggested HCPCS code on the item packaging. This is a useful aid, but the code should always be verified in the manual. Many entries in the manual also contain cross-reference information to Medicare reimbursement rules for the specific item or service.

HCPCS Level II also contains alphanumeric modifiers that can be used with either Level I CPT codes or Level II codes. The most commonly used modifiers are those that designate specific anatomical sites of procedures and non-physician provider types (Table 19-7). Many additional modifiers exist for specific Medicare

TABLE 19-6 LEVEL II HCPCS CODES	
Transportation services	A0000-A0999
Medical and surgical supplies	A4000-A7509
Miscellaneous and experimental	A9000-A9999
Enteral and parenteral therapy	B0000-B9999
Temporary hospital outpatient PPS	C0000-C9999
Dental procedures	D0000-D9999
Durable medical equipment (DME)	E0000-E9000
Procedures and services, temporary	G0000-G9999
Rehabilitative services	H0000-H9999
Drugs administered other than oral method	J0000-J8999
Chemotherapy drugs	J9000-J9999
Temporary codes for DMERCS	K0000-K9999
Orthotic procedures	L0000-L4999
Prosthetic procedures	L5000-L9999
Medical services	M0000-M9999
Pathology and laboratory	P0000-P9999
Temporary codes	Q0000-Q9999
Diagnostic radiology services	R0000-R9999
Private payer codes	S0000-S9999
State Medicaid agency codes	T0000-T9999
Vision	V0000-V2999
Hearing services	V5000-V5999

TABLE 19-7 COMMON HCPCS MODIFIERS

Modifier	Description
AH	Clinical psychologist
AJ	Clinical social worker
AS	Assistant at surgery service
CC	Procedure code change
E1	Upper left eyelid
E2	Lower left eyelid
E3	Upper right eyelid
E4	Lower right eyelid
F1	Left hand, second digit
F2	Left hand, third digit
F3	Left hand, fourth digit
F4	Left hand, fifth digit
F5	Right hand, thumb
F6	Right hand, second digit
F7	Right hand, third digit
F8	Right hand, fourth digit
F9	Right hand, fifth digit
FA	Left hand, thumb
GA	Signed advance beneficiary notice (ABN) form on file (for Medicare patients)
LT	Left side
PC	Professional courtesy
Q6	Locum tenens medical doctor (MD) service
QW	Clinical Laboratory Improvement Amendments Act (CLIA) waived test
RT	Right side
SA	Nurse practitioner with physician
SB	Nurse midwife service
TC	Technical component

Source: www.cms.gov

and Medicaid reimbursement situations. One of the most important of these is the modifier GA that indicates a Medicare Advanced Beneficiary Notice (ABN) form was signed by the patient when a covered service is expected to be denied (see ∞ Chapter 17). Through experience, medical assistants become familiar with the specific requirements for their medical office.

Ensuring Proper Reimbursement

To receive proper payment for medical services, healthcare teams must keep adequate, accurate, and complete patient medical and billing records. The adage, "If it isn't charted, it wasn't done," applies.

To keep proper medical records, medical offices must undertake accurate and comprehensive procedure coding. Proper coding begins with the right tools: an up-to-date *CPT-4* coding book, a HCPCS book, and a medical dictionary. Outdated coding tools can provide outdated codes, and outdated codes risk claim delay or denial. Once the right tools are on hand, every service or procedure must be documented in electronic or paper form, and before any claims are sent to insurance companies.

When medical assistants are asked to code charts with incomplete service or procedure documentation, those assistants must route the charts back to the healthcare providers who performed the services. While rerouting may delay insurance claim submission, in the long run it proves faster, and more effective than inaccurate or incomplete claims.

Critical Thinking Question 19-3

Assume Lydia complied with Dr. Anderson's request to bill Medicare for higher codes, what might Medicare do, and why?

In Practice

Linnea has been working in the billing office of a large pediatric practice for 11 years. She is responsible for entering the procedure codes for three of the practice's physicians. One of the physicians has left the office earlier than usual and Linnea finds that the charges were not circled on the last two patients' fee slips. Because Linnea has tomorrow off, she won't be able to ask the physician about the charges until the following week. Linnea thinks it will be all right if she guesses at the charges rather than wait until next week. What other options does Linnea have?

CPT is a registered trademark of the American Medical Association.

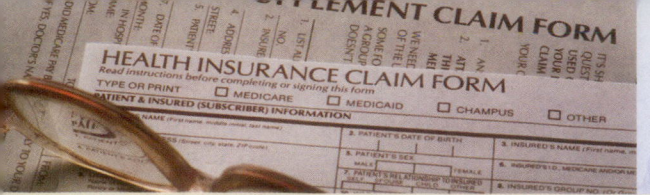

Chapter Summary

- The CPT coding book is designed to standardize the coding process by requiring healthcare providers to choose a procedure code based on the explicit description.
- Accurate CPT coding involves a number of steps, including determining correct codes via chart notes.
- Modifiers are an integral part of procedural coding, serving to add detail to procedure codes. By using modifiers, the coder is able to further identify any special circumstances that surround that particular service for that patient.
- The Health Care Common Procedure Coding System (HCPCS) provides codes for reporting nonphysician services, supplies, or durable medical equipment (DME), and certain physician services for Medicare and Medicaid.
- In all forms of coding, accurate documentation and reimbursement are tightly linked. Insurers will often request copies of patient healthcare records in order to determine the necessity of care rendered. Having accurate records of the services provided is helpful in timely and accurate payment of claims.
- Coding and billing fraud impose severe penalties. It includes falsifying medical records, billing for services not performed, and intentionally charging incorrect patients. Providers who are caught intentionally submitting fraudulent claims may be arrested and charged with crimes. In addition, they risk the loss of their licenses, practices, and preferred provider status.
- Bundling of services is the process of charging one procedure code for a group of charges that typically are performed at the same time. For bundled procedures, coders may not unbundle the charges, or charge for each procedure individually. This would be unbundling and insurance carriers consider this practice to be fraudulent.

Chapter Review

Multiple Choice

1. Procedure codes are always _____ digits long.
   a. three
   b. four
   c. five
   d. six

2. Anesthesia codes begin with
   a. 0.
   a. 1.
   a. 2.
   a. 3.

3. "Standardized" procedural coding means that every healthcare provider
   a. uses the same code to describe the same service.
   b. references the same book to look up codes.
   c. employs only registered or certified medical assistants as coders.
   d. all of the above.

4. The "CPT" acronym in the *CPT-4* code book stands for
   a. Correct Procedural Terminology.
   b. Current Procedural Terminology.
   c. Causal Procedural Terminology.
   d. none of the above.

True/False

T F 1. E&M codes are rarely used in healthcare.
T F 2. All insurance carriers today reimburse healthcare providers based on UCR charges.
T F 3. The time a physician spends with a patient is the most important factor in code selection.
T F 4. All insurance companies have the same number of followup days in their fee schedules.
T F 5. Wound repair is coded depending on the wound's location and size.

Short Answer

1. When a physician performs a procedure not found in the *CPT-4* coding book, how is that procedure billed?

2. What are the four classifications of history and physical examinations for E&M codes?

3. What are the four classifications of decision making for E&M codes?

4. Define a physical status modifier and how it is used for coding.

5. What does it mean to "unbundle" codes?

6. What are the three types of wound repairs in the CPT-4 coding book?

7. When multiple procedures are performed on the same day, how should they appear on the CMS-1500 billing form?

8. What are the four classifications of radiology codes?

9. Explain what is meant by "upcoding."

10. Describe three patient-billing situations that require modifiers.

11. Describe the relationship between accurate documentation and proper reimbursement.

Chapter Review (continued)

Research

1. Interview a person who works in the billing office of a local medical office. How does that office handle the process of procedural coding? Do the physicians assign the codes?

2. Go to your state's Department of Health Web site. What resources are available for providers who have questions about proper coding?

3. Look at your state's Medicaid Web site. What are some of the rules Medicaid applies regarding the use of procedure codes?

Externship Application Experience

Willie Harrison, a Medicare-covered patient, arrives at Dr. Annissette's office, and the physician removes two skin flaps from Willie's neck. After the procedure, the physician circles one procedure code on the superbill and writes "× 2" next to it to indicate the medical assistant should charge for two procedures. What is the proper way for the medical assistant to indicate to Medicare that the patient had two skin flaps removed?

Resource Guide

American Medical Association
515 N. State Street
Chicago, IL 60610
Phone: (800) 621-8335
www.ama-assn.org

Center for Medicare and Medicaid Services
7500 Security Boulevard
Baltimore, MD 21244
Phone: (877) 267-2323
www.cms.hhs.gov

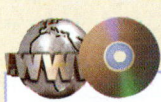

Med**Media**

http://www.MyMAKit.com

More on this chapter, including interactive resources, can be found on the Student CD-ROM accompanying this textbook and on http://www.MyMAKit.com.

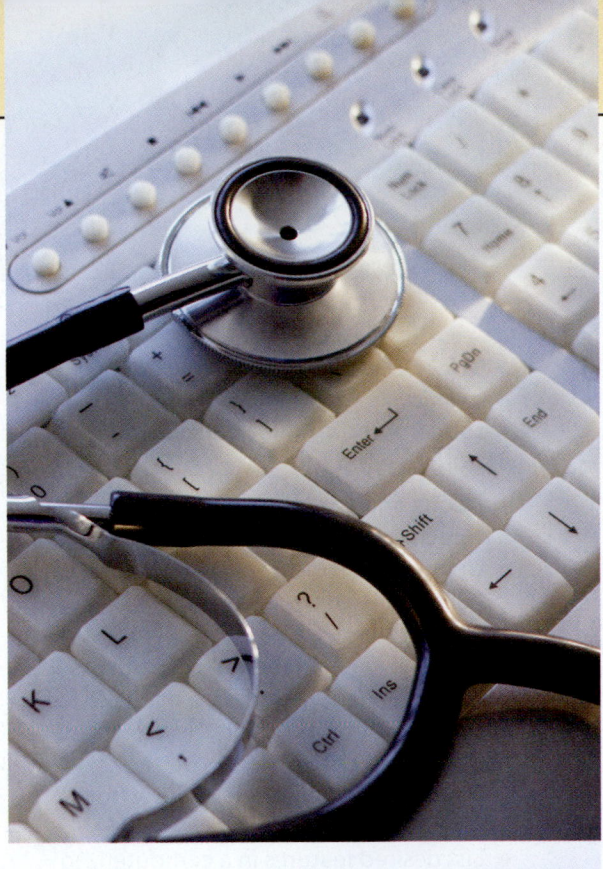

UNIT **VI**

Accounts Payable and Banking Procedures

Chapter 20   **Billing, Collections, and Credit**

My name is Amy Walter and I love my job as a medical assistant. I get to help people every day. My days consist of taking vitals, giving shots, scheduling appointments, assisting the doctor, making multiple phone calls, and sending faxes—sometimes all at once! It is a fast-paced, but rewarding job. Every day there is a new challenge that I must face. Patients come to me for help, and I do everything in my power to get them the help that they need.

I feel so lucky to be working in a large family practice with an amazing doctor. The doctor–medical assistant relationship is so important for excellent patient care. It is imperative for the medical assistant to have an open line of communication with doctors and other medical office staff. The most valuable thing I have learned working as a medical assistant is that it is okay to say "I don't know." Individuals will become better providers if they are able to admit that they don't know everything. It is okay to ask questions and look things up.

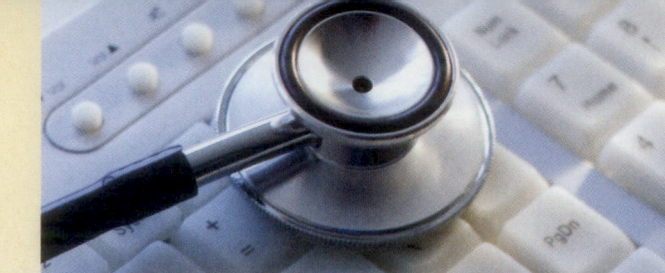

Billing, Collections, and Credit

Case Study

Millie Alonso owes $550 for services her young son received, but she has made no payments for two months. As a result, her account now appears as past due. The medical assistant must call Millie to determine when she will send payment, either in full or by installment.

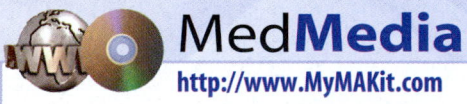

http://www.MyMAKit.com

Additional interactive resources and activities for this chapter can be found on http://www.MyMAKit.com. For a video, tips, audio glossary, legal and ethical scenarios, on-the-job scenarios, quizzes, and games related to the content of this chapter, please access the accompanying CD-ROM in this book.

Video: *Collecting Money*
Legal and Ethical Scenario: *Billing, Collections, and Credit*
On the Job Scenario: *Billing, Collections, and Credit*
Tips
Multiple Choice Quiz
Audio Glossary
HIPAA Quiz
Games: Spelling Bee, Crossword, and Strikeout

Objectives

After completing this chapter, you should be able to:

- Define and spell the key terminology in this chapter.
- Define the medical assistant's role in billing, collections, and credit.
- Identify the three types of payment typically made in the medical office.
- Describe the functions of a manual billing system, including the use of day sheets and charge slips.
- Discuss how computers are used for billing in the medical office.
- List desired features in a computerized medical billing system.
- Post payments to manual and computerized billing systems.
- Prepare an accounts receivable trial balance.
- Outline how professional fees are determined, and create a fee schedule.
- Review a managed care contract, and determine if participating would benefit the practice.
- Review the medical office's accounts receivables, and manage those accounts effectively.
- Verify patient identification.
- Create coherent collection policies in the medical office, and explain them to patients.
- Describe the various types of collection issues in managed care.
- Research collection agencies, and describe their pros and cons.
- Describe the medical assistant's role when account overpayments are made.
- Describe how small claims court works for the medical office, and discuss the pros and cons of using this method to collect past-due accounts.

✚ MEDICAL ASSISTING STANDARDS

CAAHEP ENTRY-LEVEL STANDARDS

- Perform within scope of practice (psychomotor)
- Apply ethical behaviors, including honesty/integrity in performance of medical assisting practice (affective)
- Explore issue of confidentiality as it applies to the medical assistant (cognitive)
- Respond to issues of confidentiality (psychomotor)
- Apply local, state, and federal healthcare legislation and regulation appropriate to the medical assisting practice setting (psychomotor)
- Recognize the importance of local, state, and federal legislation and regulations in the practice setting (affective)
- Use office hardware and software to maintain office systems (psychomotor)
- Document accurately in the patient record (psychomotor)
- Explain general office policies (psychomotor)
- Demonstrate telephone techniques (psychomotor)
- Explain basic bookkeeping computations (cognitive)
- Demonstrate sensitivity and professionalism in handling accounts receivable activities with clients (affective)
- Differentiate between bookkeeping and accounting (cognitive)
- Perform accounts receivable procedures (psychomotor)
- Discuss precautions for accepting checks (cognitive)
- Compare types of endorsement (cognitive)
- Differentiate between accounts payable and accounts receivable (cognitive)
- Compare manual and computerized bookkeeping systems used in ambulatory healthcare (cognitive)
- Describe common periodic financial reports (cognitive)
- Explain both billing and payment options (cognitive)
- Identify procedure for preparing patient accounts (cognitive)
- Describe the impact of both the Fair Debt Collection Act and the Federal Truth in Lending Act of 1968 as they apply to collections (cognitive)
- Discuss types of adjustments that may be made to a patient's account (cognitive)
- Utilize computerized office billing systems (psychomotor)

ABHES ENTRY-LEVEL COMPETENCIES

- Adapt to change
- Maintain confidentiality at all times
- Use appropriate guidelines when releasing records or information
- Project a positive attitude
- Be cognizant of ethical boundaries
- Evidence a responsible attitude
- Conduct work within scope of education, training, and ability
- Professional components
- Monitor legislation related to current healthcare issues and practices
- Orient patients to office policies and procedures
- Adapt what is said to the recipient's level of comprehension
- Adaptation for individualized needs
- Locate resources and information for patients and employers
- Use proper telephone techniques
- Application of electronic technology
- Apply computer concepts for office procedures
- Apply managed care policies and procedures
- Obtain managed care referrals and pre-certification
- Follow established policy in initiating or terminating medical treatment
- Establish and maintain a petty cash fund
- Perform basic secretarial skills
- Prepare a bank statement
- Reconcile a bank statement
- Maintain records for accounting and banking purposes
- Post entries on a day sheet
- Prepare a check
- Post collection agency payments
- Use manual and computerized bookkeeping systems
- Manage accounts payable and receivable
- Be courteous and diplomatic

Key Terminology

accounts receivables (AR)—money owed the medical practice

aging report—documentation of the money owed the medical office and how long accounts have been outstanding

certified letter—postal service letter that the recipient must sign for upon receipt

collection agency—company that pursues overdue accounts for a fee

community property laws—legislation that deems one spouse financially responsible for the other spouse's debts

day sheet—used with a manual pegboard system to document and track the charges and payments within the medical office

dual fee schedule—facility or healthcare provider with two fees for the same service

Fair Debt Collection Act—law that dictates how debts may be collected

fee schedule—list of services and their fees

geographical practice cost index (GPCI)—Medicare system of adjusting fees based on the area in which the healthcare provider practices

hardship agreement—agreement a patient signs to indicate an inability to pay full healthcare costs due to financial hardship

insurance fraud—illegal act by a healthcare provider involving an insurance company

ledger card—document used to track services rendered and payments made; used with manual pegboard systems

national conversion factor—number released by Medicare each year that determines fee schedules for all healthcare services

national standard—point of reference for developing charges for healthcare services used throughout the United States

Omnibus Budget Reconciliation Act (OBRA)—legislation passed by Congress in 1989 to calculate healthcare service fees by formula

patient billing statements—monthly statements sent to patients who have an outstanding balance

pegboard accounting system—manual bookkeeping system

Key Terminology *(continued)*

posting—process of adding charges or payments to a patient's account

professional courtesy—to give a patient a discount, or free service, due to the fact that the patient is a healthcare professional

relative value unit (RVU)—numeric value assigned by Medicare to formulate fee schedules for healthcare providers

superbill—document that indicates the services performed with a patient on a given visit; also called an encounter form

tickler file—tool for tracking future events, such as patient appointments

uncollectible—account believed never to be paid

write off—to remove a balance from a patient account

Abbreviations

AR—accounts receivable

CMS—Center for Medicare and Medicaid Services

CPT—Current Procedural Terminology

GPCI—geographic price cost index

HIPAA—Health Insurance Portability and Accountability Act

NCR—no carbon required

NSF—nonsufficient funds

OBRA—Omnibus Budget Reconciliation Act

RBRVS—resource-based relative value scale

RVU—relative value unit

✔ COMPETENCY SKILLS PERFORMANCE

1. Post an entry on a day sheet.
2. Prepare an accounts receivable trial balance.
3. Explain professional fees to a patient.
4. Call a patient regarding an overdue account.
5. Send a patient billing statement.
6. Post a nonsufficient funds check.
7. Post an adjustment to a patient account.
8. Post a collection agency payment.
9. Process a patient refund.
10. Process an insurance company overpayment.

Introduction

To stay in business, the medical office must be financially sound. Service fees, a vital facet of an office's success, must be in line with federal and local laws, as well as consistent from patient to patient. **Dual fee schedules**, which impose different fees on different patients, are fraudulent. In healthcare, billing, collections, and credit are best undertaken equitably and communicated about openly.

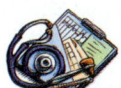

The Medical Assistant's Role in Billing, Collections, and Credit

The medical assistant is responsible for explaining fees to patients and collecting those fees when needed. Because patients may stop seeing providers due to misunderstandings with their accounts, the MA must be sure to keep miscommunication from happening in this area and always speak to patients about fees before services, especially expensive services, are performed.

Identifying Payment Basics

Patients typically make three types of payment in the medical office: (1) cash, (2) check, and (3) debit or credit card. With cash payments, medical assistants should write receipts as documents both for patients and the office. Keeping a copy of the receipt in the medical office helps discourage stealing by the office staff. With a paper trail, medical assistants or office managers can easily track all office cash.

When patients offer personal checks as payment, medical assistants must verify that the check's written amount matches the check's number amounts. Assistants must also ensure that checks are dated and signed. When assistants take checks from parties other than patients, those assistants should request the check writers' photo identification to verify the writers' identities. Many medical offices do not accept third party checks. When checks are suspicious or for large amounts, assistants should call the issuing banks to ensure funds are available. When checks are marked "Payment in Full," assistants must verify that the checks are for the full amount owed by the patient. When they are not, patients may later argue that no additional payment is required.

For the third and final payment type, debit or credit cards, providers pay bank fees in the amount of 1 to 3 percent of charges, depending on providers' credit card use when they accept credit card payments from patients. Some offices use check-verification systems that, while costly, guarantee checks. Some of these systems simply check to see if patients have written bad checks. Others are more sophisticated, holding the patient's bank funds until the check clears. As such systems become more sophisticated, however, their costs increase.

Manual Billing Systems

As most medical offices adopt computerized accounting systems, manual billing systems, also called **pegboard accounting systems**, have been losing popularity in healthcare. With pegboard systems, staff responsible for **posting** charges place **day sheets** on pegboards at the start of each business day (Figure 20-1 ◆). The day sheet is a document where the medical assistant records the charges for services and payments received throughout the day. Patients' **ledger cards**, which carry information including patients' current and previous balances, are placed on the day sheets under **superbills**. Staff write patients' charges and payment information on the ledger card, being sure to press hard enough on the no carbon required (**NCR**) paper to impact all copies. At the end of the day, or the end of the sheet if more than one sheet is used in a day, staff must total all columns to calculate the day's charges and collections. The collection total must match the bank deposit amount.

Computerized Billing Systems

With the decline of manual billing systems in the medical office, computerized systems have become the norm. While computerized systems vary, most allow staff to:

- Post charges and payments to patient accounts
- Print insurance billing forms and patient billing forms
- Create **aging reports** (documentation of the money owed the medical office and how long the account has been outstanding) that detail patients' owed amounts

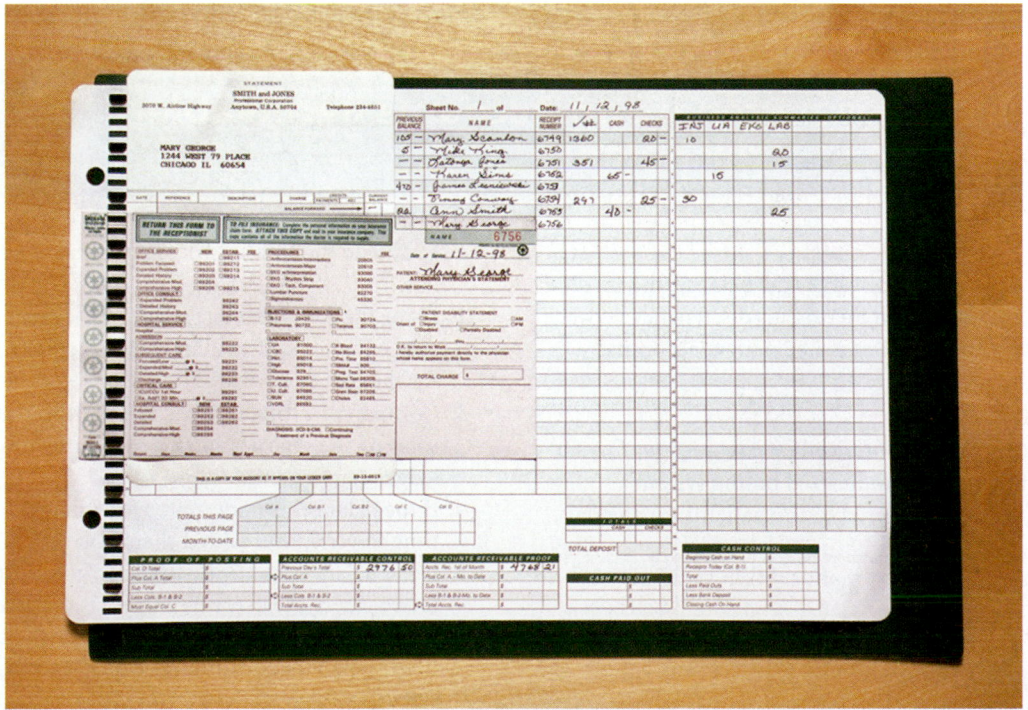

Figure 20-1 ◆ Pegboard accounting system.

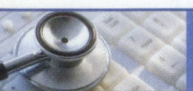

PROCEDURE 20-1 Post an Entry on a Day Sheet

Theory and Rationale

Proper use of the pegboard accounting system includes strict attention to details, such as numbers and letters. Medical assistants using the pegboard system must be able to write legibly and use a ten-key calculator skillfully.

Materials

■ Pegboard
■ Day sheet
■ Patient ledger card
■ Superbill
■ Blue or black ink pen
■ Calculator

Competency

(**Conditions**) With the necessary materials, you will be able to (**Task**) post an entry on a day sheet (**Standards**) correctly within the time allowed by the instructor.

1. Place the patient's ledger card on the day sheet.
2. Place the patient's superbill on top of the ledger card.
3. Pressing hard enough to impact all copies, enter the date, procedures, charges, and any payment in the appropriate boxes.
4. In the appropriate box, enter the new balance.
5. Verify that the entry appears on all copies.
6. File the patient's ledger card.

Most medical billing programs offer a wide variety of reports. Such reports can list information like all patients with birthdays in any given month or all female patients over age 40 who have not had a mammogram in the past year.

Billing systems with basic features like reports are affordable for most medical offices. Higher level features increase systems' prices. Some systems, for example, offer integrated electronic appointment books. Others send insurance claims electronically and receive insurance payments electronically. Some systems even allow remote access, which means healthcare teams can access their billing systems when out of their offices. To ensure that the office receives the software package it needs, the medical assistant or office manager should research a number of options. Online, the Web site www.2020software.com lists the most popular medical billing programs on the market and allows users to order demo CDs of programs at no charge.

Fee Schedules

In 1989, the U.S. Congress passed the **Omnibus Budget Reconciliation Act** (**OBRA**), in part to require that physician reimbursement for Medicare services be based on a **fee schedule** (Figure 20-2 ◆). Fee schedules set maximum amounts for services using the resource-based relative value scale (**RBRVS**), which is designed to reduce Medicare costs and establish a

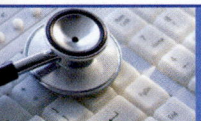

PROCEDURE 20-2 Prepare an Accounts Receivable Trial Balance

Theory and Rationale

By preparing an accounts receivable trial balance, the medical assistant is able to determine if there is any discrepancy between the daily journal and the ledger or the patient accounts.

Materials

■ Patient accounts in computerized or paper ledger format
■ Computer, if using a computerized billing system
■ Fee slips for services rendered to the patients for the day
■ Calculator
■ Pegboard system, if using a manual billing system
■ Pen

Competency

(**Conditions**) With the necessary materials, you will be able to (**Task**) prepare an accounts receivable trial balance (**Standards**) correctly within the time limit set by the instructor.

1. Calculate the total of the charges on the fee slips for the day.
2. Using the computer or the manual ledger card system, calculate the total of the charges posted to patient accounts for the day.
3. Compare the total of the charges from the fee slips to the total of the charges in the computer or on the manual ledger card system.
4. If the balances do not match, calculate the totals a second time to verify you added them correctly.
5. If the balances continue to differ, go through the fee slips to see where the error in entry has occurred.
6. Correct the entry error and calculate the totals again.
7. If the balances continue to differ, go through the above steps until they match.

AUDIOLOGY SERVICES		
Screening audio air only	92551	$ 38.00
Pure tone air	92552	$ 37.00
Pure tone air and bone	92553	$ 50.00
Comprehensive audio	92557	$101.00
Loudness balance test	92562	$ 38.00
Tone decay	92563	$ 41.00
Tympanography	92567	$ 40.00
Acoustic reflex	92568	$ 42.00
Reflex decay	92569	$ 43.00
Visual reinforced audio	92579	$ 78.00
Brain stem audiogram	92585	$327.00

Figure 20-2 ◆ Sample fee schedule.

national standard for physician payment. This national standard is itself based on the Current Procedural Coding (**CPT**) codes used for patient visits.

Medicare service fees are calculated based on the five following factors:

- Service intensity
- Time needed for the service
- Skills needed to perform the service
- Practice's overhead
- Practice's malpractice premiums

Physicians' fees are adjusted according to a **geographical practice cost index (GPCI)**, which factors in the differing healthcare costs across the United States. Together, these factors determine a healthcare provider's **relative value unit (RVU)**. The RVU was devised by the Centers for Medicare and Medicaid Services (**CMS**) as a way for physicians to create a fee schedule for the services they render. RVUs take into account three factors: how much work by the physician is involved in performing the service, what sort of expertise the physician needs to have in order to perform the service, and the cost of the physician's malpractice insurance policy.

Each year, Medicare assigns a **national conversion factor** that is added to the RVU. The national conversion factor is a number released by Medicare each year that determines fee schedules for all healthcare services. The national conversion factor is multiplied by the physician's RVU for any given service or procedure to determine the allowed fee for that service. For example, imagine CPT code 99205 has an RVU of 4.78 for a healthcare provider practicing in the Los Angeles area, and the national conversion factor is 37.5623. This would make the Medicare allowed charge for this service $179.55 (4.78 × 37.5623 = $179.55). Because most health insurance plans base their fee schedules on the Medicare fee schedule, the Medicare allowed charge is typically considered the maximum charge any insurance plan will allow for any given service or procedure.

In Practice

Dr. Bowman wants to raise his prices for certain services. He tells his medical assistant he fails to understand why insurance companies do not pay him more simply because he has begun charging more. What can the medical assistant say about fee schedule determination?

Participating Provider Agreements

Most patients with private health insurance are covered by managed care plans, which are detailed in ∞ Chapter 17. As a condition of participation, managed care plans credential healthcare providers and require those providers to apply. When providers agree to participate in managed care plans, they agree to accept predetermined fee schedules. Some managed care plans also dictate the type of medications providers can prescribe and the types of specialist referrals those providers are allowed to make.

Participating provider agreements range from several pages long to small-book size. Though it may be time consuming, physicians should read their agreements in full. Once providers have signed with plans, they are obligated to see patients with that coverage for the agreed-upon fees, which may be lower than providers are willing to accept.

The best way to review participating provider agreements is with a highlighter. Medical assistants should highlight all areas of interest or concern, especially any details about fee schedules or provider care restrictions, and then review the highlighted areas with the physicians. Objections to any item may be grounds for declining plan participation.

Credit and Collections

The best way to ensure that patients pay their bills properly is to discuss the medical office's credit and collection policies before services are rendered. Medical assistants should discuss all fees and outline all payment policies. When patients will make regular payments on their balances, for example, medical assistants should provide written contracts that stipulate the payment amounts and due dates (Figure 20-3 ◆). Such contracts avoid confusion and reduce or eliminate patient questions.

To further help ensure payment terms are clear, many medical offices include important financial information in their office brochures and send these brochures, along with registration paperwork and fee and credit policies, before patients arrive for their first visits. Figure 20-4 ◆ identifies some items that should be included in introductory brochures. Well informed patients help avoid collection problems. Copayments, for example, should be paid at visit check-in.

Each state has a statute of limitations that sets the maximum time in which healthcare providers can collect patient debts. Because Medicare and many managed care insurance companies prohibit providers from billing patients until insurance companies have issued explanations of benefits outlining the amounts patients owe, it is crucial to bill insurance providers

May 21, 2010

I, [patient's name], agree to pay Monroe Family Practice $100 every 2 weeks until my $800 balance is paid in full. I understand that finance charges will not accrue while I am making these payments and that if I stop making payments before my balance is paid in full finance charges in the amount of 12% annually will begin to accrue on the remaining balance.

Patient Signature   Date

_____

Witness Signature   Date

_____

Figure 20-3 ◆ Sample payment contract.

❑ Requirement for payment at the time of service, if any
❑ Allowable time frame for payment (e.g., "within 30 days")
❑ Guidelines for insurance claim submission on patients' behalf
❑ Time the medical office will carry an outstanding balance
❑ Credit limit extended to patients
❑ Percentage of finance charges that will accrue on a balance and when starting (e.g., after 30 days, after 60 days)
❑ Point at which accounts are turned over to collection agencies
❑ Process for assigning benefits to the provider

Figure 20-4 ◆ Payment policies in an office brochure.

soon after the service is provided so that the patient portion can be billed in a timely manner. Table 20-1 outlines the number of years from the patient's last date of service or last billing statement that a healthcare provider may send a bill to a patient.

Critical Thinking Question 20-1

Would Millie be more or less likely to have a balance due if someone in the medical office had discussed a payment plan when services were rendered? Why?

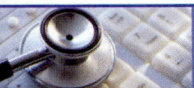

PROCEDURE 20-3 Explain Professional Fees to a Patient

Theory and Rationale

Patients who clearly understand fees for physician services are better equipped to make healthcare choices, as well as understand their bills. When patients do not understand the fees they incur in the medical facility, this confusion can lead to nonpayment of the bill.

Materials

- Patient medical record
- Copy of office fee schedule
- Blue or black pen
- Payment contract

Competency

(**Conditions**) With the necessary materials, you will be able to (**Task**) explain the physician's professional fees to a patient (**Standards**) correctly within the time limit set by the instructor.

1. Find a private location to sit with the patient.
2. Explain to the patient the procedure the physician has prescribed.
3. Explain to the patient the fee for the procedure.
4. Explain to the patient any insurance coverage for the fee.
5. Explain to the patient the payment amount and deadline.
6. Secure an agreement from the patient about the payment date.
7. Enter the payment agreement and arrangements on the payment contract.
8. On the payment contract, obtain the patient's signature and sign as the witness.
9. Answer any questions the patient may have about the fee or the procedure.
10. Place the payment agreement in the patient's financial record.

TABLE 20-1 STATUTES OF LIMITATIONS
ON HEALTHCARE DEBTS

State	Number of Years	State	Number of Years
AL	6	MT	8
AK	6	NE	5
AZ	6	NV	6
AR	5	NH	3
CA	4	NJ	6
CO	6	NM	6
CT	6	NY	6
DE	3	NC	3
D.C.	3	ND	6
FL	5	OH	15
GA	6	OK	5
HI	6	OR	6
ID	5	PA	6
IL	10	RI	15
IN	10	SC	10
IA	10	SD	6
KS	5	TN	6
KY	15	TX	4
LA	10	UT	6
ME	6	VA	5
MD	3	VT	6
MA	6	WA	6
MI	6	WI	6
MN	6	WV	10
MS	3	WY	10
MO	10		

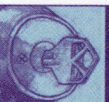

Keys to Success
INFORMATION REQUIRED ON PATIENT REGISTRATION FORMS

Medical offices should request certain pieces of information on their patient registration forms to make tracking patients, and therefore debt collection, easier. For example, offices should request patients' employers' names and telephone numbers, as well as the names and numbers of emergency contacts who do not live with the patients. Emergency contact information helps provide options for contacting the patient when patients' accounts become past due and medical assistants cannot reach patients at home.

In terms of credit, medical offices should predetermine the amounts they are willing to extend to patients, document those amounts in policies, and apply the policies equitably. The healthcare provider may not pick and choose the patients who will receive an extension of credit. The credit extension policy must apply to every patient in the facility.

Verifying Patient Identification

When new patients visit the medical office, medical assistants must copy those patients' driver's licenses and insurance cards, front and back (Figure 20-5 ◆). Such documentation confirms the patient's identity and can help the assistant track the patient for collection purposes.

Managing Accounts Receivables

Any successful medical office must manage its **accounts receivables (AR)**, which is the money owed the office from all sources, including patients, insurance companies, worker's compensation, Medicare, and Medicaid. AR management, which entails documenting how much money is owed the

office, by whom, and for how long, is a weighty task and so must be done regularly and thoroughly.

As mentioned earlier, medical billing programs can run reports, some on AR accounts. Aging reports are important to AR management for a number of reasons. When physicians wish to take business loans, for example, banks will request documentation on AR accounts. Some malpractice insurance companies are beginning to examine physicians' AR before extending policies. Physicians with high or old AR are considered greater risks to insure.

The most effective way to collect money on past due accounts is to speak with patients while they are in the office. When face-to-face communication is not possible, the next most effective method is calling patients, but from private office locations to safeguard patient confidentiality. Medical assistants making such calls must pay strict attention to the law regarding collections and document all calls and conversations, as well as any patient messages, in patients' financial records. Table 20-2 outlines procedures for telephone collection calls.

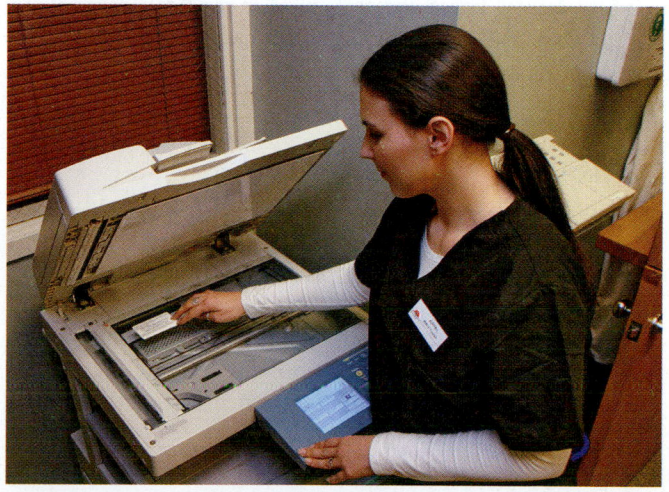

Figure 20-5 ◆ The medical assistant should make a copy of both sides of the patient's insurance card.

TABLE 20-2 DOs AND DON'Ts FOR COLLECTION TELEPHONE CALLS

Do	Don't
Call the patient from a private location in the medical office.	Call the patient from a location where other patients can overhear.
Call the patient between 8 A.M. and 9 P.M.	Call the patient despite the patient's wishes.
Verify the patient's identity.	Speak with anyone except the patient or the patient's parent or guardian about the patient's bill.
Be respectful, polite, and professional.	
Tell the patient the reason for the call.	Call repeatedly if the patient fails to answer or return messages.
Keep the conversation short and to the point.	Become angry if the emotion arises.
Document any promises the patient makes.	Make promises that cannot be kept, such as reducing the bill.
Follow up on any of the patient's promises.	Converse about topics other than the subject of the call.
	Neglect to document all parts of the conversation with the patient.

Collection in Managed Care

Some medical offices collect entire first-day visit fees from patients, but the practice is not recommended if the patient is covered by managed care. Some managed care plans strictly govern how much money, if any, providers may collect from patients. When offices participate with Medicare, for example, providers are disallowed from charging patients for covered services at the time of service. Instead, those providers must bill Medicare and then bill the patients for the portions Medicare states those patients owe.

When speaking with patients about fees or payments, it is important to remember that people tend to associate payment with value. When medical assistants act embarrassed about fees, or fail to ask for payment, they give the impression that the physician's services lack value.

Forgiving Deductibles or Copayments

It is illegal, and in fact considered **insurance fraud**, for healthcare providers to forgive patients' deductibles or copayments. When patients cannot pay their bills and physicians agree to treat them for lesser or no fees, those patients must sign and date **hardship agreement** letters for their file (Figure 20-6 ◆). Hardship letters become part of patients' permanent medical records.

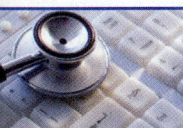

PROCEDURE 20-4 Call a Patient Regarding an Overdue Account

Theory and Rationale
Even with the most efficient administrative staff, every medical office has patients who are slow to pay and have long overdue accounts. These accounts require medical assistants to act, such as call the patients. These telephone calls must be made professionally and documented appropriately.

Materials
- Telephone
- Patient's ledger information
- Blue or black pen

Competency
(**Conditions**) With the necessary materials, you will be able to (**Task**) call a patient regarding an overdue account (**Standards**) correctly within the time limit set by the instructor.

1. Dial the patient's home telephone number.
2. If you reach the patient:
   - Identify yourself and the name of your clinic and state the reason for the call.
   - Ask the patient when payment on the outstanding bill will be made.
   - If the patient agrees to pay via credit card, take the credit card information over the telephone, verify the amount to be charged, charge the credit card, and mail the patient a receipt.
   - If the patient agrees to mail payment to the office, secure a date by which the payment is to be received and note the date in the patient's billing ledger.
   - If the patient expresses an inability to make a payment at this time, secure a date by which the patient expects to be able to make a payment and note the date in the patient's billing ledger.
3. If unable to reach the patient, leave a message that discloses no personal information about the patient's care in the office.
4. Note the message in the patient's billing ledger.

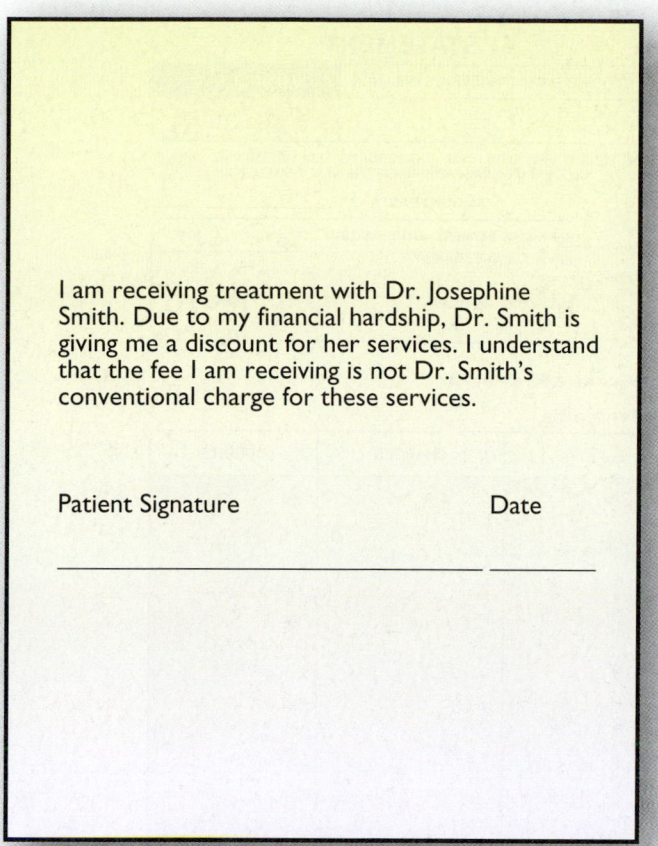

I am receiving treatment with Dr. Josephine Smith. Due to my financial hardship, Dr. Smith is giving me a discount for her services. I understand that the fee I am receiving is not Dr. Smith's conventional charge for these services.

Patient Signature   Date

_____   _____

Figure 20-6 ◆ Sample hardship agreement.

Patients Who File for Bankruptcy

Patients who are unable to pay their medical bill may file for bankruptcy. A Harvard study performed in 2005 found that inability to pay medical bills is the leading cause of bankruptcy filings, affecting nearly 2 million Americans each year. Depending upon the type of bankruptcy the patient files, the medical office may or may not be repaid any of the amount outstanding on the patient's account. Since bankruptcy is designed to protect debtors from further collection activity, the medical office may no longer contact the patient for payment of the account once the patient has filed a bankruptcy claim.

Patients may file bankruptcy of one of the five following types:

1. *Chapter 7*—All nonexempt patient assets are sold and the proceeds distributed to creditors. Secured creditors, like mortgage or car loans, are paid first; unsecured creditors, like medical providers, are paid last. This type of bankruptcy is considered complete in that most or all patient debt dissolves. If the patient's assets are less than the debts, the medical office may not receive any of the amount outstanding and may have to write off the patient's balance.
2. *Chapter 9*—Used for town reorganizations. This does not apply to medical bills.
3. *Chapter 11*—Used for business reorganizations. This does not apply to medical bills.

4. *Chapter 12*—Used by farmers who cannot meet their financial obligations. This does not apply to medical bills.
5. *Chapter 13*—Protects debtors from creditors while the debtors arrange to repay all or some of their debts over three- to five-year periods. When those periods end, the balances on most debts dissolve.

Professional Courtesy

Physicians who treat other physicians for free or at greatly reduced fees extend what is called **professional courtesy**. Such courtesy is often extended to family or friends of the physician, to the family of other physicians, or even to such professional associates as the physician's attorney or accountant.

In cases of professional courtesy, accurate patient charts are vital to avoid the appearance of fraud or impropriety. Medical assistants should have any patients in these situations sign professional courtesy agreements, such as, "I understand Dr. Jones is giving me a professional courtesy discount for services rendered."

Patient Billing Statements

Medical offices should set aside a day each month to send **patient billing statements** to patients with balances due (Figure 20-7 ◆), preferably after the first of the month when rent and mortgages are typically due. Patient billing statements that arrive mid- to late month are more likely to be paid in a timely fashion.

While patient billing statements are one means of securing patients' payment, collecting patient copays at the time of office visit is far more cost effective. Monthly billing statements have been shown to cost about $8 per month per bill. To provide incentive, healthcare providers can offer discounts, called "cash discounts," to patients who pay their bills in full. However, such discounts should not exceed 5 percent of total fees or the provider may be accused of having a dual fee schedule, which is considered insurance fraud.

? Critical Thinking Question 20-2

Should medical offices have policies to offer discounts to patients like Millie when those patients agree to pay their full bills via credit card during collection calls? Why or why not?

Collecting from patients while those patients are in the office is the most effective way to collect payment. When patients with past due accounts are due in for appointments, medical assistants should ask the receptionist to route those patients to the billing department before those patients receive treatment. In private areas out of other patients' hearing range, the assistants can then remind the patients of their balances. When patients cannot provide payment in full, the assistants should make payment arrangements with the patient.

Heritage Park Women's Clinic
14 Heritage Way
Heritage Park, IN 12345

STATEMENT

CLOSING DATE	PREVIOUS BALANCE	BALANCE DUE
10/2/09	0	20.00

NOTE: ALL PAYMENTS AND CHARGES POSTED AFTER THE ABOVE
CLOSING DATE WILL APPEAR ON THE NEXT STATEMENT.

AMOUNT PAID $ _____

BANKCARD PAYMENT AUTHORIZATION	☐ VISA	☐ M/C
VISA M/C ACCOUNT NUMBER		
CARDHOLDER SIGNATURE		EXP. DATE

Lillian Vidali
2715-16th Drive SW
Heritage Park, IN 12345

PLEASE DETACH AND **RETURN** THIS STUB WITH YOUR PAYMENT TO INSURE PROPER CREDIT

RETAIN THIS PORTION FOR YOUR RECORDS.

DATE OF SERVICE	DOCTOR / CPT CODE	DESCRIPTION	CHARGES	CREDITS
9/7/09	Wilson/99211	Office Visit	62.00	
9/20/09	Wilson	Insurance payment 9/7/09		42.00

PAST DUE					CURRENT		BALANCE DUE
0	0	0	0		20.00	▶	20.00
OVER 120 DAYS	OVER 90 DAYS	OVER 60 DAYS	OVER 30 DAYS		0 - 30 DAYS		

COMMENTS: Payment due by 11/10/09

Figure 20-7 ◆ Sample patient billing statement.

Dismissing Patients Due to Nonpayment

When patients are chronically late with payments or refuse to pay at all, providers can dismiss those patients from care via **certified letter**. Figure 20-8 ◆ provides an example of a dismissal letter to a patient. Providers must give patients at least thirty days to receive care, but after that period providers are no longer bound to provide treatment. Physicians who do not honor this commitment may be sued for patient abandonment. Patients should be dismissed only after physicians have given their consent, and a signed receipt verifying that the patient received the certified letter has been filed in the patient's permanent medical records.

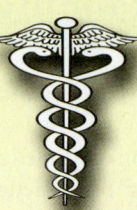

Marian Williams, MD
Markson Family Practice
2323 Front Street
Yonkers, NY 12345

Joseph Paterniti
41 Bronxville Ave
Yonkers, NY 12345

January 31, 2009

Dear Mr. Paterniti:

Our office has tried several times to contact you regarding your outstanding balance with us. Because we have failed to reach you, I must dismiss you as a patient. Please find a new physician and notify this office within 30 days if you would like your medical records transferred. If you need care within the next 30 days, you may still patronize this office. After 30 days, you will be disallowed from making another appointment with us.

Sincerely,

Marian Williams, MD

Figure 20-8 ◆ Sample dismissal letter.

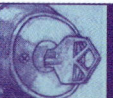

Keys to Success
BILLING FOR THE PHYSICIAN'S FRIENDS AND FAMILY

Medicare prohibits physicians from billing for the treatment they provide their relatives or household members. Immediate relatives include the physician's spouse, parent, children, siblings, grandparents, grandchildren, stepparents, stepsisters, stepbrothers, and stepchildren. Household members include anyone living in the same home as the physician, like a nanny, maid, butler, chauffer, medical caregiver, or assistant. Boarders, people who rent rooms from physicians, are not considered household members.

Charging Interest on Medical Accounts

Medical providers who wish to charge interest on past due balances must be sure to check the laws in their states. Any changes in financial policy, including the decision to charge interest on accounts, requires providers to post written notices in prominent office locations at least thirty days before the financial changes occur.

Addressing Checks That Fail to Clear

When patients provide "bounced" or nonsufficient funds (**NSF**) checks, which are checks drawn on insufficient funds, most banks charge the medical office a fee. As a result, offices can

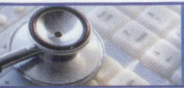

PROCEDURE 20-5 Send a Patient Billing Statement

Theory and Rationale

Nearly every medical office sends monthly billing statements to patients with outstanding balances. These billing statements must be Health Insurance Portability and Accountability Act (**HIPAA**)–compliant and sent on or near the same day each month. In order to be HIPAA compliant, the statement must be sent in a security envelope (one that does not allow for the contents to be viewed without opening the envelope).

Materials

- Computer with medical billing software
- Printer (computerized billing)
- Patient ledger card (manual billing)
- Copy machine (manual billing)

Competency

(**Conditions**) With the necessary materials, you will be able to (**Task**) send a patient billing statement (**Standards**) correctly within the time limit set by the instructor.

1. Manual billing: Make a photocopy of the patient's ledger card.
   - Make a notation on the ledger card of the date and write "Bill to Patient" on the ledger.
   - Verify that the information on the ledger is correct, including that the balance has been correctly totaled.
   - Place the copy of the ledger card in an envelope.
   - Stamp the envelope, and place it in the mail.
2. Computerized billing: Within the billing software, follow the appropriate steps to print a patient billing statement.
   - Once printed, verify the information on the bill is correct.
   - Place the copy of the ledger card into an envelope.
   - Stamp the envelope and place it in the mail.

---

legally charge patients a fee in return. Most banks redeposit NSF checks only once, so when checks cannot be redeposited, medical assistants must contact the patients to inform them of their checks' return and communicate the fee charged by the office. In such conversations, assistants should determine the date by which the patient will send a replacement payment. At the end of the interaction, assistants should make any relevant notations in the patient's billing ledger.

Contacting Nonpaying Patients

When patients fail to pay their monthly billing statements by the date due, medical assistants should try to contact the patients regarding payment. Unless patients have instructed otherwise, it is legal to contact patients at their places of employment. Once assistants reach patients, they should communicate the outstanding balance and ask when payment may be expected. When patients agree to dates and amounts, assistants should make notations in a **tickler file**. Serving as a reminder, a tickler file facilitates followup should payment fail to arrive when expected. Tickler files can be manual, as in index cards in a small box, or electronic. Many medical software programs have such reminder mechanisms.

In addition to making notes in tickler files, assistants should follow up with patients in writing. Letters should outline conversation details, including the amount owed on the account, the agreed-upon payment amount and due date, and any followup actions in the event of nonpayment. Many medical offices send a return envelope with these letters to give the patient an easy way to mail the payment to the office.

HIPAA Compliance

HIPAA regulations prevent members of the healthcare team from leaving messages with live parties or on voice mail when those messages may violate patient confidentiality. It is inappropriate, for example, to mention that a message is about a past due balance. An appropriate message is, "This is Ceila from Dr. Stewart's office. I need to leave a message for John Cooper to call me at (425) 555-9899." Document all phone calls in the patient's financial ledger.

Critical Thinking Question 20-3

Imagine that Millie agrees to pay $100 on her credit card now and $100 per month for the next four months. What is the best means the medical assistant has for tracking this agreement?

Sending Patients Collection Letters

When patients continue to be delinquent in their accounts, medical assistants can send those patients letters stating the amounts owed and any requested payment terms. Figure 20-9 ◆ gives an example. Some offices have their office managers, clinic directors, or healthcare providers try to contact the patients. Whatever procedure an office follows, the medical assistant must be sure to consistently and carefully apply the same guidelines to all patients.

When patients ignore medical offices' efforts to collect their accounts, offices may send those patients' accounts to

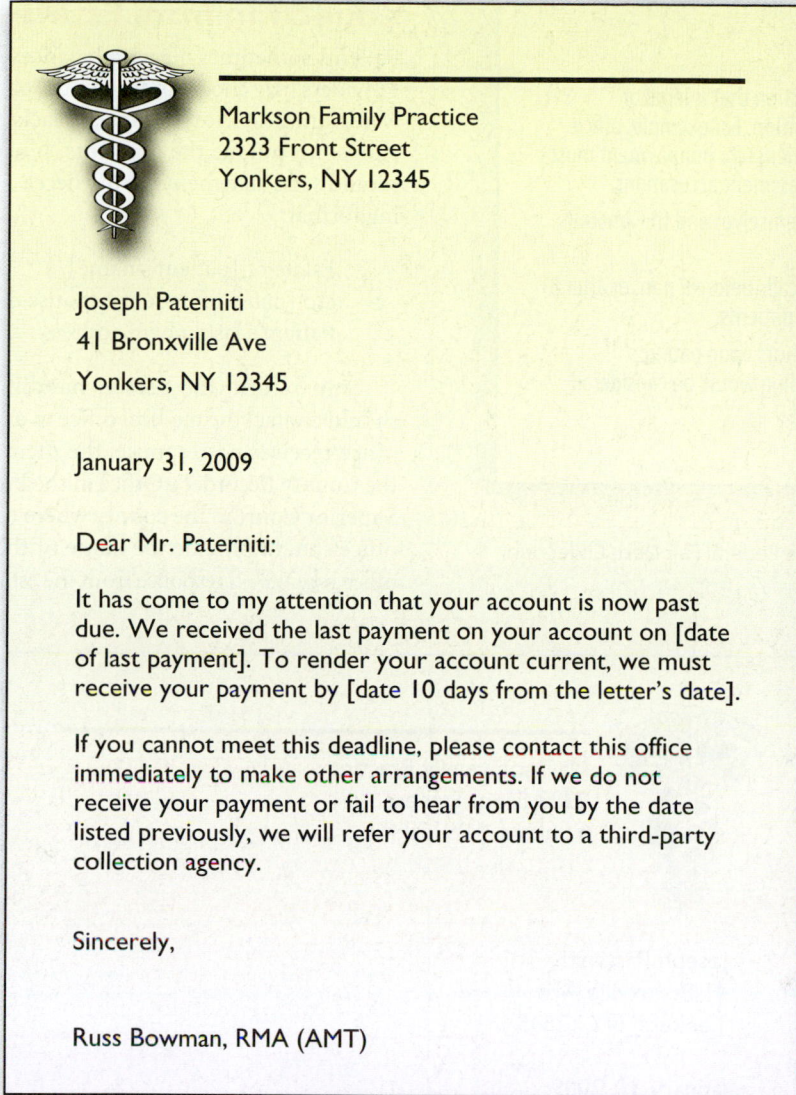

Markson Family Practice
2323 Front Street
Yonkers, NY 12345

Joseph Paterniti
41 Bronxville Ave
Yonkers, NY 12345

January 31, 2009

Dear Mr. Paterniti:

It has come to my attention that your account is now past due. We received the last payment on your account on [date of last payment]. To render your account current, we must receive your payment by [date 10 days from the letter's date].

If you cannot meet this deadline, please contact this office immediately to make other arrangements. If we do not receive your payment or fail to hear from you by the date listed previously, we will refer your account to a third-party collection agency.

Sincerely,

Russ Bowman, RMA (AMT)

Figure 20-9 ◆ Sample collection letter to a patient.

collection agencies, write off the balances, or take the patients to small claims court. All these options require the physicians' consent, however.

When offices choose **collection agencies** to collect past due accounts, those collection agencies must be reputable. Other medical offices are good sources for agency references. Collections companies should actively pursue accounts, not harass or offend patients. Such agencies must also abide by federal guidelines for debt collection (Figure 20-10 ◆). The **Fair Debt Collection Act** was enacted to eliminate abusive, deceptive, and unfair collection practices. This law applies to all consumer debt for personal, family, or household purposes.

Once accounts go to collections, offices typically write off the balances owed. Collection agencies typically charge percentage fees for their services. The standard rate is 33 percent of the amount owing. Therefore, if a patient owes $99 when

the office sends the account to collections, the provider is paid $66.00 when the collection agency collects the account in full ($99.00 − $33.00). Some collection agencies charge flat dollar amounts to collect accounts, which is most cost effective for large accounts. To maximize their collections efforts, medical offices can use multiple collection agencies.

Uncollectible Accounts

Some offices choose to **write off** accounts deemed **uncollectible** to maintain patient relations. Patients may have legitimate reasons for nonpayment, such as the death of a spouse or the loss of a job. This is legal and should only be done with the physician's approval. When medical offices choose to write off patients' owed balances, medical assistants must send the patients letters to that effect (Figure 20-11 ◆). Copies of the letters should reside in the patients' files.

Medical offices must:

❏ Threaten to take only action that is legal or intended to come to fruition. For example, offices that threaten to sue patients for nonpayment must file lawsuits or face harassment accusations.

❏ Accurately represent themselves and the amounts patients owe.

❏ Make collection phone calls before 9 p.m. or after 8 a.m. unless directed by patients.

❏ Stop calling about accounts upon patients' requests. Continued calling would be considered harassment.

Figure 20-10 ◆ Highlights of the Federal Fair Debt Collection guidelines.

Collecting from Estates

Patients sometimes die with balances owed the medical office. Providers may choose to forgive the balances when the deceased were unmarried, for example, or lacked assets. When providers choose to pursue the amounts, however, medical assistants should send statements to the deceased's estates in the following format:

> Estate of [patient's name]
> c/o [name of patient's spouse or next of kin]
> Patient's last known address

In return, the person handling the deceased's estate should contact the medical office to arrange for payment. If the office receives no response, the medical assistant can contact the County Recorder's Office in the Probate Department of the Superior Court in the county where the deceased resided. This office should provide the name of the estate's executor. If the office receives no response from the estate's executor, the assistant

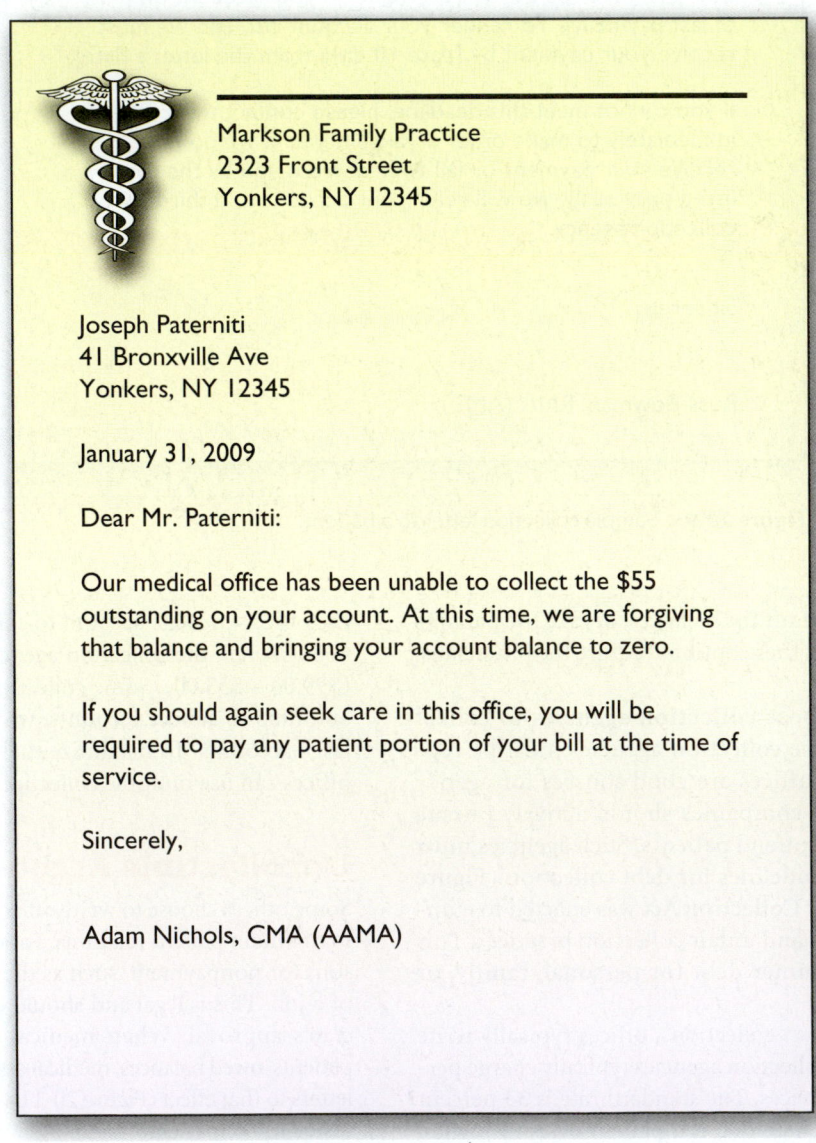

Markson Family Practice
2323 Front Street
Yonkers, NY 12345

Joseph Paterniti
41 Bronxville Ave
Yonkers, NY 12345

January 31, 2009

Dear Mr. Paterniti:

Our medical office has been unable to collect the $55 outstanding on your account. At this time, we are forgiving that balance and bringing your account balance to zero.

If you should again seek care in this office, you will be required to pay any patient portion of your bill at the time of service.

Sincerely,

Adam Nichols, CMA (AAMA)

Figure 20-11 ◆ Sample letter forgiving a patient balance.

PROCEDURE 20-6 Post a Nonsufficient Funds Check

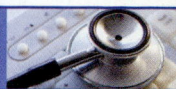

Theory and Rationale

When medical offices receive nonsufficient (NSF) checks from patients, those checks must be handled according to office policy and with respect for the patients. As with any patient conversations about finances, NSF check discussions must be clearly noted in patients' financial records.

Materials

- Check returned due to NSF
- For manual billing:
  - Patient billing ledger
  - Day sheet
  - Blue or black pen
- For computerized billing:
  - Computer with medical billing software

Competency

(**Conditions**) With the necessary materials, you will be able to (**Task**) post an NSF check (**Standards**) correctly within the time limit set by the instructor.

1. Verify that you have the correct patient ledger.
2. When billing manually:
   - Place the patient's ledger on the day sheet.
   - On the ledger card, record the NSF check and any applicable fees.
   - Calculate the new total on the account.
3. When using computer billing software:
   - Enter the NSF check and any fees into the patient's ledger.
4. Notify the patient via phone that the check was returned. Indicate any corresponding fees.
5. Secure a date by which a replacement payment will be received.
6. In the patient's financial record or ledger, note the outcome of the conversation.

should gather the proper forms from the County Clerk's office to file a claim against the estate for the amount owed. In general, medical offices have from 2 to 36 months to act. While a claim remains outstanding, the assistant should continue sending the estate's executor monthly billing statements.

Overpayment on Accounts

Account overpayments can occur for a number of reasons, including when patients overpay on their accounts or when insurance policies pay unexpectedly high amounts or when

PROCEDURE 20-7 Post an Adjustment to a Patient Account

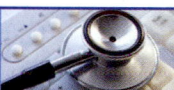

Theory and Rationale

Once medical offices have sent accounts to collection agencies, the balances of those accounts are typically written off. To effect this change, medical assistants must post adjustments to those accounts.

Materials

- For manual billing:
  - Patient's ledger
  - Day sheet
  - Blue or black pen
  - Calculator
- For computerized billing:
  - Medical billing software

Competency

(**Conditions**) With the necessary materials, you will be able to (**Task**) post an adjustment to a patient account (**Standards**) correctly within the time limit set by the instructor.

1. When billing manually:
   - Place the patient's billing ledger on the day sheet.
   - Pressing hard enough to impact all layers of paper, enter the type of adjustment on the ledger card.
   - Add or subtract adjustments as appropriate.
   - Calculate the new balance.
   - Enter the new balance on the ledger card.
2. When billing via computer:
   - Locate the correct patient ledger in the computer.
   - Enter the adjustment as a debit or a credit.
3. In the patient's financial record, note the reason for the adjustment.

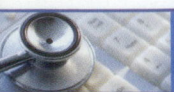

PROCEDURE 20-8 Post a Collection Agency Payment

Theory and Rationale

When collection agencies send medical offices payments on accounts, medical assistants must properly post the payments and make appropriate debit adjustments.

Materials

- For a manual posting system:
  - Day sheet
  - Ledger card
  - Pegboard
  - Calculator
  - Blue or black pen
  - Collection agency payment
- For a computerized posting system:
  - Calculator
  - Computer
  - Collection agency payment

Competency

(**Conditions**) With the necessary materials, you will be able to (**Task**) post a collection agency payment (**Standards**) correctly within the time limit set by the instructor.

1. When using a manual system:
   - Verify which patient account will receive the payment.
   - Align the patient's ledger card with the next line on the day sheet.

- In the appropriate columns, enter the patient's name, previous balance, payment date, payment amount, and name of the collection agency.
- In the checks column of the day sheet's deposit section, enter the payment amount.
- Subtract the payment from the previous patient balance.
- Record the new balance on the patient's ledger card.
- When an adjustment is to be made to the account due to collection agency fee, record the amount in brackets [ ] in the adjustment column of the ledger card and enter as the description "collection agency fee."
- Subtract the amount of the adjustment from the previous patient balance, and record the new balance on the patient's ledger card.

2. When using a computerized system:
   - Find the patient's account in the computer.
   - Verify the patient account is correct.
   - Post the payment, choosing "collection payment" as the payment source.
   - If applicable, enter any adjustment due to collection agency fee.
   - Verify the payment amount and adjustment.
   - Save all changes.

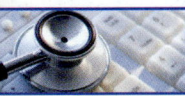

PROCEDURE 20-9 Process a Patient Refund

Theory and Rationale

When patient balances are overpaid, credit balances result. Research is needed to return credit balances to the appropriate parties. When patients are owed refunds, medical assistants must know how to post those refunds.

Materials

- For manual billing:
  - Patient ledger card
  - Day sheet
  - Blue or black pen
  - Calculator
- For computerized billing:
  - Computer with medical billing software

Competency

(**Conditions**) With the necessary materials, you will be able to (**Task**) process a refund to a patient (**Standards**) correctly within the time limit set by the instructor.

1. When billing manually:
   - Place the patient's ledger card on the day sheet.
   - Pressing hard enough to impact all copies, enter "Patient Refund" on the line.
   - Enter the dollar amount of the refund being sent to the patient.
   - Add the refund amount to the patient's balance.
   - Enter the new balance in the proper box.
2. When billing via computer:
   - Locate the proper patient ledger in the billing software.
   - Enter the refund amount.
   - Choose the adjustment code for "Refund to Patient."
3. Obtain a refund check from the physician or office manager.
4. Send the refund check to the patient.
5. In the patient ledger, note the party receiving the refund and the number of the refund check.

PROCEDURE 20-10 Process an Insurance Company Overpayment

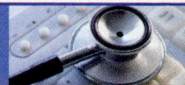

Theory and Rationale

When credits appear on patient accounts due to insurance company overpayment, medical assistants must process refunds to those companies. The medical assistant must carefully review the file to determine the appropriate insurance company to receive the refund.

Materials

- For manual billing:
  - Patient ledger card
  - Day sheet
  - Blue or black pen
  - Copies of insurance companies' explanations of benefits
- For computerized billing:
  - Computer with medical billing software
  - Copies of insurance companies' explanations of benefits

Competency

(**Conditions**) With the necessary materials, you will be able to (**Task**) process a refund to an insurance company (**Standards**) correctly within the time limit set by the instructor.

1. Using the insurance companies' explanations of benefits, determine which company is the patient's primary insurance carrier and which is secondary.
2. When billing manually:
   - Place the patient's ledger card on the day sheet.
   - Pressing hard enough to impact all copies, enter the refund amount and write "refund to insurance company." The refund amount is written in the adjustment column on the patient ledger.
   - Enter the new balance.
3. When billing via computer:
   - Find the appropriate patient ledger in the computer.
   - Using the appropriate code, enter the refund to the insurance company.
4. Obtain a refund check from the physician or office manager.
5. Send a note to the insurance company explaining the reason for the refund, as well as copies of the primary and secondary insurance companies' explanations of benefits.

---

patients have multiple policies that together pay more than owed. When overpayments occur, careful review is needed to identify the party to receive the refund.

Collections Through Small Claims Court

Small claims court is yet another option for collecting on past due accounts. To pursue a small claims suit, the patient's balance owing must fit the "small claim" criteria in the state where the provider's office is located.

Depending on the laws in the states where medical assistants work, those assistants may be able to file claims online or through the mail. Some states require claims to be filed in person at the local county courthouse. All methods incur a cost at the time of filing. Notice of the suit must be served on the

patient by someone who does not work in the medical office. Often, offices hire companies specializing in this task.

When small-claims cases enter court, staff from the medical office must appear to testify. The office representative will need a copy of the patient's account ledger and any documentation proving the healthcare provider treated the patient. Any signed documentation indicating the patient agreed to pay any outstanding bill is also important to bring. Typically, in small claims court, the healthcare provider's office need only prove that the patient was treated and that the patient knew of the charges for the service. Providers often win judgment in these cases, and patients are ordered to pay their bills.

When patients fail to pay their ordered amounts, physicians may opt to garnish those patients' wages. In states with **community property laws**, patients' spouses are also responsible for the bills. As a result, spouses' wages can also be garnished. To act appropriately, medical assistants must check the laws in their states.

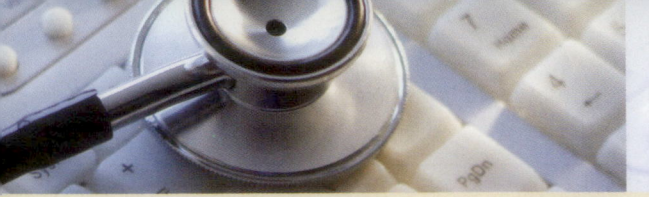

REVIEW

- A manual billing system, though used less often in the medical office, employs day sheets and charge slips to secure patient payment.
- Given their ease, accuracy, and cost effectiveness, computers are now predominantly used for medical office billing.
- The best computerized medical billing systems provide basic functionality, like payment posting and reporting, as well as any advanced features that support the office's business objectives.
- Professional fees are determined by a set of defined criteria so medical offices can operate within a fair and consistent fee schedule.
- A medical office's accounts receivables department is vital to securing payment for services rendered.

- Because fees are a crucial facet of an office's business success, collection policies are important.
- Collection agencies should be fair and equitable while being effective.
- Out of professional courtesy, physicians may sometimes treat patients they know personally without charging the patient for the service, or for a reduced fee.
- Hardship discounts are reserved for those who most need them. They are typically given to those patients who need the care but are unable to afford the cost. These cases are typically granted on a case-by-case basis.
- When otherwise able patients fail to honor their financial obligations, small claims courts can help medical offices collect their past-due accounts.

Chapter Review

Multiple Choice

1. A physician might decide to give a professional-courtesy discount to
   a. another physician.
   b. an employee of the physician.
   c. the physician's mother.
   d. all of the above.

2. Each month, each patient statement costs about $_____ to send.
   a. 5
   b. 6
   c. 7
   d. 8

3. Healthcare providers can discount their services _____ percent for patients who pay in full at the time of service.
   a. 5
   b. 10
   c. 15
   d. 20

4. The most effective way to collect money from patients who owe is
   a. over the telephone.
   b. in person in the office.
   c. through the mail.
   d. none of the above.

5. Which of the following is illegal under the Fair Debt Collection Act?
   a. Refusing to self-identify to patients
   b. Calling patients who have requested no further contact
   c. Threatening to send patients to collections with no intentions of followthrough
   d. All of the above

True/False

T F 1. Pegboard accounting systems are common in healthcare today.

T F 2. Most health insurance plans base their fee schedules on the Medicare fee schedule.

T F 3. A medical office can choose which patients will receive credit.

T F 4. Legally, healthcare providers can forgive patients' copays or deductibles.

T F 5. Dismissing patients from care due to nonpayment is legal.

T F 6. The interest rate on medical accounts is the same in all states.

T F 7. All collection agencies charge a 33 percent fee to collect accounts.

T F 8. Small claims court cases handle amounts of less than $500.

Chapter Review (continued)

Short Answer

1. What is an accounts aging report?

2. Why is it important to analyze participating provider agreements before deciding to become a participating provider?

3. What are "accounts receivables" in the medical office?

4. What is a hardship agreement, and how is it used in the medical office?

5. What is a professional courtesy?

6. What is a tickler file, and why would it be useful in a medical office?

7. What is the purpose of sending an office brochure to new patients before those patients first visit the office?

8. How should a medical office handle a situation in which a patient dies while owing the office?

Research

1. Interview a person who works in the billing office of a local medical office. What kind of training has the person had before taking the job?

2. Research the various local collection agencies in your area that handle medical accounts. How do they compare to one another?

3. Research the laws in your state regarding collecting medical debts.

Externship Application Experience

Martina Sylvan, a patient in Dr. DaSilva's office, owes $652 on her account. The medical assistant must contact Martina regarding her outstanding balance and set up a payment plan.

When the assistant reaches Martina via telephone, she says she has no extra money to pay her bill at this time. How should the medical assistant handle this situation?

Resource Guide

Federal Trade Commission
600 Pennsylvania Avenue, N.W.
Washington, DC 20580
Phone: (202) 326-2222
www.ftc.gov

Managed Outsource Solutions (provides both domestic and offshore outsourcing services)
Phone: (918) 451-8175
www.managedoutsource.com

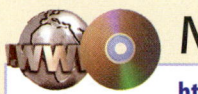

MedMedia

http://www.MyMAKit.com

More on this chapter, including interactive resources, can be found on the Student CD-ROM accompanying this textbook and on http://www.MyMAKit.com.

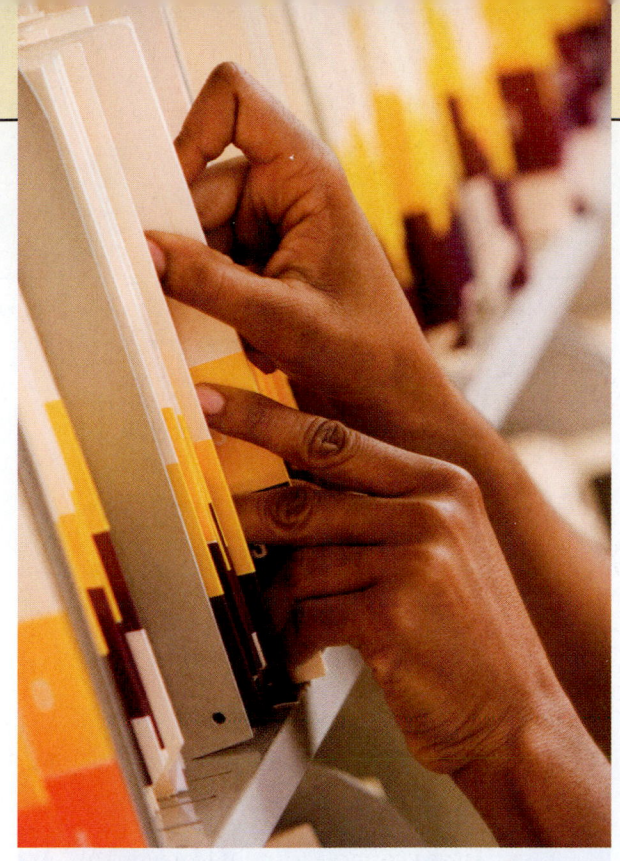

UNIT **VII**

Managing the Medical Office: Banking Procedures and Human Resources Management

Chapter 21   **Payroll, Accounts Payable, and Banking Procedures**

Chapter 22   **Managing the Medical Office**

My name is Sara Brown. Two years ago I began the process of opening a brand new primary care clinic and had the task of hiring medical assistants. I interviewed numerous applicants, some experienced, and some straight out of school.

There were several qualities I sought when hiring MAs. First, I was looking for the ability to handle change. We were going to be learning several new workflow processes and implementing new technologies; the staff I hired needed to be willing and ready to change. Second, I was looking for flexibility. We planned on running an extended hours operation, and this meant staff hours might have to change to meet the needs of the business. Finding medical assistants who had flexible work schedules and the willingness to change their hours to meet the needs of our patients was significant to our success. Third, I was looking for confidence. We needed MAs who were brave enough to try something different, but sharp enough to know when to ask a question. Since we were opening a new site there were a lot of unknowns, having confident MAs on staff gave me the piece of mind to know that our patients would be the top priority.

Some of our MAs who had come straight from school were more confident in a particular department, so I utilized their skills to encourage others to become more self-assured in that area. I am happy to say that after sixteen months, the MAs we hired right out of school are now training our new employees and working with the physicians to create a medical home for our patients.

Payroll, Accounts Payable, and Banking Procedures

Case Study

Francie, who works as the medical office's receptionist, recently married a man with three children. Francie asks the medical assistant, who is in charge of payroll, to help her change her tax deductions so that fewer taxes are taken from her paycheck.

Objectives

After completing this chapter, you should be able to:

- Define and spell the key terminology in this chapter.
- Define the role of the medical assistant as it pertains to payroll, accounts payable, and banking procedures.
- Discuss the payroll function in the medical office.
- List the pros and cons of manual and computerized payroll systems.
- Describe the function of accounts payable in the medical office.
- List the correct procedure for writing a payroll check.
- Differentiate between monthly expenses and one-time expenses.
- Name the steps to creating a deposit of payments collected in the medical office.
- List the steps to endorsing a check for deposit.
- Describe how to access bank accounts via the Internet
- Give several uses of petty cash in the medical office.
- Describe how to reconcile a monthly bank statement.

MedMedia

http://www.MyMAKit.com

Additional interactive resources and activities for this chapter can be found on http://www.MyMAKit.com. For a video, tips, audio glossary, legal and ethical scenarios, on-the-job scenarios, quizzes, and games related to the content of this chapter, please access the accompanying CD-ROM in this book.

Video: *The Petty Cash Fund*
Legal and Ethical Scenario: *Payroll, Accounts Payable, and Banking Procedures*
On the Job Scenario: *Payroll, Accounts Payable, and Banking Procedures*
Tips
Multiple Choice Quiz
Audio Glossary
HIPAA Quiz
Games: Spelling Bee, Crossword, and Strikeout

✚ MEDICAL ASSISTING STANDARDS

CAAHEP ENTRY-LEVEL STANDARDS	ABHES ENTRY-LEVEL COMPETENCIES
■ Perform within scope of practice (psychomotor) ■ Apply ethical behaviors, including honesty/integrity in performance of medical assisting practice (affective) ■ Explore issue of confidentiality as it applies to the medical assistant (cognitive) ■ Respond to issues of confidentiality (psychomotor) ■ Apply local, state, and federal health care legislation and regulation appropriate to the medical assisting practice setting (psychomotor) ■ Recognize the importance of local, state, and federal legislation and regulations in the practice setting (affective) ■ Use office hardware and software to maintain office systems (psychomotor) ■ Explain general office policies (psychomotor) ■ Demonstrate telephone techniques (psychomotor) ■ Explain basic bookkeeping computations (cognitive) ■ Differentiate between accounts payable and accounts receivable (cognitive) ■ Prepare a bank deposit (psychomotor)	■ Adapt to change ■ Maintain confidentiality at all times ■ Use appropriate guidelines when releasing records or information ■ Project a positive attitude ■ Be cognizant of ethical boundaries ■ Evidence a responsible attitude ■ Conduct work within scope of education, training, and ability ■ Monitor legislation related to current healthcare issues and practices ■ Application of electronic technology ■ Establish a petty cash fund ■ Perform basic secretarial skills ■ Prepare a bank statement ■ Reconcile a bank statement ■ Maintain records for accounting and banking procedures ■ Prepare a check ■ Use manual and computerized bookkeeping systems ■ Manage accounts payable and receivable ■ Exercise efficient time management ■ Process employee payroll

✔ COMPETENCY SKILLS PERFORMANCE

1. Create a new employee record.
2. Calculate an employee's payroll.
3. Write checks to pay bills.
4. Pay an office supply invoice.
5. Complete a deposit slip.
6. Account for petty cash.
7. Reconcile a bank statement.

Key Terminology

auditors—those who review personal or corporate bank or tax records on behalf of an agency such as the Internal Revenue Service (IRS)

charitable contributions—cash or other donations given to charitable organizations

Circular E—yearly booklet published by the IRS that outlines the federal tax deductions to be taken from individuals' wages depending on marital status and number of exemptions

deductions—number of allowances to be withheld from wages

endorsement stamp—rubber tool that imprints a receiving agency's banking information

Fair Labor Standards Act (FLSA)—law passed by U.S. Congress in 1938 to address employment issues like federal minimum wage

Federal Insurance Contributions Act (FICA)—law that addresses Social Security withholding taxes

Federal Unemployment Tax Act (FUTA)—law that addresses federal unemployment tax withholdings

garnish—to withhold wages from an employee's paycheck due to a court order

gross pay—amount earned before taxes or deductions are subtracted

net pay—amount remaining after deductions and taxes are subtracted

outsource—to send to another business for completion

overtime—wages paid beyond 40 hours in a work week, at a rate $1\frac{1}{2}$ times the normal rate for that employee

payroll—process of calculating the amounts employees receive for their work

payroll taxes—monies withheld from wages for federal income, Social Security, and Medicare obligations

personnel file—set of employment-related documents for an employee, to include an original application, federal withholding requests, and dates and copies of evaluations

quarterly payroll reports—documents that specify the taxes withheld from wages quarterly

security envelope—nontransparent envelope

Key Terminology *(continued)*

Social Security Act—law passed by the U.S. Congress in 1935 to provide workers and their families financial security post-retirement

time clock—piece of equipment that records employees' arrival and departure times for payroll purposes

unemployment insurance—program that pays employees who have lost their jobs

W-2 form—U.S. federal form that annually documents the wages employees drew the previous year

W-4 form—U.S. federal form that indicates employees' marital status and federal tax exemptions

wages—monies paid for work performed

withholding allowances—number of exemptions on federal tax forms

Abbreviations

CPR—cardiopulmonary resuscitation

FICA—Federal Insurance Contributions Act

FLSA—Fair Labor Standards Act

FUTA—Federal Unemployment Tax Act

HIPAA—Health Insurance Portability and Accountability Act

IRS—Internal Revenue Service

Introduction

In healthcare, payroll, accounts payable, and banking procedures are vital to office functioning. The payroll function involves keeping accurate records on employees. Accounts payable involves paying the office bills for rent, utilities, and supplies. Banking procedures involve balancing the office checking account and filing the appropriate quarterly and yearly statements with state and federal agencies.

Many large medical offices hire outside firms to help them complete their financial procedures; smaller offices tend to rely on their physicians or office managers for these tasks. Whether accounting, banking, and payroll procedures are outsourced or completed in house, medical assistants should understand how those procedures work.

The Medical Assistant's Role in Payroll, Accounts Payable, and Banking Procedures

The medical assistant's role in payroll, accounts payable, and banking procedures in the medical office will vary according to the type and size of the facility where employed. In smaller offices, the MA may be involved in these procedures. In larger offices, these tasks may be performed by outside agencies.

Processing Payroll

Given its role in employees' financial stability, payroll in the medical office is vital. As computer technology has advanced, payroll's function has been transformed.

The History of Payroll

When the sixteenth Constitutional Amendment passed in 1913, Congress gained the ability to impose a federal income tax on individuals and corporations. Each year when they filed their returns, employees paid the federal government directly. By 1918, the government was collecting just over $1 billion each year as a result. By 1920, that figure had risen to $5.4 billion.

When World War II launched and employment increased, taxes climbed to $7.3 billion annually.

In 1935, Congress passed the **Social Security Act** to provide workers and their families financial security. Congress followed that legislation with the **Fair Labor Standards Act (FLSA)** in 1938. This act addressed several worker-related issues, including a federal minimum wage that rises with the inflation rate. As of 2007, the federal minimum wage was $5.15. Many states choose to enforce a minimum wage that is higher than the federal minimum wage. In addition to things like minimum wage, the FLSA requires employers to pay employees **overtime** earnings of 1.5 times normal hourly wages for any work completed beyond 40 hours in 1 week.

As the years passed, the government tried to remain vigilant to workers' needs, but many employees were finding it difficult to keep up with increasing taxes. Many individual taxpayers found it tough to pay their full tax bills at the end of each year. Relief came in 1943, when withholding taxes on wages was introduced. Under this law, businesses were responsible for collecting employees' income taxes and sending those taxes to the government. Employers had to keep written records of all the taxes they withheld from employee pay, as well as records of those employees' addresses, employment dates, and wages. This legislation boosted the number of taxpayers yet further. By 1945, taxes collected had jumped to $43 billion.

Present-Day Employment Issues

Throughout the decades, the U.S. government has continued to use legislation to address employment issues. For example, the Social Security Act enacted in the mid-1930s has evolved over the years to a system that today has two main parts: (1) elderly, survivors, and disability insurance and (2) hospital insurance, known as Medicare. Two other laws address the payment of Social Security and Medicare taxes: (1) the **Federal Insurance Contributions Act (FICA)** and (2) the **Federal Unemployment Tax Act (FUTA)**. Still other laws require **unemployment insurance**, a program for which employers make quarterly payments to their state and federal governments. Employees who lose their jobs may be eligible to collect from the unemployment insurance fund while they seek new employment.

When the FICA tax started, it was set at 1 percent. In 2007, given rising inflation, it rests at 7.65 percent. Of that 7.65 percent FICA tax, employees pay 6.2 percent of their gross income for Social Security and 1.45 percent for Medicare. All employers must match the 7.65 percent amount, creating a deposit for each employee of 15.3 percent of their gross payrolls. Not all income is subject to FICA tax, however. As of 2007, only the first $90,000 of an individual's wages is subject to FICA tax. The Medicare tax has no wage limit.

The federal agency responsible for enforcing income tax laws is the Internal Revenue Service (IRS). This agency has offices in every major city and employs over 15,000 **auditors**. Auditors are responsible not only for conducting tax audits but giving taxpayers federal tax advice. The federal income taxes an employer withholds from employees' pay must be paid to the IRS each month. FICA taxes, like IRS taxes, must be deposited monthly. Every business must file quarterly payroll reports to the IRS in which they account for all monies withheld as taxes and deposits made to the IRS of those taxes (Figure 21-1 ◆).

Many states have income taxes that are separate from the federal income tax. States laws are similar to federal ones with regard to tax deductions and deposits. To comply with state tax laws, employers must withhold specified amounts and file reports quarterly.

In addition to income taxes, most states have laws that require employers to provide employees with coverage should those employees become injured on the job. This coverage, known as workers' compensation, is used for medical care, lost wages, or death benefits. In many states, the employee pays a portion of the workers' compensation premium, but the employer generally funds the larger share. Employers in high-injury-risk industries like construction or mining pay higher premiums than those in low-risk businesses like insurance processing or data entry. However, even employers in low-risk industries will pay higher premiums if many of their employees are injured on the job.

Payroll Processing

Today, **payroll** processing involves far more than paycheck issuance. Various laws and regulations govern just about every phase of payroll, from calculating employees' deductions and the taxes to be withheld from employees' **gross pay** to maintaining and reporting payroll records. The local and national laws impacting payroll practices can continue to change, so it is crucial for the staff member responsible for the medical office's payroll function to track those changes.

Many large offices now use computer software for their payroll functions, but some still calculate payroll manually. Still other offices **outsource** their payroll function to parties like accountants. In large and small medical offices alike, the member of the health care team who processes payroll is assigned a wide range of duties, including:

- Staying current with state and federal laws for **payroll taxes**
- Keeping written records of employees' hours and wages
- Computing the taxes and other **deductions** to be taken from employees' paychecks
- Documenting the **wages**, deductions, and **net pay** for each employee
- Preparing and distributing paychecks to employees
- Calculating payroll taxes and depositing the funds
- Preparing **quarterly payroll reports**

Creating New Employee Records

For each new employee, the medical office should create a **personnel file** with all of the employee's employment-related documentation, such as the job application, resume, credentials, licensing and insurance information, I-9, and references. To prove their identities at hire, all new employees must provide copies of their drivers' licenses or other photo identification, as well as copies of their Social Security cards.

Updating Employee Records

Personnel records should reflect all changes to employee employment status, such as pay raises, evaluations, disciplinary actions, marital status changes, tax exemptions, and continuing education credits, as those changes occur. Employee records should also include copies of such items as employees' cardiopulmonary resuscitation (**CPR**) certifications and malpractice insurance documents. In short, personnel records should be accurate, up-to-date pictures of employees.

Form **941 for 2008:** **Employer's QUARTERLY Federal Tax Return**
(Rev. October 2008)
Department of the Treasury — Internal Revenue Service

950108

OMB No. 1545-0029

(EIN)
Employer identification number

☐☐ – ☐☐☐☐☐☐☐

Name *(not your trade name)*

Trade name *(if any)*

Address

Number   Street   Suite or room number

City   State   ZIP code

Report for this Quarter of 2008
(Check one.)

☐ **1:** January, February, March

☐ **2:** April, May, June

☐ **3:** July, August, September

☐ **4:** October, November, December

Read the separate instructions before you complete Form 941. Type or print within the boxes.

Part 1: Answer these questions for this quarter.

1 Number of employees who received wages, tips, or other compensation for the pay period including: *Mar. 12* (Quarter 1), *June 12* (Quarter 2), *Sept. 12* (Quarter 3), *Dec. 12* (Quarter 4) **1**

2 Wages, tips, and other compensation **2**

3 Income tax withheld from wages, tips, and other compensation **3**

4 If no wages, tips, and other compensation are subject to social security or Medicare tax . ☐ Check and go to line 6.

5 Taxable social security and Medicare wages and tips:

Column 1   Column 2

5a Taxable social security wages   × .124 =

5b Taxable social security tips   × .124 =

5c Taxable Medicare wages & tips   × .029 =

5d Total social security and Medicare taxes (*Column 2*, lines 5a + 5b + 5c = line 5d) . **5d**

6 Total taxes before adjustments (lines 3 + 5d = line 6) **6**

7 **TAX ADJUSTMENTS.** Read the instructions for line 7 before completing lines 7a through 7g.

7a Current quarter's fractions of cents . . . .

7b Current quarter's sick pay . . . .

7c Current quarter's adjustments for tips and group-term life insurance

7d Current year's income tax withholding. Attach Form 941c . . .

7e Prior quarters' social security and Medicare taxes. Attach Form 941c

7f Special additions to federal income tax. Attach Form 941c . . .

7g Special additions to social security and Medicare. Attach Form 941c

7h **TOTAL ADJUSTMENTS.** Combine all amounts on lines 7a through 7g **7h**

8 Total taxes after adjustments. Combine lines 6 and 7h **8**

9 Advance earned income credit (EIC) payments made to employees . . **9**

10 Total taxes after adjustment for advance EIC (line 8 – line 9 = line 10) **10**

11 Total deposits for this quarter, including overpayment applied from a prior quarter . . . **11**

12 **Balance due.** If line 10 is more than line 11, write the difference here. **12**
For information on how to pay, see the instructions.

13 **Overpayment.** If line 11 is more than line 10, write the difference here   Check one
☐ Apply to next return.
☐ Send a refund.

▶ You **MUST** complete both pages of Form 941 and **SIGN** it.   Next ➡

For Privacy Act and Paperwork Reduction Act Notice, see the back of the Payment Voucher.   Cat. No. 17001Z   Form **941** (Rev. 10-2008)

Figure 21-1 ◆ A 941 payroll tax reporting statement.

According to the Health Insurance Portability and Accountability Act (**HIPAA**), all personal employee information in the medical office, including payroll information, must be kept confidential and in places where only healthcare staff can access it. Under no circumstances should unauthorized parties be allowed access to personal employee information. Employees, however, must be allowed to view their personnel files and to request corrections as needed.

Critical Thinking Question 21–1
What should the medical assistant do with Francie's employee file now that she has provided new information?

950208

Name *(not your trade name)*	Employer identification number (EIN)

Part 2: Tell us about your deposit schedule and tax liability for this quarter.

If you are unsure about whether you are a monthly schedule depositor or a semiweekly schedule depositor, see *Pub. 15 (Circular E)*, section 11.

14 ☐ ☐   Write the state abbreviation for the state where you made your deposits OR write "**MU**" if you made your deposits in *multiple* states.

15 Check one: ☐   **Line 10 is less than $2,500.** Go to Part 3.

☐   You were a monthly schedule depositor for the entire quarter. Enter your tax liability for each month. Then go to Part 3.

Tax liability: Month 1 ☐ . ☐

Month 2 ☐ . ☐

Month 3 ☐ . ☐

Total liability for quarter ☐ . ☐   Total must equal line 10.

☐   You were a semiweekly schedule depositor for any part of this quarter. Complete *Schedule B (Form 941): Report of Tax Liability for Semiweekly Schedule Depositors,* and attach it to Form 941.

Part 3: Tell us about your business. If a question does NOT apply to your business, leave it blank.

16 If your business has closed or you stopped paying wages . . . . ☐ Check here, and

enter the final date you paid wages   /   /

17 If you are a seasonal employer and you do not have to file a return for every quarter of the year . . ☐ Check here.

Part 4: May we speak with your third-party designee?

Do you want to allow an employee, a paid tax preparer, or another person to discuss this return with the IRS? See the instructions for details.

☐ **Yes.** Designee's name and phone number _____   ( ) –

Select a 5-digit Personal Identification Number (PIN) to use when talking to the IRS. ☐ ☐ ☐ ☐ ☐

☐ **No.**

Part 5: Sign here. You MUST complete both pages of Form 941 and SIGN it.

Under penalties of perjury, I declare that I have examined this return, including accompanying schedules and statements, and to the best of my knowledge and belief, it is true, correct, and complete. Declaration of preparer (other than taxpayer) is based on all information of which preparer has any knowledge.

X   Sign your name here

Print your name here _____

Print your title here _____

Date   /   /   Best daytime phone ( ) –

Paid preparer's use only   Check if you are self-employed . . . . ☐

Preparer's name		Preparer's SSN/PTIN	
Preparer's signature		Date / /	
Firm's name (or yours if self-employed)		EIN	
Address		Phone ( ) –	
City		State	ZIP code

Figure 21-1 ◆ (Continued)

The W-4 Form

Every new employee must complete an **IRS W-4 form**, or Employee's Withholding Allowance Certificate, which shows the employer the number of **withholding allowances** the employee is claiming (Figure 21-2 ◆). This number determines the amount, if any, to be withheld from the employee's earnings each payroll period.

? Critical Thinking Question 21-2

What does the office manager need to do to help Francie ensure that withholding allowances are processed properly?

Form W-4 (2008)

Purpose. Complete Form W-4 so that your employer can withhold the correct federal income tax from your pay. Consider completing a new Form W-4 each year and when your personal or financial situation changes.

Exemption from withholding. If you are exempt, complete **only** lines 1, 2, 3, 4, and 7 and sign the form to validate it. Your exemption for 2008 expires February 16, 2009. See Pub. 505, Tax Withholding and Estimated Tax.

Note. You cannot claim exemption from withholding if (a) your income exceeds $900 and includes more than $300 of unearned income (for example, interest and dividends) and (b) another person can claim you as a dependent on their tax return.

Basic instructions. If you are not exempt, complete the **Personal Allowances Worksheet** below. The worksheets on page 2 adjust your withholding allowances based on itemized deductions, certain credits,

adjustments to income, or two-earner/multiple job situations. Complete all worksheets that apply. However, you may claim fewer (or zero) allowances.

Head of household. Generally, you may claim head of household filing status on your tax return only if you are unmarried and pay more than 50% of the costs of keeping up a home for yourself and your dependent(s) or other qualifying individuals. See Pub. 501, Exemptions, Standard Deduction, and Filing Information, for information.

Tax credits. You can take projected tax credits into account in figuring your allowable number of withholding allowances. Credits for child or dependent care expenses and the child tax credit may be claimed using the **Personal Allowances Worksheet** below. See Pub. 919, How Do I Adjust My Tax Withholding, for information on converting your other credits into withholding allowances.

Nonwage income. If you have a large amount of nonwage income, such as interest or dividends, consider making estimated tax

payments using Form 1040-ES, Estimated Tax for Individuals. Otherwise, you may owe additional tax. If you have pension or annuity income, see Pub. 919 to find out if you should adjust your withholding on Form W-4 or W-4P.

Two earners or multiple jobs. If you have a working spouse or more than one job, figure the total number of allowances you are entitled to claim on all jobs using worksheets from only one Form W-4. Your withholding usually will be most accurate when all allowances are claimed on the Form W-4 for the highest paying job and zero allowances are claimed on the others. See Pub. 919 for details.

Nonresident alien. If you are a nonresident alien, see the Instructions for Form 8233 before completing this Form W-4.

Check your withholding. After your Form W-4 takes effect, use Pub. 919 to see how the dollar amount you are having withheld compares to your projected total tax for 2008. See Pub. 919, especially if your earnings exceed $130,000 (Single) or $180,000 (Married).

Personal Allowances Worksheet (Keep for your records.)

A Enter "1" for **yourself** if no one else can claim you as a dependent . . . . **A** _____

B Enter "1" if: {
- You are single and have only one job; or
- You are married, have only one job, and your spouse does not work; or
- Your wages from a second job or your spouse's wages (or the total of both) are $1,500 or less.
} . . **B** _____

C Enter "1" for your **spouse.** But, you may choose to enter "-0-" if you are married and have either a working spouse or more than one job. (Entering "-0-" may help you avoid having too little tax withheld.) . . . . **C** _____

D Enter number of **dependents** (other than your spouse or yourself) you will claim on your tax return . . . . **D** _____

E Enter "1" if you will file as **head of household** on your tax return (see conditions under **Head of household** above) . **E** _____

F Enter "1" if you have at least $1,500 of **child or dependent care expenses** for which you plan to claim a credit . . **F** _____
(**Note.** Do **not** include child support payments. See Pub. 503, Child and Dependent Care Expenses, for details.)

G **Child Tax Credit** (including additional child tax credit). See Pub. 972, Child Tax Credit, for more information.
- If your total income will be less than $58,000 ($86,000 if married), enter "2" for each eligible child.
- If your total income will be between $58,000 and $84,000 ($86,000 and $119,000 if married), enter "1" for each eligible child plus "1" **additional** if you have 4 or more eligible children. . . . . **G** _____

H Add lines A through G and enter total here. (**Note.** This may be different from the number of exemptions you claim on your tax return.) ▶ **H** _____

For accuracy, complete all worksheets that apply.	• If you plan to **itemize or claim adjustments to income** and want to reduce your withholding, see the **Deductions and Adjustments Worksheet** on page 2.
	• If you have **more than one job** or are **married and you and your spouse both work** and the combined earnings from all jobs exceed $40,000 ($25,000 if married), see the **Two-Earners/Multiple Jobs Worksheet** on page 2 to avoid having too little tax withheld.
	• If **neither** of the above situations applies, **stop here** and enter the number from line H on line 5 of Form W-4 below.

Cut here and give Form W-4 to your employer. Keep the top part for your records.

Form **W-4**

Department of the Treasury
Internal Revenue Service

Employee's Withholding Allowance Certificate

▶ Whether you are entitled to claim a certain number of allowances or exemption from withholding is subject to review by the IRS. Your employer may be required to send a copy of this form to the IRS.

OMB No. 1545-0074

2008

1 Type or print your first name and middle initial	Last name	2 Your social security number

Home address (number and street or rural route)	3 ☐ Single ☐ Married ☐ Married, but withhold at higher Single rate.
	Note. If married, but legally separated, or spouse is a nonresident alien, check the "Single" box.
City or town, state, and ZIP code	4 If your last name differs from that shown on your social security card, check here. You must call 1-800-772-1213 for a replacement card. ▶ ☐

5 Total number of allowances you are claiming (from line **H** above **or** from the applicable worksheet on page 2) | **5** _____

6 Additional amount, if any, you want withheld from each paycheck . . . . | **6** $ _____

7 I claim exemption from withholding for 2008, and I certify that I meet **both** of the following conditions for exemption.
- Last year I had a right to a refund of **all** federal income tax withheld because I had **no** tax liability **and**
- This year I expect a refund of **all** federal income tax withheld because I expect to have **no** tax liability.
If you meet both conditions, write "Exempt" here . . . . ▶ | **7** _____

Under penalties of perjury, I declare that I have examined this certificate and to the best of my knowledge and belief, it is true, correct, and complete.

Employee's signature
(Form is not valid unless you sign it.) ▶ _____ Date ▶ _____

8 Employer's name and address (Employer: Complete lines 8 and 10 only if sending to the IRS.)	9 Office code (optional)	10 Employer identification number (EIN)

For Privacy Act and Paperwork Reduction Act Notice, see page 2. | Cat. No. 10220Q | Form **W-4** (2008)

Figure 21-2 ◆ W-4 form.

To ensure timely payroll processing, employees must complete and sign their W-4 forms before their first payroll period. As employees experience life changes, such as marriage or children, those employees' withholding allowances will change. To keep their payrolls up to date, medical offices should require employees to notify their personnel departments or payroll staff of any such changes.

When employees wish to change their withholding allowance, they must complete and sign new W-4 forms. W-4 changes should take effect in the next payroll periods. When

medical offices outsource their payroll functions, W-4 changes may be delayed. When this is the case, offices should notify the affected employees.

Critical Thinking Question 21-3

Because the medical assistant, and not an outside agency, handles the medical office's payroll, what can the assistant tell Francie about the time it will take to change her payroll deductions?

Form W-4 (2008)   Page **2**

Deductions and Adjustments Worksheet

Note. Use this worksheet *only* if you plan to itemize deductions, claim certain credits, or claim adjustments to income on your 2008 tax return.

1 Enter an estimate of your 2008 itemized deductions. These include qualifying home mortgage interest, charitable contributions, state and local taxes, medical expenses in excess of 7.5% of your income, and miscellaneous deductions. (For 2008, you may have to reduce your itemized deductions if your income is over $159,950 ($79,975 if married filing separately). See *Worksheet 2* in Pub. 919 for details.) . . **1** $ _____

2 Enter: { $10,900 if married filing jointly or qualifying widow(er)
         $ 8,000 if head of household
         $ 5,450 if single or married filing separately } **2** $ _____

3 **Subtract** line 2 from line 1. If zero or less, enter "-0-" . . . . **3** $ _____

4 Enter an estimate of your 2008 adjustments to income, including alimony, deductible IRA contributions, and student loan interest **4** $ _____

5 **Add** lines 3 and 4 and enter the total. (Include any amount for credits from *Worksheet 8* in Pub. 919) **5** $ _____

6 Enter an estimate of your 2008 nonwage income (such as dividends or interest) . . . . **6** $ _____

7 **Subtract** line 6 from line 5. If zero or less, enter "-0-" . . . . **7** $ _____

8 **Divide** the amount on line 7 by $3,500 and enter the result here. Drop any fraction . . . **8** _____

9 Enter the number from the **Personal Allowances Worksheet**, line H, page 1 . . . . **9** _____

10 **Add** lines 8 and 9 and enter the total here. If you plan to use the **Two-Earners/Multiple Jobs Worksheet**, also enter this total on line 1 below. Otherwise, **stop here** and enter this total on Form W-4, line 5, page 1 **10** _____

Two-Earners/Multiple Jobs Worksheet (See *Two earners or multiple jobs* on page 1.)

Note. Use this worksheet *only* if the instructions under line H on page 1 direct you here.

1 Enter the number from line H, page 1 (or from line 10 above if you used the **Deductions and Adjustments Worksheet**) **1** _____

2 Find the number in **Table 1** below that applies to the **LOWEST** paying job and enter it here. **However,** if you are married filing jointly and wages from the highest paying job are $50,000 or less, do not enter more than "3." . . . . **2** _____

3 If line 1 is **more than or equal to** line 2, subtract line 2 from line 1. Enter the result here (if zero, enter "-0-") and on Form W-4, line 5, page 1. **Do not** use the rest of this worksheet . . . . **3** _____

Note. If line 1 is *less than* line 2, enter "-0-" on Form W-4, line 5, page 1. Complete lines 4-9 below to calculate the additional withholding amount necessary to avoid a year-end tax bill.

4 Enter the number from line 2 of this worksheet . . . . **4** _____

5 Enter the number from line 1 of this worksheet . . . . **5** _____

6 **Subtract** line 5 from line 4 . . . . **6** $ _____

7 Find the amount in **Table 2** below that applies to the **HIGHEST** paying job and enter it here . . . . **7** $ _____

8 **Multiply** line 7 by line 6 and enter the result here. This is the additional annual withholding needed . . **8** $ _____

9 Divide line 8 by the number of pay periods remaining in 2008. For example, divide by 26 if you are paid every two weeks and you complete this form in December 2007. Enter the result here and on Form W-4, line 6, page 1. This is the additional amount to be withheld from each paycheck . . . . **9** $ _____

| Table 1 | | | | Table 2 | | | |
| Married Filing Jointly | | All Others | | Married Filing Jointly | | All Others | |
If wages from **LOWEST** paying job are—	Enter on line 2 above	If wages from **LOWEST** paying job are—	Enter on line 2 above	If wages from **HIGHEST** paying job are—	Enter on line 7 above	If wages from **HIGHEST** paying job are—	Enter on line 7 above
$0 - $4,500	0	$0 - $6,500	0	$0 - $65,000	$530	$0 - $35,000	$530
4,501 - 10,000	1	6,501 - 12,000	1	65,001 - 120,000	880	35,001 - 80,000	880
10,001 - 18,000	2	12,001 - 20,000	2	120,001 - 180,000	980	80,001 - 150,000	980
18,001 - 22,000	3	20,001 - 27,000	3	180,001 - 310,000	1,160	150,001 - 340,000	1,160
22,001 - 27,000	4	27,001 - 35,000	4	310,001 and over	1,230	340,001 and over	1,230
27,001 - 33,000	5	35,001 - 50,000	5				
33,001 - 40,000	6	50,001 - 65,000	6				
40,001 - 50,000	7	65,001 - 80,000	7				
50,001 - 55,000	8	80,001 - 95,000	8				
55,001 - 60,000	9	95,001 - 120,000	9				
60,001 - 65,000	10	120,001 and over	10				
65,001 - 75,000	11						
75,001 - 100,000	12						
100,001 - 110,000	13						
110,001 - 120,000	14						
120,001 and over	15						

Privacy Act and Paperwork Reduction Act Notice. We ask for the information on this form to carry out the Internal Revenue laws of the United States. The Internal Revenue Code requires this information under sections 3402(f)(2)(A) and 6109 and their regulations. Failure to provide a properly completed form will result in your being treated as a single person who claims no withholding allowances; providing fraudulent information may also subject you to penalties. Routine uses of this information include giving it to the Department of Justice for civil and criminal litigation, to cities, states, and the District of Columbia for use in administering their tax laws, and using it in the National Directory of New Hires. We may also disclose this information to other countries under a tax treaty, to federal and state agencies to enforce federal nontax criminal laws, or to federal law enforcement and intelligence agencies to combat terrorism.

You are not required to provide the information requested on a form that is subject to the Paperwork Reduction Act unless the form displays a valid OMB control number. Books or records relating to a form or its instructions must be retained as long as their contents may become material in the administration of any Internal Revenue law. Generally, tax returns and return information are confidential, as required by Code section 6103.

The average time and expenses required to complete and file this form will vary depending on individual circumstances. For estimated averages, see the instructions for your income tax return.

If you have suggestions for making this form simpler, we would be happy to hear from you. See the instructions for your income tax return.

Figure 21-2 ◆ (Continued)

Recording Employees' Work Hours

To meet FLSA requirements for overtime pay, employers must accurately record the hours their employees work. For all employees, salaried and hourly, employers must also send their states premiums to cover workers' compensation insurance. Such premiums are based on the number of hours all covered employees worked in each quarter.

Calculating Payroll

Employers have varied ways to track employees' work hours. Some employers use **time clocks** that stamp employees' cards at the beginning and end of shifts (Figure 21-3 ◆). Other employers direct employees to track their hours on timesheets they submit when each pay period ends.

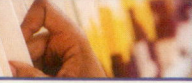

PROCEDURE 21-1 Create a New Employee Record

Theory and Rationale

As each new staff member is added to the medical facility, a new employee record must be created. Much of what is contained in the record is mandated by local and federal law. The medical assistant must be aware of the paperwork needed and must comply with all laws regarding the maintenance of these records.

Materials

- Pen
- Paper
- Employee file
- Copy machine

Competency

(**Conditions**) With the necessary materials, you will be able to (**Task**) create a new employee record (**Standards**) correctly within the time limit set by the instructor.

1. Ask the new employee to bring the following items on the first day of employment:
   a. Picture identification or other proof of ability to work in the United States
   b. Social Security card
   c. Copies of any certification or professional licenses
2. Photocopy any documents the employee has brought for the employee record.
3. Give the employee a W-4 IRS form to complete to indicate the number of exemptions to be claimed.
4. Place the employee's resume and application into the employee record.
5. Give the employee an I-9 form to complete to verify citizenship.

Employees Paid on an Hourly Basis

The gross earnings of an employee paid hourly are calculated by multiplying the number of regular hours worked by the employee's hourly rate. Any overtime hours are calculated by multiplying the overtime hours worked by 1.5 times the employee's hourly rate. When employees work partial hours, some employers round those hours to the nearest half hour; others round to the nearest quarter hour. Figure 21-4 ◆ shows how hourly payroll is calculated.

Salaried Employees

The gross earnings of a salaried employee remain the same each pay period, no matter how many hours are worked, up to 40 hours in 1 week. In general, when salaried employees work more than 40 hours in a week, they must be paid overtime for each hour over 40. Overtime pay is calculated based on an hourly rate, which is calculated by dividing the employee's salaried amount by the number of hours in the pay period. Figure 21-5 ◆ provides an example of how salaried payroll is calculated.

Computing Payroll Deductions

Some payroll deductions, like the federal withholding and FICA taxes discussed earlier, are mandated by law. Other deductions, like those for health and life insurance or disability policies, are voluntary. Medical offices should give new employees lists of voluntary deductions so those employees can choose to participate if desired.

The Circular E

When employers calculate payroll manually, medical assistants need an IRS publication called the **Circular E** (Figure 21-6 ◆).

This publication, revised annually, tells employers how much federal tax to withhold for each employee. Married and single employees appear in separate tables, as do weekly, biweekly, semimonthly, and monthly pay periods. To use the Circular E form properly, medical assistants need employees' completed W-4 forms. Table 21-1 describes how to use the Circular E tables.

To determine employees' FICA withholding amounts, medical assistants must first multiply the employees' gross earnings from regular and overtime pay by 6.2 percent for Social Security. Next, the assistants must multiply the employees' gross earnings by 1.45 percent for Medicare withholding. When assistants work in states with state and local income taxes, they will consult state and local reference tables to determine state and local taxes.

Other Deductions

To determine total deductions from employees' payrolls, amounts for items like worker's compensation insurance, health insurance, retirement plans, and **charitable contributions** must be calculated

---

TABLE 21-1 CIRCULAR E USE

Danesha is married and claims four withholding allowances from her payroll. Her gross earnings this biweekly payroll period are $855.00. To determine the federal tax to withhold from Danesha's earnings, consult the married persons, biweekly payroll period chart (Figure 21-7 ◆). Move down the left column to Danesha's wages, and then move across the row to the number for people claiming four exemptions. This amount is the federal tax to withhold from Danesha's earnings.

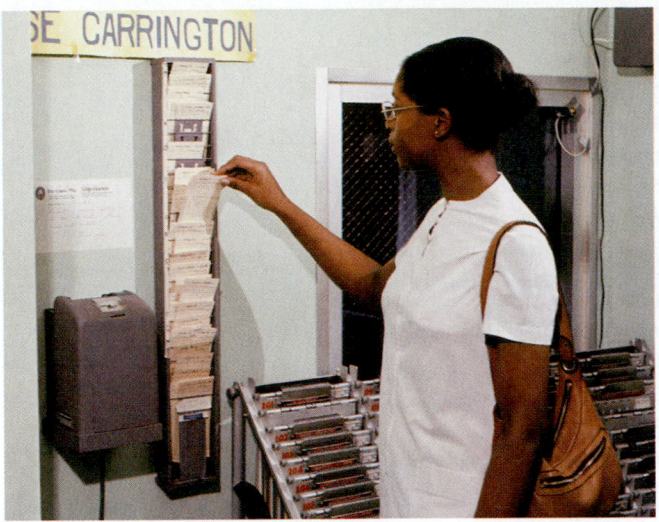

Figure 21-3 ◆ An employee uses a time clock to document the time she arrives at work.

Molly is a salaried employee paid $1,000.00 for each 2-week payroll period. In this pay period, Molly worked 85 hours. Calculating Molly's overtime pay entails first determining her normal hourly wage by dividing her $1,000.00 salary by the 80 hours in the 2-week pay period ($1,000.00/80 hours = $12.50 per hour). Next, determine Molly's overtime rate by multiplying 1.5 by her normal hourly rate (1.5 × $12.50 = $18.75) and then multiplying that figure by the 5 extra hours she worked during the pay period ($18.75 × 5 hours = $93.75). Finally, add Molly's base salary to her overtime hours to determine her gross earnings total for the pay period ($1,000.00 + $93.75 = $1093.75).

Figure 21-5 ◆ Salaried payroll calculation.

and added to federal and state or local taxes. Once all deductions are subtracted, the balance, called the net payroll or "take-home pay," is the amount the employee will receive in a check.

Using Software to Calculate Payroll

For employers who calculate payroll using computer software, payroll is far simpler than for those who choose the manual option. Although payroll software requires employers to set up each new employee, it streamlines the process of entering employees' hours and calculating employees' withholdings. Many such software packages also print payroll checks, quarterly payroll tax reports, and **W-2 forms.**

Ortiz's regular hourly rate is $15.00, and his regular hours per week are 40. In the past 2-week payroll period, Ortiz worked 84 hours. To calculate Ortiz's gross earnings, multiply his regular hours by his hourly wage (80 × $15.00 = $1,200.00). Next, calculate his overtime earnings by calculating his overtime hourly rate (1.5 × $15.00 = $22.50) and then multiply his overtime rate by his overtime hours ($22.50 × 4 = $90.00). Finally, add the amount Ortiz earned in regular hours with the amount he earned in overtime hours to determine his gross earnings for the payroll period ($1,200.00 + $90.00 = $1,290.00).

Figure 21-4 ◆ Hourly payroll calculation.

W-2 forms (Figure 21-8 ◆) outline employees' payroll information for the previous year. Because employees need these forms to file their personal taxes, federal law requires employers to send these forms to employees with no later than a January 31 postmark.

Garnishing Wages

Employees' wages may be **garnished**, or taken, for many reasons. Wages may be garnished to repay loans, honor child or spousal support, or pay monetary judgments against employees. Medical assistants who handle payroll must keep accurate records of all garnishment requests, which arise from court orders. These court orders specify the amounts to be taken from employees' gross wages, as well as the parties who are to receive those amounts. Occasionally, percentages of employees' gross wages, rather than set dollar amounts, are garnished. Separate checks for garnished amounts must be sent to the agencies on the court orders. Whenever medical assistants mail checks to agencies, insurance carriers, or patients, they should use **security envelopes** to mask the contents. When wages are garnished, corresponding deductions appear on employees' payroll sheets. The employees receive the balances of their wages, which are less other deductions and taxes.

Accounts Payable

The accounts payable function in the medical office is like the financial function most people have in their homes: Bills come in and must be paid. In the medical office, bills may include those for office rent, utilities, insurance, and supplies. Some accounts are paid in single installments, whereas others are paid monthly or on other, similarly regular schedules. The medical

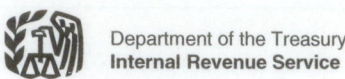

Department of the Treasury
Internal Revenue Service

Publication 15
Cat. No. 10000W

(Circular E), Employer's Tax Guide

(Including 2008 Wage Withholding and Advance Earned Income Credit Payment Tables)

For use in **2008**

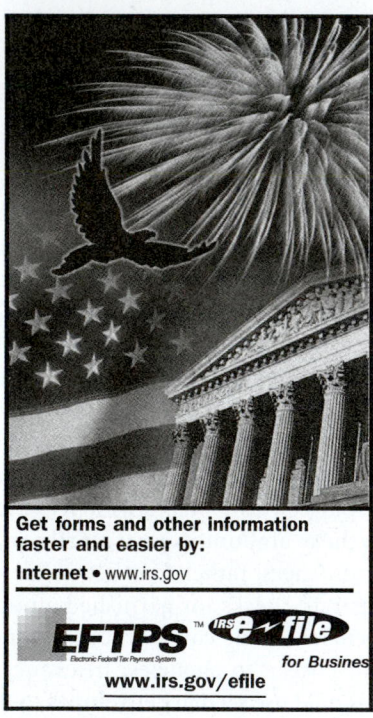

Get forms and other information faster and easier by:

Internet • www.irs.gov

EFTPS™ Electronic Federal Tax Payment System

IRS e-file for Business

www.irs.gov/efile

Contents

What's New	1
Calendar	2
Reminders	3
Introduction	7
1. Employer Identification Number (EIN)	8
2. Who Are Employees?	8
3. Family Employees	9
4. Employee's Social Security Number (SSN)	9
5. Wages and Other Compensation	10
6. Tips	13
7. Supplemental Wages	13
8. Payroll Period	14
9. Withholding From Employees' Wages	15
10. Advance Earned Income Credit (EIC) Payment	18
11. Depositing Taxes	19
12. Filing Form 941 or Form 944	25
13. Reporting Adjustments on Form 941 or Form 944	26
14. Federal Unemployment (FUTA) Tax	29
15. Special Rules for Various Types of Services and Payments	31
16. How To Use the Income Tax Withholding and Advance Earned Income Credit (EIC) Payment Tables	36
2008 Income Tax Withholding Tables:	
Percentage Method	38–39
Wage Bracket Method	40–59
2008 Advance EIC Payment Tables:	
Percentage Method	60–61
Wage Bracket Method	62–67
Index	68
Quick and Easy Access to IRS Tax Help and Tax Products	69

What's New

Social security and Medicare tax for 2008. Do not withhold social security tax after an employee reaches $102,000 in social security wages. There is no limit on the amount of wages subject to Medicare tax. Social security and Medicare taxes apply to the wages of household workers you pay $1,600 or more in cash. Social security and Medicare taxes apply to election workers who are paid $1,400 or more.

Disregarded entities and qualified subchapter S subsidiaries (QSubs). The IRS has published final regulations (T.D. 9356) under which QSubs and eligible single-owner disregarded entities are treated as separate entities for employment tax purposes. For more information, see *Disregarded entities and qualified subchapter S subsidiaries* in the Introduction.

Figure 21-6 ◆ The Circular E IRS table is used to find the correct amount of federal withholding tax for an employee.

assistant in charge of the accounts payable function must determine the accuracy of bills before making payment and keep accurate records of all checks going out.

Several suppliers offer discounts for bills paid by set dates, which are typically ten, fifteen, or thirty days after supplies ship. Other suppliers offer discounts when supplies are paid by credit card rather than invoice. To take advantage of such discounts, medical assistants should research suppliers' and vendors' policies.

The Checkbook Register

Whether medical offices keep their checkbook registers electronically or in handwritten form, those registers must be accurate and clear as to payment purpose and receiver. Clarity, like the availability of the information, is especially important when the IRS conducts audits. To ensure clarity, checkbook registers should have columns with labels such as "Utilities," "Payroll," and "Clinical Supplies." Categorized expenditures help offices track their payments. Figure 21-9 ◆ lists some common expenditure categories.

MARRIED Persons—BIWEEKLY Payroll Period
(For Wages Paid in 2008)

If the wages are—		And the number of withholding allowances claimed is—										
At least	But less than	0	1	2	3	4	5	6	7	8	9	10
		The amount of income tax to be withheld is—										
$1,380	$1,400	$132	$112	$92	$72	$54	$41	$27	$14	$1	$0	$0
1,400	1,420	135	115	95	75	56	43	29	16	3	0	0
1,420	1,440	138	118	98	78	58	45	31	18	5	0	0
1,440	1,460	141	121	101	81	61	47	33	20	7	0	0
1,460	1,480	144	124	104	84	64	49	35	22	9	0	0
1,480	1,500	147	127	107	87	67	51	37	24	11	0	0
1,500	1,520	150	130	110	90	70	53	39	26	13	0	0
1,520	1,540	153	133	113	93	73	55	41	28	15	1	0
1,540	1,560	156	136	116	96	76	57	43	30	17	3	0
1,560	1,580	159	139	119	99	79	59	45	32	19	5	0
1,580	1,600	162	142	122	102	82	61	47	34	21	7	0
1,600	1,620	165	145	125	105	85	64	49	36	23	9	0
1,620	1,640	168	148	128	108	88	67	51	38	25	11	0
1,640	1,660	171	151	131	111	91	70	53	40	27	13	0
1,660	1,680	174	154	134	114	94	73	55	42	29	15	2
1,680	1,700	177	157	137	117	97	76	57	44	31	17	4
1,700	1,720	180	160	140	120	100	79	59	46	33	19	6
1,720	1,740	183	163	143	123	103	82	62	48	35	21	8
1,740	1,760	186	166	146	126	106	85	65	50	37	23	10
1,760	1,780	189	169	149	129	109	88	68	52	39	25	12
1,780	1,800	192	172	152	132	112	91	71	54	41	27	14
1,800	1,820	195	175	155	135	115	94	74	56	43	29	16
1,820	1,840	198	178	158	138	118	97	77	58	45	31	18
1,840	1,860	201	181	161	141	121	100	80	60	47	33	20
1,860	1,880	204	184	164	144	124	103	83	63	49	35	22
1,880	1,900	207	187	167	147	127	106	86	66	51	37	24
1,900	1,920	210	190	170	150	130	109	89	69	53	39	26
1,920	1,940	213	193	173	153	133	112	92	72	55	41	28
1,940	1,960	216	196	176	156	136	115	95	75	57	43	30
1,960	1,980	219	199	179	159	139	118	98	78	59	45	32
1,980	2,000	222	202	182	162	142	121	101	81	61	47	34
2,000	2,020	225	205	185	165	145	124	104	84	64	49	36
2,020	2,040	228	208	188	168	148	127	107	87	67	51	38
2,040	2,060	231	211	191	171	151	130	110	90	70	53	40
2,060	2,080	234	214	194	174	154	133	113	93	73	55	42
2,080	2,100	237	217	197	177	157	136	116	96	76	57	44
2,100	2,120	240	220	200	180	160	139	119	99	79	59	46
2,120	2,140	243	223	203	183	163	142	122	102	82	62	48
2,140	2,160	246	226	206	186	166	145	125	105	85	65	50
2,160	2,180	249	229	209	189	169	148	128	108	88	68	52
2,180	2,200	252	232	212	192	172	151	131	111	91	71	54
2,200	2,220	255	235	215	195	175	154	134	114	94	74	56
2,220	2,240	258	238	218	198	178	157	137	117	97	77	58
2,240	2,260	261	241	221	201	181	160	140	120	100	80	60
2,260	2,280	264	244	224	204	184	163	143	123	103	83	63
2,280	2,300	267	247	227	207	187	166	146	126	106	86	66
2,300	2,320	270	250	230	210	190	169	149	129	109	89	69
2,320	2,340	273	253	233	213	193	172	152	132	112	92	72
2,340	2,360	276	256	236	216	196	175	155	135	115	95	75
2,360	2,380	279	259	239	219	199	178	158	138	118	98	78
2,380	2,400	282	262	242	222	202	181	161	141	121	101	81
2,400	2,420	285	265	245	225	205	184	164	144	124	104	84
2,420	2,440	288	268	248	228	208	187	167	147	127	107	87
2,440	2,460	291	271	251	231	211	190	170	150	130	110	90
2,460	2,480	294	274	254	234	214	193	173	153	133	113	93
2,480	2,500	297	277	257	237	217	196	176	156	136	116	96
2,500	2,520	300	280	260	240	220	199	179	159	139	119	99
2,520	2,540	303	283	263	243	223	202	182	162	142	122	102
2,540	2,560	306	286	266	246	226	205	185	165	145	125	105
2,560	2,580	309	289	269	249	229	208	188	168	148	128	108
2,580	2,600	312	292	272	252	232	211	191	171	151	131	111
2,600	2,620	315	295	275	255	235	214	194	174	154	134	114
2,620	2,640	318	298	278	258	238	217	197	177	157	137	117
2,640	2,660	321	301	281	261	241	220	200	180	160	140	120
2,660	2,680	324	304	284	264	244	223	203	183	163	143	123
2,680	2,700	327	307	287	267	247	226	206	186	166	146	126

$2,700 and over   Use Table 2(b) for a **MARRIED person** on page 38. Also see the instructions on page 36.

Figure 21-7 ◆ This chart from the Circular E shows the correct amount of withholding tax for this employee.

22222	Void ☐	**a** Employee's social security number	For Official Use Only ▶ OMB No. 1545-0008		
b Employer identification number (EIN)				**1** Wages, tips, other compensation	**2** Federal income tax withheld
c Employer's name, address, and ZIP code			**3** Social security wages		**4** Social security tax withheld
			5 Medicare wages and tips		**6** Medicare tax withheld
			7 Social security tips		**8** Allocated tips
d Control number			**9** Advance EIC payment		**10** Dependent care benefits
e Employee's first name and initial	Last name	Suff.	**11** Nonqualified plans		**12a** See instructions for box 12
			13 Statutory employee ☐ Retirement plan ☐ Third-party sick pay ☐		**12b**
			14 Other		**12c**
					12d
f Employee's address and ZIP code					

15 State	Employer's state ID number	**16** State wages, tips, etc.	**17** State income tax	**18** Local wages, tips, etc.	**19** Local income tax	**20** Locality name

Form **W-2** **Wage and Tax Statement**   **2008**   Department of the Treasury—Internal Revenue Service

Copy A For Social Security Administration — Send this entire page with Form W-3 to the Social Security Administration; photocopies are **not** acceptable.

For Privacy Act and Paperwork Reduction Act Notice, see back of Copy D.

Cat. No. 10134D

Do Not Cut, Fold, or Staple Forms on This Page — Do Not Cut, Fold, or Staple Forms on This Page

Figure 21-8 ◆ W-2 form.

Ordering and Receiving Supplies

Before ordering medical office supplies, the healthcare team should thoroughly investigate the suppliers and their policies. For example, staff should try to uncover any hidden costs, determine shipping costs, explore the possibility of bulk-rate discounts, and examine companies' return policies. For large purchases, offices may want to ask suppliers for referrals as an added investigative step.

When supplies arrive in the office, staff should check packing slips to verify the orders. Any invoices should be routed to the accounts payable office. ∞ Chapter 15 details the supply inventorying and ordering processes.

Preparing a Deposit Slip

At the end of each business day, medical offices should make deposits of their daily receipts (Figure 21-10 ◆). Such deposits include cash and personal checks collected from patients, usually for copays, and insurance and patient payments received in the mail. Patients may sometimes fund their services through traveler's checks, which are purchased while traveling as a safe alternative to cash. These are deposited with the daily receipts. Computerized offices can print their days' collections via the medical office

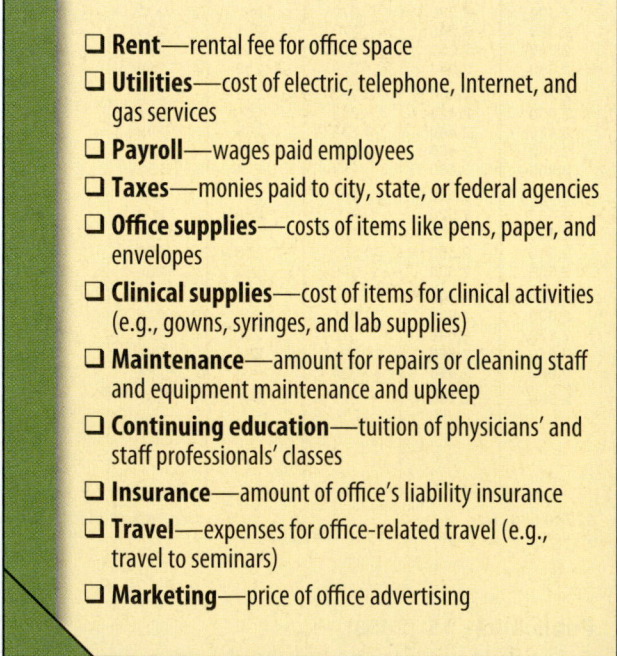

- ❑ **Rent**—rental fee for office space
- ❑ **Utilities**—cost of electric, telephone, Internet, and gas services
- ❑ **Payroll**—wages paid employees
- ❑ **Taxes**—monies paid to city, state, or federal agencies
- ❑ **Office supplies**—costs of items like pens, paper, and envelopes
- ❑ **Clinical supplies**—cost of items for clinical activities (e.g., gowns, syringes, and lab supplies)
- ❑ **Maintenance**—amount for repairs or cleaning staff and equipment maintenance and upkeep
- ❑ **Continuing education**—tuition of physicians' and staff professionals' classes
- ❑ **Insurance**—amount of office's liability insurance
- ❑ **Travel**—expenses for office-related travel (e.g., travel to seminars)
- ❑ **Marketing**—price of office advertising

Figure 21-9 ◆ Expenditure Categories.

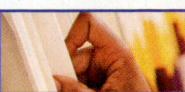

PROCEDURE 21-2   Calculate an Employee's Payroll

Theory and Rationale

Depending on the size of the medical office, the medical assistant may perform the employee payroll function. This function must be performed while paying strict attention to the state and national laws governing payroll.

Materials

- Calculator
- Employee's W-4 form
- IRS Circular E list of federal tax deduction amounts
- Record of number of hours the employee worked
- Employee's payroll record

Competency

(**Conditions**) With the necessary materials, you will be able to (**Task**) calculate the amount of an employee's payroll (**Standards**) correctly within the time limit set by the instructor.

1. Calculate the number of hours the employee worked during the payroll period.
2. For an hourly employee, calculate the employee's gross wage by multiplying the number of hours worked in the payroll period by the employee's hourly wage.

3. If the employee worked any overtime hours, first multiply the employee's hourly wage by 1.5 and then multiply that amount by the employee's overtime hours.
4. Consult the employee's W-4 form to determine filing status (i.e., married or single) and the number of deductions.
5. Consult the IRS Circular E form to determine the amount to be withheld from the employee's gross wages.
6. Deduct the federal withholding tax from the Circular E form from the employee's gross payroll.
7. Multiply the employee's gross payroll amount by 6.2 percent to determine the FICA (Social Security) to withhold from the employee's payroll.
8. Multiply the employee's gross payroll amount by 1.45 percent to determine the Medicare tax to withhold from the employee's payroll.
9. Consult the employee's file to determine any other deductions (e.g., health insurance or retirement contributions) to withhold from the employee's payroll.
10. Determine the net payroll by subtracting all deductions from the gross payroll.

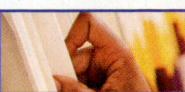

Figure 21-10 ◆ Sample deposit slip.

software. Such reports, which detail the day's receipts, should cross-check against the money to be deposited. In offices using manual bookkeeping systems, like the pegboard, staff must total payment columns and match the amount to be deposited.

The medical assistants who are responsible for preparing deposits must ensure that the amounts the computers or pegboards indicate as the daily collections match the deposit amounts. When these figures fail to match, assistants must search for and rectify the errors. Only when figures match may deposit slips be prepared.

Endorsement Stamps

Medical offices use **endorsement stamps** to endorse the backs of all checks they receive (Figure 21-11 ◆). These stamps list the offices' names, the banks' names, and the banks' account numbers. The phrase "For Deposit Only" should also appear on these stamps. Checks stamped in this manner are difficult to cash by unauthorized parties. The "deposit only" stamp is known as a restrictive endorsement.

HIPAA Compliance

Any documents with patient information, including personal checks, are considered confidential. As a result, documents like these must be kept out of the view of other patients or staff who lack the authority to access confidential patient information.

Accessing Bank Accounts via the Internet

Most banks now allow users to access their bank accounts and complete banking functions, like bill paying, via the Internet. These services are convenient, because they are available 24 hours

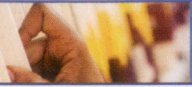

PROCEDURE 21-3 Write Checks to Pay Bills

Theory and Rationale

In the medical office, varied bills (accounts payable) must be paid in a timely manner. The medical assistant who performs this function must understand how to use the checkbook register to pay the bills, as well as the importance of accuracy in this function.

Materials

- Office checkbook register
- Bills to be paid
- Blue or black pen
- Calculator

Competency

(**Conditions**) With the necessary materials, you will be able to (**Task**) write checks in payment of office bills (**Standards**) correctly within the time limit set by the instructor.

1. Verify the bill is accurate and that the supplies or services were received.
2. Determine if the company offers a discount if the bill is paid by a certain date. If so, pay the bill by the discount due date to obtain the discount.
3. Complete the check, providing the date, name of the vendor or supplier, and check amount.
4. On the invoice, write the date, check number, and payment amount.
5. File the invoice.
6. Give the check to the physician or office manager for signature.
7. In the checkbook register, note the payment category, date, and amount of the check.

```
ENDORSE CHECK HERE

X        For Deposit Only
    Sound View Medical Center
          US Bank
         03726457809


_____

DO NOT WRITE, STAMP, OR SIGN BELOW THIS LINE
```

Figure 21-11 ◆ Sample endorsed check.

a day, 7 days a week, and medical offices may receive such payments from patients via the mail. Medical assistants should post these payments, identified with patient account or identification numbers, as they would post conventional hard-copy checks.

Petty Cash

Most medical offices keep petty cash funds, small amounts of money to fund spur-of-the-moment costs like out-of-stock office supplies or postage. Whenever monies are taken from petty cash, receipts or vouchers in the amounts paid, as well as statements of payments' reasons, should replace the monies in the funds. Each month, petty cash funds should be balanced, which entails ensuring that the total of the receipts for expenditures and the money remaining in the fund equal the petty cash fund's assumed total.

In Practice

Wendy Lu, a registered medical assistant who works for Dr. Patch, is responsible for balancing the office's petty cash fund. When Wendy tries to balance the fund today, however, she notices the account is $40 short. What should she do to find the error?

Reconciling Bank Statements

Medical assistants, physicians, office managers, or outside companies may be responsible for reconciling the medical office's bank statements. Online banking is also a convenient option in this realm, because it allows whomever is reconciling the bank statement to view the office's banking activities in real time.

PROCEDURE 21-4 Pay an Office Supply Invoice

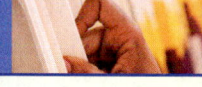

Theory and Rationale

Many suppliers ask for payment upon receipt and mark their invoices accordingly. The medical assistant must know how to pay these invoices in a timely manner.

Materials

- Office supply invoice
- Office checkbook and checkbook register
- Blue or black pen
- Calculator

Competency

(**Conditions**) With the necessary materials, you will be able to (**Task**) pay an office supply invoice (**Standards**) correctly within the time limit set by the instructor.

1. Verify that the supplies on the invoice were received, that inventory was taken of the supplies, and that the supplies were distributed in the office appropriately.
2. Determine if the supplier offers a discount if the bill is paid by a certain date. If so, pay the bill by the discount due to obtain the discount.
3. Write a check for the supplies, providing the date, supplier name, and check amount.
4. Give the check to the physician or office manager for signature.
5. In the office checkbook register, note the payment, including the supplies' category, the date, and the amount of the check
6. Mail the payment to the supplier.

Offices need not wait for statements to arrive or call banks with payment or deposit questions when using online banking.

The reconciliation of medical office bank statements resembles the reconciliation of personal bank statements. Once the office's bank statement arrives from the bank, the staff member in charge of reconciliation must check off on the office's book register the checks and deposits listed as processed on the statement. Next, staff should add the end-of-month balance on the statement to any outstanding deposits in the office's checkbook register. From that number, any outstanding checks must be deducted. The resulting number should match the amount in the office's checkbook register.

PROCEDURE 21-5 Complete a Deposit Slip

Theory and Rationale

In the medical office, part of keeping accurate records is completing the deposit slip correctly and accurately. This function is typically handled at the end of the business day so that the deposit can be taken to the bank after the office has closed.

Materials

- Calculator
- Deposit slip
- Printout from the electronic or manual billing system showing amount received for the day
- Pen
- Endorsement stamp

Competency

(**Conditions**) With the necessary materials, you will be able to (**Task**) fill out a deposit slip (**Standards**) correctly within the time limit set by the instructor.

1. Check to see that all checks have been properly endorsed.
2. Total all cash receipts.

3. On the line marked "cash" on the deposit slip, list the cash receipt total.
4. On the deposit slip, list each check individually by bank routing number or name of the patient or insurance company.
5. Total the checks.
6. On the appropriate line of the deposit slip, list the check total.
7. Total the checks and cash.
8. On the appropriate line of the deposit slip, list the checks and cash total.
9. Attach the deposit slip, cash, and checks via paperclip.
10. Place the paper clipped deposit in an envelope.
11. Take the deposit to the bank.
12. Obtain a receipt.
13. Return to the office.
14. Using the receipt, record the deposit amount in the clinic checkbook register.

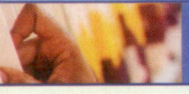

PROCEDURE 21-6 Account for Petty Cash

Theory and Rationale

Most medical offices have petty cash funds for small, unplanned purchases. Medical assistants must know how to balance these funds and should do so regularly. Petty cash funds should be balanced each month. The MA must ensure that the total of the receipts for expenditures and the money remaining in the fund equal the petty cash fund total.

Materials

- Petty cash record
- Receipts for petty cash purchases
- Blue or black pen
- Calculator

Competency

(**Conditions**) With the necessary materials, you will be able to (**Task**) balance the petty cash fund (**Standards**) correctly within the time limit set by the instructor.

1. Verify that all petty cash expenditures have been listed on the petty cash record and that each has a receipt.
2. Subtract all expenditures from the petty cash balance.
3. Enter the new balance on the petty cash record.
4. Count the money in petty cash.
5. Verify that the petty cash amount matches the resulting amount in step 2.
6. If the amounts do not match, verify that all subtraction was done accurately and that all receipts were entered in the petty cash record.
7. Once the account balances, obtain a check for the total expenditures from the physician or office manager.
8. Cash the check at the bank.
9. Enter the money in the petty cash record.

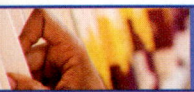

PROCEDURE 21-7 Reconcile a Bank Statement

Theory and Rationale

The medical office's bank statement must be balanced monthly to ensure the account balance is accurate and error free.

Materials

- Bank statement
- Checkbook register
- Calculator
- Blue or black pen

Competency

(**Conditions**) With the necessary materials, you will be able to (**Task**) balance the clinic bank statement (**Standards**) correctly within the time limit set by the instructor.

1. Comparing the bank statement to the checkbook register, make a check mark next to each check processed by the bank.

2. Write the ending balance on the bank statement.
3. Add any deposits made since the bank statement was printed.
4. Subtract any checks not yet processed when the bank statement was printed.
5. Add any interest awarded by the bank.
6. Subtract any bank service fees taken by the bank.
7. If the resulting balance fails to match that in the checkbook register balance, verify that steps 1 through 6 were performed correctly.
8. If the balances still do not match, check for addition or subtraction errors in the checkbook register.

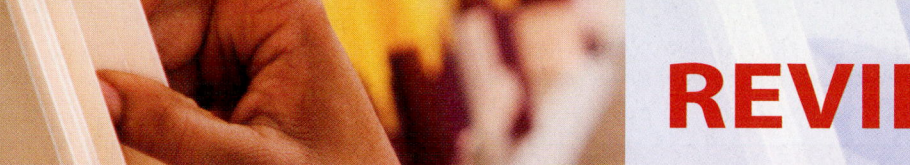

REVIEW

Chapter Review

Multiple Choice

1. In what year did Congress pass legislation requiring that federal income taxes be paid?
   a. 1893
   b. 1903
   c. 1913
   d. 1923

2. As of 2007, the federal minimum wage was
   a. $3.15.
   b. $4.15.
   c. $5.15.
   d. $6.15.

3. Worker's compensation covers
   a. work time lost due to injury.
   b. medical expenses incurred due to injury.
   c. A and B.
   d. neither A nor B.

4. Overtime is to be paid at _____ times the hourly rate.
   a. 1.25
   b. 1.5
   c. 1.75
   d. 2

True/False

T F 1. Employers use the IRS Circular E form to determine the federal withholding taxes to be withheld from employees' wages.

T F 2. Employers must track the hours their employees work, whether those employees are salaried or hourly.

T F 3. Another term for "gross pay" is "net pay."

T F 4. All employers must match the Social Security and Medicare taxes withheld from employees' payrolls.

T F 5. Medical office collections should be deposited daily.

T F 6. All states in the United States have state income taxes.

Short Answer

1. Name three items that should be in every employee's personnel file.

2. When choosing new suppliers for the medical office, what kinds of questions should be asked?

3. What does it mean to endorse a check?

4. Why is it important to endorse checks soon after they arrive in the medical office?

5. Name a common purchase made with petty cash.

6. Describe some characteristics desired in medical assistants who handle office payroll or accounts payable functions.

7. Why would patients pay for their physician's visits with traveler's checks?

8. Define the term "accounts payable."

9. Explain what it means to garnish an employee's wages.

10. Explain how a time clock is used.

Research

1. Interview the office manager of a local medical office. Ask the manager if the function of payroll is handled within the medical office or if it is handled by an outside firm.

2. Look at the IRS Web site. What information is contained there that might be helpful to the medical office with regard to processing payroll?

3. Research the laws regarding the garnishment of wages in your state.

Externship Application Experience

A recently hired medical assistant has been asked to visit the manager's office on his first day so that the manager can set up an employee file. What type of information should the assistant bring to expedite this task?

Resource Guide

Payroll-Taxes.com
14350 North 87th Street, Suite 170
Scottsdale, AZ 85260
Phone: (480) 596-1500
Fax: (480) 991-0572
www.payroll-taxes.com

Quickbooks Payroll
Phone: (888) 729-1996
www.quickbooks.com

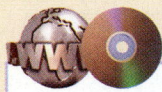

MedMedia

http://www.MyMAKit.com

More on this chapter, including interactive resources, can be found on the Student CD-ROM accompanying this textbook and on http://www.MyMAKit.com.

Objectives

After completing this chapter, you should be able to:

- Define and spell the key terminology in this chapter.
- Define the medical assistant's role in managing the medical office.
- Describe the characteristics and responsibilities of an effective office manager.
- Describe different management leadership styles.
- Explain how to conduct an effective staff meeting, how to write a staff meeting agenda, and discuss items that should be included.
- Explain the importance of a job description.
- Write effective job placement ads.
- List places where a medical office can advertise for staff.
- Describe how to lead an effective interview.
- List appropriate questions for potential employees.
- Name the steps involved in calling for employee references.
- Describe the MA's responsibility in hiring, training, and supervising staff.
- Discuss how to overcome scheduling issues.
- Explain the importance of employee evaluations.
- Discuss the steps to effectively manage medical office staff, including disciplining and terminating of staff.
- Discuss the importance of sexual harassment policy in the medical office.
- Describe employment resources available to employees.
- List the steps involved in providing employee references.
- Describe the team effort involved in improving quality and managing risk in the medical office.

Managing the Medical Office

Case Study

Juanita Ryan is the office manager at Valley View Medical Clinic, which has three physicians, one of whom arrives late every morning and returns late after lunch. Juanita has spoken with the physician, Dr. Whittier, several times. Patients are angry and frustrated by their long waits.

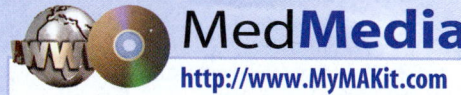

MedMedia

http://www.MyMAKit.com

Additional interactive resources and activities for this chapter can be found on http://www.MyMAKit.com. For a video, tips, audio glossary, legal and ethical scenarios, on-the-job scenarios, quizzes, and games related to the content of this chapter, please access the accompanying CD-ROM in this book.

Video
Legal and Ethical Scenario: *Managing the Medical Office*
On the Job Scenario: *Managing the Medical Office*
Tips
Multiple Choice Quiz
Audio Glossary
HIPAA Quiz
Games: Spelling Bee, Crossword, and Strikeout

Key Terminology

adverse outcome—unfavorable treatment result

agenda—list of items to be addressed during a meeting

body language—set of nonverbal actions that communicate what a person is thinking or feeling

credentials—certified documents that show an individual's certification status (CMA (AAMA) or RMA (AMT))

delegate—to assign a task to another individual

Employment Assistance Programs (EAPs)—resources for those in personal crises, such as counseling and drug or alcohol rehabilitation.

sentinel event—in healthcare, injurious or possibly injurious act

sexual harassment—unwanted sexual attention or comments in the workplace

Abbreviations

ADA—Americans with Disabilities Act

ADEA—Age Discrimination in Employment Act

EAP—Employee Assistant Program

EEOC—Equal Employment Opportunity Commission

✚ MEDICAL ASSISTING STANDARDS

CAAHEP ENTRY-LEVEL STANDARDS	ABHES ENTRY-LEVEL COMPETENCIES
■ Perform within scope of practice (psychomotor) ■ Apply ethical behaviors, including honesty/integrity in performance of medical assisting practice (affective) ■ Explore issue of confidentiality as it applies to the medical assistant (cognitive) ■ Respond to issues of confidentiality (psychomotor) ■ Explain general office policies (psychomotor) ■ Identify resources and adaptations that are required based on individual needs (cognitive) ■ Apply active listening skills (affective) ■ Demonstrate empathy in communicating with patients, family and staff (affective) ■ Use office hardware and software to maintain office systems (psychomotor) ■ Demonstrate telephone techniques (psychomotor) ■ Identify nonverbal communication (cognitive) ■ Identify styles and types of verbal communication (cognitive) ■ Recognize elements of fundamental writing skills (cognitive) ■ List and discuss legal and illegal interview questions (cognitive)	■ Adapt to change ■ Maintain confidentiality at all times ■ Use appropriate guidelines when releasing records or information ■ Project a positive attitude ■ Be cognizant of ethical boundaries ■ Evidence a responsible attitude ■ Conduct work within scope of education, training, and ability ■ Professional components ■ Maintain licenses and accreditation ■ Maintain liability coverage ■ Monitor legislation related to current healthcare issues and practices ■ Locate resources and information for patients and employers ■ Manage physician's professional schedule and travel ■ Use proper telephone techniques ■ Application of electronic technology ■ Apply computer concepts for office procedures ■ Follow established policy in initiating or terminating medical treatment ■ Exercise efficient time management ■ Receive, organize, prioritize, and transmit information efficiently ■ Fundamental writing skills ■ Orient and train personnel

✓ COMPETENCY SKILLS PERFORMANCE

1. Direct a staff meeting.
2. Write a job description.
3. Conduct an interview.
4. Call employee references.
5. Perform an employee evaluation.
6. Discipline an employee.
7. Terminate an employee.

Introduction

A skilled office manager is vital to the success of the ambulatory healthcare office. Often, office managers are medical assistants who prefer to complete administrative tasks, but it is also common to find office managers who lack clinical training. Sometimes, physicians act as their own office managers, but such arrangements fail to use physicians' time most efficiently. In some offices, clinical office managers direct the clinical portions while administrative office managers oversee administrative duties. Whatever the arrangement, as office leader, the office manager oversees and facilitates all office activities.

The Medical Assistant's Role in Managing the Medical Office

Medical assistants may desire to manage the medical office one day. This position may be held by a person with either a clinical or an administrative background. No matter what the training of the medical office manager, the individual in this role should possess good communication skills.

Characteristics of the Medical Office Manager

Successful office managers know that being a leader involves more than simply telling others what to do. Good leaders lead by example and encourage those they manage to do the best jobs they can do.

As office lead, the medical office manager must be able to multitask, which means being able to manage several people as well as several projects at the same time. Office managers must have excellent communication skills and the ability to project confidence. Figure 22-1 ◆ lists the traits office managers must possess.

Responsibilities of the Office Manager

The office manager may be called on to handle any number of situations in the medical office. Unresolvable disputes between staff are just one example. When such disputes arise, the office manager must remain objective and fair and listen to both parties in an attempt to reach a mutual and fair solution. Office managers may also be called upon to address patient complaints. To address complaints in a fair and timely fashion, the office manager needs top-notch communication skills.

In general, the medical office manager must be able to **delegate** as well as oversee tasks. One person alone cannot complete all tasks in a busy medical practice, so knowing how, and to whom, to hand off tasks is a sign of true efficiency. Figure 22-2 ◆ lists many of the responsibilities that are typically given to the medical office manager. These duties will vary depending upon the type and size of practice.

- ❏ Supervising employees
- ❏ Interviewing and hiring employees
- ❏ Scheduling staff
- ❏ Performing employee evaluations
- ❏ Disciplining and terminating employees
- ❏ Tracking the financial flow within the medical office
- ❏ Handling disputes between staff members
- ❏ Organizing and leading staff meetings
- ❏ Handling difficulties with patients
- ❏ Overseeing of the inventory and equipment maintenance within the office
- ❏ Functioning as a buffer between the physicians and the staff
- ❏ Preparing quarterly financial reports
- ❏ Preparing payroll

Figure 22-2 ◆ Responsibilities of the office manager.

In Practice

Carrie is a medical assistant working the medical office's reception desk. Mrs. Carnes enters the office and begins to loudly complain about a bill she has received. She demands that Carrie explain why the bill is so high. During the exchange, several other patients in the reception room watch Carrie for her reaction. What should Carrie do to defuse this scene?

Critical Thinking Question 22-1

As the office manager, how should Juanita address Dr. Whittier's tardiness?

Leadership Styles

Leadership takes one of three basic styles (Figure 22-3 ◆). Managers generally tailor their leadership style to the situation at hand.

It is important for medical office managers to adopt different leadership styles in response to varying situations. Constant use of the autocratic leading style, for example, may inspire staff to resign or resist making decisions on their own. The laissez-faire style, in contrast, may disorganize the office

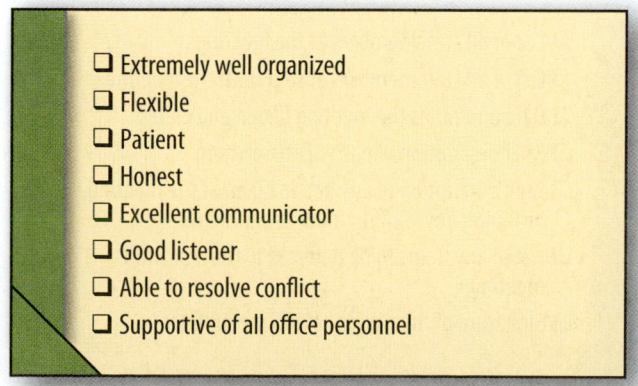

- ❏ Extremely well organized
- ❏ Flexible
- ❏ Patient
- ❏ Honest
- ❏ Excellent communicator
- ❏ Good listener
- ❏ Able to resolve conflict
- ❏ Supportive of all office personnel

Figure 22-1 ◆ Medical office manager traits.

Autocratic

The leader makes all decisions without seeking input. This style works best in emergencies, when orders must be given quickly and followed exactly.

Democratic

The leader who tends to ask for opinions and/or advice before making decisions and may seek consensus or retain sole decision-making authority.

Laissez-Faire

The leader tends to allow others to make their own decisions, becoming involved only when absolutely needed.

Figure 22-3 ◆ Leadership styles.

when used all the time. The ability to balance all these styles is critical to addressing issues on a case-by-case basis.

Conducting Effective Staff Meetings

Staff meetings should be scheduled regularly in the medical office (Figure 22-4 ◆). During the business day, staff are often too busy to communicate with each other effectively, and miscommunication and errors can result. Regular staff meetings with all staff present can help keep the lines of communication open between coworkers. When staff meetings are scheduled outside normal office hours or during lunch times, all in attendance should be compensated. Such a gesture communicates to staff that the meetings, and their time, are both valuable to the office.

Typically, office managers or physicians lead staff meetings. Some offices find that alternating the staff meeting leader encourages full staff participation, confirms that all staff are members of the healthcare team, and underscores that each staff member's participation is valuable.

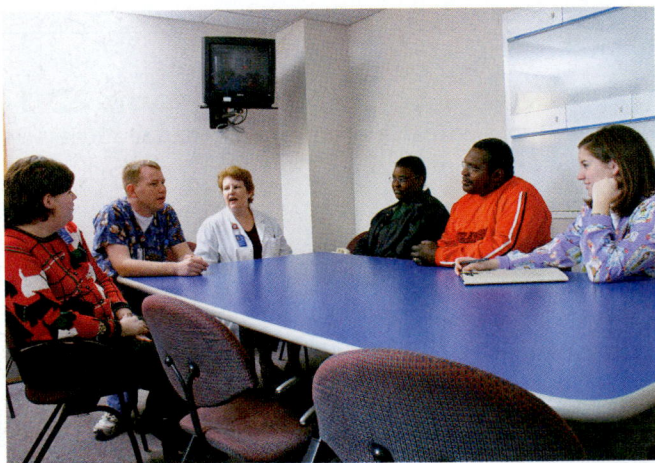

Figure 22-4 ◆ A staff meeting in the medical office.

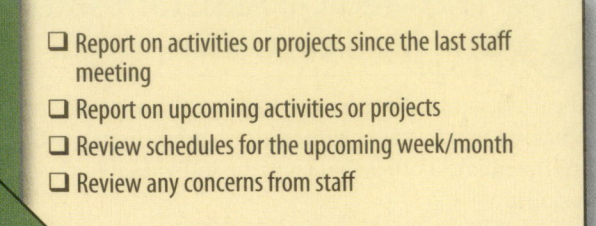

- ❑ Report on activities or projects since the last staff meeting
- ❑ Report on upcoming activities or projects
- ❑ Review schedules for the upcoming week/month
- ❑ Review any concerns from staff

Figure 22-5 ◆ Sample staff meeting agenda.

❓ Critical Thinking Question 22-2

How could Juanita use a staff meeting to address the issue of Dr. Whittier's tardiness?

Creating Staff Meeting Agendas

To be maximally effective, staff meetings should have clear start and end times and follow well-organized **agendas** that staff receive before the meetings commence (Figure 22-5 ◆). Staff-meeting agendas are designed to notify attendees of discussion topics so those attendees can come prepared to participate. Generally, meeting leaders prepare agendas, which should be followed as strictly as possible to honor time and other commitments.

Occasionally, attendees raise topics not on the agenda. When this occurs, the staff-meeting leader should determine whether there is time to discuss the topic. If not, the topic should be deferred to the next staff meeting and listed on the next agenda.

Staff Meeting Minutes

Staff-meeting minutes serve as written accounts of meeting discussions. Such accounts are important for several reasons. First, staff members who cannot attend can review them and catch up on missed material. Second, minutes are written accounts that cannot easily be misinterpreted or forgotten. Finally, staff can use meeting minutes as references when composing the agendas of subsequent meetings. Figure 22-6 ◆ outlines the items that should appear in staff-meeting minutes.

- ❑ List of all staff members at the meeting
- ❑ List of all staff members absent from the meeting
- ❑ Date and times the meeting began and ended
- ❑ Brief description of each discussed item
- ❑ Brief description of any action taken at the meeting, including any staff member assignments
- ❑ List of any items to be deferred to the next staff meeting
- ❑ Signature of the person taking the minutes

Figure 22-6 ◆ Items to include in staff meeting minutes.

Critical Thinking Question 22-3

Imagine that the chronically late physician, Dr. Whittier, fails to attend the staff meeting at which the issue is addressed. How should Juanita inform him of the staff meeting's discussion?

A person other than the staff-meeting leader should record the meeting's minutes. Like they do with leading the staff meeting, staff should take turns assuming recording duties to encourage full team participation. Whoever records a meeting's minutes should type and distribute those minutes to all staff, including those not in attendance. A copy should also appear in the office notebook as documentation of the meeting's events.

Staffing the Medical Office

One of the most important parts of the office manager's job is staffing the medical office. Staffing involves discussing staffing needs with physicians, writing job descriptions, recruiting and interviewing candidates, evaluating employees' performances, scheduling staff shifts, and handling any disciplinary or termination actions.

Writing Job Descriptions

Every position in the medical office must have a clear and concise description. A job description outlines the duties and expectations of a position and helps the office manager both interview potential employees and evaluate existing ones. Figure 22-7 ◆ identifies the items every job description should include.

- ❑ Title of the job
- ❑ Name of the supervisor for this position
- ❑ Summary of the position's duties
- ❑ Required hours for the position
- ❑ Position's location, when the business has multiple locations
- ❑ Any employment requirements (e.g., cardiopulmonary [CPR] certification or malpractice insurance)
- ❑ Any physical requirements (e.g., lifting, standing, sitting, or walking)
- ❑ Summary of the office's evaluation process

Figure 22-7 ◆ Job description items.

The job-description format may vary from office to office, but within an office that format should be consistent. Figure 22-8 ◆ shows a sample job description.

Creating Job Advertisements

Attracting and hiring the best employees starts with effective job advertisement placement. To be effective, job ads need not include in-depth information about positions. Instead, they should list a handful of the duties required, as well as any certification or experience stipulations. While many employers add terms like "friendly," "team player," and "professional" to their ads, these are characteristics to be uncovered in interviews, not necessarily items that should appear in job ads. Figure 22-9 ◆ is an effective job placement ad.

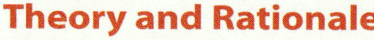

PROCEDURE 22-1 Direct a Staff Meeting

Theory and Rationale

The office manager is often responsible for directing the medical office staff meeting. The office manager should project authority while including all staff.

Materials

- Blue or black pen
- Paper
- Clock or watch to keep time
- Staff meeting agenda

Competency

(**Conditions**) With the necessary materials, you will be able to (**Task**) direct a staff meeting (**Standards**) correctly within the time limit set by the instructor.

1. Before the staff meeting, create an agenda of the meeting's discussion topics.
2. Start the meeting on time.
3. Note staff in attendance and staff who are absent.
4. Discuss the agenda items one at a time, being mindful of the time.
5. When nonagenda items arise, determine if they should be included in this meeting or moved to the next.
6. Address any issues or concerns that arise.
7. End the meeting at the prearranged time.

Administrative Medical Assistant Job Description

Administrative Duties

❑ Answers telephone calls and assesses urgency of call.

- Provides assistance or directs caller to appropriate person, contacting physician/nurse directly for urgent needs.
- Provides assistance to other receptionists in screening patient calls.

❑ Provides specialized information related to section, policies, procedures, insurance, and services.

- Assists patients with the completion of forms.
- Builds monthly provider master schedules and clinic calendars from established sources and verifies provider sessions worked. Modifies master schedules to accommodate time off, extra patients, hospital emergencies, etc.
- Creates patient bump lists as necessary due to last-minute provider callouts.
- Schedules patient appointments and resolves scheduling conflicts.
- Notifies patients of changes/cancellations and prioritizes urgency of appointments for rescheduling.
- Receives patients and visitors. Secures names and needs and directs accordingly.
- Updates patient information and verifies insurance information, level of services, and tracks referrals when necessary.
- Initiates billing process by completing patient encounter forms and accepts and processes fee-for-service payments.
- Books diagnostic tests and specialized appointments for patients at hospitals and other medical facilities and ensures that patients are provided with necessary paperwork and specialized instructions for procedures.
- Schedules surgical procedures for patients. Coordinates available dates for surgery and scheduling of pre- and postoperative exams and lab work.
- Obtains and distributes necessary paperwork and maintains system to track completion.
- Coordinates surgery schedule changes as necessary.
- Schedules and coordinates departmental meetings, classes, clinics, conferences, etc.
- Utilizes computer input and retrieves data. Merges and manipulates data to generate complex reports. Compiles and maintains clinical and patient statistical data and produces summaries and reports.
- Keyboards correspondence, clinical information, reports, publicity material, educational handouts, etc. Composes general written material.
- Obtains patient charts, medical records, and lab reports, and verifies for completeness.
- Sorts, screens, and distributes incoming mail. Prioritizes and ensures completion of medical forms by clinical staff.
- Establishes and maintains filling systems.
- Maintains inventory of administrative office supplies and educational material
- Ensures adequate coverage of reception desk.

Figure 22-8 ◆ Sample job description.

Recruiting and Interviewing Candidates

Medical offices can recruit new employees in varied ways, but the most common are local employment offices, private job-listing agencies, online employment services, and local newspapers. Many medical offices post openings with local colleges, especially those with accredited medical assisting programs.

   To collect applications from candidates, offices might ask applicants to mail or fax their resumes or submit applications online. Once offices receive applications and resumes, office managers can review them for suitability. Typically, managers will discard any applicants who fail to meet the qualifications. Because resumes and applications reflect the candidates who submit them, office managers also often discard any applications with poor grammar or typographical errors.

Certified or registered medical assistant wanted full time in busy pediatrics office. Two-plus years experience
working with children and current CMA
(AAMA) or RMA (AMT) certification
required. Position includes clinical
and administrative duties, as well as
laboratory skills. Please e-mail resume
to srangel@monroefp.com.

Figure 22-9 ◆ Sample job placement ad.

❏ Why do you want to work in this office?

❏ Do you have the skills needed to perform the job?

❏ Why did you leave your last position?

❏ How do you respond to pressure?

❏ What is your desired salary?

Figure 22-10 ◆ Interview questions for job candidates.

Once office managers have identified a pool of potential candidates, they will schedule those applicants for in-person interviews. Because first impressions are important, office managers use interviews to assess things like applicants' appearance and confidence as well as their professional qualifications. To remain consistent from candidate to candidate, managers should use preprinted lists of questions and tailor any other questions as needed. Figure 22-10 ◆ lists some common questions to ask job candidates.

Because office managers often interview multiple applicants for positions, they should take notes during interviews. In addition to observations about applicants' clothing and appearances, managers should capture applicants' responses and their positive or negative behaviors.

Avoiding Illegal Interview Questions

As the parties in charge of employment practices, office managers must know state and federal laws regulating employees, among them Title VII of the Civil Rights Act, the Americans with Disabilities Act (**ADA**), and the Age Dis-

crimination in Employment Act (**ADEA**). According to agencies like the U.S. Equal Employment Opportunity Commission (**EEOC**), which enforces many, similar laws, employers may not discriminate in their hiring, promotion, pay, benefits, retirement plan, discipline, or firing practices. When questions address employee safety or suitability, however, they are appropriate in interviews. For example, when positions will expose medical assistants to medications hazardous to unborn fetuses, employers may ask female candidates about pregnancy. Figure 22-11 ◆ provides questions to avoid in interviews.

❏ What is your race or ethnic background?

❏ What country are you from?

❏ What is/are your religion/religious beliefs?

❏ What is your gender?

❏ How old are you?

❏ Do you have any disabilities? (*Note*: Disabilities prohibiting job performance are legally addressed.)

❏ What is your marital status?

❏ What political party do you belong to, or what are your political beliefs?

❏ What is your sexual orientation?

❏ Are you pregnant or thinking of becoming pregnant? (*Note:* This question may be asked if the employee will be exposed to chemicals hazardous to an unborn child.)

Figure 22-11 ◆ Illegal interview questions.

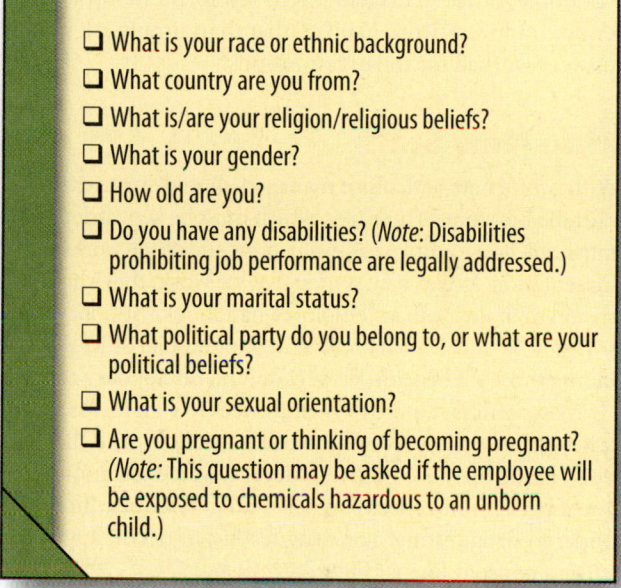

PROCEDURE 22-2 Write a Job Description

Theory and Rationale

The medical office manager must compose a job description for every position in the medical office. To avoid confusion between employer and employee, these descriptions must be accurate and thorough.

Materials

■ Computer with word-processing software
■ List of skills needed for the position
■ List of duties required for the position

Competency

(**Conditions**) With the necessary materials, you will be able to (**Task**) write a job description (**Standards**) correctly within the time limit set by the instructor.

1. Create a title for the job position.
2. List the name of the supervisor for the position.
3. Create a summary description of the position's duties.
4. List the hours required of the position.
5. List the location of the position, when it varies.
6. List any employment requirements (e.g., certification, malpractice insurance).
7. List any physical requirements for the position (e.g., lifting, excessive sitting or standing).
8. Describe the evaluation process for the position.
9. Review the job description for accuracy, as well as with the physician if needed.

Calling for Employment References

Employment references, like employee credentials, are critical tools in the staffing process. During interviews, office managers should ask applicants if they may call previous or current employers for references. Reference information usually appears on applicants' resumes or applications, but when it does not, managers should ask applicants to supply the information. Applicants who resist such requests may be hiding negative information about previous employment.

Open-ended questions, not those answered with just "yes" or "no," are appropriate when calling for employment references, because they tend to provide more useful information. For example, office managers might ask former employers to describe employees' work habits rather than simply ask if those employees worked for the organizations.

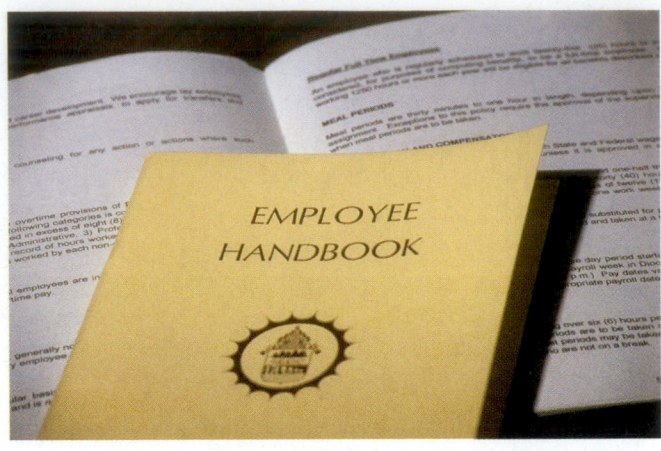

Figure 22-12 ◆ Sample employee handbook.

Hiring New Staff

Once they hire new staff, office managers should create employee files for the new hires. These files, which must be kept strictly confidential, will house employees' evaluations and other, work-related documentation. When new staff arrive for work, they should be given copies of their offices' employee handbooks or policy manuals (Figure 22-12 ◆). Such books should outline all office policies, including those for benefits, dress code, and disciplinary action.

Many offices require new employees to sign forms stating they have received copies of their offices' policies and that they agree to abide by those policies. Medical offices also often run criminal background checks on new staff and require those staff to undergo drug testing. For drug testing to occur, applicants must sign consent forms (Figure 22-13 ◆).

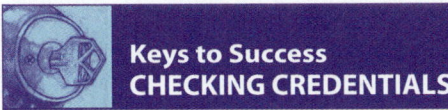

Keys to Success
CHECKING CREDENTIALS

Before applicants are offered positions in the medical office, office managers must check their **credentials** by calling state licensing agencies or certification registries. For example, certified medical assistant (CMA) (AAMA) certification status can be verified by calling (800) ACT-AAMA. Simply asking prospective employees to provide certification information fails to suffice, because some applicants will be dishonest.

I, a current employee of The Marysville Clinic ("the Company"), understand that the use of drugs, alcohol, and other controlled substances by employees creates a dangerous work environment. In consideration for my desire for a safe work environment, I give my consent for the Company to conduct the drug tests it considers necessary as outlined in its Drug Test policy. I hereby allow the Company to take the necessary specimens from me to test for any controlled substance, and I authorize the laboratory or medical personnel retained by the Company for these tests to release the results to the Company for whatever use the Company deems appropriate. Further, I release the laboratory or medical personnel conducting the drug test, the Company, and the Company's employees, directors, officers, and successors from any liabilities, claims, and causes of action, known or unknown, contingent or fixed, that may result from this drug test. I agree not to file any lawsuit or other action to assert a claim.

I have read and understood this agreement, and I sign this without any coercion or duress by any individual or institution.

_____   _____   _____

Print Name   Signature   Date

Figure 22-13 ◆ Sample consent form for drug testing.

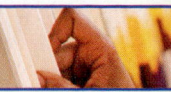

PROCEDURE 22-3 Conduct an Interview

Theory and Rationale

Medical office managers are typically responsible for interviewing prospective employees. Those managers must do so legally and with the aim of finding the best candidates.

Materials

- Pen
- Applicant's resume

Competency

(**Conditions**) With the necessary materials, you will be able to (**Task**) perform an interview (**Standards**) correctly within the time limit set by the instructor.

1. Before meeting the applicant, read the resume.
2. Highlight any areas of concern or interest on the resume.
3. Highlight resume items such as experience that apply to the position being filled.
4. Greet the applicant while making direct eye contact.
5. Use a firm handshake to shake hands with the applicant.
6. Lead the applicant to a private room.
7. Show the applicant where to sit for the interview.
8. Ask the applicant about the potential to perform the job.
9. Review any areas of concern highlighted on the resume.
10. Review the job description.
11. Verify the applicant's ability to perform the required tasks.
12. Ask the applicant if he or she has any questions about the office or physicians.
13. Take note of any pertinent information.
14. Provide a decision date for the position.
15. Thank the applicant, and escort the applicant out of the office.

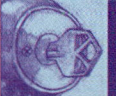

Keys to Success
CALLING THE EMPLOYEE'S CURRENT EMPLOYER

Some applicants are employed when they interview for new positions and do not notify their current employers of their plans to work elsewhere. As a result, office managers should not call applicants' current employers unless those applicants state that doing so is acceptable.

Training New Staff

As a lead employee in the medical office, the office manager may be charged with overseeing new staff training. While another staff member typically completes the training, the office manager must ensure that the training has been completed and that the new staff member is clear about employment expectations. A detailed, up-to-date office policy manual facilitates such training (Figure 22-14 ◆). ∞ Chapter 16 details the process behind creating a policy and procedure manual.

Supervising Staff

Well-trained employees who clearly understand expectations ease the office manager's task of office supervision. Depending on their work styles and personalities, staff require varying amounts of the manager's time in this arena. Some employees work well with little supervision; others require more oversight. The office manager must determine the best supervision method for each office employee.

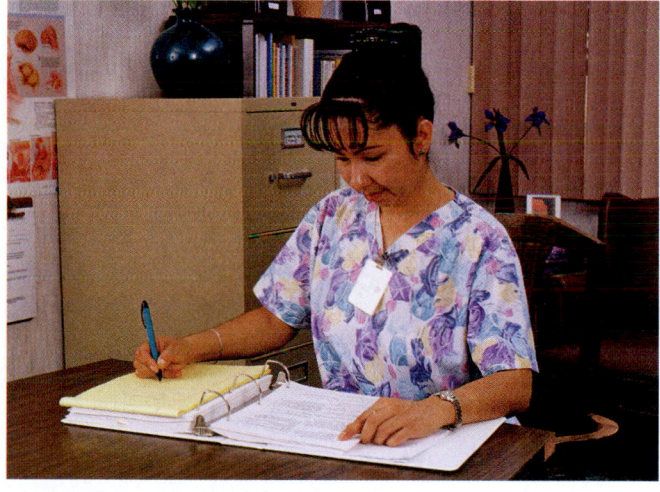

Figure 22-14 ◆ The policy and procedure manual is a valuable resource in the medical office.

Overcoming Scheduling Issues

To ensure staff are scheduled properly, and therefore patient and physician needs are met, the office manager must create and adhere to a fair policy. When employees approach office managers with schedule change requests, those managers must balance the needs of all employees when honoring such requests. To avoid miscommunication, employees should submit their time-off requests in writing within a certain time frame, such as at least two weeks prior to the time requested off. Figure 22-15 ◆ is a sample form for this task.

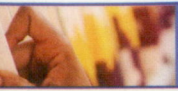

PROCEDURE 22-4 Call Employee References

Theory and Rationale

The medical office manager may uncover useful information from an employee's former employer. The key is to ask the correct questions about the employee's history with his or her previous employer.

Materials

- Telephone
- Employee resume
- Pen

Competency

(**Conditions**) With the necessary materials, you will be able to (**Task**) call for an employee reference (**Standards**) correctly within the time limit set by the instructor.

1. Call the applicant's previous employer.
2. Ask to speak with the office manager or supervisor.
3. Self-identify, and give the reason for the call.
4. Ask the previous employer open-ended questions about the employee.
5. Ask the previous employer if the employee would be eligible for rehire.
6. Ask specifics as to the employee's job duties and job performance.
7. Ask the previous employer for any other, relevant information.
8. Note all of the previous employer's statements.
9. Thank the previous employer.

REQUEST FOR TIME OFF

Date: _____

Employee: _____

Request: _____

_____

Figure 22-15 ◆ Time off request.

Performance Evaluations

To monitor employees' job performances and help employees improve as needed, the office manager should evaluate employees yearly. Yearly evaluations help keep employees apprised of job expectations and help to build and maintain confidence and morale.

New employees should be evaluated frequently in their first years, perhaps at thirty, sixty, and ninety days, and then again on their one-year anniversaries. Evaluations should be positive experiences for employees, not simply forums for raising new problems or issues. Well-managed offices bring issues to employee attention as soon after those issues arise as is possible.

To lay the groundwork for evaluations, offices should give employees self-evaluation forms to complete before the

evaluations occur. Correspondingly, office managers should prepare written evaluations and distribute copies to employees. Originals should reside in employees' files. Once evaluation meetings take place, office managers and employees should review the evaluations and discuss any areas of concern.

Typically, employee evaluations include an assessment of the employee's performance within their position in the office. This will include any attendance or tardiness issues the employee may have had since the last evaluation. The evaluation should include going over the employee's job description and analyzing how the employee is meeting the expectations outlined within. Any items the employee needs to work on should be noted in writing, and the office manager and employee should come up with an agreed-upon time frame for those issues to be resolved. The evaluation should be signed by both the office manager and the employee; a copy is given to the employee and the original goes into the employee's file. If any issues were brought up in the evaluation, the office manager and employee should meet again after the target date for improvement has passed in order to review the progress that has been made.

Disciplining and Terminating Staff

Employee handbooks should clearly identify situations mandating employee discipline. For example, patient or coworker abuse or use of an illegal substance may be causes for immediate termination. Excessive tardiness or poor job performance, in contrast, may be cause for discipline.

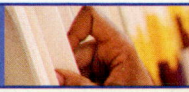

PROCEDURE 22-5 Perform an Employee Evaluation

Theory and Rationale
The medical office manager must evaluate all office employees at least once per year. Typically, evaluations fall on or near employees' anniversary dates of hire.

Materials
- Employee evaluation form
- Pen

Competency
(**Conditions**) With the necessary materials, you will be able to (**Task**) perform an employee evaluation (**Standards**) correctly within the time allowed by the instructor.

1. Before the evaluation meeting, ask the employee to complete a self-evaluation form on job performance. Be sure to include job performance goals for the next year.
2. Meet with the employee at a prearranged time and in a private room.
3. Compare the employee's self-evaluation form with your evaluation.
4. Address any discrepancies between the two evaluations.
5. Address any areas of concern in performance or behavior.
6. Review the last evaluation's goals, and discuss progress toward those goals.
7. Review the goals set for the next evaluation, and set timelines as needed.
8. Discuss any pay raise associated with employee's performance.
9. Have the employee sign the employee evaluation.
10. Place the evaluation in the employee's personnel file.
11. Raise any concerns about the performance evaluation with the physician.

When staff must be disciplined, the office manager should act as soon as possible. Delays may be viewed as endorsements of unacceptable behavior, not only by the employees committing the infractions but by the rest of the staff. Employee morale could plummet as a result. Before disciplining an employee, the office manager should gather all facts relevant to the case. When an employee has been excessively tardy, for example, the office manager should list all the dates the employee has been late.

Meetings on disciplinary issues should occur in private locations, and the office manager should remain professional and calm. First offenses may impose verbal warnings that should be noted in employee files. Serious infractions, like breaching patient confidentiality, require a written warning that outlines the offense and the action the offending employee must take (Figure 22-16 ◆). Employees should sign any written warning and receive a copy. Originals should reside in employee files.

To prepare for the often difficult task of employee termination, office managers should keep clear timelines of warnings and disciplinary actions in employees' files. These types of documents, like clear office policies, both ease the difficult event and help safeguard offices from wrongful termination lawsuits.

When employees are terminated, they should be taken to a private location and advised of the reasons. Managers should regain all keys and other office-owned items and escort employees while they obtain any personal items in the office. When all property has been properly returned, managers should escort the employees from the buildings.

Sexual Harrassment in the Medical Office

Title VII of the Civil Rights Act protects employees against sexual harassment.

Sexual harassment is legally defined as unwanted sexual advances, requests for sexual favors, and other verbal or physical conduct of a sexual nature, whether intentional or unintentional where:

- An individual's employment hinges upon participating in the sexual activity.
- The conduct of an individual causes a hostile, humiliating, or offensive work environment for another individual.

Sexual harassment is illegal in all workplaces and the medical office is no exception. In order for the conduct to be considered sexual harassment, it must be unwelcome. While there are many examples of conduct that could be construed as sexual harassment, examples include:

- Unwelcome sexual advances, including gestures, whistling, or comments
- Sexual jokes, either written or spoken
- Gossip regarding an individual's sex life
- Comments about an individual's body
- Displaying sexually explicit photographs, objects, or cartoons
- Questions about an individual's sexual experiences or activities

Date: June 21, 2010

Employee: Sara Brown

Infraction: On the following dates, the employee was more than 10 minutes late for her shift:

    5/21/10
    5/25/10
    6/10/10
    6/19/10

According to office policy regarding tardiness, any employee who is late four or more times in a month will incur disciplinary action in the form of a written warning. If, after this initial warning, the employee is more than 10 minutes late for a shift in the next 2 weeks, the employee will experience a second disciplinary action of a 1-week, nonpaid employment suspension.

Signature of Employee _____ Date_____

Signature of Office Manager_____ Date_____

Figure 22-16 ◆ Sample warning of disciplinary action.

If an employee feels he or she has been sexually harassed, he or she must bring the problem to the attention of the office manager or supervisor. The office manager or supervisor must then take immediate action to investigate the claim and take proper action by educating, disciplining, or even terminating the offender. If, after receiving a complaint and verifying the validity of the complaint, the office manager or supervisor does not take action, the complaining employee may then file a lawsuit against the employer for allowing a hostile work environment to continue.

In Practice

Gail is the office manager of a dermatology practice. Annie comes into Gail's office one morning and says, "The new medical assistant, Roger, has been making comments to me that are making me very uncomfortable." When Gail asks Annie about the comments Annie says that Roger's comments are of a sexual nature. Annie has asked Roger to stop making the comments but he has continued to make them. What should Gail do about this situation?

PROCEDURE 22-6 Discipline an Employee

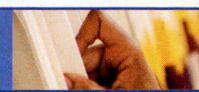

Theory and Rationale

The medical office manager must adhere to office policies for staff discipline. Staff discipline must be done in a private location, and copies of all documents must be signed by the employee and the office manager and placed in the employee's permanent file.

Materials

- Pen
- Paper

Competency

(**Conditions**) With the necessary materials, you will be able to (**Task**) discipline an employee (**Standards**) correctly within the time allowed by the instructor.

1. Verify all facts before meeting with the employee.
2. Write a disciplinary notice that contains the reason for the discipline and the action to be taken by the office and/or by the employee as a result.
3. Request a meeting with the employee.
4. Hold the meeting in a private room.
5. Let the employee know the reason for the meeting.
6. Discuss the disciplinary action being levied on the employee.
7. Discuss your expectations of the employee.
8. Discuss the outcome if the employee's behavior does not change.
9. Ask the employee to sign the disciplinary statement.
10. If the employee refuses to sign the statement, make a note on the statement of "Contents reviewed with employee. Employee refused to sign." Sign your signature and date the document.
11. Place the statement in the employee's personnel record.
12. Agree to a future date on which you will meet with the employee to discuss progress.
13. Inform the physician of the meeting's outcome.

Employment Resources

Employment Assistance Programs (EAPs), resources for those in personal crises, such as counseling and drug or alcohol rehabilitation, are common in large medical offices and hospitals. Any resources should be outlined in office policies. Office managers should keep lists of resources as added reference. While any referrals should appear in employees' personnel files, all such information must be kept confidential.

Providing Employee References

Once staff leave offices' employment, office managers may receive requests from potential employers for those former employees' references. For legal reasons, offices must follow strict, consistent policies in this arena. For example, office managers must give references for all employees, not just a select few, and they must share facts only, not speculations or opinions. Office policy should dictate what information is to be given to potential employers.

PROCEDURE 22-7 Terminate an Employee

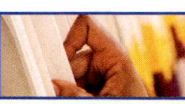

Theory and Rationale

While employee termination is generally difficult, the office manager is obligated to undertake the task professionally, respectfully, and legally.

Materials

- Pen
- Paper

Competency

(**Conditions**) With the necessary materials, you will be able to (**Task**) terminate an employee (**Standards**) correctly within the time allowed by the instructor.

1. Take the employee to a private room.
2. Discuss the reason for termination.
3. Ask the employee to return any office items, such as keys or identification badges.
4. Escort the employee to the workstation to collect personal belongings.
5. Escort the employee from the building.
6. If the employee is loud or abusive, ask the employee to leave immediately and inform the employee that personal belongings will be sent.
7. Note the meeting's outcome in the employee's personnel file.
8. Notify the physician of the meeting's outcome.

References might include only the dates employees worked in the office, the employee's job title, and any proven information in the employee's file. Managers can share when former employees have stolen, for example, but only when such events have been proven. Inaccurate information can damage former employees and subject offices to lawsuits. Similarly, positive references for undeserving employees are grounds for legal action if a potential employer hires an employee with a proven track record for stealing from the office and the office manager did not disclose that information when called for a reference.

Improving Quality and Managing Risk in the Medical Office

As healthcare consumers, patients face a wide array of choices. As in all other businesses, quality customer service is crucial to medical office success. Patients who are treated respectfully and equitably communicate positive information about the office and will likely stay with those offices long term. Research has shown that patients rate their healthcare higher simply because they felt staff cared about them and took the time to listen to their concerns. Improving quality in the medical office includes looking for ways to improve the patient's experience in the medical office. This includes making sure patients do not wait for long periods for their appointment, explaining charges to patients prior to services being performed, and maintaining patient confidentiality in all aspects of patient care.

?— Critical Thinking Question 22-4
How could Juanita communicate to the chronically tardy physician the potential impact of his actions on patient care?

Creating a Quality Improvement Program

Quality improvement programs that focus on patients' emotional and physical health are vital to the success of any healthcare practice. Such programs should be implemented whenever healthcare employees notice areas or situations that when improved would raise patient satisfaction or safety. When staff members notice broken chairs or hallway carpet that has begun to unravel, they should raise the possible safety hazard with the appropriate parties. Figure 22-17 ◆ identifies other issues that could benefit from quality improvement.

Healthcare staff should work as a team to solve problems immediately through quality improvement programs, which can be very simple. One common office problem is patient wait time. When offices receive complaints about long patient wait times, those offices should mobilize teams quickly to solve the problem by studying appointment times or discussing outcomes with physicians. When patient wait times are allowed to remain long, patients may seek care elsewhere.

❑ Long patient wait times

❑ Insurance company rejections of certain services or procedures

❑ Equipment needs

❑ Health Insurance Portability and Accountability Act (HIPAA) violations

❑ Complaints about collection practices

❑ Office remodeling

❑ Inconvenient patient flow in the office

❑ Office waste

❑ Inefficient staffing

❑ Personal use of office telephones or computers

Figure 22-17 ◆ Possible issues for quality improvement review.

Working to Ensure Patient Safety

Every member of the healthcare team is responsible for patient safety, which means medical assistants should speak up when they see potential risk factors. For example, when physicians order medications that medical assistants believe to be incorrect, those assistants are responsible for clarifying the medication orders before administration. This should only be done outside of the patient's hearing range.

Patient trust is a vital stepping stone to patient safety. Patients who trust their healthcare providers become partners in their own safety. To participate in the patient partnership, medical assistants should listen to patients' questions and learn to recognize the **body language** that alerts them to patients' unspoken messages. To make these tasks easier, assistants should sit next to patients or their families whenever appropriate (Figure 22-18 ◆) and try to anticipate patient questions. As much as possible, assistants should provide the answers to

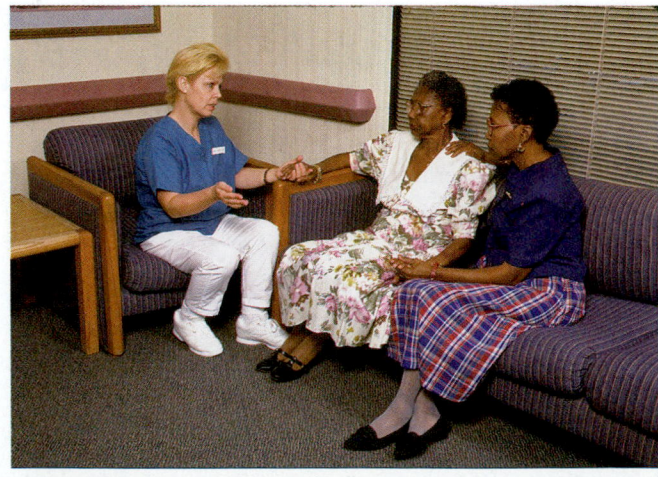

Figure 22-18 ◆ The medical assistant should be ready to speak to the patient's family if necessary.

commonly asked questions. It is also helpful for assistants to use touch appropriately to show concern and to speak in patients' native languages when possible or to arrange for interpreters if needed. To ensure communication is understood, medical assistants should ask patients and their families to repeat discussions in their own words. Respecting patients' decisions and maintaining patients' confidence are parts of advocating for patients in healthcare.

Procedures to provide a safe environment for everyone in the medical office are discussed in ∞ Chapter 23.

Reporting Office Incidents

Occasionally, **adverse outcomes,** which are events that were unexpected or that are the result of an error on the part of one or more persons on the healthcare team, occur in the medical office. Adverse outcomes that cause patient injury or could cause patient injury are called **sentinel events.** The Joint Commission on the Accreditation of Healthcare Organizations (JCAHO) describes sentinel events as ones in which injuries occurred, or could have occurred, in a medical setting. Figure 22-19 ◆ lists possible sentinel events in ambulatory care.

When sentinel events occur, the medical office must document and report those events properly, not to blame or punish employees but to aid in prevention. Offices that strive to use errors as learning experiences rather than punishment tools promote a culture in which employees feel safe enough to self-report errors.

A more detailed discussion of filing incident reports is in ∞ Chapter 23, The Clinical Environment and Safety in the Medical Office.

❑ Incorrect medication administration
❑ Patient falls in the office
❑ Missing prescription pads or medications
❑ Incorrect or absent patient instructions following procedures
❑ Needle stick injuries to staff
❑ Inappropriate handling of patient laboratory samples

Figure 22-19 ◆ Possible sentinel events in ambulatory care.

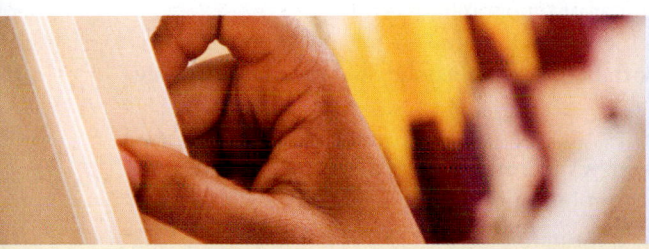

REVIEW

Chapter Summary

- An effective medical office manager demonstrates a range of high-level skills, from communication and organization and possibly clinical aptitude.
- Because healthcare situations dictate the appropriate management style, office managers must be able to assess situations and adapt accordingly.
- Effective staff meetings, often led by office managers, usually result from planning that includes detailed, accurate agendas.
- Job descriptions are important when medical offices are recruiting staff. Job descriptions include a list of the required duties the employee is expected to perform in addition to the hours and days the employee is expected to work.
- Offices can advertise for staff in a number of places, from conventional newspapers and Web sites to agencies and colleges.
- Effective job placement ads give an overview of job responsibilities.
- Effective interviews uncover the issues and characteristics untouched by resumes. These characteristics might include

noticing that an employee is nervous or overly talkative or perhaps an employee who wears unprofessional attire to the interview.
- When interviewing job candidates, employers must be careful to remain within ethical and legal boundaries.
- It is wise for hiring offices to check employees' professional credentials, as well as references.
- Once they are hired, medical office staff are effectively managed with organization, equity, and open communication.
- Employment policies that outline issues such as the terms for employee discipline or termination are valuable tools for offices.
- Employee evaluations are critical ways to ensure employees remain fulfilled and productive as they progress.
- When medical offices must provide employee references, those offices should again defer to legal boundaries to remain professional and appropriate.
- Quality improvement programs are designed to keep the medical office a high-functioning, safe entity. Quality improvement

Chapter Summary (continued)

programs include looking for ways to improve patient satisfaction in the medical office.

■ All members of the healthcare team are accountable for quality improvement and patient safety outcomes.

■ To help keep patients and healthcare staff alike safe, offices should report injury incidents properly.

Chapter Review

Multiple Choice

1. Performance evaluations should be done at what time?
   a. Yearly
   b. Weekly
   c. Monthly
   d. When there is a performance issue.

2. The _____ leader is laid back and becomes involved only when needed.
   a. autocratic
   b. democratic
   c. laissez-faire
   d. none of the above

3. What is the main purpose of reporting sentinel events in the medical office?
   a. To fire employees who were involved in the event
   b. To provide an experience for the office to learn how to prevent a similar event in the future
   c. To protect the office in the event a patient files a lawsuit
   d. All of the above

4. Why are employee evaluations necessary?
   a. To communicate with the employee any areas needing addressed
   b. To document any agreements made with the employee regarding job performance
   c. To give the employee a written document outlining their perceived performance within the medical office
   d. All of the above

5. Before conducting drug testing on employees, employers must do which one of the following?
   a. Get the employee's written permission
   b. Not charge the employee for the testing
   c. Give the employee the result of the testing
   d. All of the above

True/False

T F 1. Quality improvement programs are used to improve an office's targeted areas.

T F 2. The medical assistant is not responsible for alerting the office to a piece of broken equipment.

T F 3. When giving references for former fired employees, the office manager should tell the potential employers why the employees were fired even when lacking proof.

T F 4. To be the most effective, office managers should learn to tailor their leadership styles to situations.

T F 5. Only top-level management should attend staff meetings.

T F 6. When staff must be disciplined, the office manager should act as soon as possible.

T F 7. Each job description should outline the duties and physical requirements of the position.

T F 8. Because resumes and applications reflect employees, office managers often discard applications with poor grammar or typographical errors.

T F 9. When giving references for former employees, it is important to have a set policy and to follow it closely.

Short Answer

1. Explain why a medical office manager must have outstanding communication skills.

2. What does it mean to delegate tasks?

3. What is the purpose of a staff meeting agenda?

4. What method might an office manager use to fill a vacant position in the medical office?

5. How can an office check a medical assistant's credentials?

6. Define the term "adverse outcome."

Research

1. What classes might you take at your local community college in order to obtain the skills needed to seek employment as a medical office manager?

2. Looking at Figure 22-10, answer each of those questions as if you were interviewing for a position. How might you improve your answers?

3. What sort of information would you gather before performing an evaluation on an employee?

Externship Application Experience

While patient Monica Schneider is in Dr. Garcia's examination room, she trips over an exposed carpet seam and falls. Afterward, she complains that her knee hurts where it hit the floor.

What should the medical assistant do? What suggestions could the assistant make to prevent similar occurrences?

Resource Guide

Americans with Disabilities Act
Phone: (800) 514-0301
www.ada.gov

Centers for Medicare and Medicaid Services
7500 Security Boulevard
Baltimore, MD 21244
www.cms.hhs.gov/HIPAAGenInfo/

**Employee Assistance Programs Online
(an agency that provides links to employee
assistance programs online)**
www.eap-sap.com/

Joint Commission
One Renaissance Blvd.
Oakbrook Terrace, IL 60181
Phone: (630) 792-5000
www.jointcommission.org/SentinelEvents/

U.S. Department of Labor
Frances Perkins Building,
200 Constitution Avenue, NW
Washington, DC 20210
Phone: (866) 4-USA-DOL
www.dol.gov
www.osha.gov/SLTC/healthcarefacilities/index.html

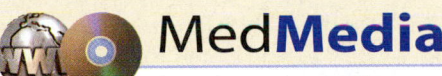

MedMedia

http://www.MyMAKit.com

More on this chapter, including interactive resources, can be found on the Student CD-ROM accompanying this textbook and on http://www.MyMAKit.com.

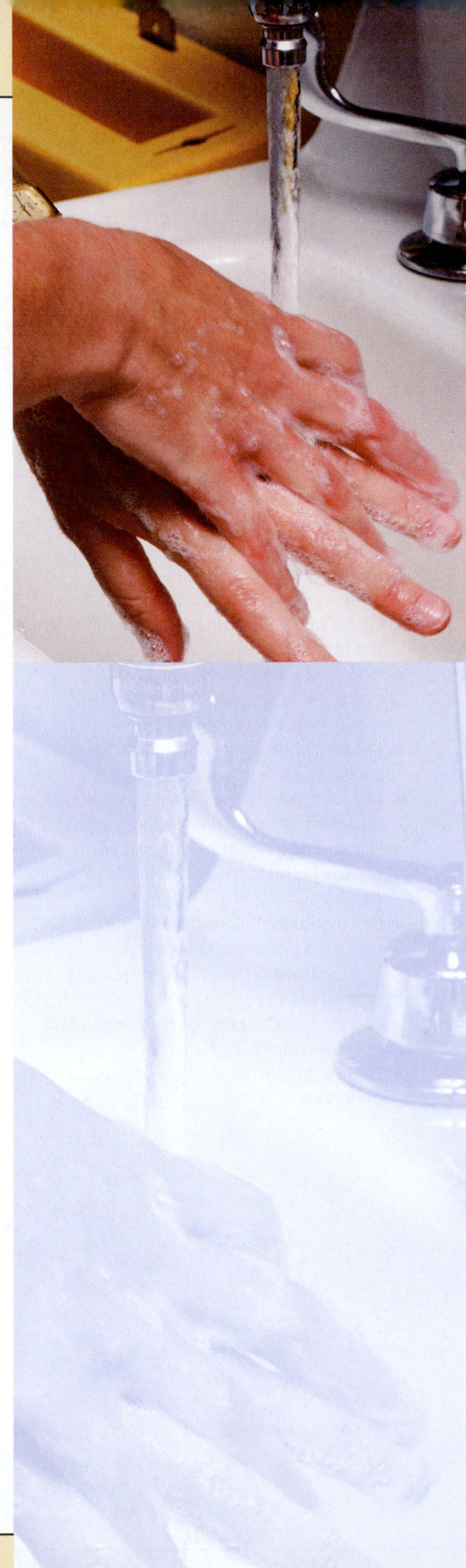

UNIT VIII

The Clinical Environment

Chapter 23   **The Clinical Environment and Safety in the Medical Office**

Chapter 24   **The Clinical Visit: Office Preparation and the Patient Encounter**

Chapter 25   **Medical Asepsis**

Chapter 26   **Surgical Asepsis**

Chapter 27   **Pharmacology and Medication Administration**

Chapter 28   **Vital Signs**

Chapter 29   **Minor Surgery**

My name is Walter R. Nicholas. At the present time I am a phlebotomist, but I am going to school to be a medical assistant. I would eventually like to become a registered nurse. What I have learned so far is that a medical assistant takes vitals signs, performs height and weight assessments, assists the physician with minor office surgery, and sets up for procedures performed in the office. The MA may also administer medications and perform intramuscular, subcutaneous, and intradermal injections.

I really like my job; it makes me feel so good when I have a patient tell me that I do my job very well. It gets stressful at times, but I just think of the patients I am helping. I think that as a healthcare professional, if you smile no matter how bad the situation is, it will become better. A person's first impression is a lasting one.

The Clinical Environment and Safety in the Medical Office

Case Study

Ian and Cora are busy completing the opening procedures for the wound care center where they work. At 5 minutes to opening time, Ian walks back through the reception area to check for wrinkles in the carpet and loose electrical cords from the lamps while Cora goes to the front door to unlock it.

As Cora walks back to the reception desk, a man stumbles through the front door, moaning, with blood running down his forehead. Just as he steps inside the door, he collapses.

Cora shouts to Ian, who is in the back. Hearing her cry for help, Ian quickly places the soda he is drinking in the mini-fridge the staff uses for injectable medications and rushes to offer assistance.

Objectives

After completing this chapter, you should be able to:

- Define and spell the key terminology in this chapter.
- Define the medical assistant's role as it relates to safety in the medical office.
- Discuss personal safety measures in the medical office.
- Discuss proper body mechanics for the medical office employee.
- Describe procedures intended to provide a safe environment for everyone in the medical office.
- Describe emergency plans for fire, electrical accidents, explosions, and workplace-related violence.
- List basic precautions to follow to secure the medical office.
- List examples of events that should be recorded on an incident report form.
- List and describe the elements of OSHA's Bloodborne Pathogen Standards.
- Discuss infection control measures with regard to patient safety.
- Discuss how to develop an exposure control plan.
- Explain standard precautions and infection control practices.
- Discuss the disposal of biohazardous materials.

Med**Media**

http://www.MyMAKit.com

Additional interactive resources and activities for this chapter can be found on http://www.MyMAKit.com. For a video, audio glossary, legal and ethical scenarios, job scenarios, quizzes, and games related to the content of this chapter, please access the accompanying CD-ROM in this book.

Audio Glossary
Legal and Ethical Scenario: *The Clinical Environment and Safety in the Medical Office*
On the Job Scenario: *The Clinical Environment and Safety in the Medical Office*
Video: *Disposing of Medical Waste*
Multiple Choice Quiz
Games: Crossword, Strikeout, and Spelling Bee
Tips
HIPAA Quiz

✚ MEDICAL ASSISTING STANDARDS

CAAHEP ENTRY-LEVEL STANDARDS	ABHES ENTRY-LEVEL COMPETENCIES
■ Perform within scope of practice (psychomotor) ■ Apply ethical behaviors, including honesty/integrity in performance of medical assisting practice (affective) ■ Apply local, state and federal health care legislation and regulation appropriate to the medical assisting practice setting (psychomotor) ■ Recognize the importance of local, state and federal legislation and regulations in the practice setting (affective) ■ Complete an incident report (psychomotor) ■ Describe standard precautions (cognitive) ■ Discuss the application of Standard Precautions (cognitive) ■ Report illegal and/or unsafe activities and behaviors that affect health, safety and welfare of others to proper authorities (pyschomotor) ■ Identify safety techniques that can be used to prevent accidents and maintain a safe work environment (cognitive) ■ Evaluate the work environment to identify safe vs. unsafe working conditions (psychomotor) ■ Demonstrate self awareness in responding to emergency situations (affective) ■ Describe fundamental principles for evacuation of a healthcare setting (cognitive) ■ Discuss fire safety issues in a healthcare environment (cognitive) ■ Identify principles of body mechanics and ergonomics (cognitive) ■ Use proper body mechanics (psychomotor) ■ Develop an environmental safety plan (psychomotor) ■ Discuss critical elements of an emergency plan for response to a natural disaster or other emergency (cognitive) ■ Identify emergency preparedness plans in your community (cognitive) ■ Discuss potential role(s) of the medical assistant in emergency preparedness (cognitive)	■ Be cognizant of ethical boundaries. ■ Exhibit initiative. ■ Adapt to change. ■ Evidence a responsible attitude. ■ Be courteous and diplomatic. ■ Conduct work within scope of education, training, and ability.

Key Terminology

decontamination—use of physical means or chemical agents to remove, inactivate, or destroy pathogens on a surface or object to the point where they are no longer capable of transmitting infectious disease, thereby rendering the surface or object safe for handling, use, or disposal.

pathogen—disease-causing microorganism

Abbreviations

ADA—Americans with Disabilities Act

AIDS—acquired immunodeficiency syndrome

HBV—Hepatitis B virus

HIV—human immunodeficiency virus

MSDS—material safety data sheet

OSHA—Occupational Safety and Health Administration

✓ COMPETENCY SKILLS PERFORMANCE

1. File a medical incident report.
2. Develop an exposure control plan.

Introduction

Safety in the medical office is the responsibility of all employees. In 1970, the Occupational Safety and Health Administration (**OSHA**) was created by Congress to establish safety and health standards and regulations in the workplace. The Occupational Safety and Health Act (1970), which established OSHA, also set regulations for exposure to toxic chemicals, lead, asbestos, cotton dust, pesticides, and noise. In 1991, OSHA's Occupational Exposure to Bloodborne Pathogens Standards were developed. A **pathogen** is a disease-causing microorganism. The standards are designed to reduce employee risk of pathogen-caused diseases such Hepatitis B and AIDS.

The Medical Assistant's Role in Office Safety

Medical assistants need to be aware of and trained in general and medical safety procedures. It is essential that MAs report any unsafe conditions to the proper person(s) immediately and follow all office safety rules. Following general and medical safety procedures will lower the potential for harm to employees and the public, and it will keep liability for injuries resulting from unsafe practices to a minimum.

Personal Safety Measures

For safety, the medical assistant should:

- Avoid loose and baggy clothing that could get caught in equipment.
- Keep jewelry to a minimum (it can get caught in equipment and may harbor bacteria).
- Wear shoes that are supportive and appropriate.
- Secure long hair back, as it can get caught in equipment.
- Store all personal items, such as your medication and jewelry, in a secure area away from patients.

Body Mechanics

Whether caring for patients or moving and lifting supplies and equipment, proper body mechanics are vital to the MA's job. The MA must know how to lift, carry, and move to protect herself from injury. The following are some guidelines for proper body mechanics.

- Before lifting, check the object to be lifted. If it is too heavy, ask for help. When items in a box are likely to shift, grasp it properly or ask for help.
- Make sure the floor is clean and dry where you are going to lift.
- Face the object; move your feet apart to a distance equal to your shoulder width, and put one foot slightly forward.

- Bend at the knees, then firmly grasp the object with both hands (Figure 23-1 ◆).
- Tighten your stomach muscles and keep your back straight.
- Lift the object with your legs. This technique uses the stronger leg muscles to lift rather than the weaker back muscles.
- If you need to turn, use your whole body. Never twist your body.
- Carry the object close to your body and close to your center of gravity. Keep your back straight (Figure 23-2 ◆).
- Bend at the knees, using the legs to balance the weight and to put the load down.
- Push, rather than lift, larger objects.

General Office Safety

In the medical office, general safety measures include the following:

- Attending to possible hazards, such as spilled fluids and electrical cords on the floor, immediately.
- Storing food separately from medication in a designated refrigerator and/or cabinet.
- Following directions for the use of office equipment and machinery.
- Removing obstructions in hallways and reception area.
- Following traffic flow patterns.

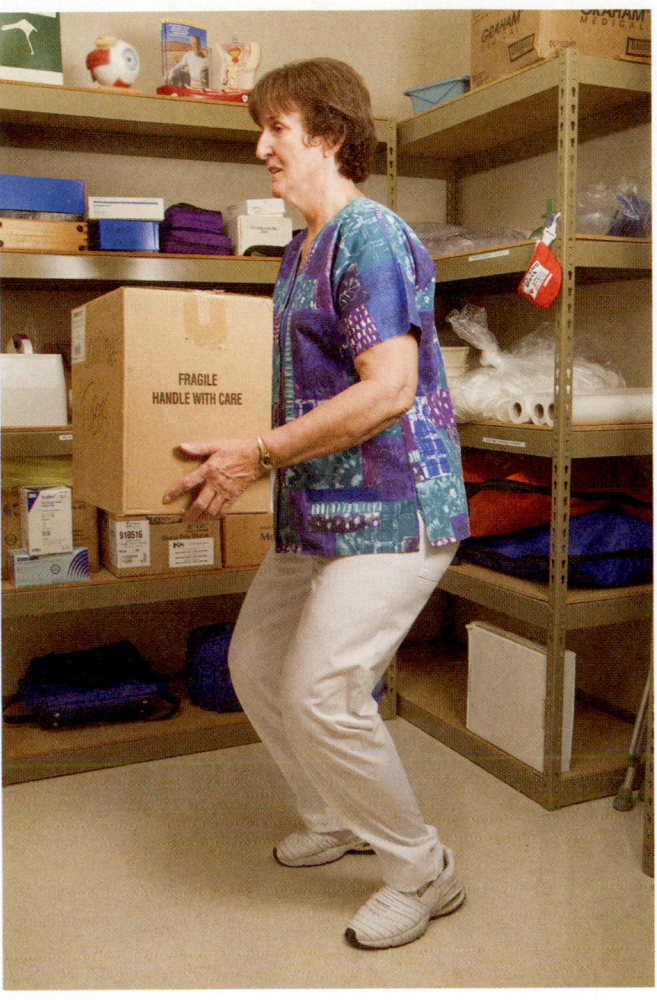

Figure 23-1 ◆ Bend at the knees, then firmly grasp the object with both hands.

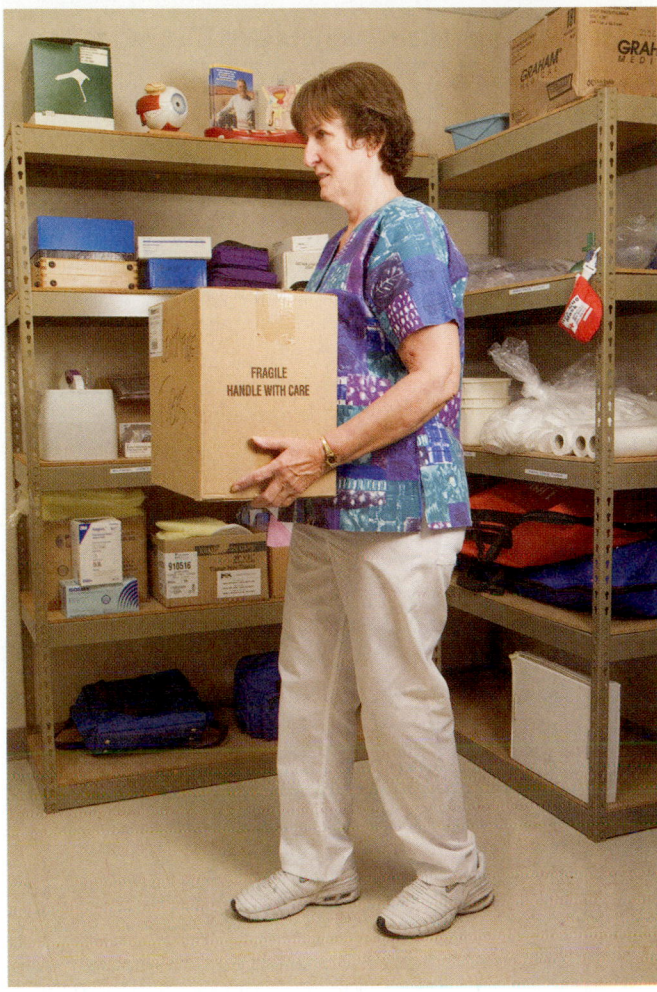

Figure 23-2 ◆ Carry the object close to your body and keep your back straight.

- Exercising caution when passing through doorways.
- Replacing light bulbs or letting the appropriate person know when a light bulb needs to be replaced.
- Keeping reception areas clean and orderly.

If the medical assistant is unable to correct a situation, he or she should bring it to the attention of the office manager or administrator.

Examination room safety includes the following:

- Keeping all medications locked in a cabinet.
- Disposing of expired medications by returning them to the manufacturer, or by crushing them and throwing them into the trash.
- Keeping floors clean, dry, and free of obstructions.
- Securing equipment, such as sphygmomanometers and otoscopes, at the proper wall height.
- Storing other equipment in appropriate drawers and cabinets.
- Performing routine surface cleaning to prevent microbial growth.
- Disposing of all medical materials in appropriate containers.
- Offering assistance to patients getting on or off the examination table.

The office should always have supplies available to maintain dry floors to prevent slips and falls.

Critical Thinking Question 23-1

Ian wants to save time and get to the reception area as quickly as possible. But what is the proper procedure for storing personal food items and medications in an office environment?

The Americans with Disabilities Act (**ADA**) of 1990 requires that every effort be taken to protect the civil rights of the disabled (Table 23-1). This includes making all areas of the office handicapped accessible. Should any barrier be brought to your attention, report it to the office manager or administrator.

The ADA is divided into five sections or titles. It is primarily intended to protect the civil rights of the disabled. It also applies to individuals who are associated with or assist persons with disabilities. Employment provisions apply to businesses of fifteen or more employees. Public accommodations apply to businesses of all sizes.

TABLE 23-1 AMERICANS WITH DISABILITIES ACT (ADA)

Title I	Employers must provide reasonable accommodations to all employees with disabilities in all aspects of pre-employment and work performance.
Title II	Public services cannot deny services to persons with disabilities that are offered to persons without disabilities.
Title III	All new construction must meet ADA requirements. Present structures must remove barriers to access if easily achievable. Included in this section are parking lot ramp requirements.
Title IV	Telecommunications telephone service to the general public must also provide relay services, such as TTY.
Title V	This section prohibits coercing, threatening, or retaliating against the disabled or those aiding persons with disabilities.

In Practice

As Melanie is putting away cleaning solutions in the medical office storage room she accidentally spills the solution. Just then, the physician calls Melanie over the paging system to join her in an exam room right away to assist with a patient. What should Melanie do?

Emergency Plans

As a new hire in a medical office, part of the MA's training must include emergency plans. These should be permanently kept in a policy or procedure manual. The MA should review this information on a regular basis.

Emergencies include fire, electrical accidents, explosions, and workplace-related violence. Disasters can be acts of nature or "acts of God." They include earthquakes, tornadoes, hurricanes, floods, snowstorms, and other weather-related events.

It is essential that the medical assistant:

- Remain calm during an emergency.
- Take care of patients first.
- Call the authorities, such as the fire department.
- Evacuate if necessary.

The MA should know where evacuation plans are posted in each room and keep hallways and exit doors free from obstructions. The office manager or administrator should be notified if an exit door is blocked or locked. It is a violation of fire codes to block exit routes. When an evacuation is announced, the MA should assist all patients from the office and/or building and know his assigned meeting place.

? —Critical Thinking Question 23-2—

Once Ian is on the scene with Cora, who is assessing the patient's vital signs and status, what should he do next?

Fire and Electrical Safety

The medical assistant should know the location of fire exits, alarms, and fire extinguishers and follow all emergency plans. The MA must keep all hallways and exit doors free from obstructions. *If a fire is discovered, pull the alarm.*

If the alarm sounds:

- Call or direct someone to call 911 (only if it is safe to do so), or call from a safe place outside the building.
- Close all doors and windows (only if it is safe to do so).
- Check bathrooms and examination rooms to make sure all patients and staff are aware of the fire alarm.
- Evacuate with patients immediately.
- Meet at an assigned place.
- Never use the building elevator during a fire, as it can stop on the floor with the fire; use the stairs.

The only time a fire extinguisher should be used is when the fire is between you and the door. If you have to use the extinguisher, use the PASS method (Figure 23-3 ◆). It is important that you know how to use the appropriate kind of fire extinguisher before trying to use it. Local fire departments generally train employees regarding fire safety in the office. Practice fire drills and emergency carries.

Electrical safety requires exercising caution. Be careful with all equipment and make sure it is in good condition before using it. Tell your office manager or administrator if you see:

- Frayed wires or cords
- Overused extension cords
- Lack of ground plugs or grounded outlets
- Cracked or broken switch or receptacle plates
- Sparking when a plug is inserted into or removed from an outlet
- Broken lights

Disasters

Learn the guidelines for specific natural disasters in your area. The director of emergency preparedness or emergency management in your community is a source for these guidelines. ∞ Chapter 41, Emergency Care, provides a detailed discussion of emergency preparedness.

If a disaster happens, the MA must remain calm. The amount of time that the MA has to prepare before a disaster strikes can vary.

- The National Oceanic and Atmospheric Administration's (NOAA) National Weather Service issues watches and warnings for weather events such as tornadoes. A *watch* means conditions are favorable for the formation of a tornado. A *warning* means a tornado has been sighted in the area and immediate action must be taken. Patients and staff must move to a safe area, such as a basement or an inner room without glass windows. Everyone must get down on the floor and cover their heads. There is usually advance warning for hurricanes, and preparations can be made before the storm arrives.

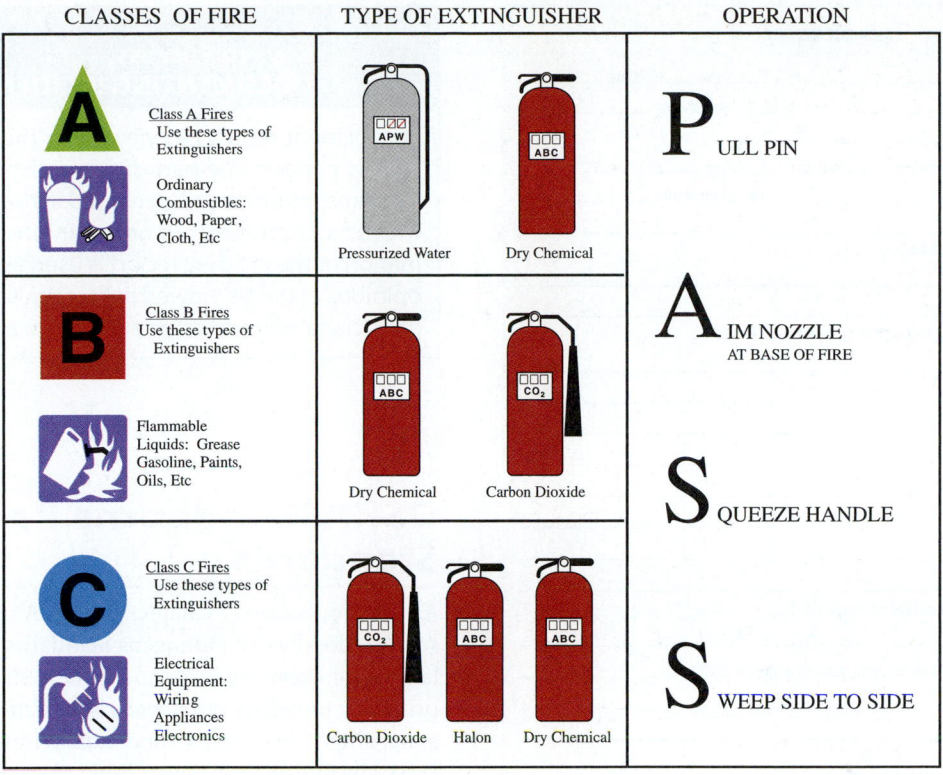

| CLASSES OF FIRE | TYPE OF EXTINGUISHER | OPERATION |

Figure 23-3 ◆ PASS method of firefighting: Pull the pin, aim at the base of the fire, squeeze the trigger, and sweep from side to side.
Source: The University of Texas Health Science Center at Houston Environmental Health and Safety Department.

■ Earthquakes usually happen without warning. The best approach is to evacuate the building, away from possible falling debris. If the MA is unable to leave the building, he should get under a heavy piece of furniture and cover his head.

The MA should be alert for secondary hazards after a disaster has occurred, such as ruptured gas or water lines, downed electrical or other wires, fires, broken pavement or earth, glass and debris, and fallen objects and trees. Common sense is the best guide before, during, and after natural disasters.

Workplace Violence

Violence in the workplace may be committed by an employee, former employee, patient, former patient, a patient's family member, or total stronger. If faced with a threatening person, the MA should speak in a calm and quiet voice and alert another staff member who can call the police.

Workplace Security

Workplace security has become an issue in recent years. Medical offices have become a target for thieves and drug addicts. Some basic precautions should be followed.

■ Doors and windows must be locked at the end of the day. Security keys or codes are usually assigned to select employees. If the MA is given keys and one is missing, she must tell the office manager or administrator. All locks must be changed when a key is lost.

■ Prescription pads should be kept out of patients' sight. The MA must account for all prescription pads at the end of the workday. If any pads are missing, an incident report should be filed and the appropriate law enforcement or drug enforcement agency notified.

Incident Reports

Incident reports are used to document unusual occurrences or accidents in the medical office (Figure 23-4 ◆). The persons involved, witnesses, a description of the event, and treatments given are among required information. Incident reports are a good tool for analyzing the event to prevent it from happening again.

Examples of events that should be recorded on an incident report form include the following:

■ Receiving a contaminated needle stick injury.
■ Discovering that a wrong medication has been given.
■ Finding a patient who has fainted in the reception area, examination room, or the parking lot.
■ Discovering that prescription pads are missing.
■ Seeing a patient or office staff member fall on a wet floor.
■ Feeling an electric shock while plugging an EKG machine into an electrical outlet.

INCIDENT REPORT

Name of injured party _____ Date _____

Address _____ Telephone _____

_____

The injured party was: ☐ Employee   ☐ Patient   ☐ Other _____

Date of accident/incident _____ Time of incident _____

Where did incident occur? _____

Names of witnesses (include titles):

_____

_____   _____

What first aid/treatment was given at the time of the incident?

_____

_____

Who administered first aid? _____

Briefly describe the incident. _____

_____

_____

_____

_____

_____

Names of employees present at time of incident/injury:

_____

Follow-up: What steps have been taken to prevent a similar accident? _____

_____

_____

_____
Date   Employee's signature

_____
Date   Supervisor's signature

Figure 23-4 ◆ An example of a typical incident report.

? Critical Thinking Question 23-3

After the situation in the reception area has been taken care of and the patient is no longer in need of medical assistance, how should the incident be recorded, and by whom?

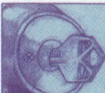

Keys to Success
DOCUMENTING INCIDENTS

The incident report is reviewed by the physician's office. It does not become part of the patient's chart, although the same information is recorded in the chart. Record only the facts. Do not record any opinions. If the chart information or the incident report is used as evidence in court, opinions could be viewed as an admission of fault by the physician's office or as an attempt to blur the facts.

OSHA Bloodborne Pathogen Standards

As mentioned in ∞ Chapter 4, OSHA's Occupational Exposure to Bloodborne Pathogens Standards are important regulations for every medical office. These standards are designed primarily to reduce employee risk of infectious diseases such as hepatitis B virus (**HBV**) and human immunodeficiency virus (**HIV**) by limiting exposure (Table 23-2). (∞ Refer to Chapter 25, Medical Asepsis, for more information on HBV and HIV.) Although the goal is employee safety, any worker or employer with potential occupational exposure must follow these standards. Failure to comply could result in a citation and a fine up to $7,000 for each violation and a maximum penalty of $70,000 for repeat violations.

According to OSHA's standards, each medical office must have a written exposure control plan that addresses:

■ Methods of compliance
■ Infection control practices
■ Housekeeping and laundry **decontamination**
■ Hepatitis B vaccinations
■ Engineering and work practice controls

PROCEDURE 23-1   File a Medical Incident Report

Theory and Rationale

In the medical office, staff members must file reports for incidents in which patients or employees are injured or could have been injured. Medical facilities that are JCAHO-certified are required to file incident reports. Medical clinics that are not JCAHO-certified may be required to do so by the Department of Health within the state where the practice is located.

Materials

■ Incident report form
■ Black or blue ink pen
■ Patient's chart

Competency

(**Conditions**) With the necessary materials, you will be able to (**Task**) fill out an incident report (**Standards**) correctly within the time allowed by the instructor.

1. Complete all areas of the incident report form using only facts, not opinions or judgments. For inapplicable areas, enter "NA" or "Not applicable."
2. Sign and date the form.
3. Give the form to the office manager or office director.
4. Participate in any educational meetings to determine how similar events could be avoided.

TABLE 23-2 POTENTIALLY INFECTIOUS (REGULATED) MATERIALS

Blood or body fluid visibly contaminated with blood
Vaginal secretions or semen
Body fluids, including cerebrospinal, peritoneal, synovial, peri-
   cardial, pleural, amniotic, and saliva in dental procedures
Pathology specimens, such as tissue culture, cells, any unfixed
   human tissue, or fluid known to be HIV infected

- Postexposure evaluation and followup
- Hazards communications
- Documentation of training and record keeping

Patient Safety

Following OSHA standards greatly reduces the risk of pathogen transmission from healthcare worker to patient. An employee who has been or is a known disease carrier and who performs high-risk procedures should know his or her HBV and HIV status. An employee with HIV or HBV should not perform patient care without first consulting a personal physician and a medical review committee. The affected employee must also tell patients of the potential risk, as appropriate. An employee with draining lesions should tell a supervisor, and patient contact will be restricted.

The Centers for Disease Control suggest TB screening of every healthcare worker. The MA should refer to state guidelines for his or her area's specific requirements. Initial screening by Mantoux skin test is usually an acceptable screening tool. The CDC also recommends that each healthcare facility have an exposure plan developed and in place. Again, the MA should refer to state and local guidelines for specific recommendations. Administrators responsible for plans should obtain medical and epidemiologic guidance from state and local health departments. Risk assessment should help to determine the types of administrative, environmental, and respiratory protection controls that are required and provide an ongoing evaluation tool of the quality of TB infection control. This assessment will also assist in the identification of any necessary improvements in infection control measures.

Exposure Control Plan

In the exposure control plan, each employee is classified according to the likelihood of exposure to blood and other potentially infectious materials. Employee categories are based on:

- Ongoing occupational exposure risk
- Accidental or potential exposure risk
- No exposure risk

For example, a medical assistant or other clinical person is at risk for ongoing occupational exposure. Custodial or laundry service staff are at risk of accidental or potential exposure to improperly discarded sharps in the trash or laundry.

The exposure control plan sets effective dates for other provisions of the standard. The plan must also establish procedures

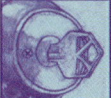

Keys to Success
WRITTEN PROCEDURES

When procedures are written for the medical office or any health-care facility, standards of performance and safety are included:

- Materials and required steps
- Personal protective equipment (PPE) required
- Instructions for proper cleaning, sterilization, or disposal of used supplies and equipment
- Description of body fluid type and approximate exposure amount during the procedure

for evaluating exposure incidents. These written procedures must be readily available to employees and to OSHA. The plan must be evaluated annually.

Standard Precautions and Infection Control Practices

Standard Precautions, including both Universal Precautions and Body Substance Isolation, are infection control guidelines established by the Centers for Disease Control and Prevention (CDC). All human blood and body fluids are considered infectious. (Refer to ∞ Chapter 25, Medical Asepsis, for more complete information on Standard Precautions.)

Engineering and Work Practice Controls

Engineering controls reduce or eliminate the risk of occupational exposure. Examples include devices that isolate or remove health hazards, such as autoclaves, biohazard containers, and safety cabinets. In November 2000, President Clinton signed the Needlestick Safety and Prevention Act, which specifies employee involvement in evaluating needle devices in current use and in the selection of better, safer needle devices. Following OSHA work practice controls also reduces the risk of exposure.

Frequent hand washing is one of the most important ways to reduce risk. Other work practice controls include the following.

1. Keep the potential for spraying, spattering, and splashing moisture droplets from blood and body fluids to a minimum.
2. Know the appropriate color coding or labeling for biohazard containers and biohazard-containing appliances

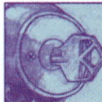

Keys to Success
GOOD SAMARITAN ACT

If a worker assists another coworker who has become ill, is this occupational exposure? The answer is no. This is considered a "Good Samaritan" act, not part of the job.

(Figure 23-5 ◆). An explanation of MSDS labeling appears in Figure 23-6 ◆.

3. Bandage open wounds on the hands.
4. Wash the hands after each glove removal.
5. Wash any skin surface immediately after contact with blood or body fluids. Flush mucous membranes with water.
6. Dispose of contaminated needles and other sharps in the appropriate puncture-resistant container after use.
7. Never eat, drink, store food, smoke, or apply cosmetics in areas where blood or body fluids are present because of potential contamination.
8. Place potentially infectious blood or tissue into containers that prevent leakage during collection, handling, processing, storage, and transport. Containers should be closed, except during collections and processing, and specially labeled or color coded as containing biohazardous materials.
9. Decontaminate equipment contaminated with blood and body fluids before it is cleaned.
10. File an incident report if an employee is exposed to a potentially infectious material. The employer must begin the exposure procedures.

Personal Protective Equipment

Personal protective equipment (PPE) is required protective wear. PPE protects healthcare employees from contact with potentially infectious blood and body fluids. Single or combined PPE may be worn depending on the degree of anticipated exposure. PPE includes:

- Gloves (for direct hand contact)
- Face shields or masks (for sprays, splashes, or droplets)

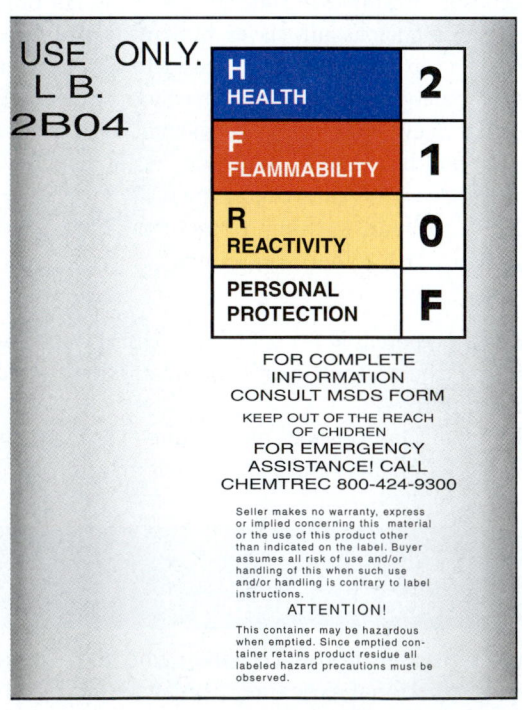

Figure 23-5 ◆ MSDS label.

BLUE-Health Risks of a Substance

4—Severe health risk could cause death or irreversible injury.

3—Could cause serious temporary or irreversible injury

2—Could cause temporary incapacitation.

1—Could cause irritation

0—No health hazard

RED-Flammability Risks of a Substance

4—Flammable vapor or gas that burns readily.

3—Flammable liquid or sold that can be readily ignited.

2—The substance must be heated for ignition.

1—The substance must be preheated before ignition.

0—No fire hazard

YELLOW-Reactivity of a Substance

4—Capable of detonation or explosive reaction.

3—May detonate when exposed to a heat or an ignition source.

2—Capable of a nonexplosive reaction.

1—May become unstable at high temperatures.

WHITE-PPE Recommendation of a Substance

A—Safety glasses

B—Safety glasses and gloves

C—Safety glasses, gloves, and apron

D—Face shield, gloves, and an apron

E—Safety glasses, gloves, apron, and a dust respirator

F—Safety glasses, gloves, apron, and a dust respirator

Figure 23-6 ◆ Explanation of MSDS labeling.
Reprinted by permission of Kristiana Routh.

- Gowns or laboratory coats (for large amounts of infectious materials)
- Masks (for airborne transmission)

OSHA requires that PPE be provided by the employer at no charge to the employee. The employer also covers the cost of replacing, maintaining, or cleaning PPE. More medical offices are using disposable items when they are more cost effective than cleaning and/or sterilizing. Examples include patient gowns and disposable suture removal sets. Gloves are *never* reused. Clothing or equipment such as masks must be strong enough that body substances do not penetrate and reach the employee's clothing, skin, or mucous membranes. Before leaving the medical office, the employee must place contaminated equipment or clothing in a designated container. (∞ Refer to Chapter 25, Medical Asepsis, for more information on PPE.)

PROCEDURE 23-2 Develop an Exposure Control Plan

Theory and Rationale

OSHA requires all medical offices to have exposure control plans that list all personal protective equipment in the office and information regarding its use, as well as information on what the employee is to do in the event of an exposure.

Materials

- List of personal protective equipment within the office
- Training manual

Competency

(**Conditions**) With the necessary materials, you will be able to (**Task**) develop an exposure control plan (**Standards**) correctly within the time allowed by the instructor.

1. List each piece of personal protective equipment in the office.
2. List the situations when each piece of equipment should/must be used.
3. Hold an in-office training session to review each item and to discuss its use.
4. Demonstrate each item's use.
5. Discuss how the office can reduce or eliminate exposures in the office.
6. Discuss the steps the employees should take in the event of exposure.
7. Document everything discussed at the meeting, and distribute copies to all staff.

Housekeeping and Laundry Decontamination

Housekeeping employees in a medical office are at risk for exposure to potentially infectious materials. They must receive OSHA-required training and offered immunization protection. All employees must follow OSHA standards regarding housekeeping and laundry decontamination procedures, which are defined by the facility. (∞ Refer to Chapter 25, Medical Asepsis, for complete information on cleanup and decontamination.)

Hepatitis B Vaccinations

OSHA requires that Hepatitis B vaccinations be offered to every healthcare worker within ten days of beginning employment. The employer must provide immunization at no charge to the employee, along with education regarding the benefits of the vaccination. The employee is given the opportunity to accept or decline immunization. If the employee declines, he or she must sign a form so indicating. The employee can later choose to accept immunization.

Hazard Communication Program

Orange or orange-red labels are required on items such as containers and refrigerators that contain regulated infectious waste (Figure 23-7 ◆). Items not labeled are to be stored and transported in red bags or containers. Decontaminated, regulated waste and tested HIV/HBV-free blood does not need to be labeled. When all specimens and all laundry are handled according to Standard Precautions, red bags or hazard labels are not needed.

Radioactive waste occurs as a by-product of nuclear medicine or radiation therapy and must be clearly labeled. It is never incinerated or poured down the drain and must be disposed of by a licensed facility.

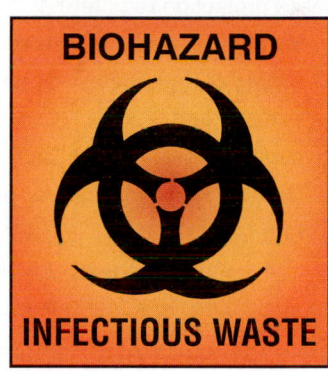

Figure 23-7 ◆ Orange or orange-red labels are required on items such as containers and refrigerators that contain regulated infectious waste.

Medical offices are required to keep an inventory of toxic substances used on the premises. The Material Safety Data Sheet (**MSDS**) (Figure 23-8 ◆) for each chemical includes such information as:

- Product name and/or synonymous (identical) names
- The manufacturer's name, address, and phone number
- Components of the chemical
- Effects of exposure to the chemical
- First aid and emergency measures for exposure
- Storage and disposal requirements
- Procedures for cleaning leaks or spills
- Use of PPE

Employees must read each MSDS. The employer must be able to provide evidence that all employees have read the MSDS. Usually, the signature or initials of each employee on the MSDS is sufficient. By signing or initialing, the employee

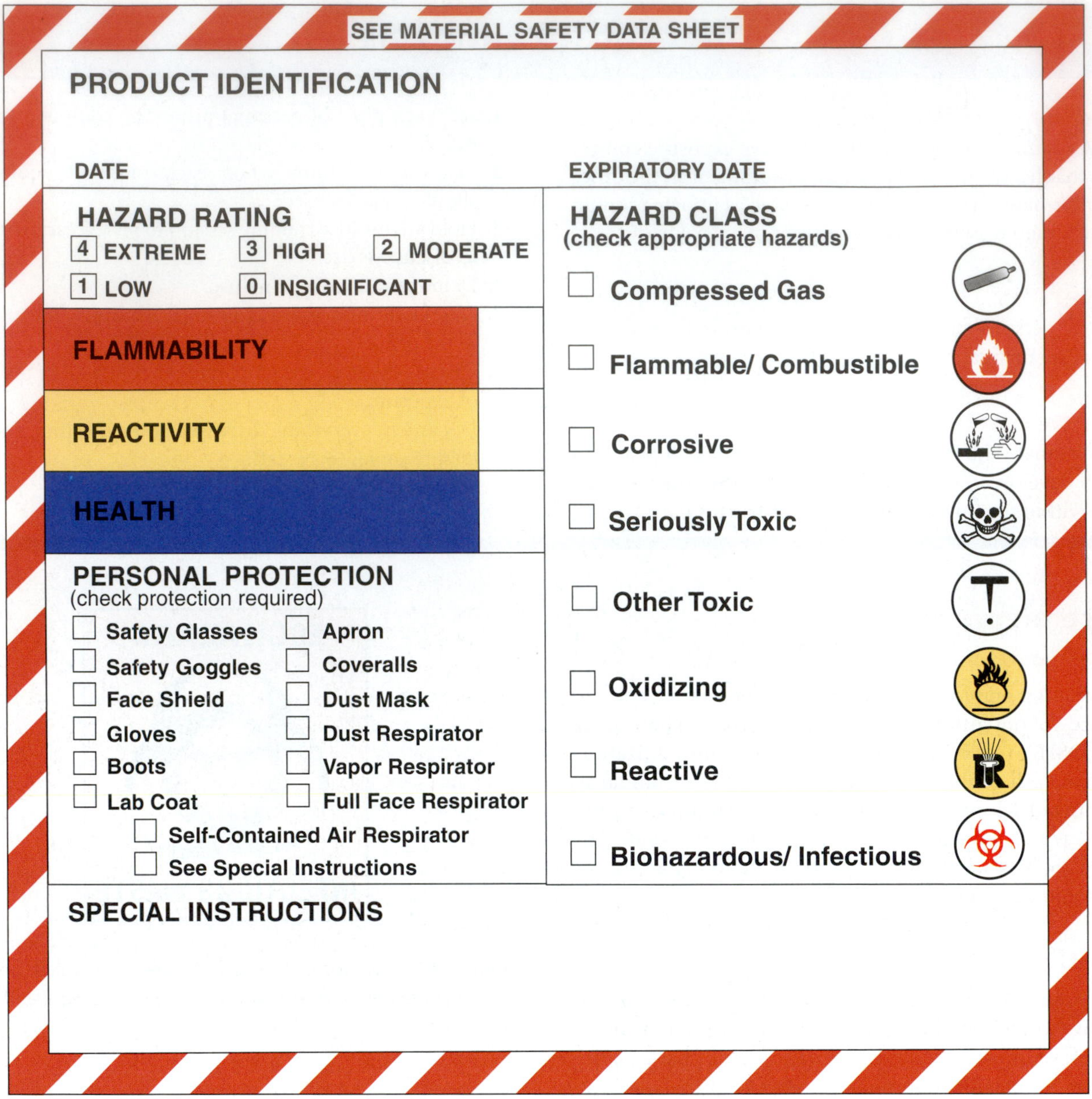

SEE MATERIAL SAFETY DATA SHEET

PRODUCT IDENTIFICATION

DATE   EXPIRATORY DATE

HAZARD RATING
[4] EXTREME   [3] HIGH   [2] MODERATE
[1] LOW   [0] INSIGNIFICANT

FLAMMABILITY

REACTIVITY

HEALTH

PERSONAL PROTECTION
(check protection required)
- Safety Glasses
- Safety Goggles
- Face Shield
- Gloves
- Boots
- Lab Coat
- Apron
- Coveralls
- Dust Mask
- Dust Respirator
- Vapor Respirator
- Full Face Respirator
- Self-Contained Air Respirator
- See Special Instructions

HAZARD CLASS
(check appropriate hazards)
- Compressed Gas
- Flammable/ Combustible
- Corrosive
- Seriously Toxic
- Other Toxic
- Oxidizing
- Reactive
- Biohazardous/ Infectious

SPECIAL INSTRUCTIONS

Figure 23-8 ◆ An example of a Material Safety Data Sheet (MSDS).

accepts responsibility for the correct handling of the hazardous substance.

Training and Record Keeping

OSHA standards require that employers provide training to employees at occupational risk of exposure to infectious body substances. Training must occur during the first ninety days of employment, then every year thereafter. The training includes information and updates on the exposure control plan and methods of compliance.

Employers must keep training records for three years after the training session. Confidential records for each at-risk medical office employee are kept for thirty years post-employment (Table 23-3).

TABLE 23-3 OSHA RECORD REQUIREMENTS

Employee Records
Name
Social security number
Hepatitis B vaccination dates
Postexposure examinations, testing, and followup (including medical evaluation and recommendations)
Copy of exposure report

Training Records
Content
Session dates
Names and qualifications of presenters
Names and titles of employee attendees

Exposure, Postexposure Evaluation, and Followup

Each medical office or other healthcare facility must have a specified procedure to be followed for exposure incidents. If an employee is exposed to a hazardous substance, an exposure report form must be filled out.

Postexposure medical evaluation and treatment are provided by the employer without charge to the employee. Employee information created by the medical evaluation must be kept confidential. The evaluation includes events of the exposure and blood testing of the source person and the employee. If consent is given, treatment and counseling are provided.

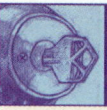

Keys to Success
THE CONTROVERSY OVER MERCURY THERMOMETERS

Exposure to even small amounts of mercury can be harmful. Swallowing mercury from a broken glass thermometer is an emergency, requiring a visit to the emergency room or a call to the poison control center. If a person with a healthy gastrointestinal (GI) tract swallows mercury, it is usually eliminated quickly, without causing symptoms. If the person has a history of gastrointestinal ulcers, fistulas, or inflammatory bowel disease, passage through the GI system is slower and exposure to the mercury is prolonged.

Mercury is a very heavy element that is not well absorbed through the skin or cuts. The most likely reaction to mercury contact is a skin rash. Mercury contact occurs mostly through inhalation of vapors with more than a one-time, short exposure. Mercury is an environmental hazard and must be disposed of properly.

If a mercury thermometer breaks, wear gloves when you clean up the spill. Mercury beads on a hard surface. It can be scooped up and lifted into a jar with stiff paper or cardboard. It can also be lifted with a small eye dropper. If mercury gets on a carpet, cut out the spot. Put the mercury or mercury-soaked carpeting in a jar and seal tightly. Never vacuum mercury, because the heat may cause it to evaporate. The objective when cleaning up is to prevent inhalation of the fumes.

Alcohol thermometers are an alternative; however, they may not be as accurate. Digital thermometers, although more costly, are becoming more common. Many facilities are removing mercury thermometers from use, and some communities have banned them.

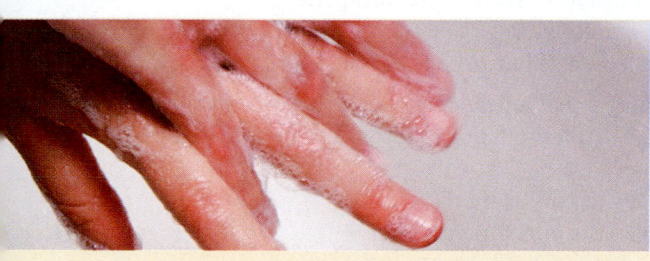

REVIEW

Chapter Summary

- In 1970, the Occupational Safety and Health Administration was created to establish safety regulations and health standards for the workplace. In 1991, Occupational Exposure to Bloodborne Standards were developed to reduce employees' risk for infectious diseases. All employees must follow these standards. Employers must provide a written exposure control plan.
- As an MA, you must always be alert to the safety of your patients, yourself, and the office.
- General office safety includes basic safety measures, such as removing hallway obstructions and exercising caution when

passing through doorways, and examination room safety, such as securing equipment and disposing of all medical materials in appropriate containers.
- The ADA requires that every effort be made to protect the civil rights of the disabled. This includes making the medical office handicapped accessible.
- Every medical office must have an emergency plan for disasters, fires, electrical problems, violence in the workplace, and security breaches. All employees must have access to the plan.

Chapter Summary (continued)

- It is most important to remain calm in an emergency. Follow all office procedures for evacuation and calling the police and fire department.
- Incident report forms must be filed for unusual occurrences and emergencies.
- The exposure control plan classifies each employee according to the likelihood of exposure to blood and other infectious materials. Included in the plan are Standard Precautions, PPE, engineering and work practice controls, housekeeping and laundry decontamination, Hepatitis B vaccinations, a hazard communication program, training, and record keeping.
- PPE protects wearers from contact with infectious blood and body fluids.
- A hazard communication program requires the proper handling and disposal of all hazardous substances, including contaminated, infectious, and radioactive wastes. Chemicals used in the medical office must have MSDSs on file and available to all employees.

Chapter Review

Multiple Choice

1. The first thing you should do before lifting is to
   a. make sure the object is not too heavy for you to lift.
   b. ask someone else to do it.
   c. move it with your foot.
   d. remove your shoes, so you have better balance.

2. When you are lifting a box, you should
   a. keep your feet together.
   b. bend at the waist.
   c. lift with your legs.
   d. loosen your stomach muscles.

3. The ADA requires that
   a. access to a public building is required, but public services can be denied.
   b. the civil rights of a person with disabilities should be protected.
   c. access to a public building can be denied, but public services are required.
   d. the civil rights of a person with disabilities be considered different from those of persons without disabilities.

4. Workplace security involves
   a. learning how to use a fire extinguisher.
   b. listening to the weather band on the radio.
   c. reporting overused electrical outlets.
   d. keeping prescription pads out of patients' sight.

5. A written exposure control plan must include information on
   a. documenting of training.
   b. types of fire extinguishers.
   c. types of security alarms.
   d. documenting disasters.

6. Which of the following measures is most important for reducing exposure risk?
   a. decontaminating equipment
   b. washing hands frequently
   c. using an autoclave
   d. labeling biohazard containers

7. OSHA requires employers to provide PPE to an employee
   a. and for the employee to pay for cleaning of the item.
   b. on a one-time basis, after which the employee is responsible for replacing an item.
   c. and for the employee to pay for the cost of replacing any worn item.
   d. and allows the employee to reuse gloves.

8. Which of the following is true about Hepatitis B vaccinations?
   a. An employee may be charged for the vaccination.
   b. An employee must be vaccinated.
   c. An employee must be offered the vaccination after three months on the job.
   d. An employee may decline being vaccinated.

9. A hazard communication program covers
   a. only bloodborne pathogens.
   b. toxic substances used in the workplace.
   c. only chemicals.
   d. regulated waste in workplace.

10. OSHA requires that a new employee at occupational risk for exposure to infectious body substances be trained within the first
    a. 110 days of employment.
    b. 100 days of employment.
    c. 90 days of employment.
    d. 120 days of employment.

True/False

T F 1. As an MA, you will need to be aware of and trained in general and medical safety procedures.

T F 2. In 1950, the Occupational Safety and Health Administration (OSHA) was created by Congress to establish safety and health standards and regulations in the workplace.

T F 3. For your safety, you should avoid loose and baggy clothing that could get caught in equipment.

Chapter Review (continued)

T F   4. The exposure control plan classifies each employee according to the likelihood of exposure to blood and other infectious materials.

T F   5. OSHA's Occupational Exposure to Bloodborne Pathogens Standards are designed to reduce employee risk of infectious diseases.

Short Answer

1. What did Joseph Lister use in 1867 to combat infections during transfusions?

2. According to OSHA, when must Hepatitis B vaccinations be offered to healthcare workers?

3. What document will give you information about chemicals used in the medical office, such as the effects of exposure as well as storage and disposal requirements?

4. What should you wear to protect yourself from contact with potentially infectious blood and body fluids?

5. Which government agency issues watches and warnings for weather events such as tornadoes?

Research

1. Does your local area have a standard 911 system, or is there another number that must be dialed?

2. List the following emergency numbers for your community:
   Hospital _____
   Fire Department _____
   Poison Control _____
   Non-emergency Transport _____
   EMT _____

Externship Application Experience

As a student in the medical office, you bring your lunch for the day. You ask the receptionist where you should put it until lunchtime. She shows you a refrigerator in the clean utility room and tells you to put it there. When you open the door, you notice that medications are being stored in this refrigerator. What do you do?

Resource Guide

Centers for Disease Control and Prevention (CDC)
Emergency Preparedness and Response
1600 Clifton Road
Atlanta, GA 30333
1-800-CDC-INFO
www.bt.cdc.gov

Federal Emergency Management Agency (FEMA)
500 C Street, SW
Washington, DC 20472
202-566-1600
www.fema.gov

Joint Commission on Accreditation of Healthcare Organizations (JCAHO)
601 13th Street, NW
Suite 1150N
Washington, DC 20005
630-792-5000
www.jcaho.org

Occupational Safety & Health Administration (OSHA)
200 Constitution Avenue, NW
Washington, DC 20210
1-800-321-OSHA (6742)
TTY 1-877-889-5627
www.osha.gov

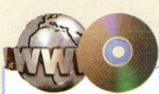

Med**Media**

http://www.MyMAKit.com

More on this chapter, including interactive resources, can be found on the Student CD-ROM accompanying this textbook and on http://www.MyMAKit.com.

The Clinical Visit: Office Preparation and the Patient Encounter

Case Study

Ali Keen, an RMA (AMT), is preparing the patient charts she will need for the day. She cannot locate the chart for her 1:00 patient. Ali looks on the physician's desk and in the vertical storage file, without luck. She then searches the computer schedule and sees that her patient came in as a walk-in appointment last week and was treated by Dr. Erin Strauser, her regular physician's partner.

Certain that Alexis, Dr. Strauser's MA, will have the chart, Ali goes to speak to her. After several minutes of shifting the clutter on Alexis's desk, she finds the chart. Ali notices that it's covered with coffee stains, which have soaked into several of the reports inside.

"Is this coffee? The chart can't be used like this," she says as she hands the chart back to Alexis.

Alexis takes the chart and hastily wipes off the cover and rips out several pages. She scribbles most of the information (incorrectly) onto new sheets and throws away the prescription refill notes. She says they are unnecessary since the medications have already been refilled and taken and the notes are more than six months old. Alexis then gives the chart back to Ali.

Objectives

After completing this chapter, you should be able to:

- Define and spell the key terminology within the chapter.
- Define the medical assistant's role in the clinical visit.
- List items commonly found in a standard examination room.
- Explain how to prepare and maintain examination and treatment room areas.
- Define triage and give examples of triage procedures in the medical office.
- Discuss the essentials of consent.
- List important elements contained in an initial patient history.
- List guidelines for charting a clinical visit.
- Explain how to chart a procedure.

MedMedia

http://www.MyMAKit.com

Additional interactive resources and activities for this chapter can be found on http://www.MyMAKit.com. For a video, audio glossary, legal and ethical scenarios, job scenarios, quizzes, and games related to the content of this chapter, please access the accompanying CD-ROM in this book.

Audio Glossary
Legal and Ethical Scenario: *The Clinical Visit: Office Preparation and the Patient Encounter*
On the Job Scenario: *The Clinical Visit: Office Preparation and the Patient Encounter*
Video: *Taking Patient Histories*
Multiple Choice Quiz
Games: Crossword, Strikeout, and Spelling Bee
Tips
HIPAA Quiz

✚ MEDICAL ASSISTING STANDARDS

CAAHEP ENTRY-LEVEL STANDARDS	ABHES ENTRY-LEVEL COMPETENCIES
■ Perform within scope of practice (psychomotor) ■ Apply ethical behaviors, including honesty/integrity in performance of medical assisting practice (affective) ■ Document patient care (psychomotor) ■ Perform patient screening using established protocols (psychomotor) ■ Recognize the role of patient advocacy in the practice of medical assisting (cognitive) ■ Explain general office policies (psychomotor) ■ Demonstrate recognition of the patient's level of understanding in communications (psychomotor) ■ Describe various types of content maintained in a patient's medical record (cognitive) ■ Apply critical thinking skills in performing patient assessment and care (affective) ■ Use language/verbal skills that enable patients' understanding (affective) ■ Demonstrate respect for diversity in approaching patients and families (affective)	■ Interview and take a patient history. ■ Prepare and maintain examination and treatment area. ■ Perform telephone and in-person screening. ■ Determine needs for documentation and reporting. ■ Document accurately. ■ Follow established policy in initiating or terminating medical treatment. ■ Operate and maintain facilities and equipment safely. ■ Orient patient to office policies and procedures.

✓ COMPETENCY SKILLS PERFORMANCE

1. Complete a patient history form.
2. Document a clinical visit and procedure.

Key Terminology

charting—documentation of all the events of a patient's visit

diagnosis—conclusion made about the patient's condition by interpretation of data

ophthalmoscope—instrument used to examine the eyes

otoscope—instrument used to examine the ears

prognosis—an outcome prediction for the course of a disease and patient recovery

sign—that which can be seen, heard, measured, or felt by the examiner

sphygmomanometer—instrument used to measure blood pressure

stethoscope—instrument used to listen to sounds within the body

symptom—a perceptible change in the body related by the patient

thermometer—instrument used to measure body temperature

triage—prioritizing patient needs by assessing symptoms, situations, and external factors and arranging patients according to most immediate need

Abbreviations

POMR—problem-oriented medical record

SOAP—subjective, objective, assessment, plan

Introduction

The patient has the right to expect a safe, clean, and orderly environment in the medical office. A physician also requires the same clean and orderly environment to provide efficient and thorough care to the patient. Convenient placement of instruments, supplies, and equipment allows the physician to make best use of time and movement in the examination or treatment areas.

As discussed in Chapter 12, carefully documented medical records are critical for patient care. Whether documenting an initial visit, patient history, or clinical visit, accuracy and attention to detail in these charts are a major responsibility in the medical office.

The Medical Assistant's Role in the Clinical Visit

Medical assistants usually do not have great input into the physical layout of a physician's office. However, the MA is responsible for providing a clean, safe environment in the examination and treatment areas. Preparing and maintaining the examination and treatment areas depend on the type of specialty practice in which the MA is employed.

Depending on the office duties assigned to the medical assistant, he or she may be involved in administrative responsibilities such as triage and preparing medical records, including consent forms, and third-party information, or in clinical responsibilities—obtaining the patient's history, taking vital signs, and updating the patient's chart.

The Standard Medical Office

The majority of office complexes are designed to provide efficiency in the physical structure with each physician using at least two examination rooms. Nearly all examination rooms and treatment areas have a sink, a small cabinet for supplies, an examination table, a stool, a writing surface, auxiliary lighting, hazardous waste and sharps containers, a chair, and possibly a telephone (Figure 24-1 ◆). An area for dressing or a screen is often provided for patient privacy. The patient's coat or clothing may be hung on a hook or placed on a chair. Sheets or paper drapes provide the patient with privacy and warmth if necessary.

The area should be well lit and easily ventilated. The walls and door of the room should be soundproof for patient privacy and confidentiality. The door should be kept closed for patient privacy. There are racks for chart holders by the door on the wall outside the room. Temperature controls should be placed so that the rooms can be kept at a comfortable temperature for the patient.

Standard equipment may include the following:

- A wall-mounted or portable **sphygmomanometer,** which measures blood pressure
- An **otoscope,** which is used to examine the ears
- An **ophthalmoscope,** which is used to examine the eyes
- An examination table with stirrups and a pull-out foot rest

- A wall-mounted X-ray view box
- Portable lighting

Depending on the specialty, other equipment may be required. Equipment to monitor vital signs includes a **thermometer,** which is used to measure patient's temperature; a **stethoscope,** which is used to listen to sounds within the body; and a sphygmomanometer. A scale to weigh and to measure the patient's height is available in the clinical area of the medical office. A Snellen eye chart is usually mounted in a hall or other location that allows the patient's vision to be tested at a distance of 20 feet.

Equipment should be checked on a regular basis to make sure it is in working condition. It is the responsibility of the MA to know how the equipment works and to be able to assist the physician in its use.

Storage for equipment and supplies includes the examination table, supply cabinet, and desk. The examination table has drawers in which to store equipment and supplies, such as patient gowns, drapes, sheets, vaginal specula, emesis basins, lubricant, and urine specimen containers. The supply cabinet is a storage unit for thermometers, alcohol prep pads, slides and specimen containers, tongue depressors, cotton-tipped applicators, a tuning fork, specula for the otoscope, disposable gloves, sterile gloves, laryngeal mirror, nasal speculum, reflex hammer, stethoscope, otoscope, ophthalmoscope, and tape measure. Tissues and writing materials are available on the small desk.

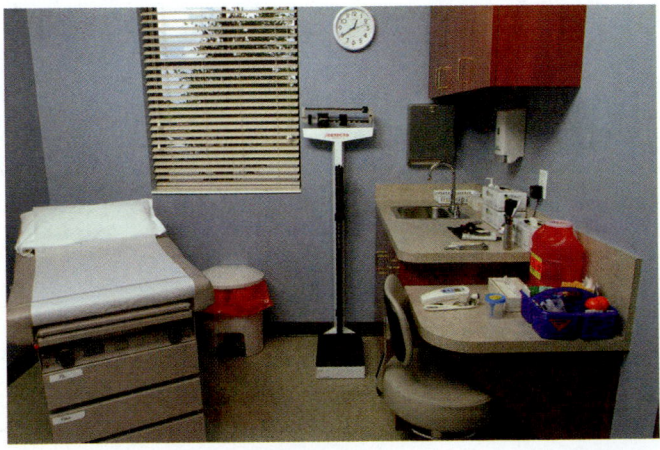

Figure 24-1 ◆ Examination room.

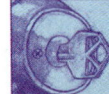

Keys to Success
EQUIPMENT MALFUNCTIONS

Do not forget or ignore broken equipment or assume someone else will take care of it. Follow office policy and take immediate steps to store the broken item in another location, label it as broken, and make repair arrangements. Also, keep a log on the item, noting labeling, removing, and repairing.

In a court of law, when involved in a legal case, it is usually a point to establish who knew about the equipment failure and when it occurred. Liability is more severe if it becomes known that staff knew of malfunctioning equipment and did not take safeguards to label and repair it.

Preparing and Maintaining Examination and Treatment Areas

At the beginning of the day, the MA should check all examination rooms to see that they are clean, free of clutter, and in order. The MA should make sure there are adequate supplies for the day and restock if necessary. Then check the patient roster for the day and why the patients are being seen. Any supplies for special examinations or procedures should be on hand in the supply area.

After the patient visit is completed and the patient has left the room, the MA must replace the examination table paper. When removing used table paper, turn all soiled surfaces inward and fold the paper into a small package for disposal (Figure 24-2 ◆). This way, hands come in contact with the clean side only. (The same principle applies to removing gloves.)

In Practice

Rocky has just finished with his last patient of the day. Since Rocky has tickets to the basketball game tonight, he wants to get out of the office as soon as possible. Rocky will be working first thing in the morning, so he thinks it will be alright if he leaves the exam rooms uncleaned until the morning. Why might this be a bad idea?

Any soiled areas are cleansed according to office protocol. Used or soiled equipment should be removed to the "dirty" area for cleansing and appropriate disinfection or sterilization. Waste receptacles should be emptied frequently. If necessary, use a disinfectant spray to combat germs and/or odor. Any spills should be cleaned immediately. Generally, professional cleaning services are contracted to maintain the floors, windows, and other structural components of the office.

At the end of the day, check all areas for cleanliness and make sure that adequate supplies are available for the next day.

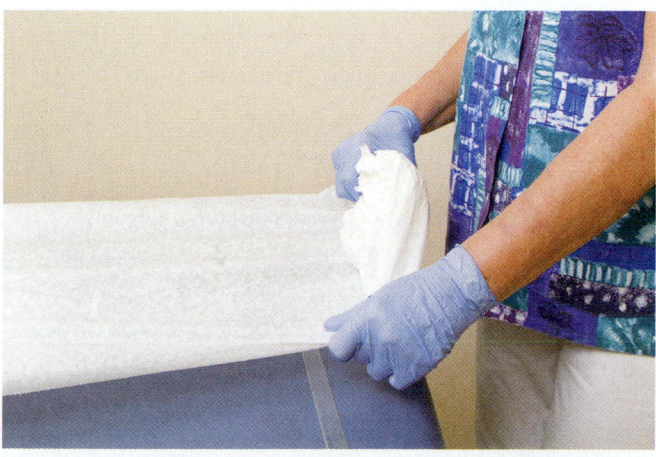

Figure 24-2 ◆ When removing used table paper, turn all soiled surfaces inward and fold the paper into a small package for disposal.

Dispose of hazardous materials according to office and OSHA guidelines. Clean and disinfect the restroom and restock it with paper supplies and urine specimen cups if necessary.

Triage

Triage is the process of prioritizing patient needs by assessing symptoms, situations, and external factors and arranging patients according to most immediate need. Triage can occur through direct patient contact to assess who is in the most immediate need of medical attention, or by phone (see ∞ Chapter 9) to assess who has the most immediate need for a return phone call. Listening to the complaint and the information imparted by the patient is of utmost importance. The MA should follow office policy or protocol concerning additional questions and the triage of critically ill or severely injured patients. The medical assistant may need to confer with an office nurse or physician for further instructions.

Critically Ill or Severely Injured Patients

Office policy should be established concerning individuals calling in or presenting with chest pain and/or difficulty breathing. Most physician offices refer patients with any chest pain or those having difficulty breathing and not present in the office to Emergency Medical Services (EMS). Depending on the situation, the patient or the caller may or may not be able to call 911. In this situation, office staff should use another phone line to call EMS while keeping the caller on the phone for additional information, including location and continuing condition. Should the patient present at the office, the MA should take him or her into a treatment room WITHOUT DELAY and have the physician notified immediately while assessing vital signs and symptoms. The physician will determine the course of treatment for these patients.

Other patients with sudden onset of severe pain should be considered emergency patients. Again, depending on office policy and the presence of the physician in the office, a patient contacting the office by phone may be instructed to call Emergency Medical Services (usually 911), proceed to an emergency facility, or come to the office as soon as possible. This patient will be taken into the treatment area upon arrival and assessed. Symptoms, including onset and location of pain, should be assessed and documented. The patient will be asked about the onset and duration of the pain, what makes it better or worse, and if it has occurred before. The MA should be aware of conditions that are considered serious or emergency conditions requiring immediate intervention. In addition to chest pain, other emergencies requiring immediate assessment or intervention include the following:

- Difficulty breathing
- Seizures
- Decreased level of consciousness
- Allergic reactions
- Diabetic reactions

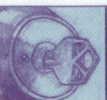

- Drug overdose
- Head injuries
- Severe lacerations and bleeding
- Sudden onset of paralysis or loss of speech
- Severe dizziness

A patient must be placed in a treatment room and the physician notified immediately for

- Sudden onset of acute pain
- Sudden acute illness
- Severe vomiting
- Poisoning
- Foreign body in the eye
- Possible fractures
- Drug overdose

All of these conditions require intervention as soon as possible. In the meantime, the MA should assess the situation and have information available for the physician on his or her arrival in the examination/treatment room.

Common sense is a good guideline for triage. Office policy is the best principle to follow in these matters. All personnel must be familiar with these policies and follow them.

Consent

As discussed in ∞ Chapter 4, Medical Law and Ethics, patients must give their consent to be examined and/or treated by the physician or healthcare provider and sign a consent form before they are accepted for care in the medical office. Many offices rely on implied consent, meaning that the patient agrees to examination and treatment when presenting for a routine visit. The contract between a physician and a patient consists of the request for service, provision of the services, and compensation for the services. The patient also has the right to expect care that is customary, reasonable, and consistent with what a prudent provider should do within the scope of his or her practice and training.

Signed consent forms are required legal documents stating that the patient is giving his or her permission for certain procedures to be performed or for information or documents to be released. A completed form must contain the patient's signature (or that of the patient's representative), date of signing, and date the consent will expire. The signatures on all consent forms must be witnessed. Often it is the MA who witnesses the signing of the consent form. The witness also signs the document, with the date. In signing, the witness merely verifies that the signature is that of the patient.

A Consent to Release of Information form is signed by a patient before the care provider can apply for third-party reimbursement (Figure 24-3 ◆). Forms to release information should include the following:

- Name of the medical facility or practice that will be releasing the information
- Name of the individual who is to receive the information
- Patient's full name, specific information to be released
- Purpose of releasing the information

Special procedures and surgical procedures require informed consent. See ∞ Chapter 4, Medical Law and Ethics, for a more detailed discussion of informed consent. See Figure 4-4 for a sample of an informed consent form.

? — **Critical Thinking Question 24-1**
What is the proper protocol for Alexis to follow after discovering the soiled chart? Who is responsible for the chart?

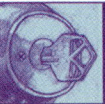

WINDY CITY CLINIC
Beth Williams, M.D.
123 Michigan Avenue
Chicago, IL 60610
(312) 123-1234

RECORDS RELEASE   Date _____

To _____
                              Doctor
_____
                              Address

I hereby authorize and request you to release

to _____
                              Doctor
_____
                              Address

all medical records in your possession concerning any examination, diagnosis, and/or treatment rendered to me

during the period from _____ to _____

_____
Signature of patient or closest relative

_____
Relationship

_____   _____
Signature of witness   Address

Figure 24-3 ◆ Consent to release information form.

Charting the Medical History and Clinical Visit

Charting is the documentation of all the events of a patient's visit. Along with the patient history, it is done by those involved with the treatment of the patient and is part of the medical record. Because it is a legal document, accuracy and correctness are critical. Unless a procedure is charted after completion, the documentation is considered incomplete by the legal system. Accurate charting requires skill and practice. Personal opinions are *never* to be charted.

Patient History

As part of the initial assessment, the medical assistant will review the patient's health history by asking specific questions about general health and previous health conditions. The physician will review this history with the patient (Figure 24-4 ◆).

A patient history should include the following:

- Personal history/social and occupational history
- Past medical or health history, including allergies and medications
- Family medical history
- Chief complaint (CC)

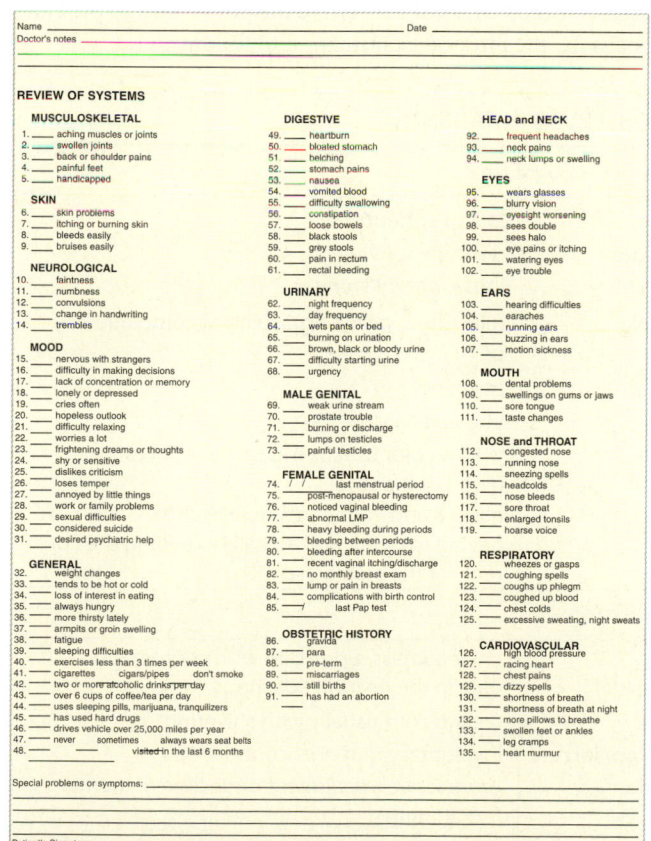

Figure 24-4 ◆ An example of a medical health history form used by the physician.
Courtesy of Bibbero Systems, Inc., Petaluma, CA; Phone: 800-242-2376
Fax: 800-242-9330; Email: info@bibbero.com; Web: www.bibbero.com

TABLE 24-1 PERSONAL HISTORY INFORMATION	
■ Lifestyle ■ Family situation ■ Living environment ■ Education ■ Military service ■ Occupation, both past and present ■ Exercise habits ■ Sleeping patterns	■ Alcohol consumption ■ Smoking or tobacco habits ■ Caffeine consumption ■ Dietary habits ■ Health habits ■ Foreign travel ■ Living arrangements ■ Seat belt use

- Present illness
- Assessment/review of body systems

Combined with diagnostic data and the physical examination, the physician draws on the history to make a **diagnosis,** which is a conclusion about the patient's condition. Finally, the physician anticipates the patient's response to treatment as well as the **prognosis,** which is a prediction of the outcome of a disease and patient recovery.

Personal History

Personal history may also be referred to as social and occupational history and includes the factors listed in Table 24-1.

Past Medical or Health History

Past medical or health history provides a background of previous or ongoing health concerns (Table 24-2).

Family Medical History

The family medical history provides the physician with an assessment of the patient's extended family health history. Questions are asked about the age, current health status, and disease occurrences of blood relatives, including parents, grandparents, siblings, and children, as well as of the spouse. If a family member is deceased, age and cause of death are noted. Some physicians have patients complete a health *genogram.* This chart, in the form of a family tree, illustrates any patterns of illnesses or health conditions in the patient's ancestors and siblings. Some diseases are genetic or hereditary, others show a familial tendency, and occasionally environmental factors affect some family members earlier or more intensely than others.

TABLE 24-2 PAST HISTORY INFORMATION	
■ Allergies ■ Past major illnesses ■ Previous hospitalizations and surgical procedures ■ Childhood diseases	■ Any injuries or accidents ■ Unusual infections ■ Immunizations ■ Previous medical tests ■ Medications, both past and present

All this information provides the physician with an insight into the patient's present condition, clues to the cause of any health-related problems, and an indication of how the patient may comply with treatment options. Some physicians are selective about the questions they prefer to be asked, and some forms are tailored to specialty practices.

Chief Complaint

An important part of any history, whether during the initial encounter or on repeat visits, is the presenting chief complaint (CC). The patient describes the symptoms causing the most trouble or the reason for the visit. **Symptoms** are changes in body functions reported by the patient and indicating the presence of disease or injury. Symptoms like pain, pruritus, vertigo, and nausea are felt only by the patient and are considered subjective in nature. It is for the medical assistant or another person to observe objective symptoms, such as rash, coughing, weight gain, edema, and cyanosis. Recording or charting the CC is essential to quality patient-centered care.

Present Illness

As the cause of the CC is explored, information about the present illness is expanded. The medical assistant should ask the patient for a detailed description of the present symptoms and illness. Open-ended questions such as "What brings you in today to see the physician?" are a good starting point. The patient's statement should be recorded in his or her own words

as closely as possible. Table 24-3 lists some of the signs and symptoms patients may describe.

The MA should try to limit the chief complaint to one or two specific symptoms. Information about the symptoms should include:

- Onset
- Duration
- Location, indicating specific area of the body
- Frequency
- Intensity of the symptoms, from just bothersome to severe and interfering with sleep and normal activities
- Any changes over time

Patients may describe pain as aching, burning, cramping, crushing, dull, sharp, shooting, squeezing, or throbbing. They may also say it is constant, intermittent, radiating, transient, localized, deep, or superficial. The MA should guide the patient with questions and write down the answers in his or her own words.

Assessment of Body Systems

The assessment of body systems is a physician review of all body systems with the patient to identify any symptoms not yet revealed. The physician asks questions regarding each body system and notes the answers on the chart. This preliminary step suggests specific areas of concern to the physician and provides a focus for the physical examination to follow.

TABLE 24-3 COMMON SIGNS AND SYMPTOMS RELATED BY AND OBSERVED IN PATIENTS

Circulatory System		Gastrointestinal System	
Angina	chest pain occurring during exertion	**Anorexia**	loss of appetite
Arrhythmia	irregular heartbeat	**Constipation**	difficulty moving the bowels
Bradycardia	slow heart rate, below 60 BPM	**Diarrhea**	loose, watery stools
Cyanosis	bluish tint to skin	**Dysphagia**	difficulty swallowing, usually accompanied by pain
Dehydration	loss of body fluids		
Edema	swelling, fluid in tissues	**Eructation**	belching
Palpitations	rapid, thumping heartbeat	**Flatus**	intestinal gas
Petechiae	small pinpoint hemorrhages on the skin	**Jaundice**	yellow color to skin and whites of eyes
		Melena	blood in the stool
Tachycardia	rapid heartbeat, over 100 BPM	**N & V**	nausea and vomiting; unpleasant sensation of
Varicosities	abnormally swollen and twisted veins, usually in legs		having to vomit and actually expelling the contents of the stomach orally
Integumentary System		**Nervous System**	
Diaphoresis	sudden onset of intense perspiration	**Ataxia**	unsteadiness, a problem with coordination
		Cephalgia	pain in the head, headache
Flushing	sudden redness to skin	**Chill**	feeling cold, usually with shivering
Pruritus	severe itching	**Convulsion/seizure**	involuntary muscular contractions
Rash	an eruption on the skin, usually red in color	**Dementia**	progressive impairment or decline of mental functioning
		Dyslexia	a learning disorder involving ability to read or write
		Fever or pyrexia	body temperature elevated above normal
		Insomnia	difficulty sleeping

TABLE 24-3 COMMON SIGNS AND SYMPTOMS RELATED BY AND OBSERVED IN PATIENTS (CONTINUED)

Integumentary System		Nervous System	
		Neuralgia	severe and sharp pain along a nerve
		Pain	unpleasant sensation
		Palsy	inability to control muscle movement, shaking
		Syncope	fainting
		Vertigo	dizziness
Reproductive System		**Respiratory System**	
Amenorrhea	absence of menses	Coughing	forceful, violent expiratory effort
Dysmenorrhea	painful menses	Cyanosis	bluish tint to skin
Erectile dysfunction	inability to achieve or maintain an erection with stimulation	Dyspnea	difficult or painful breathing
		Epistaxis	nosebleed
Menorrhagia	excessive bleeding during menses, heavy period	Laryngitis	loss of voice, hoarseness with little volume
		Orthopnea	difficulty breathing unless in a sitting position
		Rhinorrhea	runny nose
Urinary System		**Psychological or Emotional Symptoms**	
Anuria	absence of urine output	Aggression	a forceful action, physical, verbal, or symbolic
Dysuria	painful urination	Anxiety	apprehension, uneasiness
Enuresis	bedwetting	Depression	hopeless, helpless, sad feeling; crying all the time
Incontinence	inability to hold urine		
Nocturia	frequent urination during the night	Hallucinations	imaginary perceptions of visual or auditory stimuli
Oliguria	scanty urine output	Paranoia	feeling of being persecuted or pursued
Polyuria	voiding large amounts of urine		

Completing a Patient History Form

Collecting information on a patient's health history involves an oral interview. Information obtained from the health history and subsequent visits provides a complete historical record of the patient's health, including data to identify the patient, reason for the current visit, and family and patient history of disease conditions, illnesses, and hospitalizations. The physician uses past and family medical information to treat a patient for current and long-term medical conditions. The physician also uses the information to promote patient education and individual responsibility for prevention or progression of disease.

Charting a Clinical Visit

Guidelines for charting include the following.

- Select the correct chart for the patient. Verify the patient's name and, if necessary, birth date.
- Write or print legibly, using black or blue ink. Red ink is acceptable for allergies.
- Check to make sure the patient's name is on each page.
- Date and initial every entry.
- Write brief but complete entries.
- Use only accepted medical abbreviations.
- Make sure all medical terms are spelled correctly.

- *Never* erase or white-out mistakes. Draw a line through any mistake, write the word "error" above the mistake, date, and initial. Follow the mistake with the correct information and sign the completed entry.
- Document phone conversations with the patient or significant other by any staff member with action taken or recommended.
- Document all missed appointments.

As discussed in ∞ Chapter 12, charting or documenting the patient's medical record may be done in several formats.

Two primary methods are used to chart.

- The first method is chronological (Figure 24-5 ◆). It is a sheet of paper with the name at the top. Each entry is dated, vital signs are added, and reason for visit is documented.

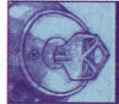

Keys to Success
OBTAINING DETAILS FOR A CC

Encourage the patient to describe the reason for the visit in his or her own words. Avoid using disease terminology. Using the patient's own words provides a more accurate picture for the physician.

PROCEDURE 24-1 Complete a Patient History Form

Theory and Rationale

The MA escorts the patient to a private area, usually the examination room, to interview him or her. Privacy encourages open communication and reduces anxiety and distractions for the patient. The MA's body language must show interest in the patient's concerns. Generally, patients respond more openly to a calm and caring approach. The medical assistant should address the patient in a formal manner unless the patient encourages a more informal manner. For the comfort of parent and child during a child's clinical visit, the MA should ask the parent or child what name the child prefers.

Materials

- Chart
- File folder for chart
- Patient history form
- Blue or black ink pen

Competency

(**Conditions**) With the necessary materials listed above, (**Task**) you will be able to complete the Patient History Form (**Standards**) following office policy and within the time and to the degree of accuracy designated by the instructor.

1. Greet the patient in a formal or age-appropriate manner.
2. Explain the health history form. Explain to the patient or parent that additional information beyond the original question is always important and can be added.

3. Observe patient's body language and respond appropriately or tactfully to encourage open sharing of medical information.
4. The order of interview for the Patient History Form follows the order of the form unless office policy dictates otherwise.
5. Instruct the patient to fill in the patient identification section. Review it to make sure the information is complete.
6. Use open-ended questions to obtain details of the patient's CC, or present illness, such as:
   - How long have the symptoms been occurring?
   - Where do the symptoms occur?
   - What activity brings on the symptoms or makes the symptoms worse?
   - Do the symptoms occur suddenly or gradually?
   - What activity helps the symptom(s) disappear or lessen?
   - When symptoms occur, how long do they last?
7. Proceed through questions about past medical history, family medical history, and social/occupational history as presented on the Patient History Form.

Patient Education

Discuss with the patient or parent the importance of complete and accurate information. Provide the patient with a pencil and paper to take notes on items that might need more information at a later or follow-up visit.

The physician adds narrative comments with each visit. New sheets of paper are added as needed.

- A second method, based on the patient's problems, is called the problem-oriented medical record (**POMR**). Information is charted by all employees providing care or treatment for the patient. All problems are recorded, and a numbered problem list is created. At each visit or encounter, information pertaining to a numbered problem is identified and recorded.

Charting for POMR is done by the subjective, objective, assessment plan (**SOAP**) method (see Figure 12-4). When problems are identified, they are documented in a systematic manner.

Patient's Name: Isabel Miranda
7/10/XX 9:30 a.m. 37-year-old Spanish-speaking female presents with a CC of sore throat, difficulty swallowing and excessive coughing, onset 3 days ago and getting progressively worse. 15-year-old daughter accompanies to translate. Skin is very warm to touch and is flushed. Patient is alert and cooperative. Nonproductive cough is noted. Vital signs: T 102.7 F, P 114, R 28, BP 140/90. Wt, 150#, Ht, 65". LMP - 7-02-02. Allergies – Penicillin. Meds, aspirin for pain, BCP, Zantac. Husband is L&W; has two other children, L&W: parents are deceased. Recently immigrated to US from Mexico for husband's employment and to be with other children. Marjorie Nelson, CMA (AAMA)

Figure 24-5 ◆ Sample completed chronological form.

S Subjective; refers to the symptoms described by the patient and/or family. It is best to record the patient's actual words in quotation marks, or write "Patient states _____."

O Objective; refers to findings elicited on the physical exam, the vital **signs,** and results of laboratory or other diagnostic testing.

A Assessment; includes the physician's diagnosis or nurse's assessment.

P Plan of action; includes any recommended treatments, additional testing, medications administered or prescribed, consultations recommended, surgery or physical therapy suggested.

In a medical office, the MA is responsible for charting the subjective and objective components. Other professionals, including physicians, nurses, laboratory technicians, and others, document some or all SOAP components, depending on the need for complete or partial documentation and established policies. Observations, test procedures, or results may be documented in partial SOAP format according to office procedures and within the scope of practice of each professional.

The MA must remember that diagnosis is not within the scope of his or her training. When charting a history, the MA must be careful not to make diagnostic statements. Occasionally a patient may suggest a diagnosis. The medical assistant should document the patient's exact words and place quotations around them.

Charting Procedures

Procedures performed on the patient are mostly charted by the MA (Table 24-4 lists commonly used abbreviations and terminology). Extensive or operative procedures are usually dictated by the physician. Procedures should be charted immediately after performing them. For legal reasons, it is important to remember that a procedure was not done unless documented in the chart. Charting before a procedure is *illegal.*

The following information must be included in chart documentation: vital signs, including temperature, pulse, respirations, and blood pressure, as well as weight and height. New pain assessment guidelines for inpatient facilities are required, and some medical offices have adopted charting this aspect of patient assessment at each visit. Medication administration, specimen collection and laboratory tests, cardiac testing, and respiratory testing are also recorded.

Documenting a Clinical Visit

In the reception room, the medical assistant should call the patient's name and ask him or her to accompany the MA the examination room or a room that is quiet and comfortable with a door that can be closed for privacy. The MA should introduce himself, verify the patient's name, offer the patient a chair, and be seated. Using professional communication skills, the MA should do the following.

- Ask the patient the name he or she prefers to be called.
- Maintain good eye contact and display a sincere interest in and concern for the patient.
- Use terminology that the patient can understand.
- Listen carefully to the patient and observe his or her nonverbal body language.
- Avoid making any judgmental comments.
- Take your time and avoid hurrying the patient.

On the progress note of the patient's chart, the medical assistant must note the date, time, and list the CC as one or two major symptoms, being brief and concise. The MA should note the patient's words in quotation marks. *What, when,* and *where*

TABLE 24-4 ABBREVIATIONS AND TERMINOLOGY COMMONLY USED TO CHART SYMPTOMS

ac	before meals	ea	each
AM	before noon	EDC	expected date of confinement
amt	amount	EENT	eyes, ears, nose, throat
ANS	autonomic nervous system	ENT	ears, nose, throat
ASAP	as soon as possible	FX,fx	fracture
ASL	American Sign Language	GI	gastrointestinal
BCP	birth control pills	GU	genitourinary
BM	bowel movement	GYN	gynecology
c̄	with	H₂O	water
CC	chief complaint	HRT	hormone replacement therapy
CMA	Certified Medical Assistant	h.s.	at bedtime
CNS	central nervous system	hx	history
c/o	complains of	Lac	laceration
CXR	chest x-ray	LMP	last menstrual period
dc	discontinue	meds	medications
DOB	date of birth	MH	marital history
DOI	date of injury	MMR	measles, rumps, rubella
DPT	diptheria, pertussis, tetanus injection	MVA	motor vehicle accident
dsg	dressing	NAD	no apparent distress

(continued)

TABLE 24-4 ABBREVIATIONS AND TERMINOLOGY COMMONLY USED TO CHART SYMPTOMS (CONTINUED)

NB	newborn	pre-op	preoperative
N/C	no complaints	prep	preparation
neg	negative	PT	physical therapy
NKA/NKDA	no known drug allergies	pt	patient
N&V	nausea and vomiting	qns	quantity not sufficient
NPO	nothing by mouth	qs	quantity sufficient
OB	obstetrics	RMA	registered medical assistant
opth	ophthalmology	ROM	range of motion
ortho	orthopedics	Rx	prescription
OPV	oral polio vaccine	s̄	without
OT	occupational therapy	S&S	signs and symptoms
OTC	over the counter	SOB	shortness of breath
OV	office visit	spec	specimen
pc	after meals	stat	immediately
peds	pediatrics	TPR	temperature, pulse, respirations
per	by or through	Tx	treatment
PM	afternoon	VS	vital signs
PNS	peripheral nervous system	V&D	vomiting and diarrhea
po	by mouth	WNL	within normal limits
post-op	postoperative		

PROCEDURE 24-2 Document a Clinical Visit and Procedure

Theory and Rationale

It is the responsibility of the medical assistant, along with other clinical staff, to document details of the clinical visit and the procedures performed. Accurate, concise, and complete documentation provides information for chart audits, medical insurance companies, courts of law, and the patient care team. If members of the healthcare team are aware of all efforts being made on the patient's behalf, efforts can be coordinated, patient teaching can be reinforced, and errors can be reduced or eliminated. Documenting observations during patient visits can inform healthcare team members whether the symptoms, illness, or patient's treatment response is progressing or regressing. As visit and procedure notes are compared, patient improvement will dictate the need for continuing or discontinuing the current treatment. Lack of patient progress or worsening symptoms will suggest the need for treatment changes.

Materials

■ Patient chart
■ Narrative or progress note forms to be added to the chart
■ Blue or black ink pen

Competency

(**Conditions**) Using the listed materials, (**Task**) you will be able to document a clinical visit or procedure (**Standards**) in the time and with a score designated by the instructor.

1. Verify that the chart is the correct one for the patient.
2. If notes are insufficient for documentation, add the appropriate form.

3. With narrative charting or SOAP charting, avoid leaving blank areas.
4. Write the date and time in the left-hand column of the notes.
5. Continue writing in the charting format used by the medical office.
6. Document immediately after performance of procedures.
7. Use only standard, accepted abbreviations and describe clinical observations during performance of the procedure.
8. Document only facts. DO NOT make diagnoses or judgmental statements.
9. Sign your name and add your title at the end of the documentation.

Patient Education

Discuss with the patient the importance of complete and accurate information. Provide the patient with a pencil and paper to take notes on items that might need more information at a later or followup visit.

Charting Example

04/28/xx 1:30 P.M. Patient returned for blood pressure follow-up. BP lying 110/60, BP sitting up 100/60, BP standing 90/60. Physician notified of blood pressures taken on left arm at 10-minute intervals. Michael Richards, RMA (AMT)

are good words with which to elicit descriptions of symptoms. The medical assistant should note the answers on the chart, thank the patient for the input, then proceed to the next step, which is usually taking vital signs. Advise the patient that the physician will be with him or her shortly. Place the patient's chart in the proper place to inform the physician that the patient is ready to be seen.

Critical Thinking Question 24-2

Do you think the situation in the case study should be reported to the office manager or physician? Why or why not?

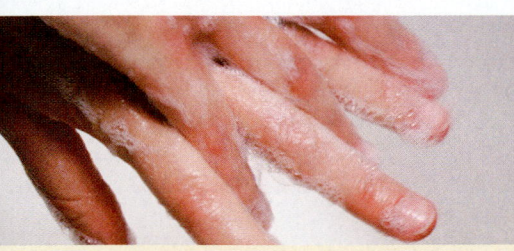

REVIEW

Chapter Summary

- Medical assistants have a primary role in the preparation and maintenance of examination and treatment areas of the medical office. In the performance of his or her duties the MA will also provide a clean, orderly, and safe clinical environment for the patient.

- Each examination room is usually soundproof or muted for confidential conversation and standardized with examination table, appropriate lighting, supply cabinets, a stool for the physician, a place for the patient to sit and to place clothes on, and a way to provide privacy for dressing/undressing. Necessary equipment includes a sphygmomanometer, stethoscope, thermometer, otoscope, ophthalmoscope, and a wall-mounted X-ray view box. The MA will ensure that all equipment is working and clean and that the examination room is adequately stocked. At the end of the clinical visit the MA will change the examination table paper and clean any soiled areas per office procedure.

- Established office triage procedures for making immediate or same-day appointments or referring patients to urgent care or emergency room for treatment may be part of the MA's job. It is important that the MA listen carefully as the patient describes symptoms over the phone or at the reception desk. It may be necessary to confer with an office nurse or physician for additional instructions. In addition to urgent or emergency conditions, patients presenting with contagious diseases will need to be removed from the reception area immediately and placed in an examination room.

- For routine office visits, patients give implied consent for treatment. A Consent to Release Information form must be signed by the patient before the information can be sent to third parties. Only the requested information is sent. Special procedures, including invasive or surgical procedures, require the patient's signature on an Informed Consent Form.

- Many forms are part of the patient's medical record. It is often the responsibility of the MA to assemble the record and add more forms when needed to continue documentation. Before or during the initial visit, the patient completes patient registration, insurance information, and a health questionnaire.

- Charting, also known as medical documentation, provides a legal document. Guidelines, including the correction of errors and writing in dark ink, are to be followed at all times. Charting is done only after a procedure is completed and is signed by the person making the entry. Chart immediately after the procedure to document accurately. If documentation is not done, the courts will assume the procedure was not performed.

- Charting usually follows one of two formats. The first is chronological, with each entry dated and vital signs or other narrative notes following. A second format uses the SOAP method. *S* refers to subjective statements made by the patient about the reason for the clinical visit. *O* refers to objective data gathered by the clinical staff, such as vital signs, laboratory data, X-rays, or observations of the patient. *A* refers to the assessment by the physician or nurse relating to the subjective and objective data. *P* refers to the plan of care based on the assessment of the patient's clinical illness or symptoms.

- The Patient History covers the following areas: personal history/social and occupational history, past medical history, family medical history, CC, present illness, and assessment and review of body systems.

- Questions should be open-ended to encourage the patient to provide all the necessary information. Sample questions include: How long have you had the symptoms? When did the symptoms start? What makes the symptoms worse? What helps to lessen the symptoms? What were you doing when the symptoms started? Generally the patient's own words are

Chapter Summary (continued)

used to describe symptoms. The MA does not make diagnostic statements because diagnosis is not in the scope of practice.

■ When communicating with the patient, the MA should use the name the patient prefers, maintain eye contact, use body language that shows interest and concern, and document the information in patient quotes as much as possible. After all information is obtained for the visit, the MA should inform the patient the physician will be in soon, and follow office procedure for informing the physician that the patient is ready to be seen.

■ The physician reviews all initial information retrieved by others before conducting a review of body systems, identifying any other symptoms or findings not yet revealed. The physician then provides the patient with a diagnosis, prognosis, and treatment plan.

Chapter Review

Multiple Choice

1. Doors to examination rooms are kept closed for
   a. equipment safety.
   b. room temperature regulation.
   c. patient privacy.
   d. storage.

2. Which of the following is a part of triage?
   a. Immediately isolating a patient with a contagious disease in an examination room
   b. Putting a patient who is calling in and experiencing chest pain on hold to talk with the physician
   c. Asking a patient who is experiencing severe pain on arrival at the office to sit in the reception area until an examination room is available
   d. Asking a patient who is in the office and experiencing chest pain to leave immediately for the emergency room because the physician is away from the office

3. A Consent to Release Information form allows a medical office to send
   a. requested information without the witness's signature.
   b. all information in the patient's medical record without signature.
   c. information without the patient's signature being witnessed.
   d. only requested information for which the patient signs.

4. It is acceptable to document allergies in
   a. black ink.
   b. blue ink.
   c. red ink.
   d. green ink.

5. Which of the following is included in a patient history?
   a. Next-of-kin phone number
   b. Insurance coverage
   c. Individual responsible for payment
   d. Military service

6. A CC is the patient's
   a. chief complaint.
   b. congestion/cough.
   c. cyanosis care.
   d. chill and cough.

7. Which of the following is an appropriate question to ask a patient about his or her symptoms?
   a. "When you cough, is it similar to COPD?"
   b. "Why didn't you phone this condition in sooner?"
   c. "Why didn't your other physician notice this symptom?"
   d. "When symptoms occur, how long do they last?"

8. When you make a mistake on a chart, you should
   a. erase it.
   b. draw a line through it.
   c. use white-out.
   d. block it out with a permanent marker.

9. Which of the following is a vital sign to be charted?
   a. Pulse
   b. Pain
   c. Weight
   d. Specimens

10. When conversing with a patient, you should
    a. avoid eye contact.
    b. avoid making any judgmental comments.
    c. automatically use a nickname for the patient.
    d. make sure you complete the process quickly.

True/False

T F 1. Whether documenting an initial visit, patient history, or clinical visit, accuracy and attention to detail are a major responsibility in the medical office.

T F 2. As an MA, you will be responsible for providing a clean, safe environment in the examination and treatment areas.

Chapter Review (continued)

T F 3. To promote efficient use of the physician's time, the MA provides expert medical advice to patients when they call and request to speak to the doctor.

T F 4. Standard equipment in an exam room may include several types of lighting.

T F 5. Charting is the documentation only of the vitals taken during a patient's visit.

Short Answer

1. What elements does a physician use to make a diagnosis about the patient's condition?

2. What is triage?

3. What is the correct procedure for a patient with a possible contagious disease?

4. List at least eight emergencies requiring immediate assessment or intervention.

5. What is the difference between implied and informed consent?

Research

1. Call five clinics in your local area. Do they use electronic charting or paper charts?

2. Research a medical malpractice case won by the plaintiff due to insufficient charting. How would you protect your physician employer from the same fate?

Externship Application Experience

1. Consider the following circumstances for triaging office appointments for the day, including room assignments. List each patient as a regular, a minor procedure, or isolation room.

   Already scheduled appointments:
   - Cast removal
   - Routine Pap
   - Well-baby check
   - Dressing change for a surgical wound
   - Recheck for respiratory TB diagnosed one week ago, on medication
   - Mole removal

   Call-ins for appointments that day:
   - HIV diagnosed patient c/o coughing and elevated temp
   - Child with suspected chickenpox, sibling diagnosed two weeks ago
   - Diagnosed hepatitis B with nausea and vomiting
   - Patient c/o possible elevated blood pressure
   - 5-year-old female with chest pain

2. Report the daily routine of checking supplies in the office where the externship experience is taking place.

Resource Guide

Center for Health Promotion and Education
Centers for Disease Control and Prevention
Building 1 South, Room SSB249
1600 Clifton Road NE
Atlanta, GA 30333
404-329-3492
www.cdc.gov

U.S. Department of Health and Human Services
200 Independence Avenue, SW
Washington, DC 20201
www.os.dhhs.gov

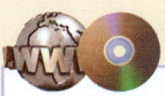

MedMedia

http://www.MyMAKit.com

More on this chapter, including interactive resources, can be found on the Student CD-ROM accompanying this textbook and on http://www.MyMAKit.com.

CHAPTER 25

Medical Asepsis

Case Study

Gloria is rushing around the office because everyone is running so far behind. It is late Friday afternoon and they have already accommodated several walk-in patients. Dr. Becan orders a throat swab from the last patient Gloria roomed to check for Strep-A. The patient presented with a fever and sore throat, and Strep-A has been a common diagnosis this winter.

In her hurry Gloria skips washing her hands when she reenters the exam room and simply dons gloves. She takes a sterile cotton applicator and begins to swab the patient's throat. The patient gags and coughs up mucus droplets on Gloria's hands.

Gloria realizes she has forgotten to bring the testing serums in the room with her, so with the swab in one hand she opens the door with her other hand and leaves the room. Still wearing the gloves, she grabs a coworker's pen and quickly jots down the patient information on the lab order form and hands it to the receptionist for coding and billing.

MedMedia

http://www.MyMAKit.com

Additional interactive resources and activities for this chapter can be found on http://www.MyMAKit.com. For a video, tips, audio glossary, legal and ethical scenarios, job scenarios, quizzes, and games related to the content of this chapter, please access the accompanying CD-ROM in this book.

Video: *Handwashing and Gloving*
Audio Glossary
Legal and Ethical Scenario: *Medical Asepsis*
On the Job Scenario: *Medical Asepsis*
Multiple Choice Quiz
Games: Crossword, Strikeout, and Spelling Bee
Tips
HIPAA Quiz

Objectives

After completing this chapter, you should be able to:

- Define and spell the key terminology in this chapter.
- Define the medical assistant's role in the promotion of infection control in the medical office.
- Explain the cycle of infection.
- Identify the body's natural defenses against infection.
- Describe the layers of the skin and their functions.
- Explain the function of the immune system.
- Explain how a person's general state of health may serve as a defense against infection.
- Identify other natural defenses against infection.
- Explain medical asepsis.
- Explain the roles of OSHA and the CDC in setting infection control guidelines.
- List and explain the importance of Universal and Standard Precautions.
- Identify the types of personal protective equipment and their uses.
- Describe hepatitis, its routes of transmission, and patient education measures.
- Describe the symptoms, diagnosis, treatment, and patient education considerations of HIV/AIDS.
- Discuss caring for the HIV/AIDS patient.
- Explain the theory of hand washing.
- Explain the theory of nonsterile gloving.
- Identify the symptoms of latex allergy and patient education measures.

➕ MEDICAL ASSISTING STANDARDS

CAAHEP ENTRY-LEVEL STANDARDS	ABHES ENTRY-LEVEL COMPETENCIES
■ Perform within scope of practice (psychomotor)	■ Project a positive attitude.
■ Apply ethical behaviors, including honesty/integrity in performance of medical assisting practice (affective)	■ Maintain confidentiality at all times.
	■ Be a "team player."
■ Apply local, state and federal health care legislation and regulation appropriate to the medical assisting practice setting (psychomotor)	■ Be cognizant of ethical boundaries.
	■ Exhibit initiative.
	■ Adapt to change.
	■ Evidence a responsible attitude.
■ Recognize the importance of local, state and federal legislation and regulations in the practice setting (affective)	■ Be courteous and diplomatic.
	■ Conduct work within scope of education, training, and ability.
■ Describe the infection cycle (cognitive)	■ Apply principles of aseptic technique and infection control.
■ Define asepsis (cognitive)	
■ Discuss infection control procedures (cognitive)	■ Dispose of biohazardous materials.
	■ Practice Standard Precautions.
■ Identify personal safety precautions as established by the Occupational Safety and Health Administration (OSHA) (cognitive)	■ Instruct patients with special needs.
	■ Teach patients methods of health promotion and disease prevention.
■ Practice Standard Precautions (psychomotor)	
■ List major types of infectious agents (cognitive)	
■ Select appropriate barrier/personal protective equipment (PPE) for potentially infectious situations (psychomotor)	
■ Compare different methods of controlling the growth of microorganisms (cognitive)	
■ Perform handwashing (psychomotor)	
■ Match types and uses of personal protective equipment (cognitive)	
■ Identify the role of the Center for Disease Control (CDC) regulations in healthcare settings (cognitive)	

✓ COMPETENCY SKILLS PERFORMANCE

1. Perform correct hand-washing procedure.
2. Demonstrate nonsterile gloving.

Introduction

The medical environment can be hazardous to a patient's health. Patients who come to a medical office may appear healthy and be well, may appear healthy but carry disease-producing organisms, or may be experiencing the symptoms of infectious or noninfectious disease. If patients or staff members are not the source of infection, the clinical environment can be. Dust harbors very tiny insects and microorganisms that carry disease.

Key Terminology

aerobe—organism able to survive and grow only in the presence of oxygen

anaerobe—organism that survives and grows in the absence of oxygen

asepsis—practice of maintaining a pathogen-free or pathogen-controlled environment to prevent the spread of illness and disease; also known as *sterile technique*

bactericidal—capable of killing or destroying bacteria

bloodborne pathogens—pathogens carried in the bloodstream

Body Substance Isolation (BSI)—procedures, equipment, and supplies used to prevent the transmission of communicable diseases by preventing direct contact with all body substances such as blood, body fluids, drainage from wounds, feces, urine, sputum, and saliva

carrier—person who has the capacity to transmit a disease and is usually unaware of infection

Centers for Disease Control (CDC)—agency of the Public Health Operating Division of the U.S. Department of Health and Human Services that studies and monitors diseases and disease prevention and works to protect public health and safety

cilia—hairlike processes projecting from the epithelial cells

contamination—making a sterile field unclean or having pathogens placed in it

dermis—middle layer of the skin

epidermis—outermost layer of the skin

epithelial—pertaining to the epithelium (cells covering the external and internal surfaces of the body)

follicle—small hollow or cavity with secretory functions (e.g., hair follicle, ovarian follicle, gastric follicle, etc.)

fomites—nonliving objects that may transmit infectious material

homeostasis—interaction between body systems that maintains optimum body function

immunity—ability to resist disease

incubation—period of time between exposure to infection and the appearance of symptoms

Key Terminology *(continued)*

infection—invasion of the body by a pathogenic microorganism

integumentary—pertaining to the skin, hair, and nails

keratinocyte—any skin cell that produces keratin, the hard protein material found in the skin, hair, and nails

medical asepsis—the practice of reducing the number of pathogens and the transmission of disease; also known as clean technique

microorganism—organism that can be viewed under a microscope, but not by the naked eye

nonpathogen—harmless organism that does not cause disease

nosocomial infection—infection resulting from the hospitalization of a patient

personal protective equipment (PPE)—protective clothing and equipment such as gloves, gowns, and masks that are worn to prevent contamination by blood and other body fluids

phagocytosis—the engulfing and destruction of microorganisms or foreign matter by phagocytic cells

prodromal—period between earliest symptoms and appearance of physical sign, such as fever or rash.

Standard Precautions—precautions that replace Body Substance Isolation and Universal Precautions in institutional healthcare settings such as hospitals and nursing homes; the first level of care combines Universal and Body Substance Isolation Precautions, and the second consists of Transmission-based Precautions

sterile—free from pathogens and all microorganisms

subcutaneous tissue—deepest layer of the skin

transmission-based precautions—care based on symptoms of disease and transmission method of the pathogen, such as contact, droplet, air, vector, or common vehicle

Universal Precautions—the CDC's original guidelines for preventing the transmission of AIDS and other bloodborne diseases

Abbreviation

ELISA—enzyme-linked immunosorbent assay

Instruments that have not been cleaned properly may harbor infectious microorganisms. Door handles may be covered with microorganisms from ill patients. To promote health and to ensure a clean and safe environment for all patients and staff, medical offices must follow infection control practices and Universal Precautions. Understanding the basics of asepsis and infection control is essential to preventing or reducing the spread of disease.

The Medical Assistant's Role in Infection Control

It is the responsibility of the medical assistant to learn and practice the measures formulated by the federal agencies OSHA and the CDC to prevent the transmission of disease in the medical setting. These measures are based on interrupting the cycle of infectious disease. They include frequent washing of the hands, correct gloving technique, using personal protective equipment, and other Universal and Standard Precautions. The MA will also instruct patients in the proper aseptic technique to follow at home.

? **Critical Thinking Question 25-1**

How do you think Gloria's actions make her patient feel? How much time do you think Gloria really saved by not washing her hands and then not removing the gloves and washing her hands again?

The Cycle of Infection

Microorganisms are organisms that cannot be seen by the naked eye but must be viewed under a microscope. All microorganisms require an optimum environment for growth. They grow well at normal body temperature (98.6 degrees F) and in the dark, moist environments of body cavities. Microorganisms also require nutrition, oxygen (**aerobes**) or the lack of oxygen (**anaerobes**), and usually a neutral pH (7.0).

Microorganisms can be pathogens or nonpathogens. Disease-producing organisms are pathogens (Figure 25-1 ◆). Harmless microorganisms are called **nonpathogens.** Bacteria, viruses, fungi, parasites, and protozoa are pathogens when disease conditions result from their presence. **Bloodborne pathogens** are disease-producing microorganisms carried in the bloodstream. Table 25-1 lists some bloodborne pathogens and diseases.

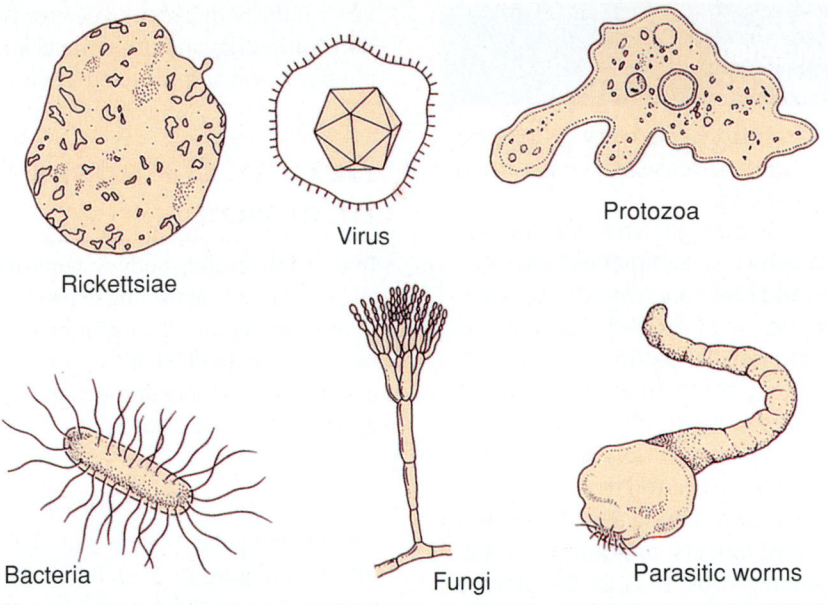

Figure 25-1 ◆ Pathogens.

Nonpathogenic microorganisms can become disease-producing pathogens when they leave their natural environments. As an example, *Escherichia coli (E. coli)* may move from its normal habitat in the colon to the urinary tract and cause a urinary tract infection. Nonpathogens can also become pathogenic when the body's immune system has been overwhelmed.

There are five elements, or links, in the cycle of infection in which pathogens are transmitted from one host to another (Figure 25-2 ◆):

- Reservoir host
- Means of exit
- Means of transmission
- Means of entrance
- Susceptible host

The cycle begins with a reservoir or **carrier** host. The host may exhibit symptoms of the disease or may be unaware that he or she may be spreading potentially pathogenic microorganisms. After a period of reproduction and **incubation,** the pathogen finds a portal of exit to leave the body. Blood and body fluids, including tears, saliva,

sputum, feces, urine, and vaginal secretions, are common vehicles of transmission. During the entry, reproduction, and incubation phases of the cycle, the patient does not experience any clinical symptoms. Next, the pathogen is transmitted to a susceptible host. Microorganisms may be transmitted by air, contact, contaminated food, human carriers, animal carriers, insects, **fomites,** and soil. They enter the portals of the respiratory, genitourinary, and gastrointestinal tracts or the eyes, ears, and open areas of the skin. Pathogens may also cross the placental barrier to infect the fetus. Effective means of interrupting the cycle of infection include wearing barrier protection and following proper cleaning procedures.

?—Critical Thinking Question 25-2-
In the case study, who has been put at risk of possible exposure to Strep A by Gloria's actions?

After the pathogenic organism reproduces in the new host, the body responds with pain, swelling, and redness at the infected sites. Other symptoms, such as higher temperature and

TABLE 25-1 BLOODBORNE PATHOGENS AND DISEASES

Arboviral infections	Herpes simplex virus
Babesiosis	Human immunodeficiency
Brucellosis	virus (HIV)
Creutzfeld-Jakob disease	Human T-lymphotrophic virus
Hepatitis A virus (HAV)	Type I
Hepatitis B virus (HBV)	Leptospirosis
Hepatitis C virus (HCV)	Relapsing fever
	Syphilis
	Viral hemorrhagic fever

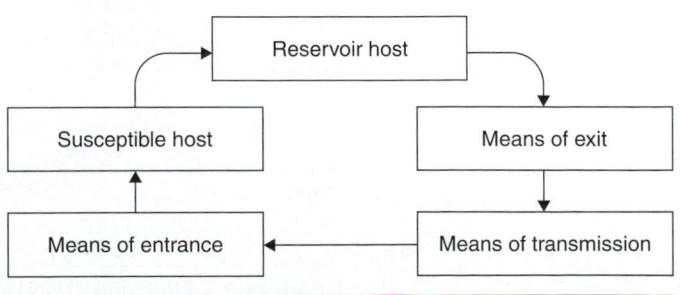

Figure 25-2 ◆ Five links in the cycle of infection.

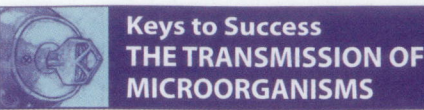

Keys to Success
THE TRANSMISSION OF MICROORGANISMS

- Vector transmission: Parasitic insects carry disease via animals. An example is Lyme disease, which is carried by a tick commonly found on deer.
- Airborne transmission: Microorganisms are moved through the air on dust particles. Examples include rubeola and varicella viruses and *Myco-bacterium tuberculosis.*
- Droplet transmission: The moist droplets from sneezing, coughing, and talking transfer pathogenic microorganisms. Respiratory infections such as the common cold and influenza are spread by droplet transmission.
- Indirect contact, also known as common vehicle transmission: Microorganisms are transferred to a susceptible host by physical contact or by touching a contaminated object such as a food tray, faucets, or equipment. HIV (human immunodeficiency virus) may be transferred from a contaminated needle to the puncture site.
- Direct contact: There is direct contact between an infected area and another skin surface or mucous membrane. Medical personnel are required to wash their hands between patients to avoid skin-to-skin transmission of microorganisms such as *Staphylococcus aureus.*

pulse rate, indicate that the patient has entered the prodromal phase of the illness. Laboratory tests will indicate an elevated white blood cell count. In the acute phase the patient experiences the strongest symptoms of the illness. In the recovery phase, the patient's symptoms diminish.

If the body's natural defenses cannot overcome the infection, antibiotics and other medications may be ordered by the physician and administered by clinical staff.

Natural Defenses Against Infection

Interactions among body systems maintain **homeostasis.** Overall health and functioning depend on the body's natural ability to resist **infection.** The integumentary system, the immune system, general good health, and specific body mechanisms such as coughing and sneezing are among the body's natural defenses against infectious disease.

The Integumentary System

The **integumentary** system (skin) is the first line of defense against infection (Figure 25-3 ◆). Intact skin serves as a barrier against invasion by the microorganisms normally present on the skin's surface. When there is a break in the skin—such as an abrasion, laceration, or surgical wound—the risk of infection increases. The skin is the largest organ in the human body. In the average person, it measures approximately 20 square feet and weighs 5.6 pounds.

The skin consists of three layers (Table 25-2).

- The outermost, protective layer is called the **epidermis.** It is made up of five stratified layers of **epithelial** cells that have been pushed up from the lowest layer, called the stratum germinativum, where **keratinocytes** are first formed. In the middle layer of the epidermis, the stratum granulosum, cells become cornified and are no longer living. These cells move upward to the outermost

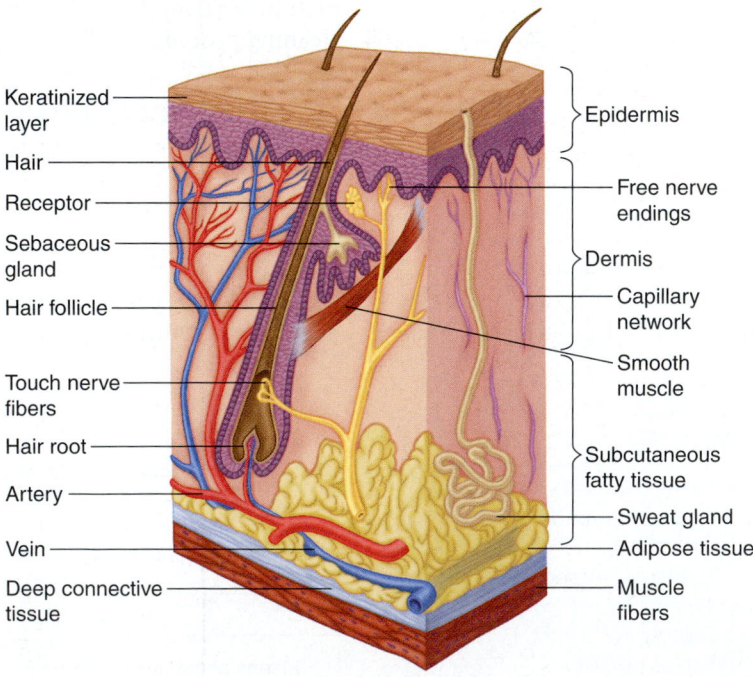

Figure 25-3 ◆ Structure of the skin.

TABLE 25-2 LAYERS OF THE SKIN
Epidermis (five sublayers)
■ stratum corneum
■ stratum lucidum
■ stratum granulosum
■ stratum malpighii
■ stratum germinativum
Dermis
Subcutaneous tissue

layer of the epidermis, the stratum corneum. This is the sloughing layer that sheds during showers or baths.

■ The middle layer is the **dermis.** It contains hair **follicles,** connective tissue, nerve endings, and sweat (sudoriferous) and oil (sebaceous) glands. Sebaceous glands secrete oil onto the skin that prevents dryness and cracking.

■ The deepest layer is the **subcutaneous tissue.** It contains fat, blood and lymph vessels, and other connective tissue. This layer helps to insulate and cushion internal organs from injury.

The Immune System

The immune system is another of the body's defenses against infection. It is a vessel system that serves as a filter for the plasma portion of the blood. **Immunity** is the ability to resist disease. There are two specific immunity defenses: cell-mediated immunity and humoral immunity.

■ T4 lymphocytes or helper cells play a dominant role in cell-mediated immunity.

■ Humoral immunity utilizes B cells, which are responsible for antibody production.

Cytokines are proteins produced by monocytes or lymphocytes that regulate other cell activities within the immune system. Immunizations assist the body in developing active and passive immunity. Active immunity develops antibodies or sensitized lymphocytes within the body that kill the infectious agent. Passive immunity utilizes previously developed antibodies for the same purpose. For further discussion of the immune system, see ∞ Chapter 38.

General Health

A person's general state of health is a third potential defense against infection and a major player in how the body fights all disease states. It is well documented that healthy individuals live longer, more productive lives. Individuals who are overweight and do not eat properly, do not exercise regularly, cannot relax, smoke cigarettes and abuse alcohol, or lead stressful lifestyles are placing extra physiological demands on their bodies. For example, if the body needs more oxygen because of improper lung functioning (as in chronic lung disease), the lungs will breathe faster and work harder to accomplish homeostasis and supply oxygen to the cells. Unhealthy lifestyles create new disease conditions or aggravate existing ones. Quick fixes such as diet fads are available, but only individual commitment over the long term provides a higher quality of health and life.

Other Natural Defenses

Other specific mechanisms in the body help to fight infection.

■ The mucous membranes lining cavities and passages serve as barriers to microorganisms and produce secretions that inhibit microbial growth.

■ **Cilia** are hairlike projections from epithelial cells that trap and prevent microorganisms from entering deeper into the body.

■ Coughing, sneezing, and the movement of the respiratory tract cilia serve to expel pathogens. Tears, sweat, urine, and vaginal secretions are other excretory mechanisms.

■ The acidic pH (lower than 7.0) of urine and vaginal secretions inhibits microbial growth. Under healthy conditions, urine is **sterile.** Urination expels microorganisms from the urinary tract and cleanses the external perineal area.

■ The acidic pH of gastric juice serves as a **bactericidal** agent.

■ The circulatory and lymphatic systems also play an important role in fighting infection. Leukocytes (white blood cells) surround and destroy pathogens in a process known as **phagocytosis** (Figure 25-4 ◆). Lymphocytes are activated to produce antibodies when antigens (foreign substances) are introduced into the body.

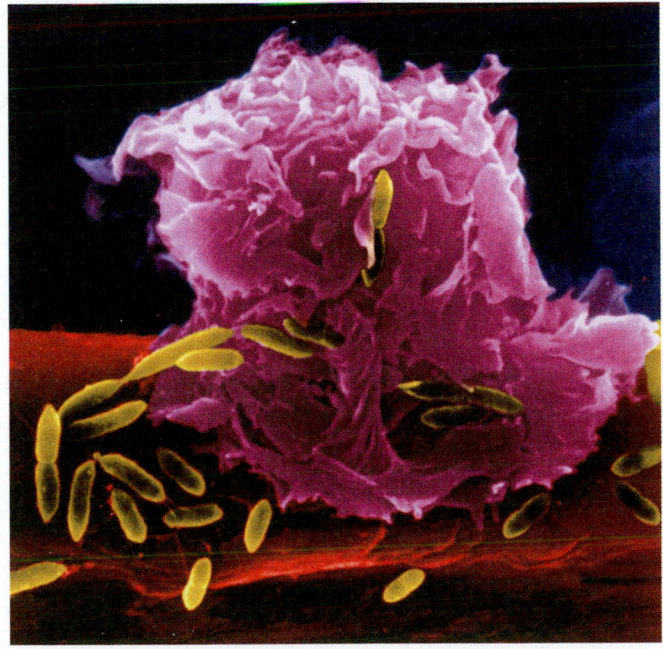

Figure 25-4 ◆ Phagocytosis
Source: Phototake.

Asepsis and Infection Control

Asepsis is defined as the practice of maintaining a pathogen-free or pathogen-controlled environment to prevent the spread of illness and disease. There are two kinds of asepsis: **medical asepsis** and surgical asepsis. Surgical asepsis requires sterile technique and is discussed in ∞ Chapter 26. Every medical office develops infection control policies and procedures to prevent the transmission of disease-causing microorganisms. Infection control consists of aseptic procedures and Standard Precautions, described in greater detail later in this chapter.

The primary purposes of medical asepsis, also known as the clean technique, are to maintain a clean environment and prevent the transmission of disease by reducing the number of pathogens. The most important procedure in the maintenance of medical asepsis is hand washing. Other practices include keeping the office free of dirt, dust, and insects; proper disposal of biological waste materials according to OSHA's Bloodborne Pathogen Standards; ensuring adequate lighting and ventilation; and wearing minimal jewelry (Figure 25-5 ◆).

Occupational Safety and Health Administration (OSHA)

The Occupational Safety and Health Administration (OSHA) was established to ensure worker safety on the job by reducing hazards in any type of work setting. It has also established and maintained health programs for employees. In the medical office setting, OSHA enforces regulations for safety and infection control practices.

The Occupational Safety and Health Administration (OSHA) was established by Congress in 1970. It is one of approximately twenty agencies of the Department of Labor. OSHA draws criticism from some businesses as an unfair regulatory agency enforcing excessive compliance, documentation,

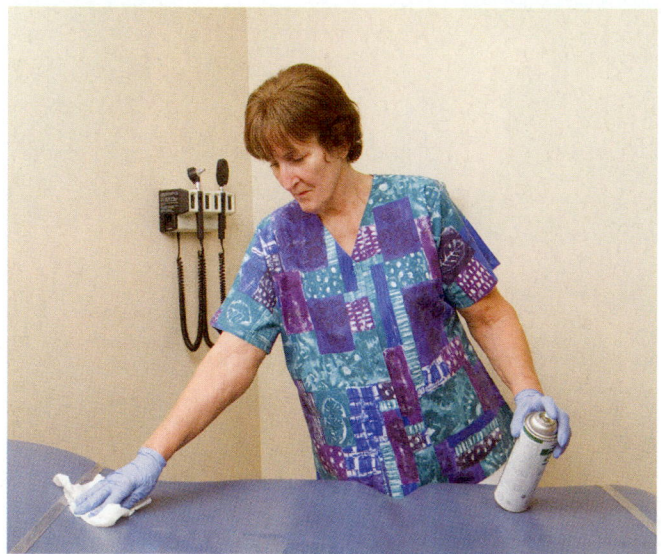

Figure 25-5 ◆ The primary purposes of medical asepsis are to maintain a clean environment and prevent the transmission of disease by reducing the number of pathogens.

TABLE 25-3 U.S. DEPARTMENT OF HEALTH AND HUMAN SERVICES	
Public Health Operating Division	**Human Services Operating Division**
National Institutes of Health	Health Care Financing
Food and Drug Administration	Administration (Medicare and Medicaid)
Centers for Disease Control and Prevention	Administration for Children and Families
Agency for Toxic Substances and Disease Registry	Administration on Aging and Prevention
Indian Health Service	
Health Resources and Services Administration	
Substance Abuse and Mental Health Services Administration	
Agency for Healthcare Research Quality	

and penalties. On the other hand, many labor groups believe it does not do enough to protect the occupational health of U.S. workers. OSHA has its headquarters in Washington, DC, and ten regional offices throughout the United States.

Centers for Disease Control and Prevention (CDC)

The **Centers for Disease Control and Prevention (CDC)** studies and monitors diseases and disease prevention and works to protect public health and safety. In addition to researching infectious disease, it provides immunization services and dispenses health information to the public and the medical community. The CDC is an agency of the Public Health Operating Division of the U.S. Department of Health and Human Services (Table 25-3).

Infection Control Precautions

OSHA requires that all health professionals follow "universal blood and body fluid precautions." **Universal Precautions** were established in 1985 by the CDC to reduce the risk of hepatitis and acquired immunodeficiency syndrome (AIDS). All blood, blood products, human tissue, and body fluids are considered potentially infectious materials. Examples include nasal and oral secretions, cerebrospinal fluid, amniotic fluid, and joint and other body cavity fluids. Sources of infectious material include pathologic waste, microbiological waste, and body tissues, cells, or fluids previously identified as infected with HIV.

It is important for all healthcare providers to consider *every* patient a potential source of AIDS, hepatitis B, or other bloodborne pathogens. OSHA suggests the following guidelines.

- Every individual, even if healthy, should be considered a potential carrier host capable of transmitting infection.
- Wash the hands before and after gloves are used.
- Change gloves after each patient contact.
- Wear personal protective barriers according to anticipated exposure to blood and body fluids. Protective barriers include gloves, face or eye shields, gowns, and masks.
- After exposure to blood or body fluids, immediately remove protective barriers and thoroughly wash your hands.
- Follow proper technique when handling, cleaning, and disposing of sharps.
- Resuscitation devices must be available for mouth-to-mouth or mouth-to-tracheostomy artificial ventilations.
- Refrain from patient care if open or weeping skin lesions are present.
- Use 10% sodium hypochlorite solution immediately to clean any blood or body fluid **contamination** on hard surfaces. To make a 10% solution, mix one part sodium hypochlorite (common household bleach) with nine parts water. Make a fresh solution daily. Do not store the mixed solution, as it may deteriorate and lose its effectiveness.
- Report all sharps injuries immediately.

In Practice

Martha Smith is in the office for her annual exam. The physician has ordered lab work and the medical assistant prepares to perform phlebotomy in order to obtain a blood specimen. After washing her hands and putting her gloves on, the patient asks why the medical assistant needs to wear gloves since she has already washed her hands. The patient insists that she is healthy. What should the medical assistant tell the patient?

If Universal Precautions are not followed when caring for an asymptomatic patient, both worker and patient may become part of the transmission of disease. Because some microorganisms may be fatal to the healthcare worker or other patients, strict adherence to universal precautions benefits the health of all medical professionals and patients.

In 1992, **Body Substance Isolation** (BSI) was developed. BSI regards all body substances as infectious materials. Under BSI precautions, all body substances of individuals seeking emergency and nonemergency medical treatment (including blood and body fluids, drainage from wounds, feces, urine, tears, sputum, and saliva) are isolated to prevent the transmission of pathogen-caused diseases. BSI went further than Universal Precautions to isolate substances not currently known to contain HIV.

Neither Universal nor Body Substance Isolation Precautions addressed the transmission of airborne droplets or contact with pathogens that may be present on dry, unbroken skin. In 1996, the original Universal Precautions were expanded by the CDC to include **nosocomial infections** and became known as **Standard Precautions,** applicable to patients receiving care in institutional healthcare settings such as hospitals and nursing homes. With broader applications, Standard Precautions are made up of two tiers:

1. Universal Precautions and Body Substance Isolation for all hospital patient care.
2. **Transmission-based precautions** for patients who are infected or suspected of being infected. Barrier protection, in addition to gloves, is based on anticipated exposure and the mode of infectious disease transmission.

Figure 25-6 ◆ lists the standard precautions recommended by the CDC.

Personal Protective Equipment (PPE)

Standard Precautions applying to **personal protective equipment** are based on actual and anticipated exposure to blood and body fluids (Figure 25-7 ◆). Correct procedures must be followed when using PPE or disease transmission will continue. For example, wearing gloves during patient contact is ineffective if the gloves are not discarded between patients and the hands are not washed. Protective clothing or equipment should be strong enough to prevent infectious material from reaching the wearer's clothing, skin, or mucous membranes. Contaminated PPE must be properly disposed of after use. Table 25-4 lists the uses for various PPE.

Hepatitis

Hepatitis, or inflammation of the liver, is usually caused by a viral infection. The severity of symptoms depends on the type of hepatitis and the health of the individual before infection. Five types of hepatitis have been identified: Hepatitis A (HAV), Hepatitis B (HBV), Hepatitis C (HCV), Hepatitis D (HDV), and Hepatitis E (HEV). New types continue to be identified. (See ∞ Chapter 42, Gastroenterology and Nutrition, for more information.)

HAV and HEV are transmitted via oral and fecal routes. HBV, HCV, and HDV are transmitted through percutaneous contact, permucosal contact, blood, products for blood transfusion, and IV drug use. Renal-dialysis and multiple-transfusion patients may also be blood transmitters. HBV can be transmitted through sexual contact. HEV occurs in areas such as Asia, India, Africa, and Central America, but may also be seen in travelers to those areas. HAV, HBV, and HCV are the most common types in the United States.

Healthcare workers are at risk for contracting hepatitis because of their daily occupational exposure to blood and body fluids. They can decrease that risk by practicing consistent hand washing and sharps precautions. Several forms of immunization for Hepatitis B are also available, including Heptavax B, developed in 1982.

Patient Education

After the first hepatitis immunization, the second dose is given one month later, and the third is given six months after the initial dose. When the immunization series has been completed,

Hand Washing

☒ Wash hands after touching blood, body fluids, secretions, excretions, and contaminated items, whether or not gloves are worn.

☒ Wash hands immediately after gloves are removed, between patient contacts, and when otherwise indicated to avoid transfer of microorganisms to other patients or environments. It may be necessary to wash hands between tasks and procedures on the same patient to prevent cross-contamination of different body sites.

☒ Use a plain soap for routine hand washing.

☒ Use an antimicrobial agent for specific circumstances, as defined by the infection-control program.

Gloves

☒ Wear gloves when touching blood, body fluids, secretions, excretions, and contaminated items.

☒ Put on clean gloves just before touching mucous membranes and nonintact skin.

☒ Change gloves between tasks and procedures on the same patient after contact with material that may contain a high concentration of microorganisms.

☒ Remove gloves promptly after use, before touching noncontaminated items and environmental surfaces, and before treating another patient.

Mask, Eye Protection, Face Shield

☒ Wear a mask and eye protection or a face shield to protect mucous membranes of the eyes, nose, and mouth during procedures and patient-care activities that are likely to generate splashes or sprays of blood, body fluids, secretions, and excretions.

Gown

☒ Wear a gown to protect skin and to prevent soiling of clothing during procedures and patient care activities that are likely to generate splashes or sprays of blood, body fluids, secretions, or excretions.

☒ Remove a soiled gown as promptly as possible.

Patient-Care Equipment

☒ Handle used patient care equipment soiled with blood, body fluids, secretions, and excretions in a manner that prevents skin and mucous membrane exposures, contamination of clothing, and transfer of microorganisms to other patients and environments.

☒ Ensure that reusable equipment is not used for the care of another patient until it has been cleaned and reprocessed appropriately.

☒ Ensure that single-use items are discarded properly.

Environmental Control

☒ Ensure that the facility has adequate procedures for the routine care, cleaning, and disinfection of environmental surfaces, beds, bedrails, bedside equipment, and other frequently touched surfaces.

Linen

☒ Handle, transport, and process used linen soiled with blood, body fluids, secretions, and excretions in a manner that prevents skin and mucous membrane exposures and contamination of clothing.

Occupational Health and Bloodborne Pathogens

☒ Take care to prevent injuries when using needles, scalpels, and other sharp instruments or devices; when handling sharp instruments after procedures; when cleaning used instruments; and when disposing of used needles.

☒ Never recap used needles, or otherwise manipulate them using both hands or use any other technique that involves directly the point of a needle toward any part of the body.

☒ Do not remove used needles from disposable syringes by hand, and do not bend, break, or otherwise manipulate used needles by hand.

☒ Place used disposable syringes and needles, scalpel blades, and other sharp items in appropriate puncture-resistant containers.

☒ Use mouthpieces, resuscitation bags, or other ventilation devices as alternatives to mouth-to-mouth resuscitation methods in areas where the need for resuscitation is predictable.

Patient Placement

☒ Place a patient who contaminates the environment or who does not or cannot be expected to assist in maintaining appropriate hygiene or environmental control in a private room.

Figure 25-6 ◆ CDC recommended standard precautions.

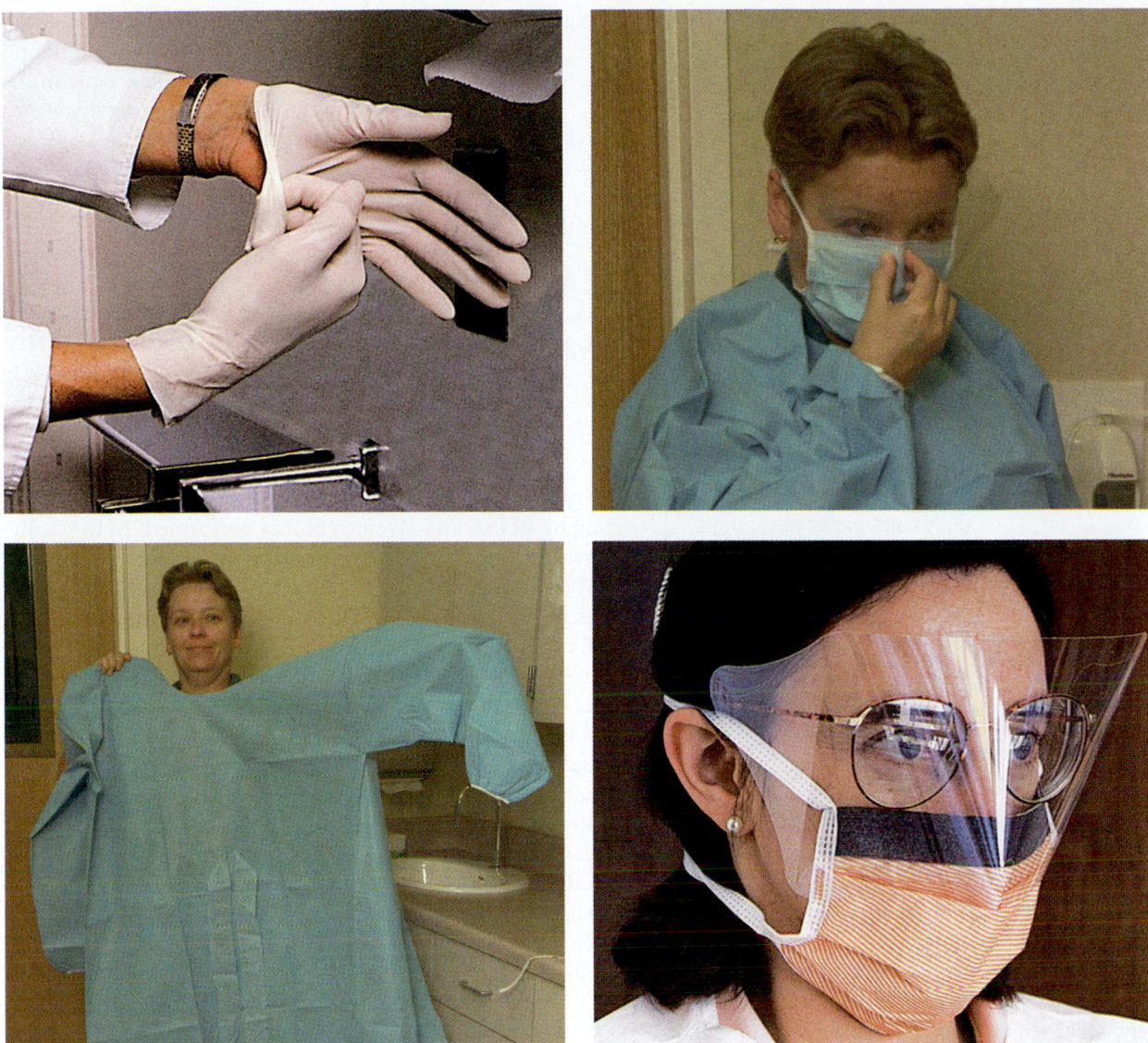

Figure 25-7 ◆ Personal protective equipment: gloves, gown, mask, and protective eyewear.

a blood sample should be tested for seroconversion. Occasionally, the injections may need to be repeated.

Patients with multiple sexual partners or a history of intravenous drug use should be advised to receive the HBV vaccination. Some states, such as Indiana, require that children receive a series of three HBV vaccinations before kindergarten.

Patients who have received blood transfusions cannot donate blood for six months. Patients who have been infected with HBV or HCV should never donate blood.

Acquired Immunodeficiency Syndrome (AIDS)

Acquired immunodeficiency syndrome, or AIDS, is a disease state caused by the human immunodeficiency virus (HIV). Approximately 1 million people in the United States are infected with HIV. Every year, 50,000 more people are infected, including 2,500 infants.

HIV can be transmitted only by contact with blood or body fluids from an infected person. The transmission is complete when the contaminated materials come in contact with the recipient's body membranes or skin breaks and then move into the bloodstream. Certain individuals or groups are at high risk of contracting HIV, including those with multiple sex partners and those who use contaminated needles. Other ways in which HIV is spread are blood transfusions, placental transfer to the fetus, and continued breastfeeding after nipples have been traumatized. Since 1985, blood transfusions in the United States have been screened for HIV antibodies, greatly reducing the risk to patients requiring blood transfusion.

There have been no documented cases of HIV infection from tears or saliva. However, during oral sex, the virus can be transferred into bleeding gums or open sores in the mouth.

TABLE 25-4 PERSONAL PROTECTIVE EQUIPMENT

PPE	When to Use
Gloves	■ Anticipated contact with blood or body fluids ■ Contact with open wounds, sores, or mucous membranes
Gowns	■ Anticipated contact with body fluid splashes or droplets ■ Contact with open wounds, sores, or mucous membranes
Masks, protective eyewear, or face shields	■ Anticipated contact with body fluid splashes or droplets ■ Anticipated droplet spread from patient's productive cough ■ Anticipated aerosol spread of body fluids or tissues during procedures
Disposable patient equipment	■ Easily transmitted infectious diseases (if disposable equipment is unavailable, disinfect and sterilize nondisposable equipment before use with another patient)

The initial infection occurs when the virus attaches to the T4 lymphocytes (helper cells) at the CD4 receptor. HIV, a retrovirus, transfers its own DNA to that of the cell it has invaded. The lymphocyte function changes to that of the invasive HIV. Reproduction ensures the survival of the HIV-trained lymphocyte and the destruction of the T4 lymphocyte and impairs the immune system's capabilities. The immune system is progressively weakened until it fails completely. In the final stages of the disease, overwhelming and often repeated opportunistic infections eventually become fatal to the patient.

The early stages of HIV infection are characterized by non-specific viral signs and symptoms such as fever, malaise, joint pain, rash, and swollen lymph glands. Many patients do not experience symptoms for years and may not be diagnosed for as long as seven to ten years after the initial infection. Even without symptoms, however, an infected individual is a carrier. Blood testing can be performed only after antibodies form, and antibodies take approximately three months to develop from the time of infection.

There are numerous ways to label or classify the progression of HIV infection to the final stage of AIDS. Most classifications of the stages of HIV infection involve the T4 count and the absence, presence, and degree of symptoms. There are four major stages in the diagnosis of HIV infection or AIDS.

Stage 1: The primary HIV infection stage may bring flu-like symptoms and last for a few weeks. Diagnosis is likely to be missed because antibodies have not yet developed.

Stage 2: The clinically asymptomatic stage may last up to ten years. The patient is likely to have swollen lymph glands, and the HIV antibody is detectable in the blood. HIV is actively replicating during this stage.

Stage 3: During the symptomatic HIV infection stage, the immune system becomes progressively impaired as it loses the struggle to replace T4 cells being destroyed by the HIV infection. Symptoms are usually mild in the beginning but worsen as the immune system deteriorates. Opportunistic infections and cancers begin during this stage.

Stage 4: During this final stage of progression from HIV infection to AIDS, the immune system is severely damaged, with a T4 count of less than 200 mm³.

A diagnosis of HIV infection is based in part on a history of high-risk factors and behaviors. Then serologic testing by **ELISA** and Western blot is performed. ELISA is the first test for HIV antibodies, but results are not specific for HIV infection alone. The Western blot test, or immunofluorescent antibody (IFA), is the second and confirming test for HIV infection. Occasionally, the Western blot is neither positive nor negative because of an error in interpretation or because testing is done too early. The test results of ELISA and Western blot can also be inaccurate if the tourniquet is applied for longer than one minute when the blood specimen is obtained. In this case the test should be repeated at intervals until results are confirmed as positive or HIV has been ruled out as a possible diagnosis. In rare cases HIV antibodies do not develop. The most recent criteria for positive diagnosis of AIDS is a CD4 or T cell count lower than 200 per cubic millimeter (mm³) of blood. The count in a healthy individual is 1000/mm³.

Other diagnostic findings include anemia, a decreased white blood cell count, and biopsies or imaging procedures that confirm involvement of opportunistic diseases in organs and systems. Home tests that use ELISA, Western blot, or IFA are identified by number only to ensure confidentiality.

The organisms of opportunistic infections are normally present in humans. But when the immune system is impaired or severely compromised, the body cannot inhibit the growth and reproduction of these organisms or of some types of cancer. During the initial and asymptomatic stages of HIV infection, the body has some immunity protection. During the symptomatic stages, the body is increasingly overwhelmed by the virus and by opportunistic infections. Table 25-5 lists common opportunistic infections and the sites they affect. Ultimately, the patient dies from repeated opportunistic infections or cancers, not from AIDS. The body fails because it cannot both fight the infections/cancers and support normal body functions.

Kaposi's sarcoma is not an opportunistic infection. It is a malignant neoplasm characterized by purplish or dark red blemishes on the skin. Biopsy confirms this clinical diagnosis. The disease spreads to other body tissues, but like opportunistic infections it is rarely the cause of death in the AIDS patient (Figure 25-8 ◆).

TABLE 25-5 COMMON OPPORTUNISTIC INFECTIONS

Organism Name	Organism Type/Infection Site
Candida albicans*	Fungus/mouth (thrush), vagina
Herpes simplex	Virus/vagina
Herpes varicella zoster (chickenpox, shingles)	Virus/skin
Cryptococcus	Fungus/liver, bone, brain
Histoplasmosis	Fungus/bone marrow, liver, lungs
Toxoplasmosis	Parasite/brain
Cryptosporidiosis	Parasite/gastrointestinal tract
Pneumocystis carinii (PCP)*	Protozoa/lungs
Salmonella	Bacteria/gastrointestinal tract
Cytomegalovirus*	Virus/eyes, gastrointestinal tract, lungs

*The most common opportunistic infections in AIDS.

This list is not inclusive. Other infecting organisms may become opportunistic in a patient with immunologic compromise.

Caring for the Patient with HIV/AIDS

There are several guidelines for caring for a patient with HIV or AIDS.

- Follow the CDC's Universal Precautions for handling blood and body fluids.
- Wear eye protection, a mask, gloves, and a gown in anticipation of contact with blood and body fluids.
- Avoid skin puncture by carefully disposing of needles in a sharps container immediately after use.
- Double-bag and label contaminated linens, equipment, and trash before processing.

- Educate the patient about the importance of frequent hand washing and avoiding oral or genital transmission of the infection.
- Instruct the significant other or the family on how to provide supportive care for symptoms the patient will experience, such as fever, anorexia, and fatigue. As the patient's outside contacts learn of the disease, the patient is likely to experience isolation. During the terminal stage, the patient enters the grieving process, experiencing anger, guilt, denial, bargaining, and depression. Family and/or significant other(s) need to be aware that these psychological needs are normal and encouraged to continue providing emotional support.
- Assist the patient by providing information about social agencies that may provide assistance with food, housing, medical costs, or hospice care.

Patient Education

For patients at risk or those with HIV infection, the following behaviors should be discussed and encouraged.

- Avoid multiple sex partners, regardless of sexual orientation.
- Avoid unprotected sex. Use latex condoms correctly and consistently. (Keep in mind, however, that it is not entirely accurate to call condom use "safe sex" as it is not 100% effective against HIV transmission.)
- Do not share IV needles.
- Avoid irresponsible behavior that passes the infection to others.

? — **Critical Thinking Question 25-3**

How would you feel if you were a patient and Gloria enters the exam room and does not wash her hands before examining you?

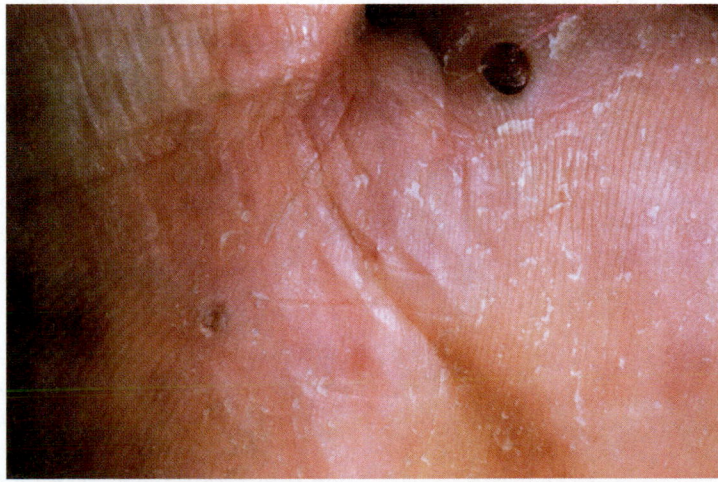

Figure 25-8 ◆ Kaposi's sarcoma found on the bottom of foot.
Courtesy of the CDC/Dr. Steve Kraus, 1981.

PROCEDURE 25-1 Perform Correct Handwashing

Theory and Rationale

You must wash your hands frequently whether you are working in the office or in the clinical areas. *Washing your hands is one of the most important ways you can prevent the transmission of disease.* Washing your hands does not sterilize them, but it reduces the number of microorganisms present on the skin. Although gloves serve as barriers to the spread of infection, *do not* use gloves without taking the extra precaution of washing your hands.

You must wash your hands before and after physical contact with every patient. Keep your hands and fingers below the elbows to prevent contaminated or dirty water from running down onto your hands and fingers from your arms. Hands must be washed for a minimum of 2 minutes before beginning to work with patients and 30 seconds following each patient contact.

There are some simple but important points to keep in mind about hand washing:

■ Hand washing with soap and water is best in situations of direct patient contact. Antiseptics that do not use water are used in certain circumstances; however, recent studies have questioned their effectiveness. Use warm water to wash the hands, as water that is too hot or cold can promote dry skin.

■ Nails should be kept short. Microorganisms on the hands are found in greatest numbers around and under the nails.

■ Jewelry should be kept to a minimum, as it creates more areas in which to trap microorganisms.

■ Lotion should be applied nightly to the hands to keep the skin from drying and cracking. Broken integrity of the skin is an open invitation to pathogens.

■ Bar soap should be avoided unless it can be rinsed and placed on a drainable soap tray.

■ Always wash your hands before and after using gloves. Gloves do not absolutely guarantee the prevention of disease transmission, as they may be torn or have holes too tiny to see.

■ Faucets are contaminated. Use paper towels when turning them on or off.

In the clinical setting, *always* wash your hands:

■ before starting and after ending the clinical day
■ before and after assisting in the performance of procedures
■ before and after physical contact with each patient
■ before and after handling potentially contaminated equipment
■ after cleaning in the medical office environment
■ after sneezing, blowing your nose, covering your mouth to cough, or using the toilet
■ before mealtimes or handling food

Materials

■ Soap (bar or pump)
■ Paper towels
■ Waste container
■ Nail brush or cuticle stick

Competency

(**Conditions**) With the necessary materials you will be able to (**Task**) wash your hands (**Standards**) following medically aseptic technique in the time designated by the instructor.

1. Remove and secure most jewelry. Wedding bands and professional watches are allowed. Push the watch higher than your wrist. Avoid touching the contaminated sink front with your uniform.

2. With a paper towel, turn on the water and adjust to a warm temperature (Figure 25-9 ◆). The water should run continuously until you have finished the procedure. Discard the paper towel.

3. With your hands and fingers lower than your elbows, wet your wrists and hands.

4. Apply soap and scrub lather over the hands and fingers, between the fingers, under and around the nails, and rinse (Figures 25-10 ◆ and 25-11 ◆). Apply soap and lather to the wrists and forearms (Figure 25-12 ◆). The purpose of this washing order is to wash the dirtiest areas first. A circular motion and friction rubbing will loosen dirt and microorganisms. If you are using bar soap, rinse it before returning it to the soap dish.

5. Use the cuticle stick or nail brush to clean your nails (Figure 25-13 ◆). If you are wearing a wedding band, scrub around it with the nail brush.

6. Rinse off the lather, keeping your hands in a downward position. Avoid splashing and touching the sink or faucets.

7. Dry your hands with a paper towel and discard it.

8. Turn off the faucet with another paper towel and discard it. Using a new paper towel prevents the contamination of clean hands.

Patient Education

Discuss with the patient and/or significant other(s) the importance of frequent hand washing. Assess for cultural, physical, emotional, or educational factors that may affect the patient's motivation or ability to learn and adjust your teaching methods accordingly.

Demonstrate hand washing technique and have the patient or significant other(s) perform a return demonstration. Document your teaching efforts.

Charting Example

01/22/xx 0900 Discussed with patient that hand washing would reduce germs that she could give to family members while she is recovering from pneumonia. Patient performed return demonstration and stated that she didn't want other family members to get sick. Alexis Smith, CMA (AAMA)

PROCEDURE 25-1 Perform Correct Handwashing *(continued)*

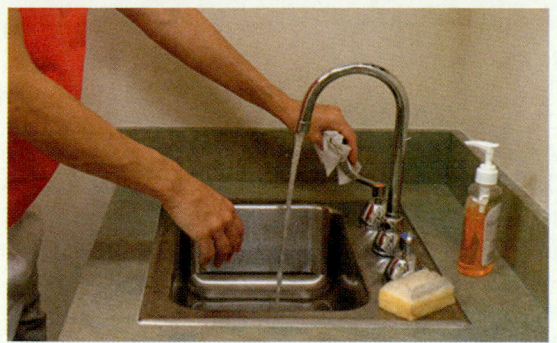

Figure 25-9 ◆ Turn on water using a paper towel.

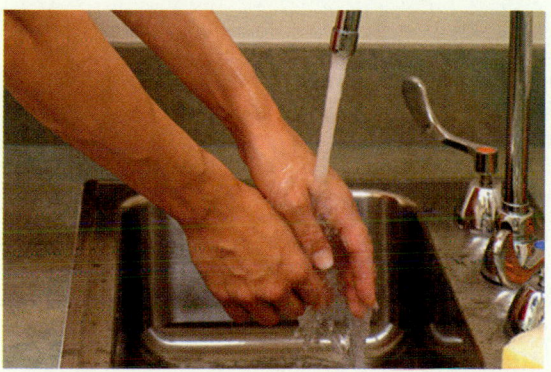

Figure 25-11 ◆ Rinse hands.

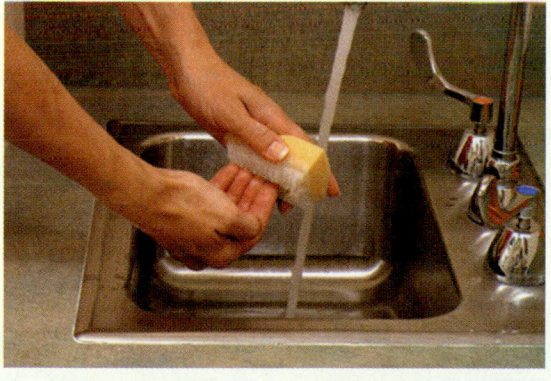

Figure 25-13 ◆ Use the nail brush to clean fingernails.

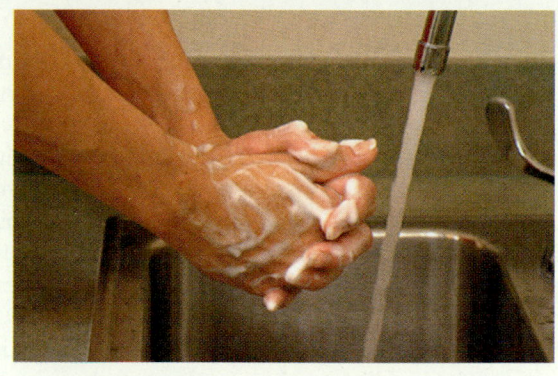

Figure 25-10 ◆ Scrub lather over the hands and fingers.

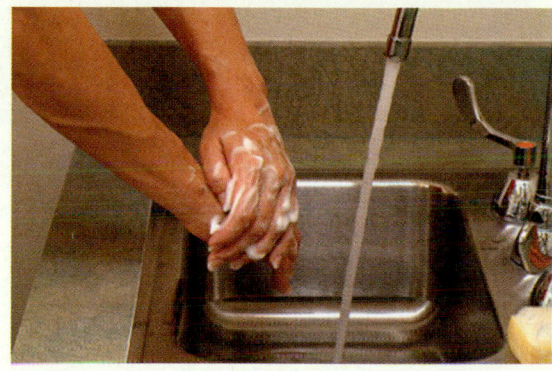

Figure 25-12 ◆ Apply soap and lather to the wrists and forearms.

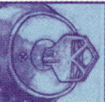

Keys to Success
JEWELRY ON THE JOB

Rings set with diamonds or gemstones are a natural breeding ground for microorganisms. During the gloving procedure, pronged settings may also catch and tear the gloves, rendering them ineffective as a protective barrier. It is best to leave most jewelry at home. In the medical office, a safety pin will secure jewelry to your uniform or scrubs.

Latex Allergy

In recent years, a growing number of healthcare workers have been affected by latex allergies. The risk for allergy extends to all others who use natural latex gloves. Latex allergies result from contact or inhalation. Natural latex is a liquid derived from rubber trees. Some synthetic rubber products are referred to as latex, but it is exposure to proteins in *natural* latex that increases the risk for allergy and the severity of symptoms.

The most common reactions to latex are irritant contact dermatitis and allergic contact dermatitis. Irritant contact

PROCEDURE 25-2 Demonstrate Nonsterile Gloving

Theory and Rationale

Nonsterile gloving is a medically aseptic procedure used in the prevention of disease transmission. It serves as a barrier tool for personal protection.

You must wash your hands even when you use gloves. Gloves create a warm, moist environment around your hands—favorable conditions for microbial growth. Perspiration mixed with the powder in most gloves also contributes to these conditions. Washing your hands reduces the number of microorganisms on your skin before you put gloves on.

Nonsterile or clean gloves are worn for direct patient contact and for handling equipment that may be contaminated by patient or secretion contact. A sequential combination of clean and sterile gloves may also be used as appropriate. For example, clean gloves may be used to remove an old dressing, and sterile gloves may be used to clean the wound and to apply a sterile dressing.

Gloves should be readily available in patient exam rooms and other work areas. They should be used only once and then discarded. Rings, except for wedding bands, should be removed to prevent the accidental puncture of the glove(s).

Materials

- Nonsterile exam gloves
- Waste receptacle

Competency

(**Conditions**) With the necessary materials you will be able to (**Task**) put on, remove, and dispose of nonsterile gloves (**Standards**) following medically aseptic technique in the time designated by the instructor.

1. Wash and dry your hands.
2. Choose gloves of the right size. They should not be so loose that they fall off during a procedure. If they are too tight, they may tear, and new gloves will have to be applied.

3. Take one glove from the box and pull it on over your hand to the wrist.
4. Take a second glove and pull it on to the wrist (Figure 25-14 ◆).
5. Adjust the gloves so that the wrists are covered.
6. To remove the first glove, grasp the outside of the glove at the wrist with the other gloved hand and pull down (Figure 25-15 ◆). This motion will keep the contaminated surface inside and is called "glove touch glove." Discard the glove immediately.
7. With your ungloved hand, reach inside the second glove (Figure 25-16 ◆). Grasp the inside of the glove and pull it down and off (Figure 25-17 ◆). This second glove removal also keeps the contaminated surface on the inside and is called "ungloved hand touch hand inside before removing." Discard the second glove immediately.
8. Wash and dry your hands.

Patient Education

Discuss with the patient and/or significant other(s) the importance of gloving and removing gloves correctly. Explain that the hands must be washed before and after glove use. Assess for cultural, physical, emotional, or educational factors that may affect the patient's motivation or ability to learn and adjust your teaching methods accordingly.

Demonstrate putting on, removing, and disposing of gloves and have the patient do the same. Document your teaching efforts.

Charting Example

01/22/xx 0915 Patient demonstrated how to glove, remove, and dispose of gloves properly. Patient washed hands after removing gloves without staff reminder. Michael Zheng, CMA (AAMA)

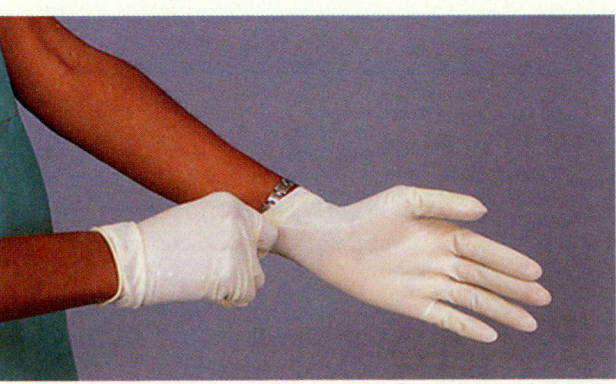

Figure 25-14 ◆ Pull the second glove on to the wrist.

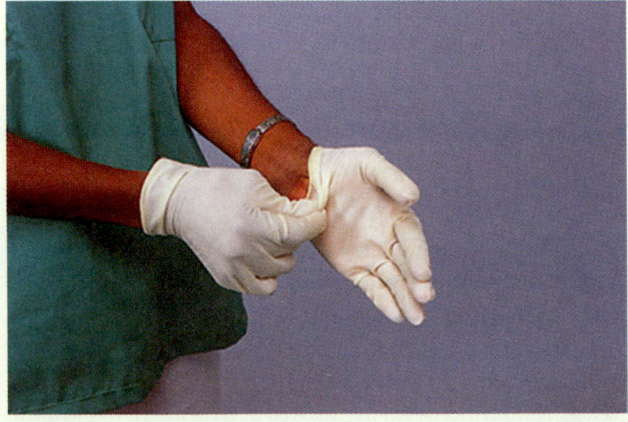

Figure 25-15 ◆ Grasp the outside of the glove at the wrist with the other gloved hand and pull down.

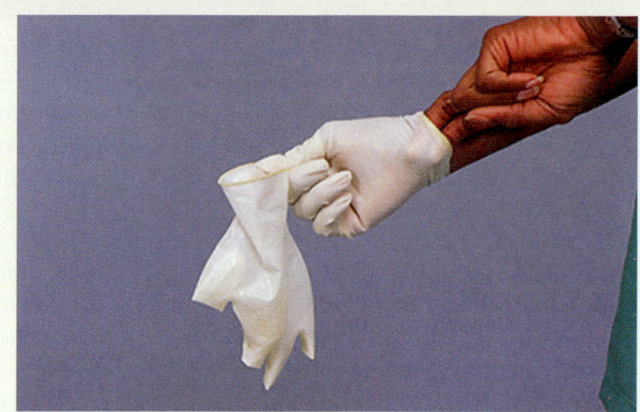

Figure 25-16 ◆ With your ungloved hand, reach inside the second glove.

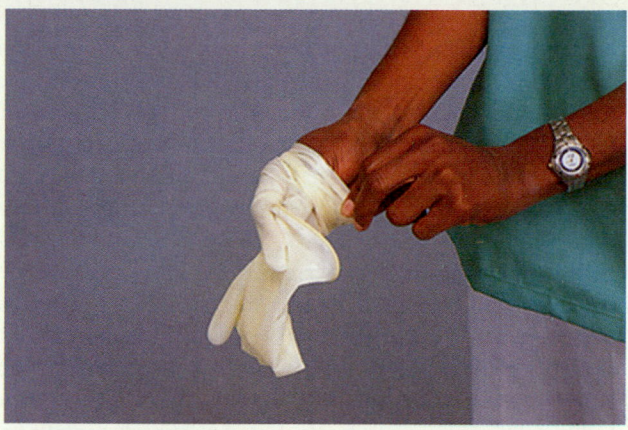

Figure 25-17 ◆ Grasp the inside of the glove and pull it down and off.

dermatitis results from exposure to the powder inside the gloves. Allergic contact dermatitis is a reaction to the chemicals added to the latex during the processing and manufacturing of the gloves.

Mild reactions can include rashes, hives, itching, and redness. Severe reactions may involve runny nose, sneezing, irritated eyes and throat, and asthma symptoms, progressing to life-threatening reactions. Reactions are not confined to the areas of contact with the skin. As powdered gloves are removed, the protein attached to airborne powder particles may be inhaled, thereby causing respiratory reactions.

Education for the Patient or Health Professional

- Use nonlatex gloves when working with noninfectious materials.

- If latex gloves are necessary, individuals with powder-related irritant contact dermatitis should use powder-free gloves. People with allergic contact dermatitis should wear hypoallergenic latex gloves to reduce the risk or severity of a reaction.
- Wash and dry your hands thoroughly after wearing latex gloves.
- Clean office areas and equipment that harbor latex-contaminated dust frequently to reduce allergens.
- Familiarize yourself with the common symptoms of latex allergy and consult a physician if symptoms arise. If latex allergy is diagnosed, wear medical alert identification and inform your friends, family members, and coworkers.
- Stay up to date about research in latex allergies.

REVIEW

- After it was scientifically established that infectious disease is caused by microorganisms, hand washing and the disinfection of instruments became the primary tools for breaking the cycle of infection. The cycle continues unless one or more of five elements are removed: the reservoir host, a means of exit, a means of transmission, a means of entrance, and a susceptible host.

- An intact integumentary system is the body's first line of defense against invasion by microorganisms, or infection. Other elements in the defense system include the immune system, a general state of good health, age, and natural mechanisms such as tears, coughing, and the acidic pH of urine. Cells in the immune system known as phagocytes engulf and digest microorganisms and foreign materials.

- Diseases such as hepatitis and AIDS place the healthcare professional at great risk because of the potential for bloodborne transmission of pathogens during patient care.

- With the rise in bloodborne diseases, the Occupational Safety and Health Administration (OSHA) and the Centers for Disease Control (CDC) have developed Bloodborne Pathogen Standards and Universal and Standard Precautions, respectively. These guidelines are designed to prevent the transmission of pathogenic microorganisms, thereby breaking the cycle of infection, and to reduce the risk of infectious disease to the healthcare professional.

- Universal and Standard Precautions are based on the assumption that all blood, blood products, human tissue, and body fluids are potentially infectious materials. They emphasize hand washing and the use of appropriate protective barriers. Gloves, gowns, and masks are examples of personal protective equipment (PPE). PPE is used for anticipated contact with blood and body fluids to prevent contact with pathogens.

- Hand washing and gloving procedures are effective only if they are performed correctly. Using gloves is not a substitute for frequent hand washing, nor does it prevent the growth or transmission of microorganisms when the hands are not washed between patient contacts.

- All professionals and patients who routinely use latex gloves should be aware of the symptoms of latex allergy and to seek treatment. Some allergy reactions are severe and can be fatal.

- In addition to medical treatment, education of the patient and significant other(s) is important to health recovery and in the prevention of disease transmission. High-risk populations, healthcare workers, and those in certain other occupations should receive the hepatitis B vaccination series.

- Following Universal and Standard Precautions is crucial. During the asymptomatic stage of infectious illness, transmission of pathogens may occur if the healthcare professional chooses not to follow precautions. It is the responsibility of healthcare professionals to stay current regarding bloodborne diseases and infection control practices. This commitment will ensure quality of care for patients and professional longevity in health-related occupations.

Chapter Review

Multiple Choice

1. The cycle of infection includes all of the following except
   a. reservoir host.
   b. means of transmission.
   c. the use of personal protective equipment (PPE).
   d. susceptible host.

2. The body's first line of defense against infection is
   a. an intact integumentary system.
   b. the immune system.
   c. mucous membranes.
   d. the acidic pH of urine.

3. The most important medically aseptic procedure in preventing the transmission of disease is
   a. dusting with a moistened cloth.
   b. hand washing.
   c. disinfecting doorknobs.
   d. wearing nonsterile gloves.

4. The common source of HBV and HIV transmission is
   a. shared use of eye drop medication.
   b. air particles.
   c. moisture droplets.
   d. blood and body fluids.

5. Personal protective equipment (PPE) prevents the transmission of infectious materials and involves wearing gloves, gowns, masks, eyewear, and/or face shields based on
   a. actual and anticipated exposure to blood and body fluids during patient care.
   b. actual exposure to blood and body fluids by direct healthcare personnel only.
   c. anticipated exposure to blood and body fluids for administrative and housekeeping personnel.
   d. anticipated exposure to airborne transmission of infectious materials.

Chapter Review (continued)

6. In the HIV-infected patient, opportunistic infections
   a. cause the immune system to intermittently become compromised and then become stronger.
   b. strengthen the immune system due to repeated exposure to infection.
   c. weaken and severely compromise the immune system.
   d. are rarely cause for concern or adjustments in treatment.

7. *Resident flora* is defined as
   a. pathogenic viruses living and thriving on equipment surfaces.
   b. pathogenic bacteria living and thriving in tissue.
   c. nonpathogenic bacteria living in tissue.
   d. none of the above.

True/False

T F 1. Door handles may be covered with microorganisms from ill patients.

T F 2. Understanding the basics of asepsis and infection control is essential to preventing or reducing the spread of disease.

T F 3. Microorganisms are organisms that can be seen by the naked eye.

T F 4. Microorganisms that require oxygen are anaerobes.

Short Answer

1. What is the difference between aerobes and anaerobes?

2. Name the five elements, or links, in the cycle of infection in which pathogens are transmitted from one host to another.

3. List six common vehicles in the transmission of microorganisms.

4. Name two microorganisms that are spread by airborne transmission.

5. What is another term for *common vehicle transmission?*

6. What is the first line of defense against infection?

7. Name the two primary purposes of medical asepsis.

8. What function do cilia perform?

9. How many cases of HIV infection from tears or saliva have been documented?

10. Name five nonspecific viral signs and symptoms of the early stages of HIV infection.

Research

1. Research the common symptoms of latex allergy. Compare the prices of latex and nonlatex gloves.

2. Where can patients in your community obtain free or low-cost HIV testing?

3. Are there HIV-specific clinics in your area that offer treatment and counseling?

Externship Application Experience

During your externship experience you observe hand-washing techniques in your assigned office. On one occasion you notice that an employee used the restroom and went back to work without washing her hands. What should you do?

Resource Guide

AIDS

National Center for HIV, STD, and TB Prevention

1600 Clifton Rd.
Atlanta, GA 30333
1-800-311-3435
www.cdc.gov/nchstp/od/nchstp.html
e-mail NCHSTP@cpsod1.em.cdc.gov
Information at this site applies to a general audience.

GOVERNMENT AGENCIES

Centers for Disease Control and Prevention (CDC)

1600 Clifton Rd.
Atlanta, GA 30333
1-800-311-3435
www.cdc.gov

Occupational Safety and Health Administration (OSHA)

Office of Public Affairs
200 Constitution Ave., Room N 3647
Washington, DC 20210
202-693-1999
www.osha.gov
For general safety and health-related inquiries, contact your OSHA area office or OSHA State Plan Office. To report emergencies, call 1-800-321-OSHA or 1-800-321-6742.

Resource Guide (continued)

LATEX ALLERGY

American Academy of Family Physicians
www.aafp.org/afp

American Latex Allergy Association
www.latexallergyresources.org/

Latex Allergy Information Service (LAIS)
176 Roosevelt Ave
Torrington, CT 06790
860-482-6869

UNIVERSAL AND STANDARD PRECAUTIONS

Centers for Disease and Control and Prevention
www.cdc.gov/ncidod/hip/BLOOD/UNIVERSA.HTM
www.cdc.gov/ncidod/hip/isolat/std_prec_excerpt.htm

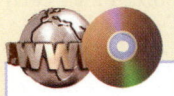

Med**Media**

http://www.MyMAKit.com

More on this chapter, including interactive resources, can be found on the Student CD-ROM accompanying this textbook and on http://www.MyMAKit.com.

Objectives

After completing this chapter, you should be able to:

- Define and spell the key terminology in this chapter.
- Describe the medical assistant's role in surgical asepsis.
- Explain the principles of aseptic technique.
- Explain the differences between sanitization, disinfection, and sterilization.
- Describe the process of sanitization.
- Discuss the different types of disinfectants and how they are used in the medical office.
- Discuss the principles of autoclave sterilization.
- Describe how to wrap instruments and prepare sterile trays using sterile technique.
- Discuss the concept of the surgical field.
- Discuss the guidelines for use of alcohol-based hand rubs.

Surgical Asepsis

Case Study

Ian is preparing to help his physician employer during an in-office surgical procedure. Ian begins by thoroughly washing the Mayo stand, letting it air-dry, and placing the proper covering on it to create a sterile field. He then carefully opens the instruments and lets them drop to the stand. Shea, a coworker, enters the room and tells Ian he has a phone call. Ian drops the last instrument on the table and leaves the room.

When Ian returns, he notices that he is one instrument short for the necessary surgical setup, so he goes to the supply cabinet to get it. Not finding it there, he checks the autoclave machine that has just been run but not emptied. Ian takes the instrument and verifies that the indicator tape has changed color. Upon opening the package, Ian notices some drops of moisture in the hinge area, so he double-checks the package. Again he verifies that the indicator tape has changed color, so he knows the autoclave was run and proceeds to place the instrument on the sterile field.

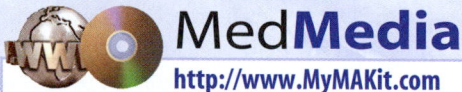

Med**Media**
http://www.MyMAKit.com

Additional interactive resources and activities for this chapter can be found on http://www.MyMAKit.com. For videos, tips, audio glossary, legal and ethical scenarios, job scenarios, quizzes, and games related to the content of this chapter, please access the accompanying CD-ROM in this book.

Audio Glossary
Legal and Ethical Scenario: *Surgical Asepsis*
On the Job Scenario: *Surgical Asepsis*
Videos: *Handwashing and Gloving; Sanitization, Disinfection, Sterilization; Surgical Scrub; Surgical Field*
Multiple Choice Quiz
Games: Crossword, Strikeout, and Spelling Bee
Tips
HIPAA Quiz

Key Terminology

asepsis, surgical—practice that keeps objects and areas sterile or free from microorganisms using sterile technique

aseptic—without germs (literally, without sepsis)

autoclave—device used to sterilize instruments under steam and pressure

autoclave load—wrapped or unwrapped instruments, packs, and supplies placed in an autoclave to be sterilized

cold sterilization—sterilization with a chemical sterilant, performed when heat cannot be used

debris—organic or inorganic extraneous material that interferes with the proper functioning or cleaning of supplies or equipment

disinfection—method of decontamination that destroys or inhibits pathogenic microorganisms but does not kill spores and some viruses; used sometimes as an alternative to autoclave sterlization

emesis—vomit

endoscope—fiber-optic instrument used to visualize the internal aspect of the GI tract

germicide—agent used to kill germs

Mayo stand—movable table used for placement of supplies and/or a sterile field during a procedure

noncritical—pertaining to objects that do not touch the patient or touch only intact skin

pH—measurement of hydrogen ion concentration in a substance or solution; a pH of 7.0 is considered neutral, below 7.0 is considered acidic, and above 7.0 is considered alkaline

sanitization—method of decontamination that reduces the numbers of microorganisms on an object or surface; removes organic material from equipment or instruments and must be performed before disinfection and sterilization

spore—capsule formed by some bacteria as a protective shell during their resting state; under favorable conditions the bacteria become active again

sterilant—chemical sterilizing agent

✚ MEDICAL ASSISTING STANDARDS

CAAHEP ENTRY-LEVEL STANDARDS	ABHES ENTRY-LEVEL COMPETENCIES
■ Perform within scope of practice (psychomotor)	■ Prepare patients for procedures.
■ Apply ethical behaviors, including honesty/integrity in performance of medical assisting practice (affective)	■ Apply principles of aseptic techniques and infection control.
■ Discuss infection control procedures (cognitive)	■ Prepare and maintain examination and treatment areas.
■ Differentiate between medical and surgical asepsis used in ambulatory care settings, identifying when each is appropriate (cognitive)	■ Prepare patient for and assist physician with routine and specialty examinations and treatments and minor office surgeries.
■ Perform handwashing (psychomotor)	■ Use quality control.
■ Prepare items for autoclaving (psychomotor)	■ Collect and process specimens.
■ Perform sterilization procedures (psychomotor)	■ Wrap items for autoclaving.
■ Apply critical thinking skills in performing patient assessment and care (affective)	■ Perform sterilization techniques.
■ Assist physician with patient care (psychomotor)	■ Dispose of biohazardous materials.
	■ Practice Standard Precautions.
	■ Operate and maintain facilities and equipment safely.

✓ COMPETENCY SKILLS PERFORMANCE

1. Demonstrate the performance of sanitization.
2. Demonstrate disinfection procedures.
3. Demonstrate how to wrap surgical instruments and prepare sterile trays for autoclave sterilization.
4. Demonstrate the correct procedure for loading and operating an autoclave.
5. Demonstrate the correct procedure for pouring sterile solution onto a sterile field.
6. Demonstrate the correct procedure for opening a sterile surgical pack to create a sterile field.
7. Demonstrate the correct procedure for using transfer forceps.
8. Demonstrate a sterile scrub (surgical hand washing).
9. Demonstrate how to glove while wearing a sterile gown.
10. Demonstrate sterile gloving and removal.

Introduction

Surgical asepsis is a very important practice for preventing the transmission of pathogenic microorganisms. Following the correct techniques for sanitization, disinfection, sterilization, and sterile technique, the medical assistant helps to ensure the patient's safety and normal healing and recovery after minor surgeries and treatments.

Key Terminology *(continued)*

sterile—free from all living microorganisms and bacterial spores

sterile field—microorganism-free environment used during procedures to prevent contamination by pathogens

sterilization—process of destroying all microbial forms of life, for which the autoclave is most commonly used

sterilization indicator—different forms of tape or inserts (strips or tubes, for example)

that provide verification of an autoclave's effectiveness

ultrasonic cleaning—use of ultrasound waves to loosen contaminants

The Medical Assistant's Role in Surgical Asepsis

During ambulatory surgery and invasive treatments, part of the medical assistant's responsibility is to remember which areas are clean and which are required to be sterile. The physician performs a surgical scrub, then dons a surgical gown, mask, and gloves. The MA usually follows clean technique and is free to obtain more supplies, open sterile supplies but not touch the inside contents of packages, place sterile contents onto the sterile field by drop or sterile transfer forceps, and perform other necessary functions, including preparing specimens for the lab.

Surgical Asepsis

The practice of **surgical asepsis** removes all microorganisms, including **spores,** from objects or designated areas. Removing all microorganisms eliminates all risk of contact with pathogens. Also known as **sterile** or **aseptic** technique, surgical asepsis is used at all times during invasive procedures and when skin integrity is or will be broken—such as during the suturing of a laceration, injections, minor surgical procedures, and the insertion of a catheter into a normally sterile environment. A sterile object remains sterile unless contaminated by violation of sterile procedure. Sterile procedure is breached when a contaminated object touches or crosses a **sterile field.**

The functions of the clinical team can be divided into clean and sterile. It is important that you and other clinical staff remember your roles as either sterile or clean and to function accordingly. (To review medical asepsis, or clean technique, see ∞ Chapter 25.) Table 26-1 compares the applications and effects of medical and surgical asepsis.

Sanitization, Disinfection, and Sterilization

Decontamination, the physical or chemical process that removes, inactivates, or destroys pathogenic microorganisms, including bloodborne pathogens, is accomplished by sanitization, disinfection, and/or sterilization.

- **Sanitization** inhibits bacterial growth or inactivates pathogens. It does not destroy microorganisms. It is used to remove organic materials from equipment or instruments.
- **Disinfection** destroys or inhibits pathogenic microorganisms but does not kill spores and some viruses. In addition to cleaning surfaces and equipment used for noninvasive procedures, it is also used to clean some

invasive equipment that may be damaged by sterilization in an **autoclave.**
- **Sterilization** destroys all living forms of microorganisms, including spores. Using a sterile field for invasive procedures creates a microorganism-free environment that prevents contamination by pathogens.

Sanitization

After each patient examination or treatment, the treatment room must be sanitized and disinfected to prevent the transfer of microorganisms to other patients. Supplies and equipment with the potential for direct or indirect patient contact are sanitized by manual scrubbing with a neutral-**pH** detergent, using a brush if necessary, followed by hot water rinsing and air drying. Items not sanitized immediately after use are soaked according to the manufacturer's directions.

TABLE 26-1 COMPARISON OF MEDICAL AND SURGICAL ASEPSIS

Medical Asepsis	Surgical Asepsis
Reduces or controls the numbers of microorganisms	Removes all microorganisms from an object or surface
Follows clean technique—using clean equipment and supplies	Follows sterile technique—using sterile equipment and supplies
Hands are washed or clean gloves worn before supplies and equipment are handled	Surgical scrub performed and sterile gloves donned before supplies and equipment are handled
Equipment and supplies placed on clean field	Equipment and supplies placed on sterile field
Used for noninvasive procedures such as taking vital signs	Used for invasive procedures such as suturing and endoscopic procedures

PROCEDURE 26-1 Demonstrate the Performance of Sanitization

Theory and Rationale

After a minor surgery or treatment, the MA should rinse or soak the instruments immediately to prevent body tissue or fluids from drying on them. The MA should take the used instruments from the treatment room to the cleaning area in a towel-covered basin, then add disinfectant to the basin after transporting the instruments to minimize spill hazards.

In compliance with OSHA's Bloodborne Pathogen Standards, the MA must wear gloves when handling contaminated instruments. Wear utility gloves over disposable gloves to protect your hands from chemicals and to add another barrier when cleaning sharp instruments.

Before using the cleaning agent or detergent, check the expiration date. An expired solution is not guaranteed to inactivate or reduce microorganisms. Read the product's MSDS safety precautions, such as the use of PPE, mixing, storage, and cleaning accidental spills. If the resulting mixture is too weak, microorganisms may not be reduced or removed effectively. If the mixture is too strong, skin contact or inhalation may be harmful.

Holding one instrument at a time, carefully use the scrubbing brush (nylon for the instrument surface and stainless steel for grooves, cracks, or serrated edges) to remove organic materials from all areas. Autoclaving does not sterilize any areas in which organic materials remain. Use a neutral-pH detergent to prevent staining the instruments. Thoroughly rinse off the detergent to prevent stains and deterioration, which could later interfere with the function of the instrument. Avoid dropping instruments, which could damage or impair their function. When the instruments are clean and dry, inspect them individually for defects and proper working function.

Materials for Manual Sanitization

- Contaminated instruments
- Basin for soaking instruments
- Examination gloves
- Utility gloves
- Neutral low-suds detergent
- Scrubbing brush
- Paper towel
- Cotton towel

Competency for Manual Sanitization

(**Conditions**) With the necessary supplies, (**Task**) you will be able to manually clean and sanitize instruments (**Standards**) correctly and safely, within the time frame designated by your instructor.

1. With examination and utility gloves on your hands, place the contaminated instruments in an empty basin, cover it with a cotton towel, and transport it to the cleaning area (Figure 26-1 ◆). Remove the towel and add disinfectant or water with detergent to the basin. After the patient is discharged, clean, disinfect, and supply the room for the next patient.
2. In the instrument cleaning area, drain off the disinfectant or detergent and remove the instruments. Carefully wipe away blood and/or any tissue **debris.** Hold the instruments by their finger openings when possible.
3. Place the instruments in a basin with the recommended amount of cleaning agent and water.
4. Cleaning one instrument at a time, use a soft brush on all serrated and smooth edges, grooves, and opened hinges (Figure 26-2 ◆).
5. Rinse all the instruments with hot water.
6. Dry each instrument with a paper towel and allow to air-dry completely on a cotton towel (Figure 26-3 ◆). Lubricate the hinges with a water-based lubricant.
7. Follow the manufacturer's directions for disposing of cleaning solution. *Do not* reuse.
8. Remove the gloves and wash your hands.
9. Inspect each instrument for defects and proper function. Package the instruments as needed to ready for sterilization.

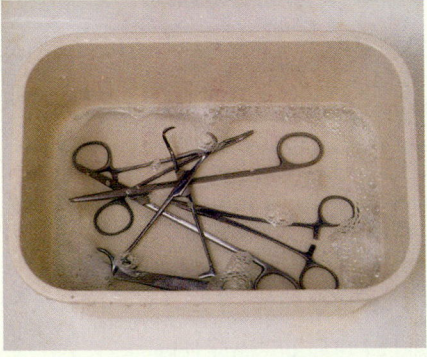

Figure 26-1 ◆ Place the contaminated instruments in an empty basin.

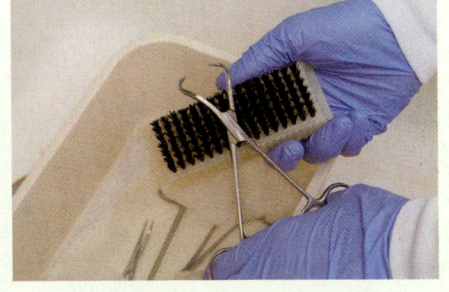

Figure 26-2 ◆ Use a soft brush on all serrated and smooth edges, grooves, and opened hinges.

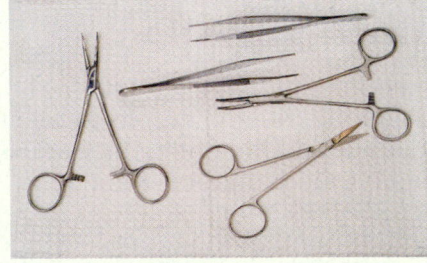

Figure 26-3 ◆ Allow instruments to air dry completely on a cotton towel.

PROCEDURE 26-1 Demonstrate the Performance of Sanitization *(continued)*

Materials for Ultrasonic Sanitization
- Ultrasonic cleaner
- Ultrasonic cleaning solution
- Examination gloves
- Utility gloves
- Paper towel
- Cotton towel

Competency for Ultrasonic Sanitization

(**Conditions**) With the necessary supplies, (**Task**) you will be able to clean and sanitize instruments with ultrasonic equipment (**Standards**) correctly and safely.

1. With examination and utility gloves on your hands, prepare the cleaning solution for the ultrasonic cleaner as directed by the manufacturer. Observe all MSDS safety and accidental spill precautions.
2. Place instruments made of different metals in separate ultrasonic cleaning loads.
3. Place the instruments in the ultrasonic cleaner with their hinges open and sharp edges not touching other instruments. Make sure that all the instruments are covered with the ultrasonic cleaning solution (Figure 26-4 ◆). Turn on the ultrasonic cleaner.
4. When the recommended cleaning time has passed, remove the instruments and rinse each one with hot tap water.
5. Dry each instrument with a paper towel and allow to air-dry completely on a cotton towel. Lubricate the hinges with a water-based lubricant.

6. Follow the manufacturer's directions for changing the cleaning solution.
7. Remove the gloves and wash your hands.
8. Inspect each instrument for defects and proper function. Package the instruments as needed to ready for sterilization.

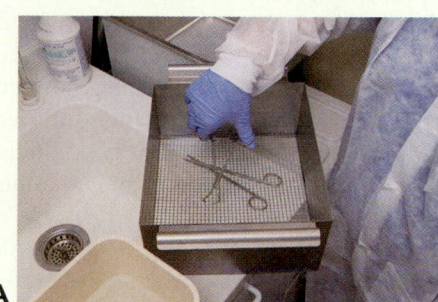
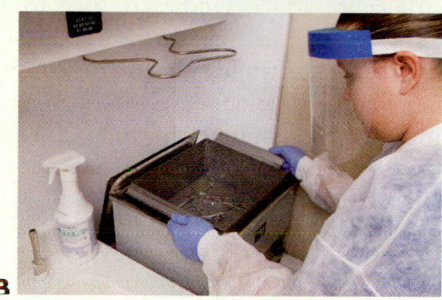

Figure 26-4 ◆ (A) Correctly position the instruments in the ultrasonic cleaner; (B) Make sure all instruments are covered in the cleaning solution.

Instruments may also be sanitized by ultrasound. In **ultrasonic cleaning,** sound waves are used to loosen contaminants, and then the articles are rinsed. Because instruments are handled less, this method may be considered safer. However, because the instruments must not touch each other and different types of metal may not be placed in the same load, fewer instruments may be sanitized at one time and the process may take longer.

Disinfection

Disinfection is the second level of microbial control and the second step of the sterilization procedure. Disinfection can destroy or inhibit pathogens but cannot kill spores and some viruses. It is accomplished by soaking in chemicals called **germicides,** by steam, or by boiling water. Chemical disinfectants are used to clean plastic and rubber items, floors, and furniture. Depending on the chemical and the manufacturer's instructions, immersion time can vary, up to several hours or more.

There are three levels of disinfection.

- Low-level disinfection kills most bacteria and viruses but does not kill microorganisms such as tuberculosis bacilli or bacterial spores. It is typically used for surfaces such as examination tables, countertops, and walls.

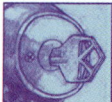

Keys to Success
CONTAMINATED OR NOT CONTAMINATED?

It is the responsibility of medical assistants and other clinical staff to consider an area or object contaminated if there is any doubt it is a sterile environment. In this situation, the correct action would be decontamination to create the required clean and/or sterile environment. To neglect action would be to risk patient and employee health.

- Intermediate-level disinfection kills mycobacteria, most viruses and bacteria, and tuberculosis bacilli, but cannot kill bacterial spores. It is used for articles that come in contact with skin but not with mucous membranes, such as blood pressure cuffs and stethoscopes.
- High-level disinfection kills all microorganisms except bacterial spores. It is used for articles that come in contact with mucous membranes, such as those in the oral cavity, throat, and vagina. Flexible sigmoidoscopes and glass thermometers require high-level disinfection.

Noncritical items are those that do not touch the patient or touch only intact skin, such as crutches, blood pressure cuffs, and gooseneck lamps. These items are not usually involved in transmitting disease. Washing noncritical items with a detergent or low-level disinfectant is sufficient. If these items are contaminated with blood or body fluids, stronger disinfection measures, sterilization, or biohazardous disposal are mandatory.

After soaking in disinfectant, items are thoroughly rinsed. Some disinfectants can only be used on inanimate objects, but alcohol and Betadine are used to disinfect a patient's skin before a procedure is performed. Chemical disinfectants for soaking or wiping include 70% isopropyl alcohol, bleach, phenol, formaldehyde, hydrogen peroxide, and soap. Items that cannot be entirely soaked, such as **endoscopes,** must be wiped with disinfectant, and removable parts must be soaked in disinfectant or sterilized according to the manufacturer's directions.

Sodium Hypochlorite

Sodium hypochlorite is also known as household bleach. It is a low-level disinfectant used mostly to disinfect surfaces. It is effective against many microorganisms, including human immunodeficiency virus (HIV) and hepatitis B virus. It is also very inexpensive to use.

Phenolics

Phenolics are used to clean countertops, walls, floors, and furniture. Because of the corrosive nature of this group, it may be necessary to wear PPE to protect the eyes and skin.

Alcohol

Two types of alcohol are used in the medical office—isopropyl alcohol and ethyl alcohol. Isopropyl is used to clean the rubber tops of vials, such as those used for medication, and for stethoscopes and percussion hammers. Ethyl alcohol is used to clean mercury glass thermometers. Stronger concentrations of alcohol are not as effective as 70% because the absence of water decreases their effectiveness. Because alcohol can dissolve the cement used to hold lenses in instruments, it should not be used to clean endoscopes.

Glutaraldehyde

Glutaraldehyde is rapid acting and requires only 10 to 30 minutes for disinfection. It is not corrosive and can be used for rubber or metal materials and for disinfecting lenses. The presence of organic material does not inactivate glutaraldehyde as it often does with other disinfectants.

Hydrogen Peroxide

Although hydrogen peroxide is used to clean wounds, it can also be used as a disinfectant for objects or surfaces that are not used for human contact. As a disinfectant it should be used with caution as it may damage some metals and some rubber or plastic surfaces.

Table 26-2 summarizes the types of disinfectant and their uses in the medical office.

TABLE 26-2 COMMON DISINFECTANTS USED IN THE MEDICAL OFFICE

Disinfectant	Level of Disinfection	Common Names and Uses
Chlorine and compounds	Low	Sodium hypochlorite, also known as household bleach. Recommended by OSHA to clean blood spills. Used also as a surface disinfectant. Usually diluted to 1 part bleach to 10 parts water.
Phenolics	Low	Carbolic acid, phenylic acid, phenyl hydroxide, phenic acid, hydroxybenzene, hexachlorophene, Lysol. Used as a surface disinfectant.
Hydrogen peroxide	Low	Hydrogen peroxide. Used to clean objects or surfaces not intended for human contact.
Alcohol		
Isopropyl	Low to intermediate	Isopropyl alcohol. Used to disinfect rubber tops of vials, stethoscopes, percussion hammers.
Ethyl	High	Ethyl alcohol. Used to clean glass thermometers.
Glutaraldehyde	High	Cidex, Cidex Plus, Glutarex, Metricide, Procide, Omnicide, Wavicide. Can also be used as a chemical sterilant. As a disinfectant, is used to clean glass thermometers and flexible sigmoidoscopes.

PROCEDURE 26-2 Demonstrate Disinfection Procedures

Theory and Rationale

All instruments to be sterilized must first undergo sanitization, then disinfection. When performed correctly, sanitization removes all organic materials and prepares instruments for effective disinfection. All organic material must be completely removed for the disinfectant to reach all areas of the article or instrument. Instruments must be dried thoroughly before they are placed in the disinfectant, as any water may dilute the chemical disinfectant.

Before proceeding with the disinfection of contaminated articles, the MA should read the MSDS for the disinfectant and look for general information regarding potential hazards, how to clean accidental spills, and which PPE to wear. Disposable gloves serve as a protective barrier against potentially infectious materials or contaminated instruments such as blood or body tissue. Additional utility gloves protect the skin from the irritating chemicals used for disinfection. Before moving the basin containing the contaminated instruments to another room, the MA should cover it with a cotton towel.

Materials
- Contaminated articles
- MSDS
- Disposable gloves
- Utility gloves
- Chemical disinfectant

- Soaking container
- Paper towels
- Cotton towel

Competency

(**Conditions**) With the necessary supplies, (**Task**) you will be able to perform the steps of disinfection (**Standards**) correctly and safely.

1. Review the MSDS, noting potential hazards, how to clean accidental spills, and whether PPE should be worn.
2. Apply disposable gloves to place the contaminated items into the basin. Then apply an additional layer of utility gloves.
3. Complete the sanitizing steps in Procedure 26-1. Remember to cover the basin of contaminated instruments with a cloth towel when you move them to the cleaning area.
4. Check the expiration date of the disinfectant and follow the manufacturer's directions for mixing and use (Figure 26-5 ◆).
5. With gloves on, completely immerse the contaminated articles in the container of disinfectant (Figure 26-6 ◆). Cover the container and soak the instruments for the length of time recommended by the manufacturer.
6. Remove and rinse each instrument thoroughly. Dry the instruments with paper towels.
7. Place the disinfected instruments on muslin or into sterilizing packets for the autoclave.

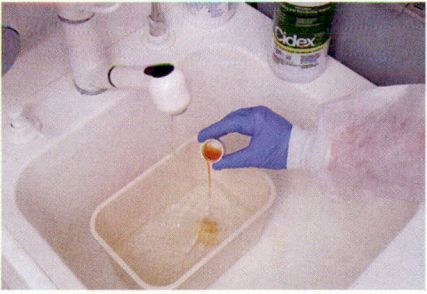

Figure 26-5 ◆ Follow the manufacturer's directions for mixing and use of the disinfectant.

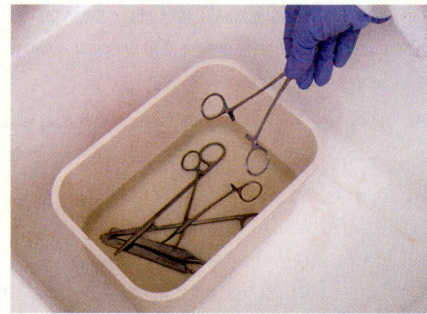

Figure 26-6 ◆ Completely immerse the contaminated articles in the container of disinfectant.

Sterilization

Sterilization is the third method of microbial control. All microorganisms, including spores, are killed by steam, dry heat, or chemical sterilization. The physical nature of the material determines the type of sterilization used. Because autoclave steam can damage certain materials, chemicals or dry heat may be used instead. In addition, some dense items require the use of dry heat. Items must first undergo sanitization and sometimes disinfection before they are sterilized.

Autoclave Sterilization

The autoclave consists of two separate compartments (Figure 26-7 ◆). An outer compartment surrounds the inner sterilizing chamber. Reducing the air in the inner chamber allows air pressure to build to 15 pounds of pressure per square inch. This pressure causes the distilled water in the chamber to reach a temperature of 250 degrees F, at which point it converts to steam. The steam penetrates the wrappers on the instruments and kills all microorganisms and bacterial spores. The high temperature

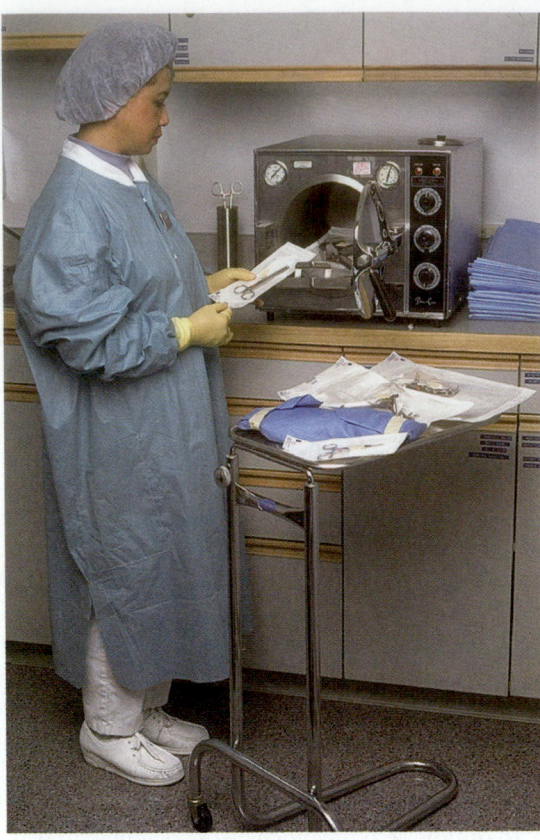

Figure 26-7 ◆ An autoclave.

TABLE 26-3 MINIMUM TIME REQUIREMENTS FOR AUTOCLAVE STERILIZATION

Time	Articles
15 minutes	Unwrapped metal instruments on open tray, hinges open
	Open glassware or metal containers
	Needles and unassembled syringes
	Unwrapped rubber tubing
20 minutes	Wrapped or covered instruments
	Muslin fabric
	Wrapped rubber products such as tubing and catheters
30 minutes	Instrument packs wrapped in muslin or paper
	Syringes unassembled and wrapped in gauze or glass tubes
	Needles packaged individually in gauze or paper
	Sutures, needles, and materials wrapped in muslin or paper
	Dressings, loosely packed
	Liquids or semiliquids

Note: These times apply to the manual operation of an autoclave.

of the steam must be maintained for over 15 minutes to assure the death of all living organism in the autoclave.

Certain guidelines for the use of autoclaves in the physician's office must be followed.

- *Location*—The autoclave must be on a level surface, close to the electrical outlet, with the front of the autoclave near the front of the support surface and providing a surface for the drain tube to drain.
- *Filling and loading*—The water must contain no minerals; therefore, distilled water is always used. The reservoir should be filled to the level indicated in the manual. Objects and packs must be properly loaded to ensure adequate steam penetration and air circulation.
- *Timing*—The processing must be timed once the desired pressure and temperature are reached. The sterilizing time is determined by the items to be sterilized (Table 26-3). Once the proper time has elapsed, the autoclave controls are turned to off and the pressure is allowed to return to normal. At that point the door of the autoclave is opened and air is allowed to circulate within the inner chamber until the items inside are dry. Then they can be safely removed and stored.

? —Critical Thinking Question 26-1—

In the case study, is the surgical instrument that Ian placed last, with noticeable moisture on it, considered sterile? Could the moisture possibly indicate that the autoclave is not working properly or that the cycle was not completed properly?

In automatic autoclaves, the sterilization countdown begins when 250 degrees F (121 degrees C) and 15 pounds of pressure per square inch have been reached.

Whether using manual or automatic settings, the MA must follow the manufacturer's directions for operation, maintenance, cleaning, and recommended sterilization times. The autoclave should be cleaned with a manufacturer-recommended detergent and rinsed thoroughly so that it is free from lint or debris before each load. The MA should check all discharge lines, valves, and vents to eliminate the possibility of obstructions, and check the seals to make sure there are no cracks. The MA should learn how to read the gauges for the outside jacket pressure, inner chamber pressure, timer, and temperature.

To ensure sterility quality, the Centers for Disease Control and Prevention (CDC) recommends keeping thorough records of all loads and quality control measures. Details of each load, such as operator, date, time, description, sterilization exposure time, and results of sterilization indicators are recorded. If there is an automatic printout for each sterilization cycle, that should be kept. Policies should also be established for regular monitoring by outside agencies—for instance, by sending samples from an **autoclave load** to a testing agency.

Other Methods of Sterilization

In addition to the autoclave, sterilization methods include the following.

- The dry heat oven is used to sterilize items that are harmed by steam or cannot be penetrated by steam. For example, steam sterilization dulls needles and sharps, erodes ground

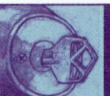

glass, and does not penetrate substances such as petroleum jelly. Dry heat ovens operate like household ovens. Items are placed in protective foil before sterilization.

- **Cold sterilization** involves immersion in a chemical agent for a specified period of time, usually 6 to 24 hours. Whenever an instrument is added, the timing must be restarted. Because cold sterilization can harm instruments and processing time must be periodically restarted, it is used only when other recommended methods of sterilization are not available.
- Radiation is used only when heat or chemical sterilizing methods cannot be used. In this method, ionizing radiation is the sterilizing agent.
- Heat-sensitive items or prepackaged instruments or equipment can be sterilized with ethylene oxide gas. These include plastic and rubber articles such as catheters and syringes. Because the process is complicated and expensive, it is not used in the medical office.

Wrapping Instruments and Preparing Sterile Trays

Procedures for wrapping instruments and preparing sterile trays vary from one medical office to another according to the clinical practice and physician preference. For example, packaging sterile

TABLE 26-4 EXAMPLES OF STERILE TRAY PACKAGING FOR DIFFERENT PROCEDURES

Incision and Drainage (I&D)	Biopsy	Vasectomy
Kelly hemostat	Hemostats	Scalpel handle and blade (no. 15)
Scalpel handle and blades (no. 11)	Scalpel handle and blades (nos. 10 and 15)	Curved mosquito forceps
Tissue forceps	Tissue forceps	Straight forceps
Thumb dressing forceps	Thumb dressing forceps	Dressing forceps
Curved iris scissors	Splinter forceps	Suture scissors
Retractor	Blunt probe	Suture materials and needles
4 × 4 gauze	Suture materials and needles	Retractor
	Needle holder	Towel clamps
	Retractor	4 × 4 gauze
	4 × 4 gauze	

hemostats and suture kits may be similar in all settings. However, some clinical settings may require sterile instrument packaging for Pap smears, and others may require sterile packaging for cataract surgery. In addition to the information in this chapter and in specialty chapters later in the text, you will incorporate specific applications in the clinical setting in which you work.

Table 26-4 lists examples of sterile tray packaging. Instruments may be wrapped individually or in packages. All instruments must be sanitized before sterilization. **Sterilization indicators** verify that a package or instrument has been placed in the autoclave, that steam heat has reached the inside of each package, and that sterilization has been achieved (Figure 26-8 ◆). Sterilizing tape is used on the outside of packages, with stripes that turn dark when a package has been sterilized.

Preparing the Surgical Field

A surgical field is an area that is considered sterile. Sterile towels or sterile drapes on a table or tray provide a sterile field on which instruments and suture material can be placed. The wrapping of a sterile surgical pack may also provide a sterile or surgical field when it is opened.

The MA will use sterile supplies to prepare a sterile field by opening the surgical pack, adding to the surgical field, and sterile gloving. It is the medical assistant's responsibility and that of others involved in the sterile procedure to follow sterile field guidelines to prevent contamination and the potential transfer of microorganisms (Table 26-5). If sterile technique is breached during an invasive procedure, the patient may be harmed and the medical office and clinical staff may be held liable.

— Critical Thinking Question 26-2 —

Ian left the room to take a phone call after dropping one last instrument on the sterile field. When he reenters the room, is the setup still considered sterile?

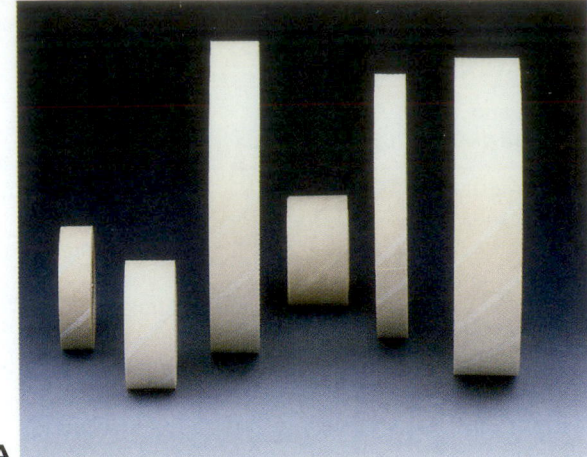

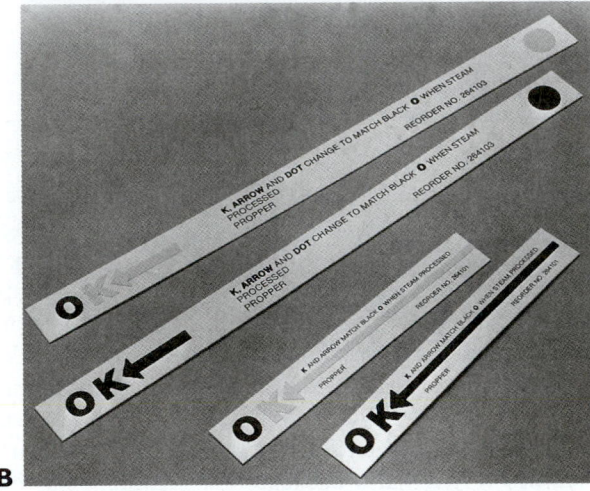

Figure 26-8 ◆ (A) Autoclave indicator tapes; (B) Sterility check strips. *Reprinted by permission of Propper Manufacturing Co., Inc.*

Sometimes sterile solutions for irrigation, infusion, or injection must be added to the sterile field, or vials must be ready for the withdrawal of medication. Certain techniques are followed for pouring solutions and withdrawing medication to prevent contamination of the sterile field.

- If a solution is to be added, the physician holds the sterile container just beyond the edge of the sterile field and the MA palms the label of the solution, pours some solution into a trash receptacle or sink, then pours the rest into the sterile container (see Figures 26-16 and 26-17). Palming the label before pouring avoids staining the label and making it difficult to read.
- If the physician needs to withdraw local anesthetic from a vial, the MA, with clean or gloved hands, uses an alcohol prep pad to clean the vial top, then holds the vial upside down just outside the sterile field with the label facing the physician so that the physician can verify it is the correct solution. The physician uses a sterile syringe and needle from the sterile field to withdraw medication.

TABLE 26-5 GUIDELINES FOR A STERILE FIELD

- Never reach, lean, or pass over a sterile field. The air above a sterile field is considered sterile.
- Sterile areas should be set up away from areas with potential air currents such as doors, windows, and fans to avoid the transfer of microorganisms.
- Never cough, sneeze, or talk over a sterile field. Moisture droplets will contaminate the sterile air and sterile field.
- Wet areas on the sterile field lead to contamination. Depending on the extent of a spill, the area may be covered or a new sterile field may need to be created.
- Movement around the sterile field should be minimal and purposeful. Always face the sterile field and keep your arms above waist level. An extra sterile drape or towel can be kept close by for those times you may have to turn your back on the sterile field or leave the room.
- Place all items toward the center of the sterile field. Anything in the 1-inch perimeter is considered contaminated because of its proximity to clothing or other nonsterile work surfaces.

In Practice

After unloading several dry packs from the autoclave, the medical assistant notes that the indicator tape color has not changed. Are the instruments located in the dry packs sterile? What should the medical assistant do?

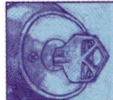

Keys to Success
THE IMPORTANCE OF CLEANING INSTRUMENTS PROPERLY

What happens when a pathogenic outbreak is identified? In cooperation with the CDC, the local Public Health Department investigates each patient history for common factors. For example, did the patients eat at the same restaurant, go to the same medical office, use the same bathroom, or receive the same procedure at the same medical office? Microorganism cultures may be taken of food samples, disinfected or sterilized medical instruments, bathroom faucets, toilet handles, and so on.

Once the cause of the outbreak is determined, actions are taken to eliminate the possibility of recurrence. This might involve, but is not limited to, temporary or permanent closing of the facility, resterilization of items thought to be sterilized, and treatment of persons who might harbor the pathogen. If patients have been harmed during A procedure, malpractice lawsuits may be filed against the facility and all persons involved in the procedure or the cleaning of instruments, including the medical assistant.

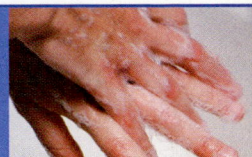

PROCEDURE 26-3 Demonstrate How to Wrap Surgical Instruments and Prepare Sterile Trays for Autoclave Sterilization

Theory and Rationale

Some instruments that are used immediately or used in procedures that do not require sterilized instruments do not require wrapping. These instruments may be placed in an autoclaving tray. For other instruments, single or variety groups must be packaged for the appropriate procedure. Whenever possible, sterilize items in small packs that steam can penetrate more easily.

Materials used to package instruments for sterilization include porous plastic, paper, and fabric. Porous materials allow the moisture and heat to penetrate and sterilize the package contents. Muslin fabric is the most commonly used wrapping material. A sealer may have to be purchased for some types of plastic packaging.

Place instruments in the center of the wrapping material and alternate with any dressing materials required for the procedure. Position the instruments in such a way as to prevent metal-to-metal contact within the pack. Hinged instruments should be slightly open to allow for steam penetration and sterilization. Place the inside sterilization indicator tape within the package before folding and/or sealing the package.

Double-back folding is an important step in wrapping. Later, when the package is opened to create a sterile field, it will provide edges to grab and help to prevent contamination. Place sterilization indicator tape across the last folded edge and write on the tape the type of tray and the expiration date. Each office has a specific policy concerning expiration dates—for example, sterilized packages may be used for up to one month after the autoclave date. Using an expired package would not guarantee sterility.

Materials

- Dry wrapping paper, muslin cloth, or sealable bags
- Sanitized and disinfected items to be sterilized
- Sterilization indicators for interior and exterior of packages
- Marker pen

Competency

(**Conditions**) With the necessary supplies, (**Task**) you will be able to package and wrap instruments and supplies to be placed in the autoclave (**Standards**) correctly, in the time designated by your instructor.

1. Place the sanitized items to be sterilized in the center of the dry wrapping paper, muslin, or sealable bag. Place an indicator strip inside the package (Figure 26-9 ◆). The sealable bag may need to be sealed if it is not manufacturer-prepared.
2. For cloth or paper packaging, fold up one corner to cover the items. Double-back a small fold to use as a pull corner for unwrapping (Figure 26-10 ◆). Do the same fold and double-back fold for the right side and left side. Fold the last side once toward the center and tuck the corner under before applying sterilization indicator tape (Figures 26-11 ◆ and 26-12 ◆).
3. Use the marker to label the tape with the date and contents.

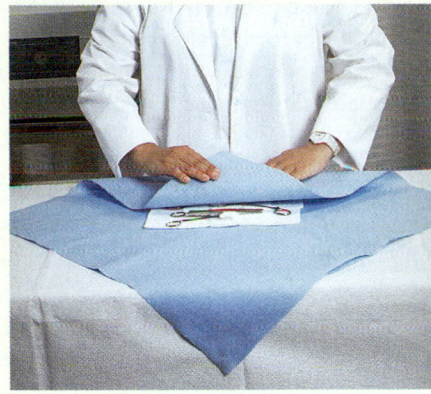

Figure 26-9 ◆ Place the sanitized items in the center of the dry wrapping paper.

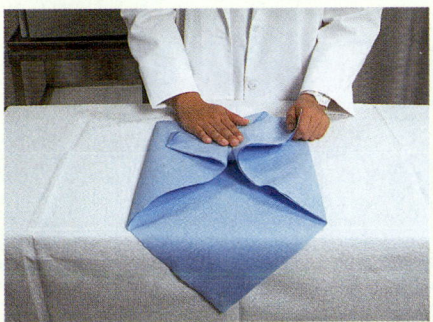

Figure 26-10 ◆ Double-back a small fold to use as a pull corner for unwrapping.

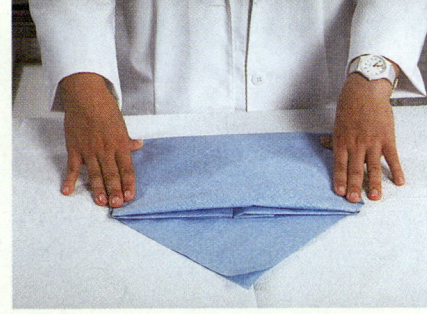

Figure 26-11 ◆ Do the same fold and double-back fold for the right side and left side.

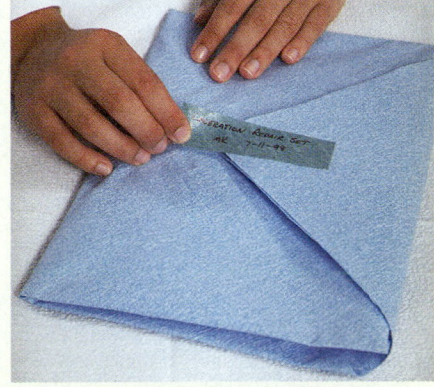

Figure 26-12 ◆ Apply the sterilization indicator tape.

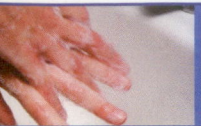

PROCEDURE 26-4 Demonstrate Correct Procedure for Loading and Operating an Autoclave

Theory and Rationale

Sanitization and disinfection remove organic and inorganic debris from instruments before sterilization in the autoclave. Sterilization is the last defense against pathogenic bacteria.

The autoclave reservoir is filled with distilled water to produce steam for sterilization. Using distilled water prevents mineral corrosion inside the autoclave and mineral deposits that might block the air exhaust valves. Air pockets, created when the autoclave reservoir is emptied of water, can reduce the temperature during the sterilization process. To prevent air pockets, it is an important daily routine to fill the reservoir at the beginning of every day or every load, depending on the frequency of autoclave use.

The autoclave must be loaded correctly to ensure steam penetration and complete sterilization. Steam must reach all surfaces for the required time and at the required temperature to kill all microorganisms. Loading guidelines include the following.

- Position packs and instruments loosely in the inner chamber to allow steam to circulate, penetrate all porous materials, and make contact with all surfaces. Larger packs should be spaced 2 to 4 inches apart, and smaller packs 1 to 3 inches apart.
- Sterilization pouches should be placed on their sides, rather than flat, to allow better steam penetration and drying. Containers should also be placed on their sides, with their lids removed to allow air to escape. Trapped air in a side-lying container would prevent the steam from reaching all surfaces. Dressing packs should be arranged in a vertical position to allow the steam to penetrate each layer.
- Avoid leaning any item against plastic, as the heat will mold the plastic to the shape of the object.

Once the autoclave has been loaded, follow the operating instructions. As a safety measure, make sure the steam pressure has been automatically or manually released before you start the autoclave. Otherwise, pressure in the inner chamber can "pop" the door open suddenly and forcefully and cause injury. Newer models are designed to keep the pressurized chamber door from opening this way. Be sure to read the instruction manual.

Sterilization time begins when the correct pressure and temperature have been reached. (See Table 26-3 for recommended sterilizing times.)

Remove the dry packs with heat-resistant gloves. Packs are considered contaminated if they are removed while wet or damp, if they are torn or have holes, or if the indicator tape color has not changed.

Materials

- Wrapped or unwrapped sanitized and disinfected instruments
- Distilled water
- Heat-resistant gloves
- Manual or automatic autoclave
- Manufacturer's instruction manual
- Sterile transfer forceps
- Storage containers or shelf areas

Competency

(**Conditions**) With the necessary supplies, (**Task**) you will be able to load and operate an autoclave correctly and safely (**Standards**) to ensure complete sterilization.

1. Wash your hands and assemble materials.
2. Check the level of distilled water in the autoclave reservoir and fill as necessary (Figure 26-13 ◆).
3. Load the autoclave, asking yourself the following questions:
   Are the autoclave trays 1 inch apart?
   Are small packs 1 to 3 inches apart?
   Are large packs 2 to 4 inches apart?
   Are any of the packs touching the inside of the autoclave chamber?
   Are glassware and jars on their sides?
   Are dressings and sterilization pouches in a vertical position, on their sides?
   Are any materials leaning against plastic items?
   For a mixed load of porous and nonporous materials, are materials such as dressings on the top shelf and instruments on the lower shelf?
4. Close and latch the door. Turn on the autoclave (Figure 26-14 ◆).
5. Sterilization time starts when the correct pressure and temperature have been reached.

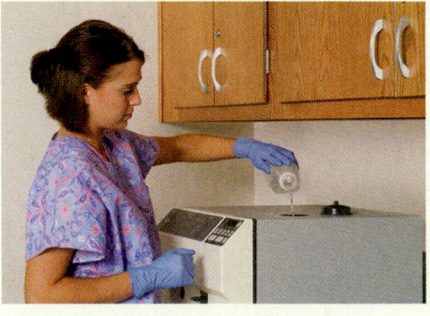

Figure 26-13 ◆ Fill the reservoir as necessary.

PROCEDURE 26-4 Demonstrate Correct Procedure for Loading and Operating an Autoclave *(continued)*

6. After steam pressure has been manually or automatically released, open the autoclave door slightly to allow the load to dry. Larger packs with dressings may take 45 to 60 minutes to dry.

7. Wearing heat-resistant gloves, remove the dry packages. Inspect for holes, tears, and indicator tape color change. Use the sterile transfer forceps to remove single instruments or items to a clean container (Figure 26-15 ◆). Place

sterile items toward the back of the stock so that the oldest dated materials are used first. Avoid storing in cool areas that may cause condensation, make the materials damp, and require additional wrapping and sterilizing.

8. Remove the gloves and wash your hands.

9. Record the date, autoclave load contents, and use of sterilization indicators and quality controls in the sterilization log book.

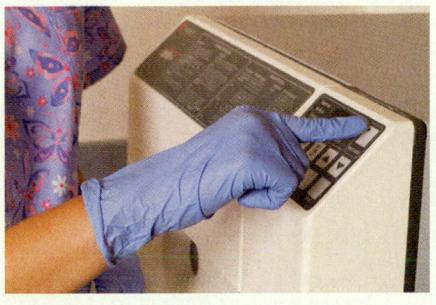

Figure 26-14 ◆ Turn on the autoclave.

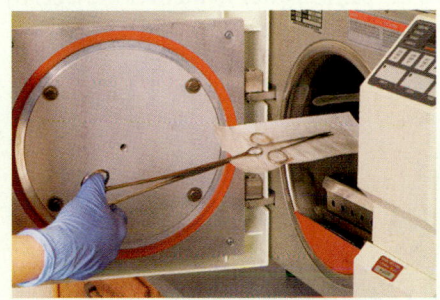

Figure 26-15 ◆ Remove instruments to a clean container using the sterile transfer forceps.

PROCEDURE 26-5 Demonstrate Correct Procedure for Pouring Sterile Solution onto a Sterile Field

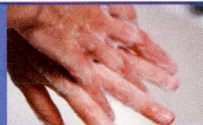

Theory and Rationale

Sterile solutions are often required during the surgical procedure to irrigate a wound. Several sterile solutions are commonly used during minor surgery procedures. These may include sterile water, normal saline (0.9%) sodium chloride, povidine-iodine solutions.

Bottles of these sterile solutions come in a variety of sizes; use the smallest size that will meet the requirement for solution needed during the procedure. This will assist in minimizing cost since any unused solution must be discarded.

Always ensure that you read the label to verify that you have the correct solution. Be certain to check the expiration date on the solution. Outdated solutions should not be used and should be discarded immediately.

When pouring the solution, cover the label of the bottle with the palm of your hand to keep the label dry and avoid staining the label making it difficult to read. Remove the cap by touching only the outside and place the cap on a flat surface

with the open end up. Placing the cap with the open end up prevents contamination of the inside of the cap by an unsterile surface. Before pouring the solution into a sterile container, pour a small amount of the liquid into a waste container to clean the lip of the bottle. Rinsing the lip washes away any microorganisms that may be on it. As you pour the solution into the sterile bowl or container, hold the bottle at an angle so that you do not reach over the sterile field. Be certain to not allow the neck of the bottle to come in contact with the sterile container, and be careful not to splash solution onto the sterile field. Solutions spilled on the sterile field may contaminate the field.

Materials

- Bottle of sterile solution
- Sterile stainless steel bowl or container
- Sterile field
- Waste container

continued

PROCEDURE 26-5 Demonstrate Correct Procedure for Pouring Sterile Solution onto a Sterile Field (continued)

Competency

(**Conditions**) With the necessary supplies, (**Task**) you will be able to pour sterile solution onto a sterile field (**Standards**) correctly within the time frame designated by your instructor.

1. Wash your hands.
2. Gather your supplies.
3. Read the label to ensure that you have the correct solution.
4. Check the expiration date on the solution.
5. Place the palm of your hand over the label to avoid staining the label (Figure 26-16 ◆).
6. Remove the cap by touching only the outside and place the cap on a flat surface with the open end up.
7. Pour a small amount of solution into a waste container to rinse the lip of the bottle.
8. Without splashing solution, pour the proper amount of solution into the sterile container located on the sterile field (Figure 26-17 ◆).
9. Replace the cap on the container without contaminating it.
10. Check the label for a final time to ensure that you have poured the correct solution.

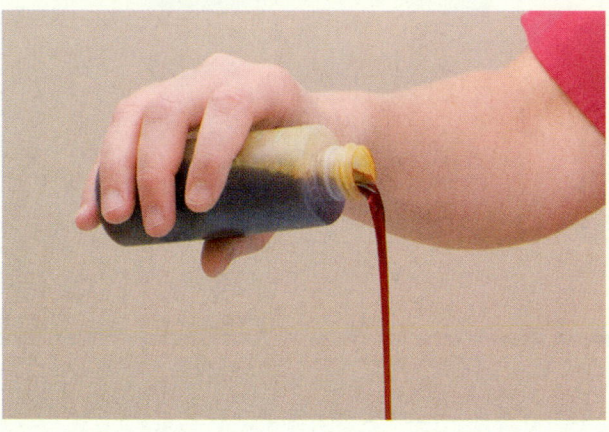

Figure 26-16 ◆ Palm the label.

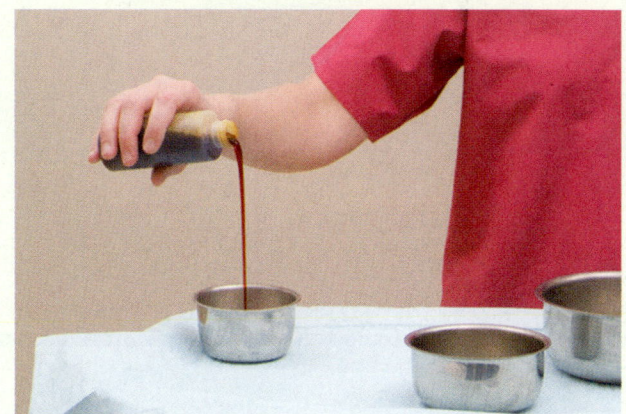

Figure 26-17 ◆ Pour the remaining solution into the sterile container.

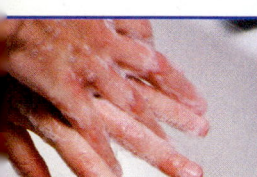

PROCEDURE 26-6 Demonstrate Correct Procedure for Opening a Sterile Surgical Pack to Create a Sterile Field

Theory and Rationale

Creating a sterile field involves using "no-touch" sterile techniques. The first step is to adjust the height of the **Mayo stand** to provide a comfortable working level, prevent back strain, and help maintain a sterile field.

After noting the expiration date on the primary sterile surgical pack and determining that it is usable, open the pack. Lift the top flap away from your body to prevent contamination from reaching or crossing over the sterile field as the rest of the flaps are opened. Next, open the side flaps, then the last flap. In addition to the surgical pack contents, you should have already gathered other supplies, such as

appropriate-size sterile gloves, suture materials, needles, instruments, dressings, and basins.

At all times during the opening and preparation of the sterile field, *do not* allow any part of your body or clothing to touch the sterile field. Touching the sterile field, even with clean clothing or skin, would result in contamination and the need to prepare a new sterile field. If additional supplies are needed, another person may open the outer pack while the sterile-gloved physician or medical assistant takes the sterile contents inside. Or the outer wrapping of the package may be opened and the items dropped on the sterile field. When all items are on the sterile field, they can be moved with transfer

PROCEDURE 26-6 Demonstrate Correct Procedure for Opening a Sterile Surgical Pack to Create a Sterile Field (continued)

forceps or sterile gloves. A sterile cotton towel or drape is used to cover the completed sterile field.

Materials
- Mayo stand
- Sterile packet(s)
- Sterile transfer forceps
- Sterile gloves
- Sterile towels or drapes
- Waste container

Competency
(**Conditions**) With the necessary supplies, (**Task**) you will be able to use sterile technique to open a sterile surgical pack for a sterile field (**Standards**) correctly within the time frame designated by your instructor.

1. Wash your hands and assemble the equipment.
2. Adjust the height of the Mayo stand to a comfortable working position.
3. Position the sterile surgical pack on the Mayo stand so that the top flap will open away from you (Figure 26-18 ◆).

4. Remove the sterilization indicator tape from the pack, note whether the appropriate color change occurred to indicate sterility, and discard.
5. Pull the top flap away from you and down to hang over the edge of the Mayo stand. Pull each of the side flaps away from the packet and over the edge (Figure 26-19 ◆).
6. Without reaching over the sterile field, bring the last flap toward you and down to hang over the edge. Do not touch your body to any part of the sterile field while opening the pack or anytime during a sterile procedure.
7. The inside of the pack is now the sterile field.
   - To move items on the sterile field, use sterile transfer forceps
   - To add items to a sterile field, open other packages without touching the inner side of the package or contents, then dump the contents on the sterile field without crossing or touching it (Figure 26-20 ◆).

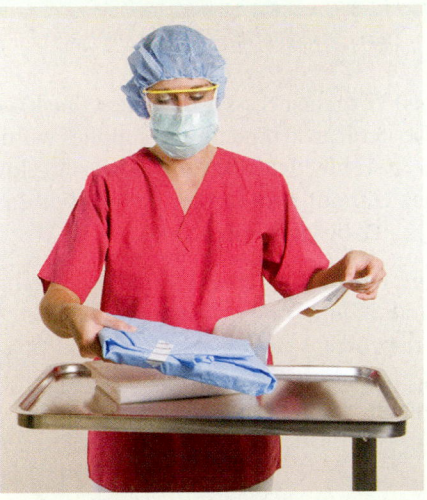

Figure 26-18 ◆ Position the sterile surgical pack on the Mayo stand.

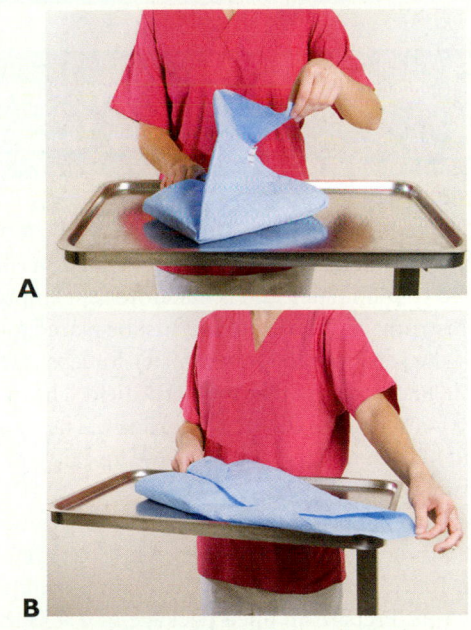

Figure 26-19 ◆ (A) Pull the top flap away from you and down to hang over the edge of the Mayo stand; (B) Pull each of the side flaps away from the packet and over the edge.

continued

PROCEDURE 26-6 Demonstrate Correct Procedure for Opening a Sterile Surgical Pack to Create a Sterile Field *(continued)*

- To open the inner package of another sterile surgical pack during the procedure, a person with clean hands may open the outer package so that a person with sterile gloves may take the inner packet of instruments and supplies (Figure 26-21 ◆).

8. Cover the tray with sterile towels or drape until ready to use. Open a pack of sterile gloves and a pack of sterile drapes or towels, then put on the sterile gloves to unfold the drape or towel over the sterile field (Figure 26-22 ◆). Some sterile packets come with material for draping the sterile field.

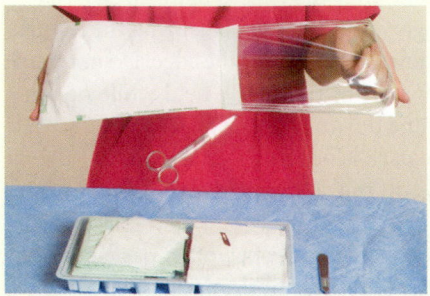

Figure 26-20 ◆ Place the contents of another package on sterile field without crossing or touching it.

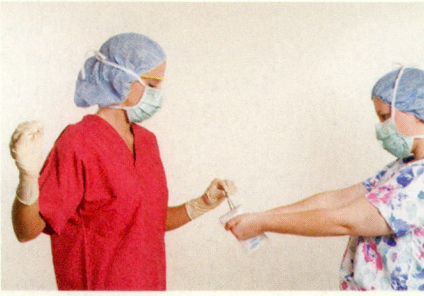

Figure 26-21 ◆ Another person wearing sterile gloves takes inner packet of instruments out.

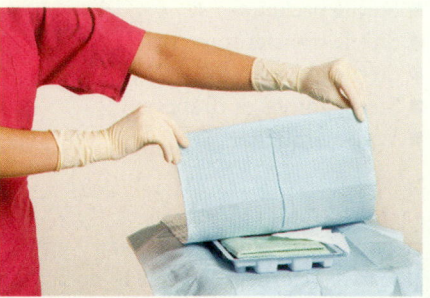

Figure 26-22 ◆ Place the drape or towel over the sterile field.

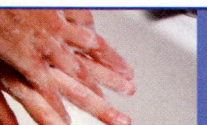

PROCEDURE 26-7 Demonstrate the Correct Procedure for Using Transfer Forceps

Theory and Rationale

The 1-inch perimeter around the outside of a sterile field is considered contaminated and is therefore kept empty of supplies or instruments. Sterile items must be placed toward the center of the sterile field. Only transfer forceps can be used to move items onto or within the sterile field. The forceps are kept in a container of chemical **sterilant.** The handles are clean and may be touched, but the jaws and tips are considered sterile.

Remove the transfer forceps vertically from the container, holding the handles firmly while keeping the tips together. Touching the sides of the container could contaminate the tips. Prepare an open package of 4 × 4s to dry the transfer forceps by contact and prevent dripping onto the sterile field. Transfer forceps must be cleaned and autoclaved weekly. The sterilant solution should also be changed weekly.

Materials

- Transfer forceps
- Sterile tray set up on a Mayo stand
- Forceps container 2/3 full of Cidex or other sterilant
- Sterile 4 × 4 gauze package
- Instrument or supply pack for use with sterile transfer forceps

Competency

(**Conditions**) With the necessary supplies, (**Task**) you will be able to move sterile instruments and supplies within a sterile field, onto a sterile field, or into a sterile gloved hand (**Standards**) without contaminating and within the time frame designated by your instructor.

1. Open the 4 × 4 gauze package using sterile technique and lay it on the countertop or Mayo stand.
2. Grasp the forceps handles, keeping the tips together. Remove the forceps vertically from the container without touching the sides (Figure 26-23 ◆).

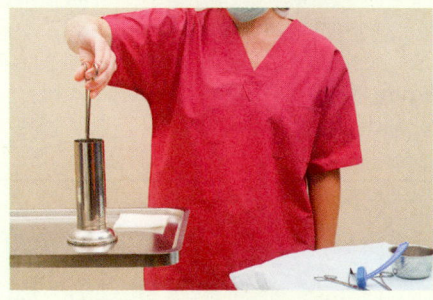

Figure 26-23 ◆ Remove forceps from the container without touching the sides.

PROCEDURE 26-7 Demonstrate the Correct Procedure for Using Transfer Forceps *(continued)*

3. Touch the forceps tips to the 4 × 4s to dry them. Do not allow the forceps to touch the sterile field. Holding them vertically, pick up and move an item from the open pack to the sterile field. To move a sterile item on the sterile field, keep the forceps vertical, pick up the item, and lift it to the desired location without touching the sterile field (Figure 26-24 ◆).
4. Place the transfer forceps back into the standing container without touching the sides.

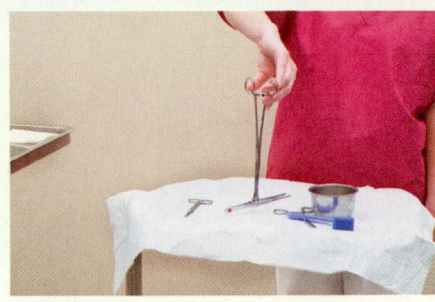

Figure 26-24 ◆ Keep the forceps vertical, pick up the item, and lift it to the desired location without touching the sterile field.

PROCEDURE 26-8 Demonstrate a Sterile Scrub (Surgical Hand Washing)

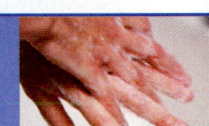

Theory and Rationale

Medical hand washing, recognized simply as hand washing, is required for most procedures in the clinical setting. Hand washing reduces the numbers of microorganisms and the possibility of cross-infection between staff and patients. For example, it is performed first thing in the morning before patient care, between patients, and after using the bathroom. Some procedures, because of their invasive nature or the lowered immunity of the patient, require surgical hand washing, or a sterile scrub.

Before beginning a sterile scrub, gather supplies. Open the sterile towel pack away from the splash area of the faucets to prevent moisture contamination of the sterile towel that you will use to dry your hands after the second rinse. You will need a clock or watch to time the first and second scrubs—5 minutes and 3 minutes respectively for each hand. Remove all jewelry. Microorganisms are likely to hide around jewelry sites, under the fingernails, and between the fingers. (It is best to leave jewelry at home; however, you may secure it to your uniform top.)

The general order of the procedure is:

■ Wetting
■ Scrubbing
■ Rinsing
■ Second scrubbing
■ Second rinsing
■ Drying

Start with your fingers and proceed to your hands, wrists, and lower arms. The second scrub and rinse are a precautionary measure to ensure the elimination of as many microorganisms as possible. To prevent chapping and cracking, use warm, not hot, water. Breaks in skin integrity could harbor microorganisms that may be transferred to patients. Keep the hands pointed upward and rinse them from fingertips to elbows to prevent contaminating the hands. Turn off the water only *after* you have dried your hands with the sterile towel. Use the towel to prevent contact between your hands and the faucet handles when you turn off the water. Touching the handles without a barrier would contaminate your hands and would require starting the sterile scrub from the beginning. Some sinks are equipped with knee handles or foot pedals that eliminate the possibility of hand contamination.

Materials
■ Germicidal liquid soap in dispenser
■ Large wall clock
■ Sink with hand, knee, or foot on/off controls
■ Sterile towel packet
■ Sterile scrub sponge
■ Orangewood stick or nail file

Competency
(**Conditions**) With the necessary supplies, (**Task**) you will be able to perform surgical hand washing using sterile technique (**Standards**) correctly within the time frame designated by your instructor.

1. Without touching the inside, open the sterile towel packet some distance from potential water spray.
2. Remove all jewelry from your hands and wrists. Use an orangewood stick or nail file to remove dirt from under your fingernails.
3. Turn on the water with hand, knee, or foot controls and adjust the temperature. Wet your arm from the fingertips to the elbows (Figure 26-25 ◆).

continued

PROCEDURE 26-8 Demonstrate a Sterile Scrub (Surgical Hand Washing) *(continued)*

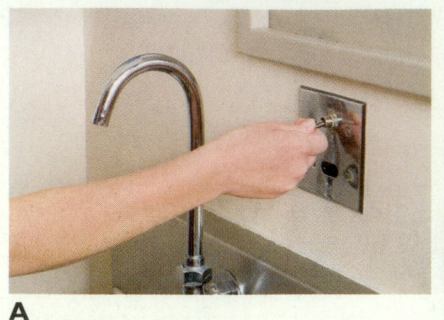 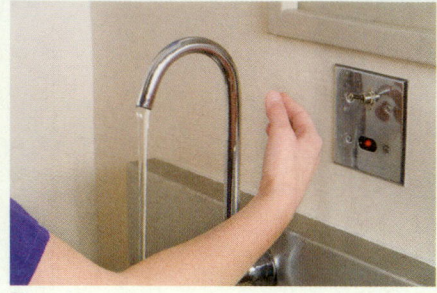 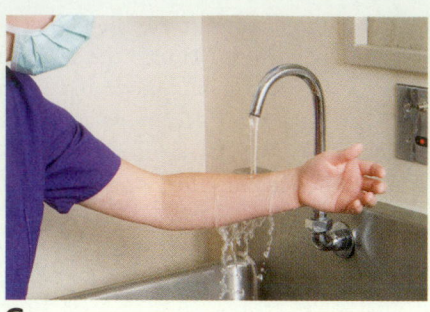

A   B   C

Figure 26-25 ◆ (A) Turn on the water with the hand, knee, or foot controls; (B) Adjust the temperature; (C) Wet your arms from the fingertips to the elbows.

4. Apply liquid soap to your hands and lower arms. For 5 minutes, use a circular motion to create lather, starting from the fingertips and working toward and including the elbows (Figure 26-26 ◆). Be sure to wash between the fingers and under the fingernails.

5. Rinse the lather from your arm, beginning at the fingertips and proceeding to the elbows. Keep your hands above your elbows.

6. Repeat the process, applying liquid soap to your hands and lower arms. Scrub from the fingertips to the elbows with the sponge for 3 minutes (Figure 26-27 ◆).

7. Rinse thoroughly and leave the water running. Use a sterile towel to dry your hands (Figure 26-28 ◆).

8. Use the towel to turn off a hand-controlled faucet or, if necessary, use your elbow. Otherwise release the foot pedal or move the knee control to turn off the water.

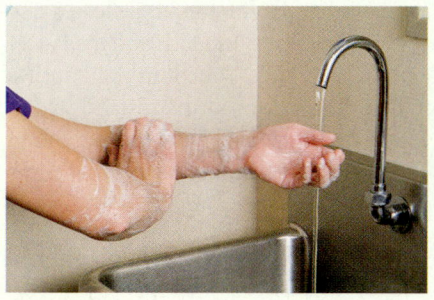 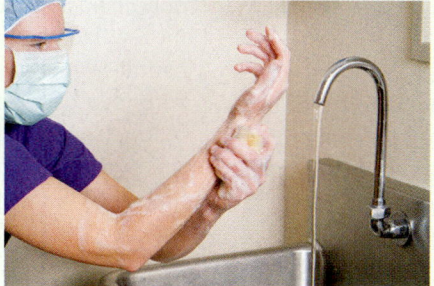 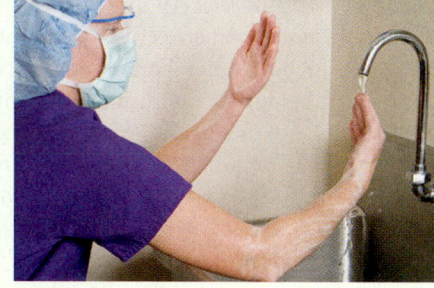

Figure 26-26 ◆ Use a circular motion to create lather, starting from the fingertips and working toward and including the elbows.

Figure 26-27 ◆ Scrub from the fingertips to the elbows with the sponge for 3 minutes.

Figure 26-28 ◆ Rinse thoroughly and leave water running.

Alcohol-Based Hand Rubs

The Centers for Disease Control and Prevention has presented new guidelines on the use of alcohol-based hand rubs, which suggest that these hand rubs can be used at the times usually required for hand washing.

The guidelines state that rings, watches, and bracelets should be removed before beginning the surgical hand scrub, and debris should be removed from underneath the fingernails using a nail cleaner under running water. Hands and forearms should be prewashed with a non-antimicrobial soap and then dried completely before using the alcohol-based surgical hand scrub product. When decontaminating hands with the alcohol-based surgical hand rub and following the manufacturer's instructions, apply the product to the palm of one hand and rub hands together, covering all surfaces of the hands and fingers (Figure 26-29 ◆). Apply the hand rub to the forearms as well and scrub persistently (Figure 26-30 ◆).

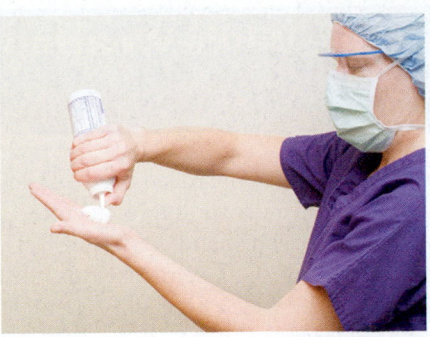

Figure 26-29 ◆ Apply the product to the palm of one hand and rub hands together, covering all surfaces of the hands and fingers.

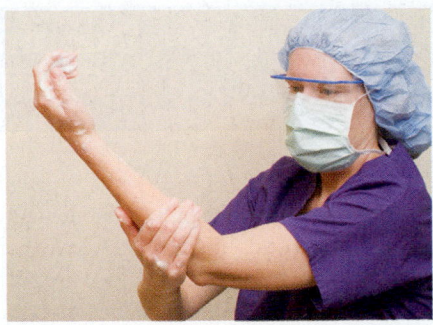

Figure 26-30 ◆ Apply the hand rub to the forearm.

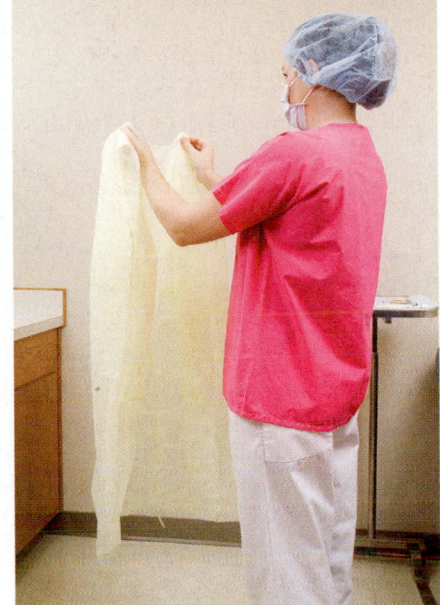

Figure 26-31 ◆ Pick up the gown by the inner neckline.

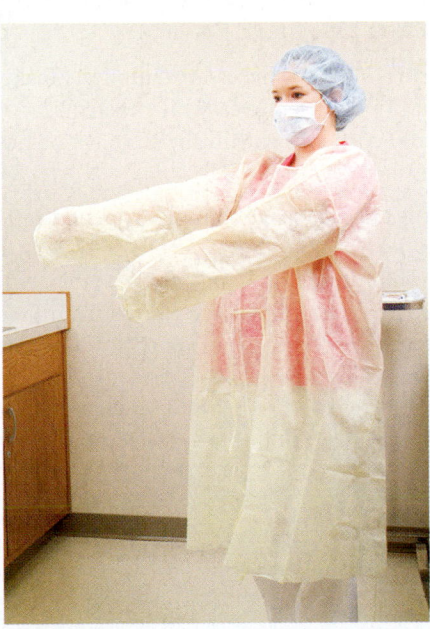

Figure 26-32 ◆ Insert arms into sleeves one at a time without touching the outer surface.

Keys to Success
STERILE GOWNING

The outer surfaces of uniforms, scrub suits, and gowns harbor microorganisms that can contaminate a sterile surgical field. For some procedures it is necessary to cover this clothing with a sterile coverup or gown. Sterile gowns may be made of washable cloth or disposable material. Disposable gowns have a protective moisture barrier on the inner surface and are more commonly used. Remember that nonsterile hands or surfaces must never touch the sterile gown's outer surface. The inner surface of the gown may be touched as it is considered contaminated.

A sterile gown may be donned mostly on one's own or with assistance.

1. After applying a surgical mask and hair cover, perform a surgical scrub. Pick up the gown by the inner neckline and hold it away from your body, high enough that the bottom does not touch the floor (Figure 26-31 ◆).
2. Insert your arms into the sleeves one at a time without touching the outer surface of the gown. Depending on how the sterile gloves are to be donned, you may or may not pull your hands completely through the sleeves (Figure 26-32 ◆). If you are donning the gown unassisted, your hands will advance only as far as the cuffs of the gown, and you will handle the gloves from within the cuffs. This takes a great deal of practice. If you are being assisted, you may pass your hands through the cuffs, making sure you touch nothing until you are assisted in the application of the sterile gloves.
3. The back of the gown is considered contaminated and you will need someone to tie the ties.
4. After gowning is completed, keep your hands above the waistline to prevent contamination.

You should receive specialized training in donning a sterile gown before you are required to do so in a surgical procedure.

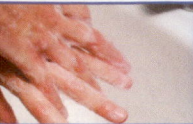

PROCEDURE 26-9 Demonstrate How to Glove While Wearing a Sterile Gown

Theory and Rationale

In order to prevent the transfer of pathogenic material to the patient, a sterile gown and gloves must be worn and special caution must be taken to avoid contamination of these sterile garments. There are certain rules that must be observed while wearing a sterile gown and gloves. These rules include:

- Keep sterile gloved hands above the waist at all times; do not let hands drop below the waist.
- Keep your hands within full view at all times; do not place hands behind back or tuck under arms.
- Never reach across an unsterile area for an item.
- Never touch an unsterile object or item with sterile gloved hands.
- Never touch the sterile gown above the area of the axillae or below the waist.
- The stockinette cuff of the sterile gown is not considered sterile and must be covered by sterile gloves.
- If the sterile gown or gloves become contaminated, discard and replace the gown and gloves.

The danger of contamination to sterile gloves is reduced with sterile gowns in place since the skin surfaces of the hands are not exposed. The gloves are applied with the hands covered by the sterile gown to avoid contamination. Remember that the mask, goggles, and hair cover are not sterile and should be donned before the sterile gown and gloves.

Materials

- Sterile gloves, opened on a sterile field
- Sterile gown (already donned), mask, goggles, hair cover

Competency

(**Conditions**) With the necessary supplies, (**Task**) you will be able to apply sterile gloves while wearing a sterile gown (**Standards**) correctly within the time frame designated by your instructor.

1. A sterile glove package should be opened and placed on a sterile field.
2. Using your dominant hand, and keeping it within the cuff of the left sleeve, pick up the glove, from the inner wrap of the glove package, by grasping the folded cuff with your thumb and forefinger.
3. Place the glove in the palm of your nondominant hand, with glove fingers pointing to the elbows (Figure 26-33 ◆).

4. With both hands, pinch the rolled edges of the glove and stretch the glove up and over the gown cuff.
5. Pull the glove over your hand as you push through the gown cuff (Figure 26-34 ◆). Remember that the bare hand will only touch the inside of the glove. Gently slide your fingers in the glove.
6. Unroll the glove cuff so that it covers the stockinette sleeve cuff.

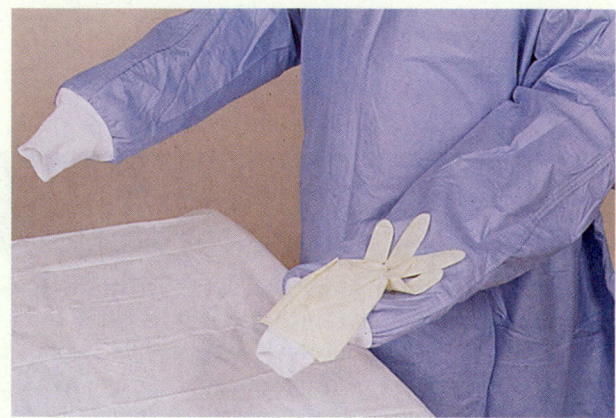

Figure 26-33 ◆ Place the glove in the palm of your nondominant hand, with glove fingers pointing to the elbows.

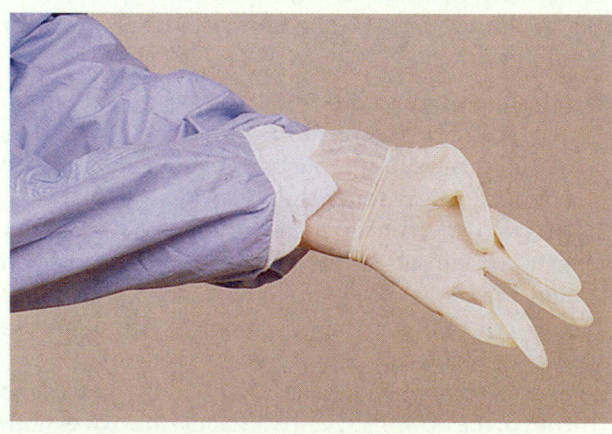

Figure 26-34 ◆ Pull the glove over your hand as you push through the gown cuff.

PROCEDURE 26-9 Demonstrate How to Glove While Wearing a Sterile Gown (continued)

7. With your nondominant hand gloved, place your fingers under the cuff of the second glove.
8. Pull the glove over your hand as you push through the gown cuff (Figure 26-35 ◆).
9. Adjust the cuffs and make sure that each gown cuff is secured and covered completely by the cuff of the glove. Last, adjust the fingers of the glove as necessary so that they fit snugly.

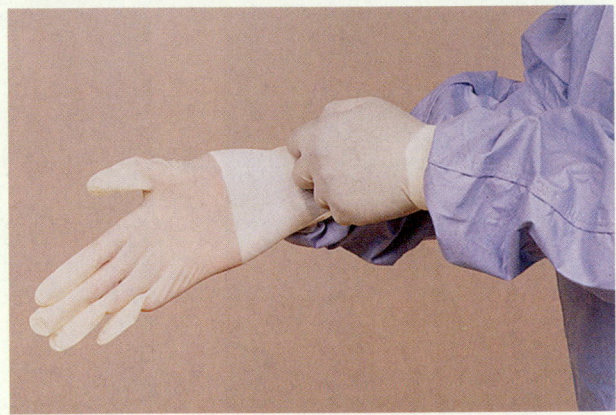

Figure 26-35 ◆ Place your fingers under the cuff of the second glove and pull the glove over your hand as you push through the gown cuff.
Source: Kozier/Fundamentals of Nursing.

PROCEDURE 26-10 Demonstrate Sterile Gloving and Removal

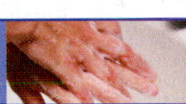

Theory and Rationale

When you first learn to don and remove sterile gloves, you are likely to make errors that result in contamination. To help reduce errors, remember this phrase: skin to skin, sterile to sterile. For example, if you have the first sterile glove halfway on your hand, use the fingers of your other hand to pinch the inside or skin-side of the glove to pull it up further. Do *not* attempt to skin-touch the sterile glove fingers for proper fit at this time. Let them dangle and proceed with using the sterile portion of the glove to help get the other sterile glove on. Once both sterile gloves are on, you can adjust the fit by using the sterile surface of one to maneuver the sterile surface of the other.

Occasionally, one sterile-gloved hand could be contaminated while the other remains sterile. It takes a great deal of concentration to remember which hand can be used in the sterile procedure, and this situation should be avoided. You will also learn which size glove to use for yourself and for the physician and how to adjust an improperly fitting sterile glove.

Place the gloves on a flat surface at waist height with the cuff end of the gloves facing toward you. Remember if a sterile glove is punctured or if you touch the outside of the glove with your hand, it is considered nonsterile. Ensure that you do not reach over the inner wrapper or touch the inside of the wrapper.

Materials

- Sterile glove pack in correct size

Competency

(**Conditions**) With the necessary supplies, (**Task**) you will be able to apply gloves using sterile technique (**Standards**) correctly within the time frame designated by your instructor.

1. Open the pack of sterile gloves, touching only the outside of the pack. Touching only the outside of the inner packet, turn the cuff end toward you.
2. Open the inner packet by pulling each edge to the side. The gloves will be lying on the sterile field created by opening the inner pack (Figure 26-36 ◆). *Do not* touch the inside of the inner pack.
3. Perform a sterile scrub (see Procedure 26-8).
4. The following directions are for a right-handed person. Perform the opposite actions if you are left-handed. With the thumb and fingers of the left hand, grasp only the folded-back cuff area (skin to skin: your skin touches what is to be the inside of the glove). While dangling the glove with the left hand, carefully slide the right hand in (Figure 26-37 ◆). *Do not* touch the outside of the glove with your ungloved hand. Keep your hands above your waist and in front of you.

continued

PROCEDURE 26-10 Demonstrate Sterile Gloving and Removal *(continued)*

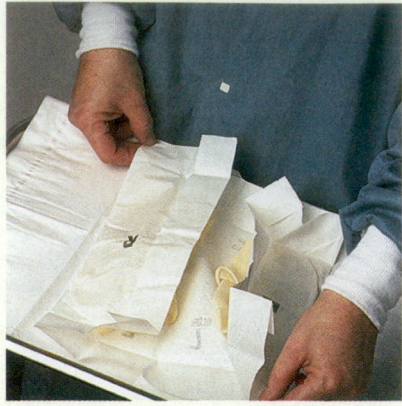

Figure 26-36 ◆ Open the inner packet.

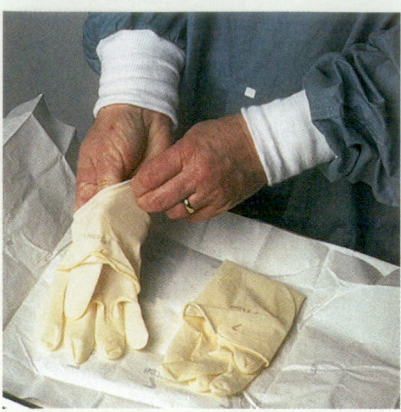

Figure 26-37 ◆ Carefully slide the right hand in.

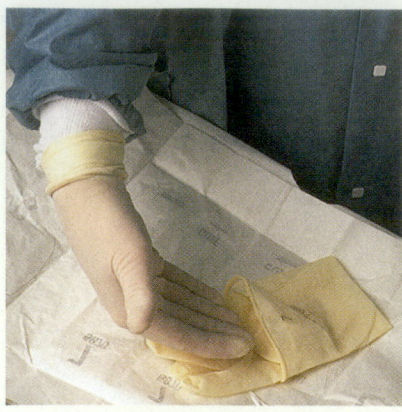

Figure 26-38 ◆ To don the second glove, slide the fingers of your gloved hand under the cuff.

5. To don the second sterile glove, slide the fingers of your gloved hand under the cuff (sterile to sterile: the outside of the gloved hand is sterile against the sterile outside of the second glove) (Figure 26-38 ◆). With the second glove "hooked" by the fingers of your gloved hand, slide your second hand into the glove (Figure 26-39 ◆). Continue to keep your hands above your waist and in front of you.
6. Adjust the finger and thumb fit of the gloves (sterile to sterile).

7. To remove the gloves, use the fingers of one gloved hand to grasp the other glove at the wrist. Pull the glove over itself and hold it in the palm of the gloved hand. Slide the fingers of the ungloved hand under the cuff of the remaining glove, grasp the inside, and pull it down over the glove and off the hand (Figures 26-40 ◆ and 26-41 ◆).
8. Discard the gloves in a biohazard waste receptacle.

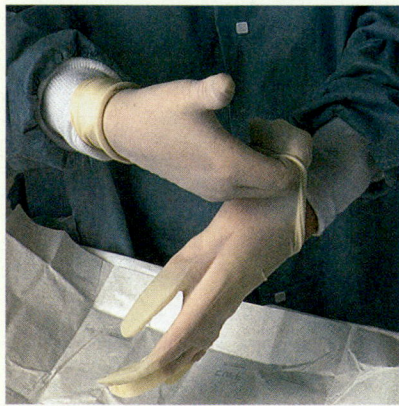

Figure 26-39 ◆ Slide your second hand into the glove.

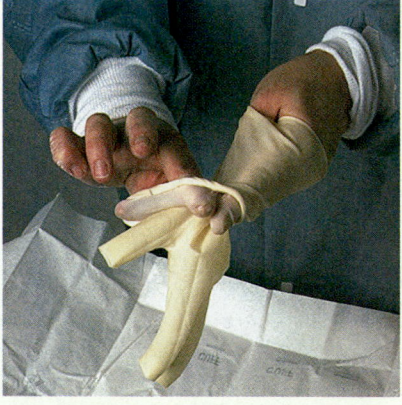

Figure 26-40 ◆ Use the fingers of one gloved hand to grasp the other glove at the wrist.

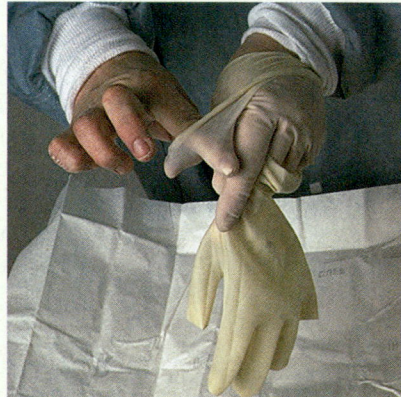

Figure 26-41 ◆ Pull the cuff of the remaining glove down over the glove and off the hand.

REVIEW

Chapter Summary

- Medical asepsis is used during clean procedures. Surgical asepsis, also known as sterile or aseptic technique, is used when assisting with minor surgery and treatment procedures. Surgical asepsis removes all microorganisms from an object or surface using sterile technique and sterile supplies. A sterile item that touches or is touched by a nonsterile or contaminated area or object is also contaminated. The medical assistant must be able to distinguish clean, sterile, and contaminated areas.

- Decontamination removes, inactivates, or destroys pathogens on a surface or object. Three methods of decontamination are sanitization, disinfection, and sterilization. Sanitization inhibits bacterial growth or inactivates pathogens. It is used to remove organic material from instruments and equipment. Disinfection destroys some microorganisms, inhibits others, but does not destroy spores and some viruses. Disinfection is used to clean surfaces and some noninvasive equipment. Sterilization is the only method that destroys all microorganisms, including spores and viruses. It is most commonly performed with the steam autoclave, although dry heat, chemical sterilization, and radiation are also used for specific materials. Individual and packaged instruments and supplies used in a sterile field must be sterilized.

- Supplies and equipment are sanitized by manual scrubbing, hot water rinsing, and air drying. Ultrasonic cleaning is another method of sanitization.

- Disinfection is accomplished by the use of germicides, steam, or boiling water. There are three levels of disinfection: low level, intermediate level, and high level. Commonly used chemical disinfectants are 70% isopropyl alcohol, sodium hypochlorite (bleach), phenol, formaldehyde, hydrogen peroxide, and soap.

- An autoclave consists of an inner sterilizing chamber and an outer compartment. Distilled water is heated to create steam, which, under pressure, sterilizes implements and supplies. Items for sterilization may be wrapped in procedure packs. Sterilization time varies according to the materials being processed and the size of the pack. It begins when a temperature of 250 degrees F (121 degrees C) inside the autoclave has been reached.

- Other methods of sterilization include the dry heat oven, cold sterilization, radiation, and ethylene oxide gas.

- Instruments are sanitized and sometimes disinfected before sterilization to remove all debris. They are wrapped individually and in procedure packs, with sterilization indicators inside each pack and dated autoclave tape on the outside. Each autoclave load must be correctly positioned. Some packs should be vertically placed, open containers should be placed on their sides, and packs should be 1 to 4 inches apart. Hinges of instruments are left open and dressings are layered to allow for more thorough steam penetration. At the end of the recommended sterilization time, any package whose indicators and tape have not changed color should not be used, because the sterility of the instruments and supplies cannot be guaranteed.

- The CDC requires that autoclave results be recorded. Culture samples may be sent to an outside agency to monitor quality control.

- To create a sterile field, follow sterile procedure to open sterile surgical packs, gloves, or individual dressings or instruments. The outer 1 inch of a sterile field is considered contaminated, so all instruments must be kept toward the center and within the sterile area. Open the surgical pack by pulling the first flap away from you, then opening the side flaps, then pulling the last flap toward you. This practice avoids crossing over the newly created sterile field and should be followed throughout the procedure to prevent contamination. The sterile glove package is opened by touching only the inner and outer wraps. It helps to remember "skin to skin" and "sterile to sterile" as you put on the gloves. Move items on the sterile field wearing sterile gloves or using transfer forceps. Single items may be added by spreading packages open and carefully dropping the items onto the sterile field.

- The manufacturer's directions must be followed when using chemical solutions or equipment for sanitization, disinfection, or sterilization. Diluting chemicals decreases their effectiveness and creates infection control hazards.

Chapter Review

Multiple Choice

1. During ambulatory surgery and invasive treatments, part of the medical assistant's responsibility is to
   a. remember which areas are porous.
   b. remember which areas are safe for chlorine disinfectant.
   c. remember which are required to be sterile.
   d. remember which areas are nonporous.

2. The area that is considered contaminated on a sterile field is
   a. There is no contaminated area on a sterile field.
   b. 1/2 inch around the outer edge.
   c. only the outer edge not covered by the sterile drape.
   d. 1 inch around the outer edge.

Chapter Review (continued)

3. The CDC requires that autoclave results be
   a. recorded.
   b. faxed in daily.
   c. mailed in monthly.
   d. none of the above.

4. To open a sterile packet you should
   a. don latex gloves, then open the package.
   b. don sterile gloves, then open the package.
   c. open the flaps away from your body and let them drop to the table.
   d. open the package with flaps toward you so you are less likely to drop the item.

5. Once you have donned a sterile gown and gloves, you should keep your hands
   a. above the height of the surgical table.
   b. above your waistline.
   c. at shoulder level.
   d. at your sides, provided you do not touch anything.

6. If you must reach across a sterile field, you should
   a. never reach across for any reason.
   b. make certain your sterile gown does not touch the table.
   c. make certain you only reach across with sterile gloves on.
   d. not worry about it if you are already sterile.

7. When performing a surgical hand scrub, you should
   a. turn off the water using a disposable paper towel before you have dried your hands with a sterile towel.
   b. turn off the water before you have dried your hands with the sterile towel.
   c. turn off the water using a disposable paper towel after you have dried your hands with a sterile towel.
   d. turn off the water only after you have dried your hands with the sterile towel.

8. In ultrasonic cleaning, sound waves are used to
   a. loosen contaminants after the articles are rinsed.
   b. loosen contaminants before the articles are rinsed.
   c. disinfect the instruments.
   d. sanitize the instruments.

9. If a solution is to be added to the sterile field, the physician holds the sterile container
   a. over a biohazard container.
   b. over the sink.
   c. just beyond the sterile field.
   d. over the transfer container.

10. For the pouring procedure on a sterile field, the MA palms the label of the solution then
    a. pours some solution into a trash receptacle or sink, then pours the rest into the sterile container.
    b. pours the solution directly into the sterile container, holding it beyond the sterile field.
    c. pours the solution directly into a sterile transfer container, holding it over a sink, then transfers it to the sterile field.
    d. pours the solution into a sterile specimen cup to be placed on the sterile field.

True/False

T F 1. To place sterile contents correctly onto a sterile field, you must drop them or use sterile transfer forceps.

T F 2. To perform a sterile pour, you should place the rim of the solution bottle on the container the solution is being transferred to in order to prevent droplets from splashing onto the sterile field.

T F 3. Surgical asepsis is used at all times during invasive procedures and when skin integrity is or will be broken.

T F 4. Pasteurization, a heat process for killing bacteria in milk, is named for Joseph Lister, who discovered that many diseases are caused by bacteria.

T F 5. Louis Pasteur, an English surgeon, discovered that carbolic acid killed germs.

Short Answer

1. What two procedures must be performed on all instruments before they are sterilized?

2. In what type of procedure are sound waves used to loosen contaminants?

3. What are the two types of alcohol used in the medical office, and what are they used to clean?

4. What is cold sterilization?

5. What are sterilization indicators?

6. What is the second step of the sterilization procedure?

7. How does disinfection differ from sterilization?

8. Name three ways disinfection can be accomplished.

9. Why should you never reach, lean, or pass over a sterile field?

10. What instrument should you use to move items onto or within a sterile field?

Research

1. In your local area, do the clinics use autoclaves or do they send items out for sterilization?

2. How many hospitals in your community use gas sterilization for beds, wheelchairs, and other large equipment?

Externship Application Experience

You are assisting the clinical medical assistant in unloading the autoclave. She accidentally drops a sterile packet on the floor. She picks it up and puts it in the storage cabinet. What do you do?

Resource Guide

American Hospital Association
One North Franklin
Chicago, IL 60606
312-422-300
www.aha.org

Association of Surgical Technologists
7108-C South Alton Way, Suite 100
Englewood, CO 80112
1-800-637-7433
www.ast.org

Liaison Council on Certification for the Surgical Technologist
7790 East Arapahoe Road, Suite 240
Englewood, CO 80012-1274
(303) 694-9264
(800) 707-0057
www.lcc-st.org

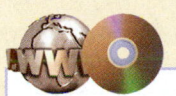

Med**Media**

http://www.MyMAKit.com

More on this chapter, including interactive resources, can be found on the Student CD-ROM accompanying this textbook and on http://www.MyMAKit.com.

CHAPTER 27

Pharmacology and Medication Administration

Case Study

Heidi has been a CMA for Dr. Wittig, a GI specialist, for six months. A patient, Claire, calls to say that she is now seven months pregnant and suffering from horrible heartburn. This is not a new medical condition for Claire. Heidi reads in her chart that Claire has suffered heartburn for several years and takes 150 mg of Zantac twice a day. Claire states that she has been taking her Zantac regularly and would like to know if she can increase the dose because the pregnancy is causing more heartburn. Heidi notes that Claire missed her regular six-month follow-up appointment with Dr. Wittig. In fact, she has not been seen in the office for ten months now but has been continuing to get medication refills.

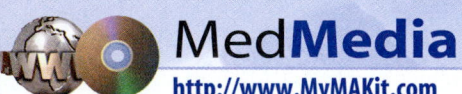

MedMedia

http://www.MyMAKit.com

Additional interactive resources and activities for this chapter can be found on http://www.MyMAKit.com. For videos, tips, audio glossary, legal and ethical scenarios, job scenarios, quizzes, games, and virtual tours related to the content of this chapter, please access the accompanying CD-ROM in this book.

Audio Glossary
Legal and Ethical Scenario: *Pharmacology and the Administration of Medications*
On the Job Scenario: *Pharmacology and the Administration of Medications*
Videos: *Pharmacology, Injections; Syringe Prep*
A & P Quizzes: *The Skeletal System; The Muscular System; Body Structure and Function*
Multiple Choice Quiz
Games: Crossword, Strikeout, and Spelling Bee
3D Virtual Tour: Muscular System: Hand and Forearm, Hip and Thigh
Drag and Drop: Muscular System: Muscles of the Posterior; Muscles of the Anterior; Interior Muscle Structure
Tips
HIPAA Quiz

Objectives

After completing this chapter, you should be able to:

- Define and spell the key terminology in this chapter.
- Discuss the medical assistant's role in administering and dispensing drugs.
- Explain the basic actions of drugs in the body.
- Differentiate the various types of effects of drugs in the body.
- List the basic functions of drugs.
- Explain the differences between prescription and over-the-counter drugs.
- List and describe the three names every drug is assigned.
- List the main drug reference resources.
- Describe the various drug classifications and give examples of each.
- Explain the legal guidelines for prescribing and administering controlled substances.
- Explain how drugs are measured and conversions are calculated.
- Explain how drug dosages are calculated.
- List safety guidelines that must be followed when drugs are administered.
- Describe the parts of a prescription.
- Explain how and why prescription pads should be safeguarded.
- Identify and describe the forms and routes of drug administration.
- Discuss the parenteral administration of medications.
- Discuss intravenous therapy.

MEDICAL ASSISTING STANDARDS

CAAHEP ENTRY-LEVEL STANDARDS	ABHES ENTRY-LEVEL COMPETENCIES
■ Perform within scope of practice (psychomotor)	■ Project a positive attitude.
■ Apply ethical behaviors, including honesty/integrity in performance of medical assisting practice (affective)	■ Maintain confidentiality at all times.
■ Explore issue of confidentiality as it applies to the medical assistant (cognitive)	■ Be a "team player."
■ Respond to issues of confidentiality (psychomotor)	■ Be cognizant of ethical boundaries.
■ Apply local, state and federal health care legislation and regulation appropriate to the medical assisting practice setting (psychomotor)	■ Exhibit initiative.
■ Recognize the importance of local, state and federal legislation and regulations in the practice setting (affective)	■ Adapt to change.
■ Document accurately in the patient record (psychomotor)	■ Evidence a responsible attitude.
■ Demonstrate knowledge of basic math (cognitive)	■ Be courteous and diplomatic.
■ Prepare proper dosages of medication for administration (psychomotor)	■ Conduct work within scope of education, training, and ability.
■ Verify ordered doses/dosages prior to administration (affective)	■ Practice Standard Precautions.
■ Apply mathematical computations to solve equations (cognitive)	■ Use quality control.
■ Identify measurement systems (cognitive)	■ Dispose of biohazardous materials.
■ Define basic units of measurement in metric, apothecary and household systems (cognitive)	■ Prepare and administer oral and parenteral medications as directed by the physician.
■ Select proper sites for administering parenteral medication (psychomotor)	■ Maintain medication and immunization records.
■ Convert among measurement systems (cognitive)	
■ Practice standard precautions (psychomotor)	
■ Select appropriate PPE for potentially infectious situations (psychomotor)	
■ Administer oral medications (psychomotor)	
■ Administer parenteral medications (psychomotor)	
■ Identify both abbreviations and symbols used in calculating medication dosages (cognitive)	
■ Identify the classifications of medications including desired effects, side effects and adverse reactions (cognitive)	
■ Apply critical thinking skills in performing patient assessment and care (affective)	

Key Terminology

chemical name—official pharmaceutical name for a drug based on its chemical composition

contraindication—reason or condition for which a drug should not be administered, e.g., pregnancy

controlled substance—drugs that have a potential for being addictive or abused

drug—any substance capable of producing a change in function when administered to a living organism; commonly, a term for a substance used to treat or prevent disease; in the medical office, synonymous with the term *medication*

generic (nonproprietary) name—pharmaceutical name for a medication, often a shortened chemical name; used by all manufacturers that produce the medication; never capitalized

over-the-counter (OTC) medications—nonprescription medications that can be purchased anywhere without a physician's prescription; examples include antacids, cold remedies, and aspirin

pharmacology—the study of drugs and their effects on the human body

side effect—effect other than the therapeutic effect

therapeutic effect—the desired or intended effect

toxic effect—potential harmful or life-threatening effect

trade (brand, proprietary) name—name registered by a manufacturer for use only by that manufacturer; has a registered trademark symbol; first letter is always capitalized

Abbreviations

CSA—Federal Controlled Substances Act

DEA—Drug Enforcement Administration

OTC—over-the-counter

PDR—Physician's Desk Reference

USP-NF—U.S. Pharmacopeia and National Formulary

MEDICAL ASSISTING STANDARDS (CONTINUED)

CAAHEP ENTRY-LEVEL STANDARDS	ABHES ENTRY-LEVEL COMPETENCIES
■ Describe the relationship between anatomy and physiology of all body systems and medications used for treatment in each (cognitive) ■ Discuss all levels of governmental legislation and regulations as they apply to medical assisting practices, including FDA and DEA regulations (cognitive)	

 COMPETENCY SKILLS PERFORMANCE

1. Demonstrate safety measures to prepare, administer, and document medication.
2. Demonstrate the preparation of a prescription for the physician's signature.
3. Demonstrate withdrawing medication from an ampule.
4. Demonstrate withdrawing medication from a vial.
5. Demonstrate the reconstitution of a powdered drug for injection administration.
6. Demonstrate the administration of medication during infusion therapy.
7. Demonstrate the preparation and administration of oral medication.
8. Demonstrate the administration of a subcutaneous injection.
9. Demonstrate the administration of an intramuscular injection to adults and children.
10. Demonstrate the administration of a Z-track injection.

Introduction

Pharmacology is the study of **drugs** and their effects on the human body. It is a complex area of study that incorporates the chemical structure of a drug, its chemical action within the body, the desired or intended effects of treatment, and potential undesirable effects. Drug forms and methods of administration are part of pharmacology. Medical professionals who dispense and administer medications must have an understanding of pharmacological basics. They must also take into account the present functioning state of the healthy or diseased body and such factors as the individual's absorption, distribution, metabolism, and excretion capabilities.

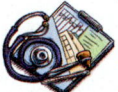 The Medical Assistant's Role in Administering and Dispensing Drugs

Drug therapy is a major part of medical care today, and medical assistants must be familiar with medications administered in or prescribed by the medical office. The MA must be familiar with the legal guidelines set by the Drug Enforcement Agency (**DEA**), a branch of the Department of Justice. Responsibilities of the MA will include reading medication orders or prescriptions, administering medications, being aware of possible side effects, recognizing side effects, instructing patients, and consulting reference resources for additional information.

Upon the physician's order and following state law and office protocol, the MA may give the patient a supply of drugs for self-administration. The medical assistant must obtain verification from another clinical staff person that the correct drug is being dispensed in the correct amount. All drugs must be clearly and completely labeled prior to dispensing. The MA will need to document the dispensing of any medication, including samples from pharmaceutical companies.

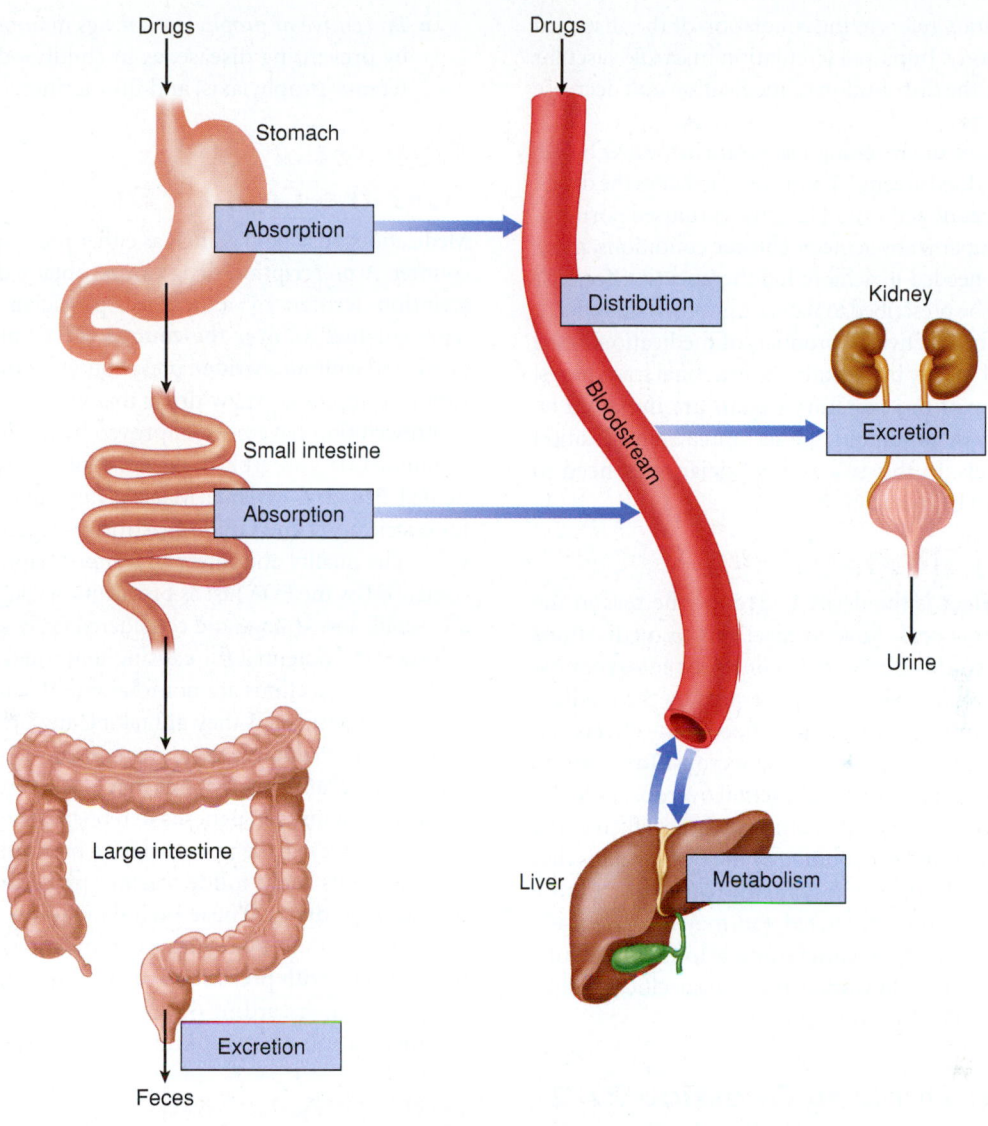

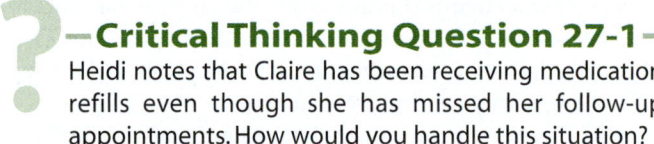

Figure 27-1 ◆ The four processes of drug movement.

?—**Critical Thinking Question 27-1**—
Heidi notes that Claire has been receiving medication refills even though she has missed her follow-up appointments. How would you handle this situation?

Basic Pharmacology

Pharmacology studies the biological and chemical interactions between drugs and bodily organs and processes. The basic actions of drugs in the body are absorption, distribution, metabolism, and excretion (Figure 27-1 ◆).

Absorption refers to the time and process whereby a drug reaches the cells and produces the desired action. For example, oral tablets are absorbed slowly because digestion must take place before the medication can be absorbed into the bloodstream. Oral liquid medication passes through the digestive system more quickly, while intravenous medication is absorbed immediately into the bloodstream. The absorption time of medications absorbed through the mucous membranes (sublingual or buccal

tablets, vaginal or rectal suppositories) is between that of oral and intravenous medications because these medications do not undergo digestion but pass easily through the membranes and directly into the circulatory system. Table 27-1 lists and compares the factors that affect absorption.

TABLE 27-1 FACTORS THAT AFFECT ABSORPTION

Concentration (dose) of administered drug	Genetics
Frequency of drug dosing	Excretion rate (rate of elimination)
Food-drug interactions	Half-life ($t_{1/2}$) of administered drug
Drug-drug interactions	
Absorption rate	Changing medical condition (liver or kidney disease)
Metabolic rate (lower in children and elderly patients)	

Source: Holland, Norman; Adams, Michael Patrick, Core Concepts in Pharmacology, *2nd ed. © 2007. Reprinted by permission of Pearson Education, Inc. Upper Saddle River, NJ.*

Drug *distribution* refers to the circulation of the absorbed drug through the body. Impaired circulation in cardiovascular disease may impede the distribution of medication and decrease its therapeutic effects.

Drug *metabolism,* or processing, takes place in the liver before or after entering the bloodstream. This process facilitates the drugs' chemical and therapeutic action and inactivates unused portions. If liver function is impaired by acute or chronic conditions, more medication may be needed to achieve full therapeutic effects, or less medication may be prescribed to reduce unwanted side effects.

Excretion of the inactivated products of medication in the system is performed mostly by the kidneys, intestinal tract, lungs, and skin. When any of the excretory organs are impaired by acute or chronic disease conditions, the accumulated medication can reach toxic levels. In this case the physician may need to decrease the amount of medication.

The General Effects of Drugs

The **therapeutic effect** is the desired effect or the reason the drug is being administered. Adverse reactions to medications may be classified as side effects, toxic effects, or idiosyncratic reactions. **Side effects** are the effects generated by the medication other than the intended or desired effects. Side effects can be therapeutic, nontherapeutic, or even dangerous. **Toxic effects** result from prescription overdose, accidental overdose, allergic reactions, interactions between two or more drugs taken at the same time, or the impaired functioning of the body organs that metabolize or excrete the drug. Idiosyncratic reactions are those that cannot be explained or predicted and may be genetically determined. Most drugs have **contraindications,** or reasons against prescribing and administering them to specific patients. A common contraindication is pregnancy.

? — Critical Thinking Question 27-2 —

Claire has not been seen in Dr. Wittig's office for the past ten months and is now seven months pregnant. Dr. Wittig may not be aware that Claire is pregnant and has continued taking Zantac, which may be contraindicated during pregnancy. Now that Heidi is aware of this situation, how should she proceed?

The Basic Functions of Drugs

Treatment with drugs serves five basic functions.

- *Therapeutic drugs* treat and relieve symptoms in a disease process, as in pain relief, anesthesia, improved GI function, and stimulation of the pancreas to secrete insulin.
- *Diagnostic drugs* assist in the diagnosis of disease, as in the use of contrast materials in imaging studies and the assessment of endocrine hormones.
- *Curative drugs* intervene in the disease process and improve the patient's quality of life, as in the treatment of infections with antibiotic and antimicrobial agents.
- *Replacement drugs* restore a normal body substance, element, or chemical that is deficient in the body, as in insulin replacement and thyroid hormone replacement in hypothyroidism.

- *Preventive or prophylactic drugs* maintain a healthy state by preventing disease, as in childhood immunizations, tetanus prophylaxis, and flu vaccines.

Prescription Versus Over-the-Counter Drugs

Medications may be classified as either prescription or over-the-counter. A prescription drug can be obtained only with a prescription written by a licensed physician or a physician's representative. An **over-the-counter (OTC) medication** may be purchased without a written prescription for the self-treatment of various symptoms. Many drugs that were once obtainable only by prescription have been approved by the FDA for OTC sale. Common OTCs are aspirin, Tylenol, Motrin, Aleve, Advil, Sudafed, Actifed, Benadryl, Mylanta, Maalox, Tums, and other medications for gastric upset and GERD (gastroesophageal reflux disease).

The quality and safety of nonprescription substances are controlled by the FDA just as prescription drugs are. These drugs are usually low-dosage and considered fairly safe, although they still have the potential for causing unwanted side effects, especially when directions are not followed. It is important that the MA ask all patients if they are taking any OTC drugs, as many people do not consider them medications to be reported to the physician. Because interactions may occur between medications, the MA must instruct patients to report to the physician any use of OTCs to reduce the potential for a harmful reaction.

Patients must follow certain precautions when taking prescription drugs. These include reading and following all printed directions, following recommended dosages, not combining OTCs with prescribed medications unless approved by the physician, discarding outdated medications, and not using any medication a patient knows he or she is allergic to.

Drug Nomenclature

Drug nomenclature (the way drugs are named) comprises three general names: the *chemical name, generic name,* and *brand name.*

- A drug's **chemical name** is its official pharmaceutical name and is based on its chemical composition. The chemical name identifies the exact chemicals in the drug along with its molecular structure.
- The **generic or nonproprietary name,** also called the common name, is assigned to the drug by the manufacturer who first seeks approval of the drug by the FDA (Food and Drug Administration). The generic name is a pharmaceutical name, often a shortened chemical name, used by all manufacturers that produce the medication. It is never capitalized.
- The **trade, brand,** or **proprietary name** is registered by a manufacturer for use only by that manufacturer. It is used with a registered trademark symbol, and the first letter is always capitalized. The chemical and generic names of the drug are listed in the *Pharmacopoeia/National Formulary* (USP/NF) as the official name of the drug.

The manufacturer who originally proposes the drug to the FDA for approval and clinical trial owns exclusive rights to produce the drug for twenty years after the initial proposal.

After that time, other manufacturers may produce the drug under other brand names, but it must have the same generic name and chemical structure. Generic forms of the drug are usually less costly than the brand-name or proprietary drug.

Drug Reference Sources

The MA assisting the physican to fill out prescriptions, calling in prescriptions, and administering medications in the medical office should know how to use drug reference books and materials.

The *U.S. Pharmacopeia and National Formulary* (**USP-NF**) and the *Physician's Desk Reference* (**PDR**) are two standard drug reference books. As the recognized official source of drug standards, the USP-NF lists and describes all accepted therapeutic drugs and their chemical formulas. The PDR, published annually, contains information about approximately 2,500 drugs. It is one of the most widely used medical references and is available in most healthcare settings. Categories of information include classification, generic names, recommended uses, and listings by manufacturer's name or trade name. Color photos assist in the identification of many drugs. A PDR supplement listing OTC medications is published every year.

Other sources of drug information are the package inserts that accompany medications and the computer-generated printouts dispensed by the pharmacy with every prescription.

Drug Classifications

Drugs are classified according to function and the area of the body they affect. Some drugs affect specific organs or tissues, while others have a more general effect.

Many drug formulas are based on the functions of the autonomic nervous system (ANS). Understanding the normal functions of the sympathetic and parasympathetic divisions of the autonomic nervous system is essential to understanding the drugs that mimic these functions. Drugs that mimic the sympathetic nervous system are known as sympathomimetic.

The nervous system is divided into two general anatomical areas or systems, the central nervous system and the peripheral nervous system. (The nervous system is more fully discussed in ∞ Chapter 46.) The central nervous system comprises the brain and spinal cord. The peripheral nervous system is composed of all nervous system structures outside the brain and spinal cord and includes twelve pairs of cranial nerves, thirty-one pairs of spinal nerves, peripheral smaller branching nerves, and the autonomic nervous system (Figure 27-2 ◆).

The brain is composed of different areas that exert control over conscious and unconscious actions of the body. The cerebrum or forebrain is responsible for cognitive functions,

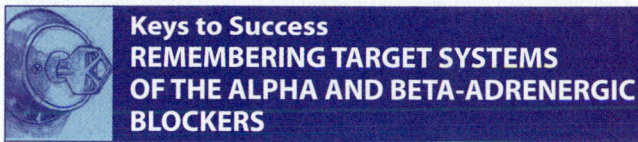

Keys to Success
REMEMBERING TARGET SYSTEMS OF THE ALPHA AND BETA-ADRENERGIC BLOCKERS

An easy way to remember target systems of the alpha and beta-adrenergic blockers is to think of it in this way. *Alpha* blockers exert activity on the *arteries*, *beta₁* blockers on the heart (the body has only *one* heart), and *beta₂* blockers on the lungs (the body has *two* lungs).

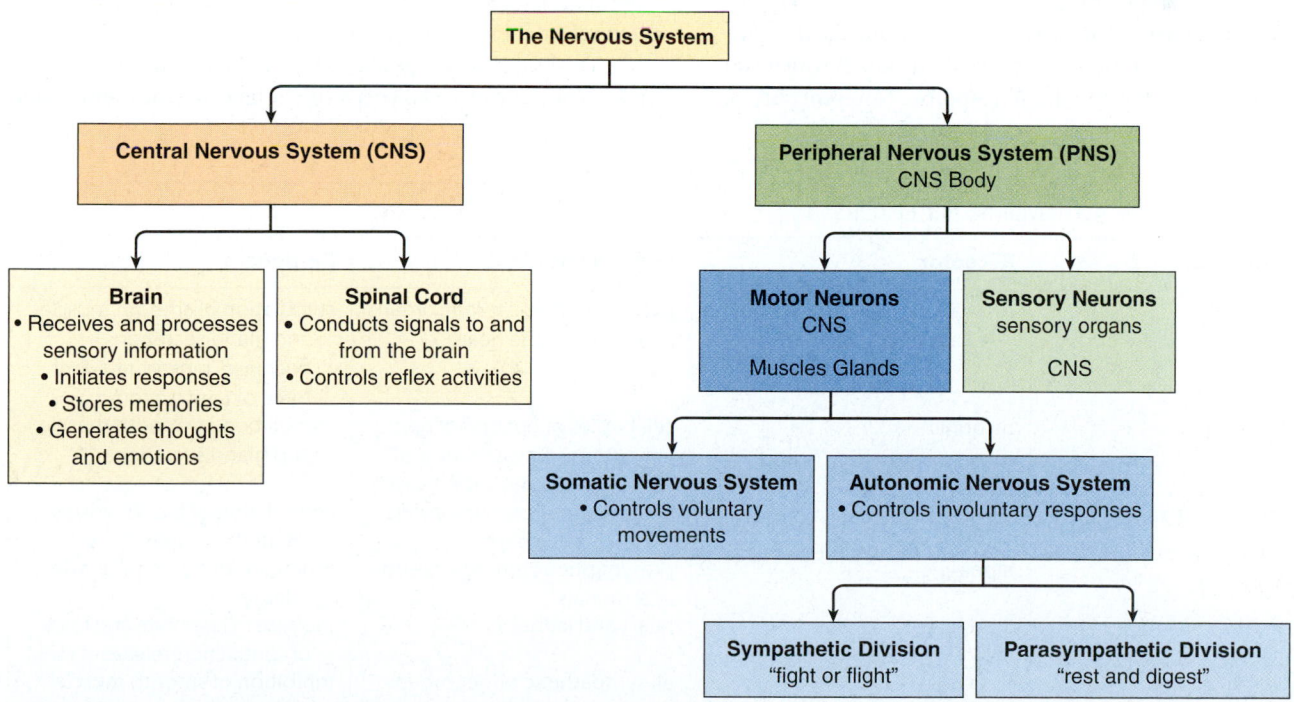

Figure 27-2 ◆ Functional divisions of the nervous system.

Source: Holland, Norma; Adams, Michael Patrick, Core Concepts in Pharmacology, 2nd ed. © 2007. Reprinted with permission of Pearson Education, Inc. Upper Saddle River, NJ.

TABLE 27-2 AUTONOMIC NERVOUS SYSTEM REACTIONS

Body System or Organ	Adrenergic Agonists, Sympathomimetics	Cholinergic Agonists, Parasympathomimetics
Vessels	Constrict	Dilate
Heart	Speeds up rate and increases contractility	Slows down rate and decreases contractility
Respiratory	Constricts bronchioles	Dilates bronchioles
GI tract	Slows peristalsis	Increases peristalsis
Urinary tract	Relaxes the bladder, contracts the sphincter	Contracts the bladder, relaxes the sphincter
Eyes	Dilates pupils (mydriasis)	Constricts pupils (myosis)

including thinking, reasoning, hearing, talking, seeing, and motor activities. The cerebellum is concerned primarily with balance, coordination, and equilibrium. The midbrain acts as a relay station as well as an area where the cerebrospinal fluid is managed. The brain is connected to the spinal cord through the medulla oblongata and the pons. The spinal cord and peripheral nerves transport impulses to and from the brain for interpretation and response.

The autonomic system is made up of two divisions, the sympathetic and parasympathetic nervous systems. The sympathetic nervous system initiates the body's response to threat or danger. This is often referred to as the "fight-or-flight" response. Because the body cannot survive in the emergency state of response for extended periods of time, the parasympathetic nervous system applies the "brakes" to bring body functioning back to normal. The sympathetic nervous system's response is termed *cholinergic*, and that of the parasympathetic nervous system is *anticholinergic* (Table 27-2).

The neurotransmitters responsible for activities in the ANS are epinephrine, norepinephrine, and acetylcholine. Epinephrine and norepinephrine, adrenergic agonists, stimulate the sympathetic system in the event of a perceived threat to the organism and cause the typical fight-or-flight response. Norepinephrine,

of the sympathetic nervous system, can be further divided into alpha and beta receptors. Acetylcholine is the main parasympathetic or cholinergic neurotransmitter that acts as a "housekeeping" agent to restore body systems to normal function. Sympathetic and parasympathetic agonists mimic the actions of the two systems, adrenergic and cholinergic, respectively. The sympathetic nervous system response can be inhibited by adrenergic blockers (alpha and beta-blockers) and the parasympathetic system can be inhibited by cholinergic blockers, or anticholinergics (alpha and beta-blockers) (Table 27-3).

Central nervous system drugs generally affect the whole system, although some target only one area. CNS drugs may help to reduce pain (analgesics), eliminate pain during surgical procedures (anesthetics), reduce elevated body temperature (antipyretic agents), prevent or stop seizures (anticonvulsants, antiepileptics), sedate or induce sleep (hypnotics/sedatives), reduce anxiety (antianxiety agents), help to relieve symptoms of Alzheimer disease, treat symptoms of depression (antidepressants), and treat psychotic disorders (antipsychotic drugs). Antianxiety, antipsychotic, and antidepressant medications are often referred to as psychotropic agents.

Analgesics are drugs that help to reduce pain without altering level of consciousness. They work by blocking the transmission

TABLE 27-3 TYPES OF AUTONOMIC RECEPTORS

Neurotransmitter	Receptor	Primary Locations	Responses
Acetylcholine (cholinergic)	muscarinic	parasympathetic target: organs other than the heart	stimulation of smooth muscle and gland secretions decrease in heart rate and force of contraction
	nicotinic	cell bodies of postganglionic neurons (sympathetic and parasympathetic pathways)	stimulation of smooth muscle and gland secretions
Norepinephrine (adrenergic)	alpha$_1$	all sympathetic target organs except the heart	constriction of blood vessels, dilation of pupils
	alpha$_2$	presynaptic adrenergic neuron terminals	inhibition of norepinephrine release
	beta$_1$	heart and kidneys	increase in heart rate and force of contraction; release of renin
	beta$_2$	all sympathetic target organs except the heart	inhibition of smooth muscle

Source: Holland, Norman and Adams, Michael Patrick, Core Concepts in Pharmacology, *2nd Edition © 2007. Reprinted with permission of Pearson Education, Inc. Upper Saddle River, NJ.*

of pain impulses to the brain or blocking the interpretation of pain impulses by the brain. Some analgesic drugs also have an antipyretic effect. Analgesics are normally classified as narcotic or non-narcotic. Narcotic analgesics are either derivatives of opium or synthetic opioids.

Anesthetic medications are available in two forms, general and local. General anesthetics achieve total loss of sensation in the body by inducing loss of consciousness. Local anesthetics provide a temporary loss of sensation from specific areas of the body. Anesthetics are used during surgical procedures to remove the sensation of pain and allow the procedure to progress in a therapeutic and humane manner.

Anti-inflammatory drugs may be corticosteroids or NSAIDs (non-steroidal anti-inflammatory drugs). Corticosteroids are prescribed when the inflammatory process is severe and immediate reversal of the condition is indicated. These drugs often have serious side effects and are avoided whenever possible. NSAIDs help to relieve common inflammation, including arthritis and other chronic inflammatory conditions. Frequent blood studies are indicated to check for liver and kidney injury.

Cardiovascular drugs are used to treat conditions of the heart and blood vessels. (The cardiovascular system is discussed in ∞ Chapter 35.) This family of drugs includes cardiac glycosides, antiarrhythmic agents, anticoagulants, platelet inhibitors, hemostatic agents/coagulants, thrombolytic agents, vasoconstrictors, vasodilators, and antihypertensive drugs. Cardiac glycosides are used in the treatment of congestive heart failure to slow and strengthen the heartbeat. Antiarrhythmic drugs help to restore the heart rhythm to normal. Anticoagulants and platelet inhibitors are used in the treatment of clot formations or any condition in which clot formation is likely. The function of hemostatic drugs is to treat uncontrolled bleeding and hemorrhage. Thrombolytics, often referred to as "clot busters," dissolve existing clots and restore blood flow. Vasoconstrictors are administered to treat shock by constricting blood vessels and maintaining a viable blood pressure. Vasodilators have the opposite effect—they dilate the vessels—and are used to treat arterial spasms, angina (chest pain), and certain vascular disorders. The antihypertensive group of drugs is used in the treatment of hypertension, or high blood pressure. Drugs used to treat hyperlipidemia or to lower cholesterol and triglyceride levels are often also classified as cardiovascular drugs.

Drugs that affect the gastrointestinal (GI) system can be classified according to the part of the system they target: the esophagus, the stomach, the small intestine, or the large intestine. Other GI drugs may be classified according to their specific action, such as laxatives, anti-flatulence drugs, or proton-pump inhibitors.

Antiinfective agents are used to treat infections caused by bacteria, viruses, parasites, fungi, or protozoa. A culture and sensitivity test is often performed to determine the optimum drug for the particular infective microorganism.

Respiratory system drugs include antihistamines, antitussives, bronchodilators, decongestants, and expectorants. Antihistamines help to relieve nasal congestion. Antitussive medications, both narcotic and non-narcotic, help to relieve coughing. Bronchodilators are used in the treatment of asthma and other obstructive airway conditions. Decongestants help to relieve congestion in the upper respiratory region and are helpful in treating the common cold, sinusitis, and rhinitis. Expectorants help to liquefy respiratory mucous membrane secretions and promote the expectoration of mucus.

Medications prescribed for common disorders of the endocrine system include drugs used to treat diabetes mellitus and thyroid disorders. Drug therapy prescribed for the reproductive system, whose functions are related to those of the endocrine system, has its own categories. Contraceptive drugs, hormone replacement drugs, and erectile dysfunction agents are the drugs most frequently prescribed for reproductive conditions. Contraceptives are available in oral, intradermal, and injectable form. Hormone therapy is often prescribed for women who have experienced natural or early surgical menopause.

Urinary system drugs include diuretics, which increase urine production and excretion; antibiotics and antiseptics to treat UTIs; analgesics; and drugs that relax bladder muscles. Conditions affecting the prostate gland in men, including urinary retention, frequency, and urgency, may be successfully treated with drug therapy.

Miscellaneous drugs include neoplastic agents, used to treat cancers and neoplastic disease; antihistamines, used to treat allergic reactions; and antiallergic drugs, used as a prophylactic measure to prevent allergic attacks.

Table 27-4 lists and briefly describes the various drug classifications.

Controlled Substances

Drugs with a potential for abuse have been identified in the Federal Controlled Substances Act (**CSA**), which is enforced by the DEA (Table 27-5). The CSA sets guidelines for the storage, record keeping, and safekeeping of these **controlled substances,** also called *schedule drugs.* Drugs with the potential for abuse include narcotics; drugs that are potentially addictive or habit-forming, such as depressants and stimulants; and drugs with hallucinogenic properties. The potential for abuse must be established before a drug is placed on the list.

All drugs must be accounted for at all times. Records concerning the purchase and management of controlled substances must be maintained for two years, kept in an area separate from the patient chart, and available for inspection by DEA personnel at any time. Any controlled substance administered to a patient must be recorded in a log with the date, time, patient name, dosage, and amount discarded, if appropriate. The controlled substance log is required in addition to documentation in the patient chart.

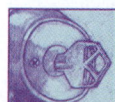

Keys to Success
THE TOP 50

An excellent way to stay current in pharmacology is to find out which drugs are most commonly prescribed. *Pharmacy Times* publishes a list of the fifty most frequently prescribed drugs in its April issue each year. Peruse the list, check previous years' lists, and see if you can spot any trends. This will give you a snapshot of where drug therapy has been and where it is now.

TABLE 27-4 DRUG CLASSIFICATIONS

Classes and Examples	Main Functions
Alzheimer treatment: Cognex, Aricept	Stimulate nerve transmitters as a means of improving memory and behavior.
Analgesics, narcotic: morphine, Demerol, codeine, oxycontin, diladid, Duragesic, Darvon	Relieve severe pain, including postoperative pain, myocardial pain, pain from trauma and terminal illness.
Analgesics, non-narcotic or non-opioid: acetaminophen, aspirin, ibuprofen, naproxen	Relieve minor to moderate pain and chronic pain.
Antiallergic: cromolyn (Intal)	Used prophylactically to prevent asthma attacks and associated bronchospasms, coughing, and wheezing.
Antianxiety: Valium, Xanax, Ativan, Tranxene	Relieve anxiety, some psychosomatic disorders, muscle tension, nausea and vomiting.
Antiarrhythmic agents: atenolol (Tenormin), propanolol (Inderal), verapamil (Isoptin, Calan), Topril	Treat arrhythmias and restore normal heartbeat.
Antibiotics: penicillin (ampicillin, amoxicillin, Staphcillin, Unipen, Geocillin, Pipracil); cephalosporins (Duricef, Keflex, Cecloe, Suprax, Rocephin); aminoglycosides (Amikin, Garamycin, Nebcin); tetracyclines (Vibramycin Terramycin, Minocin); sulfonamide antimicrobials (Sulfonamide, Sulamyd, Gantanol, Gantrisin); macrolides (erythromycin, Zithromax, Biaxin, Dynabac); fluroquinolone antimicrobials (Cipro)	Treat bacterial infections.
Anticoagulants: dicumarol, warfarin sodium (Coumadin), heparin sodium	Prevent or delay blood clots from forming. Also prescribed to treat deep vein thrombosis and other thrombosis conditions.
Anticonvulsants, antiepileptics: Dilantin, Zarontin, Tegretol, phenobarbital, Valium, Depakene, Mysoline, Klonopin, Neurontin, Keppra, Zarontin, Lyrica	Prevent seizures, treat and halt seizures in progress. Barbiturates used in all forms of epilepsy; Dilantin, Keppra, Neurontin for grand mal seizures; Zarontin for petit mal seizures. Neurontin also used to treat post-herpetic neuralgia and some nerve pain.
Antidepressants, tricyclic agents: Elavil, Triavil, Trifanil, Pamelor; **SSRI,** Prozac, Paxil, Zoloft; **MAO inhibitor,** Nardil	Treat depression; often referred to as mood elevators.
Antiemetics: Phenergan, Tigan, Reglan, Compazine, Zofran	Prevent vomiting, relieve nausea.
Antifungal: fluconazole (Diflucan), Monistat 3, Mycelex vaginal tabs, Vagistat-1, griseofulvin (Grisactin), tolnaftate (Tinactin)	Treat candidiasis, coccidiodomycosis, tinea capitis, tinea pedis, and other miscellaneous fungal infections.
Antihistamines: diphenhydramine (Benadryl), chlorpheniramine (Chlor-Trimeton), clemastine (Tavist), fexofenadine (Allegra), loratadine (Claritin), cetirizine (Zyrtec). (See Histaminic II blockers)	Relieve symptoms of allergic response by blocking histamine reactions in tissue. Often used to treat runny nose and watery eyes connected with hay fever and other allergies.
Antihyperlipidemic or hypolipidemic drugs: simvastin (Zocor), pravastatin (Pravachol), atorvastatin (Lipitor), ezetimibe (Zetia)	Treat hyperlipidema by reducing blood cholesterol levels; statin drugs may reverse some plaque accumulation in blood vessels.
Antihypertensive agents: ramipril (Altace), doxazosin (Cardura), benzothiazepine (Cardizem), clonidine (Catapres), methyldopa (Aldoril)	Treat hypertension. Altace inhibits angiotension-converting enzymes; Cardura dilates vessels.
Anti-inflammatory agents: *NSAIDS:* aspirin, acetaminophen (Tylenol), ibuprofen (Motrin, Advil), naproxen (naprosyn, Aleve), nabumetone (Relafen), celecoxib (Celebrex), valdecoxib (Bextra). *Steroids:* prednisone	Treat conditions caused by inflammation of the muscles and joints.
Antineoplastic agents: fluorouracil (5-FU), cyclophosphamide (Cytoxan), methotrexate (Folex)	Chemotherapy prescribed to treat cancer and inhibit growth of neoplasms. Often used before surgery or radiation to shrink tumors or as adjunct therapy with surgery or radiation.
Antiparasitic: Vermox, Biltricide, Antiminth, Pin-Rid, Mintezol	Treat parasitic worm infections.
Anti-Parkinson's drugs: Symmetrel, Sinemet, Cogentin, Kemadrin, Artane	Treat symptoms of Parkinson's by increasing level of dopamine or dopaminergic activity. Anticholinergic drugs reduce activity of ACH. Goal is to stop or moderate tremors, muscle spasms, and muscle rigidity.
Antipruritic: diphenhydramine (Benadryl), calamine lotion, corticosteroid ointments and creams, hydroxyzine HCl (Atarax), clemastine (Tavist)	Treat itching. Some used directly on skin, others systemic.

TABLE 27-4 DRUG CLASSIFICATIONS (CONTINUED)

Classes and Examples	Main Functions
Antipsychotic drugs: Thorazine, Haldol, Eskalith, Risperdal, Mellari, Prolixin	Treat symptoms of psychosis and severe neurosis. Lithium levels must be routinely monitored. Eskalith is a lithium preparation used to treat bipolar disorders.
Antipyretic agents: acetaminophen, aspirin, ibuprofen, naproxen	Lower elevated body temperature.
Antispasmodics: atropine, belladonna, Robinul, Pro-Banthine, Bentyl, Zelmac	Treat hypermotility in GI tract.
Antitussive drugs: codeine sulfate, dextromethorphan (Romilar, Robitussin DM, Benylin, Triaminic)	Treat or suppress cough.
Antiulcer treatment: Biaxin, Amozil	Peptic ulcer treatment; eliminates *H. pylori* from stomach
Antivirals: amantadine, rimantadine, ganciclovir, ribravirin, acyclovir, famciclovir, trifluridine, valacuclovir, vidarabine; **for HIV,** didanosine, delavirdine, nelfinavir, nevirapine, zalcitabine	Treat viral infections including influenza, CMV retinitis, RSV syncytial virus infections, herpes zoster, genital herpes, herpes simplex, keratitis, HIV (drugs used to treat HIV are fairly new; success uncertain).
Asthma prophylactics: cromolyn sodium	Used before exposure to allergen to prevent allergic reaction.
Bronchodilators: Proventil, Theo-Dur	Relax smooth muscle in bronchi and slow or stop bronchial spasm.
Cardiac glycosides: digitoxin (Digitoline, Crystodigin), digoxin (Lanoxin)	Slow and strengthen the heartbeat. Used in treatment of congestive heart failure.
Cathartics and laxatives: CoLyte, mineral oil, citrate of magnesia, Dulcolax, castor oil, Surfak, Serutan	Stimulate evacuation of the bowel.
Contraceptives: Ovral, Triphasic	Prevent pregnancy.
Decongestants: Afrin, Sudafed	Used to constrict the nasal membrane to open air passageways. Constricts nasal mucosal vessels.
Diuretics: Lasix, Bumex, HydroDIURIL	Used to treat fluid retention, CHF, hypertension.
Expectorants: Robitussin, Organidin	Increases respiratory secretions, liquefies secretions for easier expectoration.
General anesthetics: thiopental Na (Pentothal), midazolam (Versed), methohexital (Brevital)	Produce loss of sensation for surgical, dental, and other procedures. General anesthesia induces loss of consciousness.
Hemostatic/coagulants: menadiol sodium (Synkavite), phytonadione (AquaMEPHYTON, vitamin K)	Increase coagulating ability of blood, treat hemorrhage and excessive or uncontrolled bleeding.
Histaminic II blockers (antagonists): Tagamet, Axid, Zantac, Pepcid	Treat peptic ulcers; also reduce gastric acid secretion by blocking histaminic II receptors.
Hormone replacement therapy: Premarin, Estrace, Provera, Prempro	Treat symptoms of menopause.
Hypoglycemic agents: Glucotrol, Glynase, Diabeta, Glucophage	Stimulate production of insulin by pancreas.
Hypnotics/sedatives: Amytal, Seconal, Noctec, Dalmane, Halcion, Ambien, Restoril, Lunesta	Promote rest and sleep.
Insulin: NPH, Humulin	Replaces insulin not produced by pancreas.
Local anesthetics: lidocaine (Xylocaine), procaine (Novocaine), bupivacaine (Marcaine)	Produce regional or local anesthesia for specific area of body.
Platelet inhibitors: aspirin, dipyridamole (Persantine), clopidogrel (Plavix)	Prevent platelet aggregation. Usually prescribed in combination with aspirin for better effect.
Proton pump inhibitors: Prilosec, Prevacid, Nexium, Aciphex	Treat peptic ulcers; reduce gastric acid secretion by blocking enzyme responsible for secreting hydrochloric acid.
Thrombolytics: alteplase (Activase), streptokinase (Streptase), tenectoplase (tissue plasminogen activator, TPA)	Dissolve blood clots, especially in MIs and CVAs.
Thyroid medications: antithyroid (Tapazole, propylthiouracil) and thyroid replacement (Synthroid)	Inhibit production of thyroid hormone when too much is produced; replacement therapy when inadequate amounts are produced.
Vasoconstrictors: norepinephrine (Levophed), epinephrine (Adrenalin)	Treat shock; primary action is constriction of vessels.
Vasodilators: nitroglycerin (Nitro-stat), isoxsuprine (Isordil), hydralazine (Apresoline), sodium nitroprusside (Nipride)	Treat angina and hypertensive crisis.

TABLE 27-5 SCHEDULE OF CONTROLLED SUBSTANCES

Schedule I Substances (C-I): Substances with no accepted medical use in the United States and high potential for abuse. Illegal to obtain or prescribe for use in the United States.
- Narcotics, including heroin
- Stimulants, including amphetamine variations and Ecstasy
- Depressants
- Hallucinogens, including LSD, mescaline, peyote
- Cannabis, including marijuana

Schedule II Substances (C-II): Substances with accepted medical use and high potential for abuse. No refills without a new physician-written prescription.
- Narcotics, including Demerol, morphine, codeine, Dilaudid, Oxycodone
- Amphetamines, including Dexadrine, Ritalin
- Cocaine
- Short-acting barbiturates, including phenobarbital, Amobarbital, Seconal

Schedule III Substances (C-III): Substances with accepted medical use and lower abuse potential than Schedule I or Schedule II controlled substances. Prescriptions may be refilled five times within six months with physician authorization.
- Combination drugs containing lower amounts of narcotics or stimulants, including Tylenol with codeine

Schedule IV Substances (C-IV): Substances with accepted medical use and less potential for abuse than Schedule III substances. May be refilled five times within six months with physician authorization.
- Antianxiety drugs including Xanax, Valium, Librium
- Sedative hypnotics including Dalmane, Restoril, Halcion, Ambien, Versed

Schedule V Substances (C-V): Substances with accepted medical use and limited abuse potential. Prescription must be authorized by physician, and patient must be 18 years old and show identification.
- Cough medicines with codeine, antidiarrheal medication such as Lomotil

Schedule drugs must be stored in a safe or in a locked box inside another locked box that is securely fastened to the wall. The drugs must be counted by two staff members whenever keys are transferred. Two staff members must document any discrepancy in the drug count. Missing drugs must be reported immediately to the DEA and the local law enforcement agency. An investigation must also be initiated per established office policy. The disposal of an unused portion of a controlled substance must be witnessed by two staff members and documented on the controlled substance inventory form. All scheduled drugs must be returned to the pharmacy to be destroyed. Schedule II drugs must be counted by a licensed pharmacist, and that number verified by the office staff prior to being destroyed.

Medication Measurement and Conversion

Different systems are used to measure drugs before they are administered. Historically, narcotics, barbiturates, aspirin, acetaminophen, atropine, and thyroid hormone replacements have been prescribed in apothecary and metric dosages. The apothecary system of weights is rarely used today. The metric system is the most widely used measurement system. Other systems are medication-specific: mEq for electrolytes (e.g., potassium), units (e.g., insulin), inches (Nitrobid paste), and drops (liquid medication administered by dropper). Percentages are used to measure the mixtures used in intravenous solutions or ointments. Household measurements (teaspoon, tablespoon, etc.) cannot be standardized and are therefore not used often. When medication dosage is ordered in teaspoons, the pharmacy includes a standardized medication cup or spoon with the teaspoon level clearly marked.

The units of apothecary measurement include the minim (or drop), grain, and dram. The grain unit is based on the weight of one grain of wheat. The metric equivalent of one grain (gr i) is 60 milligrams (60 mg). One dram (dr i) equals 4–5 milliliters (4–5 ml), or one teaspoon (1 tsp). Apothecary dosages are written with the unit first, followed by a Roman numeral—for example, gr iv, meaning 4 grains.

Medical assistants should have a basic understanding of the apothecary system, because some physicians still write orders with these abbreviations. It is also important to remember that similarities between some abbreviations may cause inaccurate dosage administration. For example, the symbol for dram is ℨ, and the symbol for ounce is ℥. A medication error occurs if a patient receives an ounce (30 ml) when a dram (4–5 ml) was ordered. Another error is mistaking gr (grain) for gm (gram).

Metric measurements consist of units of length (meter), volume (liter), and weight or mass (gram). The first step in studying the metric system is to memorize the order of the metric prefixes: kilo-, hecto-, deka-, deci-, centi-, milli-, and micro-. Then pair the numerical value with the prefix: kilo- = 1000, hecto- = 100, and so forth. Converting from one metric unit to another is a matter of moving the decimal a specific number of places in one direction or the other. For example, 1 liter becomes X milliliters by moving three decimal places to the right: 1000.0 milliliters. To convert 1 liter to X kiloliters, move the decimal three places to the left: 0.001 kiloliters. Because of the extra three digit places between milli- and micro- units, an extra three decimal places would need to be added or subtracted, depending on the direction of the conversion.

The MA uses only some of the basic metric units for conversion: kilogram, meter, liter, gram, centimeter, millimeter, milliliter, milligram, and microgram. The other units are used more commonly in scientific research.

Table 27-6 lists the most common metric and apothecary/metric equivalents. Printed conversion charts are posted in most medication preparation workstations. Be sure to double-check any conversion you have calculated against the printed chart.

Table 27-7 lists abbreviations and symbols used in medication dosing.

Dosage Calculation

Dosage calculations are based on adult dosages, pediatric dosages, or the patient's weight in pounds or kilograms.

TABLE 27-6 COMMON METRIC AND APOTHECARY/METRIC EQUIVALENTS

	Metric
Weight	1 kilogram (kg) = 2.2 pounds (lb)
	1 kilogram (kg) = 1000 grams (gm)
	1 gram (gm) = 1000 milligrams (mg)
	1 milligram (mg) = 1000 micrograms (mcg)
Length	1 inch (in) = 2.5 centimeters (cm)
Volume	1 liter (L) = 1000 milliliters (ml) or 1000 cubic centimeters (cc)*
	Apothecary/Metric
Weight	1 ounce (oz) = 30 grams (gm)
	1 gram (gm) = 15 grains (gr)
	1 grain (gr) = 60 milligrams (mg)
	1/2 grain (gr) = 30 milligrams (mg)
Volume	1 gallon (4 quarts) = 4000 milliliters (ml)
	1 quart (2 pints or 32 fluidounces) = 1000 milliliters (ml)
	1 pint (16 fluidounces) = 500 milliliters (ml)
	1 cup (8 fluidounces) = 250 milliliters (ml)
	1 fluidounce (8 fluidrams) = 30 milliliters (ml)
	1 fluidram (60 minims) = 4 milliliters (ml)
	1 milliliter (ml) = 15 minims

cc and ml are used interchangeably (e.g., 1 cc = 1 ml)

Although most drugs have standard adult dosages, other factors may need to be considered for the elderly, the extremely thin, the young, and patients with illness or disease conditions. The concentration of the drug is another factor that may enter into the calculation.

TABLE 27-7 ABBREVIATIONS AND SYMBOLS USED IN MEDICATION DOSING

Symbol/Abbreviations		Meaning
gtt	Drop	drop
℞	Min	minim
ℨ	dr	dram
flℨ	fl dr	fluid dram
℥	oz	ounce
fl℥	fl oz	fluid ounce
	gr	grain
	gr ss	1/2 grain
	gr xv	15 grains
mcg	μ	Microgram
mg		Milligram
gm		Gram

- It is important to note that some abbreviations are being phased out of medication dosing in accordance to standards set forth by the Joint Commission on the Accreditation of Healthcare Organizations.
- Medical offices often determine which symbols are allowable for use in their offices.

As an example, consider the following scenario. A patient weighs 110 pounds. The medication dosage to be given is 4 mg/kg. The medication comes in a vial of 200 mg/ml.

1. Convert pounds to kilograms if necessary. To convert pounds to kilograms, *divide* the patient's weight by 2.2. To convert kilograms to pounds, *multiply* the patient's weight by 2.2. When converting pounds to kilograms, you should always end with a smaller number. When converting kilograms to pounds, your final answer should always be larger than your starting number. To convert 110 pounds to kilograms: 110/2.2 = 50 kilograms. To convert 50 kilograms to pounds: 50 × 2.2 = 110 pounds.
2. Calculate the medication for the kg weight of the patient. The dosage to be given is 4 mg/kg.

$$\frac{X \text{ mg}}{50 \text{ kg}} = \frac{4 \text{ mg}}{1 \text{ kg}}$$

Cross-multiply and divide as above to find the unknown.

$$200 \text{ mg/kg} = X \text{ mg/kg}$$
$$200 \text{ mg} = X \text{ mg}$$
$$200 = X$$

The answer is 200 mg.

3. Calculate the amount of tablets or solution to be given to the patient.

$$\frac{100 \text{ mg}}{1 \text{ ml}} = \frac{200 \text{ mg}}{X \text{ ml}}$$

Cross-multiply and divide as above to find the unknown.

$$100 \text{ mg/}X \text{ ml} = 200 \text{ mg/1 ml}$$
$$100 \text{ mg} = 200 \text{ mg}$$
$$100 X = 200$$
$$X = 2$$

The amount to be given to the patient for the correct amount of medication in this scenario is 2 ml.

Keep in mind that the physician will likely order the amount to be given based on his or her knowledge of the standard dose. If the MA is unfamiliar with the standard dose, he should look up the standard dose or the amount to be given per weight in kilograms and calculate as a double-check.

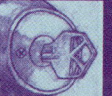

Keys to Success
REMEMBER THE GRAIN

The grain is a unit of measurement that is sometimes used in medication dosing. The grain measures weight, similarly to a milligram. Roman numerals are most often used with grain measurements. When writing a grain measurement, the abbreviation **gr** always precedes the Roman numeral value. For instance on a prescription, five grains would be written as **gr v.**

Remember that most medication errors occur because of shortcuts or omission in following the rights of medication administration.

It is possible to calculate dosages easily using a formula. To determine the amount of the drug needed, set up the following formula:

Calculation formula:

$$\frac{\text{Available strength}}{\text{Ordered strength}} = \frac{\text{available amount}}{\text{amount to give}}$$

Available strength is the strength of the drug in stock. The available amount is the amount of drug in the container. The ordered strength is the physician's order, and the amount to give is the unknown quantity (the *x*).

For example, the physician order is to give 500 mg of a drug, and there is a vial that contains 1000 mg/mL.

Calculation formula:

$$\frac{\text{Available strength}}{\text{Ordered strength}} = \frac{\text{available amount}}{\text{amount to give}}$$

strength of the drug in the vial = 1000 mg/mL

Available amount = 1 mL

Ordered strength = 500 mg

Amount to give = x

$$\frac{1000 \text{ mg}}{500 \text{ mg}} = \frac{1 \text{ mL}}{x}$$

$$1000 \times x = 500 \times 1$$

$$1000x = 500$$

$$\frac{1000x}{1000} = \frac{500}{1000}$$

$$1x = 5/10 = \tfrac{1}{2} \text{ mL} = 0.5 \text{ mL}$$

You would fill the syringe with 0.5 mL of liquid to give you the physician's order of 500 mg of medication. To solve a problem using other forms of medications, such as tablets, use the same formula:

Physician's order: Give 10 grains of medication.
Available: Tablets containing 2.5 grains each.

Calculation formula:

$$\frac{\text{Available strength}}{\text{Ordered strength}} = \frac{\text{available amount}}{\text{amount to give}}$$

$$2.5 \text{ gr} = 1 \text{ tablet}$$

$$10 \text{ gr } x \text{ (number of tablets)}$$

$$2.5 \times x = 10 \times 1$$

$$2.5x = 10$$

$$\frac{2.5x}{2.5} = \frac{10}{2.5}$$

$$1x = 4 \text{ tablets}$$

Another formula that is frequently used is $D/H \times Q$, where

D = desired or ordered dose
H = supply on hand or available supply
Q = quantity available

Problem: The physician ordered penicillin 250 mg. The bottle from the supply cabinet is labeled "Penicillin 500 mg per mL."

Solution: Set up the formula

$$\frac{\text{Desired}}{\text{Hand}} \times \text{Quantity}$$

The physician's order is placed in the Desired (*D*) space and the supply you have on hand is placed in the Hand (*H*) space. The quantity per mL is placed in the Quantity (*Q*) space:

$$\frac{D}{H} \times Q = \frac{250}{500} \times 1$$

Divide 250 by 500 $\times \dfrac{1}{1} = 0.5$ mL

The answer is 0.5 mL or $\tfrac{1}{2}$ mL.

Metric and Household Systems of Measurement

The MA may use one of two types of measurement in the medical office to calculate medication dosage: metric or household measurements. Although household measurements are approximate and used infrequently in the medical office, the MA should still be familiar with them. The metric system, considered the official measurement for scientific purposes, is used more frequently. Table 27-8 lists common household measurements. Metric measurements and their equivalent household measurements are listed in Table 27-9.

The MA will likely be required to calculate dosages using metric measurements. For example, the doctor orders 0.2 grams of Gatifloxacin for a patient. The medication is available in 400 mg tablets. Begin with an equation using proportions, or ratios.

1. 1000 mg : 1 gm = X mg : 0.2 gm

    This equation is read as "1000 milligrams is to 1 gram as X milligrams is to 0.2 grams." Always make certain you have an equal equation: mg : gm = mg : gm.

2. Solve for the unknown by multiplying the means by the means and the extremes by the extremes. The means of a proportion are the inner two numbers, and the extremes are the outer two numbers. In the equation above, 1 gm and X mg are the means and 1,000 mg and 0.2 gm are the extremes.

$$1 \text{ gm} \times X = 1X$$
$$1000 \times 0.2 = 200$$
$$1 X = 200$$
$$X = 200 \text{ mg}$$

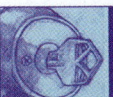

Keys to Success
ZERO VERSUS 0

When dosage is communicated verbally, the word *zero* must be used rather than number 0 to avoid confusion with the letter O. For example, 0.05 mg is said as "zero point zero five milligrams." Likewise, a decimal point should always be preceded by a zero (for example, 0.3 mg, or "zero point three milligrams," not .3).

TABLE 27-8 COMMON HOUSEHOLD MEASUREMENTS

60 drops* = 1 teaspoon (tsp)
3 tsp = 1 tablespoon (tbsp)
2 tbsp = 1 ounce
8 ounces = 1 regular glass or cup
16 tbsp = 1 cup
2 cups = 1 pint (pt)
2 pints (pt) = 1 quart (qt)
4 quarts (qt) = 1 gallon (gal)

The approximate measurement of drops depends on the thickness of the liquid and the opening in the dropper.

3. Now calculate the number of tablets to be given.

Known unit on hand : known dosage form = dose ordered : unknown amount to be given
400 mg : 1 tablet = 200 mg : X tablets
400 : 1 = 200 : X

4. Multiply the means by the means and the extremes by the extremes.

$$400 \times X = 400X$$
$$1 \times 200 = 200$$
$$400X = 200$$
$$X = 0.5 \,(1/2 \text{ of a } 400 \text{ mg tablet})$$

Calculating Pediatric Dosages by Body Weight

According to the Institute of Medicine, 7,000 patients are killed and 375,000 are injured every year due to prescription error. Many medications, especially in the pediatric setting, are given in doses based on a patient's weight. In the past, Clark's and Fried's methods of calculations were used to determine what percent of an adult dose was appropriate for a child. But because children do not develop and grow in steady, predictable patterns, these calculations are no longer used.

TABLE 27-9 METRIC AND HOUSEHOLD MEASUREMENTS: APPROXIMATE EQUIVALENTS

Metric	Household
1 gm	1/4 tsp
15 gm	1 tbsp
30 gm	1 ounce
1 kg	2.2 lbs
1 mL	15 drops
5 mL	1 tsp
15 mL	1 tbsp
30 mL	1 fl. oz.
500 mL	1 pt
1,000 mL	4 cups (1 qt)
2.5 cm	1 inch

There are two ways to determine the exact dosage of medication for a child: according to body weight or according to body mass (BSA). The calculation based on body weight is the most widely used, and most people find it easier to calculate correctly. BSA calculations require the use of a formula and a nomogram.

As an example of body weight calculation, the doctor orders medication at 15 mg/kg/day for a young patient. The patient is to take the medication with a meal three times per day for 30 days, then be reevaluated. You weigh the patient before beginning your calculations. She weighs 55 pounds.

1. Convert pounds to kilograms.

$$55 \text{ lbs} \div 2.2 = 25 \text{ kg}$$

2. Calculate the dosage (15 mg/kg/day) for the client's weight, or 15 mg/25 kg/day.

$$15 \text{ mg} \times 25 = 375 \text{ mg/day}$$
$$375 \text{ mg/day} \div 3 \text{ doses/day} = 125 \text{ mg per dose}$$

3. The patient should take 125 mg of medication with each meal for the next 30 days.
4. The total number of 125 mg tablets needed to fill the prescription would be 3 tablets per day × 30 days = 90 tablets.

Young's Rule Young's rule is used for children who are over 1 year of age. The formula used for Young's rule is: Pediatric dose =

$$\frac{\text{child's age in years}}{\text{child's age in years} + 12} \times \text{adult dose}$$

To use this formula, divide the child's age in years by the same number plus 12. Multiply this number by the adult dose to determine the correct pediatric dosage.

West's Nomogram The two methods most commonly used for calculating pediatric dosages are body weight (such as mg/kg), and body surface area (BSA). The West's nomogram is the preferred method for sick and underweight children. It can be used for both infants and children. The chart is frequently found in pediatric offices, medical textbooks, and dictionaries.

West's nomogram is the preferred method of pediatric calculation particular for oncology and critical care patients because it is based on the calculation of the body surface area of the child. The body surface area (BSA) is based on a calculation of the child's height and weight, and is expressed as m^2. The chart has three columns (see Figure 27-3 ♦). To calculate the child's BSA, a straight line is drawn from the patient's height in inches or centimeters across the columns to the patient's weight in kilograms or pounds. The straight line will intersect on the BSA column. This point will give the BSA average. Once a BSA average is calculated, it is applied to the following formula:

$$\text{Pediatric dose} = \frac{\text{BSA of child}}{1.73 \text{ square meters}} \times \text{adult dose}$$

1.73 meters is the standard adult BSA.

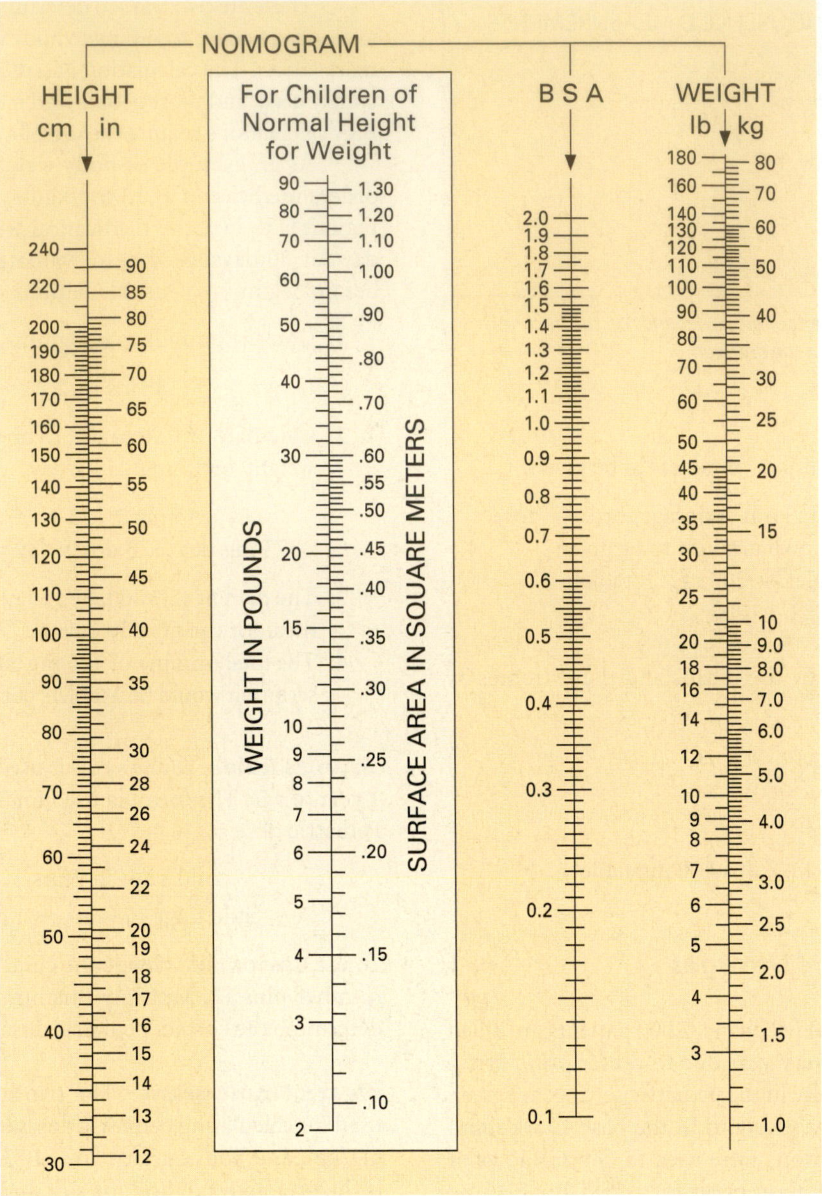

Figure 27-3 ◆ Nomogram chart.

Safety Guidelines for Administering Medications

Medications should be prepared in a well-lit environment with a minimum of distraction. Always wash your hands before beginning the procedure. Always practice the "six rights" and the three label checkpoints when preparing any medication. These factors are as follows:

1. Right patient:
   ■ Identify the patient by asking him or her to state name.
2. Right drug (medication):
   ■ Dispense or administer only medications you have prepared yourself.
   ■ Compare the medication with the physician's order three times:
   • when removing the medication from the storage area
   • before taking the medication from the container
   • before returning the medication to the storage area or disposing of the empty container
3. Right dose:
   ■ Confirm the adult or child dosage.
   ■ Verify the accuracy of your dosage calculation with another clinical staff member.
4. Right route:
   ■ Confirm the route on the physician's order.
   ■ Use the correct site for parenteral medication.
5. Right time: Confirm the specified time with the physician's order.
6. Right documentation:
   ■ Record the date, time, name, dosage, and administration route of the medication on the patient chart. All

documentation must be signed by the individual dispensing or administering the medication.

- If the medication is an injection, record the site.
- For immunizations and allergy medications, also document the lot number and expiration date.
- If the medication is not given, document the reasons and report to the physician.

The Prescription

The physician is responsible for prescribing medications, either in written form (physician's order or prescription) or verbally. A prescription is a legal document and should be typed or written in ink. Depending on state practice acts, the MA may complete a prescription blank according to the physician's order and have him or her sign it. All Schedule II, III, and IV drug prescriptions must be signed by the physician. Office protocol must be followed in every case. The MA may call a prescription in to a pharmacy, except for controlled substances.

A written prescription is usually a preprinted form with the physician's name, address, phone number, and DEA number (Figures 27-4 ◆ and 27-5 ◆). Some physicians write prescriptions on hospital or clinic forms printed with the hospital or clinic name and information. Prescription forms for controlled substances are printed on special paper that identifies any alterations to the prescription, especially attempted erasures.

In addition to the physician's data, the customary parts of a prescription are the following:

1. The patient's name and address, and the prescription date
2. Superscription: the symbol Rx, which means "take"
3. Inscription (main part of the prescription): drug name, form, and strength

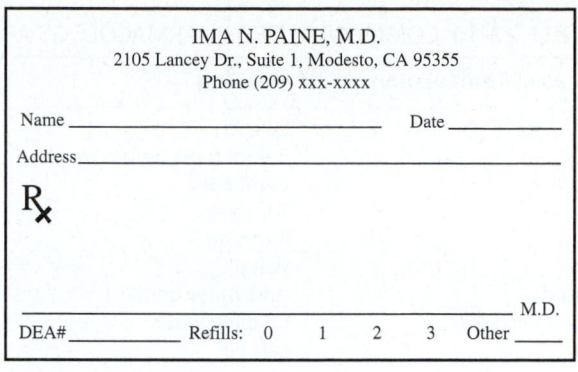

Figure 27-4 ◆ Example of a prescription form used in a medical office.

4. Subscription: directions to pharmacist for amount of drug to be dispensed
5. Signature: patient instructions (Sig:) to be placed on label
6. Refill information ("REPETATUR 0 1 2 3 PRN"): refill instructions for the physician to circle
7. Physician's signature and "Dispense as written" or "Substitute generic medication"

Some preprinted prescriptions feature a box with the word "Label," which instructs the pharmacist to label the prescription container.

Table 27-10 lists the most common pharmacology abbreviations used in prescriptions and other medical forms. In May 2005, in order to reduce the number of medical errors related to the incorrect use of terminology, The Joint Commission on Accreditation of Healthcare Organizations (JCAHO) issued a

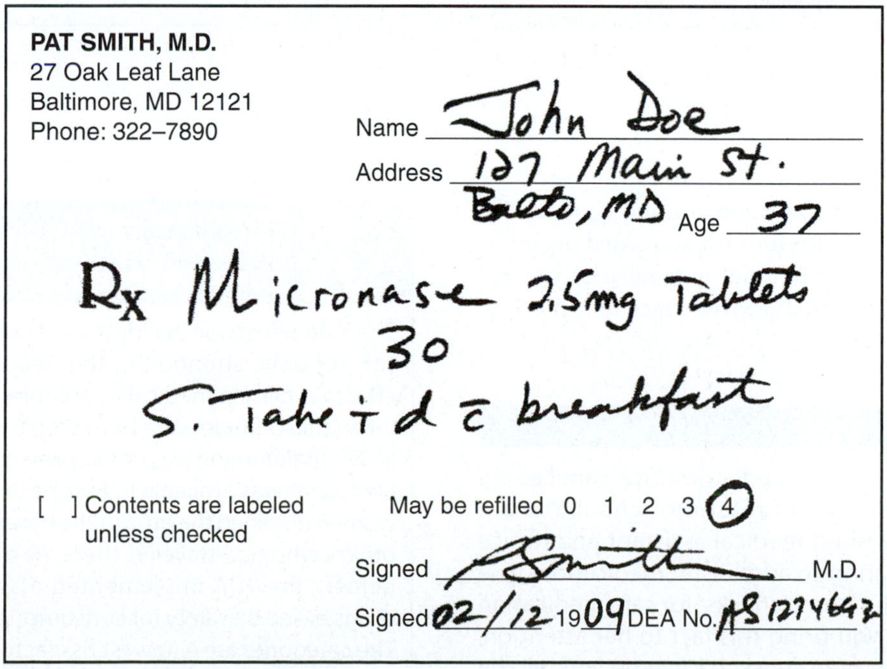

Figure 27-5 ◆ Example of a completed prescription.

TABLE 27-10 COMMONLY USED PHARMACOLOGY ABBREVIATIONS

Medical Abbreviation	Meaning	Medical Abbreviation	Meaning
a.a. or aa	Of each	LIQ	Liquid
a.c.	Before food, before meals	mcg.	Microgram
a.d.	Right ear	mEq.	Milliequivalent
ad	To, up to	mg.	Milligram
a.m.	Morning	ml.	Milliliter
Aq	Water	NS	Normal saline
aq. ad	Add water up to	o.d.	Right eye
Aqua. Dist., DW	Distilled water	o.s.	Left eye
a.s	Left ear	OTC	Over-the-counter
a.t.c.	Around the clock	o.u.	Each eye
a.u.	Each ear	p.c.	After food, after meals
b.i.d	Twice a day	PDR	Physician's Desk Reference
c̄	With	p.o.	By mouth
Caps	Caplets, capsules	p.r.n.	As needed
CSA	Federal Controlled Substances Act	q	Each, every
		q.h.	Each hour
DEA	Drug Enforcement Administration	q.i.d.	Four times a day
		q.s.	A sufficient quantity
dil.	Dilute	q.s. ad	Add a sufficient amount to make
disp.	Dispense		
div.	Divide	s	Without
d.t.d.	Give of such doses	SC, subc, subq, s	Subcutaneously
Elix.	Elixir	ss	Half
f, fl.	Fluid	Stat.	Immediately
f, ft.	Make, let it be made	Supp.	Suppository
g., G, gm	Gram	Syr.	Syrup
gtt.	Drops	Tab	Tablet
h	Hour, at the hour of	tbsp.	Tablespoon
h.s.	At bedtime, at hour of sleep	t.i.d.	Three times a day
i.m., IM	Intramuscular	top	Topically
Inj., INJ	Injection	tsp.	Teaspoon
i.v., IV	Intravenous	Ung	Ointment
i.v.p., IVP	Intravenous push	USP-NF	U.S. Pharmacopeia and National Formulary
IVPB	Intravenous piggyback		
l	Left	ut dict., u.d	As directed
L	Liter		

"do not use" list of abbreviations, acronyms, and symbols. The abbreviations must be included on each accredited organization's "do not use" list. It is important to familiarize yourself with this list, which can be viewed at www.jointcommission.org/PatientSafety/DoNotUseList/.

In Practice

You are employed with a busy pediatric office. Families are preparing for their children to return to school. You are working with a newly hired medical assistant and notice that while she is preparing to administer medications, she neglects to perform the "three checks" for safe medication administration. When you bring this fact to her attention, she asks "What are the three checks?" What do you tell the new medical assistant?

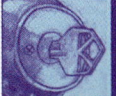

Keys to Success
PRESCRIPTION DRUGS TAKEN DURING PREGNANCY

The side effects of thalidomide taken during pregnancy called public attention in the 1960s to the teratogenic effects of certain medications. Babies whose mothers had taken thalidomide were born with partial or undeveloped limbs. Thalidomide was not approved for use in the United States but was available in Europe as a sedative. Pregnant women obtained the drug while traveling in Europe or from others who had traveled there. As a result of these birth defects, the FDA implemented a system for classifying drugs based on safety for consumption during pregnancy. The categories are A (lowest risk factor), B, C, D, and X (highest risk factor). Package inserts identify the level of risk.

PROCEDURE 27-1 Demonstrate Safety Measures to Prepare, Administer, and Document Medication

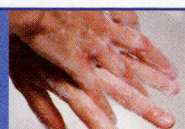

Theory and Rationale

To ensure patient safety in medication administration, the medical assistant must follow certain guidelines every time a medication is ordered. The medical assistant must practice medical asepsis by washing hands before and after administering medication. Verification of the drug order requires ensuring that the medical order is legible and can be read and clearly understood.

Materials

- written medication order, including name of patient, drug name, strength, dose, and route of medication
- *Physician's Desk Reference (PDR)* or drug package insert
- container of ordered medication
- correct supplies for administering the drug
- gloves
- patient chart

Competency

(**Conditions**) With the necessary materials you will be able to (**Task**) safely prepare, administer, and document medication (**Standards**) correctly within the time frame designated by the instructor.

1. Read the medication order and clarify the medication order with the physician, if needed.
2. If unfamiliar with the drug, refer to the *PDR* or the package insert to determine the medication's function, usual dose, side effects, and any pertinent precautions or contraindications. Follow the "six rights" to prevent errors.
3. Based upon the information on the medication order and the medication on hand, calculate the dosage to match the medication order. Confirm the answer with the physician if you have any questions.
4. Wash your hands.
5. Dispense the medication in a well-lit, quiet, low-traffic area.
6. Perform the three checks to prevent errors:
    a. Compare the written label with the label on the medication container or vial when you remove it from storage. Check the expiration date and properly dispose of any expired medication.
    b. Compare the written order with the label on the medication container or vial before dispensing or drawing

up medication. Ensure that the strength on the label matches the medication order and that you dispense the correctly calculated dose.
    c. Compare the written order and the label on the medication container or vial before returning it to storage or discarding.
7. If at any time you have any doubts about the function of the medication, the dosage, route of medication, or the possibility of an allergic reaction, *immediately* consult the physician.
8. Identify the patient and escort him to the treatment area. Verify allergy information in the chart and ask the patient if he has any allergies.
9. Wash your hands and put on gloves.
10. Administer the medication according to the medication order, following the "six rights" to prevent errors, and using Occupational Safety and Health Administration (OSHA) precautions.
11. Provide patient education on the function of the drug administered, typical side effects, and dosage and storage recommendations, if applicable. Refer to the physician if additional information is needed.
12. Document the procedure. Include the date, time, medication, route, and amount administered. Follow office policy for recording the expiration date and lot number.

Patient Education

If office policy or potential side effects dictate that the patient wait in the reception area for a specified period of time, explain the reasons for the waiting period. Be prepared to explain side effects that the patient should be alert for and report. Instruct the patient to report any sudden reactions to the medication, whether local or general.

Charting Example

6/8/xx 3:50 pm Mantoux TB Test 0.1 ml given intradermally in R anterior forearm. Lot # MF16290D, exp. 4/xx. Patient tolerated procedure well. Patient instructed to return to office in 48 hours to have test results read and documented. Kelly Clinton, RMA (AMT).

Safeguarding Prescription Pads

The potential for theft and substance abuse exists in every medical office. The MA and other medical office staff are responsible for the safekeeping of prescription pads. The following guidelines help to prevent theft and drug abuse.

- Prescription blanks and preprinted prescriptions should be stored in a locked area. They must never be left lying around in the office.
- The physician should use one prescription pad at a time.
- Prescription blanks should be numbered and used in numerical order.

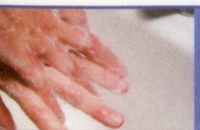

PROCEDURE 27-2 Demonstrate the Preparation of a Prescription for the Physician's Signature

Theory and Rationale

In compliance with the Controlled Substance Act of 1970, all physicians who prescribe any type of drug, either over-the-counter or controlled, must register with the DEA. Every physician must fill out a registration form, renewable every three years, with his or her state license number and signature. Physicians who write prescriptions in different states must be registered in each state. Physicians who practice in multiple locations in the same state must register each address. The certificate of approval from the DEA must be kept at each registered location and be available for inspection by officials.

Every prescription must bear the physician's name, address, and DEA number in permanent ink so that it can be traced back to the physician who authorized the medication. There is no approved medical use for Schedule I drugs, so prescriptions for these drugs are prohibited. Schedule II medications are controlled substances for which a written prescription is required. As refills for these drugs are not allowed, the patient must obtain a new prescription whenever additional medication is needed. In cases of emergency, the DEA allows for a one-time limited amount of Schedule II medications to be phoned in by the physician, with the signed, written prescription to be delivered to the pharmacy within 72 hours.

Once a prescription is filled, all identifying information, including an assigned prescription number, is entered into a computer. The paper version of the prescription is then filed and kept for a minimum of seven years. The pharmacy may file prescriptions according to schedule (II through V).

Materials

- physician's order for medication
- patient chart
- ink pen or computer if Rx is typed
- blank prescription

Competency

(**Conditions**) With the necessary materials, you will be able to (**Task**) write a prescription (**Standards**) correctly within 10 minutes.

1. Gather the equipment.
2. Obtain the prescription information (name, dose, amount, frequency, refills) from the physician.
3. Correctly write out the prescription according to the information received from the physician.
4. Check for accuracy and present the prescription to the physician for signature.
5. Document the procedure. Include the date, time, medication, strength, dose, frequency, and refills allowed. Many offices will want a photocopy of the written Rx.

Patient Education

If office procedures indicate the need, instruct the patient when and how to obtain refills if any are needed. Some offices prefer that the patient call the pharmacy directly with the refill request, some have dedicated prescription refill lines, and others prefer to fax requests.

Charting Example

01/26/XX 8:00 am Patient received written prescription for Ambien 10mg #30 for treatment of idiopathic insomnia. Sig: Take 1 tablet by mouth 30 minutes prior to sleep on nights that are available to dedicate to a full 8 hours of sleep. No refills issued. Patient instructed to avoid taking medication on nights when 8 hours of sleep are not available and to watch for side effects, such as but not limited to hypersomnia. Photocopy of prescription filled in chart under medication flow sheet. Juanita Hernandez, RMA (AMT)

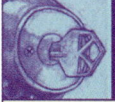

Keys to Success
AVOIDING MEDICATION ERRORS

Medication errors can be easily avoided by strictly observing the Six Rights of Medication Administration. The Six Rights are as follows: right patient, right time, right dose, right route, right drug, and right documentation. In the event that you make an error when administering medications, it is important to alert the physician immediately, then document the error and any corrective actions in the patient's chart. Be sure to follow the office procedure for filing an incident report.

Forms and Routes of Medication Administration

Medications may be administered in several different forms. Solid forms include tablets (chewable, sublingual, enteric coated, and plain), capsules (sustained release and caplet form), lozenges, suppositories (vaginal, rectal, or urethral), and dermatological forms (creams and ointments, transdermal patches). Liquid forms include elixirs, solutions, suspensions, syrups, sprays, and tinctures. Injectables are available in powder form (to be mixed prior to administration) or in commercially prepared, ready-to-use liquid form.

Medications may also be administered via a number of routes: oral (swallowing), sublingual (under the tongue), transdermal, parenteral (intradermal, subcutaneous, intramuscular, and intravenous, buccal, inhalation, irrigation, instillation, rectal, topical). See Figures 27-6 ◆ and 27-7 ◆ and Table 27-11.

The form of medication prescribed for specific patients may be affected by certain factors. For example, if a patient is unable to take the oral form of digoxin, it may be administered intravenously. A physician may also prescribe the intravenous route to obtain rapid therapeutic action and later prescribe the oral form for daily use. Other factors in the choice of medication form and route include the present functioning of the healthy or diseased body as well as the patient's absorption, distribution, metabolism, and excretion capabilities. Age is another factor. In the elderly, medication is generally absorbed, distributed, metabolized, and excreted more slowly. Dosages may also be smaller because of the potential for toxicity.

The oral route is the safest route of administration, because the medication can be retrieved, if necessary, in the immediate minutes after administration. Emesis can be induced and the drug expelled from the body. IV administration requires complete accuracy in administration because once the medication is injected into the bloodstream, its action is permanent and retrieval is not possible. The rapid action of sublingual and buccal medications is essential in emergency situations, but again, the action usually cannot be halted.

Medications administered by different routes are absorbed by the body at different rates, as follows.

1. **Oral**—Depending on the medication type (tablet, capsule, liquid, etc.) and whether the medication is to be taken on a full stomach, oral medications can take 10 to 30 minutes to be absorbed and distributed in the body. Most oral medications are absorbed through the wall of

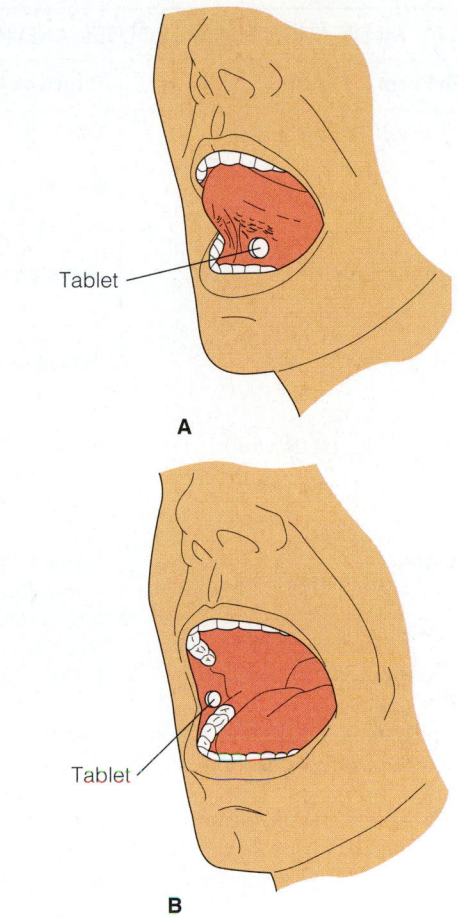

Figure 27-6 ◆ (A) Sublingual administration; (B) Buccal administration.

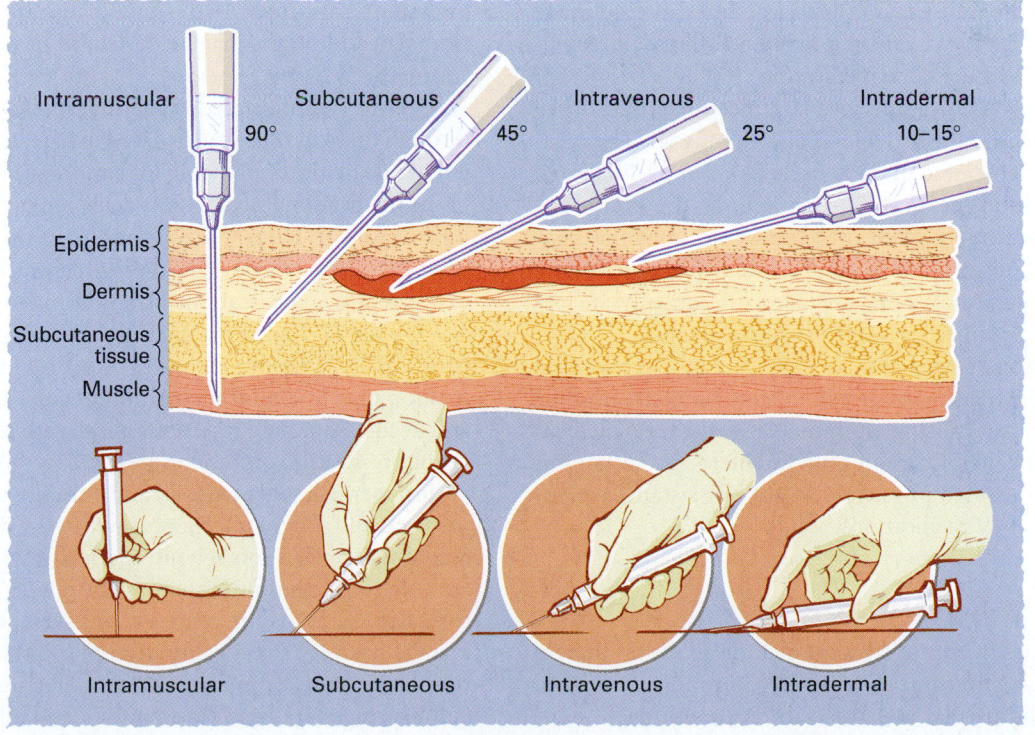

Figure 27-7 ◆ Parenteral drug administration: Intramuscular, subcutaneous, intravenous, and intradermal.

TABLE 27-11 MEDICATION FORMS, ROUTES, AND PROCEDURES FOR ADMINISTERING

Medication Form	Route of Administration	Procedure
Capsule, pill, tablet, spansule, liquid, solution	Oral	Medication is given orally and swallowed.
Tablet	Buccal (oral cheek space)	The tablet is placed between the gums or teeth and the cheek and is absorbed as it dissolves.
Tablet, liquid, or solution	Sublingual	Medication is placed under the tongue for absorption through the oral mucous membrane.
Aerosol, mist, spray, or stream	Inhalation	Equipment (inhalation device, nebulizer, or ventilator) dispenses the medication in a mist or liquid form for inhalation.
Liquid medication in solution form	Irrigation	Solution is passed through a cavity or over a membrane, then allowed to drain.
	Instillation	Medication is released into a body cavity for absorption by tissue.
Sterile solution	Injection (intradermal, subcutaneous, or intramuscular)	Medication is injected into body tissue.
	Intravenous (infusion or injection)	Medication is injected or instilled into a vein.
Solution or suppository	Rectal	Medication is introduced into the rectum for absorption.
Cream, dermal patch (transdermal), lotion, spray, tincture, powder, and ointment	Topical	Medication is applied to the skin with gloved hands. Dermal patches are self-adhering.
Suppository, cream, ointment, foam, solution and liquid	Vaginal	Medication is introduced into the vagina by insertion, application, or irrigation.

the small intestine, which accounts for the delay in absorption time. The oral route is the route most often prescribed because it is quick, easy, and can be done at home, which is convenient for patients who require multiple doses of the same medication.

2. **Injection**—Medications given by injection are absorbed quickly, due to the high blood flow in muscles. The medication is absorbed in the muscle fibers and transferred to the bloodstream, then throughout the body. The injectable route is often used for medications that may cause GI upset and possibly interfere with absorption, and for medications that are taken infrequently, such as monthly B_{12} injections for pernicious anemia.

3. **Intravenous**—Medications given via IV have a rapid onset. The medication is administered directly into the bloodstream, causing an immediate effect. IV medications are generally given only in emergency situations and by a trained physician. Medical assistants cannot administer IV medications.

Parenteral Administration

Parenteral routes of administration include all routes that do not involve the gastrointestinal tract. Common parenteral routes are intramuscular injections, intravenous injections or infusions, subcutaneous injections, inhalation, and topical or

dermal application. Drugs administered through the GI tract usually have a slower onset of action than those administered by parenteral route. Also, some drugs are irritating to the stomach, and others may be destroyed or inactivated by gastric acids.

Drugs administered via dermal application are absorbed through the skin. The drugs placed in dermal patches have different release times, allowing for a more consistent blood level of the medication. Medications delivered by this route include cardiovascular drugs (Nitroderm), pain medications (Duragesic, Lidoderm patches), hormones (contraceptives and HRT), and antinausea medications (Transderm scop).

Table 27-12 describes various types of parenteral administration by injection. Figure 27-8 ◆ provides an example of rotation sites. Injectable medications require the use of a syringe and needle. Although injections may be administered by intravenous route, the common routes used in the physician's office are intradermal, subcutaneous, and intramuscular. The different methods and sites of injection, as well as the different types and amounts of medication, require a variety of syringes and needles.

Syringes commonly used in the physician's office include the tuberculin, insulin, and 3 cc/ml syringe. The tuberculin syringe has very small calibration markings that allow injection of amounts as minute as 0.1 cc (Figure 27-9 ◆). Tuberculin syringes are used for Mantoux and allergy tests via the intradermal route. Insulin is administered with insulin syringes,

TABLE 27-12 TYPES OF INJECTIONS

	Intradermal	Subcutaneous	Intramuscular
Purpose	Allergy tests and Mantoux testing	Quick bloodstream absorption of medication	Gradual and maximum blood-stream absorption of medication
Sites	Distal to the antecubital space of the anterior aspect of the forearm	Outer aspect of the upper arm, abdomen, and anterior thigh	Dorsal aspect of the gluteus, deltoid, vastus lateralis of the thigh, and ventral aspect of the gluteus
Amount	0.1 to 0.3 ml	Less than 2 ml	2 to 5 ml. Dosages above 4 ml should be divided and administered at two different sites.
Needle Length and Size	1–1/2" to 5/8" length, 25 to 27 gauge	5/8" to 1" length, 22 to 27 gauge	1–1/2" to 2" length, 14 to 22 gauge

usually U50 or U100 marked, via the subcutaneous route (Figure 27-10 ◆). The 3 cc/ml syringe (Figure 27-11 ◆) is used most often for intramuscular injections. If the amount of medication is greater than the size of the syringe, the dosage may be split and administered in different sites with two syringes.

Needle sizes vary according to the type and depth of tissue to be injected. Tuberculin and insulin syringe needles, which are used for intradermal and subcutaneous administration, respectively, are smaller than the needles used for intramuscular injections. Intradermal and subcutaneous injections are administered into the most exterior layers of the skin. Intramuscular injections penetrate into the deeper tissues below the skin.

Always follow safety procedures and universal precautions when handling sharps. Avoid recapping needles unless

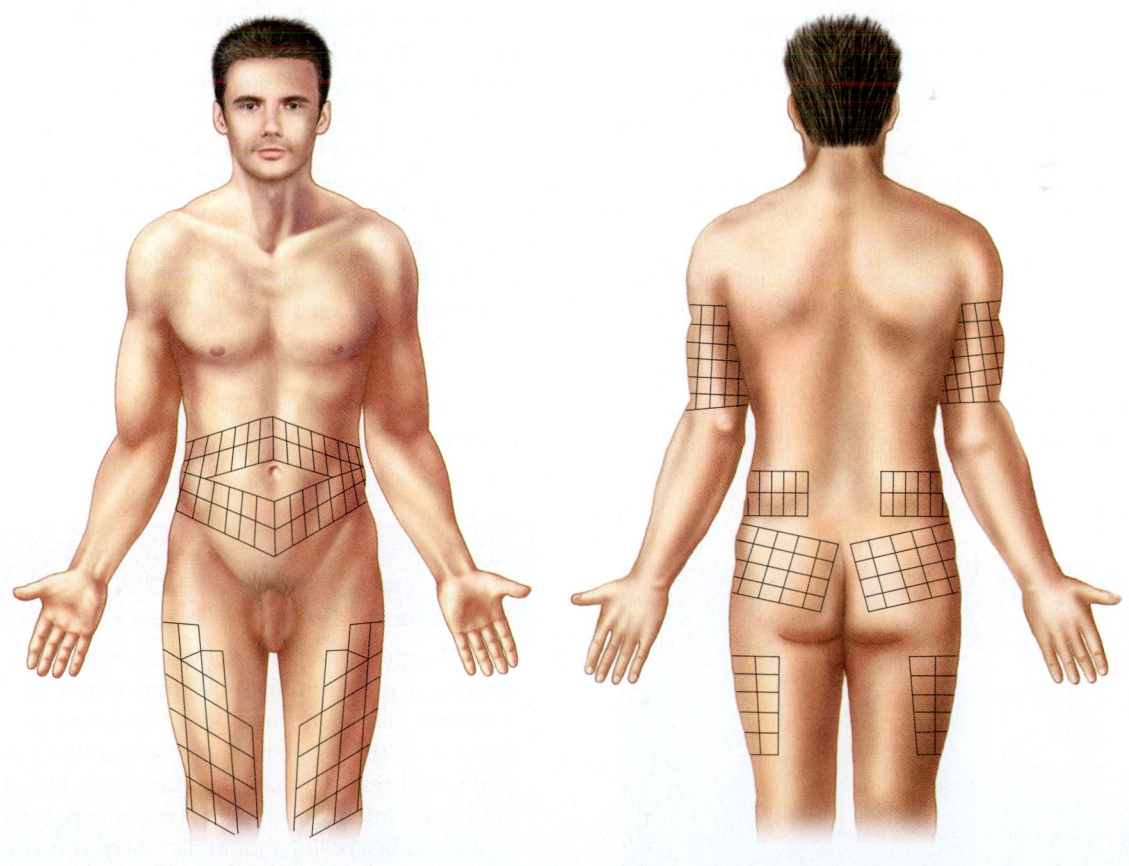

Figure 27-8 ◆ Example of rotation sites.

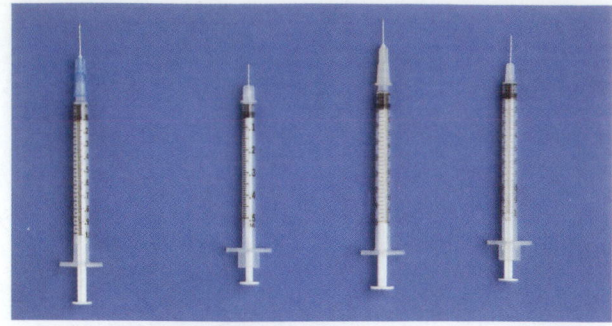

Figure 27-9 ◆ Tuberculin syringes.

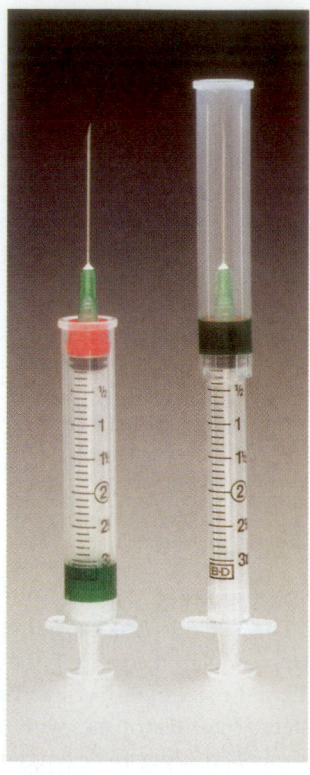

Figure 27-11 ◆ 3 cc/ml syringes.

you use a slide cap procedure. In this method, you slide the exposed needle into the cap before lifting the syringe/needle combination to an upright position or to another surface before injection. Do not anchor the cap tightly to the syringe. A tight cap would be hard to remove and increase the risk of needle injury during removal. (Newer safety syringes have safety guards that prevent needle stick injury.) After use, dispose of syringe/needle combinations and other sharps, such as glass ampules, into the nearest sharps container. (∞ See Chapter 23 for more information concerning the use and disposal of sharps.)

Ampules and Vials

Medication for parenteral administration comes in ready-to-use liquid form in vials and ampules and in powdered form for reconstitution. Ampules and vials are available in small and large sizes and in clear or darkened glass. Some medications are stored in plastic vials. Storage in a glass ampule prevents a chemical reaction with other materials, such as the rubber stopper of a vial or the plastic of a pre-filled syringe. An ampule also ensures sterility.

An ampule removed from storage or packaging may have fluid in the top portion above the neck or breaking line. Tapping lightly with a fingertip may be enough to release the fluid into the bottom portion. If bubbles develop, however, the final dosage amount may be affected. Another method is to hold the top of the ampule and twirl it so that the medication slides into the bottom.

Most ampules are painted with a break line at the upper portion of the neck, marking the expected break and weakest point of the glass. Breaking the top of the ampule usually requires only an alcohol pad to protect you. Safety ampule breakers are also available. For a larger ampule, wipe the neck with an alcohol wipe, then use 2 × 2 gauze to snap off the top. Discard the top into a sharps container. Using a filtered needle to withdraw medication will prevent glass fragments from entering the syringe. If it is necessary to invert the ampule to withdraw medication, note that the fluid will not drain because of the air pressure outside the ampule pushing up on the liquid at the smaller ampule neck. Do not inject air into the ampule while it is upside down, as this will force medication or diluent to drain. After the medication has been withdrawn, pull the

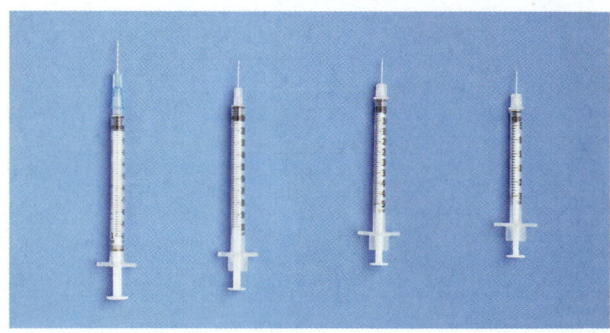

Figure 27-10 ◆ Insulin syringes.

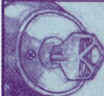

Keys to Success
GLOVING PROTOCOL FOR INJECTIONS

The CDC does not have regulations pertaining to the wearing of gloves during injections. When administering intramuscular or subcutaneous injections, OSHA recommends that gloves are not necessary, as long as bleeding that could result in hand contact with blood or other potentially infectious materials is not expected.

Each office policy should dictate gloving protocol for injections, since the practice of whether to wear gloves for IM or subcutaneous injections is in transition.

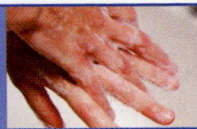

PROCEDURE 27-3 Demonstrate Withdrawing Medication from an Ampule

Theory and Rationale

An ampule is a single-use, single-dose, sterile glass container of liquid medication. Many prepackaged surgical sets, such as disposable Thorascopy tray sets, contain Xylocaine or another medication in an ampule as part of the kit.

Materials

- sterile filter needle/syringe set
- ampule of medication
- sterile gauze 2 × 4s or 4 × 4s or safety ampule breaker
- alcohol wipes
- gloves
- sharps container
- patient chart

Competency

(**Conditions**) With the necessary materials, you will be able (**Task**) to withdraw medication from an ampule (**Standards**) correctly within 15 minutes.

1. Wash your hands and gather equipment.
2. Check to make sure the medication matches the physician's order. Calculate the dosage, if necessary. Look up information relating to the medication's function, usual doses, and side effects. Check for patient allergies.
3. Check the medication label a second time against the physician's order. Verify the medication, expiration date, and medication quality following the six rights.
4. Identify the patient and escort her to the treatment area. Verify allergy information in the chart and ask the patient if she has allergies.
5. Put on your gloves.
6. Dislodge any medication that may be trapped in the ampule neck by holding the ampule by the neck and quickly flicking your wrist in a downward motion.
7. Disinfect the ampule with an alcohol swab and check the label again for correct medication and dosage.
8. Completely wrap the neck of the ampule with the sterile cotton gauze and snap off the top by pulling it toward you (Figure 27-12 ◆). Discard the top in a sharps container.
9. With a filtered needle, withdraw the necessary medication amount. You can withdraw the medication with the ampule inverted or not (Figure 27-13 ◆).
10. Change needles and discard the filtered needle into a sharps container.
11. Identify the patient, if you have drawn up the medication in a separate room. If the medication will affect driving, verify patient has a driver or ride home.
12. Administer the medication according to the physician's orders.
13. Discard the used needle into the sharps container.
14. Remove the gloves and wash your hands.
15. Document the procedure. Include date, time, site, medication, route, and amount administered. Follow office policy for recording the expiration date and lot number.

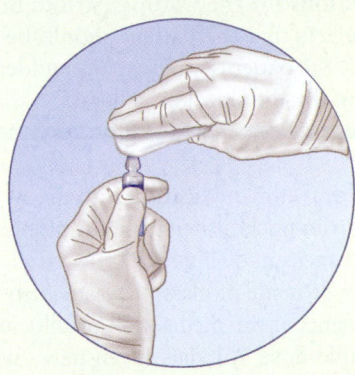

Figure 27-12 ◆ Wrap the neck of the ampule with the sterile cotton gauze.

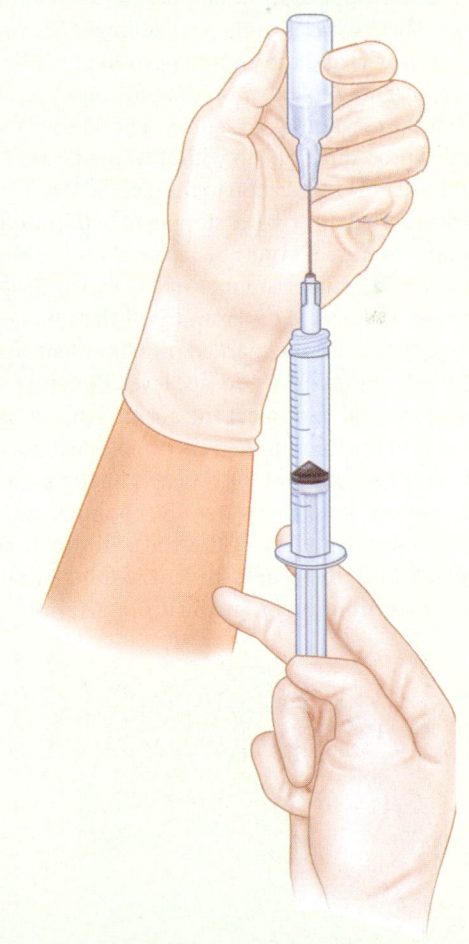

Figure 27-13 ◆ Withdraw the necessary medication amount with the ampule inverted or not.

continued

PROCEDURE 27-3 Demonstrate Withdrawing Medication from an Ampule *(continued)*

Patient Education

If office policy or potential side effects dictate that the patient wait in the reception area for a specified period of time, explain the reasons for the waiting period. Be prepared to explain side effects that the patient should be alert for and report. Instruct the patient to report any sudden reactions to the medication, whether local or general.

Charting Example

04/18/XX 9:35 AM Phenergan 25mg injection administered to patient in the left ventrogluteal area for leg pain. Patient was instructed to wait in the exam room for 20 minutes for observation and was released. Dennis Benson, CMA (AAMA)

plunger back to draw the medication into the syringe. Tap any bubbles to the top air pocket, then push the plunger up until the correct dosage is measured (Figure 27-14 ◆).

A vial may be made of glass or plastic, depending on the storage requirements of the medication or diluent, and may be single- or multiple-dose. All vials (even new ones) should be cleaned prior to use. When using a multiple-dose vial, always wipe the rubber stopper with an alcohol wipe before withdrawing the medication or diluent. Repeated use of a multiple-dose vial can damage the rubber stopper. If the stopper has been damaged or you can see rubber particles in the vial, follow office procedure for disposal of the vial and the unused portion of medication.

It is important to follow procedure for injecting air into a vial to prevent the creation of a vacuum. The MA will need two needles for this procedure, one to withdraw medication and the other to administer the medication to the patient. When you force the first needle through the rubber stopper to withdraw the medication, the tip is dulled and must be replaced for the injection.

First clean the rubber stopper of the vial and allow it to air-dry. Remove the needle cover and pull the plunger of the empty syringe back until the marked measurement side of the rubber stopper is at the correct dosage level. Puncture the rubber stopper of the vial and inject the air into the air space. (If air is injected into the fluid in the vial, bubbles will form. Bubbles may affect the accuracy of the dosage.) Keeping the syringe and needle in place, hold the vial with the index and second fingers of the other hand. Invert the vial with the needle and syringe in place. Keep the needle under the fluid level to withdraw the correct amount of medication. Aspirate a small

amount of medication above the correct amount and withdraw the needle from the vial. With the needle pointing up, pull the plunger back to create an air pocket at the top of the barrel. Tap all air bubbles to the air pocket. Push the plunger to move the stopper to the correct dosage level. Slide the needle into a cap cover if not administering the medication immediately.

Some medications must be mixed prior to administration because the solution does not remain chemically stable or evenly mixed for extended periods of time. Powdered medication is mixed with a diluent such as sterile saline or water. Diluents are stored in ampules or vials. It is important to follow procedures for removing the correct amount of diluent from a vial or ampule. Using the correct amount ensures correct dilution and the correct dosage as ordered by the physician. To calculate the amount required for the dosage ordered by the physician, use the strength of the correctly mixed medication. For example, after a medication is reconstituted correctly according to directions, the strength is 50 mg/ml. The physician has ordered 75 mg. Therefore the correct amount of medication to administer is 1.5 ml.

Intravenous Therapy

Medications or therapeutic solutions may be injected directly into the bloodstream for immediate circulation and use by the body. State practice acts designate which healthcare professionals can initiate intravenous (IV) fluid therapy and medication administration. Medical assistants must consult their state practice act before attempting any intravenous procedure. In some states the medical assistant may start IV fluid therapy with advanced training and physician supervision. Medical assistants should be aware of the dangers of administering medications by the intravenous route and recognize they do not have the training necessary to push IV medications (bolus). *The following information is provided only to acquaint you with the IV therapy process and should not be considered a competency.*

Generally, intravenous fluids are administered to replenish body fluid supply and electrolytes, most commonly solutions of 5% dextrose, normal saline, 45% normal saline, or 5% dextrose with normal saline. Dextrose contributes glucose to meet energy needs and saline contributes sodium, an electrolyte that maintains fluid balance and cellular functions. In addition, blood products, including packed cells or plasma; hyperalimentation (designed for patients too sick to meet their own nutritional needs); and medications may be administered by the IV route.

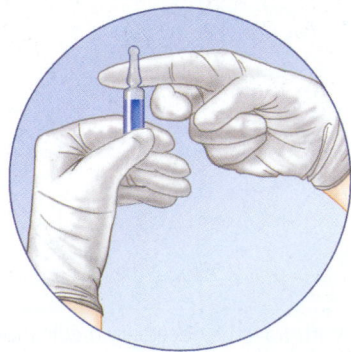

Figure 27-14 ◆ Tap syringe to remove any air bubbles.

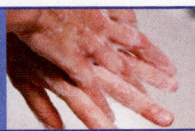

PROCEDURE 27-4 Demonstrate Withdrawing Medication from a Vial

Theory and Rationale

Medication comes in a variety of containers, and liquid medications are often supplied in vials made of glass or plastic, depending on the requirements of the medication.

Materials

- alcohol wipes
- two appropriate-sized needles and a syringe
- vial of medication
- bandage strips
- sharps container
- patient chart

Competency

(**Conditions**) With the necessary materials, you will (**Task**) withdraw a medication for injection from a vial (**Standards**) correctly within 15 minutes.

1. Wash your hands and gather the equipment.
2. Select the correct-size needle to withdraw the medication. Viscous medications require a greater needle gauge.
3. Check the vial label against the physician's medication order (Figure 27-15 ◆).
4. Remove the plastic cap from the vial if necessary. If the vial has already been used, wipe the rubber stopper with an alcohol wipe (Figure 27-16 ◆).
5. Inject air into the vial in an amount equal to the medication being removed.
   - Place the vial on a firm surface and insert the needle through the rubber stopper.
   - Inject air into the vial.
   - Invert the vial with the needle tip under the surface of the medication to avoid getting air into the syringe (Figure 27-17 ◆).
   - Pull back the plunger to withdraw the necessary amount of medication (Figure 27-18 ◆).
   - If air bubbles are present, tap firmly on the syringe to release the bubbles and reinject them into the vial (Figure 27-19 ◆).
   - Check the level of medication in the vial and withdraw more if needed.
   - Withdraw the needle from the vial and replace the cap.

6. Remove the needle and discard it in a sharps container.
7. Replace the needle with a sharp, sterile needle of appropriate size.
8. Inject the medication at the appropriate site.
9. Document the procedure. Include the date, time, medication, site, route, and amount administered. Follow office policy for recording the medication expiration date and lot number.

Patient Education

See Procedure 27-1.

Charting Example

02/22/XX 4:45 PM Patient received monthly injection of B12, cyanocobalamin crystalline, for anemia. Maintenance dose of 100mcg (1 mL) administered subcutaneously in the right ventrogluteal area. Patient was observed in the waiting area for 20 minutes and told to report any unusual effects immediately. Elaine Rodgers, RMA (AMI)

continued

PROCEDURE 27-4 **Demonstrate Withdrawing Medication from a Vial** (continued)

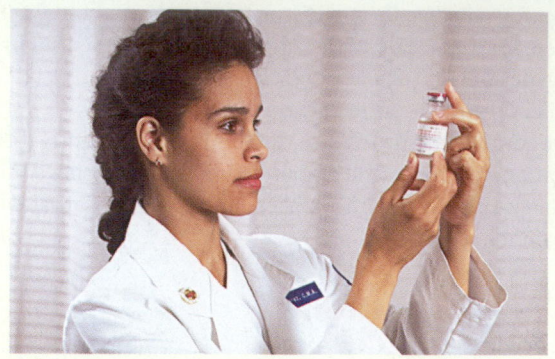

Figure 27-15 ◆ Check the vial against the physician's order.

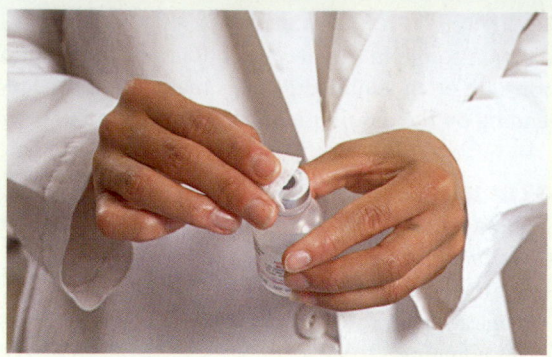

Figure 27-16 ◆ Wipe the rubber stopper with an alcohol wipe.

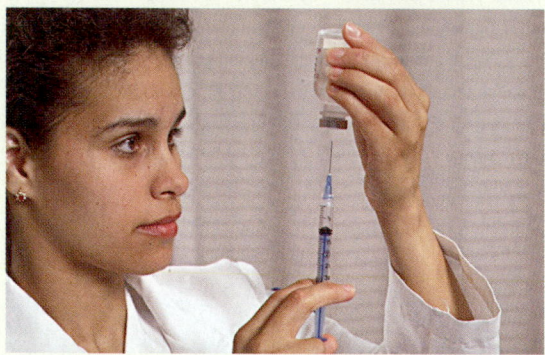

Figure 27-17 ◆ Invert the vial with the needle tip under the surface of the medication to avoid getting air into the syringe.

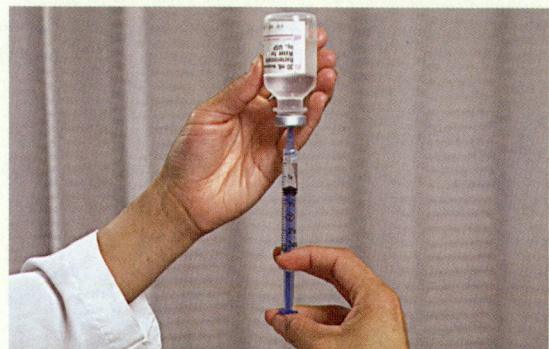

Figure 27-18 ◆ Pull back the plunger to withdraw the necessary amount of medication.

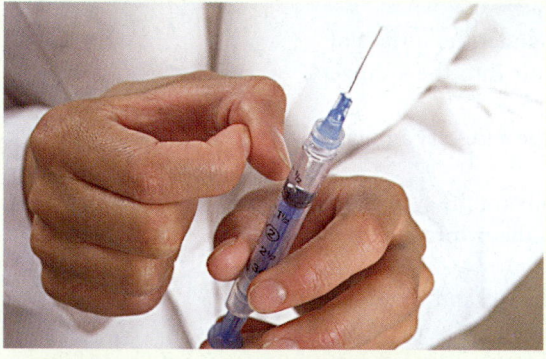

Figure 27-19 ◆ Tap firmly on the syringe to release air bubbles.

PROCEDURE 27-5 Demonstrate the Reconstitution of a Powdered Drug for Injection Administration

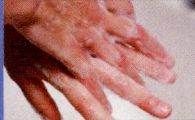

Theory and Rationale

When an injectable medication is supplied as a powder, it must first be reconstituted into liquid form, usually with a sterile diluent such as water or saline. A sterile water vial is cleaned and the correct amount is injected into the vial containing the powdered medication and mixed. It is important to read the inserts that come with powdered medications. Many of these medications have a rapid expiration time, beginning as soon as the powder is mixed into liquid form. When mixing the solution, gently roll the vial between the palms of your hands. Do not shake or jolt the container, which would cause bubbles to form in the solution.

Materials

- gloves
- alcohol wipes
- two appropriate-size syringes with needles
- vial of medication
- sterile water
- sharps container
- fine-tip permanent marker
- patient chart

Competency

(**Conditions**) With the necessary materials, you will be able to (**Task**) reconstitute a powdered medication for injection (**Standards**) correctly within 15 minutes.

1. Wash your hands and gather the equipment.
2. Check to make sure the medication matches the physician's order. Calculate the dosage if necessary. Look up information relating to the function of the medication, usual dosage, and side effects. Follow the six rights.
3. Check the medication label again against the physician's order to make sure it is the right medication.
4. Put on gloves.
5. Remove the protective tops from the diluent (sterile water) and medication and wipe both with alcohol.
6. Insert one needle into the diluent, making certain to inject an amount of air equal to the amount of solution you are removing. Withdraw the necessary amount of diluent.
7. Inject the diluent into the powdered medication vial.
8. Discard the used needle in the sharps container.
9. Roll the vial containing the diluent and powder between your palms. It may take several minutes to mix the solution thoroughly. Avoid shaking the vial.
10. If the medication will not be used immediately, label the vial with the date and time prepared, your initials, and the expiration date/time.
11. With the second needle, draw up the correct amount of prepared medication to give to the patient.
12. Remove your gloves and wash hands.
13. Document the procedure. Include the date, time, medication, site, route, and amount administered. Follow office policy for recording the medication expiration date and lot number.

Patient Education

See Procedure 27-1.

Charting Example

04/28/XX 2:45 PM Patient came in for her monthly injection of Xolair (Omalizumab) 375 mg to be administered by subcutaneous injection as determined by serum total IgE level and patient weight. Xolair chart consulted for appropriate dose assignment. Medication prepared per manufacturer administration guidelines. The medication was administered with a 25-gauge needle, subcutaneous injection. Patient is familiar with common side effects and was given the package insert for reference and instructed to call if any unusual effects should occur. David Johnson, RMA (AMI)

PROCEDURE 27-6 Demonstrate the Administration of Medication during Infusion Therapy

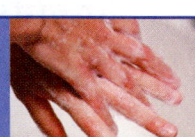

Theory and Rationale

Depending on state regulations, a CMA or RMA may be allowed to administer medication to a patient during IV therapy under the supervision of a registered nurse and/or physician. There are several methods for administering medication to a patient receiving infusion therapy. Medications may be added to the primary infusate container, although this is rarely done because pharmacists perform this function in the pharmacy under strict asepsis to ensure proper mixing and prevent the drug from infusing in the base of the container and being delivered as a bolus dose to the patient. The medication may also be administered directly into a vein that is not being used

continued

PROCEDURE 27-6 Demonstrate the Administration of Medication during Infusion Therapy *(continued)*

in the IV therapy. In the most common method, the medication is added through an injection port using the "S-A-S" method described below. Normal saline is injected into the cannula port to ensure the lock is clear ("S"). Then the medication is administered as prescribed by the physician into the cannula port ("A"), followed by more saline to ensure that the full amount of medication has cleared the lock ("S").

Materials

- three syringes with needles
- medication to be administered
- normal saline (0.9%) 4 mL
- alcohol wipes
- gloves
- sharps container
- patient chart
- artificial IV therapy arm, or vein block stimulator

Competency

(**Conditions**) With the necessary materials, you will be able to (**Task**) administer medication (**Standards**) through an intermittent infusion device correctly within 15 minutes.

1. Wash your hands and gather equipment.
2. Check to make sure the medication matches the physician's order. Calculate the dosage, if necessary. Look up information relating to the medication's function, usual doses, and side effects. Check for patient allergies by verifying in chart *and* asking the patient.
3. Check medication compatibility with the infusion product being used.
4. Put on gloves.
5. Disinfect the cannula port with the alcohol wipe.
6. Verify that the cannula and vein are freely open, with no blockages.
7. With the first of the three syringes, slowly inject 2 mL of the normal saline into the cannula port.
8. With the second syringe, administer the medication as prescribed by the physician into the cannula port.
9. With the final syringe, inject 2 mL of normal saline into the cannula port.
10. Remove the gloves and wash your hands.
11. Document the procedure. Include date, time, site, medication, route, and amount administered. Follow office policy for recording the expiration date and lot number.

Patient Education

Be prepared to explain side effects the patient should be alert for and report. Instruct the patient to report any sudden reactions to the medication, whether local or general.

Charting Example

04/18/XX 9:35 AM Injection of medication XXXXX given to patient via cannula port. Injections of 2 mL of normal saline used to ensure cleared lock before and after injection of medication. Infusion therapy continues in the cephalic vein above right dorsal venous arch. Patient reports that the vein is slightly "sore" but he reports he is in no significant pain. 2/10 on the pain scale. Sage Wade, RMA (AMT)

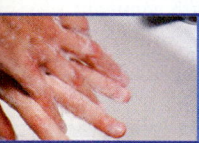

PROCEDURE 27-7 Demonstrate the Preparation and Administration of Oral Medication

Theory and Rationale

The preferred route for administering medications is the oral route. Oral medications can be self-administered by the patient at home. The oral route is used when rapid absorption is not necessary and the medication is not destroyed by the gastrointestinal tract before absorption. Patients are more compliant when their medications can be swallowed and can be scheduled around other activities of the day—for example, before or after meals or at bedtime. Patients are also more compliant because of the relatively low cost of oral medications compared to that of other types of medication.

Medications packaged in single-use containers can be checked three times per standard routine and returned to storage if for some reason the medication is not used or the package has not been opened. Medications prepared as stock medications must be poured from the original container according to the prescribed dosage. Whether you are pouring tablets, pills, capsules, liquids, or suspensions, be careful to avoid contaminating the bottle against the container for the patient. Maintaining a small distance between the containers while pouring prevents contamination and enables the continued clean storage of the medication for later use by other patients. Some liquid suspensions separate during storage and must be shaken gently until thoroughly mixed to ensure an accurate dosage of all components. When pouring any liquid medication, hold the container with the palm covering the label. This action will prevent spills or drips from making the label illegible for future use.

PROCEDURE 27-7 **Demonstrate the Preparation and Administration of Oral Medication** (continued)

Materials
- vial of medication
- gloves
- patient chart

Competency
(**Conditions**) With the necessary materials, you will be able to (**Task**) administer oral medication (**Standards**) correctly within 15 minutes.

1. Wash your hands and gather equipment.
2. Put on gloves.
3. Check to make sure the medication matches the physician's order. Calculate the dosage, if necessary. Look up information relating to the medication's function, usual doses, and side effects. Check for patient allergies by asking patient and verifying in the chart. Always follow the six rights of medication administration.
4. Check the medication label a second time against the physician's order.
5. Identify the patient and escort him to the treatment area.
6. Pour the correct amount of medication.
   - *For pills, capsules, and tablets:* Pour the correct amount from the container directly into a medicine cup.
   - *For liquids and suspensions:* If the ingredients are not evenly mixed, shake the bottle gently but thoroughly. Allow time for any bubbles to disappear. When pouring, hold the medication bottle with your palm over the label and hold the medicine cup at eye level.
7. Check a third time to match the medication against the physician's order.
8. If at any time you have doubts about the function of the medication, the dosage or route of administration, or the possibility of an allergic reaction, *immediately* consult the physician.
9. Give the medicine cup to the patient. Have drinking water available for pills, capsules, and tablets, as well as for liquids or suspensions, if necessary.
10. Observe as the patient takes the medication to ensure that it is swallowed completely, without difficulty.
11. Dispose of the used medication cup and preparation supplies. Remove your gloves and wash your hands. Return the multiple-use medication bottle to the storage shelf.
12. Document the procedure. Include date, time, site, medication, route, and amount administered. Follow office policy for recording the expiration date and lot number.

Patient Education
If office policy or potential side effects dictate that the patient wait in the reception area for a specified period of time, explain the reasons for the waiting period. Be prepared to explain side effects the patient should be alert for and report. Instruct the patient to report any sudden reactions to the medication, whether local or general. Make sure the patient has a ride home if necessary.

Charting Example
04/18/XX 9:35 AM Tylenol #3, two tablets given as ordered by mouth for lt. knee pain. Patient denies any allergy to the Tylenol or codeine components of the medication. Appointment made for follow-up X-ray of left knee upon arrival at the hospital X-ray department because of lingering pain and inability to use non-prescription pain medications. Julia Sanchez, CMA (AAMA)

The intravenous administration of medications or solutions may be per unit dosage or may be continuous. Examples of unit dosage are bolus, IV push, or scheduled intermittent administration by heparin lock or piggyback medication into an IV port. An example of continuous dosage is an IV drip that may last several hours or around the clock. The flow rate of intravenous lines is regulated by a flow clamp or infusion pump.

Intravenous administration requires extra knowledge and precautions because of the direct access to the bloodstream. Adverse reactions, which can be fatal, may be caused by the specific medication, too many fluids administered too rapidly into the body, violation of any of the medication rights of administration, or certain pre-existing medical conditions. Nonfatal reactions include necrosis of tissue (sometimes a reaction to chemotherapy) or swelling or infiltration through the blood vessel into the tissue, obstructing IV flow. Any office in which IV fluid therapy is performed must have emergency equipment, emergency medical access, and established office policies for routine administration, dealing with adverse reactions, and the handling of emergencies. The patient and the infusion site must be assessed regularly during the infusion for signs of adverse reactions.

Starting an IV requires preparation. Before an intravenous site is chosen, tubing is selected and connected to the correct solution container, following sterile technique. The tubing is flushed to remove all air. Tape and dressing supplies for the site must also be prepared beforehand. A preparation tray with appropriate IV starter materials and the prepared IV is taken to the patient. An intravenous pole is used to hang the IV solution on.

The intravenous site and the appropriate size and type of catheter are selected. The IV is generally started in the arm, although different medical scenarios may require other sites. The intravenous catheter includes an outer cannula to thread into the vein and an inner needle to serve as a guide for insertion and then to be removed. A constricting tourniquet is placed above the site. The skin is cleansed and the catheter is

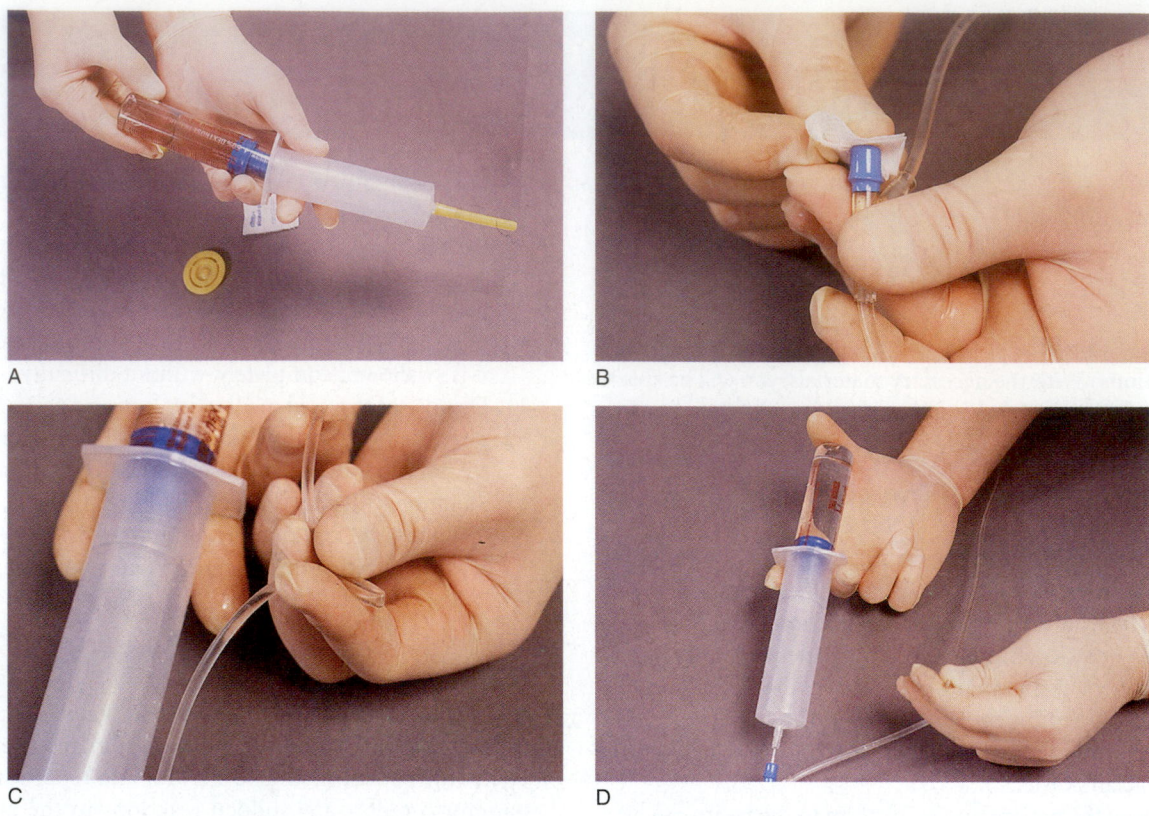

Figure 27-20 ◆ IV setup and initiation: (A) Prepare the drug; (B) Clean the administration port; (C) Pinch the line; (D) Administer the drug.

introduced into the vein to obtain an open blood supply. The tourniquet is released and removed. The plastic cannula is advanced into the vein and the needle is removed. To reduce the patient's anxiety, it is important to mention that the needle has been removed and that only the plastic cannula remains. As soon as the needle is removed and blood supply has been established, the site is anchored with tape, the IV tubing is connected, and dressing of the site is completed. The IV is regulated with flow clamps or IV pump as prescribed by the physician. Gloves are worn during the procedure as part of standard precautions. All needles and biohazard materials are disposed according to office policy and OSHA standard precautions. Figure 27-20 ◆ illustrates the setting up and initiating of an IV.

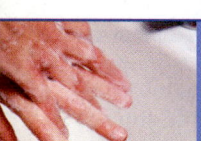

PROCEDURE 27-8 Demonstrate the Administration of a Subcutaneous Injection

Theory and Rationale

When a medication is administered by subcutaneous injection, it is absorbed quickly into the bloodstream. Sites for this injection are the outer upper arm, the scapular area of the back, the abdomen, and the anterior thigh. The scapular area is generally used by clinical staff because it is too hard for the patient to reach. A syringe that can hold 2 ml of solution and a needle that is 25 to 27 gauge and 5/8 inch long are used. Before the medication is injected, aspiration is performed to determine if the needle is within a blood vessel. If there is no blood in the syringe when aspiration is performed, the medication is administered. Medication injected when blood is aspirated would be detrimental to the patient because the medication would be administered directly into the bloodstream, with overly rapid, adverse effects.

Materials

- gloves
- alcohol wipes
- syringe with needle
- vial or ampule of medication
- Bandage strip(s)
- sharps container
- patient chart

PROCEDURE 27-8   Demonstrate the Administration of a Subcutaneous Injection *(continued)*

Competency

(**Conditions**) With the necessary materials, you will be able to (**Task**) administer a subcutaneous injection (**Standards**) correctly within 15 minutes.

1. Wash your hands and gather the equipment.
2. Check to make sure the medication matches the physician's order. Calculate dosage if necessary. Look up information relating to the function of the medication, usual dosage, and side effects. Always follow the six rights to medication administration.
3. Check the medication label again against the physician's order to make sure it is the right medication.
4. Identify the patient and escort to treatment area. Verify the patient's allergies by asking the patient and checking the chart.
5. Select the subcutaneous site. Put on gloves.
6. Loosen the cap of the needle so that you can drop it on the counter just before you withdraw medication from the ampule or vial. Cleanse the skin site with an alcohol wipe and allow it to thoroughly air-dry.
7. Withdraw the correct amount of medication. If necessary, cover the needle by the slide cap method. Otherwise, if the patient is nearby, do *not* recap the needle.
8. Check a third time to match the medication against the physician's order.
9. If you have any doubts, consult the physician immediately before administering the medication. If you must leave the room, bring the medication with you.
10. Grasp the skin immediately surrounding the injection site with your nondominant hand (Figure 27-21 ◆).
11. Quickly insert the needle at a 45-degree angle. Hold the barrel of the syringe with your nondominant hand and pull (aspirate) the plunger with your dominant hand. If no blood appears in the syringe barrel, move your nondominant hand to the skin position and hold the syringe with your dominant hand. Push the plunger down with your index finger.
12. Withdraw the needle and blot the area gently with an alcohol wipe. Discard the syringe into the sharps container. Apply a bandage strip to protect the patient's clothing.
13. Remove the gloves and wash your hands.
14. Document the procedure. Include the date, time, medication, site, route, and amount administered. Follow office policy for recording the medication expiration date and lot number.

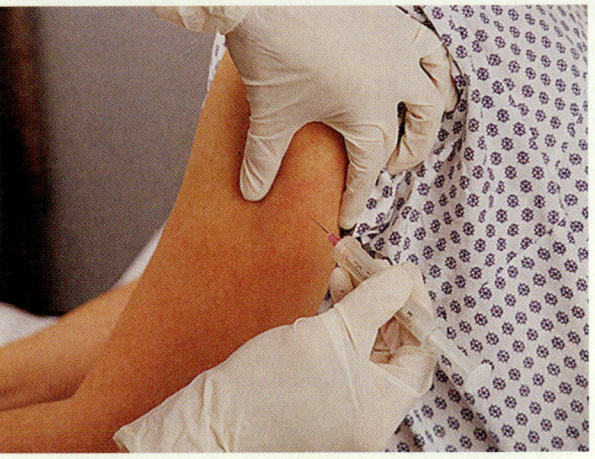

Figure 27-21 ◆ Grasp the skin immediately surrounding the injection site with your nondominant hand.

Patient Education

See Procedure 27-1.

Charting Example

03/28/XX 2:45 PM Regular insulin (20 units given) subcutaneous as ordered by the physician into rt. arm, directly above tricep muscle, for a blood sugar of 180. Patient has been diabetic for five years and states knowledge of low blood sugar symptoms. Pt instructed to report to laboratory for fasting glucose and glucose tolerance testing at 7 AM at the hospital outpatient area. Patient states awareness of nothing to eat or drink past midnight for the blood testing. Dwayne Lincoln, RMA (AMT)

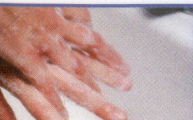

PROCEDURE 27-9 Demonstrate the Administration of an Intramuscular Injection to Adults and Children

Theory and Rationale

Medication administered by intramuscular injection is gradually absorbed into the bloodstream. Sites are the deltoid, vastus lateralis of the thigh, dorsogluteal, and ventral gluteal muscles. Although all these sites may be used for adults, the vastus lateralis is used in children under 3 years old. The dorsogluteal site is not used until after the child has been walking for at least one year.

Syringe and needle size are different for adults and children.

■ For adults, injections of 2 to 5 ml can be given, although any dose 4 ml or above should be divided and administered as two injections. Needle size should be 22 gauge and 1 to 1-1/2 inches long, depending on the size of the patient. The needle gauge may have to be larger (smaller number) when more viscous medications are administered.

■ For young children, the medication amount should not exceed 1 ml because of the size of the vastus lateralis muscle. The needle size for an infant injection should be 25 gauge and one inch long, but may vary according to the size of the child and the viscosity of the medication.

As with a subcutaneous injection, aspiration is performed before an intramuscular injection is performed to determine if the needle has entered a blood vessel. If you are giving a medication injection to a child, there are additional forms that must be filled out prior to the administration of the medication. A consent form must be signed and a medication information form including common side effects, and pros and cons of the medication must be given to the parent for review.

Materials

■ gloves
■ alcohol wipes
■ syringe with needle
■ vial or ampule of medication
■ bandage strips
■ sharps container
■ patient chart

Competency

(**Conditions**) With the necessary materials, you will be able to (**Task**) administer an intramuscular injection to an adult or child (**Standards**) correctly within 15 minutes.

1. Wash your hands and gather the equipment.
2. Check to make sure the medication matches the physician's order. Calculate dosage if necessary. Look up information relating to the function of the medication, usual dosage, and side effects. Always follow the six rights to medication administration.
3. Check the medication label again against the physician's order to make sure it is the right medication.
4. Identify the patient and escort to treatment area. Ask parents to identify the child patient.
5. Select the intramuscular site. Put on the gloves.
6. Loosen the cap of the needle so that you can drop it on the counter just before you withdraw medication from the ampule or vial. Cleanse the skin site with an alcohol wipe and allow it to thoroughly air-dry.
7. Follow the procedure for withdrawing medication from a vial or ampule. Withdraw the correct amount. If necessary, cover the needle by the slide cap method. Otherwise, do *not* recap the needle.
8. Check a third time to match the medication against the physician's order.
9. If you have any doubts, consult the physician immediately before administering the medication.

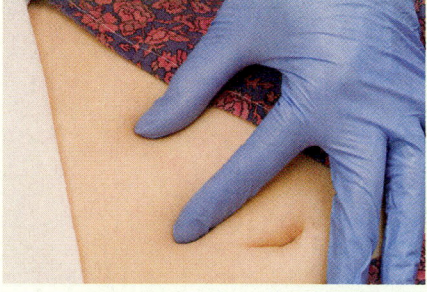

Figure 27-22 ◆ Stretch the skin with your nondominant hand.

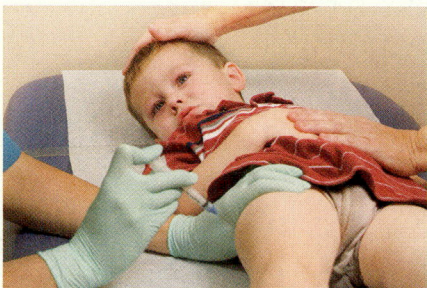

Figure 27-23 ◆ For a small child, grasp the upper outer quadrant area of the vastus lateralis muscle.

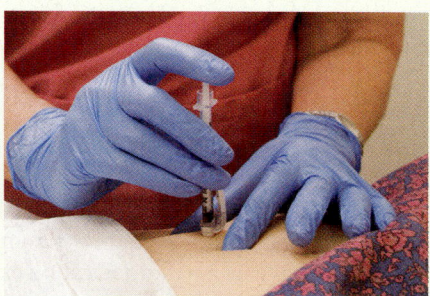

Figure 27-24 ◆ Push the plunger down with your index finger.

PROCEDURE 27-9 Demonstrate the Administration of an Intramuscular Injection to Adults and Children *(continued)*

10. Lightly stretch the skin immediately surrounding the injection site with your nondominant hand (Figure 27-22 ◆). For a small child, ask another clinical staff person to hold the child, then grasp the upper outer quadrant area of the vastus lateralis muscle (Figure 27-23 ◆).

11. Quickly but lightly thrust the needle at a 90-degree (perpendicular) angle. Hold the barrel of the syringe with your nondominant hand and with your dominant hand pull (aspirate) the plunger. If no blood appears in the syringe barrel, move your nondominant hand to the skin position and hold the syringe with your dominant hand. Push the plunger down with your index finger (Figure 27-24 ◆).

12. Withdraw the needle and apply pressure with an alcohol wipe. Massage the muscle unless contraindicated. Discard the syringe into the sharps container. Apply a bandage strip to protect the patient's clothing.

13. Remove the gloves and wash your hands.

14. Document the procedure. Include the date, time, medication, site, route, and amount administered. Follow office policy for recording the medication expiration date and lot number.

Patient Education
See Procedure 27-1.

Charting Example
10/13/XX 2:43 PM Demerol 50 mg given into rt. dorsogluteal site as ordered by physician for complaints of severe pain. Patient and significant other state awareness that patient is not to drive for 24 hours. Patient and significant other have been instructed to seek continued emergency room evaluation for potential hospital admission for kidney stones. At time of discharge, additional written instructions given to significant other for kidney stone diagnosis and treatment. Janet Wahl, RMA (AMT)

PROCEDURE 27-10 Demonstrate the Administration of a Z-Track Injection

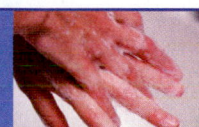

Theory and Rationale
The Z-track method, a type of intramuscular injection, is used when medication should not leak into subcutaneous tissues, when total intramuscular absorption of the medication is required, or when medication would discolor the tissue. The dorsogluteal site is preferred for the Z-track method, although the ventral gluteal and vastus lateralis sites may be also used. The medication is drawn into the syringe with 0.2 to 0.4 ml of air. When the injection is given, the additional air allows the medication to fully clear the needle and enter the muscle tissue. The needle should be 22 gauge and 1-1/2 to 2 inches long. The needle gauge may be larger (smaller number) if the medication is viscous. The skin is pulled laterally before the needle is inserted. When the needle is removed, a Z-track is left that allows the subcutaneous tissue to cover the muscular injection site.

Medications administered by this method include Vistaril, iron dextran, gamma globulin, antibiotics, narcotics, estrogen and testosterone, Procaine, and Imferon.

Materials
- gloves
- alcohol wipes
- tuberculin syringe with needle
- vial of medication
- bandage strips
- sharps container
- patient chart

Competency
(**Conditions**) With the necessary materials, you will be able to (**Task**) administer a Z-track injection (**Standards**) correctly within 15 minutes.

1. Wash your hands and gather the equipment.
2. Identify the patient and escort to the treatment area.
3. Select the appropriate intramuscular site. Put on the gloves.
4. Cleanse the skin with an alcohol wipe and allow to thoroughly air-dry.
5. Cleanse the top of the medication vial with an alcohol wipe and allow to air-dry. Withdraw the correct dosage from the vial and hold the syringe in your dominant hand.
6. With your nondominant hand, pull the skin laterally toward the side opposite the site (Figure 27-25 ◆).

continued

PROCEDURE 27-10 Demonstrate the Administration of a Z-Track Injection *(continued)*

7. Quickly but lightly thrust the needle into the site at a 90-degree (perpendicular) angle. While still holding the skin away from the needle site, inject the medication and wait for 10 seconds (Figure 27-26 ◆).
8. After 10 seconds, quickly withdraw the needle and allow the skin to track back over the original injection site.
9. Blot the area gently with an alcohol wipe. Discard the syringe into the sharps container. Apply a bandage strip to protect the patient's clothing.
10. Do not massage the injection site.
11. Document the procedure. Include the date, time, medication, site, route, and amount administered. Follow office policy for recording the medication expiration date and lot number.

Patient Education

See Procedure 27-1.

Charting Example

03/27/XX 2:40 PM 2 ml of Vistaril given via Z-track injection per office procedure into the left dorsogluteal area. Patient and significant other state awareness that patient is not to drive for 24 hours. Patient and significant other have been instructed to seek continued emergency room evaluation if discussed potential side effects occur. Anthony Laden, CMA (AAMA)

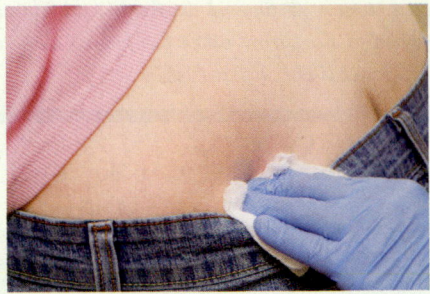

Figure 27-25 ◆ Pull the skin laterally toward the opposite side of the site.

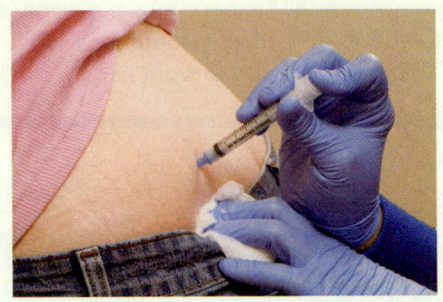

Figure 27-26 ◆ Inject the medication.

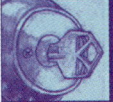

Keys to Success
LOW-INCOME PATIENTS AND THE COST OF MEDICATIONS

People with limited or fixed incomes often face the dilemma of deciding between paying for basic necessities such as food and heat and purchasing prescription drugs. Some lower-income patients choose to take intermittent or split dosages to make the medication last longer. Often the result is a decline in the patient's condition. Many people have turned to foreign sources, such as Canada or Mexico, for prescription medications at a reduced cost. However, drugs from outside the United States are not subject to FDA standards.

The medical community, including medical offices, hospitals, and clinics, provides some assistance through complimentary drug samples left by pharmaceutical sales representatives. The medical office may refer patients to free clinics, social service agencies, community trustees, or pharmaceutical programs. Recent Medicare reform includes a provision for prescription coverage to ease the financial burden of the elderly and chronically disabled.

REVIEW

Chapter Summary

- Pharmacology is a study of drugs and their effects on the human body. It focuses on the chemical structure of a drug, the chemical action within the body, the therapeutic effects of treatment, and potential side effects.

- A medical assistant's responsibilities in the physician's office include reading medication orders, ordering prescriptions, administering medications, using reference resources, recognizing side effects, and providing patient instruction.

- Drug absorption, distribution, metabolism, and excretion are factors that affect the biological and chemical reactions of medications within the body. Other factors, such as the patient's present state of health, medical conditions, and age, also require consideration before the physician prescribes medication.

- Drugs perform five basic functions: therapeutic, diagnostic, curative, replacement, and preventive.

- Drugs can be obtained with a physician's prescription or without prescription (over-the-counter). It is important to obtain information from the patient about nonprescription and prescription medications to prevent potential drug interactions.

- Drug classifications include (but are not limited to) the following categories.
  - Analgesics—relieve pain
  - Anesthetic medications—decrease or eliminate sensation or pain
  - Antianxiety medications—for emotional, behavior, or sleep deprivation or for treatment of seizures
  - Antiinflammatory drugs—decrease inflammation
  - Cardiovascular drugs—treat various heart and circulatory conditions
  - Gastrointestinal medications—treat conditions of the esophagus, stomach, small and large intestines
  - Anti-infectives—treat various system and organ infections
  - Respiratory medications—treat upper and lower, acute and chronic lung conditions
  - Endocrine drugs—replace or control hormones and hormonal reactions
  - Urinary system drugs—increase urine output, treat urinary infections and other kidney and bladder conditions

- Controlled substances, or schedule drugs, have a higher potential for abuse, and are classified into five categories by the Federal Controlled Substances Act. All schedule drugs are prescribed, administered, and monitored according to strict legal requirements.

- Every drug has three names: a chemical name, a generic name, and a trade name. The *Physician's Desk Reference* and the *U.S. Pharmacopeia and National Formulary* are important resources for information about drugs.

- The physician's prescription functions to communicate to the pharmacist the name and amount of the prescribed drug, directions for dispensing, instructions to the patient, the number of refills, and permission to use generic forms of the medication. Prescription pads must be kept in a secure, locked location.

- To eliminate the possibility of medication errors, it is important to follow the safety guidelines for administration ("six rights"): right patient, right drug, right dose, right route, right time, and right documentation.

- Metric, apothecary, and household measurement systems are used in the administration of medication. The metric system is used most often. Conversion equivalents can be used to convert one system to another when the medication order does not match the concentration of the medication available. The medical assistant must be able to use conversion tables and calculate dosages.

- Medications for oral routes of administration are available as liquids or solids. Other routes of administration include suppositories, dermatological, and parenteral routes.

- Needle gauge (size) and length are determined by the type and amount of medication to be administered. The type of medication administered results in immediate (intravenous), time-controlled (subcutaneous, intramuscular), or skin reaction (intradermal) absorption.

- The intravenous route is used primarily to replenish fluids, electrolytes, and blood products, but may also be used to administer medications. Intravenous medications may be administered only by designated licensed personnel.

Chapter Review

Multiple Choice

1. The effect of a drug other than the intended therapeutic effect is known as a
   a. toxic effect.
   b. side effect.
   c. therapeutic effect.
   d. pharmacology effect.

2. The time and process whereby a drug reaches the cells and produces the desired action is known as
   a. reception.
   b. distribution.
   c. elimination.
   d. absorption.

Chapter Review (continued)

3. The circulation of an absorbed drug throughout the body is called
   a. metabolism.
   b. distribution.
   c. absorption.
   d. reception.

4. Drugs that treat and relieve symptoms in a disease process are
   a. curative.
   b. diagnostic.
   c. therapeutic.
   d. preventive.

5. Drugs prescribed to improve a patient's quality of life by intervening in the disease process are
   a. curative.
   b. therapeutic.
   c. diagnostic.
   d. prophylactic.

6. Common OTC drugs include all of the following except
   a. Aleve.
   b. Pepcid AC.
   c. Claritin.
   d. Visteril.

7. Which common medication is not produced synthetically today?
   a. Salicylates
   b. Penicillin
   c. Digoxin
   d. Bovine insulin

8. Which of the following is not a neurotransmitter responsible for activities in the ANS?
   a. Acetylcholine
   b. Epinephrine
   c. Norepinephrine
   d. Adrenergic agonists

9. Which of the following drugs help restore heart rhythm to normal?
   a. Antiarrhythmic
   b. Glycosides
   c. Anticoagulants
   d. Hemostatic agents

10. Which drug is used to treat shock?
    a. Vasodilator
    b. Antihypertensive
    c. Vasoconstrictor
    d. Cardiac glycosides

True/False

T F 1. Anti-inflammatory drugs may be corticosteroids or NSAIDs.

T F 2. Glycosides are administered to quicken the heart rate of patients with congestive heart failure.

T F 3. Thrombolytics dissolve existing blood clots but do not restore blood flow.

T F 4. Hemostatic drugs are used to control bleeding and hemorrhage.

T F 5. A laxative is considered a gastrointestinal drug.

T F 6. A vasodilator dilates vessels to control arterial spasms but has no effect on angina.

T F 7. Anti-infective agents are used to prevent infections caused by bacteria, viruses, and parasites.

T F 8. Drugs with potential for abuse are identified by the DEA, which is controlled by the CSA.

T F 9. Schedule I drugs include Ritalin, narcotics, barbiturates, and other drugs with a high potential for abuse.

T F 10. If a physician signs the Rx line "Substitute generic medication," the patient can still state he or she would like brand-name medications only.

Short Answer

1. Name four sources from which drugs can be derived.

2. What is the difference between analgesic and anesthetic drugs?

3. What is the function of thrombolytic drugs?

Research

1. Your patient cannot remember the name of the medication she is taking but knows the shape and color and says she would recognize it if she saw it or heard the name. She has no idea what the medication does for her. How can you verify what medication she is taking?

2. A patient states that every time he gets an antibiotic for an infection he "saves" some of the pills for future use. What can happen to the pathogen that causes the infection if the antibiotic is not taken at the prescribed strength for the correct duration of treatment?

Externship Application Experience

The physician has asked you to write a prescription for 25 mcg of Synthroid, "dispense 30." You write it for 25 mg of Synthroid. What are the possible implications if this error is not caught by the pharmacist? What is your response when the pharmacist calls the physician to report the error?

Resource Guide

Drug Enforcement Administration
Office of Diversion Control
2401 Jefferson Davis Highway
Alexandria, VA 22301
1-800-882-9539
www.dea.gov

Medline Plus
National Library of Medicine
National Institutes of Health
www.nlm.nih.gov/druginformation.html

Pharmacy Times
241 Forsgate Drive
Jamesburg, NJ 08831
www.pharmacytimes.com

RX List: The Internet Drug Index
www.rxlist.com/top200.htm

U.S. Pharmacopeia
12601 Twinbrook Parkway
Rockville, MD 20852
1-800-822-8772
www.usp.org

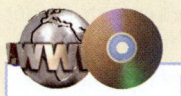

Med**Media**

http://www.MyMAKit.com

More on this chapter, including interactive resources, can be found on the Student CD-ROM accompanying this textbook and on http://www.MyMAKit.com.

CHAPTER 28

Vital Signs

Case Study

Chelsea has been working with Dr. Sevigney, a pulmonologist, for only a few weeks. Recently, while taking a patient's blood pressure, she was uncertain about what she was hearing. Chelsea first heard the blood pressure in the right arm at 130/110. Then she measured the blood pressure in the left arm and heard two distinct blood pressure starts and stops. She heard the first blood pressure sounds at 160/140 and then at 130/110 in the same arm.

Objectives

After completing this chapter, you should be able to:

- Define and spell the key terminology for this chapter.
- Define the medical assistant's role in the initial clinical visit.
- Explain the principles of vital signs and state normal values for various age groups.
- Explain the significance of changes in body temperature.
- Define *pulse* and explain the factors that affect pulse rates.
- Discuss the importance of respirations in patient assessment.
- Discuss blood pressure and its role in patient assessment.
- Describe the five phases of Korotkoff sounds.
- Explain the significance of weight and height measurements in a patient's health status.
- Explain the medical assistant's role in patient preparation, including gowning, positioning, and draping.
- Describe the methods of assessment used during a medical examination.
- Explain the ways in which the medical assistant assists the physician during the medical examination.
- Discuss the medical assistant's role during recurrent clinical visits.

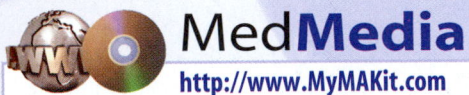

Med**Media**
http://www.MyMAKit.com

Additional interactive resources and activities for this chapter can be found on http://www.MyMAKit.com. For videos, tips, audio glossary, legal and ethical scenarios, job scenarios, quizzes, games, and virtual tours related to the content of this chapter, please access the accompanying CD-ROM in this book.

Audio Glossary
Legal and Ethical Scenario: *Vital Signs*
On the Job Scenario: *Vital Signs*
Videos: *Exam Room Preparation; Vital Signs*
Multiple Choice Quiz
Games: Crossword, Strikeout and Spelling Bee
3D Virtual Tour: Lungs; Cardiovascular System: Heart; Ear: The Ear
Tips
HIPAA Quiz

✚ MEDICAL ASSISTING STANDARDS

CAAHEP ENTRY-LEVEL STANDARDS	ABHES ENTRY-LEVEL COMPETENCIES
■ Perform within scope of practice (psychomotor) ■ Apply ethical behaviors, including honesty/integrity in performance of medical assisting practice (affective) ■ Explore issue of confidentiality as it applies to the medical assistant (cognitive) ■ Explain the rationale for performance of a procedure to a patient (affective) ■ Perform handwashing (psychomotor) ■ Assist physician with patient care (psychomotor) ■ Document accurately in the patient record (psychomotor) ■ Obtain vital signs (psychomotor) ■ Identify nonverbal communication (cognitive) ■ Identify styles and types of verbal communication (cognitive) ■ Explain general office policies (psychomotor) ■ Apply active listening skills (affective) ■ Use language/verbal skills that enable patients' understanding (affective)	■ Prepare and maintain examination and treatment area. ■ Apply principles of aseptic techniques and infection control. ■ Take vital signs. ■ Prepare patient for and assist with routine and specialty examinations. ■ Dispose of biohazardous materials. ■ Practice Standard Precautions. ■ Determine needs for documentation and reporting. ■ Document accurately. ■ Operate and maintain facilities and equipment safely. ■ Orient patient to office policies and procedures.

✔ COMPETENCY SKILLS PERFORMANCE

1. Obtain an oral temperature with an electronic digital thermometer.
2. Obtain an axillary temperature with an electronic digital thermometer.
3. Obtain a rectal temperature with an electronic digital thermometer.
4. Obtain an aural temperature with a tympanic thermometer.
5. Obtain a dermal temperature with a disposable thermometer.
6. Perform a radial pulse count.
7. Perform an apical pulse count.
8. Perform a respiration count.
9. Perform a blood pressure measurement.
10. Obtain weight and height measurements.
11. Demonstrate patient positions used in medical examinations.
12. Prepare the patient for medical examination and assist the physician.

Introduction

The medical assistant plays an integral role in assisting the physician and caring for the patient. The physician needs basic information about the patient to make an informed diagnosis. The patient history and vital signs provide the physician with an initial picture of the patient's general health status. This information establishes a baseline for future comparison of health status and an assessment of treatments. Medical assistants assist during the physical examination by providing the physician with assessment equipment and supplies, by positioning and draping the patient to facilitate a thorough examination, and by performing and documenting vital signs.

Key Terminology

accommodation—the adjustment of the lens of the eye to various distances

anthropometry—the science of size, proportion, weight, and height.

apical—at the apex of the heart

aural—pertaining to the ear

auscultation—listening to various areas of the body

axillary—under the arm

blood pressure—pressure the blood exerts on the vessel walls as a result of the pumping action of the heart

conduction—heat transfer by direct contact through fluids, solids, or other substances

convection—heat transfer by air

diaphoresis—profuse sweating

diastole—the relaxation phase of the heart muscle; lowest reading of the blood pressure

expiration—exhalation of carbon dioxide by physical or therapeutic means

hypertension—elevated blood pressure

hypotension—below-normal blood pressure

inspection—visual examination of both the external surface of the body and the interior portions of body cavities

inspiration—inhalation of atmosphere air or oxygen by physical or therapeutic means

malignant hypertension—rapidly developing, severe elevation of blood pressure, often fatal

mensuration—measurement

oral—by mouth

palpation—examination involving touch; examiner uses the hands and fingers to feel both the surface of the body (for abnormalities or irregularities) and various organs (for size, location, and tenderness) and feel generally for masses or lumps and assessing the texture and temperature of the tissue

percussion—examination consisting of tapping the fingertips lightly but sharply against the body to assess the size and location of underlying organs

pulse—the regular, palpable beat of the arteries caused by the contractions of the heart

radial—at the wrist over the radial artery

Key Terminology *(continued)*

rhythm—time interval between pulses or breaths

sublingually—under the tongue

systole—the contraction phase of the heart; highest reading of the blood pressure

temperature—measurement of body heat produced and lost during metabolism,

respiration, elimination, and environmental fluctuation

turgor—normal appearance of the skin and its ability to return to normal after being pinched

vital signs—signs that measure the patient's general state of health, include temperature, pulse, respirations, and blood pressure

Abbreviations

BPM—beats per minute

CV—cardiovascular

TPR—temperature, pulse, respirations

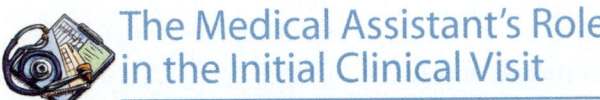

The Medical Assistant's Role in the Initial Clinical Visit

The medical assistant working in the clinical area of the medical office has many responsibilities in patient assessment. Before the physician begins the examination, a thorough patient history is essential. (Refer to ∞ Chapter 24 for information on taking a patient history.) As the MA records the history and obtains vital signs, she will use observational skills to assess the patient's general condition, including cooperation, skin condition, alertness, level of consciousness, and apparent presence of pain.

Vital signs include temperature, pulse, respirations, and blood pressure. Height and weight measurements are two important measurements that may also be taken by the MA during the initial clinical visit. These measurements are called anthropometric measurements, since they relate to **anthropometry**, which is the science of size, proportion, weight, and height. A visual and auditory examination may also be required as part of the assessment. After vital signs and a patient history have been taken, the MA will prepare the patient for the physical examination by gowning, draping, and positioning. The MA may also assist the physician during the examination and when it is completed, will assist the patient to dress, then prepare the room for the next patient.

Vital Signs Measurement

Vital signs measure the patient's general state of health and include temperature, pulse, respirations, and blood pressure (**TPR** and BP). TPR and BP, along with weight and height, are usually measured and recorded at each visit. The physician compares these findings to normal ranges to help determine a diagnosis, prognosis, and course of treatment for the patient. Vital signs are also taken during the course of treatment to evaluate the patient's reaction to any procedure or medication.

Temperature

Temperature is the measurement of body heat produced and lost during metabolism, respiration, elimination, and environmental fluctuation. Changes in a patient's body temperature may be an indication of a change in health status or illness.

The temperature is regulated by several organs and processes.

- In the hypothalamus, various mechanisms regulate heat production and loss.
- In the metabolic process, glucose from food is oxidized in body cells, producing heat. This heat is distributed throughout the body by the blood and blood vessels.
- As blood vessels pass near the body's surface, heat is lost through the skin by **conduction**, **convection**, radiation, and evaporation of perspiration.
- Heat is lost through respiration and the elimination of urine and feces.

Taking the Temperature

Body temperature is measured by either the Fahrenheit or Celsius scale (Table 28-1). It may be assessed in different ways, according to the patient's age and physical status.

- The **oral** method of temperature measurement is most commonly used. The thermometer probe is placed under

TABLE 28-1 TEMPERATURE CONVERSION

- To convert Celsius to Fahrenheit:
  Fahrenheit degrees = (Celsius degrees × 9/5) + 32
- To convert Fahrenheit to Celsius:
  Celsius degrees = (Fahrenheit degrees − 32) × 5/9
  Examples of Celsius and Fahrenheit readings in degrees:

Celsius (C)	Fahrenheit (F)
35.0	95.0
35.5	95.9
36.0	96.8
36.5	97.7
37.0	98.6 (normal oral)
37.5	99.5
38.0	100.4
38.5	101.3
39.0	102.2
39.5	103.1
40.0	104.0
40.5	104.9
41.0	105.8

the tongue until the reading is obtained. The patient must be alert, cooperative, and cognizant of the process.

- For patients who are unconscious, uncooperative, or too young, a digital thermometer probe may be placed in the **axillary** space under the arm or in the rectum. The axillary temperature is considered less accurate because the thermometer has less direct contact with the body's blood circulation (skin instead of mucous membranes).
- **Aural** thermometers read the temperature of the tympanic membrane. Dermal devices measure the temperature of the skin.
- Mercury thermometers are still used in some facilities; however, many states have passed laws that limit or prevent new production of mercury-containing equipment along with more stringent standards for disposal.
- A newcomer on the thermometer scene is the alcohol thermometer. It is calibrated like a mercury thermometer and works on the same principle.

Normal temperatures vary according to the method used to obtain them (Table 28-2). An **oral** temperature of 98.6 degrees F (Fahrenheit) or 37 degrees C (Celsius) is considered normal. A rectal temperature is considered normal at 99.6 degrees F or 37.6 degrees C. A normal axillary temperature is

TABLE 28-2 NORMAL TEMPERATURE RANGES (FAHRENHEIT)

Routes	Normal Ranges
Oral	97.6–99.6
Rectal	98.6–100.6
Axillary	96.6–98.6
Tympanic	similar to rectal range

97.6 degrees F or 36.4 degrees C. Historically, the oral temperature reading has been considered the baseline for normal at 98.6 degrees F. Rectal temperature readings are usually a degree warmer because of the internal environment of the rectum. Axillary temperatures are usually considered a degree lower than oral temperatures because the axilla is more exposed to air.

Rectal temperatures are considered the most accurate; however, particularly with small children, there is a risk of perforating the rectal wall with the thermometer. At present, rectal temperatures are rarely taken in medical offices or hospitals. Many pediatricians prefer to have patients' temperatures obtained by the axillary or aural method.

Many factors influence changes in body temperature. An elevated temperature may occur as a result of bacterial infection, increased food intake, physical activity, exposure to heat, metabolism-raising drugs, pregnancy, stress, or emotional reactions. Some women experience a slight increase in body temperature during ovulation. Age is a variable as well; an infant's or young child's body temperature may be one or two degrees higher than that of adults.

There are several kinds of abnormally elevated temperature, or fever:

- *Continuous:* Body temperature remains fairly constant and above the patient's normal baseline
- *Remittent:* Fluctuating body temperature remains above normal
- *Intermittent:* Fluctuating body temperature returns to normal, then rises again
- *Relapsing:* Fever returns after an interval of several days of normal temperature

Lowered body temperatures may result from viral infections, fasting, decreased muscular activity, exposure to cold, metabolism-lowering drugs, depression, hemorrhage, dehydration, and severe central nervous system insults. In the elderly, decreased metabolic and physical activity lowers the body temperature.

Time of day is another factor. The temperature is usually at its lowest early in the day, following rest, and during decreased activity and sleep. Muscular and metabolic activity throughout the day usually raises the body temperature, which reaches its peak in the evening.

In Practice

Mrs. Gonzalez calls the office to schedule an appointment because she believes that her 15-month-old daughter has a fever. She tells the medical assistant that she took her daughter's temperature using a rectal thermometer and the temperature was 100.6 degrees F. Her husband came home and took the child's temperature using an aural thermometer and he said that the child's temperature is only 98.6 degrees F and is normal. What should the medical assistant tell the mother about the differences in temperature readings? Should the medical assistant schedule the child for an appointment?

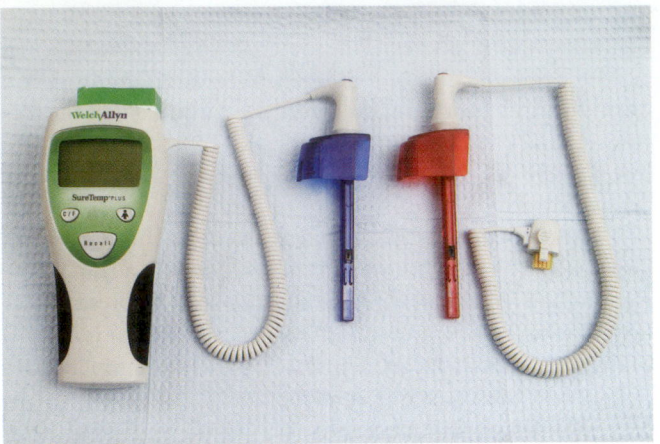

Figure 28-1 ◆ Electronic thermometers come with two different probes; one for oral and axillary routes and the other for the rectal route.

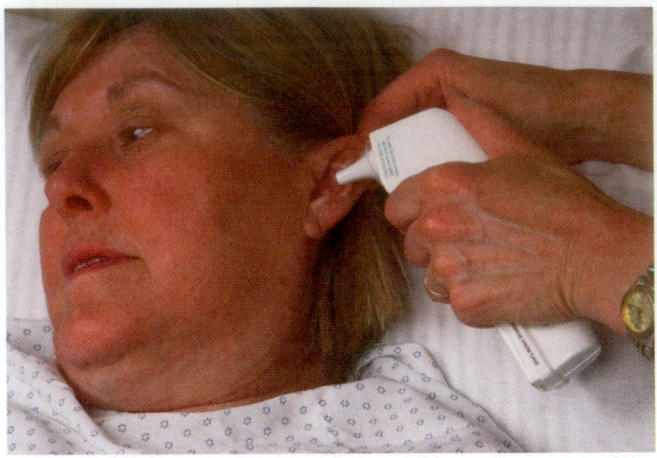

Figure 28-2 ◆ Position client so ear canal is easily seen and pull pinna back and up.

Thermometers

Thermometers are used to measure body temperature.

- The traditional glass thermometer contains mercury, which expands and elevates in the column as it warms. There are glass thermometers for oral, rectal, and axillary routes. The thermometer used to take oral and axillary temperature has a slender, longer bulb, while the thermometer designed for rectal use has a short, round bulb. Both types are marked with both Fahrenheit and Celsius calibrations, and elevations are usually marked in red. Traditional mercury thermometers are no longer recommended for use in the medical setting, because the biohazards of mercury outweigh any of its benefits. Some professionals are also questioning the safety of glass thermometers now that alternative methods are readily available. Alcohol thermometers, like mercury thermometers, may be placed under the tongue, under the arm, or in the rectum.

- Battery-operated electronic thermometers allow a much more rapid reading. They come with two different probes, one for oral and axillary routes and the other for the rectal route, as well as disposable covers for the probes (Figure 28-1 ◆).

- Aural thermometers come with either a disposable or reusable ear speculum and give a reading within 3 seconds (Figure 28-2 ◆).

Pulse

The **pulse** is the regular, palpable beat of the arteries caused by the contractions of the heart. It is an indication of the pressure

---

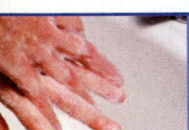

PROCEDURE 28-1 **Obtain an Oral Temperature with an Electronic Digital Thermometer**

Theory and Rationale

Before taking the temperature, ask the patient if he or she has smoked or had any hot or cold liquids immediately before coming to the medical office. Taking a temperature under those conditions could yield inaccurate results. Install a cover on the electronic thermometer probe to allow multiple patient uses and prevent cross-contamination. Place the thermometer **sublingually** next to the frenulum linguae. Heat transferred by conduction from the blood supply under the tongue to the thermometer is measured as the patient's temperature.

Instruct the patient to keep the mouth closed while taking an oral temperature. Breathing through the mouth may transfer heat by convection and result in an altered temperature. The thermometer should remain in place until beeping indicates that the temperature has been measured.

You must remain in the room while an oral temperature is taken. You may need to help the patient hold the thermometer in the correct position in the mouth. If you are not doing that, you can count the radial pulse and respirations while waiting for the temperature to register.

Materials

- electronic digital thermometer
- thermometer probe covers
- watch with second hand (for pulse and respiration count)
- examination gloves

Competency

(**Conditions**) With the necessary supplies, (**Task**) you will be able to measure oral temperature (**Standards**) accurately and in the time designated by the instructor.

1. Identify the patient, escort to the examination room, and offer a place to sit on a chair or the examination table.

PROCEDURE 28-1 Obtain an Oral Temperature with an Electronic Digital Thermometer *(continued)*

2. Wash your hands and apply gloves.
3. Ask the patient if he or she has had hot or cold drinks or food or smoked a cigarette within the last 10 minutes. If so, wait 10 minutes. If not, proceed with taking the oral temperature.
4. Remove the electronic thermometer from its charge base and place a cover on the probe (Figure 28-3 ◆).
5. Place the probe under the tongue near the frenulum linguae. Instruct the patient to close the mouth around the thermometer.
6. Explain to the patient that the thermometer will need to stay in place until the beep sounds. You may count pulse and respirations now (see Procedures 28-6 through 28-8) or after the temperature is taken.
7. When the beep sounds, remove the thermometer from the patient's mouth, note the temperature, and discard the probe cover in a waste receptacle (Figure 28-4 ◆).
8. Remove the gloves and wash your hands. Return the thermometer to its charge base (Figure 28-5 ◆).
9. Record the temperature, pulse, and respirations in the appropriate place on the chart. Return the thermometer to its designated storage location.

Patient Education

Remind the patient that cold or hot substances that have been in the mouth shortly before the temperature is measured will affect the accuracy of the temperature. It is also important for the patient to hold the thermometer in the "pocket" on either side of the frenulum linguae.

Charting Example

10/11/XX 10:45 AM T 98.6°F, P 76, regular and strong, R 20. Patient states purpose of visit is for annual physical. Taylor Furber, RMA (AMT)

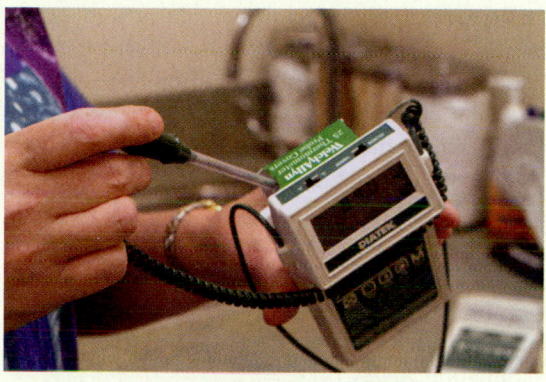

Figure 28-3 ◆ Place a cover on the probe.

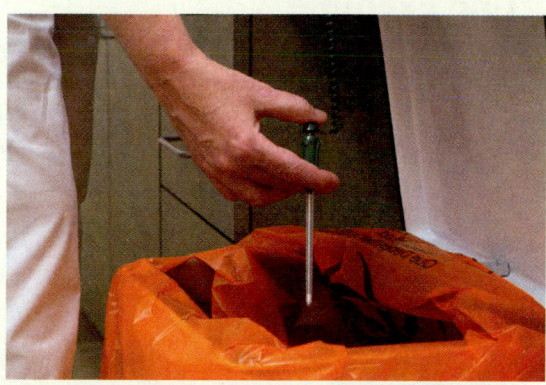

Figure 28-4 ◆ Discard the probe cover.

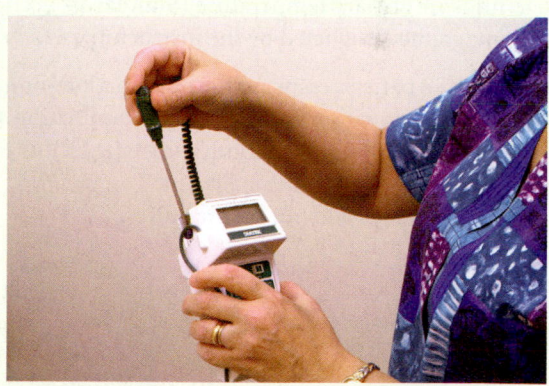

Figure 28-5 ◆ Return the thermometer to its charge base.

PROCEDURE 28-2 Obtain an Axillary Temperature with an Electronic Digital Thermometer

Theory and Rationale

The axillary method of taking the temperature is recommended for mouth-breathing patients or for patients who have had oral surgery, trauma, or inflammation. It is also recommended for infants, toddlers, and preschoolers who are too young to hold the thermometer in their mouths. Parents can hold a sick child close and provide comfort while an axillary temperature is taken.

It may be necessary to remove clothing from the arm and shoulder area to allow correct placement of an axillary thermometer. Because diaphoresis may affect the measurement, the area should be gently patted dry. Rubbing the area to dry it stimulates local skin circulation, which may in turn raise the temperature. Once the thermometer is placed in the center of the axilla, in direct contact with the skin, the patient lowers the arm to the side and brings the forearm against the chest. This position reduces air currents to the thermometer.

Materials

- electronic digital thermometer
- thermometer probe cover
- watch with second hand (for pulse and respiration count)
- examination gloves

Competency

(**Conditions**) With the necessary supplies, (**Task**) you will be able to measure axillary temperature (**Standards**) accurately in the time frame designated by the instructor.

1. Identify the patient, escort to the examination room, and offer a place to sit on a chair or the examination table. Have the patient either unbutton or take off his or her shirt to allow access to the axilla.
2. Wash your hands and put on the gloves.

3. Observe the axillary area for dryness or **diaphoresis**. Pat the area dry with a washcloth or towel if it is diaphoretic.
4. Remove the electronic thermometer from its charge base and place a cover on the probe.
5. Ask the patient to raise an arm. Place the thermometer in direct contact with the skin of the axilla and have the patient lower the arm against the side of the chest (Figure 28-6 ◆). Explain that the thermometer will need to stay in place until the beep sounds. You may count pulse and respirations now or after the temperature is taken.
6. When the beep sounds, remove the thermometer and discard the probe cover in a waste receptacle.
7. Remove the gloves and wash your hands. Return the thermometer to its charge base.
8. Record the temperature (Figure 28-7 ◆), pulse, and respirations in the appropriate place on the chart. Write "A" after the temperature to indicate that the axillary route was used.
9. Return the thermometer to its designated storage location.

Patient Education

Inform the patient that the underarm must be dry and that the arm should be held against the side and chest for an accurate reading. Patients who take their own temperature at home should always report the route to the medical office staff because an axillary temperature is considered one degree higher than an oral temperature.

Charting Example

10/11/XX 11:00 AM T 101.4°F A, P 110. Unable to obtain respirations due to fussiness of 6-month-old. Mom states child has been fussy on and off for two days. Takes formula when Motrin brings fever down. Has had fever for one day. Philip Romo, CMA (AAMA)

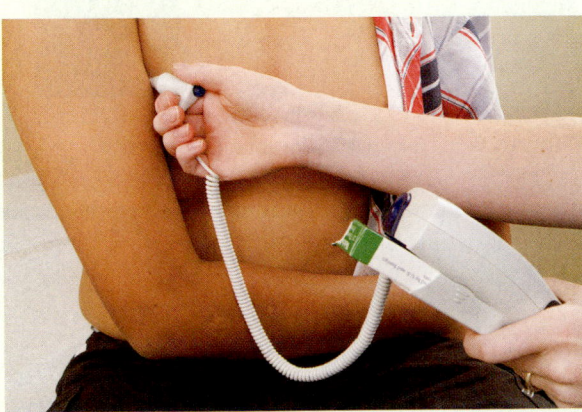

Figure 28-6 ◆ Place the thermometer in direct contact with the skin of the axilla.

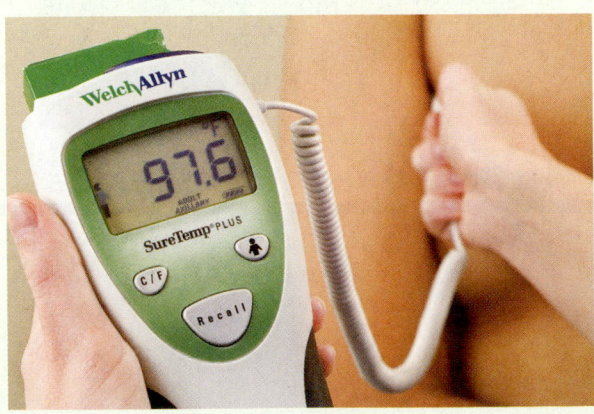

Figure 28-7 ◆ Record the temperature.

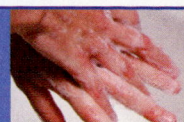

PROCEDURE 28-3 Obtain a Rectal Temperature with an Electronic Digital Thermometer

Theory and Rationale

The rectal temperature is considered more accurate than both oral and axillary temperatures because the thermometer is in direct contact with mucous membranes rather than potentially exposed to the air. With the advent of the tympanic thermometer, this method is rarely used today, especially in the physician office. However, it can be used with unconscious patients, mouth-breathing patients, and small children. There may be a safety concern with patients who cannot lie still during the taking of a rectal temperature. The distal end of the thermometer probe stem must be held throughout the procedure. To avoid perforating the bowel, do *not* insert the thermometer if there is any possibility of an obstruction.

Safety note: Prepare equipment and place it in reaching proximity before positioning the patient. A young, old, or seriously ill patient may be at risk for falling from the examination table and should *not* be left in position before or during the procedure.

Materials

- electronic digital rectal thermometer and probe covers
- lubricant and tissue
- examination gloves

Competency

(**Conditions**) With the necessary supplies, (**Task**) you will be able to measure rectal temperature (**Standards**) accurately in the time designated by the instructor.

1. Identify the patient and escort to the examination room. Assist the patient in removing clothing from the waist down. Keeping the patient draped, assist him or her into a left side-lying position (Sim's position) on the examination table. Drape for exposure of the buttocks only.
2. Wash your hands and apply gloves.
3. Remove the electronic thermometer from its charge base and place a cover on the probe.
4. Place a small amount of lubricant on a tissue next to the patient. Dip the tip of the probe cover in the lubricant.
5. Inform the patient of procedure before you insert the rectal probe. For an adult, insert the lubricated probe cover approximately 1-1/2 inches into the anus (Figure 28-8 ◆). For an infant, insert it 1/4 to 1/2 inch, and for a child, 1/2 to 1 inch.

6. Hold the thermometer in place until it beeps. Remove the thermometer and discard the probe cover in a waste receptacle.
7. Remove the gloves and wash your hands. Return the thermometer to its charge base.
8. Record the temperature in the appropriate place on the chart. Write an "R" after the measurement to indicate the rectal route.
9. Return the thermometer to its designated storage location.

Patient Education

Rectal temperatures are taken only when the patient's medical condition dictates and with controls for safety concerns. Assure the patient that you will hold the rectal thermometer during the procedure.

Charting Example

11/13/XX 1330 T 102.6° R, P 100, R 40. Temperature taken rectally because patient had breathing difficulty and extreme diaphoresis. The head of examination table was raised about 30 degrees during the procedure. After temperature completed, patient was assisted to sitting position for remainder of office visit. McKenzie Adams, RMA (AMT)

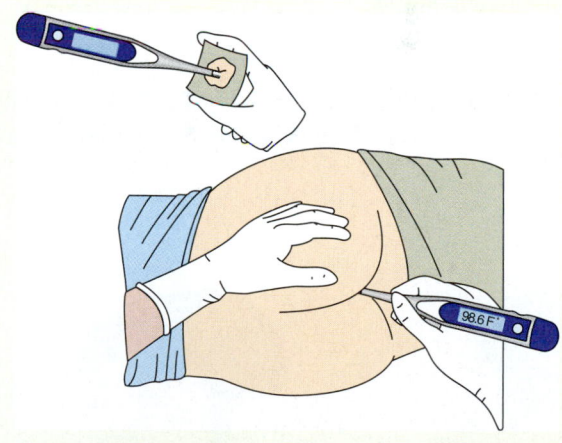

Figure 28-8 ◆ Insert the probe cover approximately 1-1/2 inches into the anus.

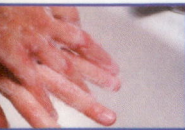

PROCEDURE 28-4 Obtain an Aural Temperature with a Tympanic Thermometer

Theory and Rationale

Aural temperatures with an electronic tympanic thermometer are taken when a rapid temperature reading is needed and the patient's comfort is an issue. This method works well with pediatric patients. The parent or other family member can hug the child snugly and hold the child's head while the medical assistant takes the aural temperature.

The tympanic or aural thermometer measures the temperature of the warmth within the ear canal and the tympanic membrane with infrared light. The tympanic membrane reflects the central core temperature of the body and provides readings close to the temperature of the pulmonary artery. The tympanic thermometer is considered an accurate alternative to the mercury thermometer.

Because of the anatomical differences in the ear canal between the adult and the infant or child, the canal must be positioned differently to obtain the most accurate aural temperature. With an adult, gently pull the outer ear upward. With an infant or child, pull the outer ear downward. With your other hand insert the tympanic thermometer to obtain the reading. As the thermometer is inserted, the ear canal is closed to air currents that would affect the accuracy of the aural temperature.

Materials

- tympanic thermometer and probe covers
- examination gloves

Competency

(**Conditions**) With procedure materials, (**Task**) you will be able to perform an aural temperatures (**Standards**) accurately, according to the patient's age, within the time designated by the instructor.

1. Identify the patient, escort to the examination room, and offer a place to sit on a chair or the examination table. If the patient is a child, encourage the parent to sit and hold the child.
2. Wash your hands and apply the gloves.
3. Explain the basic procedure to the patient or parent. Assess whether the patient has had an aural temperature before. Depending on the patient's age and previous experience or knowledge of the procedure, you may need to assure him or her that the procedure is painless or demonstrate on the parent before taking a child's temperature.
4. Remove the tympanic thermometer from its charge base and place a cover on the probe.
5. For an adult, pull the outer ear in an upward direction. For a child or infant, pull the outer ear in a downward direction.
6. With your hand insert the probe-covered earpiece of the thermometer into the ear canal and press the scan button to obtain the temperature reading (Figure 28-9 ◆).
7. When the thermometer beeps, withdraw it from the patient's ear and pop the probe cover into the waste receptacle. Read the temperature reading in the thermometer's display window (Figure 28-10 ◆).
8. Remove the gloves and wash your hands. Return the thermometer to its charge base.
9. Record the temperature on the patient's chart, followed by a "T" to indicate tympanic temperature.
10. Return the tympanic thermometer to its designated storage location.

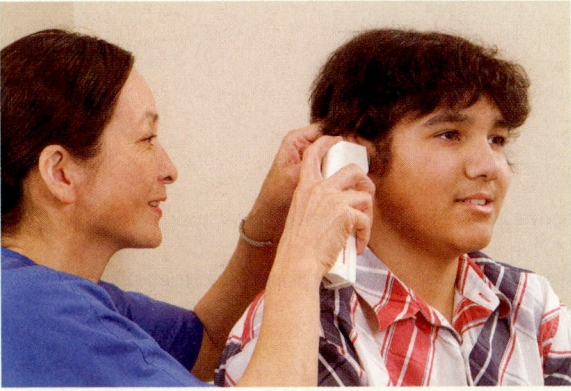

Figure 28-9 ◆ Insert the probe-covered earpiece of the thermometer into the ear canal.

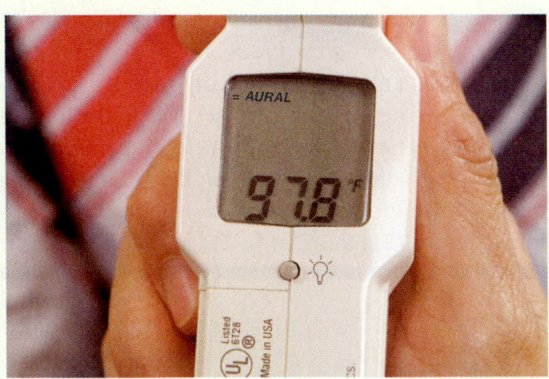

Figure 28-10 ◆ Read the temperature in the display window.

PROCEDURE 28-4 Obtain an Aural Temperature with a Tympanic Thermometer (continued)

Patient Education

Explain to the patient or parent the reason for pulling the outer ear upward for the adult patient or downward for the infant or child. Emphasize that a different probe cover should be used each time for the same person or for different persons within the same household to prevent the reintroduction of microorganisms.

Charting Example

10/23/XX 0935 AM Mother brings child to office. Child has runny nose, which mom states has been present for one week. Mother states that child has had on and off fever for three days and appetite has decreased. Aural temperature obtained, 97.8°F Wallace Banks, CMA (AAMA)

PROCEDURE 28-5 Obtain a Dermal Temperature with a Disposable Thermometer

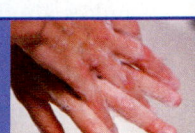

Theory and Rationale

Chemical thermometers can be either oral or dermal. Both types are single-use and consist of chemical reactant dots or tape that respond to heat by changing color. Chemical thermometers are generally used only in the home. Although they are not considered as accurate as other thermometers, they do provide a general assessment of the patient's temperature patterns.

Like electronic thermometers, disposable oral thermometers are placed under the tongue and left in place for about 60 seconds. Dermal thermometers are disposable strips that are held on the forehead for about 15 seconds. For both types, the last color change is the temperature reading.

Because these thermometers react chemically to heat and to the heat generated by light, they should be stored in a cool, dark place. Unwrap and handle them carefully to avoid touching the chemical dots.

Materials

- disposable dermal strips
- clean, dry washcloth
- examination gloves

Competency

(**Conditions**) With the necessary supplies, (**Task**) you will be able to measure dermal temperature (**Standards**) accurately in the time designated by the instructor.

1. Identify the patient, escort to the examination room, and offer a place to sit on a chair or the examination table.
2. Wash your hands and apply gloves.

3. Observe the forehead for dryness or diaphoresis. Pat the area dry with a washcloth if it is diaphoretic.
4. Carefully unwrap the dermal strip without touching the chemical dots and place it on the forehead.
5. Leave the strip on the forehead for the length of time recommended by the manufacturer, usually about 15 seconds.
6. After noting the temperature of the last color-changed dot, remove and dispose of the dermal thermometer in a waste receptacle.
7. Remove the gloves and wash your hands.
8. Record the temperature on the patient's chart, followed by the word "dermal."

Patient Education

Instruct the patient or parent to avoid touching the chemical dots because the temperature reading could be affected. Reinforce that the last dot affected indicates the temperature. The same procedure should be followed whenever the temperature is taken so that temperatures can effectively be compared. Patting the forehead dry allows the dermal temperature strip to stick for the required time.

Charting Example

11/11/XX 11:00 AM T 101.4 dermal, P 110. Unable to obtain respirations due to fussiness of 6-month-old. Temperature has been as high as 102 last midnight. Mother states infant has had three watery stools and has taken only 4 ounces of formula since midnight. Patricia Davis, RMA (AMT)

exerted by the blood flow during the contraction (systole) phase of the heartbeat. Assessing the patient's pulse provides a rapid picture of the heart's pumping action, including rate, rhythm, and volume. It is also an indicator of the patient's response to treatments and medications as well as general cardiac status.

A normal heart beats 60 to 100 times a minute, or **BPM** (beats per minute). Table 28-3 lists normal pulse ranges. The **rhythm** is regular and is normally felt as strong. Deviations are called *arrhythmias* and are often indicative of underlying cardiac conditions (refer to ∞ Chapter 35 for a discussion of cardiac arrhythmias).

In a medical office the most common site for obtaining a pulse is the **radial** artery in the wrist (radial pulse). Other sites where a pulse may be palpated include the brachial, temporal, facial, carotid, pedal, popliteal, and femoral sites (Figure 28-11 ◆). The carotid and femoral pulses are used to assess cardiac function in a critically ill adult patient, and the brachial site is used in a critically ill infant or child.

An **apical** pulse is the pulse or heartbeat heard through a stethoscope at the apex of the heart. The apical pulse is counted for a full 60 seconds and is the most accurate assessment of the heartbeat. Apical pulses are usually taken on infants, individuals taking certain heart medications, and patients who are critically ill.

Occasionally an apical-radial pulse rate may be required. The preferred method involves one practitioner taking the apical pulse and another taking the radial pulse at the same time. The person timing the minute usually lifts a finger to indicate when to begin counting, then lowers the finger when the minute has elapsed. Any difference in the pulse rates obtained is termed a *pulse deficit*.

Volume, or the pressure of the blood against the arterial walls, may range from normal, strong, or bounding to weak, feeble, or thready. The volume felt by the fingertips provides a general assessment of the strength or weakness of cardiac muscle effort during the contraction phase of the heartbeat. Factors affecting the strength of the heartbeat include the amount of blood in the **CV** system (which may be influenced by dehydration), the forcefulness of the heart contraction, and the condition of the arterial walls. Further assessment of volume may be made by the appropriate professional.

It is possible to assess both the rate and rhythm of the heartbeat with the pulse. The rate is the beats per minute.

![Points on the human body where pulse may be taken with labels: Carotid, Apical, Brachial, Ulnar, Radial, Femoral, Popliteal, Posterior Tibia, Dorsalis Pedis]

Figure 28-11 ◆ Points on the human body where pulse may be taken.

Rhythm is defined by the regularity or irregularity of the pulsation felt by fingertips or sounds heard with the stethoscope and is an indicator of cardiac condition. Many factors affect rate and rhythm (Table 28-4).

Respirations

Oxygen is necessary for life. The body breathes oxygen in and exhales carbon dioxide. Respiration, the act of breathing, includes inspiration and expiration (see Figure 36-1, the respiratory system, on p. 772). **Inspiration** is the inhalation of atmospheric air or oxygen by physical or therapeutic means.

TABLE 28-3 AVERAGE PULSE RANGES BY AGE	
Newborns	130–160 BPM
Infants	110–130 BPM
Children 1–7 years	80–120 BPM
Children over 7 years	80–90 BPM
Adults	60–80 BPM
Elderly adults	50–70 BPM

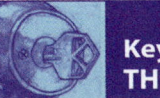

Keys to Success
THE PATIENT ON DIGITALIS

When teaching a patient who is taking digitalis how to take an apical pulse, emphasize that the pulse should be counted for one full minute to ensure accuracy. The pulse should be measured prior to the administration or ingestion of the digitalis.

TABLE 28-4 FACTORS THAT AFFECT HEART RATE AND RHYTHM

Age	Infants and children normally have a more rapid heartbeat than adults. It is not unusual for a newborn to have a heart rate of 160 BPM. Likewise, it may be normal for an elderly individual to have a heart rate of 50–60 BPM.
Gender	Females tend to have a faster heartbeat than males, usually by about 10 BPM.
Exercise/physical activity	Since increased activity requires more oxygen and nutrition to be delivered to the cells, the heart rate temporarily increases 20–30 BPM to accommodate for the greater need.
Size	Larger individuals usually have a slower heartbeat than smaller persons.
Physical condition	People who exercise vigorously and regularly tend to have heartbeats that are slower than normal. It is not unusual for an individual who runs on a regular basis to have a heartbeat in the range of 48–56 BPM.
Medications	Medications may either raise or lower the heart rate. Drugs that raise the heart rate include stimulants (caffeine), sympathetic agents (epinephrine, albuterol, terbutaline), and ACE inhibitors. Drugs that slow the heart rate include cardiac glycosides (digitalis), beta blockers (propanolol and atenolol), and parasympathetic drugs. Refer to ∞ Chapter 27 for drugs that affect the heart rate.
Presence of disease or illness	The raised metabolic rate of an individual experiencing illness or disease usually causes the heart to beat faster.
Anxiety, fear, anger	Any highly emotional state that causes an increase in sympathetic nervous system activity tends to raise the heart rate.
Depression	Depressed individuals tend to have a slower heart rate.
Increased intracranial pressure	This lowers the heart rate.
Thyroid disease	Hypothyroidism slows the heart rate. Hyperthyroidism causes a rapid heartbeat.
Shock	Shock speeds up the heart rate as the body attempts to compensate for dilated blood vessels.

PROCEDURE 28-6 Perform a Radial Pulse Count

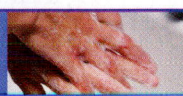

Theory and Rationale

Taking a baseline pulse is important for monitoring changes in the patient's condition. The radial pulse is measured at a resting rate. Ask the patient about activity levels and smoking, which may increase the pulse rate above the baseline resting rate. Use only your fingertips when taking the pulse. If you use your thumb, you are likely to feel your own pulse as well as that of the patient. Do not apply too much pressure when palpating for the radial pulse, as you may close off the artery and the pulse will not be palpable.

Materials

■ watch with second hand

Competency

(**Conditions**) With the necessary supplies, (**Task**) you will be able to perform a radial pulse count (**Standards**) accurately within the time frame designated by the instructor.

1. The patient has been identified, escorted to the examination room, and offered a place to sit on a chair or the examination table.
2. Wash your hands (unless you have already done so prior to taking the temperature).
3. Explain the procedure to the patient (unless you have already done so prior to taking the temperature). Do *not* mention that you will be counting respirations after taking the pulse.
4. Position the patient's arm at about heart level, with the palm facing down. Identify the radial artery with the three middle fingertips by feeling pulsation through the arterial wall (Figure 28-12 ◆).

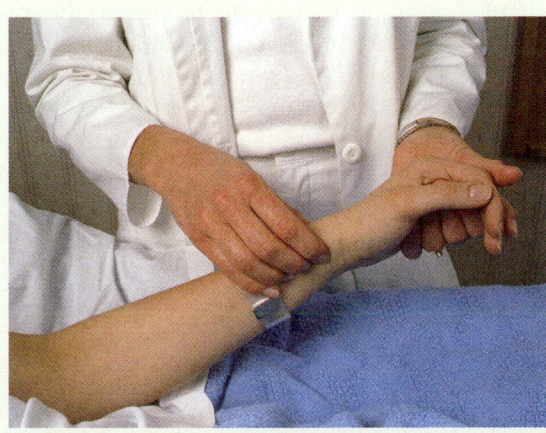

Figure 28-12 ◆ Obtaining a radial pulse count.

continued

PROCEDURE 28-6 Perform a Radial Pulse Count *(continued)*

5. Palpate for the pulsation of the radial artery on the inside of the wrist below the thumb. Note the strength and rhythm of the pulse. Do *not* palpate the pulse with your thumb.

6. Looking at your watch, start counting the pulse beats when the second hand is at 3, 6, 9, or 12. Count for one full minute.

   While still holding the wrist, observe the patient's respiratory efforts and count as instructed in Procedure 28-8.

7. Document the rate, strength, and rhythm of the pulse on the chart.

8. Wash your hands.

Patient Education

Teach the patient or significant other to feel for the radial artery with the fingertips rather than the thumb. The pulse should be counted for one full minute, and the strength, rhythm, and rate should be noted. Ask the patient or significant other to demonstrate how to take the radial pulse. Make sure the patient or significant other realizes that learning to perform a radial pulse may be challenging for some and easy for others. Be supportive and encouraging. Secondary arrangements may have to be made for monitoring the pulse. The patient or significant other should keep a record of daily pulse counts to show the physician at each visit.

Charting Example

11/15/XX 1425 Patient has been placed on digoxin for irregular heartbeat. She has seen video on taking pulse and has demonstrated correctly with fingertips how to take her own pulse. Patient verbalizes she will call the doctor's office if her pulse rate is less than 60 before she takes her medicine. Andrea Thomson, CMA (AAMA)

PROCEDURE 28-7 Perform an Apical Pulse Count

Theory and Rationale

An apical pulse is usually taken when the patient is on heart medication for an irregular or weak pulse or an abnormal heart rate. The apical pulse is also taken on babies and critically ill patients.

The apical pulse is most audible at the apex of the heart and can be found at the fifth intercostal space below the midclavicular line. Count five rib spaces down from where the ribs join the sternum. In that intercostal space, imagine a line drawn down from the middle of the clavicle at the top of the left shoulder. The apex of the heart is anatomically just below the left nipple.

Before counting the apical pulse, wipe the earpieces and diaphragm of the stethoscope to prevent the transfer of microorganisms to the staff or the patient. If the chestpiece of the stethoscope (the part containing the diaphragm and bell) is cold, hold it in your hands for a short period. Placing a cold chestpiece on the patient may speed up the heartbeat from its normal resting state. If a second person is measuring the radial pulse at the same time, use one watch to count both. The person with the watch should indicate when the counting starts and stops to help ensure the accuracy of the pulse deficit.

Materials
■ stethoscope
■ alcohol prep
■ watch with a second hand

Competency

(**Conditions**) With the necessary supplies, (**Task**) you will be able to perform an apical pulse count (**Standards**) accurately within the time frame designated by the instructor.

1. The patient has already been identified, and you have washed your hands to obtain vital signs.

2. Explain the procedure to the patient. Do *not* mention that you will be counting respirations after you have noted the apical pulse.

3. Wipe the stethoscope earpieces with the alcohol prep. With the earpieces pointed toward the nose, place the stethoscope earpieces in your ears Place the bell or diaphragm on the patient's chest in the area of the apex of the heart (Figure 28-13 ◆).

4. Begin counting heartbeats (each "lub-dub" counts as one heartbeat) when the second hand of the watch is at 3, 6, 9, or 12.

5. Count for one full minute. Note the quality and regularity of the heartbeat.

6. Chart the rate, rhythm, and any other pertinent information. If the radial pulse is also documented, write "RP" before the radial pulse rate and "AP" before the apical pulse rate.

PROCEDURE 28-7　Perform an Apical Pulse Count *(continued)*

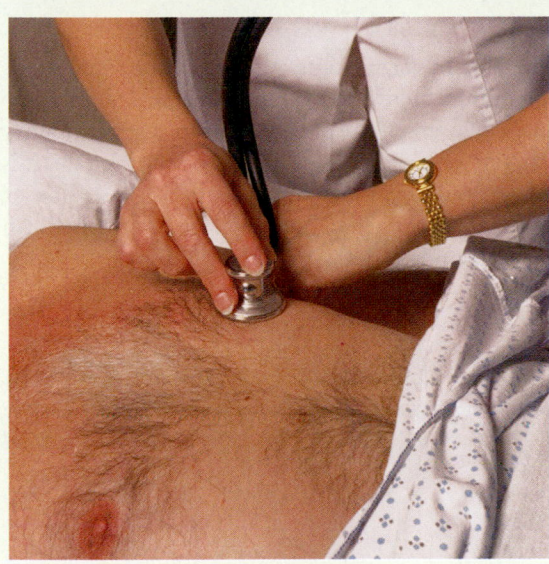

Figure 28-13 ◆ Place the bell or diaphragm on the patient's chest.

Patient Education

Instruct patients that the apical pulse and the different sounds of the heart often give the physician important medical information. The patient and/or family should keep a record of the daily apical pulse to show the physician at each visit.

Charting Example

10/23/XX 2 PM 55-year-old male patient is visiting physician because of recent frequent episodes of chest pain and SOB that are relieved by periods of rest. T 98.6°F, RP 90, AP 110, R 24. Thomas Medley, RMA (AMT)

Expiration is the exhalation of carbon dioxide by physical or therapeutic means. For most people the act of breathing is an "autonomic" body function that does not require thought. However, it is controlled by the medulla oblongata of the brain, the diaphragm, and acid-base balance factors. Due to the process of acute or chronic illness, some individuals require assistance with breathing—by mask, nasal cannula, or ventilator.

A rapid assessment of a patient's respiratory function is accomplished by counting the number of breaths taken in one minute and noting the depth and regularity of the respiratory pattern. Rate, depth, and regularity of breathing affect the amount of oxygen inhaled and the amount of carbon dioxide exhaled. These two factors and additional factors listed below ultimately affect the patient's overall health status and ability to adjust to temporary healthy conditions or to chronic medical conditions. For example, breathing fast during a race is healthy and serves to bring more oxygen to the tissues. Breathing fast may also reflect an attempt by the body to lower abnormally high carbon dioxide levels caused by respiratory or other medical conditions. The examiner uses the assessment of rate, depth, and rhythm to request more definitive testing, make a diagnosis, and prescribe appropriate treatment.

Factors that affect the respiratory rate include the following:

- Allergic reactions
- Disease
- Exercise
- Excitement, anger
- Stimulation of peripheral nervous system (PNS)
- Fever, deviations from normal body temperature
- Hemorrhage
- High altitude
- Medications, drugs
- Obstruction of airway
- Pain
- Shock
- Decrease or increase of CO_2 in blood

Blood Pressure

Blood pressure is the measurement of circulating blood pressure exerted on vessel walls by the pumping action of the heart. The pressure varies with the contraction and relaxation phases of the heartbeat. **Systole** refers to the contraction phase, and **diastole** refers to the relaxation phase.

Blood pressure readings provide the examiner with a quick overview of the patient's circulatory status. Excessive or abnormally low pressure on the vessel walls from high or low blood pressure, respectively, may lead to complications or

PROCEDURE 28-8 Perform a Respiration Count

Theory and Rationale

Assessment of the rate, rhythm, and depth of respirations is an essential part of taking vital signs. The respiratory rate is usually counted immediately after the radial or apical pulse is measured. Keep your hand on the patient's wrist after the radial pulse count (or the stethoscope on the chest after the apical pulse count), but glance toward the chest to observe and count respirations. The patient should be unaware that respirations are being counted. Otherwise, he or she may consciously try to control the breathing, which will affect the resting respiratory count.

Materials

■ watch with second hand

Competency

(**Conditions**) With the necessary supplies, (**Task**) you will perform a respiration count (**Standards**) accurately, in the time designated by the instructor, making sure the patient is unaware that you are doing so.

1. This procedure is a continuation of the radial or apical pulse count. The patient has been identified and you have washed your hands.
2. After counting the radial or apical pulse and mentally noting the rate, continue holding the patient's wrist or holding the stethoscope chestpiece in place.
3. Watch the patient's chest rise (inspiration) and fall (expiration) and count the respiratory cycles for 30 seconds. Observe the regularity and depth of the respirations (Figure 28-14 ◆). Make a mental note of the respiratory rate.
4. Multiply the 30-second count by two and record that figure as the respiratory rate. Record the pulse as well. Add any appropriate comments about the regularity or depth of the respirations on the chart.

Patient Education

Instruct the patient's significant other to count respirations for one full minute following the radial or apical pulse, while the patient is unaware. If the patient is aware, the respiratory count could increase or decrease above the resting rate. It is also important to determine if the respirations are shallow or deep. The significant other should describe to the physician any abnormal sounds heard with the respirations.

Charting Example

09/21/XX 1530 Daughter states that patient has been getting weaker and breathing has been getting more difficult for the patient. T 99.6°F, P 100, R 28, B/P 140/90. Emeka Wright, CMA (AAMA)

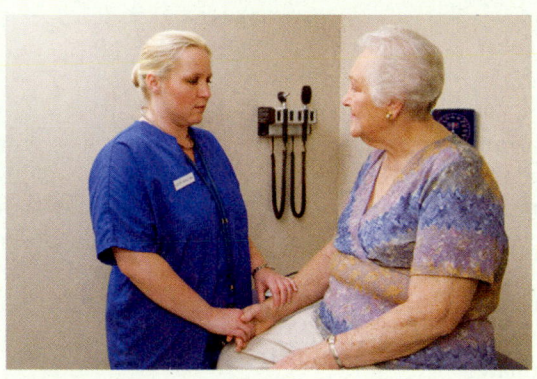

Figure 28-14 ◆ Performing a respiration count.

---

related medical conditions. Deviations in blood pressure readings (high or low) provide information with which to formulate a possible diagnosis and treatment.

A sphygmomanometer is used to measure blood pressure in millimeters of mercury (mm Hg)—either in a calibrated column of mercury or with an aneroid dial (Figures 28-15 ◆ and 28-16 ◆). Mercury has been found to pose serious health risks, and thus mercury sphygmomanometers are being eliminated. Restrictions vary from state to state, so some offices may still have them in use. A stethoscope is used in conjunction with the sphygmomanometer to hear systolic and diastolic pressure, which are represented by the two numerical values in a blood pressure measurement.

■ *Systolic pressure* is the period of highest pressure. It represents the force of the blood pushing against arterial walls when the ventricles of the heart are contracting.
■ *Diastolic pressure* is the period of lowest pressure, when the ventricles relax.

A blood pressure reading is recorded as a fraction, with systolic over diastolic pressure. A normal blood pressure reading for an adult is 120/80—120 is systolic and 80 is diastolic (Table 28-5). The numerical difference is called the *pulse pressure*. Normal pulse pressure is 40 points. Pulse pressure lower than 30 points or greater than 50 points is considered abnormal and an indication of an underlying problem.

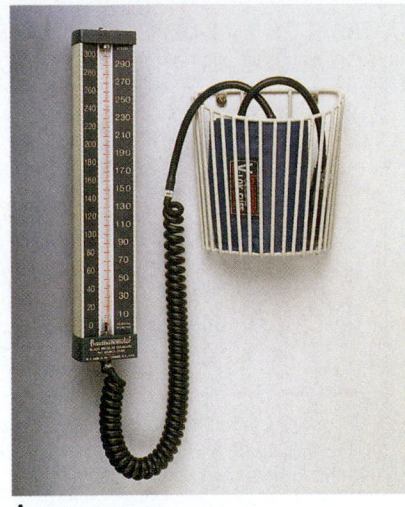 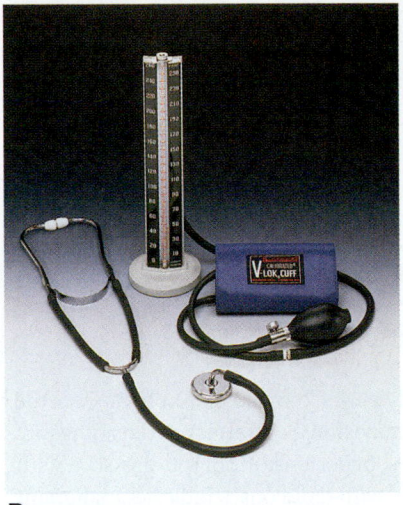

A   B

Figure 28-15 ◆ (A) Wall-mounted mercury sphygmomanometer; (B) Portable mercury sphygmomanometer. Note that mercury sphygmomanometers are being eliminated, as mercury has been found to pose serious health risks.
Reprinted with permission of W. A. Baum.

? —Critical Thinking Question 28-1-

Knowing that a normal pulse pressure is between 30 mm Hg and 50 mm Hg, what should Chelsea do next?

Korotkoff Sounds

Korotkoff sounds are the sounds actually heard as the arterial wall distends during the compression of the blood pressure cuff. The sounds were first classified into five different phases by Russian neurologist Nicolai Korotkoff.

When the blood pressure cuff is first inflated, no sound can be heard because the brachial artery is compressed. As air is slowly removed from the cuff during deflation, the Korotkoff sounds become audible. The deflation of air should be at the rate of 2 to 3 mmHg per heartbeat. The medical assistant should practice taking blood pressure readings slowly in order to be able to identify each phase. The systolic pressure is the first distinct clear tapping sound that is heard, and the diastolic pressure is the pressure at which the last sound is heard. Some facilities and physicians measure the diastolic pressure at the fourth Korotkoff phase where the sound changes from a clear tapping or thumping sound to a more muffled softer sound. When the fourth sound is used as the diastolic pressure, three readings are often made: systolic, first diastolic (fourth Korotkoff sound), and second diastolic (last sound). Korotkoff sounds are described in Table 28-6.

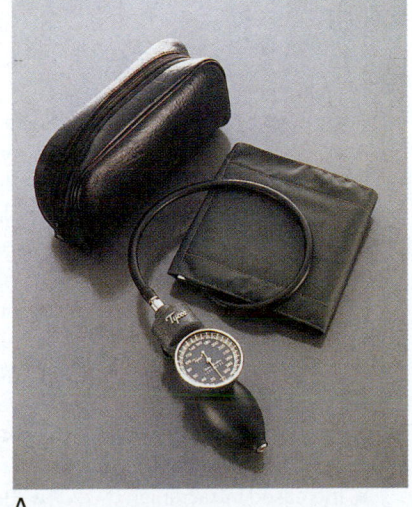 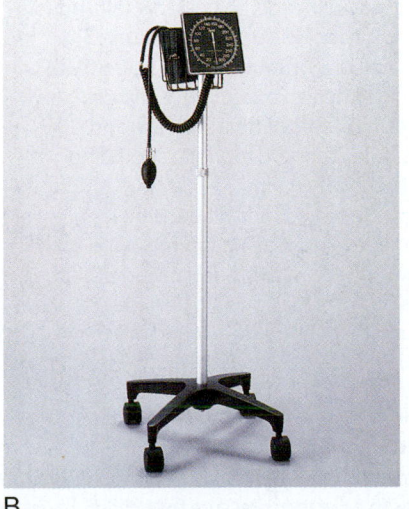

A   B

Figure 28-16 ◆ (A) Portable aneroid sphygmomanometer; (B) Portable aneroid sphygmomanometer on wheels.
Courtesy of Welch Allyyn, Inc.

TABLE 28-5 AVERAGE SYSTOLIC/DIASTOLIC VALUES FOR BLOOD PRESSURE BY AGE

Newborn	80/50 mm Hg
Infant	90/60 mm Hg
Child, 3 years	100/60 mm Hg
Child, 6 years	100/60 mm Hg
Child, 10 years	110/60 mm Hg
Child, 14 years	120/60 mm Hg
Adult	120/80 mm Hg
Elderly > 60 years of age	155/95 mm Hg

Blood pressure consistently elevated by 20 to 30 points over the baseline BP is termed **hypertension**. Several elevated readings are required for a diagnosis of hypertension. Blood pressure with significant elevation, usually with rapid onset, indicates **malignant hypertension**, and immediate intervention is required.

The American Heart Association issued the following guidelines concerning classifications of hypertension (Table 28-7): "The classifications in the table below are for people who aren't taking antihypertensive (blood pressure-lowering) drugs and aren't acutely ill. When a person's systolic and diastolic pressures fall into different categories, the higher category is used to classify the blood pressure status. Diagnosing high blood pressure is based on the average of two or more readings taken at each of two or more visits after an initial screening."

TABLE 28-7 CLASSIFICATION OF BLOOD PRESSURE FOR ADULTS AGE 18 YEARS AND OLDER

Category	Systolic (mm Hg)		Diastolic (mm Hg)
Normal*	less than 120	and	less than 80
Prehypertension	120–139	or	80–89
Hypertension:			
Stage 1	140–159	or	90–99
Stage 2	160 or higher	or	100 or higher

Unusually low readings should be evaluated for clinical significance.
Reproduced with permission www.americanheart.org. © 2006, American Heart Association, Inc.

Readings 20 to 30 points *below* normal are indicative of **hypotension**. A sudden, significant drop in pressure is indicative of shock, and immediate intervention is required to prevent circulatory collapse. (See ∞ Chapter 41 for information on emergency intervention.)

Table 28-8 lists the causes of abnormally elevated and lowered blood pressure.

TABLE 28-6 FIVE PHASES OF KOROTKOFF SOUNDS

Phase I	This is the first faint sound heard as the cuff is deflated. Record this reading as the systolic pressure reading. The cuff must be inflated to a high enough level to hear this first sound during relaxation.
Phase II	The second phase occurs as the cuff continues to be deflated and blood flows through the artery. This sound has a swishing quality. The cuff has to be slowly deflated in order to hear this soft sound. An auscultary gap is said to have occurred if there is a total loss of sound at this stage that then reoccurs later. An auscultary gap can occur in certain cases of heart disease and hypertension. An auscultary gap should be reported to the physician.
Phase III	During this phase the sound will become less muffled and develop a crisp tapping sound as the blood flow moves easily through the artery. If the BP cuff was not inflated enough to hear the Phase I sound, then the Phase III sound may be heard and incorrectly stated as the systolic reading.
Phase IV	The sound will now begin to fade and become muffled. The American Heart Association, which believes Phase IV is the best indicator of the diastolic pressure, recommends the reading at this phase be recorded as the diastolic pressure for a child.
Phase V	Sound will disappear at this phase. Some physicians want both Phase IV and Phase V recorded for the diastolic pressure reading (for example, 120/78/74 rather than 120/74).

TABLE 28-8 CAUSES OF VARIATIONS IN BLOOD PRESSURE

Increased or Elevated Blood Pressure	Decreased or Lowered Blood Pressure
■ Exercise	■ Weak heart
■ Stress, anxiety, excitement, fear	■ Massive heart attack
■ Pain	■ Hemorrhage
■ Increased arterial blood volume	■ Shock and vascular collapse
■ Loss of vessel elasticity as blood vessels age	■ Dehydration
■ Increased peripheral resistance, narrowing of blood vessels	■ Adrenal insufficiency
■ Endocrine disorders	■ Certain drug therapies
■ Smoking	■ Disorders of the nervous system
■ Renal disease	■ Hypothyroidism
■ Liver disease	■ Sleep
■ Heart disease	■ Infections, fevers
■ Right arm higher than left arm	■ Cancer
■ Certain drug therapies	■ Anemia
■ Increased intracranial pressure	■ Approaching death
■ Late pregnancy	■ Middle pregnancy
■ Obesity	■ Pain
■ Time of day	■ Starvation
	■ Sudden postural changes
	■ Time of day

?—Critical Thinking Question 28-2-
Chelsea heard two distinct blood pressure readings in the same arm. How should she record this in the patient's chart?

Errors in Blood Pressure Readings

Factors that contribute to errors in blood pressure readings include the following:

- Using a cuff of incorrect size
- Air leaks in the valve
- Failing to uncover the patient's arm (not rolling up the sleeve, etc.) before applying the cuff
- Incorrectly positioning the patient's arm
- Applying the cuff too loosely
- Not centering the cuff over the brachial artery
- Not securing the end of the cuff properly
- Allowing the stethoscope tubing to touch something else
- Improperly positioning the stethoscope earpieces in the ears
- Placing the bell or diaphragm incorrectly over the brachial artery
- Not inflating the cuff to 20 mm above the normal pressure
- Closing the thumbscrew incompletely, allowing air to escape from the cuff
- Deflating the cuff too rapidly
- Retaking the blood pressure before waiting a minute or retaking the pressure in the same arm more than twice
- Failing to calibrate the sphygmomanometer
- Upset, anxious, or shaking patient

Weight and Height

The **mensuration,** or measuring of a patient's weight and height, establishes baseline information for future comparison and helps in the assessment of health status and response to illness and/or treatment. These measurements are used to diagnose obesity and aid in the management of conditions such as diabetes and congestive heart failure. Medication dosages are prescribed on the basis of weight. Children are weighed and measured on a routine basis to assess their growth.

Weight

An individual's weight is another valuable tool for assessing health status. Weight measurements are used to monitor the growth of an infant or child. The weight of any patient, child or adult, is an important factor in calculating drug dosages as well as the effectiveness of drug and nutritional therapies. Physicians use daily weight measurements as an assessment tool in

---

PROCEDURE 28-9 Perform a Blood Pressure Measurement

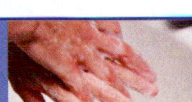

Theory and Rationale

Blood pressure is measured as part of vital sign assessment during most patient visits to the medical office. The usual inflation is a minimum of 20 mm of mercury above the previous reading or to a level of 180 mm Hg as the starting point. The stethoscope tubing should not be touching anything during the procedure because the added noises may affect the accuracy of the measurement.

The width of the blood pressure cuff is important. To obtain an accurate reading, the cuff must fit the limb. Appropriate cuff widths are:

Newborns of average size:	2.5 cm (1 inch)
Children 1–4 years of age:	6 cm (2.3 inches)
Children 4–8 years of age:	9 cm (3.5 inches)
Adults:	13 cm (5.1 inches)
Obese adults:	20 cm (8 inches)

Routine blood pressure is measured in the sitting position. If it is measured while the patient is standing or lying down, note that on the chart.

Materials

- stethoscope
- 70% isopropyl alcohol wipes
- sphygmomanometer (aneroid or mercury)

Competency

(**Conditions**) With the necessary supplies, (**Task**) you will obtain an accurate blood pressure reading (**Standards**) accurately within the time frame designated by the instructor.

1. Wash your hands and assemble the equipment. Squeeze the bladder of the sphygmomanometer cuff to make sure it is completely deflated.
2. Identify the patient and escort to a central area or patient examination room. Have the patient sit either on a chair or on the examination table. Explain the procedure to the patient.
3. Cleanse the earpieces, diaphragm, and bell of the stethoscope with the alcohol wipes.

continued

PROCEDURE 28-9 Perform a Blood Pressure Measurement (continued)

4. Expose the patient's upper arm and ask the patient to extend the arm with the palm facing upward. You may have to assist the patient in rolling up the sleeve.
5. Place the sphygmomanometer cuff around the patient's upper arm and secure it snugly, centering over the brachial artery (Figure 28-17 ◆).
6. Palpate the brachial pulse.
7. Hold the arm with the attached sphygmomanometer at heart level.
8. Place the sphygmomanometer gauge where you can monitor it easily or ask the patient to hold it (Figure 28-18 ◆).
9. Place the stethoscope earpieces in your ears. Place the diaphragm of the stethoscope over the location where you felt the brachial pulse. Hold the bell of the stethoscope in place with the thumb of your nondominant hand while supporting the elbow with your fingers (Figure 28-19 ◆).
10. With your dominant hand, close the thumbscrew on the hand bulb by turning it clockwise. Quickly and evenly pump the bulb to inflate the cuff.
11. Slowly turn the thumbscrew counterclockwise, releasing air at approximately 2–3 mm per second.
12. Listen and mentally note when you hear the first pulsation. Slowly continue to release air until the pulsation sounds cease, and make a mental note of that reading.
13. Quickly release the rest of the air, deflating the cuff. Remove the cuff.
14. If it is necessary to check the blood pressure reading because of an error in the procedure or an abnormally high or low reading, wait one minute before retaking the blood pressure on the same arm.
15. Clean the earpieces and diaphragm with 70% ethyl alcohol. Return the sphygmomanometer and stethoscope to their usual storage places.
16. Wash your hands.
17. After recording the date and time, document the first pulsation sounds as systolic and the last sounds as diastolic readings. Write the systolic over diastolic readings in fraction format. If the blood pressure was taken with the patient standing or lying down, specify the position in the chart. If the patient asks for the reading and office policy allows it, you may inform the patient of the reading.

Patient Education

Patients and significant others generally go to a medical supply or department store to buy a sphygmomanometer. Emphasize the importance of seeking help to find a properly fitting cuff. Kits are often available with a stethoscope but are also sold separately. The entire arm should be level with the heart during the procedure. Demonstrate ways to do this, such as placing the arm on a higher countertop or holding the arm elevated. Because of the potential for impairing circulation, instruct the patient never to inflate the cuff more than twice on the same arm. The patient or significant others should keep records of the blood pressures for the next medical office visit. This information will be used to adjust, add, or delete medications and evaluate the status of acute and chronic medical conditions.

Charting Example

06/29/XX 8:30 AM T 98.6 P 94 R 24 B/P 160/110. Patient states narrowly missed being in an auto accident before coming for office appointment. Carol Herns, RMA (AMT)

06/29/XX 8:50 AM P 88 R 20 B/P 140/90. Carol Herns, RMA (AMT)

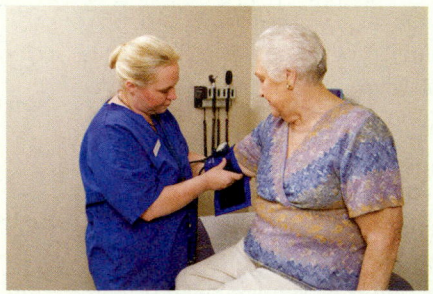

Figure 28-17 ◆ Place the sphygmomanometer cuff around the patient's upper arm.

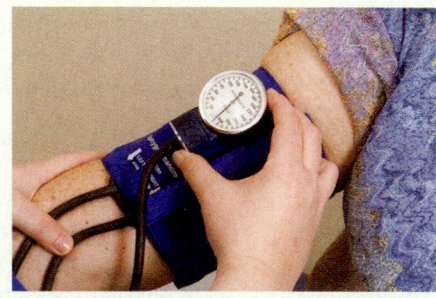

Figure 28-18 ◆ Place the sphygmomanometer gauge where you can monitor it easily.

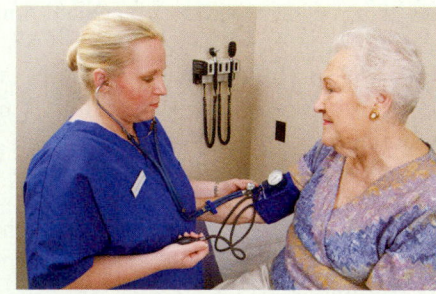

Figure 28-19 ◆ Hold the bell of the stethoscope in place with the thumb of your nondominant hand.

the treatment of specific diagnoses. Patients with congestive heart failure or renal failure may require daily weighing. For example, rapid weight gain would indicate the need for additional diuretics or dialysis treatments.

While there are standard guidelines for normal weight based on height, variations are to be expected. An "ideal weight" must be individualized for body type, age, and health status. Being either underweight or overweight can have serious implications for the patient's well-being. An underweight individual may be experiencing nutritional problems or metabolic disorders. An overweight individual may also be experiencing nutritional or metabolic problems, but with the added complication of hypertension, heart disease, or diabetes.

The patient is usually weighed at every visit. On the initial visit the weight establishes a baseline for future comparison. It is good practice during the initial assessment to ask the patient what his or her usual weight is and whether the current weight is significantly different. The MA should be alert to any changes and call them to the physician's attention.

Some patients are very sensitive about their weight and do not want anyone to know what it is. Scales should be kept in a private area. When weighing the patient, the MA should not comment on the weight. Chart the results, return the balance weights to the zero position before the patient steps down from the scales, and escort the patient back to the examination room. If the patient is accompanied by another individual or support person, try to keep the weight a confidential matter between the physician and the patient.

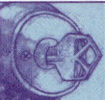

Keys to Success
POUNDS AND KILOS

Most scales measure weight in pounds and ounces. Canadian clients are used to measuring their weight in kilograms. To convert pounds to kilograms, divide the weight in pounds by 2.2. For example, 180 pounds is 81.8 kilos. To convert kilograms to pounds, multiply the weight in kilograms by 2.2. Patients from the United Kingdom may express their weight in stones. One stone is equal to 14 pounds, so a 126-pound woman weighs 9 stone.

Height

Like weight, height is a valuable tool in assessing the status of a patient's health. Height measurements are used to monitor the growth of an infant or child. Failure to grow is ascertained in a child or infant who shows little or no change in height. During the aging process, individuals may begin to lose height because of spinal compression or other disease processes.

Measurements of height or length are usually reported in feet and inches. However, some practitioners may prefer the metric system of measurement and report the measurement in meters and centimeters.

PROCEDURE 28-10 Obtain Weight and Height Measurements

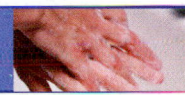

Theory and Rationale

The measurement of weight and height is considered part of the routine that includes the taking of temperature, pulse, respirations, and blood pressure. The following procedural steps are for patients who can stand and follow directions, and step on and off the scales with or without assistance. (Measuring the length, weight, and head circumference of infants is covered in ∞ Chapter 45.)

The patient is weighed at each visit, initially to determine a baseline weight, and on following visits to observe for trends or sudden changes. You can measure a patient's weight quickly if the patient knows approximately what he or she weighs. The scales should be balanced to zero before the patient is weighed. On electronic models this calibration may be done with a button; on manual models a screw on the upper arm of the scale is loosened or tightened until the scale is balanced. To maintain patient confidentiality and privacy, the scales should be kept in a private area away from other patients. Return the weight to zero after you record the patient's results. Height is measured as the last step, and then the patient is returned to the examination room.

When measuring height and weight, note whether the patient is wearing shoes with thick soles or heels. Note on the chart any added height from shoes. If the patient has removed the shoes, note that on the chart. The same concept applies to clothing. Some offices prefer that the patient remove coats or bulky jackets and/or shoes before weighing. Other heavy or bulky clothes should be noted on the chart. If possible, ask patients to remove keys and other heavy objects from their pockets. Common sense should prevail in these situations.

Whether a patient's weight is measured in the office or at home, the same standards should be followed—for example, if shoes and/or socks are worn during weighing in the office, they should be worn for weighing at home. Other standards include wearing clothing or minimal clothing, weighing at the same time every day, and using the same scales. A change greater than three to five pounds in one day should be called in to the medical office.

The physician generally reads the weight figure when he or she looks over the entire set of vital sign measurements. If necessary, you can share weight results with the physician out of the patient's sight and hearing.

continued

PROCEDURE 28-10 Obtain Weight and Height Measurements *(continued)*

Materials

- upright balance scales with height bar
- paper towel

Competency

(**Conditions**) With the necessary supplies, (**Task**) you will be able to obtain weight and height measurements (**Standards**) accurately within the time frame designated by the instructor.

1. Identify the patient and escort him or her to the examination room.
2. Wash your hands.
3. Explain the procedure to the patient. Explain that most personal items may be left in the room, although a female patient may want to take her purse. Escort the patient to the scales.
4. Balance the scales to read zero.
5. Instruct the patient to step on the scales. You may need to place a paper towel on the scale for patients who wish to remove their shoes. Assist the patient onto the scales and provide support as needed.
6. Instruct the patient to stand still. Move the weights until the scale balances (Figure 28-20 ◆).
7. Note the weight and return the balance weights to zero.
8. Ask the patient to step off the scales, assisting as necessary.
9. Help the patient to step on the scales backwards so that his or her back is against the scale. Ask the patient to stand erect, eyes looking ahead.
10. Raise the height bar in a collapsed position above the patient's head (Figure 28-21 ◆). Extend the bar and slowly bring it down until it touches the top of the patient's head (Figure 28-22 ◆). Note the height.
11. Raise the entire height bar up over the patient's head, collapse it, and return it to its original position.
12. Ask the patient to step off the scales, assisting as necessary.
13. Record the height and weight on the patient's chart.

Patient Education

Instruct the patient or significant other to follow the same weighing procedure every day: weigh at the same time, use the same scales, wear shoes or not, wear regular or minimal clothing. The patient should also keep a daily record and call the physician about any weight changes greater than three to five pounds in one day.

Charting Example

08/23/XX 1120 Patient called to state that weight has been increasing by approximately a pound a day. Patient reports a 3-pound weight gain today. Physician informed. Lasix dosage has been increased from 10 to 20 mg/day by mouth and prescription has been called to Wellbetter Pharmacy as requested by patient. William Martinez, CMA (AAMA)

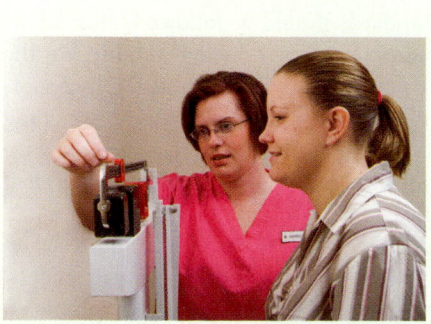

Figure 28-20 ◆ Move weight to balanced position.

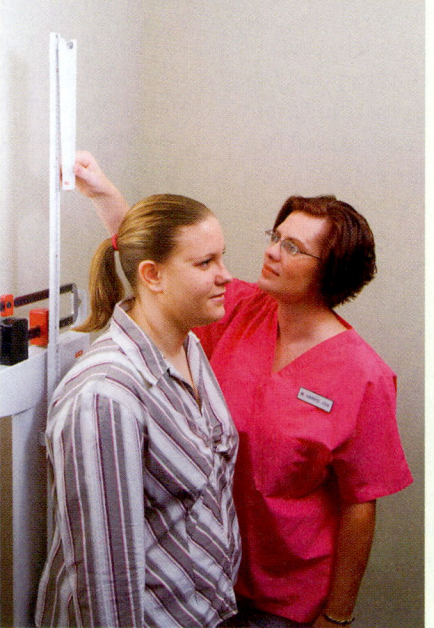

Figure 28-21 ◆ Raise the height bar in a collapsed position above the patient's head.

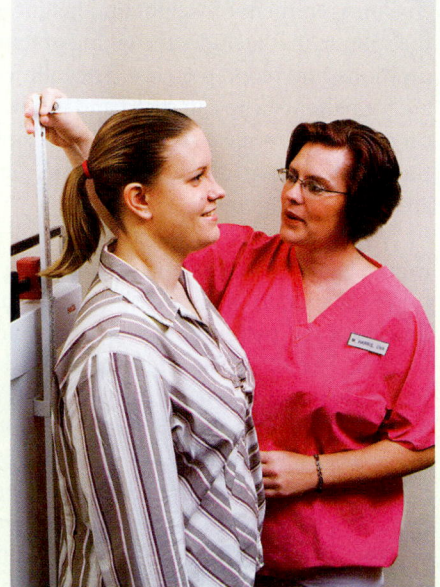

Figure 28-22 ◆ Bring the bar down until it touches the top of the patient's head.

Visual Acuity

Visual acuity is an assessment of the acuteness or clarity of the patient's vision. This is an easy test to perform and is often included in a pre-employment physical. Visual acuity testing is part of the application for certain drivers' licenses. (Refer to ∞ Chapter 37 for detailed information and skills proficiency on visual acuity screening.)

Hearing Assessment

Hearing assessment includes an evaluation with a tuning fork. An audiometer may be used for a more thorough and complete assessment of an individual's hearing range. (Refer to ∞ Chapter 37 for additional information on hearing assessment.)

Preparing the Patient for a Physical Examination

The physician must be able to easily access the part of the body to be examined. The patient is asked to remove clothing as necessary and to don a patient gown, pants, or drape. Draping provides for modesty, comfort, and warmth. The patient is then properly positioned, usually on the examination table, for the physical examination.

Gowning

In preparation for examination by the physician, the MA will instruct the patient regarding the removal of clothing and donning the patient gown. During a complete physical examination, the physician visually inspects the entire body. The patient may need to remove all clothing and wear a gown, usually with closure in the back. Depending on the thoroughness of the examination, undergarments may be left on. However, if the examination or procedure includes exposure of the pelvic cavity, rectum, or chest/breast areas, undergarments will need to be removed and a gown with front closure worn.

Gowns are made of cloth or paper, with ties or snaps for closure. Half-paper gowns cover only the chest, and paper or cloth sheets allow for privacy and draping (Figure 28-23 ◆).

Draping

Draping involves covering any area that may be exposed during the examination. A sheet over the legs is the usual drape for a patient in a sitting position. (Positions are described in the following section.) A sheet over the torso and legs is the usual drape for a patient in a lying position, both supine and prone. A sheet is placed over the lower torso and can be draped over the legs of a patient in lithotomy position. For a patient in the knee-chest position, a sheet is placed over the posterior torso and can be draped over the buttocks. Similarly, a sheet is draped over a patient in Sims' position, and the edge can be lifted to provide access to the buttocks and rectal region.

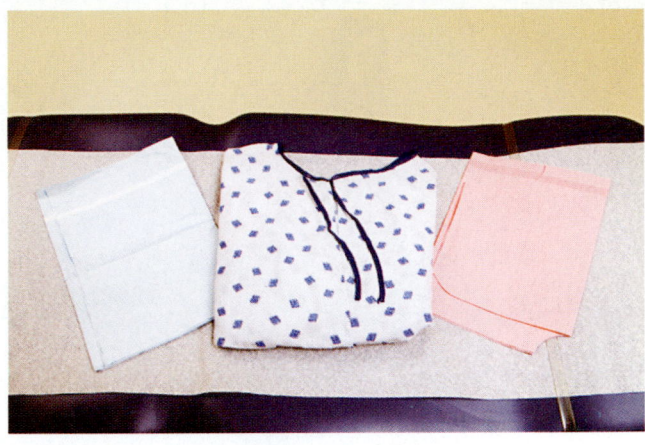

Figure 28-23 ◆ Types of gowns.

Positioning the Patient

Patient positioning for the examination is usually done by the medical assistant. A common position for the beginning of an examination is to have the patient sit upright on the exam table. As the examination progresses, the MA will assist the patient into various positions, depending on the area of the body being examined. Positions include the following:

- Anatomical—standing
- Sitting—sitting upright with the legs hanging over the side of the examination table (Figure 28-24 ◆)
- Fowler's—sitting erect on the table with the legs extended in front and the back rest at a 90-degree angle (Figure 28-25 ◆)
- Semi-Fowler's—sitting on the table with the legs extended and the back rest at 45 degrees (Figure 28-26 ◆)
- Supine—lying flat on the back
- Dorsal recumbent—lying flat on the back with the knees bent and the feet flat on the table (Figure 28-27 ◆)
- Prone—lying on the abdomen with the head to one side (Figure 28-28 ◆)
- Trendelenburg—lying flat on the back with the head lower than the feet (Figure 28-29 ◆)
- Knee-chest—kneeling on the table with the buttocks raised and the head and chest on the examination table (Figure 28-30 ◆)
- Jackknife—lying with the abdomen on the table, the knees on the table step, and the buttocks extended (Figure 28-31 ◆)
- Lithotomy—lying on the back in dorsal recumbent with the feet on the corners of the table or in the stirrups (Figure 28-32 ◆)
- Left lateral recumbent—lying horizontal on the left side
- Right lateral recumbent—lying horizontal on the right side
- Sims'—right or left lateral recumbent with the upper leg flexed (Figure 28-33 ◆)

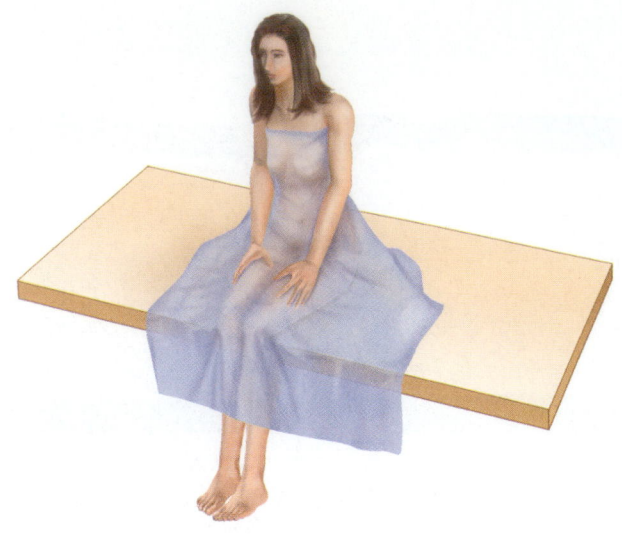

Figure 28-24 ◆ Sitting position.

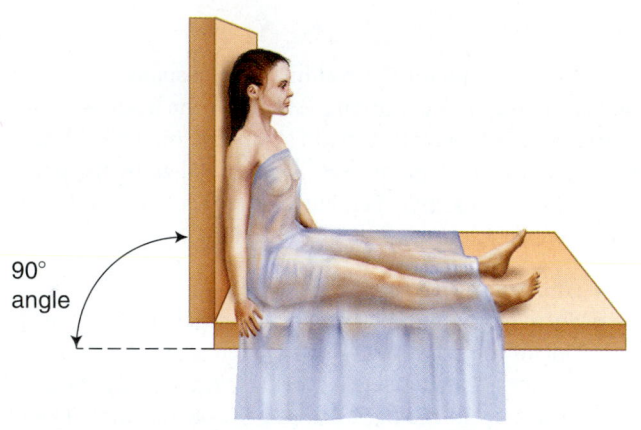

90°
angle

Figure 28-25 ◆ Fowler's position.

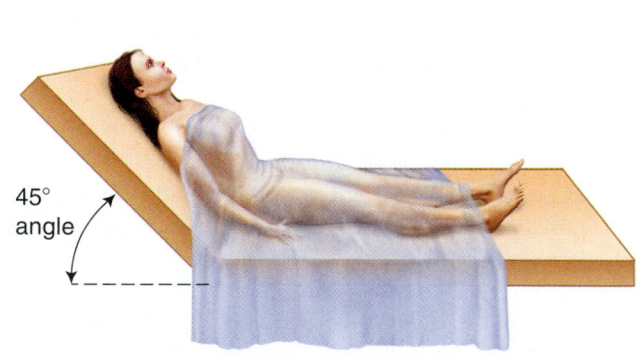

45°
angle

Figure 28-26 ◆ Semi-Fowler's position.

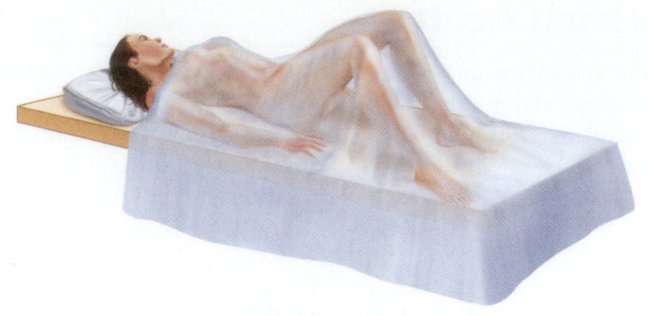

Figure 28-27 ◆ Dorsal recumbent position.

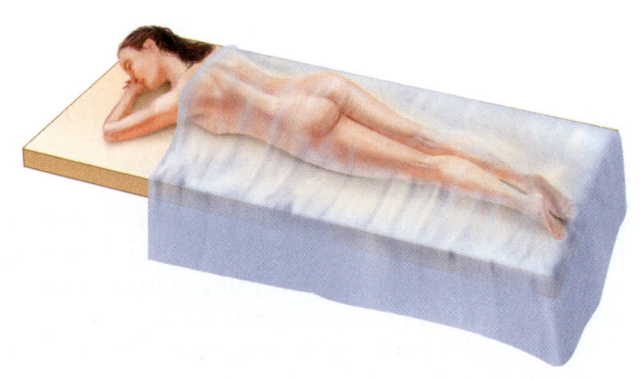

Figure 28-28 ◆ Prone position.

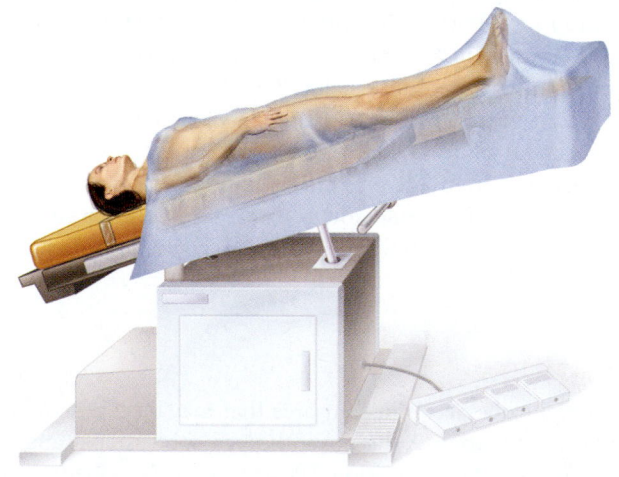

Figure 28-29 ◆ Trendelenburg position.

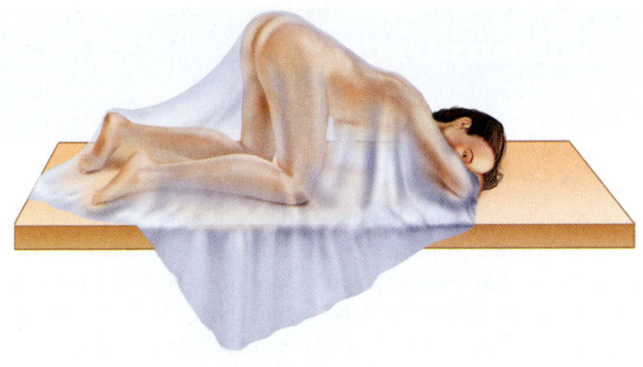

Figure 28-30 ◆ Knee-chest position.

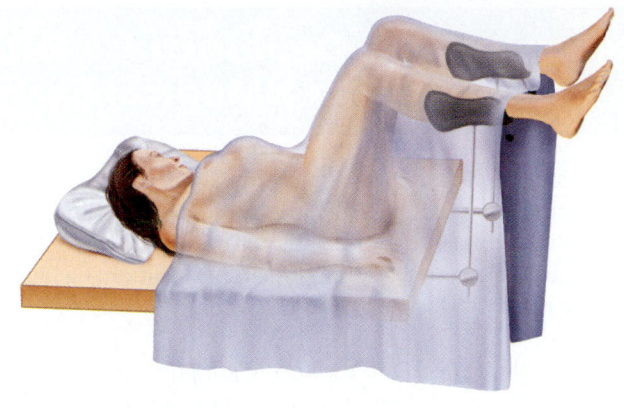

Figure 28-32 ◆ Lithotomy position.

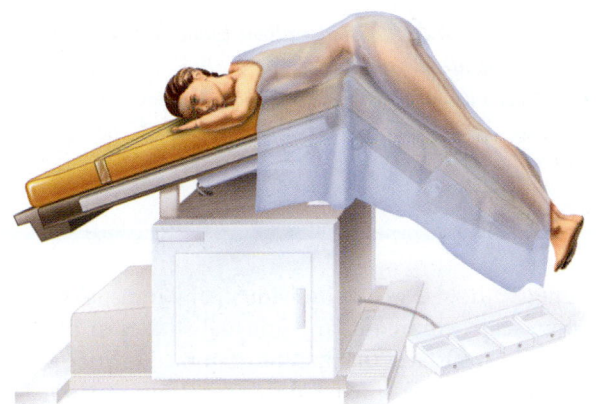

Figure 28-31 ◆ Jackknife position.

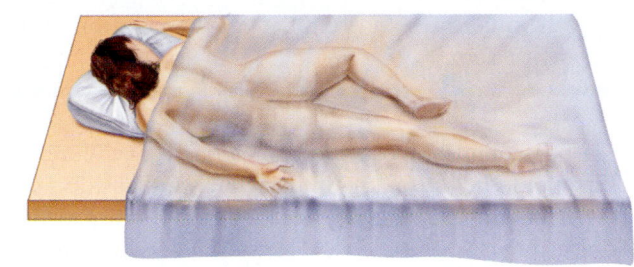

Figure 28-33 ◆ Sims' position.

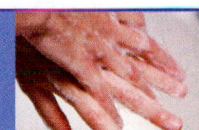

PROCEDURE 28-11   Demonstrate Patient Positions Used in a Medical Examination

Theory and Rationale

When positioning the patient, some factors to be considered are the patient's range of motion, the patient's comfort, and the length of time the position will be maintained. You should not place the patient in any position other than sitting or lying until the examination or procedure is ready to begin. Children and the elderly should never be left alone. The patient should be covered with a drape that is lifted only when the body part is being examined.

Depending on the type of examination, the physician will have the patient shift from a sitting position to other positions. For a pelvic examination and Pap smear, the patient is moved from sitting to supine, then dorsal recumbent, and last to the lithotomy position. A patient experiencing shortness of breath should be placed in a Fowler's position to facilitate breathing. As you may not be present for the entire examination, it is important that you anticipate draping and positioning needs based on the patient's reason for visiting the medical office.

Materials

■ patient gown, pants, and drapes
■ examination table paper

Competency

(**Conditions**) With the necessary supplies, (**Task**) you will be able to assist the patient into the sitting, supine, Sims', prone, dorsal recumbent, lithotomy, Fowler's, semi-Fowler's, and Knee-chest positions (**Standards**) correctly within the time frame designated by the instructor.

1. Identify the patient and escort to examination room.
2. Wash your hands and gather drape materials.
3. Explain the procedure to the patient. Ask the patient to completely undress and to put on a patient gown. For a breast examination, instruct the patient to tie the gown in front.
4. Instruct the patient to sit on the examination table, assiting as necessary. Cover the patient with the drape.
5. Assist the patient into the Fowler's position.
6. Assist the patient into the semi-Fowler's position.

continued

PROCEDURE 28-11 Demonstrate Patient Positions Used in a Medical Examination *(continued)*

7. Assist the patient into the supine position.
8. Assist the patient into the dorsal recumbent position.
9. Assist the patient into the lithotomy position.
10. Assist the patient back into the supine position, then into the prone position.
11. Assist the patient into the Sims' position.
12. Assist the patient into the knee-chest position.
13. Assist the patient into the sitting position and stepping off the examination table.
14. After the examination has been completed and the physician has discussed the procedure with the patient, clean the examination room. Remove the used paper from the examination table and replace it with clean paper for the next patient.
15. Wash your hands and complete documentation in the patient's chart.

Patient Education

Explain to the patient that he or she will be assisted/directed through change of positions for the examination. Provide reassurance that modesty will be provided. Inform patient that some discomfort may be experienced, but encourage patient to verbalize any additional needs that may need to be addressed throughout the examination.

Charting Example

12/05/XX 9:30 AM Assisted patient turning from supine to left-lateral position for rectal examination. Patient tolerated examination without discomfort. Danica Verdo, RMA (AMJ)

Upon completion of the examination or procedure, the patient should be assisted to an upright sitting position and observed for any signs of light-headedness. Then the patient is assisted to a standing position and assisted to dress if necessary.

Assessment Methods Used in an Examination

Physicians use a variety of assessment methods during a physical examination: inspection, palpation, auscultation, percussion, and, in some instances, mensuration.

Inspection is the visual examination of both the external surface of the body and the interior portions of body cavities (Figure 28-34 ◆). The external surface is examined for asymmetry, the size of the individual, any unusual breaks in the skin, scars, color, and any unusual shapes or positions. Internal cavity surfaces that may be examined include the eyes, throat, nares, ears, vaginal walls, cervix, and rectum. These examinations require the use of certain instruments.

Palpation is an examination involving touch (Figure 28-35 ◆). The examiner uses the hands and fingers to feel both the surface of the body (for any abnormalities or irregularities) and various organs (for size, location, and tenderness). In addition to assessing the texture and temperature of the tissue, the examiner palpates for lumps or masses.

Auscultation consists of listening to various areas of the body (Figure 28-36 ◆). It is possible to assess the status of the heart, lungs, and gastrointestinal tract by auscultation. The valves of the heart make a particular sound when they are

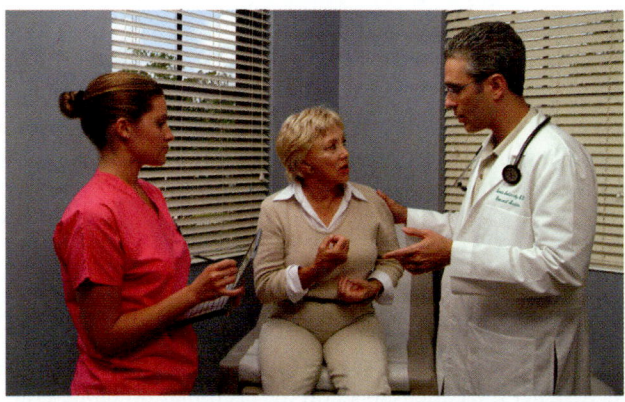

Figure 28-34 ◆ Inspection is an assessment method used by the physician.

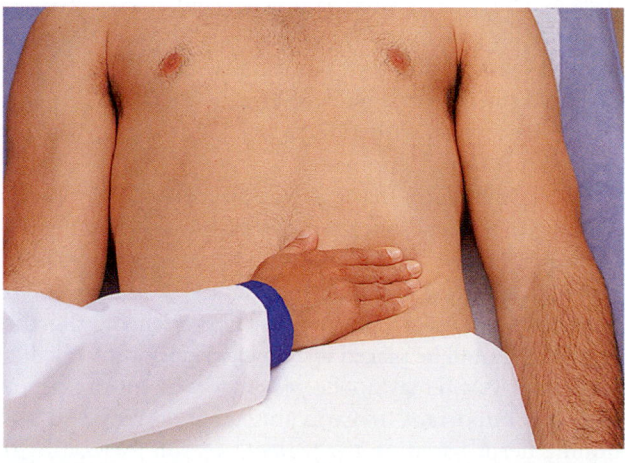

Figure 28-35 ◆ An example of palpation of the abdomen.

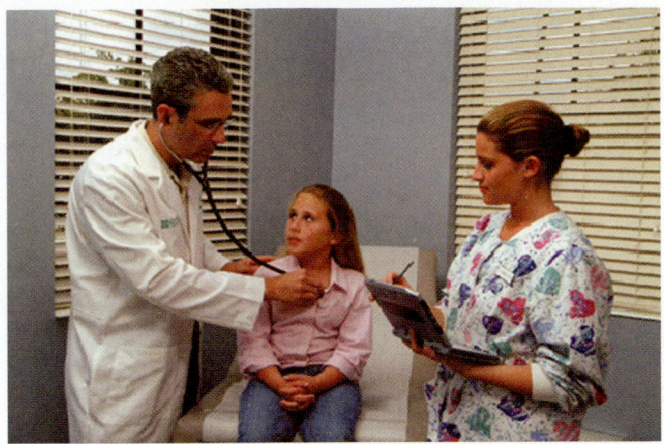

Figure 28-36 ◆ Auscultation consists of listening to various areas of the body.

healthy and a different sound in the presence of disease or irregularity. Breath sounds are assessed for depth and texture. Fluid in the chest cavity can be detected during auscultation. The presence, absence, strength, and quality of bowel sounds aid in detecting problems within the GI tract. The examiner usually uses a stethoscope for auscultation, although some breath sounds are audible without it.

In **percussion,** the examiner taps the fingertips lightly but sharply against the body to assess the size and location of underlying organs (Figure 28-37 ◆). The technique involves placing two fingers of one hand on the patient's skin and gently striking those fingers with the index and middle fingers of the other hand. Training allows for differentiation of the sounds of the percussion. For example, a deviation from normal may lead the examiner to suspect fluid or pus in a cavity or a change in the density of an organ. Another percussion method involves the use of a percussion hammer to test tendon reflexes.

Mensuration is the measurement of certain parts of the body or the length and height of the individual. Tissue calipers measure the size of certain tissues. A tape measure is used to

measure the circumference of the head, neck, chest, abdomen, legs, ankles, arms, and wrists. A standing scale with a height measurement bar is used to measure height, except for infants, whose length is measured with a tape measure.

The medical assistant uses assessment tools to some extent. For example, taking blood pressure involves palpation of the brachial artery as well as auscultation with a stethoscope. The MA always uses the inspection method and documents and reports abnormal findings. If you are not sure if a finding is abnormal, ask the physician and/or nurse.

When the initial examination is complete, the physician may order diagnostic testing. It is the MA's responsibility to schedule the tests and coordinate the time with the patient. The MA will give the patient instructions for the tests as well as directions to the testing facility (unless testing is to be done in the office). The MA will note on the chart when to schedule a return appointment and assist the patient in doing so. (Refer to ∞ Chapter 30 for more information on scheduling diagnostic testing.)

Assisting the Physician During the Examination

Most complete physical examinations begin at the head and proceed downward. The skin is observed for color, warmth, moisture, and **turgor**. The physician notes the patient's level of consciousness, demeanor, and cooperativeness. Examination of the head includes the eyes, ears, nares, and oral cavity. The eyes are normally examined for pupil equality, reaction to light, and **accommodation**. Ocular muscle activity or coordination may also be assessed with an ophthalmoscope. The ears are examined with an otoscope, usually with a disposable speculum. A wider speculum may be added to the otoscope for examination of the nares. The otoscope may be used as a light source to examine the oral cavity. A tongue depressor is used to hold the tongue in place while the examiner visualizes the throat. It also aids in the inspection of the buccal surface of the cheeks and the teeth.

The examiner palpates the neck for any masses or abnormalities. Usually the patient is asked to grip the examiner's fingers and squeeze as an evaluation of muscle and nerve strength of the arms and hands. The carotid arteries in the neck are palpated for texture and lumps, then auscultated for any bruits or unusual sounds. A visual examination of the anterior chest wall will reveal any abnormalities, including asymmetrical rise and fall of the rib cage as well as any sternal retraction. The posterior chest is visually inspected, followed by auscultation of the chest cavity for any abnormal breath sounds or heart tones.

This portion of the examination is usually completed with the patient in a sitting position with the legs extending over the side of the exam table. The examiner may check knee reflexes, pedal pulses, and swelling of the ankles and feet as well as any other aspect of the legs and feet.

Examination of the abdomen requires that the patient lie down on the exam table. The examiner visually inspects the

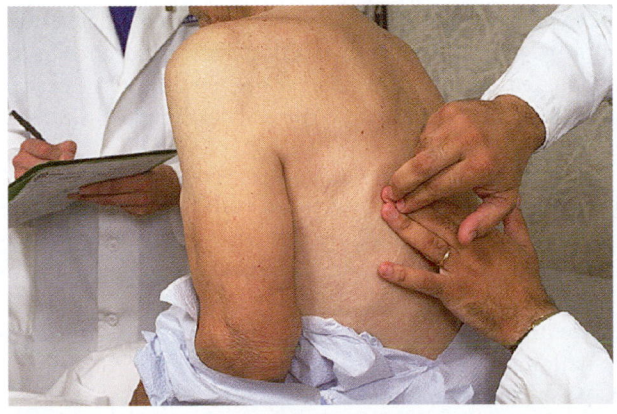

Figure 28-37 ◆ The physician uses percussion to assess the size and location of underlying organs.

skin of the abdomen and observes for any unusual movement under the surface of the skin. This is usually followed by auscultation of the abdominal region—listening for bowel sounds with a stethoscope. The abdomen is usually palpated for masses, tenderness, and guarding. Palpation begins in the right upper quadrant and progresses clockwise through the right lower quadrant, left lower quadrant, left upper quadrant, and back to the starting point.

The pelvic region may be palpated for masses and tenderness just above the pubic bone. If the patient complains of midback or flank region pain, the examiner may palpate the area over the kidneys and just under the ribs posteriorly to ascertain tenderness and pain.

For a pelvic exam and Pap smear, the patient is assisted into stirrups and the lithotomy position. The patient may be placed in a knee-chest or Sim's position for a rectal examination. Other specialty examinations will be addressed in the appropriate chapters.

The patient may be asked to walk in the examination room so that the examiner can assess gait, posture, and any spinal abnormalities.

When the examination is complete, you assist the patient to dress, if necessary, and provide any other assistance the patient needs.

Recurrent Clinical Visits

On recurrent clinical visits, the medical assistant will escort the patient to the appropriate examination room and obtain a brief history, including the reason for the visit, any changes noted since the last visit, and an update on medications. The MA will measure vital signs, including weight and height, and update the chart to reflect the observations and findings. Then the MA will prepare the patient for the physical examination in the usual manner.

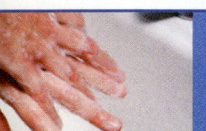

PROCEDURE 28-12 Prepare the Patient for Medical Examination and Assist the Physician

Theory and Rationale

Physical examinations require more of the physician's and medical assistant's time. Each medical office has an established protocol for blocking time for physical examinations. Depending on the patient's age, gender, and medical condition, you may leave or be required to stay during all or part of the physical examination.

The patient must disrobe completely or almost completely for this procedure. Some patients are very modest, and are resistive to completely undressing. Patients who are concerned about the cool temperature of the examination room may be allowed to wear underwear until it needs to be removed. Provide these patients with extra draping or cover. Protect the patient's dignity with draping and provide assurance by explaining the basic components of the procedure.

Throughout the procedure, observe the patient's body language for any signs of discomfort or anxiety. Before the procedure begins, ask if the patient needs to use the bathroom. Emptying the bladder helps the patient feel more comfortable during the physical examination. If a urine specimen is required, it can be obtained at this point.

Materials

- examination table with clean covering (sheet) and stirrups if pelvic examination is to be performed
- patient gown and appropriate drapes
- pillow with disposable cover
- scales with height rod
- Snellen chart and color vision charts
- disposable gloves
- lubricant and tissues
- emesis basin

- alcohol swabs
- laryngeal mirror
- nasal and ear speculums
- ophthalmoscope and otoscope
- pen light
- reflex hammer
- sphygmomanometer and stethoscope
- tape measure
- thermometer
- tongue depressors
- tuning fork
- urine specimen container
- gooseneck lamp

Competency

(**Conditions**) With the necessary supplies, (**Task**) you will be able to prepare the clinical room with the appropriate examination supplies, provide instruction and reassurance to the patient, and assist the physician as needed during the examination procedure (**Standards**) correctly within the time frame designated by the instructor.

1. Equip each examination room with the necessary supplies, equipment, and instruments. Ensure that instruments are in working order and the room temperature is comfortable.
2. Identify the patient and escort him or her to the examination room.
3. Wash your hands.
4. Obtain the patient's weight and height, usually in a semi-private but central location in the clinical area.
5. Obtain vital signs and pain assessment.

PROCEDURE 28-12 Prepare the Patient for Medical Examination and Assist the Physician (continued)

6. Instruct the patient to remove necessary clothing and to put on the gown or cover. Offer to assist the patient if necessary and explain where to place removed clothing.
7. Instruct the patient to sit on the examination table and provide a drape.
8. Obtain the patient history through interview and review of the completed forms (Figure 28-38 ◆).
9. Gather the instruments the physician will need.
10. Notify the physician that the patient is ready.
11. When the physician is ready, assist with positioning the patient and the physical examination. Be prepared to gather additional supplies and assist the physician with any instruments or supplies necessary for the examination.
12. Upon completion of the examination, assist the patient from the examination table.
13. Prepare specimens for examination and/or transport by labeling and completing appropriate forms.
14. Remove soiled instruments and equipment to the utility room for cleaning.
15. Clean the room and dispose of any waste. Wash your hands.
16. Prepare the room for the next patient.

Patient Education

Instruct the patient on the importance of accurate information. If the patient is unable to answer questions, reassure him or her that the information can be documented when the patient remembers. If the patient has specific questions for the physician and is worried about forgetting, provide a pen and paper for the patient to make notes while waiting.

Charting Example

04/27/XX 2:30 PM T 98.6°F, P 86, R 20. B/P 126/80. Pt states this is a routine physical. Medical history forms reviewed and completed with assistance from patient. Linda Anderson, RMA (AMT)

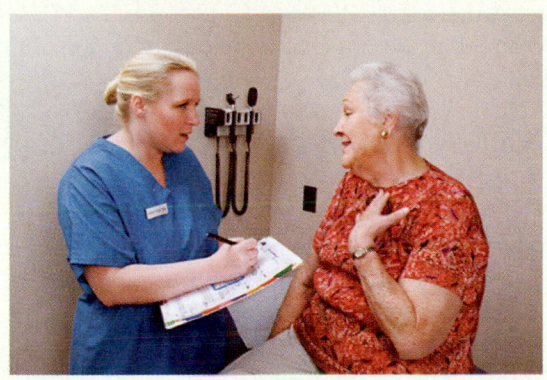

Figure 28-38 ◆ Taking the patient's history.

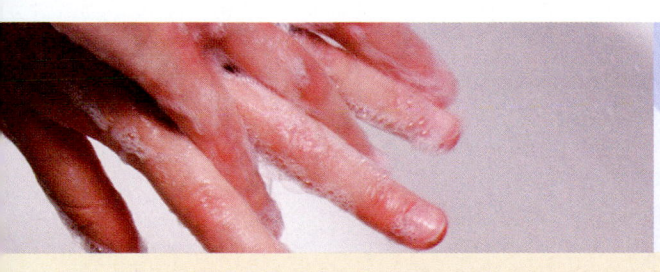

REVIEW

Chapter Summary

■ Vital signs establish baseline values for present and future medical assessment and treatment. They vary according to age but are specific to the individual because of medical condition(s), medications and medication interactions, and other factors such as obesity or exercise level.

■ Body temperature is generally lower in the morning before activity. Fever is an elevation of temperature and often indicates an infectious disease process that may or may not require antibiotic therapy.

■ Deviations from average pulse or respiration rates may indicate a normal physiological reaction, such as during and immediately after exercise, or may indicate a disease process of the cardiovascular and/or respiratory systems.

■ Blood pressure is the pressure the blood exerts on vessel walls during cardiac contraction and relaxation. The patient's baseline blood pressure and family and past medical history are useful in the diagnosis and treatment of medical conditions such as hypertension.

Chapter Summary (continued)

- Korotkoff sounds are the sounds that are actually heard as the arterial wall distends during the compression of the blood pressure cuff. The MA should practice taking blood pressure readings slowly in order to be able to identify each phase.
- Weight and height measurements are used as guidelines to diagnose obesity, but are also used to adjust medication dosages and dietary management for medical conditions such as diabetes mellitus.
- The medical assistant prepares the examination room and anticipates the physician's needs during the physical examination. The MA also prepares the patient by providing instruction and assistance in gowning, positioning, and draping. Draping protects the patient's modesty and provides warmth and comfort.
- The physician performs patient assessment using the tools of palpation, percussion, auscultation, and inspection during the medical examination.
- Recurrent patient visits include taking vital signs and preparing the patient and the examination room for the anticipated procedure.

Chapter Review

Multiple Choice

1. The appropriate cuff width for a child 1 to 4 years old is
   a. 6 cm.
   b. 9 cm.
   c. 2.5 cm.
   d. 13 cm.

2. Heat is lost through the skin by
   a. respiration.
   b. contraction.
   c. conduction.
   d. elimination.

3. The body temperature is lowest
   a. in the evening.
   b. 10 minutes after consuming food or a beverage.
   c. in the afternoon.
   d. in the morning.

4. An oral temperature is not contraindicated when
   a. the patient is an infant.
   b. the patient is elderly.
   c. the patient is combative.
   d. the patient is unconscious.

5. The skin is not observed for which of the following?
   a. elasticity
   b. color
   c. warmth
   d. turgor

6. A blood pressure reading of 110/60 mm Hg is an average normal reading for a child who is
   a. 6 years old.
   b. 3 years old.
   c. 10 years old.
   d. 14 years old.

7. When taking a tympanic temperature on an adult, you should
   a. not move the ear at all.
   b. pull the ear downward.
   c. pull the ear upward and forward.
   d. pull the ear upward.

8. When taking a tympanic temperature on a child, you should
   a. pull the ear upward and forward.
   b. pull the ear upward.
   c. pull the ear downward.
   d. not move the ear at all.

9. The measurement of weight and height is considered part of the routine that also includes all of the following except
   a. chest circumference.
   b. temperature.
   c. pulse.
   d. respirations.

10. Breathing is regulated by the
    a. hypothalamus.
    b. medulla oblongata.
    c. pituitary gland.
    d. thyroid.

True/False

T F 1. Temperature is the measurement of body heat produced and lost during metabolism, respiration, elimination, and environmental fluctuation.

T F 2. Most complete physical examinations begin at the head and proceed downward.

T F 3. The skin is observed for color, warmth, moisture, and turgor.

T F 4. The eyes are examined with an otoscope.

T F 5. Fluid in the chest cavity can be detected during palpation.

Chapter Review (continued)

Short Answer

1. Name and describe the four different types of fever.
2. Define *pulse.*
3. For a pelvic exam and Pap smear, the patient is assisted into which position?
4. What blood pressure readings are indicative of hypotension?
5. List at least six factors that affect the respiratory rate.

Research

1. Research common vital signs and symptoms of patients with known cardiac conditions such as hypertension, CAGB, and so on. How do these conditions affect the vital sign readings?
2. Research common vital signs and symptoms of patients with known pulmonary conditions such as COPD, emphysema, and so on. How do these conditions affect the vital sign readings?

Externship Application Experience

A patient has come to the office for her annual pelvic exam and Pap smear. This is her first physical examination since her left radical mastectomy. She appears anxious. Describe psychological support that you might give her during both preparation and procedure.

Resource Guide

U.S. Department of Health and Human Services
200 Independence Avenue, SW
Washington, DC 20201
1-877-696-6775
www.os.dhhs.gov

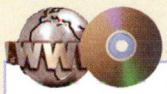

Med**Media**

http://www.MyMAKit.com

More on this chapter, including interactive resources, can be found on the Student CD-ROM accompanying this textbook and on http://www.MyMAKit.com.

CHAPTER 29

Minor Surgery

Case Study

Latesha is a new RMA in the office and Gwen, the office manager, is showing her the office protocol for nonroutine surgeries. First on the list of things to do is to check that a consent form has been signed and is available in the chart. When Latesha looks for it, she cannot find it and lets Gwen know. "Oh, I know it was signed. It just hasn't been filed yet. I'll bring it to you later," Gwen replies.

Next, Gwen takes Latesha to the room the surgery will be performed in. Latesha notices that the table paper is crinkled and a laryngoscope has been left on the counter. Latesha observes Gwen quickly change the table paper and place the laryngoscope back in its case and under the counter. Gwen does not use a disinfectant or sterilize any of the surfaces.

Objectives

After completing this chapter, you should be able to:

- Define and spell the key terminology in this chapter.
- Define the medical assistant's role in medical office surgery.
- List and describe surgeries performed in the medical office.
- Explain the essentials of consent.
- Discuss preoperative care of the patient in the medical office.
- Discuss how to set up the room for surgery in the medical office.
- Identify the types and functions of instruments used during surgery in the medical office.
- Explain the principles of positioning and draping for minor surgical procedures.
- List the types of anesthesia used during surgery in the medical office.
- Discuss the ways in which the MA assists the physician during minor surgery.
- Describe the suture materials used in minor surgery.
- Discuss recovery and postoperative care of the patient following surgery in the medical office.
- Describe postoperative patient teaching and discharge.
- Describe the stages of wound healing.
- Discuss the types of dressings used in medical office surgical procedures.

MedMedia
http://www.MyMAKit.com

Additional interactive resources and activities for this chapter can be found on http://www.MyMAKit.com. For videos, tips, audio glossary, legal and ethical scenarios, job scenarios, quizzes, games, and activities related to the content of this chapter, please access the accompanying CD-ROM in this book.

Video
Audio Glossary
Legal and Ethical Scenario: *Minor Surgery*
On the Job Scenario: *Minor Surgery*
Multiple Choice Quiz
Games: Crossword, Strikeout and Spelling Bee
Drag and Drop: Integumentary System: Organization of the Body
Tips
HIPAA Quiz

✚ MEDICAL ASSISTING STANDARDS

CAAHEP ENTRY-LEVEL STANDARDS	ABHES ENTRY-LEVEL COMPETENCIES
■ Perform within scope of practice (psychomotor) ■ Apply ethical behaviors, including honesty/integrity in performance of medical assisting practice (affective) ■ Explore issue of confidentiality as it applies to the medical assistant (cognitive) ■ Explain the rationale for performance of a procedure to a patient (affective) ■ Perform handwashing (psychomotor) ■ Assist physician with patient care (psychomotor) ■ Document accurately in the patient record (psychomotor) ■ Apply critical thinking skills in performing patient assessment and care (affective) ■ Practice Standard Precautions (psychomotor) ■ Perform sterilization procedures (psychomotor) ■ Show awareness of patients' concerns regarding their perceptions related to the procedure being performed (affective)	■ Maintain confidentiality at all times. ■ Be cognizant of ethical boundaries. ■ Exhibit initiative. ■ Adapt to change. ■ Evidence a responsible attitude. ■ Be courteous and diplomatic. ■ Conduct work within scope of education, training, and ability. ■ Be attentive, listen, and learn. ■ Be impartial and show empathy when dealing with patients. ■ Adapt what is said to the recipient's level of comprehension. ■ Adaptation for individualized needs. ■ Prepare patients for procedures. ■ Apply principles of aseptic techniques and infection control. ■ Wrap items for autoclaving. ■ Perform sterilization techniques. ■ Dispose of hazardous materials. ■ Practice Standard Precautions. ■ Prepare and maintain examination and treatment area. ■ Assist physician with examination and treatments. ■ Use quality control. ■ Collect and process specimens.

✔ COMPETENCY SKILLS PERFORMANCE

1. Prepare the skin for surgical procedure.
2. Set up a sterile tray and assist the physician with minor surgical procedures.
3. Assist the physician with suturing.
4. Assist the physician with suture or staple removal.
5. Change a sterile dressing.

Introduction

Changes within the insurance reimbursement system, along with advances in medical technology and surgical procedures, have resulted in many surgeries now being performed as outpatient procedures. Often referred to as ambulatory, minor, or office surgery, outpatient surgeries may range from a simple 10-minute procedure, such as the removal of a skin lesion, to the 23-hour outpatient stay for a surgical clinic procedure, such as disk repair and patient recovery time.

Key Terminology

abrasion—scraping away of the surface such as skin or teeth, by friction; an abrasion can be the result of injury or by mechanical means, as in dermabrasion for scar removal

anesthesia—partial or complete loss of sensation

approximation—joining together of surgical wound edges

avulsion—process of forcibly tearing off a part or structure of the body, such as a finger or a toe

biopsy—the obtaining of a representative tissue sample for microscopic examination, usually to establish a diagnosis

cannula—tube or sheath

closed wound—wound that involves trauma to the underlying tissue without a break in the skin or mucous membrane or exposure of the underlying tissue

colposcopy—the examination of vaginal and cervical tissue by means of a colposcope

contraction—process of drawing up or thickening of a muscle fiber

cryosurgery—the use of extremely cold probes to destroy unwanted, cancerous, or infected tissues

cutting—using a knife or surgical scissors to separate or divide tissues

debridement—the removal of foreign material and dead, damaged tissue from a wound using sterile technique

dissection—cutting into smaller parts for study and analysis of each part

distal—away from the center

drainage—the flow or withdrawal of fluids from a wound or cavity, such as pus from a cavity or wound

elective surgery—a treatment or surgical procedure not requiring immediate attention and therefore planned for the patient's or provider's convenience

electrocautery—cauterization using a variety of electrical modalities to create thermal energy, including a directly heated metallic applicator or bipolar or monopolar electrodes

emergency surgery—any urgent condition perceived by the physician as requiring immediate medical or surgical evaluation or treatment

Key Terminology *(continued)*

granulation—fleshy projections formed on the surface of a gaping wound that is not healing by first intention or indirect union

hemostat—instrument used to stop blood flow

incision—a cut made with a knife, electro-surgical unit, or laser especially for surgical purposes

inflammatory—an immunological defense against injury, infection, or allergy, marked by increases in regional blood flow, immigration of white blood cells, and release of chemical toxins

intraoperative—pertaining to patient care during surgery

laceration—a wound or irregular tear of the flesh

local anesthesia—absence of feeling or pain in a localized area of tissue without the loss of consciousness

Mayo stand—stand that holds a flat metal tray for setting up a sterile field for instruments and supplies; usually has an open side that allows it to be moved over a gurney or table

open wound—break in the skin or mucous membrane that exposes underlying tissues

optional surgery—the patient is given the option of surgery; surgery is not medically relevant, denial for surgery will have no adverse effects on the patient's health

postoperative (post-op)—pertaining to patient care following surgery

preoperative (pre-op)—pertaining to preparation before surgery

puncture—a hole or wound made by a sharp pointed instrument

Abbreviations

D & C—dilatation and curettage

I & D—incision and drainage

The Medical Assistant's Role in Office Surgery

The medical assistant's role in office surgery can cover scheduling through the completion of the procedure and dismissal of the patient. Individual responsibilities may include obtaining precertification approval, making sure the consent form is signed, ordering supplies, and cleaning and/or sterilizing instruments.

The term **preoperative** pertains to the period of preparation time before surgery. **Intraoperative** pertains to the period during surgery. **Postoperative** refers to the period involving patient care following surgery. Preoperative, intraoperative, and postoperative duties may include the following:

- Setting up the room for surgery
- Prepping the patient
- Assisting the physician during the treatment or minor surgical procedure
- Labeling and transporting any specimens
- Applying dressings
- Recovering the patient
- Providing reassurance to the patient
- Filing the insurance claim
- Transcribing dictation

The physician explains the nature of the procedure and associated potential risks to the patient and also answers the patient's questions. Patient teaching by an MA, under the direction of the physician, can include wound care, signs of infection, postoperative activity level, and prescriptions.

During the actual surgical procedure, the MA may be involved in two different roles—scrub assistant or circulating assistant. The scrub assistant is responsible for setting up the sterile field and assisting the physician in sterile procedures. Other responsibilities may include performing a 5-minute surgical scrub, sterile gowning, and gloving or assisting the physician with sterile gowning or gloving. During the surgical procedure, the scrub assistant hands instruments and other supplies to the physician and may also perform draping and cut sutures.

In some offices a circulating assistant is called a float assistant. The circulating assistant is considered "clean" rather than "sterile" and is responsible for obtaining supplies, equipment, and sterile packets for the "sterile" team. The circulating assistant completes any necessary requisitions, identifies specimens, and sends them to the laboratory. Positioning the patient and adjusting the surgical light are other duties. Occasionally, an assistant may wear sterile gloves to assist with cutting sutures and applying dressings.

Occasionally, the physician is the only one who scrubs, and one assistant may prepare the sterile field and assist the physician as needed. Cleaning the treatment room after the procedure, washing instruments, and discarding any disposables are also responsibilities of the scrub assistant.

Surgeries Performed in the Medical Office

Surgeries performed in a physician's office usually take 15 to 60 minutes. They include the following, also summarized in Table 29-1.

- **Biopsies** may be done with a needle, by shaving off a small area of the tissue, by punch, or by excision of the tissue.
- **Colposcopy** allows the physician to visually examine the vagina and cervix using light and magnification. During this procedure the physician may remove cells for biopsy.

TABLE 29-1 SIMPLE SURGICAL PROCEDURES THAT MAY BE PERFORMED IN A MEDICAL OFFICE OR SURGICAL CLINIC	
Arthroscopies	Laceration repair
Biopsy specimen collection	Laparoscopic procedures
Cataract and other surgical eye procedures	Laser surgery
	Mastectomies
Colposcopy	Nail or part of nail removal
Cryosurgery	Orthopedic repairs
Disk repairs	Prostate biopsies
D&Cs (dilatation and curettage)	Puncture wound irrigation and cleansing
Electrocauterization	Small growth, lesion, or cyst removal
Endoscopic procedures	
ENT (ear, nose, and throat) procedures	Suture and staple removal
	Tubal ligations
Foreign body removal	Vasectomies
Incision and drainage	Wound cleansing and debridement
Ingrown toenail excision	

- **Cryosurgery**—freezing abnormal tissue and destroying abnormal cells—may be performed in combination with colposcopy.
- **Debridement** is the removal of foreign material and dead, damaged tissue from a wound using sterile technique.
- **Electrocautery** is the use of high-frequency alternating electric current to destroy, cut, or remove tissue and coagulate small blood vessels.
- **Incision** and **drainage** (**I & D**) involves draining pus from abscesses caused by infection. I & D relieves pain and pressure.
- Foreign bodies embedded in soft tissue may be surgically removed.
- Growths and tumors are often excised in the medical office.
- Suture and staple removal, while not a surgical procedure, requires sterile technique.
- Suturing lacerations and other wounds requires cleansing, **approximation** (joining together surgical wound edges), and sterile technique.
- Vasectomies are regularly performed as outpatient surgeries in a medical office.

More complex procedures, while still considered ambulatory, are more often performed in a surgi-center or an outpatient surgical clinic. Most of these facilities are situated close to a hospital or in the same complex as the physician's office. Some can accommodate a 23-hour outpatient procedure, meaning the patient stays less than 24 hours without an overnight stay. Although these facilities employ MAs, advanced training is necessary for these positions.

Another way to classify surgeries is elective, emergency, or optional. An **elective surgical procedure** is considered medically necessary but may be performed at the patient's convenience. Surgery that must be performed immediately is considered an **emergency surgery**. An **optional surgery** is

not medically necessary but is one the patient wishes to have done.

Implied and Informed Consent

As you learned in ∞ Chapters 4 and 24, patient consent is required before all medical treatment. When a patient visits the physician's office, he or she "implies" consent for routine examination and procedures by body language or action. For example, a patient who sits on the examining table and raises her arm for blood pressure to be taken or lowers her arm for venipuncture is giving implied consent.

For a nonroutine procedure, however, informed consent is required. Special procedures and surgical procedures usually require a signed consent form. The physician must discuss with the patient details of the procedure, the expected outcome, the risks involved, and possible negative outcomes.

Preoperative Care and Patient Preparation

In some cases, preoperative care may start a week before the scheduled procedure. Preoperative care includes the following:

- Obtaining the necessary laboratory tests.
- Instructing the patient in both preoperative preparation and postoperative care.
- Informing the patient about the time to arrive for the procedure.
- Instructing the patient to have someone available to drive him or her home after the procedure.

As with other patient teaching, both oral and written instructions should be given. It is good practice to include a family member or significant other(s) in the teaching process, both in the preoperative preparation and in the postoperative release. The patient and/or significant other(s) should be advised concerning diet and any other preoperative requirements. Postoperative instructions may also be given at this time. The patient should be instructed to notify the office if he or she develops a fever or any other illness the day of the scheduled surgery.

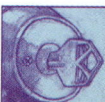

**Keys to Success
SIGNING THE CONSENT FORM**

Some physicians place a statement at the bottom of the consent form: "To assure that you have understood the information presented, please copy the following statement in your own handwriting: 'I understand the information presented and am willing to accept the fact that this procedure is not 100 percent guaranteed for success.'" This statement is usually specific to the procedure and may list possible unsuccessful results. It is meant to ensure that a patient reads and fully understands the consent he or she has given for surgery, including the risks.

Critical Thinking Question 29-1

Latesha cannot locate the signed informed consent paperwork that Gwen "knows" she had the patient sign and that she promised to bring to Latesha later. How should Latesha handle this situation?

Setting Up the Room

For each surgical procedure, nonsterile surgical supplies must be gathered and arranged in an area separate from the sterile field. The MA should review the procedure book or card to see what supplies are necessary and in what order they will be used. Before setting up any supplies or equipment, the MA should confirm that the room is clean and that all surfaces are disinfected. The MA should place clean table paper on the examination or surgical table and check the sterilization dates on all sterile packets. Changes in JCAHO and AAMI standards reflect that sterility is event-related and not time-related. Packages that have not been compromised are now considered sterile indefinitely. The standard expiration date depends on the type of package; however, many offices will adhere to the following guidelines:

- 30 days for packages enclosed with non-woven paper
- 3 weeks for packages enclosed with muslin
- 9 to 12 months for packages enclosed in disposable pouches

Gather any necessary equipment or supplies.

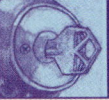

Critical Thinking Question 29-2

Latesha observed Gwen cleaning the room but not sanitizing it or confirming that the counters were disinfected. What should Latesha do?

Keys to Success
EASING A PATIENT'S ANXIETY AND FEARS

As an MA, you play an important role in helping to ease a patient's fears and anxieties. An informed patient is usually a less anxious patient. Some facilities mail or give printed materials to a patient when the procedure is scheduled. These materials provide instructions for any preoperative preparations, diet, or testing that is to be done, as well as instructions for the day of the surgery. Many are procedure-specific, explaining the procedure, the anesthesia, the recovery time and process, and anticipated activity restrictions.

If the procedure is done during an office visit as the result of findings during that office visit, you should be prepared to answer questions as you are prepping the patient. Should there be a question beyond your scope of training or knowledge, you should refer it to the physician before the start of the procedure. Remain calm and answer all questions honestly and confidently.

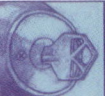

Keys to Success
PROCEDURE CARDS AND BOOKS

To provide quality care and continuity, most facilities have procedure cards or books that list each procedure, the required supplies and equipment, and step-by-step instructions.

Wash your hands before setting up the sterile field on a **Mayo stand**(s). Open the sterile packets and drop sterile instruments and supplies on the field without contaminating them. Cover or drape the sterile field with a sterile cloth and push the Mayo stand to the side out of the traffic pattern.

Instruments

Surgical instruments are classified by function, such as clamping, cutting, dilating, dissecting, grasping, probing, suturing, and visualization. Specialty areas, such as ear, nose, and throat (ENT), gynecology, neurology, obstetrics, orthopedics, proctology, and urology require special instruments. Some instruments are named for the surgeon who developed them. Most are made of steel and are rustproof, stainproof, heat-resistant, and durable. They are delicate and expensive and must be handled with care.

The tray for a minor surgical procedure usually includes a scalpel with or without a blade, scissors, **hemostat,** and needle holder (Figure 29-1 ◆). The physician indicates what type of blade and suture will be used. A syringe and needle are dropped on the sterile field for the physician to use for the local anesthesia. The physician may use a larger gauge needle to draw up the anesthetic and then change to a smaller-gauge needle for the injection.

Clamping and Grasping

Forceps are two-pronged instruments used to grasp tissue (Figure 29-2 ◆). Some are hinged at one end with a spring-type hinge and can be opened and closed with the fingers and

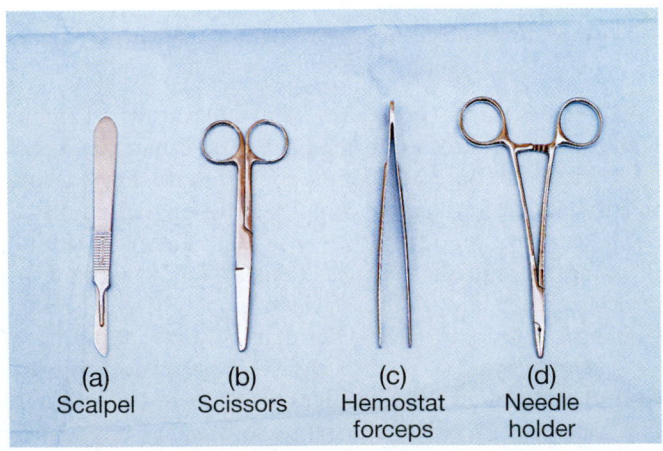

(a) Scalpel   (b) Scissors   (c) Hemostat forceps   (d) Needle holder

Figure 29-1 ◆ Tray for a minor surgical procedure.

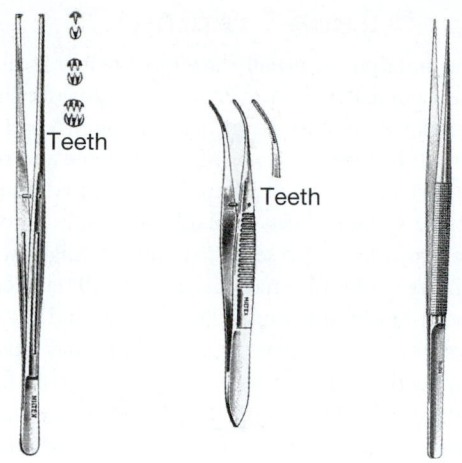

Figure 29-2 ◆ Types of forceps.

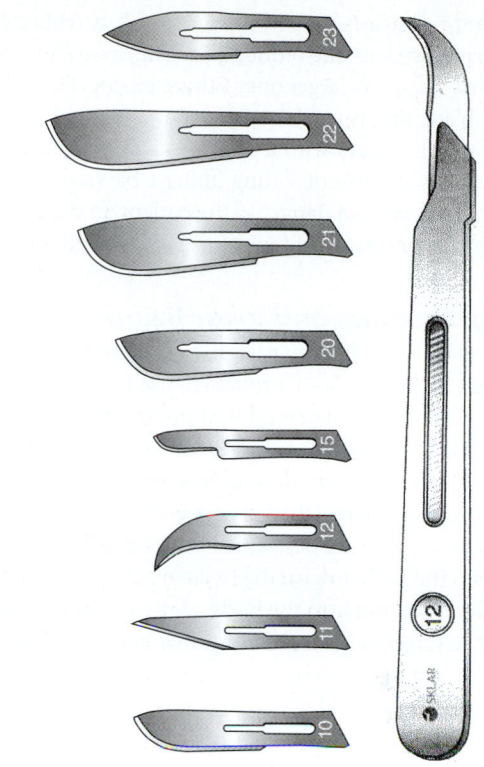

Figure 29-3 ◆ Scalpels and blades.

thumb. They may have either a smooth mouth or teeth to help with grasping.

Ring or sponge forceps have hinges farther down on the shanks, similar to scissors hinges. These forceps may be straight or curved and may have teeth or be smooth. A ratchet on the handle allows for securing or fastening the forceps. The operator end has a ring-like structure for a finger and a thumb. These forceps include Allis tissue forceps, small mosquito hemostats, longer Kelly hemostats, even longer hemostats, and hemostats with ring-like structures to grasp sponges. Hemostats are used specifically to clamp blood vessels.

Needle holders hold the needle for suturing. Like hinged hemostats, needle holders are hinged, usually close to the working end. There are grooves on the inner part of the holder shank to secure the needle. Placement of the needle is important. The needle holder should grasp the needle toward the eye, one-third of the length of the shaft. Care must be taken to face the needle in the correct direction for a right-handed or left-handed physician.

Towel clamps have sharp points to hold towels and drapes in place.

Cutting

Cutting is using a knife or surgical scissors to separate or divide tissues. Scalpels are knives with different types and sizes of blades. They may consist of one piece and be disposable or have a reusable handle and a disposable blade (Figure 29-3 ◆). Surgical blades come in various sizes and shapes. Some are longer than others, some have straight blades, and others have curved blades. The physician indicates his or her choice by number. Scalpels and blades must be handled carefully and are disposed of as sharps.

Scissors are used for dissecting as well as for cutting (Figure 29-4 ◆). **Dissection** is the process of cutting into smaller parts for study and analysis. Scissors may have sharp (pointed) or blunt tips, and straight or curved blades.

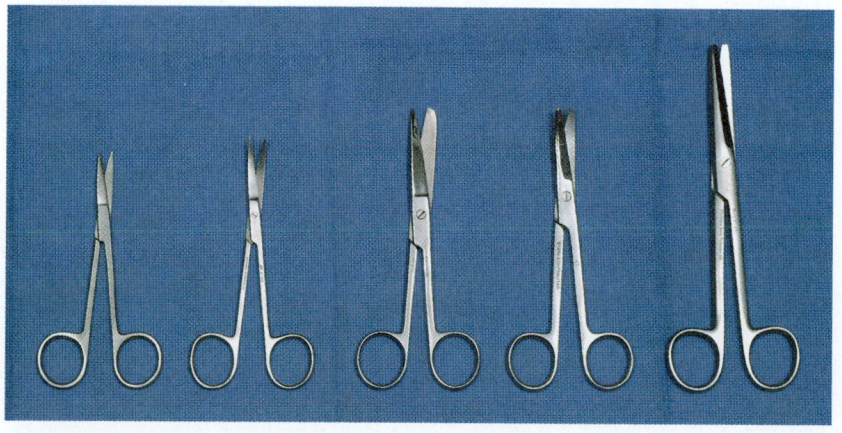

Figure 29-4 ◆ Types of scissors.

Operating scissors have two sharp blades, two blunt blades, or one sharp blade and one blunt blade. They range in size from very small iris scissors to larger ones. Suture scissors have a hooked tip on one blade that is used to slip under a suture to clip it for removal. Angled scissors with a blunt tip on the longer end are bandage scissors, capable of sliding under a bandage or dressing and cutting it off without danger to the patient. In dissecting scissors both blades are blunt and may be either straight or curved.

Dilating, Probing, and Visualizing

Instruments used for dilating may also be used for probing and visualization (Figure 29-5 ◆). Probes are used to explore wounds and cavities. They have a curved blunt point for easier insertion. A trocar is a hollow **cannula** inserted into a body cavity to withdraw fluids. Punches are used to remove small samples of tissue for examination and detection of cancerous cells.

Various types of scopes, which are usually lighted, may be inserted into the body to visualize a cavity. A speculum may be opened after insertion into the body cavity to visualize the area or to remove samples of tissue for additional examination.

Positioning and Draping

Positioning and draping usually take place before local anesthesia is administered. Positioning provides support for the patient and proper exposure of the surgical area. The MA will assist the patient onto the examination or operating table and make him or her comfortable, use small pillows to provide additional comfort and place a drape, sheet, or blanket over any exposed areas to provide warmth and preserve the patient's dignity. If a general anesthesia is administered, the patient will be asleep before the final positioning and draping. The MA should pay attention to any disabilities or special needs the patient may have.

Draping the patient and the area provides a sterile field for the procedure. The physician can work without contaminating instruments or equipment, which helps to prevent microorganisms from entering the wound.

Drapes are made of sterile muslin cloth or sterile paper, often with a vinyl or plastic backing. They come in various sizes and colors. The choice depends on the physician's preference. Drapes called *fenestrated drapes* have a slit or hole that exposes the surgical area.

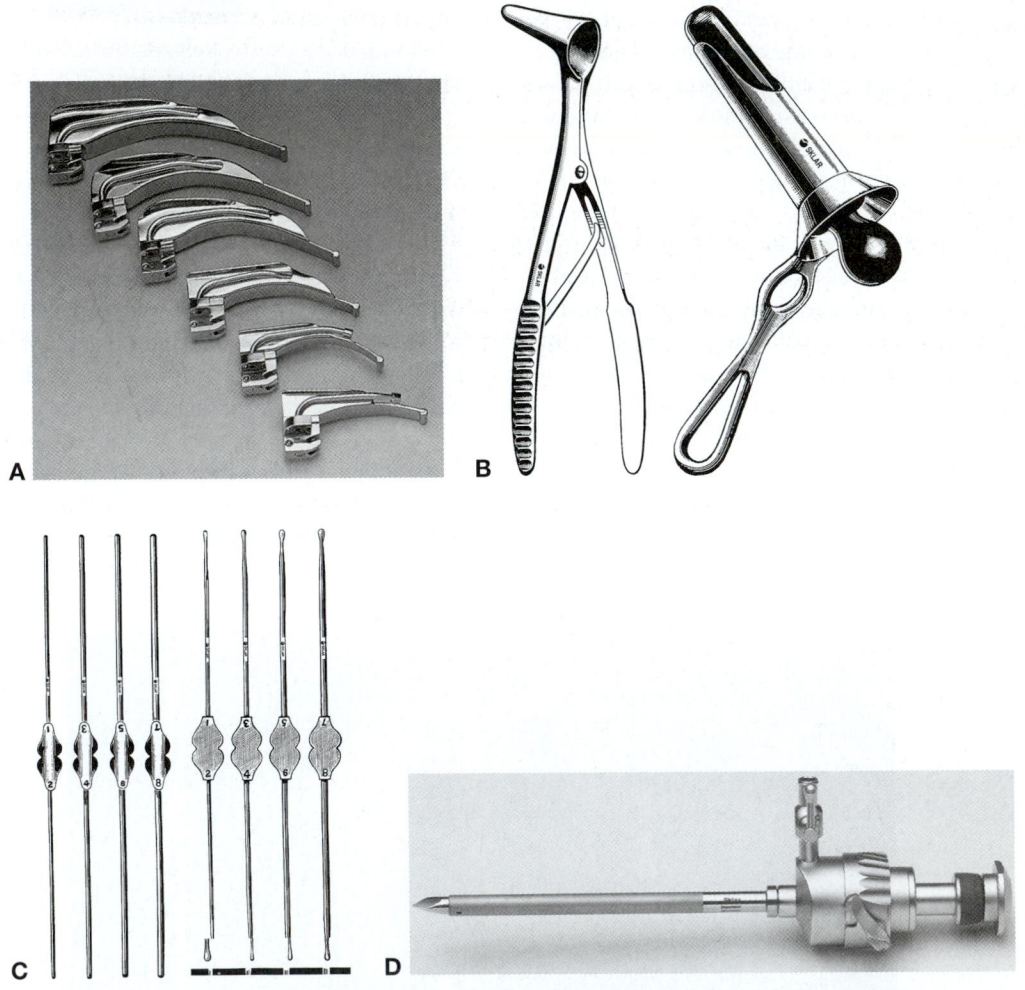

Figure 29-5 ◆ (A) Scopes; (B) speculums; (C) probes; (D) trocar.

PROCEDURE 29-1 Prepare the Skin for Surgical Procedure
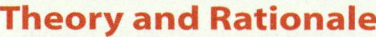

Theory and Rationale

Proper skin preparation, including cleansing, disinfecting, and applying antiseptic, is critical to prevent contamination by microorganisms and lower the potential for infection during surgical procedures. The area prepped must be at least 2 inches beyond the surgical field or the area exposed by drapes. A plastic-backed drape is placed under the portion of the patient's body to be prepped in order to absorb or contain any liquids.

The basic skin prep consists of three steps:

1. Shaving, if necessary.
2. Scrubbing and rinsing with an antiseptic soap.
3. Applying antiseptic to the surgical area.

Sterile sponges held by sterile forceps or sterile gloved hands are used for each of these steps and for each area cleansed. Applying the sponges in concentric circles from the center outward removes microorganisms from the immediate surgical area. Most physicians prefer a 5-minute scrub of the area. Should the prep area be a hand or foot, the entire appendage must be cleansed, particularly between the fingers or toes, to remove microorganisms from crevices or folds.

Hair is considered a contaminant and may need to be removed from the surgical site by shaving. If shaving is required, a disposable razor is used to shave the hair from the cleansed area in the direction of growth.

The next step of the skin prep involves application of an antiseptic solution, such as Povidone iodine, chlorhexidine gluconate, or benzalkonium chloride. It is important to confirm that the patient is not allergic to iodine solutions before applying. The antiseptic solution is applied in the same manner as the cleansing process or may be applied with cotton-tipped applicators. The area is allowed to air-dry so that the disinfectant has time to reduce and kill microorganisms.

Either you or the physician places sterile drapes over the area until the procedure begins. Dispose of contaminated supplies and instruments used during skin preparation and tray setup. This keeps the procedure area organized and the clean, dirty, and sterile areas defined.

After the procedure, dispose of soiled dressings and material. Remove your gloves and place one hand inside an empty plastic bag. With this hand pick up and place all soiled materials in a bag. With the other hand pull the outside of the bag over the soiled dressings and material. Dispose of gloves and soiled materials in a biohazard bag or container.

Materials

- shave prep kit, including razor, sterile basin pack, antiseptic germicidal soap, sterile 4 × 4s, sterile applicators, sterile sponge forceps
- Mayo stand or side tray
- sterile water or saline
- waste receptacle
- hazardous waste container
- plastic bags for disposal of contaminated material
- sterile gloves
- sterile towels
- sterile drapes
- antiseptic

Competency

(**Conditions**) With the necessary materials, you will be able to (**Task**) prepare the patient's skin for a surgical procedure with a surgical scrub and shave (**Standards**) correctly, within the time designated by your instructor.

1. Wash your hands thoroughly. Gather equipment and supplies.
2. Identify the patient and guide him or her to the treatment area. Explain the entire procedure to the patient.
3. Instruct the patient to void if necessary.
4. Have the patient remove appropriate clothing and wear a patient gown until it is time for positioning and draping.
5. Wash your hands and apply non-sterile gloves. Position the patient and remove the gown as necessary.
6. Unwrap the outer wraps of all packs. Unwrap the basin pack.
7. Following correct technique for pouring liquids in a sterile field, pour germicidal soap into one basin, sterile water or saline into the second basin, and germicidal solution into the third basin (Figure 29-6 ◆).
8. You may need to shave the area before it is surgically scrubbed. If so, apply soap solution to the area.
9. Remove the razor from the shave prep pack that has been placed outside the sterile field.
10. Pull the skin gently taut at the surgical site. Shave in the direction of hair growth (Figure 29-7 ◆).
11. Rinse the skin with sterile saline or water in an outward circular motion, then pat the area dry.

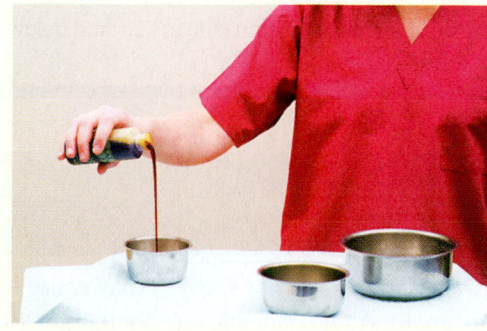

Figure 29-6 ◆ Pour germicidal soap into one basin, sterile water or saline into the second basin, and antiseptic into the third basin.

continued

PROCEDURE 29-1 Prepare the Skin for Surgical Procedure (continued)

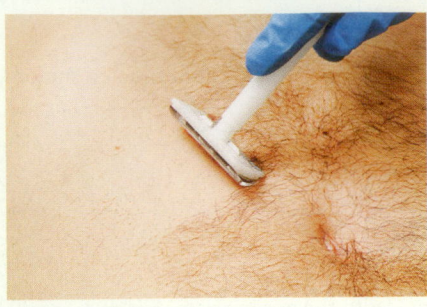

Figure 29-7 ◆ Shave in the direction of hair growth.

12. Wash your hands and put on sterile gloves.
13. Apply soapy solution to the patient's skin in a circular motion with a sterile sponge, starting at the center of the surgical site and moving outward (Figure 29-8 ◆). During the application the circles should not overlap each other or repeat over the same area.
14. Rinse the area in the same circular manner with new sterile sponges.
15. Allow area to air dry.
16. Apply germicidal solution in concentric circles with a sterile sponge or cotton-tipped applicators.

17. After allowing the prep area to completely air-dry, drape 3 to 5 inches above and below the surgical site with sterile towels (Figure 29-9 ◆).
18. Drape the prepared surgical site with a sterile towel (Figure 29-10 ◆). If the patient must be left unattended at any time after the surgical scrub, another medical assistant or scrub float will need to cover the prepped area with a sterile towel.
19. If the physician did not participate in the patient prep or setting up the surgical tray, alert him or her that the patient has been prepped.
20. Document the scrub procedure with patient education notes.

Patient Education

The patient should be instructed not to touch the prepped area. The patient should understand that the prepping procedure reduces the risk for infection by setting up a sterile surgical field.

Charting Example

03/17/xx 8:30 a.m. Right lower-quadrant prepped and draped for mole excision. Disinfected with Betadine. Patient instructed not to touch area. Patient nodded agreement. Richard McNeal, CMA (AAMA)

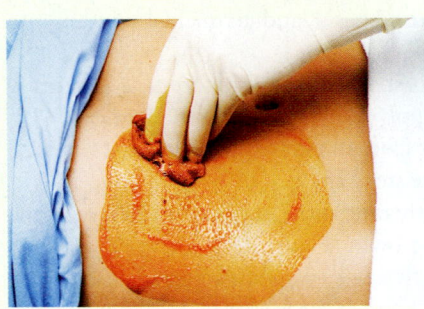

Figure 29-8 ◆ Apply soapy solution to the patient's skin in a circular motion with a sterile sponge.

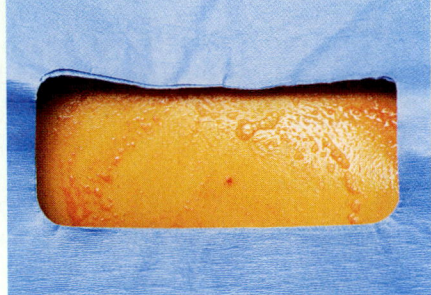

Figure 29-9 ◆ Drape 3 to 5 inches above and below the surgical site with sterile towels.

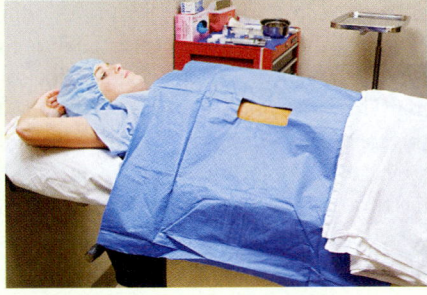

Figure 29-10 ◆ Drape the prepared surgical site with a sterile towel.

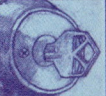

Keys to Success
SHAVING

Some practitioners feel that shaving may cause minute nicks or breaks in the skin, leaving open areas that are prone to infection. It is the policy of some physicians not to shave the area, or they may do it themselves, especially when areas of the scalp near the face are involved. Others may request that excess hair be carefully removed by trimming it close with scissors.

Anesthesia

Anesthesia is the partial or complete absence of sensation. During many procedures, usually surgical procedures, anesthetic medications are administered to relieve the patient of feelings of pain. Sometimes an additional amnesiac drug or muscle relaxant may be needed. In most office procedures local anesthetics are used to achieve a painless state, with the patient alert during the procedure. Occasionally, an anesthesiologist may administer a general anesthesia that induces loss of consciousness.

When drugs are administered to alter the patient's level of consciousness, the patient is placed on a cardiac monitor or a pulse oximeter. Emergency equipment and supplies, including oxygen, an Ambu bag, and a crash cart or emergency drug box, are all in close range of the anesthesiologist, who monitors the patient's vital signs throughout general anesthesia.

Local Anesthesia

Local anesthesia induces the absence of sensation in a specific area of tissue without the loss of consciousness. Table 29-2 lists some of the medications used in the three methods of administering local anesthesia. The physician determines which local anesthetic to use based on the patient's medical condition, history, and other medications the patient takes. The physician may also consider longer-lasting anesthesia to provide the patient with greater comfort during the procedure.

Local anesthesia in topical form may be a cream, gel, liquid, or spray. It may be used on children or on small lacerations in adults and reduces or eliminates the pain caused by injected local anesthesia. It takes topical anesthesia 15 to 20 minutes to anesthetize an area. Liquid anesthesia is applied to a wound with a sterile cotton applicator in repeated applications until the area loses feeling. The patient should be advised that it may sting or burn briefly when it is first applied to an open wound. Epinephrine in the preparation causes constriction of the vessels and an obvious blanching (whitening) of the tissue where it is applied.

Injected local anesthesia may also contain epinephrine, a drug with vasoconstricting (reducing blood flow to the area) properties. In addition to increasing the duration of action of the anesthetic, it prevents extra blood from entering the surgical field and improves visualization for the physician. However, certain precautions must be taken when epinephrine is used with a local anesthesia. Because of its vasoconstricting properties, it must not be used in procedures on fingers, toes, nose, ears, penis, or any area where local blood supply would be compromised. Also, caution should be used with patients with heart or respiratory disease.

The MA may often assist the physician in drawing up the local anesthesia. The physician wears sterile gloves and takes a sterile syringe from a sterile field or from an opened, sterile package that the MA is holding with contaminated edges folded back. After checking that he has chosen the correct vial of local anesthesia, the MA will cleanse the rubber stopper of the vial with 70% isopropyl alcohol. Holding the vial firmly in one hand while supporting his wrist with his other hand, the MA will extend the rubber stopper end toward the physician. The physician must be able to read the label and confirm it is the correct medication. The physician inserts the needle into the rubber stopper, injects air from the syringe, and withdraws the desired amount of anesthesia medication. Occasionally, the physician may change needles to a smaller gauge before injecting into the tissue.

Injected local anesthetics tend to burn for approximately 10 seconds after the injection. It is good practice to prepare the patient for the initial unpleasant sensation.

Nerve blocks may be administered for procedures that are more involved than simple laceration repair. Depending on the location of the nerve to be blocked, either the physician or the anesthesiologist may administer it.

Before any anesthetic is administered, the patient *must* be questioned about allergies and any previous reaction to local anesthetic. Questions about any cardiac problems or disease and any respiratory difficulties must also be asked. Patient reactions to local anesthetics may be as severe as anaphylactic shock. In an office where minor surgical procedures are performed, one of the MA's responsibilities will be to maintain the emergency drug box or cart and to see that it is within easy reach of rooms where surgical procedures are performed.

Assisting During Minor Surgery

The MA may assist the physician during minor surgical procedures by performing preoperative, intraoperative, and postoperative duties. The MA will also provide emotional support for the patient. On the day of the procedure the medical assistant will ask the patient again about allergies to medications, especially to anesthesia. The MA will assess and record vital signs. If the patient expresses any concern or has any questions, the physician should be advised.

Passing instruments to the physician is a skill developed over time. If the scrub assistant is sterile, the instruments may be passed directly into the physician's extended hand. The scrub assistant grasps the working end of the instrument with care and firmly places the operator end in the physician's palm. It is not necessary to "slap" the instrument into the physician's hand but only to firmly place it there.

Should the physician be the only one with sterile gloves, the MA will open the sterile packaging of the instrument, folding it back over his or her hand. The MA must be sure to open the package at the handle or operator end. The MA will extend the operator end of the sterile instrument to the physician, who will grasp and remove it without touching the nonsterile outside of the package.

TABLE 29-2 TYPES OF LOCAL ANESTHESIA	
Method	**Pharmaceutical Example**
Topical or surface anesthesia (painted or sprayed on the skin or mucous membranes)	Lidocaine 4% Ethyl chloride spray, external only Cocaine with or without epinephrine
Nerve block	Procaine 1%–2% Lidocaine 1%–2%
Infiltration or injection	Procaine (Novocaine) 1%–2% Lidocaine (Xylocaine) 1%–2% Tetracaine (Pontocaine) 0.2, 0.3, & 1% Bupivacaine (Marcaine) 0.25–0.75% Lidocaine with epinephrine

PROCEDURE 29-2 **Set Up a Sterile Tray and Assist the Physician with Minor Surgical Procedures**

Theory and Rationale

Preoperative, intraoperative, and postoperative duties may include setting up the room for surgery, prepping the patient, assisting the physician during the procedure, labeling and transporting any specimens, applying dressings, and re-covering the patient. As an MA, you will likely assume the role of circulating assistant during minor surgery.

As a circulating assistant, you will add sterile supplies by folding back edges of packages and dropping items onto the sterile field. The sterile wrapper edges must hang over the edge of the Mayo stand to protect both the sterile field and the operator from contamination. Using sterile transfer forceps, place instruments in the correct position on the sterile field according to the physician's preference and clinical protocol. *Avoid reaching across the sterile field for any reason during the procedure.* Crossing over a sterile field can contaminate it, in which case a new sterile tray setup will be required.

Upon completion of the procedure, you will cleanse and dress the operative area as directed. Wearing gloves, you will place any specimens or tissue in the appropriate container(s), label for the laboratory, and store in the appropriate area. Once the specimens have been collected, while you are still wearing gloves, you may cover the surgical tray, as it may be disturbing for some patients to view the used/blood-tinted surgical equipment. You should remove your gloves and wash your hands.

Next you should assist the patient with re-dressing as appropriate and provide education of what to expect in the days following the surgery. Once the patient has been removed from the surgical area, you may don the appropriate PPE and clean the surgical area by placing the disposable items in the biohazard containers and taking the nondisposable items to be sterilized in the appropriate area. Without leaving the patient, you will begin cleaning the area by gathering instruments and supplies used during the procedure. You will place any specimens or tissue in an appropriate container and label it for the laboratory.

Patient teaching concerning the procedure and postoperative care is usually your responsibility. Under the direction of the physician, you will give instructions regarding wound care, signs of infection, activity level, prescriptions, and so on. Simple procedures usually only require repeating postoperative instructions, reviewing printed instructions with the patient and/or family or significant other(s), and confirming follow-up appointments. More complex procedures may require a recheck of vital signs and having the patient upright for a short time to make sure he or she is clinically stable enough to leave.

Materials

- sterile surgical pack, including two pairs of sterile gloves, towel pack, 4 × 4 sponge pack, sterile drapes, needle pack and suture materials, sterile instrument pack, sterile syringe pack, two sterile surgical basins, and sterile specimen containers
- Mayo stand and/or a surgical instrument table
- transfer forceps and holder
- waste container lined with plastic bag
- sharps disposal container
- biohazard waste container
- local anesthetic
- alcohol preps

Competency

(**Conditions**) With the necessary materials, you will be able to (**Task**) assist the physician with minor surgery by preparing for the procedure, anticipating physician needs, and providing or reinforcing instruction to the patient or significant other(s) (**Standards**) correctly and within the time designated by the instructor.

1. Determine scrub and float assistant staffing needs for the procedure.
2. Wash your hands.
3. Sanitize and disinfect a Mayo instrument stand by using a 4 × 4 gauze square that has been soaked in 70% isopropyl alcohol. Starting from the middle of the tray, use a circular motion to cleanse the entire tray, including the rim (Figure 29-11 ◆).
4. If your place of employment uses sterile disposable drapes, place the package on a counter and carefully peel back the top layer to expose the fan-folded drape. Grasping only the corner of the drape with your thumb and forefinger, raise it quickly to a height that allows it to carefully unfold, *without* touching the countertop, or any portion of your body. If your place of employment uses sterile towels, they will be folded in the same manner and placed inside towel canisters. Sterile towels will be removed the same way.

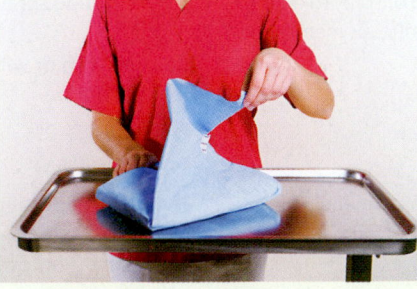

Figure 29-11 ◆ Open the sterile packs on the Mayo stand or surgery table.

PROCEDURE 29-2 Set Up a Sterile Tray and Assist the Physician with Minor Surgical Procedures *(continued)*

5. With the drape held firmly with the thumb and forefinger of one hand well above waist level, take your other hand and pinch the opposite corner of the drape between your thumb and forefinger. Both corners along the shortest side of the drape are now firmly held.

6. With the drape held above waist level, carefully reach over the Mayo stand and pull the drape toward you as you lay it on the stand. It is critical that the bottom edge of the drape does not touch the stand as you are reaching across. The drape must also not swing and touch any portion of your body at any time.

7. At this point in the procedure the tray is now considered sterile. It must not be left unattended, reached over, or touched. If the sterile drape needs to be adjusted, you may reach under and use the draping portions to make minor adjustments.

8. Gather the appropriate supplies needed for the procedure. If you gather items that are wrapped twice, you must apply them in a sterile manner:
   - Position the package in your nondominant hand with the flap facing up. The package should look like an envelope, with the envelope opening on top and toward your fingertips. You may adjust the package as needed at this point, as this outer wrapping is not sterile and neither is your hand.
   - Pull open the top flap by gently grasping it with your other hand and pulling it up and underneath, tucking it into the fingers of the nondominant hand.
   - Follow the same procedure, pulling the right flap to the right and the left flap to the left, without crossing over your nondominant hand. Rationale: This method allows the inner package to remain sterile while it is being exposed for removal. Gathering the loose ends into your fingers prevents them from being dragged across the sterile field or folding back onto the sterile package before it is placed on the tray.
   - Carefully apply the package to the sterile field by holding it well above the tray and letting it carefully fall onto the tray.

   Items that have been sterilized in plastic pouches must also be applied in a sterile manner:
   - Carefully peel apart the package and allow the instrument to fall onto the sterile field.
   - Do not allow the package to touch the sterile field and do not allow the instruments to slide or bounce as they land on the tray.

9. Once all items have been applied to the sterile field, you may wash your hands using a surgical scrub and apply sterile gloves. With sterile gloves on you may open the previously applied sterile package and verify its contents. You may also arrange the items on the tray according to

physician preference. Note: If you drop your hands below your waist or touch any item outside of the sterile area, you are once again contaminated. You must also pay very close attention to your clothes as scrubs that are worn too loosely will fall forward and contaminate the sterile tray. Once you have verified that all items are present and arranged according to physician preference, you must cover the sterile tray. To cover the sterile tray follow the instructions for setup, but instead of crossing over the field and pulling the drape to you, you must hold the drape in front of you at a level so that the top towel and bottom towel are even and carefully lay it over the tray.

10. Identify the patient and guide him or her to the treatment area. Explain the entire procedure to the patient.

11. Instruct the patient to void if necessary.

12. Provide draping or a gown for the patient as required for the procedure. Sometimes patients disrobe and gown in another room before entering the treatment area.

13. Assist the patient onto the examination table.

14. Perform a skin prep as described in Procedure 29-1.

15. Assist the physician in scrubbing, gowning, and gloving as needed.

16. The physician may want you to open the packet of sterile gloves for him or her and place the packet where it can be easily accessed at the start of the procedure. (Depending on the duties of the scrub assistant during the procedure, you may be designated to scrub, and to gown, mask, and glove.)

17. When the physician is ready to proceed, he or she may remove the drapes from the tray setups without contaminating the trays or the sterile field. If you are directed to do this, grasp the towel or drape at the **distal** corners (away from the center) (Figure 29-12 ◆). Lift the towel toward you without reaching over the tray and unprotected sterile field.

18. In anticipation of soiled dressings, place a bag or container to the side for the physician to discard them into.

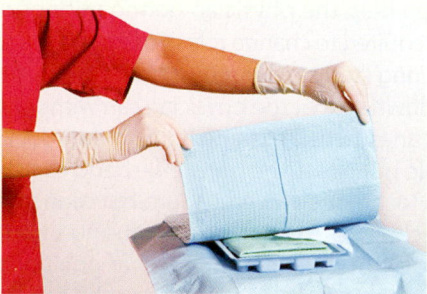

Figure 29-12 ◆ Grasp the towel or drape at the distal corners.

continued

PROCEDURE 29-2 Set Up a Sterile Tray and Assist the Physician with Minor Surgical Procedures *(continued)*

19. Observe closely and anticipate the physician's needs.
    - If a specimen container is needed, hold it to receive a specimen.
    - *Note:* You may fulfill the role of scrub assistant or circulating assistant, depending on the procedure and the needs of the physician.
20. In most cases the physician will prefer to apply the first sterile dressing but occasionally may direct the scrub to do it. You will reinforce or anchor the dressing.
21. When the procedure has been completed, collect all soiled instruments in a basin and remove them from the patient's view. Dispose of soiled dressings in biohazard containers.
22. Remove your gloves and discard.
23. Wash your hands.
24. If specimen containers have been contaminated, use clean gloves to place and tighten lids on them.
25. Label and bag specimens before transporting or sending them to the lab.
26. Obtain and chart vital signs following office policy and document your recovery observations, including mental status, changes in drainage and size of drainage on dressings, and ability to ambulate and urinate. (Observation requirements may vary according to the medical office specialty.)
27. Review your observations with the physician.
28. When the physician determines discharge readiness, he or she discusses care instructions with the patient and significant other(s).
29. Give the patient a printed copy of the physician's discharge instructions, and review and reinforce them with the patient. Before the patient leaves the facility, help with any additional paperwork, such as follow-up appointments.
30. Assist or transport the patient to significant others or, in some cases, to the car.
31. Chart the results of patient instruction immediately.
32. Don appropriate PPE to clean and sanitize the treatment room for the next patient.
33. Wash your hands.

Patient Education

It is important to inform the patient of each step of the procedure. A simple explanation about why a particular step or technique is performed decreases the patient's anxiety and ensures cooperation. Follow-up instruction is also vital. Ask the patient or significant other(s) to repeat discharge instructions to make sure of understanding and compliance.

Charting Example

04/29/xx 10:30 a.m. Discharge instructions reviewed with the patient and family. Patient displays some facial expression of pain. Wife able to verbalize correctly how to administer pain medication and antibiotic. Wife states correctly the signs of infection to report if they occur. Carlos Lopez, RMA (AMI)

NOTE: The physician will also chart about the procedure and his or her observations immediately after the procedure.

Sutures and Suture Removal

Sutures, or "stitches," hold the edges of tissue together as a wound heals. The wound may be accidental or intentional, such as a surgical incision. Sutures are also used in the ligation of vessels to stop bleeding.

Most suture material comes prepackaged with attached needles called *swaged needles*. Other sutures must be threaded into a needle. When opening prepackaged swaged sutures, grasp the needle with the needle holder and remove it first while grasping the suture close to the needle and guiding it through the thumb and finger. This will help straighten the suture as it is removed (Figure 29-13 ◆). Care must be taken not to contaminate the entire length of suture material.

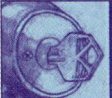

**Keys to Success
CHANGING ROLES**

When you help the physician during minor surgery, you may be required to change roles. For example, a scrub assistant wearing sterile gloves must hold a bottle of lidocaine upside-down so that the physician can withdraw some for the local anesthetic. The hand holding the lidocaine is now nonsterile but clean. The nonsterile hand can still be used for clean technique and procedure, but cannot be used for sterile technique. This can be a confusing situation, as the scrub assistant must remember that one hand is sterile and the other is clean and that he or she cannot pass the nonsterile hand over sterile areas.

Remember that sterile gloves can be used for clean gloves when clean gloves are unavailable. However, clean gloves *cannot ever* be used as sterile gloves.

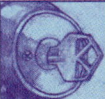

**Keys to Success
LEAVING THE TREATMENT ROOM**

Should you leave the treatment room once the sterile trays have been set up? The answer is no. For legal purposes, you are responsible and accountable for keeping the sterile field in sterile condition. You cannot guarantee that the sterile field remains sterile if you leave the room and the setup unattended.

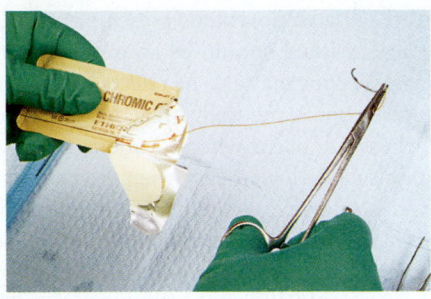

Figure 29-13 ◆ Remove the swaged needle from the package with the needle holder.

Suture material is either absorbable or nonabsorbable. Absorbable suture material is dissolved by body fluids and does not need to be removed. It is usually absorbed five to twenty days after insertion. Absorbable suture is used on internal organs, including the intestines, bladder, and subcutaneous tissue, and to tie off blood vessels. It is occasionally used for skin sutures as well. Surgical gut (catgut) and synthetic materials, including polyglycolic acid and polyglactin 910, are types of absorbable suture material. Nonabsorbable sutures include sutures made of silk, nylon, steel, and other materials that cannot be absorbed. These sutures are often used in deep tissues to permanently hold tissue in place. They are also used for skin repair and must be removed. (See Procedure 29-4.)

The size or gauge (diameter) of suture material is designated by numbers ranging from 0, the thickest, to 11-0 (00000000000), the smallest. On the delicate tissue of the face and neck, 5-0 or 6-0 is generally used. Areas where the skin or tissue is stronger and exposed to movement are usually sutured with 2-0 or 3-0; 10-0 and 11-0 may be used in neurological, possibly microscopic, surgery to suture very tiny vessels. In physician offices, other than ophthalmology or other specialty practices, only 1-0 to 6-0 size sutures are normally used.

Straight needles are used for suturing that passes directly through the tissue in a straight line. Curved needles allow for easier maneuvering in small spaces. The swaged needle, in which the suture and needle are one unit, is most commonly used as it causes the least amount of trauma to the tissue.

The physician assesses the wound and tissue before selecting the suture material and needle (Figure 29-14 ◆). A taper

point needle, which tapers to a sharp point, is used on easily penetrated tissue and causes less trauma to the tissue. A cutting needle, which has at least two sharp edges, is used on tougher or stronger tissue that may be difficult to penetrate.

Other wound closure materials include wire staples and adhesive skin closure strips. Wire staples are considered the fastest way to close long incisions and wounds with approximated edges (Figure 29-15 ◆). Because the tissue is handled less, there is also less tissue trauma. The staples are inserted with a special staple gun and must be removed with a staple remover. Staplers containing a cartridge of staples may be disposable or reusable.

Nonallergenic sterile strips of adhesive material may be used to hold the edges of a wound in place as healing takes place (Figure 29-16 ◆). The strips are often used in areas where there is little tension on the skin edges—for example, a laceration on the arm where no movement or stress is likely to occur. After the area is cleansed, the strips are applied crossways to bring the skin edges together. The advantages of adhesive skin closures are that local anesthetic is unnecessary, application and removal are easy, and less scarring usually results.

Suturing

The physician may require the MA's help when suturing a simple repair of a laceration or tear. Suturing may also follow removal of a lesion or I & D of an infected wound. Assistance may include assembling supplies and equipment, setting up the sterile field, applying a dressing, gloving, passing instruments, and cutting sutures. Regardless of the complexity of the procedure, sterile technique must be maintained at all times.

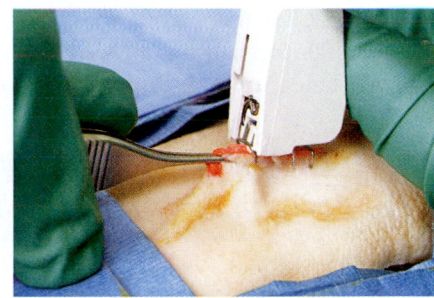

Figure 29-15 ◆ Physician stapling wound closed.

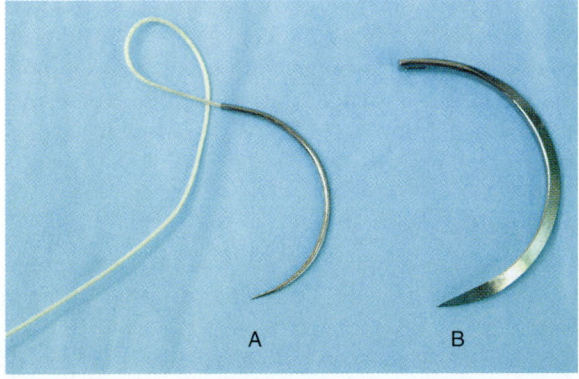

Figure 29-14 ◆ (A) Taper point needle; (B) Cutting point needle.

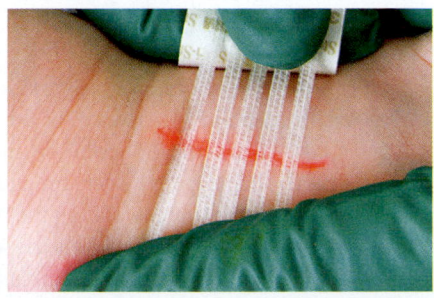

Figure 29-16 ◆ An example of the proper application of adhesive strips.

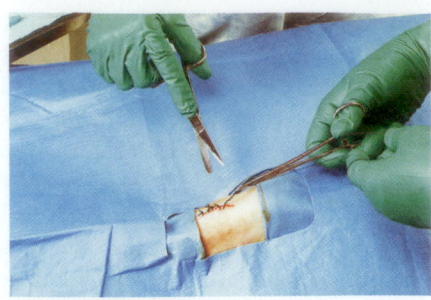

Figure 29-17 ◆ The proper way to hold scissors in a surgical procedure.

When assisting the physician in a surgical procedure, the MA will be required to cut excess suture material after the suture is placed. The MA will wear sterile gloves and pick up sterile surgical scissors. The best way to hold and control the scissors is to place the thumb in one hole and the ring finger in the other. Placing the index finger on the hinge of the scissors allows excellent control of any downward movement of the scissors tips (Figure 29-17 ◆).

Recovery/Postoperative Care

Once the surgical procedure is complete, the patient may be moved to a recovery area. If a relatively simple procedure was done under local anesthesia, the MA will be responsible for cleansing the skin, applying pressure as directed, and then dressing the site with a sterile dressing. While doing this, the MA will observe the patient for any signs of reaction, dizziness, or lightheadedness. The patient will need to be checked for orthostatic hypotension. The physical symptoms of orthostatic hypotension consist of dizziness, faintness, or lightheadedness that appear when the patient stands up. The symptoms of orthostatic hypotension are caused by low blood pressure. Another condition that the medical assistant should be aware of is vasovagal syncope. Vasovagal syncope may also be referred to as fainting, neurocardiogenic syncope, or neurally mediated syncope. Vasovagal syncope is believed to occur when a patient sits down and the blood flow pools in the lower legs; when the patient stands, the trapped blood is returned to the heart, resulting in a fainting spell. Neither vasovagal syncope or orthostatic hypotension are life-threatening conditions, but the patient must be monitored so that he or she does not fall, causing other injuries. The MA will assist the patient in sitting up on the side of the table until he or she has determined that the patient is stable enough to stand. If indicated by the procedure and by office policy, vital signs should be taken and recorded.

While the patient is sitting up, the MA should review the physician's instructions with the patient and family member or significant others and provide them with a written copy. The patient should be assisted in dressing if clothing was removed for the procedure. During the entire time, the MA will use observation skills to assess any possible reaction to the procedure. The MA will schedule the next appointment and dismiss the patient, who is usually escorted by a family member or significant other.

For more complex procedures and those performed with general anesthesia, vital signs are assessed and recorded. When general anesthesia has been administered, the level of consciousness and time of response to verbal stimuli are charted. Vital signs should be monitored and recorded every 15 minutes for the first hour, every 30 minutes for the next hour, then hourly until dismissal. Any nausea and vomiting are reported to the physician. Medication may be given for pain control and for prevention or control of nausea and vomiting. The patient is dismissed following facility guidelines when fully awake and able to ambulate. As with the less complicated ambulatory surgery, instructions are given and a follow-up appointment scheduled.

PROCEDURE 29-3 Assist the Physician with Suturing

Theory and Rationale

Any break in the skin may allow the entry of microorganisms into the tissue and subsequent infection. Most wounds and incisions require repair and closure to prevent infection, stop bleeding, promote healing, and reduce pain in the area. Sterile technique is required to achieve this goal.

In addition to passing instruments during the procedure, you may be required to sponge the area to clear any drainage and to keep the area visually clear. In anticipation of the physician's need for the scalpel, you will put the desired blade on the handle with a hemostat. Using the hemostat is a safety precaution to prevent cutting the fingers when manually adding the blade to the handle. As an additional safety precaution, pass the scalpel handle and blade to the physician carefully and with the blade edge down. If the edges of the wound need grasping, anticipate the physician's need for toothed forceps. Throughout the entire procedure, observe and reassure the patient.

When suturing is complete, each suture will extend 1/8 to 1/4 inch above the knot. This ensures that the knot is secure, visible, and easy to remove. As soon as the procedure is finished, soak the used instruments in disinfectant solution to remove residual tissue or body fluids. If debris is not removed, the contaminated, unclean portions are not sterilized during the sterilization process.

Materials

- sterile packs, including patient drapes, towels, and 4 × 4s, scalpels with blades (size according to physician's preference)
- suture and needle pack (according to physician's preference)

PROCEDURE 29-3 Assist the Physician with Suturing *(continued)*

- sterile suture pack, including scalpel handle, thumb forceps, needle holder, scissors, hemostats
- Mayo stand and side stand or table
- anesthetic (usually local)
- sterile transfer forceps and holder
- sterile basins
- sterile saline or water
- sterile gloves
- needle and syringe pack
- waste container with plastic bag liner
- biohazard waste container
- sharps container

Competency

(**Conditions**) With the necessary materials, you will be able to (**Task**) demonstrate sterile technique when assisting with suture repair of an incision (**Standards**) correctly and within the time frame designated by your instructor.

1. Wash your hands.
2. Identify the patient and guide him or her to the treatment area. Explain the entire procedure to the patient.
3. Position the patient on the exam table so that the area to be sutured is exposed.
4. Drape to cover the patient's clothing.
5. Follow the guidelines for prepping the skin and draping it for minor surgery.
6. Perform a 5-minute sterile scrub.
7. Put on sterile gloves.
8. Take a position standing opposite the physician.
9. Place two sterile sponges near the wound site. Have additional sponges ready as needed.
10. Pass instruments to the physician as requested, with a firm "snap" into the palm of the physician's hand.
11. Prepare a scalpel handle with blade according to the physician's preference. Pass the scalpel to the physician when necessary (Figure 29-18 ◆).
12. Sponge the area as necessary and as directed by the physician.
13. Pass other instruments, such as toothed forceps, as necessary (Figure 29-19 ◆).
14. Place the needle in the needle holder. Pass the needle holder, needle, and suture to the physician, keeping the suture material within the sterile field.
15. Keep a hold on the distal end of the suture until the physician sees it and takes it.
16. With suture scissors, cut sutures as directed by the physician 1/8 to 1/4 inch above the knot (Figure 29-20 ◆).
17. Sponge the closed wound during suturing and discard the soiled sponges (Figure 29-21 ◆).

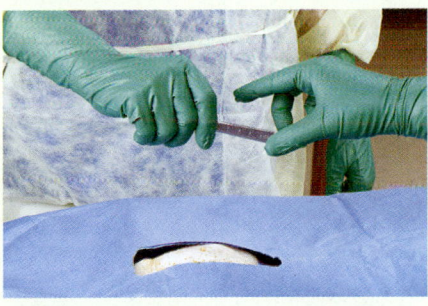

Figure 29-18 ◆ Pass the scalpel to the physician when necessary.

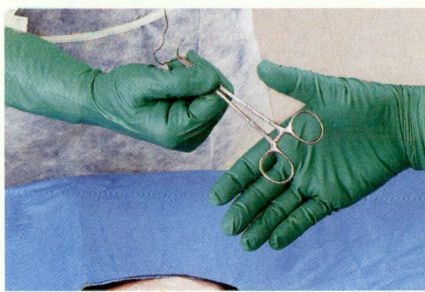

Figure 29-19 ◆ Pass other instruments as necessary.

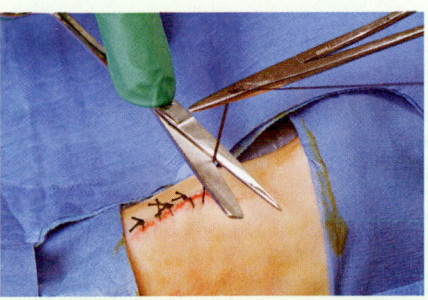

Figure 29-20 ◆ Cut sutures as directed by the physician, 1/8 to 1/4 inch above the knot.

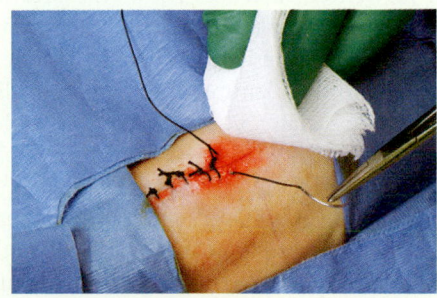

Figure 29-21 ◆ Sponge the wound during suturing.

continued

PROCEDURE 29-3 Assist the Physician with Suturing *(continued)*

18. Place used instruments in a disinfectant-filled instrument basin immediately.
19. Add unused sterile instruments to the disinfectant at the same time, or use another disinfectant-filled instrument basin.
20. Remove the gloves and discard. Wash your hands.
21. Apply dressings as instructed by the physician.
22. Help the patient into a comfortable position. Monitor vital signs according to office procedures.
23. Provide the patient with both oral and written postoperative instructions, including the date and time of the follow-up appointment.
24. Make sure the patient is stable for discharge.
25. Complete requisitions for specimens. Transport them to the laboratory or secure them for courier transport to the laboratory.
26. Clean, sanitize, and sterilize the instruments. Inspect them for residual tissue or body fluids and remove any you discover.
27. Clean and sanitize the room for the next patient.
28. Wash your hands.

Patient Education

Explain the basic elements of the procedure to the patient before the procedure begins. Explain that he or she should remain calm and still during the procedure. Follow-up instructions for the patient and/or significant others are also vital.

Charting Example

06/11/xx 11:00 a.m. Reviewed discharge instructions with patient. She verbalized the return appointment date and time and any signs of infection that should be reported. B/P 120/80, T 97.6°F, P 88, R 20. Ambulates steadily with husband escorting. Denies any nausea at time of discharge. Osi Kiwanuka, RMA (AMT)

NOTE: The physician will also document the procedure and any observations immediately after the suturing procedure.

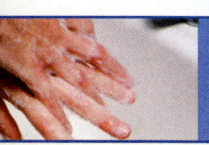

PROCEDURE 29-4 Assist the Physician with Suture or Staple Removal

Theory and Rationale

Nonabsorbable suture materials are used on external surfaces and must be removed when they are no longer needed to support a healed and intact incision line. The healing rate of the sutured tissue depends on the blood supply to the area. Face and head tissue generally heals more quickly than tissue lower in the body. Depending on the location of the sutures, removal is directed by the physician, usually in three to five days on the face and head and five to ten days on the rest of the body. Nonabsorbable suture materials include cotton, silk, nylon, and stainless steel wire. Metal skin clips or "staples" may also be used.

Before discharge, the physician informs the patient, verbally and in written instructions, of the return date for removal of sutures or staples. During the return office visit, the physician assesses the condition of the incision area and may direct you to remove the sutures or staples. Immediately after treatment, the physician and/or you must document observations of the approximated incision line, removal of suture materials, and instructions given to the patient.

To prevent the possibility of infection, antiseptic must be used before and after sutures or staples are removed. Use sterile saline or hydrogen peroxide to remove exudate and prevent the introduction of bacteria into the tiny open areas left by the sutures or staples. Another infection control measure is to cut one side of the suture as closely as possible to the skin, which reduces the amount of exposed suture material that is pulled through the skin.

Materials

■ suture removal kit, including suture scissors, thumb forceps, and sterile 4 × 4 gauze, *or* staple removal kit, including staple remover and sterile 4 × 4 gauze
■ antiseptic swabs
■ sterile 4 × 4 gauze
■ gloves
■ surgical tape
■ biohazard waste container
■ sharps container, if necessary

Competency

(**Conditions**) With the necessary materials, you will be able to (**Task**) demonstrate the procedure for removal of sutures or staples (**Standards**) correctly and within the time frame designated by the instructor.

1. Wash your hands.
2. Identify the patient and guide him or her to the treatment area. Explain the entire procedure to the patient.
3. Describe the sensation of pulling or tugging normally felt as the sutures or staples are removed.
4. Apply gloves.

PROCEDURE 29-4   Assist the Physician with Suture or Staple Removal *(continued)*

5. Remove any dressing present. Moisten adhered dressing with sterile saline or hydrogen peroxide before removal, if necessary.
6. Grasp the edge of the dressing and lift it halfway to the point of the suture line. Then lift the other edge in the same manner. Once the dressing is free of the suture area, it can be disposed of in a biohazard container.
7. Cleanse the suture or staple area and surrounding skin.
8. Open the sterile suture or staple removal kit.
9. Wash your hands and put on sterile gloves.

For Sutures

1. With the thumb forceps, grasp the suture knot. Gently lift the knot upward.
2. With your other hand, slip the notched edge of the suture scissors under the suture as close to the skin as possible. Close the scissors to cut the suture (Figure 29-22(a) ◆).
3. Gently pull on the knot and pull the unexposed suture through the skin (Figure 29-22(b) ◆). Place it on the 4 × 4 gauze.
4. Continue until all the sutures are removed. Check the patient chart for total number of sutures applied to verify that all sutures have been removed. If the count is inconsistent you must report this to the physician for further instructions.

5. Cleanse the skin with an antiseptic swab.
6. Allow the skin to air-dry and apply adhesive skin closures or dressing as the physician directs.

For Staples

1. Slide the bottom jaw of the staple remover under the staple (Figure 29-23 ◆).
2. Squeeze the staple remover handles together. The staple will bend slightly into a "V" shape.
3. Carefully lift the staple from the skin. Place it on the 4 × 4 gauze (Figure 29-24 ◆).
4. Continue the process until all the staples are removed.
5. Cleanse the skin with antiseptic swab.
6. Allow the skin to air-dry and apply adhesive skin closures or dressing as the physician directs.

Clean-up for Both Procedures

1. Dispose of contaminated materials in a biohazard or sharps container as appropriate.
2. Remove the gloves and discard.
3. Wash your hands.
4. Document the procedure.

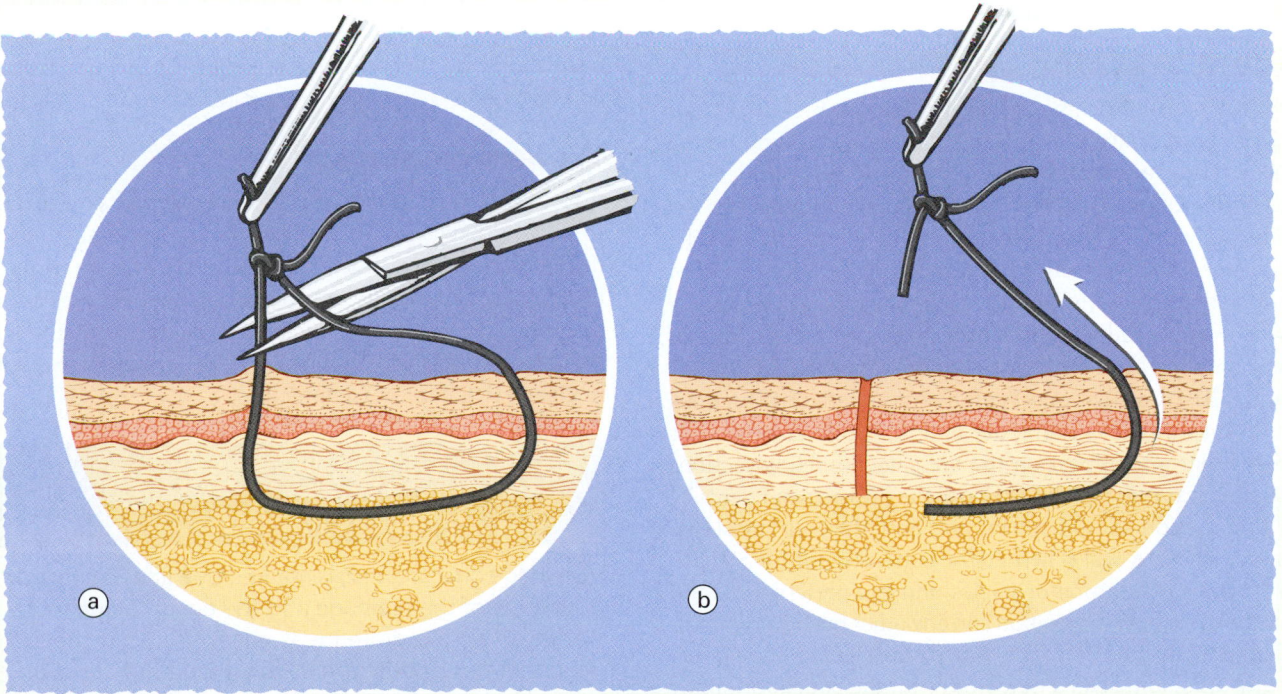

(a)   (b)

Figure 29-22 ◆ Removal of sutures.

continued

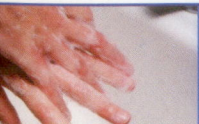

PROCEDURE 29-4 Assist the Physician with Suture or Staple Removal *(continued)*

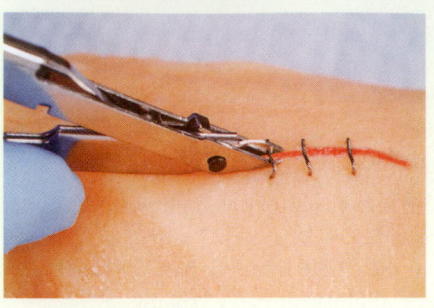

Figure 29-23 ◆ Slide the bottom jaw of the staple remover under the staple.

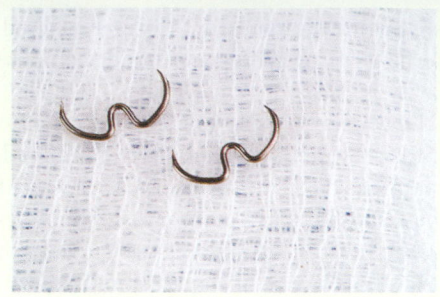

Figure 29-24 ◆ Place the staple on the 4 × 4 gauze.

Patient Education

The patient is usually allowed to shower after suture or staple removal, but check with the physician to confirm this before discussing it with the patient. To avoid irritation, the patient should pat the area dry rather than rub it. If the physician requires a dressing or adhesive skin closures, review and have the patient demonstrate correct application. The patient should be given both verbal and written wound care instructions and a list of signs to look for that may indicate a possible infection.

Charting Example

07/01/xx 9:30 a.m. Sutures intact and surgical incision approximated without signs of infection. Suture area cleansed with iodine and sutures × 15 removed from the abdominal incision per sterile technique. Iodine reapplied and allowed to air-dry before dressing applied. Incision and dressing care reviewed. Patient verbalized correct instructions for dressing changes. Abby McNair, CMA (AAMA)

Patient Teaching and Dismissal

As with all patient teaching, feedback is important. Instructions are given both orally and in printed form. Depending on the nature of the procedure the MA will go over the postoperative instructions either with the attending family members or the patient individually. The patient or family member should be able to repeat the instructions or provide other demonstration of understanding. If the MA gives the postoperative instructions to a family member he should ascertain that a release of information has been signed prior to the conversation to comply with HIPAA regulations. Typical postoperative instructions include keeping the dressing dry and reporting any blood or drainage that may appear on the dressing. Some instructions give a time frame in which to remove the dressing and describe how the incision should appear and how the area should be cleansed. The MA will schedule the appointment for recheck and/or removal of sutures or staples, and give prescriptions and instructions for pain medication and any other medications indicated to the patient or the family member. The MA should discuss any other anticipated outcomes with the patient or family member.

The medical assistant will chart the patient's vital signs (if indicated), the patient's condition and apparent understanding of instructions, the method of discharge (ambulatory or wheelchair), and the person accompanying the patient.

Wound Healing

A wound is an insult or damage to an external skin surface or to the internal aspect of tissue. A wound is classified as accidental or intentional, and open or closed. An **open wound** is a break in the skin or mucous membrane that exposes underlying tissues. Open wounds include **abrasions, avulsions,** incisions, **lacerations,** and **punctures.** (Open wounds are discussed in greater detail in ∞ Chapter 41.)

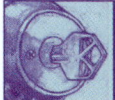

Keys to Success
MARKING DRAINAGE

Drainage on a dressing is marked by a line drawn around the edge of the drainage and the time the line is drawn. At intervals the drainage is checked and, if the area is expanding, another line is drawn and marked with the time by the patient or health-care person caring for the patient after dismissal. The physician will provide instructions as to when the office should be alerted.

In Practice

Michelle Johnson returns to the office for a wound check after having sutures placed on a laceration of her left hand. The medical assistant observes the skin and notes that the wound has begun to form a scar. What phase of normal healing is this?

A **closed wound** is a wound that involves trauma to the underlying tissue without a break in the skin or mucous membrane or exposure of the underlying tissue. Closed wounds include contusions, or bruises. Tissues under the skin are injured, blood vessels rupture, and blood seeps into the tissue, resulting in the bluish color of a bruise.

A wound must be cleansed and repaired to prevent infection, arrest any bleeding, promote healing, and reduce pain. The healing process begins with inflammation, which increases blood circulation to the wounded area to destroy the invading microorganisms. There are three phases in the process of normal healing: the inflammatory, granulation, and contraction phases (Table 29-3).

Dressings and Bandages

Dressings and bandages are used to cover wounds. Dressings also serve to:

- Act as a protective barrier against infection.
- Keep the surrounding skin clean and dry by absorbing drainage from wounds or surgical incisions.

TABLE 29-3 THE PHASES OF NORMAL HEALING

Phase	Process
Inflammatory phase	■ Blood serum and cells form a network of fibrin in the wound. ■ A clot forms, filling in the wound and bringing the edges together with shreds of fibrin. ■ A scab begins to form.
Granulation phase (also called fibroblastic phase)	■ A network of granulation tissue absorbs fluid. ■ Epithelial cells begin to form from the edge of the wound. ■ A scar begins to form.
Contraction phase (also called maturation phase)	■ Small blood vessels are absorbed and fibroblasts contract. ■ The scar shrinks and becomes lighter in color.

- Reduce discomfort by restricting the movement of tissue surrounding the wound and by preventing irritation from clothing against the skin.

Bandages are also used to anchor dressings. Applying or changing a dressing allows for inspection of the wound. Observations of color, inflammation, edema, drainage, and healing stage should be noted and charted.

PROCEDURE 29-5 Change a Sterile Dressing

Theory and Rationale

Practicing sterile technique when applying or changing a dressing helps to reduce the chance of infectious organisms entering the body. The dressing must cover the wound but not be so large as to catch other materials. It is secured in place with tape or bandages. Gauze dressings come in various sizes, primarily 2×2, 3×3, and 4×4. The 4×4 is the most commonly used. Larger absorbent dressings are called ABD dressings.

As the wound drains, the gauze dressing absorbs the drainage. However, as the drainage dries, the gauze adheres to the wound. To prevent this, a nonadherent dressing is often used.

When the dressing is removed, you will assess the wound for color, inflammation, edema, drainage, and approximation. Document and report your observations to the physician to ensure proper treatment and continued healing.

After applying the appropriate dressing, secure it with either tape or a bandage. Tape can be used to make a complete seal around the dressing when you want to prevent drainage from leaking beyond the dressing onto other parts of the skin. Microbial growth can occur with a moist dressing or moist drainage beyond a dressing. When you remove or change a dressing, gently loosen the tape by applying slight fingertip pressure against the skin with one hand and using the other hand to pull up the tape perpendicular to the skin.

Materials

- prepackaged dressing pack, including sterile gauze or sponges, sterile thumb forceps, sterile dressings, adhesive tape (or tape most appropriate for skin condition and dressing function)
- Mayo stand and side tray
- antiseptic solution
- sterile transfer forceps
- sterile gloves
- scissors
- sterile basins

continued

PROCEDURE 29-5 Change a Sterile Dressing *(continued)*

- thumb forceps
- disposable gloves
- waste container with plastic bag liner
- biohazard waste container

Competency

(**Conditions**) With the necessary materials, you will be able to (**Task**) demonstrate a sterile dressing change (**Standards**) correctly within the time frame designated by the instructor.

1. Identify the patient and guide him or her to the treatment area. Explain the entire procedure to the patient.
2. Wash your hands.
3. Assemble the equipment on the Mayo stand or side table, using aseptic technique.
4. Apply nonsterile gloves and remove the dressing by pulling it in the direction of the wound.
5. Place the removed dressing into a biohazard bag, without touching the outside of the bag. Be careful not to pass it over your sterile tray.
6. Inspect the patient's wound and make a mental note to later document in the chart. A description of the wound size, shape, and any indication of infection, such as pus or inflammation, should be noted.
7. Removed your soiled gloves.
8. Hold the antiseptic container with your palm covering the label. Pour some of the antiseptic into a sink or waste container. As the solution flows across the edge of the container, the edge will be disinfected. Pour the antiseptic into the sterile basin.
9. Wash your hands with a surgical scrub and apply sterile gloves.
10. Using sterile forceps and sterile cotton balls or sterile gauze pads, depending on the size of the wound, cleanse the wound. Disposable materials can be discarded in biohazard, and reusable items will be cleaned at the end of the procedure.
11. Cleanse the wound by moving from the inside to the outside, wiping from the top of the wound to the bottom, one time. The cotton ball must be changed with each stroke (Figure 29-25 ◆).
12. Apply the sterile dressing to the wound and remove your gloves. Verify that your patient does not have an allergy to adhesives. If an allergy is present, secure the dressing with non-adhesive disposable bandage wrap such as Coban.
13. Secure the dressing with adhesive tape. Tape should not cover the entire dressing or be wrapped completely around the extremity.
14. Provide the patient with written and verbal instructions on wound care, signs of infection, and when he or she should follow up with the physician.
15. When the patient has exited the procedure area you may apply nonsterile gloves and clean the room in preparation for the next patient.
16. Remove your gloves and wash hands.
17. Chart the procedure, including the date, time, location, and condition of the wound. Chart and describe any drainage noted.

Patient Education

Instruct the patient and the patient's family or significant other(s) about the signs of infection: redness, increasing amount and odor of drainage, warmth, and hardness of the surgical site. Emphasize the importance of keeping the dressing dry to prevent the moist conditions in which microorganisms grow and reproduce. Ask the patient or significant other to verbalize the signs of infection. If dressings are to be changed as needed at home, it may be necessary to schedule a return visit to direct the patient or significant other through a supervised dressing change. Encourage the patient and/or family member or significant other to call the medical office if questions or problems arise.

Charting Example

05/01/xx 10:15 a.m. ABD drsg changed with sterile technique. Sutured wound was clean without signs of redness, swelling, or drainage. Patient asked when she could take showers. Reinforced physician's verbal instructions about waiting for showers until a few days after sutures were taken out. Return appointment scheduled for sutures to be taken out on 05/27/XX. Patient verbalized she would wait to take shower until after her next appointment. Joy Jones, CMA (AAMA)

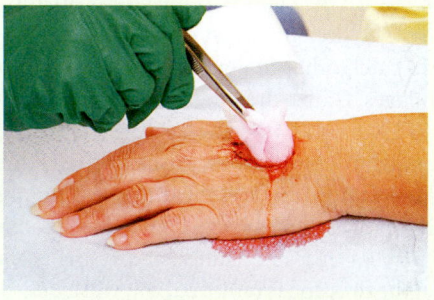

Figure 29-25 ◆ Clean the wound from the top downward or from the center outward.

REVIEW

Chapter Summary

- Minor surgeries range from a simple 10-minute procedure to 23-hour outpatient stay.
- As an MA, you could be responsible for any of the following.
  - scheduling outpatient testing and surgical procedures
  - assisting physician in the procedure
  - providing instructions
  - dismissing patients
  - obtaining insurance precertification and consent signature
  - ordering supplies for future surgeries
  - preparing instruments by cleaning, disinfecting, and sterilizing
  - setting up the room or treatment area
  - preparing the patient
  - properly handling specimens
  - processing insurance claims
- The scrub assistant sets up the sterile field and maintains sterile working conditions while assisting the physician during the procedure. The circulating assistant obtains supplies for the sterile team and performs all other procedures in which sterile procedure is not required.
- Many surgeries are performed in the medical office setting, including biopsy, colposcopy, cryosurgery, electrocautery, incision and drainage, removal of foreign bodies, suturing of lacerations, and suture or staple removal.
- Regardless of the type of minor surgery, implied or informed consent must be given by the patient. A patient must completely understand the procedure and risks before signing the consent form. A signed consent form is mandatory.
- Preoperative patient care involves instructing the patient about the procedure, time, diet, and someone to drive him or her home if necessary; obtaining laboratory tests; and easing the patient's concerns about the surgery. Setting up the room, positioning and draping the patient, taking vital signs, and assisting the physician with anesthesia are also part of preoperative care.
- Instruments are classified as clamping, cutting, dilating, dissecting, grasping, probing, suturing, and visualization. Forceps, scissors, scalpels, needle holders, and trocars are examples of surgical instruments.

- During the setup of sterile trays and during the procedure, it is important to know which areas are sterile, clean, and dirty. By remembering whether an instrument, dressing, or step in a procedure is sterile, clean, or dirty, the medical assistant can move around and maintain a sterile field during the performance of all actions. It is critical that you *never* reach over the sterile field.
- In the preparation of the surgical area, it is very important to follow cleaning from the surgical site outward and to use a separate sponge for each concentric circular area.
- Anesthesia used in the medical office is generally local anesthesia, in topical form or as an injection. The MA assists by holding the vial while the physician draws the medication into a syringe for injection.
- Intraoperative care varies according to the type of minor surgery and the physician's preference. Usually, the MA is trained to perform all procedures related to minor surgery, including dressing changes, suturing, and suture removal.
- In a wound, whether caused by trauma or surgery, the skin surface is broken. Wounds may be open, such as abrasions, avulsions, incisions, lacerations, and punctures, or closed, such as contusions. The phases of healing are the inflammatory, granulation, and contraction phases. You should be able to identify signs of wound infection, including redness, heat, and/or pain.
- Applied correctly, dressings protect a wound site from further trauma and can protect it from infection.
- During postoperative recovery, the MA is responsible for performing and monitoring patient vital signs and observing patient progress. Any abnormalities should be reported to the physician. When the patient is ready for discharge or dismissal, you will give verbal and written instructions as directed by the physician.
- Documentation is another important aspect of minor surgery. Records of the procedure, outpatient testing, patient education, and patient progress are among the required documentation in the patient chart.

Chapter Review

Multiple Choice

1. The circulating assistant's role is to
   a. assist with a 5-minute surgical scrub.
   b. position the patient.
   c. hand instruments to the physician.
   d. assist the physician with sterile gloving.

2. Which of the following is most likely to involve a 23-hour outpatient procedure?
   a. cyst removal
   b. abscess incision and drainage
   c. D & C
   d. staple removal

Chapter Review (continued)

3. Which of the following should you do after setting up the sterile field?
   a. Cover or drape the sterile field with a sterile cloth.
   b. Leave the room to get patient drapes.
   c. Leave the sterile field uncovered, ready for surgery.
   d. Push the Mayo stand next to the examination table.

4. Forceps are used for
   a. cutting.
   b. dissecting.
   c. grasping.
   d. probing.

5. A trocar is used for
   a. cutting.
   b. dissecting.
   c. grasping.
   d. probing.

6. When shaving a patient for surgery, you should
   a. shave the surgical site in the direction opposite that of hair growth.
   b. shave the surgical site in the direction of the hair growth.
   c. use antiseptic in concentric circles before shaving.
   d. avoid using germicidal soap because it causes irritation.

7. Which of the following is used as a local anesthesia?
   a. Ether
   b. Heroin
   c. Ethyl chloride spray
   d. Procaine

8. If a local anesthetic is used during surgery, you should
   a. hold the vial upside down with the label facing the physician.
   b. hold the vial upright with the label facing you.
   c. insert the needle into the rubber stopper and withdraw the desired amount.
   d. insert the needle into the rubber stopper, inject air from the syringe, and withdraw the desired amount.

9. A suture should be cut
   a. 1/16 inch above the knot.
   b. 1/4 inch above the knot.
   c. 1/2 inch above the knot.
   d. 1 inch above the knot.

10. Which of the following procedures should be done when changing a sterile dressing?
    a. Cleanse the wound from the center inward.
    b. Cleanse the wound from the bottom of the wound to the top.
    c. Cleanse the wound from side to side.
    d. Cleanse the wound from the top of the wound to the bottom.

True/False

T F 1. The term *preoperative* refers to the period during a surgery.

T F 2. The term *intraoperative* means "before surgery."

T F 3. The postoperative period follows a surgery.

T F 4. A scrub assistant is also known as a float or "clean" assistant.

T F 5. A scrub assistant may be responsible for setting up the sterile field and assisting the physician in sterile procedures.

T F 6. Optional surgery is medically necessary but can be done when it is most convenient for the patient.

T F 7. Elective surgery is not medically necessary and is only done when the patient requests it.

T F 8. Emergency surgery is performed when there is an immediate need.

T F 9. If a patient is having a nonroutine procedure, an informed consent is not needed.

T F 10. A circulating assistant can obtain supplies and sterile equipment for the "sterile team."

Short Answer

1. List the types of surgery.

2. Name a medically necessary surgery that can be done at the patient's convenience.

3. What must patients sign before all nonroutine procedures?

4. What is an I & D procedure? Why is it performed?

5. What is the difference between a closed wound and an open wound?

Research

1. In your local area, how many women have elective C-sections?

2. In your community, are there any outpatient surgery centers? Or are all surgeries, regardless of length and type, performed in a hospital?

Externship Application Experience

It is your second externship day in the office, and a mole removal is scheduled for a patient. You are to observe the procedure so that you can assist on the next scheduled minor surgery. As an MA is opening the sterile packet, you notice she reaches across the sterile field on several occasions. How do you handle the situation?

Resource Guide

Allegiance Healthcare Corporation
1430 Waukegan Road
McGaw Park, IL 60085-6787
1-800-964-5227
www.cardinal.com

Miltex Instrument Company, Inc.
700 Hicksville Road
Bethpage, NY 11714
1-800-645-8000
www.miltex.com

SAMBA: Society for Ambulatory Anesthesia
520 N. Northwest Highway
Parkridge, IL 60068-2573
847-825-5586

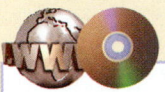

Med**Media**

http://www.MyMAKit.com

More on this chapter, including interactive resources, can be found on the Student CD-ROM accompanying this textbook and on http://www.MyMAKit.com.

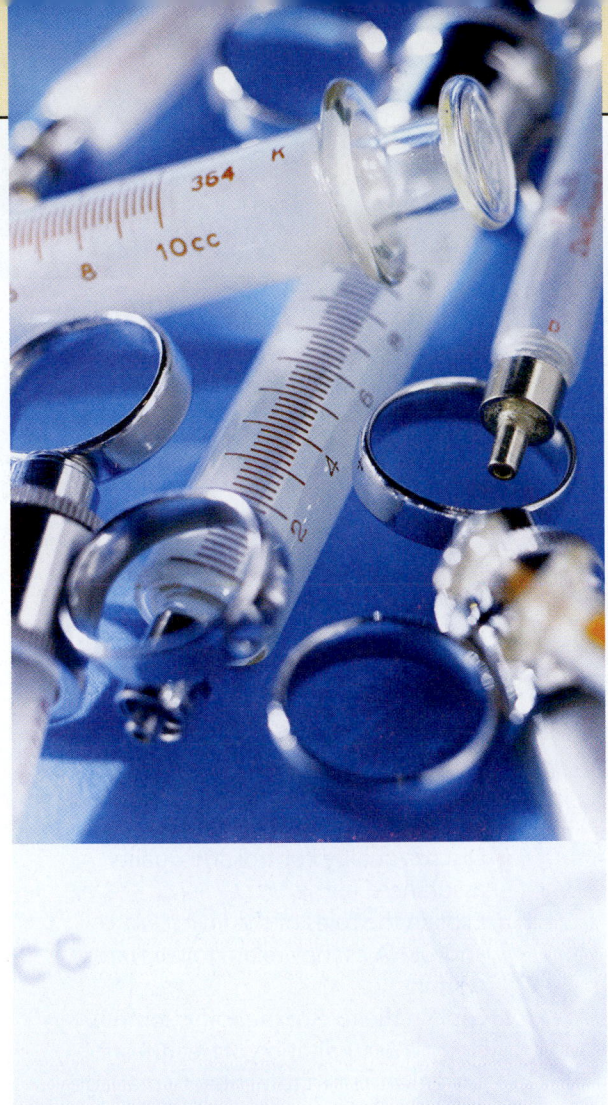

UNIT IX

Diagnostic Testing in the Medical Office

Chapter 30   **Diagnostic Procedures**
Chapter 31   **Microscopes and Microbiology**
Chapter 32   **Hematology and Chemistry**

My name is Glenda Gibson. I became a Medical Assistant in 1983. At the time, I was working at a semi-decent job, but it was one that had no future of growth or advancement. Then one day when I was watching television, I saw a commercial for the Missouri School for Doctor's Assistants. It sounded like just the right thing for me. I called and got an interview with the school director and signed up for classes.

My first job was at an internist's office. Here, the staff was responsible for performing EKGs on all new patients. We also set up and assisted in EKG stress testing. Since it was my first job, I had a lot to learn about drawing blood—drawing blood well was my biggest challenge. With all the practice I obtained, I turned out to be very good at drawing blood. The internist office's also had its own lab. It was part of my job to run protime, do CBCs, and get the lab ready for the morning lab person to come in and start testing. For a first-time job, this job really incorporated all aspects of my medical assistant training.

Now I am working for a large laboratory company. In the office where I am currently located, I am the only person working at the site. I use all skills from answering phone calls to coding diagnoses with my ICD-9 knowledge. I get a lot of satisfaction from doing my job well. The customers who come to my site appreciate the work I do. These customers tell me that I have great phlebotomy and front office skills.

Medical assisting has been a great career for me. Now I am looking for future advancement by going back to school and getting certifications in Medical Office Administrator and Advanced Medical Coding, as well as a B.S. in Social Work. My long-term goal is to run a medical office.

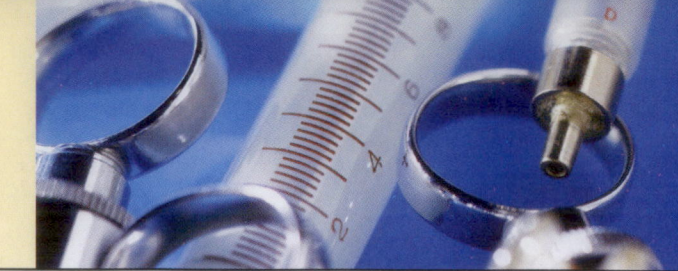

CHAPTER 30

Diagnostic Procedures

Case Study

Jason, a medical assistant, is busy working in a medical facility that utilizes an in-clinic laboratory. Some of the tests he has learned to perform are urine pregnancy tests, simple gross urinalysis, and glucose screening.

Objectives

After completing this chapter, you should be able to:

- Define and spell the key terminology in this chapter.
- Define the medical assistant's role in diagnostic procedures and the laboratory.
- Explain the role of Clinical Laboratory Improvement Amendments (CLIA) in setting standards for laboratory testing.
- Explain the differences between waived, PPMP, moderate-complexity, and high-complexity tests.
- Discuss quality control and quality assurance.
- Explain the roles of the FDA, EPA, and OSHA as they relate to laboratory testing.
- Explain the role of the Joint Commission on Accreditation of Healthcare Organizations in total quality management within the hospital setting.
- Discuss the Safe Medical Devices Act.
- Describe diagnostic testing in hospital laboratories.
- Identify equipment found in a physician office laboratory (POL).
- Explain how the physician's order is transmitted to the testing facility.
- Discuss the importance and process of obtaining precertification when required.
- Explain the procedure for scheduling diagnostic tests with outside agencies.
- Discuss the screening and following up of test results.

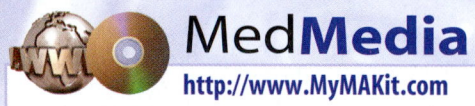

MedMedia

http://www.MyMAKit.com

Additional interactive resources and activities for this chapter can be found on http://www.MyMAKit.com. For videos, tips, audio glossary, legal and ethical scenarios, job scenarios, quizzes, games, and virtual tours related to the content of this chapter, please access the accompanying CD-ROM in this book.

Audio Glossary
Legal and Ethical Scenario: *Diagnostic Procedures*
On the Job Scenario: *Diagnostic Procedures*
Video
Multiple Choice Quiz
Games: Crossword, Strikeout, and Spelling Bee
Tips
HIPAA Quiz

✚ MEDICAL ASSISTING STANDARDS

CAAHEP ENTRY-LEVEL STANDARDS	ABHES ENTRY-LEVEL COMPETENCIES
■ Perform within scope of practice (psychomotor) ■ Apply ethical behaviors, including honesty/integrity in performance of medical assisting practice (affective) ■ Apply local, state and federal health care legislation and regulation appropriate to the medical assisting practice setting (psychomotor) ■ Recognize the importance of local, state and federal legislation and regulations in the practice setting (affective) ■ Explore issue of confidentiality as it applies to the medical assistant (cognitive) ■ Document accurately in the patient record (psychomotor) ■ Perform handwashing (psychomotor) ■ Practice Standard Precautions (psychomotor) ■ Perform quality control measures (psychomotor) ■ Screen test results (psychomotor)	■ Project a positive attitude. ■ Maintain confidentiality at all times. ■ Be a "team player." ■ Be cognizant of ethical boundaries. ■ Exhibit initiative. ■ Adapt to change. ■ Evidence a responsible attitude. ■ Be courteous and diplomatic. ■ Conduct work within scope of education, training, and ability. ■ Interview and take a patient history. ■ Prepare patients for procedures. ■ Apply principles of aseptic techniques and infection control. ■ Prepare and maintain examination and treatment area. ■ Collect and process specimens. ■ Perform selected CLIA waived tests that assist with diagnosis and treatment. ■ Dispose of biohazardous materials. ■ Practice standard precautions.

✓ COMPETENCY SKILLS PERFORMANCE

1. Check the accuracy of glucometer results using quality control methods.
2. Screen and follow up test results.

Introduction

Diagnostic testing is essential for a complete picture of the patient's health status. It also provides the physician with feedback concerning the effectiveness and proper dosage of prescribed medications.

A physician has two choices for laboratory testing—a reference laboratory or a physician office laboratory **(POL).** Both types of laboratories are governed by the same regulations and guidelines. A reference laboratory is independently owned and operated by an outside source and can perform high-level testing unavailable in the POL. Many reference labs have contracts with insurance providers and managed care providers.

One advantage of the POL is immediate testing, results, and treatment while the patient is still in the office. Other advantages are convenience and reduced time and travel for the patient.

The Medical Assistant's Role in Diagnostic Testing

The MA working in a hospital or reference laboratory may schedule tests, maintain or file records of results, record or log calibrations, assist with quality control records, and obtain specimens. Depending on state regulations, and with immediate supervision, the MA may be able to perform a simple gross urinalysis and certain mechanized tests, procure capillary and venipuncture specimens, centrifuge urine and blood specimens, and plate specimens for culture. Also, depending on state and facility guidelines, the medical assistant may be able to transmit test results to the physician's office.

The MA working in a POL may perform waived tests, provide patient education about obtaining specimens, and collect specimens within the scope of training and physician supervision. Specimens that might be obtained include urine, stool, cultures, and venous and capillary blood. The MA may set up certain microscopic tests; however, the physician must make the microscopic diagnosis. In some states the MA may read the microscopic results with further specialized training and with physician supervision and responsibility. The MA should check state practice acts where he or she will be employed for what the medical assistant is specifically and legally allowed to do in a POL.

When using equipment, the MA will be required to follow OSHA and Clinical Laboratory Improvement Amendments (**CLIA**) guidelines. In all procedures the MA must exercise caution to prevent accidents and exposure to biohazardous and chemical waste, and follow all OSHA, CLIA, and manufacturer's instructions when disposing of biohazardous and chemical waste.

Clinical Laboratory Improvement Amendments (CLIA)

Accurate laboratory testing has been recognized as a critical element of correct diagnosis in medical office visits and in life-threatening situations. Decisions about diagnosis, care, medication, dosages, and procedures are based on the results of these tests.

In 1988, U.S. Congress passed the Clinical Laboratory Improvement Amendments (CLIA), establishing quality standards for all laboratory testing. Implementation of CLIA was the responsibility of the Health Care Financing Administration (**HCFA**). The goal of CLIA is "to ensure the accuracy, reliability and timeliness of patient test results regardless of where the test was performed." Certification by the Secretary of Health and Human Services is "required for all laboratories that examine materials derived from the human body fluids for diagnosis, prevention, or treatment purposes." Test categorization and CLIA studies are the responsibility of the CDC.

Quality standards are specified for proficiency testing (PT), quality control, quality assurance, patient test management, and personnel qualifications. The regulations are based on the complexity of the test method. The more complicated the test is, the more stringent the requirements. Tests fall into three categories:

- Waived complexity
- Moderate complexity, which includes the subcategory of provider-performed microscopy procedures (**PPMP**)
- High complexity

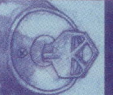

Keys to Success
TYPES OF CLIA CERTIFICATES

Certificate of Waiver—issued to a laboratory that performs only waived tests

Certificate for PPMP (Provider-Performed Microscopy Procedures)—issued to a laboratory in which a physician, midlevel practitioner, or dentist performs no tests other than microscopic tests; the laboratory may also perform waived tests

Certificate of Registration—issued to a laboratory that conducts moderate- and/or high-complexity laboratory testing until it is determined that the laboratory complies with CLIA regulations

Certificate of Compliance—issued to a laboratory after an inspection that confirms the laboratory complies with all applicable CLIA requirements

Certificate of Accreditation—issued to a laboratory on the basis of the laboratory's accreditation by an HCFA-approved accreditation organization.

Adapted from HCFA guidelines.

There are also specific cytology requirements.

Enrollment in the CLIA program requires several steps. Laboratories must complete an application for registration, pay applicable fees, be surveyed, and, when necessary, become certified. Full-service providers (those performing moderate- and high-complexity tests) are surveyed routinely. Laboratories performing waived and PPMP testing may apply directly for the certificate and are not subject to routine inspections.

Waived Tests

Waived tests are the least complex tests to perform, so there is little danger of error or risk to the patient. Many of these tests have been approved by the FDA for patient use at home, such as blood glucose screening and urine pregnancy tests. Most waived tests are performed by physicians (MDs/DOs), registered nurses (RNs), licensed practical nurses (LPNs), and medical assistants (MAs). Very few medical technologists (MTs) and medical laboratory technicians (MLTs) regularly perform waived tests. Reading and following the manufacturer's instructions are required for any waived test.

Laboratories performing waived tests only, including POLs, apply for a Certificate of Waiver. The certificate exempts them from meeting various CLIA 1988 standards that apply to the other types of tests.

PPMP Tests

A waived laboratory with a PPMP certificate can perform tests using a microscope. Such tests are done during a patient visit on a specimen that is not easily transportable (Figure 30-1 ◆). Included in PPMP tests are pinworm examination, microscopic urinalysis, fecal leukocyte examination, and semen analysis

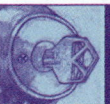

Keys to Success
CLIA WAIVED TESTS

1. Dipstick of tablet reagent urinalysis for:
   bilirubin
   glucose
   hemoglobin
   ketone
   leukocytes
   nitrite
   pH
   protein
   specific gravity
   urobilinogen
2. Fecal occult blood
3. Urine pregnancy tests: visual color comparison tests
4. Ovulation tests: visual color comparison tests for luteinizing hormone
5. Blood glucose using FDA approved glucose monitoring devices
6. Hemoglobin: copper sulfate, non-automated
7. Erythrocyte sedimentation rate, non-automated
8. Hemoglobin using single analyte instruments
9. Spun microhematocrit

(presence and/or motility of sperm, excluding the Huhner test, a postcoital test on cervical mucus).

Moderate-Complexity Tests

A moderate-complexity test is also simple to perform, but it may involve a more serious risk to the patient if results are inaccurate. Blood chemistries, red and white blood cell counts, **hemoglobin, hematocrit,** and urine cultures are categorized as moderate-complexity tests. Although many chemistries are performed with automated instruments, training beyond the MA level is required to perform these tests. Normal values as

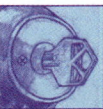

Keys to Success
PATIENT EDUCATION FOR HOME TESTS

Although normally accurate, testing at home can have some risk for error. For example, a home glucose monitor error can put an insulin-dependent diabetes mellitus (IDDM) patient at risk for overdose, insulin shock, and possibly death. A false negative result for a home pregnancy test could jeopardize fetal health if the mother takes certain drugs or practices behaviors with known adverse effects on a developing fetus.

Patient education includes instructing the patient to follow the manufacturer's instructions for home testing exactly as written to reduce the potential for inaccurate results. The patient should contact the office with any questions.

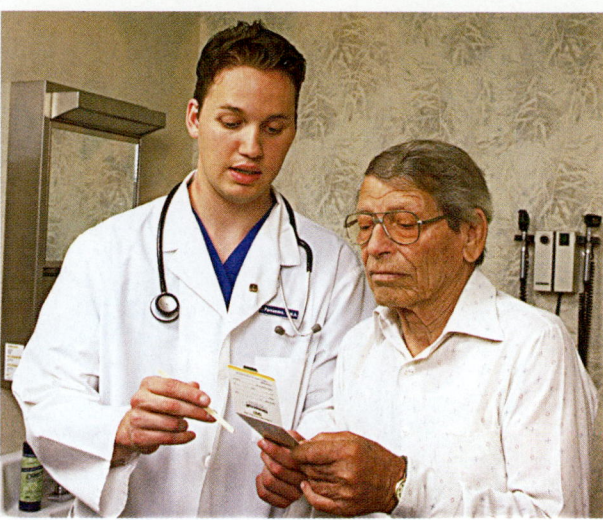

Figure 30-1 ◆ The MA explains to the patient how to use a collection specimen kit.

indicated in printed lab reports are variable according to the reference laboratory's values. (Where applicable, chemistries are discussed or listed in later chapters with the disease or condition to which they apply.)

High-Complexity Tests

A high-complexity test is complicated to perform and poses considerable risk to the patient if results are inaccurate. Bone marrow evaluations, immunoassays, flow cytometry, and electrophoresis are high complexity. These tests require sophisticated instrumentation and must be overseen by a pathologist or PhD-level scientist.

Quality Control and Quality Assurance

The objective of quality control is to ensure reliable and valid test results by applying the correct methods and detecting or eliminating errors. Quality control is essential for the physician to properly diagnose and treat a patient. Patient preparation and specimen collection, handling, transport, and testing are elements of quality control.

Quality control before testing includes confirming that the patient has followed the required preparation and selecting the appropriate container or system (Figure 30-2 ◆). The container is labeled with the patient's name, any identification number, the date, and the technician's initials.

Quality control methods used in testing involve the following:

- Checking dated supplies and discarding outdated reagents.
- Calibrating and performing function checks on equipment.
- Maintaining equipment and documenting maintenance.
- Running and documenting control samples of each test for consistency.

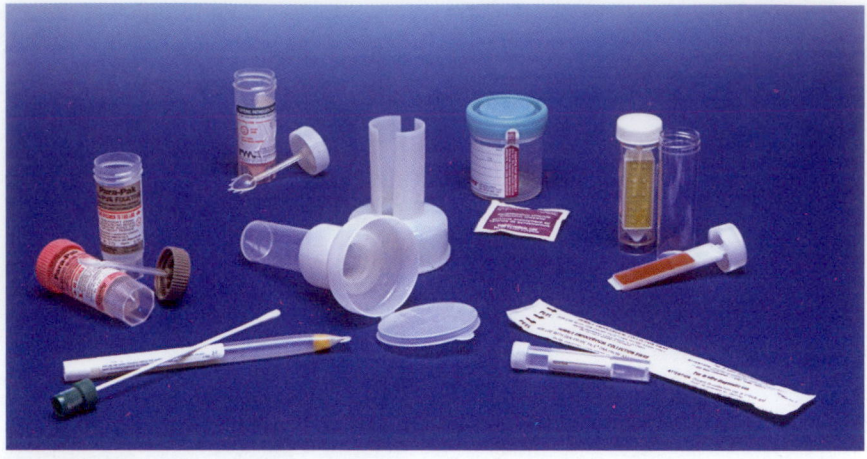

Figure 30-2 ◆ Specimen collection containers.

Quality assurance is a type of outcome assessment. Monitoring laboratory testing begins at the start of the process, continues through the process, and ends with the results of the process. Each step in the process requires following instructions and methodology to ensure quality. Information, test results, and data are then assembled and reviewed. The data is compared to acceptable standards for testing. Services provided as well as results are compared. Written policies and documentation of the results are completed.

In Practice

It is the beginning of the day and you are checking office equipment for accuracy using quality control methods. The office glucometer is tested daily for accuracy according to manufacturer recommendations and office policy. After three separate readings, it is noted that the control readings are abnormal. Can the equipment be used for the day's testing? If not, what can you as the medical assistant do?

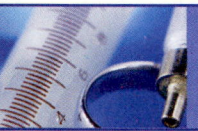

PROCEDURE 30-1 Check the Accuracy of Glucometer Results Using Quality Control Methods

Theory and Rationale

Quality control is performed to ensure standardized and accurate results of all manual and automated tests. A glucometer is used in the medical office and by patients at home to measure blood glucose, with immediate and accurate results. Whether performed at home by the patient or at the medical office, quality control requires keeping records of control testing, cleaning, equipment maintenance, and repairs. You will need to educate the patient on the importance of quality control at home because it directly affects the amount of insulin administered.

Materials

■ quality control log book
■ glucometer
■ quality controls specific to brand of glucometer

Competency

(**Conditions**) With the necessary materials, you will be able to (**Task**) perform quality control testing of the glucometer (**Standards**) within the time and to the degree of accuracy designated by the instructor.

1. Wash your hands and assemble materials.
2. Perform control testing as recommended by the manufacturer and per office policy.
   - Check unsealed quality control vials and test strips for open and discard dates and expiration dates. Label the control vials and test strips if you are opening them for the first time.
   - If you are changing code strips, calibrate and change the number per manufacturer's instructions.
3. Record the test results in a quality control log (Figure 30-3 ◆). If control results are abnormal, report them to the supervisor. Label the glucometer "Repair" and remove it from the clinical area to prevent other staff from using it. Return the glucometer to the clinical area only after the problem has been corrected.
4. Dispose of waste materials in the appropriate container.
5. Wash your hands and return the glucometer and quality test control equipment to the designated storage area.

Patient Education

Emphasize the importance of glucometer quality control in the treatment of diabetes. Instruct the patient in how to perform quality control tests, and have the patient do a

PROCEDURE 30-1   Check the Accuracy of Glucometer Results Using Quality Control Methods (continued)

return demonstration. Include instruction on keeping logs for quality control testing.

Charting Example

10/30/XX 11:45 A.M. Patient demonstrated quality control testing correctly and verbalized understanding of how to keep log records. Return appointment scheduled for one month to review logs of quality control testing and of blood glucose monitoring results. Patient verbalizes understanding of Regular Insulin sliding scale for elevated blood glucose and recording additional insulin on the glucose monitoring log. LaDanian Miller, CMA (AAMA)

Sample Form: Quality Control for Glucometer

Goal: Perform quality control testing and ensure accuracy of patient test results for blood glucose monitoring.

Glucometer serial number: _____

Code strip number: _____

Test strip lot number: _____

Check strip acceptable value range: _____

Low control solution lot number: _____

Low control solution expiration date: _____

Low control solution acceptable value range: _____

High control solution lot number: _____

High control solution expiration date: _____

High control solution acceptable value range: _____

*Mark opened vials of low and high control solution with "open" and "discard" dates.

Year/Month/Day	Low Solution Test Results	High Solution Test Results	Check Strip Test Results	Action taken if control test results abnormal	Initials

Use back of sheet for additional information, if necessary. Date and initial each entry.

Figure 30-3 ◆ Sample form for quality control.

Regulations and Laboratory Safety

The Food and Drug Administration (FDA) and the Environmental Protection Agency (EPA) are the two federal agencies that enforce safety standards. The FDA evaluates equipment for clinical performance, medical relevance, and safety. The Safe Medical Devices Act of 1990 monitors and evaluates incidents involving equipment. The EPA enforces legal and proper disposal of hazardous chemical and biological materials. OSHA rules protect patients and healthcare workers by mandating employee use of personal protective equipment (PPE) during blood and specimen collection. OSHA requires that MSDS sheets for all chemical substances be available in the medical office.

Joint Commission on the Accreditation of Healthcare Organizations

The Joint Commission on the Accreditation of Healthcare Organizations (JCAHO), a private, nongovernmental agency, has established guidelines regarding the quality of care in hospitals and healthcare agencies, including laboratories. JCAHO provides accreditation for healthcare agencies that establish a proven record of monitoring, evaluating, and implementing policies and procedures for quality assurance in patient care. Departments such as laboratories are required to identify indicators of high-risk and high-volume procedures, establish minimal baselines for acceptable quality of care, and gather monitored data. When necessary, the healthcare institution has to demonstrate a plan of correction, communication about the plan, and the effectiveness of correction. An accredited hospital laboratory or POL has demonstrated an effective quality assurance plan and established a high standard for patient care.

Safe Medical Devices Act

The Safe Medical Devices Act of 1990 was implemented to protect patients, visitors, and healthcare facilities staff. The act requires anyone using a medical device to report to the manufacturer and/or the FDA any incidents that reasonably suggest that a medical device caused or contributed to a serious injury to or death of a patient. The act defines an injury or illness as "either permanent impairment of bodily function or permanent damage to a bodily structure or one that necessitates immediate medical or surgical intervention to preclude permanent impairment of a bodily function or permanent damage to a bodily structure." It also provides for enforcing the use of safe medical devices when drawing blood or handling blood or other body fluids, such as syringes or vacuum tube holders with retractable needles. Inspections and the training of employees in the use of these medical devices are mandatory. A log must be maintained to record any incidents regarding medical devices, and an exposure plan should be in place and reviewed on a periodic basis.

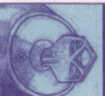

Keys to Success
GENERAL GUIDELINES FOR LABORATORY SAFETY

1. *Always* wash your hands before and after all procedures.
2. Use PPE as required by OSHA and department policy. This includes gloves, gowns, and eye and face protective wear.
3. Avoid wearing loose clothing and wear long hair pulled back to prevent entangling it in the laboratory equipment.
4. Wear shoes that cover the entire foot and have slip-resistant soles to prevent injury from spills or falls.
5. *Always* walk or walk quickly, but never run.
6. *Never* recap needles. Put used needles immediately in a sharps container. Use caution when handling or transporting sharp instruments.
7. Cover biological specimens at all times when transporting and centrifuging.
8. Dispose of biological specimens, such as blood, urine, and tissue, in biohazardous waste containers.
9. Decontaminate specimen collection, preparation, and processing areas following procedures.
10. Use caution when handling chemicals to avoid eye splash.
11. Follow OSHA standards for cleaning accidental chemical or biological specimen spills.
12. Report all equipment or lighting malfunctions.
13. Keep traffic areas clear of debris and obstructions.
14. *Never* eat, drink, smoke, or place any item in the mouth while in the medical laboratory.
15. *Never* apply makeup, lipstick, or contact lenses in the medical laboratory.
16. *Never* store personal food or drinks in the laboratory specimen refrigerator.

Hospital Laboratory Setting

The hospital laboratory setting provides for both inpatient and outpatient diagnostic testing. It is divided into functional areas for clinical analysis and surgical and anatomical pathology analysis (Table 30-1).

Blood chemistry tests include electrolyte levels (sodium, potassium, chloride, and carbon dioxide or CO_2); lipid studies, including cholesterol and triglycerides; creatinine; blood urea nitrogen (**BUN**); uric acid; liver and cardiac enzymes; serum protein; bilirubin; and blood glucose (Figure 30-4 ◆). Automated testing procedures are generally used, thereby ensuring better quality assurance and a more efficient, standardized level of testing.

Hematology and coagulation studies include the complete blood count (**CBC**) with its component parts as well as

TABLE 30-1 HOSPITAL LABORATORY FUNCTIONAL AREAS	
Clinical	**Surgical and Anatomical**
■ Hematology and coagulation studies ■ Microbiology ■ Virology ■ Toxicology ■ Immunology ■ Serology ■ Blood bank ■ Urinalysis	■ Surgical biopsy ■ Surgical histology ■ Cytology ■ Autopsy

erythrocyte sedimentation rate (**ESR**); partial thromboplastin time (**PTT**); prothrombin time (**PT**); coagulation studies; and reticulocyte counts. A CBC with differential includes a red blood cell count (**RBC**), white blood cell count (**WBC**), hematocrit (**Hct**), hemoglobin (**Hgb**), platelet count, and differential white blood cell count (**diff**).

The microbiology department identifies the microorganisms in specimens such as blood, urine, stool, nose and throat tissues or mucus, other body fluids, and wound drainage. It then tests the microorganism sensitivity to various antibiotics to determine which medication is most effective for treatment. This procedure is referred to as culture and sensitivity (**C & S**). Bacteriology, virology, and mycology are part of the microbiology department.

Blood serum studies to determine antigen–antibody reaction are conducted in the immunology area of the laboratory. The serology area conducts tests for diseases associated with immune disorders, including AIDS, HIV, syphilis,

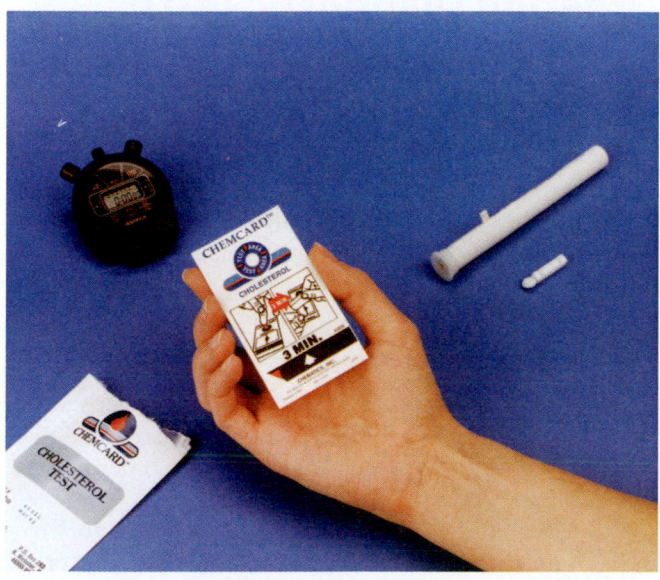

Figure 30-4 ◆ Chemcard™ cholesterol test.
Courtesy of Chematics, Inc.

rheumatoid arthritis, and mononucleosis. Tests on RBCs and serum, blood typing, compatibility, cross matching, and antibodies are performed in the blood bank area of the laboratory. Three forms of urinalysis tests are performed—physical, chemical, and microscopic—usually in a special area designated for urine studies.

Autopsies to determine the cause of death are performed in the surgical and anatomical pathology department of the laboratory. The surgical or histology area conducts tests on tissue specimens removed during surgical procedures. Histology tests help in the diagnosis of disease. In the cytology area of the laboratory, tests are conducted on cells from body fluids or tissues to determine the presence of abnormalities.

The Physician Office Laboratory

Physician office laboratories, or POLs, are small laboratories located in physicians' offices to provide a convenient place to perform simple tests on human specimens. According to CLIA regulations, these tests are classified as waived complexity because they require no interpretation and can be performed by medical assistants. Tests of higher complexity may be performed in the POL, but by a medical laboratory technician or medical technologist.

POL Equipment

Users must be trained in the operation of equipment in a POL. Training is a combination of formal education in the classroom, on-the-job training, and specific training by a sales representative for the equipment. Safety and CLIA guidelines are covered.

Equipment used in the laboratory includes centrifuges, microscopes, autoclaves, and electronic equipment, such as analyzers and measurement tools.

Centrifuge

The **centrifuge** is an instrument that separates specimens into their components using a rapid spinning action (Figure 30-5 ◆). Centrifugal force separates solids from liquids. For example, a centrifuge separates a blood specimen into red cells, white cells, and plasma, the lightest part of the blood. The heavier RBCs settle to the bottom of the tube, then a layer of WBCs, then the plasma on top. Urine specimens are also centrifuged to separate and obtain the portion required for microscopic study.

Microscope

A microscope is an optical instrument that magnifies minute objects (Figure 30-6 ◆). It is used in a POL to examine blood smears, perform microscopic blood cell counts, and identify

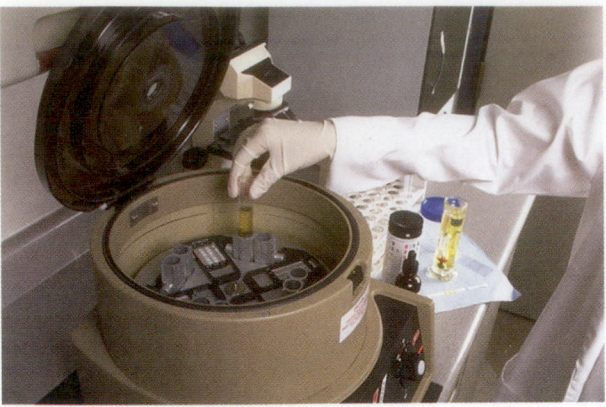

Figure 30-5 ◆ Example of a centrifuge used for blood and for urine.

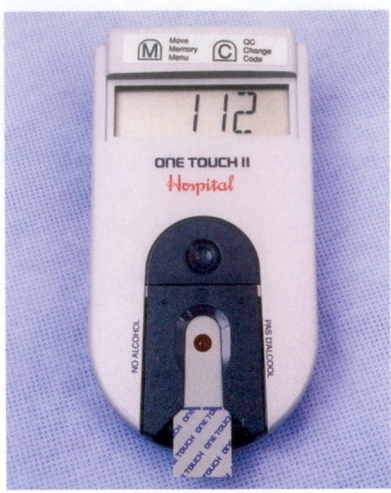

Figure 30-7 ◆ The glucose meter will display the glucose reading.

microorganisms in body fluid samples. The optical microscope is the type most frequently used in the POL. Light is concentrated through a condenser to focus through the object being examined and project an image. A compound microscope contains two lenses that magnify the image created by the condensed light. Specimen slides and cover slips are used with the microscope.

Electronic Equipment

Electronic equipment in a POL may include various types of automated analyzers that permit the rapid and accurate

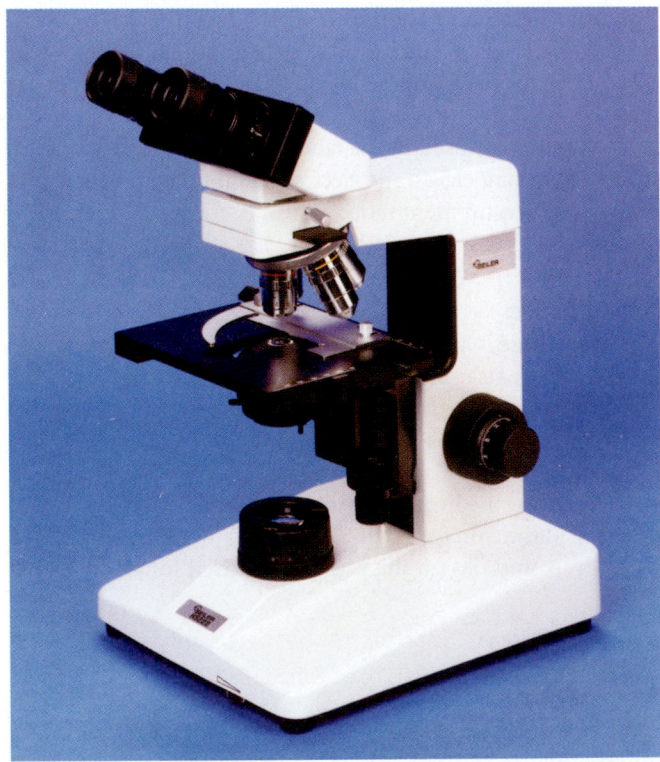

Figure 30-6 ◆ Clinical binocular microscope.
Courtesy of Seiler Instrument.

analysis of a specimen. Calibration for quality control must be conducted on a daily basis. Preventive maintenance must also be scheduled on a routine basis. Calibration testing, preventive maintenance, and unscheduled maintenance must be documented.

A **glucometer** is a small, handheld electronic instrument used to measure glucose levels in blood samples (Figure 30-7 ◆). Several types are available; most provide a reading using a drop of blood. Usually the results are available on a screen in less than 60 seconds. A glucometer uses a **photometer**, a common electronic component in laboratory equipment, to reflect light and assist in the measurement of blood glucose levels.

Other types of electronic equipment are instruments that count red or white blood cells and complex chemical analyzers.

Ordering Diagnostic Tests

The physician initiates orders for diagnostic testing as needed. The medical assistant then calls third-party providers for precertification to initiate the process of obtaining financial reimbursement for the tests. The MA will also schedule in-house and outside-agency diagnostic testing. When test results are returned to the medical office, the MA will compare the normal values to the patient's values and forward abnormal values to the physician for follow-up.

The Physician's Order

Although physicians often give verbal orders for diagnostic testing, the orders must be in writing. If the physician or the office calls an order in to a reference laboratory, the order must be signed within 30 days.

Medical offices use preprinted forms or laboratory requisitions for common tests (Figure 30-8 ◆). The name of the test is circled, underlined, or checked. The patient's name, date of birth (**DOB**), and insurance information are entered on the form, which must be signed by the physician or the physician's representative (MA, RN, or LPN). In some states the encounter

LABORATORY REQUISITION FORM

ORDER DATE: _____

COLLECTION DATE/TIME/BY: _____

FASTING
Y ☐ N ☐

Patient Name: _____ SS# _____ Sex: M ☐ F ☐ D.O.B _____
Address: _____ Parent/guarantor: _____
Ordering Physician: _____ Bill to: Patient ☐ or Insurance ☐
Insurance Company: _____ Policy Number: _____
Medicare number: _____ Medicaid Number: _____

Medicare Only Covers Medically Necessary Lab Tests

Narrative Diagnosis:
_____
_____
_____

Tests Performed At: _____

☐ ALBUMIN	☐ CPK	☐ MONO SCREEN
☐ ALKALINE PHOSPHATASE	☐ CREATININE	☐ PLATELET COUNT
☐ ALT (SGPT)	☐ GLUCOSE	☐ POTASSIUM
☐ AMYLASE	___ MEAL ___ GLUCOLA	☐ PROTEIN TOTAL
☐ AST (SGOT)	☐ GLUCOSE	☐ PROTIME WITH INR
☐ BETA HCG, QUAL (PREGNANCY)	___ 1 HR PP ___ 2 HR PP	☐ RSV
___ SERUM ___ URINE	☐ GTT (ORAL)	☐ SED RATE, WESTERGREN
☐ BILIRUBIN	___ 2 HR ___ 3 HR (PREGNANCY)	☐ SODIUM
___ TOTAL ___ DIRECT ___ NEWBORN	☐ HEMATOCRIT	☐ TROPONIN (FINGERSTICK)
☐ BUN	☐ HEMOGLOBIN	☐ UA URINE DIP/REFLEXED MICROSCOPIC
☐ CALCIUM	☐ INFLUENZA A & B	☐ URIC ACID
☐ CBC/AUTOMATED DIFF	☐ KOH PREP	☐ URINALYSIS, COMPLETE
☐ CBC/NO DIFF (HEMOGRAM)	☐ LDH	☐ WET PREP
☐ CHLORIDE	☐ LIPASE	
☐ CK-MB	☐ MAGNESIUM	

Tests Performed At: _____

☐ ALPHA FETO PROTEIN	☐ DRUG ABUSE SCREEN, URINE	☐ PROSTATIC SPECIFIC ANTIGEN (PSA)
(Complete separate form)	___ WITH ETOH	___ DIAGNOSTIC ___ SCREEN
☐ ANTIBODY SCREEN	___ WITH CONFIRMATION	___ FREE & TOTAL
☐ ASO SLIDE 0 WITH REFLEXED TITER	☐ ESTRADIOL	☐ PTT (PARTIAL THROMBOPLASTIN TIME)
☐ BETA HCG, QUANT	☐ FERRITIN	☐ RETICULOCYTE COUNT
☐ CA-125	☐ FOLATE	☐ RH IMMUNE GLOBULIN
☐ CARCINOEMBRYONIC ANTIGEN (CEA)	☐ GLYCOSOLATED HEMOGLOBIN (A1C)	☐ RA WITH REFLEXED TITER
☐ CHOLESTEROL	☐ HEPATITIS B SURFACE ANTIBODY	☐ RPR
☐ HDL CHOLESTEROL ☐ LDL DIRECT	☐ HEPATITIS B SURFACE ANTIGEN (w/conf)	___ WITH FTA CONFIRMATION
☐ CORTISOL, SERUM	☐ HIV SCREEN WITH CONFIRMATION	☐ T4 ☐ T3 UPTAKE ☐ T4, FREE
___ AM ___ PM ___ RANDOM	☐ IRON	☐ THEOPHYLLINE
☐ DIGOXIN	☐ IRON BINDING CAPACITY	
☐ DILANTIN	☐ LITHIUM	
☐ DIRECT COOMBS	☐ PHOSPHORUS	

PANELS:

☐ COMPREHENSIVE PANEL: ALB, ALK PHOS, ALT, AST, T BIL, BUN, CA, CREAT, GLUC, CO2, NA, K, CL, TP	☐ TYPE AND RH
	☐ VITAMIN B12
☐ BASIC METABOLIC: GLUC, BUN, CREAT, NA, K, CL, CO2, CALCIUM	☐ LIPID PANEL: CHOL, TRIG, HDL, CALCULATED LDL, CHOL: HDL
☐ HEPATIC FUNCTION: T BILI, D BILI, ALBUMIN, ALK PHOS, AST, ALT, TOTAL PROTEIN	☐ HEPATITIS PANEL: HBSAG, HB CORE, HEP A, HEP C
☐ ELECTROLYTES	☐ PRENATAL PROFILE 1 (OB PANEL): CBC/HISTO DIFF, RUBELLA, TYPE & RH, ANTIBODY SCREEN, RPR, HBSAG, GLUCOSE
☐ THYROID STIMULATING HORMONE (TSH)	☐ PRENATAL PROFILE 2: CBC/NO DIFF, RPR, ANTIBODY SCREEN, GLUCOSE
☐ TRIGLYCERIDES	
☐ TRIPLE SCREEN *(Complete separate form)*	☐ RENAL FUNCTION PANEL: ALB, CA, CO2, CL, CREAT, GLUC, PHOS, NA, K, BUN
☐ TROPONIN	

Physician's Signature: _____ Date: _____

White copy • Medical record   Yellow copy • Lab testing dept.   Pink copy • Coding (attach to fee ticket)

Figure 30-8 ◆ Sample diagnostic test request form.

form or a prescription blank may be used to document the order in writing if a form is unavailable. The prescription blank must be printed with the physician's name, address, phone number, and other pertinent information. Office staff transcribing the order enter the patient's name, DOB, and the diagnostic procedure ordered.

Many insurance companies, as well as Medicare and Medicaid, require a diagnosis and the *International Classification of Diseases, 9th Revision, Clinical Modification* (ICD-9-CM) code on the order. Following the practice guidelines of the specific state in which the practice is located, a designated staff member signs or stamps the physician's name, then signs his or her own name or initials. The completed order is given to the patient to take to the laboratory. It is accepted practice in most areas to fax a copy of the order to the diagnostic facility. The procedure

is coded using the Physician's Current Procedural Terminology (CPT) and must agree with the diagnosis for the patient as listed by the ICD-9-CM code. For example, a CBC or EKG is not acceptable for a patient with a primary diagnosis of diabetes. A second diagnosis of anemia would justify a CBC, and chest pain or complaints of palpitations would justify the EKG.

In-House Ordering

With a POL in the office, the physician may have certain routine tests performed on patients. An example is checking the urine sample of a pregnant patient for glucose and protein. This would be considered a standing order and would be conducted before the patient is seen by the physician. Other diagnostic tests may be performed after the patient sees the physician,

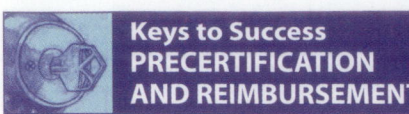

Keys to Success
PRECERTIFICATION
AND REIMBURSEMENT

Reimbursement is often based on precertification. Payment for services can be denied if precertification is not obtained, in which case either the patient or the ordering physician is held responsible for paying the charges. *All* required precertifications *must* be obtained and documented on the patient's chart.

while the patient waits for the results, or before the patient leaves the office. If the patient leaves before the physician knows the results, the patient is contacted for follow-up.

Standing orders are signed by the physician and placed in the patient's chart. Billing third-party providers requires a diagnosis appropriate for the test, test documentation, results, and any follow-up treatment or additional testing.

Precertification

Many third-party providers, or insurance carriers, require precertification for diagnostic testing. It is good policy to establish and maintain a file containing precertification requirements and guidelines for various third-party providers. Many providers contract with specific facilities to provide the services at a reduced rate for guaranteed reimbursement.

Precertification by Telephone

Before scheduling a diagnostic test, the medical office must contact the insurance carrier to confirm coverage and the facilities where the test may be performed. See ∞ Chapter 17 for more detailed information on obtaining authorizations from insurance companies.

Scheduling with Outside Agencies

Since not all diagnostic tests can be performed in the office, the MA will be responsible for coordinating test ordering and scheduling (Figure 30-9 ◆). Factors to consider when scheduling include the patient's condition, the timely or urgent need for diagnostic information, the patient's employment schedule, home and family responsibilities, and transportation availability. These factors should be discussed with the patient before the MA contacts the outside agency for scheduling.

?—**Critical Thinking Question 30-1**—
Jason is scheduling a patient for a laboratory procedure to be done at another location. He has offered the patient several appointment times, but she has rejected each one, saying she has too many other things she needs to do. How should Jason handle this?

The MA should have the following information before scheduling procedures with outside agencies: the patient's name, address, phone number, DOB, social security number (**SSN**), insurance or financial responsibility, type of test to be ordered, precertification requirements, and individuals or agencies to whom the results are to be released. Once the test is scheduled, it must be confirmed with the patient both verbally and in writing.

The MA should provide the patient with directions, verbally and in writing, to the testing facility. The MA should instruct the patient on what to do before the test, again verbally and in writing, with understanding confirmed verbally. The patient chart should document precertification, arrangements made, directions given to which facilities, instructions given for tests, and that instructions were verbal and written.

Screening and Follow Up of Test Results

Diagnostic reports on studies done in reference laboratories are returned to the physician office by telephone, fax, email, and U.S. mail. When these reports arrive, the MA will look at the results and compare them to normal values (norm) for the test. The MA will flag any abnormal results to call them to the physician's attention and record any intervention ordered by the physician and contact the patient for follow-up.

An easy way to keep track of patient follow-up is to maintain a tickler card file that alerts you when to contact the patient. Document contact with the patient in the chart and make a note on the card for further follow-up if necessary.

Once all reports are reviewed and the physician has completed or delegated all necessary communication, the reports are filed with the patient chart (Table 30-2). Some offices file the reports in a special section identified as laboratory reports.

Diagnostic test results are an integral part of the physician's diagnosis and treatment. Communicating test results to the patient enhances his or her active participation in the treatment plan.

?—**Critical Thinking Question 30-2**—
Jason has called the patient several times this week to make a follow-up appointment to review test results. The physician has specified that she does not want the patient to receive the test results over the phone. But the patient has not returned any of Jason's calls. What can he do?

Lab Services

IMPORTANT
Patient instructions and map on back

PHYSICIAN ORDERS

Patient ______ Last Name ______ First ______ M.I. ______ D.O.B. ______ M F ☐ Patient ☐ SS# ___ — ___ — ___

Address ______ City ______ Zip ______ Phone # ______

Physician ______ ATTACH COPY OF INSURANCE CARD

Diagnosis/ICD-9 Code ______ (Additional codes on reverse)

Date & Time of Collection: ______ Drawing Facility ______

☐ 789.00 Abdominal Pain
☐ 285.9 Anemia (NOS)
☐ 414.9 Coronary Artery Disease (CAD)
☐ 250.0 DM (diabetes mellitus)
☐ 780.7 Fatigue/Malaise
☐ 272.0 Hypercholesterolemia
☐ 244.9 Hypothyroidism
☐ 272.4 Hyperlipidemia
☐ 401.9 Hypertension
☐ 483.9 URI (upper respiratory infection)
☐ ROUTINE ☐ ASAP ☐ STAT
☐ PHONE RESULTS TO: # ______
☐ FAX RESULTS TO: # ______
☐ COPY TO: ______

HEMATOLOGY
☐ 1021 CBC, Automated Diff (incl, Platelet Ct.)
☐ 1023 Hemoglobin/Hematocrit
☐ 1020 Hemogram
☐ 1025 Platelet Count
☐ 1150 Pro Time Diagnostic
☐ 1151 Pro Time, Therapeutic
☐ 1155 PTT
☐ 1315 Reticulocyte Count
☐ 1310 Sed Rate/ Westergren

URINE
☐ 1059 Urinalysis
☐ 1082 Urinalysis w/Culture if indicated
Urine-24 Hr ______ Spot ______ Ht. ______ Wt. ______
☐ 3033 Creatinine
☐ 3036 Creatinine Clearance (also requires blood)
☐ 3095 Protein
☐ 3096 Sodium/Potassium
☐ Microalbumin 24 Hr ______ Spot ______

SEROLOGY
☐ 8020 ANA (Antinuclear Antibody)
☐ 8040 Mono Spot
☐ 3494 Rheumatoid Factor
☐ 8010 RPR
☐ 5365 Rubella

CHEMISTRY
☐ 5550 Alpha Fetoprotein, Prenatal
☐ 3000 Amylase
☐ 3153 B12/Folate
☐ 3156 Beta HCG, Quantitative
☐ 3321 Bilirubin, Total
☐ 3324 Bilirubin, Total/Direct
☐ 3009 BUN
☐ 3159 CEA
☐ 3348 Cholesterol
☐ 3030 Creatinine, Serum
☐ 3509 Digoxin (recommend 12 hrs, after dose)
☐ 3515 Dilantin
☐ 3168 Ferritin
☐ 3193 FSH
☐ 3066 ▼ Glucose, Fasting
☐ 3061 Glucose, 1st Post 50 g Glucola
☐ 3075 ▼ Glucose, 2nd Post Glucola
☐ 3060 Glucose, 2nd Post
☐ Prandial (meal)
☐ 3049 ▼ Glucose Tolerance Oral GTT
☐ 3047 ▼ Glucose Tolerance
☐ Gestational GTT
☐ 3650 Hemoglobin, A1C

CHEMISTRY
☐ 5232 HBsAg
☐ 3175 HIV (Consent required)
☐ 3581 Iron & Iron Binding Capacity
☐ 3195 LH
☐ 3590 Magnesium
☐ 3527 Phenobarbital
☐ 3095 Potassium
☐ 3689 Pregnancy Test Serum (HCG, qual)
☐ 3653 Pregnancy Test, Urine
☐ 3197 Prolactin
☐ 3199 PSA
☐ 3339 SGOT/AST
☐ 3342 SGPT/ALT
☐ 3093 Sodium/Potassium, Serum
☐ 3510 Tegretol
☐ 3551 Theophylline
☐ 3333 Uric Acid

MICROBIOLOGY
Source ______
☐ 7240 Culture, AFB
☐ 7200 Culture, Blood x ______
☐ Draw interval ______
☐ 7280 Culture, Fungus
☐ Culture, Routine
☐ 7005 Culture, Stool
☐ 7010 Culture, Throat
☐ 7000 Culture, Urine
☐ 7300 Gram Stain
☐ 7353 Occult Blood x ______
☐ 7365 Ova & Parasites x ______
☐ 7400 Smear & Suspension (includes Gram Stain/Wet Mount)
☐ 7060 Rapid Strep A Screen (____)
☐ 7065 Rapid Strep A Screen only
☐ 7030 Beta Strep Culture
☐ 5207 GC by DNA Probe
☐ 5130 Chlamydia by DNA Probe
☐ 5555 Chlamydia/GC by DNA Probe
☐ 7375 Wright Stain, Stool

Additional Tests ______

PANELS & PROFILES
☐ ✗ 3309 CHEM 12 Albumin, Alkaline Phosphatase, BUN, Calcium, Cholesterol, Glucose, LDH, Phosphorus, AST, Total Bilirubin, Total Protein, Uric Acid
☐ ▼ 3315 CHEM 20 Chem 12, Electrolyte Panel, Creatinine, Iron, Gamma GT, ALT, Triglycerides
☐ ▼ 3357 CARDIAC RISK PANEL Cholesterol, HDL, LDL, Risk Factors, VLDL Triglycerides
☐ ✗ 3042 CRITICAL CARE PANEL BUN, Chloride, CO2, Glucose, Potassium, Sodium
☐ 3046 ELECTROLYTE PANEL Chloride, CO2, Potassium, Sodium
☐ ▼ 3399 EXECUTIVE PANEL Chem 20, Iron, Cardiac Risk Panel CBC, RPR, Thyroid Cascade
☐ 5242 HEPATITIS PANEL, ACUTE HAVIgMAb, HBsAg, HBsAb, HBcAb, HCVAb
☐ ▼ 3355 LIPID MONITORING PANEL Cholesterol, Triglycerides, HDL, LDL, VLDL, ALT, AST
☐ 3312 LIVER PANEL Alkaline Phosphatase, AST, Total Bilirubin, Gamma GT, Total Protein, Albumin ALT
☐ ✗ 3083 METABOLIC STATUS PANEL BUN, Osmolality (calculated), Chloride, CO_2 Creatinine, Glucose, Potassium, Sodium, BUN/Creatinine, Ratio, Anion Gap
☐ ✗ 3376 PANEL B Chem 12, CBC, Electrolyte Panel
☐ ▼ 3382 PANEL D Chem 20, CBC, Thyroid Cascade
☐ ✗ 3385 PANEL F Chem 12, CBC, Electrolyte Panel, Thyroid Cascade
☐ ▼ 3391 PANEL G Chem 20, Cardiac Risk Panel, CBC, Thyroid Cascade
☐ ▼ 3393 PANEL H Chem 20, CBC, Cardiac Risk Panel, Rheumatoid Factor, Thyroid Cascade
☐ ▼ 3397 PANEL J Chem 20, Cardiac Risk Panel
☐ 5351 PRENATAL PANEL Antibody Screen, ABO/Rh, CBC Rubella, HBsAg, RPR 1059 with Urinalysis Routine 1062 with Urinalysis w/Culture if indicated
☐ ✗ 3102 RENAL PANEL Matabolic Status Panel, Calcium, Phosphorus
☐ 3188 THYROID CASCADE TSH, Reflex Testing

▼ - patient **required** to fast for 12-14 hours
✗ - patient recommended to fast 12-14 hours

LAB USE ONLY
☐ SST ☐ PURPLE ☐ YELLOW ☐ BLUE ☐ GREEN ☐ GREY ☐ URINE ☐ BLACK ☐ OTHER:
☐ PLASMA ☐ SERUM ☐ SWAB ☐ SLIDES ☐ DNA PROBE ☐ B. CULT BTLS
RECV. SPECIMEN: ☐ AMBIENT ☐ FROZEN ☐ ON ICE

Special Instructions/Pertinent Clinical Information ______

Physician's Signature ______ Date ______

These orders may be FAXed to: 449-5288 LAB 7060-500 (7/96)

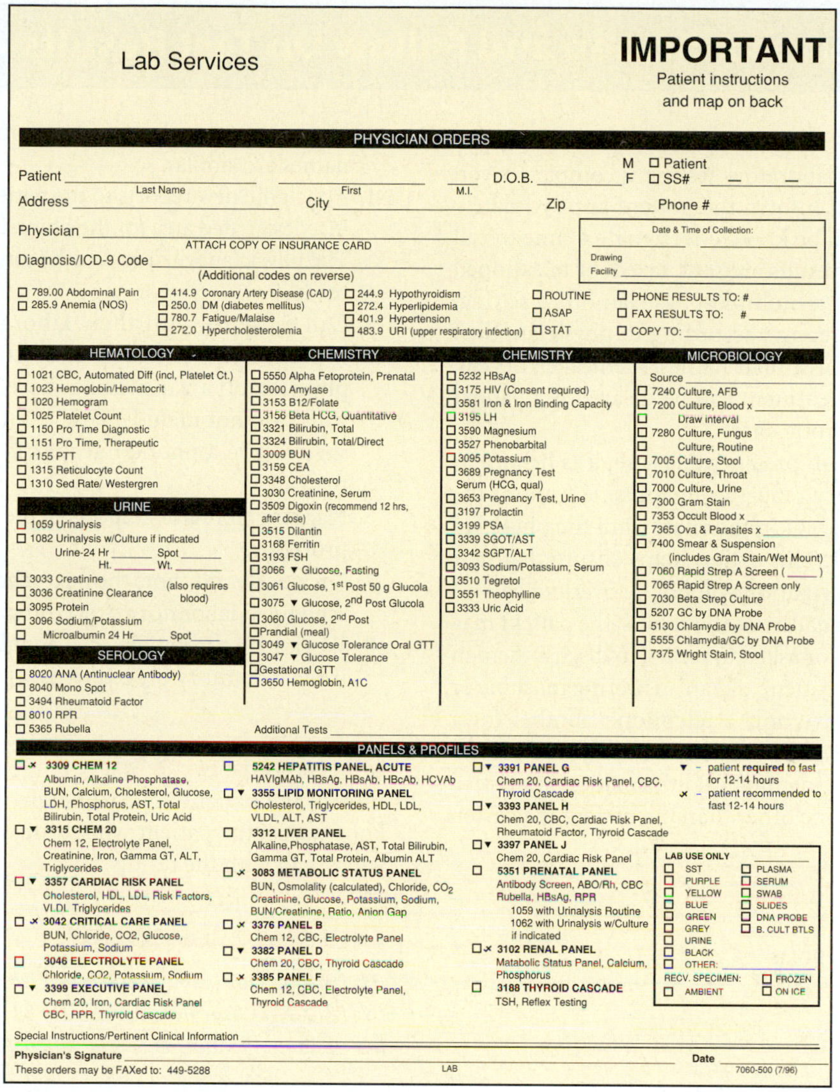

Figure 30-9 ◆ Requisition form for outside laboratory.

TABLE 30-2 INFORMATION ON A DIAGNOSTIC TEST REPORT

1. Diagnostic facility name, address, telephone number, fax number, and any identification number.
2. Ordering physician's name, address, telephone number, and other information
3. Patient name, address, telephone number, and other information
4. Patient's ID number
5. Date specimen was received by facility
6. Date of report of test results
7. Tests performed
8. Test results
9. Normal values or range for tests performed

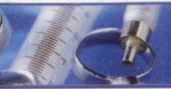

PROCEDURE 30-2 Screen and Follow Up Test Results

Theory and Rationale

When the procedure or laboratory testing is completed, you or other office staff will inform the patient approximately when the test results will be known. Designate a time to call the patient. Laboratory results are sent, faxed, or telephoned to the medical office. In a multiple-physician office setting, sort mailed laboratory reports according to physician, then alphabetically. Be alert for similar names. Medical errors can occur and therapeutic treatment can be delayed if a patient report is placed in the wrong chart.

Unless the physician prefers otherwise, it is helpful to attach the new laboratory report to the outside front of the patient chart. Do *not* place it in the chart until the physician has read and initialed it. This action helps ensure that new and critical medical information will not be overlooked.

Depending on the nature of the results, the patient may be called with the results or asked to return to discuss them in the office. If you call the patient and an answering machine or voicemail comes on, leave only a telephone number for a return call. Do *not* leave any patient information on the answering machine. Leaving medical information is a risk to confidentiality, as someone other than the patient may listen to the message.

Materials

- returned laboratory reports
- patient chart
- blue or black ink pen
- telephone

Competency

(**Conditions**) With procedure materials, you will be able to (**Task**) screen and follow up on returned laboratory results (**Standards**) within the time and to the degree of accuracy designated by the instructor.

1. Sort lab reports according to physician.
2. Sort the reports according to last name, first name, and initial for each physician.

3. Match patient identification numbers in cases where names are similar.
4. Attach the new reports to the patient chart and place them in a designated area for the physician to read and interpret. The physician will initial each laboratory test that he or she reads.
5. Call patients with their laboratory results or set up appointments to discuss the results as designated by the physician. If an answering machine or voicemail is activated, do not include patient information in your message. Leave a phone number for the patient to return the call.
6. Place the laboratory reports in the chart according to office procedure.
7. On a tickler file, note the next scheduled date for routinely scheduled laboratory procedures.
8. Work with the patient to schedule the next appointment if the laboratory procedure is weekly or monthly.

Patient Education

Inform the patient approximately when the results will be known. Ask the patient what time of day would be best for you to call with the results.

Charting Example

07/19/XX 1:00 p.m. Results of Hgb and Hct performed on 07/18/XX within normal limits. Pt notified per physician's instructions. Jordan Leonard, CMA (AAMA)

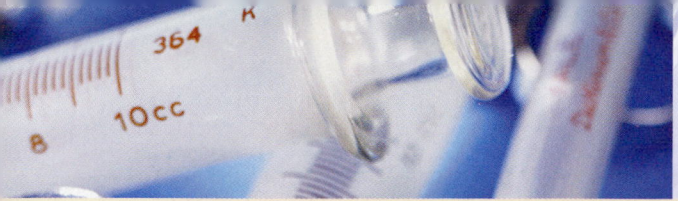

REVIEW

- Diagnostic test information plays an important role in the diagnosis and confirmation of disease or wellness. Laboratory testing is done in either a POL or an independently owned and operated reference laboratory. The main advantage of POLs is quick testing and results. The primary advantage of reference laboratories is their capacity to perform higher-complexity tests.

- As an MA, you will perform waived testing. In some states, with supervision and training, you may be able to perform duties related to preparing specimens or doing mechanized testing.

- CLIA, a federal act, established quality standards for laboratory testing. The accuracy of laboratory testing affects diagnosis, treatment, medication, and dosages. Three categories of tests have been established: waived tests, moderate complexity-tests, and high-complexity tests. Quality standards are specified for proficiency testing (PT), quality control, quality assurance, patient test management, and personnel qualifications. Regulations affecting laboratory procedures are increasingly more stringent as tests become more complex to perform.

- Quality control ensures that test results are valid and reliable. It is the goal of quality control to detect and eliminate errors that may interfere with accurate test results.

- Quality assurance is a form of outcomes assessment that reviews documentation of test results, services provided, and other recorded data. This information is compared with acceptable standards of testing.

- A hospital usually has two laboratory divisions. One is the clinical division, which performs numerous diagnostic tests such as hematology and serology. The other is the surgical and anatomical laboratory, which performs autopsies, biopsies, surgical histology, and cytology. JCAHO has established guidelines regarding quality of care by hospitals and healthcare agencies, including laboratory settings.

- FDA, EPA, and OSHA are federal agencies that regulate the safety of patients and healthcare employees. The Safe Medical Devices Act of 1990 requires reporting to the manufacturer and/or the FDA any incidents that reasonably suggest that a medical device caused or contributed to a serious injury to or death of a patient. It also requires enforcing the use of safe medical devices when drawing or handling blood or other body fluids.

- Equipment used in the laboratory includes centrifuges, microscopes, autoclaves, measurement tools, and electronic equipment such as analyzers. Training in the use of laboratory equipment includes safety and CLIA guidelines.

- The physician writes an order for laboratory testing on a laboratory request or prescription form. Demographic and insurance data, along with ICD-9-CM and CPT codes, are included on the forms.

- Precertification is often required to ensure insurance provider payment. Some orders for laboratory testing within the physician's office are routine and are called standing orders. Preprinted standing orders are placed in the patient chart for signing later by the physician. Precertification must be obtained or insurance claims filed for standing orders.

- As an MA, you may need to schedule procedures or laboratory testing outside the physician's office. When diagnostic reports are returned to the physician's office, you will review and compare the results against norms and flag abnormal results for the physician. The physician will give you directions for following up test results with the patient or in some cases may personally call the patient. Diagnostic reports are placed in the chart and follow-up is documented.

Chapter Review

Multiple Choice

1. Which of the following is true about a reference laboratory?
    a. It is convenient for the patient.
    b. It performs high-level testing.
    c. Test results are returned more quickly than from a POL.
    d. The regulations are different for a reference lab than for a POL.

2. As an MA working in a POL, you may obtain a(n)
    a. biopsy.
    b. bone marrow specimen.
    c. immunoassay.
    d. capillary specimen.

3. Quality assurance is a type of
    a. methodology.
    b. outcome assessment.
    c. instruction.
    d. calibration.

4. The FDA oversees
    a. evaluation of medical equipment.
    b. disposal of biohazardous waste.
    c. disposal of chemical waste.
    d. evaluation of PPE.

Chapter Review (continued)

5. If a medical device may cause serious injury to a patient, it should be reported to
   a. FDA.
   b. OSHA.
   c. EPA.
   d. HCFA.

6. A physician order to a reference laboratory must be signed within
   a. 5 days.
   b. 30 days.
   c. 10 days.
   d. 20 days.

7. After precertification has been granted by an insurance company, you should receive a(n)
   a. treatment location.
   b. set of forms.
   c. set of labels for charts.
   d. assigned number.

8. In a POL, a standing order is a
   a. high-complexity test.
   b. routine test.
   c. prescription form.
   d. third-party billing form.

9. In a multiple-physician office, which of the following is the first step in handling laboratory reports?
   a. Sorting reports by physician
   b. Sorting reports by alphabetical order
   c. Sorting reports by similar names
   d. Sorting reports by size

10. Which of the following should you do when contacting a patient by phone about his or her test results?
    a. Leave a detailed message on the answering machine if the patient is not at home.
    b. Leave a detailed message with whoever answers the phone if the patient is not at home.
    c. Leave a phone number for a return call.
    d. Leave no message and call back at a later date.

True/False

T F 1. When using equipment, you are required to follow OSHA and Clinical Laboratory Improvement Amendments (CLIA) guidelines.

T F 2. Blood glucose and urine pregnancy tests have been approved by the FDA for patients to use at home.

T F 3. Blood chemistries and urine cultures are categorized as moderate-complexity tests.

T F 4. Quality control before testing means only checking that the patient has used the appropriate container for collection.

T F 5. A high-complexity test is so named because it takes longer to perform than a moderate- or low-complexity test.

Short Answer

1. What is quality control?

2. Name the two federal agencies that enforce safety standards.

3. What are waived tests? Name several examples.

4. What is the purpose of autopsies?

5. What is the function of a glucometer?

Research

1. Are medical assistants allowed to perform capillary and venipuncture mechanized tests in your local area?

2. Are MAs in your state allowed to centrifuge urine and blood specimens?

Externship Application Experience

As an extern, you are observing an MA in the office as she performs a glucose test using a glucometer. The quality control log specifies daily quality control checks on the glucometer. While cleaning and organizing the area after the test, however, you notice that no quality control checks have been logged in the past two days. What should you do?

Resource Guide

Environmental Protection Agency (EPA)
1200 Pennsylvania Ave., NW
Washington, DC 20460
www.epa.gov

Food and Drug Administration
5600 Fishers Lane
Rockville, MD 20857-0001
1-888-463-6332 (1-888-INFO-FDA)
www.FDA.gov

Centers for Medicare and Medicaid Services (CMS)
7500 Security Boulevard
Baltimore, MD 21244
www.cms.hhs.gov

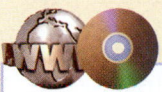

Med**Media**

http://www.MyMAKit.com

More on this chapter, including interactive resources, can be found on the Student CD-ROM accompanying this textbook and on http://www.MyMAKit.com.

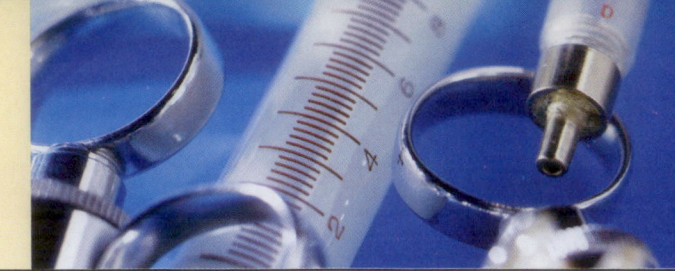

CHAPTER 31

Microscopes and Microbiology

Case Study

Irene has been working in a clinical laboratory for several months and is very comfortable obtaining specimens and using the microscopes. Irene has received several samples from a local physician's office. The first sample is from a patient who has been complaining of urinary frequency, burning and the inability to fully empty the bladder. Irene identifies the organism as *Escherichia coli*. The next sample she tests is from a toddler. The parents state that the little girl has had a runny nose for more than ten days and developed a rash with a crust over it directly under her nose. The doctor wants to check the toddler for impetigo, which is caused by *Staphylococcus aureus*, which Irene will be able to easily identify by shape.

Objectives

After completing this chapter, you should be able to:

- Define and spell key terminology in this chapter.
- Define the medical assistant's role in microbiological testing and specimen collection.
- Identify various types of microscopes and explain when each is used.
- Identify the structures of a microscope and the function of each.
- Explain how to use and maintain a microscope.
- Discuss bacterial nomenclature and grouping.
- Describe the normal flora present in the body.
- Discuss how bacteria, parasites, and viruses cause disease.
- Explain how to prepare a specimen smear.
- Define gram staining and discuss when it is used.
- Explain the three ways to prepare wet mount slides.
- Discuss the role of stool specimens in the diagnosis of disease and how they are obtained.
- Explain culture and sensitivity testing.
- Describe how urine culture specimens are collected.

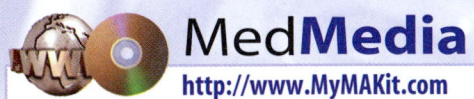 **MedMedia**
http://www.MyMAKit.com

Additional interactive resources and activities for this chapter can be found on http://www.MyMAKit.com. For a video, tips, audio glossary, legal and ethical scenarios, job scenarios, quizzes, and games related to the content of this chapter, please access the accompanying CD-ROM in this book.

Video: *Specimens*
Audio Glossary
Legal and Ethical Scenario: *Microscopes and Microbiology*
On the Job Scenario: *Microscopes and Microbiology*
Multiple Choice Quiz
Games: Crossword, Strikeout, and Spelling Bee
Tips
HIPAA Quiz

✚ MEDICAL ASSISTING STANDARDS

CAAHEP ENTRY-LEVEL STANDARDS	ABHES ENTRY-LEVEL COMPETENCIES
■ Perform within scope of practice (psychomotor) ■ Apply ethical behaviors, including honesty/integrity in performance of medical assisting practice (affective) ■ Apply local, state and federal health care legislation and regulation appropriate to the medical assisting practice setting (psychomotor) ■ Recognize the importance of local, state and federal legislation and regulations in the practice setting (affective) ■ Explore issue of confidentiality as it applies to the medical assistant (cognitive) ■ Document accurately in the patient record (psychomotor) ■ Perform handwashing (psychomotor) ■ Practice Standard Precautions (psychomotor) ■ Perform quality control measures (psychomotor) ■ Screen test results (psychomotor) ■ Assist physician with patient care (psychomotor) ■ Obtain specimens for microbiological testing (psychomotor) ■ Identify disease processes that are indications for CLIA waived tests (cognitive) ■ Perform CLIA waived microbiology testing (psychomotor) ■ Display sensitivity to patient rights and feelings in collecting specimens (affective) ■ Prepare a patient for procedures and/or treatments (psychomotor) ■ Explain the rationale for performance of a procedure to the patient (affective) ■ Document patient care (psychomotor) ■ Document patient education (psychomotor)	■ Project a positive attitude. ■ Maintain confidentiality at all times. ■ Be a "team player." ■ Be cognizant of ethical boundaries. ■ Exhibit initiative. ■ Adapt to change. ■ Evidence a responsible attitude. ■ Be courteous and diplomatic. ■ Conduct work within scope of education, training, and ability. ■ Practice Standard Precautions. ■ Use quality control. ■ Collect and process specimens. ■ Dispose of biohazardous materials. ■ Obtain throat specimen for microbiological testing. ■ Perform wound collection procedure for microbiological testing. ■ Perform microbiology testing. ■ Instruct patients in the collection of fecal specimen.

✓ COMPETENCY SKILLS PERFORMANCE

1. Demonstrate correct use of the microscope.
2. Prepare a specimen smear for microbiologic examination.
3. Prepare a gram stain.
4. Instruct the patient in the collection of a fecal specimen for occult blood or culture testing and develop the fecal occult blood test.
5. Perform a wound or throat culture collection using sterile swabs.
6. Perform Rapid Group A strep testing.

Key Terminology

binocular—having two eyepieces (on a microscope)

eukaryotes—group of microorganisms, such as fungi and parasites, that have organized nuclear material and organelles to assist in reproduction

microbiology—the study of microorganisms

monocular—having one eyepiece (on a microscope)

morphology—the study of shape or form; in microbiology, a method of classifying bacteria according to shape

mycology—study of fungi, such as yeast and molds

normal flora—generally harmless microorganisms common in the human body

ocular—pertaining to the eye; also, the microscope's eyepiece

opportunistic pathogen—normally nonpathogenic microorganism that causes disease in a host whose immune resistance has been lowered by certain disorders or treatments

organelle—a very small organ-functioning unit within a living cell; mitochondria organelles are responsible for the metabolism of lipids and the synthesis (building) of proteins

parasitology—branch of biology that studies parasites

pathogenicity—ability of an organism to cause disease

prokaryotes—group of microorganisms, such as bacteria, that lack an organized nucleus and cytoplasmic organelles

serology—laboratory science in which blood serum is tested for the presence of antibodies

staph—*Staphylococcus*

strep—*Streptococcus*

ultramicroscopic—requiring magnification with an electron microscope to be seen

virology—specialized branch of microbiology that studies viruses and associated diseases

viruses—ultramicroscopic, nonliving organisms classified as microorganisms because they contain DNA or RNA and are capable of parasitic metabolism and reproduction

Abbreviations

KOH—potassium hydroxide   **QS**—quantity sufficient   **UTI**—urinary tract infection
QNS—quantity not sufficient

Introduction

The microscope is used to magnify and examine blood and urine specimens to detect the presence of pathogenic organisms. The diagnosis of an illness is not always clear based on the patient's complaints or symptoms and may require diagnostic testing using the microscope. Each step in preparing a slide for microscopic examination is time sensitive and critical to proper diagnosis.

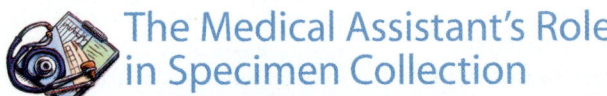

The Medical Assistant's Role in Specimen Collection

The physician will require the MA's assistance in preparing the patient, collecting the specimen, and processing and/or transporting the specimen. With classroom training and competency completion, the MA will help with microbiology testing by preparing the specimen for examination under the microscope. The medical assistant will also be involved in patient education when the patient collects the specimen, as in the case of urine collection. Laboratory results are only as accurate as the specimen provided.

Microscopes

In 1665, in his work *Micrographia,* Robert Hooke published intricate, highly accurate drawings of tiny creatures such as fleas that he had observed through an early microscope. Based on his work, Anton van Leeuwenhoek (1632–1723), a Dutch lens maker, proposed that illness and disease were caused by something too small to be seen with the naked eye. In an effort to see these mysterious entities, he invented the first light microscope. He examined water from a local pond and saw tiny, motile organisms living in it. His invention was a startling breakthrough for the scientific community and was the foundation for the field of **microbiology,** the study of microorganisms.

Types of Microscopes

Five kinds of microscopes are routinely used in laboratories (Table 31-1). The type of microscope used is determined by the specimen and the particular examination the physician requests.

Structure and Parts of a Microscope

The magnification of an object by a microscope is accomplished by the interaction of visible light and the lens systems. The lenses of a microscope are convex (curved outward in the middle). The curvature refracts, or bends, the light waves as they pass through the lenses. Lens sizes and degree of curvature are directly related to the degree of magnification. When an object

is illuminated by the light source, the light goes through the lens system and forms an optical replica from the refracted light. The real image is projected and magnified, forming a virtual image that is the reverse of the real image. The virtual image is the one the user sees.

The component parts of an optical microscope include the **oculars,** objectives (lenses), oil immersion objective, arm and focus controls, light source, stage, and substage (Figure 31-1 ◆).

Oculars

The microscope may be **monocular** (one eyepiece) or **binocular** (two eyepieces). The eyepieces on binoculars can be adjusted to compensate for differences in the visual acuity of the user's eyes

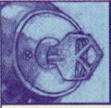

Keys to Success
OTHER TYPES OF MICROSCOPES

- The dissection microscope is used to look at larger specimens but cannot examine single cells because of its low magnification.
- In a confocal microscope, a laser light scans the specimen and the image appears on a computer screen for examination.
- Scanning electron and transmission electron microscopes use electron illumination for high magnification and 3D or 2D images, respectively. They are used in pathology examination and research.

TABLE 31-1 TYPES OF MICROSCOPES

Type	Use	Magnification	Light	Stain
Compound or bright field	Most common type. Specimen is dark against an illuminated background.	Two magnification systems 100X to 1000X	Located below the specimen	Stained and unstained
Phase contrast	Thickness provides the contrast needed to see the live specimen. Thin areas are light; thick areas are dark. Background is dark.	100X to 1000X	Passes through or is deflected by the specimen	Unstained
Dark field	Light is deflected from the specimen, so the image is seen on a dark background.	100X to 1000X	Light source is projected from below. Condenser does not allow light to pass through the specimen. Light is directed at an angle.	Unstained
Fluorescence compound	Light rays are directed through a tube, a series of filters, a mirror, then through the ocular lens system, which illuminates the specimen on a black background.	100X to 1000X	Mercury lamp emits light rays.	Stained with special fluorescent stains. Colors range from bright yellow to orange to lime green.
Electron	Used to view ultramicroscopic organisms or individual cellular components. Image is formed on a screen, as in a television.	Up to 100,000 times normal size	Power source excites electrons through an electromagnetic field.	Stained and unstained

and to comfortably fit the distance between the eyes. A magnifying lens mounted at the top of the tube magnifies the image ten times and is called a 10X lens.

Objectives

The tube of the microscope contains a series of mirrors that reflect light and the image to be viewed. At the end of the tube is a revolving nosepiece that houses the objectives. Objectives include 10X (low power), 40X (high dry), and 100X (immersion oil) lenses. Total magnification of the microscope is the ocular magnification multiplied by the objective used. For example, if viewing an object with the 40X objective, you have a total magnification of 400X, or ocular × objective (10 × 40 = 400). Other objectives may be added for special applications.

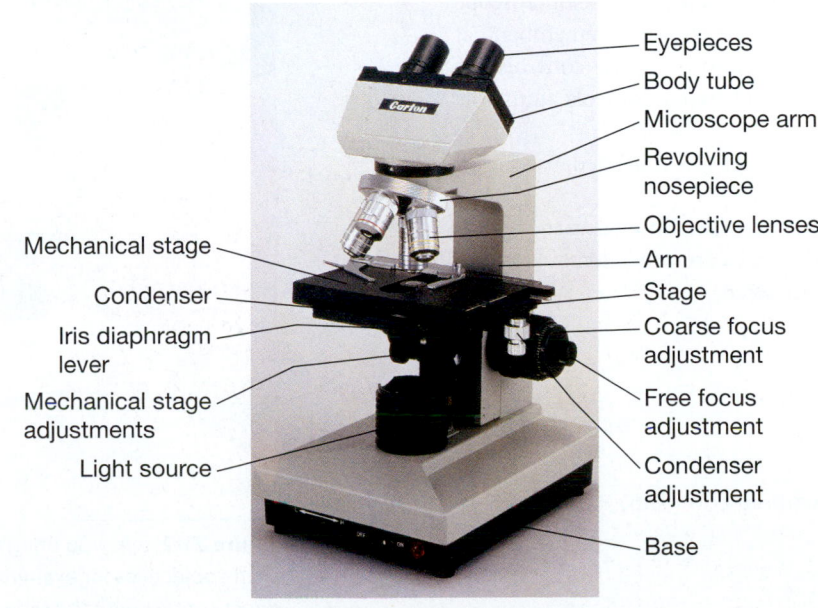

Figure 31-1 ◆ Binocular microscope with parts labeled.

Labels: Eyepieces, Body tube, Microscope arm, Revolving nosepiece, Objective lenses, Arm, Stage, Coarse focus adjustment, Free focus adjustment, Condenser adjustment, Base, Mechanical stage, Condenser, Iris diaphragm lever, Mechanical stage adjustments, Light source

Oil Immersion Objective

Immersion oil must be used with the 100X lens to increase the resolution, or clarity. Higher resolution clarifies and sharpens the image. The oil fills the space between the slide and the objective, decreasing the number of deflected rays and wavelength changes that occur after the light passes through the specimen.

Arm and Focus Control

The arm is used to mount the focusing system and to suspend the ocular system over the stage area. Focus adjustment knobs are located on the arm near the base. Microscopes have fine and coarse adjustment knobs. One knob assembly often houses both. Coarse adjustment knobs are on the outside diameter, and fine focus knobs are contained in the inside diameter.

Light Source

The light source, the condenser, and the diaphragm are located under the mechanical stage. The condenser directs light rays from the light source through the diaphragm. The diaphragm is adjustable, which allows the user to increase or decrease the amount of light from the source lamp. The microscope base contains a power cord, a tungsten lamp light source, and an on/off switch.

Stage

The mechanical stage is a flat surface on which specimens are placed. Stage clips hold the specimen slide in place. It can be moved forward or to the right or left so that the user can view the entire slide. An opening in the stage allows light to be directed through the condenser and diaphragm to illuminate the slide.

Substage

The condenser is located below the stage on the substage, where it directs concentrated light through the specimen. The iris, below the substage, opens and closes like a camera shutter, controlling the amount of light that illuminates the specimen.

Using the Microscope

The proper use of a microscope is crucial to examining specimens successfully. Remember that you are viewing the image in reverse and upside down. You turn the stage focus knob left to move the slide to your right. To move the image up or down, you turn the adjustment knob clockwise or counterclockwise. You can adjust the amount of light by opening the diaphragm, closing the diaphragm, adjusting the condenser, or, with some microscopes, using the built-in light adjustment system.

Medical assistants are responsible for cleaning, maintaining, and operating the microscope. When not in use, the microscope must be covered. Unplug the cord and wrap it

---

PROCEDURE 31-1 Demonstrate Correct Use of the Microscope

Theory and Rationale

As you bring the slide closer to the objectives for examination, avoid direct contact with the slide or cover slip (Figure 31-2 ◆). Otherwise, the specimen will be contaminated and a new one would have to be prepared. When you prepare the microscope and specimen for examination by the physician, remember that the objectives increase magnification, the iris controls the amount of light, and the fine and coarse controls adjust the clarity.

If magnification greater than 45X is needed, use the oil immersion lens.

Note the date and time on the maintenance log whenever a light bulb is replaced, repairs are needed, maintenance is called, and repairs are completed.

Materials

- microscope
- lens paper
- lens cleaner
- prepared slide (with or without cover slip)
- immersion oil
- disposable gloves
- tissues

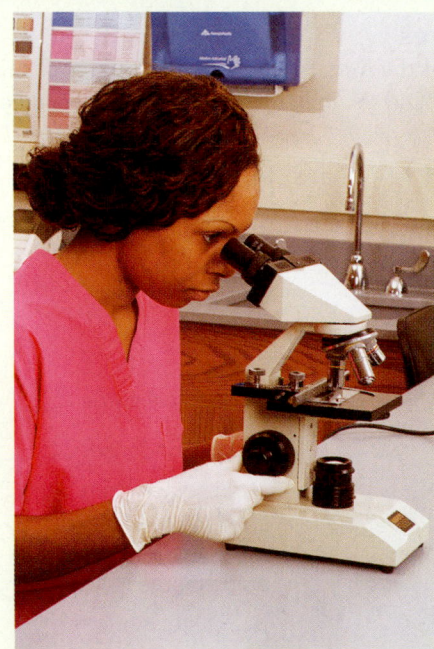

Figure 31-2 ◆ As you bring the slide closer to the objectives for examination, avoid direct contact with the slide or cover slip.

PROCEDURE 31-1 Demonstrate Correct Use of the Microscope *(continued)*

Competency

(**Conditions**) With the necessary materials, you will be able to (**Task**) demonstrate how to use the microscope and focus all three objectives (**Standards**) correctly within 30 minutes.

1. Wash your hands and put on disposable gloves.
2. Remove the cover from the microscope.
3. Check that the microscope is clean and in working order. Replace the light bulb if necessary.
4. Turn the light off until you are ready to focus the objectives on the specimen slide.
5. Clean the lenses and eyepieces (oculars) with lens paper. Use lens cleaner as necessary, but do *not* oversaturate the glue holding the lens in place.
6. Secure the slide on the stage with the slide clips.
7. Revolve the low-power objective into place until it is seated or you hear a click.
8. Adjust the oculars so that you see only one field rather than separate left and right views.
9. Using the coarse adjustment control knob, raise the body tube of the microscope, and swivel the 10X objective into place.
10. Turn the light on.
11. Lower the body tube with the coarse adjustment control knob to bring the slide into general focus.
12. With the iris controls, adjust the light to cover the slide. It is not important at this point to achieve clear focus.
13. Observing from the side, lower the body tube to bring the objective closer to the slide without touching it.
14. Look through the oculars, using the coarse adjustment to bring the specimen into focus. Adjust the iris if you need more light.
15. Observing from the side, switch to the high-power objective without touching the slide. The body tube may need to be adjusted during this process.
16. When the high-power objective (40X) is in place, adjust the fine focus controls to bring the specimen into clear focus (Figure 31-3 ◆).
17. If the slide specimen is dry and does not have a cover slip, apply a drop of oil and turn the oil immersion objective into place. Lower the objective until it is covered with oil.
18. After the specimen has been examined, lower the stage.
19. Remove the slide specimen and dispose of it in a biohazard waste receptacle.
20. Turn off the light.
21. Clean the lenses with lens cleaner and lens paper. Clean the stage.
22. Rotate the objectives to return the low-power objective directly above the stage.
23. Cover the microscope.
24. Clean the work area.
25. Dispose of the gloves and wash your hands.

Patient Education

Generally, the patient does not receive instruction on how to operate a microscope, although you might give a basic explanation of how some of the tests ordered by the physician are conducted with the microscope.

Charting Example

Operating the microscope is not documented in the patient chart. Maintenance, cleaning, and repairs are documented in the log.

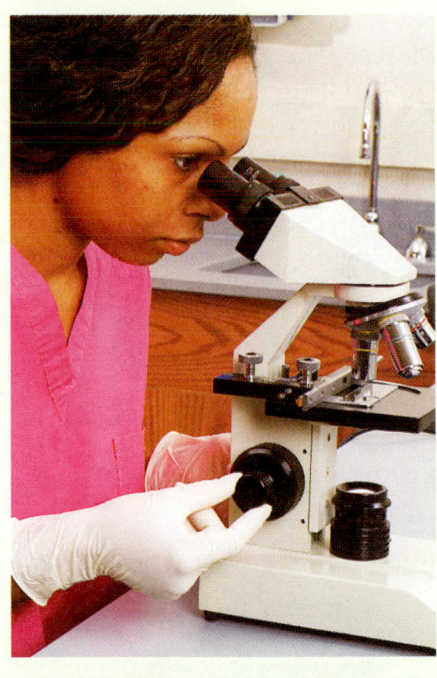

Figure 31-3 ◆ Adjust the fine focus.

---

loosely around the microscope. When you move it, hold it by the arm, supporting it at the base.

Microscope Maintenance

The lens systems are the most important part of a microscope. Proper cleaning is essential to their proper operation. Artifacts such as eye makeup, eyelashes, and skin oil are often left on the oculars, and specimens and oil can leave residue on the stage or objectives, particularly the oil objective. Fibers may also be left behind when tissue paper or paper towels are used to clean the lenses.

After use, all lenses must be cleaned. Wipe the stage with lint-free cloth or paper to remove any oil or dirt. Then return the stage to its original position. Cover the microscope to keep it free of dust.

Microbiology

Microbiology is an area of biology focusing on organisms that are not visible to the naked eye but can be seen only with magnification. Many diseases and syndromes are the direct result of infection by a microorganism.

Microbiological testing in the medical office gives the clinician information with which to make a diagnosis. Some tests, such as direct gram stains and wet preps (wet mounts), may be processed before a patient leaves the office, while others, such as culture and sensitivity (C & S) tests, may require incubation of two or more days.

Scientific Nomenclature and Morphology

Microorganisms are classified into three major groups:

- **Prokaryotes** lack an organized nucleus and cytoplasmic **organelles.** Bacteria are the most important group of prokaryotic organisms (Figure 31-4 ◆).
- **Eukaryotes** are cells surrounded by a membrane. They have a nucleus and organelles that assist in reproduction. Fungi and parasites are eukaryotic organisms (Figure 31-5 ◆).
- **Viruses** are **ultramicroscopic,** nonliving organisms that are classified as microorganisms because they carry DNA or RNA and are capable of parasitic metabolism and reproduction (Figure 31-6 ◆).

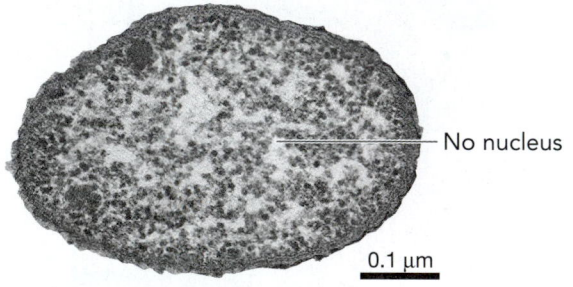

Figure 31-4 ◆ A prokaryotic cell.

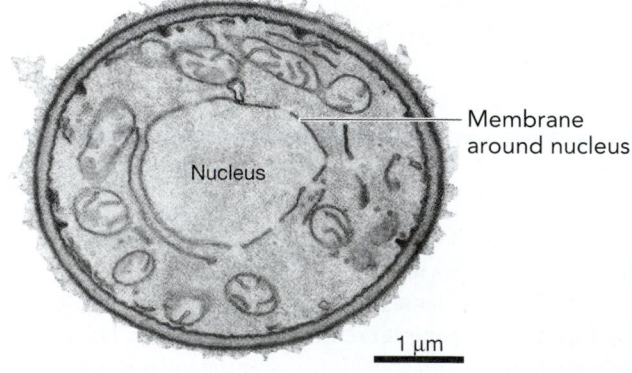

Figure 31-5 ◆ A eukaryotic cell.

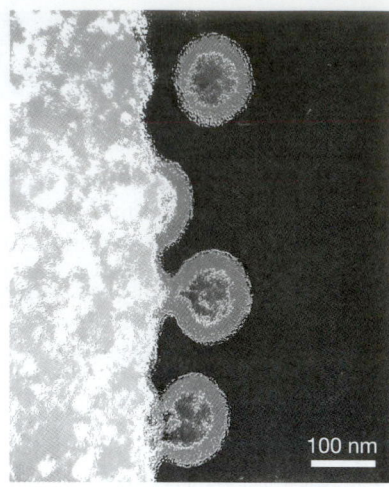

Figure 31-6 ◆ Viruses.

All organisms are classified using scientific nomenclature. In the laboratory, a binomial system (two names) is used for prokaryotic and eukaryotic microorganisms. Each microorganism is named according to its genus and species. The first name represents the genus name and is capitalized. The second name is the species name and is always in lowercase letters. Both names are italicized. For example, in the name *Staphylococcus aureus*, the genus is *Staphylococcus* and the species is *aureus*.

Normal Flora

Normal flora are generally harmless but potentially pathogenic microorganisms that colonize in the human body (Table 31-2). Although normal flora inhabit every nonsterile major body

TABLE 31-2 NORMAL FLORA IN BODY SYSTEMS		
Skin	**Respiratory Tract**	**Gastrointestinal Tract**
Staphylococcus aureus (**staph**)	*Micrococcus* species	*Escherichia coli*
Staphylococcus epidermidis	*Peptostreptococci*	*Enterococcus* species
Corynebacterium species	*Neisseria* species (other than *Neisseria gonorrhoeae*)	*Lactobacillus* species
Alpha (α) *Streptococcus* (**strep**)	*Corynebacterium* species	α *Streptococcus*
Bacillus species	α *Streptococcus*	*Pseudomonas aeruginosa*
Micrococcus species	*Candida albicans*	*Staphylococcus* species
Aerotolerant anaerobes, such as *Proprionibacterium* acnes	*Haemophilus parainfluenzae*	*Candida albicans*
	Many anaerobic organisms	*Bacteroides* species
		Clostridium species
		Klebsiella species
		Proteus species
		Enterobacter species
		Many other bacteria

TABLE 31-3 SOME COMMON PATHOGENS

Upper Respiratory Tract	Lower Respiratory Tract	Gastrointestinal Tract
Streptococcus pyogenes Candida albicans *Eikenella corrodens* Actinomyces *israelii*	*Streptococcus pneumoniae* Enterobacteriaceae *Haemophilus influenzae* *Mycobacterium tuberculosis* Fungi	*Salmonella* species *Shigella* species *Aeromonas* species *Campylobacter* species *Clostridium difficile*

TABLE 31-4 CLASSIFICATION OF BACTERIA ACCORDING TO MORPHOLOGY

Bacteria	Shape	Appearance	Examples
Coccus (plural: cocci)	Spherical	Often exist in pairs, groups, tetrads, or chains	*Staphylococcus* species *Streptococcus* species *Neisseria* species
Bacillus (plural: bacilli)	Rod-shaped	Parallel sides; different lengths and thickness depending on genus-specific characteristics	*Escherichia* species *Proteus* species *Campylobacter* species
Spirochetes	Spiral or cork-screw-shaped	Vary in length and thickness	*Treponema* species *Borrelia* species

system, these microorganisms can cause disease if they are transferred to another part of the body.

Pathogens

Pathogens are microorganisms capable of causing disease (Table 31-3). They possess a virulence factor that damages host cells directly or indirectly through the production of toxins. **Pathogenicity** refers to the ability of an organism to cause disease. True pathogens cause disease whenever they are introduced into a living system. Microorganisms that cause disease only when the patient's immune system is compromised are called **opportunistic pathogens.**

Bacteria

Bacteria are classified in two ways:

1. By **morphology** or shape (Table 31-4)
2. By gram reaction (the result of staining the organism)

A gram stain is a simple diagnostic test that identifies types of bacteria by positive or negative classification (Table 31-5). Bacteria varieties stain or do not stain depending on the compounds in their cell walls. Gram-positive organisms retain the color reaction to the stain procedure and are seen as blue/purple under a microscope. Gram-negative organisms lose the primary stain and retain the red/pink secondary stain. Bacteria are the only organisms that stain well with this procedure. Its reliability is more limited with other organisms because of their complex cellular structure. Although yeast and fungi are not classified as bacteria, they stain positive.

Staphylococcus aureus is a gram-positive pathogen capable of causing a variety of infections: skin infections such as boils, carbuncles, and furuncles; subcutaneous infections such as cellulitis or abscesses; other infectious disease conditions such as osteomyelitis, foodborne illnesses, conjunctivitis, toxic shock syndrome, urinary tract infections (**UTIs**), septicemia, and pneumonia (Figure 31-7 ◆). *Staphylococcus aureus* is found on the skin, in water and soil, and can live for long periods of time on inanimate objects. *Staphylococcus epidermidis* is associated with infections caused by prosthetic devices.

? —Critical Thinking Question 31-1—

The sample of *Staphylococcus aureus* taken from the toddler's rash confirms the physician's diagnosis of impetigo. Irene knows what the pathogen will look like and that it will be gram-positive even before she begins the microscopic exam. How does she know this?

Enterococcus faecalis is a gram-positive organism that causes infections such as UTIs, wound infection, and septicemia. *Streptococcus pyogenes* or *Group A Streptococcus* is the causative agent of strep throat. Other diseases associated with *Group A strep* infections include scarlet fever, pyelonephritis, rheumatic fever, pneumonia, wound infections, cellulitis, osteomyelitis, flesh-eating disease, and impetigo.

TABLE 31-5 CLASSIFICATION OF MICROORGANISMS ACCORDING TO GRAM REACTION

Gram-positive	Gram-negative
Enterococcus faecalis *Streptococcus pyogenes* or Group A Streptococcus *Staphylococcus epidermidis* *Streptococcus agalactiae* or Group B Streptococcus *Streptococcus pneumoniae* *Listeria monocytogenes* *Clostridium perfringens*	*Escherichia coli* *Pseudomonas aeruginosa* *Klebsiella* species *Salmonella* species *Shigella* species *Campylobacter* species *Bacteroides* species *Fusobacterium* species

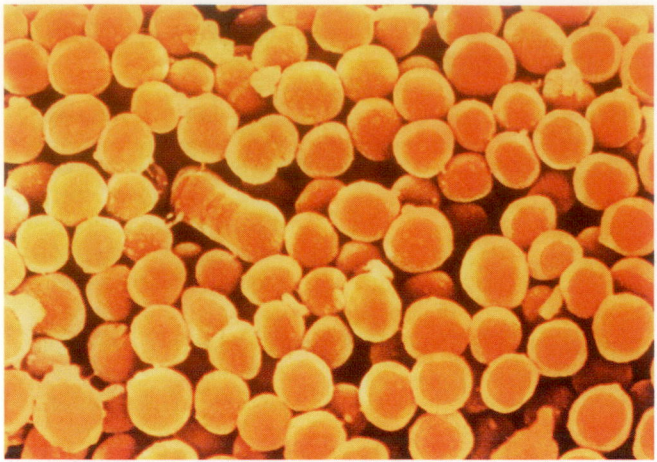

Figure 31-7 ◆ A microscopic view of staph.
Source: Phototake NYC.

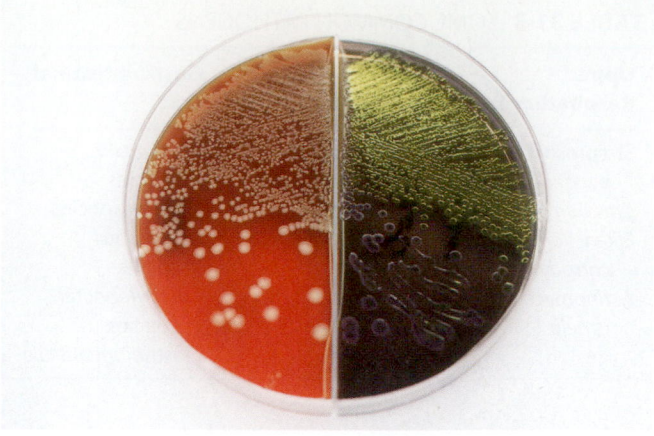

Figure 31-8 ◆ A microscopic view of a mold.

Streptococcus agalactiae or *Group B Streptococcus* is mainly associated with neonatal infections, vaginal infections, UTIs, and wound infections. *Streptococcus pneumoniae* is the primary cause of community-acquired (but not hospital-acquired) pneumonia. *Listeria monocytogenes* causes septicemia in postnatal women. *Clostridium perfringens* is an anaerobic organism that causes gas gangrene. It is found in wound cultures, gunshot wounds, and other trauma-induced injuries.

Escherichia coli (*E. coli*) is the most common gram-negative pathogen. It is the primary cause of UTIs. Other diseases caused by *E. coli* include bacteremia, wound infections, pneumonia, foodborne illnesses, and abscesses. It is normally found in feces and can also inhabit the vaginal area. *Pseudomonas aeruginosa* causes many hospital-acquired or nosocomial infections such as pneumonia, UTIs, and wound infections, as well as folliculitis and external ear infections. It is often seen in cystic fibrosis patients.

? — Critical Thinking Question 31-2 —

Irene confirms that the patient is positive for an *E. coli* infection in her bladder. What are some possible causes for the bladder infection?

Other pathogenic gram-negative organisms include *Klebsiella* species, *Proteus* species, and *Enterobacter* species. These organisms are commonly associated with UTIs, wound infections, and pneumonia. *Salmonella* species, *Shigella* species, and *Campylobacter* species are causative agents in gastroenteritis and foodborne illnesses. *Bacteroides* and *Fusobacterium* species are anaerobic organisms often isolated from abscesses and trauma wounds.

Fungi

Yeast, molds, and other fungi are also capable of causing disease in humans (Figure 31-8 ◆). The study of these organisms is called **mycology.** Common mycological infections include oral thrush, vaginal yeast infections, and fungal infections of the hair, skin, and nails. Fungi are opportunistic pathogens that cause disease only when the normal balance of flora in the body is upset by traumatic injury, poor hygiene, or a compromised immune system. Treatment of fungal infection ranges from normal flora replacement to therapy with antifungal antibiotics.

Parasites

Parasitology is the study of parasites, organisms that infect living hosts and live at the expense of their hosts without contributing to their survival (Figure 31-9 ◆). Human parasites include protozoa, helminths, and arthropods. Pathogenic intestinal protozoa are transmitted through contaminated drinking water, animals, and poor hygiene. Transmission requires three elements:

1. A source of infection
2. A mode of transmission
3. A susceptible host

Parasites take vital nutrients from the host. Damage to the host is caused by the invasion or destruction of host cells,

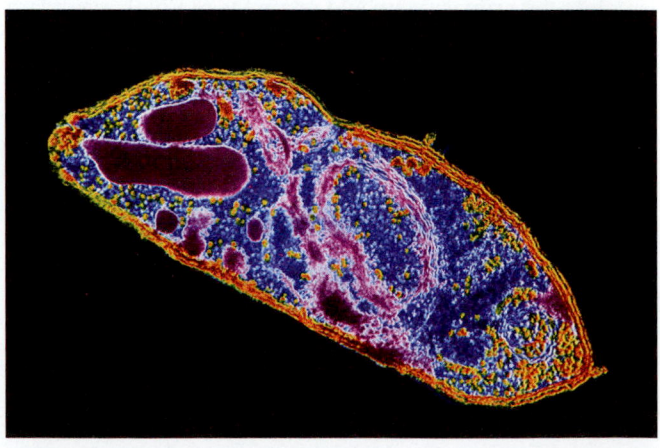

Figure 31-9 ◆ A microscopic view of a parasite.
Source: Phototake NYC.

usually the intestinal mucosa, or by the inflammatory response. Diarrhea and abdominal discomfort are the most common symptoms of intestinal parasites. Treatment ranges from no treatment, if the infection is self-limiting, to antiparasitic drugs.

Viruses

Virology is a specialized branch of microbiology that studies viruses and resulting diseases (Figure 31-10 ◆). Although classified as microorganisms, viruses are actually nonliving organisms that cannot reproduce without invading host cells. Viruses cause hepatitis A, B, and C, and the human immunodeficiency virus (HIV) causes acquired immunodeficiency syndrome (AIDS).

Once a virus locates a target cell, it attaches itself to the cell, penetrates the cell membrane, and takes control of the nucleus. It uses the cell's resources to self-replicate, severely damaging and often killing the host cell in the process.

Diagnosis of a viral infection is generally done through indirect **serology** testing. Serum from the patient's venous blood specimen is tested for the presence of antibodies. The amount and type of antibody present can indicate disease progression to the physician. If necessary, direct specimens (tissue or secretions obtained by invasive or noninvasive techniques) may be tested for the presence of viral agents. Commercially available kits allow for testing for influenza virus in respiratory specimens, for example.

Preparing Specimens for Microscopic Examination

Microbiological specimens must be properly prepared on a slide before they can be examined under the microscope. The MA will be responsible for procuring the specimen, processing some

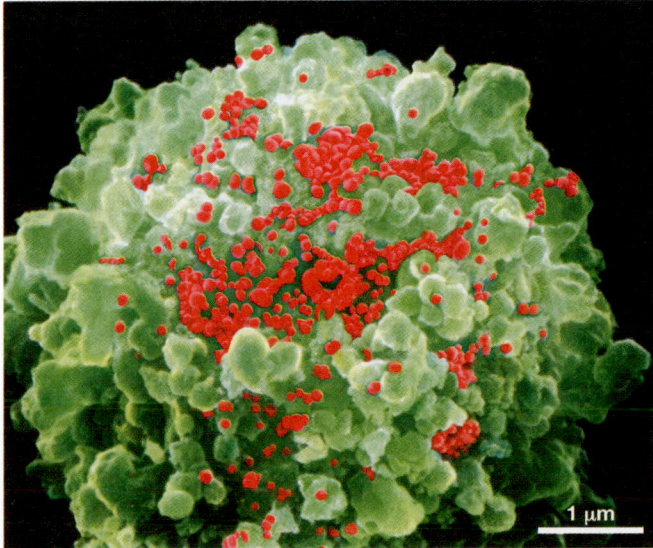

Figure 31-10 ◆ The human immunodeficiency virus (HIV).
Source: Photo Researchers, Inc.

slides, and preparing the microscope. The laboratory technician or physician develops slides and examines them under the microscope. Many slides require cover slips, which prevent contamination of the microscope by the specimen. Specimens that are stained or are examined with an oil immersion lens do not require cover slips.

Preparing a Specimen Smear

The gram stain, used to identify gram-negative and gram-positive microorganisms, is performed on a slide containing a thin smear of specimen.

Performing a Gram Stain

Hans C. J. Gram (1853–1928), a Danish physician, developed the gram stain procedure in the late 1800s. To this day, the gram stain is used to help identify bacteria, which are very small and almost colorless. The different appearances of colorized bacteria determine not only their gram-positive or gram-negative status but also their shape and grouping. With this information, the physician can make an initial diagnosis and determine the appropriate medication until the diagnosis is confirmed by a C & S test.

The gram stain procedure consists of four basic steps:

1. The cells are colorized with crystal violet, a primary stain.
2. A mordant (chemical fixative), Gram's iodine, is added.
3. The cells are decolorized with an alcohol/acetone mixture.
4. The last stain is safranin, a counterstain that provides contrasting color to cellular components not previously visible from the first stain.

Preparing Wet Mounts

A wet mount slide is another way to examine microorganisms under a microscope. There are three methods of preparing a wet mount slide:

- Normal saline (NS)
- Potassium hydroxide (**KOH**)
- India ink

Saline

A saline mount involves placing a specimen smear on the slide, adding and mixing a drop of saline into the smear, placing a cover slip over it, and examining it immediately under the microscope. *Trichomonas vaginalis*, a sexually transmitted pathogen, is identified in this manner.

Potassium Hydroxide

Some microorganisms, such as fungi, are masked in a specimen because of the amount of protein they contain. Potassium hydroxide added to the specimen smear and left sitting at room temperature for 30 minutes dissolves the protein and makes fungal spores or hyphae visible under the microscope. Vaginal yeast infections are diagnosed with this method.

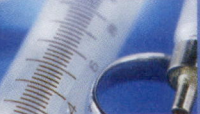

PROCEDURE 31-2 Prepare a Specimen Smear for Microbiological Examination

Theory and Rationale

A frosted-edge slide is easier to grasp during preparation and to label with patient information. Patient identification must be done with a labeling pen. Do not use felt-tip markers that might run during the staining procedure.

Specimens for smear preparation can be from a culture swab, a culture growing in a petri dish, or a liquid source. Spread the smear thinly to allow for better microscopic examination and faster air-drying time.

Heat fixation is performed to make sure the cells stick to the slide during the staining process. Heat also kills the microorganisms, thus lowering the possibility of disease transmission during slide preparation and handling. The slide should not become too hot to hold, as excess heat could damage the specimen and alter test results.

Materials

- glass slide (preferably with frosted edge)
- disposable gloves
- sterile distilled water
- inoculating loops or specimen swabs
- flame source
- biohazardous waste container
- sharps container

Competency

(**Conditions**) With the necessary materials, you will be able to (**Task**) prepare a slide (**Standards**) correctly for microscopic examination within 30 minutes.

1. Wash your hands.
2. Gather equipment and supplies.
3. Wash your hands again and put on disposable gloves.
4. Write the patient information on the frosted edge of the slide.
5. Prepare a thin film, or smear, on the slide.
   For a specimen from a swab: Roll and turn the swab across the slide (Figure 31-11 ◆).
   For a specimen from a Petri dish (Figure 31-12 ◆):
   - Gather sterile distilled water with a sterile inoculating loop and place it on the slide.
   - Use the inoculating loop to gather the microbial specimen, without gathering any culture medium.
   - Mix the specimen into the distilled water on the slide.
   - Sterilize the loop over the flame.
   For a specimen from a liquid (Figure 31-13 ◆):
   - Dip the inside of the sterile inoculating loop in the culture until it appears covered with a film.
   - Touch the film to the center of the slide.
   - Allow the specimen on the slide to air-dry completely.
   - Hold and pass the slide through the flame several times. The slide is now ready to stain.
6. Clean the work area.
7. Dispose of the gloves and wash your hands.

Charting Example

Document in the designated log any quality control or safety measures you followed, such as looking at expiration dates or correctly storing the specimen.

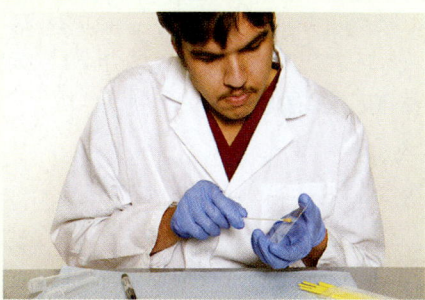

Figure 31-11 ◆ Roll and turn the swab across the slide.

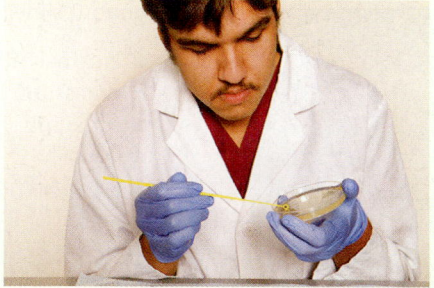

Figure 31-12 ◆ Using a loop with a Petri dish.

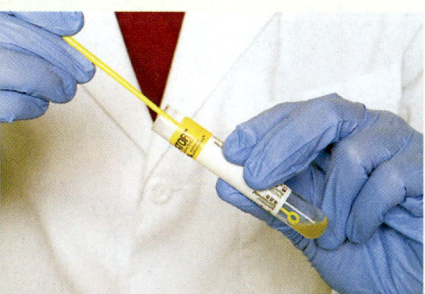

Figure 31-13 ◆ Using a loop with a liquid.

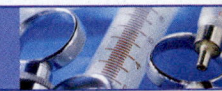

PROCEDURE 31-3 Prepare a Gram Stain

Theory and Rationale

Timing and rinsing techniques are critical to the correct identification of gram-positive or gram-negative bacteria. Stains are left on the slide for a period based on institution procedure and the manufacturer's directions and may be a minimum of 30 seconds or as long as 2 minutes.

It is important to rinse correctly but not excessively for the cells to retain the dye color. Excessive rinsing during the crystal violet phase can remove too much purple from gram-positive cells. After the Gram's iodine is added, the purple color remains to identify the gram-positive bacteria (Figure 31-14 ◆). During decolorization, the color must be removed according to the manufacturer's directions; otherwise it may also remove a degree of crystal violet from gram-positive cells. Organisms from which the primary stain is removed by decolorization exhibit a pink color from the safranin dye (Figure 31-15 ◆).

Materials

- disposable gloves
- slide with fixed smear
- crystal violet dye
- Gram's iodine
- alcohol/acetone mixture
- safranin dye
- wash bottle filled with distilled water
- rack and tray for slide staining
- forceps
- paper towel
- biohazardous waste container
- sharps container

Competency

(**Conditions**) With the necessary materials, you will be able to (**Task**) prepare a slide for microscopic examination of gram-negative and gram-positive bacteria (**Standards**) correctly, within 15 minutes.

1. Wash your hands.
2. Gather equipment, supplies, and the prepared slide (see Procedure 31-2).
3. Wash your hands again and put on disposable gloves.
4. Lay the slide on the slide rack and tray.
5. Pour crystal violet on the slide and allow it to stain for 1 minute.
6. Rinse the slide gently with water from the wash bottle.
7. Lay the slide on the slide rack and tray.
8. Pour Gram's iodine, also known as mordant, on the slide. Allow it to stain for 2 minutes.
9. Lift the slide diagonally with the forceps and rinse gently with water from the wash bottle.
10. Maintaining the vertical hold, gently pour the acetone/alcohol decolorizing mixture over the slide. Pour until the runoff is clear (approximately 1 minute).
11. Lay the slide on the slide rack and tray.
12. Pour safranin dye on the slide and allow it to stain for 30 seconds.
13. Lift the slide angled vertically with the forceps and rinse gently.
14. Let the slide air-dry vertically, or blot—do not wipe—the stained area with a paper towel.
15. Mount the slide on the microscope for examination.
16. Return supplies to storage.
17. Clean the work area.
18. Dispose of biohazardous waste and sharps in the appropriate containers.
19. Dispose of the gloves and wash your hands.

Charting Example

Document in designated logs any quality control or safety measures you followed, such as looking at expiration dates of dyes or other supplies; correct storage of specimen or prepared slide; or following OSHA precautions. The technician or physician performing the microscopic examination will document the results of the gram staining.

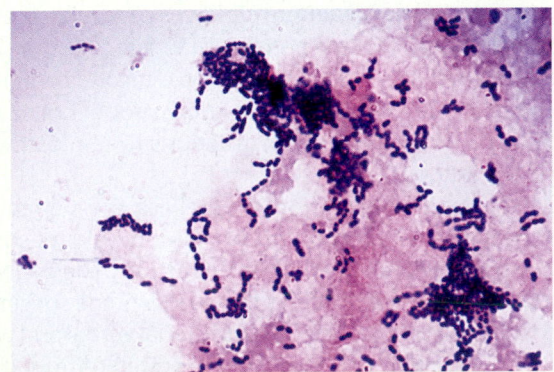

Figure 31-14 ◆ Gram-positive *Streptococcus pyogenes* bacteria in chains.

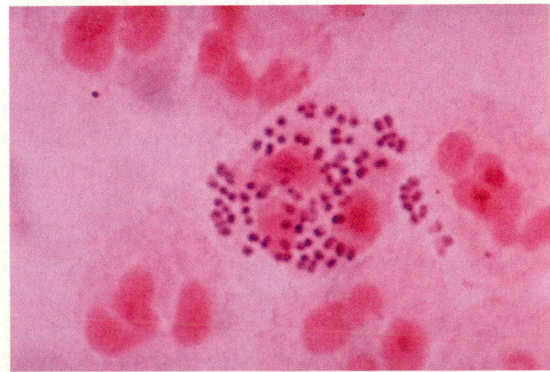

Figure 31-15 ◆ Gram-negative *N. gonorrhoeae.*
Source: Visuals Unlimited.

India Ink

India ink is used to visualize *Cryptococcus neoformans* in spinal fluid. After centrifugation, a drop of sediment and a drop of India ink are placed together on a slide.

Specimen Collection, Storage, and Transport

"Garbage in, garbage out." The quality of a test is only as good as the specimen submitted. Although this applies to all specimen collection, quality and procedural standards are especially important in microbial testing. There are several important considerations to keep in mind when you collect a specimen.

- A specimen should be collected before treatment has begun to ensure correct diagnosis.
- A specimen must measure "quantity sufficient" (**QS**) to ensure that all requested tests can be performed. If the quantity is not sufficient (**QNS**), more specimen will be needed.
- A specimen must be placed in a sterile collection device or sterile container.
- Specimens should be labeled at the time of collection with the patient's name (first and last), date of collection, time of collection, and body area or fluid source.
- Collection devices should be appropriate for the source to be cultured.
- When transport to the testing area is not immediate, transport media and packaging must be used. These ensure optimal recovery as well as the safety of transporting and testing personnel.

Collection of Stool Specimens

The physician may ask a patient to collect a stool specimen, or a series of three stool specimens, for a number of reasons, including microscopic examination for enteric pathogens, ova and parasite examination, and occult blood detection. Naturally passed stool is the preferred source for each specimen. Any stool for testing must be collected in a clean, dry container, free from urine contamination, and transported to the testing area in a container with a tight-fitting lid. One specimen per 24 hours is the standard for stool cultures. Some physicians may request that three specimens be collected on the same day, if possible; others may request one specimen a day for three consecutive days.

Fecal Culture Testing for Ova, Parasites, and Other Infectious Organisms

Stool specimens for culture must be processed within one hour of collection or placed in appropriate transport media to recover enteric (intestinal) pathogens (such as Carey-Blair media) (Figure 31-16 ◆). Stool in transport media is viable for up to 24 hours. Follow the manufacturer's recommendations for transport times.

Stool specimen collection for ova and parasites is identical to collection for culture. A different type of transport media—a two-vial system—is used if the patient cannot return the specimen within one hour of collection. One vial contains PVA, a preservative used to permanently stain the specimen. The other vial contains formalin for preparing wet mounts of the specimen. All stools for ova and parasite examination are stained and examined on wet mounts to ensure the detection of all life stages of amoebae, helminths, and pathogenic protozoa. Specimens in

---

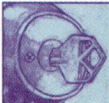

Keys to Success
PATIENT RIGHTS AND FEELINGS: SENSITIVITY DURING SPECIMEN COLLECTION

It is important to remember that when collecting specimens the MA should always take the patient's feelings into consideration. For invasive procedures such as venipuncture, a patient may be very apprehensive. It may be beneficial to have the patient lie down during the procedure and speak to them in a calm and quiet voice. Other procedures such as collecting a urine or fecal sample can be embarrassing for patients. In these instances it important to reassure the patient that his or her privacy and confidentiality is of the utmost importance.

Patients also have the right to deny a procedure. In such circumstances, it is important to inform the physician immediately of the patient's wishes. Most often, a patient will have to sign a waiver stating that he or she is refusing a procedure. This will protect both the medical office and its staff from liability.

Keys to Success
INSTRUCTING THE PATIENT FOR SPECIMEN COLLECTION

Your role in specimen collection is extremely important. Whether you are assisting the physician in collection, collecting the specimen yourself, or instructing the patient in proper collection, you must follow strict guidelines to ensure accurate results. When the patient is collecting any specimen, verbal instructions must be clear and complete. Do *not* assume the patient will know proper collection technique. Provide written instructions to reinforce verbal information.

After explaining the procedure, ask the patient to describe what he or she has understood. Ask questions and encourage the patient to ask questions. The patient's level of understanding affects the quality of the specimen and the results of the test. Give additional verbal and written instructions if the specimen requires refrigeration and/or transport. Any specimen that is not collected, stored, and transported correctly must be discarded. Having to repeat the specimen collection delays diagnosis and treatment.

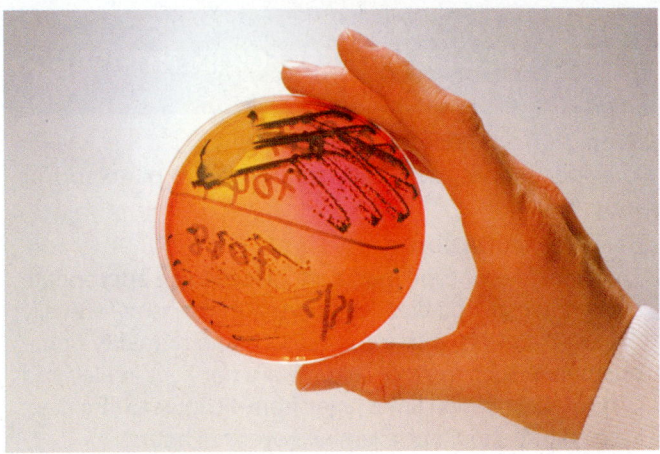

Figure 31-16 ◆ Petri dish containing fecal bacterial cultures.
Source: Jim Varney.

this type of transport system are acceptable for testing for up to three days. Many physician offices and hospital laboratories do not perform ova and parasite examination on site because it requires extensive training. Specimens are usually referred to a reference laboratory. The patient is given verbal and written instructions for transferring the specimen to the vials.

Fecal Occult Blood Testing

Fecal occult blood testing, or stool guaiac, detects the presence of blood in the stool. The patient follows a modified diet for three days, then collects three different specimens. Because dietary guidelines may vary between test kits, it is important to follow the manufacturer's directions. Many foods, and even aspirin, can cause false positive results. A list of foods and medications to avoid is included in each kit.

Specimen collection for fecal occult blood testing can be done in the same manner as for an unpreserved stool culture. In the test preparation area, a clean, dry fecal specimen is taken from the container and placed on a testing card. An alternative method allows the patient to collect the specimen at home and place a smear directly on the testing card. The card is labeled with first and last name and the date and time of collection. The specimen is usable for testing for 14 days.

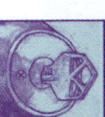

Keys to Success
PATIENT INSTRUCTIONS BEFORE SPECIMEN COLLECTION FOR CULTURE

- Obtain a clean, dry specimen.
- Alert the medical office if it will take more than one hour to transport the specimen to the laboratory, as this will require a different container to preserve the organisms.
- Obtain only one specimen in a 24-hour period.
- Do not take a stool specimen for 72 hours after a barium or radiology test.
- Do not use a urine-contaminated specimen.
- Do not use a specimen from a diaper.

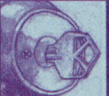

Keys to Success
PEDIATRIC STOOL COLLECTION

Stool specimens taken from diapers are not acceptable for culture because of the absorbency of the material. If the diaper is lined with a nonabsorbent material, however, a specimen may be taken and placed in a container or transport device.

Rectal swabs may be collected in the physician's office. Lay the child on his or her stomach, carefully insert the transport swab 1 to 1-1/2 inches into the rectum. Rotate the swab and withdraw. Place it in a transport sheath, label it with patient information, and send it to the testing area.

Fecal specimens may be collected for cultures or to examine for the presence of occult blood. While these tests are different in purpose, the specimen collection process is similar, and they are discussed together in the procedure.

Culture and Sensitivity Testing

The term *culture* refers to a process in which a direct specimen of tissue or secretion is cultivated in prepared media. When the specimen has grown, it is examined for pathogenic

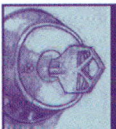

Keys to Success
PATIENT INSTRUCTIONS FOR SPECIMEN COLLECTION FOR FECAL OCCULT BLOOD TESTING

Follow the guidelines listed below for three days before the first specimen and until all three specimens have been obtained. These guidelines must be followed for accurate test results and comparisons.

- Do not take medications containing aspirin, iron, steroids, or Vitamin C. Your physician has reviewed the medications that you are taking and will let you know which ones not to take until after all specimens have been collected. Inform your physician of any other medications or nutritional supplements he or she may not already be aware of.
- Do not eat rare or red meat, liver or processed meats, cauliflower, broccoli, turnips, radishes, horseradish, or melons.
- Do eat well-cooked pork, chicken, or fish; a variety of raw and cooked vegetables (except for cauliflower, broccoli, turnips, radishes, and horseradish); a variety of fruits, other than melons; and a variety of high-fiber foods.
- Do *not* collect any specimens for testing in the presence of hemorrhoidal bleeding. For female patients, do not take any specimens during and for three days following a menstrual period.
- Store the three test slides at room temperature until you use them.

bacteria. Specific protocols are set up for each specimen type to maximize the recovery of these organisms. Special media are used to inhibit the growth of normal flora, allow for visual differentiation of bacteria groups, allow the pathogen to be easily recognized, and aid in the recovery of fastidious organisms (microorganisms that require special conditions and nutrients for culture, such as anaerobic bacteria, which grow only in the absence of oxygen). The medical assistant will obtain the specimen and the laboratory technician will process the culture by inoculation, incubation, inspection, and identification.

Once identification is made, sensitivity testing may follow. Sensitivity testing determines which antimicrobial medication would be effective against the pathogen. Some organisms follow very predictable patterns and do not require routine testing. Others must be tested to ensure proper treatment. The organism is tested for sensitivity to selected drugs by either disc diffusion or broth dilution methods. Effectiveness is measured by the drug's ability to stop or inhibit the organism's growth in a controlled situation.

With the Kirby-Bauer disc diffusion (KBDD) method of sensitivity testing, the organism is designated as susceptible, intermediate, or resistant to particular concentrations of antibiotic. Microscan plates are manufactured to perform culture and sensitivity (C & S) or just sensitivity tests.

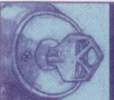

Keys to Success
CULTURE PROCESS FOR IDENTIFICATION OF MICROORGANISMS

Step 1: Inoculation
The specimen is aseptically transferred to plate and/or tube media.

Step 2: Incubation
The plate and/or tube media are placed in an appropriate environment to optimize the recovery of organisms—usually 35° to 37° Celsius, with increased CO_2 and humidity. Some exceptions, such as stool cultures, are not kept in elevated CO_2. Total incubation times range from 48 hours to four days. Each culture should be examined every 24 hours.

Step 3: Inspection
After the initial incubation of 24 hours, each plate is visually examined and any suspected pathogen is subcultured for purity and prepared for Step 4.

Step 4: Identification
Any suspected pathogen must be identified. A variety of manual and automated methods can be used to identify organisms to genus and species levels. Gram staining is an important part of this procedure. Enzymatic testing, carbohydrate assimilation testing, and antigen detection tests are other ways to identify organisms.

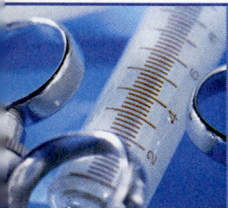

PROCEDURE 31-4 Instruct a Patient in the Collection of a Fecal Specimen for Occult Blood or Culture Testing and Develop the Fecal Occult Blood Test

Theory and Rationale
Fecal occult blood testing is important to the early diagnosis and treatment of colon cancer. The patient must follow dietary modifications and medication adjustments for three days. Specimens should not be collected during the active bleeding of menstruation or hemorrhoids. Always check the expiration date of the test kit, as chemical changes may affect the accuracy of results.

Fecal culture testing for ova, parasites, or other infectious organisms plays a role in the diagnosis of intestinal infestation or infection. The patient often experiences symptoms of abdominal pain, diarrhea, and vomiting caused by new, transient organisms that upset the balance of normal flora in the intestinal tract. For accurate test results and appropriate diagnosis and treatment, it is important that the fecal specimen is obtained without urine and that storage and transport are in line with institutional policy and the manufacturer's directions (Figure 31-17 ◆). Because certain microorganisms' growth and death are affected by temperature, oxygen, and nutrition, be

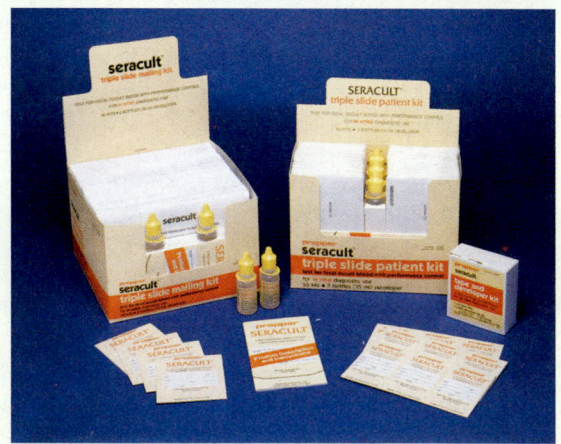

Figure 31-17 ◆ Test for occult blood.
Courtesy of Propper Manufacturing Company.

PROCEDURE 31-4 **Instruct a Patient in the Collection of a Fecal Specimen for Occult Blood or Culture Testing and Develop the Fecal Occult Blood Test** *(continued)*

sure to follow standard procedure and the manufacturer's guidelines for specimen storage and processing to accurately reflect the microbial population at the time the specimen is obtained. Fecal testing for occult blood does not require live cells; therefore, the patient may complete the fecal occult blood sample cards at home and bring them to the office.

Materials

Fecal Occult Blood

- patient chart
- testing kit
- clean and dry large-mouth container with spatula
- patient label and laboratory requisition form, if needed
- disposable gloves
- black ink pen

Fecal Culture Testing

- patient chart
- specimen container for transport
- spatula
- patient label and laboratory requisition form, if needed
- disposable gloves
- black ink pen

Developing the Fecal Occult Blood Test

- disposable gloves
- prepared occult blood slides
- developing solution
- patient chart
- waste container

Competency: Instructing the Patient

(**Conditions**) With the necessary materials, you will be able to (**Task**) provide verbal and written instruction to the patient (**Standards**) correctly within 30 minutes.

1. Wash your hands.
2. Gather supplies.
3. Check the kit to make sure it has not expired.
4. Greet and identify the patient. Escort him or her to the examination room.
5. Ask the patient what he or she understands about the reason(s) for the test. Clarify the information as needed to help the patient understand.
6. Inform the physician if further discussion would benefit the patient.
7. Provide verbal instructions for fecal occult blood or culture testing. Reinforce them by giving the patient a writ-

ten copy of the instructions and the appropriate test kit supplies, lab requisitions, and patient identification labels.
8. For *fecal occult blood specimen collection,* instruct the patient as follows.
    - Using the spatula provided for each slide, place a thin smear over the first square (labeled A).
    - Take a small specimen from a different area and smear it over the second square (labeled B).
    - Close the flap covering the slide.
    - Allow the slide to air-dry.
    - Repeat these steps for the remaining two slides, according to the physician's order.
    - Return the three slides to the medical office as soon as possible.
9. For *fecal culture specimen collection,* instruct the patient as follows.
    - After collecting the specimen in a clean, dry container, tighten the container lid.
    - Transport the specimen immediately or transfer it to a preservative container.
10. Document on the chart the instructions you gave and the patient's understanding.
11. Wash your hands.

Competency: Developing the Fecal Occult Blood Test

(**Conditions**) With the necessary materials, you will be able to (**Task**) prepare and develop a fecal occult blood test (**Standards**) correctly within 10 minutes.

1. Wash your hands.
2. Gather your supplies.
3. Check the developing solution bottle to make sure it has not expired.
4. Put on disposable gloves.
5. Open the back flap of the cardboard slides.
6. Apply 2 drops of the developing solution to the guaiac test paper directly over each smear.
7. Read the results within 60 seconds. Any trace of blue on or at the edge of the smear is positive for occult blood.
8. Perform the quality control procedure to ensure the accuracy and reliability of the test results.
9. Dispose of the fecal occult blood test in a regular waste container.
10. Remove your gloves and sanitize your hands.
11. Document on the chart the results of the test including the date and time, the brand name of the test, and the test results for each slide.

(continued)

PROCEDURE 31-4 Instruct a Patient in the Collection of a Fecal Specimen for Occult Blood or Culture Testing and Develop the Fecal Occult Blood Test *(continued)*

Patient Education

Fecal Occult Blood Specimen: Inform the patient that testing for fecal occult blood is performed to diagnose the cause of rectal and/or intestinal bleeding. Rectal bleeding is symptomatic of many disease conditions, including hemorrhoids, gastrointestinal tract ulcers, diverticulosis/itis, polyps, and colorectal cancer. Following the instructions for testing correctly will help to eliminate false results. If results indicate bleeding, there will be further diagnostic procedures, diagnosis, and treatment.

   Culture for Ova, Parasites, or Other Infectious Organisms: Inform the patient that stool culture testing is performed to diagnose ova, parasites, or other organisms that cause intestinal infestation or infection. Abdominal pain, diarrhea, and vomiting are symptoms. Although the intestinal tract contains normal, resident microorganisms, it is newly hosted, transient microorganisms or parasites that cause symptoms. Following the instructions for testing correctly will help to eliminate false results and assist in the accurate diagnosis and treatment of the pathogen.

Charting Example

Document in designated logs any quality control or safety measures you followed, such as looking at expiration dates of the developer or other supplies used; correct storage and disposal of specimen or prepared slide; or OSHA precautions taken. The medical assistant will document the results of the fecal occult blood test in the patient's chart.

11/22/xx 9:30 a.m. Pt given verbal and written instruction for collection of fecal occult testing specimens. Pt able to state correctly in own words the importance of following instructions. Lea Harden, CMA (AAMA)

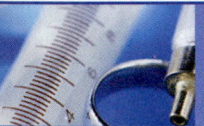

PROCEDURE 31-5 Perform a Wound or Throat Culture Collection Using Sterile Swabs

Theory and Rationale

For a wound culture, collect the exudate (pus or fluid accumulation) by removing the coating of the lesion and inserting a syringe with needle to aspirate the fluid. After a specimen is obtained, detach and dispose of the needle, cover the syringe end, and label the specimen with the patient's first and last name and the date and time of collection. Transport the syringe to the testing area immediately for processing.

   If aspiration is not possible, a swab can be inserted into the lesion to collect the exudate or drainage. Label the swab and transport it to the testing area as soon as possible.

   If no exudate is present, roll the swab over the surface of the uncovered lesion and place it in transport media.

   Specimens on aerobic swabs are acceptable for culture for approximately 12 to 16 hours after collection. Specimens in syringes should be processed within one hour to optimize the recovery of anaerobic organisms. Use anaerobic transport media and swabs if inoculation of the specimen must be delayed for longer than an hour. A double-swab system is best

for wound specimen collection if both a direct gram stain and a culture are both anticipated. Always check institutional procedure and the manufacturer's directions before proceeding with specimen collection.

   Throat specimens can be obtained by using two swabs instead of one if the physician orders both Rapid Strep and C&S testing. Use a noncotton swab, such as Dacron®, to collect the throat specimen. Instruct the patient to open the mouth widely by saying "Ahh." Hold the tongue down with a clean tongue depressor to clear a path to the posterior pharynx. Being careful not to touch the inside of the mouth, the teeth, or the tongue, wipe the opened swabs against the throat and tonsil area in a circular or figure "8" pattern to collect a representative sample of microorganisms. Gather specimens only from the infected area, not the area surrounding it. Remove the swab carefully, without touching other parts of the oral cavity. Following procedure, place the swabs in a collection container, usually a tube with culture media, and transport them to the processing area.

PROCEDURE 31-5 Perform a Wound or Throat Culture Collection Using Sterile Swabs *(continued)*

Materials

Wound

- patient chart
- single- or double-swab collection device (one swab for culture inoculation and one for gram stain)
- setup for anaerobic culture (for nonsuperficial wound, if physician ordered)
- specimen label
- disposable gloves

Throat

- patient chart
- tongue depressor
- sterile swab and transport device
- specimen label
- disposable gloves

Competency

(**Conditions**) With the necessary materials, you will be able to (**Task**) perform swab culture collection and prepare it (**Standards**) correctly for transport and processing within 15 minutes.

1. Wash your hands.
2. Gather equipment and supplies.
3. Identify and greet the patient, then escort him or her to the examination room. Explain the process of specimen collection.
4. Wash your hands again and put on disposable gloves.
5. Wound specimen collection:
   - Mentally note the type and amount of drainage; any redness, warmth, or swelling in the surrounding area; any other abnormalities.
   - Swab the inside of the wound (Figure 31-18 ◆). Do not swab the surrounding skin area.
   - Place the swab in the transport container and medium, if used (Figure 31-19 ◆).

Throat culture specimen collection:
   - Ask the patient to open the mouth wide and extend the tongue forward.
   - Examine the throat and observe for redness, swelling of throat tissue, amount and type of drainage, or the presence of white patches or pustules.
   - Place the tongue depressor firmly on the tongue and press down.
   - Swab the posterior pharynx between the tonsillar pillars. Place the swab in the transport container and medium, if used (Figure 31-20 ◆).
6. Label the container with the patient's name (first and last), date and time of collection, and source of specimen.
7. Dispose of any waste materials in the appropriate container(s).
8. Remove and dispose of gloves. Wash your hands.
9. Transport the specimen to the testing area.
10. Perform the required charting or laboratory documentation relating to specimen collection.

Patient Education

Ask the patient to verbalize his or her understanding of why the test was performed. Usually the physician prescribes an antibiotic based on clinical symptoms and the usual microorganisms present in a wound or throat infection. If so, reinforce medication instructions. Inform the patient that C & S results usually take three days, but this can vary depending on the type of pathogen present. The test results will determine if the patient will remain on the same antibiotic or receive another prescription for a more effective medication.

Charting Example

9/30/xx 9:30 a.m. Throat culture specimen obtained per office procedure. Specimen placed in culturette tube and transported to laboratory immediately. Pt medication instructions reviewed. Pt repeated back medication instructions correctly. Pt informed that he would be called with results, and adjustments in treatment would be made, if necessary, in 3-4 days. Kirk Peters, RMA (AMI)

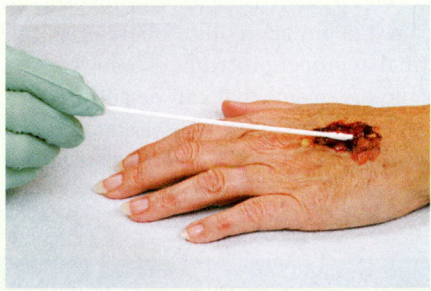

Figure 31-18 ◆ Swab the inside of the wound.

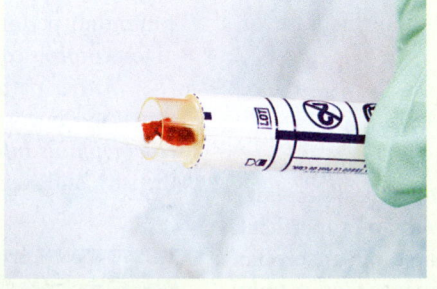

Figure 31-19 ◆ Place the swab in the specimen container.

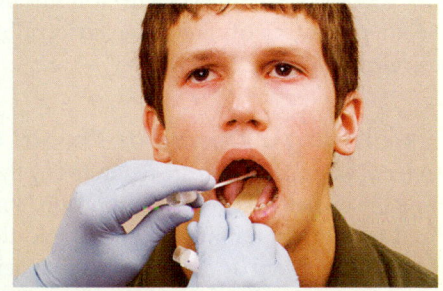

Figure 31-20 ◆ Swab the posterior pharynx between the tonsillar pillars.

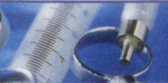

PROCEDURE 31-6 Perform Rapid Group A Strep Testing

Theory and Rationale

Group A Streptococcus (*Streptococcus pyogenes*) is one of the most common bacterial causes of sore throat and upper respiratory infections. Streptococcus pharyngitis, or strep throat, primarily affects children and young adults. It is a potentially serious condition, and rapid diagnosis is necessary in order to begin appropriate treatment. Many immunoassay kits are available to test quickly for Group A beta-hemolytic streptococcus. If the test result is positive, treatment can begin at once. Specific instructions are included with every commercially available antigen identification test.

Materials

- labeled throat specimen
- Group A strep kit (controls may be included, depending on the kit)
- personal protective equipment
- timer
- biohazard waste container

Competency

(**Conditions**) With the necessary materials, you will be able to perform (**Task**) rapid Group A strep testing (**Standards**) correctly within 15 minutes.

1. Wash your hands and gather supplies.
2. Verify that the name on the specimen container and the laboratory requisition form are the same.
3. Put on your personal protective equipment.
4. Label one extraction tube with the patient's name, one for the positive control, and one for the negative control.
5. Follow the directions for the kit according to the manufacturer's instructions.

6. Add the appropriate reagents and drops to each of the extraction tubes.
7. Insert the patient's swab into the labeled extraction tube and add the appropriate controls to each of the labeled extraction tubes.
8. To ensure accuracy, set the timer for the appropriate time.
9. Add the appropriate reagent and drops to each of the extraction tubes.
10. Mix the reagents with the swab and add three drops from the well-mixed extraction tube to the sample window of the Strep A test unit. Repeat this procedure for each control.
11. Set the timer for the time indicated by the manufacturer.
12. A positive or negative result appears within 5 minutes. Refer to the directions in the kit to differentiate between a negative or positive result.
13. Properly dispose of the equipment and supplies in a biohazard waste container.
14. Remove your personal protective equipment and wash your hands.
15. Document the procedure and results in the patient chart.
16. Sanitize the area.

Patient Education

See Procedure 31-5.

Charting Example

12/23/xx 4:50 p.m. QuickVue One Step Strep A test performed according to manufacturer's guidelines. Test results positive. Patient medication instructions reviewed. Pamela King, CMA (AAMA)

Broth dilution, or minimum inhibitory concentration (MIC) testing, is more specific. The results indicate the lowest dilution of the drug that stops the growth of the organism. Results are reported with a numerical MIC value and the interpretation of that value (susceptible, intermediate, or resistant).

Performing a Wound or Throat Culture

Bacterial wound cultures are requested by the physician to determine the causative agent of an infection. Some typical sites cultured are abscesses, animal bites, diabetic ulcers, and superficial skin wounds. Deep wounds require both aerobic and anaerobic cultures, but superficial wounds and skin infections require only aerobic cultures.

Throat cultures aid in the diagnosis of *Group A strep,* the main pathogen implicated in pharyngeal infections. Identification

of the *Streptococcus* organism is important because of other disease conditions that can result, such as rheumatic fever, endocarditis, or acute glomerulonephritis. Rapid antigen testing (Rapid Strep testing) for the bacteria *Group A Strep* (*Streptococcus pyogenes*) is a commonly performed test in physician office laboratories. Built-in test controls confirm that proper procedure is followed.

Other pathogenic organisms that can be cultured from throat specimens include *Bordetella pertussis* (whooping cough), *Haemophilus influenzae* (epiglottitis), *Candida albicans* (oral thrush), and *Neisseria gonorrhoeae* (oral gonorrhoeae).

In Practice

Paul Richardson is a new patient who is complaining of a fever, sore throat, and difficulty eating for the past 2 days. He states that he knows that he has "strep throat" because his daughter was just seen in the office three days ago and diagnosed with the infection. He wants to know if the doctor will call in a prescription for him so that he doesn't have to come to the office. What should the medical assistant tell the patient? What organism might be responsible for the pharyngeal infection?

Urine Cultures

Specimens for urine culture are obtained from clean-catch or voided-midstream urine and catheterized urine (Figure 31-21 ◆). Random urine specimens commonly used for routine urinalysis tests are not used for cultures as they may be contaminated.

A clean-catch or voided-midstream specimen is obtained when the patient voids into a sterile container. The container is labeled with the patient's full name, the date and time of collection, and the type of specimen collected. It is transported to the testing area or stored appropriately until testing is completed.

Before collecting a urine specimen for culture, the patient must clean the urogenital area with cleansing towelettes or sterile gauze, soap, and water. A female patient must cleanse the labia majora, labia minora, and vaginal area from front to back, then repeat the procedure two more times to remove normal flora. A male patient cleanses the urethral opening and foreskin, if present, using the three cleansing wipes provided.

After cleansing, the patient holds the vaginal folds (female) or foreskin (male) away from the urethral opening, then begins urinating in the commode. After a few seconds the patient stops the urine flow, positions the sterile container, and begins urinating again, catching approximately 20 to 50 ml of urine. The patient may then finish voiding in the commode. The container must be closed securely with a lid. The patient must not touch the inside of the lid.

For a patient unable to provide a specimen, a nurse or physician performs a catheterization. The catheter is inserted through the urinary meatus and passed through the urethra into the bladder. Catheterization requires sterile technique to avoid introducing bacteria into the urinary tract.

Catheters can be temporary or indwelling. Straight (temporary) catheterization, or "in and out catheter," involves threading the catheter into the bladder, collecting the urine in a sterile container, and removing the catheter. Indwelling catheters are anchored in the bladder, and urine is continuously collected in an attached bag. A specimen collected from

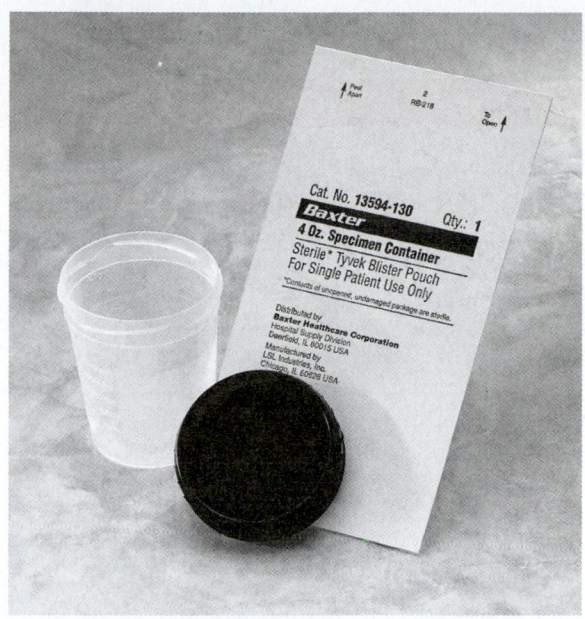

Figure 31-21 ◆ Container for clean-catch urine specimen. *Image courtesy of Cardinal Health, Inc. or one of its subsidiaries.*

an indwelling catheter must be taken from the port of the tubing. First, the catheter tubing must be drained of all urine. Then it is bent just below the withdrawal port, the port is cleaned with an alcohol swab, and a specimen is aspirated with a syringe and needle.

Small infants and toddlers in diapers pose a greater challenge. Special sterile collection devices can be used in place of straight catheterization. After the urogenital area is cleaned, a urine bag or "wee" bag is placed over the child's external genitals and secured with an adhesive. After the child urinates, the device is removed and placed in a sterile container for transport to the testing laboratory.

Storage and Transport of Urine Specimens

Unrefrigerated urine should be received in the testing area within one hour of collection. When this is not possible, urinalysis specimens may be refrigerated for up to four hours and urine culture specimens for up to 24 hours without compromising results. If specimens must be transported to an outside facility and constant refrigeration is impossible, special transport devices containing preservatives and buffers keep the pH stable and bacteria recoverable without refrigeration.

REVIEW

Chapter Summary

- The invention of the microscope greatly advanced the study and discovery of the causes of disease. The microscope helps to identify the tiny, pathogenic microorganisms that cause many diseases. Although there are five basic types of microscopes, the compound microscope is the one most commonly used.
- As an MA, you will prepare specimens for microscopic examination, assist in instructing and preparing the patient for specimen collection, and maintain logs related to laboratory testing in the medical office or laboratory setting.
- In the field of microbiology, it is important to differentiate between normal, resident flora and pathogenic, or disease-causing, microorganisms. Bacteria, fungi, parasites, and viruses are microorganisms.
- Bacteria are classified in two ways—by morphology and by gram stain reaction. Based on morphology, they are grouped into cocci, bacilli, and spirochetes. Based on gram stain reaction, they are either gram-positive or gram-negative. Bacteria generally have a genus name (beginning with a capital letter) and a species name (in lowercase). *Staphylococcus aureus* is an example.
- Specimen collection before treatment with antibiotics helps in the identification of causative pathogens. The accuracy of any test and of the resulting diagnosis depends on the quality and quantity of the specimen collected.
- When clinical symptoms are present, wet mounting and gram staining are two methods of examining specimens for pathogens before the patient leaves the medical office. Wet mount slide preparation usually involves placing a saline drop on a specimen smear and covering it with a cover slip before examining it under the microscope. Gram staining identifies whether pathogens are gram-positive or gram-negative.
- Many pathogens are common to specific infections, such as gram-positive *Staphylococcus aureus* (skin infections and abscesses), and gram-negative *E. coli* (urinary tract infections). An antibiotic is usually prescribed by the physician during the office visit to treat the suspected gram-negative or gram-positive organism. Later, if culture and sensitivity testing indicates there is a more effective medication, the physician changes the treatment.
- If specimen collection requires patient preparation and instruction, the MA provides verbal and written instructions. Reinforce to the patient that following the instructions exactly will ensure accurate, timely results and appropriate medical treatment.
- Throat, wound, urine, and stool specimens are used in C & S testing as appropriate to the clinical symptoms.

Chapter Review

Multiple Choice

1. Which of the following objectives requires oil immersion?
   a. 10X
   b. 100X
   c. 20X
   d. 40X

2. When cleaning a lens, you should
   a. use lens paper.
   b. use a disposable paper towel.
   c. completely soak the lens with lens cleaner.
   d. completely soak the lens with distilled water.

3. A eukaryote has
   a. organelles but no organized nucleus.
   b. no organized nucleus or organelles.
   c. organelles and a cell nucleus surrounded by a membrane.
   d. a cell nucleus surrounded by a membrane but no organelles.

4. Which of the following is bacteria?
   a. Yeast
   b. *Listeria monocytogenes*
   c. Protozoa
   d. Hepatitis A

5. The leading cause of UTIs is
   a. *Staphylococcus aureus.*
   b. *Clostridium perfringens.*
   c. *Pseudomonas aeruginosa.*
   d. *Escherichia coli.*

6. The gram-stained color of gram-positive pathogens is
   a. purple.
   b. blue.
   c. red.
   d. yellow.

7. When applying heat fixation to a specimen smear, you should
   a. keep the slide over the flame until it is hot.
   b. blow on the slide to cool it after heating.
   c. pass the slide through the flame.
   d. refrigerate it immediately.

8. Sensitivity testing is used to
   a. identify the causative pathogen.
   b. verify the gram staining procedure.
   c. decolorize the pathogen for identification.
   d. determine the most effective medication for treatment.

Chapter Review (continued)

9. How long after a radiology procedure with barium salt can a stool specimen be collected?
   a. 8 hours
   b. 72 hours
   c. 24 hours
   d. 48 hours

10. Without compromising the results, a urinalysis specimen may be refrigerated for up to
   a. 6 hours.
   b. 8 hours.
   c. 4 hours.
   d. 24 hours.

True/False

T F 1. The lenses of a microscope are concave.

T F 2. Objectives on the microscope include 10X, 20X, 40X, and 100X power lenses.

T F 3. Using immersion oil with the 100X lens makes items clearer.

T F 4. The light source, the condenser, and the diaphragm are located under the mechanical stage.

T F 5. Normal flora inhabit every nonsterile major body system.

Short Answer

1. What is a dissection microscope used for?

2. What are the three classifications of bacteria according to morphology?

3. What is pathogenicity?

4. Why are viruses classified as microorganisms?

5. Why are fungi considered opportunistic pathogens?

Research

1. Are there wound-care centers in your community designed specifically for the treatment of patient wounds and/or identification of infectious pathogens?

2. Research a type of Group A Strep known as "flesh-eating disease." How is it contracted? How is it treated? What is the mortality rate?

Externship Application Experience

A wound drainage specimen obtained by syringe was not processed within the recommended hour after collection. You are aware of this because the specimen was marked as 12/16/XX 6 A.M., and it is now 10 A.M. Why is it important to process a syringe specimen within the hour time frame, and what do you do?

Resource Guide

American Association of Blood Banks (AABB)
8101 Glenbrook Road
Bethesda, MD 20814-2749
301-907-6977
www.aabb.org

American Medical Technologists (AMT)
710 Higgins Road
Park Ridge, IL 60068
847-823-5169
www.amt1.com

American Society for Clinical Laboratory Science
6701 Democracy Blvd., Suite 300
Bethesda, MD 20817
301-657-2768
www.ascls.org

American Society for Clinical Pathology (ASCP)
2100 West Harrison St.
Chicago, IL 60612
312-738-1336
www.ascp.org

National Accrediting Agency for Clinical Laboratory Sciences (NAACLS)
8410 W. Bryn Mawr Ave., Suite 670
Chicago, IL 60631
773-714-8880
www.naacls.org

National Credentialing Agency for Laboratory Personnel (NCA)
PO Box 15945-289
Lenexa, KS 66285-5935
913-438-5110
www.nca-Info.org

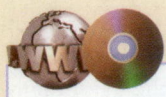

Med**Media**

http://www.MyMAKit.com

More on this chapter, including interactive resources, can be found on the Student CD-ROM accompanying this textbook and on http://www.MyMAKit.com.

Objectives

After completing this chapter, you should be able to:

- Define and spell the key terminology in this chapter.
- Define the medical assistant's role in blood specimen collection in the POL.
- Describe the components of blood.
- Explain how blood cells are formed.
- Define immunohematology.
- Identify the equipment used in blood collection.
- Explain the importance of following the correct order of draw.
- Describe the differences between venipuncture and capillary puncture.
- List important considerations in the transport of blood specimens.
- Identify and describe basic hematology tests.
- Explain the use of chemistry analyzers in common blood chemistry tests.
- Discuss the basics of blood typing.

Hematology and Chemistry

Case Study

Kathleen is working in a medical laboratory as part of her externship and does a lot of routine blood draws. She is running behind, and many patients are getting angry because of the long wait time. While setting up to perform a CBC, CMP, and prothrombin time, Kathleen gathers the vacutainers, alcohol wipes, cotton balls, and tourniquets. She cannot find a disposable gown to wear and decides to perform the draw without it.

Kathleen begins to perform the tests, but one of the tubes, the light blue one, has a faulty vacuum and isn't filling properly. She didn't bring extra blue tubes to the station, so she quickly grabs the extra "brick-top" tube to collect the sample. After she completes the draw, Kathleen notices that some blood has spilled on her uniform shirt.

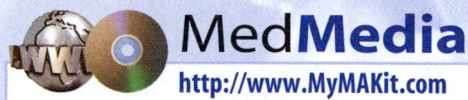

MedMedia
http://www.MyMAKit.com

Additional interactive resources and activities for this chapter can be found on http://www.MyMAKit.com. For videos, tips, audio glossary, legal and ethical scenarios, job scenarios, quizzes, games, and activities related to the content of this chapter, please access the accompanying CD-ROM in this book.

Audio Glossary
Legal and Ethical Scenario: *Hematology and Chemistry*
On the Job Scenario: *Hematology and Chemistry*
Videos: *The Basics of Blood Tests; Venipuncture & Capillary Puncture Demonstration*
Multiple Choice Quiz
Games: Crossword, Strikeout, and Spelling Bee
Drag and Drop: Circulatory System: Blood Types; Circulatory System: Blood Cells; Circulatory System: Circulatory System
Tips
HIPAA Quiz

Key Terminology

agglutination—process in which platelets clump or aggregate together to form a plug or clot

anticoagulant—substance that inhibits blood clot formation

coagulation—blood clot formation

diluent—diluting agent

dyscrasia—abnormal blood or bone marrow condition, such as leukemia

erythrocytes—red blood cells; contain hemoglobin, which carries oxygen from the lungs to the body's cells

hematology—study of blood

hemostasis—process by which the body spontaneously stops bleeding and maintains the blood in a fluid state within the vascular compartment

immunohematology—study of antigens, antibodies, and their interactions

leukocytes—white blood cells; different types of cells that protect against bacterial infection and other foreign invaders

phagocytic—having the ability to ingest particulate material, such as bacteria

phlebotomist—individual trained to draw blood

phlebotomy—process of blood collection, sometimes defined as "an incision into a vein"

plasma—liquid portion of anticoagulated blood

serum—liquid portion that remains when the blood has been allowed to clot

spectrophotometric—measurement or estimate of the amount of color in a solution

thrombocytes—platelets; smallest cells found in blood

venipuncture—method of obtaining venous blood for analysis of hematology and chemistry studies

✚ MEDICAL ASSISTING STANDARDS

CAAHEP ENTRY-LEVEL STANDARDS	ABHES ENTRY-LEVEL COMPETENCIES
■ Perform within scope of practice (psychomotor) ■ Apply ethical behaviors, including honesty/integrity in performance of medical assisting practice (affective) ■ Apply local, state and federal health care legislation and regulation appropriate to the medical assisting practice setting (psychomotor) ■ Recognize the importance of local, state and federal legislation and regulations in the practice setting (affective) ■ Explore issue of confidentiality as it applies to the medical assistant (cognitive) ■ Document accurately in the patient record (psychomotor) ■ Display sensitivity to patient rights and feelings in collecting specimens (affective) ■ Explain the rationale for performance of a procedure to the patient (affective) ■ Use language/verbal skills that enable patients' understanding (affective) ■ Perform handwashing (psychomotor) ■ Practice Standard Precautions (psychomotor) ■ Screen test results (psychomotor) ■ Describe the normal function of each body system (cognitive) ■ Identify common pathology related to each body system (cognitive) ■ Apply critical thinking skills in performing patient assessment and care (affective) ■ Assist physician with patient care (psychomotor) ■ Perform hematology testing (psychomotor) ■ Perform quality control measures (psychomotor) ■ Perform chemistry testing (psychomotor) ■ Perform venipuncture (psychomotor) ■ Perform capillary puncture (psychomotor) ■ Identify disease processes that are indications for CLIA waived tests (cognitive) ■ Prepare a patient for procedures and/or treatments (psychomotor) ■ Document patient care (psychomotor)	■ Project a positive attitude. ■ Maintain confidentiality at all times. ■ Be a "team player." ■ Be cognizant of ethical boundaries. ■ Exhibit initiative. ■ Adapt to change. ■ Evidence a responsible attitude. ■ Be courteous and diplomatic. ■ Conduct work within scope of education, training, and ability. ■ Interview and take patient history. ■ Prepare patients for procedures. ■ Apply principles of aseptic techniques and infection control. ■ Prepare and maintain examination and treatment areas. ■ Use quality control. ■ Collect and process specimens. ■ Perform selected tests that assist with diagnosis and treatment. ■ Screen and follow up patient test results. ■ Dispose of hazardous materials. ■ Practice Standard Precautions. ■ Perform venipuncture. ■ Perform hematology.

Abbreviations

CLIS—Clinical and Laboratory Standards Institute

FBS—fasting blood sugar

Hgb—hemoglobin

MCH—mean corpuscular hemoglobin; a measure of the average hemoglobin content of RBCs

MCHC—mean corpuscular hemoglobin concentration; a measure of the concentration of hemoglobin in the average RBC

MCV—mean corpuscular volume; a measure of the average volume (size) of RBCs in cubic microns

PMN—polymorphonuclear WBCs

✔ COMPETENCY SKILLS PERFORMANCE

1. Perform a butterfly draw using a hand vein.
2. Demonstrate a venipuncture using the evacuation system.
3. Demonstrate a venipuncture using the syringe method.
4. Perform a capillary puncture.
5. Perform a WBC and platelet count with a Unopette vial and hemacytometer.
6. Prepare a blood smear for a differentiated cell count.
7. Prepare a smear stained with Wright's stain.
8. Perform a microhematocrit by capillary tube.
9. Perform a hemoglobin test using a hemoglobulinometer.
10. Perform an ESR using the Westergren method.
11. Measure blood glucose using the Accu-Chek™ Glucometer.
12. Perform a blood cholesterol measurement using the ProAct testing device.
13. Perform a test for infectious mononucleosis.

Introduction

Hematology is the study of blood. **Phlebotomy** is the process of blood collection, the surgical opening of a vein to withdraw blood. Properly collected, labeled, and transported blood samples are the basis for accurate laboratory results. It is the role of the **phlebotomist** to make sure that appropriate blood samples are collected and properly processed.

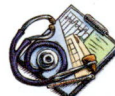

The Medical Assistant's Role in Hematology and Chemistry

Medical assistants must be familiar with the basic anatomy and physiology of the blood and veins to perform phlebotomy. MA training in phlebotomy will cover various methods of **venipuncture** and capillary blood collection. Responsibilities include properly identifying the patient, reviewing the physician's order, completing the laboratory requisition, and knowing which tubes to use and how much blood to collect.

The MA must wear the PPE required by OSHA for blood collection, particularly gloves. Snugly fitting latex gloves are most commonly used. Gloves made of other materials, such as polyethylene or nitrile, are available for healthcare professionals and patients who are allergic to latex. If there is a possibility that blood will be spilled or will contaminate clothing, a water-repellent coat may be required. In some situations, such as working with isolation patients, the MA will need to wear special protective gowns and masks.

The Anatomy and Physiology of Blood

There are five to six liters of blood in the body of an average adult. Blood consists of **plasma** and cellular components. Solids (formed cells) comprise approximately 45 to 50 percent of blood, and plasma comprises approximately 50 to 55 percent. Approximately 90 percent of plasma is water. Formed elements include **erythrocytes, leucocytes,** and **thrombocytes**. Erythrocytes account for most of the 45 to 50 percent of blood volume; leucocytes and thrombocytes, also referred to as the buffy coat, account for less than 1 percent.

Plasma

Plasma is the liquid portion of blood and comprises approximately 55 to 65 percent of the blood volume. Plasma consists of a high percentage of water. Other components are sugars, salts, gases, hormones, antibodies, minerals, vitamins, **coagulation** factors, and waste products. Plasma appears light yellow in color when it is separated from the cells by centrifugation.

Plasma is the liquid portion of blood in its unclotted or anticoagulated state; **serum** is the liquid portion that remains when the blood has been allowed to clot. Some laboratory tests require serum and others require plasma, so it is important to understand the difference.

Blood Cells

The cellular components of blood include the red blood cells, white blood cells, and platelets.

Red Blood Cells

Red blood cells (also called RBCs or erythrocytes) contain the pigment hemoglobin (**Hgb**), which provides the blood's reddish color (Figure 32-1 ◆). Oxygen from the lungs is bound to hemoglobin and transported through the blood to the tissues, where it is released to the cells. Carbon dioxide (CO_2) is a waste product that is picked up by the blood and carried back to the lungs. RBCs are produced in the bone marrow and live approximately 120 days.

Hemoglobin blood test results are directly proportional to the oxygen-carrying capacity of the red blood cells. Because RBCs may have varying amounts of hemoglobin, the number of RBCs does not accurately indicate the blood's hemoglobin content. Hematocrit indirectly measures red blood cell mass by comparing packed red blood cell volume to the volume of whole blood in the test specimen.

White Blood Cells

Five types of white blood cells (WBCs or leukocytes) are found in normal blood. The type can be identified by performing a WBC differential. In this procedure, a stained blood smear is examined under a microscope, 100 WBCs are counted, and each WBC is identified. The differential is often performed by an automated analyzer that flags abnormal results for a technologist's review. WBCs and platelets appear as a white layer

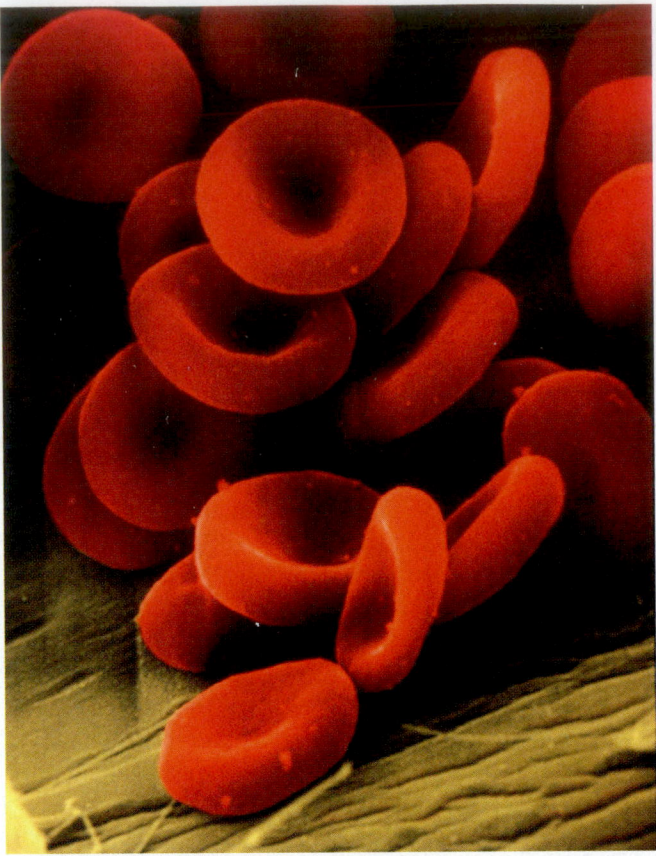

Figure 32-1 ◆ Red blood cells (RBCs) as seen under a microscope. *Source: Dennis Kunkel/Phototake NYC.*

(buffy coat) between the plasma and RBCs when whole blood is centrifuged.

The five types of WBCs are neutrophils, lymphocytes, monocytes, eosinophils, and basophils.

■ Neutrophils (polymorphonuclear white blood cells, also known as **PMNs** or segs and bands) are the most common WBCs and function to defend the body against infectious diseases, especially bacterial diseases (Figure 32-2 ◆).

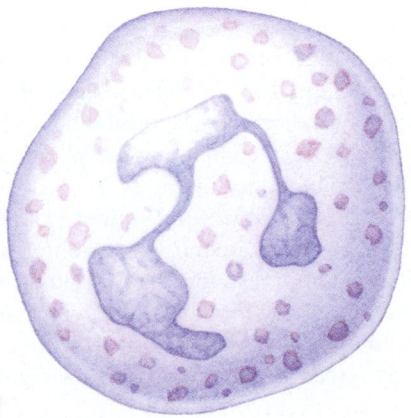

Figure 32-2 ◆ Neutrophil. *Source: Dorling Kindersley*

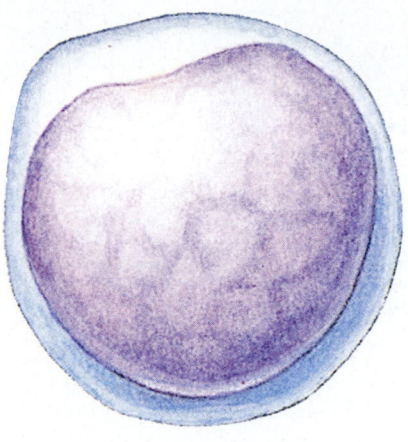

Figure 32-3 ◆ Lymphocyte.
Source: Dorling Kindersley

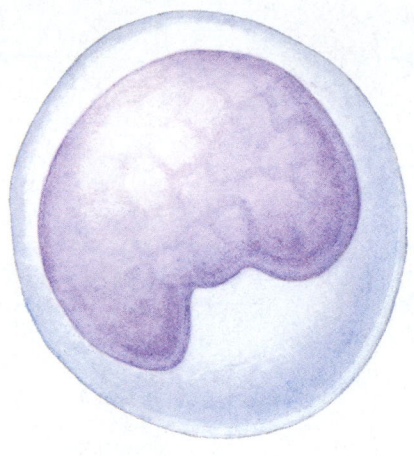

Figure 32-4 ◆ Monocyte.
Source: Dorling Kindersley

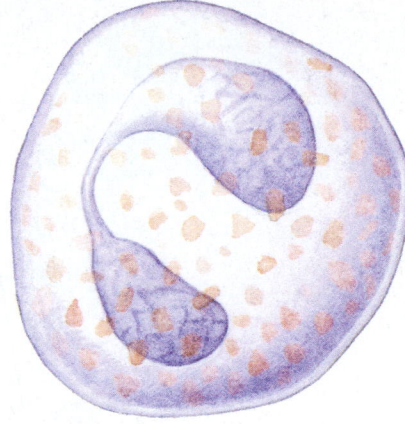

Figure 32-5 ◆ Eosinophil.
Source: Dorling Kindersley

- Lymphocytes are the second most common WBCs in adults, and often the most common in children (Figure 32-3 ◆). The primary role of lymphocytes is to aid in the immune defense of the body and to respond to viruses.
- Monocytes are the largest cells in normal blood, two or three times the diameter of erythrocytes (Figure 32-4 ◆). Monocytes are **phagocytic** cells and play a role in cell-mediated immunity.
- Eosinophils are similar in size to neutrophils (Figure 32-5 ◆). They function mainly in allergic or inflammatory responses, but also increase in some types of parasitic infections.
- Basophils are the least numerous WBCs, with a normal range of 0 to 2 percent (Figure 32-6 ◆). They contain histamine and appear to react in allergic states.

Platelets

Platelets (thrombocytes) are the smallest cells found in blood, ranging in size between 2 and 4 microns in diameter (Figure 32-7 ◆). Platelets function in **hemostasis**, during which the body spontaneously stops bleeding and maintains the blood in a fluid state within the vascular compartment. Platelets are an important factor in coagulation, which is the formation of blood clots that occurs when a blood vessel is damaged. A patient with a very low platelet count usually bleeds for an extended period, so extra care must be taken when performing venipunctures. **Agglutination** is the term for the process in which platelets clump or aggregate together to form a plug or clot.

Blood Cell Formation

The hematopoietic system is responsible for the production and maturation of all blood cells. This process takes place in the red bone marrow and other body tissues and organs. All blood cells start as stem cells that grow into blast cells (immature cells). The blast cells then differentiate by function to become mature erythrocytes, platelets, or leukocytes. The five basic kinds of leukocytes, or WBCs, are neutrophils, eosinophils, and basophils, which are all granular, and lymphocytes and monocytes, which are agranular. Agranulocytic monocytes, or mobile, immature, phagocytic leukocytes, circulate in the blood, migrate into the

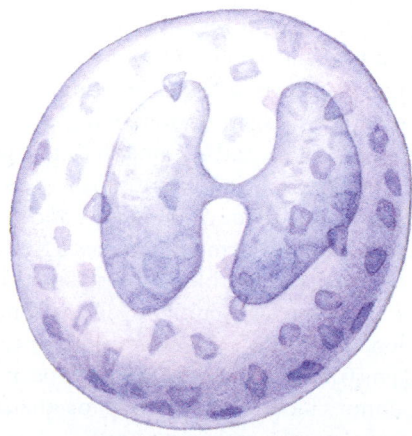

Figure 32-6 ◆ Basophil.
Source: Dorling Kindersley

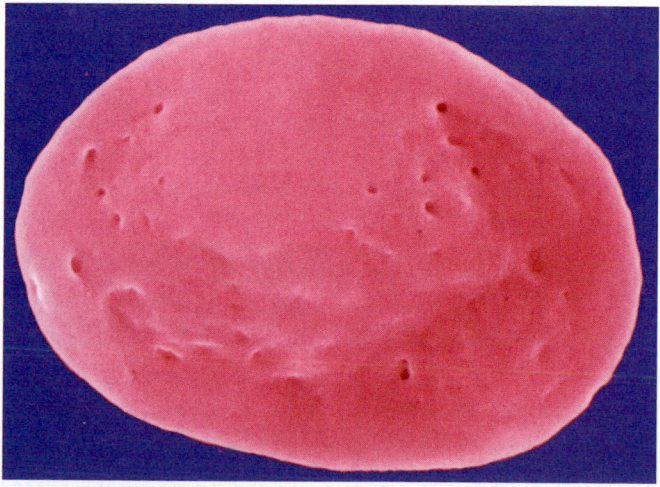

Figure 32-7 ◆ Platelet (thrombocyte).
Source: Phototake NYC

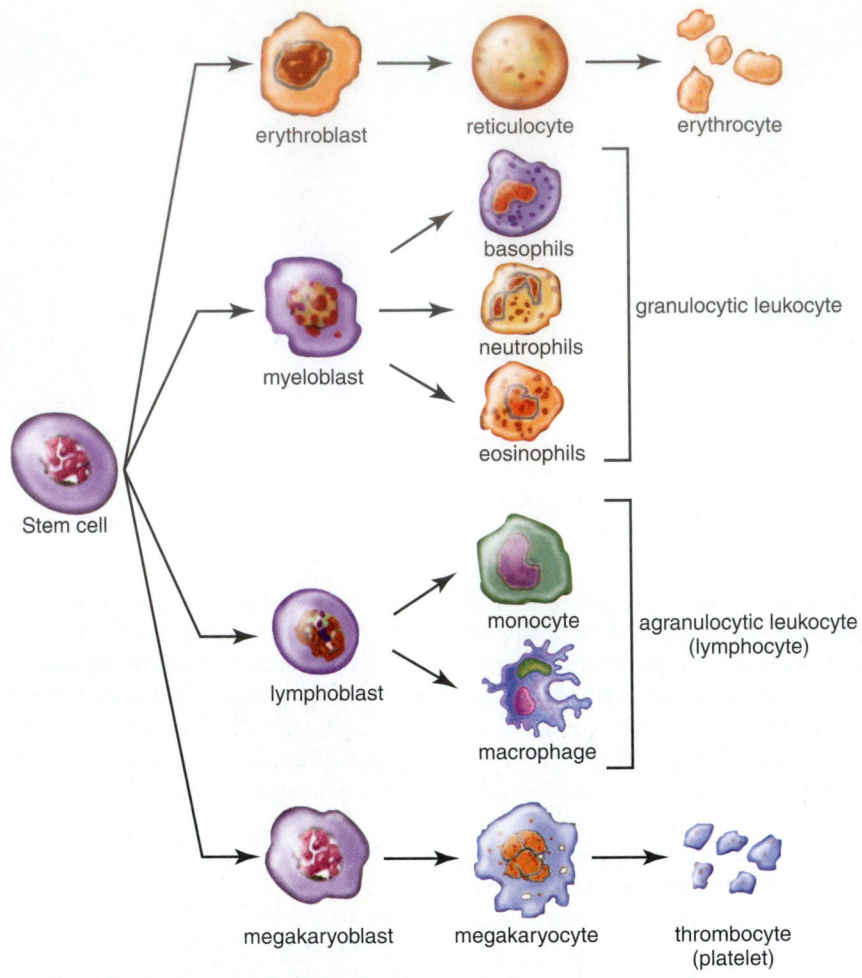

Figure 32-8 ◆ Diagram of differentiation of stem cells.

tissues, and become nonmobile, mature, phagocytic macrophages. Some cells are also designed to become precursor lymph cells that later develop into B- and T-lymphocytes, which help the body's immunological defenses. A **dyscrasia**, or blood disorder, can develop from aberrations in the blood cell differentiation and development process. Figure 32-8 ◆ illustrates some simplified examples of how a stem cell can differentiate into one of several different types of mature cell.

Altered functioning of the body's hematopoietic system affects CBC laboratory results. For example, an elevated RBC count indicates a different disease diagnosis than an elevated reticulocyte (an earlier stage of RBC development) count.

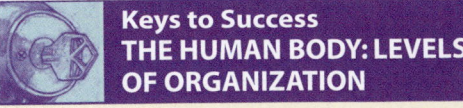

Keys to Success
THE HUMAN BODY: LEVELS OF ORGANIZATION

The human body is organized in different levels (Figure 32-9 ◆). These include atoms (the smallest unit), molecules, cells, tissues, organs, systems, and finally the body. As you study the body, you will find that organ systems often depend on each other, or at least assist each other in completing the required functions for a healthy life.

Immunohematology

Immunohematology is the study of antigens, antibodies, and their interactions. Antigens recognize foreign substances or organisms and stimulate an antibody reaction and the production of lymphocytes, granulocytes, and monocytes. Most clinical laboratories work with RBC antigen/antibody systems only. Immunology testing procedures with WBCs and platelets are often quite complicated and are most commonly performed by specially trained technologists in the blood bank area of the laboratory.

Knowledge of antigen-antibody reactions is important in the treatment of allergies, organ donation and transplantation, blood typing (A, B, AB, and O), and Rh factor (positive or negative). For example, A (blood type) positive (Rh factor) blood has antigen markings for A blood type and positive Rh factor to stimulate antibody formation against a transfusion of B negative blood. An A positive blood transfusion to a patient with A positive blood prevents antibody formation, prevents antibody reaction, and prevents blood transfusion reaction, in that order. Administration of the wrong blood type or Rh factor may cause the donor's blood cells to clump together, plug vital blood vessels, and cause the recipient's death.

Blood group antigens consist of protein molecules with specific groups of sugar molecules attached in precise locations.

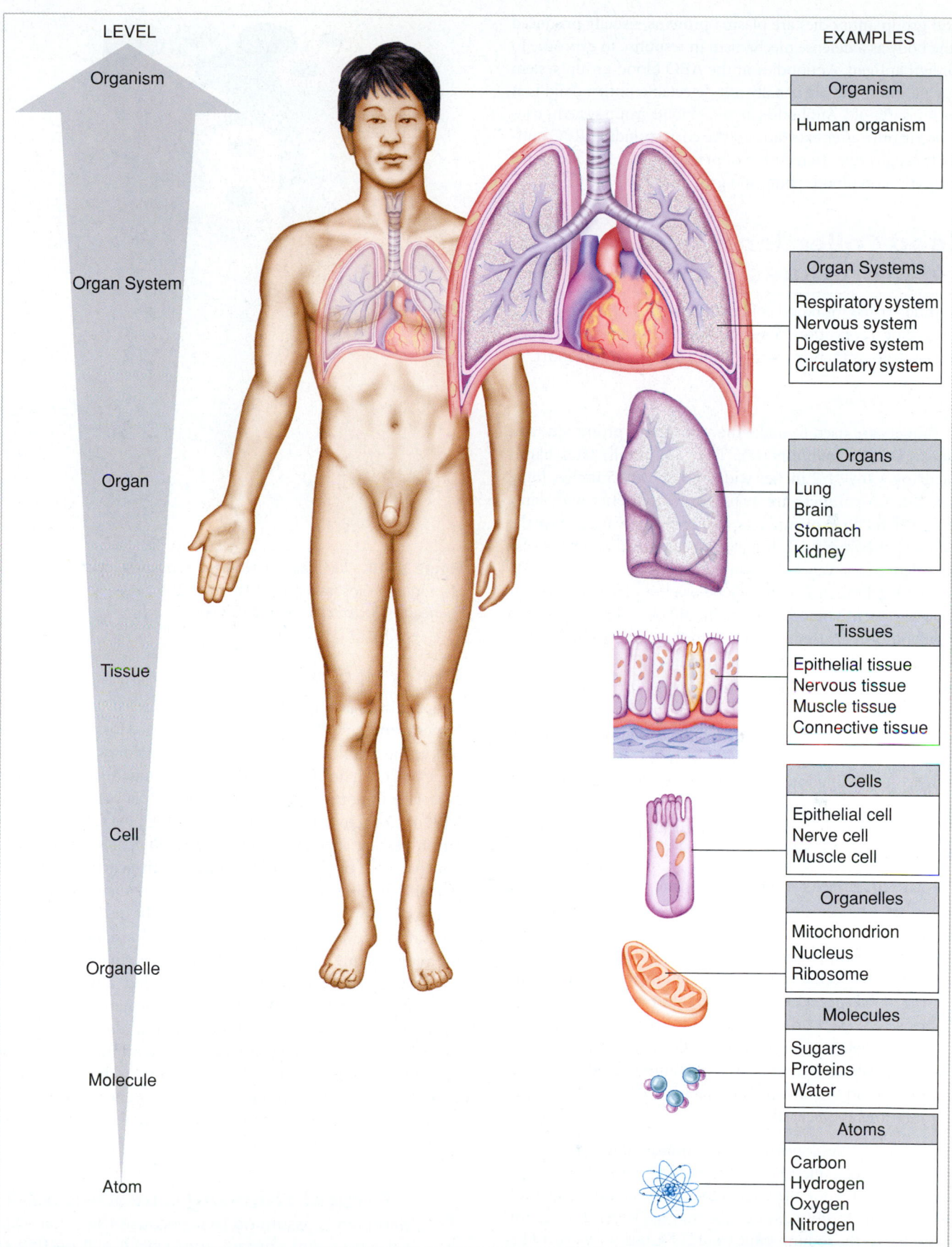

Figure 32-9 ◆ Organization of the human body.

Blood group antibodies are plasma proteins, usually produced by the body as a defense mechanism in response to exposure to a foreign antigen. Antibodies in the ABO blood group system occur naturally but are usually not detectable until a child is at least 3 months old. Antibodies in other blood group systems usually occur only after exposure to the corresponding RBC antigens, through either transfusion or pregnancy. ∞ For additional information on blood typing and grouping, see page 649.

Blood Collection Equipment and Procedures

Equipment used for blood collection includes tourniquets and various blood collection tubes and devices. Procedures include order of draw, puncture methods, and specimen transport.

Tourniquets

Tourniquets are used to make the veins more prominent and easier to find for venipuncture. They are usually latex bands measuring 1 to 1 1/2 inches wide and about 15 inches long. Latex-free tourniquets are available for patients with latex allergy. Velcro-type tourniquets, also commonly used, have the advantage of being quick and easy to apply and allow for easy adjustment of the venous pressure.

A blood pressure cuff may be used in place of a tourniquet. The patient's blood pressure should be taken first. During the phlebotomy procedure, maintain the cuff pressure below the level of the patient's diastolic pressure.

Blood Collection Tubes

Evacuated or vacuum tubes are used for laboratory blood collection. Vacutainer tubes are the type most commonly used, but the color coding for each tube type is consistent across all brands (Figure 32-10 ◆).

The color of the tube stopper indicates which additive, if any, is present in the tube. Additives include the following:

- **Anticoagulants**—contained in most blood collection tubes; each type of anticoagulant works to prevent clotting in a specific way.
- Clot activators—substances that produce clot formation within a specific time frame when mixed properly with the blood specimen; examples are citrate-phosphate-dextrose (CPD), acid-citrate-dextrose (ACD), oxalates, citrates, ethylene-diamine tetra-acetic acid (EDTA), heparin.
- Preservatives—substances that maintain blood cell components in the "drawn" and stable state by decreasing cellular metabolic activity.

Table 32-1 describes the most common tube types according to stopper color. Plasma collected in tubes with different types of anticoagulant is not interchangeable. For instance, plasma collected in a blue sodium citrate tube may *not* be used for chemistry studies, as the sodium value would be grossly elevated. Other types may be required by reference laboratories for specific tests. Sterile tubes containing a nutrient broth or enrichment media are required for blood cultures in cases of suspected septicemia.

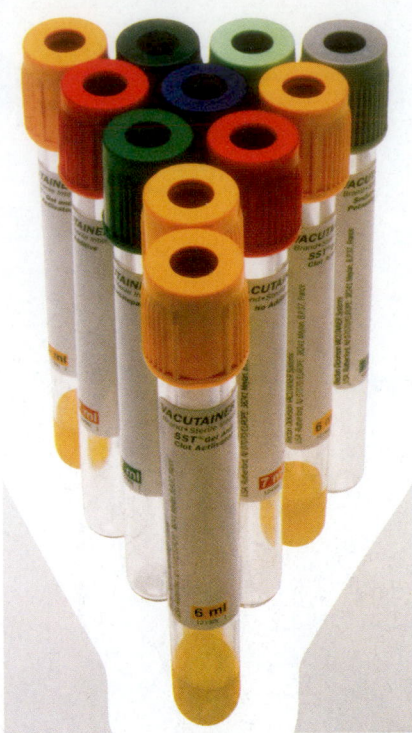

Figure 32-10 ◆ Vacutainer evacuated specimen tubes with Hemogard™ Closure blood collection tube.
Courtesy of © Beckton, Dickinson and Company.

Order of Draw

Order of draw is important and is determined by the lab tests to be performed and the type of tubes to be used for collecting and processing the blood specimen. Blood being drawn for cultures must be drawn first to prevent contaminating the specimen. It is especially important that no tube containing other anticoagulants or clot activators be drawn before the blue tube, as coagulation testing is very sensitive to even small amounts of anticoagulant or clot activator. Any additive carryover has the potential to cause inaccurate results. It is recommended that when only a blue-top tube is drawn, a red-top tube be drawn first and set aside to prevent thromboplastin release from the cells during the venipuncture, which would contaminate the blue-top tube and skew the results of the coagulation testing. The Clinical and Laboratory Standards Institute (**CLIS**), formerly the National Committee for Clinical Laboratory Standards (NCCLS), has instituted a recommended order of draw to minimize the effects of additive carryover (Table 32-2). Protocols for the proper order of draw may vary by manufacturer, the CSLI, and individual laboratories. The medical assistant should adhere to the protocols established by his or her facility.

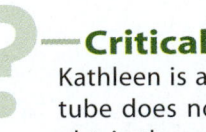

Critical Thinking Question 32-1

Kathleen is assuming that because the "brick-top" tube does not contain additives, it will be fine to obtain the prothrombin time sample in. Why is this incorrect?

TABLE 32-1 ADDITIVES FOR BLOOD SPECIMEN VACUTAINER TUBES

Color of Stopper	Additive	Description and Use	Special Requirements
Red, large glass	No additive or clot activator	15 ml red-top tube used when serum is required for: ■ Chemistry testing ■ Blood bank testing ■ Immunology ■ Many reference lab tests	No mixing required.
Blue	Sodium citrate	Used primarily for coagulation tests (PT, PTT, D-dimer, fibrinogen). Sodium citrate prevents coagulation by binding calcium. Correct blood volume is required for accurate coagulation test results. *Never* use a blue tube as the first tube in an evacuated tube draw as there may be some fluid contamination from surrounding tissues. Draw 2 to 3 ml of blood in a tube containing no additives before drawing the blue tube.	Gently mix 8 to 10 times.
Red, small plastic	Clot activator	Small 7 ml red-top tube. The serum may be used for chemistry and immunology testing.	Gently mix 8 to 10 times.
Red, black mottled (also called serum separator tubes or SST brand) tubes	Clot activator and serum gel separator	Separator consisting of an inert gel works as a barrier by settling between the clot and the serum during centrifugation. This tube is especially useful for "send out" tests, as the serum does not need to be transferred to another tube. Serum may be used for most chemistry and immunology testing but is not recommended for blood bank antibody testing.	Gently mix 8 to 10 times.
Green	Heparin	Heparin is a natural anticoagulant that inhibits thrombin and thus prevents fibrin formation from fibrinogen. Plasma and whole blood are collected in these tubes and are often used for routine chemistry testing, as heparin does not interfere with common blood chemistry elements.	Gently mix 8 to 10 times.
Lavender	EDTA	Used for most hematology testing (CBC, reticulocyte count, sedimentation rates) and for some specialized testing. The anticoagulant EDTA binds the calcium needed for clot formation.	Gently mix 8 to 10 times.
Gray	Sodium fluoride and potassium oxalate	Sodium fluoride is A preservative that inhibits glycolytic action, and potassium oxalate is an anticoagulant that binds calcium. These tubes are usually used to collect specimens for glucose and lactic analysis.	Gently mix 8 to 10 times.

Venipuncture

There are three basic means of collecting venous blood samples:

■ Evacuated tube system
■ Syringe and needle
■ Winged infusion set (butterfly) method

These methods allow for a choice of needle gauge and length. *Needle gauge* refers to the diameter of the needle. The larger the gauge number, the smaller the needle diameter. A needle gauge of 21 to 23 is most commonly used for routine blood collection. Needle length is usually 1 to 1 1/2 inches. Deeper veins may require longer needles.

Evacuated Tube

The evacuated tube system consists of a plastic holder, attachable needles of various gauges, and vacuum tubes (Figure 32-11 ◆). The needle screws into the holder and has two pointed ends. The longer, beveled end is used for venipuncture. The short end

TABLE 32-2 ORDER OF DRAW

1. Blood cultures (yellow) SPS sterile; sometimes a non-additive discard tube
2. Light blue (sodium citrate tube)
3. Red (plain) or Tiger-Top mottled red (gel separator tube)
4. Green and light green (heparin tubes)
5. Lavender (EDTA)
6. Pink or white (EDTA)
7. Gray (sodium fluoride/oxalate)
8. Dark blue (FDP)
9. Royal Blue last

2003 CLIS/NCCLS recommendation.

is covered with a retractable sheath that is pushed into the tube stopper and allows blood to flow into the vacuum tube when venipuncture is performed. This is the fastest and most efficient system for venous blood collection.

Needle and Syringe

The needle and syringe are used if the veins are fragile or if there is concern that the vein may collapse with the pressure of the evacuated tube system (Figure 32-12 ◆). A needle of the appropriate gauge is attached to a syringe of the desired size. The basic phlebotomy steps are followed and the blood is transferred from the syringe to the appropriate tubes.

Winged Infusion (Butterfly)

The winged infusion or butterfly set consists of a very small needle attached to a length of tubing (Figure 32-13 ◆). This device is used on very small or fragile veins. A syringe is attached to the tubing.

Patient Reactions to Venipuncture

The patient may have significant reactions to the phlebotomy procedure such as dizziness, light headedness, fainting, upset stomach, and even vomiting. The medical assistant must be aware that the potential for these problems exists and must take adequate steps for patient safety. Some patients who come in for a

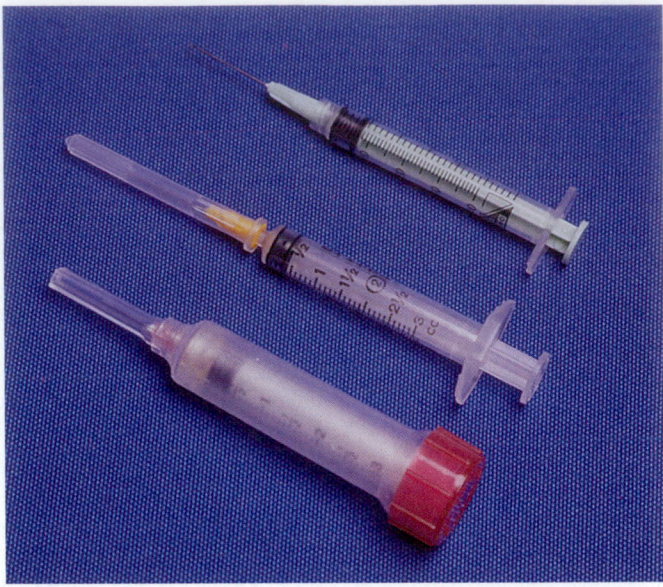

Figure 32-12 ◆ Disposable plastic syringes and needles: *Top,* with syringe and needle exposed; *Middle,* with plastic cap over the needle; *Bottom,* with plastic case over the needle and syringe. *Photographer: Elena Dorfman*

blood draw will have been fasting for several hours per physician instructions. These patients will have a greater likelihood of adverse reactions such as fainting due to low blood sugar.

The best way to protect the patient from an adverse effect is to be prepared for the possibility that something will happen. Most phlebotomy stations come with a phlebotomy chair that includes a padded cross bar that is lowered across the patient's lap. In the event that the patient faints, the padded bar will prevent him or her from slipping out of the chair or striking the head.

No matter how many times patients report they have had their blood drawn, they should be instructed to take several slow deep breaths and move from the phlebotomy station only when they feel comfortable enough to do so. Rushing patients before they are ready increases the likelihood that they will become dizzy and fall.

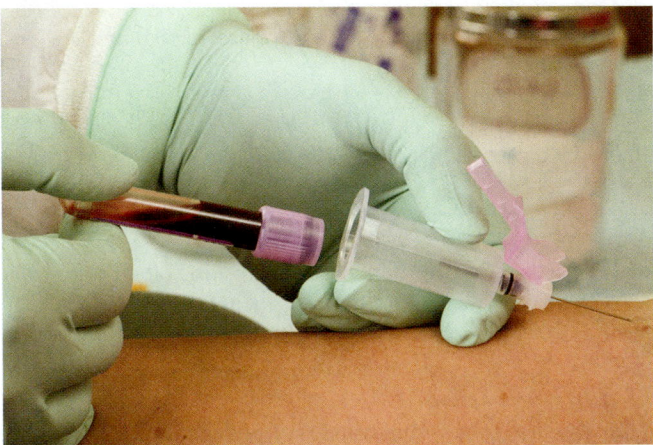

Figure 32-11 ◆ Traditional components of the evacuated tube system.

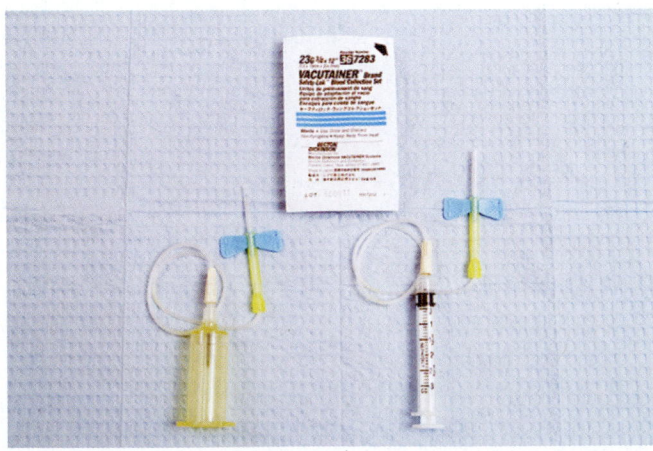

Figure 32-13 ◆ Winged infusion or butterfly set.

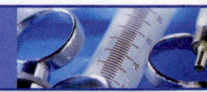

PROCEDURE 32-1 Perform a Butterfly Draw Using a Hand Vein

Theory and Rationale

For patients with weak or compromised veins, or veins that are not easily seen or felt, venous blood specimens can be drawn more easily with a butterfly needle (winged infusion) system. This system can be used with a vacutainer or syringe. Veins that are weak or compromised are at risk for collapse under the strong pressure caused by an evacuated tube system, so syringes are generally used. The sites most commonly chosen for the butterfly method are the back of the hand or the antecubital space in the arm. If you are obtaining a blood sample from the back of the hand, always use a syringe to collect the blood sample with the winged infusion system to prevent vein collapse. Also, have a variety of bandages available. Some patients may be allergic to the adhesives in bandage strips or paper tape, or they may have fragile skin that will tear easily with adhesives. For these patients make sure you have Coban, an adhesive-free self-adhering wrap, or a similar material available.

Materials

- gloves
- sterile butterfly package
- cotton balls
- tourniquet
- vacutainer or syringe
- bandage, Coban, or paper tape
- alcohol
- sharps container
- permanent pen for marking lab sample
- patient chart

Competency

(**Conditions**) With the necessary materials, you will be able to (**Task**) obtain a venous blood specimen from the back of the hand using a butterfly system (**Standards**) correctly within 15 minutes.

1. Wash your hands and gather the equipment.
2. Identify the patient and escort him or her to the treatment area.
3. Select the appropriate hand site. Put on gloves.
4. Cleanse the skin with alcohol.
5. Open the sterile butterfly package and stretch the tubing slightly to prevent it from recoiling when you begin the blood draw.
6. Apply the tourniquet to the patient's wrist area, proximal to the wrist bone, at least 3 inches above the injection site.
7. Have the patient make a fist or hold a stress ball or roll of gauze to slightly elevate the hand.
8. Enter the vein with the needle. The bevel should face upward, at a 30-degree angle to the skin. Advance the needle into the vein (Figure 32-14 ◆). Some people prefer to pinch the wings upward to hold the needle, while others prefer to hold just one wing from the side. If you enter the vein correctly, you will see blood "flash" into the hub of the needle, occasionally

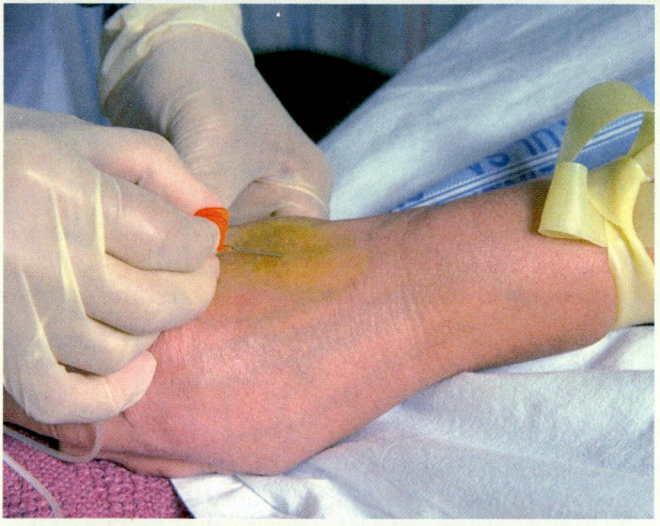

Figure 32-14 ◆ Insert needle at 30-degree angle through skin below selected vein.

into the tubing. Hand veins have a tendency to roll, so you may want to do a single-finger or double-finger anchor.

- Single-finger anchor: With your thumb, pull the skin taut toward the patient's knuckles to hold the vein in place. Do not put excessive pressure on the vein, as it will collapse and be difficult to enter.
- Double-finger anchor: Place your thumb below the puncture site and pull the skin toward the knuckles. Place the index finger of the same hand above the puncture site with slight pressure. You will insert the needle between your two fingers, so take great care to avoid an accidental needle stick.

9. When blood appears in the tubing, release the tourniquet.
10. With the needle secured in the vein, pull back on the plunger to obtain the necessary amount of blood for testing. If you are taking blood from the anetcubital space with a vacutainer, advance the tube onto the collection hub with your other hand, using the wings for support.
11. When you have obtained the correct amount of blood, break the suction of the vacutainer by removing the tube. (If you are using a syringe, there is no suction.)
12. Place a cotton ball or gauze pad over the puncture site without pressure and remove the needle.
13. Discard the needle and butterfly collection tubing into a sharps container.
14. Bandage as necessary.
15. Remove gloves and wash hands.
16. Label the blood specimen and fill out the laboratory paperwork.

continued

PROCEDURE 32-1 Perform a Butterfly Draw Using a Hand Vein (continued)

Patient Education

Inform the patient about puncture site care and when to expect to receive test results, if required by your medical office.

Charting Example

12/16/XX 10:48 AM Venous blood sample obtained from back of patient hand, left, through butterfly collection. Blood specimen sent to laboratory for CBC, CMP, and LFTs. Patient was told to keep bandage over puncture site for approximately 10 minutes and report any unusual bleeding, swelling, or bruising. Blake Singer, RMA (AMT)

Venipuncture Sites

The antecubital fossa, a triangular area below the elbow, is the most commonly used venipuncture site (Figure 32-15 ◆). The veins here are usually larger, better supported by surrounding tissue, and less painful to puncture than any other site. The median cubital vein is the vein of choice because it is large and well anchored. The cephalic vein may be more difficult to find and has a tendency to move. Extreme care must be taken if the basilic vein is used because of its proximity to the brachial artery.

Dorsal wrist and hand veins are also acceptable sites for venipuncture. Alternate sites, such as ankle or lower extremity veins, may be used when the usual sites are difficult to access. The physician's permission may be required in these cases.

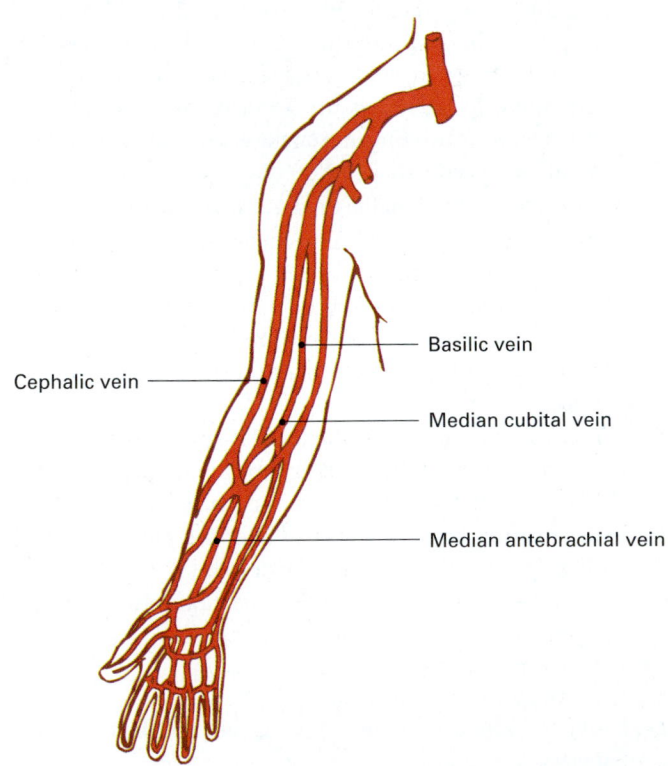

Figure 32-15 ◆ The antecubital fossa is the most commonly used venipuncture site.

Cephalic vein

Basilic vein

Median cubital vein

Median antebrachial vein

Using the Evacuation System

Before proceeding with the actual venipuncture, be sure to follow the appropriate preparation steps: verifying the physician's orders, preparing the laboratory requisition, checking availability of supplies, identifying the patient, verifying patient preparation, and comfortably and securely seating the patient.

Verifying the Orders

The MA must verify that the physician's orders for laboratory tests are legible and contain all the necessary information since the healthcare organization may be subject to legal action if laboratory tests are performed based on incomplete orders (Figure 32-16 ◆). Transcribing the physician's order for tests may involve entering the orders into a computerized laboratory information system or writing the information on a laboratory form. The MA must always order tests accurately to avoid having the patient return because of laboratory personnel errors. If possible, the MA should have someone else check the test orders for accuracy before collecting the blood sample.

When assigned to complete a lab requisition for a patient to take to a laboratory, the MA must complete all required information: the patient's name, date of birth, insurance, and contact information; the ordering physician's name and contact information; and the tests ordered and the diagnosis or reason for the test, usually in ICD-9-CM codes. Additionally, a notation

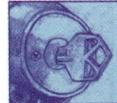

Keys to Success
VENIPUNCTURE SITES TO AVOID

Do *not* draw blood:

- Above an IV, as IV fluid dilution or contamination may yield inaccurate results that may lead to misdiagnosis.
- From the side on which a mastectomy was performed, because of the potential harm to the patient from lymphostasis.
- Near hematomas, as specimens may yield erroneous results.
- Near burned areas, which are very susceptible to infection.
- From an area reserved for dialysis access.
- Near an area with edema, as the specimen may be diluted with tissue fluids that could affect the test results.

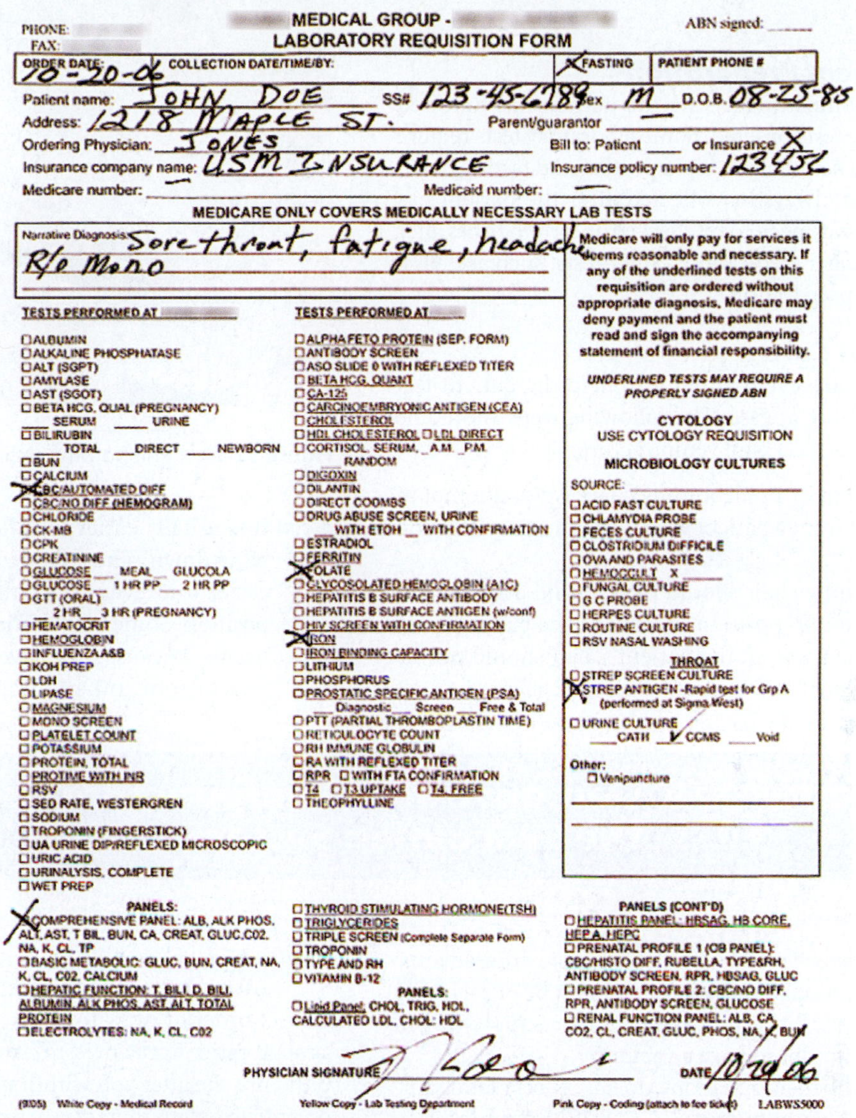

MEDICAL GROUP -
LABORATORY REQUISITION FORM

PHONE:
FAX:
ABN signed: _____

ORDER DATE: 10-20-06   COLLECTION DATE/TIME/BY: X FASTING   PATIENT PHONE #

Patient name: JOHN DOE   SS# 123-45-6789   Sex M   D.O.B. 08-25-85
Address: 1218 MAPLE ST.   Parent/guarantor
Ordering Physician: JONES   Bill to: Patient ___ or Insurance X
Insurance company name: USM INSURANCE   Insurance policy number: 123452
Medicare number: ___   Medicaid number: ___

MEDICARE ONLY COVERS MEDICALLY NECESSARY LAB TESTS

Narrative Diagnosis: Sore throat, fatigue, headache
R/o Mono

Medicare will only pay for services it deems reasonable and necessary. If any of the underlined tests on this requisition are ordered without appropriate diagnosis, Medicare may deny payment and the patient must read and sign the accompanying statement of financial responsibility.

UNDERLINED TESTS MAY REQUIRE A PROPERLY SIGNED ABN

CYTOLOGY
USE CYTOLOGY REQUISITION

TESTS PERFORMED AT ___

☐ ALBUMIN
☐ ALKALINE PHOSPHATASE
☐ ALT (SGPT)
☐ AMYLASE
☐ AST (SGOT)
☐ BETA HCG, QUAL (PREGNANCY)
    SERUM ___ URINE
☐ BILIRUBIN
    ___ TOTAL ___ DIRECT ___ NEWBORN
☐ BUN
☐ CALCIUM
X CBC/AUTOMATED DIFF
X CBC/NO DIFF (HEMOGRAM)
☐ CHLORIDE
☐ CK-MB
☐ CPK
☐ CREATININE
☐ GLUCOSE ___ MEAL ___ GLUCOLA
☐ GLUCOSE ___ 1 HR PP ___ 2 HR PP
☐ GTT (ORAL)
    ___ 2 HR ___ 3 HR (PREGNANCY)
☐ HEMATOCRIT
☐ HEMOGLOBIN
☐ INFLUENZA A&B
☐ KOH PREP
☐ LDH
☐ LIPASE
☐ MAGNESIUM
☐ MONO SCREEN
☐ PLATELET COUNT
☐ POTASSIUM
☐ PROTEIN, TOTAL
☐ PROTIME WITH INR
☐ RSV
☐ SED RATE, WESTERGREN
☐ SODIUM
☐ TROPONIN (FINGERSTICK)
☐ UA URINE DIP/REFLEXED MICROSCOPIC
☐ URIC ACID
☐ URINALYSIS, COMPLETE
☐ WET PREP

TESTS PERFORMED AT ___

☐ ALPHA FETO PROTEIN (SEP. FORM)
☐ ANTIBODY SCREEN
☐ ASO SLIDE 0 WITH REFLEXED TITER
☐ BETA HCG, QUANT
☐ CA-125
☐ CARCINOEMBRYONIC ANTIGEN (CEA)
☐ CHOLESTEROL
☐ HDL CHOLESTEROL ☐ LDL DIRECT
☐ CORTISOL, SERUM, ___ A.M. ___ P.M.
    ___ RANDOM
☐ DIGOXIN
☐ DILANTIN
☐ DIRECT COOMBS
☐ DRUG ABUSE SCREEN, URINE
    ___ WITH ETOH ___ WITH CONFIRMATION
☐ ESTRADIOL
☐ FERRITIN
X FOLATE
☐ GLYCOSOLATED HEMOGLOBIN (A1C)
☐ HEPATITIS B SURFACE ANTIBODY
☐ HEPATITIS B SURFACE ANTIGEN (w/conf)
☐ HIV SCREEN WITH CONFIRMATION
X IRON
☐ IRON BINDING CAPACITY
☐ LITHIUM
☐ PHOSPHORUS
☐ PROSTATIC SPECIFIC ANTIGEN (PSA)
    ___ Diagnostic ___ Screen ___ Free & Total
☐ PTT (PARTIAL THROMBOPLASTIN TIME)
☐ RETICULOCYTE COUNT
☐ RH IMMUNE GLOBULIN
☐ RA WITH REFLEXED TITER
☐ RPR ☐ WITH FTA CONFIRMATION
☐ T4 ☐ T3 UPTAKE ☐ T4, FREE
☐ THEOPHYLLINE

MICROBIOLOGY CULTURES

SOURCE: ___

☐ ACID FAST CULTURE
☐ CHLAMYDIA PROBE
☐ FECES CULTURE
☐ CLOSTRIDIUM DIFFICILE
☐ OVA AND PARASITES
☐ HEMOCCULT X
☐ FUNGAL CULTURE
☐ G C PROBE
☐ HERPES CULTURE
☐ ROUTINE CULTURE
☐ RSV NASAL WASHING

THROAT
☐ STREP SCREEN CULTURE
X STREP ANTIGEN -Rapid test for Grp A
    (performed at Sigma West)

☐ URINE CULTURE
    ___ CATH ✓ CCMS ___ Void

Other:
☐ Venipuncture

PANELS:
X COMPREHENSIVE PANEL: ALB, ALK PHOS. ALT, AST, T BIL, BUN, CA, CREAT, GLUC, CO2, NA, K, CL, TP
☐ BASIC METABOLIC: GLUC, BUN, CREAT, NA, K, CL, CO2, CALCIUM
☐ HEPATIC FUNCTION: T. BILI, D. BILI, ALBUMIN, ALK PHOS, AST, ALT, TOTAL PROTEIN
☐ ELECTROLYTES: NA, K, CL, CO2

☐ THYROID STIMULATING HORMONE (TSH)
☐ TRIGLYCERIDES
☐ TRIPLE SCREEN (Complete Separate Form)
☐ TROPONIN
☐ TYPE AND RH
☐ VITAMIN B-12

PANELS:
☐ Lipid Panel: CHOL, TRIG, HDL, CALCULATED LDL, CHOL: HDL

PANELS (CONT'D)
☐ HEPATITIS PANEL: HBSAG, HB CORE, HEP A, HEP C
☐ PRENATAL PROFILE 1 (OB PANEL): CBC/NO DIFF, RUBELLA, TYPE&RH, ANTIBODY SCREEN, RPR, HBSAG, GLUC
☐ PRENATAL PROFILE 2: CBC/NO DIFF, RPR, ANTIBODY SCREEN, GLUCOSE
☐ RENAL FUNCTION PANEL: ALB, CA, CO2, CL, CREAT, GLUC, PHOS, NA, K, BUN

PHYSICIAN SIGNATURE ___   DATE 10-24-06

(9/05)   White Copy - Medical Record   Yellow Copy - Lab Testing Department   Pink Copy - Coding (attach to fee ticket)   LABWS5000

Figure 32-16 ◆ Physician's order for lab test.

should be entered if fasting is required, along with the length of the fasting period prior to the test. Any other pertinent information should also be included.

Obtaining Supplies

The MA should make sure all routine phlebotomy supplies are readily available and avoid searching for supplies while the patient is sitting in the phlebotomy chair. Lack of preparation can make the patient anxious and does not reflect well on the institution or the medical assistant.

Some tests require special tubes that may need to be obtained from a different storage area within the laboratory or from the reference laboratory. The MA should check to see if special handling is required for the ordered tests. For instance, ammonias should be transported on ice; cold agglutinins should be allowed to clot in a 37°C heat block.

Blood draws are usually performed using evacuated, or vacuum, tube systems. The needle for puncture and procurement of the blood specimen is attached securely to a holder, and the different evacuated tubes are placed in and removed from the holder in correct order of draw. This method is preferred because it eliminates the possibility of cell hemolysis, prevents clot adherence to the wall of the collection container, and reduces the chances of needle injury and exposure to blood that occur during other types of blood draw. A butterfly needle is used if the blood specimen is more difficult to collect, as in the case of some pediatric, geriatric, and cancer patients. The butterfly needle can be secured to the holder for evacuated tubes or to a syringe for later placement in an evacuated tube.

Identifying the Patient

In a doctor's office or hospital outpatient setting, the MA should ask the patient for his or her name. The MA should avoid asking questions such as "Are you Susie Smith?" There may be other patients nearby and enough sound interference to make it difficult for the patient to hear clearly. The patient may say yes out of confusion. The MA should also check the birthdate. It is common to have two patients with the same name but different birthdates.

Verifying Patient Preparation

Medical assistants must make sure the patient has followed instructions for the tests ordered. Some laboratory tests require special preparation beforehand. Lipid profiles and fasting blood sugars (**FBS**) must always be collected after the patient has fasted. Drug levels may need to be checked at certain times after the patient has taken a medication. Other tests, such as CBCs, require no special preparation.

Proper Patient Care

The MA should make every attempt to help the patient feel comfortable and more at ease. The following steps should be followed to ensure a successful venipuncture:

- Seat the patient in a phlebotomy chair. *Never* attempt to collect blood from a patient who is standing or sitting on a high stool.
- The phlebotomy chair should have a solid armrest that can be locked into position in front of the patient. Supported by the armrest, the patient's arm should not be significantly bent at the elbow (Figure 32-17 ◆).

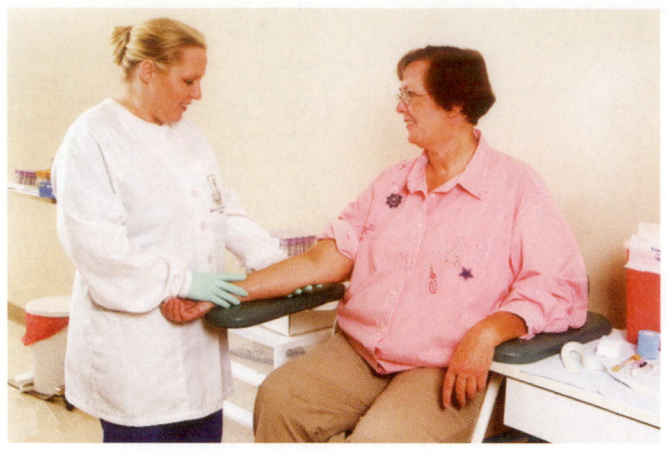

Figure 32-17 ◆ Phlebotomy chair.

- It is usually easier to collect blood from a child who is lying down. The child feels more comfortable, and it is easier to prevent the child's arm from moving in that position. Some adult patients may also need to lie down, usually because they have previously experienced faintness or some other difficulty with blood collection.

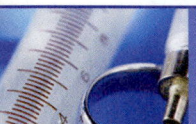

PROCEDURE 32-2 Demonstrate a Venipuncture Using the Evacuation System

Theory and Rationale

Make sure the proper tubes are available for the ordered tests. For backup, it is a good idea to keep an extra tube of each type in your lab coat pocket or in a venipuncture supply tray in case a tube is found not to have a vacuum.

In routine inpatient situations, do *not* collect blood samples from patients without hospital identification bracelets. Ask the nursing staff to attach an identification bracelet to the patient before you collect blood. In a true emergency, such as with an ER trauma patient, there may not be time for a hospital bracelet. In this case, ask the patient to tell you his or her name or have the patient identified by the nurse.

Test result accuracy and patient comfort are your main concerns when applying the tourniquet. Prolonged application can result in the formation of a hematoma as blood infiltrates the tissue and can alter some test results. Leave the tourniquet on as briefly as possible, preferably no longer than one minute per application. The tourniquet may need to be applied twice, once before the procedure to select the vein, then just before the vein is punctured.

Verify that the patient does not have latex allergies. If the patient indicates a possible latex allergy, use a latex-free tourniquet and gloves.

Asking the patient to make a fist will help to make the veins more prominent and prevent them from rolling.

Cleanse the site with an antiseptic, usually 70 percent isopropyl alcohol. *When you collect blood for blood alcohol levels, you must use an aqueous, not alcohol-based, antiseptic to ensure valid results.*

After performing the venipuncture, fill the tubes in the correct order of draw to ensure the proper blood-to-anticoagulant ratio. Apply pressure and monitor bleeding from the puncture site after you withdraw the needle. A patient who is on anticoagulant therapy, such as Coumadin or heparin, may bleed from the venipuncture site for longer than normal. You can ask an able patient to apply pressure to the site. Make sure that bleeding has completely stopped before bandaging the site. Firmly apply an adhesive bandage over the pressure gauze to ensure continued clotting.

Materials

- phlebotomy tray *or* individual items (antiseptic pads, appropriate vacutainers, holder, and needle)
- tourniquet
- handwritten or preprinted specimen labels
- disposable gloves
- sharps container

Competency

(**Conditions**) With the necessary materials, you will be able to (**Task**) demonstrate a venipuncture using an evacuation system (**Standards**) correctly within 15 minutes.

1. Review the physician's order. Verify that the order is legible, includes a diagnosis and other necessary information,

PROCEDURE 32-2 Demonstrate a Venipuncture Using the Evacuation System *(continued)*

and is signed by the physician or his or her assigned person. If any test order is not legible, or if there is any confusion about which test has been ordered, contact the physician or the office nurse for confirmation. Document on the physician's order the correct tests and the name of the person who confirmed the order.

2. Wash your hands.
3. Prepare the laboratory requisition from the physician's order.
4. Make sure all routine and special supplies are available for venipuncture and transporting the specimen.
5. Identify the patient and escort him or her to the treatment area.
6. Verify that the patient has been properly prepared.
7. Position and reassure the patient.
8. Wash your hands and put on disposable gloves.
9. Prepare the needle.
   For evacuated tubes and holder: Thread the appropriate needle into the holder until it is secured, using the needle sheath as a wrench (Figure 32-18 ◆).
   For a syringe: Insert the needle into the syringe (Figure 32-19 ◆). Move the plunger within the barrel to check movement.
10. Apply the tourniquet. Wrap it around the patient's upper arm 3 to 4 inches above the antecubital fossa (Figure 32-20 ◆). Cross the ends of the tourniquet and pull them snugly against the patient's arm (Figure 32-21 ◆). With your thumb and forefinger, hold the tourniquet in place while pulling a loop of one end behind the joined area (Figure 32-22 ◆).
11. Select the venipuncture site.
12. Ask the patient to make a fist.
13. Palpate the antecubital area with your index finger to determine the exact vein location and needle entry site.
14. Clean the antecubital area (or other selected site) with an antiseptic wipe, cotton ball soaked in antiseptic, or alcohol wipe. Use a circular motion from the venipuncture site outward.
15. Allow the site to air-dry, or dry it with a clean gauze pad.
16. Insert the blood collection tube into the holder and onto the needle up to the recessed guideline on the needle

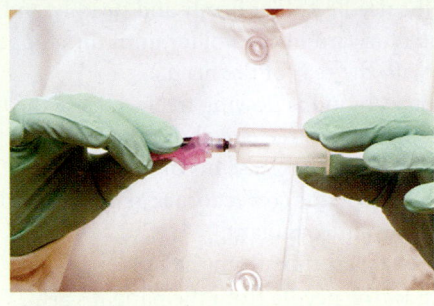

Figure 32-18 ◆ Thread the appropriate needle into the holder.

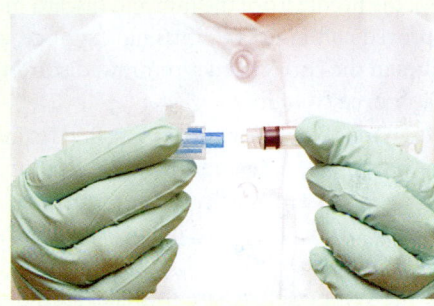

Figure 32-19 ◆ Insert the needle into the syringe.

holder. Avoid pushing the tube beyond the guideline to prevent loss of vacuum.
17. Remove the plastic protective cover from the needle.
18. To perform the venipuncture:
    - Make sure the patient's arm (or other venipuncture site) is in a downward position to prevent reflux or backflow.
    - Grasp the patient's arm firmly but gently.
    - Draw the patient's skin taut with your thumb to anchor the vein.
    - Line the needle bevel-up with the vein.
    - With a single, direct puncture, enter the vein at a 15- to 30-degree angle.

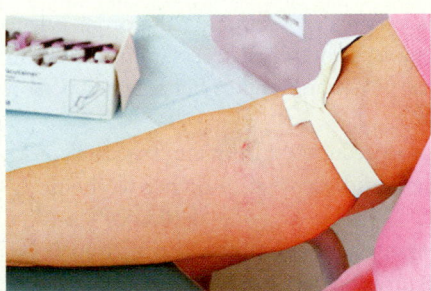

Figure 32-20 ◆ Apply the tourniquet around the patient's upper arm 3 to 4 inches above the antecubital fossa.

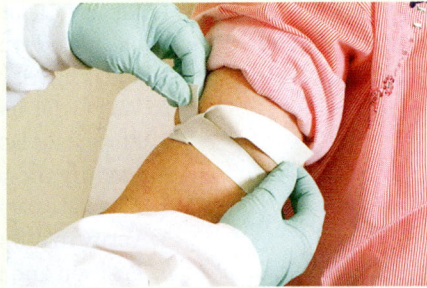

Figure 32-21 ◆ Cross the ends of the tourniquet and pull them snugly against the patient's arm.

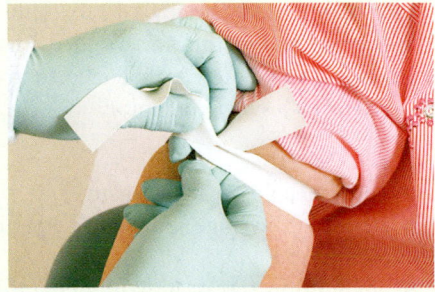

Figure 32-22 ◆ Form the tourniquet loop.

continued

PROCEDURE 32-2 Demonstrate a Venipuncture Using the Evacuation System *(continued)*

19. Hold the needle holder firmly and steadily, and then push the tube forward in the holder until the stopper is punctured with the rear of the needle.
20. As soon as blood is flowing freely, release the tourniquet by pulling on the free end above the loop.
21. Ask the patient to release his or her fist.
22. Fill the tubes in the correct order of draw. Invert any tubes containing anticoagulant.
23. Remove the last tube from the holder.
24. Withdraw the needle from the patient's arm.
25. Immediately place a clean gauze pad over the site. Apply pressure or instruct the patient to apply pressure.
26. Remove the needle from the hub and discard the needle in an approved container. Or, if using a syringe, after filling the tubes in the correct order of draw, discard the syringe in an approved container.
27. Label each tube with the patient's first and last name, identification number, date and time of collection, and your initials or identifying code. *Or,* if preprinted computer labels are available, initial each label and attach the labels to the appropriate tubes.
28. Check the venipuncture site to make sure bleeding has stopped, and bandage it. Instruct the patient to leave the bandage on for at least 15 minutes.
29. Remove and dispose of your gloves. Wash your hands.

30. Evaluate the patient for signs of faintness or color loss. If the patient appears stable, thank the patient for cooperating and escort him or her back to the waiting room.

Patient Education

Instruct the patient beforehand in the general procedure. Do *not* promise the patient that the procedure will not hurt. It is more tactful to say that it might feel like a "brief sting." Let the patient know when the actual puncture is about to happen. As necessary, provide information about how long the results will take and how they will be transmitted to the patient.

Charting Example

Sometimes charting may not be required for phlebotomy procedures because laboratory processing documentation is sufficient. If charting is required, it might look like this:

08/25/XX 7:30 a.m. Pt anxious about phlebotomy procedure. General explanations given before each step. Pt voiced concern over the amount of pain she would experience and that her veins were hard to get blood from. Venous specimen obtained for a CBC, Na, K, and Cl with appropriate tubes. Pt held pressure gauze onsite, site was bandaged, and pt was instructed to leave the bandage in place for 15 minutes. Pt escorted to the exit. Decon Ramirez, CMA (AAMA)

PROCEDURE 32-3 Demonstrate a Venipuncture Using the Syringe Method

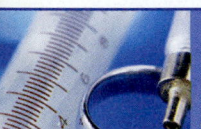

Theory and Rationale

The evacuation method is not always the best choice for performing venipuncture. The needle and syringe method is often used when very small or fragile veins are involved. The vacuum created when the collection tube is pressed over the needle point can cause damage to the tissue or collapse of the vein. The size of the syringe will vary according to the amount of blood needed. Usually a 10 to 20 ml syringe is used when several vacutainer tubes are needed. Ensure that venous specimen is immediately transferred to appropriate vacutainer tubes using a syringe adaptor.

Materials

- sterile needle (21- or 22-gauge)
- 10 to 20 ml syringe and syringe adaptor to transfer to vacutainer tubes
- phlebotomy tray or individual items (antiseptic or alcohol pads, appropriate vacutainers, sterile gauze)
- tourniquet
- handwritten or preprinted specimen labels
- disposable gloves

- sharps container
- nonallergic tape or bandage

Competency

(Conditions) With the necessary materials, you will be able to **(Task)** demonstrate a venipuncture using the syringe method **(Standards)** correctly within 15 minutes.

1. Review the physician's order. Verify that the order is legible, includes a diagnosis and other necessary information, and is signed by the physician or his or her assigned person.
2. Wash your hands.
3. Prepare the laboratory requisition from the physician's order.
4. Identify the patient and escort him or her to the designated area.
5. Verify that the patient has been properly prepared.
6. Position and reassure the patient.
7. Wash your hands again and put on disposable gloves.
8. Insert the needle into the syringe. Move the plunger within the barrel to check movement.
9. Apply the tourniquet. Wrap it around the patient's upper arm 3 to 4 inches above the antecubital fossa (Figure 32-23 ◆).

PROCEDURE 32-3 Demonstrate a Venipuncture Using the Syringe Method *(continued)*

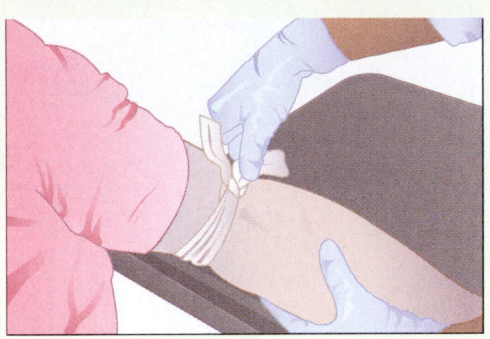

Figure 32-23 ◆ Apply the tourniquet 3 to 4 inches above the antecubital fossa.

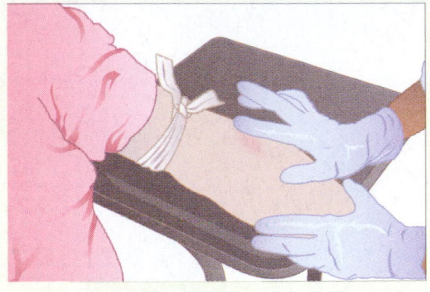

Figure 32-24 ◆ Palpate the antecubital area to determine the exact vein location and needle entry site.

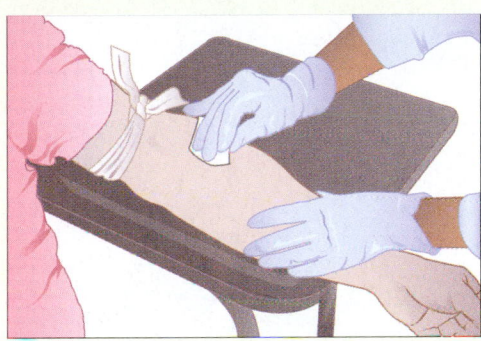

Figure 32-25 ◆ Clean the selected site with an antiseptic or alcohol wipe.

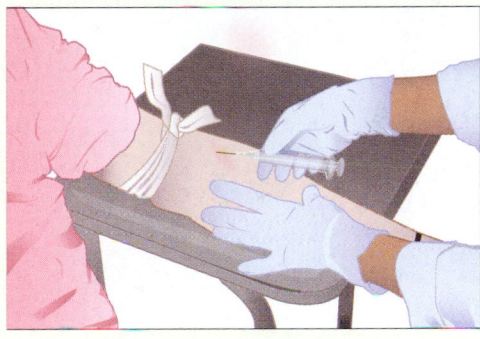

Figure 32-26 ◆ Enter the vein at a 15- to 30-degree angle.

Cross the ends of the tourniquet and pull them snugly against the patient's arm. With your thumb and forefinger, hold the tourniquet in place while pulling a loop of one end behind the joined area.

10. Select the venipuncture site.
11. Ask the patient to make a fist.
12. Palpate the antecubital area with your index finger to determine the exact vein location and needle entry site (Figure 32-24 ◆).
13. Clean the antecubital area (or other selected site) with an antiseptic or alcohol wipe (Figure 32-25 ◆).
14. Allow the site to air dry, or dry it with a clean gauze pad.
15. Hold the syringe with your dominant hand. Remove the plastic protective cover from the needle.
16. To perform venipuncture:
    - Make sure the patient's arm is in a downward position to prevent reflux or backflow.
    - Use your thumb to draw the skin taut to anchor the vein.
    - Line the needle bevel-up with the vein.
    - With a single, direct puncture, enter the vein at a 15- to 30-degree angle (Figure 32-26 ◆).
    - Observe for a "flash" of blood in the hub of the syringe.
    - Have the patient release his or her fist.
17. Slowly pull back the plunger of the syringe (Figure 32-27 ◆). Be certain that you do not move the needle after entering the vein. Fill the barrel to the needed volume.
18. Release the tourniquet when you have obtained the appropriate volume and venipuncture is complete (Figure 32-28 ◆).
19. Immediately place a sterile gauze pad over the site and withdraw the needle from the patient's arm (Figure 32-29 ◆).
20. Apply pressure or instruct the patient to apply pressure on the puncture site with sterile gauze.
21. Transfer the blood immediately to the required tube(s) using the syringe adaptor. Invert the tubes after the addition of the blood.
22. Discard the syringe in an approved container.
23. Use the preprinted labels or label each tube with the patient's first and last name, identification number (if applicable), date and time of collection, and your initials.
24. Check the venipuncture site to make sure bleeding has stopped, then bandage it. Instruct the patient to leave the bandage on for at least 15 minutes (Figure 32-30 ◆).

continued

PROCEDURE 32-3 Demonstrate a Venipuncture Using the Syringe Method *(continued)*

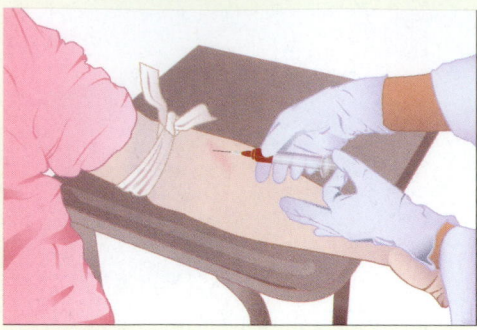

Figure 32-27 ◆ Slowly pull back the plunger of the syringe.

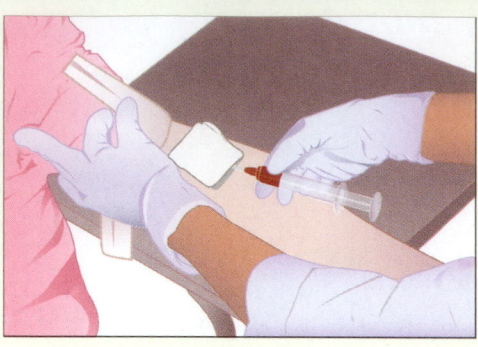

Figure 32-28 ◆ Release the tourniquet.

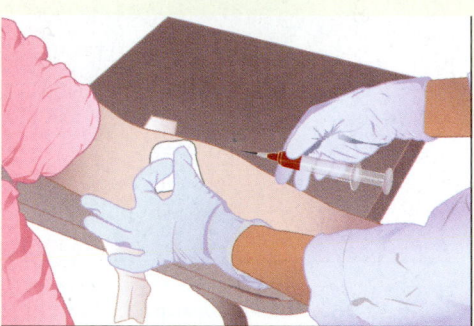

Figure 32-29 ◆ Immediately place a sterile gauze pad over the site and withdraw the needle from the patient's arm.

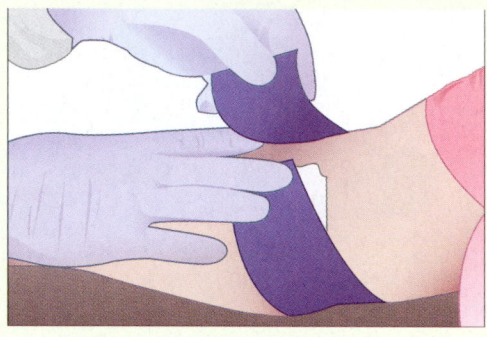

Figure 32-30 ◆ Bandage the site.

25. Remove and dispose of gloves.
26. Wash your hands.
27. Evaluate the patient for signs of faintness or color loss.
28. Complete the laboratory requisition form and route the specimen to the proper place.
29. Record the procedure in the patient's chart.

Patient Education

Instruct the patient beforehand of the general procedure. Do not promise the patient that the procedure will not hurt. It is more tactful to say that it may feel like a brief "sting." Let the patient know when the actual puncture is about to happen to avoid movement. As necessary, provide information about how long the results will take and how they will be transmitted to the patient.

Charting Example

Sometimes charting may not be required for phlebotomy procedures because laboratory processing documentation is sufficient. If charting is required, it might look like this:

6/8/XX 8:50 a.m. Pt appears calm but states that she has been told that she has small and fragile veins. General instructions given before each step. Venous specimen obtained using needle and syringe method. Obtained 15 ml of venous specimen and transferred to appropriate tubes. Pt. held pressure gauze on site, site bandaged, and pt. instructed to leave bandage in place for 15 minutes. Pt. escorted to waiting area. Maria Hernandez, CMA (AAMA)

■ Try to make unthreatening, professional statements such as "I need to collect a blood sample," rather than "I need to stick you to get some blood." Avoid telling the patient, especially a child, that the venipuncture will not hurt. Instead, use minimizing phrases such as "This will sting for a moment."

Capillary Puncture Collection

Capillary or dermal puncture collection is used with infants or small children and, in certain cases, with adults (Figure 32-31 ◆). It is performed with special lancets, usually disposable self-contained lancets with a trigger that releases the actual puncturing device. A capillary tube (stoppered with clay sealant after the specimen has been collected), microcontainer with scoop, or micropipette with dilution system may also be used to collect the specimen.

Performing a Capillary Puncture

A dermal (capillary) collection is performed when only a small amount of blood is required for testing, or when venipuncture is not appropriate, such as with infants, small children, or adults whose veins are difficult to find. Dermal collections are also recommended for burned or scarred patients, patients being monitored with a glucose monitoring device, patients with thrombotic tendencies, or patients whose veins must be saved for chemotherapy or dialysis. Skin puncture blood is a mixture of blood from arterioles, venules, capillaries, and some cellular fluids. Some chemical blood elements may differ significantly between venous and capillary blood, so it is important to document on the report whether a capillary collection was performed.

If the MA or another employee is accidentally exposed to a needle stick or puncture the directions for institutional post-exposure follow-up testing should be followed. Employers are required to provide this service. The CDC bases its recommendations for better safeguards on statistics from new disease or clinical information.

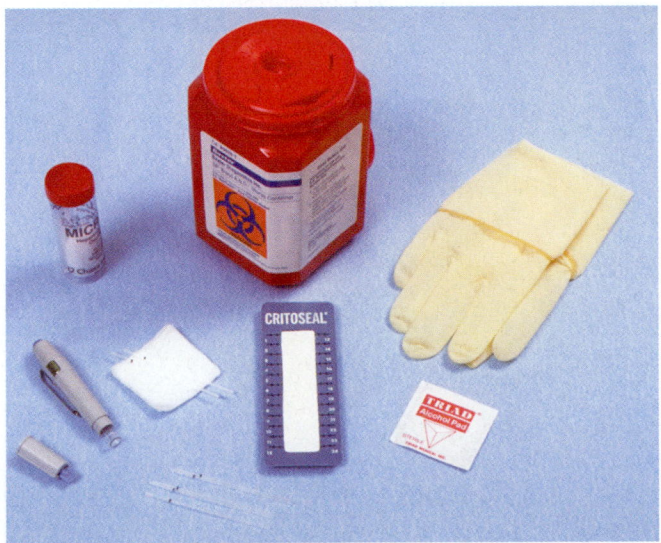

Figure 32-31 ◆ Capillary puncture equipment.

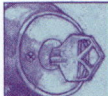

Keys to Success
SPECIAL-NEEDS BLOOD TESTING

Special considerations or adaptations of procedure should be made for the following patients.

- **Diabetics:** Before you take a blood specimen, ask the patient when he or she took diabetic medication last, and the name and dosage of the medication. Note this information on the laboratory requisition. Take blood specimens only from patients who have fasted. This is based on the fact that the test deals with glucose content of the blood. CBC, blood type, and other tests that normally do not require fasting may be drawn on a diabetic who has eaten. Ascertain whether you will need to help the patient obtain food after the test.

- **Children:** Probably the most important step is to reassure the child and parents or guardian and be truthful about the minor discomforts of the procedure. Allow parental involvement in reassuring and immobilizing the child. If the parents are more of a hindrance than a help, escort them to an adjacent room, if possible, and explain tactfully that the procedure will be less stressful for the child if they are not present. They will likely feel less anxious if they are close by.

- **Elderly patients:** Always consider how the individual has been affected by age. The patient may need assistance with transfer and ambulation. Proceed cautiously with venipuncture, as the veins may be more fragile or scarred. Smaller needles, such as the butterfly, are used more often with elderly patients, and the tourniquet may not be necessary. Elderly patients should be encouraged to carry a current list of medications and dosages with them.

- **"Bleeders":** A patient who is a hemophiliac or on anti-coagulant therapy or chemotherapy will often tell you. However, it is a good habit to scan each patient's diagnosis information before the procedure. Note on the laboratory requisition any medications, last time/dosage taken, or diagnoses that indicate bleeding tendencies. Plan extra time for pressure on and observation of the venipuncture site.

- **Difficult or other emotionally needy patients:** Start by asking the patient to state why he or she is refusing to have blood drawn. While listening to the response, remain nonjudgmental. If the patient knows the reason and it can be resolved, you will likely gain the patient's cooperation. If the patient remains difficult and uncooperative, request assistance from the supervisor or a physician. Remember, performing venipuncture on an unwilling patient would be considered battery.

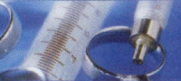

PROCEDURE 32-4 **Perform a Capillary Puncture**

Theory and Rationale

Select an age-appropriate dermal puncture site where there is no danger of contact with bone. For an infant less than 1 year old, use the medial and lateral areas of the heel (Figure 32-32 ◆). For safety and convenience, an infant should be on his or her back in a bassinet. Hold the foot firmly to avoid any sudden movement.

The preferred site for finger sticks is the middle or ring finger, halfway between the center of the ball of the finger and its side (Figure 32-33 ◆). Avoid the thumb and index finger, as the thumb has a pulse and the index finger may be more sensitive or callused. The patient must be sitting or lying down for finger sticks.

If possible, warm the puncture site. Warming increases the capillary blood flow and makes blood collection much more efficient.

After cleansing the puncture site, allow the antiseptic to dry or wipe it with clean, dry gauze. Failure to dry properly may contaminate the specimen with antiseptic, hemolyze or destroy the blood cells, or cause stinging at the puncture site.

The device used to puncture the skin is the lancet. Lancets may be either manual or automatic. The automatic lancet is designed with a spring-loaded mechanism that controls the depth of puncture, causing less pain to the patient. Choose a capillary puncturing device in an age-appropriate size. There are different sizes for infant heel sticks and for finger sticks. After a lancet is used, it should never be reused and should be immediately discarded in a sharps container.

The order of draw for capillary puncture is different than for venipuncture: lavender, other additive tubes, and red. Fill the tubes to the appropriate fill line using the collection scoop. Do not squeeze the heel or finger to obtain the sample, as squeezing releases tissue that may dilute the blood and lead to inaccurate results. Lightly touching the underside of the blood drop will prompt the blood to flow through the scoop and into the collection tube. Gently tap the tubes containing anticoagulant after each drop of blood to ensure adequate mixing. Invert each tube eight to ten times after filling.

Materials

- phlebotomy tray *or* individual items (antiseptic pads and capillary puncture and collection devices)
- handwritten or preprinted specimen labels
- disposable gloves
- sharps container

Competency

(**Conditions**) With the necessary materials, you will be able to (**Task**) demonstrate a capillary puncture (**Standards**) correctly within 15 minutes.

1. Review the physician's order (see Procedure 32-1) and prepare the laboratory requisition.
2. Gather the supplies for capillary puncture and specimen transport.

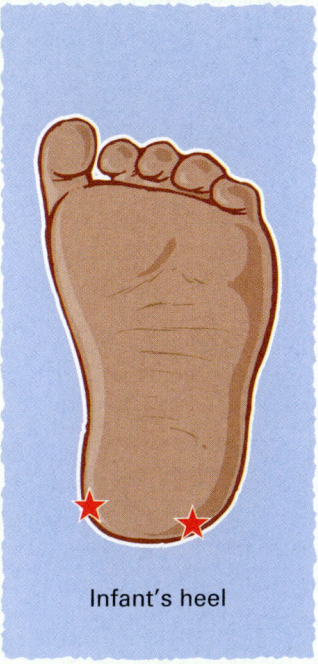

Figure 32-32 ◆ Capillary puncture site: infant's heel.

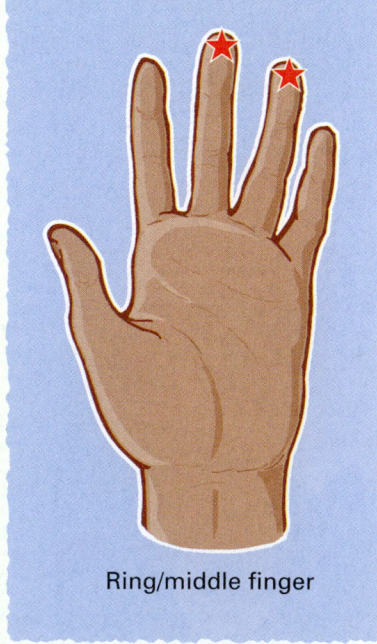

Figure 32-33 ◆ Capillary puncture site for adult: middle or ring finger.

PROCEDURE 32-4 Perform a Capillary Puncture *(continued)*

3. Wash your hands.

4. Ask the patient to state his or her name. Ask the parents or guardian of babies or young children for identification information. Escort the patient or the parent/guardian with the child to the treatment area.

5. Verify that the patient has followed test preparation instructions such as changing the diet or taking special medications and is not allergic to latex.

6. Position and reassure the patient.

7. Select an age-appropriate dermal puncture site where there is no danger of contact with bone.

8. If possible, warm the site with a warming device or a warm, moist cloth (no warmer than 40°C/105°F) for three minutes.

9. Wash your hands and put on disposable gloves.

10. Clean the site with an antiseptic wipe, usually 70 percent isopropyl alcohol. Allow the area to thoroughly air-dry, or dry it with clean gauze.

11. Choose a puncturing device of the appropriate size. Remove the safety indicator and discard it in the appropriate biohazardous waste container.

12. Place the puncturing device firmly on the prepared skin surface, so that the lancet cuts across the grooves of the finger or heel print. Press the safety trigger to release the puncturing lancet (Figure 32-34 ◆).

13. For a finger stick, massage gently from the hand to near the puncture site, keeping the hand below elbow level to obtain the required blood sample.

14. Wipe away the first drop of blood with clean gauze. The first drop contains tissue fluids and may contaminate the blood sample (Figure 32-35 ◆).

15. Follow the correct order of draw for capillary puncture specimens to fill the tubes to the fill line: lavender, the other additive tubes, then red.

16. Collect the specimen by holding the scoop of the micro-collection tube directly beneath the puncture site. Apply gentle pressure at the puncture site ends, opening the puncture slightly to maximize blood flow. (For a finger stick, apply gentle, intermittent pressure on the entire finger to allow the capillaries to refill with blood and to help ensure continuous blood flow.) (Figure 32-36 ◆)

17. Lightly touch the collection scoop to the underside of the drop of blood so that the blood flows through the scoop and into the collection tube.

18. Gently tap each tube containing anticoagulant after the addition of each drop of blood to ensure that the blood falls to the anticoagulant/blood mixture.

19. After filling the tube, invert it back and forth eight to ten times.

20. When the blood collection is complete, wipe the site dry and apply pressure with clean gauze until the bleeding stops.

21. Apply a cloth tape bandage to the puncture site.

22. Dispose of all used sharps and biohazardous waste in the appropriate containers.

23. Label each tube with the patient's first and last name, identification number, date and time of collection, and your initials or identifying code. Or, if preprinted computer labels are available, initial each label and attach the labels to the appropriate tubes.

24. Remove the disposable gloves and discard appropriately. Wash your hands.

25. Instruct the patient, or the patient's parent or guardian, to remove the bandage after at least 15 minutes. Thank the patient or parent/guardian for cooperating or assisting.

26. Escort the patient to the waiting room for further instructions.

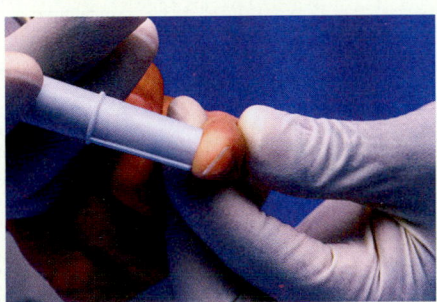

Figure 32-34 ◆ Place the injector against the site.

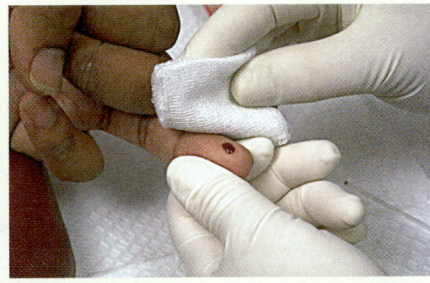

Figure 32-35 ◆ Wipe away the first drop of blood with clean gauze.

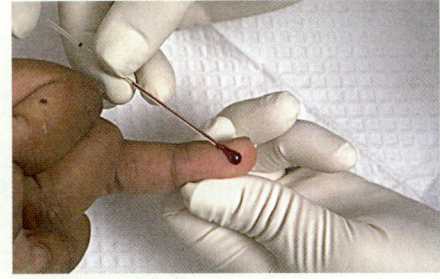

Figure 32-36 ◆ Collect the specimen using the microcollection tube.

continued

PROCEDURE 32-4 **Perform a Capillary Puncture** (continued)

Patient Education

Instruct the patient beforehand in the general procedure. Do *not* promise the patient that the procedure will not hurt. It is more tactful to say that it might feel like a "brief sting." Let the patient know when the actual puncture is about to happen. As necessary, provide information about how long the results will take and how they will be transmitted to the patient.

Charting Example

Sometimes charting is not required for phlebotomy procedures because laboratory processing documentation is sufficient. If charting is required, it might look like this:

08/25/XX 9:30 A.m. Hgb, Hct capillary specimen obtained from the ring finger of the patient's hand. Pressure applied, site checked and absent of bleeding, and bandage applied. Joan Houston, RMA (AMI)

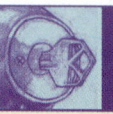

Keys to Success
MAINTAINING PATIENT CONFIDENTIALITY

Regardless of the kind of test involved, a breach of confidentiality concerning lab test results is considered *negligence*. Testing could include standard CBCs and urinalysis, but it could also include tests relating to illegal drug use or HIV. Treat all testing with the same high standard of confidentiality. All patient or employee results, chart information, and verbal and nonverbal communication must be kept between the patient and employee and/or the physician.

Keys to Success
DIAGNOSIS FROM BLOOD TESTING

Diagnostic tests such as CBC, electrolytes, and many others measure present values in the patient's venous or arterial blood. These are compared to normal blood values, which are often stated on the same laboratory report. In addition to the patient complaint associated with the office visit and the physician's examination of the patient, laboratory results confirm or rule out the presence of particular diseases. If lab results do not yield diagnostic answers, the physician may order further tests.

Also, the disease process can be monitored for progress or relapse, and treatment can be monitored for effectiveness with blood tests. For example, an antibiotic is given to treat a particular infection. A WBC can determine if the disease is present or if it is reacting correctly to the antibiotic. Drug levels can be monitored to determine if they are at therapeutic level. Other tests, such as BUN and creatinine, can determine if the treatment is affecting kidney function. (See Appendix F for Normal Blood Values/Disease Conditions evaluated for abnormal values.)

Transporting Specimens

Blood specimens are placed in an approved leakproof container, such as a sealed biohazard bag, before transport to the laboratory. The MA should be attentive to any time constraints or special handling. For instance, sedimentation rates should be performed within two hours of collection. Place the specimens in the designated location in the laboratory and make sure that laboratory staff are aware they have been delivered.

Performing Basic Laboratory Testing

The MA working in a hospital laboratory will usually be responsible only for blood collections. An MA in a physician's office laboratory will often be required to perform some basic laboratory testing. Each laboratory has a written procedure for every test performed in that laboratory. It is essential that the tests be performed *exactly* as written.

Every laboratory has its own set of reference values, sometimes referred to as "normal values," based on the patient population in its area. In addition to reference values, each laboratory also has critical values, formerly referred to as panic values, for many tests. Critical values are abnormal values that indicate a possible threat to the patient's

health status. They must be immediately communicated to the physician or healthcare professional responsible for the patient's care.

It is the responsibility of the medical assistant performing laboratory tests to make sure that any applicable quality control has been performed and that all reagents are "in date," meaning their expiration dates have not passed. Quality control is necessary to assure results as accurate as possible for all tests performed. All facets of laboratory activity must be monitored from specimen collection to processing, testing, and reporting the results. Quality control assessment includes checks of supplies, reagents, personnel, machinery, and test performance. The results of all quality control procedures must be recorded and maintained.

Basics of Hematology Testing

Basic hematology testing includes WBC counts, RBC counts, hemoglobin, hematocrit (Hct), RBC indices, and platelet counts. WBC differentials are often considered basic tests as well.

Hemoglobin and hematocrit measurements are helpful to the physician in diagnosing many conditions. An abnormally high hemoglobin value may be indicative of dehydration, and an abnormally low value may indicate anemia. Other possible implications include but are not limited to high concentration or value: polycythemia, congestive heart failure, chronic obstructive lung disease, high altitudes, or severe burns. Likewise, other possible implications include but are not limited to low concentration or value: kidney disease, excessive IV fluids, cancers, and Hodgkin's disease. Normal values for adult males are 13.5 –18 g/dL, and for adult females 12–16 g/dL.

Hematocrit values, expressed as a percentage, indicate the concentration of packed red blood cells in 100 ml of blood. Normal values for the adult male are 40–54% and for the adult female 36–46%. Decreased percentages are indicative of but not limited to acute blood loss, anemia, leukemia, Hodgkin's disease, multiple myeloma, malnutrition, bone marrow failure, chronic renal disease, vitamin B and C deficiencies, cirrhosis of the liver, pregnancy, peptic ulcer, rheumatoid arthritis, and SLE. Increased percentages are indicative of but not limited to dehydration, polycythemia vera, eclampsia, trauma, pulmonary emphysema, hypovolemia, severe diarrhea, diabetic acidosis, surgery, trauma, and transient ischemic cerebral accident (TIA).

Most POLs have an automated cell counter (Figure 32-37 ◆). This device accurately counts and sizes cells by detecting and measuring changes in electrical resistance when a cell, in a conductive liquid, passes through a small aperture. Hemoglobin concentration is determined by **spectrophotometric** methods. Hematocrit, **MCHC**, and **MCV** are calculated based on the measured RBC count, **MCH**, and hemoglobin. When using an automated counter, it is important to follow institutional as well as manufacturer's guidelines for maintenance, calibration, and quality control.

Manual Tests

The following procedures may be performed manually in a POL:

- A WBC and platelet count with a Unopette vial and hemacytometer
- A blood smear for a differentiated cell count
- A microhematocrit
- An erythrocyte sedimentation rate (ESR) using the Westergren method

Performing a WBC and Platelet Count with a Unopette Vial and Hemacytometer

When an automated counter or analyzer is not available, the MA may have to rely on manual methods to do cell counts and hematocrits. Manual cell counts are performed with a hemacytometer, a heavy glass slide with a depressed central area of precise volume

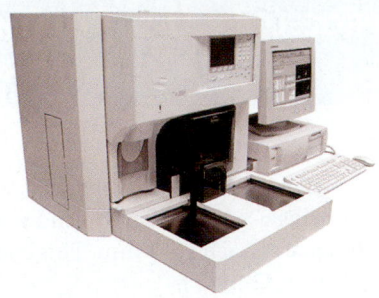

Figure 32-37 ◆ Sysmex™ automated cell counter.
Courtesy of Sysmex America.

specifications. Unopettes are vials that contain **diluent** solutions and are used to prepare blood dilutions for manual WBC and/or platelet counts. This test is no longer done on a regular basis in physician office labs. However, the basics are presented here for the practitioner who does not have access to an automated counter or analyzer.

White Blood Cell Differential

WBC differentials (diff) are a very useful diagnostic tool. Many disease states are diagnosed by the presence of certain WBC populations. For instance, increased polys and bands are found in cases of bacterial infections, appendicitis, and other disorders; infectious mononucleosis is characterized by increased numbers of atypical lymphocytes; allergy patients have higher levels of eosinophils; and, of course, immature and abnormal white blood cells are found in patients with leukemia.

In a manual diff, a drop of capillary or well-mixed EDTA anticoagulated blood is placed at the end of a glass microscope slide. A second slide is used to "push" the blood evenly to cover approximately three-quarters of the slide. The end of the blood smear must have a "feathered edge," where the blood is one cell thick (Figure 32-38 ◆). After the blood has dried, the slide is stained with Wright's stain and allowed to dry. The slide is then examined under a microscope with either the 50X or 100X oil objective. The technologist first counts 100 white blood cells as a group and then counts the 100 WBCs by type.

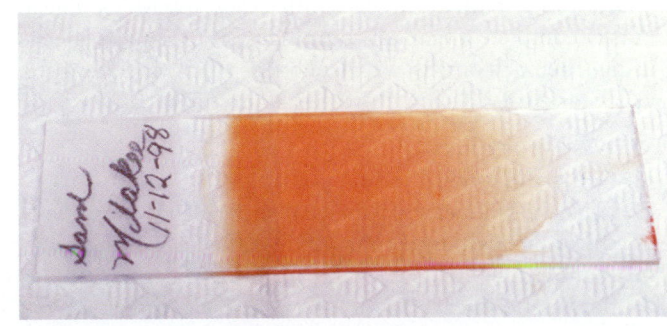

Figure 32-38 ◆ Blood smear on a slide, with feathered edge.

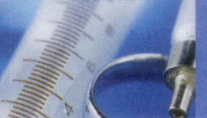

PROCEDURE 32-5 Perform a WBC and Platelet Count with a Unopette Vial and

Theory and Rationale

Most hemacytometers use the Neubauer ruling, which consists of a square measuring 3×3 mm (9 mm²) and subdivided into nine secondary squares, each 1×1 mm. This counting area is 0.1 mm deep (Figure 32-39 ◆).

When counting the WBCs and platelets, use the average count in the calculation formula. To ensure standardization and accurate results, check the laboratory's standard policy regarding the similarity of the side count numbers. Laboratory policy usually dictates that the side count numbers vary by less than 10 to 15 percent.

The 10/9 in each of the following formulas is a correction factor for the depth of the hemacytometer. For a healthy individual, the normal values of white blood cells range between 4,000 and 10,500 per cubic millimeter (mm³), and platelets range between 150,000 and 450,000/mm³.

The white blood cell calculation formula is: average count $\times$ 10/9 $\times$ 100 = WBC/mm³. For example:

$$\text{Side } 1 = 90$$
$$\text{Side } 2 = 88$$
$$\text{Average} = 89$$
$$89 \times 10/9 \times 100 = 9888.9/\text{mm}^3 \text{ or } 9.8 \times 10^3/\text{mm}^3$$

The platelet calculation formula is: average count $\times$ 9 $\times$ 10/9 $\times$ 100 = PLT/mm³. For example:

$$\text{Side } 1 = 490$$
$$\text{Side } 2 = 510$$
$$\text{Average} = 500$$
$$500 \times 9 \times 10/9 \times 100 = 500,000/\text{mm}^3$$

Materials

- Unopette vial and pipette unit
- hemacytometer with Neubauer ruling
- petri dish
- sterile gauze squares
- disposable gloves
- sharps container
- biohazardous waste container

Competency

(**Conditions**) With the necessary materials, you will be able to (**Task**) complete a manual counting of WBCs and platelets using a hemacytometer with Neubauer ruling and Unopette vial (**Standards**) accurately within 30 minutes.

1. Wash your hands.
2. Gather equipment and supplies.
3. Place the Unopette vial on a flat surface. Push the pipette shield through the diaphragm into the neck of the vial.
4. Remove the pipette assembly from the vial, then remove the pipette shield.

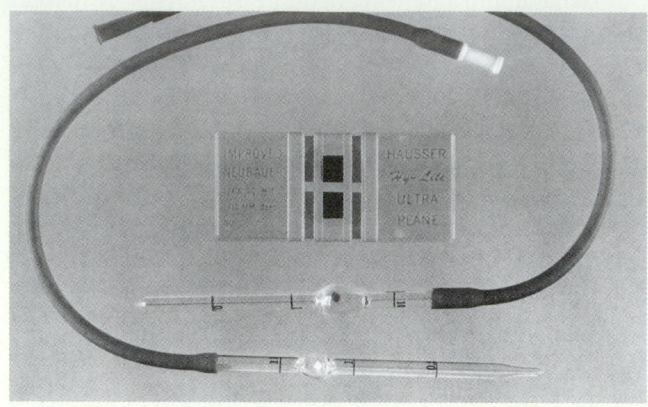

Figure 32-39 ◆ Hemacytometer.

5. Holding the pipette horizontally, touch the tip to the blood sample—venous, mixed EDTA anticoagulated, or capillary. The capillary action filling the pipette will stop when the blood reaches the capillary bore end in the pipette neck.
6. Clean any blood from the outside of the pipette, being careful not to remove any blood from the pipette bore.
7. Squeeze and maintain a slight pressure on the Unopette vial to force out air but not the liquid.
8. With your index finger, cover the opening of the pipette overflow chamber. Insert the pipette into the punctured neck opening of the Unopette vial.
9. Remove your index finger from the pipette opening. The resulting negative pressure draws blood into the diluent.
10. Rinse the capillary pipette bore by gently squeezing the vial two or three times. Thoroughly mix the blood and diluent by swirling the vial.
11. Leave the vial standing for 10 minutes to hemolyze the red blood cells.
12. Invert the vial to thoroughly remix and suspend the cells in the fluid.
13. Convert to a dropper assembly by withdrawing the pipette from the reservoir and reseating it in the reverse position.
14. Gently squeeze the sides of the vial and discard the first three or four drops. Fill the chamber of the Neubauer hemacytometer with the diluted blood.
15. Place the hemacytometer on moistened paper in a petri dish. Cover the petri dish and leave it standing for 10 minutes so the cells settle.
16. Count and calculate for WBCs and platelets:
    - For WBCs, examine under 40X microscope power with lower light. Count all the white blood cells in the nine large squares of the counting chamber. Count the opposite side in the same manner. Add both sides and divide by two to obtain the average.

PROCEDURE 32-5 Perform a WBC and Platelet Count with a Unopette Vial and Hemacytometer *(continued)*

Calculation formula: average count × 10/9 × 100 = WBC/mm³

- For platelets, examine under 40X microscope power with lower light. Count all the platelets in center secondary square of the Neubauer ruling of the counting chamber. Count the opposite side in the same manner. Add both sides and divide by two for the average.
  Calculation formula: average count × 9 × 10/9 × 100 = PLT/mm³

17. Dispose of all used sharps and biohazardous waste in the appropriate containers.
18. Remove the disposable gloves and discard appropriately. Wash your hands.

Patient Education

Instruct the patient beforehand in the general procedure. Do *not* promise the patient that the procedure will not hurt. It is more tactful to say that it might feel like a "brief sting." Let the patient know when the actual puncture is about to happen. As necessary, provide information about how long the results will take and how they will be transmitted to the patient.

Charting Example

Sometimes charting may not be required for phlebotomy procedures because laboratory processing documentation is sufficient. If charting is required, it might look like this:

08/25/XX 7:30 a.m. Pt anxious about phlebotomy procedure. General explanations given before each step. Pt voiced concern over the amount of pain she would experience and that her veins were hard to get blood from. Venous specimen obtained for a CBC, Na, K, and Cl with appropriate tubes. Pt held pressure gauze onsite, site was bandaged, and pt was instructed to leave the bandage in place for 15 minutes. Pt escorted to the exit. Barbara Nelson, CMA (AAMA)

PROCEDURE 32-6 Prepare a Blood Smear for a Differentiated Cell Count

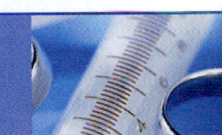

Theory and Rationale

It is important to be precise at each step of this procedure. Accurate technique ensures that the blood smear is only one cell thick, which is ideal for microscopic analysis. High-quality smears have a feathered edge without lines, holes, or ridges. Low-quality smears result from failing to spread the smear before the blood dries, using a blood drop that is too large, or smearing the specimen with a cracked or chipped slide. Resist the temptation to blow on the specimen to dry it, as this could spread biological materials into the air or affect the quality of the smear. Because fingerprints could obscure a damp smear, the slide should be labeled after the specimen has air-dried. The dry, labeled slide is placed in a protective folder and transported to the laboratory. The medical technologist evaluates the slide for quality and performs staining procedures with Wright's stain.

Materials

- materials for venipuncture or capillary puncture
- microscope
- two glass slides
- gauze squares
- disposable gloves
- sharps container
- biohazardous waste container

Competency

(**Conditions**) With the necessary materials, you will be able to (**Task**) prepare a blood smear slide for microscopic examination (**Standards**) correctly within 10 minutes.

1. Wash your hands.
2. Gather equipment and supplies.
3. Ensure that the microscope is clean and working properly.
4. Greet and the identify patient and escort him or her to the laboratory draw area.
5. Wash your hands and put on disposable gloves.
6. Obtain a drop of blood by any one of the following methods. Place the blood drop 1/2 to 1 inch from the label end of the slide (Figure 32-40 ◆).
   For a capillary puncture:
   - Puncture the skin per the capillary puncture method.
   - Wipe the first drop of blood away with a sterile gauze square.
   - Lightly touch the second drop of blood to a slide.
   For a fresh venous specimen:
   - After you withdraw the needle from the venipuncture site, immediately touch the drop of blood lightly to a slide.
   For a venous specimen from a vacutainer:
   - Place a capillary tube in the vacutainer. It will automatically draw the correct amount of blood.

continued

PROCEDURE 32-6 **Prepare a Blood Smear for a Differentiated Cell Count** (continued)

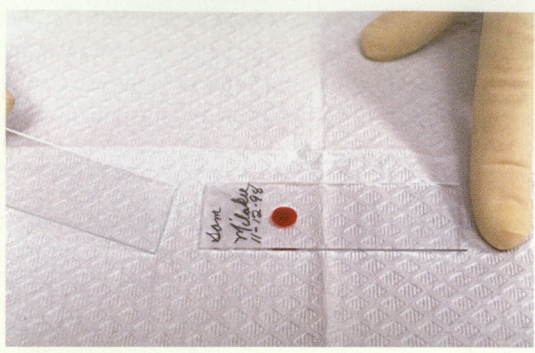

Figure 32-40 ◆ Place the blood drop 1/2 to 1 inch from the label end of the slide.

- With sterile gauze, wipe away any blood from the outside of the tube, being careful not to remove the blood from the tip.
- Lightly touch the drop of blood from the capillary tube to a slide.

7. Place the second slide lengthwise, in front of, and in contact with the drop of blood (Figure 32-41 ◆). Allow the blood to spread along the edge of the slide by capillary action.

8. At a 30-degree angle and applying only light pressure, pull the second slide toward the opposite edge of the first slide (Figure 32-42 ◆). After approximately 1 inch and as the specimen is feathering, lift the second slide in a sliding arch away from the first slide.

9. Allow the slide to air-dry.

10. Label the slide and place it next to the microscope for examination.

11. Follow institutional procedure for the cell count, which is performed by a designated individual.

12. Dispose of all used sharps and biohazardous waste in the appropriate containers.

13. Remove the disposable gloves and discard appropriately. Wash your hands.

14. Document the procedure in the chart or log per institutional procedure.

Patient Education

Instruct the patient beforehand in the general procedure. Do *not* promise the patient that the procedure will not hurt. It is more tactful to say that it might feel like a "brief sting." Let the patient know when the actual puncture is about to happen. As necessary, provide information about how long the results will take and how they will be transmitted to the patient.

Charting Example

Sometimes charting may not be required for phlebotomy procedures because laboratory processing documentation is sufficient. If charting is required, it might look like this:

08/25/XX 7:30 a.m. Pt anxious about phlebotomy procedure. General explanations given before each step. Pt voiced concern over the amount of pain she would experience and that her veins were hard to get blood from. Venous specimen obtained for a CBC, Na, K, and Cl with appropriate tubes. Pt held pressure gauze onsite, site was bandaged, and pt was instructed to leave the bandage in place for 15 minutes. Pt escorted to the exit. Shawna Phillips, RMA (AMT)

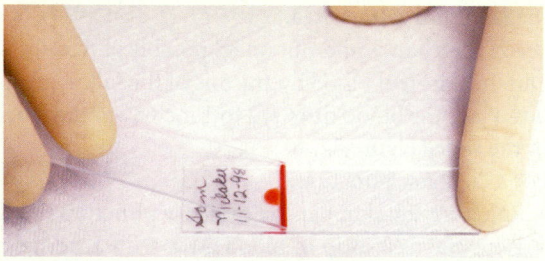

Figure 32-41 ◆ Place the second slide lengthwise, in front of, and in contact with the drop of blood.

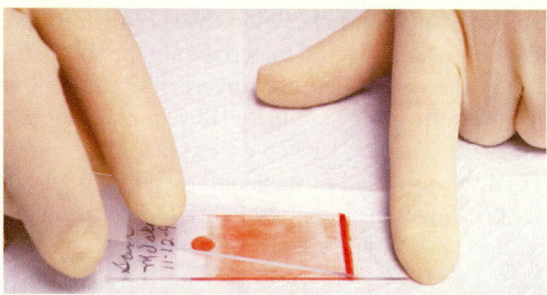

Figure 32-42 ◆ Pull the second slide toward the opposite edge of the first slide.

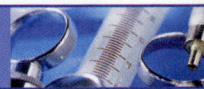

PROCEDURE 32-7 Prepare a Smear Stained with Wright's Stain

Theory and Rationale

Performing a blood smear allows the technician to view the cellular components of a blood specimen. Different stains dye different cell components different colors. Most stains contain methylene blue, a blue stain, or eosin, a red-orange stain. When the cells are stained, their structures can be easily visualized and differentiated. Wright's stain is the most commonly used differential blood stain.

Label the thick end of the smear with a pencil, not a pen. Labeling the thick end will ensure that the name does not wash off in the staining process.

Materials

- clean glass slides (more than needed, in case of a break)
- transfer device, either a pipette or a capillary tube
- blood specimen
- Wright's stain
- disposable gloves

Competency

(**Conditions**) With the necessary materials, you will be able to (**Task**) prepare a blood smear stained with Wright's stain (**Standards**) correctly within 15 minutes.

1. Have all the necessary materials in your laboratory workstation.
2. Wash your hands and put on the gloves.
3. Mix the blood sample. If it has separated, gently swirl it in the tube.
4. With a pipette, take a small sample of the blood and drop it on the slide, approximately 1/4 inch from the end of the slide.
5. Hold the end of the slide with one hand. With your other hand, place the other slide directly in front of the blood specimen at a 30-degree angle.
6. Pull the spreader slide back into the drop of blood, just until contact is made. This will cause the blood to spread out along the edge of the slide in a thin line. You should be pulling the blood back toward the closer end of the slide.
7. To avoid air bubbles, push the spreader slide back toward the opposite end of the slide in a quick, smooth motion, being careful to maintain the 30-degree angle.
8. Allow the slide to dry.
9. When the slide is dry, label the thick end of the smear with a pencil.
10. Place the slide on a staining rack with the blood side up (Figure 32-43 ◆). Flood the smear with Wright's stain (Figure 32-44 ◆).
11. Follow the instructions for the waiting time, generally 1 to 3 minutes.
12. Add a buffer in an amount equivalent to the Wright's stain. Mix the stain and buffer and blow gently on the mixture for several minutes until a green, metallic sheen appears.

13. Rinse the slide completely with distilled water (Figure 32-45 ◆).
14. Allow the excess water to drain off the slide and stand it on end to allow it to dry.

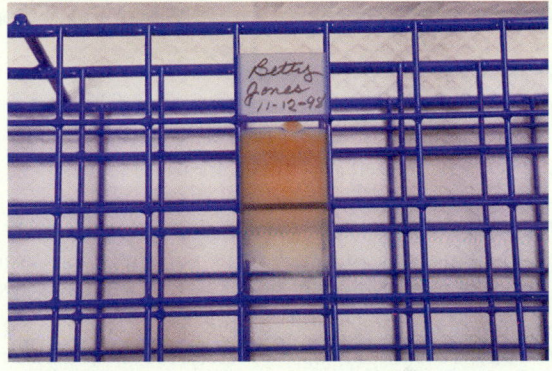

Figure 32-43 ◆ Place the slide on a staining rack with the blood side up.

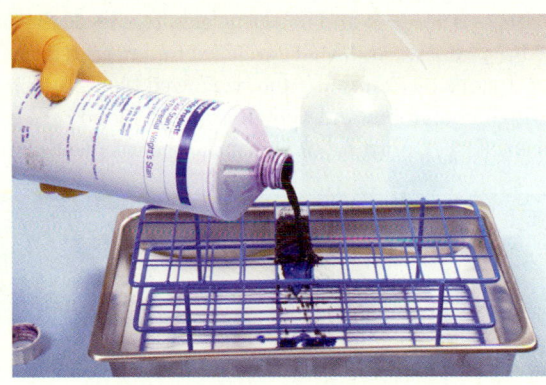

Figure 32-44 ◆ Flood the smear with Wright's stain.

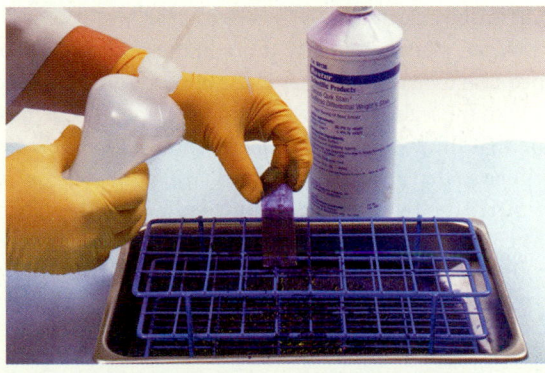

Figure 32-45 ◆ Rinse the slide with distilled water.

continued

PROCEDURE 32-7 Prepare a Smear Stained with Wright's Stain (continued)

Patient Education

Let the patient know that although the staining will be done immediately, the results will not be available until they have been reviewed by the physician. Give the patient a time frame in which to expect the test results.

Charting Example

09/05/XX 12:05 PM Wright's stain prepared for examination using 2-step method. Ellen Woods, CMA (AAMA)

Preparing a Blood Smear

Blood smears are made from venous or arterial blood for the purpose of examination under the microscope. Fresh drops of blood or anticoagulated specimens are used.

Manual Hematocrit

A blood hematocrit is defined as the volume of erythrocytes (RBCs) in a given volume of blood and is usually measured as a percentage of the total blood volume. A hematocrit is a quick, easy test and is commonly used to screen for anemia. In a manual hematocrit, a blood-filled capillary tube is rapidly centrifuged, which packs the erythrocytes at the bottom.

The patient's age affects normal values for hematocrit. Adults have higher values than children. Normal values vary among institutions, but the generally accepted range for hematocrits in normal adult females is 36–46% and in normal adult males 40–54%.

MCV, MCHC, and MCH are used to differentiate specific types of anemia by examining the size of red blood cells and by measuring hemoglobin and hematocrit. Red blood cells can be macrocytic (large), normocytic (normal), and microcytic (small).

RBCs with normal amounts of hemoglobin and normal color are normochromic. In anemic states, RBCs may be hypochromic (having less than normal color). MCV indicates the size of the red blood cells, MCHC measures the average RBC hemoglobin concentration, and MCH measures the average hemoglobin weight in each red blood cell. The MCHC is considered most accurate because both hemoglobin and hematocrit are used in the calculation of the diagnostic value. Types of anemia include pernicious anemia, with macrocytic RBCs; aplastic anemia, with normocytic, normochromic RBCs; and iron deficiency anemia, with microcytic RBCs.

Erythrocyte Sedimentation Rate

The ESR or sed rate is useful in monitoring the progression of disease processes. The blood test results are standardized by using calibrated Wintrobe tubes and mixing the anticoagulated blood specimen before the procedure. When well-mixed blood is placed in a vertical tube, erythrocytes settle out or "sediment." The sedimentation process in the healthy person is slow, but the sedimentation rate increases at an accelerated rate in disease processes, depending on the severity of the disease. A greater

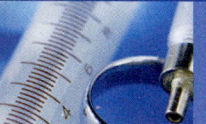

PROCEDURE 32-8 Perform a Microhematocrit by Capillary Tube

Theory and Rationale

The centrifuged capillary tube is placed on a reading device and the volume of packed red blood cells is compared to the total amount of blood (RBC, WBC, platelets, and plasma) in the tube. There are several microhematocrit methods; the following is one example.

When placing capillary tubes in the centrifuge, counterbalance each tube with another in the opposite position. Place the tubes with the sealant side away from the center. These measures ensure that the specimen is properly spun. Close the lid of the centrifuge so that any accidental breakage of tubes is contained.

After the two- to five-minute spin, turn the centrifuge off. After it has stopped spinning, open the lid. Read the results from the line created between the plasma and the blood cells.

Materials

- heparinized capillary tubes
- microhematocrit centrifuge
- microhematocrit reader
- tube sealer or sealing clay
- gauze squares
- disposable gloves
- sharps container
- biohazardous waste container

Competency

(**Conditions**) With the necessary materials, you will be able to (**Task**) perform a microhematocrit (**Standards**) correctly within 15 minutes.

PROCEDURE 32-8 Perform a Microhematocrit by Capillary Tube *(continued)*

1. Wash your hands.
2. Gather equipment and supplies.
3. Greet and identify the patient and escort him or her to the laboratory draw area. Explain the procedure.
4. Wash your hands and put on disposable gloves.
5. Perform a capillary puncture or venipuncture.
6. Fill a capillary tube with capillary or well-mixed anticoagulated blood approximately three-quarters full.
7. Wipe excess blood off the outside of the tube.
8. Repeat steps 6 and 7. You will use the second tube as a counterbalance weight in the centrifuge or as a second test to confirm the accuracy of the results (Figure 32-46 ◆).
9. Holding each capillary tube by its sides, place the blood-filled end in the sealing clay to form a plug. Pull the tube straight up and out of the sealing clay.
10. Place the capillary tubes in the microhematocrit head grooves opposite each other. Make sure the sealed ends of the tubes face away from the center of the centrifuge and are touching the outside rim of the centrifuge head.
11. Attach and secure the lid of the centrifuge.
12. Centrifuge the capillary tubes at 12,000 RPM for the optimum time stated on the instrument, usually 2 to 5 minutes.
13. Remove the capillary tubes after the centrifuge has stopped spinning.
14. Place one centrifuged capillary tube into the groove on the clear plastic piece of the microhematocrit reader with the plug end toward the reader bottom center. The reference line near the top of the groove should be under the separation line in the capillary tube where the clay plug and the RBCs meet.
15. Rotate the bottom of the reader plate so that the metal stop on the outer rim makes contact with the left edge of the grooved piece.
16. Holding the bottom plate steady, rotate the top plate to align the outer edge of the spiral line with the outer edge of the plasma meniscus.
17. Rotate the entire bottom portion of the reader clockwise until the spiral line intersects the line separating the buffy coat and plasma layer.
18. Read the results on the ruled scale where the red line intersects it.
19. Dispose of all used sharps and biohazardous waste in the appropriate containers.
20. Remove the disposable gloves and discard appropriately. Wash your hands.
21. Document the percentage results on the laboratory requisition or other designated area of the chart.

Patient Education

Instruct the patient beforehand in the general procedure. Do *not* promise the patient that the procedure will not hurt. It is more tactful to say that it might feel like a "brief sting." Let the patient know when the actual puncture is about to happen. As necessary, provide information about how long the results will take and how they will be transmitted to the patient.

Charting Example

Sometimes charting may not be required for phlebotomy procedures because laboratory processing documentation is sufficient. If charting is required, it might look like this:

08/25/XX 7:30 a.m. Pt anxious about phlebotomy procedure. General explanations given before each step. Pt voiced concern over the amount of pain she would experience and that her veins were hard to get blood from. Venous specimen obtained for a CBC, Na, K, and Cl with appropriate tubes. Pt held pressure gauze onsite, site was bandaged, and pt was instructed to leave the bandage in place for 15 minutes. Pt escorted to the exit. Kelly Abrams, CMA (AAMA)

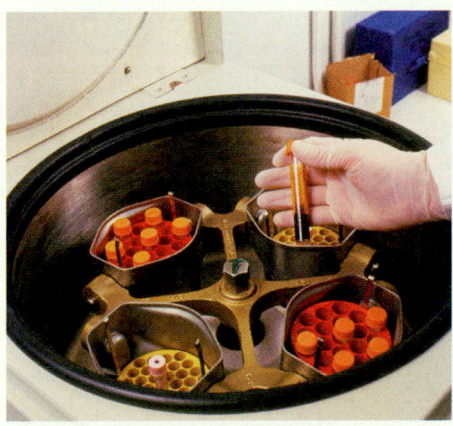

Figure 32-46 ◆ Loading a centrifuge.

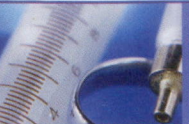

PROCEDURE 32-9 Perform a Hemoglobin Test Using a Hemoglobulinometer

Theory and Rationale

Hemoglobin (Hgb) is the functioning unit of the red blood cell. There are millions of hemoglobin molecules in each RBC. Hemoglobin testing provides the physician with information regarding the amount of hemoglobin that is present in the blood sample. The normal range for hemoglobin is 13 to 18 g/dl (or g/100 mL) in men and 12 to 16 g/dL in women. A low Hgb may indicate iron-deficiency anemia.

Materials

- hemoglobinometer
- applicator sticks
- whole blood sample (by capillary puncture)
- gloves
- biohazard waste container
- patient record

Competency

(**Conditions**) With the necessary materials, you will be able to (**Task**) perform a hemoglobin test using a Hemoglobinometer (**Standards**) correctly within the time designated by your instructor.

1. Wash your hands and assemble equipment and supplies.
2. Put on gloves.
3. Obtain a blood specimen from the patient by capillary puncture following the steps outlined in Procedure 32-4.
4. Place well-mixed whole blood into the hemoglobinometer chamber as described by the manufacturer.

5. Slide the chamber into the hemoglobinometer.
6. Remove gloves and discard.
7. Wash your hands.
8. Record the hemoglobin level in the patient's record.

NOTE: This procedure will vary with the instrument. Always follow the manufacturer's instructions exactly to ensure adherence to the appropriate testing guidelines. In addition to the hemoglobinometer, there are other point-of-care methods approved for hemoglobin testing such as the HemoCue System Hemoglobin Analyzer.

Patient Education

Instruct the patient beforehand of the general procedure. Do not promise the patient that the procedure will not hurt. It is more tactful to say that it may feel like a "brief sting." Let the patient know when the actual puncture is about to happen to avoid movement. As necessary, provide information about how long the results will take and how they will be transmitted to the patient.

Charting Example

Sometimes charting may not be required for phlebotomy procedures because laboratory processing documentation is sufficient. If charting is required, it might look like this:

6/26/XX 1:50 p.m. Capillary puncture L ring finger. Patient tolerated procedure well. Hgb 13 g/DL. Dr. Jones notified of results. Rita Wilson, RMA (AMT)

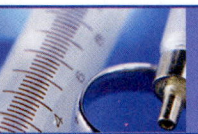

PROCEDURE 32-10 Perform an ESR Using the Westergren Method

Theory and Rationale

A well-mixed anticoagulated blood sample is drawn into a Westergren tube and left upright for an hour. The full length of red cells from the top of the column in that hour is the erythrocyte sedimentation rate, or sed rate. Reference ranges vary among institutions, but the generally accepted reference range is 0 to 20 mm/hr for women and 0 to 15 mm/hr for men.

Materials

- ESR kit (Sediplast ESR System)
- EDTA anticoagulated patient blood sample
- gauze square
- disposable gloves

- biohazard waste container
- sharps container
- patient record

Competency

(**Conditions**) With the necessary materials, you will be able to (**Task**) demonstrate performing an ESR using the Westergren method (**Standards**) correctly in one hour.

1. Wash your hands.
2. Gather equipment and supplies.
3. Greet and identify the patient and escort him or her to the laboratory draw area. Explain the procedure.

PROCEDURE 32-10 Perform an ESR Using the Westergren Method *(continued)*

4. Wash your hands and put on your gloves and PPE.

5. Perform a venipuncture and obtain an EDTA-anticoagulated tube of patient blood; gently mix the anticoagulation tube for 2 minutes.

6. Remove the stopper on the prefilled vial included with the Sediplast ESR System. Fill the vial to the indicated line with blood.

7. Replace the stopper and invert several times to mix.

8. Insert the pipette through the pierceable stopper, and push down until the pipette touches the bottom of the vial. The pipette will autozero the blood and any excess with flow into the closed reservoir compartment.

9. Let the pipette stand for one hour, then read the numerical results of the ESR.

10. Dispose of all used sharps and biohazardous waste in the appropriate containers.

11. Remove the disposable gloves and discard appropriately. Wash your hands.

12. Document the sed rate in mm/hr on the laboratory requisition or other designated area of the chart.

Patient Education

Instruct the patient beforehand in the general procedure. Do *not* promise the patient that the procedure will not hurt. It is more tactful to say that it might feel like a "brief sting." Let the patient know when the actual puncture is about to happen. As necessary, provide information about how long the results will take and how they will be transmitted to the patient.

Charting Example

Sometimes charting may not be required for phlebotomy procedures because laboratory processing documentation is sufficient. If charting is required, it might look like this:

08/25/XX 7:30 a.m. Pt anxious about phlebotomy procedure. General explanations given before each step. Pt voiced concern over the amount of pain she would experience and that her veins were hard to get blood from. Venous specimen obtained for a CBC, Na, K, and Cl with appropriate tubes. Pt held pressure gauze onsite, site was bandaged, and pt was instructed to leave the bandage in place for 15 minutes. Pt escorted to the exit. Robert Larin, RMA (AMT)

---

tendency of the RBCs to sediment is commonly found in inflammatory disorders such as subacute bacterial endocarditis, rheumatic fever, rheumatoid arthritis, and pelvic inflammatory disease, as well as in other disease conditions such as respiratory infections, pulmonary embolism, and cancer. There are several methods for performing sed rates, including some automated methods. Manual methods include the Westergren method, the Zeta sedimentation rate, and the Wintrobe method.

Blood Chemistry Testing

There are hundreds of blood chemistry tests that aid in clinical diagnosis. The most commonly performed are tests for blood glucose levels, glycosylated hemoglobin, electrolytes (sodium, potassium, chloride, and CO_2), creatinine, BUN, total protein, albumin, and bilirubin levels. Some tests are very useful as a relatively rapid diagnostic tool, such as those for CPK and troponin I, which are elevated in cases of heart attack. Liver function tests and lipid profiles are also considered important in the diagnosis or monitoring of diseases. These tests and the importance of their values are discussed in appropriate chapters. It is important to remember that reference laboratories have different values for the testing they do. Suggested values will be referenced in chapters in which the disease or condition applicable to them are discussed.

Laboratories often combine commonly ordered groups of tests into a chemistry panel. For instance, glucose, electrolytes, BUN, and creatinine may be combined into a test panel called a basic metabolic panel. Test panels may also be organized based on organ function. For example, a liver function panel could consist of total bilirubin, serum glutamic oxaloacetic transaminase (SGOT), and serum glutamic pyruvic transaminase (SGPT).

Automated Chemistry Analyzers

A wide variety of automated chemistry analyzers are available. Many are programmed to perform specific organ panels or chemistry profiles, or individual chemistry tests on each sample. These analyzers are designed for use in hospital or reference laboratory settings and require sophisticated calibration and quality control protocols. They are maintained and operated by trained technologists.

Other analyzers are designed to perform a single test and can be operated by a patient or MA at the patient's bedside (point-of-care testing). A glucometer is the most common point-of-care analyzer, and you will be expected to know how to operate it. Portable cholesterol monitors are also commonly used and are operated in much the same way glucometers are.

Measuring Blood Glucose

Many types of glucometers are available for patient use. The timing of each step in the procedure contributes to the accuracy of the test results. Some monitors require waiting for the blood to soak into the test strip before placing it in the glucometer for reading. With other glucometers there is a waiting period as the blood moistens and reacts with the strip, and then excess blood is

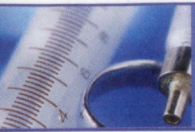

PROCEDURE 32-11 Measure Blood Glucose Using Accu-Chek™ Glucometer

Theory and Rationale

The light of the glucometer passes through the test strip to read the blood glucose level. Do not let the strip touch the patient's skin when you obtain the specimen, because oils from the skin may affect the test results. Also, to maintain accuracy, make sure the blood drop completely covers the specimen square on the strip.

Some patients may complain of pain after the capillary puncture. To ease discomfort, instruct the patient to hold a 2 × 2 gauze firmly against the site for a few minutes. Normal values vary among institutions, but the generally accepted normal range for adults is 70–110 mg/dl, and 30–70 mg/dl for newborns.

New glucometers appear on the market frequently. Newer models can process testing faster, use less blood supply, and store results in memory. Glucometers also store memory of the patient test strips used. Whichever model is used at home or in the POL, the glucometer must be calibrated and tested for accuracy with control solutions and calibration test strips. In your patient instruction, reinforce the importance of following the manufacturer's directions to ensure accuracy. Following instructions becomes even more important if the patient changes glucometer models.

Materials

- Accu-Chek™ glucometer
- Accu-Chek™ test strips
- glucose control solutions
- puncture device
- sterile 2 × 2 gauze
- disposable gloves
- sharps container
- biohazardous waste container

Competency

(**Conditions**) With the necessary materials, you will be able to (**Task**) measure blood glucose with a glucometer and record patient results (**Standards**) correctly within 15 minutes.

1. Wash your hands.
2. Gather equipment and supplies.
3. Verify that calibration and quality control have been performed and are acceptable.
4. Greet and identify the patient and escort him or her to the laboratory draw area. Explain the procedure.
5. Wash your hands and put on disposable gloves.
6. Check the expiration date on the test strip bottle. Obtain a different bottle if the expiration date has passed.
7. Turn on the glucometer by pressing the ON button (Figure 32-47 ◆).
8. Follow the manufacturer's directions for entering the three-digit test-strip code in the display if the glucometer code does not match the code on the test strip bottle (Figure 32-48 ◆).
9. Enter the patient identification number. (Home glucometers may not require this information.)
10. Wait for the indicator that the monitor is ready for a test strip. Within the short time frame specified by the glucometer model, insert one test strip as directed into the monitor (Figure 32-49 ◆).
11. Remove the monitor from the charging station.
12. Obtain a capillary blood specimen from the patient following standard procedure for capillary blood collections. Venous or arterial specimens may also be used.
13. Touch the edge of the test strip to the drop of blood. The blood will be pulled into the strip. Fill the target area of the strip completely (Figure 32-50 ◆).
14. The glucose result will appear in the time frame specified by the manufacturer, usually within 30 seconds (Figure 32-51 ◆).
15. Remove the test strip and discard in a biohazard container. Dispose of the lancet or blade in the sharps container.
16. Return the monitor to the charging/storage unit.
17. Remove the disposable gloves and discard appropriately. Wash your hands.
18. Document the date, time, finger used, patient's tolerance of the procedure, and results in the designated area of the chart.

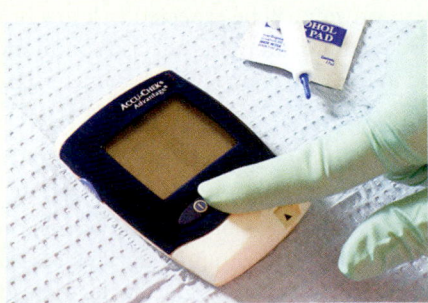

Figure 32-47 ◆ Turn on the glucometer.

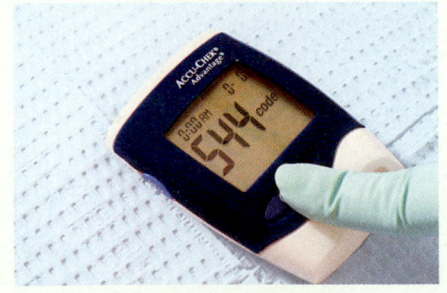

Figure 32-48 ◆ Enter the three-digit test code.

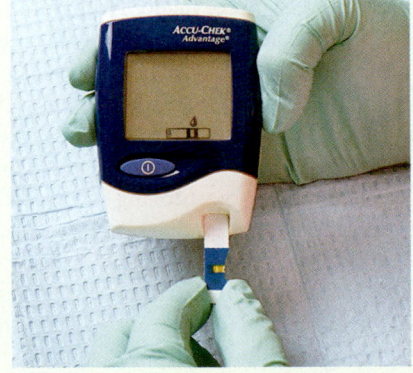

Figure 32-49 ◆ Insert one test strip into the monitor as directed.

PROCEDURE 32-11 Measure Blood Glucose Using Accu-Chek™ Glucometer (continued)

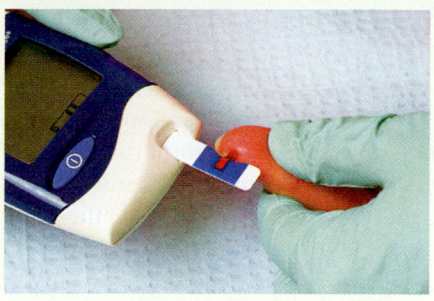

Figure 32-50 ◆ Touch the edge of the test strip to the drop of blood.

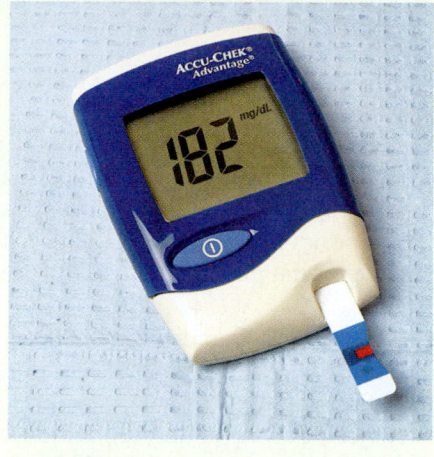

Figure 32-51 ◆ Glucose results.

Patient Education

Instruct the patient beforehand in the general procedure. Do *not* promise the procedure will not hurt. It is more tactful to say that it might feel like a "short sting."

Teach the patient to keep a record of home testing with the glucometer or to monitor the stored results in the memory of the glucometer. The patient should document the date, time, results, and symptoms if the results are above or below normal limits. The physician will refer to these records at the next office visit to make any necessary insulin or dietary adjustments.

Charting Example

Sometimes charting may not be required for phlebotomy procedures because laboratory processing documentation is sufficient. If charting is required, it might look like this:

08/25/XX 8:30 a.m. General explanation given before each step. Glucometer screening completed as ordered by physician. Capillary puncture left middle finger. Results of fasting blood sugar: 60 mg/dL. Physician notified. Gregory Fuller, RMA (AMT)

PROCEDURE 32-12 Perform a Blood Cholesterol Measurement Using the ProAct Testing Device

Theory and Rationale

High cholesterol levels have been linked to stroke and heart disease. As part of their overall health maintenance, patients should understand the importance of regular cholesterol testing. They should know their cholesterol numbers, including HDL and LDL, and how to improve them.

In 2001, in response to continuing high rates of heart disease, the National Heart, Lung and Blood Institute of the National Institutes of Health issued new guidelines for cholesterol levels. According to the new guidelines, total cholesterol is less important than HDL and LDL cholesterol numbers.

Materials

■ ProAct testing device
■ capillary tube containing lithium heparin
■ lancet device
■ 2 × 2 gauze pads, sterile
■ alcohol pads
■ disposable gloves
■ patient's chart

Competency

(**Conditions**) With the necessary materials, you will be able to (**Task**) measure cholesterol level using a ProAct testing device (**Standards**) correctly within 15 minutes.

1. Wash your hands and put on the gloves.
2. Verify the physician's order and the patient's identity. Explain the procedure to the patient.
3. Load the lancet device according to the directions.
4. Choose a puncture site free of broken skin or bruising.

continued

PROCEDURE 32-12 Perform a Blood Cholesterol Measurement Using the ProAct Testing Device *(continued)*

5. Wipe the patient's finger with an alcohol wipe and allow to dry.

6. Puncture the finger and wipe away the first drop of blood that forms with the sterile gauze.

7. Hold the capillary tube horizontal to the patient's finger, making sure no air bubbles enter the tube. If air bubbles enter, you must throw away the tube and start over again.

8. When the tube has filled, remove it and have the patient put pressure on the puncture site with a sterile gauze square.

9. Remove a testing strip from the container and peel away the protective foil. Place the strip on a hard work surface.

10. Attach the filled capillary tube to the pipette.

11. Without touching the tip of the capillary tube to the testing strip, place one drop in the center of the application zone (Figure 32-52 ◆).

12. Allow the blood droplet to soak into the testing mesh for 15 to 20 seconds.

13. Place the strip in the ProAct device port (Figure 32-53 ◆). The device will start to count down approximately 160 seconds.

14. While the machine is running, clean the test area. Throw the pipette and capillary tube into a sharps container.

15. When the LED screen indicates, remove the test strip and observe it for uneven color development. (If the color is uneven, you will need to perform the entire test again.)

16. Discard the test strip into a biohazardous container.

17. Record the test results as displayed in the patient's chart.

Patient Education

Give the patient the cholesterol results after the physician has reviewed them, along with verbal and written dietary recommendations to help improve the patient's overall cholesterol numbers.

Charting Example

09/05/XX 12:05 PM Cholesterol level obtained using ProAct device. Patient reported no additional bleeding from puncture site and a pain level of 1/10. Cholesterol level reported to physician for analysis and lab report letter sent to patient with dietary recommendations. Jackie Chin, CMA (AAMA)

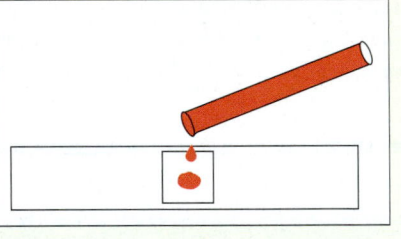

Figure 32-52 ◆ Place one drop in the center of the application zone.

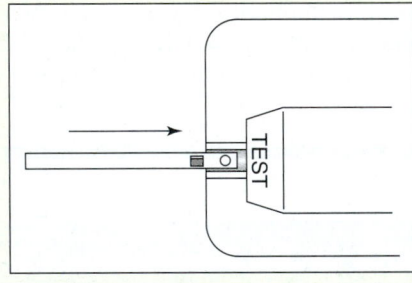

Figure 32-53 ◆ Place the strip in the ProAct device port.

removed before the strip is placed in the glucometer. Because of these timing and procedural differences, always follow the manufacturer's directions for the particular model you are working with.

General instructions for an Accu-Chek™ glucose monitor are given in the Procedure 32-11. Follow the quality control and calibration guidelines of your healthcare institution before using any glucometer. Perform calibration each time a new lot number of test strips is put into use. Refer to the user's manual for calibration and quality control instructions as well as for care and maintenance recommendations.

Measuring Blood Cholesterol

Cell membranes hold a fatty substance known as cholesterol. Cholesterol is a substance necessary for the formation of bile

acids and hormones. Diet, caloric intake, physical activity, and family heritage all play a factor in the amount of cholesterol formed in the body. It is important for patients to understand that there are different types of cholesterol: the type that comes from the foods we eat and the type that is produced in the body. LDL cholesterol is considered "bad" cholesterol, and lower blood levels indicate a lower risk of heart disease. When too much LDL cholesterol builds up, it sticks to the walls of the arteries, decreasing the blood flow to the heart and brain. HDL cholesterol is "good" cholesterol, and higher levels are beneficial to health. HDL cholesterol binds to LDL cholesterol, moves it away from the heart and brain, and deposits it in the liver, where it can be processed and passed from the body. Too low a level of HDL cholesterol indicates a greater risk of heart attack.

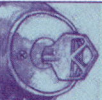

Keys to Success
HOME DISPOSAL OF SHARPS

Instruct a patient using puncture devices and syringes at home that these devices must be disposed of carefully, in a strong, puncture-resistant container. A hard plastic detergent container is an example of a safe container.

TABLE 32-3 BLOOD GROUP INTERPRETATION OF SLIDE REACTIONS

Anti-A	Anti-B	Blood Group
Negative	Negative	O
Positive	Negative	A
Negative	Positive	B
Positive	Positive	AB

In Practice

Karen Smith states that she was recently at a health fair at the mall and she had her cholesterol checked and it was 310. She wants to know what the difference is between "good" and "bad" cholesterol. She also wants to know what she can do to lower her cholesterol. What type of patient education information should you as the medical assistant provide?

Blood Typing and Grouping

When a blood group antigen and its corresponding antibody unite, agglutination (clumping) is the result. This reaction is the basis for the blood typing procedure. Commercially available antiserum (antibody) is mixed with whole blood. Agglutination is considered a positive reaction; it indicates that the antigen corresponding to the antiserum is present on the tested red blood cells. The absence of agglutination is considered a negative reaction, indicating that the antigen corresponding to the testing antiserum is absent on the RBCs.

Transfusions are compatible when the recipient's blood does not have antibodies that interact with the donor's blood antigens. Type A blood has A antigens and anti-B antibodies. If type A blood were given to a patient with type B blood, the antibodies present would cause a transfusion reaction. Similarly, Type B blood contains B antigens and anti-A antibodies. If type B blood were given to a patient with type A blood, the anti-A antibodies would cause a transfusion reaction. Type AB blood has both A and B antigens but lacks antibodies and is known as the "universal recipient." A transfusion patient with type AB blood can receive any blood type. Type O blood has neither the A nor B antigen, but it does have anti-A and anti-B antibodies. Type O blood is known as "universal donor" because it can be transfused to any receiving patient regardless of blood type—it lacks antigens to interact with antibodies in type A, B, or AB blood.

Most immunohematology testing is performed in laboratories by specially trained technologists. Some office laboratories, however, offer slide blood typing. Table 32-3 includes blood group interpretation of slide reactions.

Immunology Testing

Test kits are used in immunology testing, including tests for infectious mononucleosis, rheumatoid arthritis, and antistreptolysin O (ASO). One of the most commonly requested immunology tests is that for infectious mono.

PROCEDURE 32-13 Perform a Test for Infectious Mononucleosis

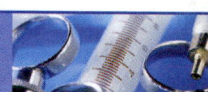

Theory and Rationale
Once called the "kissing disease," mononucleosis is an acute infectious disease caused by the Epstein-Barr virus (EBV). EBV is a common virus worldwide. It is a member of the herpes virus family, although it has nothing to do with cold sores or genital herpes. A person can contract EBV and never have been infected with any other herpes virus. EBV most frequently infects people between 10 and 25 years of age. Symptoms such as swollen tonsils, sore throat, fever, and swollen lymph nodes that may last only a few days are often indistinguishable from those of other mild illnesses. For this reason, EBV infection is not always recognized. Infectious mononucleosis is almost never fatal but can lead to serious complications such as heart problems or swollen spleen and liver.

Materials
■ Mono-Test kit
■ nonsterile disposable gloves

■ blood serum or plasma
■ disposable capillary tube

Competency
(**Conditions**) With the necessary materials, you will be able to (**Task**) test for infectious mononucleosis (**Standards**) correctly within 15 minutes.

1. Bring all liquid reagents to room temperature. Check the expiration date of all reagents in the kit.
2. Wash and dry your hands and put on disposable gloves.
3. After obtaining a blood sample from the patient and processing it to separate the serum, fill the capillary tube to the marked line with the serum.
4. Using the glass slide and rubber bulb in the kit, place a small drop of the specimen serum in the first of the three circles on the slide.
5. Place a single drop of the negative control in the second circle on the slide.

continued

PROCEDURE 32-13 Perform a Test for Infectious Mononucleosis *(continued)*

6. Place a single drop of the positive control in the third circle.

7. Holding the bottle of Mono-Test reagent upright between your palms, gently roll it back and forth, making certain that the reagent RBCs that have settled in the tube are mixed thoroughly.

8. Hold the dropper 1 inch above the slide and place one drop of reagent into each of the three circles. Make certain the dropper does not come into contact with the slide and become contaminated.

9. Using the enclosed stirrers, one for each circle, quickly and thoroughly mix each area and spread it out to the full 1-inch diameter of the circle.

10. Observe the slide as you rock it back and forth gently for exactly 2 minutes.

11. Agglutination is a positive test result; no agglutination is negative. Verify the test results by comparing them to the positive and negative controls on the slide.

12. Clean the work area, disposing of the test in a biohazardous container. Wash your hands.

13. Record the test results.

Patient Education

If the test results are positive, the patient should know what to expect over the standard course of infectious mononucleosis. Advise the patient to get plenty of rest, use throat lozenges to soothe sore throat, and take acetaminophen (such as Tylenol) or ibuprofen (such as Advil) to reduce fever and relieve sore throat and headaches, as prescribed by the physician. The feeling of weakness and fatigue may take weeks to subside and for some people can last several months. The patient should avoid heavy lifting and excessive physical activity until energy levels return to normal.

Charting Example

04-8-XX 4:28 p.m. Patient presented with acute fatigue, swollen lymph nodes, and aching muscles. Mono-Spot test was ordered and results were positive for EBV. Patient was given written and verbal instructions for care and released. Beth Loman, RMA (AMT)

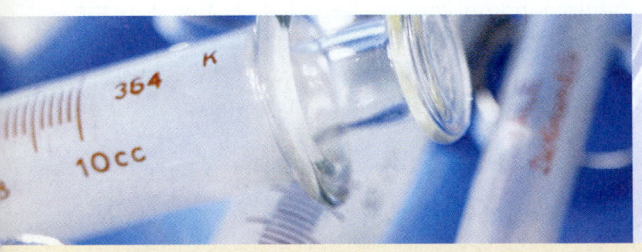

REVIEW

Chapter Summary

- A medical assistant plays a vital role in the laboratory. Key preparation steps before blood collection include checking the doctor's orders for clarity and completeness, preparing the laboratory requisition, checking supplies, identifying the patient, verifying patient preparation, and seating the patient.

- Blood consists of plasma and cellular elements: RBCs, WBCs, and platelets. The RBCs contain hemoglobin, which transports oxygen through the body. The RBCs are also the site of the blood group antigens. WBCs play an important role in the body's immune defenses and in the defense against infectious disease. Platelets function primarily in blood clotting. A variety of blood chemistry, immunology, and coagulation tests may be performed with plasma or serum.

- There are several types of blood collection tubes. The type of anticoagulant contained in each tube is indicated by the color of the stopper and written on the label. The order of collection using these tubes is important, as there may be some carryover from one tube to the next that could result in erroneous lab results. Different types and sizes of puncture devices are used in blood collection, depending on the size and accessibility of the patient's veins and the amount of blood required.

- The most common venipuncture site is the antecubital fossa. Other sites are hand veins and sometimes foot veins. In some cases blood may be collected from finger sticks, or heel sticks in infants.

- Key steps in actual blood collection are to make the patient as comfortable as possible, wash your hands, use appropriate personal protection equipment, and prepare the appropriate collection device. Apply the tourniquet, select the actual site, clean the venipuncture site with antiseptic and avoid retouching the site before sticking, fill tubes in the correct order of draw, mix tubes containing anticoagulant, release the tourniquet before removing the needle, and apply firm pressure to

Chapter Summary (continued)

the site until the bleeding stops. Dispose of all sharps immediately and appropriately. Similar steps are followed for capillary punctures. Label all tubes with the patient's name, date and time of collection, and your initials. Some laboratories require the patient's medical record number on each tube as well.

■ A hemacytometer is used for a manual WBC and platelet count. A microhematocrit is performed by spinning capillary tubes in a centrifuge and placing them on a reading device. The ESR can be measured using the Wintrobe method. A glucometer is a hand-held chemistry analyzer used by the patient at home and by healthcare professionals. Automated cell counters and chemistry analyzers reduce the chances of human error and are preferred over manual methods of testing.

■ Every laboratory or medical office has specific written procedures in place for each test it performs. It is important to follow each laboratory's procedure exactly as written for specimen quality, test standardization, accurate results, and the health and safety of patient and personnel.

Chapter Review

Multiple Choice

1. The most common WBCs are
   a. PMNs.
   b. lymphocytes.
   c. eosinophils.
   d. basophils.

2. The main function of platelets in blood is to
   a. ingest bacteria.
   b. transport oxygen.
   c. form blood clots.
   d. respond to allergies.

3. Which of the following tubes must be drawn first because of potential anticoagulant carryover?
   a. Green top
   b. Blue top
   c. Red top
   d. Lavender top

4. It is safe to leave a tourniquet on a patient for
   a. 3 minutes.
   b. 5 minutes.
   c. 6 minutes.
   d. 1 minute.

5. Which of the following methods for collecting blood is the best to use with infants?
   a. Capillary puncture
   b. Winged infusion
   c. Needle and syringe
   d. Evacuated tube

6. The preferred site for a finger stick is the
   a. thumb.
   b. index finger.
   c. little or pinkie finger.
   d. middle finger.

7. Normal values for hematocrit in adults range from
   a. 10 to 20 percent.
   b. 32 to 48 percent.
   c. 60 to 65 percent.
   d. 21 to 26 percent.

8. The ESR is used most commonly for
   a. diagnosing allergies.
   b. detecting anemia.
   c. monitoring disease progression.
   d. diagnosing bacterial infections.

9. Which of the following blood groups tests positive for both anti-A and anti-B reagents?
   a. AB
   b. A
   c. B
   d. O

10. When collecting blood from an elderly person, you should
    a. use smaller needles because the veins may be more fragile.
    b. securely tighten the tourniquet because the arm is smaller.
    c. do the procedure as quickly as possible.
    d. avoid requesting a list of medications.

True/False

T F 1. RBCs may have varying amounts of hemoglobin.

T F 2. Hematocrit is the protein-iron bond substance in red blood cells that carries oxygen from the lungs to the cells and transports carbon dioxide from the cells to the lungs.

T F 3. Vacutainer collections are recommended for burned or scarred patients.

T F 4. Dermal collections are recommended for children and the elderly.

T F 5. You can obtain a blood sample from the side on which a mastectomy was performed.

T F 6. You cannot obtain a blood sample from or near burned areas, which are very susceptible to infection.

T F 7. Plasma appears light yellow when it is separated from the cells by centrifugation.

T F 8. Unopettes are vials that contain diluent solutions and are used to prepare blood dilutions for manual WBC and/or platelet counts.

Chapter Review (continued)

T F 9. An abnormally high hemoglobin value may be indicative of dehydration, and an abnormally low value may be indicative of anemia.

T F 10. A glucometer is the most common point-of-care analyzer.

Short Answer

1. How is Type O blood different from other blood types in terms of antigens and antibodies?

2. Name the cellular elements in blood.

3. What do hematocrit values indicate?

4. Why should the thumb and forefinger be avoided for finger sticks?

5. What is the ESR or sed rate used for?

Research

1. What are the five vacutainer tubes most commonly used in phlebotomy?

2. What is the normal range of RBCs in men and women? What factors influence that number?

Externship Application Experience

As an extern, this is the first day you will perform phlebotomy in the laboratory section of this clinical site. You observe that the MA is not following the order of draw that you have been taught. What should you do?

Resource Guide

American Academy of Family Physicians
Office Lab Proficiency Testing
1-800-274-7911
www.aafp.org/pt.xml

American Diabetes Association
ATTN: National Call Center
1701 North Beauregard Street
Alexandria, VA 22311
1-800-DIABETES
www.diabetes.org/

American Medical Technologists
710 Higgins Road
Park Ridge, IL 60068
1-800-275-1268
www.amt1.com

Clinical Laboratory Improvement Amendments
www.cms.hhs.gov/clia/

National Accrediting Agency for Clinical Laboratory Sciences
8410 W. Bryn Mawr Ave. Suite 670
Chicago, IL 60631
www.naacls.org

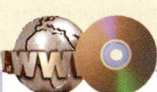

Med**Media**

http://www.MyMAKit.com

More on this chapter, including interactive resources, can be found on the Student CD-ROM accompanying this textbook and on http://www.MyMAKit.com.

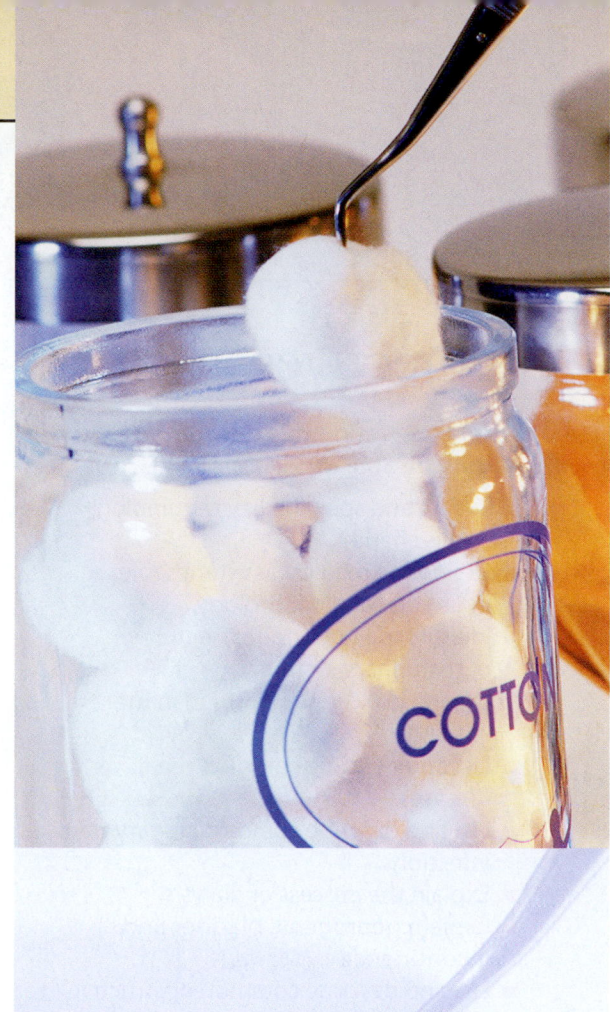

UNIT **X**

Medical Specialties and Testing

Chapter 33   **Urology and Nephrology**

Chapter 34   **Medical Imaging**

Chapter 35   **Cardiology and Cardiac Testing**

Chapter 36   **Pulmonology and Pulmonary Testing**

Chapter 37   **EENT**

Chapter 38   **Immunology and Allergies**

Chapter 39   **Dermatology**

Chapter 40   **Endocrinology**

Chapter 41   **Emergency Care**

Chapter 42   **Gastroenterology and Nutrition**

Chapter 43   **Orthopedics and Physical Therapy**

Chapter 44   **Obstetrics and Gynecology**

Chapter 45   **Pediatrics**

Chapter 46   **Neurology**

Chapter 47   **Mental Health**

Chapter 48   **Oncology**

Chapter 49   **Geriatrics**

My name is April Minger and I currently work for a medical group where I have the opportunity to work for seven physicians and two physician's assistants. I have a lot of responsibility working for a medical group; working with so many different physicians means being flexible and able to multitask and think on your feet. I perform EKGs, treadmill stress tests, and placement of Holter monitors on a regular basis. I schedule patients for surgical procedures such as heart catheters and pacemakers. I also aid physicians with pre- and postoperative procedures. I prepare numerous laboratory specimens for the physicians. I perform many urinalyses and give countless injections such as hepatitis A and B, tetanus, TB skin test, vitamin B-12, and many more.

Being a medical assistant is both rewarding and challenging. The gratification I feel from knowing that I have in some small way touched the life of someone else, just by doing what I love to do, is remarkable.

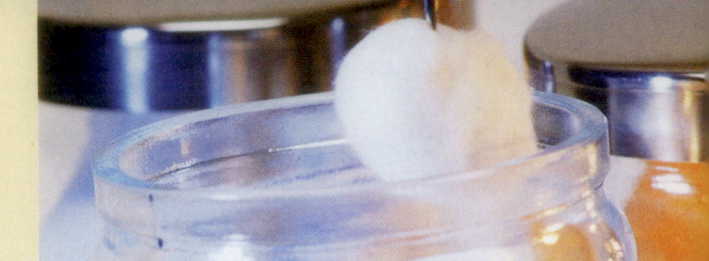

CHAPTER 33

Urology and Nephrology

Case Study

Gina has been given instructions that each of the pregnant women at her externship site are to leave a clean-catch urine sample prior to being seen by the doctor. It is Gina's responsibility to ask each patient to leave a sample after checking in and to give them collection instructions. One patient mentions that she has experienced greater urinary frequency in the last two weeks than during the rest of her pregnancy and that it has become painful to empty her bladder. She also admits that she is nervous about telling anyone because she thinks she may have caused it and that there will be no safe treatment for her due to the pregnancy.

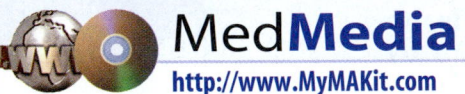

MedMedia

http://www.MyMAKit.com

Additional interactive resources and activities for this chapter can be found on http://www.MyMAKit.com. For a video, tips, audio glossary, legal and ethical scenarios, job scenarios, quizzes, games, virtual tours, and activities related to the content of this chapter, please access the accompanying CD-ROM in this book.

Video: *Urinalysis*
Audio Glossary
Legal and Ethical Scenario: *Urology and Nephrology*
On the Job Scenario: *Urology and Nephrology*
Tips
A & P Quiz: *The Urinary System*
Multiple Choice Quiz
Games: Crossword, Strikeout and Spelling Bee
3D Virtual Tour: Reproductive System: Male Reproductive System; Urinary System: The Urinary System
Drag & Drop: Urinary System: Kidney Structure
HIPAA Quiz

Objectives

After completing this chapter, you should be able to:

- Define and spell the key terminology in this chapter.
- Define the medical assistant's role in urology and nephrology.
- Identify the important structures of the urinary system.
- Explain how urine is formed in the kidneys.
- List and describe common renal diseases.
- List and describe common urinary tract infections.
- Explain the process of dialysis.
- Explain neurogenic bladder and incontinence.
- List and describe common obstructive disorders of the urinary system.
- Discuss the procedures used in the diagnosis of urinary diseases and disorders.
- Explain the methods of urine specimen collection.
- List the characteristics of a normal physical urinalysis.
- Explain the principles of the chemical test strips used in urinalysis.
- Discuss the findings of the microscopic examination of urine.
- Identify the important structures of the male reproductive system.
- List and describe the diseases and disorders of the male reproductive system.

✚ MEDICAL ASSISTING STANDARDS

CAAHEP ENTRY-LEVEL STANDARDS	ABHES ENTRY-LEVEL COMPETENCIES
■ Perform within scope of practice (psychomotor) ■ Apply ethical behaviors, including honesty/integrity in performance of medical assisting practice (affective) ■ Explore issue of confidentiality as it applies to the medical assistant (cognitive) ■ Document accurately in the patient record (psychomotor) ■ Display sensitivity to patient rights and feelings in collecting specimens (affective) ■ Explain the rationale for performance of a procedure to the patient (affective) ■ Perform handwashing (psychomotor) ■ Practice Standard Precautions (psychomotor) ■ Perform chemistry testing (psychomotor) ■ Screen test results (psychomotor) ■ Prepare a patient for procedures and/or treatments (psychomotor) ■ Describe the normal function of each body system (cognitive) ■ Identify common pathology related to each body system (cognitive) ■ Analyze pathology as it relates to the interaction of body systems (cognitive) ■ Discuss implications for disease and disability when homeostasis is not maintained (cognitive) ■ Describe implications for treatment related to pathology (cognitive) ■ Apply critical thinking skills in performing patient assessment and care (affective) ■ Perform urinalysis (psychomotor) ■ Perform quality control measures (psychomotor) ■ Perform CLIA waived microbiology testing (psychomotor)	■ Project a positive attitude. ■ Maintain confidentiality at all times. ■ Be a "team player." ■ Be cognizant of ethical boundaries. ■ Exhibit initiative. ■ Adapt to change. ■ Evidence a responsible attitude. ■ Be courteous and diplomatic. ■ Conduct work within scope of education, training, and ability. ■ Practice Standard Precautions. ■ Use quality control. ■ Collect and process specimens. ■ Dispose of biohazardous materials. ■ Collect and process specimens. ■ Instruct patients in the collection of a clean-catch midstream urine specimen.

✓ COMPETENCY SKILLS PERFORMANCE

1. Demonstrate patient instruction for collecting a clean-catch urine specimen.
2. Demonstrate patient instruction for collecting a 24-hour urine specimen.
3. Perform catheterization of a female patient.
4. Perform catheterization of a male patient.
5. Measure urine specific gravity with a refractometer.
6. Perform urinalysis using chemical test strips.
7. Perform a multidrug screen urine test using the Instant-View Multi-Drug Screen Test.
8. Demonstrate patient instruction for testicular self-examination.

Key Terminology

aliquot—representative sample of a well-mixed specimen

anuria—absence of urine

bilirubin—substance formed by breakdown of hemoglobin

cryptorchism (also cryptorchidism)—a condition in which one or both of the testes fail to descend into the scrotal sac during fetal development

cystitis—inflammation of the urinary bladder

dialysis—cleansing of waste products from the blood with a dialysis machine, or dialyzer

distal tubule—farthest tubule from the glomerulus

electrolytes—ionized substances in blood, cells, and tissues

fistula—abnormal tubelike structure connecting one body structure to another or to the surface of the body

flank—region in the lateral aspect of the midback, between the ribs and the upper border of the ilium

glomerulonephritis—inflammation and possible infection of the glomerulus

glomerulus—tuft or cluster of capillaries inside the capsule of the nephron

hematuria—blood in the urine

hydronephrosis—enlargement of the kidney caused by retention of urine due to an obstruction

incontinence—involuntary leakage of urine or feces

jaundice—yellow color in the skin and mucous membranes

kidney—one of two bean-shaped organs located retroperitoneally that filter blood, remove waste products, and manufacture urine

lithotripsy—breaking up a renal calculus with ultrasound waves aimed at the calculus from outside the body

nephrologist—physician specializing in the treatment of kidney diseases and conditions

nephrology—study of the kidney and the diseases that affect it

nephrons—microscopic tubular structures of the kidney

nocturia—increased urine output at night

oliguria—diminished urine output, less than 400 ml per day

periorbital edema—abnormal, excessive fluid surrounding the eye that usually occurs in the morning upon waking

Key Terminology *(continued)*

plasmapheresis—daily replacement of blood plasma in the body with other fluids or donated plasma for two or more weeks

polyuria—excessive urine production and frequent, urgent, and excessive urinary output

prodromal—pertaining to the initial stage of a disease, before symptoms appear

prostatitis—inflammation and/or infection of the prostate gland

proteinuria—presence of abnormally large amounts of protein in the urine

proximal tubule—tubule closest to glomerulus

pyelonephritis—inflammation of the pelvis or the kidney

pyuria—pus in the urine

renal—pertaining to the kidney

renal calculus (plural: calculi)—kidney stone

sequela (plural: sequelae)—outcome

testis (plural testes, also called testicle)—oval structure in the scrotal sac that produces sperm

trigone—triangular area in floor of urinary bladder where ureters enter and urethra exits

turbidity—cloudiness, lack of clarity

ureter—tube leading from the kidney to the urinary bladder

urethra—tube leading from urinary bladder to outside the body

urinalysis—visual and chemical examination of the urine

urinary bladder—receptacle for urine that has been manufactured by the kidneys

urinary meatus—external sphincter of the urethra

urobilinogen—derivative substance formed by conversion of direct bilirubin by bacteria in the intestinal tract

urologist—physician who specializes in treating urinary system diseases and conditions, as well as conditions involving the male reproductive system

urology—study of the urinary system in males and females and the diseases that affect it

Abbreviations

BPH—benign prostatic hypertrophy
DRE—digital rectal examination

ESRD—end stage renal disease
UA—urinalysis

UTI—urinary tract infection

Introduction

A combined urology and nephrology practice treats patients with any disease or disorder of the urinary system and kidneys. **Urology** is the study of the urinary system and diseases that affect it; the **urologist** specializes in treating urinary system diseases and conditions as well as conditions involving the male reproductive system. **Nephrology** is the study of diseases of the kidney; a **nephrologist** is a physician specializing in diseases and disorders of the kidney.

Urinary system diseases and disorders include changes in the structure and function of the kidneys; problems arising in the ureters, bladder, and urethra; chemical or traumatic insult to any parts of the system; and the effects of other disease processes on the urinary tract. Disorders of the male reproductive system include fertility problems, erectile dysfunction, prostate conditions, and sexually transmitted diseases. Infectious processes can affect both systems.

Urinalysis (UA), the physical and chemical examination of urine, provides physicians with information not only about a patient's **renal** function but also about his or her physiology. Although urine is a fluid that is easy to collect and examine, tests must be performed carefully and under controlled conditions to ensure accurate results.

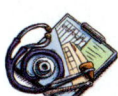

The Medical Assistant's Role in Urology and Nephrology

The MA in the urology/nephrology office will encounter patients of all ages. Some may present with seemingly minor or trivial problems, while others may have life-threatening conditions. The medical assistant will obtain a medical history, especially relating to the current complaint; vital signs; and specimens, as indicated. The MA will assist the physician. After proper training, the MA will perform chemical strip testing and some microscopic examination of specimens. Advanced training is required for catheterization.

The Anatomy and Physiology of the Urinary System

The urinary system is composed of four primary structures: the **kidneys, ureters, urinary bladder, urethra** (Figure 33-1 ◆). The human kidney is fist-sized and bean-shaped. Kidneys are well supplied with blood from the renal arteries. Blood circulating through the kidneys is filtered to remove toxins, water, sugar, urea, and certain salts. Each kidney is divided into:

- An outer layer, the cortex, where the bulk of the urine-forming tissue is located
- An inner medulla, where the urine is collected for drainage to the urinary bladder

Urine is produced from blood plasma by a system of **nephrons,** microscopic processing tubules in each kidney. Each kidney contains approximately one million nephrons. Once formed, the urine is collected by a system of internal pipes, the collecting ducts, and drained by another pipe, the ureter. The ureters deliver the urine to the urinary bladder for storage. The urine enters the bladder at the **trigone,** where both ureters enter and the urethra exits the bladder. When the smooth muscle of the bladder contracts, usually under the voluntary control of the central nervous system, the urine is delivered to the external environment through the urethra and the **urinary meatus.**

Kidney Function

In addition to the excretion of waste molecules, the kidneys have three other important physiological functions:

1. Maintaining the body's water balance by adjusting the amount of water in the urine.

2. Maintaining the acid-base balance of the body by adjusting the amount of acid.
3. Producing two internal regulatory substances, erythropoietin and renin.

The kidneys are secondary endocrine organs. Erythropoietin is a hormone that stimulates the red bone marrow to generate more red blood cells. Individuals with serious kidney disease often develop secondary anemia because the damaged kidneys do not produce adequate amounts of erythropoietin. Renin is an enzyme that activates angiotensin, a hormone involved in a complex regulatory process that maintains adequate blood volume and blood pressure.

Nephrons

The nephron (Figure 33-2 ◆) is a microscopic tubular structure connected at one end to the arterial blood supply of the kidney, and at the other end to the urine drainage system. Each nephron consists of five structural parts:

- The **glomerulus,** tuft or cluster of capillaries inside the capsule of the nephron, also called Bowman's capsule
- The **proximal tubule,** the tubule closest to the glomerulus
- The loop of the nephron, also called the loop of Henle
- The **distal tubule,** the tubule farthest from the glomerulus
- The collecting ducts

Each region of the nephron plays a major role in the kidney formation of urine. The three major activities of the nephron in the formation of urine are filtration, reabsorption, and secretion. Filtration of substances from the blood, including water, takes place in the glomerulus. The proximal tubule begins the reabsorption process by reabsorbing water,

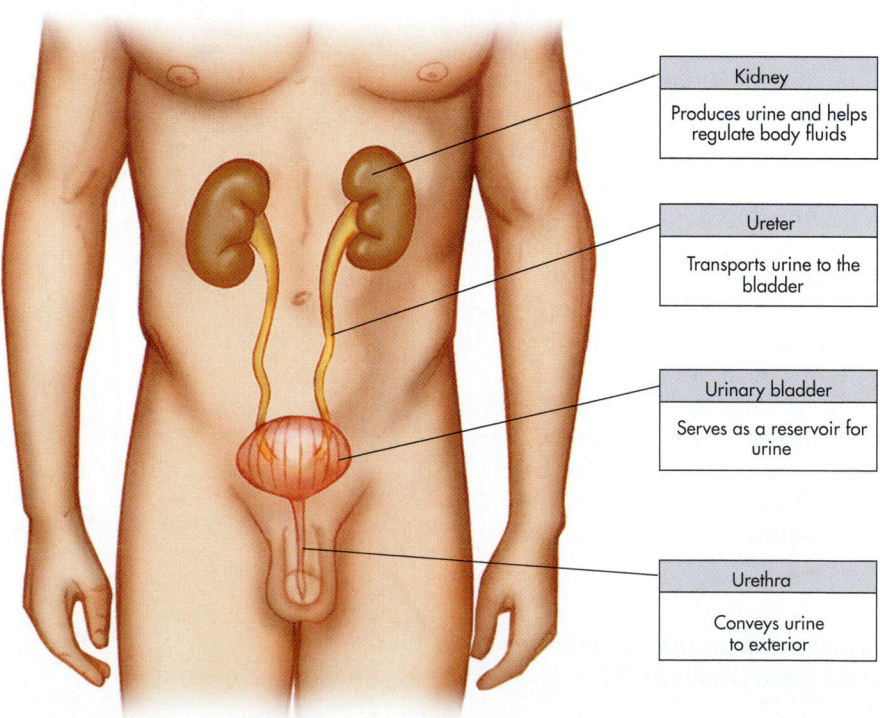

| Kidney |
| Produces urine and helps regulate body fluids |

| Ureter |
| Transports urine to the bladder |

| Urinary bladder |
| Serves as a reservoir for urine |

| Urethra |
| Conveys urine to exterior |

Figure 33-1 ◆ The urinary system.

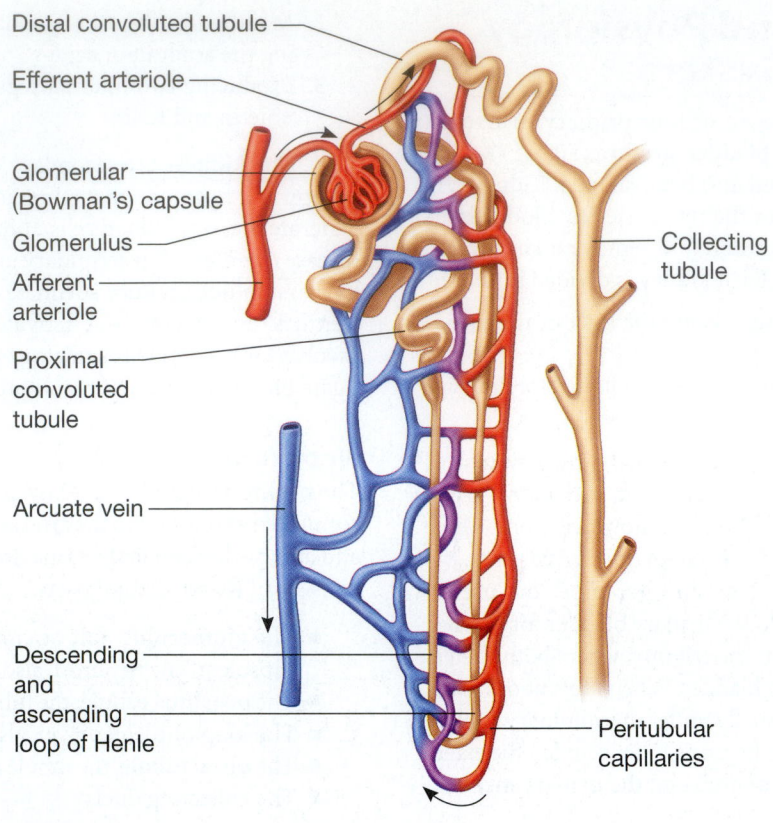

Figure 33-2 ◆ The structure of a nephron.

sodium ions, and chloride ions. Glucose, other simple sugars, amino acids, potassium, vitamins, calcium magnesium bicarbonate, phosphates, urea, and lipid soluble materials are also absorbed. Secretion of hydrogen ions, ammonium ions, and creatinine occurs in the proximal tubule. The loop of the nephron continues the reabsorption of water and sodium and chloride ions. A small amount of water is reabsorbed in the distal tubule, along with some sodium, chloride, and bicarbonate ions. Secretion of hydrogen ions, ammonium ions, creatinine, some drugs, and toxins occurs in the distal tubule. The collecting ducts continue reabsorption of water, sodium ions, bicarbonate ions, and urea under the stimulation of ADH (anti-diuretic hormone). Potassium and hydrogen ions are secreted in the collecting ducts.

Specific types of hematology testing (blood studies and chemistries) can reflect kidney function by measuring the reabsorption of certain components. Conversely, urine testing can reflect kidney function by measuring amounts of certain components that are excreted rather than reabsorbed.

Urine Formation

Urine formation is a complex process that can be broken down into five contributing functions (Figure 33-3 ◆):

1. Renal blood supply
2. Glomerular filtration

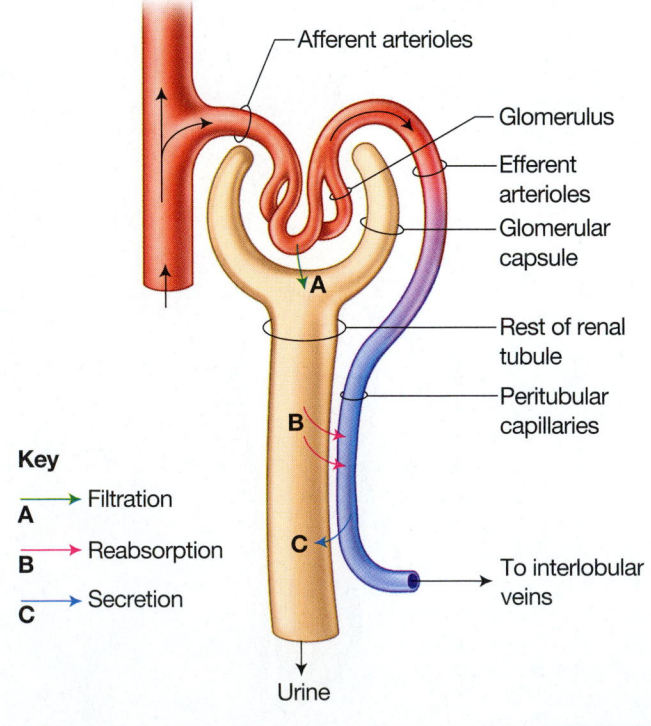

Key

A → Filtration

B → Reabsorption

C → Secretion

Figure 33-3 ◆ Schematic view of urine production: (a) filtration; (b) reabsorption; (c) secretion.

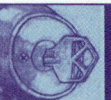

Keys to Success
USING FUNCTIONING NAMES

The structures sometimes called the loop of Henle and Bowman's capsule were named after the physicians who identified them. Modern science has dropped this naming convention and these structures are now referred to as the loop of the nephron and the glomerular capsule. The trend in medicine today is to refer to anatomical structures, equipment, or accessories by their functioning names.

3. Tubular reabsorption
4. Tubular secretion
5. Water conservation

In reality, all these functions operate at the same time and influence one another. The kidneys are capable of self-regulation at the level of the cells of the nephron, but they also receive regulatory commands from the central nervous and endocrine systems.

The wastes carried by urine are individual molecules dissolved in water. The major types of waste found in urine are molecules absorbed from meals that were of no use to the body or were in excess of the body's nutritional needs or generated as metabolic byproducts of the many biochemical pathways of the body.

Some of these molecules are charged ions, termed salts or **electrolytes.** Examples are hydrogen, sodium, potassium, calcium, chloride, bicarbonate, sulphate, and phosphate ions. Other excreted molecules are organic, carbon-based compounds, such as sugars, amino acids, vitamins, hormones, organic acids, and alkaloids. One special group of important compounds is nitrogenous wastes, metabolic byproducts of protein and nucleic acid breakdown. The four main nitrogenous waste compounds are:

■ Urea
■ Uric acid
■ Creatinine
■ Ammonium salts

Measured over the course of a day and with adequate water intake, a normal person produces approximately 1-1/2 to 2 liters of urine. Heavy physical exertion, exposure to a hot environment, or fever can lead to unusual water loss by profuse sweating. Also, illness with vomiting and/or diarrhea can cause water loss. These conditions might reduce urinary output by 90 percent, generating as little as 150 ml of urine in a day, and still maintain a satisfactory water balance. The kidneys do their job and are not overly stressed. If water loss exceeds a person's ability to replenish lost water, the kidneys attempt to conserve water by lowering the urine volume even more. Kidney damage may occur alongside the negative consequences of dehydration.

Urinary System Infections

The urinary system is a common site for infectious processes (Table 33-1). Many infections of the urethra and bladder migrate upward to the pelvis of the kidney, causing **pyelonephritis.** In the female patient, **cystitis** may be caused

TABLE 33-1 INFECTIONS OF THE URINARY SYSTEM

Infection	Symptoms	Diagnosis	Treatment
Urethritis ■ Infection of urethra ■ Usually transmitted by sexual contact ■ In males, gonococcus is frequent source of infection ■ Often accompanied by cystitis in females	■ Frequent and painful urination ■ Pus in urine ■ Penile discharge in males	■ Patient presenting symptoms ■ Urinalysis	■ Antibiotics to treat infection
Cystitis ■ Inflammation of urinary bladder caused by bacteria ■ More commonly found in women because of shorter urethra and proximity of meatal opening to vagina and rectum, which tends to increase risk of contamination ■ Common source is *E. coli,* which is spread through fecal matter in the process of wiping after a bowel movement ■ Sexual intercourse is another source of infection	■ **Polyuria** ■ **Pyuria** ■ Hematuria ■ Malodorous urine ■ Burning during urination ■ Pressure in lower abdomen ■ Lower back pain	■ Patient presenting symptoms ■ Urinalysis ■ Blood test	■ Antibiotics for infection ■ Eight glasses of water per day to lower urine concentration ■ Voiding after sexual intercourse to eliminate microorganisms from lower urinary tract ■ Wiping from front to back after urination to prevent spread of fecal matter to urethera

continued

TABLE 33-1 INFECTIONS OF THE URINARY SYSTEM (CONTINUED)

Infection	Symptoms	Diagnosis	Treatment
Acute pyelonephritis/ nephritis ■ Infection of renal medulla and upper urinary tract ■ Develops from untreated bladder infections, usually in women, which progress upward to involve renal pelvis but rarely invade nephrons ■ Recurrences are common	■ Frequent urination ■ **Flank** and lumbar back pain ■ Pyuria ■ Cloudy urine ■ High fever ■ Chills ■ Burning during urination	■ Patient presenting symptoms ■ Patient history ■ Urinalysis ■ Microscopic examination	■ Antibiotics for infection
Chronic pyelonephritis ■ Long-standing infection of renal medulla and upper urinary tract ■ Untreated, may involve nephrons and urine-collecting duct system and progress to uremia and renal failure ■ Scarring of kidneys may occur, reducing overall kidney function	■ Frequent urination ■ Flank and lumbar back pain ■ Cloudy urine ■ Blood in urine ■ High fever ■ Chills ■ Burning during urination ■ Hypertension	■ Patient presenting symptoms ■ Patient history ■ Urinalysis ■ Microscopic examination ■ Blood test ■ Intravenous pyelogram (IVP) ■ CT scan of abdomen	■ Long-term antibiotic treatment to prevent kidney damage
Uremia ■ Toxic condition resulting from kidney failure or insufficiency ■ Kidneys do not remove nitrogenous substances from blood	■ Nausea ■ Vomiting ■ Diminished vision ■ Coma, convulsions, stupor ■ Elevated blood pressure ■ Urine odor in breath ■ Dry skin ■ Oliguria	■ Patient presenting symptoms ■ Reduced amounts of urea in urine	■ Dialysis

by the introduction of bacteria following sexual relations or by incorrect cleansing after a bowel movement (the correct way is front from the meatus back toward the rectum). Females are more prone to urinary tract infections (**UTIs**) than males due to the close proximity of the urinary meatus to the rectum. In both male and female patients, UTIs may be the result of sexually transmitted diseases. UTIs could also be the result of being prone to them, poor hygiene, or sexual activity not associated with STDs.

Critical Thinking Question 33-1
When Gina's patient mentions her urinary frequency and painful urination, what can Gina do to relieve some of her nervousness?

Renal Diseases

Many factors, including infection, trauma, obstructions, and autoimmune disorders, cause diseases of the renal system (Table 33-2). Most renal diseases occur commonly, but some are fairly rare.

Chronic renal failure is the end-stage outcome of all the chronic disorders described in Table 33-2. Patients develop uremia, loss of concentration, **nocturia, oliguria,** or **anuria,** and the prognosis is poor. Acute renal failure has the same symptoms but results from a different set of causes, such as sudden shocks to the kidney that weaken or destroy functional tissue, sudden loss of blood supply, exposure to toxic agents, trauma, surgical shock or injury, burns, transfusion reactions, and other episodes of significant intravascular hemolysis. Prognosis depends on both the cause and the effectiveness of the treatment.

Blood studies and chemistries ordered in kidney diseases include the CBC (including hemoglobin and hematocrit), electrolytes, creatinine levels, and blood urea nitrogen (BUN). The patient's total clinical picture must be considered when deviations from normal in any of these tests occur. Repeat studies are used to monitor levels and the progress of the disease. (The MA should refer to a reference lab in his or her community for suggested normal levels.)

The list of important renal diseases is much longer than that in Table 33-2, but little information is derived from the routine urinalysis to assist in their diagnosis. These diseases

TABLE 33-2 RENAL DISEASES

Disease	Symptoms	Diagnosis	Treatment
Acute glomerulonephritis ■ May occur one to two weeks after an infection, commonly after a streptococcal sore throat ■ Usually no permanent tissue damage	■ Oliguria ■ **Hematuria** ■ **Periorbital edema**	■ Patient presenting symptoms ■ Urinalysis ■ Microscopic examination	■ Restriction of salt and water to reduce fluid retention and swelling ■ Dietary changes to restrict protein but maintain high calories ■ Hypertension medication if cause is not an infection ■ Antibiotics if cause is infection ■ Bed rest in certain cases
Crescentic (rapidly progressive) glomerulonephritis ■ Also called Goodpasture's syndrome ■ Acute onset progresses to oliguria and renal failure, which have a poor prognosis unless diagnosed early	■ Urine: blood, decreased output, dark color ■ Cough with bloody sputum ■ Weakness	■ Patient presenting symptoms ■ Urinalysis ■ Microscopic examination	■ Corticosteroids and anti-inflammatory drugs to reduce immune response ■ **Plasmapheresis** to slow the disorder ■ Dialysis if kidney is not functioning properly ■ Kidney transplant
Chronic glomerulonephritis ■ Membranous **glomerulonephritis:** generally occurs in patients over 40; slow progression; remission sometimes occurs but about one-third of patients eventually progress to nephrotic syndrome or chronic renal failure	■ Swelling ■ Weight gain ■ Protein in urine ■ Hypertension ■ Usually associated with other diseases: infections (hepatitis B, syphilis), connective tissue diseases (systemic lupus erythematosus, sarcoidosis), cancers, drug side effects (gold, mercurial compounds, penicillin)	■ Patient presenting symptoms ■ Patient history ■ Urinalysis ■ Microscopic examination	■ Early diagnosis critical to preventing more serious complications ■ Medication for hypertension ■ Dietary changes to reduce amount of protein, salt, and phosphate
■ Membrano-proliferative glomerulonephritis: each variety (Types I, II, and III) has a different characteristic change in microscopic anatomy of glomerulus; Type I is most common form; disease occurs mainly in people under 30 years old; prognosis extremely poor for young adults and children; patients often die within five years of diagnosis, although among children spontaneous remission may occur	In children and adolescents: ■ Protein in urine ■ Abnormal immune response ■ Antibodies in the kidney ■ Edema ■ Hypertension	■ Patient presenting symptoms ■ Patient history ■ Urinalysis ■ Microscopic examination	■ Steroids and cytotoxic agents for symptoms ■ Dietary changes to restrict sodium, fluids, and protein intake ■ Antihypertensive medications to control hypertension ■ Diuretics to reduce edema ■ Dialysis or kidney transplant when necessary
Acute renal failure ■ Sudden onset ■ Caused by decreased blood flow to kidneys post surgical shock, traumatic shock, severe dehydration, poisoning, and kidney disease ■ May be result of incompatible blood transfusion	■ Sudden drop in urine output ■ Headache ■ GI distress ■ Odor of ammonia on breath ■ Altered LOC	■ Hyperkalemia ■ Elevated serum creatinine levels ■ Elevated BUN	■ Identification of cause and attempt to correct ■ Restoration of blood volume ■ Dialysis ■ Monitor intake and output

continued

TABLE 33-2 RENAL DISEASES (CONTINUED)

Disease	Symptoms	Diagnosis	Treatment
Chronic renal failure ■ Irreversible loss of nephrons ■ Progressive ■ Gradual onset of uremia ■ Systemic effects in most or all body systems	■ Progressive weakness ■ Edema ■ Muscle weakness ■ Dyspnea	■ Elevated creatinine ■ Elevated BUN ■ Hyperkalemia ■ Decreased hemoglobin and hematocrit levels ■ 24-hour urine studies ■ Radiographic studies	■ Identification of cause and attempt to correct ■ Diet modification to control protein and sodium intake ■ Diuretic medications ■ Antihypertensive drug therapy ■ Dialysis ■ Monitor intake and output ■ Supportive care ■ Kidney transplant
Nephrotic syndrome ■ Generally develops when worsening glomerulonephritis is accompanied by circulatory problems, such as hypertension ■ Often progresses to chronic renal failure	■ Edema ■ Elevated serum lipids ■ Proteinuria ■ Poor appetite	■ Patient presenting symptoms ■ Patient history ■ Urinalysis ■ Microscopic examination	■ Prednisone to decrease protein content ■ Dietary changes to restrict sodium, fluids, and protein intake ■ Diuretics to reduce edema
Polycystic kidney disease ■ Slowly progressive disease that affects both kidneys and occurs when multiple cysts form on dilated nephrons and collecting ducts, resulting in enlarged kidneys ■ Most cases are inherited, but may be acquired following long-term chronic kidney disease and/or dialysis ■ No cure	■ Lumbar pain ■ Hematuria ■ Hypertension	■ Patient presenting symptoms ■ Physical examination	■ Supportive care for patient and family ■ Dialysis ■ Kidney transplant ■ Hypertension and infection management
Diabetic neuropathy ■ Often a **sequela** to diabetes mellitus ■ Cellular membranes of glomeruli harden or sclerose; deterioration in filtration system is the result of hypertension and elevated blood glucose levels ■ Infectious process often involved	■ Decrease in urine output ■ Nausea ■ Vomiting ■ Vision problems ■ Decreased mental alertness ■ Convulsions ■ Coma	■ Patient presenting symptoms ■ Physical examination ■ Urinalysis	■ Blood pressure and blood glucose controlled to forestall long-term effects ■ Supportive care ■ Dialysis ■ Kidney transplant is only long-term option

include inborn errors of renal metabolism, defects in specific tubular reabsorptive or secretive functions, congenital malformations, progressive wasting diseases, and many more.

Dialysis

When a patient is diagnosed with end stage renal disease (**ESRD**), the first option of treatment is one of two forms of **dialysis.**

■ Hemodialysis is the cleansing of urea and other chemical substances from the blood with a dialysis machine, or dialyzer (Figure 33-4 ◆). Joining an artery and a vein, usually in the arm or leg, surgically creates an access, or **fistula.** Two needles are inserted into the fistula, one to remove blood from the body and the other to return it. The blood that is removed passes on one side of a membranous filter while the dialysis solution is on the other side. Although the blood and the solution do not mix, urea and other waste products pass across the membrane into the dialysis solution. A pump keeps the blood flowing through the machine and then back into the body. Patients usually require hemodialysis three times a week, and the procedure takes from three to five or eight to twelve hours. Although there are special centers equipped for hemodialysis, some patients opt for home dialysis. Family members or the patients themselves are trained to maintain the equipment as well as perform the procedure at home.

■ In peritoneal dialysis, the peritoneal membrane acts as the filter. Dialyzing fluid is infused into the peritoneum through a catheter. Wastes accumulate in the fluid, which

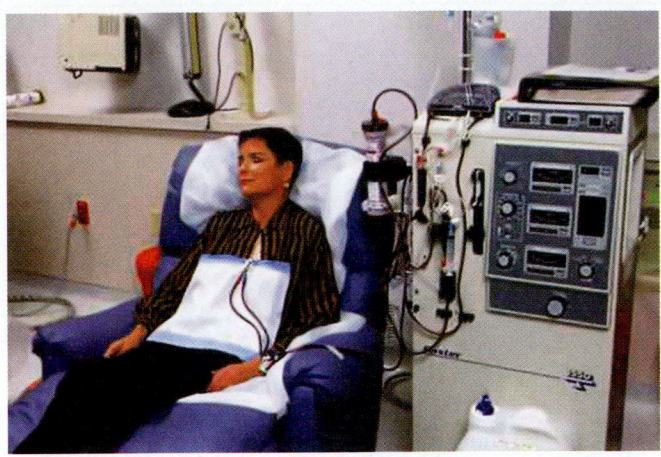

Figure 33-4 ◆ A patient on dialysis.
Source: Michal Heron Photography.

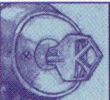

Keys to Success
STRESSING DIETARY TREATMENT

Patients with kidney disease should be made aware of the importance of diet in their treatment. Protein- and sodium-restricted diets are usually indicated when kidney function is compromised. Referral to a dietician may be indicated.

is drained and replaced by clean fluid. The procedure can be performed in three different ways for the patient's comfort and mobility.

- Continuous ambulatory peritoneal dialysis is done three to five times a day and at night. The solution is drained into a bag the patient wears around the waist.
- Continuous cycling peritoneal dialysis (CCPD) is done by a machine while the patient sleeps.
- Intermittent peritoneal dialysis is usually done three to five times a week in a clinic and requires several hours to complete.

Both forms of dialysis are treatments, not cures, intended to be replaced when a suitable donor is found and the diseased kidney can be replaced by transplant.

Neurogenic Bladder and Urinary Incontinence

Neurogenic bladder is usually the result of an insult to the nerves supplying the bladder. The patient may have difficulty starting a stream of urine or emptying the bladder or, conversely, be unable to control the release of urine (**incontinence**). Incontinence may also be caused by nerve damage, especially in the lower spinal cord. The perineal sphincter muscles may be weak. Pregnancy and childbirth may be contributing factors in the female patient.

When the bladder becomes full, the patient usually experiences pain. Treatment may involve exercises to strengthen the perineal sphincter muscle to help with pain and incontinence. Other treatments are self-catheterization and pressing on the lower abdomen over the bladder to force stored urine out of the bladder. If the leaking of urine cannot be controlled, the patient may have to wear an absorbent pad to protect clothing.

Obstructive Conditions

Obstructive disorders that prevent urine from flowing down the urinary tract to be eliminated from the body may involve one or both kidneys (Table 33-3). **Hydronephrosis** is a condition in

TABLE 33-3 OBSTRUCTIVE CONDITIONS			
Condition	**Symptoms**	**Diagnosis**	**Treatment**
Renal calculi ■ Stones may be single or multiple, large or small, and of a variety of compositions, such as uric acid, calcium salts, and cholesterol; may be round and smooth, sharp with rough edges, or, as "staghorn" stones, may take on form of renal pelvis ■ Obstruction must be relieved in approximately eight weeks to avoid permanent damage	■ Pain beginning in flank and moving downward to groin, vulva, or testicle as stone moves ■ Renal colic (severe pain in lower back over kidney) ■ Persistent urge to urinate ■ Blood in urine ■ Nausea or vomiting ■ Chills ■ Fever ■ Family or personal history	■ Patient presenting symptoms ■ Urinalysis ■ Radiographs (flat plate KUB, IVP, or CT scan)	■ Eight glasses of water per day to dilute the urine ■ Analgesics for pain ■ Dietary changes ■ **Lithotripsy,** less invasive treatment to remove the stones (Figure 33-5 ◆) ■ Surgery
Bladder calculi (bladder stones) ■ Diagnosed almost solely in men ■ Stones formed in bladder when urine is concentrated and materials crystallize ■ Obstruction must be removed to avoid permanent damage to bladder or kidneys	■ Frequent and difficult urination ■ Pain in abdomen and/or penis ■ Blood in urine ■ Abnormal color to urine	■ Urinalysis ■ Urine culture ■ Bladder x-ray ■ Cystoscopy	■ Eight glasses of water per day to dilute the urine ■ Lithotripsy to remove stones ■ Cystoscopy to remove stones and examine bladder

continued

TABLE 33-3 OBSTRUCTIVE CONDITIONS (CONTINUED)

Condition	Symptoms	Diagnosis	Treatment
Cysts ■ Noncancerous lesions of the kidney ■ Commonly found in patients over 50 ■ Large cysts can impair renal function	■ Blood in urine ■ Flank pain	■ Patient presenting symptoms ■ MRI, CT scan, or ultrasound examination	■ Surgery or needle aspiration to remove pressure or pain and prevent kidney damage
Kidney or ureter cancer ■ Several types ■ Tumors sometimes erode walls of blood vessels, producing small to moderate hemorrhages of blood into the urine ■ Cancer hastens destruction of surrounding kidney tissue and alters ability of involved kidney(s) to form urine	■ Blood in urine ■ Flank pain ■ Abdominal mass ■ Weight loss ■ Intermittent fever ■ Fatigue	■ Patient presenting symptoms ■ Patient history ■ Ultrasound examination ■ CT scan or MRI	■ Removal of mass at early stage of development to prevent spreading ■ Removal of kidney and possibly lymph nodes to prevent spreading ■ Radiation therapy to prevent spreading ■ Chemotherapy or immunotherapy at more advanced stages
Bladder cancer ■ Men more likely than women to develop ■ Occurs rarely in people under 40 ■ Early detection critical for favorable prognosis	■ Blood in urine ■ Difficulty voiding ■ Pelvic pain	■ Patient presenting symptoms ■ Patient history ■ Cystoscopy ■ IVP ■ CT scan or MRI	■ Tumor removal at early stage to prevent spread ■ Cancer drug infusion into bladder to reduce likelihood of recurrence ■ Bladder removal to prevent spread ■ Removal of prostate for men and of ovaries, uterus, and part of the vagina for women, to prevent spread ■ Chemotherapy at later stages

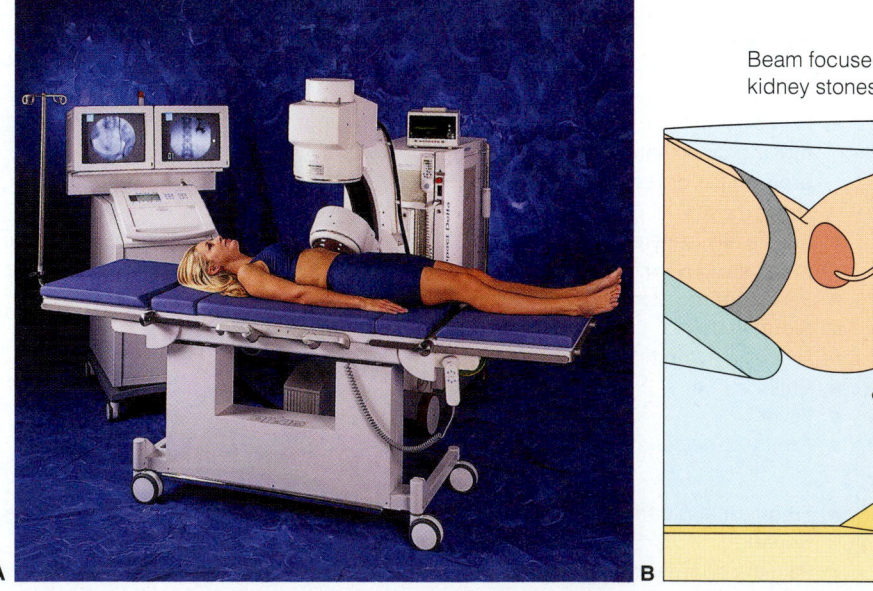
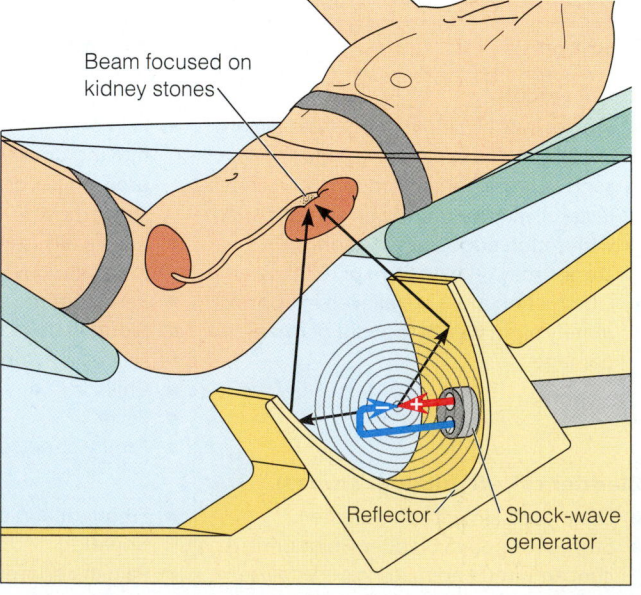

Figure 33-5 ◆ Extracorporeal shock-wave lithotripsy: (A) A shock-wave generator that does not require water immersion; (B) water immersion lithotripsy procedure.

which the kidney becomes dilated and enlarged with urine during an obstructive condition. Once the obstruction is relieved, the kidney usually returns to its normal status.

A frequent obstruction that affects one kidney is the **renal calculus** (kidney stone). Carcinoma (cancer) of the renal pelvis may also be extensive enough to cause an obstruction. An enlarged prostate is a common obstruction in older males. Cancer of the bladder is less common and occurs more frequently in males than in females.

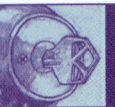

Keys to Success
PATIENT INSTRUCTIONS
FOR INTRAVENOUS PYELOGRAM (IVP)

In an intravenous pyelogram (IVP), the kidneys are examined by X-ray for renal stones. IVPs are also used to diagnose disease conditions that cause hematuria, frequent urination, and side, abdominal, and lower back pain, as well as enlarged prostate; kidney, ureter, or bladder tumors; and trauma from an accident.

A contrast medium is used to enhance details of the kidneys, ureters, and bladder. Because of potential allergies to the contrast medium, tell your physician and/or clinical staff of any medication allergies that you have. Also inform your physician and clinical staff if you are diabetic or pregnant. Special accommodations will be made if you are diabetic, and if you are or may be pregnant, the physician will likely postpone the IVP or discuss other procedures to help diagnose and treat your symptoms.

1. On the day before the procedure, the physician will prescribe a laxative medication for you. Your prescriptions for the procedure and the times for taking them are as follows: _____

   _____
2. On the day before the procedure, your dietary instructions are as follows: _____.
   Do not eat or drink or take medication after midnight.
3. On the day of the procedure and before the procedure, you may take the following medications with only sips of water: _____

   _____

   You will receive instructions for resuming the other medications after the procedure.
4. On the day of the procedure, please leave valuables at home.
5. Go through the admissions area, and you will be escorted to the radiology department. After you change into a gown, the radiologic technician will take a "before" X-ray.
6. The contrast media will be given through an IV and a series of X-rays will be taken at intervals.
7. Because individuals are different, the process of taking radiographic films after the contrast medium has been administered may take one-half to three or four hours. Please be patient. The time will go faster if you bring some reading materials.

Diagnostic Procedures

Laboratory tests for diagnosing renal diseases are invasive or noninvasive. Urinalysis testing is the most common noninvasive test. A clean-catch midstream urine test is used to diagnose the causal microorganism of urinary tract infections. Some invasive tests may be ordered to assist the physician in making or confirming a diagnosis. The invasive tests described in the following boxes are usually performed in a specialized area with radiography.

Urinalysis

A routine urinalysis tests certain aspects of the first three functions of the kidney—waste excretion, acid-base balance, and water balance—but not the fourth function, endocrine regulatory activity. Measurements of various endocrine activities of the kidneys require specialized urine testing that is usually performed in a reference lab.

Urinalysis Specimen Collection

Different types of urine specimens are required for different testing goals.

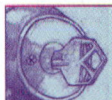

Keys to Success
PATIENT INSTRUCTIONS
FOR CYSTOSCOPY

Your physician has ordered a cystoscopy to look inside your bladder. This procedure is done to assess the size and condition of the prostate gland in males or to look for obstructions, stones, tumors, and other abnormalities. Other conditions that warrant a cystoscopic examination include hematuria, frequent UTIs, incontinence or overactive bladder, painful urination, or the need of a catheter for urination. Stones or tumors are sometimes removed or a biopsy sample is obtained during this procedure. The physician uses a gel to numb the urethra, and it is rare that any other type of anesthesia is needed.

1. On the day before the procedure, do not eat or drink or take medication after midnight. Exceptions, if any, are as follows: _____

   _____
2. On the day of the procedure, please go to the admissions area and you will be escorted to the ambulatory outpatient department. You will be asked to change into a gown.
3. A nurse or technician will apply a numbing gel (local anesthetic) to the urethral opening.
4. The physician will give you instructions and information during the procedure. You may feel some discomfort and the urge to urinate during the procedure, particularly as the bladder is filled with sterile water or saline and stretched for better visualization.
5. The examination usually lasts only 15 to 20 minutes, but additional procedures, such as removal of stones or biopsy, will make it longer.

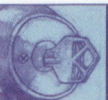

Keys to Success
PATIENT INSTRUCTIONS FOR VOIDING CYSTOGRAM

Your physician has ordered a voiding cystogram to look inside your bladder for obstructions, stones, tumors, or other abnormalities. If you are a female patient, this procedure is not done during your menstrual period.

1. On the day before the procedure, do not eat or drink or take medication after midnight. Exceptions, if any, are as follows: _____

   _____

2. On the day of the procedure, please go to the admissions area and you will be escorted to the radiology department. You will be asked to change into a gown.
3. A radiography film will be taken of your bladder before the procedure.
4. You will be asked to lie on the X-ray table for placement of a urinary catheter into the bladder.
5. A liquid contrast medium will be inserted via the catheter, and the catheter will then be removed.
6. When your bladder feels full, X-rays will be taken at intervals and you will be asked to turn from side to side. After X-rays are completed, you will be allowed to empty your bladder and a final X-ray will be taken.

1. A random voided specimen is adequate for routine screening.
2. A first morning specimen is best for routine screening, pregnancy tests, cytology (to detect abnormal cells), or orthostatic protein determination.
3. A fasting sample is required for diabetic monitoring. This is not the first but the second morning specimen, which eliminates much of the urine accumulated in the bladder overnight.
4. A midstream clean-catch is also appropriate for routine screening and best for a bacterial culture.
5. Timed or 24-hour specimens are required for quantitative analyses.
6. A catheterized specimen is sometimes requested for bacterial culture.
7. A suprapubic needle aspiration is rarely required for a bacterial culture (especially if anaerobes or other problem organisms must be identified) or for cytological examination for abnormal cells, such as cancer cells. Needle aspiration may be necessary for some pediatric specimens when a true sterile collection is required.
8. Pediatric specimens are difficult to obtain, particularly in clean-catch form. Plastic bags with adhesive may be used but require care.
9. Urine for drug testing must be collected in a very specific manner, according to the clinic's policy. Some clinics will place color altering tablets in the toilet water to verify urine has been expelled, check for warmth (to verify the urine was not brought in prepackaged), and check for concentration (to verify the patient is not attempting to "flush" his or her

system). Always check with your clinic's drug-testing policies before attempting a patient's urine drug screening test.

Urine Containers

It is important to handle containers and specimens properly and to follow each collection procedure carefully for accurate results. Three major rules apply to containers.

- They vary according to the type of specimen required.
- They must be clean, dry, and of sufficient volume to hold the routine urinalysis sample.
- They must be sterile when a microbial culture and sensitivity is ordered.

If the specimen is to be transported, it should be placed in a proper biohazard bag to ensure it does not leak. Single specimens of 50 to 100 ml are typically adequate for testing. Twenty-four-hour specimens usually require at least a one-gallon or three-liter bottle, usually made of rigid plastic or glass (Figure 33-6 ◆).

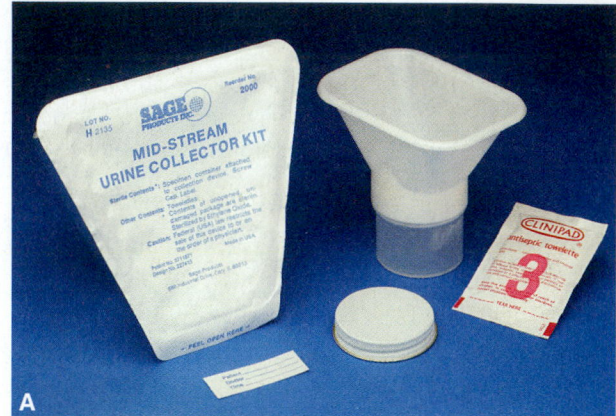

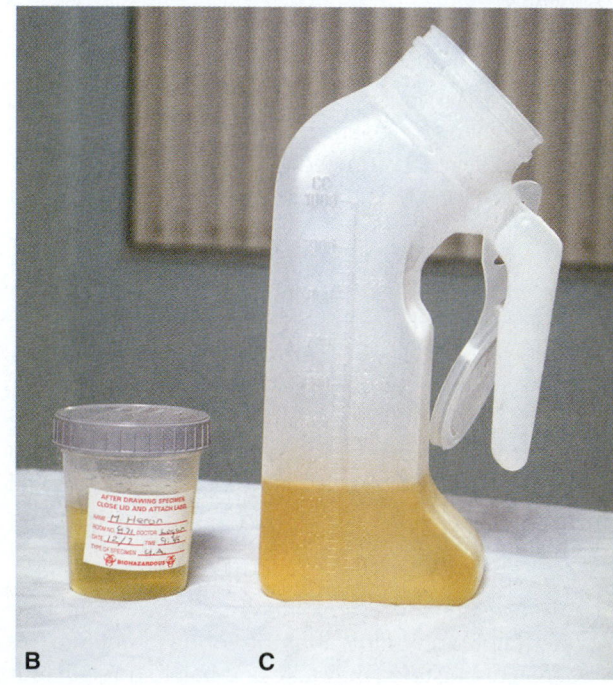

Figure 33-6 ◆ Urine specimen containers: (A) midstream clean-catch container; (B) urine collection cup; (C) 24-hour urine container.

General Specimen Handling

Correct and complete labeling is essential. At the minimum, the MA must include the patient's name and the date and time of day of collection. In a hospital, a patient's hospital number may also be mandatory. Any unlabeled or incompletely labeled container should be considered unsatisfactory, such as a container with a requisition slip around or under it. The requisition slip may be moved or stained with urine and difficult to read. The label must be affixed to guarantee the identification of the specimen source.

The most accurate results come from testing fresh urine. If the test must be delayed, the specimen should be refrigerated. Some values begin to change immediately if testing is delayed. All values are likely to be altered, some markedly, after 24 hours. The urine specimen should be allowed to come to room temperature and should be well mixed before testing.

The specimen should be delivered promptly, then either refrigerated or frozen immediately, have an appropriate preservative added immediately, or tested within one to two hours. There are many types of urine preservatives. Most are antimicrobial compounds, such as benzoic acid, boric acid, chloroform, formaldehyde, and preservative tablets with a mix of compounds. These compounds may also preserve cells, or alcohol can be mixed with the urine in equal portions for the same purpose.

Preservation kits are also available for transporting specimens to other facilities. Since preserved specimens are usually transferred to reference laboratories for special testing, follow the written procedures provided by the reference laboratory to prepare the specimen. Urine standing unpreserved at room temperature begins to change immediately, and test results will be less accurate. If the urine is to be preserved by refrigeration or chemical means, it should be done quickly.

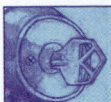

Keys to Success
UNDERSTANDING CHANGES IN UNPRESERVED URINE SPECIMENS

1. Exposure to light decreases **bilirubin** and **urobilinogen**.
2. Exposure to the atmosphere decreases CO_2. This raises the pH; permits nitrogen gas to evolve from dissolved nitrites, lowering nitrite levels; and permits volatiles to escape, such as acetone and other ketones. Evaporative water loss is only rarely significant.
3. Microbial growth:
   - breaks down urea to ammonia, raising the pH
   - changes the odor and perhaps the color
   - oxidizes urobilinogen to urobilin
   - decreases glucose and ketone bodies, lowering the pH
   - reduces nitrates by converting them into nitrites
   - increases the **turbidity**
   - alters the proportions of organisms
4. Changes in pH can:
   - precipitate crystals or dissolve crystals already present
   - break down or alter chemical constituents, and perhaps urine color
   - disintegrate cells and casts that were present (casts are discussed later in this chapter)

Clean-Catch Urine Specimen Collection

Although the bladder and urethra are normally sterile, a urine specimen can be contaminated with microorganisms from the lower portion of the urethra and the meatus. After proper training, the MA will teach the patient how to obtain a clean-catch specimen. Thorough instruction will ensure that the collected specimen is not contaminated.

PROCEDURE 33-1 **Demonstrate Patient Instruction for a Clean-Catch Urine Specimen**

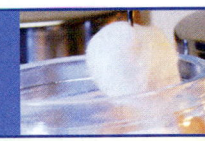

Theory and Rationale

Proper instruction keeps the patient from returning to the medical office to repeat the test. The specimen is tested immediately or refrigerated, or preservative is added. Remind the patient not to touch the inside of the container or lid to prevent contamination of the specimen. Voiding some urine into the toilet before voiding into the specimen cup will wash microorganisms away from the meatus and will also prevent contamination of the specimen.

Materials

- sterile specimen container
- label
- antiseptic wipes
- chart
- requisition slip, if necessary

Competency

(**Conditions**) With the necessary materials, (**Task**) you will be able to instruct the patient on obtaining a clean-catch specimen (**Standards**) correctly within the time frame designated by the instructor.

1. Wash your hands. Gather equipment and supplies.
2. Identify the patient and guide him or her to the treatment area.
3. Instruct the patient to:
   - Label the container, not the lid, with his or her first and last name
   - Wash the hands.
   - Open the sterile urine container and place the lid on a flat area with the inside facing up.
   - Open the antiseptic wipes and place them on top of their packaging.

continued

PROCEDURE 33-1 Demonstrate Patient Instruction for a Clean-Catch Urine Specimen *(continued)*

- If male: Retract the foreskin, if present. Cleanse the glans penis with the antiseptic wipes with a circular motion from the meatal opening and proceeding outward. Repeat, using all the antiseptic wipes.
- If female: Spread the labia apart with one hand. Wipe from front to back. Use one wipe to cleanse one side, then discard the wipe. Cleanse the other side with a new wipe and discard it. Finally, with a new wipe, cleanse down the middle across the meatus, and discard the wipe.

4. After cleansing, the patient should:
   - Discard all the used wipes in an appropriate waste container.
   - Void some urine into the toilet and stop (an uncircumcised male should also bring the foreskin forward)
   - Restart voiding to half-fill the sterile container.
   - Finish voiding into the toilet.
   - Wash the hands.
   - Put the lid on the container without touching the inside of the lid.
   - Place it in the designated receiving site.
5. Wash your hands.

6. Chart your observations of the urine specimen as well as the date, time collected, and tests ordered.
7. If the specimen is to be tested at another laboratory, complete a laboratory requisition slip. Take the specimen to the lab or refrigerator or add preservative.

Patient Education

Ask the patient to repeat his or her instructions to verify understanding. Inform the patient that the physician will review the results and call if additional or new treatment is needed. Instruct the patient to call the medical office if symptoms worsen or if he or she would like to know more about the test results.

Charting Example

03/11/XX 8:30 a.m. Pt instructed on how to obtain clean-catch midstream. Pt expressed understanding of procedure and left the labeled specimen in the bathroom. Cloudy specimen was taken to the lab at 0840 and placed in the refrigerator. Megan Steed, CMA (AAMA)

24–Hour Specimen Collection

A 24-hour specimen is performed to measure specific urine components. Calcium, potassium, creatinine, urea nitrogen, protein, and lead levels are affected by hydration, activity and exercise, and metabolic rate and can vary throughout the day. Because of these fluctuations, a 24-hour specimen gives a more accurate picture of the composition of the urine. It may also be ordered to determine the content of existing kidney stones or ways to prevent further kidney stone formation.

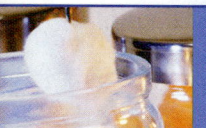

PROCEDURE 33-2 Demonstrate Patient Instruction for Collection of 24-Hour Urine Specimen

Theory and Rationale

A large container of 3000 ml, often with preservative, is used to collect a 24-hour urine specimen. The urine must be refrigerated or kept in a portable cooler to prevent deterioration and other changes. The patient should be advised to moderate fluid and alcohol intake to avoid producing more urine than the collection container can hold. The physician will evaluate the medications the patient is taking to decide if any can be discontinued for a short period. Some medications can alter the test results.

The test is started *after* the patient's first morning void and continued for the next 24 hours. If any portion of the 24-hour urine is not placed in the collection container, the results of the test are invalid and the test must be started again. The 24-hour specimen is returned to the medical office or laboratory the same morning the test is completed.

Materials

- 24-hour specimen container
- smaller collection container
- patient instruction sheet
- chart
- requisition slip

Competency

(**Conditions**) With the necessary materials, (**Task**) you will be able to instruct the patient to obtain a quality 24-hour specimen for accurate testing, diagnosis, and treatment (**Standards**) correctly within the time frame designated by the instructor.

1. Wash your hands. Gather equipment and supplies.
2. Identify the patient and guide him or her to the treatment area.

PROCEDURE 33-2 Demonstrate Patient Instruction for Collection of 24-Hour Urine Specimen *(continued)*

3. Instruct the patient to:
   - Label the container, not the lid, with first and last name.
   - Wash the hands.
   - Void into the toilet upon arising.
   - Record the time (from this time and for the next 24 hours, all urine will go into the 24-hour collection container).
   - Void all urine into the smaller collection container to pour into the larger container.
   - Each time wash, rinse, and air-dry the smaller container.
   - After each specimen is placed in the larger specimen container, screw the lid tightly and put it in the refrigerator or portable cooler.
   - At the end of the 24-hour period, bring the large container to the medical office or laboratory. (The first voided specimen of the second morning is the last specimen to be added to the container, ending the collecting period.)
4. Ask the patient if any problems occurred during the specimen collection. If too much urine was collected or if some was spilled during collection, tell the patient a new collection must be started.
5. Fill out a lab requisition slip for the specimen when it is brought to the office or taken directly to an outside laboratory.
6. Chart your observations of the urine specimen, the date, time collected, tests ordered, and any other pertinent information.

Patient Education

Ask the patient to repeat his or her instructions to verify understanding. For the test to be accurate, *all* urine after the initial morning void must go into the collection container. Inform the patient that the physician will review the results and call if additional or new treatment is needed. The patient should call the medical office if symptoms worsen or if he or she would like to know more about the test results.

Charting Example

03/13/XX 11:30 a.m. Pt said he understood the process of collecting all urine within the 24-hour period. Written instructions also sent with patient. Ivory Smith, RMA (AMT)

03/15/XX 9:00 a.m. Pt started 24-hour urine collection after 8:00 a.m. voiding on 3/14. Pt stated that urine has been kept in portable cooler during that time and that all urine has been collected. Lab requisition prepared for calcium, potassium, creatinine, urea nitrogen, and protein. Specimen sent via courier to the lab for testing. Ivory Smith, RMA (AMT)

Specimen Collection by Catheterization

For certain procedures and tests, a thin tube (catheter) is inserted into the urinary bladder to withdraw urine. The three most common reasons a catheterization is performed are the relief of urinary retention, the need for a sterile urine sample, and the need to instill a medication directly into an empty bladder. Catheterization may also be done to empty the bladder prior to a surgical procedure and to measure the amount of residual urine in the bladder of individuals with bladder-emptying problems. The collected urine can be tested for a variety of microorganisms and used in a number of tests.

Physical Urinalysis

A number of physical components are determined in a routine urinalysis: appearance (color and clarity), odor, pH, specific gravity, and many others, summarized in Table 33-4.

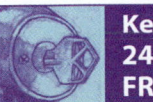

Keys to Success
24-HOUR URINE COLLECTION FROM A CHILD

If a child patient wets the bed, the 24-hour collection must begin again with a new collection container. The 24-hour specimen must consist of *all* the urine voided by the child in a 24-hour period.

TABLE 33-4 CHARACTERISTICS OF A NORMAL URINALYSIS

Appearance	Normal pigments color the urine yellow. Clear urine is normal, although turbid (cloudy) urine is not necessarily a sign of pathology. The lighter the color of the urine, the greater the patient's degree of hydration. The darker the urine, the lower the patient's degree of hydration. Color can range from pale yellow to amber.
Odor	Normal fresh specimens have a faint, characteristic odor.
pH	5.0–8.0 normal < 7.0 acid urine > 7 alkaline urine
Specific gravity	1.016–1.030
Protein	0
Glucose	None present
Ketones	None present
Bilirubin	0
Urobilinogen	2
Blood	None detected
Leukocytes	None detected
Nitrite	None

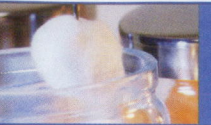

PROCEDURE 33-3 Perform Catheterization of a Female Patient

Theory and Rationale

Catheterization ensures a sterile sample but is not always the ideal method of obtaining a sample. Because a foreign object is introduced into the body, there is the possibility of also introducing pathogens. It is imperative, especially when catheterizing female patients, that the surrounding area be appropriately and thoroughly cleaned.

Materials

- lighting source, preferably a gooseneck lamp
- sterile specimen container
- sterile drapes
- sterile catheterization kit or straight catheter
- sterile K-Y gel or other lubricant
- sterilized Mayo stand
- sterile gloves, two pairs
- nonsterile latex gloves
- biohazardous waste receptacle
- several 2 × 2 sterile gauze squares (minimum of 6)
- Betadine or other iodine solution
- maxipad or pantyliner
- patient chart
- lab order forms

Competency

(**Conditions**) With the necessary materials, (**Task**) you will be able to catheterize a female patient (**Standards**) correctly within the time frame designated by the instructor.

1. Gather all needed supplies to bring into the room. Generally, the patient will already be disrobed and covered with a drape. Bringing all supplies into the room on one trip avoids opening the door more than once while your patient is in a potentially embarrassing position.
2. Explain the procedure to the patient and obtain verbal permission to begin touching her.
3. If the patient is not unclothed, explain the correct dorsal recumbent position and draping.
4. Position the gooseneck lamp so that it is directed at the genital area, but do not turn it on, as it may heat up quickly and make the patient uncomfortable.
5. Wash your hands and put on nonsterile gloves. Open the catheterization kit.
6. Ask the patient to keep her knees apart and take slow deep breaths while lifting her hips off the table surface.
7. When her hips have cleared the surface, slide a sterile drape beneath her by encircling the corners with your hands. Avoid touching the patient or the table with your hands.
8. Open a second sterile drape and place it over the patient's genital area, making sure that the vulvar area is exposed.

9. Place the insertion portion of the kit on the sterile drape you placed under the patient's hips, between her knees.
10. Remove the gloves and wash your hands.
11. Following sterile technique, put on sterile gloves.
12. Soak the 2 × 2 gauze pads in Betadine or other iodine solution.
13. Open the sterile lubricant and place it on the sterile field on the Mayo stand. Open the remaining items, including the sterile container, and place them on the tray.
14. Cleanse the patient with the Betadine-soaked gauze squares. Separate the labia with the thumb and index finger of your nondominant hand (Figure 33-7 ◆). With your other hand, take a gauze square and wipe one side of the labia from top to bottom in *one pass*. Throw the square away (Figure 33-8 ◆). Take another square, repeat on the other side, and discard. Do not let the hand that is separating the labia touch and thereby contaminate your other hand.
15. With a third gauze square, cleanse the urinary meatus with a circular motion, working from the inside to the outside. Discard the square.
16. With your dominant hand, pick up the catheter, your thumb and index finger approximately 3 inches from the end to be inserted.
17. Dip the insertion end of the catheter into the sterile lubricant. Make sure the opposite end of the catheter is in the collection portion of the kit's tray.
18. Thread the catheter into the urinary meatus approximately 2 to 3 inches, until urine begins to flow into the collection tray.

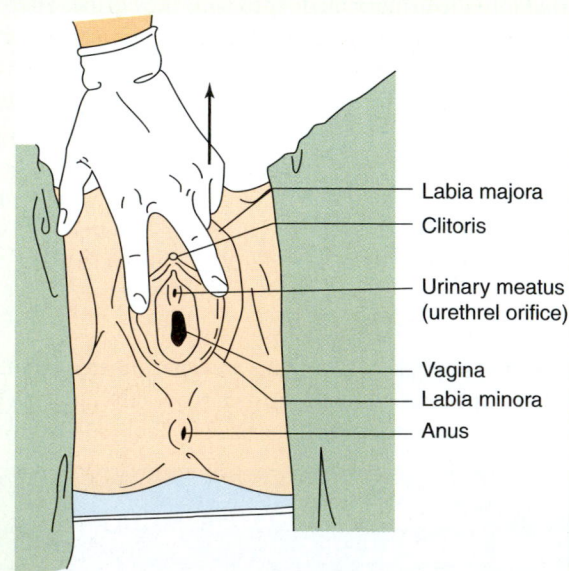

Labia majora
Clitoris
Urinary meatus (urethrel orifice)
Vagina
Labia minora
Anus

Figure 33-7 ◆ Separate the labia with the thumb and index finger of your nondominant hand.

PROCEDURE 33-3 Perform Catheterization of a Female Patient *(continued)*

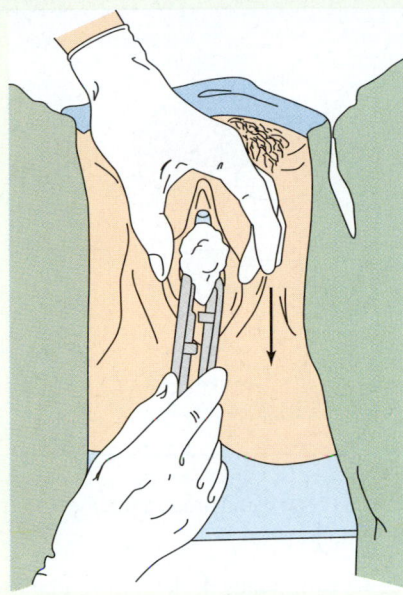

Figure 33-8 ◆ When cleansing the urinary meatus, move the swab downward.

19. If you meet resistance when threading the catheter, do not force it in. Resistance can be an indication of a problem. Remove the catheter and notify the physician.
20. After a small amount of the urine has flowed into the collection tray, move the end of the catheter into the sterile collection container.
21. Measure the urine that has flowed from the bladder. Emptying more than 500 ml at one time may cause the bladder

to spasm. If more than 500 ml has been released, clamp the catheter, wait 10 to 15 minutes, and release the remainder of the urine.
22. When the bladder is completely empty, gently remove the catheter.
23. Secure the collection container's lid in place and prepare the paperwork for laboratory testing.
24. Remove all supplies and dispose of them in a biohazardous container.
25. Assist the patient in sitting up and dressing if necessary.
26. Inform the patient that the Betadine used to cleanse the labia may stain her undergarments, and offer her a maxi-pad or pantyliner to protect her clothing.
27. Document the procedure in the patient's chart.

Patient Education

The patient should feel no discomfort or pain after the catheter is removed. Instruct her to report any discomfort, pain with urination, stinging, irritation, or fever. Also advise her to avoid using perfumed toiletries such as soaps, tissues, and tampons. Female patients should also avoid wearing overly tight pants and nylon underwear, which traps moisture and heat in the genital area.

Charting Example

05/23/XX 9:25 a.m. Sterile urine sample obtained through catheterization. Patient tolerated procedure well and does not report any pain, tingling, or burning. Urine sample sent to laboratory for culture and sensitivity testing. Mary Brady, CMA (AAMA)

PROCEDURE 33-4 Perform Catheterization of a Male Patient

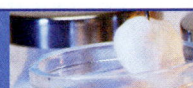

Theory and Rationale

As with a female patient, it is imperative that the male patient's genital area be appropriately and thoroughly cleaned before catheterization to prevent the introduction of pathogens.

Materials

- lighting source, preferably a gooseneck lamp
- waterproof underpad
- sterile specimen container
- sterile catheterization kit or straight catheter

- sterile drapes
- sterile K-Y gel or other lubricant
- sterilized Mayo stand
- sterile gloves, 2 pairs
- nonsterile latex gloves
- biohazardous waste receptacle
- several 2 × 2 sterile gauze squares (minimum of 6)
- Betadine or other iodine solution
- fenestrated drape
- patient chart
- lab order forms

continued

PROCEDURE 33-4 Perform Catheterization of a Male Patient (continued)

Competency

(**Conditions**) With the necessary materials, (**Task**) you will be able to catheterize a male patient (**Standards**) correctly within the time frame designated by the instructor.

1. Wash your hands. Collect all the needed supplies and bring into patient's room.
2. Explain the procedure to the patient and explain that it will be necessary to remove all articles of clothing from the waist down.
3. Assist the patient, if needed, into the supine position.
4. Wash your hands and put on nonsterile gloves.
5. Following sterile technique, open the catheterization kit and place the items on the sterile field on the Mayo stand.
6. Wrap the corners of the sterile underpad over your hands and place it over the patient's thighs, sliding it under the penis (Figure 33-9 ◆).
7. Remove the gloves, wash your hands, and put on sterile gloves.
8. Being careful not to touch the patient or the table, place a fenestrated drape over the genital area so that the penis is exposed (Figure 33-10 ◆).

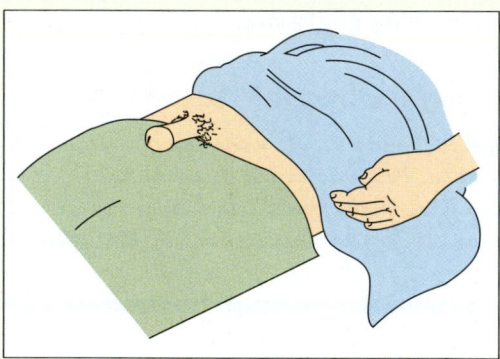

Figure 33-9 ◆ Place the sterile underpad over the patient's thighs, sliding it under the penis.

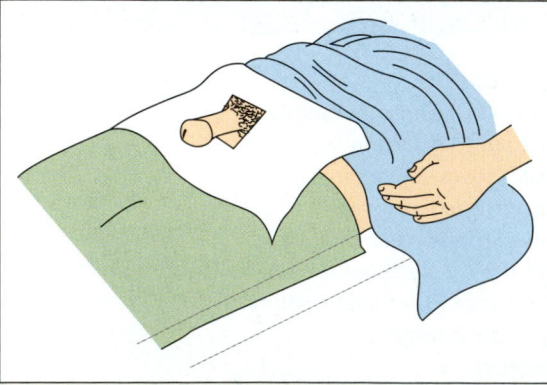

Figure 33-10 ◆ Place a fenestrated drape over the genital area so that the penis is exposed.

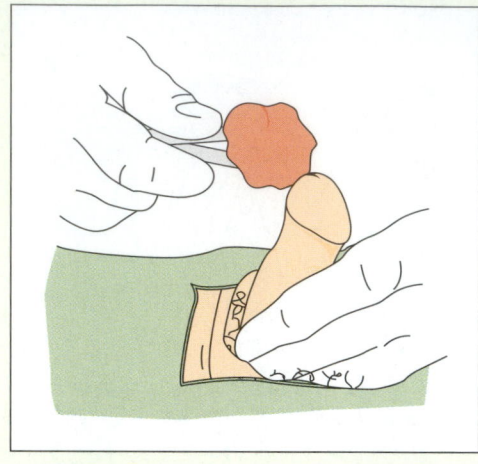

Figure 33-11 ◆ Clean around the meatus in a circular motion.

9. Soak the 2 × 2 gauze pads in Betadine and place them on the patient's thighs for easy access.
10. With your nondominant hand, grasp the penis below the glans and hold it upright. If the patient is uncircumcised, retract the foreskin to expose the meatus.
11. With your dominant hand, cleanse the meatus with a gauze square in a circular motion, working from the inside to the outside (Figure 33-11 ◆). Discard the gauze.
12. Repeat step 11 a total of three times, using a fresh gauze square each time you cleanse.
13. Dip the insertion tip of the catheter into lubricant to cover the 7 or 8 inches that will be inserted into the penis. Place the opposite end of the catheter in the collection tray.
14. Hold the penis firmly at a straight, upward angle to straighten the urethra for easier insertion.
15. Ask the patient to constrict the penis muscles in the same manner as when trying to urinate. While he is doing this, gently thread the catheter into the penis until urine begins to flow, generally 6 to 8 inches (Figure 33-12 ◆).
16. *Never* force the catheter. If you meet resistance, discontinue the procedure and notify the physician.
17. After a small amount of the urine has flowed into the collection tray, move the end of the catheter into the sterile collection container.
18. Measure the urine that has flowed from the bladder. Emptying more than 500 ml at one time may cause the bladder to spasm. If more than 500 ml has been released, clamp the catheter, wait 10 to 15 minutes, and release the remainder of the urine.
19. When the bladder is completely empty, gently remove the catheter.
20. Secure the collection container's lid in place and prepare the paperwork for laboratory testing.
21. Remove all supplies and dispose of them in a biohazardous container.

PROCEDURE 33-4 Perform Catheterization of a Male Patient *(continued)*

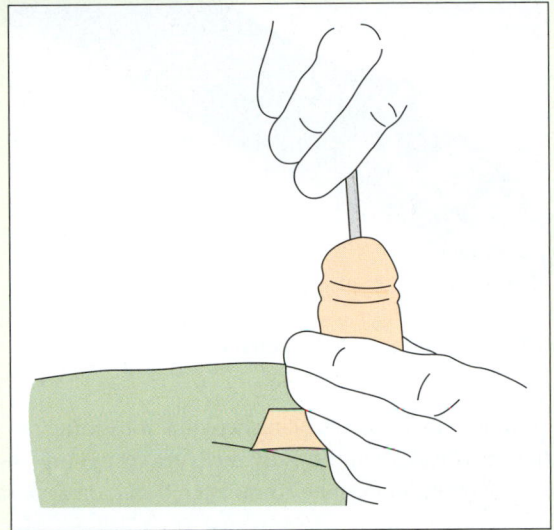

Figure 33-12 ◆ Gently thread the catheter into the penis until urine begins to flow, generally 6 to 8 inches.

22. Assist the patient in sitting up and dressing if necessary.
23. Inform the patient that the Betadine used to cleanse the glans may transfer to his undergarments and stain them.
24. Document the procedure in the patient's chart.

Patient Education

The patient should feel no discomfort or pain after the catheter is removed. Instruct him to report any discomfort, pain with urination, stinging, irritation, or fever. Remind the patient of the importance of voiding when the urge is present, as waiting stresses and irritates the bladder. The patient should also drink plenty of fluids to flush the urinary system and avoid caffeine, which may also irritate the bladder.

Charting Example

04/04/XX 9:25 a.m. Sterile urine sample obtained through catheterization. Patient tolerated procedure well and does not report any pain, tingling, or burning. Urinary sample sent to laboratory for culture and sensitivity testing. Joseph Baker, RMA (AMT)

Appearance

The color of the urine should be determined by looking down into the sample against a white background and with a good light source. Yellow is the normal color of urine (Figure 33-13 ◆). Urochrome, the pigment that colors urine, is derived from urobilin, a brown pigment. Intensity of color is usually related to the degree of concentration or dilution of the urine.

The following colors may indicate a possible disorder.

- Red or red-brown is the most common set of abnormal shades. A pink cast can be caused by several foods, such as beets or rhubarb, certain dyes, and drugs. Although hematuria, which is the introduction of RBCs, can be caused by menstrual flow, more serious conditions are likely.

- Yellow-brown or green-brown usually develops because of the presence of bile pigments, especially bilirubin (Figure 33-14 ◆). Severe **jaundice** may be accompanied by dark green urine. Other greens and blue-greens may

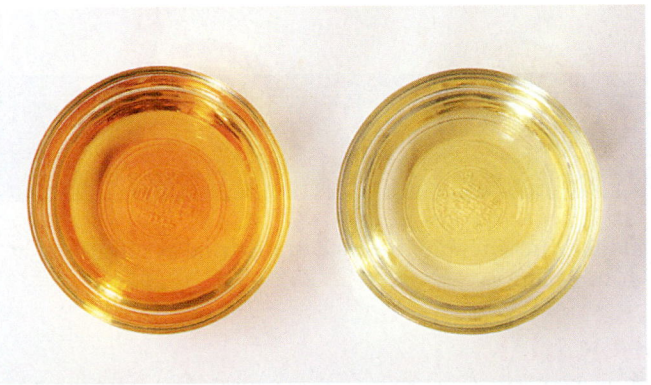

Figure 33-13 ◆ Pale yellow urine alongside a glass of concentrated urine with a dark yellow color.
Source: Dorling Kindersley.

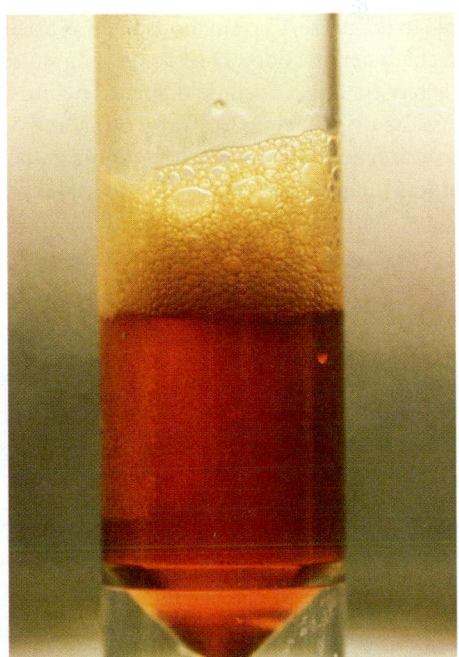

Figure 33-14 ◆ The deep yellow color of this urine is due to an excess of bilirubin, a bile pigment in the body.
Source: SPL/Photo Researchers, Inc.

be caused by pigmented microbes, such as *Pseudomonas,* or pigments in foods or drugs.

- Orange-red or orange-brown urine typically has large quantities of urobilin.
- Dark brown or black urine is usually the result of hemoglobin darkening upon standing, or more rarely a genetic disease, alkaptonuria.

Turbid or cloudy urine generally contains some sort of suspended particulate or cellular material. The urine may be treated with acid, heat, or a lipid solvent to help identify the specific source of turbidity.

- Leukocytes can form a white cloud that is not eliminated by the addition of acid. High numbers of neutrophils are indicative of pyuria. Bacteria or yeasts in high numbers create an opalescent turbidity. Hematuria may produce a turbid or smoky appearance.
- Prostatic fluid or mucus may produce a whitish turbidity. Small renal calculi or bladder stones, nicknamed "gravel," produce turbidity, as can fecal contamination. Larger material, or "clumps," can be created by pus, fecal contamination, calculi, or menstrual discharge. Contamination with powders and some antiseptics can produce turbidity. Emulsified paraffin from some vaginal creams can produce a milky appearance.
- Very rarely there may be leakage of lymph into the urine. Lipoproteins may also enter the urine in nephrosis and in some crush injuries.

Odor

Normal fresh specimens have a faint, characteristic odor. Upon standing, bacterial metabolism may impart an odor of rotting or ammonia to the urine. Certain foods, such as asparagus, give the urine a characteristic odor. Disease-causing states that produce characteristic odors include diabetes mellitus, in which ketones give the urine a sweet or fruity odor, and a variety of hereditary amino acid disorders. Urine odors associated with these disorders include "sweaty feet," "maple syrup," "cabbage hops," "mousy," "rotting fish," and "rancid."

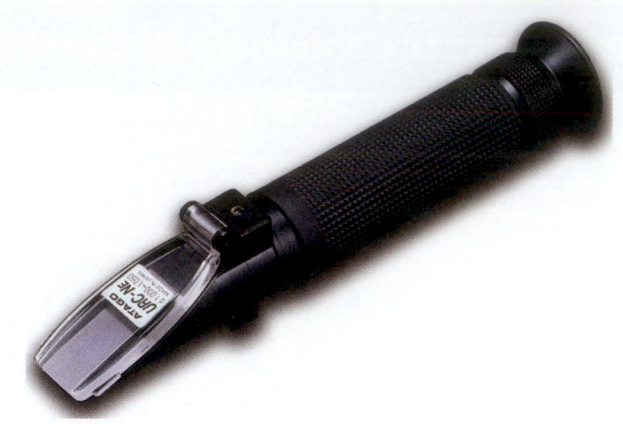

Figure 33-15 ◆ Portable digital refractometer.

Amino acid disorders, being hereditary, are quite rare, and detection is critical when the individuals are very young, so that appropriate treatment can be administered as soon as possible.

Specific Gravity

Specific gravity is the measurement of a specific volume of urine to an equal volume of water. Solutes in the urine contribute to the measurement. The concentrating and filtrating status of the kidneys, as well as the body's hydration status, are assessed by measuring urine specific gravity.

The normal range of specific gravity of urine for adults with normal diets and normal fluid intake is moderately concentrated, from 1.016 to 1.022, compared with the specific gravity of blood plasma, which remains very close to 1.010 at all times. In conditions such as diabetes insipidus, in which the urine is more dilute, the specific gravity is lower. In conditions such as diabetes mellitus, in which the urine is more concentrated, the specific gravity is higher.

The specific gravity of urine can be measured with a refractometer (Figure 33-15 ◆) (also called a hydrometer), or a chemical test strip. Urinometers are now used infrequently, as other devices, such as dipsticks, are easier and more accurate. Some PLOs prefer to use the refractometer.

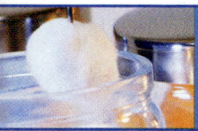

PROCEDURE 33-5 Measure Urine Specific Gravity with a Refractometer

Theory and Rationale

Specific gravity measures the kidney's ability to concentrate or dilute urine in relation to plasma. Because urine is a solution of minerals, salts, and compounds dissolved in water, the specific gravity is greater than 1.000. The more concentrated the urine, the higher the urine specific gravity. An adult's kidneys have a remarkable ability to concentrate or dilute urine. In infants, the range for specific gravity is less because immature kidneys are not able to concentrate urine as effectively as mature kidneys.

Materials

- urine specimen (at room temperature)
- urinary refractometer
- disposable pipette
- distilled water (if calibration of refractometer is required)

PROCEDURE 33-5 Measure Urine Specific Gravity with a Refractometer *(continued)*

- biohazard waste container
- patient chart or laboratory report form

Competency

(**Conditions**) With the necessary materials, (**Task**) you will be able to measure urine specific gravity with a refractometer (**Standards**) correctly within the time frame designated by the instructor.

1. Wash your hands and gather equipment and supplies.
2. Apply gloves and protective clothing and check the specimen container for proper labeling.
3. Mix the urine specimen in the urine collection container.
4. Confirm that the refractometer has been calibrated according to manufacturer specifications. Record the calibration values in the quality control log.
5. Open the hinged lid of the refractometer.
6. Draw up a small amount of the specimen into the pipette. Discard the pipette in a biohazard waste container.

7. Place one drop of the specimen under the cover and close the lid.
8. Turn on the light or point the device toward a light source. Read the specific gravity value on the scale.
9. Discard the urine specimen appropriately.
10. Remove the gloves and wash your hands.
11. Record the specific gravity value on the laboratory report form.
12. Clean the instrument according to the manufacture's guidelines.

Charting Example

Document in designated logs any quality control or safety measures you followed, such as calibration of the refractometer, correct storage and disposal of specimen, or OSHA precautions taken. The medical assistant will document the results of the urine specific gravity in the patient's chart.

Urinalysis with Chemical Test Strips

The presence of abnormal body processes that affect the metabolism of carbohydrates, acid-base balance, and liver and kidney functions can be determined by testing the urine with chemical reagent test strips, or dipsticks (Figure 33-16 ◆). The same test is also used to detect infections or assess for drugs.

Each reagent pad on a test strip is saturated with chemicals that react with urine components to produce a predictable color change. The color can be observed with the naked eye and compared to color change charts and graphics provided by the manufacturer. Results are reported on standardized forms or entered into computer databases. Test strips may also be read by specially designed instruments that recognize and measure the same color changes that the human eye detects. This method is referred to as *reflectance spectrophotometry*. Each manufacturer

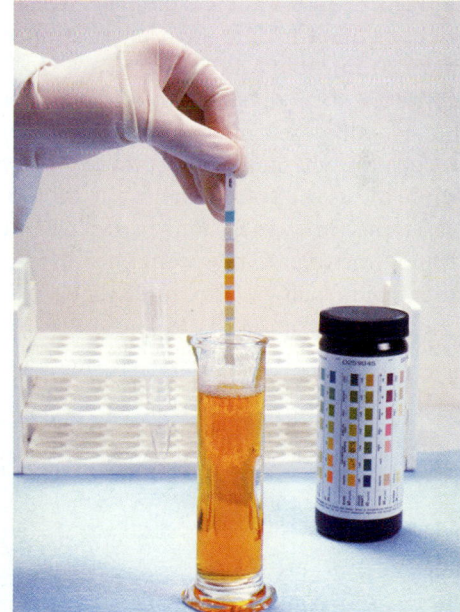

Figure 33-16 ◆ Chemical test strips.

may place the reagent pads in its own specific order; verify order and results with manufacturer's instructions.

The test strip is immersed for one second in the urine. The back of the strip is wiped against a blotter, such as a paper towel, then turned at a right angle to drain excess urine (Figure 33-17 ◆).

Strip reactions occur rapidly and should be read quickly after the appropriate incubation time, which ranges from

Keys to Success
CHECKLIST FOR URINE SPECIMEN EVALUATION

1. Is the specimen properly labeled?
2. Is it the proper type of specimen for the requested test?
3. Is the specimen properly preserved, if necessary?
4. Has the specimen been received in a timely fashion?
5. Are there any signs of contamination?
6. If the specimen is for multiple tests, has the bacteriologic examination been done first?
7. How many **aliquots** must be taken?

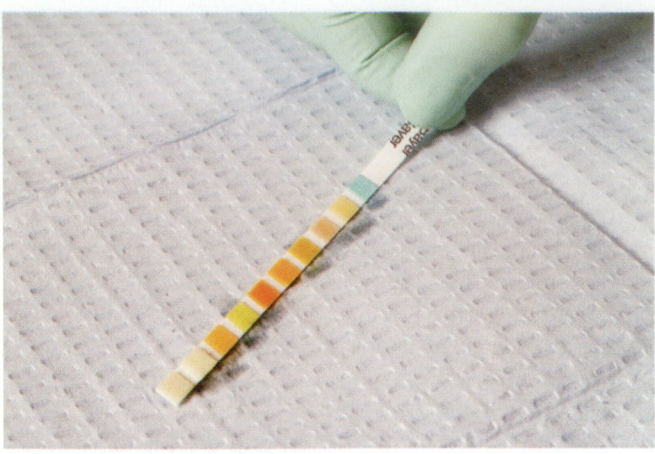

Figure 33-17 ◆ The back of the strip is wiped, then turned at a right angle to drain excess urine.

30 seconds (bilirubin and glucose) to 2 minutes (leukocytes). The test strip pad is designed so the user can begin reading with the glucose and bilirubin pads at the grip end and finish with the leukocytes pad at the tip.

To read the test strip manually, simply hold it close to the manufacturer's color chart on the side of the container or on a separate sheet and read the color change under a bright white light source (Figure 33-18 ◆). If an automated reader is available, simply insert the strip onto the reader tray after blotting and allow the instrument to read the results.

Urinalysis test strips should always be kept tightly sealed in their containers, at room temperature, until use. Discolored pads indicate damage and should be discarded. CLIA 1988 regulations require the use of a positive and a negative or normal control at least once in each 24-hour period when testing is performed and whenever a new container of dipsticks is opened. Patient and quality control results must be recorded

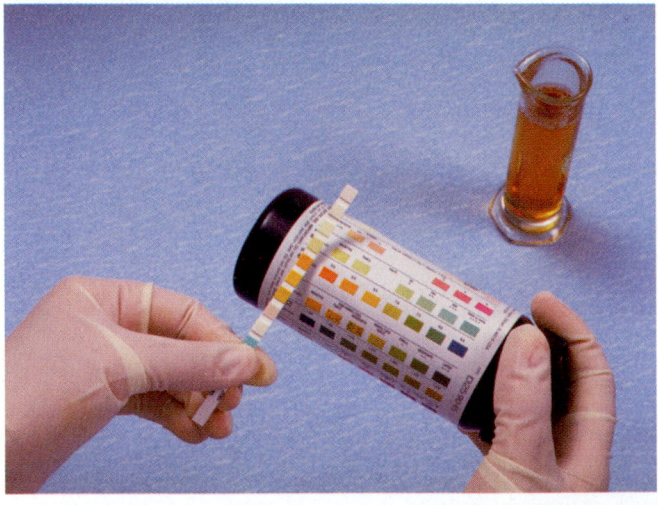

Figure 33-18 ◆ Hold the test strip next to the color chart and take the reading.

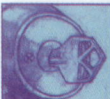

Keys to Success
TESTING STRONGLY PIGMENTED URINE

A strong abnormal color to the urine, regardless of the shade, may interfere with the accurate reading of some or all of the test strip pad reagent reactions, whether the reading is done visually or by instrument. Multistix® 10 SG Reagent Strips read visually or on the Clinitek® 50 instrument are waived under CLIA guidelines.

and maintained for reference. Factors that affect test strip testing are summarized in Table 33-5.

The chemical tests typically performed in a routine urinalysis are pH, specific gravity, protein, glucose, ketones, bilirubin, urobilinogen, blood, leukocytes, and nitrite.

pH

Normal urine pH ranges from moderately acidic (pH 5) to moderately alkaline (pH 8). Most individuals produce a slightly acidic urine (pH 5.0–6.0). Compounds in the diet have a great influence on urine pH, as do a variety of drugs. The pH reaction should be read at 60 seconds. No pH reading from a test strip indicates an abnormal situation by itself. There are no conditions that produce a false positive (pH result too high or alkaline) on the pH pad. However, improperly stored urine may have a genuine change of pH to the alkaline because of bacterial conversion of urea to ammonia. A false negative pH (pH result too low or acid) can occur in the presence of runoff of the acid buffer in the adjacent protein pad. This can be prevented by proper blotting.

Specific Gravity

No specific gravity reading with a dipstick indicates an abnormal situation by itself because other factors, such as exercise or high fluid intake before the test, can affect the results.

Protein

The normal level of urinary protein is insignificant. The urine dipstick is adjusted so that this normal background protein does not trigger a reaction on the pad. A positive reaction indicates clinically a significant increase in urine proteins. Normal individuals may experience **proteinuria** after strenuous exercise or other circumstances that create a transient dehydration through sweating, such as fevers or prolonged exposure to a hot environment.

Glucose

The normal urinary glucose level should be zero because normally all the glucose filtered at the glomerulus is rapidly reabsorbed in the proximal tubule. Occasionally, after a very rich meal, a normal individual may have a transient blood glucose level high enough to be read; otherwise, glucose enters the urine only if the patient is consistently hyperglycemic.

TABLE 33-5 FACTORS THAT AFFECT TEST STRIP TESTING

Test	Renal Disease	Systemic Disease	False Positives	False Negatives
Specific gravity	Urine-concentrating disorder	Fluid status changes	Proteinuria	Alkaline urine
pH	Renal tubular acidosis	Acid-base disorders	None	None
	UTIs may produce alkaline pH			
Protein	Glomerular disease	Infection	Alkaline pH	Dilute urine
	Infection	Exercise-caused transient	Detergents	Bence-Jones
	Tubular disorders	proteinuria		protein
		Bence-Jones protein in myeloma and related disorders		
Microalbumin	Early renal disease	(See protein)	Timing errors	Timing errors
Glucose	Rarely increased in tubular disorders	Diabetes mellitus	Detergents	Vitamin C
			Hypochlorite	Aspirin
			Peroxide	
Ketones	None	Ketotic states	L-Dopa	Old specimens
Blood	Any site of bleeding in urinary tract (glomerulo-nephritis, tumor, stones, infection)	Coagulopathy	Colored meds	Vitamin C
		Hemoglobinuria in hemolysis		Exposure to air
		Myoglobinuria with muscle damage		
Ascorbic acid	None	Treatment with vitamin C	Other reducing substances	None
Bilirubin	None	Liver and biliary disease	Colored meds	Light exposure
Urobilinogen	None	Hemolysis	Colored meds	Light exposure
		Cirrhosis		Nitrite
				Formalin
Nitrite	Infection with most gram-negative organisms	None	Colored meds	Vitamin C
Leukocyte esterase	Infection of genitourinary system	None	Oxidizing detergents	Glucose
	Interstitial nephritis			Protein
				High specific gravity

Ketones

Acetacetic acid, B-hydroxybuteric acid, and acetone are normal intermediary metabolites of fat metabolism, termed ketones or "ketone bodies." Ketones are normally recycled by the liver into other usable organic nutrient compounds. Small quantities are normal in the blood and may spill over into the urine. They become markedly increased and of clinical significance in uncontrolled diabetes mellitus, particularly in diabetic ketoacidosis; in starvation or the temporary starvation that accompanies disorders whose symptoms include severe vomiting and/or diarrhea; and in acute febrile illnesses.

Bilirubin and Urobilinogen

Bilirubin levels rise in the blood and other body fluids, including urine, under three main conditions:

- Any major hemolytic episode in which blood escapes into a tissue space and must be broken down
- Liver disease
- Obstructions

Blood

The test strip pad for blood responds not only to intact RBCs but also to free hemoglobin and free myoglobin suspended in the specimen. Blood in the urine may indicate conditions such as hemorrhagic tissue injury, infection, coagulation disorder, kidney disorders, certain drug responses, and cancer.

Leukocytes

With their ability to use ameboid movements, leukocytes can enter the urinary tract anywhere along its length. A few leukocytes in anyone's urine specimen are considered normal. Increased leukocytes, however, are an excellent indicator of an inflammatory process occurring somewhere within the urinary tract. A positive result on the test strip leukocytes pad should be confirmed and compared to urine microscopy results.

Nitrite

The presence of nitrite in the urine is strong indirect evidence of bacteria in the urine. Nitrite is the metabolic product of the enzyme nitrate reductase. Although not all bacterial species capable of causing a urinary tract infection (UTI) produce nitrate reductase, most of the common ones do.

Critical Thinking Question 33-2

Given the patient's complaint, what tests do you think Gina should prepare to perform?

Sediment Examination

Before proceeding with a microscopic urinalysis, the specimen should be spun in a centrifuge. Centrifuging separates the sediment, which is the insoluble material, from the soluble material. Sediment settles to the bottom of the test tube after centrifuging.

The centrifuged urine sediment is examined with a standard bright field microscope with a low-power (10X) and high-power (40X) objective. Stains that color cellular structures, such as the Sternheimer-Malbin stain, are often used to assist in identification.

The formed elements that can be viewed under the microscope consist of the following:

crystals	bacteria
yeast and fungi	protozoa
parasites	epithelial cells
renal tubular epithelial cells	RBCs
WBCs	sperm cells
casts	artifacts

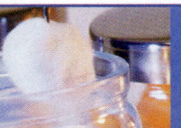

PROCEDURE 33-6 **Perform Urinalysis Using Chemical Test Strips**

Theory and Rationale

Check the expiration date of the chemical test strips to ensure accurate test results. Keep the test strips dry and avoid touching the reactive reagent materials on the strips. Tighten the lid of the bottle immediately after removing a strip.

The test strip must be immersed completely to cover all the reagent squares. To prevent dilution of the chemicals and inaccurate results, pull out the strip in less than one second and remove excess urine. Hold the strip carefully above but close to the color chart. Any urine from the strip that touches the bottle could affect the colors of the chart. Finally, read the test strip areas at the correct times to ensure accuracy. The time for reading results ranges from 30 seconds to 2 minutes.

Although used less commonly, Acetest® (for ketones) and Clinitest® (for glucose) tablets may be used in urine testing of the diabetic.

Materials

- chemical reagent urine test strips
- blotting paper
- urine container
- centrifuge and test tubes
- microscope
- slide and cover slip
- pipette
- disposable gloves
- biohazardous waste receptacle
- urinalysis report form

Competency

(**Conditions**) With the necessary materials, (**Task**) you will be able to perform a urinalysis with chemical test strips (**Standards**) correctly.

1. Wash your hands. Gather equipment and supplies. Check the expiration date on the reagent strip container.

2. Identify the patient and guide him or her to the treatment area.

3. Provide the patient with a labeled urine container. Instruct the patient on how to obtain the specimen and where to leave it.

4. Wash your hands. Put on disposable gloves.

5. After the patient leaves the specimen in the designated area, move it to the testing area.

6. Observe and describe the urine's color, quantity, and odor. Inform the physician that the sample is ready for viewing.

7. Remove one reagent strip and recap the bottle tightly and immediately. Do not touch the test area of the strip. If necessary, place the strip temporarily on a dry paper towel while you open the urine specimen container.

8. Dip the test strip briefly in the urine, making sure to cover all testing areas (Figure 33-19 ◆). Pull the strip gently back against the inner edge of the container mouth, then place the length of the strip at a right angle to the blotting paper to remove excess urine.

9. Hold the reagent test areas of the strip next to, but not touching, the matching areas on the test strip bottle. Note the reaction reading at the time mentioned on the bottle for each square of reagent.

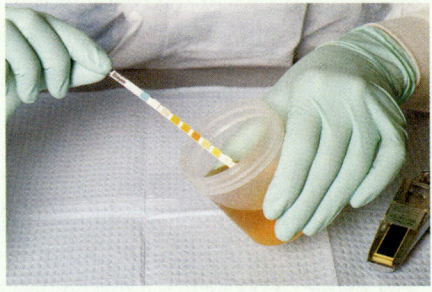

Figure 33-19 ◆ Dip the test strip into urine, covering all testing areas.

PROCEDURE 33-6 Perform Urinalysis Using Chemical Test Strips *(continued)*

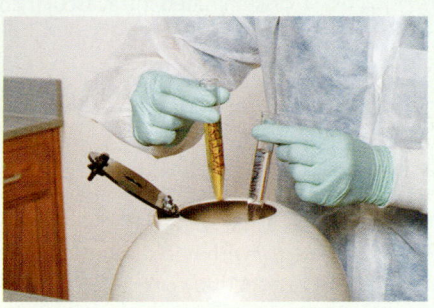

Figure 33-20 ◆ Load the centrifuge.

10. Dispose of the urine test strip in the biohazardous waste container.
11. Prepare urine for microscopic examination by the physician.
    - Put approximately 10 cc in a tube on one side of the centrifuge, and on the opposite side an equal amount of liquid in another tube (Figure 33-20 ◆).
    - Run the centrifuge for 5 minutes.
    - Pour out most of the liquid (supernatant) from the tube, but keep the sediment (Figure 33-21 ◆).
    - Mix the remaining liquid with the sediment and pipette a couple of drops of moistened sediment onto a slide (Figure 33-22 ◆).
    - Cover with a cover slip. Position and focus the slide under the lighted microscope.
12. Remove the gloves and discard in proper container. Wash your hands.

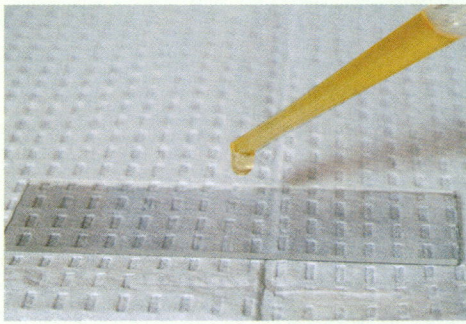

Figure 33-22 ◆ Place the urine sample on the slide.

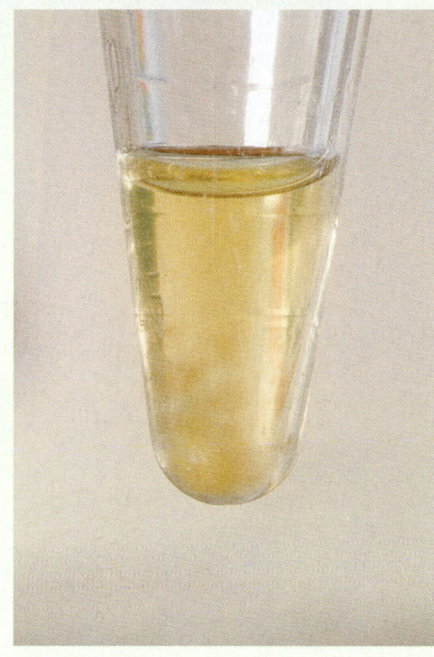

Figure 33-21 ◆ Pour out most of the liquid (supernatant) from the tube, but keep the sediment.

13. Chart the results on the reporting urine lab slip immediately, including the date, time, and urine test strip brand name. Record the color, odor, volume, and cloudiness or sediment.
14. On the patient's chart, chart the date and time of specimen collection and procedure performance.
15. Return to the microscope examination area for cleaning and disposal.

Patient Education

Inform the patient that urine test strip testing will identify components in the urine and that the physician will review the results and call if additional or new treatment is needed.

Charting Example

04/8/XX 1:30 p.m. Routine urinalysis specimen provided by pt. Immediate testing showed traces of protein and glucose. Information placed in chart and physician notified. Jennifer Wilson, CMA (AAMA)

Table 33-6 lists significant microscopic findings that may be found in urine by the medical technologist or physician. The physician may examine the centrifuged specimen under the microscope, record his or her observations, diagnose the problem, and prescribe treatment and medication while the patient is still in the office. The information in the table is useful for a basic understanding of the correlation between the report and the diagnosis and treatment.

Crystals

Crystals form in the urine as salts (Figure 33-23 ◆) and can be found in the urine of a healthy patient. The number of crystals

TABLE 33-6 SIGNIFICANT MICROSCOPIC FINDINGS IN URINE

Finding	Normal	Urinary Tract Disease	Systemic Disease
RBCs	3/high power field; higher in menstruating women	Glomerular injury Nephrolithiasis Inflammation (especially hemorrhagic cystitis) Neoplasms	Rarely with sickle cell anemia, disseminated intravascular coagulation
WBCs	3–5/high power	Infections of bladder or kidney Interstitial nephritis (eosinophils)	Infection of prostate, cervix, or vagina
Hyaline casts	After exercise, dehydration stress	Any cause of proteinuria, especially glomerular disease	Dehydration, fever, other causes of proteinuria, such as diabetes
Granular casts	Similar to hyaline casts	Heavy proteinuria Pigmented granular casts with acute tubular necrosis	Rarely with non-glomerular causes of proteinuria
Cellular casts	Not found	RBC casts in glomerulonephritis WBC casts in pyelonephritis	Not commonly found
Epithelial cells	Squamous, transitional epithelial cells	Renal tubular cells with tubular injury (tubular necrosis, transplant rejection)	None
Crystals	Uric acid, calcium oxalate, triple phosphate	Cystine in some tubular disorders Uric acid, calcium oxalate rarely with nephrolithiasis	Congenital aminoacidurias, drug crystals
Organisms	Present from contamination or prolonged storage before examination	Cystitis Pyelonephritis	Prostatitis may also give positive culture

(A) Crystals in Acid Urine

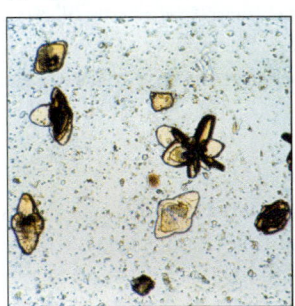 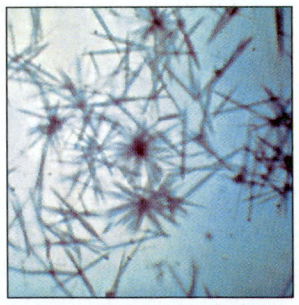 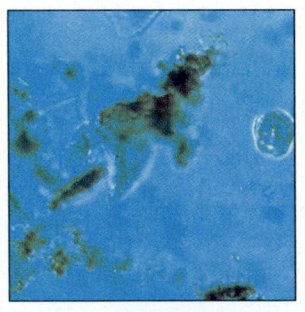 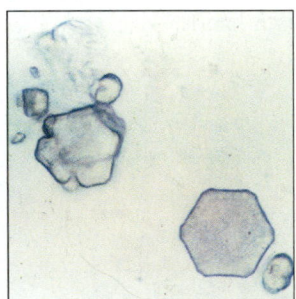

(B) Crystals in Alkaline Urine

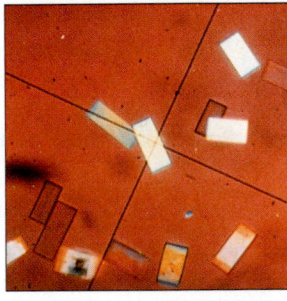 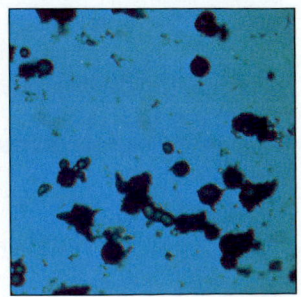 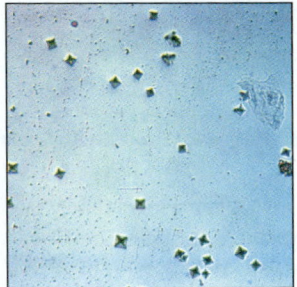

Figure 33-23 ◆ (A) Crystals in acid urine; (B) Crystals in alkaline urine.
Courtesy of Bayer Diagnostic

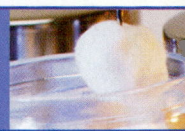

PROCEDURE 33-7 Perform a Multidrug Screen Urine Test Using the Instant-View Multi-Drug Screen Test

Theory and Rationale

Urine drug testing kits are available for testing urine specimens in the physician office laboratory (POL). The most commonly abused drugs are usually tested with the current urine drug screening tests. The drugs often targeted include amphetamines, barbiturates, cocaine, benzodiazepines, marijuana, opiates, PCP, and methadone. The usual procedure for urine drug testing involves screening the specimen and confirming positive results with more specific urine tests. The results are read according to the manufacturer's instructions. A chain of custody must be followed exactly and any alteration will result in a break in the chain. The chain-of-custody process is used to maintain and document the history of the specimen and ensures that the sample has been in the possession of, or secured by, a responsible person at all times.

Materials

- Instant-View Multi-Drug Screen Urine Test in a sealed pouch
- freshly voided urine sample
- timer
- biohazard waste container

Competency

(**Conditions**) With the necessary materials, you will be able to (**Task**) perform a Multi-Drug Screen Test (**Standards**) correctly within the time designated by your instructor.

1. Wash your hands and put on your gloves and PPE.
2. Assemble the equipment and urine specimen. Ensure that the test kit has not expired. Expired test kits should be discarded immediately.

3. Determine the urine temperature (within 4 minutes of voiding). The temperature should range between 90 degrees F and 100 degrees F.
4. Remove the device from the foil patch and label it with the patient's identification information.
5. Remove the cap from the urine specimen cup and dip the device into the specimen for 10 seconds. The surface of the urine must be above the sample well and below the arrowheads in the window.
6. Recap the urine specimen.
7. Set the timer for 4 to 7 minutes. Do not read the results after 7 minutes.
8. Interpret the results according to the manufacturer's guidelines.
9. Discard all biohazard waste in the appropriate container.
10. Remove your gloves and mask.
11. Wash your hands.
12. Record the results in the patient's chart.

Patient Education

Inform the patient that medication (both prescription and nonprescription) will show up in the test results; therefore, it is important for the patient to disclose the names and types of all substances consumed in the last 30 days, including what was taken and how much. This information can be disclosed on a drug screen consent form.

Charting

5/16/xx 10:15 am Instant-View Multi-Drug Screen Test performed and results read according to manufacturer's instructions. Screening test result negative. Consent formed signed by patient and chain-of-custody followed without any alteration. Derrick Joshua, CMA (AAMA)

---

in a urine specimen is affected by cooling and by aging. After a specimen has been collected and begins to cool, especially if it is refrigerated, additional crystals may form that were not present in the fresh specimen. On the other hand, as a urine specimen ages and the pH changes, crystals that were initially present in the fresh specimen may degrade or even disappear. The addition or degradation of crystals affects the accuracy of the test results. Assessing crystal formation helps in the diagnosis and treatment of disorders.

A given patient specimen may contain several different kinds of crystals in various proportions. Normal crystals tend to form in neutral to alkaline urines. All the abnormal crystals of significance generally tend to form in acid urines. They include certain amino acids, such as cystine, leucine, and tyrosine, which are observed in some renal tubular

disorders. Bilirubin and cholesterol are two other abnormal crystals.

A variety of drugs, such as sulfonamides, penicillins, and cephalosporins, form abnormal crystals when the urine is concentrated and the pH is favorable for crystallization. Drug crystals take a variety of forms and are difficult to identify without the patient's medication records for confirmation.

The Male Reproductive System

The male reproductive system uses part of the urinary tract in its function. The urological medical office is where male reproductive system disorders are often treated. These include prostate disorders, fertility problems and disorders, testicular disorders, and sexually transmitted diseases.

Anatomy and Physiology

The male reproductive system is composed of two major external structures and several internal structures (Figure 33-24 ◆). The penis and the scrotum are the external structures.

Penis

Tubular in shape and hollow, the penis provides a route for sperm to leave the male reproductive system and be directed into the female reproductive system. Arteries in the penis engorge with blood during sexual stimulation, promoting an erection. The firmness of the penis allows penetration into the vagina. Ejaculation releases sperm into the vagina; the sperm meet with and fertilize the ovum. The reproductive function of the penis is secondary to the excretion of urine from the urinary bladder through the urethra.

Scrotum

The scrotum contains two walnut-sized ovoid structures, the **testes** or **testicles.** Each testicle is made up of fibrous tissue and many lobes containing small tubes, the seminiferous tubules. Sperm cells, or spermatozoa, develop in these tubes. Testosterone is also produced in the testes. Secondary sex characteristics are stimulated by testosterone. Located posterior to each testicle is the epididymis. The tubules from the testicle join to form efferent tubules that open into the epididymis. Sperm is stored here to mature before moving on in the system. Spermatozoa are sensitive to heat and are destroyed by normal body temperature; therefore, the testes are suspended down from the body in a cooler environment.

All males should be taught and encouraged to perform routine self-examination of the testicles after puberty.

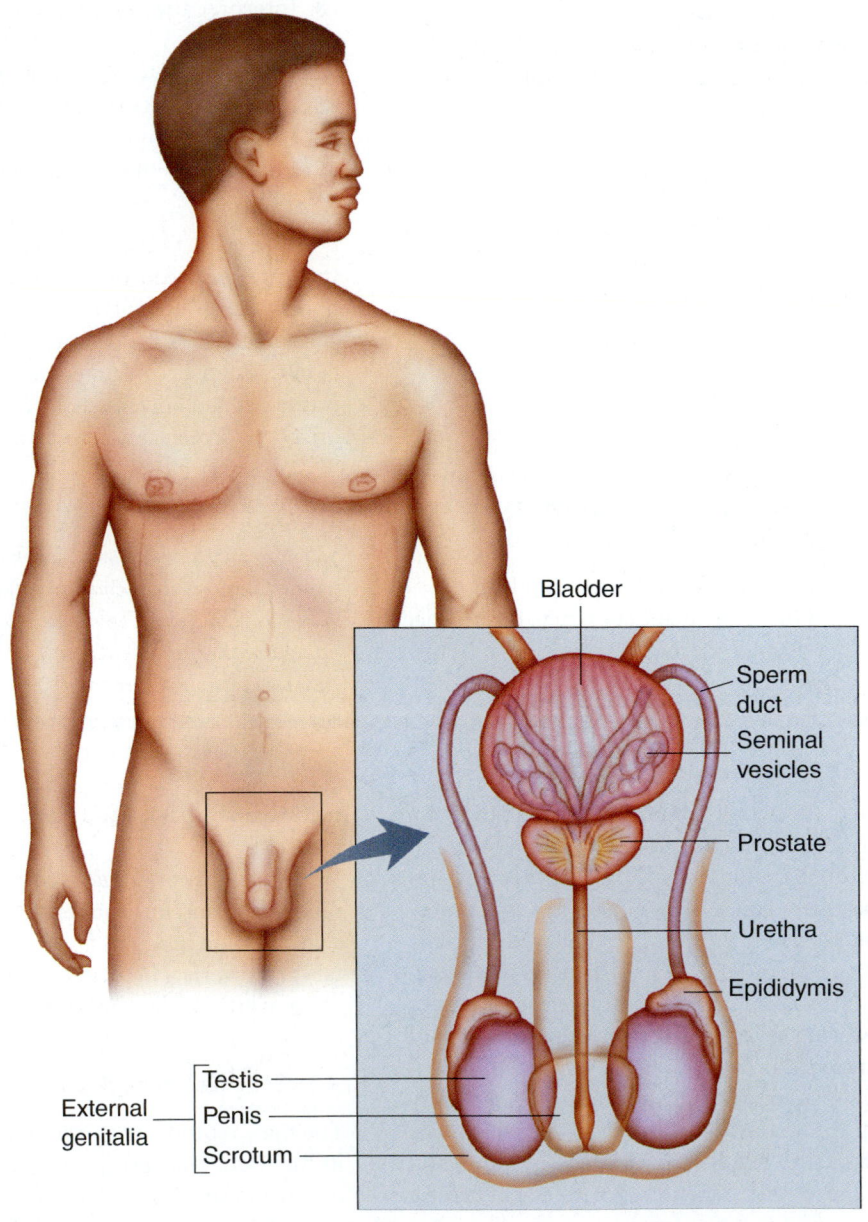

Figure 33-24 ◆ Diagram of the male reproductive system.

In Practice

Christopher King presents to the medical office for a routine checkup. After his exam, the physician requests that the medical assistant provide patient instruction for the testicular self-examination. Why is testicular self-examination important?

Internal Structures

Internal structures ascend into the anterior pelvis as the epididymis transforms into the vas deferens. The vas deferens passes over the bladder and descends posterior in another tubular structure, the seminal vesicle. The seminal vesicles produce an alkaline fluid that becomes the semen that transports the sperm. The seminal vesicle descends and makes an anterior turn to pass through the posterior portion of the prostate gland to join at an approximate midpoint, the prostatic urethra that has descended from the urinary bladder. The urethra continues anterior and then descends down the penis to exit at the urinary meatus. The bulbourethral gland lies under the prostate gland and connects to the urethra as the urethra descends from the prostate gland. These glands, also called Cowper's glands, produce a mucus-type fluid that becomes part of semen, the product ejaculated during intercourse.

PROCEDURE 33-8   Demonstrate Patient Instruction for Testicular Self-Examination

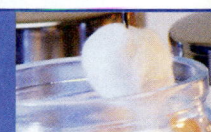

Theory and Rationale

Examination of a man's testicles should be part of a general physical exam. The American Cancer Society (ACS) recommends a testicular exam as part of a routine cancer-related checkup. The ACS advises men to be aware of testicular cancer and to see a doctor right away if a mass is found. Identifying masses promptly is an important factor in getting early treatment, and it is recommended that all men do monthly testicular self-exams after puberty.

　　The patient should be aware that each normal testis has an epididymis, which appears as a small "bump" on the upper or middle outer side of the testis. Normal testicles also contain blood vessels, supporting tissues, and tubes that conduct sperm. Other noncancerous conditions, such as hydroceles and varicoceles, can sometimes cause enlargement or lumpiness around a testicle. Some men may confuse these with cancer. If the patient has any doubts, he should speak with the doctor. Whether the abnormality is a possible tumor or another condition, early treatment is often less complicated and severe.

Materials

■ Pamphlet with instructions for performing an at-home testicular exam.

Competency

(**Conditions**) With the necessary materials, (**Task**) you will be able to instruct the patient on performing a testicular self-examination (**Standards**) correctly within the time frame designated by the instructor.

1. Wash your hands. Gather equipment and supplies.
2. Identify the patient and guide him to the treatment area.

3. Instruct the patient to:
   - Take a warm bath or shower to relax the scrotum. In the clinical setting, the patient should take several deep breaths.
   - Observe the contour of the scrotum. If one testicle is slightly larger or lies somewhat lower than the other, this is considered normal (Figure 33-25 ◆).

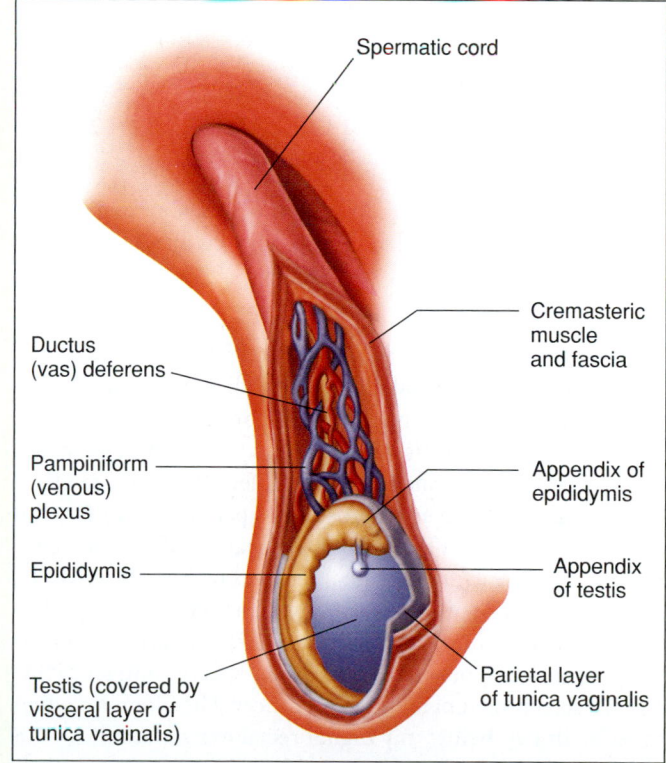

Figure 33-25 ◆ Illustration of normal scrotum.

continued

PROCEDURE 33-8 Demonstrate Patient Instruction for Testicular Self-Examination *(continued)*

- Elevate the right leg to the level of a toilet, chair, or bed to expose the right testicle.
- With the left hand, lightly support the right testicle. With the right hand, palpate the right testicle for hardness, lumps, or anything unusual (Figure 33-26 ♦).
- Reverse the process by elevating the left leg to examine the left testicle. Support the left testicle with the right hand and, with the left hand, palpate the left testicle.

4. If the patient finds any abnormalities or has any questions, he should contact the physician.

Patient Education

Ask the patient to repeat the instructions to verify that he understands them. Provide him with written instructions, if available.

Charting Example

02-28-XX 9:25 a.m. Patient given written and verbal testicular self-exam instructions. Patient demonstrated correct technique and understanding of the importance of monthly self-examinations. Erin Janson, RMA (AMT)

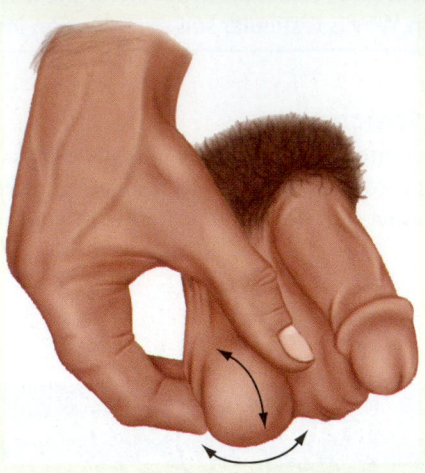

Figure 33-26 ♦ Palpate the testicle for hardness, lumps, or anything unusual.

Diseases and Disorders of the Male Reproductive System

Diseases and disorders of the male reproductive system include not only reproductive and fertility conditions but often urinary conditions as well.

Diseases and Disorders of the Prostate

The prostate gland is located just below the male urinary bladder and encircles the urethra. Any condition affecting the prostate gland may cause enlargement, followed by pain and urinary retention. Conditions that affect the prostate gland include **prostatitis,** benign prostatic hypertrophy (**BPH**), and cancer (carcinoma) (Table 33-7). Evaluation of prostate conditions usually includes a digital rectal examination (**DRE**) by the physician. The prostate gland is palpated by inserting a finger into the rectum and evaluating for size, tenderness, and any nodules or lumps present. The prostate-specific antigen (PSA) test is a screening tool for prostate cancer. The blood for a PSA must be drawn before any digital rectal examination. A DRE can cause the prostate gland to release PSA into the bloodstream, resulting in an inaccurate value.

Male Reproductive Disorders

Sexually active couples who do not conceive after one year of unprotected sexual intercourse are considered to have a fertility problem. The urologist may be involved in diagnosing and treating male fertility disorders (Table 33-8). Evaluation of the male reproductive system involves a thorough medical history, physical examination, and evaluation of semen for sperm count and

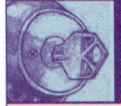

Keys to Success
VALUES FOR PROSTATE-SPECIFIC ANTIGENS (PSAS)

The PSA test is recommended annually for males over age 50. It is important for men to establish a baseline at some point between the ages of 40 and 50. Any sudden elevation in the value requires further evaluation. A continuous climb in values is a good indication of the presence of carcinoma. Fluctuations up and down indicate BPH or prostatitis. Patients should be cautioned that the PSA test is a screening tool and that the DRE is a major part of the diagnosis.

TABLE 33-7 DISEASES AND DISORDERS OF THE PROSTATE

Disease or Disorder	Symptoms	Diagnosis	Treatment
Prostatitis ■ Inflammation of the prostate gland ■ Can be acute bacterial, chronic bacterial, or chronic noninfectious in nature. Causative agents in both bacterial forms commonly are *E. coli* and Proteus ■ Bacterial condition usually affects younger males and is often recurrent	Acute: ■ Fever ■ Chills ■ Rectal, low back, or perineal pain Chronic bacterial: ■ Recurrent UTIs ■ Dysuria ■ Genital and ejaculatory pain Chronic nonbacterial: ■ Chronic pelvic pain ■ Ejaculatory pain	■ Patient presenting symptoms ■ Urinalysis ■ Digital rectal examination (DRE)	■ Antibacterial medications ■ Anti-inflammatory drugs, alpha blockers, and allopurinol for inflammatory condition ■ 20-minute hot sitz baths two or three times a day to help relieve pain of inflammatory conditions ■ Application of ice two to three times a day for 20 minutes to help relieve pain of inflammatory conditions when sitz baths fail ■ Increased fluid intake (especially water) to dilute urine ■ Avoidance of caffeine-containing beverages to avoid dehydration
Benign prostatic hypertrophy (BPH) ■ Progressive enlargement of prostate gland that eventually causes obstruction of urethra and interferes with urination ■ Common in older men with increasing age ■ Cause is unknown	Hematuria Urination: ■ Frequent ■ Difficulty starting ■ Decreased force ■ Dribbling after voiding ■ Feeling bladder is not empty after voiding	■ Patient presenting symptoms ■ Physical examination ■ DRE ■ Urinalysis ■ Urine culture ■ Bladder X-ray ■ Cystoscopy	■ Drug therapy to relax neck of bladder and possibly shrink prostate ■ Laser treatment less invasive treatment to remove offending tissue ■ Cystoscopy for transurethral resection less invasive treatment with cystoscope, which is passed up the urethra; portions of prostate gland are shaved off and flushed from bladder ■ Surgery to remove enlarged gland through incision in lower abdomen, just above pelvis
Cancer (Carcinoma) ■ Second most common cause of male cancer deaths ■ Has a tendency to metastasize ■ Prostate feels hard and lumpy on palpation during a DRE	■ Similar to BPH ■ Elevated PSA	■ Patient presenting symptoms ■ DRE ■ Biopsy	■ Radiation ■ Chemotherapy ■ Hormonal drug therapy ■ Surgery (side effects of radical surgical excision include urinary incontinence, erectile dysfunction, and/or impotence) ■ Treatment factors include patient's age and physical condition, treatment side effects, and extent of cancer

motility. Causes of problems in the male include structural anomalies, low sperm count and motility, trauma to the perineum and testicles, exposure to radiation, previous infectious diseases of the system, hormonal imbalances, and stress. Treatment depends on the cause, and not all male fertility problems can be corrected.

Patient Education

African American males are at greater risk for prostate and bladder cancers. The importance of routine PSA screenings and DREs should be stressed in public awareness campaigns and in patient education in the medical office.

TABLE 33-8 MALE REPRODUCTIVE DISORDERS

Disease or Disorder	Symptoms	Diagnosis	Treatment
Erectile dysfunction ■ Inability to achieve erection with stimulation and maintain it for ejaculation ■ Experienced by most men at some time in their lives ■ Caused by failure of arteries that supply blood to penis to dilate and engorge penis; by nerve damage to spinal cord or other nerves supplying penis; by medical conditions such as diabetes, hyper-tension, heart disease; by drugs for these conditions; by alcohol consumption, smoking, stress	■ Failure to achieve erection	■ Patient presenting symptoms	■ Vasodilator such as sildenafil citrate (Viagra®) ■ Penile implants and suction pumps for artificial erection ■ Counseling for couples
Cryptorchism ■ One or both testes fail to descend into scrotal sac during fetal development ■ Must be treated in first year of child's life to prevent infertility and possible predisposition to tumors later in life	■ Undescended testes	■ Examination of scrotal sac after birth and at well-baby checkups	■ Hormone injections to help testes descend ■ Orchidopexy, RA surgical procedure to move testes to scrotal sac
Torsion of the testicles ■ Spermatic cord is twisted, resulting in diminished venous flow ■ Often result of traumatic insult to scrotum and testicles or result of congenital problem	■ Severe pain ■ Swelling ■ Redness ■ Tenderness	■ Patient presenting symptoms ■ Physical examination	■ Surgery if problem does not resolve on its own
Testicular cancer ■ Leading cancer in males 25 to 40 ■ Risk factors: family history, age under 40, Caucasian, undescended testes at birth, history of testicular infections ■ Painless lump in testicle is often first indication ■ Favorable outcome if discovered early and treated aggressively	■ Presence of lump	■ Physical examination ■ Biopsy	■ Surgery to remove lump ■ Radiation ■ Chemotherapy

Testicular disorders include but are not limited to **cryptorchism,** torsion of the testicles, and cancer of the testicles.

Sexually Transmitted Diseases

Sexually transmitted diseases (STDs) or infections take many forms (Table 33-9). Common STDs in men include chlamydia, gonorrhea, syphilis, genital herpes, genital warts (*Condylamata acuminata*) and trichomoniasis. Many of these conditions present no symptoms at the onset. STDs are transmitted not only through sexual contact but by blood and body fluids. Untreated STDs are spread unknowingly, can cause sterility, and may even become life-threatening.

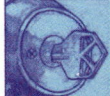

Keys to Success
THE SIDE EFFECTS OF VIAGRA

Viagra (sildenafil citrate) is a vasodilator with specific activity directed to the penile arteries and has some dangerous side effects. Men with a history of cardiovascular disease, cerebral vascular accident, hypo- or hypertension, angina, or glaucoma should not take Viagra. Vascular dilation could be life-threatening in men with these disorders.

TABLE 33-9 SEXUALLY TRANSMITTED DISEASES IN MALES

Disease	Symptoms	Diagnosis	Treatment
Chlamydia ■ Caused by *Chlamydia trachomatis* ■ Often no symptoms until irreversible damage has occurred	■ Frequent and painful urination ■ Pus in urine ■ Penile discharge	■ Patient presenting symptoms	■ Antibiotics (other than penicillin) for bacterial infections ■ Abstinence or protected (safe) sex for prevention
Gonorrhea ■ Caused by *Neiserria gonorrhoeae* ■ Transmitted by sexual contact ■ May become systemic	■ Pus or purulent discharge from urethra	■ Patient presenting symptoms ■ Physical examination	■ Antibiotics: penicillin, tetracycline, and ceftriaxone ■ Abstinence or protected (safe) sex for prevention
Syphilis ■ Caused by *Treponema pallidum;* can become systemic if undiagnosed and untreated ■ Transmitted by sexual contact; contagious in first and second stages ■ May go dormant for a number of years but remains in bloodstream ■ At end stage, cannot be reversed	■ First stage: ulcer or chancre on genital area ■ If untreated, second stage: rash appears on any part of body ■ If still untreated, damage to cardiovascular system, cerebral areas, and nervous system	■ Patient presenting symptoms ■ Physical examination	■ Antibiotics: Penicillin G and others ■ Abstinence or protected (safe) sex for prevention
Genital herpes ■ Ulcerative infection of genital skin ■ Caused by *Herpes simplex* virus type 2 ■ Contagious not only when lesions are present, but also in **prodromal** period ■ No cure at present	■ Blister-like eruptions ■ Systemic flu-like symptoms: fever, headache, general aching ■ Dysuria	■ Patient presenting symptoms ■ Physical examination	■ Antiviral drugs, acyclovir and valacyclovir, shorten duration and severity and reduce frequency of outbreaks ■ Abstinence or protected (safe) sex for prevention ■ Stress reduction to reduce frequency
Genital warts (Condylamata acuminata) ■ Caused by human papillomavirus ■ Transmitted by sexual contact ■ Recurrence is common	■ Raised growths on perineal region, in or near rectum	■ Patient presenting symptoms ■ Physical examination	■ Chemical or surgical removal to symptoms remove growths ■ Abstinence or protected (safe) sex for prevention
Trichomoniasis ■ Protozoal infection of genitourinary tract ■ Caused by *Trichomonas vaginalis*	■ Itching ■ Painful urination ■ Possibly urethritis	■ Patient presenting symptoms ■ Physical examination ■ Wet prep test of male urethral discharge	■ Antiprotozoal medications such as Flagyl® to treat both or all partners ■ Abstinence or protected (safe) sex for prevention

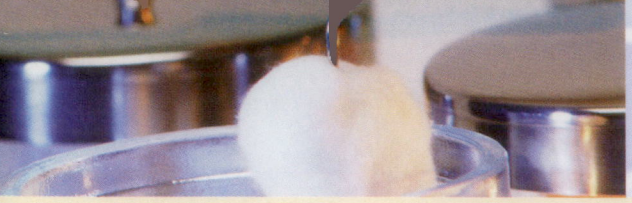

REVIEW

Chapter Summary

- Urinalysis is an important diagnostic tool that provides information about a patient's physiology and renal function. Proper standards and procedures must be followed to ensure accurate results.

- You have a vital role in the urology and nephrology medical office. Key instructions for the patient include obtaining a clean-catch urine specimen, preparing for a urological procedure, and what to expect during the procedure. You may be trained to test or microscopically examine urine. With more extensive training you may be asked to catheterize a patient.

- The urinary system consists of two kidneys, two ureters, a urinary bladder, and a urethra. Urine is formed in the kidneys, passes through the ureters to the bladder, then passes through the urethra to exit the body at the meatus. Urine is a combination of waste molecules and water. Some of the excreted molecules are electrolytes, sugars, amino acids, vitamins, hormones, organic acids, alkaloids, and nitrogenous wastes.

- In addition to the excretion of waste products, the kidneys have three other important physiological functions: (1) maintaining the water balance of the body; (2) maintaining the acid-base balance; and (3) producing the hormones erythropoietin, to stimulate the bone marrow to generate more red blood cells, and renin, to assist angiotensin to maintain adequate blood volume and blood pressure.

- Urinalysis provides information about waste excretion, acid-base balance, and water balance. Diagnostic information gained from the waste products in urine can give clues to different disease processes, such as glomerulonephritis, renal failure, nephrotic syndrome, pyelonephritis, and kidney stones.

- A routine urinalysis requires a clean container, a clean-catch requires a sterile container, and a 24-hour requires a large container that must be kept cold as the specimen is collected. A routine urinalysis and clean specimen require a freshly voided specimen.

- All urine, if not tested immediately, must be protected from deterioration, which affects the accuracy of results. Deterioration or other changes in urine occur if the specimen is not refrigerated or frozen or if preservative is not added. Specimens of 50 to 100 ml are adequate for testing; 12 ml or cc is the typical standardized amount for specific testing. The total volume of urine is important in qualitative and quantitative measurements and in the analysis of results.

- A routine, or normal, urinalysis consists of physical observation, chemical testing, and microscopic analysis. Chemical testing involves the use of reagent test strips or tablets. A rapid urine culture test, a chemical reagent test strip, is performed to immediately determine if a urinary tract infection is present. If results are positive, a culture and sensitivity test or gram stain is performed to identify the causative organism.

- Chemical reagents used for testing must be kept in tightly sealed containers and at room temperature. The expiration date must always be checked. CLIA 1988 regulations require that controls be run to ensure accuracy and that records be kept and monitored.

- The specific gravity of urine can be measured with chemical test strips, a urinometer, or a refractometer.

- Microscopic analysis involves spinning a specimen in the centrifuge and preparing a slide for the physician, who will examine the specimen for RBCs, white blood cells, casts, crystals, epithelial cells, mucus, bacteria, parasites, yeast, and sperm cells.

- The function of the male reproductive system is to produce, store, and transfer sperm cells to the female. Diseases and disorders of the male reproductive tract include prostate disorders, fertility problems and disorders, testicular disorders, and STDs. Conditions that affect the prostate gland include prostatitis, benign prostatic hypertrophy, and prostate cancer. The DRE is a common diagnostic procedure performed by the physician to differentiate the particular prostate condition.

- Male fertility disorders include erectile dysfunction and testicular disorders—cryptorchism, torsion of the testes, and testicular cancer. Monthly self-examination of the testes is recommended for all males aged 15 to 40.

- Sexually transmitted diseases are transmitted not only through sexual contact but by blood and body fluids. Common STDs include chlamydia, gonorrhea, syphilis, genital herpes, genital warts (*Condylomata acuminata*), and trichomoniasis. Untreated STDs can cause sterility and even become life-threatening.

Chapter Review

Multiple Choice

1. Which of the following structures contains the nephrons?
   a. Ureter
   b. Kidney
   c. Urinary bladder
   d. Urethra

2. Cystitis is a(n)
   a. disorder of the kidneys.
   b. infection of the nephritis.
   c. inflammation of the bladder.
   d. obstruction of the ureter.

Chapter Review (continued)

3. Which of the following disorders is diagnosed almost solely in men?
   a. Bladder calculi
   b. Kidney cysts
   c. Ureter cancer
   d. Renal colic

4. An unpreserved urine specimen is likely to show a(n)
   a. decrease in turbidity.
   b. increase in cells and casts.
   c. increase in nitrates.
   d. decrease in glucose and ketone bodies.

5. Normal urine has a(n)
   a. faint, characteristic odor.
   b. opalescent turbidity.
   c. yellow-brown color.
   d. pH greater than 7.

6. In a urinalysis, pH reactions should be read at
   a. 20 seconds.
   b. 35 seconds.
   c. 60 seconds.
   d. 40 seconds.

7. When you examine a urine specimen under a microscope, motile bacteria may appear as
   a. RBCs.
   b. rods.
   c. gel.
   d. sand.

8. Abnormal crystals form in
   a. alkaline urine.
   b. nephrons.
   c. urinary tract mucus.
   d. acid urine.

9. Cryptorchism is normally diagnosed in
   a. men over the age of 50.
   b. men over the age of 60.
   c. infants.
   d. teenagers.

10. Which of the following is the cause of genital herpes?
   a. A bacterium
   b. A virus
   c. A protozoan
   d. A parasite

True/False

T F 1. Nephrology is the study of diseases of the bladder.

T F 2. Angiotensin is an enzyme that activates renin, a hormone involved in a complex regulatory process that maintains adequate blood volume and blood pressure.

T F 3. Each kidney contains approximately 1 million nephrons.

T F 4. For a 24-hour urine sample, the patient should collect each void, starting with the very first one in the morning.

T F 5. To calibrate a refractometer, you may use distilled or tap water.

T F 6. The human kidney is walnut-sized and bean-shaped.

T F 7. Urine enters the bladder at the trigone.

T F 8. The loop of Henle and Bowman's capsule were named after the physicians who identified them.

T F 9. A normal person produces approximately 1-1/2 to 2 liters of urine per day.

T F 10. Neurogenic bladder is usually the result of an insult to the nerves supplying the bladder.

Short Answer

1. Name the four primary structures of the urinary system.

2. What are the main symptoms of neurogenic bladder?

3. What are the uses of an IVP?

4. Which three kidney functions can a routine urinalysis be used to test?

5. What does light-colored urine indicate? What about darker-colored urine?

Research

1. In what states are MAs allowed to perform catheterization on patients?

2. What are the best exercises women can perform after childbirth to recondition the pelvic floor muscles?

Externship Application Experience

1. You have been assisting another office MA during a test strip procedure on a patient's urine specimen. She has given the report to the physician. You notice the date on the test strip container and realize the expiration date was six months ago. How do you handle this situation?

2. As a female MA, you are bringing an elderly male to the examination room. You note on the chart this is a return visit to discuss drug therapy prescribed for erectile dysfunction. During the usual assessment, you inquire about the reason for the visit. The patient appears embarrassed and reluctant to answer your questions. How do you proceed?

Resource Guide

American Association of Clinical Urologists
1111 North Plaza Drive, Suite 550
Schamburg, IL 60173
www.aacuweb.org

American Foundation for Urologic Disease
1128 North Charles Street
Baltimore, MD 21201
1-800-242-2383
www.afud.org

American Society of Nephrology
2025 M Street NW, Suite 800
Washington, DC 20036
1-202-367-1190
www.asn-online.org

American Society of Transplantation
17000 Commerce Parkway, Suite C
Mt. Laurel, NJ 08054
1-856-439-0500
www.a-s-t.org

American Urological Association, Inc.
1120 North Charles Street
Baltimore, MD 21201-5559
1-410-727-1100
www.auanet.org

National Kidney Foundation (NKF)
30 East 33rd Street
New York, NY 10016
1-800-622-9010
www.kidney.org

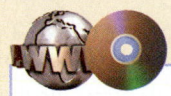 Med**Media**

http://www.MyMAKit.com

More on this chapter, including interactive resources, can be found on the Student CD-ROM accompanying this textbook and on http://www.MyMAKit.com.

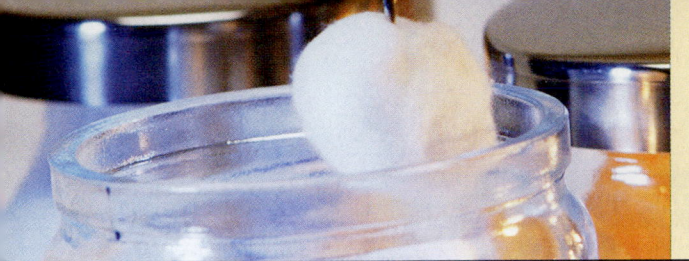

Objectives

After completing this chapter, you should be able to:

- Define and spell the key terminology in this chapter.
- Define the medical assistant's role in medical imaging.
- Describe X-rays and how they function in radiology.
- Describe the information obtained from radiography and contrast studies, fluoroscopy, computed tomography, magnetic resonance imaging, sonography, and nuclear medicine.
- Describe the equipment used in medical imaging.
- Identify safety guidelines that protect both patient and technician during radiographic procedures.
- Define limited-scope radiography.
- Explain how radiographs are scheduled.
- Discuss how to prepare the X-ray room for a radiographic procedure.
- Define the terms commonly used in radiology procedures.
- Discuss patient preparation and instructions for contrast upper GI, lower GI, IVP, cholecystogram, and mammography procedures.
- Describe patient positioning for various chest X-ray projections.

Medical Imaging

Case Study

Olivia is excited to begin work in a radiology facility, which is her first MA job since graduation. During her externship, Olivia worked in a pulmonology office where she was taught how to instruct patients in preparing for simple X-rays. At her new job, Olivia has a chance to practice with different types of medical imaging. Her orientation included learning more than fifteen different types of tests and the safety precautions for each.

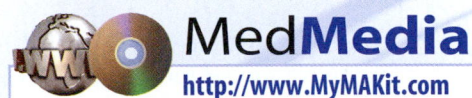

Med**Media**

http://www.MyMAKit.com

Additional interactive resources and activities for this chapter can be found on http://www.MyMAKit.com. For a video, tips, audio glossary, legal and ethical scenarios, job scenarios, quizzes, games, and activities related to the content of this chapter, please access the accompanying CD-ROM in this book.

Video
Audio Glossary
Legal and Ethical Scenario: *Medical Imaging*
On the Job Scenario: *Medical Imaging*
Multiple Choice Quiz
Games: Crossword, Strikeout, and Spelling Bee
Drag and Drop: Skeletal System: The Skeleton; Skeletal System: The Skull; Skeletal System: Long Bone
Tips
HIPAA Quiz

Key Terminology

angiography—radiograph of the vessels usually with contrast medium

arthrography—radiographic examination of a joint

cholecystography—radiograph of the gallbladder, using oral contrast; often referred to as gallbladder series

echocardiogram—type of sonogram used to study the internal structures of the heart

fluoroscopy—radiographic study in which structures are visualized in motion

mammogram—radiograph of breast tissue

myelography—radiographs of the spinal cord using a contrast medium

radiation—radiant energy

radiology—medical specialty that uses radiant energy forms, ultrasound, and magnetic waves to study, diagnose, and treat disease and injury

radiologist—physician who specializes in radiology

radiograph—developed X-ray film

radiography—study or practice of radiology using X-rays

radiolucent—easily penetrated by X-rays

radiopaque—capable of obstructing the passage of X-rays

sonography—use of ultrasound waves to view internal body structures

ultrasound—use of high frequency sound waves being projected and bounced back to the transmitter resulting in an image being projected

X-rays—form of electromagnetic radiation that travels in waves at the speed of light and can penetrate matter and produce a visible image on film

Abbreviations

ALARA—as low as reasonably achievable

AP—anteroposterior view; central ray is directed from front to back

CAT—computerized axial tomography

CT—computed tomography

IVP—intravenous pyelogram

LL—left lateral view; left side of the body faces the film

MRI—magnetic resonance imaging

PA—posteroanterior view; central ray is directed from back to front

PET—positron emission tomography

RL—right lateral view; right side of the body faces the film

✚ MEDICAL ASSISTING STANDARDS

CAAHEP ENTRY-LEVEL STANDARDS	ABHES ENTRY-LEVEL COMPETENCIES
■ Perform within scope of practice (psychomotor) ■ Apply ethical behaviors, including honesty/integrity in performance of medical assisting practice (affective) ■ Apply local, state and federal health care legislation and regulation appropriate to the medical assisting practice setting (psychomotor) ■ Recognize the importance of local, state and federal legislation and regulations in the practice setting (affective) ■ Explore issue of confidentiality as it applies to the medical assistant (cognitive) ■ Document accurately in the patient record (psychomotor) ■ Use language/verbal skills that enable patients' understanding (affective) ■ Practice Standard Precautions (psychomotor) ■ Instruct patients according to their needs to promote health maintenance and disease prevention (psychomotor)	■ Project a positive attitude. ■ Maintain confidentiality at all times. ■ Be a "team player." ■ Be cognizant of ethical boundaries. ■ Exhibit initiative. ■ Adapt to change. ■ Evidence a responsible attitude. ■ Be courteous and diplomatic. ■ Conduct work within scope of education, training, and ability. ■ Prepare patients for procedures. ■ Prepare and maintain examination and treatment area. ■ Practice Standard Precautions. ■ Document accurately. ■ Use appropriate guidelines when releasing records or information.

✔ COMPETENCY SKILLS PERFORMANCE

1. Perform the general procedure for an X-ray examination.
2. File and loan radiographic records.

Introduction

Medical imaging is a specialty that today encompasses radiology, sonography, fluoroscopy, computed tomography (**CT**), magnetic resonance imaging (**MRI**), and nuclear medicine. **Radiology** traditionally has involved the use of **radiographs,** or developed X-ray film, to produce images of bones and internal body structures. Computers have made it possible to scan a body part in dissecting planes or "slices," then assemble them to produce a three-dimensional, 360-degree image—a process called computed tomography. An MRI also produces a three-dimensional view, using magnetic fields rather than radiation. Medical imaging is an invaluable diagnostic tool for the physician.

The Medical Assistant's Role in Medical Imaging

The MA's role will involve patient education, preparation, and positioning, and following safety precautions. The MA may be required to schedule X-ray studies. Advanced training is required to become a radiology technician (rad tech) or radiographer. A radiographer maintains and uses radiology and imaging equipment in a safe manner to produce images of the body on X-ray film or screens, including fluoroscopic and CT screens. Advanced training is also required for the performance of MRIs, CT scans, mammograms, and ultrasound examinations. Nuclear medicine technologists are specialists who aid the physician in nuclear medicine procedures, and **radiation** therapy technologists assist in the delivery of radiation therapy.

Radiology

Radiology uses radiant energy—**X-rays**—to view body parts and functions. This specialty is an important aid in the study, diagnosis, and treatment of disease. There are several methods, or modalities, for visualizing the human body through diagnostic imaging. They include **radiography,** contrast studies, **fluoroscopy,** computed tomography, MRI studies, **sonography,** and nuclear medicine. Although they do not involve radiant energy, MRI (magnetic fields) and sonography (**ultrasound** waves) are usually considered part of the radiology department. Every specialty requires the core knowledge and skills common to all **radiologists.**

X-rays

X-rays are a form of electromagnetic radiation, similar to light rays but invisible to the human eye. They travel in waves at the speed of light, are capable of penetrating most matter, and can be directed through the body to record an image on radiographic film. The four different tissue densities—air, fat, water, and bone—develop on the film in different shades of black and white. Air, the least dense, is easily penetrated by X-rays (**radiolucent**) and shows on the film as very dark. Bone, a very dense, calcium-containing substance, is much harder to penetrate. It is **radiopaque** and appears white on X-ray film. Physicians, especially radiologists, are trained to identify the structures of the body by studying the dark areas, lighter areas, and shadows.

 **Critical Thinking Question 34-1**

Olivia's previous experience with X-rays has made her comfortable with patient preparation, gowning, and draping instructions. The X-ray technician has been ordered to take chest X-rays of a female patient who is believed to have pneumonia. The patient is elderly and has come to the appointment alone. She needs help removing her clothing and getting the drape set up and is not steady enough on her feet to stand alone in the X-ray room. What instructions or assistance should Olivia give her?

The discovery of the X-ray revolutionized the diagnosis of disease. Today, X-ray machines are technologically advanced and many are designed to work with computers to produce digital images of the body.

Radiographs and Contrast Studies

Diagnostic radiography allows the radiologist to view internal body structures and aids physicians in disease diagnosis and treatment. Common procedures include the following:

- Venous studies
- Trauma procedures
- Head, neck and spinal studies
- Bone and joint studies
- Chest, abdomen, pelvic studies
- KUB (kidneys, ureters, bladder) radiography/urinary system studies, including retrograde pyelography
- Surgical procedures
- Myelography

Flat-plate, or plain film, X-rays are taken of the chest, abdomen, skull, skeleton (including long bones and spine), and the kidneys, ureters, and bladder (KUB) (Table 34-1).

A contrast medium is a radiopaque substance. It provides a more accurate visualization of the internal body organ(s) and

TABLE 34-1 FLAT-PLATE RADIOGRAPHY FINDINGS		
Anatomical Structure	**Normal Findings**	**Examples of Abnormal Findings**
Chest	Normal bony structure and lung tissue	Pneumonia, TB, atelectasis, pneumothorax, tumor, abscess, sarcoidosis, sarcoma, incidental findings of scoliosis and kyphosis
Heart	Normal shape and size of heart and blood vessels	Cardiomegaly, aneurysms, and aortic anomalies
Abdomen	Normal size and shape of abdominal structures, including gallbladder, liver, stomach, pancreas, spleen, and small and large intestines; normal gas patterns	Abdominal masses, intestinal obstructions, abdominal tissue trauma, ascites, blood in the peritoneal space
Kidney, ureters, bladder (KUB)	Normal size and structure of the kidneys, ureters, and bladder	Abnormal size and structure of kidneys, ureters, and bladder, renal calculi, masses, obstructions, urinary system abscesses
Skull	Normal structures	Intracranial pressure caused by fluid and swelling, cranial vault fractures, bone defects, congenital anomalies
Skeleton	Normal structures	Fractures, osteomyelitis, arthritic conditions, bone growth

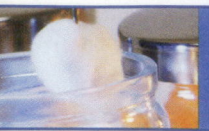

PROCEDURE 34-1 Perform the General Procedure for an X-ray Examination

Theory and Rationale

X-rays are used to view the body's bony and soft structures on flat film. The patient's reproductive organs must be protected from radiation with a lead apron. You should also avoid unnecessary exposure by wearing the proper protective garments and a dosimeter badge and remaining behind a lead wall whenever possible.

Materials

- physician's order
- patient chart
- dosimeter badge
- X-ray film
- X-ray film holder
- X-ray machine
- processing machine
- lead aprons for MA and patient
- paper drapes, as needed

Competency

(**Conditions**) With the necessary materials, (**Task**) you will be able to X-ray a patient (**Standards**) correctly within the time frame designated by the instructor.

1. Verify the patient's identity and the physician's order.
2. Check the X-ray equipment.
3. Explain the procedure to the patient.

4. Instruct the patient to remove the appropriate clothing for the X-ray. Provide paper drapes for modesty. For chest and neck X-rays, the patient should remove all jewelry and large hair bands, which may obstruct the view of the structures.
5. Position the patient according to the X-ray view(s) required (Figure 34-1 ◆).
6. Set the controls with the X-ray tube and cassette at the proper distance (Figure 34-2 ◆).
7. If necessary, ask the patient to take a deep breath and hold it.
8. Stand behind the lead wall or shield to take the X-ray.
9. Instruct the patient to adjust to a comfortable position while you develop the X-rays and have them reviewed. The patient should not dress or leave the X-ray suite until the physician has indicated that the X-rays are satisfactory.
10. With the physician's approval, assist the patient in dressing, if necessary.
11. Label the X-ray and X-ray sleeve according to office procedure.
12. Document the procedure in the patient's chart.

Patient Education

To ensure that the patient goes to the correct place and follows the correct pre-exam procedures, instructions should be given both verbally and in written form. Following instructions correctly saves time and money by preventing the need to reschedule or perform the tests more than once. The patient should be aware

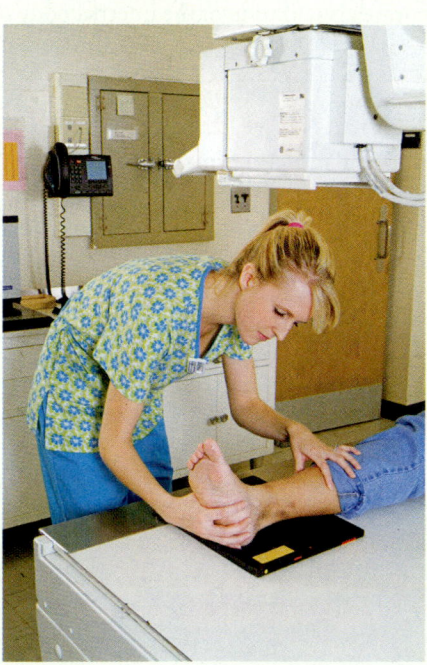

Figure 34-1 ◆ Position the patient properly.

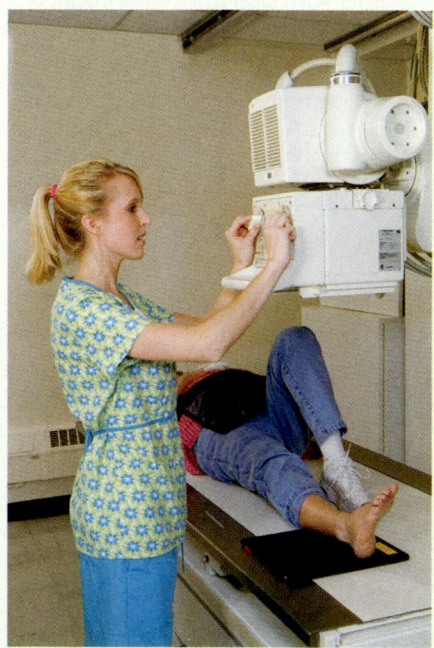

Figure 34-2 ◆ Align the X-ray tube to the cassette at the correct distance.

PROCEDURE 34-1 Perform the General Procedure for an X-ray Examination *(continued)*

of when the results will be available. You may see abnormalities on the film as soon as it is developed, but be careful not to give the patient any advice without the physician's direct permission.

Charting Example

02/14/XX 4:25 p.m. Anterioposterior views obtained through X-ray as ordered. Candace Jones, RMA (AMT)

tissues adjacent to the point of interest (Table 34-2). The contrast medium may be a gas, such as air, oxygen, or carbon dioxide; the heavy metal barium sulfate; or organic iodine, either oil based or water-soluble. Contrast media may be administered orally, parentally, or via enema. Each one is specific for the examination of a particular organ or tissue (Figure 34-3 ◆).

Specialized radiographic examinations include mammography, angiography, arthrography, and cholecystography.

Mammography

A **mammogram** is an X-ray of the breast tissue taken to detect possible abnormalities, such as tumors, cysts, or malignant tissue (Figure 34-4 ◆). Two views are taken of each breast. When lesions without clinical symptoms are detected, early treatment leads to a higher survival rate. Regular mammograms are usually part of a woman's routine gynecological examination. However, men who may require mammograms to detect breast cancer or trauma injury are often overlooked.

A mammographer is a technologist who specializes in the imaging of the breast. He or she must be knowledgeable in breast anatomy, mammography equipment and procedure, the correct positioning of the breast, and quality assurance related to patient care. An advanced certification examination given by the American Registry of Radiologic Technologists (ARRT) is required for employment as a mammographer.

Angiography

Angiography, an invasive examination of the blood vessels, helps in the evaluation of the patency of vessels and in the

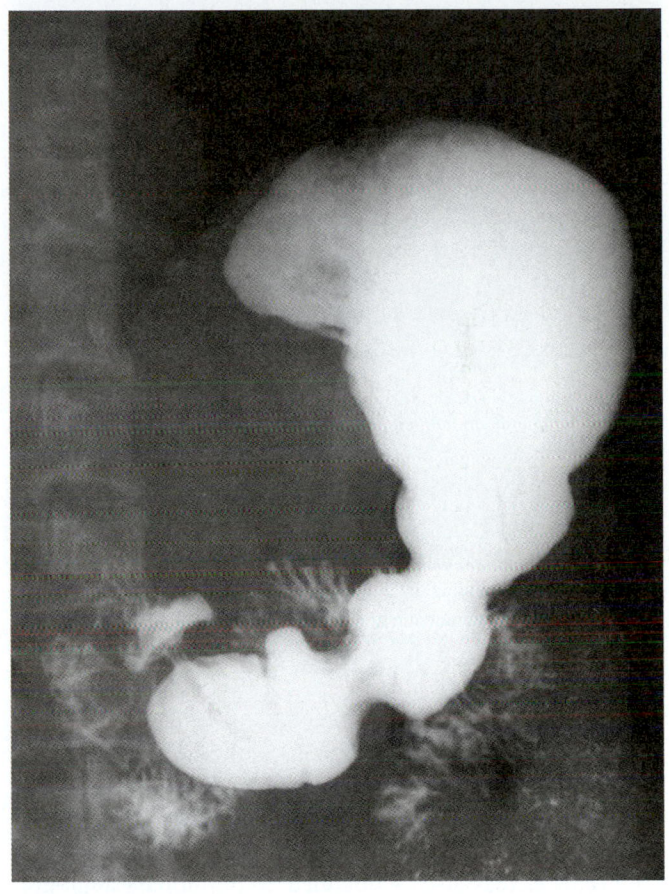

Figure 34-3 ◆ Upper GI series.
Source: Phototake NYC.

TABLE 34-2 COMMON CONTRAST STUDIES

Contrast Study	Systems Examined	Reason for Examination
Upper GI, small bowel series, barium swallow	Upper GI tract including esophagus, stomach, small intestines	To diagnose ulcers, tumors, obstructions, hiatal hernia, or esophageal varices; to study size and shape of organs and structures
Lower GI, air contrast colon study or barium enema	Large intestines	To examine for disease or disorders of the large intestine and to diagnose conditions such as polyps, diverticuli, obstructions, tumors, and lesions
Cholecystogram or gallbladder series	Gallbladder	To diagnose disease or disorders such as blockage, tumors, calculi, and inflammation
Intravenous pyelogram (IVP)	Urinary tract including kidneys, ureters, urinary bladder, and urethra	To diagnose disease or disorders such as obstruction, narrowing, tumors, and calculi; to study size of organs and structures

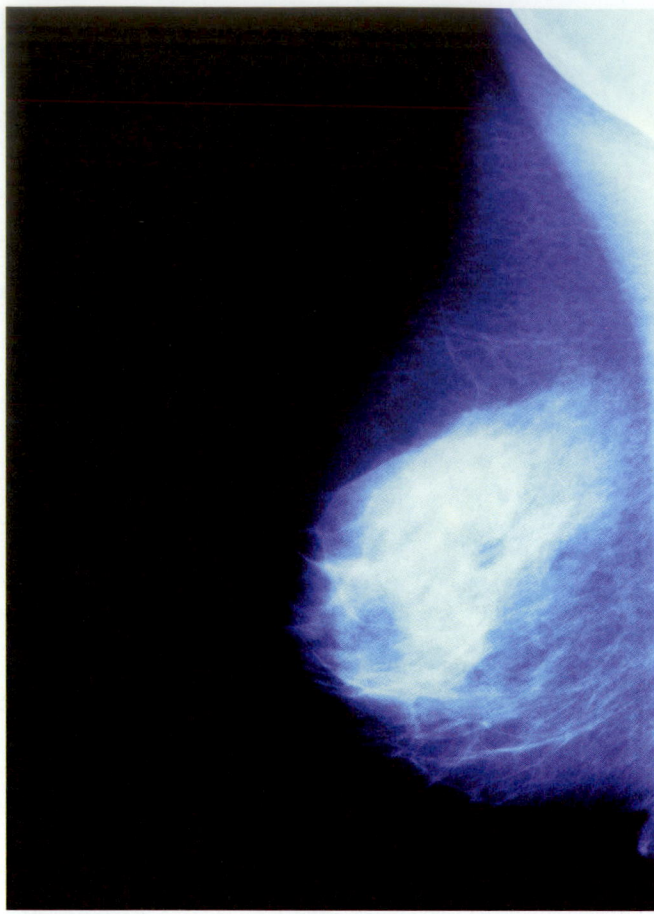

Figure 34-4 ◆ Normal mammogram.
Source: Photo Researchers, Inc.

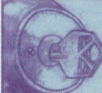

Keys to Success
PREVENTING ALLERGIC AND MEDICAL REACTIONS

Before administering any contrast medium, question the patient about allergies and any medications being taken. Iodine can cause reactions from mild to severe to life-threatening. Mild reactions include the following:

nausea and vomiting	coughing	headache
dizziness	pallor	flushing
anxiety	itching	altered taste
shaking	chills	sweating
rash	nasal stuffiness	

More serious reactions include the following:

cardiovascular: pulse changes, hypotension, hypertension
respiratory: dyspnea, wheezing, bronchospasm, laryngospasm

Life-threatening reactions include the following:

unresponsiveness	convulsions	serious
anaphylactic shock	cardiopulmonary arrest	arrhythmias

Medications with the potential to interact with iodine and cause serious reactions include beta-blockers, calcium channel blockers, and metformin (Glucophage®). A patient with diabetes who takes metformin (Glucophage®) to control non-insulin-dependent diabetes mellitus (NIDDM) is at risk for developing lactic acidosis if iodine contrast is administered within 48 hours of the last metformin dose. The next metformin dose must be withheld for 48 hours following the administration of iodine. Many physicians prefer to avoid the risk and order ultrasound examinations or CT scans, neither of which requires a contrast medium.

identification of abnormal vascularization, a possible result of tumors (Figure 34-5 ◆). In cerebral angiography, the carotid and vertebral arteries are outlined by injected dye. Information about the circle of Willis and small cerebral arterial branches may also be obtained. In pulmonary angiography, injected dye helps to visualize pulmonary vessels. Renal angiography is used to view and evaluate renal circulation and to find causes for hypertension such as thrombi, vascular stenosis, and lesions. Angiography is also employed in cardiac catheterization.

Arthrography

In **arthrography,** the radiographic examination of a joint, air and dye are injected into the joint space so that it can be viewed before an arthroscopic procedure.

Cholecystography

Cholecystography, sometimes referred to as a gallbladder series, is an examination of the gallbladder using oral (swallowed) contrast to provide a visual picture of the gallbladder. It is used in the diagnosis of gallstones or obstruction of the cystic duct. For further diagnosis, IV cholangiography may be performed.

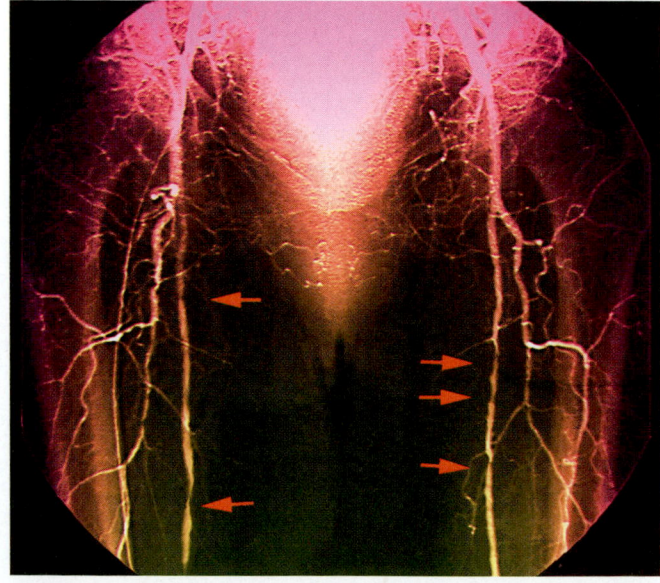

Figure 34-5 ◆ Digital angiogram of the lower limbs, front view, showing atheromatous stenoses of the femoral arteries.
Source: Phototake.

Fluoroscopy

A fluoroscopy procedure studies internal organ(s) as they function—for instance, the heart, stomach, intestines, and fallopian tubes (Figure 34-6 ◆). An X-ray instrument, a fluoroscope, projects visual images on a fluorescent screen rather than on a film. The radiographic tilt table is used for this procedure. The technician can view internal structures on a monitor as well as take pictures for diagnosis or documentation.

Myelography uses both fluoroscopic and radiographic means to examine the spinal subarachnoid space. Air and a contrast medium are injected into the space at the lumbar region so that any abnormalities in that space, such as herniated intervertebral disks, can be viewed. MRIs have replaced most myelography procedures. However, MRIs cannot be performed on patients with metal implants or pacemakers, and for these patients myelograms are the preferred diagnostic procedure.

Computed Tomography

Until the 1970s, only two-dimensional X-rays were available for viewing the internal human body. A new technique, the computer tomography scan (CT scan, formerly called computerized axial tomography or **CAT** scan), is a nonharmful procedure that provides tomographic information far superior to that obtained by serial sectioning. Tomography allows for a specific level or plane of the body to be imaged by removing images of the tissue above and below the selected plane. Two issues influence its scientific usefulness: the clarity of image resolution and the tissue density of the image illuminated by the X-ray beam.

This technique rotates a specific plane of an internal object as it is illuminated by a narrow X-ray beam. By sequentially merging many two-dimensional radiographs of an internal structure, a three-dimensional image can be recorded for further study (Table 34-3).

Magnetic Resonance Imaging

Magnetic resonance imaging (MRI) is used primarily in a medical setting to produce high-quality images of the inside of the human body (Figure 34-7 ◆). A CT scan specializes in larger images, whereas MRI images are smaller. MRI uses wavelengths of energy to produce the images based on spatial variations in the phase and frequency of the radio frequency energy absorbed and emitted by the imaged object. Abscesses, aneurysms, thrombi, congenital heart disease, cysts, edema, hemorrhage, infarctions, multiple sclerosis, muscular disease, skeletal abnormalities, thrombosis, and vascular plaque formation are all clinical problems that can be detected with MRI.

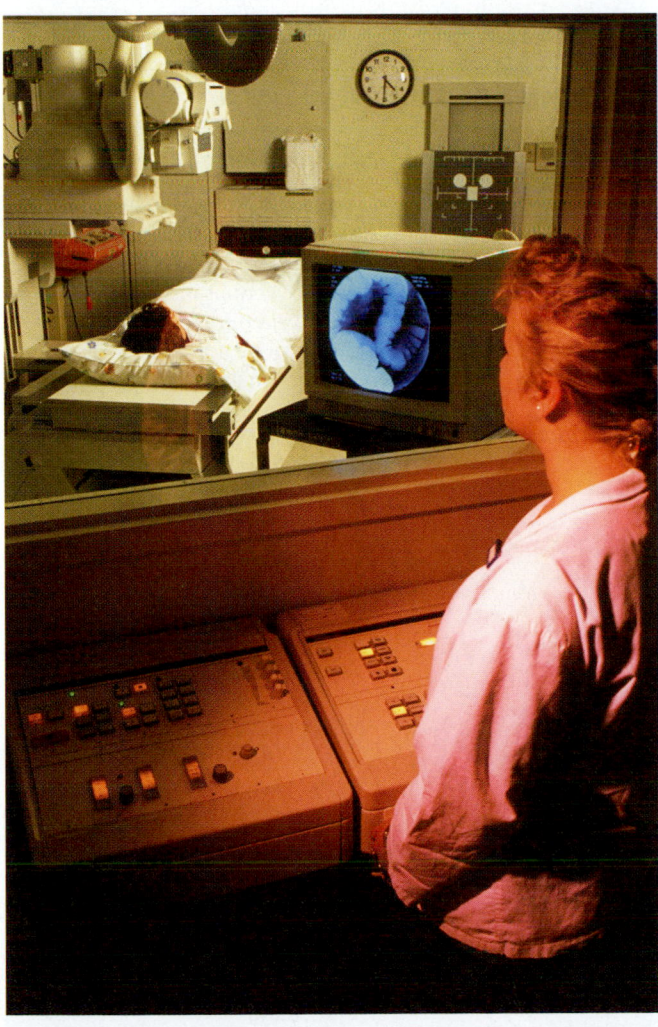

Figure 34-6 ◆ A fluoroscopic unit with upper GI study on screen
Source: The Stock Connection.

TABLE 34-3 CT FINDINGS

Anatomical Structure	Examples of Abnormal Findings
Head	Abscess, atrophy, cysts, edema, hematomas, hydrocephalus, infarction, tumors
Abdomen	
Adrenal	Tumors
Biliary	Obstructions due to calculi
Kidney	Abscesses, calculi, congenital anomalies, cysts, perirenal hematomas, tumors
Liver	Abscesses, cirrhosis with ascites, cysts, hematomas, tumors
Pancreatic	Acute and chronic pancreatitis, pancreatic lesions including abscesses, pseudocysts, and tumors
Chest and thorax	Aortic aneurysm, abscesses, cysts, tumors, pleural effusion, enlarged lymph nodes in the mediastinum
Spine	Herniated intervertebral disks, congenital spinal anomalies, tumors, paraspinal cysts, vascular malformations

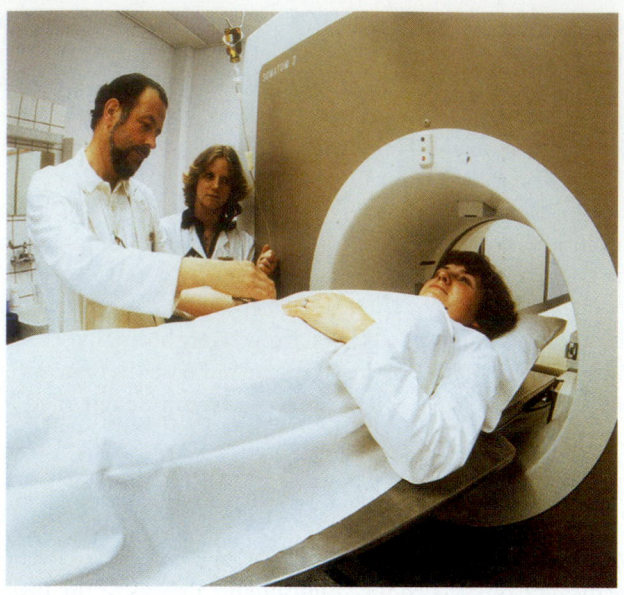

Figure 34-7 ◆ A patient undergoing an MRI.

MRIs cannot be performed on patients with pacemakers, metal hardware, metal staples in the chest, or metal foreign bodies in the eye. The magnetic field may damage a pacemaker or disrupt its settings and pacing. Metal implants may be dislocated and would contribute to artifact, rendering the MRI inaccurate.

CAT scans and MRIs are used for similar tissue studies. Often the physician's choice depends on the contrast medium required for the procedure. Patients occasionally exhibit an allergic response to contrast medium, so the physician decides which procedure is least harmful and has the most diagnostic benefits for those patients. The magnetic field in an MRI is negatively affected by a patient with:

- Any type of metal implant or metal surgical clip, which can get hot.
- A pacemaker and/or aneurysm clips.
- Body tattoos made with dye containing metal.

Sonography

In sonography, very high-frequency sound waves are bounced off internal body structures (Figure 34-8 ◆). An echo is passed back to the monitor and recorded, forming a composite picture. Ultrasounds also display movement of the structure at the time of examination (Table 34-4).

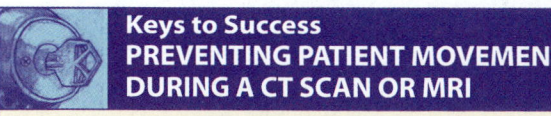

Keys to Success
PREVENTING PATIENT MOVEMENT DURING A CT SCAN OR MRI

Both CT scans and MRIs involve surrounding the patient with a circular camera. Some patients experience claustrophobia during the procedure, and a sedative may have to be administered before the procedure is performed. Even children may require sedation, as any motion causes a distortion of the image and the reading may not be accurate.

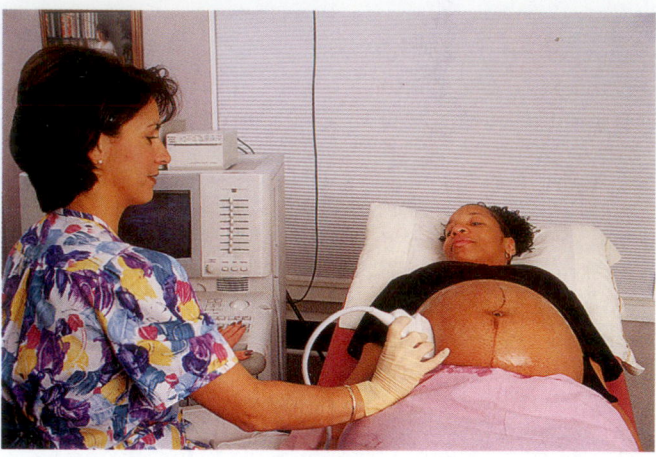

Figure 34-8 ◆ Ultrasound scanning.

Ultrasound is performed on pregnant women to assess fetal growth and size, the number of fetuses, placental location, and possible birth defects (Figure 34-9 ◆). Ultrasound is considered safe for both mother and child. Newer ultrasound equipment shows a three-dimensional view of the fetus (3-D ultrasound).

TABLE 34-4 SONOGRAPHIC FINDINGS

Anatomical Structure	Abnormal Findings
Abdominal aorta	Aortic aneurysm, aortic stenosis
Arteries and veins	Arterial occlusion (partial or complete), arterial trauma, chronic venous insufficiency, deep vein thrombosis (DVT)
Brain	Intracranial hemorrhage, hydrocephalus, lesions (tumors or abscesses)
Gallbladder	Acute cholecystitis, biliary obstruction, cholelithiasis
Heart	Cardiomegaly, aortic stenosis and insufficiency, congenital heart disease, mitral valve stenosis, pericardial effusion
Kidney	Acute glomerulonephritis, acute pyelonephritis hydronephrosis, renal cysts and tumors, perirenal abscesses, renal calculi
Liver	Hepatomegaly, abscesses, hepatic cysts, hepatic metastasis, hepatocellular disease
Pancreas	Acute pancreatitis, pancreatic tumors, pseudocysts
Pelvic, uterus, and/ or pregnant uterus	Uterine fibroids, uterine tumors, fetal death, abruptio placenta, placenta previa, breech fetal presentation, fetal hydrocephalus
Spleen	Splenomegaly, abscesses, splenic cysts, tumor
Thyroid	Lesions (benign or malignant), goiters, cysts

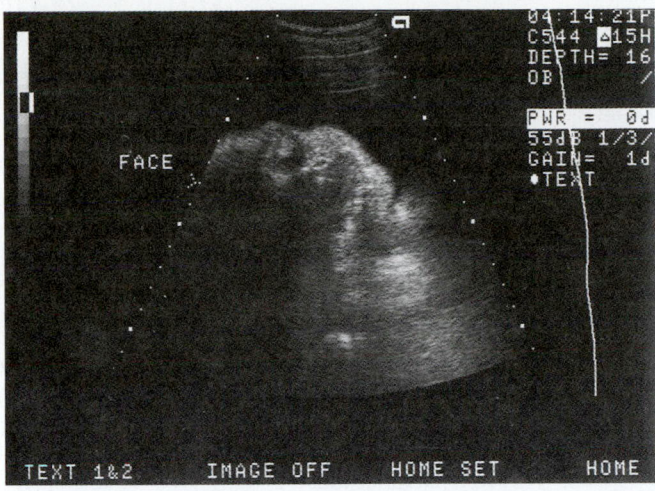

Figure 34-9 ◆ Ultrasound of the fetal face.

An **echocardiogram** is a type of sonogram that can detect abnormalities in the internal structures of the heart. It is used to assess general anatomy, valve function, myocardial function, blood flow, and heart chamber size. A transducer is passed over the chest, and an ultrasonic echo is displayed on a monitor called an oscilloscope. An ultrasonic gel is applied to the skin under the transducer to ensure a clearer projection.

Ultrasounds are considered a low risk to the patient. Patients who cannot undergo contrast studies because of allergies or other risks often have ultrasound examinations instead. Although an ultrasound is effective at ruling out a defect, it is less effective at identifying one. A video film of the ultrasound procedure is made for more thorough examination by the radiologist and cardiologist.

Nuclear Medicine

In nuclear medicine, the patient either swallows or is injected with a radioactive material called a tracer that is absorbed by the target tissue or organ. A special scanner then detects the tracer and provides information about the function, chemical activity, or metabolism of the tissue or organ.

Positron emission tomography (**PET**) is a nuclear medicine technique that produces three-dimensional, multicolored scans with radioisotopes and a computer. PET scanning is used to identify amyloid plaques and tangles that are believed to cause Alzheimer's disease. Before the PET scan was available, Alzheimer's could be truly identified only through autopsy. Identifying the disease with a PET scan is critical to tracking the progression of dementia and planning its treatment.

Nuclear medicine treatments for cancer include brachytherapy and teletherapy. Both techniques use radiation to damage cancer cells during frequent cellular division. Because normal cells undergo a lower division rate, radiation kills the cancer cells and causes less harm to surrounding healthy tissues. In brachytherapy, also called internal radiation therapy, small radioactive materials are implanted within or near the malignant tumor. In teletherapy, or external beam radiotherapy, radiation is directed at the malignancy from outside the body.

Equipment

The equipment used in radiology is complicated and expensive. It is used primarily by physicians with many years of education and training and the support of trained technicians.

The X-ray machine consists of four major components.

- Tube: The cylindrical radiographic glass tube contains a vacuum that produces radiation.
- Table: The X-ray table comes in many shapes and sizes to meet the needs of an office, clinic, or diagnostic center (Figure 34-10 ◆). Some tables tilt to aid the patient in a fluoroscopy procedure, and some have a floating tabletop that is helpful in positioning the patient. All tables contain a Bucky tray, which holds the film cassette and

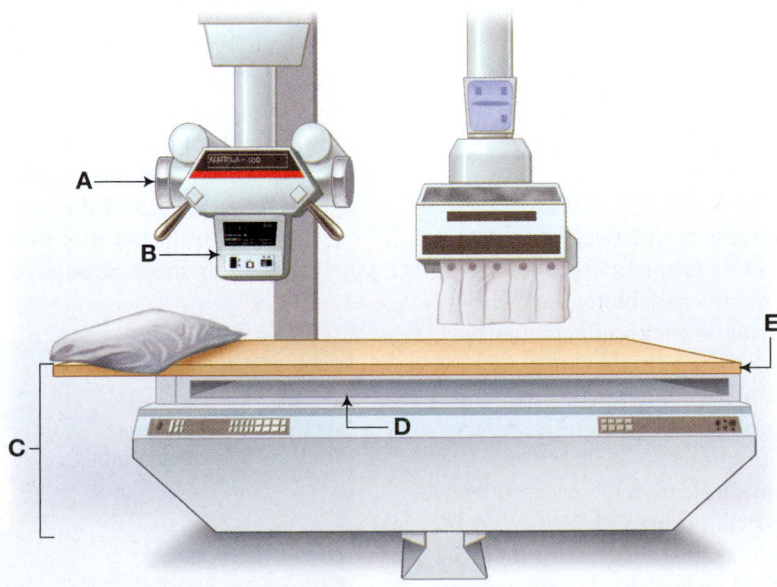

Figure 34-10 ◆ Diagram of the X-ray table: (A) X-ray tube; (B) collimeter; (C) radiographic table; (D) Bucky tray for cassette and film; (E) movable table.

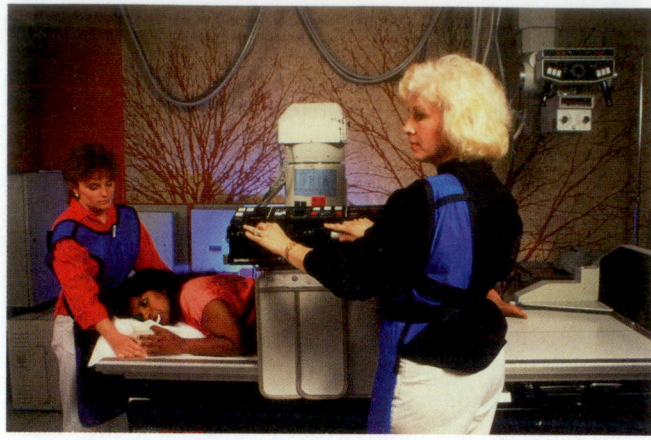

Figure 34-11 ◆ A fluoroscope and portable equipment.
Source: The Stock Connection.

TABLE 34-5 SAMPLE SOURCES OF RADIATION		
Natural		
Internal (occur naturally in the human body)	**External**	**Artificial**
Potassium Carbon	Cosmic rays— radiation emitted from the sun Terrestrial— radiation produced in the earth, such as from uranium Radionuclides— interact with cosmic rays	Medical and dental X-rays Nuclear power Mining Radiopharmaceutical isotopes

can be moved from one end of the table to the other. A lead strip around the top of the table helps absorb the scatter radiation between the patient and the film.

- Control panel: Unless the X-ray equipment is a mobile unit that takes portable images, the control panel is inside a lead-lined area with a lead-treated observation window. Control panels vary, depending on the manufacturer, but all operate on the same basic concepts: quantity (milliamperes, or mA), quality (kilovoltage, or KVP), and time (milliampere seconds, or mAS).
- Generator: This is the source of power for the equipment.

Portable or Fluoroscopic Equipment

Portable equipment is mounted on large wheels and can be rolled to the patient's bedside (Figure 34-11 ◆). The fluoroscopic camera is mounted on a C arm. When portable or fluoroscopic films are being exposed, the technicians, physicians, and other staff present in the room wear lead aprons and gloves for protection against radiation exposure.

Safety Precautions and Patient Protection

Because the effects of radiation are cumulative, it presents a potential hazard to anyone who is frequently exposed to it (Table 34-5). Excessive exposure can cause biological changes, including cell and tissue destruction, with effects that may include temporary or permanent damage to the skin, eyes, thyroid gland, and blood-forming and reproductive organs. X-rays may also be harmful to developing embryos or fetuses, damage germ cells, and cause genetic mutations.

All radiation exposure must be kept as low as reasonably achievable (**ALARA**). The physician must weigh the risks of radiation exposure to the patient against the benefits that will be derived. The procedure should be explained to the patient and adequate preparation should be performed to eliminate any repeat exposure.

The patient must always be protected. Before any exposure to X-rays, females of childbearing age must be asked if they could be pregnant. Follow the ten-day rule: A woman in her childbearing years can be safely X-rayed during the first ten days following the onset of her menses.

Three primary principles govern radiation exposure for the radiography technician and the patient:

- Time: The length of exposure should be kept as short as possible.
- Distance: The distance between the technician and the radiation source should be the maximum distance at all times.
- Shielding: Lead aprons, lead gloves, and thyroid shielding should be worn to protect the reproductive organs at all times by the employee and the patient. A radiation exposure badge (dosimeter badge) must also be worn at all times by all employees who are required to spend time in radiation areas (Figure 34-12 ◆).

An ambulatory patient may require assistance onto the table. The MA should always offer a hand to the patient as he or she sits on the table and help the patient lift the feet and legs up on the table, moving them together as a unit rather than separately. The MA should offer the same consideration when the procedure is over and the patient is getting off the table.

Respect for the patient's modesty and privacy is important. Blankets or sheets should cover legs and exposed body

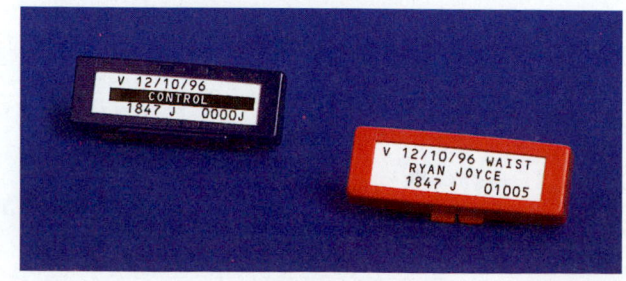

Figure 34-12 ◆ A radiation exposure badge (dosimeter badge).

parts when it is not necessary to view them. The MA should provide a pillow if possible for comfort as well as blankets for warmth if they are needed.

Radiation Shields

A variety of shields containing 1/16 inch of lead equivalent is available for both patient and technician (Figure 34-13 ◆):

- Full aprons (cover the breasts and abdominal–pelvic areas)
- Half aprons (cover the abdominal–pelvic area)
- Gonadal shields
- Thyroid shields
- Eye shields

Full aprons should be worn by both males and females when the extremities are X-rayed, half aprons when the chest is X-rayed, and gonadal shields when the abdomen is X-rayed. Thyroid shielding is worn primarily for skull X-rays and eye shields for lower jaw or larynx X-rays. Lead gloves should be worn to protect the hands when they may be exposed to radiation (Figure 34-14 ◆).

Personnel or family members who assist with patients should be provided with lead aprons, gloves, and thyroid shields.

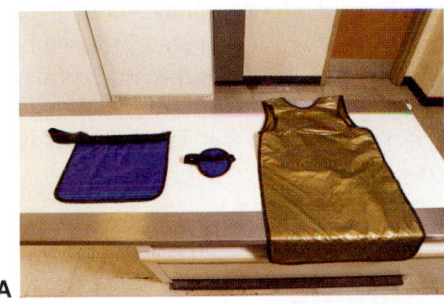

A

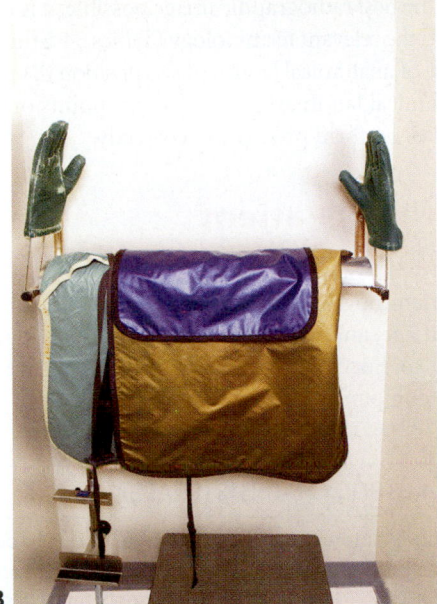

B

Figure 34-13 ◆ (A) A variety of shields: half apron, gonadal shield, and apron; (B) Storage rack for aprons and gloves.

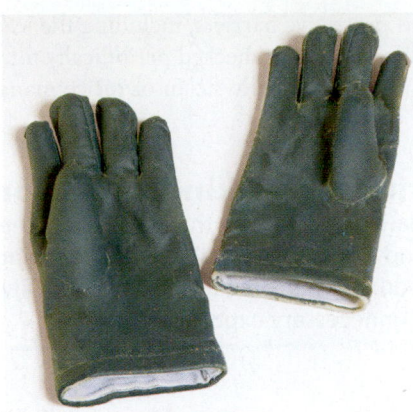

Figure 34-14 ◆ Lead gloves.

If someone must remain in the room when a radiograph is performed, the person should be positioned to the back of the tube.

The room where the X-rays are taken is also protected. Walls painted with lead equivalent (usually 1/16 inch) thick capture any bouncing radiation in the room and absorb radioactive ions that may scatter from the primary beam. A lead strip at the base of the wall and a strip around the X-ray tabletop absorb scattered radiation as well. Using grids in the film cassette and reducing the field size protect the patient further.

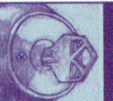

Keys to Success
RADIATION EXPOSURE TIME

A good way to keep a patient safe from radiation is to remember the acronym ALARA—as low as reasonably achievable. Maintain the shortest exposure time, the lowest radiation strength, and the greatest distance possible from the source of radiation to achieve the required X-ray results.

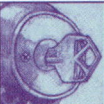

Keys to Success
MEDICAL PRACTICE ACTS

You must be aware of medical practice acts in your community and state regarding limited-scope radiography. In some states MAs are allowed to perform this activity, but other states prohibit it. Some state statutes prohibit the presence of students other than radiology students in a room where radiographs are exposed.

Current licensure information can be obtained from the American Registry of Radiologic Technologists (AART). In order to comply with states' current regulations regarding the dispensing of ionizing radiation, schools that provide training for limited-scope radiology must be officially recognized by each individual state. The state certification exam is customized in each state. After successful completion of training and examination, the limited-scope radiographer may seek employment. Continuing education is mandatory to maintain certification.

All lead protective barriers, including the lead strips on the X-ray table, should be checked periodically for cracks and signs of wear. Inform the physician or office manager of any wear.

> **? Critical Thinking Question 34-2**
> The patient tells Olivia that she is not steady on her feet and would like Olivia's assistance during the X-ray procedure. What precautions should Olivia take to avoid unnecessary exposure to radiation?

Limited-Scope Radiography

Some physicians have equipment in the office with which to perform simple X-ray procedures. After the appropriate training and depending on state regulations, the MA may be asked to expose and develop film in addition to preparing the patient. Limited-scope radiography allows the MA to perform limited numbers and types of X-ray procedures, typically upper and lower extremities, chest, and some skull procedures. As a limited-scope radiographer the MA is subject to state regulations.

Scheduling Radiographs

Some radiology testing can be performed in the medical office. Otherwise, it is scheduled with a radiology facility in a clinic, freestanding facility, or hospital radiology department.

- On-site: If the procedure is not performed immediately in the office, the physician writes an order for one. An appointment is scheduled, and an appointment card and verbal and written instructions are given to the patient.
- Off-site: After the physician writes the order, the patient is asked to confirm whether his or her insurance covers the suggested facility. If so, the order is relayed to the facility, usually by phone. An appointment date and time are confirmed with the patient. The facility then relays preparation instructions, which are given in verbal and written form to the patient along with an appointment card containing the name, address, and phone number of the facility. Transportation requirements may need to be discussed, and written directions are provided as necessary to the patient or patient's family member or caregiver.

Assisting with an X-ray

Simple X-rays may be performed in a physician's office depending on the office location and the availability of radiographic equipment. X-rays of limbs and appendages are often taken in an office where the physician treats fractures and simple trauma. Chest X-rays may be taken when the physician needs a rapid diagnosis of a respiratory complaint or condition. Podiatrists often take X-rays of the feet as a diagnostic tool. A flat plate or plain film radiograph of the abdomen or a KUB may be taken if a radiology facility is not readily accessed. Many physicians' offices are located in clinic complexes where the patient may have an X-ray taken, then return to the medical office for treatment.

Patient Preparation and Instructions

Any female of childbearing age must be asked if she could be pregnant. Usually, signs are posted in radiology departments instructing female patients to inform the technician or staff if they are or think they may be pregnant.

Jewelry and any metal objects must be removed from the area to be filmed and stored in a secure place. Any clothing or undergarments with metal closures must also be removed. Metal objects may interfere with the accuracy of the radiographic results.

Preparation of the X-ray Room

Preparation for the X-ray room is minimal. A film cassette is stored upright, on its end, in a cabinet. It should *never* be stored flat or on its side. All film is stored flat in a dark cabinet. X-ray accessories, such as calipers, foam spacers, and risers, are kept in a place that is convenient for the technician but away from patients' reach.

Nothing should be kept in the X-ray room except the equipment to be used. The X-ray table should be cleaned with a mild disinfectant after each patient. Be careful not to damage the lead strip that surrounds the table as this could interfere with the capture of scattered radiation. Clean the chin rest as well as anything else that a patient may have touched after each use.

Terminology and Landmarks for Positioning

To obtain the best radiographic image possible, it is important to understand the relevant terminology (Tables 34-6 through 34-10) and the use of anatomical landmarks to position the patient properly. Anatomical landmarks are reference points or body structures used to perform procedures correctly.

Preparing a Patient for a Mammogram

Baseline mammograms are recommended for women around 35 years of age, and yearly mammograms for women over 40 (see Keys to Success box, page 724). Medicare and most insurance companies cover the procedure.

TABLE 34-6 · BODY HABITUS (SHAPE)	
Sthenic body habitus	Average body shape and size
Hyposthenic body habitus	Tall and slender body shape
Asthenic body habitus	Extremely tall and slender body shape
Hypersthenic body habitus	Short and stout body shape

TABLE 34-7   RADIOGRAPHIC POSITIONING TERMS

Projection	Path of the central rays from the source though the object
Tangential	Describing the path of the central ray along a body part as the part is seen in profile
Axial	Describing the path of the central ray along the long axis of the body part
Axillary	Describing the path of the central ray toward the axilla (underarm)
Cephalic	Describing the central ray toward the head
Caudal	Describing the central ray toward the feet
View	How the image is seen from the image receptor; the opposite of projection
Anteroposterior view (**AP**)	Central ray is directed from front to back
Posteroanterior view (**PA**)	Central ray is directed from back to front
Right lateral view (**RL**)	Right side of the body faces the film
Left lateral view (**LL**)	Left side of the body faces the film

TABLE 34-8   BODY PLANES (FIGURE 34-15 ◆)

Midsagittal plane	Division of the body into equal right and left halves
Sagittal plane	Vertical division of the body or body part into equal or unequal right and left sections
Coronal plane	Division of the body into front and back portions
Horizontal or transverse plane	Horizontal division of the body into upper and lower portions

TABLE 34-9   BODY POSITIONS

Position	Placement of the body or body part
Erect	Sitting or standing
Recumbent	In a reclining position or lying down
Decubitus	Lying down position
Left decubitus	Lying on the left side, recumbent
Right decubitus	Lying on the right side, recumbent
Supine or dorsal recumbent	Lying face up
Prone or ventral recumbent	Lying face down
Left lateral recumbent	Lying on the left side
Right lateral recumbent	Lying on the right side
Lateral	Body or body part placed at a 90-degree angle
Oblique	Body or body part placed at less than a 90-degree angle

TABLE 34-10   BODY MOVEMENTS

Flexion	Decreasing the angle between two bones; bending at the joint
Extension	Increasing the angle between two bones; straightening at the joint
Adduction	Moving a body part away from the midline of the body
Abduction	Moving a body part toward the midline of the body
Eversion	Turning a body part toward the outside
Inversion	Turning a body part toward the inside
Supination	Turning the palm of the hand upward
Pronation	Turning the palm of the hand downward

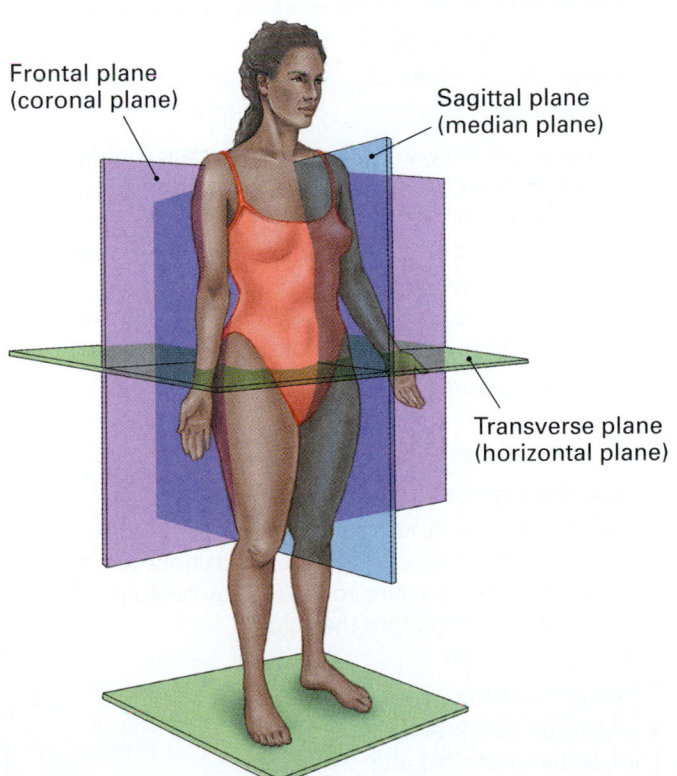

Frontal plane (coronal plane)

Sagittal plane (median plane)

Transverse plane (horizontal plane)

Figure 34-15 ◆ Planes of the body.

Preparing the Patient for Abdominal Contrast Studies

Patients may require radiographs made with a contrast medium, such as upper GI and intravenous pyelogram (**IVP**) (see the following boxes). Preparation for radiographic examinations of organs in the trunk area includes evacuation of GI contents. Failure to comply with these instructions and complete the prep may result in X-rays that do not supply adequate information for diagnosis. The entire procedure, including prep, may have to be repeated, resulting in additional stress on the patient as well as additional expense.

In Practice

The physician has requested that the medical assistant schedule Ms. James for her annual mammogram. The patient informs the medical assistant that she has never had a mammogram and has heard that it hurts. She also tells the medical assistant that her best friend was just diagnosed with breast cancer after having a mammogram and that she is afraid that the same might be true for her. What should the medical assistant tell the patient? How can the medical assistant prepare the patient for the mammogram?

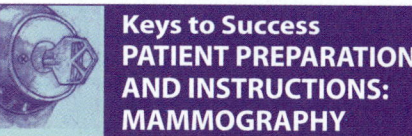

Keys to Success
PATIENT PREPARATION AND INSTRUCTIONS: MAMMOGRAPHY

Purpose: Radiographic examination of both breasts to detect any disease or disorders such as lesions, tumors, or cysts.

Patient preparation:

- The patient should make an appointment for one week after the menses, when the breasts are less tender.
- Mammography does not require GI tract preparation.

Day of procedure:

- The patient will undress from the waist up and wear a gown.
- The patient should wear no lotions, powders, perfume, or deodorant under the arms.

Procedure steps:

- Both breasts are X-rayed.
- The patient is placed in several positions with the breast placed between two plastic plates.
- Two views are routinely taken of each breast.

Scheduled time: 30 to 40 minutes

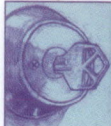

Keys to Success
PATIENT PREPARATION AND INSTRUCTIONS: UPPER GI (BARIUM SWALLOW)

Purpose: Radiographic examination of the esophagus, stomach, and small intestines for diagnosis of ulcers, tumors, obstructions, hiatal hernia, or esophageal varices.

Patient preparation:
Day before procedure:

- Light evening meal.
- NPO 12 hours prior to X-rays.

Post-procedure:

- Increase fluid intake.
- Laxative if prescribed.

Procedure steps:

- The patient drinks a barium mixture (chalky mixture) while standing in front of the fluoroscope.
- The radiologist observes and X-rays the passage of the fluid through the digestive tract as the patient turns in various positions.

Scheduled time: 1 hour to 1-1/2 hours

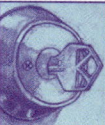

Keys to Success
PATIENT PREPARATION AND INSTRUCTIONS: LOWER GI SERIES (BARIUM ENEMA)

Purpose: A radiographic examination of the large intestines for disease or disorders such as polyps, obstructions, tumors, and lesions.

Patient preparation:
Day before procedure:

- Clear liquids only, such as coffee, tea, clear gelatin, broth, and carbonated beverages.
- No milk or milk products.
- In late afternoon or early evening, drink 3.2-oz bottle of magnesium citrate.
- In early evening, prescribed laxative and NPO except water 12 hours before procedure.

Day of procedure:

- NPO.
- Cleansing enema if needed.

Procedure steps:

- The colon is filled with a barium sulfate mixture.
- The patient is moved into various positions to allow barium to fill the entire colon. Air may be used to push the barium further into the colon.
- X-rays are taken.

Post-procedure:

- Increase fluid intake.
- Laxative if needed after 24 hours.

Scheduled time: 2 hours

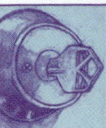

Keys to Success
PATIENT PREPARATION AND INSTRUCTIONS: INTRAVENOUS PYELOGRAM (IVP)

Purpose: Radiographic examination of the urinary tract to diagnose disease or disorders such as blockage, narrowing, tumors, and calculi

Precautions: A contrast medium of iodine is used to view the urinary tract. Warn the patient of a warm flushed sensation when the medium is injected into the bladder and a possible metallic taste for several hours after the procedure. This procedure should not be performed on a patient who is allergic to iodine or shellfish. The physician may order an ultrasound study of the kidneys if the patient cannot tolerate the iodine.

Patient preparation:
Day before procedure:

- Light evening meal.
- Prescribed laxative in the early evening.
- NPO except water for 12 hours before exam.

Day of procedure:

- Enema in the a.m. if necessary.

Procedure steps:

- The patient is asked to dress in a patient gown and to urinate, to ensure his or her comfort while lying still during the procedure.
- An initial X-ray may be taken with the patient in a supine position.
- An IV is started and contrast medium injected.
- X-rays are taken.
- The patient is asked to urinate again, and a final X-ray is taken.

Post-procedure:

- Increase fluid intake.

Scheduled time: 45 minutes to 1 hour

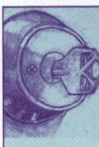

Keys to Success
PATIENT PREPARATION AND INSTRUCTIONS: CHOLECYSTOGRAM (GALLBLADDER)

Purpose: Radiographic examination of the gallbladder to diagnose disease or disorders such as blockage, tumors, calculi, and inflammation.

Precautions: Iodine is taken the night before the examination. If the patient is allergic to iodine or shellfish, another type of examination, such as ultrasound, should be performed. Warn the patient of a metallic taste after the medication is taken.

Patient preparation:
Day before procedure:

- Light, fat-free meals.
- Take iodine tablets with water after dinner.
- Laxative if prescribed.
- NPO except for water after iodine tablets are taken.

Day of procedure:

- NPO before procedure.

Procedure steps:

- X-rays are taken of the gallbladder.
- A fatty meal is given to stimulate the gallbladder.
- X-rays are taken again.

Post-procedure:

- Increase fluid intake.

Scheduled time: approximately 30 minutes

Filing and Loaning Radiographic Records

Maintaining X-rays is the same as maintaining any other medical record. The original transcription report of the X-ray is kept in the facility and a copy sent to the primary physician. Mammograms are generally kept for ten years, minor injury X-rays for five years, and asbestos X-rays permanently.

The procedure for loaning X-rays may differ with each facility. The general procedure must include the verbal and written consent of the patient. The patient or another facility can usually check out any X-ray for up to thirty days. The hospital, diagnostic center, or clinic may also copy an X-ray for another facility and charge the cost to the owner of the record.

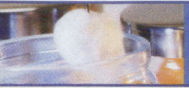

PROCEDURE 34-2 File and Loan Radiographic Records

Theory and Rationale

When X-ray films are taken by the patient to another facility or physician, notation must be made on the patient record along with the name of the receiving physician. All films leaving the department are recorded in a log or file along with the time, date, patient's name, and physicians' names.

Most radiology facilities require a written request from the requesting facility before releasing any X-ray films. The patient must sign a consent form as well. The films are placed in a large envelope or jacket labeled with the patient's name, DOB, physician's name, and the date when the films were taken.

Materials

- X-ray films
- consent form
- larger envelope or film jacket
- labels

Competency

(**Conditions**) With the necessary materials, you will be able to (**Task**) file and loan X-rays (**Standards**) correctly.

1. Place the films in a large film envelope labeled with the patient's name, DOB, date of procedure, and physician's name (Figure 34-16 ◆). The films will be taken to a radiologist to be read.
2. If the films are to be taken by the patient to another facility or physician, note the destination and receiving physician's name on the patient record.
3. Record the transfer of all films in a log or file, along with the time, date, patient's name, destination, and receiving physician.
4. Obtain the patient's signed consent for any films the patient takes from the ownership facility to another physician or diagnostic center.

Patient Education

Instruct the patient that the receiving or reviewing site returns most loaned X-rays. In other cases the patient has to hand-carry the X-rays back to the loaning facility.

Charting Example

8/24/XX 1:30 p.m. Bilateral mammography X-rays released to patient after signing consent for release for consultation with Dr. Brown. Simon Allen, CMA (AAMA)

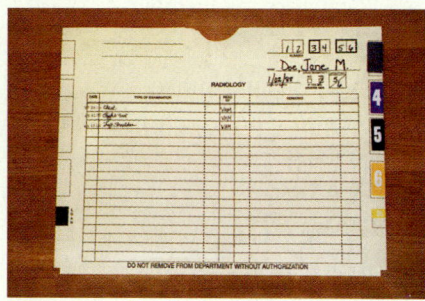
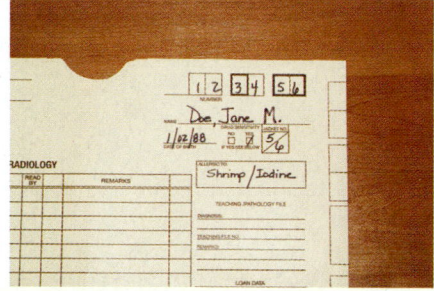

Figure 34-16 ◆ A correctly labeled X-ray envelope, front and back.

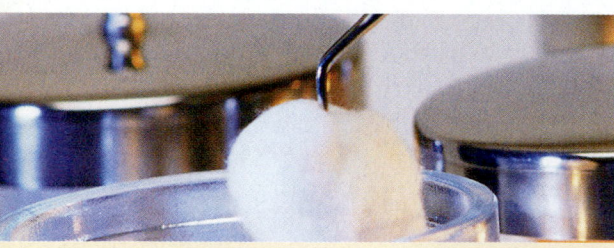

REVIEW

Chapter Summary

- Medical imaging encompasses radiology, sonography, and magnetic resonance imaging. Radiographs or X-rays produce images of bones and internal body structures. CT scans produce images of a specific body part by dissecting planes and reassembling them to produce a 360-degree image. MRIs produce 360-degree images with the use of magnetic fields rather than radiation.

- Radiologists are physicians who specialize in radiology. Radiology procedures include several specialty areas such as diagnostic radiology, fluoroscopy, mammography, computer tomography, radiation therapy, and nuclear medicine.
- X-rays can penetrate matter. They pass through the body to a specialized radiographic film, where images of light/dark contrast are recorded.

Chapter Summary (continued)

- Flat plate films are taken of the chest, abdomen, skull, skeleton (including long bones and spine), and the kidneys, ureters, and bladder. Contrast studies focus on the functioning of the GI tract, urinary tract, gallbladder and biliary system, circulatory system, cerebrospinal canal, and circulation of cerebral fluid in the brain.
- X-ray equipment includes the X-ray table, X-ray tube, and control console. The X-ray table can usually be tilted or moved from side to side. All equipment, unless portable, is housed in a lead-lined room for safety.
- Excessive exposure to radiation can cause harmful biological changes, including cell and tissue destruction. Harmful effects may include temporary or permanent damage to skin, eyes, thyroid, blood-forming and reproductive organs, and germ cells.
- The patient must be protected at all times. All females of childbearing age must be asked if they may be pregnant. According to the "ten-day rule," radiographs should be taken in the ten days following the onset of menses.
- Shields are used to protect both patient and worker against radiation. Full aprons, half aprons, gonadal shields, and eye and thyroid shields protect specific parts of the body; lead gloves should always be worn when there is a possibility of radiation exposure to the hands. A radiation detection badge must be worn at all times.
- Limited-scope radiology such as simple X-rays may be performed in the physician's office. Typical X-rays include the upper and lower extremities, chest, and some skull films. Depending on state statutes defining practice acts, medical assistants may be able to expose and develop film after preparing the patient for the procedure. Current licensure from AART is also recommended.
- Diagnostic modalities include venous studies; trauma procedures; head, neck, and spinal studies; bone and joint studies; chest, abdomen, and pelvic studies; KUB (kidneys, ureters, and bladder) and urinary system studies; surgical procedures; and myelography. Contrast media include air, oxygen, carbon dioxide, barium sulfate, and organic iodine.
- Before administering any contrast media, medication history and information about allergies must be obtained. Iodine can cause serious allergic reactions. Certain medications such as beta-blockers, calcium channel blockers, and metformin (Glucophage®) may cause potentially lethal reactions.
- Fluoroscopy employs a screen rather than a photographic plate to obtain images. Internal organs are observed in motion. The patient's position may be changed while the physician views the movement of the organs on the screen.
- Computer tomography (CT) is a noninvasive and nondestructive means of studying internal structures of the human body. With sequential merging of two-dimensional "slices." a 360-degree image of the body part can be viewed.
- Magnetic resonance imaging (MRI) is similar to CT scanning in its sequential merging of "slices" into a 360-degree image. MRIs use a magnetic field to obtain the image, so the patient is not exposed to radiation. Contrast media may be used to define specific areas.
- Sonography facilitates the viewing of internal body structures by projecting very high-frequency sound waves into the body and recording the echo passed back to the monitor. Ultrasound studies are used to determine fetal age and position and in echocardiograms to study the internal structures of the heart.
- PET scans use radioisotopes and a computer to produce three-dimensional multicolored scans.
- The MA may be called on to assist with patient preparation and instruction for radiography in the medical office. Documentation of film transfer may also be the MA's responsibility.
- Scheduling X-rays with outside agencies should be done with the patient present. Insurance coverage is verified, any necessary preauthorization is obtained and charted, and verbal and written instructions are given to the patient.
- Positioning is important in radiography. You must be familiar with the terminology of positioning and body movement.

Chapter Review

Multiple Choice

1. Bone, a dense calcium-containing substance, appears on an X-ray film as a shade of
   a. light gray.
   b. white.
   c. dark gray.
   d. black.

2. Flat-plate X-rays that do not require a contrast are taken of the
   a. skull.
   b. urinary tract.
   c. gallbladder.
   d. GI tract.

3. ALARA is the acronym for
   a. as low as reasonably accurate.
   b. as long as reliably accurate.
   c. as long as reliably applied.
   d. as low as reasonably achievable.

4. Which of the following is a more serious reaction to a contrast medium?
   a. Itching
   b. Pallor
   c. Pulse changes
   d. Headache

Chapter Review (continued)

5. Which of the following medical imaging is done while the structure is functioning?
   a. CT scan
   b. Fluoroscopy
   c. MRI
   d. X-ray

6. How long should a female patient wait after her menstrual period to have a mammogram?
   a. Three days
   b. Four days
   c. Five days
   d. One week

7. The day before a lower GI series, a patient may consume
   a. clear liquids only.
   b. milk and yogurt.
   c. a light evening meal.
   d. a full evening meal.

8. Which of the following is the standard maximum time a patient or facility can check out an X-ray?
   a. 60 days
   b. 30 days
   c. 90 days
   d. 120 days

True/False

T F 1. X-rays are a form of electromagnetic radiation and can be seen with the naked eye.

T F 2. Flat-plate or plain film can be used to view KUB.

T F 3. Arthrography is an invasive examination of the blood vessels.

T F 4. CT scans specialize in smaller images, whereas MRI images are larger.

T F 5. Both CT scans and MRIs involve surrounding the patient with a circular camera.

Short Answer

1. What is an echocardiogram?

2. Which nuclear medicine technique is used to identify Alzheimer's disease?

3. What type of radiation shield should be worn by a patient when the extremities are X-rayed? What about when the abdomen is X-rayed? The skull?

4. Generally, how long are mammograms kept as part of a patient's medical record?

Research

1. In recent years, lung cancer was a focus of media attention with the deaths of Peter Jennings and Dana Reeve. What is the survival rate of patients diagnosed with lung cancer?

2. In your state, are medical assistants allowed to perform limited radiographs? What must you do to qualify?

Externship Application Experience

As a student, you are asked to assist with a limited radiographic procedure. What are your duties and responsibilities to ensure patient safety and comfort as well as your own safety?

Resource Guide

American Board of Radiology (ABR)
5255 E. Williams Circle, Suite 3200
Tucson, AZ 85711
520-790-2900
http://theabr.org

American Registry of Radiologic Technologists (ARRT)
1255 Northland Drive
St. Paul, MN 55120-1155
651-687-0048
www.arrt.org

American Society of Radiologic Technologists
15000 Central Ave. SE
Albuquerque, NM 87123-3917
505-298-4500
www.asrt.org

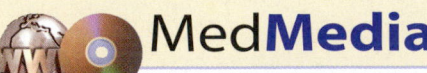

Med Media

http://www.MyMAKit.com

More on this chapter, including interactive resources, can be found on the Student CD-ROM accompanying this textbook and on http://www.MyMAKit.com.

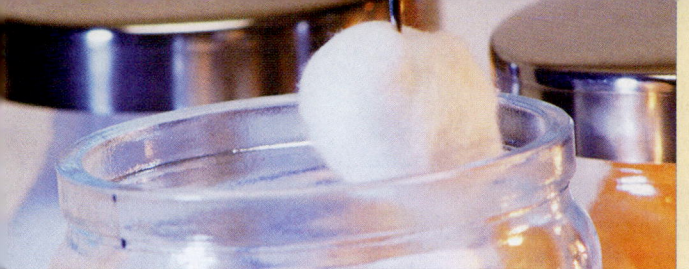

Objectives

After completing this chapter, you should be able to:

- Define and spell the key terminology in this chapter.
- Define the role of the medical assistant in a cardiology practice.
- Describe the anatomy and physiology of the heart.
- Explain the electrical conduction system of the heart.
- Discuss coronary artery disease.
- Describe the symptoms of and treatment for angina.
- Explain the symptoms, causes, and treatments for myocardial infarction.
- Describe sudden cardiac arrest.
- Explain the symptoms, causes, diagnosis and treatment of hypertension.
- Discuss congestive heart failure.
- Discuss pulmonary edema.
- Explain the symptoms, causes, diagnosis, and treatment of cardiomyopathy.
- Discuss cardiac arrhythmias and their various classifications.
- Compare the infective heart disorders: endocarditis, myocarditis, pericarditis, and rheumatic fever and rheumatic heart disease.
- Compare the various valvular disorders.
- Compare the vascular disorders, including embolisms, arteriosclerosis, aneurysms, phlebitis, thrombophlebitis, deep-vein thrombosis, Raynaud's disease, and Buerger's disease.
- Explain the electrocardiogram and its importance in cardiology.
- Explain the Holter monitor and discuss its importance in cardiology.
- Discuss stress testing and its function in cardiology.
- Explain the echocardiogram and its importance in cardiology.
- Explain the thallium scan.
- Describe a MUGA scan.
- Identify important arrhythmias.

Cardiology and Cardiac Testing

Case Study

Rachel is checking on a patient, Ray, who has come to the office for his regular appointment to follow up on his cardiac surgery. Ray mentions that he almost canceled this appointment because he thinks he may have the flu. He complains of a sudden onset of fatigue, weakness, and a fever that comes and goes. He also mentions that he has been really tired the last couple of days and has had no appetite. He even canceled a dental appointment to get a tooth abscess that has been bothering him for a while taken care of.

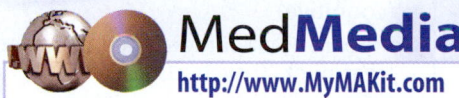

Med**Media**
http://www.MyMAKit.com

Additional interactive resources and activities for this chapter can be found on http://www.MyMAKit.com. For videos, audio glossary, legal and ethical scenarios, job scenarios, quizzes, games, tips, virtual tours and activities related to the content of this chapter, please access the accompanying CD-ROM in this book.

Audio Glossary
Legal and Ethical Scenario: *Cardiology and Cardiac Testing*
On the Job Scenario: *Cardiology and Cardiac Testing*
Video: *The Electrocardiogram and Holter Monitor*
A&P Quiz: The Circulatory System
Multiple Choice Quiz
Games: Crossword, Strikeout, and Spelling Bee
3D Virtual Tour: Cardiovascular System: Head & Neck; Cardiovascular System: Chest & Abdomen; Cardiovascular System: Arm & Shoulder; Cardiovascular System: Leg; Virtual Tour of the Heart: Heart
Drag and Drop: Circulatory System: Circulatory System; Circulatory System: Brain Blood Vessels; Circulatory System: Digestive Blood Vessels; Cardiovascular System: Anterior & Posterior of the Heart; Cardiovascular System: Interior of the Heart
Tips
HIPAA Quiz

Key Terminology

amplitude—abundance, amount, extent, fullness, or size

aneurysm—weakening and dilation of an artery

angina—left-sided chest pain brought on by exertion

angioplasty—procedure in which a balloon on the distal aspect of a cardiac catheter is inflated to compress plaque against coronary artery walls, increasing the lumen of the artery

anterior—toward the front

apex—pointed end of the ventricles

arrhythmia—absence of rhythm

arteriosclerosis—arterial hardening caused by the buildup of atherosclerotic plaque

artifact—appearance of electrical activity or waveforms from sources outside the heart

asystole—absence of cardiac activity; cardiac standstill, without systole

atherosclerosis—buildup of plaque in the arteries over a period of years

atrium (plural: atria)—right or left upper chamber of the heart

augmented lead—unipolar lead, one positive electrode; has very low voltage and must therefore be augmented by the electrocardiograph to equal the voltage of the other leads

automaticity—ability of the heart to initiate and maintain rhythmic activity without the nervous system

bradycardia—heart rate below 60 beats per minute (BPM)

cardiac catheterization—diagnostic procedure in which a catheter is threaded through a major artery back to the heart through the aorta; catheter may be threaded into the left ventricle or into the coronary arteries

cardiomegaly—enlarged heart

cardiomyopathy—diseases of the myocardium

conduction system—wiring and paths that initiate and maintain rhythmic contraction of the myocardium

conductivity—ability of a cardiac cell to transfer impulses to the next cell, allowing all areas of the heart (myocardium) to depolarize at one time

 MEDICAL ASSISTING STANDARDS

CAAHEP ENTRY-LEVEL STANDARDS	ABHES ENTRY-LEVEL COMPETENCIES
■ Perform within scope of practice (psychomotor) ■ Apply ethical behaviors, including honesty/integrity in performance of medical assisting practice (affective) ■ Explain the rationale for performance of a procedure to the patient (affective) ■ Use language/verbal skills that enable patients' understanding (affective) ■ Perform handwashing (psychomotor) ■ Screen test results (psychomotor) ■ Describe the normal function of each body system (cognitive) ■ Identify common pathology related to each body system (cognitive) ■ Analyze pathology as it relates to the interaction of body systems (cognitive) ■ Discuss implications for disease and disability when homeostasis is not maintained (cognitive) ■ Describe implications for treatment related to pathology (cognitive) ■ Apply critical thinking skills in performing patient assessment and care (affective) ■ Explore issue of confidentiality as it applies to the medical assistant (cognitive) ■ Prepare a patient for procedures and/or treatments (psychomotor) ■ Document patient education (psychomotor) ■ Document accurately in the patient record (psychomotor) ■ Perform electrocardiography (psychomotor)	■ Interview and record patient history. ■ Prepare patients for procedures. ■ Apply principles of aseptic techniques and infection control. ■ Take vital signs. ■ Recognize emergencies. ■ Perform first aid and CPR. ■ Prepare and maintain examination and treatment area. ■ Prepare patient for and assist physician with routine and specialty examinations and treatments and minor office surgeries. ■ Use quality control. ■ Collect and process specimens. ■ Screen and follow up patient test results. ■ Prepare and administer oral and parenteral medications as directed by physician. ■ Maintain medication and immunization records. ■ Dispose of biohazardous materials. ■ Practice Standard Precautions. ■ Perform electrocardiograms. ■ Perform respiratory testing. ■ Perform telephone and in-person screening.

 COMPETENCY SKILLS PERFORMANCE

1. Perform an electrocardiogram.
2. Demonstrate the application of a Holter monitor.

Key Terminology *(continued)*

contractility—ability of the heart muscle to shorten or reduce in size

coronary artery bypass—surgery in which the ischemia or obstruction in the coronary arteries is bypassed with a graft of a vessel

coronary artery disease—condition in which the coronary arteries are narrowed by constriction caused by plaque buildup

depolarization—condition in which the cardiac cell environment becomes positive

diastole—period of ventricular relaxation

dysrhythmia—abnormal, irregular, or disturbed heart rhythm

ejection fraction—measurement of the fraction of the total amount (volume) of blood filling the ventricle that is ejected during the ventricular contraction

embolism—condition in which an embolus that is moving through the vascular system becomes lodged in a vessel

embolus (plural: emboli)—mass of material or tissue in a vessel; may be a blood clot, air, fat, bone fragments, bacterial clumps, amniotic fluid, or other materials

endocarditis—inflammation of the endocardium

excitability—response of cardiac cell to electrical stimulus

fibrillation—irregular contractions of the heart; ECG shows waveforms without definite pattern or shape. Atrial fibrillation: Atria are quivering and do not have a forceful beat to push blood into ventricles. Ventricular fibrillation: Lethal arrhythmia; ventricles are quivering and do not

contract with force to push blood into aorta. Rhythm is chaotic, with no recognizable P waves, QRS complexes, or T waves; without immediate intervention and conversion of rhythm, asystole will follow.

focus (plural: foci)—specific site; the origin of an electrical cardiac impulse

hemoptysis—coughing up blood from the respiratory tract

interatrial septum—wall between the right and left atria

internodal pathway—the three tracts that carry the electrical impulse as it leaves the SA node, transmit the impulse to the AV node, and distribute it throughout the atria; the three divisions are the anterior, middle, and posterior divisions

interventriclular septum—wall between the right and left ventricles

isoelectric line—flat, horizontal line on an ECG strip representing the beginning and ending point of all waves of the ECG cycle

mitral valve prolapse—valvular disorder in which cusps of mitral valve prolapse into right atrium, failing to close and resulting in back pressure into left atrium

multifocal—originating from more than one area or focus

myocardial infarction—death of myocardial tissue due to obstructed blood supply to the tissue

myocarditis—inflammation of the myocardium

palpitations—irregular and often erratic heartbeats felt by the patient

pericarditis—inflammation of the pericardium

precordial lead—ECG lead that views the heart in a horizontal plain

premature ventricular contraction—a beat that comes early in the cardiac cycle, is not preceded by a P wave, and has a widened and distorted QRS complex; sometimes referred to as premature ventricular complex or premature ventricular beat (PVB)

repolarization—return of the cardiac cell to the resting state

sinoatrial node—pacemaker of the heart

stenosis—narrowing or constriction of a passage

stent—device implanted in a vessel to maintain its patency (openness)

systole—contraction of the myocardium

tachycardia—heart rate above 100 beats per minute (BPM)

thromboembolism—obstruction of a blood vessel by a thrombus

thrombosis—condition of having a blood clot in a blood vessel

thrombus (plural: thrombi)—blood clot in the vessel that can form an obstruction in the vessel

unifocal—originating from same area or focus

ventricle—right or left lower chamber of heart

Abbreviations

ABG—arterial blood gases

A-fib—atrial fibrillation

AV—atrioventricular node

BBB—bundle branch block

CAB—coronary artery bypass

CABG—coronary artery bypass graft

CAD—coronary artery disease

CHF—congestive heart failure

DVT—deep-vein thrombosis

ECG/EKG—electrocardiogram

EF—ejection fraction

MI—myocardial infarction

MVP—mitral valve prolapse

NSR—normal sinus rhythm

PR—P-R interval in the complex

PVC—premature ventricular contraction

QRS—QRS interval or waveform in the complex

SA—sinoatrial

ST—S-T interval or waveform in the complex

V-fib—ventricular fibrillation

V-tach—ventricular tachycardia

Introduction

The medical assistant in a cardiology office encounters many types of heart disease. A significant complaint is chest pain. Patients who complain of irregular heartbeats, shortness of breath (SOB), tissue swelling (edema), and exhaustion or fatigue are also treated on a regular basis. Complaints of nausea, excessive sweating, and denial of possible heart attack are serious symptoms that demand immediate intervention.

A variety of diagnostic tests are used in a cardiology office to identify possible cardiac disorders. An ECG measures the electrical activity of the myocardium (heart muscle). A Holter monitor 24-hour test is ordered if an electrocardiogram does not show significant findings and the patient is having persistent symptoms. An echocardiogram provides a visual concept of the heart structures coordinated with the conduction system and the contractility of the myocardium. Other diagnostic tests include stress tests, thallium scans, and MUGA scans.

Patients who have experienced a myocardial infarct, with subsequent cardiac arrest and resuscitation with CPR and/or automatic defibrillation are sometimes given follow-up care in the medical office, as are some patients who have had coronary artery bypass surgery. Patients with congestive heart failure, pulmonary edema, hypertension, arrhythmias, cardiomyopathy, cardiomegaly, vascular disorders, valve disorders, and inflammatory or infectious conditions are also treated in the cardiology office. Cardiologists perform cardiac catheterizations, angioplasty, and stent insertions in the hospital setting.

The Medical Assistant's Role in Cardiology

Diagnostic procedures in cardiology include blood testing and various electronic assessments of the cardiovascular system, such as electrocardiograms (ECG or EKG), echocardiograms, the Holter monitor, stress testing, thallium scans, and MUGA scans. A newer procedure involves a three-dimensional view of the coronary arteries by MRI. Many offices now assess cardiac functioning by evaluating the oxygenation of the blood with a pulse oximeter (discussed in ∞ Chapter 36 on respiratory testing). Medical assistants are trained to perform ECGs and in some offices may be responsible for Holter monitor application. With specialized training, they may assist in advanced procedures.

Medical assistants routinely perform ECGs, especially in a cardiology office. It is therefore important that the MA understand not only the anatomy and physiology of the heart, including the electrical conduction system, but the interpretation of rhythm strips as well.

The MA is responsible for having the patient gowned and properly draped for a cardiac examination. The room temperature should be at a comfortable level and privacy should be afforded to the patient and the physician or any technicians. An electrocardiograph may need to be moved into the room and calibrated. The physician may select his or her personal stethoscope to assess heart tones or may expect one to be available. Supplies for the ECG, including leads, sensors, and paper, should be readily available in the room or in the ECG cart. If office protocol includes an O_2 saturation, this is obtained with the pulse oximeter and recorded for the physician to note. All necessary supplies should be available in the room so that the MA does not have to leave during the procedure.

Anatomy and Physiology of the Heart

The heart is a muscle that pumps the blood throughout the body (Figure 35-1 ◆). Deoxygenated blood enters the right **atrium,** the upper right chamber of the heart, through two large veins, the *inferior* and *superior vena cava.* The blood passes through the tricuspid valve into the right **ventricle,** the lower right chamber of the heart, then through the pulmonary valve into the pulmonary arteries. The pulmonary arteries transport the oxygen-poor blood to the lungs, where a gas exchange takes place by way of the pulmonary alveolar-capillary network. In the alveoli, oxygen is transferred to the blood and carbon dioxide is removed, to be exhaled through the lungs. The oxygen-rich blood then returns through the pulmonary veins to the left atrium, or left upper chamber of the heart. From there the

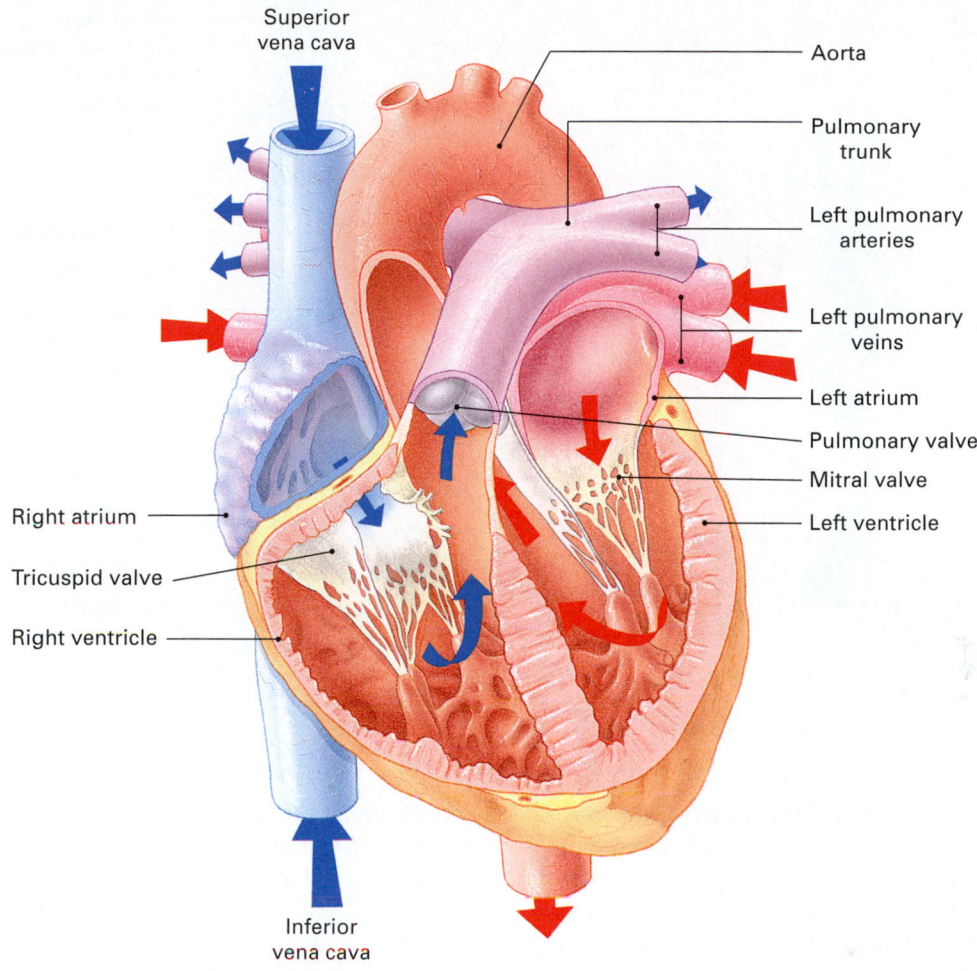

Superior
vena cava

Aorta

Pulmonary
trunk

Left pulmonary
arteries

Left pulmonary
veins

Left atrium

Pulmonary valve

Mitral valve

Left ventricle

Right atrium

Tricuspid valve

Right ventricle

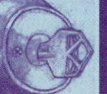

Inferior
vena cava

Figure 35-1 ◆ Blood flow through the heart.

blood is pumped through the bicuspid or mitral valve into the left ventricle, or left lower chamber of the heart. The blood then passes through the aortic valve into the aorta to be transported to the coronary arteries of the heart, the carotid arteries of the head, and other major arteries of the circulatory system. Blood then returns to the right atrium via the superior and inferior vena cava.

From outside to inside, the heart consists of three layers (Figure 35-2 ◆):

- Pericardium
- Myocardium
- Endocardium

The myocardium of this two-sided pump contains contractile filaments in each cardiac muscle cell. When the contractile filaments are stimulated by the conduction system, the healthy heart muscle contracts and relaxes 60 to 100 times a minute. Blood flow from the heart is generated by the physical contraction of the myocardial tissue.

Heart Conduction

An electrical **conduction system** within the myocardium regulates the pumping action of the heart. The pacemaker cells, specialized cellular units of the cardiac conduction system,

Keys to Success
HEART VALVES

Here's a memory aid to help you remember which side of the heart the tricuspid and bicuspid (mitral) valves are on. The right lung has three lobes. The valve between the right atrium and right ventricle has three cusps and is called the tricuspid valve. The left lung has two lobes. The valve between the left atrium and left ventricle has two cusps and is known as the bicuspid (mitral) valve.

control the rate and rhythm of the heart and are also responsible for the generation and conduction of the electrical impulses that cause the myocardium to contract. Cardiac muscle cells have the unique characteristics of **excitability, conductivity, contractility,** and **automaticity.** In addition, neurological stimulation of cardiac muscle cells, and the resulting mechanical cardiac function, are affected by abnormally high or low electrolyte levels.

Electrolyte imbalance influences both mechanical and electrical cardiac functions. Potassium, sodium, calcium, and magnesium affect the cardiac cycle. When the cardiac cell is at

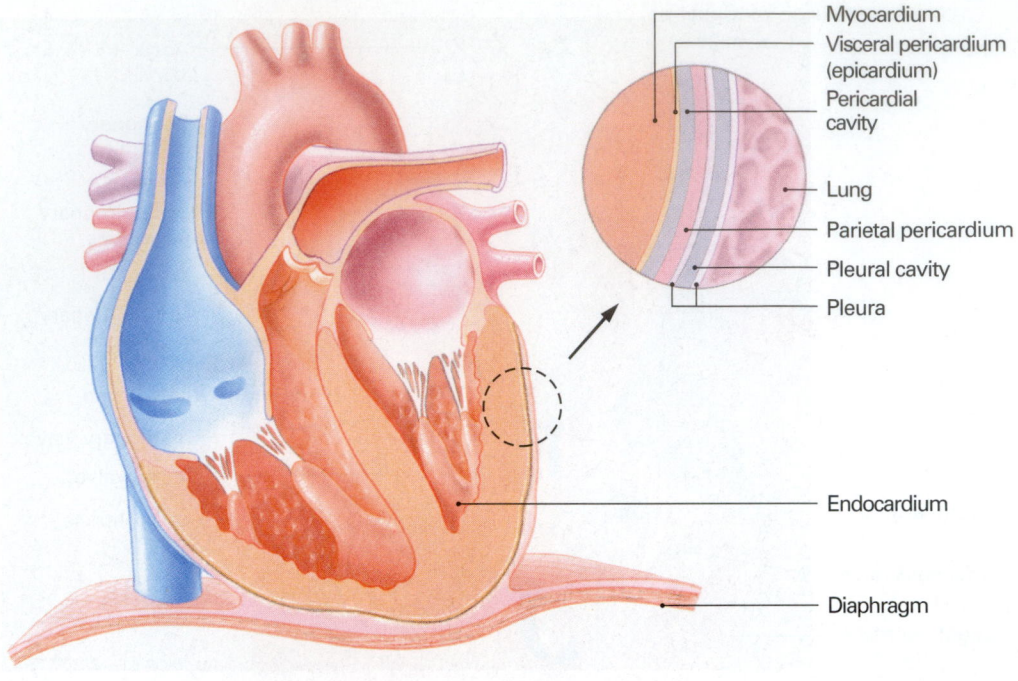

Figure 35-2 ◆ Layers of the heart.

rest, the concentration of potassium is greater inside the cell than outside the cell wall, while the concentration of sodium is greater outside the cell wall. Using the sodium–potassium exchange pump process, sodium and potassium ions are moved in and out through the cell wall. Venous blood samples measure extracellular amounts of electrolytes.

Cardiac **depolarization** and **repolarization** occur when a conduction impulse develops and spreads through the myocardium. Depolarization occurs as sodium ions rush into the myocardial cell and calcium slowly enters the cell; potassium exits the cell, resulting in the contraction of the cell. This process

is followed by potassium returning to the cell and sodium exiting the cell. Repolarization, which is slower than depolarization, returns the cell to a recovered state. The next step in the progression of cardiac muscle cell activity is a refractory or total relaxation of the myocardial cell. After this period of rest, the myocardial cell is ready for the cycle to continue.

The conduction system originates in the **sinoatrial (SA) node,** also known as the pacemaker (Figure 35-3 ◆). The SA node initiates the impulse. When it fails to do so, lower pacemaker cells can initiate the conduction as a "survival" effort. The impulse travels the **internodal pathway** through the right

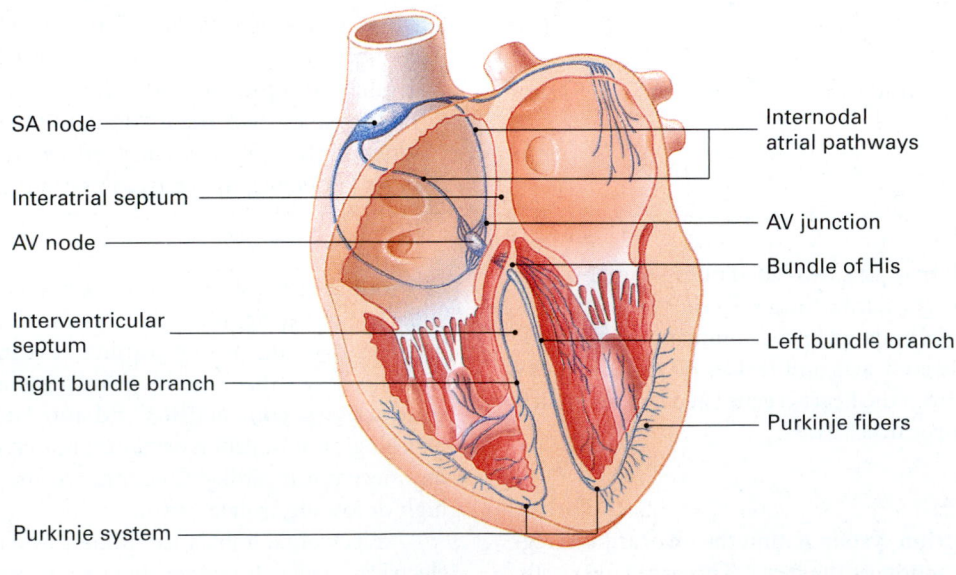

Figure 35-3 ◆ Cardiac conduction system.

atrium to the atrioventricular (**AV**) node and through Bachmann's bundle in the **interatrial septum** to the left atrium. The impulse then travels through the bundle of His (AV bundle) to the right and left branches of the bundle of His, the **interventricular septum,** and then on to the Purkinje fibers in the ventricular myocardium. As the impulse travels through the conduction system, depolarization and repolarization take place, resulting in the contraction, or **systole,** and relaxation, or **diastole,** of the myocardium. The atrial stimulation causes the initial contraction of myocardial cells of the atria, allowing blood from the atria to be pumped into the ventricles. The sequential stimulation of the ventricular myocardium then causes the ventricles to contract, sending the blood into the pulmonary and general circulation of the body.

Diseases and Disorders of the Heart

Coronary Artery Disease

Coronary artery disease (**CAD**) is the result of plaque buildup, or **atherosclerosis,** in the arteries over a period of years. The plaque causes the arteries to harden, a condition called **arteriosclerosis,** and to become weak in some areas and thick in others. The arteries become narrow or are partially obstructed, and blood flow to the surrounding tissue is reduced. Consequently, oxygen and nutrition to the tissue are also reduced (ischemia), causing cramping of the myocardium and discomfort in the form of pain. If the condition is severe enough, complete obstruction and an infarction of the myocardial tissue result. Depending on the size of the infarction, the damage may affect a small area or may be catastrophic enough to cause sudden death.

Symptoms of CAD include angina-type pain, shortness of breath, weakness or dizziness, rapid heartbeat, **palpitations,** nausea, and perspiration.

Coronary artery disease may result in two forms of "heart attack":

- Myocardial ischemia: This type of "heart attack" is the result of reduced blood flow to the myocardium, which causes angina-type pain. It may be reversed if circulation is restored to the tissue within the six-hour time frame before tissue death, or infarction, results.
- Sudden cardiac death: The second type of "heart attack" occurs when the conduction system suffers an insult. In addition to **arrhythmias** caused by coronary artery obstruction, lethal arrhythmias may be caused by electrocution, trauma, and drug overdose. Sudden cardiac death may also be the result of respiratory arrest, drowning, or massive hemorrhage. (See *Myocardial Infarction, Arrhythmias,* and *Sudden Cardiac Arrest* below for additional information.)

Risk factors for coronary artery disease are classified as nonmodifiable and modifiable. The risk factors over which the individual has no control include a family history of heart disease at an early age, male gender, postmenopausal female, age over 45 years. Risk factors that can be reduced by the individual include smoking, high blood cholesterol levels, hypertension, blood glucose levels, lack of exercise, excess weight, and stress.

Angina

The patient experiencing **angina** will complain of pressure-like pain, usually in the chest region, possibly radiating down the left arm, to the left jaw, and to the right chest and arm. This discomfort is generally experienced on exertion and ceases after a few minutes of rest. Until it is confirmed that the pain is angina, the patient is considered to be in an emergency state with possible impending MI. Immediate assessment and intervention are essential. When such a patient presents in the office, the physician is notified and assessment is begun immediately. (∞ Refer to the section on triage in Chapter 41.) If the patient calls from home, he or she is usually instructed to call 911 or to be transported to an emergency facility with cardiac resuscitation capabilities. Once the pain has been established as anginal, intervention may be in the form of a vasodilator such as nitroglycerin (Nitro-stat) or a calcium-channel blocker such as verapamil (Calan, Isoptin), diltiazem (Cardizem), or nifedipine (Procardia). Modifications in lifestyle, including diet, activity, and stress relief, are helpful in the course of treatment.

Myocardial Infarction

Myocardial infarction (**MI**) results when an obstruction to the myocardial tissue is followed by ischemia over a period of approximately six hours. The ischemia may be caused by plaque buildup in the arteries, spasm of the arteries, or a **thrombus** that has broken loose from an arterial wall or has formed and moved from the left atrium or ventricle. Intervention with **angioplasty, stent** insertion, or coronary artery bypass surgery may prevent permanent damage.

Post-Myocardial Infarction

Post-MI patients are seen in the office for followup care or possible referral to a cardiovascular surgeon. As with all cardiac patients, ECGs, vital signs, oxygen saturation levels, and body weight are important components of the office visit. Diagnostic procedures may be ordered and any previous diagnostic results may be discussed. Patient signs are assessed and symptoms or complaints are recorded. The physician reviews the chart and listens to (auscultates) the heart and breath sounds. The feet and legs are examined for edema and detection of pedal pulses. The color, temperature, and moistness of the skin are noted. (Examples: Skin warm, pink, and dry, or skin pale and dusky, cool, and slightly moist.) Pulse oximeter readings are recorded. The patient is scheduled for followup appointments and rehabilitation is discussed and scheduled. It is important to realize there may be a psychological factor involved for the post-CAB patient, whose heart has been stopped and restarted during the procedure.

Sudden Cardiac Arrest

Sudden cardiac arrest occurs when the conduction system of the myocardium sustains a massive insult. This can be the result of ischemia in the area of essential cardiac conduction path, a lethal arrhythmia that causes cardiac standstill, electrocution, major trauma to the chest and heart, massive hemorrhage, or drug overdose. Respiratory arrest and drowning may also lead to sudden cardiac death. Immediate intervention with CPR and automated external defibrillator (AED) may successfully resuscitate the victim. (∞ Refer to Chapter 41 for additional information on CPR and AED.)

Hypertension/Hypertensive Heart Disease

Hypertension is often referred to as "high blood pressure." It is also called "the silent killer" because so many people who have hypertension are unaware of it. The blood pressure range accepted as normal by the American Heart Association is less than 120 systolic and less than 80 diastolic. A reading of 120–139 systolic and 80–89 diastolic is considered prehypertension. For a diagnosis of hypertension to be made, blood pressure readings over a period of time must be persistently elevated. Many patients experience what has been called "white coat syndrome"—a high initial blood pressure in the medical office due to the patient's anxiety. For this reason, many physicians prefer to have a second blood pressure reading taken close to the end of the visit, before any procedures or before the patient is dismissed.

An elevated blood pressure makes the heart work harder to pump blood through constricted vessels. The constriction may be caused by arteriosclerosis, atherosclerosis, or renal disease. Stress is considered a factor in hypertension, as is being overweight (Table 35-1).

Essential hypertension results when a prolonged state of elevated blood pressure develops without apparent cause. With an insidious onset, it is possible for the disease process to be in an advanced state by the time it is diagnosed, as many individuals are asymptomatic. The condition may go undetected until a blood pressure reading is elevated. Symptoms include lightheadedness, headaches, dizziness, syncope, tinnitus, nosebleeds, palpitations, and malaise. Malignant hypertension may follow essential hypertension, with extreme stress often being the precipitating factor.

There is no cure for essential hypertension. Treatment is lifelong and involves decreasing the heart's workload and dilating the vascular system. The first line of defense and treatment is the modification of risk factors. Dietary changes to reduce salt and fat intake are helpful in controlling hypertension. Cessation of smoking, increased activity and exercise, weight reduction, and stress reduction are also helpful. If these lifestyle modifications do not help, drug therapy is prescribed. Drugs for hypertension include diuretics, vasodilating drugs, ACE inhibitors, and beta-blocking drugs.

Congestive Heart Failure

The patient with congestive heart failure (**CHF**) complains of shortness of breath, weight gain, swelling (edema), and possibly exhaustion. He or she will exhibit fluid retention, possibly with swollen feet and hands and facial puffiness, and may report difficulty putting on shoes and rings. These symptoms usually have an insidious onset; the dyspnea gradually increases to a severe state. Other signs include distended neck veins, respiratory distress, and pitting edema of the legs, ankles, and feet. Radiographs of the chest are taken to assess the size of the heart and are compared with previous films to measure the progression of enlargement.

Treatment of CHF includes drug therapy to reduce the workload of the heart. Additional drugs such as cardiac glycosides and digitalis preparations (Lanoxin) slow and strengthen the heartbeat, making it more efficient. Diuretics reduce blood volume and decrease the fluid in the tissues. Vasodilators reduce vascular pressure. Fluid and sodium intake is restricted. Daily weight and apical pulse assessments are also part of the treatment.

Pulmonary Edema

Pulmonary edema follows CHF as the lungs fill with interstitial fluid and pressure builds in the lung tissue, increasing the workload of the heart. Left-sided heart failure, mitral valve disorders, hypertension, renal failure, and cardiac arrhythmias may also cause pulmonary edema. The patient experiences shortness of breath, dyspnea, and coughing. Bloody, frothy sputum may be present. The symptoms often worsen at night after the patient has gone to bed and is in a reclining position.

Treatment is aimed at decreasing the fluid levels in the lung tissue, with subsequent reduction of cardiac workload. Drug therapy includes diuretics, Lanoxin, vasodilators, and bronchodilating drugs. Most patients require aggressive treatment in a hospital environment.

TABLE 35-1 RISK FACTORS IN HYPERTENSION	
Nonmodifiable Risk Factors	**Modifiable Risk Factors**
Family history of hypertensive disease	Chronic stress
	Obesity
Being of African American descent	Diet high in salt and fat
	Oral contraceptives
Older age	Sedentary lifestyle
Diabetes	Smoking
Kidney disease	

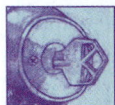

Keys to Success
BLOOD PRESSURE THERAPY IS FOR LIFE

Individuals taking medications to control their blood pressure must understand that drug therapy will be necessary for the rest of their lives. Often, because the medications lower their blood pressure, patients may believe the problem has been solved and they no longer need to take the medications. Patient education includes emphasizing the importance of regular blood pressure monitoring and consistently taking medications.

Cardiomyopathy

Cardiomyopathy, a noninflammatory disease of the myocardium, often has no identifiable cause. The muscle thickens, possibly as a result of hypertension and increased workload, and its ability to pump blood is affected.

In *dilated cardiomyopathy,* as the workload of the myocardium increases, the heart muscle fibers are stretched, the chambers are dilated, and the walls become weaker and thinner. The heart compensates and the chambers enlarge and stretch more, a condition called **cardiomegaly.** The thinning walls of the heart can no longer keep up with the circulatory demands of the body. Symptoms may be insidious or may appear fairly rapidly. They are similar to those of CHF, including fatigue, weakness, shortness of breath, edema of the legs and feet, and respiratory congestion. Diuretics are prescribed to decrease fluid volume and thus reduce the workload of the heart. Digitalis helps to strengthen and slow the heartbeat. Vasodilators help to reduce the workload by reducing the resistance of constricted vessels. If arrhythmias occur, they are controlled with antiarrhythmic drugs, including beta-blockers and calcium-channel blockers. When drug therapy is no longer effective, a heart transplant is the only solution.

Another form of cardiomyopathy is termed *hypertrophic cardiomyopathy.* The fibers of the myocardium exhibit abnormal growth and arrangement and the wall of the heart thickens, mostly in the left ventricle. As the wall thickens, it loses the ability to contract and relax completely. Blood flow diminishes, causing a breathless feeling. The patient experiences fainting, or syncope, as the brain receives inadequate blood supply. Chaotic heartbeats may occur, occasionally resulting in sudden cardiac death. Hypertrophic cardiomyopathy is often diagnosed in young asymptomatic males when exertion from exercise causes the symptoms and an awareness of the condition.

Echocardiograms and auscultation of heart sounds aid in the diagnosis of this condition. The treatment objective is to prevent lethal arrhythmias. Antiarrhythmic drugs and diuretics are usually prescribed, and exercise is limited in some cases.

Arrhythmias

Arrhythmias may be classified in different ways: by disturbance of impulse formation or origin, by disturbance of conduction, by consistency of the point of origin, and by prognosis.

The heart is autorhythmic—it initiates the impulse. This impulse normally originates in the SA node and travels through the atrium to the AV node, down the septal wall by way of the bundles of His to the Purkinje fibers. Various conditions may cause the impulse not to originate in the SA node or cause interruptions in the pathway of the impulse through the heart. Areas of ischemic or infarcted tissue block the pathway of the impulse.

Arrhythmias Resulting from Impulse Formation or Origin

The SA node normally generates rhythmic impulses at the rate of 60 to 100 per minute. When the impulse originates in the atrium at a normal rate and travels the normal pathway through the conduction system, it is called a normal sinus rhythm (**NSR**). Common cardiac arrhythmias resulting from impulse formation are categorized by the point of origin (Table 35-2).

Arrhythmias Resulting from Conduction Disturbances

Conduction disturbances refer to abnormal delays or blocks in the conduction of the cardiac impulse from the SA node through the AV node, the bundle of His, and the Purkinje fibers. Common cardiac arrhythmias resulting from conduction disturbances are listed in Table 35-3. Blocking of the impulse results in first-degree, second-degree, Mobitz second-degree, and third-degree heart blocks. Drugs and chemicals can also cause irregular impulses. Impulses may originate in other areas of the myocardium and are often identified relative to this point of origin.

Arrythmias Classified According to Consistency of Point of Origin

Another origin categorization relates to the consistency of the point of origin. **Unifocal** impulses have the same point of origin, while **multifocal** rhythms have various points of origin. Multifocal rhythms are potentially life-threatening and are identified on an ECG. Additionally, the SA node may not fire every time, causing a delayed complex or interval.

Atrial rhythms have their origin in the atria. Sinus rhythms originate in the SA node, nodal rhythms in the area of the AV node, and ventricular rhythms in the ventricles.

Arrhythmias Classified According to Prognosis

Another method of general classification is by the degree of seriousness of the arrhythmia or the prognosis of the condition

TABLE 35-2 TYPES AND EXAMPLES OF ARRHYTHMIAS RESULTING FROM IMPULSE FORMATION			
Sinoatrial Arrhythmias	**Atrial Arrhythmias**	**AV Nodal (Junctional) Arrhythmias**	**Ventricular Arrhythmias**
Sinus **tachycardia**	Premature atrial contraction	Premature junctional contractions	Premature ventricular contractions
Sinus **bradycardia**	Paroxysmal atrial tachycardia	Paroxysmal junctional tachycardia	Ventricular tachycardia
Sinus arrhythmia	Atrial flutter	Nonparoxysmal junctional tachycardia	Ventricular fibrillation
Wandering pacemaker	Atrial **fibrillation**		
Sinoatrial arrest	Atrial standstill		

TABLE 35-3 TYPES AND EXAMPLES OF ARRHYTHMIAS RESULTING FROM CONDUCTION DISTURBANCES

Sinus or Atrial	Atrioventricular Node	Ventricular
Sinoatrial block	First-degree AV block Second-degree AV block Mobitz, Type I Mobitz, Type II Third-degree (complete) AV block	Bundle-branch blocks, right or left Bilateral bundle-branch blocks Ventricular standstill

(Table 35-4). This group includes minor arrhythmias that usually do not lead to more serious arrhythmias and do not affect the circulation. Major arrhythmias may lead to the onset of lethal arrhythmias and often have serious effects on the circulation. Death-producing arrhythmias require immediate and aggressive intervention.

Medical assistants are expected to recognize potentially lethal rhythms when performing an ECG or if the patient is on a cardiac monitor. If these rhythms appear, immediate assistance is required and must be requested. The physician must be notified immediately so that aggressive intervention may be instituted.

Treatment

Once arrhythmia is diagnosed, antiarrhythmic drugs are prescribed. The patient is assessed frequently during the first few months until the heart rhythms return to near-normal status or the patient is asymptomatic. The drugs do not cure the underlying cause of the arrhythmias but are used to control them. Patients with potentially life-threatening arrhythmias may require implants of cardiac pacemakers or internal automatic defibrillators. Some cardiology offices assist pacemaker clinics in the monitoring and control of these devices.

Infective Heart Disorders

Infective and inflammatory disorders of the heart include endocarditis, myocarditis, pericarditis, and rheumatic heart disease

resulting from rheumatic fever. The causative agents of these disorders may be bacterial, viral, fungal, or parasitic. These cardiomyopathies often lead to cardiomegaly and heart failure and require aggressive treatment, including IV antibiotics and cardiac and oxygen saturation monitoring.

Endocarditis

Endocarditis, an inflammation of the lining of the heart chambers and valve surfaces, is usually the result of a bacterial infection. Pyogenic bacteria such as *Staphylococci* and *Streptococci* are often the source; viruses and trauma are other possible sources. The majority of these infections occur in the left side

TABLE 35-4 CLASSIFICATION OF ARRHYTHMIAS ACCORDING TO PROGNOSIS

Type of Arrhythmia	Examples
Minor Arrhythmias	Sinus bradycardia
	Sinus tachycardia
	Wandering pacemaker
	Premature atrial contractions
	Premature junctional contractions
Major Arrhythmias	Sinus bradycardia consistently <50 BPM
	Sinus tachycardia consistently >100 BPM
	Sinoatrial arrest
	Sinoatrial block
	Atrial tachycardia
	Atrial flutter
	Atrial fibrillation
	Paroxysmal junctional tachycardia
	Premature ventricular contractions >6 BPM or in pairs
	Ventricular tachycardia
	First-, second-, and third-degree heart block
	Bundle-branch block
Lethal Arrhythmias	Ventricular fibrillation
	Ventricular standstill

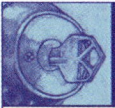

Key to Success
EINTHOVEN'S TRIANGLE

Willem Einthoven (1860–1927) introduced the concept that, when properly applied, leads I, II, and III have a relationship in which they form a triangle over the body. Limb leads are placed on the right and left arms and the left leg, forming a triangle, called Einthoven's triangle (Figure 35-4 ◆). Einthoven's Law states the following equation: lead I + lead III = lead II. The height and depth of the recordings in lead I added to those of lead III are equal to the height and depth of lead II. When the P wave is positive in lead II, it should be negative in leads I and III. Also, the height of the QRS wave in lead I plus the height of the QRS in lead III is equal to the height of the QRS wave in lead II.

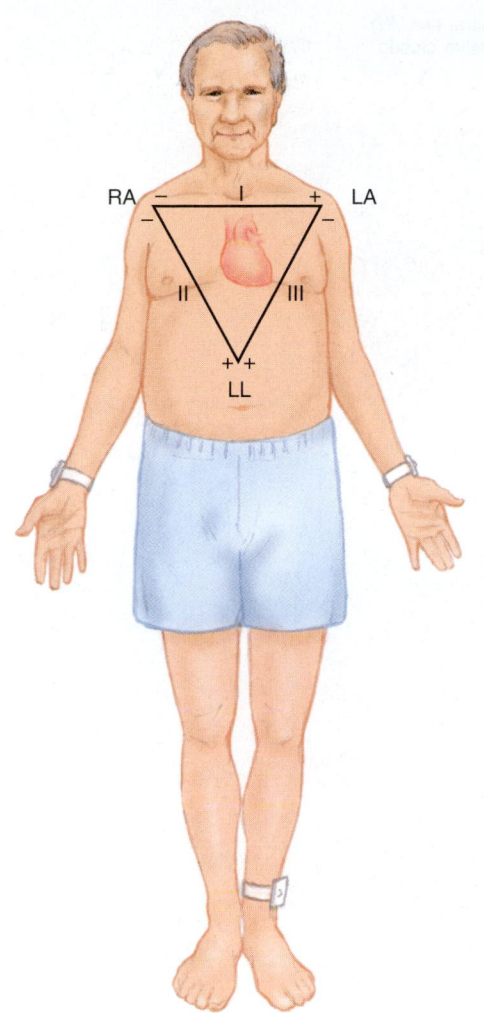

Figure 35-4 ◆ Einthoven's triangle.

of the heart. Valvular involvement results in surface defects on the valves, followed by scarring and stiffness. **Stenosis** is the narrowing or constriction of a passage.

The inability of the valve leaflets to close completely results in a murmur that may be detected during auscultation of heart sounds. Depending on the extent of the condition, the individual displays sudden onset of a febrile illness with symptoms that include chills, intermittent fever, weakness, anorexia, and fatigue. In addition, thrombi may form on the valves or chordae tendineae and eventually break loose, becoming emboli. These emboli not only have the potential for occluding a vessel but may also carry the infection to other parts of the body.

Sources of the invading bacterium may be a respiratory infection, tooth abscess, urinary tract infection, or skin infection. Individuals with a history of rheumatic fever, valvular difficulties, cardiac surgery, and extensive orthopedic surgeries are at risk for this type of infection. Therefore, prior to any dental procedure, prophylactic antibiotics are administered. Treatment involves aggressive therapy with antibiotics.

Critical Thinking Question 35-1

Knowing that Ray has a history of cardiac surgery and is planning to have dental surgery, what should Rachel's response to his presenting symptoms be?

Myocarditis

Myocarditis is an inflammation of the cardiac muscle caused by a virus, bacteria, or parasite. Vague symptoms, including mild fever, dyspnea, shortness of breath, palpitations, fatigue, and tachycardia are exhibited. Blood studies indicate an elevated WBC, increased ESR, and elevated cardiac enzymes. A chest X-ray shows left-sided cardiac enlargement, and the ECG is abnormal. Treatment includes antibiotics for infection and medication to control arrhythmias.

Pericarditis

Pericarditis is an inflammation of the pericardium, the outer surface or sac covering of the heart. The pericardial space between the pericardium and the myocardium normally contains a small amount of lubricating pericardial fluid that allows the myocardium to move within the sac during heartbeats. Pericarditis results from infection, inflammation, or other conditions in the body. Signs and symptoms include fever, chills, chest pain, dyspnea, and malaise. A friction rub may be heard during auscultation. Elevated WBC and ESR and echocardiogram abnormalities help confirm the diagnosis. Treatment includes pain relief and addressing the underlying cause.

Rheumatic Fever and Rheumatic Heart Disease

Rheumatic fever and the resulting rheumatic heart disease follow a sore throat caused by Group A beta-hemolytic *Streptococcus.* The endocardium and valves become inflamed. The bacteria settle on the valves and grow into vegetations that scar the endocardial tissue. This scarring leads to valvular insufficiency and/or stenosis.

A history of recent upper respiratory infection, sore throat, and fever followed by inflamed, painful joints leads to suspicion of strep infection. Patients have an elevated temperature and complain of joint pain and swelling, especially in the fingers, knees, and ankle joints. They may also experience weight loss, loss of appetite, malaise, weakness, and a rash on the trunk. Often a cardiac murmur is heard. Diagnosis is confirmed by taking a culture.

Prevention is the best strategy. To prevent rheumatic fever, a Rapid Strep test should be performed on children with sore throats. If the causative agent is Group A beta-hemolytic *Streptococcus,* an intense regimen of antibiotic therapy is instituted. Bed rest is helpful, along with analgesics for the pain and antipyretics for the fever.

Valvular Disorders

The heart has four valves: the tricuspid, pulmonary, mitral or bicuspid, and aortic (Figure 35-5 ◆). Any of the valves may be

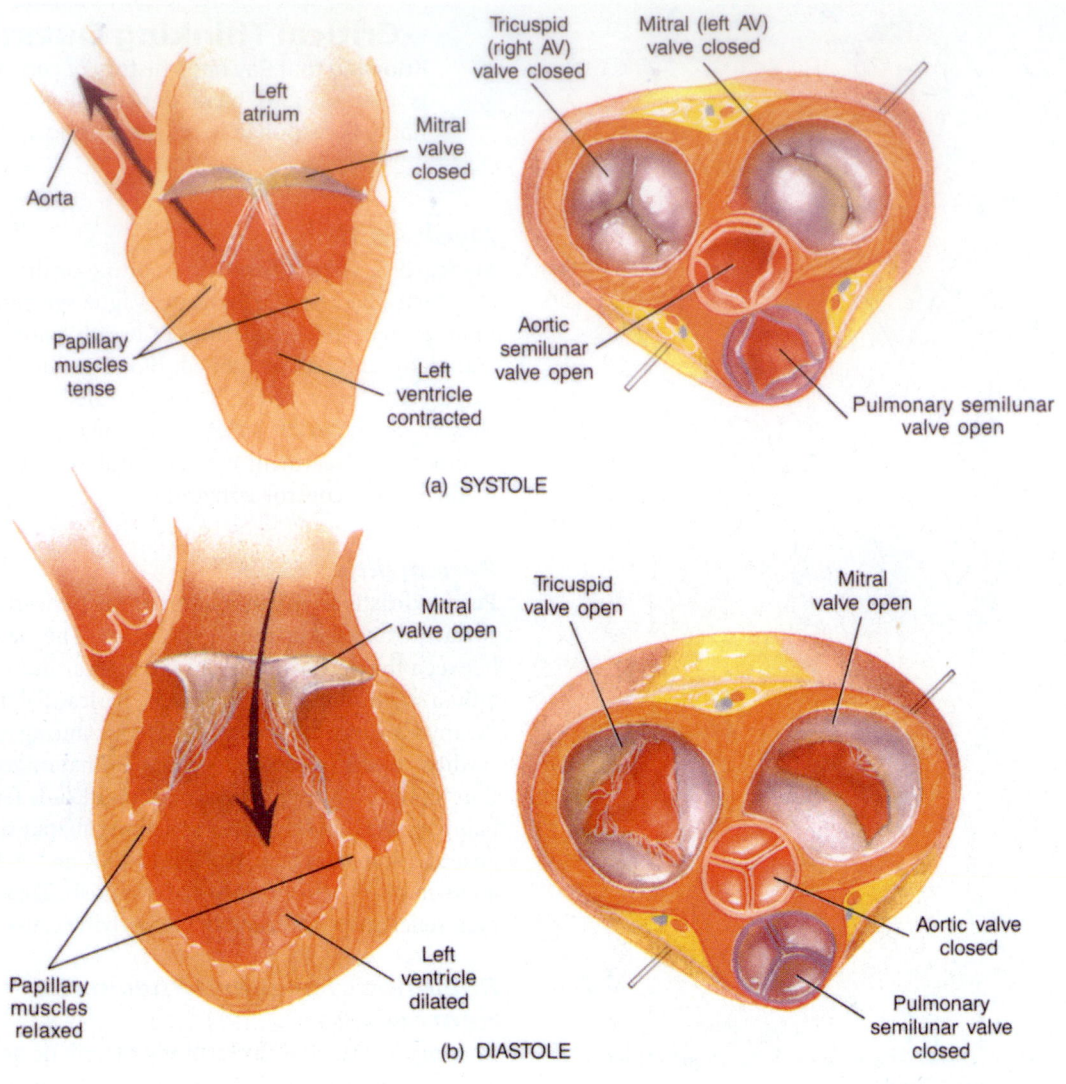

Tricuspid
(right AV)
valve closed

Mitral (left AV)
valve closed

Left
atrium

Mitral
valve
closed

Aorta

Papillary
muscles
tense

Left
ventricle
contracted

Aortic
semilunar
valve open

Pulmonary semilunar
valve open

(a) SYSTOLE

Mitral
valve open

Tricuspid
valve open

Mitral
valve open

Papillary
muscles
relaxed

Left
ventricle
dilated

Aortic valve
closed

Pulmonary
semilunar valve
closed

(b) DIASTOLE

Figure 35-5 ◆ Valves of the heart.

affected by disease or disorder. When a valve fails to close completely, it is termed *insufficient.* Blood flows back into the previous chamber, creating a back pressure on that chamber. When the valve fails to open completely because of a constriction, the condition is called stenosis. As the blood slows in the narrowed or "hardened" valve, a back-pressure is also created in the previous chamber. Heart murmur may be detected in the presence of these valvular conditions. Diagnosis may be made with the aid of ECG, echocardiogram, radiograms of the chest, and cardiac catheterization.

The mitral valve is the valve most often affected. The bacteria responsible for rheumatic heart disease migrate to the mitral valve and vegetations develop, scarring the valve cusps and preventing the valve from either completely closing or completely opening. Patients experience symptoms similar to those of many heart disorders, including dyspnea, shortness of breath, and occasionally cyanosis. Patients with mitral stenosis may experience **hemoptysis.**

Treatment of valvular conditions includes reduction of the workload of the heart with bed rest and fluid restriction or administration of diuretics. Oxygen therapy is helpful in some cases. Antibiotics are often prescribed to slow or halt any infectious process. In mitral stenosis, a surgical procedure, commissurotomy, may be performed to free up the cusps and allow the blood to flow through more easily. Valve replacement may be required in severe cases.

Table 35-5 describes common valvular disorders.

Vascular Disorders

Phlebitis

Phlebitis, an inflammatory condition of the veins, usually occurs in the deep veins of the lower limbs. Tenderness in the affected area often alerts the individual to the condition. Increasing pain with redness and swelling follow, signaling advancement of the condition. A history of insult to the tissue along with possible stasis of the blood is another indication of phlebitis. Analgesic medications are given and the individual is instructed not to rub or massage the area, as massage could stimulate clot formation or release emboli that have already formed into the

TABLE 35-5 VALVULAR DISORDERS

Valvular Disease	Physiology	Diagnosis	Treatment
Mitral insufficiency	Mitral valve does not close completely, allowing blood to flow back into left atrium. Extra workload results in increased volume of blood and elevated pressure in left atrium, leading to hypertrophy of the left atrium and right ventricle, with possible right ventricular failure.	*Symptoms:* dyspnea, fatigue, orthopnea, palpitations *Signs:* rales, peripheral edema, distended neck veins, hepatomegaly *Diagnostic tests:* cardiac catheterization, radiographs, ECG, echocardiogram	Valvotomy and repair or valve replacement. As with other cardiac conditions, symptoms are treated with diuretics to reduce blood volume and drug therapy to strengthen heartbeat.
Mitral stenosis	Mitral valve does not open completely, causing the blood to flow slowly into the left ventricle. The results are the same as for mitral insufficiency.	*Symptoms, signs, and diagnostic tests:* see Mitral insufficiency.	See Mitral insufficiency.
Mitral valve prolapse (MVP)	Chordae tendineae, either too long or too short, prevent mitral valve from closing completely, allowing blood to flow back into left atrium. As left ventricle contracts, blood regurgitates into left atrium.	*Symptoms:* Usually asymptomatic; otherwise chest pain, dizziness, syncope, dyspnea, fatigue *Signs:* Murmur heard on ascultation leads to further investigation.	Asymptomatic patient: no treatment required. Symptomatic patient: beta blockers, avoidance of caffeine and large, heavy meals *Diagnostic tests:* echocardiogram
Aortic insufficiency	Blood flows back into left ventricle, causing ventricle to enlarge and eventually leading to left ventricular failure. Condition may be result of rheumatic fever, endocarditis, hypertension, or syphilis. As ventricular failure occurs, CHF and pulmonary failure begin.	*Symptoms:* angina, syncope, fatigue, dyspnea, palpitations *Diagnostic tests:* ECG, echocardiogram, cardiac catheterization, radiogram	Progress of condition is monitored to note when surgical intervention with valve replacement is necessary
Aortic stenosis	Blood flow into aorta is compromised, causing increased pressure in left ventricle and subsequent enlargement that eventually leads to left ventricular failure. May be result of infectious process or may be congenital.	*Symptoms, signs, and diagnostic tests:* see Aortic insufficiency	See Aortic insufficiency.
Tricuspid insufficiency	Tricuspid valve unable to close completely, forcing blood back into right atrium. Condition may be result of rheumatic heart disease and right-sided heart failure.	*Symptoms:* Initial symptoms include dyspnea and fatigue, followed by peripheral edema, distended neck veins, hepatomegaly, and ascites; systolic murmur is present. *Diagnostic tests:* cardiac catheterization, radiogram, ECG, echocardiogram	Valvular replacement may be only treatment option. Treatment of symptoms is helpful for patient.
Tricuspid stenosis	Tricuspid valve fails to open completely, so blood remains in right atrium. Condition often associated with mitral valve disease.	*Symptoms:* Initial symptoms include dyspnea and fatigue, followed by peripheral edema and distended neck veins; diastolic murmur is present. *Diagnostic tests:* cardiac catheterization, radiogram, ECG, echocardiogram	See Tricuspid insufficiency.

continued

TABLE 35-5 VALVULAR DISORDERS (CONTINUED)

Valvular Disease	Physiology	Diagnosis	Treatment
Pulmonic insufficiency	Blood flows back into right ventricle, creating increased pressure. This is followed by right ventricular hypertrophy and right-sided heart failure. Condition a result of pulmonary hypertension.	*Symptoms:* chest pain, fatigue, syncope, dyspnea *Signs:* distended neck veins, peripheral edema, hepatomegaly; diastolic murmur may be present. *Diagnostic tests:* cardiac catheterization, radiogram, ECG, echocardiogram	When symptoms are controlled, no intervention may be necessary. Surgical intervention includes valve reconstruction or replacement.
Pulmonic stenosis	Blood flow into pulmonary artery is obstructed, creating increased pressure in right atrium. Pulmonic stenosis is followed by right ventricular hypertrophy and right-sided heart failure.	*Symptoms:* chest pain, fatigue, syncope, and dyspnea *Signs:* distended neck veins, peripheral edema and hepatomegaly; systolic murmur may be present *Diagnostic tests:* echocardiogram, cardiac catheterization (including digital angiography)	See Pulmonic insufficiency.

bloodstream. Treatment involves analgesics for pain and avoiding stimulation, such as massage, to the affected area.

Thrombophlebitis

Thrombophlebitis, an inflammatory condition, occurs in a vein where a thrombus has formed on the wall. Blood flow in the vein is compromised and edema occurs. Insult to the vessel, particularly to the walls, venous stasis, and hypercoagulating blood are all causes of thrombophlebitis. The individual experiences systemic chills and fever, as well as pain, edema, warmth, and redness in the area. Tenderness is exhibited with palpation of the affected area. These symptoms, along with swelling of the affected limb, lead to diagnosis, which is confirmed by venograms and ultrasound. Treatment involves immobilization of the affected limb and the administration of anticoagulant drugs and antibiotics.

Embolisms, Deep-Vein Thrombosis, and Thromboembolism

An **embolus** is a mass of material that forms an obstruction, or **embolism,** in a blood or lymphatic vessel (Figure 35-6 ◆). The material or mass may be solid, such as a blood clot (thrombus); liquid, such as amniotic fluid; gaseous, such as an air bubble; or it may be composed of fat, bone tissue, bacteria, tumor cells, or any material that may be in the bloodstream. Emboli (more than one embolus) occlude the vessel, resulting in infarction of the tissue supplied by that vessel. Many emboli are thrombi that travel from the deep vessels of the legs to the lungs, where they become pulmonary embolisms.

Deep-vein **thrombosis (DVT)** is frequently the result of stasis of the blood in the deep vessels of the legs due to inactivity. Other causes include an insult to the endothelial tissue and blood that has a tendency to clot quickly. Individuals at risk for developing emboli or thrombi are those who have experienced recent trauma or surgical procedures (especially those involving knee, hip, and prostate), CHF, severe infections, or malignancies, or who are inactive, obese, or pregnant, taking oral contraceptives, or over the age of 50. A **thromboembolism** occurs when the thrombus occludes the vessel. For those who travel great distances or for long periods of time, moving the legs frequently is a good preventive measure.

Patients with DVT usually complain of pain and tenderness in the affected leg, which may be swollen and warm to the touch. Many patients, however, are asymptomatic.

Diagnostic studies include contrast venography, Doppler ultrasound, real-time ultrasound, and clotting and coagulation blood studies. Treatment includes drug therapy to prevent enlargement of the thrombus, placement of inferior vena caval barriers, thrombolytic drug therapy, and immobilization of the affected part. Prevention is the best strategy with DVT.

Progression to pulmonary embolism is extremely serious. Aggressive intervention should be instituted as soon as possible.

Arteriosclerosis and Atherosclerosis

Arteriosclerosis is a condition, usually part of the aging process, in which the arterial walls lose elasticity. As the vessels harden, their ability to expand is compromised. Another condition affecting the internal lumen of the arteries is atherosclerosis. Deposits of plaque of saturated lipids, cholesterol, and other debris from the bloodstream adhere to the internal vessel walls, causing the walls to thicken and narrow (Figure 35-7 ◆). The cerebral and coronary vessels are most likely to be affected. Risk factors for both conditions include lipid accumulation, possibly due to lack of exercise, a diet high in saturated lipids, diabetes mellitus, obesity, hypertension, a sedentary lifestyle, smoking, and trauma to the vessels.

Many individuals are asymptomatic. The first sign of arteriosclerosis or atherosclerosis may be angina or transient ischemic attacks, precursors to acute myocardial

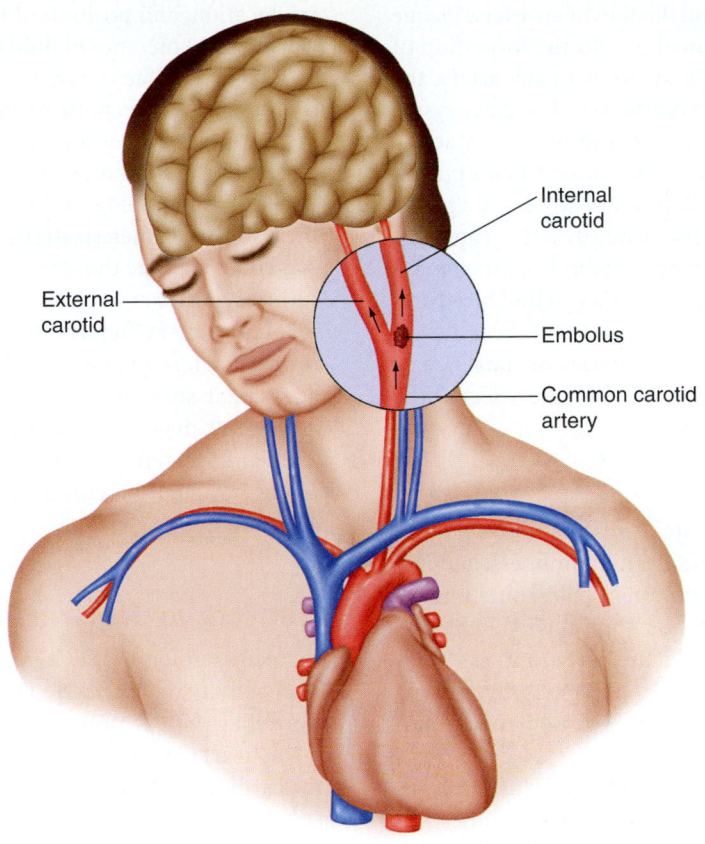

Figure 35-6 ◆ Embolus.

infarction or cerebral vascular accident. Less dramatic symptoms include elevated blood pressure, dizziness, and shortness of breath. Doppler studies aid in verifying the diagnosis of atherosclerosis.

A change in dietary habits, especially a lower intake of saturated fats, lipids, and high-cholesterol foods, is one way to manage progression of the condition; another is giving up smoking. Hyperlipidemic drugs are often prescribed, and hypertension and diabetes mellitus must be controlled.

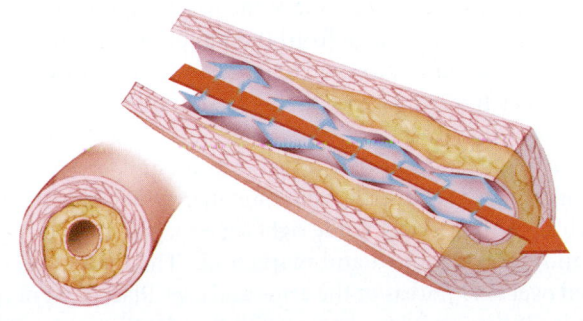

Figure 35-7 ◆ Arteriosclerosis and atherosclerosis.

Keys to Success
TEDS® ANTIEMBOLISM STOCKINGS

Teds are often prescribed for patients who have had pelvic trauma, hip replacement, or knee replacement surgeries or other surgeries or illness that require immobilization in bed for long periods. These stockings may also be used on cardiac patients. Teds exert uniform pressure on the venous system of the legs, promoting circulation to the heart. They help to prevent venous stasis and dependent edema in the lower extremities.

Teds come in various lengths and calf sizes. Patient teaching in their use is often necessary. The patient should be in a recumbent position so the vessels in the legs are not distended. The Teds are pulled over the toes and gently worked over the heels up to the knee or groin area, depending on their length. Any wrinkles must be smoothed out to prevent uneven pressure on the legs. The stockings should be removed daily to assess skin condition and to provide any necessary skin care. Sometimes the stockings are removed for an hour or so while the patient is resting and not ambulatory or sitting with the legs down.

Aneurysms

An **aneurysm** is the weakening and dilation of an artery. Plaque buildup from atherosclerosis contributes to the formation of an aneurysm. While aneurysms may occur in any artery, the usual sites are the aorta and cerebral arteries. Aneurysms develop over a period of time. It is common for an aortic aneurysm to be found on physical examination when a pulsating mass is observed and palpated. In some instances, a previously undetected aneurysm is discovered when it ruptures, causing severe pain and loss of blood. Cerebral aneurysms are usually undetected until a rupture causes a cerebral bleed and the resulting cerebral vascular accident. Many of these bleeds, whether in the aorta or in the cerebral arteries, are fatal. Treatment consists of surgical intervention to repair the defect before the aneurysm ruptures.

Raynaud's Disease

Raynaud's disease results when small vessels in the fingers, hands, toes, and feet spasm, causing pain, numbness, and tingling. These areas frequently become very pale, sometimes to the point of blanching, because of the compromised blood flow. The condition is aggravated by cold and stress, and as it progresses, the affected areas turn blue. As spasms subside, the areas turn purple, then red. Women are more likely than men to suffer from Raynaud's disease.

Application of mild warmth provides relief as the vessel spasms subside. Prevention is important and includes not smoking. The hands and feet should be protected from sudden exposure to very cold temperatures with warm gloves, socks, and heavy shoes.

Buerger's Disease (Thromboangiitis Obliterans)

Buerger's disease, or thromboangiitis obliterans, is an inflammation of the peripheral vessels of both arteries and veins, with possible clot formation in the extremities. Smoking is a primary causative factor, and males who smoke are at greatest risk. Exercise tends to initiate severe pain in the legs and feet. Rest usually relieves the pain.

Arteriograms and ultrasound studies showing the site of the clot or obstruction confirm the presence of the disease. Aggressive intervention is important to preserve the integrity of the tissue supplied by the vessels. The obstruction should be resolved before permanent damage develops. Failure to intervene can lead to tissue necrosis, followed by amputation of the affected limb.

Diagnostic Tests

Assessment of all cardiology patients includes vital signs (T, P, R, BP, and weight). Many physicians prefer an apical pulse and notations regarding strength and rhythm of the heartbeat. Notations are made of any irregularities, gasping or rapid breathing, pedal edema, and the color, temperature, and moisture content of the skin. It is customary to check for the presence and strength of pedal pulses.

Radiographs, usually chest X-rays, are done to assess the size, location, and position of the heart in the chest (pleural) cavity and the presence of fluid in the lungs. Blood tests including a CBC, cardiac enzymes, electrolytes, and, on occasion, **ABGs** are done. The pulse oximeter provides a rapid and noninvasive evaluation of the oxygen saturation of arterial blood. Coagulation studies often are performed.

Some cardiology offices are located close to facilities where cardiac catheterizations, including angiocaths, are performed to evaluate the status of the coronary arteries. These facilities perform angioplasties and/or stent insertions. **Coronary artery bypass (CAB)** procedures, also known as coronary artery bypass graft (**CABG),** are referred to a cardiovascular surgeon. Treatment for post-MI or impending MI patients may include cardiac catheterization with angioplasty and/or stent insertion. When this type of intervention cannot be achieved, coronary artery bypass surgery may be performed.

Electrocardiogram

An electrocardiogram (**ECG** or **EKG**) is a recording of the electrical activity of the heart. This record is a tool the clinician uses, along with symptoms and signs, to assess the condition of the heart. The ECG often indicates ischemic areas of the myocardium, information useful in the diagnosis of cardiac pathology.

An electrocardiograph is used to perform the ECG (Figure 35-8 ◆). This machine amplifies low-voltage electric impulses detected on the skin and provides a printed record of that electrical activity. A cardiac monitor displays the heart's electrical impulses on a screen called an *oscilloscope*. Electrodes—adhesive pads containing a conductive gel—are placed on the patient's skin. They are attached to color-coded wires called *leads* that connect to the electrocardiograph. Three leads—a positive, a negative, and a ground lead—are required to transmit the electrical activity to the electrocardiograph.

A 12-lead ECG provides images of the various planes of the heart (Table 35-6). Lead II is usually used for the rhythm strip on a monitor because of its ability to show P waves. (P waves are discussed below.) Leads I, II, and III are often referred to as limb leads (Figure 35-9 ◆). Additional limb leads are the **augmented leads,** aVL, aVR, and aVF (Figure 35-10 ◆). The **precordial leads** V1, V2, V3, V4, V5, and V6, placed on the chest in a semicircular pattern around the heart, provide a horizontal plane view of the heart (Figure 35-11 ◆). Lead II provides an image from the upper area of the heart where cardiac conduction starts. Chest leads V5 and V6 provide images from the lower area as conduction approaches the **apex** of the heart.

Wires are identified or coded by color and lead number. The right arm lead is usually white and marked RA; the left arm lead, black and marked LA: the right leg lead, green and marked RL: and the left leg, red and marked LL. The limb leads are placed over fleshy areas of the arms and legs. Placement of the chest leads (brown wires) begins with the identification of the third intercostal space and the sternum.

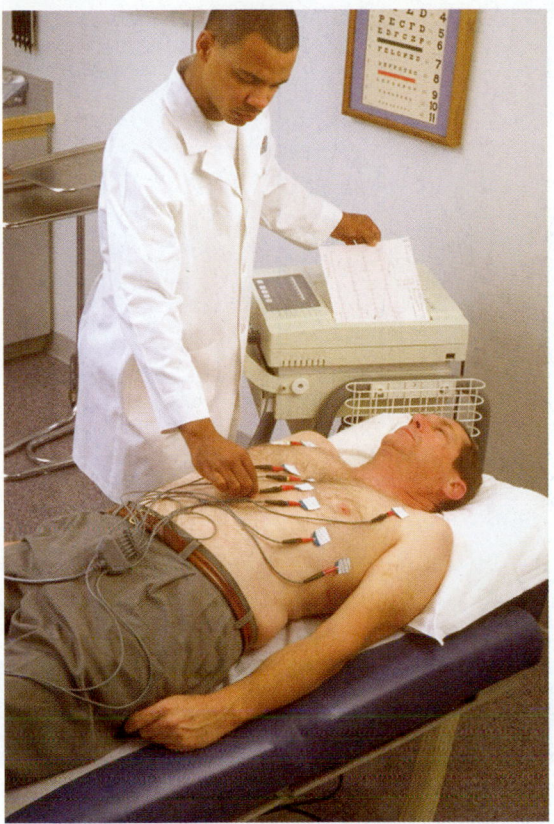

Figure 35-8 ◆ Electrocardiograph.

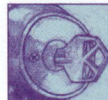

Keys to Success
UNDERSTANDING CARDIAC PROCEDURES

During a **cardiac catheterization,** a catheter is threaded through an artery in the arm or groin to the aorta and the coronary vessels. Dye is injected into the vessels, and the radiologist and cardiologist assess the circulation through the coronary arteries. Dye can also be injected into the chambers of the heart to view valve and myocardial function.

If narrowing of the arteries is detected, angioplasty may be attempted. A balloon near the distal end of the catheter is expanded, compressing the plaque against the arterial walls and thereby expanding the lumen of the vessels and allowing for increased blood flow. Stents are often inserted into the arteries after angioplasty to maintain the wider lumen. The location and extent of the occlusion or partial occlusion determine if angioplasty and/or stent insertion should be attempted. Aspirin and other anticoagulant medications are prescribed following stent insertion.

When angioplasty and/or stent insertion cannot be performed, coronary artery bypass (CAB) is done. During this surgical procedure, arteries (mammary) or veins from the legs are grafted to bypass the narrowed or occluded artery. This revascularization procedure reestablishes circulation to the compromised areas of the myocardium.

TABLE 35-6 ECG LEADS

Limb Leads

Lead I: Records electrical activity from right arm to left arm

Lead II: Records electrical activity from right arm to left leg

Lead III: Records electrical activity from left arm to left leg

Augmented Leads

aVR: Records electrical activity away from midpoint between left arm and left leg to left arm (across heart to right shoulder)

aVL: Records electrical activity from midpoint between right arm and left leg to left arm (across heart to left shoulder)

aVF: Records electrical activity from midpoint between right arm and left arm to left leg (across heart toward feet)

Chest or Precordial Leads

V1: Records electrical activity between center of heart and the chest wall where V1 electrode is placed

V2: Records electrical activity between center of heart and chest wall where V2 electrode is placed

V3: Records electrical activity between center of heart and chest wall where V3 electrode is placed

V4: Records electrical activity between center of heart and chest wall where V4 electrode is placed

V5: Records electrical activity between center of heart and chest wall where V5 electrode is placed

V6: Records electrical activity between center of the heart and chest wall where V6 electrode is placed.

In Practice

Michael Taylor, 38 years old, is at the office because he has been experiencing chest pain for two days. He states that the pain comes and goes and that he is not currently experiencing the pain. The physician orders an ECG. As she begins to prepare for the procedure, the patient asks the medical assistant what an ECG is. What should the medical assistant tell the patient?

- V1 is placed over the fourth intercostal space and to the right of the sternum (right sternal margin).
- V2 is placed over the fourth intercostal space and to the left of the sternum (left sternal margin).
- V3 is placed midway over the fourth and fifth intercostal spaces and halfway between the base of the sternum and the nipple (midway between leads 2 and lead 4).
- V4 is placed over the fifth intercostal space and in line with the nipple (junction of midclavicular line).
- V5 is placed in the same line midway between the nipple and midpoint of the axilla, **anterior** to the midaxillary line.
- V6 is placed over the intercostal space at the axilla midpoint (left midaxillary line).

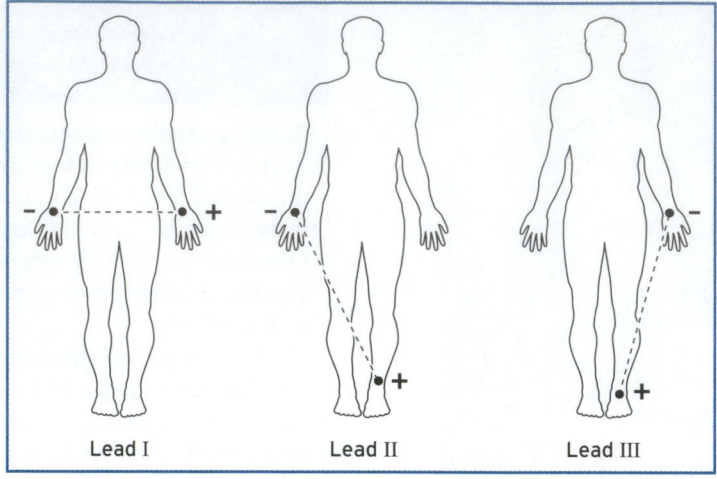

Figure 35-9 ◆ The bipolar leads.

Interpreting Waveforms on the ECG Tracing

ECGs are printed on special standardized graph paper (Figure 35-12 ◆). The paper travels through the electrocardiograph at a speed of 25 millimeters per second. The horizontal line measures time, and the vertical line measures **amplitude** or voltage. The ECG paper is divided, both vertically and horizontally, into squares 5 millimeters in width and height, each representing a time interval of 0.20 second. It is further divided into smaller squares 1 millimeter wide, each representing a time interval of 0.04 second. Proper interpretation of cardiac rhythms depends on understanding the time represented on the ECG paper.

The second aspect of the ECG is the waveform. The electrical impulse originates in the SA node and produces a waveform on the graph paper. The resting state of the myocardial cells is depicted by a baseline or **isoelectric line,** which is a straight line on the ECG strip. The beginning and ending point of all waves is represented by this line. There are five major

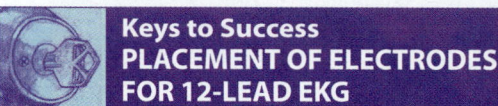

Keys to Success
PLACEMENT OF ELECTRODES FOR 12-LEAD EKG

A 12-lead ECG uses only ten electrodes because limb electrodes are used for limb and augmented leads. It provides a record of electrical activity for leads I, II, III, aVR, aVL, aVF, V1, V2, V3, V4, V5, and V6. Refer to Figures 35-9, 35-10, and 35-11 to identify the placement of the ten electrodes.

waves during a cardiac cycle: the P wave, the Q, R, and S waves, and the T wave (Figure 35-13 ◆).

■ The cardiac cycle begins with the firing of the SA node and is characterized by a P wave on the ECG. Representing the depolarization of both the right and left atria, the P wave is approximately 0.10 second in length and appears as a smooth, upward deflection.

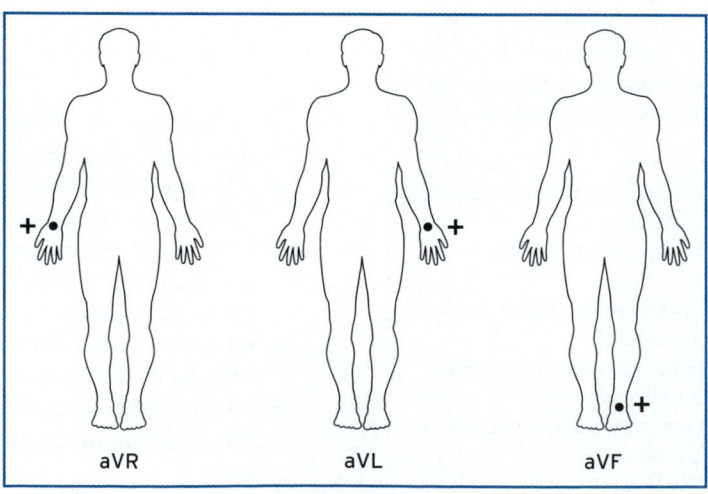

Figure 35-10 ◆ The augmented leads.

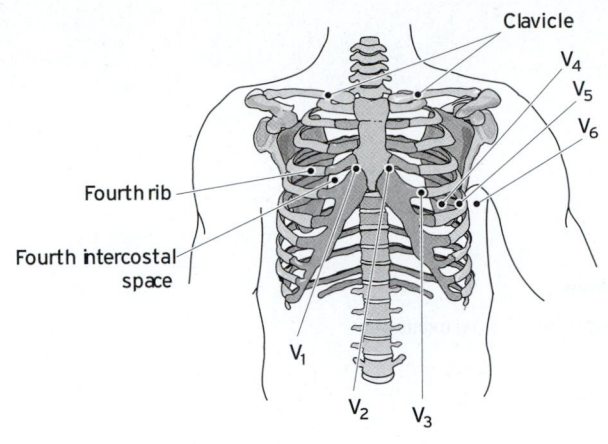

Figure 35-11 ◆ The precordial leads.

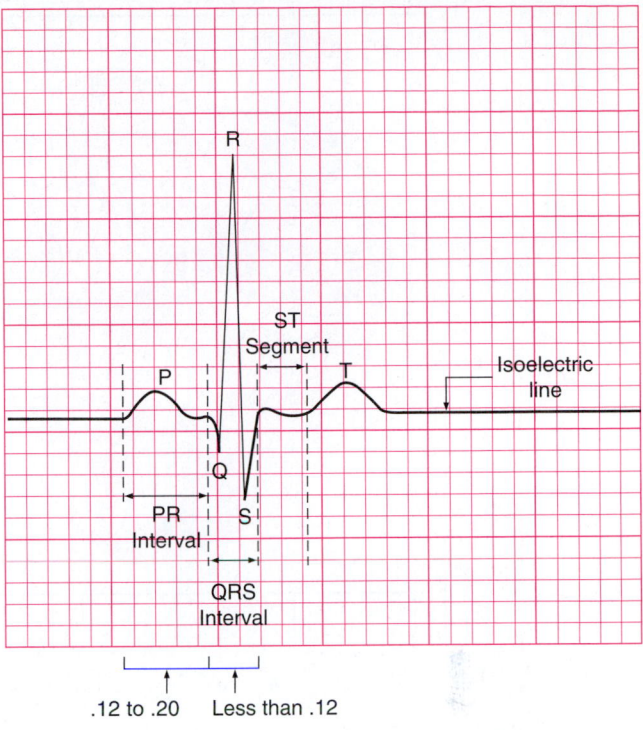

Figure 35-13 ◆ ECG waveforms.

■ The time interval during which the impulse travels from the SA node through the atria to the ventricles is the **PR** interval. The time from the beginning of the P wave to the beginning of the next complex (QRS) should measure three to five small squares or 0.12 to 0.20 second (Figure 35-14 ◆). If the SA node does not initiate the impulse, lower pacemaker cells can initiate the conduction as a "survival" effort. These impulses are termed *ectopic*.

■ The next portion of the waveform is the **QRS** complex— the Q, R, and S waves representing the conduction of the impulse from the bundle of His through the ventricles. The Q wave deflects down from the baseline, and the R wave follows with an upward deflection and reflects the patient's heart rate. The downward deflection following is the S wave. The QRS complex is measured from the beginning of the Q wave to where the S wave meets the baseline. The QRS complex normally measures less than 0.12

second or less than three small squares (Figure 35-15 ◆). There may be variations in the waves of the QRS complex among individuals, and all three waves are not always present.

■ During the **ST** segment, the ventricles are depolarized and repolarization begins. Usually, the ST segment is isometric.

■ The final portion of the waveform is the T wave, which indicates the repolarization or recovery phase of the ventricles. The normal shape of the T wave is slightly asymmetrical, slightly rounded, with a positive deflection (Figure 35-16 ◆). The T wave is the "resting phase" of the cardiac cycle, during which the heart is most vulnerable to impulses that may lead to arrhythmias.

Artifacts

An **artifact** is any electrical activity on an ECG that is noncardiac in origin and represents unwanted marks on the ECG paper. There are two types of artifacts.

■ Intentional artifacts include standardization marks and pacemaker spikes (Figure 35-17 ◆).

■ Unintentional interferences (Figure 35-18 ◆) may be caused by loose, corroded, or dirty electrodes, broken cables or wires, improper grounding, or the patient's muscular tremors, movement, talking, or nervous disorder. In addition, 60-cycle interference is caused by alternating current of electrical equipment such as IV pumps, ventilators, or electric beds. Changing outlets or moving to a different location may alleviate this type of interference.

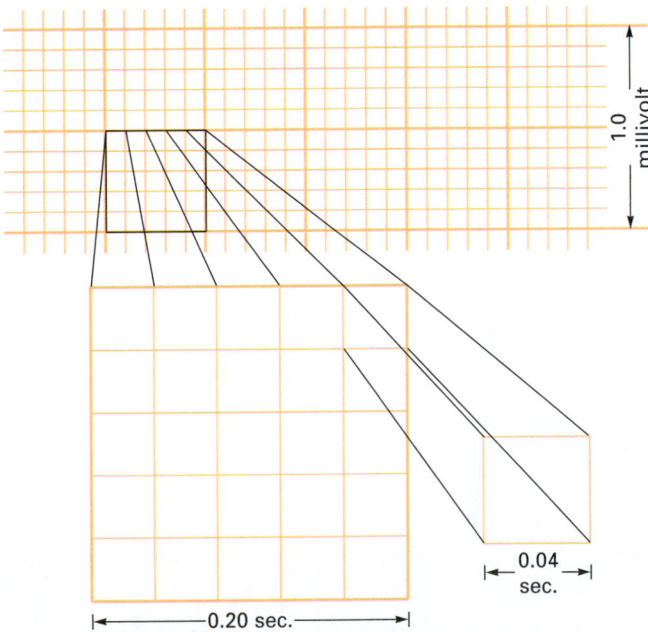

Figure 35-12 ◆ ECG paper and markings.

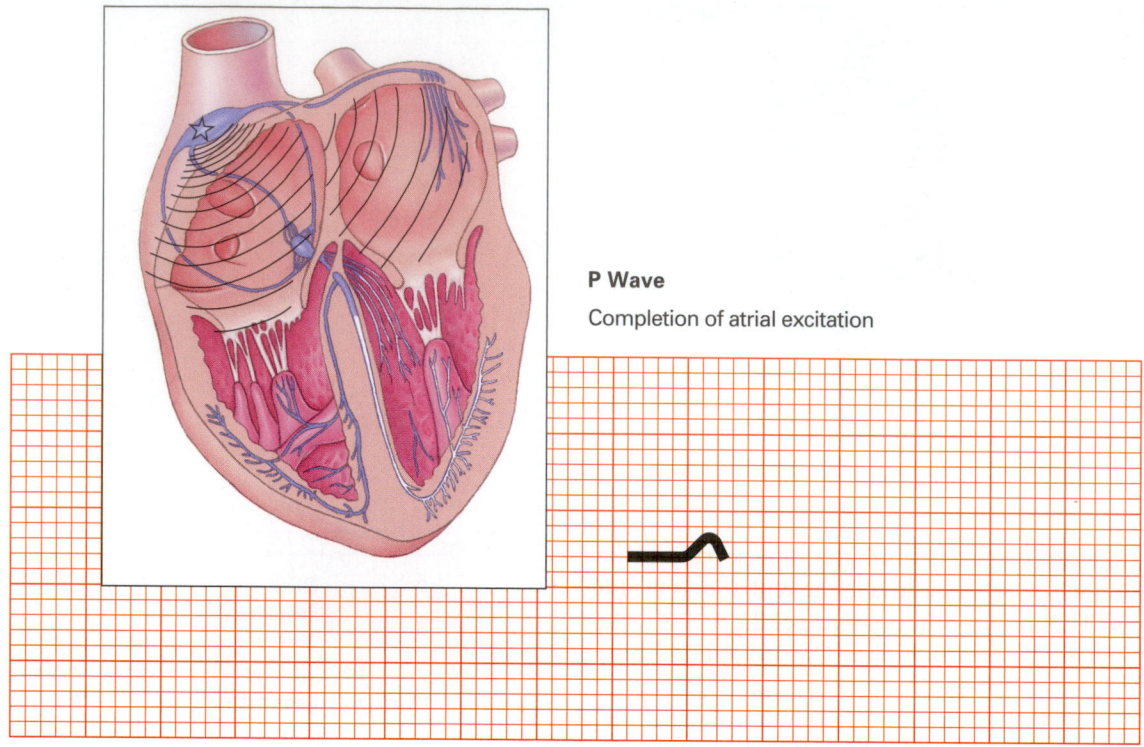

P Wave

Completion of atrial excitation

Figure 35-14 ◆ P wave.

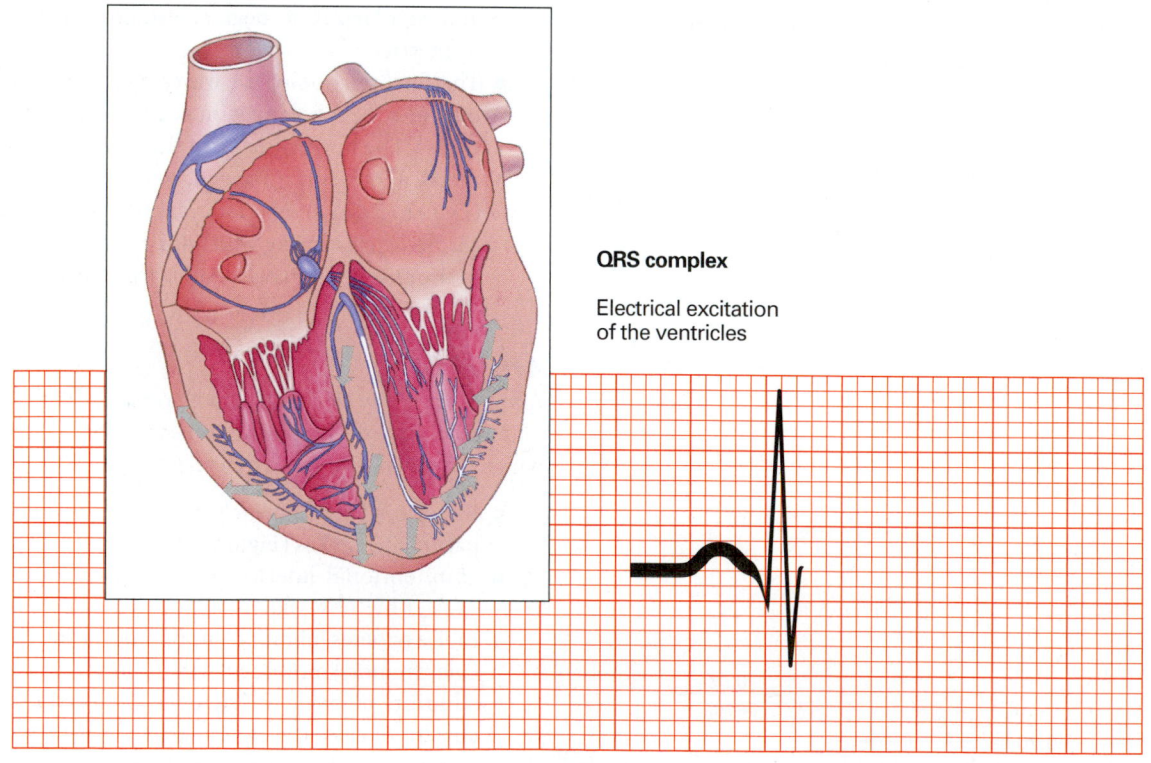

QRS complex

Electrical excitation
of the ventricles

Figure 35-15 ◆ QRS complex.

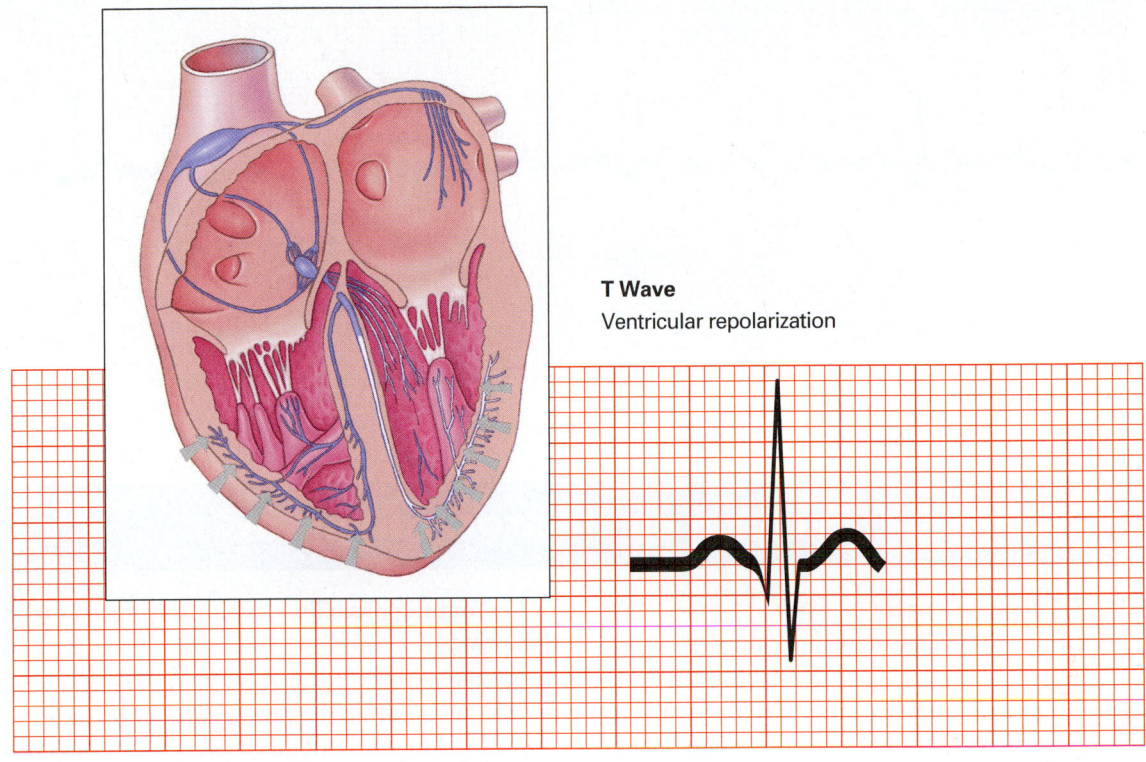

T Wave
Ventricular repolarization

Figure 35-16 ◆ T wave.

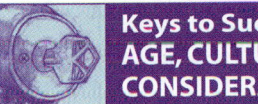

Keys to Success
AGE, CULTURAL, AND DISABILITY CONSIDERATIONS

The elderly are sometimes fearful of electrocardiographs. Assess the patient's facial, behavioral, and verbal expressions as you explain the procedure. Body language or conversation may indicate a fear of electrocution or even death. Ask the patient to restate what is involved, and clarify any misconceptions.

A patient with bilateral above-knee amputation (AKA) needs a preoperative ECG. Where are the leg electrodes placed? How would they be placed for a right AKA? In both cases, the leg electrodes are placed on the upper thigh areas. When they cannot be placed in the correct position, they must be directed away from the heart.

Holter Monitor

Many ECGs are recorded using three seconds of electronic cardiac monitoring. It is possible for **dysrhythmias** not to occur during this brief period. The physician may therefore order a portable form of monitoring, called the Holter monitor, that allows noninvasive recording of the patient's cardiac condition over a 24-hour period. This testing is useful in identifying events and unexplained symptoms in patients with arrhythmias and in monitoring the effectiveness of current medications or pacemaker function. The clinician can observe cardiac rhythms over a period of time while the patient engages in the normal activities of daily living. A 48-hour Holter monitor test may be ordered when the physician wants a longer time frame for evaluation.

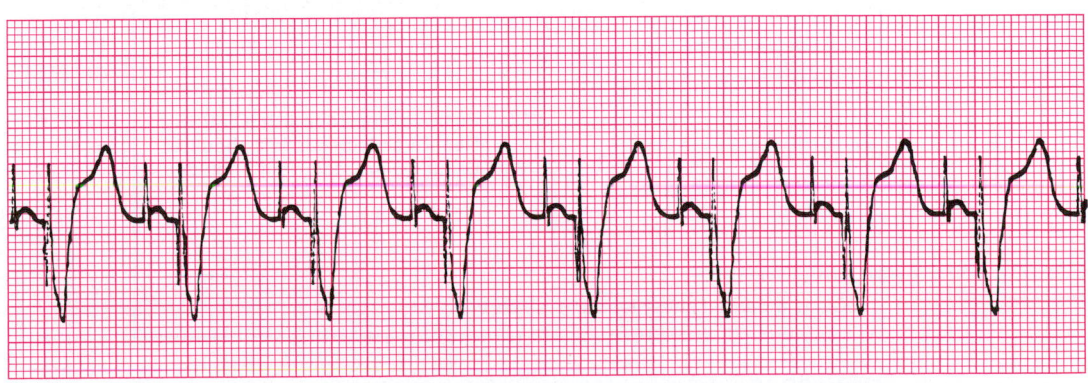

Figure 35-17 ◆ Intentional artifacts include standardization marks and pacemaker spikes.

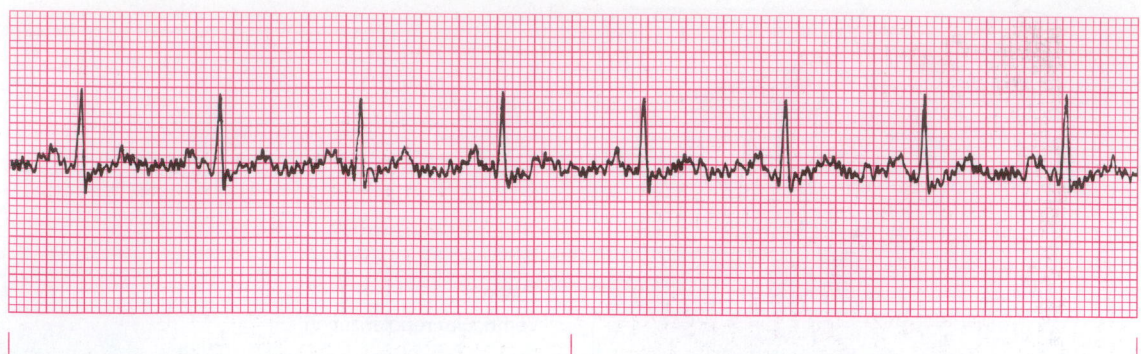

Figure 35-18 ◆ Artifact.

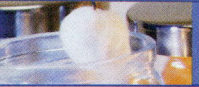

PROCEDURE 35-1 Perform an Electrocardiogram

Theory and Rationale

An electrocardiogram is used in conjunction with other diagnostic testing and physical assessment to establish baseline and medical information about the patient. To reduce patient nervousness or movement that could affect the quality of the electrocardiogram, it is important to provide a relaxing, calm, and warm environment. You can alleviate any patient anxiety by explaining the basic procedure. Some patients are unaware that an ECG records electrical activity already present in the heart and may fear that the electrocardiogram may cause shock and pain. Watch the patient's facial expressions to assess understanding or fear, and encourage the patient to ask questions or describe previous experiences with the same kind of procedure.

Your responsibilities during the procedure include the following:

■ Prevent unnecessary electrical-interference artifacts on the ECG by pointing the power cord away from the patient. Avoid taking the cord under the bed to the electrical outlet.

■ Cleanse any oils from the skin and dry it thoroughly for better contact with the electrodes. Remove the adhesive backing and place each electrode on the skin with the tab pointing toward the cable of the ECG machine. This will minimize the "pull" on the electrodes and the potential for artifacts.

■ Use anatomical landmarks (intercostal spaces, midclavicular line, midaxillary line, etc.) to place the electrodes in the correct positions (Figure 35-19 ◆).

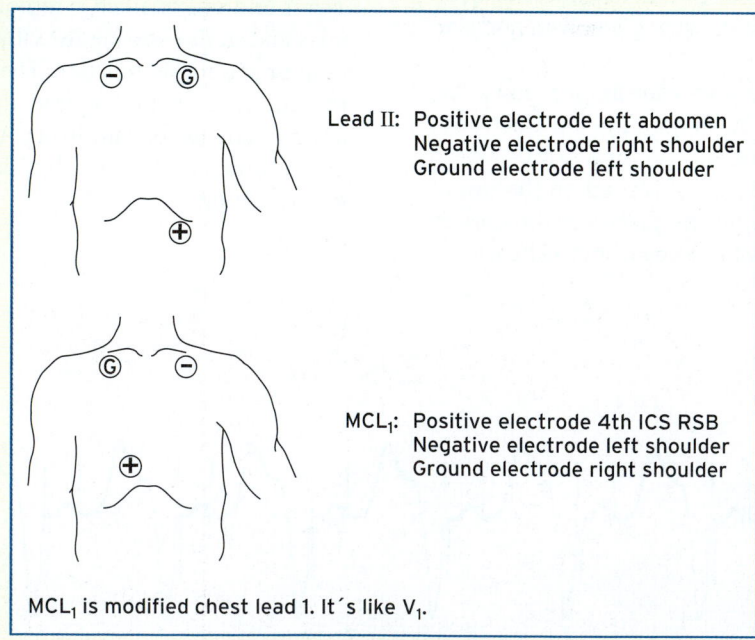

Lead II: Positive electrode left abdomen
Negative electrode right shoulder
Ground electrode left shoulder

MCL$_1$: Positive electrode 4th ICS RSB
Negative electrode left shoulder
Ground electrode right shoulder

MCL$_1$ is modified chest lead 1. It´s like V$_1$.

Figure 35-19 ◆ Anatomical landmarks for electrode placement.

PROCEDURE 35-1 **Perform an Electrocardiogram** (continued)

- Attach the lead wires only after the electrodes are in place. Reduce the potential for artifacts by laying the wires along body contours.
- Before beginning the procedure, you will need to calibrate the ECG machine. This process, also called standardization, verifies that the machine deflects 10 mm in response to 1 mv of electricity in sensitivity 1. With older machines this may have to be done manually, but newer models calibrate automatically before the electrocardiogram is printed. The paper moves 25 mm per second, and the recording stylus moves the same distance.
- Older machines do not automatically identify which lead is being recorded. In this case, you will be expected to identify each lead strip with a specified marking (Table 35-7).
- The ECG should not leave the testing area without patient identification. With newer electrocardiograph models the patient's name, age, height, weight, sex, and current medications can be entered into the machine before the procedure begins. With older models you may need to write the patient data on the ECG after it has been printed out.
- If the quality of the electrocardiogram is poor, you will need to run a second one. You should look for and correct the reasons for the poor ECG quality. Explain the problem to the patient to ensure cooperation and ease the patient's anxiety.

Materials
- electrocardiograph with wires, electrodes, and ECG paper
- patient gown and drape as necessary for privacy and warmth
- alcohol pads
- supplies for shaving, if needed

Competency
(**Conditions**) With the necessary materials, (**Task**) you will be able to perform a 12-lead ECG (**Standards**) correctly within the time frame designated by the instructor.

1. Wash your hands. Assemble the equipment and supplies.
2. Identify the patient and escort him or her to the patient examination room.
3. Explain the procedure to relieve the patient's apprehension.
4. Ask the patient to disrobe from the waist up. Assist the patient into a gown, with the opening in front. Assure the patient that his or her privacy will be respected.
5. Help the patient recline on the examination table or bed where the procedure will be performed.
6. Cover the patient with the drape, leaving the arms and legs exposed. You may need to raise pant legs to expose the calves of the lower legs.

7. Cleanse the skin with alcohol pads where the electrodes will be applied. If chest hair will interfere with contact between the electrodes and the skin, remove the hair with soap and/or shaving cream and a disposable razor.
8. Apply the electrodes in the correct positions, making sure the wires do not touch the cart or examination table and that they follow the normal contours of the body (Figure 35-20 ◆). The power cord should not cross under the examination table or bed.
9. Explain to the patient that the electrocardiograph is a sensitive machine and that he or she must remain as still as possible during the procedure.
10. Calibrate the electrocardiograph and run the ECG (Figure 35-21 ◆). Mark the leads if necessary.
11. When the ECG is complete, remove the electrodes and cleanse any residual conduction gel from the patient's skin.
12. Assist the patient in dressing. Discard the gown, if it is disposable; otherwise, place it in a laundry hamper.
13. Cleanse the equipment. Sanitize the leads by wiping them with antiseptic solution, then store them in the appropriate compartment of the electrocardiograph cart. Replace any necessary supplies. Wash your hands.
14. Label the electrocardiograph paper with the patient's name, DOB, and the date and time. Document the patient's tolerance of the procedure.
15. Per physician preference, instruct the patient to wait to discuss the test with the physician or make a followup appointment.

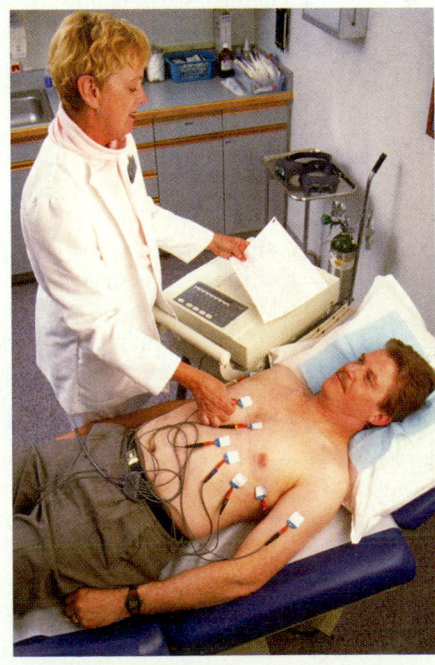

Figure 35-20 ◆ Apply the electrodes in the correct position.

continued

PROCEDURE 35-1 Perform an Electrocardiogram *(continued)*

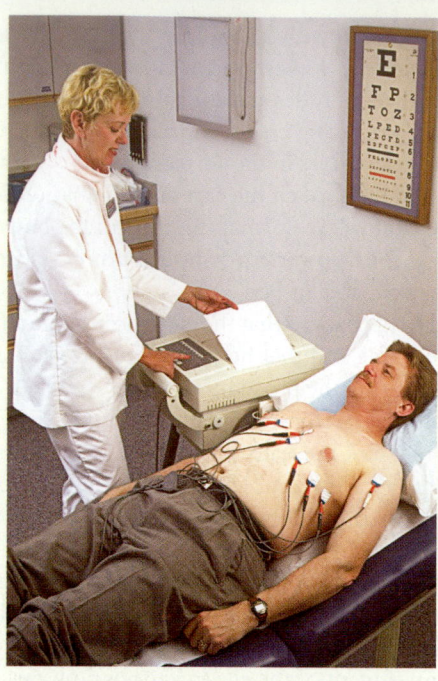

Figure 35-21 ◆ Calibrate the ECG.

Patient Education

If it is not an emergency electrocardiogram, the patient should bathe or shower beforehand. Clean skin will ensure good contact with the electrodes for a quality ECG.

The patient should be informed that the procedure—taking a "picture" of the electrical activity of the heart—is painless. Instruct the patient to remain still during the procedure and to ask for an extra cover if he or she feels cold.

If it is necessary to run a second ECG, instruct the patient on how to help and explain that the second run is not an indication of medical problems.

Charting Example

11/25/XX 2:30 PM 12-lead ECG performed with patient cooperation. States recent episodes of chest pain occurring after stressful events at work. Daniel Trees, CMA

11/25/XX 3:30 PM Physician ordered additional study of Holter monitor. Holter monitor attached and patient instructions given orally and in written handout. Patient verbalized understanding of instructions and phone number if there are questions. Daniel Trees, CMA (AAMA)

TABLE 35-7 SENSOR (LEAD) PLACEMENT AND MARKING CODES

Limb Leads	Placement	Abbreviation	Marking Code
Lead I	Right arm to left arm	RA-LA	•
Lead II	Right arm to left leg	RA-LL	• •
Lead III	Left arm to left leg	LA-LL	• • •
Augmented Leads			
aVR	RA-midpoint (LA-LL)	(LA-LL) RA	-
aVL	LA-midpoint (RA-LL)	(RA-LL) LA	- -
aVF	LL-midpoint (RA-LA)	(RA-LA) LL	- - -
Chest Leads	**Placement**		**Marking Code**
V1	4th intercostal space, right sternal border		- •
V2	4th intercostal space, left sternal border		- • •
V3	Midway between V2 and V4		- • •
V4	5th intercostal space, mid-clavicular left		- • • • •
V5	Left anterior axillary fold horizontal to V4		- • • • • •
V6	Left mid-axillary horizontal to V4 and V5		- • • • • • •

Note: The right leg is never used for the tracings, but is an electrical ground.

Source: Fremgen, Bonnie F. Essentials of Medical Assisting, 1st Edition © 1998. Reprinted by permission of Pearson Education, Inc., Upper Saddle River, NJ.

The patient may continue with daily activities except for bathing, showering, or swimming to keep monitor and electrodes dry. A diary is given to the patient with instructions to record the times of all activities for the next 24 hours, including bowel and bladder elimination, emotional changes or stressful situations, smoking, drinking caffeinated beverages, taking medications, sexual intercourse, rest or sleeping periods, and

clinical symptoms, such as chest pain and shortness of breath. The patient is also instructed to briefly push the event button of the monitor to mark the strip for later correlation of activities and times.

A return appointment is made for 24 hours later, when the monitor is turned off and the leads are removed. The strip is removed from the monitor, labeled, and correlated with

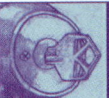

Keys to Success
INTERPRETING DYSRHYTHMIAS

When interpreting dysrhythmias, the most important component is the patient's clinical appearance. A dysrhythmia without clinical symptoms may or may not need treatment, depending upon the diagnosis.

patient information, date, and time. It is attached to the diary and forwarded to the cardiologist for interpretation. The patient is instructed as to a return visit and a discussion of the test results. The lead wires and the recorder are cleaned according to the manufacturer's guidelines and the Holter monitor is returned to the proper storage place. The recorder cartridge is removed and attached to the diary.

PROCEDURE 35-2   Demonstrate the Application of a Holter Monitor

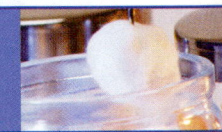

Theory and Rationale

The Holter monitor is battery-powered and has a strap for the patient to place over the shoulder. The medical assistant's role in Holter monitoring includes the application and removal of the monitor leads, identification of the monitor strip, and patient instruction. Applying the monitor leads is very similar to applying ECG leads. The skin must be clean, dry, and shaved for optimum contact with the electrodes. A new battery and a blank magnetic tape should be installed in the recorder before each patient use (Figure 35-22 ◆).

It is very important to test the Holter monitor before the patient leaves the office to ensure that waveforms are clear and artifacts are minimal or absent. The monitor should be kept in its case. Electrodes should not be touched to avoid causing interference and degrading the quality of the information obtained.

Materials

- medical order for the Holter monitor
- Holter monitor
- ECG electrodes
- ECG
- recording cassette
- fresh batteries (or recharged batteries)
- patient gown and drape as necessary for privacy and warmth
- supplies for shaving if needed
- alcohol pads
- 4 × 4 gauze pad

- liquid abrasive
- adhesive tape
- patient diary
- patient chart
- gloves

Competency

(**Conditions**) With the necessary materials, (**Task**) you will be able to apply a Holter monitor (**Standards**) correctly within the time frame designated by the instructor.

1. Run a test of the equipment to make sure it is functioning properly and that the batteries are fresh.
2. With the patient sitting on the exam table, explain the procedure while showing the patient the equipment (Figure 35-23 ◆).
3. Instruct the patient to remove all clothing from the waist up. If the exam room is cool, offer the patient a blanket.
4. Because the electrodes of the Holter monitor must be in constant contact with the skin, you may have to shave the electrode sites. If so, explain the reason for shaving before you begin.
5. Wash your hands and put on gloves.
6. Cleanse the skin with alcohol wipes to remove all lotions, cologne or perfume, and body oil.
7. Moisten a 4 × 4 gauze with liquid abrasive and abrade the skin at the electrode sites until it is slightly red to ensure the electrodes adhere (Figure 35-24 ◆).

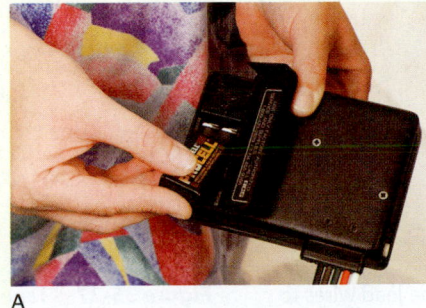

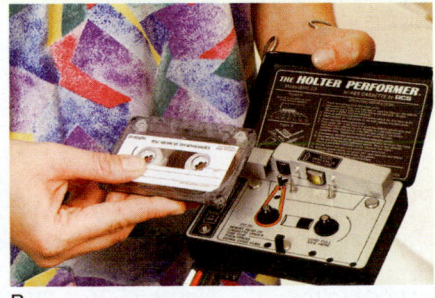

A   B

Figure 35-22 ◆ (A) Install a new battery into the Holter monitor. (B) Install a blank tape.

continued

PROCEDURE 35-2 Demonstrate the Application of a Holter Monitor *(continued)*

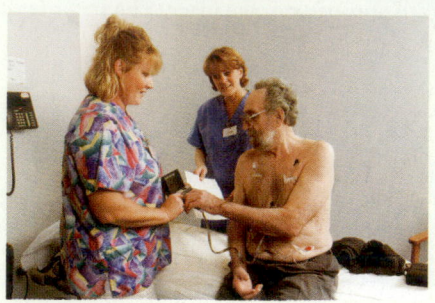

Figure 35-23 ◆ Explain the unit to the patient.

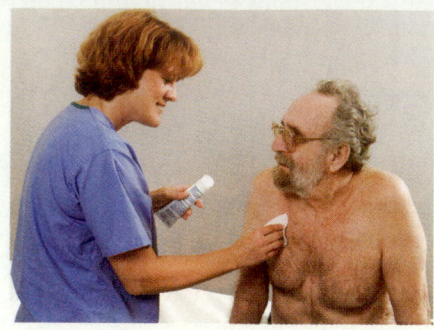

Figure 35-24 ◆ Abrade the electrode site.

8. Take the electrodes from their packaging and remove the adhesive covering from each one.
9. Check for moist gel on each electrode and apply the adhesive side to the skin site, using circular pressure from the center outward (Figure 35-25 ◆).
10. Attach the lead wires to the electrodes and tape a loop of the electrode wires to the skin (Figures 35-26 ◆, 35-27 ◆).
11. Cover each electrode site with nonallergenic tape, which will remain in place over the next 24 hours.
12. Verify the correct electrode placement by connecting the electrodes to the ECG machine and obtaining a test strip.
13. Help the patient to dress, if necessary, being careful not to disturb any of leads.
14. Test the Holter monitor by placing a cassette into it and making certain it runs smoothly. Plug the electrode cable into the recorder, and note the starting time in the patient diary and patient chart.
15. Make an appointment for 24 hours later to review the monitor and remove the electrodes.
16. Document the procedure in the patient's chart.

Patient Education

Explain to the patient the importance of keeping an activities diary in a simple spiral-bound notebook. Any activities such as eating, sleeping, and exercising must be noted, as well as changes in energy level or breathing and feelings of chest discomfort. The exact time of each occurrence should be reported so the physician can review it simultaneously with the cardiac readout from the Holter monitor.

Charting Example

11/25/XX 3:30 PM Physician ordered additional study of Holter monitor. Holter monitor attached and patient given instructions orally and in written handout. Patient verbalized understanding of instructions and phone number if there are questions. Darren Brimsek, RMA (AMI)

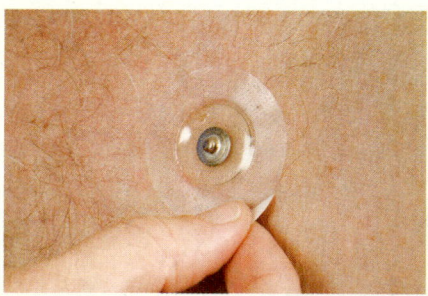

Figure 35-25 ◆ Apply electrode to the skin.

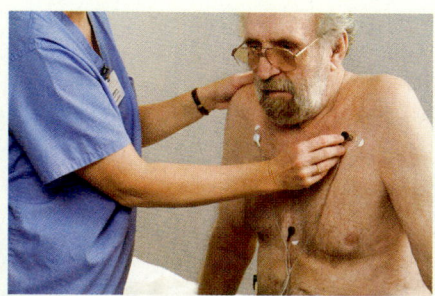

Figure 35-26 ◆ Attach the lead wires to the electrodes.

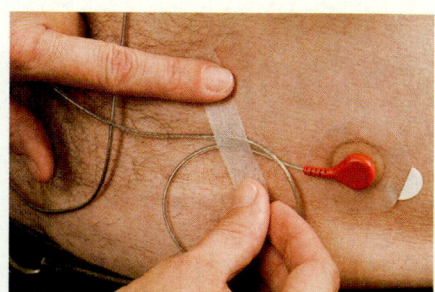

Figure 35-27 ◆ Tape a loop of the electrode wires to the skin.

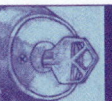

Keys to Success
KEEPING UP WITH TECHNOLOGY

Thanks to recent advancements in technology, cardiac monitoring is now possible via telephone transmission from a device called an event monitor. The patient wears a monitor for an extended period (two weeks to 30 days) and presses a record button whenever he or she feels a cardiac event occurring. Most monitors record the 30 seconds prior to the event and the 60 seconds after the event button is pressed. After a certain number of recorded events, the patient calls a service that downloads the recordings via telephone and sends the rhythm strips to the patient's physician for interpretation. If a critical event is noted, the physician is contacted immediately.

Stress Testing

After an electrocardiogram, the physician may need additional diagnostic information about the patient's cardiac status. The treadmill stress test, also known as stress or exercise testing, provides valuable information about how the patient's heart reacts to moderate, controlled exercise on a treadmill or stationary bicycle (Figure 35-28 ◆). Stress testing is used to evaluate patients with a cardiac history and those who have had cardiovascular surgery or a heart attack.

A 12-lead ECG is done prior to the treadmill exercise. Blood pressure readings are taken both prior to and during the test. Respiratory efforts are monitored. The leads on the patient are connected to a monitor during the test to monitor and record the heart's electrical activity in response to the exercise. The speed and incline of the treadmill are gradually increased. The test is terminated either when the patient can no longer tolerate the activity or when the goal of the test has been achieved. Should the patient complain of chest pain, the test is terminated immediately.

If the patient is unable to engage in routine stress testing because of a physical disability, dipyridamole or adenisene may be administered to simulate physical stress without the exercise.

The physician is present during the test. The medical assistant's role is to assist the technician in patient preparation. The MA will instruct the patient beforehand to wear comfortable walking shoes and loose-fitting clothes. Female patients should wear a blouse that opens in the front. During the test, it will be the MA's responsibility to check all equipment and make sure the crash cart and emergency medications are in the procedure room. The MA will assist the physician by monitoring the patient and taking vital signs, and you may also operate the treadmill as directed by the physician. If the patient reaches a target heart rate or exhibits abnormal symptoms (chest pain, severe weakness or tiredness) or abnormal arrhythmias (displayed on the ECG machine), the test is stopped. The patient is observed and the physician provides appropriate medical intervention. It is important to document accurately and thoroughly during the procedure. After the procedure, the patient is monitored per office protocol. Then the electrodes are removed.

Cardiac patients can be very apprehensive about performing the stress test because of a previous heart attack or the potential medical risks. The medical office gives patients printed preparation instructions as well as verbal instructions because anxious patients may not remember verbal directions. Patients who know what to expect during the procedure and what to report feel less anxiety and a greater sense of control.

When giving verbal and printed instructions, focus on these major points:

1. Instruct the patient to wear comfortable clothing and shoes for the procedure.
2. Inform the patient about normal symptoms: sweating, slight shortness of breath, some increase in pulse rate, and some fatigue.
3. Emphasize that the patient should report abnormal symptoms and may stop the procedure if he or she experiences chest pain or severe weakness or tiredness.
4. Inform the patient of safety precautions followed during the procedure. The physician is present to monitor the patient's condition and provide any necessary emergency treatment, and emergency equipment is close at hand in the testing area.

Review any further physician instructions with the patient and make followup appointments as directed.

Echocardiogram

An echocardiogram is an examination of the cardiac structure using ultrasound (acoustic imaging). It allows the clinician to measure and define the size, shape, thickness, position, and movements of various cardiac structures, including the valves, myocardial walls, septum, and chambers. The arteries and veins, aorta, pulmonary veins and arteries, and superior vena cava are also viewed in an echocardiogram (Figure 35-29 ◆).

Echocardiograms are noninvasive tests. A transducer with conductive gel is placed on the chest wall over the ribs near the sternum, directed toward the heart. Sound waves are sent into the chest cavity by the transducer and bounced off the heart walls and valves. Images of the moving heart and its structures

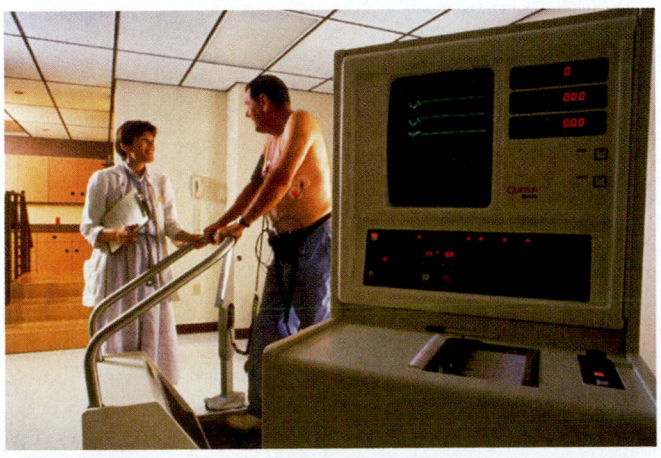

Figure 35-28 ◆ Treadmill stress test.
Source: David Scott Smith.

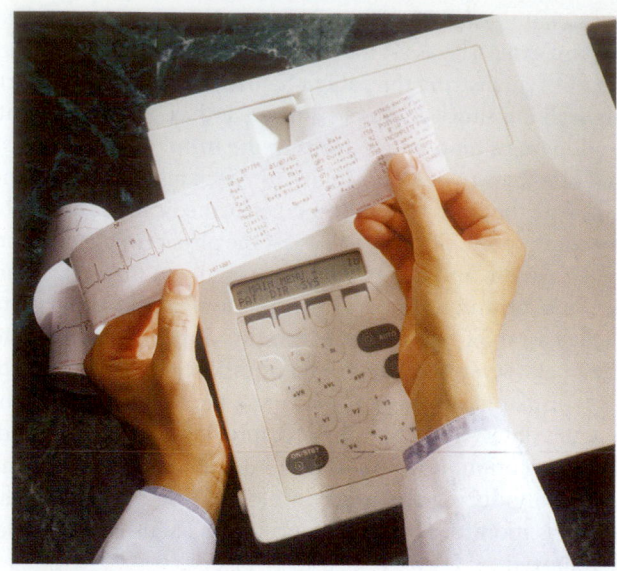

Figure 35-29 ◆ Single-channel echocardiograph.

are transmitted to an oscilloscope and recorded on paper and videotape. The Doppler measures the direction and velocity of the blood through the heart. This measurement—the fraction of blood ejected from the left ventricle with each heartbeat—is referred to as the **ejection fraction** (**EF**). Normal EF is 55%. Abnormal EF results from abnormal contractions of the heart muscle and the changing velocity of blood through the heart. Cardiac muscle enlargement and valve malfunctioning are among the structural or functional abnormalities that may be diagnosed.

Medical assistants will not perform echocardiograms unless specifically trained as an echocardiographic technician. The MA's role is to provide information to the patient and the patient's family and provide assistance to the technician.

The patient is asked to lie still, but may be asked to make minor adjustments to help the technician obtain additional information or a clearer picture. The technician applies a clear gel to the transducer, which is then applied to the chest, over the heart. The patient should be forewarned that the first touch of gel to the chest will be cold but that the sensation is temporary.

Patient Preparation and Instructions

The MA will prepare the patient room and provide patient care and support during the procedure. The MA will explain to the patient that the procedure examines the structure and function of the heart and will help the physician prescribe the most appropriate medical treatment, if any is required. Inform the patient that no preparation is necessary for the procedure. Mention that it is a painless procedure, although there might be some minor discomfort from lying still for approximately an hour. Document vital signs, observations, and the patient's tolerance of the procedure. Emphasize the need for a followup appointment as directed by the physician to discuss the test results. The physician may request that preprinted or internally developed written materials be given to the patient to reinforce verbal instructions.

Thallium Scan

In a thallium scan, an IV infusion of the radioisotope thallium-201 is used to assess myocardial perfusion. First, the patient is stressed on a treadmill. At the peak of stress, the thallium is infused and is taken up by the myocardium. The patient is then placed under a gamma camera and pictures are taken of the heart. Healthy tissue absorbs the thallium, but ischemic areas or areas of coronary artery disease do not absorb the isotope immediately and are thus identified. Infarcted areas never absorb the isotope, so the location and extent of myocardial ischemia or infarction can be identified as well. A thallium scan may also be used to determine the possible prognosis of a myocardial condition.

MUGA Scan

MUGA (multiple gated acquisition, also multinucleated gated angiography) scans assess the function of the left ventricle and identify abnormalities of the myocardial walls. Following injection of an isotope, a series of images are taken that show left ventricular function and allow the calculation of the ejection fraction.

A summary of cardiac diagnostic tests is given in Table 35-8.

Blood Studies

Blood studies aid the physician in the diagnostic process. Table 35-9 lists blood diagnostic tests often ordered by physicians to assess various stages of cardiac conditions.

Identifying Arrhythmias/Dysrhythmias

Anyone performing an ECG must recognize which arrhythmias, also known as dysrhythmias, are usual or unusual and which are life-threatening. Although atrial arrhythmias may cause symptoms of light-headedness or weakness, they usually are not life-threatening. Arrhythmias originating in the ventricles may be more serious, however, and some are considered life-threatening. The healthcare professional performing an ECG must recognize waveforms and rates and be able to rapidly interpret irregularities in order to alert the physician when necessary.

■ Rhythms originating in the SA node with normal conduction through the heart are called sinus rhythms. They may be within normal time limits (normal sinus rhythm, NSR), fast, or slow.

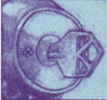

Keys to Success
CONSENT

Some cardiac procedures, such as stress tests or thallium scans, may cause serious arrhythmias as the need for oxygen and nutrition to the myocardium increases. An informed consent should therefore be signed, witnessed, and placed in the chart.

TABLE 35-8 CARDIAC DIAGNOSTIC TESTS

Diagnostic Test	Indications	Clinical Notes
ECG/EKG	Records electrical activity of the heart	■ Noninvasive study ■ May indicate need for Holter monitor testing
Holter monitor	Arrythmias of undetermined cause and abnormal ECG/EKG	■ Detects abnormal cardiac rhythm over a 24-hour period ■ Noninvasive study ■ Patient records activities in a diary
Echocardiogram	Visual diagnostic study to examine various structures, size, and cardiac output of the heart	■ Noninvasive study ■ Uses ultrasound with transducer Doppler
Stress test(s)	Assess cardiac response to stressors, including exercise	■ Usually noninvasive test using treadmill ■ May include thallium scan ■ Medications can be given to a patient physically unable to tolerate activity on the treadmill
Angiogram	Patency and structure of blood vessels	■ Invasive imaging study ■ May indicate and include angioplasty and stent
Cardiac catheterization	Patency and structure of blood vessels; also heart structure and size, cardiac and pulmonary vascular pressures	■ Invasive imaging study ■ May indicate and include angiogram, angioplasty, and stent insertion
Chest X-ray	Determines heart size and condition of lungs	■ Noninvasive radiation exposure ■ Two views

■ Rhythms originating in the AV node are called junctional or nodal rhythms and usually proceed through the conduction system from that point. If the conduction system is blocked for some reason, rhythms take a detour around the damaged tissue that is causing the block and are blocking-type rhythms.

■ Rhythms originating in the ventricles present a danger and may cause the heart to stop beating in some cases. **PVCs, or premature ventricular contractions,** originate in the ventricle and not the pacemaker cells of the heart. They prevent the atria from filling with blood, and when they cause the ventricles to contract, no blood is pumped out of

TABLE 35-9 BLOOD STUDIES

CBC (complete blood count)	Detects anemias, blood cell changes, or infections	■ Specimens must be obtained in an EDTA tube ■ Platelet count ■ Includes measurement of RBCs, WBCs, Hgb, Hct, MCV, MCH, MCHC
Cholesterol	Screen tool used for family or medical history of heart disease	■ Serum required for test ■ NPO for 12 hours pretest ■ HDL:LDL ratio provides confirmation of cholesterol screening ■ Elevated levels are precursor to diagnosis of atherosclerosis
Triglycerides	Screening tool used for arterial diseases	■ As triglycerides increase, LDL also increases
Coagulation studies	Screening tool for thromboembolic conditions and medication adjustment	■ Include PTT or PT ■ Used to adjust medication regime
Cardiac enzymes	Chest pain, myocardial status	■ CPK (CK), LDH, AST (SGOT) ■ Elevations occur after cardiac trauma, including MI ■ For additional studies, isoenzymes are ordered

the ventricle. This phenomenon may be what a patient refers to as a "skipped beat." The danger arises when there are more than six PVCs in one minute, when they occur in pairs or every other beat, or when they arise from different foci in the ventricle. Unifocal PVCs originate from the same **focus** (site) in the ventricle, whereas multifocal PVCs arise from different foci. This can be a life-threatening arrhythmia that demands immediate intervention.

The various cardiac rhythms are described in Table 35-10. The medical assistant performing ECGs must know when to alert the physician to an abnormal ECG or a life-threatening situation. The MA must therefore be familiar with waveforms and rates and be able to rapidly interpret irregularities.

Using ECG calipers, the MA will measure P-to-P or R-to-R intervals to determine if atrial (P waves) and ventricular (QRS complexes) rhythms are regular. The MA will calculate measurements of the PR interval (normal range 0.12 to 2.0 seconds) and QRS complex (normal range less than 12 seconds). Atrial and ventricular rates are both calculated because the rates may be different with some cardiac arrhythmias. If P waves or QRS complexes are not visible, the MA will not be able to calculate atrial and ventricular rates, respectively, by multiplying each number in a six-second strip × 10. If the MA is unable to identify QRS complexes, the patient is in a life-threatening clinical situation or an electrode and wire have become disconnected. *Always* check the patient for clinical signs and symptoms of cardiac and respiratory arrest, and look for signs of disconnection between the ECG, the electrodes, or the wires before initiating CPR.

The following are additional considerations when analyzing ECG conduction patterns.

1. Are some QRS complexes wider, premature to the regular rhythm, or different in appearance? Is there a pattern to the irregular, premature QRS complexes?
2. With the ECG calipers, measure the PR interval. Multiply the number of small squares by 0.4 seconds. Is the measurement within or outside the normal range of 0.12 to 0.20?

(text continues on p. 765)

TABLE 35-10 CARDIAC RHYTHMS

Normal sinus rhythm (NSR)	P wave originates in SA node, measures 0.12 to 2.0 seconds. QRS complex has normal waveform and is complete in less than 0.12 seconds. T wave has a positive deflection. Beats per minute (BPM) are 60–100 (Figure 35-30 ◆).
Sinus bradycardia	Normal waveform and complex, only less than 60 BPM (Figure 35-31 ◆).
Sinus tachycardia	Normal waveform and complex, only greater than 100 BPM (Figure 35-32 ◆).
Atrial fibrillation (**A-fib**)	Irregularly spaced QRS complexes with noticeable absence of P waves, replaced by F waves (Figure 35-33 ◆)
Atrial flutter	Electrical impulses are generated at a rapid rate in a single irritable source in the atria. Normal P waves are not present with F waves; flutter or sawtooth patterns instead (Figure 35-34 ◆).
Supraventricular tachycardia (SVT)	Encompasses all tachycardias originating above the ventricle with BPM over 100: sinus tachycardia, atrial tachycardia, paroxysmal atrial tachycardia, paroxysmal supraventricular tachycardia, paroxysmal junctional tachycardia, and junctional tachycardia.
Paroxysmal atrial tachycardia (PAT)	Atrial tachycardia with sudden onset.
Premature atrial contractions (PACs)	Occur when a single electrical impulse originates outside the SA node (Figure 35-35 ◆).
Premature junctional rhythm (PJC)	Electrical impulse originates from a single site in the AV junction and earlier than the next expected complex (Figure 35-36 ◆).
Bundle branch block (**BBB**)	Normal P wave. QRS complex is notched.
First-degree AV block	PR interval is greater than 0.20 second (Figure 35-37 ◆).
Second-degree heart block I, Mobitz Type I	P:P waves are normal interval, but R:R intervals are irregular. There is a progressive lengthening of the PR interval until a QRS complex is not conducted or present (Figure 35-38 ◆).
Second-degree heart block II, Mobitz Type II	More P waves than QRS complexes, but the PR wave has a constant interval, resulting in a slowed ventricular rate (Figure 35-39 ◆).
Third-degree heart block	No consistent relationship between P waves and QRS complexes (Figure 35-40 ◆).
Premature ventricular contractions (PVCs)	Individual complexes, not a rhythm, originate from an ectopic or irritable focus in the ventricle. No blood is pumped from the heart during a PVC, and the individual feels as if the heart is "skipping a beat."
Unifocal PVCs	PVC arises from the same focus each time, and the complexes are uniform in shape or appearance (Figure 35-41 ◆).
Multifocal PVCs	PVCs arise from different foci in the ventricle and have different shapes or configurations (Figure 35-42 ◆).
Ventricular tachycardia (**V-tach**)	Three or more PVCs in a sequence with a rate of more than 100 BPM (Figure 35-43 ◆).
Ventricular fibrillation (**V-fib**)	Often described as a fatal arrhythmia; contains no coordinated atrial or ventricular contractions and no palpable pulse (Figure 35-44 ◆).
Asystole	Straight line, cardiac standstill. No atrial or ventricular activity is present (Figure 35-45 ◆).

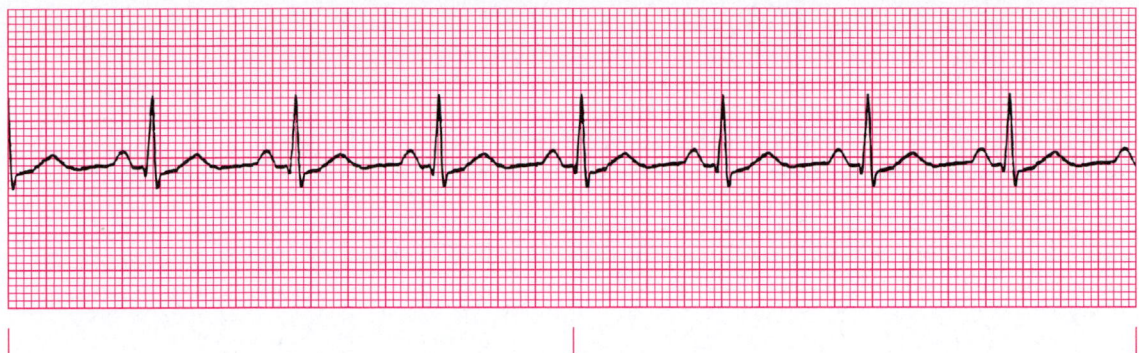

Figure 35-30 ◆ Normal sinus rhythm.

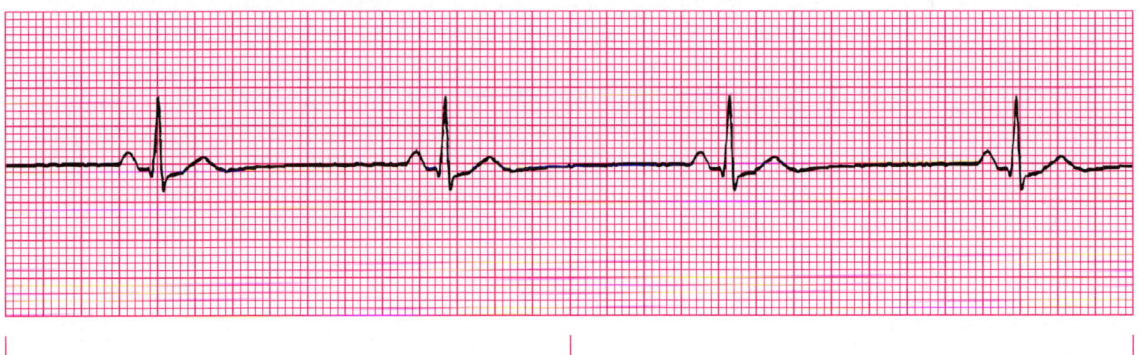

Figure 35-31 ◆ Sinus bradycardia rhythm.

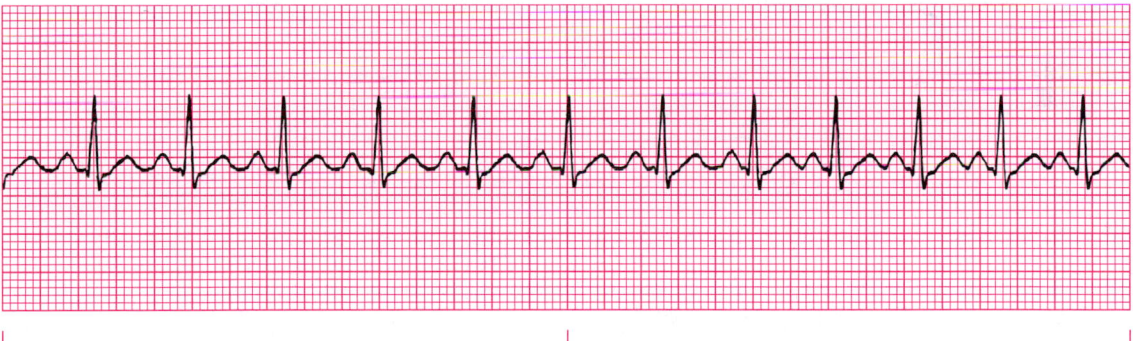

Figure 35-32 ◆ Sinus tachycardia rhythm.

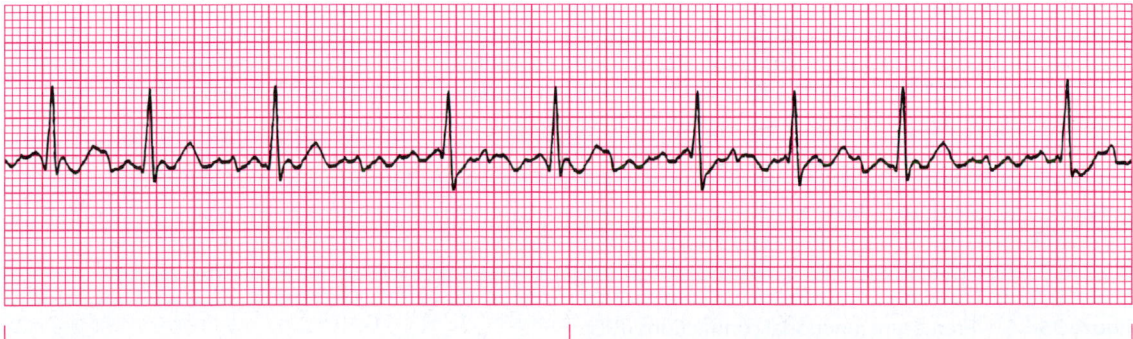

Figure 35-33 ◆ Atrial fibrillation (A-fib).

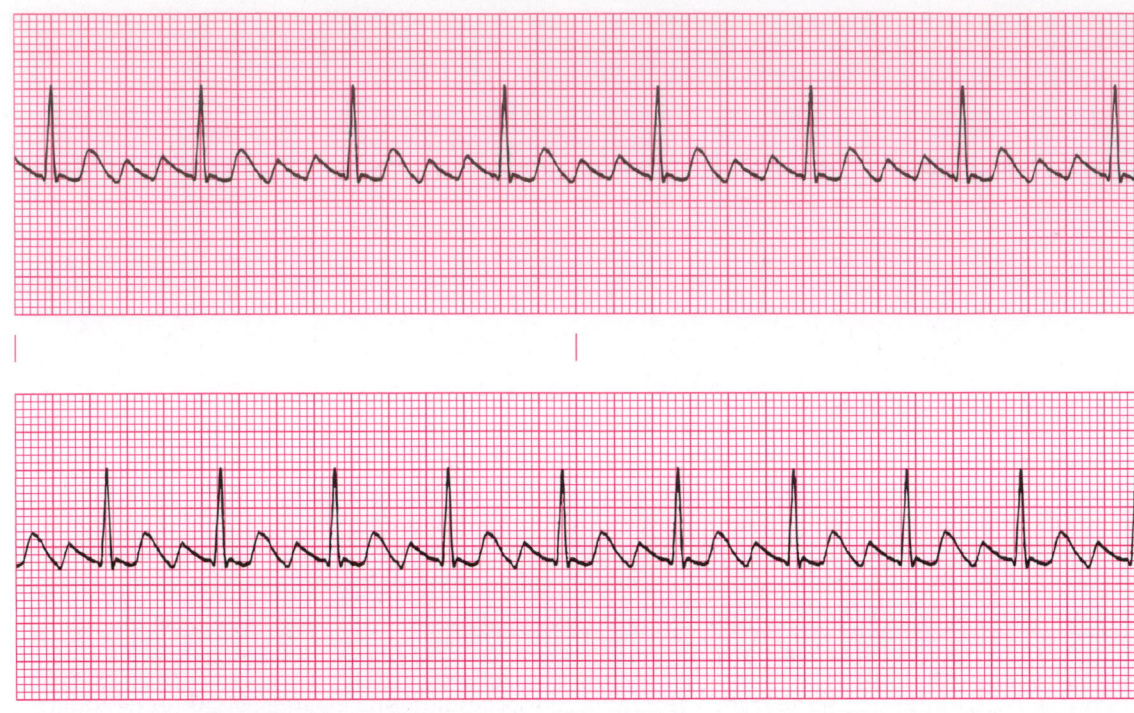

Figure 35-34 ◆ Atrial flutter.

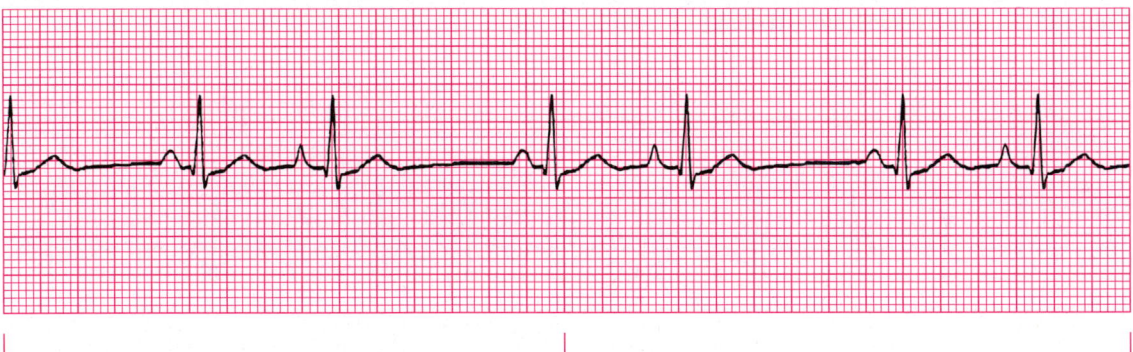

Figure 35-35 ◆ Premature atrial contractions (PAC).

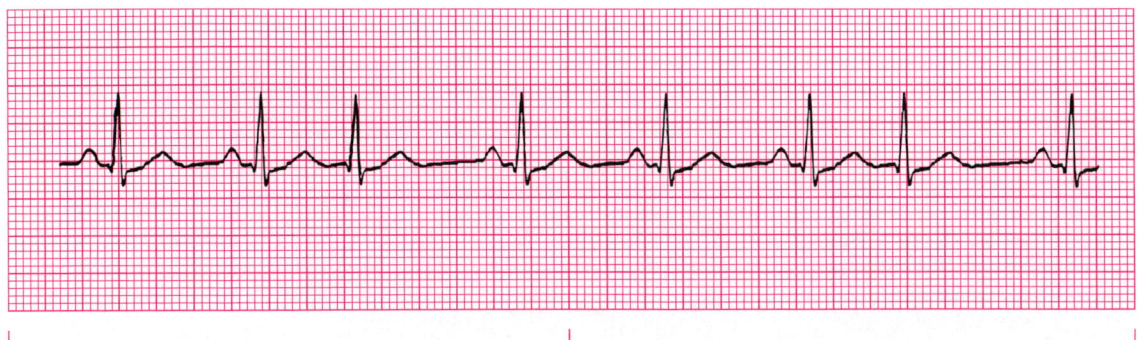

Figure 35-36 ◆ Premature junctional contractions (PJC).

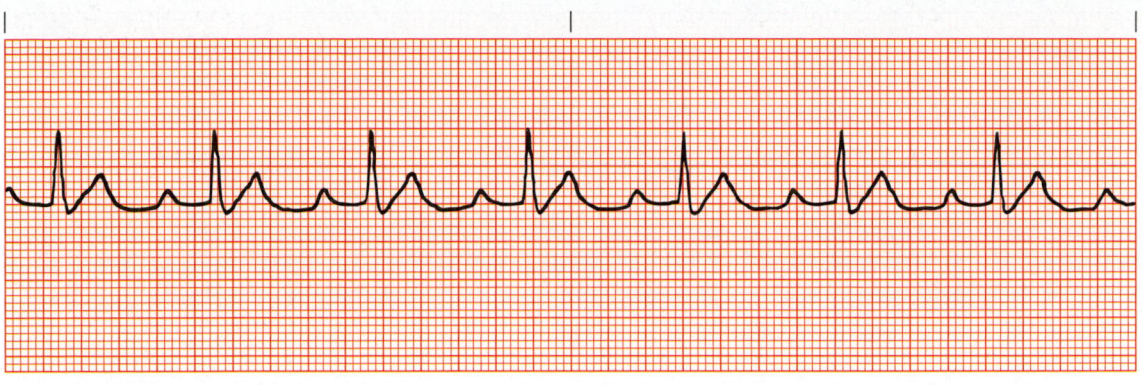

Figure 35-37 ◆ First-degree AV block.

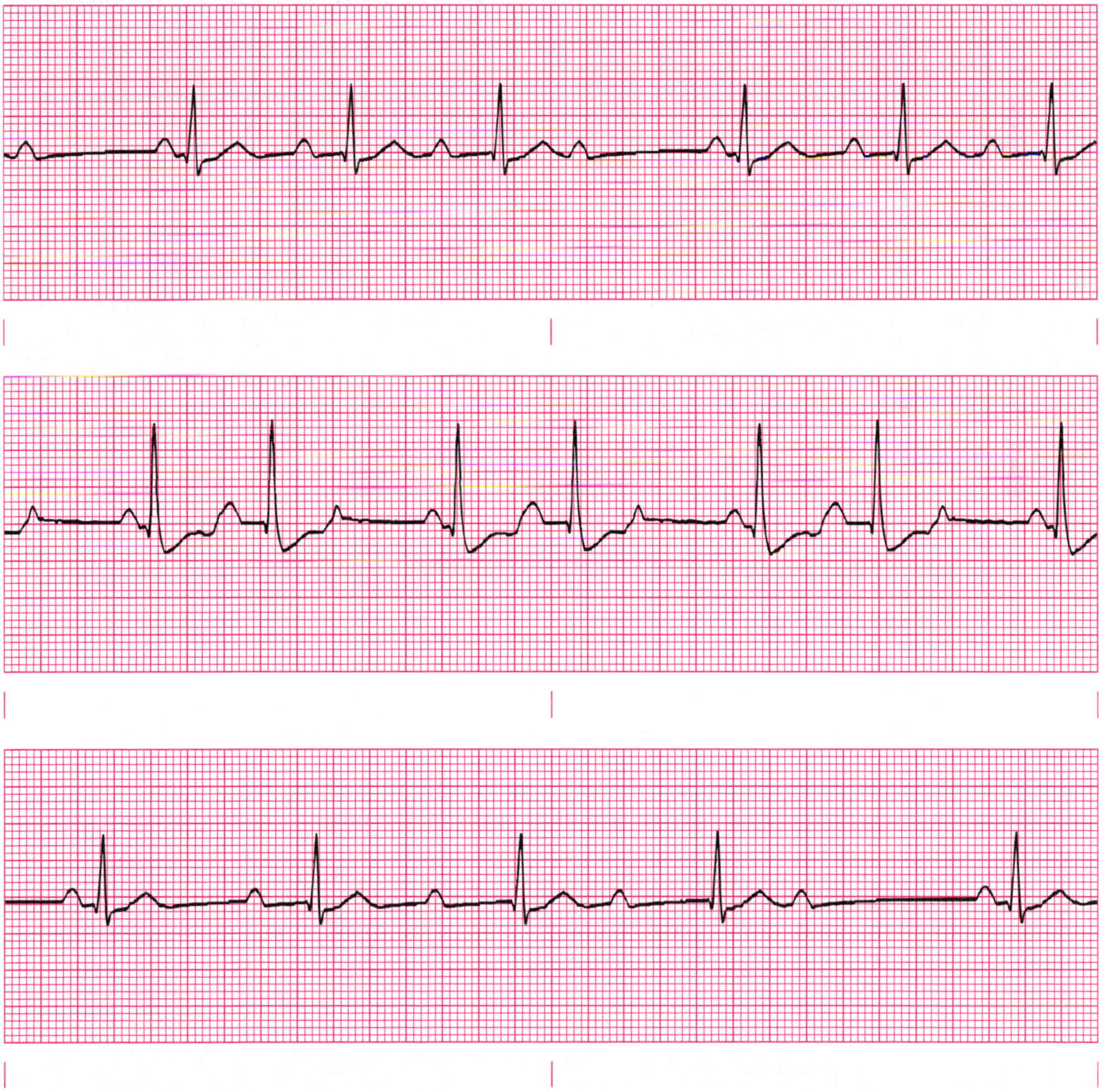

Figure 35-38 ◆ Second-degree heart block I, Mobitz Type I.

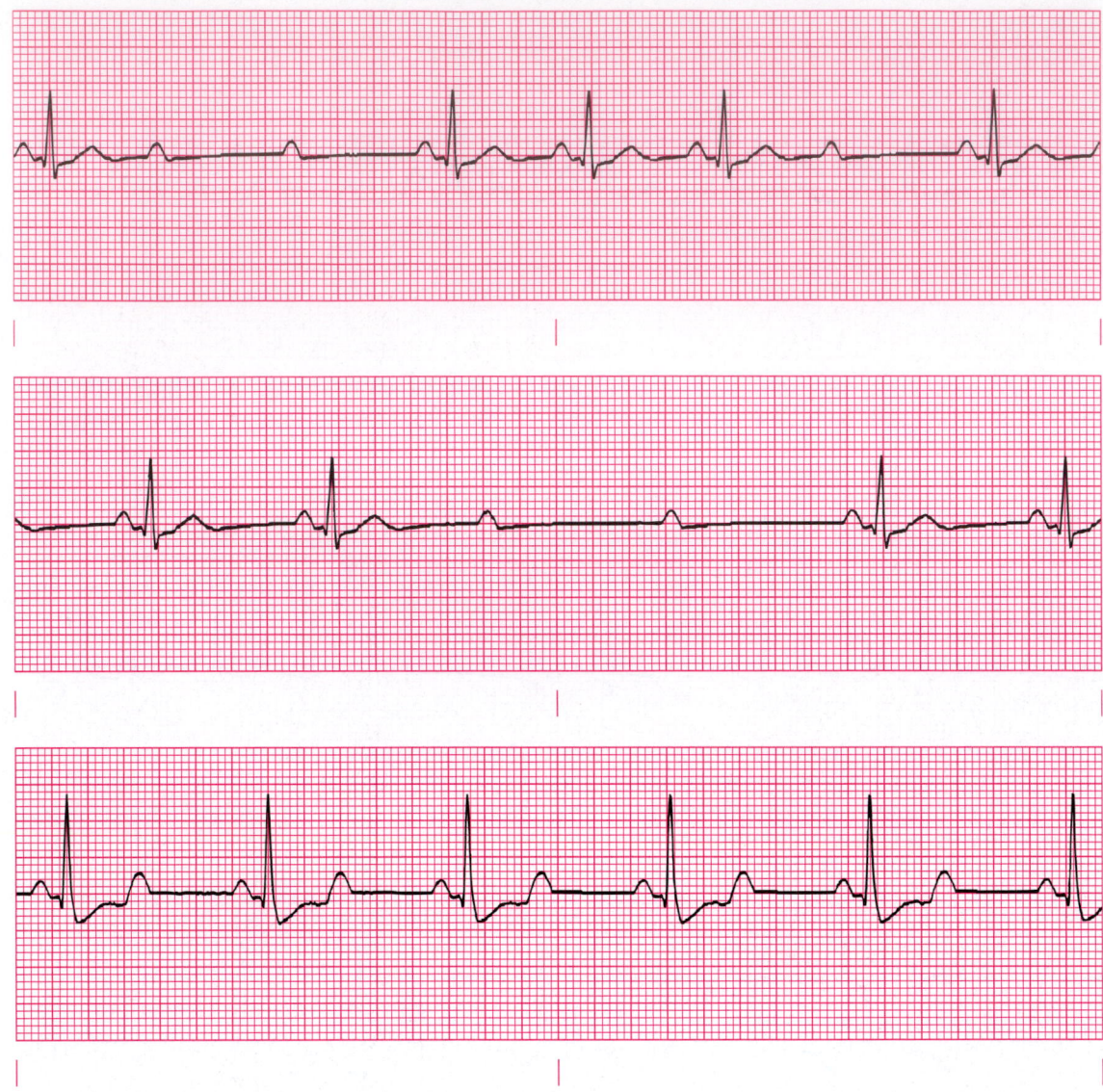

Figure 35-39 ◆ Second-degree heart block II, Mobitz Type II.

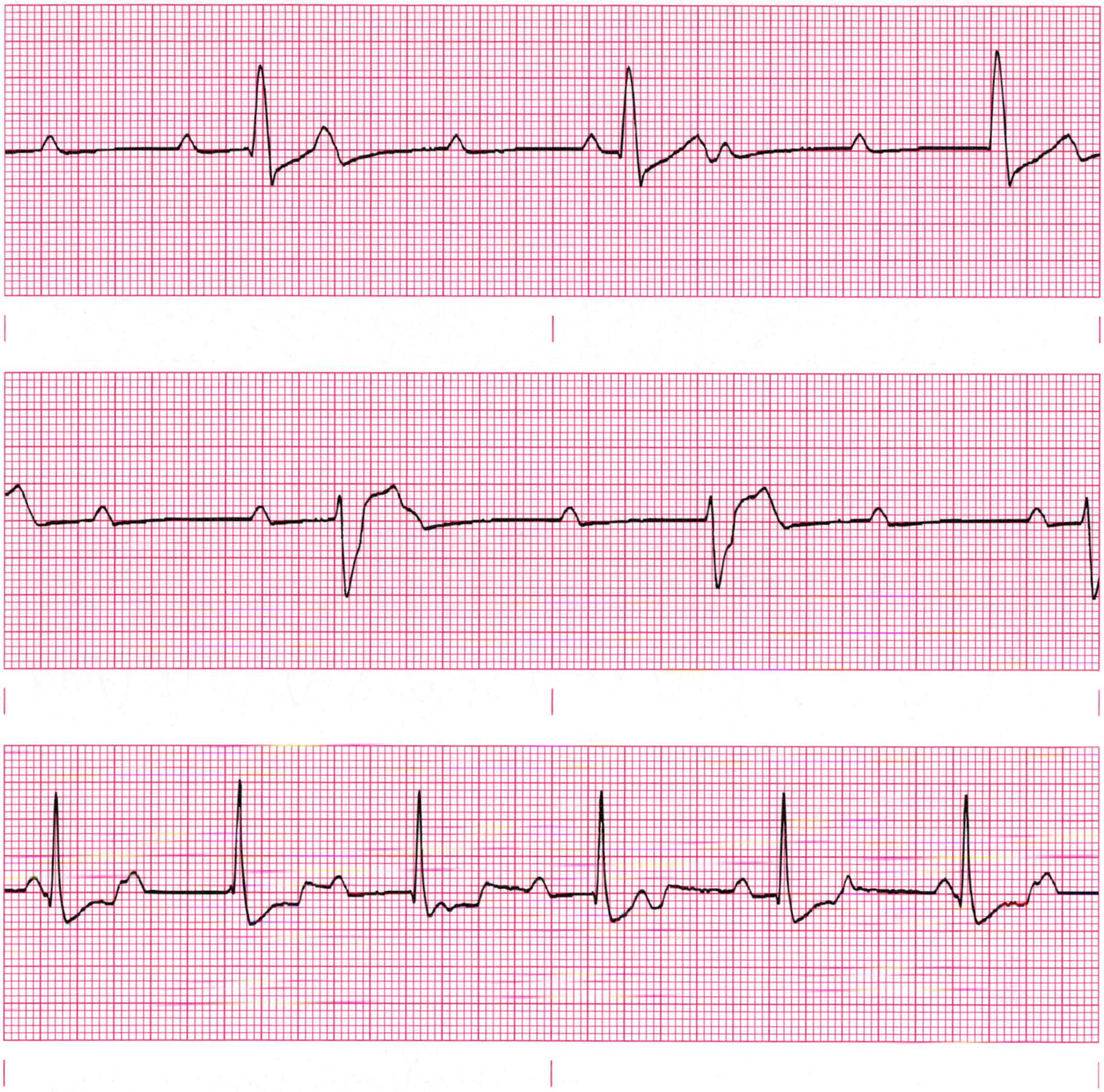

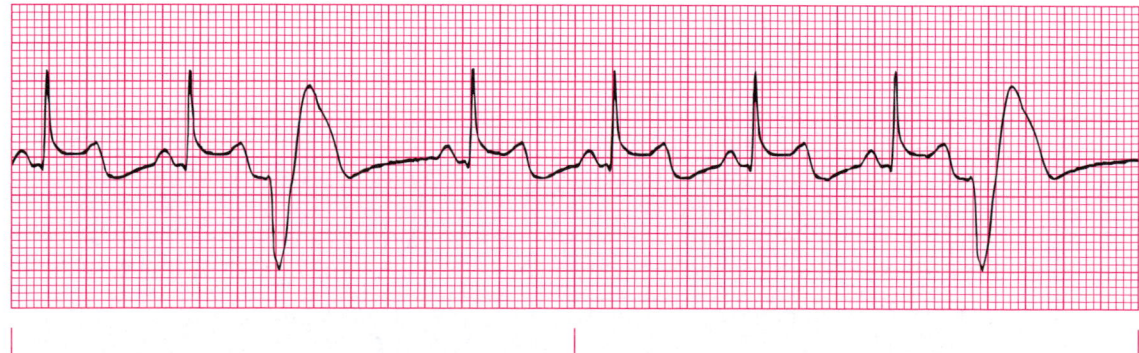

Figure 35-40 ◆ Third-degree heart block.

Figure 35-41 ◆ Unifocal PVCs (premature ventricular contractions).

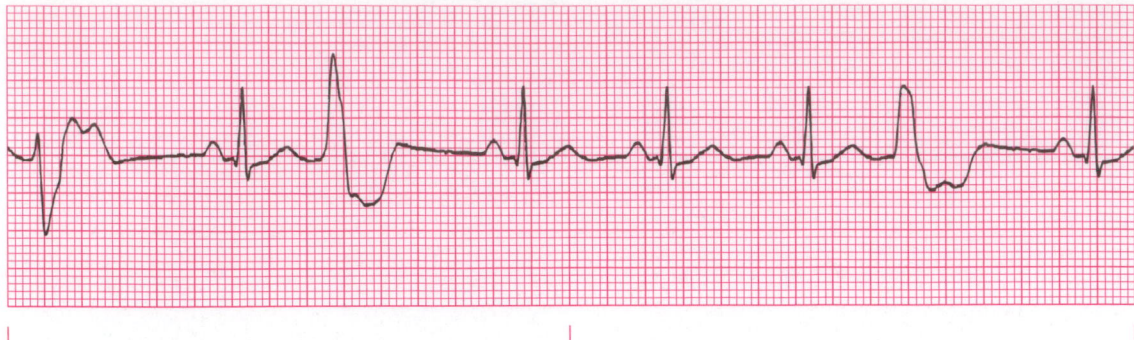

Figure 35-42 ◆ Multifocal PVCs (premature ventricular contractions).

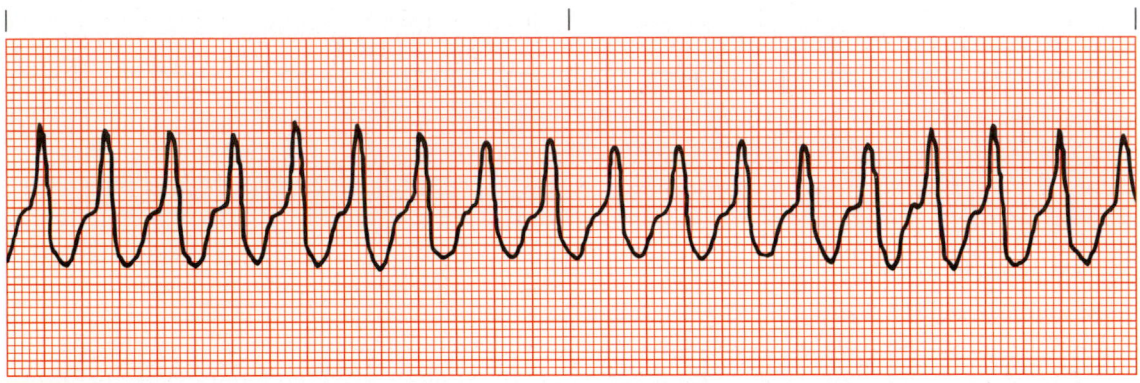

Figure 35-43 ◆ Ventricular tachycardia (V-tach).

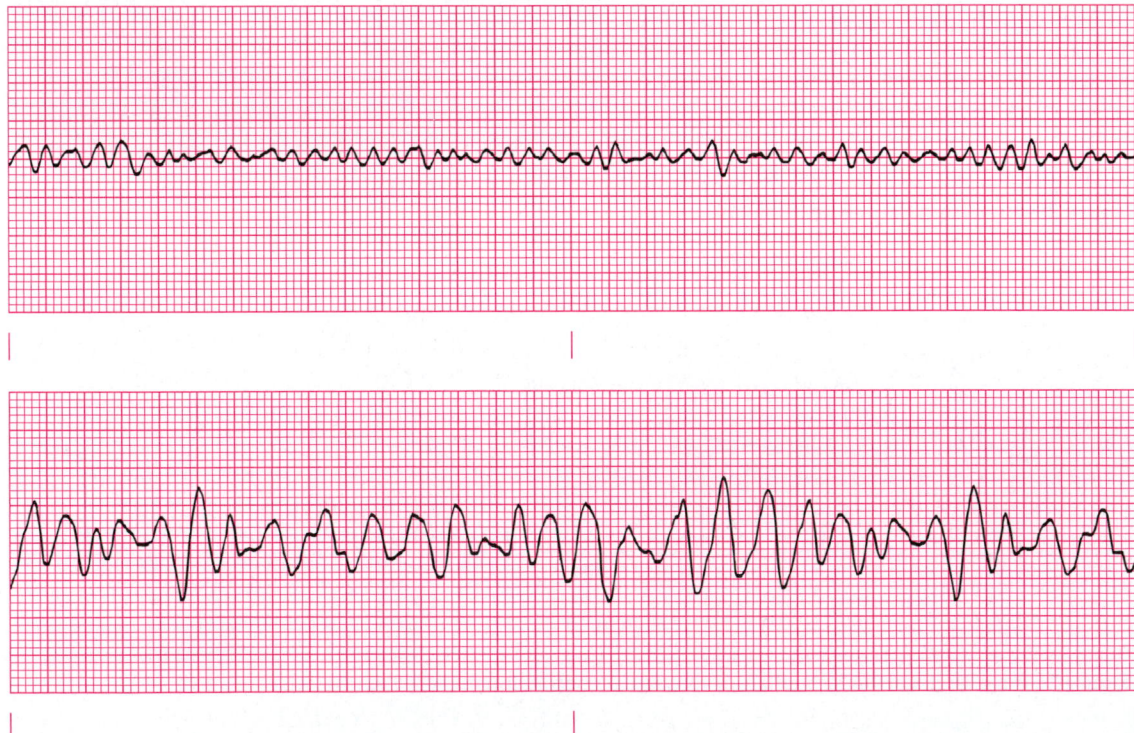

Figure 35-44 ◆ Ventricular fibrillation (V-fib).

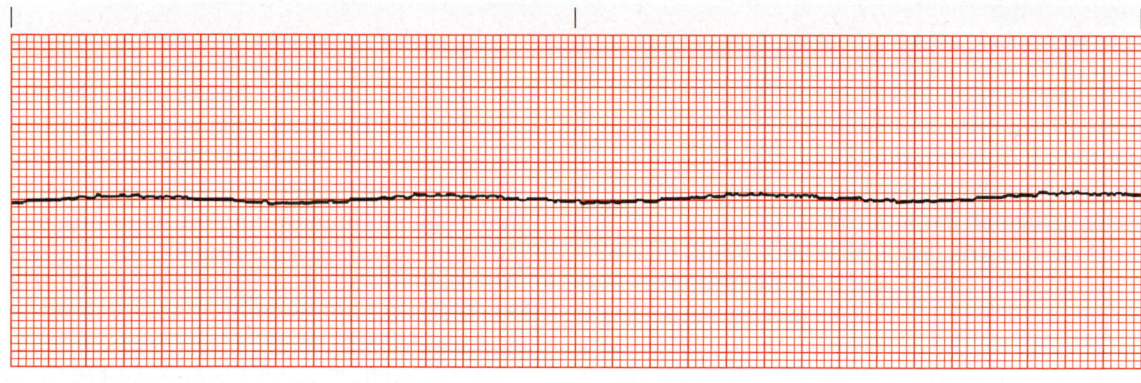

Figure 35-45 ◆ Asystole.

3. Present your ECG calculations to the physician for further analysis and interpretation. If the clinical condition of the patient changes and deteriorates rapidly, take the ECG to the physician and report signs and symptoms immediately.

As an example, the abnormal P waves, or flutter waves, of atrial flutter occur at a much faster rate. The high rate of P wave conduction is blocked along the conduction pathway to the ventricles. Therefore, the reduced number of conducted impulses to the ventricles, or number of QRS complexes, is less than the atrial rate or P wave count. The P-to-P and R-to-R intervals are both regular. The QRS complex may be normal, wider, or have a "rabbit ear" appearance due to past or current cardiac events.

All ECGs are given to the physician for interpretation. The measurements of the PR interval and QRS complex and the shape of all waveforms or segments may be within normal limits or may be affected by medications or past and current history of cardiac disease or heart attack. Some ECG equipment automatically provides an interpretation, but the physician analyzes, interprets, and verifies the programmed findings. ECGs are kept together in the same area of the patient chart so the physician can compare present and past electrocardiograms.

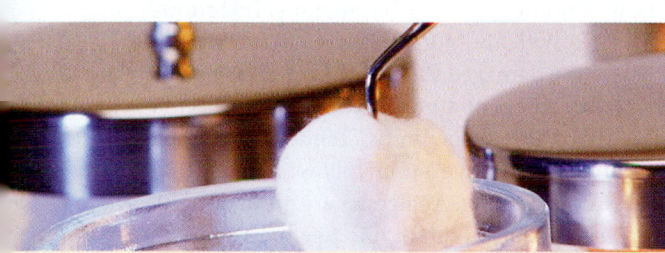

REVIEW

Chapter Summary

- Medical assistants in a cardiology office perform selected procedures and assist with others. Assessment of the cardiac patient includes taking vital signs, measuring height and weight, and assisting with ECG, rhythm assessment, and evaluation of various pulse points.
- Understanding heart anatomy and conduction is crucial to performing or assisting with cardiac testing. Deoxygenated blood enters the right atrium, passes through the tricuspid valve to the right ventricle, and continues to the lungs, where it is oxygenated. The blood then passes to the left atrium, through the left ventricle, and to all parts of the body. After the blood circulates oxygen and other nutrients to the cells, it returns to the right atrium, deoxygenated.
- The heart is a mechanical pump that is stimulated to contract by the sinoatrial node. If the SA node does not initiate the impulse, lower pacemaker cells in the heart can do so as a "survival" effort. The conduction of a healthy heart originates at the SA node of the right atrium and spreads through each atrium to the atrioventricular node, the bundle of His, and the Purkinje fibers in each ventricle. Many factors can affect the function of the mechanical and electrical systems of the heart. Electrolyte imbalance, previous or current cardiac history, and other existing medical conditions can cause or predispose a patient to cardiac events.
- Cardiac patients often complain of chest pain, irregular heartbeats, dyspnea, edema, and fatigue. Complaints of nausea, sudden onset of extensive sweating, and denial of heart attack are symptoms of an impending MI and demand immediate intervention.
- Coronary artery disease is the result of plaque buildup, or atherosclerosis that causes the coronary arteries to harden (arteriosclerosis). Blood flow is impeded to the point of complete obstruction. Pain results as oxygen and nutrition to the myocardium are denied; when deprivation is severe, the tissue

Chapter Summary (continued)

dies, causing a myocardial infarct and possible death. There are two forms of "heart attack." One occurs when the reduced blood flow to the myocardium causes anginal pain and myocardial ischemia. The second type occurs when the conduction system suffers an insult. Arrhythmias may be caused by coronary artery obstruction. Lethal arrhythmias may be caused by electrocution, trauma, and drug overdose.

■ Angina is a pressure-like pain, usually in the chest region, the left arm, possibly the left jaw, occasionally the right chest and arm. It is generally experienced on exertion and ceases a few minutes after rest. Until angina is confirmed, the patient must be treated as if experiencing an impending heart attack. The physician must be notified immediately. Vasodilating drugs and calcium channel blocking drugs are used to treat angina.

■ Myocardial infarction demands immediate intervention to restore blood flow to the myocardium. Angioplasty, stent insertion, and coronary artery bypass surgery are invasive techniques used to reverse the blockage. Post-myocardial patients are often treated in the cardiology office.

■ Sudden cardiac arrest occurs when the conduction system of the heart fails, often following a sudden and severe occlusion of the coronary arteries. It may also be the result of respiratory arrest, drowning, or massive hemorrhage. Immediate intervention consists of CPR and AED.

■ Hypertension, or high blood pressure, occurs when blood pressure readings are consistently over 140/90. Elevated blood pressure increases the workload of the heart as it pumps blood through constricted vessels. Arteriosclerosis, atherosclerosis, and renal disease often are precursors to hypertension and hypertensive heart disease. Stress and being overweight are contributing factors. Essential hypertension is chronic hypertension with no identifiable cause. There is no cure, and drug therapy with diuretics, vasodilating drugs, ACE inhibitors, and beta-blocking agents must be continued for life. Nondrug therapy includes stress reduction, weight reduction, dietary changes, and exercise.

■ A patient with congestive heart failure (CHF) complains of shortness of breath (SOB), weight gain, edema, and possibly exhaustion. Symptoms have an insidious onset and dyspnea becomes severe. Pitting edema, distended neck veins, and respiratory distress are other signs. Radiographs of the chest are helpful in the diagnosis. Treatment includes diuretics, cardiac glycosides, vasodilators, restriction of fluid and sodium intake, and daily weighing.

■ Pulmonary edema follows CHF as fluid fills the lungs, increasing the workload of the heart. Dyspnea and coughing of frothy, bloody sputum occur, especially at night. Treatment is aimed at decreasing fluid in the lungs with diuretics, Lanoxin, vasodilators, and bronchodilating drugs.

■ Cardiomyopathy is a noninflammatory disease of the myocardium often with no identifiable cause. The muscle in the heart wall thickens, with resulting inefficiency of the heartbeat. The only treatment may be a transplant.

■ Arrhythmias, or irregular heartbeats, are classified in different ways: by disturbances of impulse formation, by disturbances in conduction, or according to prognosis. When the impulse does not originate in the SA node, it is a disturbance in origin. When the impulse does not follow the normal pathway through the conduction system (SA node, AV node, bundle of His, and Purkinje fibers), it is a disturbance in conduction.

■ Infective and inflammatory diseases of the myocardium include rheumatic heart disease, endocarditis, myocarditis, and pericarditis. These diseases may lead to cardiomyopathies and cardiomegalies. Rheumatic heart disease is a sequela to rheumatic fever, which is a sequela to a Group A beta-hemolytic *Streptococcus* infection of the throat. Aggressive drug therapy with antibiotics is the usual course of action.

■ Valvular diseases occur on any of the four heart valves. Inflammation and infectious processes in the endocardium may result in scarring of the valves. If the valve fails to open completely, as in stenosis, not all the blood is emptied into the next chamber, and pressure increases in the previous chamber. If the valve fails to close completely, blood is forced back into the previous chamber, also increasing the pressure in that chamber. Symptoms include dyspnea, shortness of breath, and sometimes cyanosis. ECGs, echocardiograms, radiographs of the chest, and cardiac catheterization are used to diagnose valvular conditions. Treatment includes bed rest, fluid restriction, diuretics, and oxygen therapy. Infectious processes are treated with antibiotics. Surgery to free up the stenosis or replace the damaged valve may be performed.

■ Phlebitis, an inflammatory condition of veins, usually occurs in the deep veins of the lower limbs. Tenderness in the affected area is often the first symptom, followed by increasing pain, redness, and swelling. Analgesics are given and the individual is instructed not to rub or massage the area.

■ Thrombophlebitis, an inflammatory condition, occurs in a vein where a thrombus has formed on the wall. Blood flow in the vein is compromised and edema occurs. The individual experiences pain, edema, warmth, redness in the area, systemic chills, and fever. Insult to the vessel, particularly to the walls, venous stasis, and hypercoagulating blood are all causes. Venograms and ultrasound confirm diagnosis. Treatment involves immobilization of the affected limb and administration of anticoagulant drugs and antibiotics.

■ An embolus is a mass of material that forms an obstruction, or embolism, in a blood or lymphatic vessel. Emboli that occlude the vessel cause infarction of the tissue supplied by that vessel. Deep-vein thrombosis is often the result of stasis of the blood in the deep vessels of the legs brought on by inactivity. Other causes include blood that has a tendency to clot quickly, insult to the vessels, and surgery such as hip and knee replacement and prostate surgery.

■ Conditions of the peripheral vessels of the hands and feet include Raynaud's disease and Buerger's disease. Raynaud's occurs when the small vessels in the extremities spasm as a result of exposure to cold or stress. Cigarette smoking aggravates

Chapter Summary (continued)

the condition. Buerger's disease affects mainly males and results from inflammation of the vessels of the legs and feet. Obstruction of the vessels may lead to clot formation and severe pain in the extremities. Smoking is a primary causative factor.

■ The 12-lead ECG takes a short snapshot of the electrical activity of the heart from different angles of the conduction system. A Holter monitor allows for a 24-hour study of the conduction system.

■ The echocardiogram is a noninvasive ultrasound that examines the movements and anatomical structures of the heart while the patient rests. Stress testing is performed while the patient is exercising, usually on a treadmill or stationary bicycle. Thallium and MUGA scans are invasive tests that identify damaged, unhealthy areas of the heart.

■ Procedures performed on cardiac patients include cardiac catheterization to evaluate the status of the coronary arteries. Stent insertion may follow angioplasty to help keep the coronary artery lumen patent. Coronary artery bypass graft surgery is performed when other attempts to maintain patent coronary arteries will not achieve the goal.

■ MAs play an important role in cardiac testing. They perform procedures such as blood testing or assist with ECGs, echocardiograms, Holter monitor recording, stress testing, thallium scans, and MUGA scans. The MA must be able to identify and alert the physician to abnormal electrocardiograms.

Chapter Review

Multiple Choice

1. The mitral valve is located between the
   a. left atrium and right atrium.
   b. left atrium and respiratory circulation.
   c. left ventricle and right ventricle.
   d. left atrium and left ventricle.

2. Cardiac muscle cells have all the following properties except
   a. reproductivity.
   b. excitability.
   c. automaticity.
   d. contractility.

3. The pacemaker of the heart is the
   a. atrioventricular node.
   b. sinoatrial node.
   c. ventricular node.
   d. bundle node.

4. Angina-type pain, shortness of breath, weakness or dizziness, rapid heartbeat, palpitations, nausea, and perspiration are symptoms of
   a. hypertension.
   b. sinus bradycardia.
   c. coronary artery disease.
   d. phlebitis.

5. Myocardial infarction occurs because of
   a. opening blood flow from coronary bypass surgery.
   b. obstruction of blood flow, ischemia, and resulting death to tissues.
   c. a change in heart rate or respiratory rate.
   d. a change to reduce cardiac risk factors.

6. Treatment for congestive heart failure includes
   a. diuretics, digitalis preparations, and vasodilators.
   b. diuretics, digitalis preparations, and sodium-enriched diet.
   c. diuretics, vasodilators, and laxatives.
   d. none of the above.

7. Arrhythmias usually result from
   a. normal activities of daily living.
   b. maintaining a healthy lifestyle.
   c. reducing cardiac risk factors.
   d. disease conditions that impair the normal electrical conduction of the heart.

8. In sinus bradycardia, the heart rate is abnormally slow and the electrical impulse originates in the
   a. sinojunctional node.
   b. sinus of the left atrium.
   c. sinoatrial node.
   d. sinus of the right atrium.

9. The causative agent of endocarditis, myocarditis, and pericarditis is
   a. caffeine-containing substances.
   b. viral, fungal, bacterial, or parasitic.
   c. working and living in smoke-filled environments.
   d. working without personal protective equipment (PPE).

10. Rheumatic heart disease is caused by
    a. bacterial infection.
    b. fungal infection.
    c. viral infection.
    d. parasitic infestation.

Chapter Review (continued)

True/False

T F 1. Nausea, excessive sweating, and denial of a possible heart attack should be taken seriously.

T F 2. An ECG measures the electrical activity of the myocardium.

T F 3. Arteries (except the pulmonary arteries) carry oxygenated blood and veins carry deoxygenated blood.

T F 4. A healthy heart contracts and relaxes no more than 60 times per minute.

T F 5. The AV node is known as the "pacemaker" of the heart.

Short Answer

1. What is the difference between arteriosclerosis and atherosclerosis?

2. What are the two kinds of risk factors for coronary artery disease?

3. Describe pulmonary edema.

4. Name two dietary changes that are helpful in controlling hypertension.

5. What is the function of a Holter monitor?

Research

1. Are MAs in your state allowed to assist in a thallium scan? If so, what is their role in the procedure?

2. Are MAs in your state allowed to assist in a treadmill stress test? If so, what is their role?

Externship Application Experience

What would you do if a flat line appeared on the screen while you were performing an ECG? A flat line means that the electrocardiograph is not receiving any record of cardiac electrical activity. Does this mean that your patient has had cardiac arrest? What should you do? What should you not do?

Resource Guide

American College of Cardiology
9111 Old Georgetown Road
Bethesda, MD 20814
1-800-253-4636
www.acc.org

American Heart Association
7272 Greenville Ave.
Dallas, TX 75231
1-800-AHA-USA1
www.amhrt.org

American Red Cross
www.redcross.org

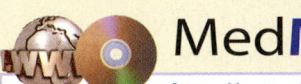 Med**Media**

http://www.MyMAKit.com

More on this chapter, including interactive resources, can be found on the Student CD-ROM accompanying this textbook and on http://www.MyMAKit.com.

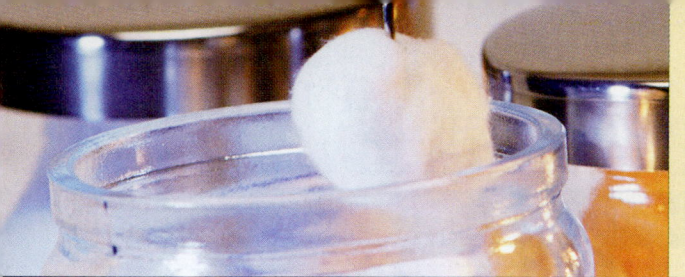

Objectives

After completing this chapter, you should be able to:

- Define and spell the key terminology in this chapter.
- Define the medical assistant's role in a pulmonology practice.
- Identify lower airway structures and their functions.
- Discuss lung and chest mechanics and the gas mechanics of respiration.
- Describe the symptoms, causes, and treatments for obstructive respiratory conditions, infectious and inflammatory pulmonary conditions, pulmonary malignancies, and mechanical insults.
- Describe breathing patterns and other signs and symptoms of pulmonary disorders.
- List pulmonary function tests that may be performed in a medical office.
- Discuss the role of inhalers and nebulizers in pulmonary treatment.
- Explain oxygen therapy and how it is administered.

Pulmonology and Pulmonary Testing

Case Study

Keera is assigned to work in a pulmonology office as part of her externship. Since she started working, she has learned to take patients' vital signs and chief complaints and perform spirometry and peak flow testing. Today her preceptor is teaching her how to obtain a sputum sample from a patient and give inhaler instructions for several new types that have come on the market.

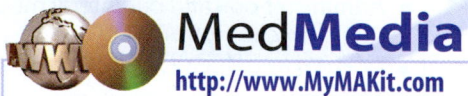

MedMedia

http://www.MyMAKit.com

Additional interactive resources and activities for this chapter can be found on http://www.MyMAKit.com. For videos, tips, audio glossary, legal and ethical scenarios, job scenarios, quizzes, games, virtual tours, and activities related to the content of this chapter, please access the accompanying CD-ROM in this book.

Audio Glossary
Videos: *Spirometer; TB Testing and Analysis*
Legal and Ethical Scenario: *Pulmonology and Pulmonary Testing*
On the Job Scenario: *Pulmonology and Pulmonary Testing*
Tips
A & P Quiz: The Respiratory System; TB Testing & Analysis
Multiple Choice Quiz
Games: Crossword, Strikeout, and Spelling Bee
3D Virtual Tours: The Respiratory System: Respiratory System
Drag & Drop: Respiratory System: Interior of the Lung; Respiratory System: The Lungs; Respiratory System: Diaphragm
HIPPA Quiz

Key Terminology

alveolus (plural: alveoli)—microscopic air sacs that are the primary unit of gas exchange in the lungs

asthma—lung disease characterized by wheezing and shortness of breath; often caused by an allergic response; also known as reversible airway obstruction

bronchiole—airway less than 1 mm in diameter

bronchitis—lung disease characterized by large volumes of pulmonary secretions and air trapping; can be chronic or acute in nature

bronchodilator—medication that dilates the walls of the bronchi

bronchus (plural: bronchi)—one of two primary airways that branch into the lungs

diaphragm—primary muscle of breathing; separates chest and abdominal cavities

dyspnea—difficult breathing

emphysema—disease of chronic airway obstruction (COPD) in which air is trapped; usually caused by either smoking or heredity

eupnea—normal breathing

hemopneumothorax—accumulation of blood and air in the pleural cavity, resulting in the partial or complete collapse of the lung

hemoptysis—coughing up sputum containing blood

hemothorax—accumulation of blood and fluids in the pleural cavity that limit the expansion of the lung

hepatotoxicity—harmful effect of drugs on the liver

immunocompetence—body's ability to fight infection; capacity for normal immune response

intradermal—between the layers of the skin

noninvasive—pertaining to a procedure or technique that does not require entry into the body by incision or inserting an instrument

orthopnea—ability to breathe only in a standing or upright sitting position

ototoxicity—harmful effect of drugs on the nerves or organs in the ear

pneumothorax—the collection of air or gas in the pleural cavity that causes the lung to partially or completely collapse

pulmonary function testing—testing performed to evaluate airflow and lung volume

septum—a thin wall dividing the two sides of the interior nose

tachypnea—rapid breathing

 MEDICAL ASSISTING STANDARDS

CAAHEP ENTRY-LEVEL STANDARDS	ABHES ENTRY-LEVEL COMPETENCIES
■ Perform within scope of practice (psychomotor) ■ Explore issue of confidentiality as it applies to the medical assistant (cognitive) ■ Apply ethical behaviors, including honesty/integrity in performance of medical assisting practice (affective) ■ Explain the rationale for performance of a procedure to the patient (affective) ■ Use language/verbal skills that enable patients' understanding (affective) ■ Describe the normal function of each body system (cognitive) ■ Identify common pathology related to each body system (cognitive) ■ Analyze pathology as it relates to the interaction of body systems (cognitive) ■ Discuss implications for disease and disability when homeostasis is not maintained (cognitive) ■ Describe implications for treatment related to pathology (cognitive) ■ Apply critical thinking skills in performing patient assessment and care (affective) ■ Prepare a patient for procedures and/or treatments (psychomotor) ■ Perform handwashing (psychomotor) ■ Screen test results (psychomotor) ■ Perform pulmonary function testing (psychomotor) ■ Administer oral and parenteral medications (psychomotor) ■ Document patient care (psychomotor)	■ Project a positive attitude. ■ Maintain confidentiality at all times. ■ Be a "team player." ■ Be cognizant of ethical boundaries. ■ Exhibit initiative. ■ Adapt to change. ■ Evidence a responsible attitude. ■ Be courteous and diplomatic. ■ Conduct work within scope of education, training, and ability. ■ Interview and take a patient history. ■ Prepare patients for and assist physician with routine and specialty examinations and treatments and minor office surgery. ■ Apply principles of aseptic techniques and infection control. ■ Prepare and maintain examination and treatment area. ■ Collect and process specimens. ■ Dispose of biohazardous materials. ■ Practice Standard Precautions. ■ Prepare and administer oral and parenteral medications as directed by the physician. ■ Maintain medication and immunization records. ■ Perform respiratory testing.

 COMPETENCY SKILLS PERFORMANCE

1. Demonstrate performance of spirometry.
2. Demonstrate performance of measuring oxygen saturation using a pulse oximeter.
3. Demonstrate performance of peak flow testing.
4. Demonstrate performance of the Mantoux test by intradermal injection.
5. Demonstrate patient instruction in the use of an inhaler.
6. Demonstrate patient instruction in the use of a nebulizer.

Abbreviations

ABG—arterial blood gases

AFB—acid-fast bacillus

BCG—bacillus Calmette-Guérin

COPD—chronic obstructive pulmonary disease

ENT—ear, nose, and throat

MDI—metered dose inhaler

O₂ sat—oxygen saturation

PaCO₂—partial pressure of carbon dioxide

PaO₂—partial pressure of oxygen

PEF—peak expiratory flow

PFT—pulmonary function testing

PPD—purified protein derivative

TB—tuberculosis

Introduction

Pulmonary testing is performed to decide which part of the pulmonary system is involved in a disorder. Testing includes determining

- The patient's ability to move air in and out of the upper airway.
- The compliance of the patient's lungs.
- The effectiveness of bronchodilators and other medications.
- Therapy treatments.

A licensed respiratory care practitioner usually evaluates and analyzes pulmonary disorders.

The Medical Assistant's Role in Pulmonology

Respiratory disorders are divided according to the part of the system affected: the upper or lower area. An ear, nose, and throat (**ENT**) specialist usually treats upper respiratory disorders. Pulmonologists treat lower pulmonary, or lower respiratory, disorders. Medical assistants in the pulmonology office help patients by giving emotional support, carrying out or assisting the physician with treatments, and giving educational support to the patient as directed by the physician and respiratory technicians.

State practice acts must be followed regarding the procedures MAs can do.

The Anatomy and Physiology of the Pulmonary System

The respiratory tree consists of the lungs, air passages serving the lungs, and anatomical structures of the thoracic and abdominal cavities that surround the lungs (Figure 36-1 ◆). Each structure is dependent on the others to function.

The Upper Airway

The upper airway consists mainly of the nose, but also includes the adjacent zone structures of the pharynx, where the nasal, oral, and laryngeal cavities meet. The two sides of the interior nose are separated by the nasal **septum.** (Refer to Chapter 37, EENT, for a more detailed discussion of the anatomical structures of the upper airway.)

The Lower Airways

The lungs are located inside the thoracic cavity (chest) in a sealed system with only one opening—the upper airway. Twelve pairs of ribs surrounding the entire cavity protect the lungs.

The ribs also aid in the respiratory process as the muscles surrounding them bring air into and out of the lungs during contraction and relaxation. The **diaphragm** forms the bottom of the pleural cavity and also aids in respiration. As it rises, it helps push the air out of the lungs; as it retracts, it makes the pleural cavity larger, allowing air to enter the lungs.

The area containing the heart, lungs, and trachea is called the pleural cavity. The right lung, with three lobes, is slightly larger than the left lung, which has two. The heart is nestled in a sulcus, or fold, of the left lung. Each lung has a double-folded membranous covering, called a pleura. The inside layer is the visceral pleura, and the outer aspect is the parietal pleura. A serous, watery substance acts as a lubricant between the two layers.

The trachea is the beginning of the lower airway. The trachea divides into two branches, the right and left bronchi. The **bronchi** lead to the right and left lungs, dividing into smaller and smaller tubelike structures, eventually becoming **bronchioles.** At the end of the bronchioles are clusters of air sacs called **alveoli.** The alveolar walls are only one cell thick, facilitating the exchange of gas with surrounding capillaries. Capillary blood absorbs

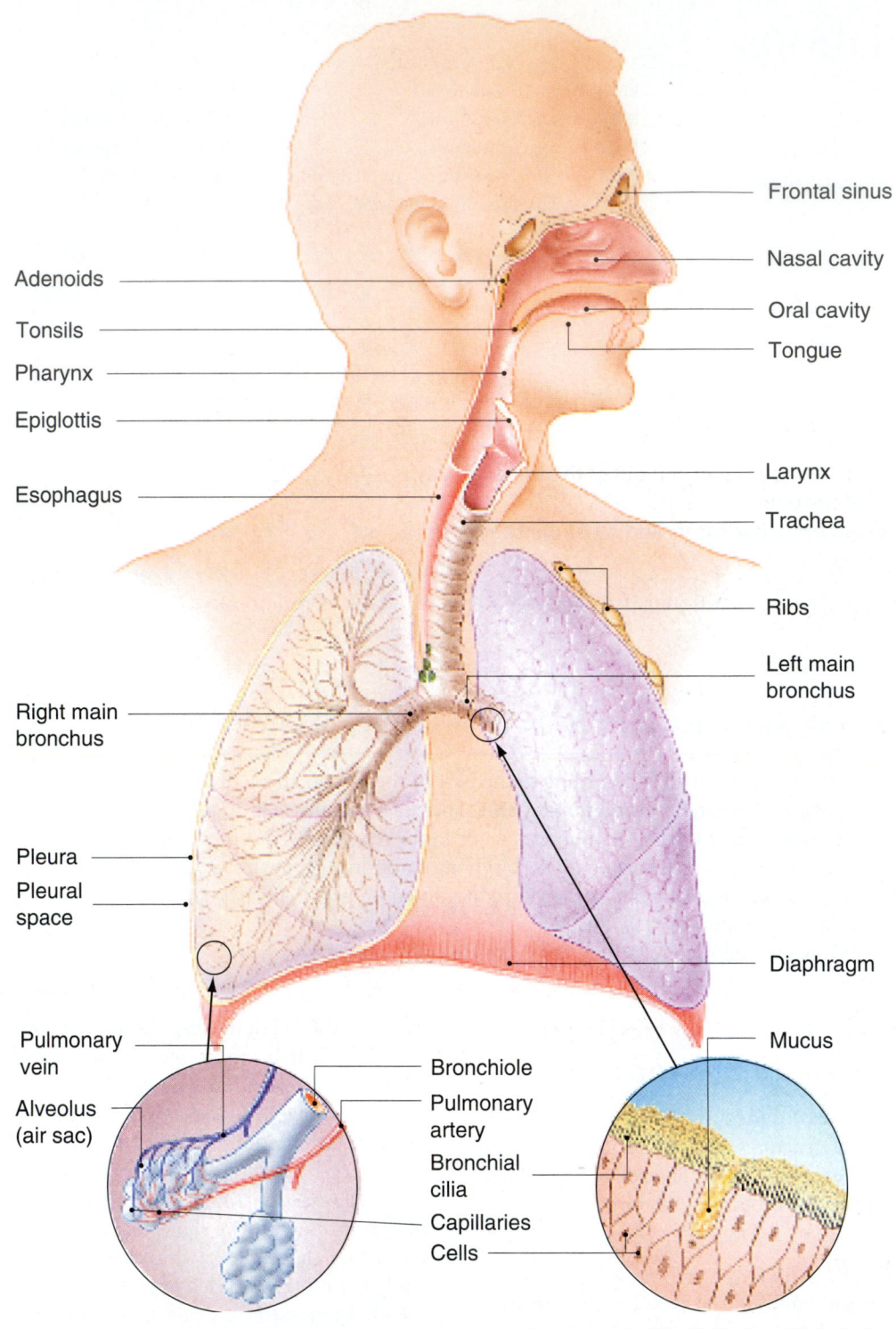

Frontal sinus

Nasal cavity

Oral cavity

Tongue

Adenoids

Tonsils

Pharynx

Epiglottis

Esophagus

Larynx

Trachea

Ribs

Left main bronchus

Right main bronchus

Pleura

Pleural space

Diaphragm

Pulmonary vein

Mucus

Alveolus (air sac)

Bronchiole

Pulmonary artery

Bronchial cilia

Capillaries

Cells

Figure 36-1 ◆ The respiratory system.

inhaled oxygen from the alveoli while exchanging carbon dioxide (CO_2), which is then exhaled from the lungs.

Pulmonary Physiology

Pulmonary physiology can be separated into lung tissue elasticity, chest mechanics, and gas exchange.

The physical mechanics of respiration are divided into inhalation and exhalation. Lungs are elastic—they return to their normal shape after being stretched. When the diaphragm falls, or relaxes, the lungs expand, creating a negative or lower pressure in the airways and cellular lung tissue. Oxygen-rich atmospheric air, of higher pressure, enters and expands the lungs. This is inhalation. This is followed by a contraction of the

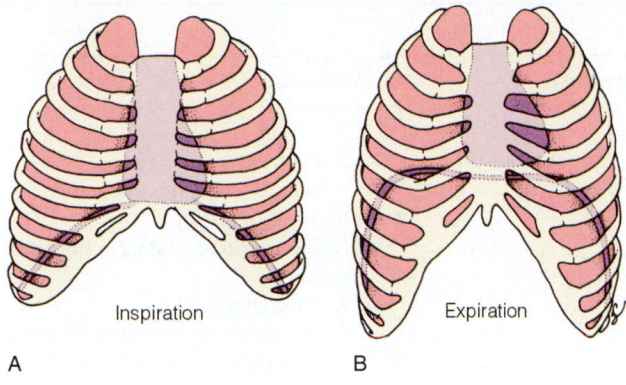

Inspiration   Expiration

A   B

Figure 36-2 ◆ (A) Inhalation (B) Exhalation.

diaphragm and thoracic muscles, which raise and squeeze lung tissue, creating higher lung pressure and lower atmospheric pressure. CO_2-laden is exhaled (Figures 36-2 ◆).

Patients with obstructive lung disease, such as **emphysema, bronchitis,** and **asthma,** have less elastic (more compliant) lungs. They can inhale fairly easily; however, their lungs do not return to their normal shape, and they trap the air.

On the other hand, some patients have more difficulty expanding their lungs. This means their lungs are more elastic (less compliant) and hold less air. Restrictive lung diseases include pulmonary edema, pneumoconiosis (also called *black lung*), and asbestosis. Black lung disease is often associated with coal miners.

Both conditions, the inability to expand the lungs or the inability to expel air, cause the patient to suffer apnea—the inability to breathe. Long-term episodes of apnea lead to hypoxemia, which may cause dizzy spells.

The Mechanics of Gas Exchange
Gases move from point to point because of the physical law of diffusion. Diffusion occurs when molecules move across a membrane from an area of high concentration to an area of low concentration. The process requires no energy expenditure. Oxygen and carbon dioxide are exchanged in the lungs through the process of diffusion.

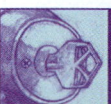

**Keys to Success
COAL MINER'S HEALTH SAFETY ACT**

"Black lung" is the common term for pneumoconiosis or anthracosis. This chronic disease is caused by breathing coal dust over an extended period and is aggravated by cigarette smoking. The Coal Miner's Health and Safety Act of 1969 was enacted to ensure the safety of coal miners, whose livelihood exposes them daily to the risk of black lung. Under the Act, coal miners must be compensated for the permanent lung damage they suffer on the job. The claim filing process requires a skilled medical claims filer in the medical office.

Blood from the right side of the heart that circulates to the lungs is oxygen-poor and carbon-dioxide-rich. As this blood enters the lung during inhalation, the available oxygen from inhalation diffuses into the blood and raises the oxygen level to 100 mmHg. The extra carbon dioxide from the blood diffuses into the lung and is exhaled. As the blood leaves the lungs, it is ready for transport to the rest of the body, replenished with oxygen and holding normal amounts of carbon dioxide. This oxygen-rich blood returns to the left side of the heart to be pumped to the heart muscle, to the head, and to all of the organs and tissues of the body.

Diseases and Disorders of the Pulmonary System

Upper respiratory disease conditions, such as acute rhinitis (common cold), rhinitis (hay fever), sinusitis, pharyngitis, and laryngitis, involve the nose and throat. The common cold is the most common upper respiratory infection and is usually caused by a viral group known as rhinovirus. (∞ See Chapter 37, EENT, for further discussion of upper respiratory diseases.)

Diseases that affect the lower respiratory system can be broadly classified into obstructive diseases, infection and inflammatory diseases, malignancies, and mechanical insults.

Lower Respiratory Obstructive Diseases

Chronic obstructive pulmonary disease (**COPD**) is the collective name for lung diseases characterized by long-term, steadily worsening airway blockage. COPD is most often caused by smoking, but long-term exposure to chemicals, fumes, or organic dust is another causative factor. Air pollution worsens symptoms. Chronic bronchitis and emphysema are the most common diagnoses linked to COPD; some patients suffer from both. Treatment includes oxygen therapy, medications, preventing infection, and quitting smoking.

Other obstructive diseases of the lower respiratory system include asthma, acute bronchitis, and pneumonoconiosis (Table 36-1). All these conditions involve airway obstruction at the bronchi, bronchioles, or alveoli.

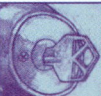

**Keys to Success
THE EFFECTS OF SMOKING**

- Physical and psychological addiction to nicotine.
- Decreased growth of lung tissue.
- Increased respiratory and cardiac symptoms and diseases.
- Higher risk of premature and low-weight births.
- Higher risk of different types of cancer.
- Shorter life expectancy.

TABLE 36-1 LOWER RESPIRATORY OBSTRUCTIVE DISEASES

Disease	Symptoms	Diagnosis	Treatment

Asthma
■ Lung disease also called bronchial asthma
■ Leading cause of childhood illness and school absences
■ Asymptomatic unless triggered by individual specific allergen or non-allergen factors
■ Attacks vary in severity
	■ SOB
	■ Wheezing
	■ Productive or nonproductive cough
	■ Leaning forward over chair, table, or counter to use accessory muscles for exhaling
	■ Skin pale and moist
	■ Cyanosis of nail bed in severe attacks
		■ Patient presenting symptoms
		■ PFT
			■ Avoid triggers
			■ Inhaler for preventive use and at onset of attack
			■ Nebulizer (used mainly in hospital setting)
			■ Asthma triggers
			  1. Allergens including mold, animal dander, dust, cockroach excrement, various foods, pollen, and household mites
			  2. stress and/or anxiety
			  3. infection
			  4. inhalation of allergens
			  5. exercise and/or overexertion
			  6. exposure to cigarette smoke
			  7. aerosol sprays or perfume

Emphysema ■ Chronic lung disease ■ Caused by trapped air in overextended, inflated alveoli	■ Mucus ■ Able or unable to cough ■ Thin, barrel-chested body type ■ Leaning forward (see "Asthma" above)	■ Patient presenting symptoms ■ Physical examination ■ Testing: PFT, chest X-rays, blood tests	■ Mucolytic agents to liquefy and loosen mucus in pulmonary airways, along with **bronchodilator,** steroid, and antibiotic medications ■ Quitting smoking, for medical reasons and for safety when using oxygen ■ "Pursed-lip" breathing to push trapped air out of the alveoli ■ Frequent, small meals and snacks to maintain health. ■ Mental health counseling and support group access when physical condition worsens and patient becomes more disabled and dependent
Acute bronchitis ■ Lung disease resulting from severe cold, flu, or no clear cause ■ Short in duration, usually lasting about 10 days ■ May progress farther down bronchial tree to bronchioles and air sacs, resulting in bronchopneumonia	■ Mucus ■ Cough ■ Possible chest pain and fever	■ Patient presenting symptoms ■ Physical examination ■ PFT	■ Rest to ease fatigue and strengthen immune system ■ Staying inside during cold weather to help prevent coughing ■ High fluid intake to thin mucous secretions and promote productive cough to clear airways ■ Avoiding cough suppressants except to allow rest. ■ Expectorants to help loosen mucus and promote productive cough ■ Antibiotics if sputum changes from gray to yellow or yellow-green, indicating possible bacterial infection ■ Quitting smoking

TABLE 36-1 LOWER RESPIRATORY OBSTRUCTIVE DISEASES (CONTINUED)

Disease	Symptoms	Diagnosis	Treatment
Chronic bronchitis ■ Lung disease resulting from repeat attacks of acute bronchitis, prolonged chemical inhalation, or cigarette smoking (main cause) ■ Occurs yearly and lasts a few months or more	■ Increase in mucus ■ Swelling and narrowing of airways ■ Chronic cough ■ Decreased ability to cough mucus from narrow airways ■ Possible increase in dyspnea ■ Greater risk for hypoxia ■ Bacterial infections possible	■ Patient presenting symptoms ■ Physical examination ■ PFT	■ See "Acute Bronchitis" ■ Yearly flu vaccination ■ Pneumonia vaccination ■ Supplemental oxygen as necessary. ■ Bronchodilators or steroids orally or via inhaler or nebulizer ■ Long-term medical management and psychological counseling
Bronchiectasis ■ Lung diseases that occur when bronchial tube walls enlarge and obstruct airway, and distended pockets below develop into sites of infection ■ May be a result of immunologic deficiency, cystic fibrosis, pneumonia-related, or obstruction ■ May progress to pneumonia	■ Productive cough with yellow or green sputum ■ Possible hemoptysis ■ Halitosis	■ Physical examination ■ Patient presenting symptoms ■ Sputum culture ■ PFT ■ Chest X-ray ■ CT scan ■ Bronchoscopy ■ Other testing (sweat test or Mantoux test)	■ Bronchodilators ■ Antibiotics ■ Postural drainage (support person helps place patient in upside-down position, so fluids drain to trachea) ■ Pulmonary percussion (support person massages patient by striking body part with light rapid blows) ■ Surgery to remove affected portion of lung
Pneumonoconiosis ■ Group of chronic obstructive lung diseases caused by inhaling dust: anthracosis or "black lung" (coal dust), silicosis (silicon), asbestosis (asbestos fibers) ■ Takes 2 to 20 years to develop; average is after 10 years of continuous exposure ■ Often considered occupational disease ■ No cure	■ Dyspnea ■ Dry cough ■ Bronchitis, asthma, and emphysema may be sequelae	■ Radiographs ■ PFT ■ ABGs	■ Avoiding exposure to causative agents with mask or respirator ■ Support treatment ■ Causative agents 　1. cigarette smoking 　2. air pollution 　3. chronic bronchitis/repeated respiratory tract infections 　4. long-term exposure to chemical irritants 　5. inhalation of corrosive gases 　6. family tendency

Infectious and Inflammatory Conditions

Infectious and inflammatory conditions include pneumonia, influenza, histoplasmosis, pulmonary tuberculosis, Legionnaire's disease, and pleuritis (Table 36-2). In these conditions, infection and inflammation are usually caused by pathogenic microorganisms, usually bacteria or viruses.

Malignancies

Respiratory system malignancies include cancer of the lung(s) and larynx. Often these malignancies show symptoms of an obstructed airway because tumor growth in any respiratory area reduces the amount of oxygen flow. A patient at risk for cancer, such as one who smokes or has a family history, needs constant support and encouragement to practice a healthier lifestyle. (∞ For further discussion of cancers related to the respiratory system, see Chapter 48, Oncology.)

Mechanical Insults

Mechanical insults include pulmonary emboli, atelectasis, and the symptoms of **hemoptysis** (Table 36-3). Major traumatic insults to the chest may cause pneumothorax, hemothorax, or hemopneumothorax. **Pneumothorax** is a condition of air in the pleural cavity that causes the lung to partially or completely collapse. **Hemothorax** is an accumulation of blood and fluids in the pleural cavity that limit the expansion of the lung. **Hemopneumothorax** is an accumulation of both blood and air in the pleural cavity, resulting in the partial or complete collapse of the lung. Depending on the severity of the condition, the patient will require observation and immediate or emergency

TABLE 36-2 INFECTIOUS AND INFLAMMATORY CONDITIONS OF THE PULMONARY SYSTEM

Disease	Symptoms	Diagnosis	Treatment
Pneumonia ▪ Lung disease with lower respiratory inflammation of bronchioles and alveoli resulting from infection ▪ Can be fatal ▪ Bilateral pneumonia affects both lungs; lobar pneumonia affects particular lobe or lobes ▪ Tuberculous pneumonia caused by *Mycobacterium tuberculosis* ▪ Secondary pneumonia is complication of another medical problem	▪ Chills ▪ Fever ▪ Chest pain or aching ▪ Cough ▪ Weakness ▪ SOB	▪ Patient presenting symptoms ▪ Physical examination ▪ Chest X-ray ▪ Sputum culture	▪ Antibiotics ▪ Rest to ease fatigue and strengthen immune system ▪ Higher fluid and calorie intake to strengthen immune system ▪ Oxygen as needed ▪ Analgesics as needed ▪ Pneumonia vaccination for prevention
Legionellosis/Legionnaire's disease ▪ Form of pneumonia caused by infection with the bacteria *Legionella pneumophila* ▪ Acute respiratory tract infection ▪ Identified after epidemic occurred at the 1976 American Legion convention in Philadelphia; over 200 people contracted the disease and 34 died as a result of the infection. ▪ Bacteria live and grow in warm aquatic environments such as cooling towers, aerosolized droplets from air conditioners, spas, and showers.	▪ Initial generalized flu-like symptoms include malaise, cough, headache. ▪ Pneumonia-like symptoms, including fever, chills, dyspnea, chest pain, anorexia, vomiting, diarrhea	▪ Radiographs of the chest ▪ Sputum cultures positive for *Legionellosis pneumophila* ▪ Elevated WBC, elevated liver emzyme levels	▪ Antibiotic therapy ▪ Antipyretics ▪ Fluid replacement if indicated ▪ Oxygen therapy
Influenza ▪ Upper respiratory viral infection that affects lungs ▪ Many varieties of virus ▪ Virus spread by moisture droplets from sneezing, coughing, or by contact with contaminated articles, such as facial tissue ▪ May put patient at risk for secondary pneumonia	▪ Cough ▪ Sore throat ▪ Sneezing ▪ Runny nose ▪ Fever ▪ Chills ▪ Muscle aches ▪ Headache ▪ Gastrointestinal symptoms (vomiting and diarrhea)	▪ Patient presenting symptoms ▪ Physical examination	▪ Rest ▪ Higher fluid intake ▪ Analgesics for pain ▪ Antipyretics to reduce fever ▪ Yearly influenza vaccination to prevent most likely flu strain(s) for that year
Histoplasmosis ▪ Fungal infection of lungs ▪ May progress to pneumonia ▪ When symptoms appear, fungus has already spread through lung tissue	▪ Weakness ▪ SOB ▪ Fever	▪ Patient presenting symptoms ▪ Chest X-ray ▪ Skin test ▪ Blood test ▪ Sputum or other tissues	▪ Antifungal medication if needed ▪ Other supportive measures and medications as needed
Pulmonary tuberculosis (TB) ▪ Infection of lung tissue, usually by *Mycobacterium tuberculosis* ▪ Spread by moisture droplets from sneezing, coughing, or contact with contaminated facial tissue; can also be inhaled through dust carrying inactive bacteria, which become active when moistened	▪ Loss of appetite, energy, and weight ▪ As infection progresses, other symptoms include dyspnea, fever, productive cough, night sweats	▪ Patient presenting symptoms ▪ Physical examination ▪ Chest X-ray ▪ Sputum test ▪ Blood test ▪ Mantoux test	▪ Preventive antibiotics when patient has been exposed to TB but does not have the active disease. (Note: Hearing and liver function must be monitored because of **ototoxicity** and **hepatotoxicty** of many anti-tuberculosis drugs)

TABLE 36-2 INFECTIOUS AND INFLAMMATORY CONDITIONS OF THE PULMONARY SYSTEM (CONTINUED)

Disease	Symptoms	Diagnosis	Treatment
Pulmonary tuberculosis (TB) ■ Although incidence of TB has been greatly reduced in the United States, case numbers are rising again			■ Antibiotics (after a prescribed period of time, patient on antibiotic therapy is no longer contagious) ■ In countries where TB is prevalent, bacillus Calmette-Guérin (**BCG**) vaccine is administered
Extrapulmonary tuberculosis ■ Disease that affects tissues and organs outside of the lungs. ■ Causative organism travels to other oxygen- and blood-rich areas of the body via lymphatic or circulatory systems ■ Accounts for about 15% of patients affected by TB ■ Other nonpulmonary organs or tissues that can be infected include bones and joints, lymph nodes, pleural space surrounding lungs, meninges surrounding brain and spinal cord, peritoneum covering abdominal organs, reproductive organs, and urinary tract	■ Symptoms relate to organ being affected	■ Patient presenting symptoms ■ Physical examination	■ TB medications ■ Other supportive measures
Pleuritis (also called pleurisy or pleuritis) ■ Lung disease with inflammation of visceral pleura membranes caused by infection, trauma, or tumor ■ Usually a secondary result of pneumonia or another infection	■ Sharp chest pains on inhaling and/or coughing	■ Patient presenting symptoms ■ Patient history ■ Physical examination ■ Auscultation of rubbing sounds ■ Chest X-ray	■ Pain medication as needed ■ Antibiotics ■ Heat compresses ■ Encircling chest bandages to decrease chest movement and pain

treatment. (∞ Other emergency respiratory conditions are discussed in Chapter 41, Emergency Care.)

Pulmonary Assessment and Diagnosis

Patients with pulmonary conditions exhibit one or more of a variety of symptoms.

- Sounds: wheezing (continuous musical sound), rales (crackles), rhonchus (wheeze, snore, or chest squeak heard on auscultation), or stridor (high-pitched, harsh sound)
- Cyanosis: a symptom of hypoxemia; often accompanies breathing difficulty or shortness of breath over a long period
- Cough: productive (with sputum) or nonproductive (dry)
- Sputum: may be blood-tinged (hemoptysis) or yellow/green (indicates infection)

- Chronic respiratory conditions: clubbing (abnormal curvature of the nail bed), barrel chest appearance, using accessory muscles (muscles that aid in a secondary way) to make up for weakened respiratory muscles and help with breathing

Respiratory breathing patterns are classified as follows:

- **Eupnea:** normal breathing
- **Dyspnea:** difficult breathing
- **Orthopnea:** breathing in a standing, or upright sitting position
- **Tachypnea:** rapid breathing

Pulmonary Function and Other Common Diagnostic Testing

Pulmonary function testing (PFT), an assessment of the performance level of respiratory system structures, is done to confirm that a patient has lung disease or to evaluate and manage

TABLE 36-3 MECHANICAL INSULTS TO THE PULMONARY SYSTEM

Mechanical Insult	Symptoms	Diagnosis	Treatment
Pulmonary embolus ■ Obstruction of pulmonary artery circulation usually caused by thrombus formed in deep veins of legs but also by foreign matter such as a piece of fat, air bubble, amniotic fluid, tumor cells, piece of bone marrow ■ Requires immediate emergency treatment (death may be sudden without treatment)	■ Usually sudden, severe chest pain ■ Cough, possibly producing bloody sputum ■ SOB ■ Tachypnea ■ Syncope ■ Skin possibly cool and clammy, pale, or cyanotic ■ Blood pressure drop ■ Rapid, weak pulse ■ Anxiety ■ Oxygen SAT drop	■ Patient presenting symptoms ■ Patient history ■ Radiograph of chest ■ Perfusion scan ■ Pulmonary angiogram ■ Doppler ultrasound studies of deep leg veins for deep vein thrombosis (DVT)	■ Supplemental oxygen ■ Thrombolytic and anticoagulant drugs to ease fatigue and strengthen immune system ■ Anti-embolism (TED™) stockings after surgery or during inactivity ■ Ambulation as soon as possible after surgery ■ Blood coagulation studies ■ Activity to avoid lengthy periods of sitting ■ Quitting smoking, especially females using hormonal birth control
Atelectasis ■ Partial lung collapse that affects alveoli ■ Caused by obstruction in airway, such as mucus plug, tumor, or foreign body ■ Possible complication following surgery ■ Requires rapid and/or emergency treatment	■ Dyspnea ■ SOB ■ Rapid heartbeat ■ Diaphoresis ■ Cyanosis ■ Substernal retraction	■ Auscultation ■ Radiographs ■ Bronchoscopy ■ CT examination	■ Suction, coughing, or bronchoscopy to remove obstruction ■ Antibiotics for infection ■ Surgery to remove any tumor ■ Preoperative deep breathing (incentive spirometry) and deep cough training for the immediate postoperative period
Hemotypsis ■ Consequence of disease process or trauma to respiratory tract ■ Causes include respiratory infection, trauma, drug abuse, especially cocaine, vascular disorders, bronchitis, inhaled foreign bodies, blood clotting disorders ■ Copious amounts of blood may be life threatening	■ Blood in sputum (bright red, dark red, or pink-tinged) ■ Spitting up blood ■ Coughing up blood ■ Pain possible	■ Patient presenting symptoms ■ Patient history ■ Physical examination ■ Imaging studies ■ Bronchoscopy	■ Intervention to halt blood flow ■ Removal of foreign bodies ■ Cauterization or ligation of blood vessels
Sleep apnea ■ Intermittent cessation of breathing ■ Usually caused by relaxation of tongue muscles, allowing tongue to fall back into oral pharynx and block airway ■ Apneic periods may last 60 to 90 seconds and occur 30 to 500 times during 7-hour sleep cycle ■ Condition may lead to heart attacks and strokes ■ Sleepiness may cause motor vehicle accidents and other accidents involving machinery	■ Excessive daytime sleepiness ■ Restless sleep ■ Snoring with apneic spells ■ Memory loss ■ Nighttime chest pain ■ Hypertension ■ Choking sensation during sleep ■ Depression ■ Morning headaches	■ Polysomnography (sleep studies)	■ Continuous positive airway pressure (CPAP) to keep airway open ■ Surgery (uvulopalatopharyngoplasty [UPPP] or radio frequency ablation, both of which have limited success) ■ BiPAP

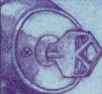

**Keys to Success
MUCUS OR MUCOUS?**

It is important that you use the terms *mucus* and *mucous* correctly.

- *Mucus* is a noun. It refers a thick fluid secreted by the mucous membranes of the respiratory, gastrointestinal, reproductive, and urinary tracts. Mucus serves as a lubricant and contains substances that slow microbial growth.
- *Mucous* is the adjective form of *mucus* and is used to describe a noun—for example, mucous membrane.

diagnosed pulmonary disorders. PFT is not used to identify a specific respiratory disease but to measure the effects of disease. There are several types of PFTs, including spirometry, lung volume, and diffusion capacity.

- Spirometry, a noninvasive test, measures the exhalation capacity of the lungs and is very helpful in tracking the progression of acute or chronic respiratory conditions such as asthma, COPD, and respiratory infections or the effects of asthma medication. Spirometry is also used as a postoperative treatment.
- Lung volume measures the inhalation capacity of the lungs, such as in emphysema.
- Diffusion capacity measures the amount of test-administered carbon monoxide absorbed in one cycle of inhalation and exhalation. The difference between the amount of carbon monoxide inhaled and the amount exhaled is an estimate of how long it takes inhaled gas to travel from the lungs to the capillary system. Adult Respiratory Distress Syndrome (ARDS) is an example of a traumatic respiratory condition that severely affects gas diffusion capabilities.

Other common diagnostic studies include chest X-ray, arterial blood gases, pulse oximetry, methacholine challenge, sputum collection for cytology and for culture and sensitivity, sweat test, and bronchoscopy.

- Chest X-rays are a **noninvasive** tool for diagnosing or screening for respiratory infections (including pneumonia, tuberculosis, and lung abscess), lung tumors, or conditions of sudden respiratory distress, such as pneumothorax (Figure 36-3 ◆). They are contraindicated for pregnant women.
- Arterial blood gases (**ABGs**) are used to analyze the acid/base balance of blood in chronic respiratory and acute respiratory, metabolic, and traumatic conditions. Examples of these conditions include COPD, ARDS, emphysema, pulmonary embolism, pneumonia, bronchitis, anxiety, fever, and diabetic ketoacidosis. ABGs also measures oxygen saturation and the carbon dioxide level of the arterial blood. Arterial blood gases are drawn from an artery, often a painful procedure. Pressure must be maintained on the puncture site for at least 3 to 5 minutes to seal the arterial wound and prevent bleeding.

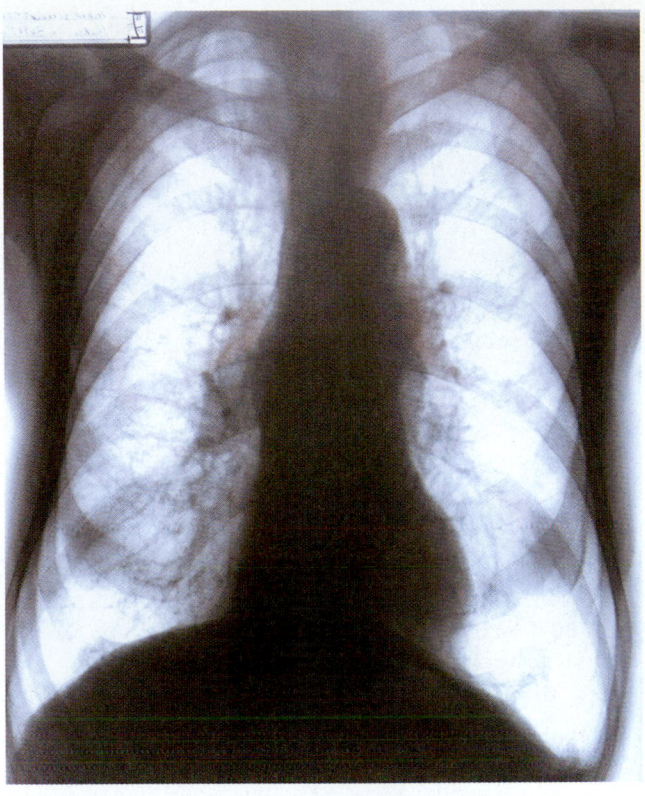

Figure 36-3 ◆ Chest X-ray of a patient with emphysema.
Source: Scott Camazine, Photo Researchers, Inc.

After an arterial blood sample is obtained, the sealed tubes containing the arterial blood are placed in a container of ice and must be transported to a laboratory and processed immediately. The laboratory values direct the treatment procedures, which are directed largely toward returning the values of pH, pCO_2, pO_2, and HCO_3 to normal for the patient.

- Pulse oximetry is an early, noninvasive screening test of blood gas status or oxygen saturation (**O_2 sat**) of tissues (Figure 36-4 ◆). It is used to analyze symptoms of cardiac, circulatory, or respiratory distress such as chest pain, dyspnea, nasal flaring, decreased consciousness, wheezing, skin color changes (paleness or cyanosis); clinical signs of shock; and symptoms following exposure to intense heat, smoke, or flame. Pulse oximetry has replaced ABGs to some extent.
- The methacholine challenge test is used in the diagnosis and treatment of asthma. The patient inhales periodic and increasing amounts of the medication methacholine and undergoes PFTs to assess the reaction of the bronchial airways and the effect on the respiratory system. Patients with certain medical conditions—including a known history of aneurysm, heart attack, stroke, chronic uncontrolled hypertension, myasthenia gravis, or who are presently pregnant or nursing—are advised not to take the methacholine challenge.
- Sputum cultures obtained by a respiratory therapist are used to diagnose respiratory infections, such as pneumonia. A deep pulmonary sputum sample is obtained by deep

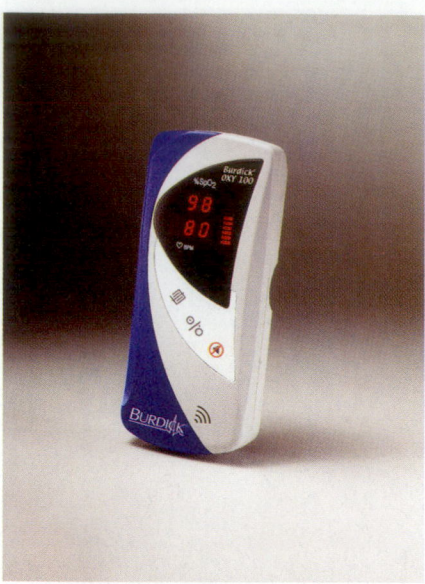

Figure 36-4 ◆ Burdick pulse oximeter.
Courtesy of Cardiac Science Corp.

thoracic coughing, stimulation, or suctioning. A specimen of saliva, rather than sputum, obtained by any individual not trained in sputum collection procedures may yield inaccurate test results. Sputum collection is beyond the scope of training of medical assistants.

- Sputum samples for cytology are used to diagnose lung carcinoma (malignant tumor). A deep pulmonary sputum sample is obtained by deep thoracic coughing, stimulation, suctioning, or during a bronchoscopy.
- Sputum samples for acid-fast bacilli (**AFB**) are used in culture testing for pulmonary tuberculosis.
- Blood tests for theophylline level reveal inadequate, excessive, or toxic medication levels within the bloodstream.
- A sweat test is performed to confirm diagnosis of cystic fibrosis. Parents often bring a child to the medical office stating that the child tastes like salt when kissed. A colorless, odorless chemical is applied to the child's skin and a sweat collection device is attached for 30 minutes to one hour. The sweat specimen is analyzed for sodium and chloride. The initial diagnosis is based on several symptoms, including foul-smelling, frothy stool; heavy pulmonary

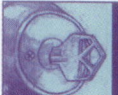

Keys to Success
SPUTUM SPECIMEN

Saliva is a clear fluid secreted from the salivary glands into the mouth to begin digestion. Sputum is material that is coughed up from the lungs and expectorated through the mouth. When obtaining a sputum specimen, ask the patient to take a deep breath and cough up secretions from deep within the lungs. This lessens the chance of getting a "spit" or saliva specimen.

secretions; and other GI symptoms. The sweat test is not a primary diagnostic test.

- Bronchoscopy is a tool for visualizing the bronchial tree, clearing mucous obstructions, and obtaining a biopsy. It is an invasive procedure that requires operative consent. It may be performed under a general or local anesthetic. Patients are required to take nothing by mouth (NPO) for at least 8 hours before the test. They are also restricted from drinking or eating until the gag reflex has returned (usually about 8 hours postprocedure).
- Other diagnostic tests include the peak flow test and Mantoux test, which are discussed in greater detail later in this chapter.

Critical Thinking Question 36-1

Keera has been given the directions for obtaining a sputum sample and has observed the technique being performed. Now that it is her turn, what precautions should she take?

In Practice

The physician orders spirometry testing for Tony Rodriquez, a 10-year-old who has a history of asthma. The patient's mother states that her son just started wheezing, and she is concerned that his medication is not working. She thinks that Tony needs an X-ray and doesn't understand why the doctor has ordered spirometry testing. What should you as the medical assistant tell the mother?

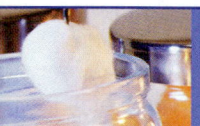

PROCEDURE 36-1 Demonstrate Performance of Spirometry

Theory and Rationale

With spirometry PFT, baseline information can be obtained about a patient's normal breathing, deep inhaling, or exhaling. The patient should be instructed not to eat a large meal or smoke for 4 to 6 hours before the PFT. The physician will also order bronchodilator drugs to be used during testing.

A nose clip helps focus the patient's efforts on sealing his or her lips around the mouthpiece and prevents air leaks from the nostrils. Make sure the patient puts forth the greatest possible effort for the best results.

During the PFT you will stay with the patient to instruct and provide emotional coaching. Your presence can decrease the patient's anxiety.

PROCEDURE 36-1 Demonstrate Performance of Spirometry *(continued)*

Materials
- spirometer
- disposable mouthpiece and tubing
- nose clip
- chart
- forms and lab slips for documentation and testing

Competency
(**Conditions**) With the necessary materials, (**Task**) you will be able to assist the patient in the performance of spirometry testing (**Standards**) correctly within 30 minutes.

1. Wash your hands. Gather equipment and supplies.
2. Identify the patient and guide him or her to the treatment area.
3. Record the patient's history and main complaint. Explain the entire procedure.
4. If the patient is chewing gum, ask him or her to dispose of it (to prevent choking during the test). If a female patient is wearing lipstick, ask her to remove it to create a tight seal.
5. Ask the patient to place the mouthpiece in his or her mouth and to close the lips tightly around the mouthpiece to make a good seal (Figure 36-5 ◆).
6. Place the nose clips on the patient's nose, sealing the nostrils closed (Figure 36-6 ◆).
7. Ask the patient to inhale as deeply as he or she possibly can and hold the breath for a short time. Then tell the patient to blow the air out into the mouthpiece as hard and as fast as possible—until he or she cannot blow out any more air (Figure 36-7 ◆).
8. Repeat this procedure two more times, giving the patient a few minutes in between.
9. The electronic equipment will usually "select" the best of the three breathing tests.
10. Document patient compliance with and tolerance of the testing procedure.
11. Follow cleaning procedures to prepare the equipment and the area for the next patient.
12. Wash your hands.

Patient Education
Explain to the patient that the purpose of the procedure is to monitor the progress of a disease or how well treatment is working and that medical treatment is based on the findings of regularly scheduled PFTs. Encourage the patient to tell the physician if the treatment is not working.

Charting Example
08/12/XX 9:00 a.m. Pt stated that last meal was at 6:00 a.m.— one egg, one toast slice, and one cup coffee. Pt stated physician wanted no bronchodilator medication until after the test. Pt followed test instructions with slight shortness of breath, but recovered within 2 minutes to repeat. Results given to physician for evaluation. Margaret Jones, CMA (AAMA)

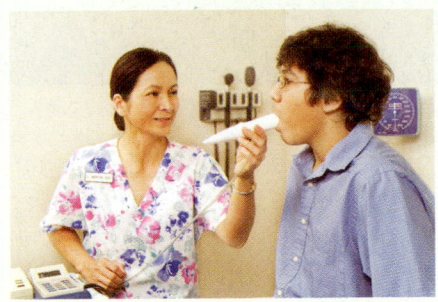

Figure 36-5 ◆ The patient should close the lips tightly around the mouthpiece.

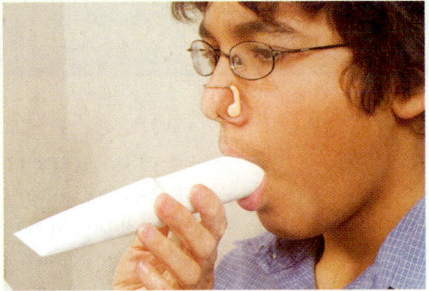

Figure 36-6 ◆ Place the nose clips on the patient's nose.

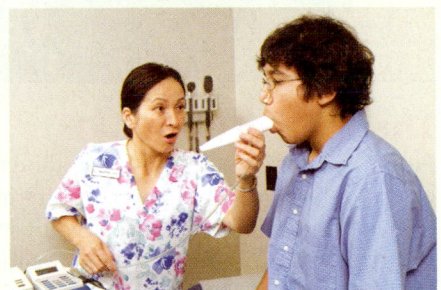

Figure 36-7 ◆ Direct the patient to blow the air out into the mouthpiece as hard and as fast as possible.

ABGs and Pulse Oximetry
It is critical to determine a patient's oxygen status. In an acute care setting, an invasive procedure known as arterial blood gas (ABG) analysis has been widely used. An ABG measures oxygen status (PaO_2 values), acid-base status (pH values), the body's ability to expel cellular waste products ($PaCO_2$ values), and possible causes of respiratory disease (Table 36-4). The information

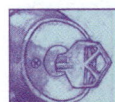

Keys to Success
COMPLIANCE VERSUS COMPLIANCE

When referring to the lungs, *compliance* means the elasticity of the lungs for breathing. When referring to the patient, *compliance* means ability to follow instructions.

TABLE 36-4 NORMAL VALUES FOR ABGS

ABG	Normal Range
Arterial pH	7.35–7.45 ■ <7.35 indicates acidosis ■ >7.45 indicates alkalosis
Arterial $PaCO_2$	35–45 mm Hg ■ When CO_2 is abnormal, the condition has a respiratory cause and the HCO_3 is normal.
Arterial HCO_3	22–26 mEq/L ■ When HCO_3 is abnormal, the condition has a metabolic cause and the pCO_2 is normal. ■ This value reflects the metabolic function of the kidneys.
Arterial PaO_2	80–100 mm Hg ■ If pO_2 is < 50 mm Hg, oxygen therapy is required
Arterial O_2 sat	95% or greater

from this study reveals how well the lungs are functioning to meet the body's oxygen needs. Only specially trained professionals can perform ABGs. The MA should check the practice acts in his or her state.

A newer, noninvasive method called pulse oximetry has gained popularity in both medical offices and acute care settings.

Although it measures oxygen saturation (SAT) indirectly rather than by blood sample analysis, pulse oximetry is a fairly simple procedure for testing a patient's oxygen status. In the clinical setting, the abbreviated terms "pulse ox" or "O_2 sat" may be used to refer to this procedure.

Pulse oximeters light up the tissues with infrared light. Oxygen-rich tissues emit a different wavelength of light than oxygen-poor tissues, and oxygen saturation is measured with these wavelengths. The lower limit of acceptable oxygen saturation is 85 percent. A patient with saturations below this level requires oxygen from a supplemental source.

Attachment points for pulse oximetry include the fingertip (most common site), earlobe, and tip of the toe. Wherever it is attached, the oximeter must fit securely. On a fingertip, nail polish, poor fit or contact with the sensor, very low blood pressure, severe anemia, or a poorly calibrated pulse oximeter can have a negative affect on a pulse oximetry reading.

Peak Flow Testing

Peak flow testing measures a patient's maximum ability to exhale (pulmonary airflow). It is one of a variety of pulmonary function tests that measures air capacity of the lungs (spirometry). Peak flow, or air flow, rates are also used to monitor the effectiveness of medication or determine the need for different medical treatment. Peak flow rates change according to the patient's medical condition, body frame, and age, as well as the time of the day the test is taken.

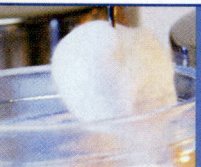

PROCEDURE 36-2 Demonstrate Performance of Measuring Oxygen Saturation Using a Pulse Oximeter

Theory and Rationale

Pulse oximetry is a noninvasive method to measure the oxygen saturation of hemoglobin in arterial blood. The pulse oximeter is a handheld device used by many medical facilities to assess a patient's oxygenation status with such respiratory disorders as pneumonia, bronchitis, emphysema, and asthma. The pulse oximeter sensor can be placed on a patient's finger, earlobe, toe, or bridge of the nose. An appropriate site can be selected by assessing capillary refill in the patient's toe or finger. If the patient has poor circulation in his fingers or toes, then use the bridge of the nose or an earlobe. Nail polish can alter results and must be removed.

The pulse oximeter uses a beam of infrared light to pass through the tissue, and the device measures the pulse and the amount of light absorbed by the hemoglobin, which is displayed as a percentage on the screen. Instruct the patient to breathe normally during the procedure. A normal pulse oximeter reading is greater than or equal to 95%. Any reading less than 95% could indicate hypoxemia and may require some type of intervention or treatment such as oxygen or bronchodilator therapies.

Materials

- pulse oximeter
- alcohol wipe
- nail polish remover as needed
- patient chart

Competency

(**Conditions**) With the necessary materials, (**Task**) you will be able to measure oxygen saturation using a pulse oximeter (**Standards**) within 30 minutes.

1. Wash your hands and gather equipment and supplies.
2. Identify the patient and guide him or her to the treatment area.
3. Explain the procedure to the patient.
4. Select the appropriate size sensor (pediatric, small, or large).
5. Instruct the patient to breathe normally.
6. Prepare the selected site (earlobe or finger) (Figure 36-8 ◆). Remove nail polish or earrings if necessary.
7. Wipe the selected site with alcohol and allow to air dry.

PROCEDURE 36-2 Demonstrate Performance of Measuring Oxygen Saturation Using a Pulse Oximeter *(continued)*

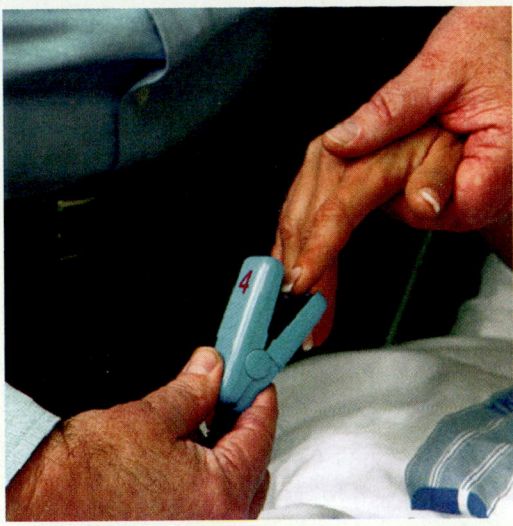

Figure 36-8 ◆ Pulse oximeter: The sensor probe is applied securely, flush with skin, making sure that both sensor probes are aligned directly opposite each other.

8. Attach the sensor to the site and connect to the pulse oximeter. Turn on the pulse oximeter and listen to the tone.
9. Read the saturation level and document it in the patient's chart. Report to the physician readings that are less than 95%.

Patient Education

Discuss the procedure with the patient beforehand. Instruct patient to limit movement throughout procedure since patient movement may be interpreted as arterial pulsations. Inform patient to alert the healthcare provider or medical assistant if he or she begins to experience respiratory distress or difficulty breathing.

Charting Example

5/12/xx Pt. Instructed to limit movement and alert medical assistant of any respiratory difficulty. Pulse oximeter was placed on left middle finger. Blood Saturation Level 96%. Michele Carpenter, RMA (AMI)

Airflow rate is measured with a peak flow meter after the patient has inhaled as deeply as possible and then exhaled as rapidly and fully as possible (Figure 36-9 ◆). The test is repeated at least three times for accuracy.

A peak flow meter measures liters per second or liters per minute. Because there are many types of peak flow meters, it is important to use the same kind for each patient to maintain uniform and accurate tests results. These meters can be mechanical or computerized.

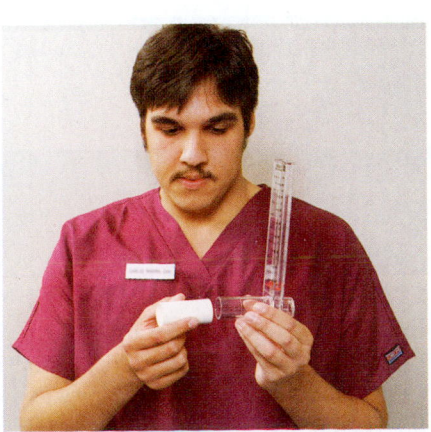

Figure 36-9 ◆ Peak flow meter.

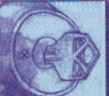

Keys to Success
PATIENT REASSURANCE

A patient who is dependent on supplemental oxygen and must undergo PFT can be very frightened. The thought of having the oxygen flow interrupted and not being able to breathe is very difficult to handle. To calm the patient:
■ Explain the entire procedure.
■ Explain that you will be there throughout the entire testing procedure and an oxygen supply will be available.
■ Stay with the patient until the procedure is complete.
■ Help the patient to restore the supplemental oxygen flow.

Mantoux Test

The Mantoux test is used to screen patients for contact with or presence of the active disease state of **TB.** Each positive result is followed by another Mantoux test and/or chest X-ray to

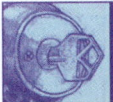

Keys to Success
INTRADERMAL TESTING

Intradermal injection is used in allergy testing as well as in the Mantoux test. For allergy testing, a permanent marker is used to label each site after the allergy substance is injected.

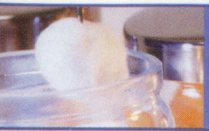

PROCEDURE 36-3 Demonstrate Performance of Peak Flow Testing

Theory and Rationale

A peak flow meter can detect an asthma attack before symptoms occur. This information allows the patient to prevent symptoms or reduce their effect. Peak flow testing gives the patient greater control over monitoring and managing the condition.

Taking peak flow readings under different conditions, such as before and after exercise, after exposure to pets, or after exposure to tobacco smoke or allergens, makes the symptoms easier to identify. If an asthma attack occurs, the patient and/or medical staff can make decisions based on the readings about whether the patient can manage the situation at home or will require emergency medical treatment at the hospital.

Materials

- peak flow meter
- patient log or diary of peak flow readings
- patient chart

Competency

(**Conditions**) With the necessary materials, (**Task**) you will be able to assist the patient in the performance of peak flow testing (**Standards**) correctly within 30 minutes.

1. Wash your hands completely. Gather equipment and supplies.
2. Identify the patient and guide him or her to the treatment area.
3. Instruct the patient to take as deep a breath as possible, place the mouthpiece just in front of the teeth, then use his or her lips to make a complete seal. Ask the patient to exhale as hard and as fast as possible (Figure 36-10 ◆).
4. Have the patient repeat step 3 three times.
5. If test results also need to be taken after medication, allow the patient to rest. Administer the medication, then repeat the test.
6. Clean the equipment and dispose of contaminated materials appropriately.

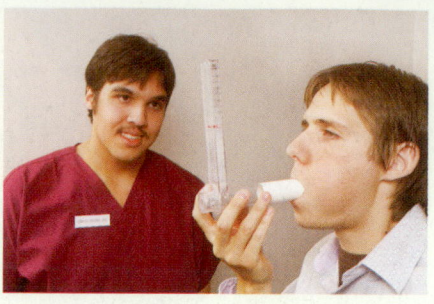

Figure 36-10 ◆ Ask the patient to exhale as hard and as fast as possible.

7. Wash your hands.
8. Record the results. Compare the results with previous readings.

Patient Education

The physician determines the pattern for peak flow testing. He or she may require that the patient be tested after awakening, before going to bed, before and after taking medications (such as inhalers), or in the presence of asthma attack triggers.

Stress to the patient the importance of following the testing schedule and the proper procedure. Give the patient a form to keep track of peak expiratory flow (**PEF**) readings, which measure highest rate of airflow that can be forced during expiration. Instruct the patient to bring the form to medical office visits and to keep and carry a medication list for medical visits or emergencies.

Charting Example

01/27/XX 12:30 p.m. ↑ shortness of breath & asthma attacks. Pt states ↑ in asthma attacks are probably due to additional emotional stress at work. A copy of the pt's PEF readings attached for physician review. John Banks, RMA (AMT)

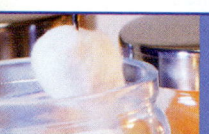

PROCEDURE 36-4 Demonstrate Performance of the Mantoux Test by Intradermal Injection

Theory and Rationale

Find a site on the patient's lower forearm without hair or blemishes. Because the medication's composition may be affected by exposure to light, prepare the medication syringe immediately prior to administration. The administration of a PPD via intradermal injection is a uniquely different method of injection and has rules for administration that vary greatly from all other types of injections. It is important that alcohol is not used to cleanse the skin prior to the application of the PPD. Alcohol, even when allowed to dry on

PROCEDURE 36-4 Demonstrate Performance of the Mantoux Test by Intradermal Injection *(continued)*

the skin, has been shown to alter the reaction of the medication. The skin can be cleansed by scrubbing with sterile water and cotton balls or gauze pads. Unlike other types of injections, the administration of PPD also specifies that the medical assistant should not aspirate; doing so will cause skin and tissue damage. The final unique difference with PPD application is that a bandage must not be applied over the administration site. The bandage can create pressure, expelling the solution from the wheal, invalidating the test results. If the patient has slight bleeding, a small cotton ball can be placed directly above the site but should not be allowed to wick any of the medication from the wheal. Preparing the medication immediately before administering it also helps to maintain the needle's sterility and allows you to proceed without recapping the needle.

After administration of the Mantoux, a return visit is scheduled so that test results may be measured and documented. Only induration, not redness, is measured. Usually, an induration less than 2 millimeters (mm) across is considered a negative result. An induration greater than 2 mm must be reported to the local health department.

Materials
- patient chart
- disposable gloves
- sterile water and cotton balls
- sharps container
- tuberculin syringe and needle unit with safety device
- vial of medication
- bandage strips

Competency

(Conditions) With the necessary materials, **(Task)** you will be able to perform the Mantoux test **(Standards)** correctly within 15 minutes.

1. Wash your hands and gather the equipment.
2. Identify the patient and guide him or her to the treatment area.
3. Wash your hands again and put on disposable gloves.
4. Ask the patient to reach out with one hand and turn the palm upward. Find a site without hair or blemishes on the forearm.
5. Cleanse the top of the PPD vial with an alcohol wipe and allow it to air-dry (Figure 36-11 ◆). Withdraw 0.1 cc from the vial and hold it in your dominant hand.

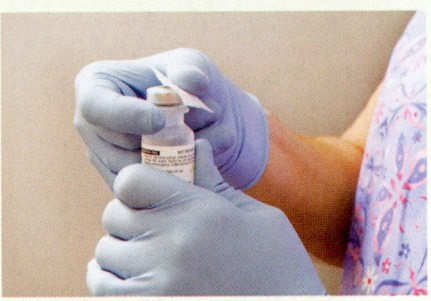

Figure 36-11 ◆ Clean the top of the medication vial.

6. Place your nondominant hand under the patient's forearm and gently pull the skin tight. Ask the patient to keep the arm still. Insert the needle bevel just into and under the skin at a 10- to 15-degree angle (Figure 36-12 ◆).
7. Inject the medication slowly to create a raised blister, or wheal (Figure 36-13 ◆).
8. Release the skin, then withdraw the needle and blot the area gently with an alcohol wipe.
9. Discard the syringe in the sharps container.
10. Make an appointment for the patient to return and have the injection site checked after 48 to 72 hours.
11. Document the procedure, including a description of the Mantoux test site.
12. When the patient returns, measure only the induration, *not* the redness. For positive results, measure in millimeters (mm) and follow local public health guidelines for reporting.

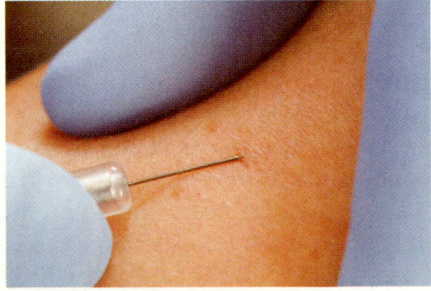

Figure 36-12 ◆ Insert the needle bevel just into and under the skin of the patient's forearm.

continued

PROCEDURE 36-4 Demonstrate Performance of the Mantoux Test by Intradermal Injection *(continued)*

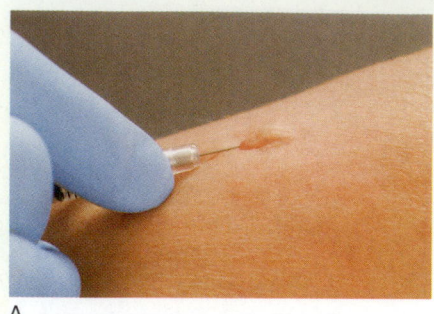
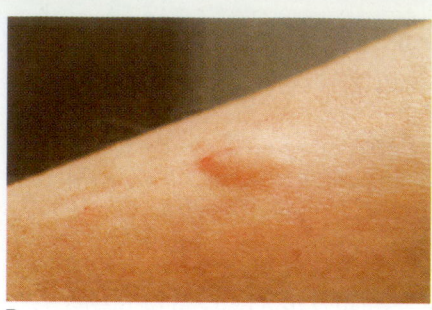

A   B

Figure 36-13 ◆ (A) Inject the medicine slowly to create a raised blister, or wheal (B) Wheal on patient's arm.

Patient Education

Discuss the procedure with the patient beforehand, including what to expect afterwards and on the return visit. Tell the patient not to irritate the test site by scratching or wearing scratchy clothing. Explain that some redness is to be expected and that a return check will be necessary to measure the induration, if any, and to observe the test site.

Charting Example

03/27/XX 2:40 p.m. Mantoux test was given following office procedure into pt's R forearm area. The pt was instructed to make a return appointment 48 to 72 hours after the test for observation and test results. Michelle Carter, RMA (AMT)

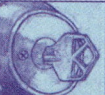

Keys to Success
VACCINATIONS

Pneumonia immunization can prevent pneumonia-related deaths and is generally recommended once for elderly patients over 65 and nursing home patients. It is also suggested for patients with chronic illness(es), a compromised immune system, or organ transplant(s).

Influenza vaccinations are recommended yearly for elderly patients, patients with chronic illnesses, and healthcare workers. Flu shots should not be given to individuals who are sensitive or allergic to eggs because the vaccination is made from viruses grown in eggs. Any allergic reaction usually occurs immediately after the injection. It is also common to experience mild flu symptoms, such as malaise, fever, and muscle pain, after immunization.

The BCG (bacillus Calmette-Guérin) vaccine is used for TB prevention in countries outside of the United States. The effectiveness varies from zero to 80 percent. Once the vaccination is given, the patient shows a positive reaction to tuberculin skin testing and needs chest X-rays to diagnose or rule out TB. The Centers for Disease Control (CDC) has guidelines for the use of the BCG vaccination for specific groups in the United States.

negate or confirm the earlier results. Positive results indicate only that the patient carries the TB bacteria. It does not indicate an active TB disease process. *(Note:* The first Mantoux test may not yield a reaction in a patient with lowered immunity and a more severe infection. Later, as the patient regains **immunocompetence,** repeated Mantoux testing with PPD will cause the expected induration at the injection site.)

The Mantoux test is administered by **intradermal** injection of purified protein derivative (**PPD**). Institutions such as nursing and retirement homes require repeat testing before admitting a patient. A positive reaction occurs more slowly in an elderly person and may not show unless a repeat test is given.

Inhalers and Nebulizers

Inhalers and nebulizers are devices used to treat obstructive airway conditions. Patient and caregiver teaching are essential to successful treatment with either device.

Inhalers are pocket-sized, portable devices for the self-administration of medication directly into the respiratory system. In addition to portability, inhalers have several advantages. They are available in many different medications. They deliver a consistent, metered dose of medication to the airways. Proper technique is very important, however, and the oral route must be easily accomplished by the patient. Another drawback is the high out-of-pocket cost per dose.

? **—Critical Thinking Question 36-2—**

Keera has just instructed the patient in the correct way to use a metered dose inhaler (**MDI**). What other instructions or methods should she mention to the patient?

The nebulizer delivers fine particles of medication to the patient via compressed air or oxygen through tubing and a mask (Figure 36-14 ◆). This delivery method is effective even if the patient has a severe problem with breathing. Nebulizers are used mainly in hospitals, but can also be used in outpatient or ambulatory care settings. With its reusable mouthpiece and mask, the nebulizer is a good alternative for those who have difficulty using inhalers. The mask is the easiest delivery route for pediatric patients. The major disadvantage of nebulizers has been that they are difficult to carry; however, a battery-operated nebulizer without a mask has recently been developed.

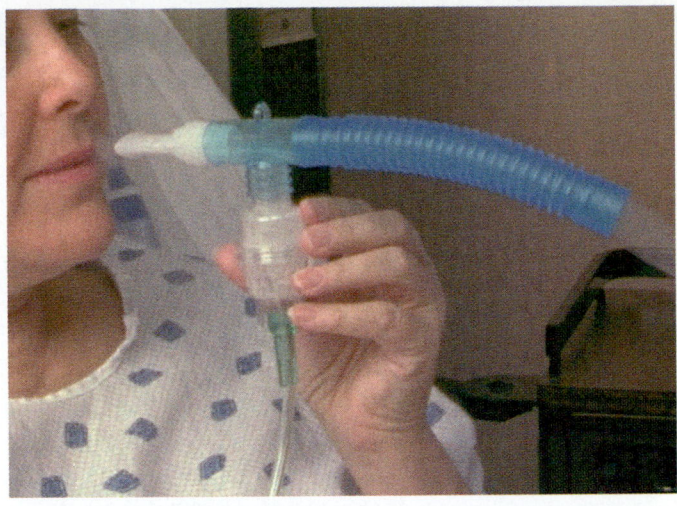

Figure 36-14 ◆ Nebulizer.

PROCEDURE 36-5   Demonstrate Patient Instruction in the Use of an Inhaler

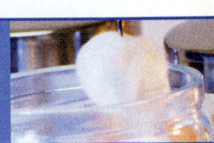

Theory and Rationale

When you instruct a patient in the use of an inhaler, keep these points in mind:

- Take note of any physical problems that may prevent correct handling. For example, a patient with arthritic hands may not be able to use an inhaler.
- The inhaler canister should be thoroughly shaken to mix the medication particles evenly.
- Holding the canister in the upright position (not at an angle) ensures that the metered dose is delivered correctly.
- The patient must inhale slowly and as deeply as possible and hold the breath to ensure that the medication penetrates deeply into the bronchial tree and lungs.

Materials

- patient's prescription inhaler
- patient's chart

Competency

(**Conditions**) With the necessary materials, (**Task**) you will be able to instruct and/or help the patient use an inhaler for the first time (**Standard**) correctly within one hour.

1. Wash your hands and gather the equipment.
2. Identify and guide the patient to the treatment area.
3. Give the patient the following instructions.
   - Shake the canister thoroughly.
   - Hold the canister upright within 2 inches of the mouth. Place the mouthpiece in your mouth, sealing the opening with your lips (Figure 36-15 ◆).

- Activate the inhaler (usually by pressing the canister down) to spray (Figure 36-16 ◆). Breathe slowly but deeply after the medication is delivered.
- Hold your breath for as long as possible, up to 10 seconds.

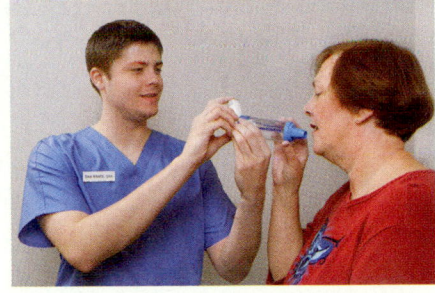

Figure 36-15 ◆ Patient with inhaler held upright.

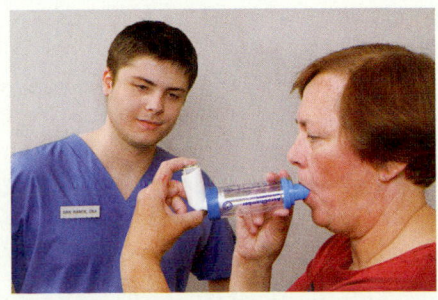

Figure 36-16 ◆ Activate the inhaler.

continued

PROCEDURE 36-5 Demonstrate Patient Instruction in the Use of an Inhaler *(continued)*

- Begin breathing normally again.
- Follow the physician's instructions for immediate repeat use.

4. Document the patient's ability to follow instructions. Inform the physician if the patient has any problems with self-administration. Give the patient backup written instructions.

Patient Education

Inform the patient about the side effects of the medication at normal prescription levels and the consequences of overuse.

Tell the patient to call the physician if the medication appears not to help or if symptoms worsen.

Charting Sample

11/23/XX 2:30 p.m. Pt demonstrated correct use of the inhaler with instruction. Written instructions were given with the office's phone number. Pt states that medication has helped make breathing easier. Parker Clay, CMA (AAMA)

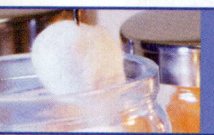

PROCEDURE 36-6 Demonstrate Patient Instruction in the Use of a Nebulizer

Theory and Rationale

Nebulizer treatments may be given after baseline PFT. Testing is then repeated to measure the patient's response to medications in the nebulizer. Medications (usually premixed) are placed in the nebulizer, which is then attached to a compressor source, and an aerosol mist is produced for the patient to inhale through a mask.

Materials

- compressor
- nebulizer with mask and tubing
- medications
- patient's chart

Competency

(Conditions) With the necessary materials, **(Task)** you will be able to assist the patient in the use of a nebulizer **(Standards)** correctly within 30 minutes.

1. Wash your hands. Gather equipment and supplies.
2. Identify the patient and guide him or her to the treatment area.
3. Obtain vital signs.
4. Wash your hands again.
5. Prepare the nebulizer cup with medication(s) as ordered and/or prescribed (Figure 36-17 ◆).
6. Turn on the compressor (Figure 36-18 ◆).
7. Instruct, or help, the patient to hold the mask while the medication is being delivered.
8. Continue treatment until no medication remains in the nebulizer. Monitor the patient's pulse every 5 minutes throughout the treatment (Figure 36-19 ◆). If the pulse

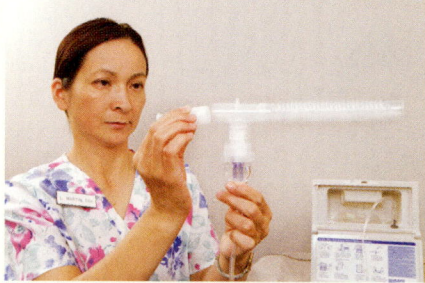

Figure 36-17 ◆ Prepare the nebulizer cup with medication(s) as ordered and/or prescribed.

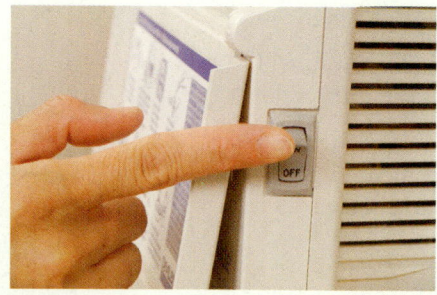

Figure 36-18 ◆ Turn on the compressor.

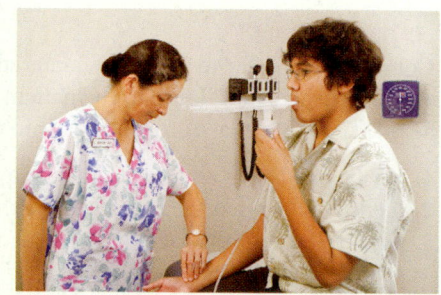

Figure 36-19 ◆ Monitor the patient's pulse.

PROCEDURE 36-6 Demonstrate Patient Instruction in the Use of a Nebulizer *(continued)*

rises to 120 beats per minute or the patient's condition worsens, *stop the treatment and tell the physician.*

9. Dispose of used materials in the appropriate containers.
10. Wash your hands.
11. Document the patient's vital signs at the beginning, middle, and end of the treatment. Also describe patient signs and symptoms at beginning and end of treatment.

Patient Education

Instruct the patient or significant other in how to do this procedure at home, and how often. After you demonstrate the procedure, have the patient or significant other return the demonstration and show you how to monitor the pulse during the procedure. If the pulse rises above 120 beats per minute, the treatment should be stopped. The physician will have to change the medication or adjust the dosage or frequency.

Charting Example

12/27/XX 2:45 p.m. Instructions given to pt's wife to perform the nebulizer treatment. She demonstrated the procedure correctly. She described the correct frequency and symptoms to observe and demonstrated the correct procedure for counting a radial pulse. Susan Tucker, RMA (AMT)

Oxygen Therapy

Oxygen therapy is administered for three primary reasons:

■ To decrease the work of breathing
■ To decrease the work of the heart
■ To reverse or prevent low blood oxygen levels

In an outpatient setting, the oxygen is usually delivered by way of a nasal cannula (also called *nasal prongs*) (Figure 36-20 ◆). The patient is attached by tubing to a portable oxygen concentrator or oxygen tank. The oxygen can also be delivered by mask.

Oxygen is a prescription drug that is administered only after a physician has written an order describing the method and concentration of oxygen delivery—for example: "Oxygen via nasal cannula at 2 liters per minute." The patient should be instructed *not* to change the flow rate without the physician's permission or direction. Doing so may worsen the patient's medical condition. The patient should be taught how to pad the skin where the oxygen tubing may rub against it and cause irritation.

The MA should instruct the patient in the safe use of oxygen. Although oxygen does not burn or explode, it can "fuel" a small spark or flame. The patient should be told that when oxygen is being used to avoid substances considered flammable, such as oil-based lubricants, smoking materials, open gas, or heat sources. If a patient tries to smoke in the medical office

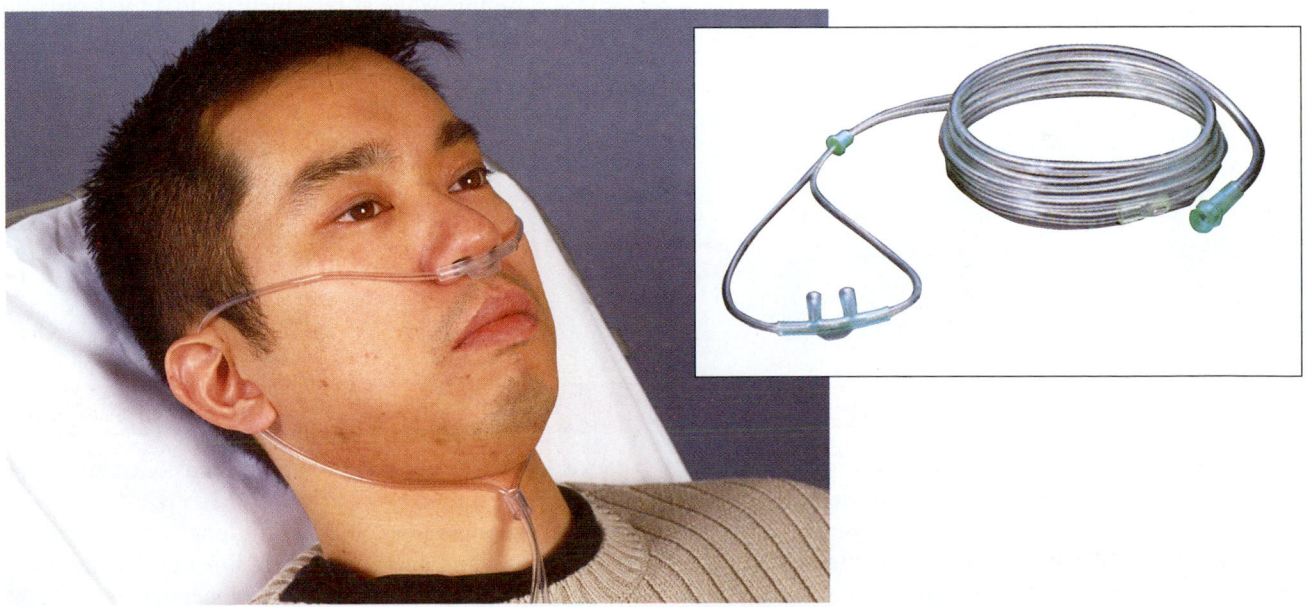

Figure 36-20 ◆ Nasal cannula.

with oxygen running, no-smoking office policies should be reinforced. If a patient is smoking, the oxygen flow should be stopped and the patient asked to put out the cigarette. Oxygen should be restarted only after the cigarette is put out. If the patient needs to moisten dry lips or nostrils caused by oxygen therapy, *only* a water-soluble lubricant may be used.

Traveling requires additional preparation. The patient should be informed to always carry his or her oxygen prescription. Before flying, the patient should check with the airline about proper procedures to follow. The physician should be alerted as well. He or she will provide the patient with specific instructions about oxygen flow rate during the high-altitude phases of the trip.

Common Oxygen Therapy Equipment

The following are different types of oxygen therapy equipment:

Oxygen tanks—Oxygen tanks come in a variety of sizes according to use and need for portability.

E tank—Small tank that holds approximately 500 liters of oxygen for patient home use in the event of power failure.

H tank—Kept in the medical office and holds approximately 6900 liters of oxygen. Used for in-office emergencies and testing patient's need for oxygen therapy.

C tank—This is a standard size, small portable tank that the patient may use for short trips away from the home. This tank holds approximately 240 liters of oxygen.

Liquid oxygen—Liquid oxygen is also commonly referred to as cryogenic liquid, its scientific name. When oxygen is liquefied it will have a boiling point of −297.3°F (−183.0°C). Although great care must be taken in the storage system of liquid oxygen, it is much less bulky than in gas form and therefore costs much less to store. A typical storage system consists of a cryogenic storage tank constructed much like a metal thermos container with inner and outer shells, one or more vaporizers, a pressure control system, and all piping necessary for the fill, vaporization, and supply functions.

Conserving device—During normal inhalation and exhalation a shift in pressure in the diaphragm occurs. This shift in pressure sends a signal that travels through the nasal cannula to a pressure sensor in the conserving device. An electronic circuit then opens an electrical valve to deliver a precisely metered dose of oxygen that has been prescribed by a physician. After the initial dose of oxygen is delivered, the system will automatically reset in anticipation for the next inhalation from the patient. Oxygen does not continue to flow when the patient is exhaling so there is much less oxygen wasted.

Concentrator—If oxygen is ordered for home use, the medical assistant will order a concentrator that runs off electricity and makes its own oxygen without the need for refilling.

Tubing—Oxygen can be delivered to the patient via a nasal cannula, which is disposable, lightweight, and easily slips into the nasal openings, or a full face mask. The face mask is used much less often because it is cumbersome, uncomfortable, and can give the patient a sense of being smothered, causing anxiety.

Typical flow rate—A patient's oxygen is ordered as a flow rate per liters in minute increments. For example, a patient who requires 2 liters of continuous oxygen will have a prescription that may read: Oxygen: 2 lpm via nasal cannula/continuous. Oxygen can be ordered as a supplement when the patient is being physically active, at rest, at night, or continuous. Individual diagnoses will determine the amount of oxygen ordered and for what extent of time. Patients may also have multiple orders for oxygen therapy, such as 2 liters per minute while at rest, increase to 4 liters per minute with exertion.

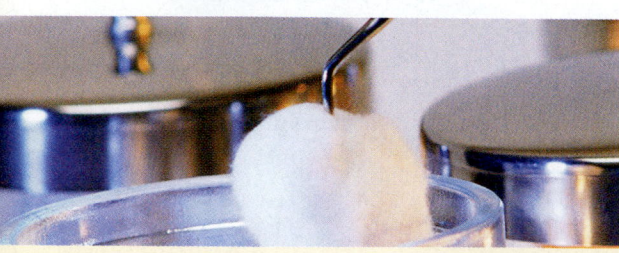

REVIEW

Chapter Summary

- Pulmonary testing measures the patient's lung elasticity and ability to breathe and has an impact on medications and treatment.
- Upper respiratory diseases are usually treated by an ENT. Lower respiratory disorders are treated by a pulmonologist. As a medical assistant you will assist with examinations, perform treatments, and provide emotional and educational support to the patient.
- The respiratory tree comprises the lungs, air passages serving the lungs, and anatomical structures of the thoracic and abdominal cavities that surround the lungs.

Chapter Summary (continued)

■ In the respiration process, oxygen is inhaled and carbon dioxide is exhaled. Blood from the right heart is oxygen poor and carbon dioxide rich. As this blood enters the lungs, oxygen diffuses into the blood and raises the oxygen level to 100 mmHg.

■ Pulse oximetry is a noninvasive form of testing that measures the oxygen content of the blood. Peak flow testing examines pulmonary airflow by measuring rapid, full, forced exhaling. It is used to evaluate pulmonary conditions or the medical management of those conditions.

■ Respiratory breathing patterns include eupnea, dyspnea, orthopnea, and tachypnea.

■ Obstructive diseases of the lower respiratory system include asthma, acute bronchitis, chronic bronchitis, emphysema, and bronchiectasis. In these conditions, the bronchial tree or portions of the alveoli are obstructed, decreasing oxygen to the body tissues.

■ Inhalers are portable devices for the self-administration of medication directly into the respiratory system. Nebulizers are used to treat respiratory conditions when oral medications or inhalers do not produce the required results. Oxygen therapy helps patients who use their accessory muscles to breathe by decreasing the workload of a weakened heart and preventing or reversing low blood oxygen levels.

■ Infectious and inflammatory pulmonary conditions include pneumonia, influenza, histoplasmosis, pulmonary tuberculosis, and pleuritis. In these conditions, infection and the resulting inflammation are usually caused by bacteria or viruses.

■ Mechanical insults include pulmonary emboli, atelectasis, and the signs and/or symptoms of hemoptysis (spitting or coughing up blood).

Chapter Review

Multiple Choice

1. The lower airways begin at the
   a. nose.
   b. true vocal cords.
   c. upper palate.
   d. sinuses.

2. Pulse oximetry is gaining use over arterial blood gas tests because it is
   a. noninvasive.
   b. invasive.
   c. more accurate.
   d. more mechanical.

3. The lowest acceptable oxygen sat limit for a patient is
   a. 55 percent.
   b. 65 percent.
   c. 75 percent.
   d. 85 percent.

4. Peak flow testing is used to measure a patient's
   a. maximum ability to inhale.
   b. minimum ability to exhale.
   c. maximum ability to exhale.
   d. minimum ability to inhale.

5. Nebulizer treatment must be stopped immediately and the physician alerted if the patient's pulse is
   a. higher than 120 beats per minute.
   b. 90 beats per minute.
   c. 100 beats per minute.
   d. lower than 110 beats per minute.

6. When oxygen therapy is ordered for a patient for home use, he or she would use
   a. an E tank
   b. a C tank
   c. liquid oxygen
   d. all of the above

7. Which of the following is acceptable for use during oxygen therapy?
   a. Water-based lubricants
   b. Hairspray
   c. Cigarette
   d. Oil-based lubricants

8. Which of the following steps is used to reduce the patient's bleeding after an intradermal test?
   a. Pulling the patient's forearm skin more tightly before removing the needle.
   b. Injecting the site on the patient's forearm without gently pulling it tight.
   c. Selecting a site on the patient's forearm with hair.
   d. Releasing the patient's forearm skin gently before removing the needle.

9. An induration is a
   a. rash.
   b. scratch.
   c. swelling.
   d. cut.

10. Which of the following is a mechanical insult?
    a. Pneumonia
    b. Pulmonary embolism
    c. TB
    d. Asthma

Chapter Review (continued)

True/False

T F 1. The upper airway includes the pharynx and the nasal, oral, and laryngeal cavities.

T F 2. The lungs are in a sealed system with only one opening.

T F 3. The right lung has more lobes than the left lung.

T F 4. The diaphragm is located in the chest cavity, above the pleural cavity.

T F 5. The trachea branches into several different branches like a tree.

Short Answer

1. Describe the condition of the lungs in obstructive lung disease.

2. Describe the condition of the lungs in pulmonary edema.

3. What is a sweat test used to confirm?

4. What is the function of the Mantoux test?

5. What does lung volume measure?

Research

1. Find a "float diagram" for MDI inhaler use. It will show your patients a quick and easy method for seeing how much medication is left in the inhaler.

2. Do some research to find patient instructions on how to correctly use an MDI inhaler, a spacer device, and a disc inhaler.

Externship Application Experience

A patient using supplemental nasal oxygen starts to light a cigarette in the medical office. As a medical assistant, what should you do?

Resource Guide

American Lung Association
61 Broadway, 6th Floor
New York, NY 10019
1-800-586-4872
www.lungusa.org

Committee on Accreditation of Respiratory Care (COARC)
1248 Harwood Rd.
Bedford, TX 76021-4244
817-283-2835
www.coarc.com

National Board for Respiratory Care (NBRC)
8310 Nieman Rd.
Lenexa, KS 66214-1579
913-599-4200
www.NBRC.org

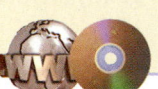

MedMedia

http://www.MyMAKit.com

More on this chapter, including interactive resources, can be found on the Student CD-ROM accompanying this textbook and on http://www.MyMAKit.com.

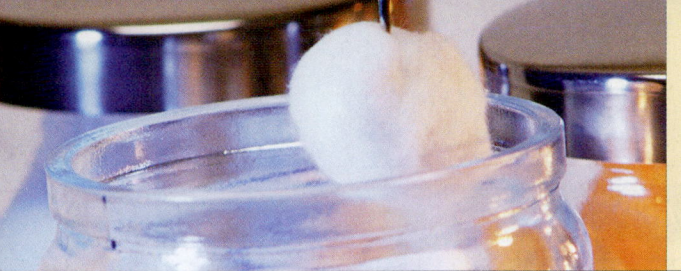

Objectives

After completing this chapter, you should be able to:

- Define and spell the key terminology in this chapter.
- Define the medical assistant's role in the EENT office.
- List and describe the roles of EENT healthcare providers.
- Describe the anatomy and physiology of the eye.
- List and discuss diseases and disorders of the eye.
- Discuss diagnostic procedures and assessments related to the eyes.
- Describe the anatomy and physiology of the ear.
- List and discuss diseases and disorders of the ear.
- Discuss diagnostic procedures and assessments related to the ears.
- Describe the anatomy and physiology of the nose and nasal passages.
- List and discuss diseases of the nasal passages and sinuses.
- Describe the anatomy and physiology of the throat.
- List and discuss diseases of the throat.

EENT

Case Study

Stacy has a busy day ahead of her at the EENT office where she is finishing her externship. First on the list of patients is a 4-year-old girl who got sand in her right eye after falling off the swing at the school playground. Next is a college student who must take a Snellen eye test for her sports physical. The receptionist has just alerted Stacy that a mother is bringing in her 3-year-old son, who stuck a small toy in his nose and then pushed it up too far for his mother to retrieve with her finger.

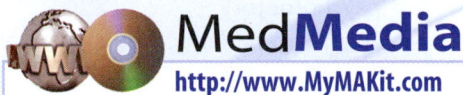

Med**Media**

http://www.MyMAKit.com

Additional interactive resources and activities for this chapter can be found on http://www.MyMAKit.com. For a video, tips, audio glossary, legal and ethical scenarios, job scenarios, quizzes, games, virtual tours and activities related to the content of this chapter, please access the accompanying CD-ROM in this book.

Video: *Pediatrics*
Audio Glossary
Legal and Ethical Scenario: *EENT*
On the Job Scenario: *EENT*
Multiple Choice Quiz
Games: Crossword, Strikeout, and Spelling Bee
3D Virtual Tours: Ear: The Ear; Eye: The Eye
Drag & Drop: Ear; Eye
Tips
HIPAA Quiz

Key Terminology

acuity—keenness or sharpness

audiologist—professional trained to assess hearing levels

audiometry—measuring and testing hearing acuity

cerumen—earwax; waxy substance secreted in external ear canal

decibel—unit for measuring the intensity of sound

degenerative—impaired in function or condition over time

intraocular—within the eye

laryngologist—physician specializing in disorders and diseases of the throat

nasal septum—cartilage wall that divides the nasal cavity

ophthalmologist—physician who specializes in the treatment of eye diseases and disorders

optician—trained professional who grinds lens, inserts the lens into frames, and fits the patient's glasses

optometrist—licensed professional (Doctor of Optometric Medicine) who examines eyes, tests for visual acuity, and prescribes and adapts lens for patients

otic—pertaining to the ear

otologist—physician who specializes in the treatment of ear diseases

otolaryngologist—physician who specializes in the treatment of ear and throat diseases

otorhinolaryngologist—physician who specializes in ear, nose, and throat diseases

purulent—containing pus

rhinologist—physician who specializes in the treatment of nasal passage and sinus diseases

tinnitus—ringing in the ears

vertigo—dizziness

Abbreviations

dB—decibels

EENT—eye, ear, nose, and throat

FB—foreign body

OD—right eye

OS—left eye

✚ MEDICAL ASSISTING STANDARDS

CAAHEP ENTRY-LEVEL STANDARDS	ABHES ENTRY-LEVEL COMPETENCIES
■ Perform within scope of practice (psychomotor) ■ Explore issue of confidentiality as it applies to the medical assistant (cognitive) ■ Apply ethical behaviors, including honesty/integrity in performance of medical assisting practice (affective) ■ Explain the rationale for performance of a procedure to the patient (affective) ■ Use language/verbal skills that enable patients' understanding (affective) ■ Describe the normal function of each body system (cognitive) ■ Identify common pathology related to each body system (cognitive) ■ Analyze pathology as it relates to the interaction of body systems (cognitive) ■ Discuss implications for disease and disability when homeostasis is not maintained (cognitive) ■ Describe implications for treatment related to pathology (cognitive) ■ Apply critical thinking skills in performing patient assessment and care (affective) ■ Prepare a patient for procedures and/or treatments (psychomotor) ■ Perform handwashing (psychomotor) ■ Screen test results (psychomotor) ■ Obtain vital signs (psychomotor) ■ Obtain specimens for microbiological testing (psychomotor) ■ Administer parenteral medications (psychomotor) ■ Document patient care (psychomotor)	■ Project a positive attitude. ■ Maintain confidentiality at all times. ■ Be a "team player." ■ Be cognizant of ethical boundaries. ■ Exhibit initiative. ■ Adapt to change. ■ Evidence a responsible attitude. ■ Be courteous and diplomatic. ■ Conduct work within scope of education, training, and ability. ■ Interview and take a patient history. ■ Prepare patients for and assist physician with routine and specialty examinations and treatments and minor office surgery. ■ Apply principles of aseptic techniques and infection control. ■ Prepare and maintain examination and treatment area. ■ Collect and process specimens. ■ Dispose of biohazardous materials. ■ Practice Standard Precautions. ■ Prepare and administer oral and parenteral medications as directed by the physician. ■ Maintain medication and immunization records. ■ Obtain throat specimen for microbiological testing.

✓ COMPETENCY SKILLS PERFORMANCE

1. Measure distance visual acuity with a Snellen chart.
2. Perform the Ishihara color vision test.
3. Perform eye irrigation.
4. Perform instillation of eye medication.
5. Perform simple audiometry.
6. Perform ear irrigation.
7. Perform instillation of an ear medication.
8. Assist with the nasal examination and obtain nasopharyngeal specimen.

Introduction

Physicians who specialize in eye, ear, nose, and throat conditions include the following:

- **Ophthalmologist**—eye diseases and conditions
- **Otorhinolaryngologist**—ear, nose, and throat diseases and conditions
- **Otolaryngologist**—ear and throat diseases and disorders
- **Laryngologist**—throat diseases and disorders
- **Rhinologist**—nose diseases and disorders
- **Otologist**—ear diseases and disorders

Optometrists and **opticians** are not physicians, although an optometrist (Doctor of Optometric Medicine) may refer a patient to an ophthalmologist for evaluation if a condition or disease is noted. Optometrists are trained to examine eyes, test visual **acuity,** and prescribe adaptive lenses and contact lenses. Opticians are trained to grind lenses, insert lenses into frames, and fit eyeglasses.

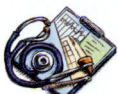

The Medical Assistant's Role in an EENT Practice

The medical assistant may use skills and knowledge in an **EENT** practice by:

- Obtaining and recording vital signs and patient history.
- Testing visual acuity.
- Performing **audiometry.**
- Performing eye and ear irrigations and instillations.

The MA may be offered additional specialty training that will enable him or her to do advanced audiometric exams and fit glasses.

The Anatomy and Physiology of the Eye

The eye is the organ of sight. It is protected by the eyebrows, lids that open and close, eyelashes, and the frontal orbital sockets of the skull (Figure 37-1 ◆). The conjunctiva, the mucous membrane covering the eyeball and lining the eyelid, moistens the eye.

The eyeball is made of three concentric (having a common center) layers of tissue: the sclera, the choroid, and the retina.

- The sclera is a tough white fibrous tissue that covers the outside of the eyeball. The extrinsic muscles that move the eye are attached to the sclera. A clear or transparent area of the sclera, the cornea, is located in the frontal portion of the eye and is covered with delicate epithelium.
- The middle layer of the wall of the eyeball is the choroid or vascular tunic. This layer contains numerous blood vessels, lymphatics, and the intrinsic eye muscles. The iris, the ciliary body, and the choroid are all contained in the middle layer. Functions of the choroid include regulating the amount of light entering the eye, supplying a route for blood vessels that provide nourishment and oxygen to the eye, secretion, and absorption.
- The retina, the innermost layer of the eye, contains sensory receptors called rods and cones. The cones are responsible mainly for color vision and daytime vision, and the rods are responsible for black and white vision and vision in dim light. The area of sharpest or most distinct vision is a concentration of cones in a small depression in the center of the posterior portion of the retina called the fovea centralis. Images are transmitted from the retina to the brain by the optic nerve.

The globe of the eye is filled with humors, watery fluids that help maintain the eye's internal pressure. Aqueous humor fills the space before the lens, and vitreous humor fills the space behind the lens. The lens lies at the rear of the anterior chamber of the eyeball.

The iris, the colored part of the eye, regulates the amount of light that enters the eye. The black spot in the middle of the iris is the pupil. Bright light reduces pupil size as the circular muscle of the iris contracts. The pupil dilates in the dark or in dim light as those muscles relax.

Vision is the result of light refraction (bending from a straight path). Light enters the sclera at the transparent cornea (the first part of the eye that refracts light). It then passes through the pupil. It is kept from scattering in the choroid. The rod and cone cells of the retina receive the light refraction image. The optic nerve at the back of the eye transmits the image through the thalamus (a division of the brain) and ends in the vision region of the cerebral cortex. At first the image is upside down. The cerebral cortex inverts it, and the image becomes what people see (Figure 37-2 ◆).

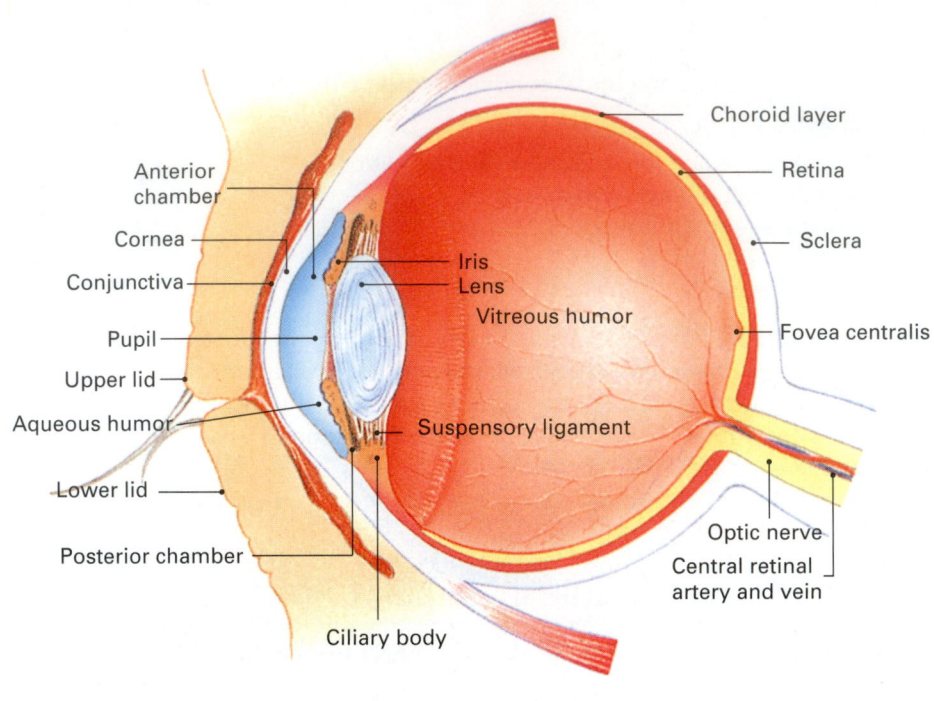

Figure 37-1 ◆ Anatomy of the eye.

Intrinsic muscles within the eye are the iris (colored membrane) and the ciliary muscle. The iris controls the size of the pupil and the amount of light that reaches the retina. The ciliary muscle changes the shape of the lens and how light is refracted to the retina.

Six extrinsic (outside) muscles control the movement of each eye:

■ Superior rectus muscle: moves the eye to look upwards
■ Inferior rectus muscle: moves the eye to look down

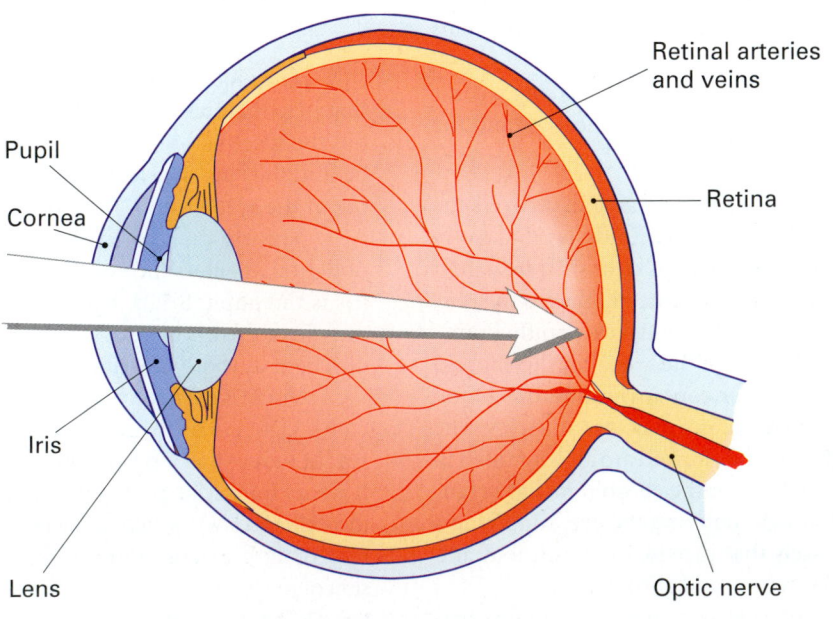

Figure 37-2 ◆ Light entering the eye.

■ Lateral rectus muscle: moves the eye laterally (corner to corner)
■ Medial rectus muscle: moves the eye medially (to the middle)
■ Superior oblique muscle: rolls the eye as it looks down and to the side
■ Inferior oblique muscle: rolls the eye as it looks up and to the side

Disorders and Diseases of the Eye

Common problems affecting vision and the eyes can be broadly classified as refractive, infectious, or **degenerative,** with additional disorders resulting from injury or foreign bodies in the eye.

■ Refractive disorders: As light passes through the eye to the retina, a break in the direct path may occur, with the result that the image is not focused directly on the retina. This change in the path of the image is a refractive error. There are four variations from normal—myopia, hyperopia, astigmatism, and presbyopia.
■ Infectious disorders: These include conjunctivitis, keratitis, blepharitis, and styes (Figures 37-3 ◆ through 37-6 ◆).
■ Degenerative disorders: Include cataracts (Figure 37-7 ◆), diabetic retinopathy, macular degeneration, strabismus, nystagmus, and glaucoma. As a patient ages, visual acuity typically becomes impaired. The condition may result in blindness.
■ Other disorders: Retinal detachment may be the result of a degenerative process or a traumatic insult. Regardless of the cause, medical care is necessary to prevent permanent vision loss. Foreign bodies (**FB**) are a common cause of eye injuries.

Table 37-1 summarizes common eye diseases and disorders in these categories.

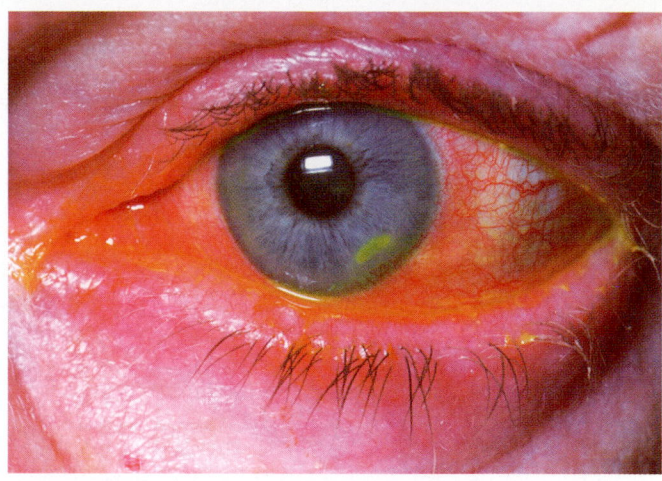

Figure 37-4 ◆ Eye with keratitis.
Source: Photo Researchers, Inc.

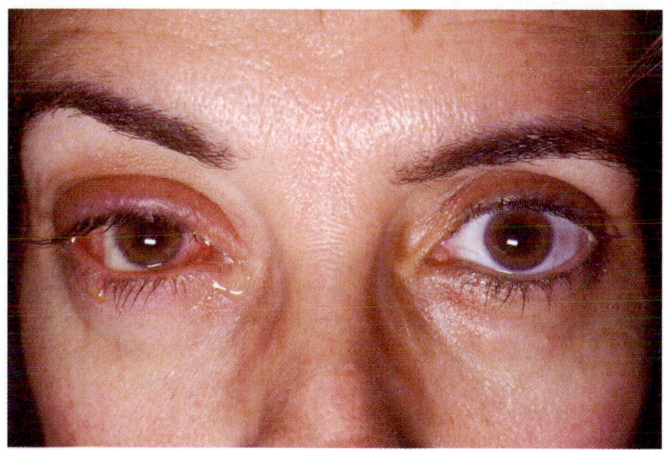

Figure 37-5 ◆ Eye with blepharitis.
Source: Phototake NYC.

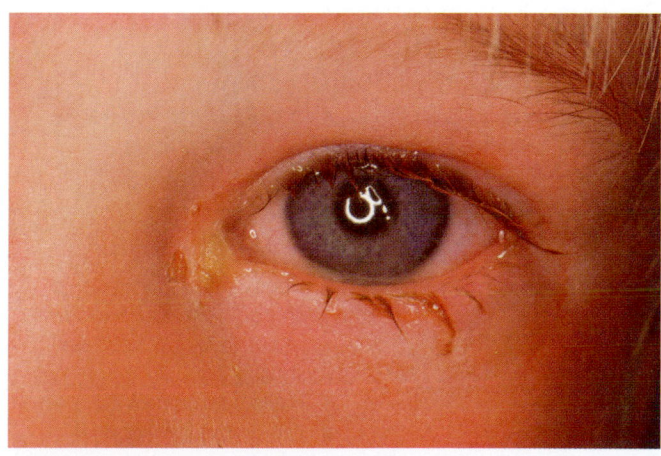

Figure 37-3 ◆ Eye with conjunctivitis.
Source: Dorling Kindersley Media Library.

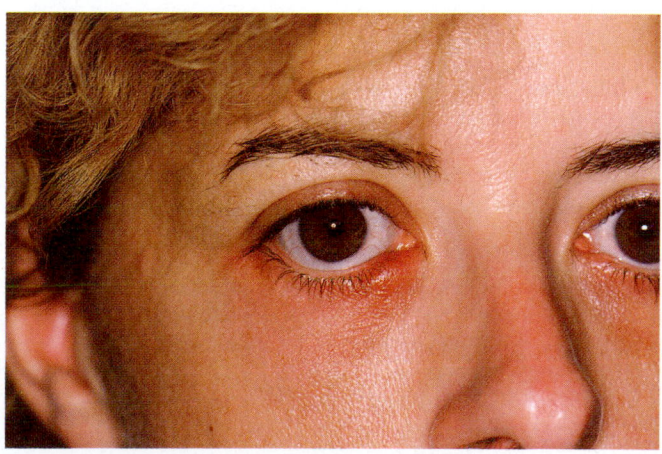

Figure 37-6 ◆ Eye with stye.
Source: Phototake NYC.

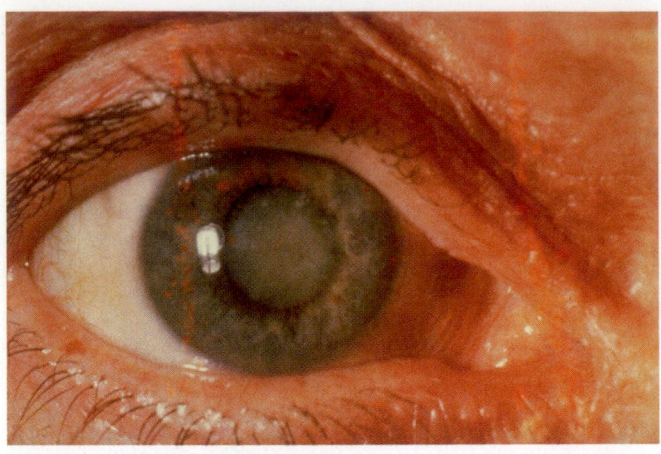

Figure 37-7 ◆ Eye with cataract.
Source: Photo Researchers, Inc.

Diagnostic Procedures

The eyes are examined with a variety of instruments, including the following:

- Ophthalmoscope: used to examine the retina and other internal structures of the eye (Figure 37-8 ◆)
- Slit lamp: used to examine and perform specialized procedures within the front structures of the eye (Figure 37-9 ◆)
- Eye spud: used to remove a foreign particle or rust ring from the cornea
- Tonometer: used to measure **intraocular** pressure (Figure 37-10 ◆)

Visual Acuity

A patient's visual acuity is measured in his or her ability to read letters on a special chart at a specific distance. Testing is performed

TABLE 37-1 DISEASES AND DISORDERS OF EYE

Disorder or Disease	Symptoms	Diagnosis	Treatment
Astigmatism ■ Eyeball is shorter than normal and image focuses behind retina	■ Inability to focus on objects (blurry vision)	■ Ophthalmologic exam ■ Astigmatoscopy ■ Jaeger chart ■ Snellen chart	■ Corrective lens
Blepharitis ■ Inflammation and infection of hair follicles and glands at margins of eyelids ■ Caused by virus, bacterial infection (*Staphylococcus*), allergic response, exposure to irritants	■ Red, tender, sore eyelids with sticky drainage ■ Watering of eyes ■ Possible eyelid inversion ■ Possible loss of eyelashes	■ Patient presenting symptoms	■ Moist heat to provide relief ■ Ophthalmic drops or ointment ■ Patient care
Cataract ■ Condition of lens of eye that develops slowly ■ As cataract becomes opaque, vision diminishes ■ Onset usually occurs with aging	■ Impaired vision ■ Eventual blindness	■ Patient presenting symptoms	■ Surgical removal ■ Lens implant
Chalazion ■ Small, localized, hard cystic mass on the eyelid ■ Caused by blockage of a meibomian gland on eyelid	■ Usually painless but if infected may be swollen, inflamed, and painful	■ Observation of mass on the eyelid and patient history	■ Watchful waiting if no symptoms present ■ Surgical removal may be indicated
Conjunctivitis ■ Inflammation and infection of conjunctiva ■ Infection may be viral or bacterial ■ Inflammation caused by allergens or irritations from chemicals and UV light	■ Conjunctiva red and swollen ■ Infection may cause **purulent** drainage	■ Patient presenting symptoms	■ Gentle cleansing of discharge from eyelid and eyelashes (eye may be sealed shut) ■ Moist heat to provide relief ■ Antibiotics for bacterial infection

TABLE 37-1 DISEASES AND DISORDERS OF EYE (CONTINUED)

Disorder or Disease	Symptoms	Diagnosis	Treatment
Diabetic retinopathy ■ Caused by diabetes ■ Causes microaneurysms (microscopic abnormal expansion of blood vessels) and hemorrhages (blood loss) in vessels of retina ■ Retinal veins become dilated and new blood vessels develop near optic disk	■ Painless ■ Blurred vision	■ Patient presenting symptoms ■ Ophthalmic examination	■ Laser surgery
Foreign bodies in eye ■ Include dust, insects, metal particles, wood splinters, or any small, airborne objects ■ Cause eye to tear in an effort to wash out offending substance	■ Pain ■ Decreased visual acuity ■ Photophobia ■ Feeling that something is under eyelid or stuck in cornea	■ Examination under eyelids	■ Irrigation with normal saline solution ■ Fluorescein to stain eye and help detect any corneal damage ■ Grinding (used when foreign body is metal and leaves a rust ring; eye and eye spud are anesthetized and rust ring is ground away)
Glaucoma ■ Increased fluid pressure within eye ■ Two forms: acute (closed angle) and chronic (open angle) ■ Causes damage to optic nerve and eventual blindness, if untreated ■ If aqueous humor does not drain due to obstruction, pressure is created in eye ■ Visual loss results from death of nerve cells	■ Visual loss	■ Patient presenting symptoms ■ Ophthalmic examination	■ Medication to release fluid ■ Laser surgery ■ Early detection, diagnosis, and treatment vital to save vision
Hyperopia (farsightedness) ■ Eyeball is shorter than normal and image focuses behind retina	■ Inability to focus on close objects	■ Ophthalmologic exam ■ Astigmatoscopy ■ Jaeger chart ■ Snellen chart	■ Biconvex (convex on both sides) lens in front of eye to focus image on retina
Keratitis ■ Inflammation and ulceration of surface of cornea ■ Caused by infection (bacterial, fungal, or viral), corneal trauma, or exposure to light from welding	■ Pain ■ Photosensitivity ■ Tearing ■ Impaired vision	■ Patient presenting symptoms	■ Eye drops ■ Ointments ■ Systemic antibiotics if necessary ■ Eye patch to protect eye from further damage

continued

TABLE 37-1 DISEASES AND DISORDERS OF EYE (CONTINUED)

Disorder or Disease	Symptoms	Diagnosis	Treatment
Macular degeneration ■ Gradual destruction of sharp central vision ■ Progressive disease related to aging ■ No cure	■ Painless ■ Blind spot in middle of visual field ■ Distorted vision; straight lines appear crooked	■ Ophthalmic examination ■ Patient presenting symptoms ■ Two types: dry and wet	■ Laser photocoagulation (allows limited improvement)
Myopia (nearsightedness) ■ Eyeball is longer or deeper than normal and image focuses in front of retina	■ Inability to focus on objects in distance	■ Ophthalmologic exam ■ Astigmatoscopy ■ Jaeger chart ■ Snellen chart	■ Biconcave (concave on both sides) lens in front of eye to focus image on retina
Nystagmus ■ Involuntary, repetitive, rhythmic movements of the eyes ■ May be caused by lesions in the brain or inner ear	■ Horizontal, vertical, or circular movement of one or both eyes ■ Possible blurred or impaired vision	■ Ophthalmologic exam	■ Treatment of underlying cause
Presbyopia ■ Focusing of light rays is delayed due to aging of structures in eye	■ Eyes take longer to focus	■ Ophthalmologic exam ■ Astigmatoscopy ■ Jaeger chart ■ Snellen chart	■ Corrective lens
Retinal detachment ■ Occurs when retina separates from choroids ■ May be result of traumatic insult to head or eye, or may be spontaneous	■ Floaters ■ Light flashes ■ Dark shadow appearing and progressing upward or to one side of visual field ■ Sudden, painless onset	■ Ophthalmologic examination to confirm separation ■ May follow cataract surgery	■ Photocoagulation (use of laser to treat detachment and retinal bleeding) ■ Cryotherapy
Strabismus ■ Failure of the eyes to focus on the same position at the same time. ■ Exotropia: when one or both eyes turn outward. Esotropia: when one or both eyes turn inward.	■ One or both eyes turning inward or outward ■ Possible double vision	■ Patient presenting symptoms	■ Corrective glasses ■ Eye exercises ■ Surgery
Stye (hordeolum) ■ Inflammation of one or more sebaceous (oil-secreting) glands of eyelid ■ Caused by bacterial infection	■ Redness ■ Pain ■ Purulence	■ Patient presenting symptoms	■ Moist heat to provide relief ■ Antibiotics

to assess degree of eye injury or disease process. It establishes baseline information, monitors the effectiveness of a treatment, or monitors the progression of chronic eye conditions.

Snellen charts are used to measure distance visual acuity. They are available in different forms—for English-speaking patients, non-English-speaking patients, and pediatric patients (Figure 37-11 ◆). The Jaeger chart is used to measure near-vision acuity (Figure 37-12 ◆). In patient documentation, the right eye is referred to as **OD,** the left eye as **OS.**

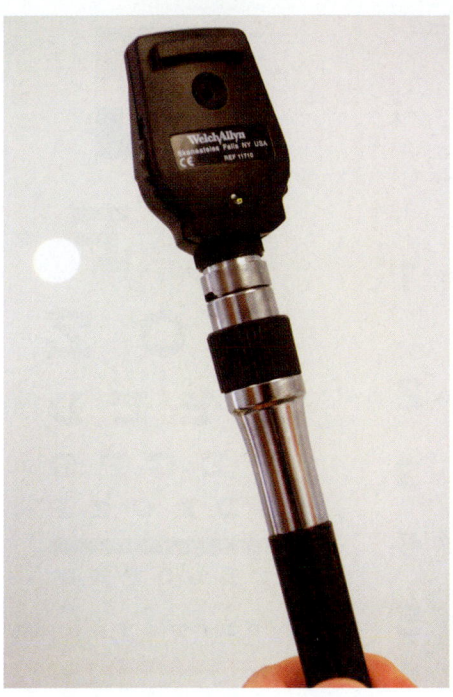

Figure 37-8 ◆ Ophthalmoscope.

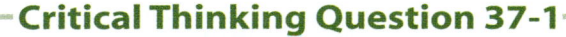

?

─Critical Thinking Question 37-1─

The college student who has come in for a Snellen test wears contact lenses. With her left eye, the patient can read to the 20/20 line, making only two errors. With her right eye, she can only read to the 20/40 line and makes three errors. How should Stacy record these results?

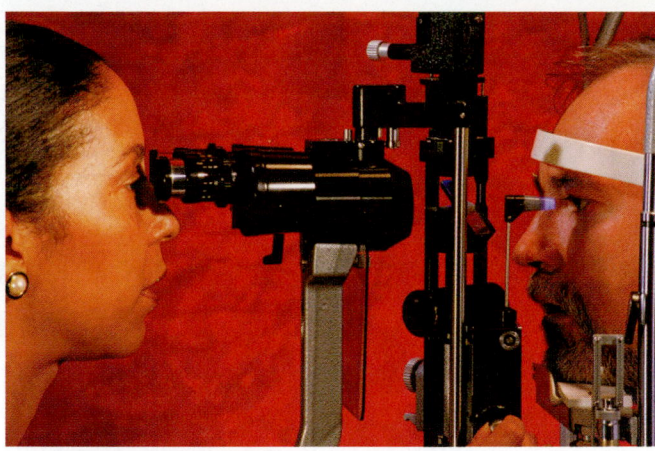

Figure 37-10 ◆ Tonometer.
Source: Photo Researchers, Inc.

Color Blindness

Color blindness (also called color deficiency) is an abnormal condition characterized by an inability to identify one or more primary colors. It is an inherited trait found mostly in males and results from a deficiency of or defects in the cones of the retina. There are two types of color blindness: achromatic vision and Daltonism. Achromatic color blindness is very rare. The affected individual cannot see any color at all, only shades of black, white, and gray. People with Daltonism, a more common disorder, cannot distinguish between red and green.

In addition to the two types of color blindness, there are three types of color deficiency: deuteranopia, protanopia, and tritanopia. Individuals with deuteranopia have difficulty distinguishing among neutral shades, bluish reds, and different shades of green. Protanopia, or "red blindness," is characterized

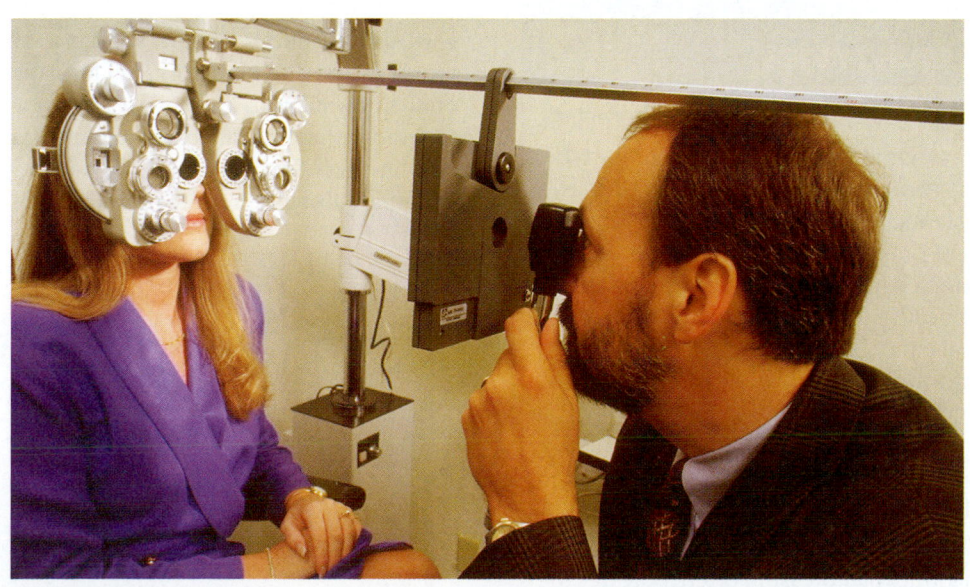

Figure 37-9 ◆ Slit lamp.

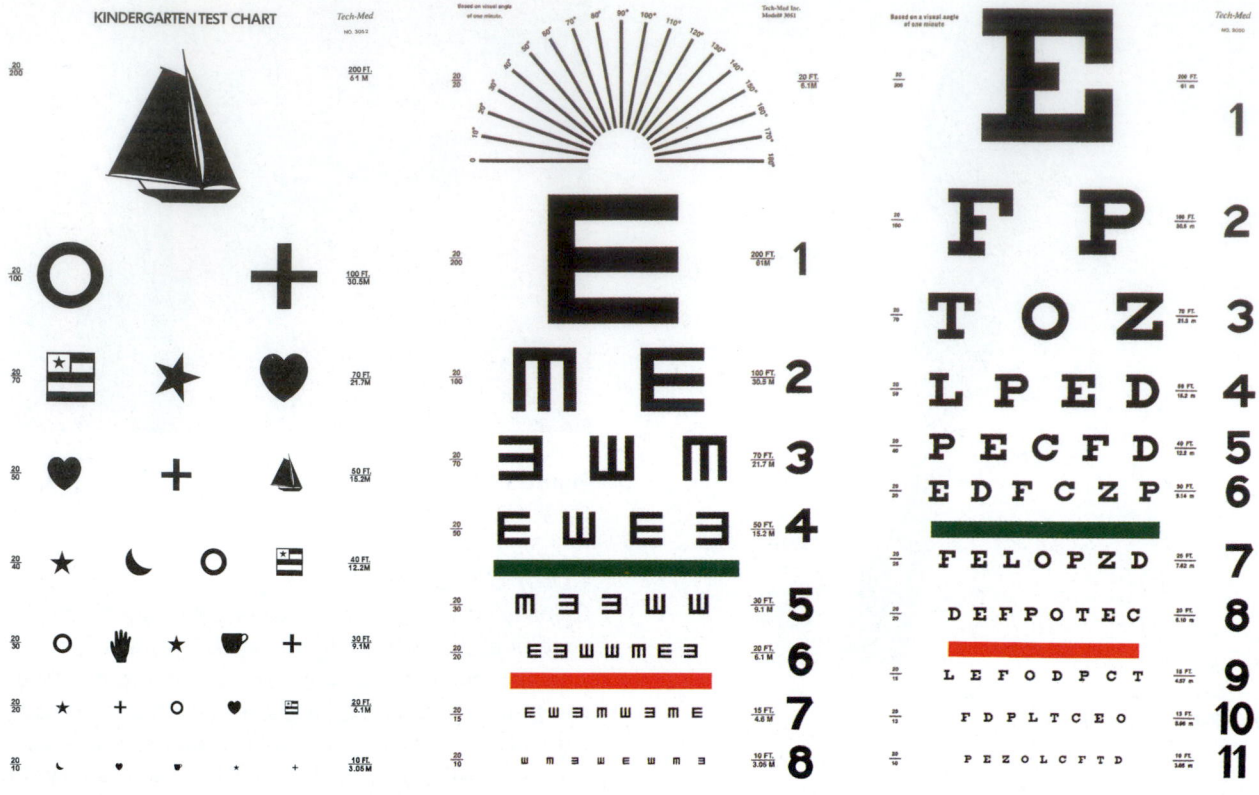

Figure 37-11 ◆ Various types of Snellen charts.

by difficulty seeing reds or, occasionally, the difference between yellows and greens. Tritanopia, or "blue blindness," is the rarest condition, in which the individual is unable to see any shade of blue.

Medical assistants may be asked to do color blindness testing with Ishihara color plates. The Ishihara book contains fourteen images of colored dots arranged in the shape of a numeral set against a background of dots in a contrasting color. Patients with color blindness have difficulty distinguishing the numerals from the background.

Eye Treatments

Dust, dirt, chemicals, or other substances may get onto the surface of the eye and can be difficult for patients to safely remove on their own. Eye irrigations are an easy and comfortable way to remove these substances in the medical office. The procedure involves flowing a fluid across the eye and flushing the irritating substance from the surface.

Keys to Success
USING A TONOMETER

Eye care professionals use different types of tonometers.

- The mechanical tonometer is the most accurate type. After the eye is anesthetized with eye drops, the eye care professional touches the cornea with the tonometer. The amount of pressure needed to make an indentation on the cornea is measured and recorded. Caution must be taken because the eye is numb and therefore at risk for corneal injury until the anesthetic wears off.
- The noncontact tonometer blows a puff of air across the eye as the individual looks into the tonometer. The cornea is flattened slightly to obtain a reading. The "air-puff" or "puff-of-air" test involves no contact with the cornea, is painless, and does not require a local anesthetic in the eye.

An increase in intraocular pressure often indicates the onset of glaucoma. Any tonometer reading above 21 mm is considered elevated, but not necessarily a diagnosis of glaucoma.

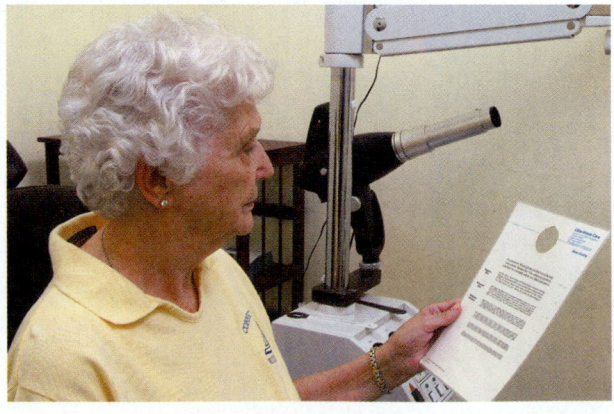

Figure 37-12 ◆ A patient using a near-vision acuity card.

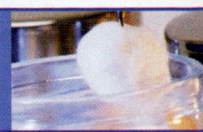

PROCEDURE 37-1 **Measure Distance Visual Acuity with a Snellen Chart**

Theory and Rationale

A line is marked on the floor 20 feet from the wall where a Snellen chart hangs. The patient stands, toes at the line, and is instructed to cover one eye with an occluder (spatula or card if an occluder is not available) to test the vision of the uncovered eye. The covered eye must be kept open to prevent squinting. If the patient tilts the head, tears, or squints during the test, he or she likely has vision problems. Note this on the patient's chart. Also note whether the patient performed the test with or without glasses or contact lenses.

Record the lowest readable level for each eye. Measurements are recorded as a fraction with the number 20 first or on top. The first number indicates the chart was 20 feet away from the patient. The second or bottom number indicates normal, uncorrected vision. For example, a score of 20/30 indicates that the patient is able to read at 20 feet what a person with normal vision could read at 30 feet.

Materials

■ Snellen chart
■ occluder, spatula, or card
■ patient chart

Competency

(**Conditions**) With the necessary materials, (**Task**) you will be able to assist the patient in testing the visual acuity of both eyes (**Standards**) correctly within 30 minutes.

1. Wash your hands. Gather equipment and supplies.
2. Identify the patient and guide him or her to the treatment area.
3. Record the patient's history and main complaint. Explain the entire procedure to the patient.
4. Position the patient, standing or sitting, at the 20-foot line. Give the patient the occluder. Observe patient during the procedure for head tilting, squinting, and tearing.

5. Ask the patient to cover the left eye, keeping it open, and to read aloud from the top line to the smallest line of readable letters.
6. Record the right-eye vision with the number of errors. For one or two errors, record the vision fraction and minus one or two. For more than two errors, record the vision fraction as noted one line above on the Snellen chart. For example, if the patient reads the 20/40 line with the right eye and two errors, the result is recorded as OD 20/40-2. If the patient reads the 20/40 line with the right eye and three errors, the result is OD 20/50, or one line above the 20/40 line.
7. Next, ask the patient to repeat the procedure, covering the right eye and reading with the left.
8. Record the left-eye vision with the number of errors.
9. Wash your hands and report the results to the physician.

Patient Education

Explain to the patient that the procedure is done with both eyes open, even though one will be covered. Tell the patient that reading the Snellen chart should not be painful, but to report any symptoms during the procedure. If the patient does not speak English and is being tested with the Snellen E chart, have the patient practice pointing his or her fingers in the direction of each E before testing begins.

Charting Example

01/23/XX 9:30 a.m. Pt tested with corrective glasses. OS reading was 20/30 −2. OD reading was 20/40. Observed the pt squinting during the testing of OD. Patient referred by physician to local optometrist. Grant Reilly, RMA (AMT)

Eyewash stations may also be used in the removal of dust, dirt, and debris. See ∞ Chapter 41 for more information on eyewash stations (page 906).

In the treatment of eye disorders, as well in preparation for eye examinations, a variety of topical drugs may be administered. Make sure that any medication you instill in a patient's eye is labeled "For Ophthalmologic Use."

■ Local anesthetics are often dropped onto the surface of the eye before a procedure. They also are used to relieve pain from a foreign body or abrasion of the cornea. Tetracaine 0.5 percent ophthalmologic is a local anesthetic.

■ Fluorescein ophthalmologic drops or strips are used to stain the eyes.
■ Mydriatic eye drops dilate the pupils.
■ Miotic medications cause the pupils to constrict.
■ Other medications are prescribed to treat conditions such as glaucoma, infections, and corneal abrasions.

Critical Thinking Question 37-2

The young girl with sand in her eye is frightened about having her eye flushed. She squeezes her eye shut and will not hold still. What are Stacy's options?

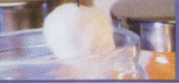

PROCEDURE 37-2 Perform the Ishihara Color Vision Test

Theory and Rationale

The ability to see colors is a function of the cones of the retina. People who can no longer see color or who have never seen color most likely have defective cones or no cones at all. If the color blindness is not congenital, it may indicate damage to or disease of the retina, optic nerve, or even the thyroid.

The Ishihara test should be administered in a well-lit room out of direct sunlight.

Materials

- Ishihara color plates book
- pen
- patient chart

Competency

(**Conditions**) With the necessary materials, (**Task**) you will be able determine color vision acuity using Ishihara color plates (**Standards**) correctly within the time frame designated by the instructor.

1. Explain the procedure to the patient.
2. Follow the physician's directions for administering the total book or in sections.
3. Ask the patient to identify the number in each plate with both eyes.
4. Have the patient cover the left eye and read the book again, then the right eye.
5. Write down the page number of any plates the patient misses. (The correct answer is on the back of each page.)
6. Follow the directions on the last page of the book to determine the level of color blindness, if any.
7. Document the procedure in the patient's chart.

Patient Education

A patient who reads ten Ishihara plates correctly is considered to have normal color vision (Figure 37-13 ◆). A patient who reads seven plates or fewer correctly has color vision abnormalities and is referred to an optometrist or ophthalmologist for further review and treatment.

Charting Example

11/25/XX 3:30 PM Ishihara color plates examined by patient. No visual abnormalities noted. Shannon Reese, RMA (AMI)

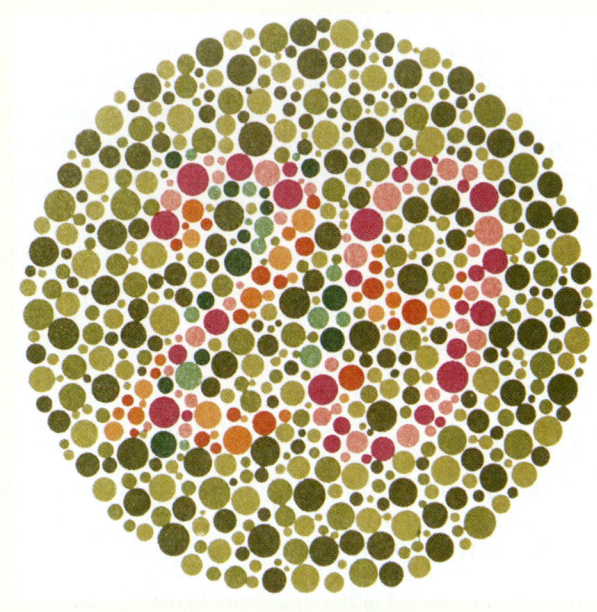

Figure 37-13 ◆ Color vision plate.
Source: Photoedit, Inc.

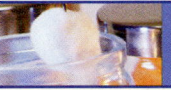

PROCEDURE 37-3 Perform Eye Irrigation

Theory and Rationale

Eye irrigation may be performed on one or both eyes with a sterile solution. As with any medication or solution used for treatment, check the label when removing the medication from the storage shelf, immediately before using, and against the physician's order. Wear protective gear—gown, face shield, and disposable gloves—to protect against possible splashing.

The solution is irrigated from the center of the face or the inner corner of the eye to the outside. This prevents cross-contamination and the movement of the foreign substance or infectious material to the other eye. The patient helps by lying or sitting and turning the head toward the eye to be irrigated. It is also important that you irrigate toward the inside of the lower eyelid, or conjunctival sac. To avoid force and trauma to the eye, do *not* irrigate directly at the corneal surface.

For safety reasons, have the patient lie or sit still during the procedure. Be sure to ask the patient about medication allergies, and check the chart as well.

Materials

- irrigating solution
- sterile basin

PROCEDURE 37-3 **Perform Eye Irrigation** (continued)

- irrigating syringe
- protective gear (gown, face shield, disposable gloves)
- towels
- kidney-shaped basin
- tissues
- patient chart

Competency

(**Conditions**) With the necessary materials, (**Task**) you will be able to irrigate the patient's eye (**Standards**) safely and correctly within 30 minutes.

1. Wash your hands. Gather equipment and supplies.
2. Identify the patient and guide him or her to the treatment area.
3. Record the patient's history and main complaint.
4. Review the physician's order for the patient's name, the volume and name of the irrigating solution, and which eye to irrigate.
5. Ask the patient about medication allergies. Explain the entire procedure.
6. Check the label of the irrigating solution against the physician's order before pouring it into the sterile basin for irrigation.
7. Wash your hands.
8. Put on the gown, face shield, and gloves before proceeding with irrigation.
9. Ask the patient to lie or sit down with the head tilted toward the eye to be irrigated. Place a towel and the kidney-shaped basin next to the patient's face to catch irrigating fluid.
10. With your dominant hand, fill the irrigating syringe with the prescribed irrigating solution.
11. With your nondominant hand, press with a tissue against the patient's cheekbone beneath the eye to expose more of the eye surface.
12. While holding the syringe approximately 1/2 inch from the eye, gently direct the fluid toward the inside surface of the lower conjunctiva and from the inner to outer corner of the eye (Figure 37-14 ◆).
13. Continue irrigating until the prescribed volume is used. Depending on the cause and symptoms, the physician may order further irrigation.
14. When irrigation is complete, dry the area around the affected eye with tissues.
15. Remove your protective clothing and place it in the proper laundry and waste containers.

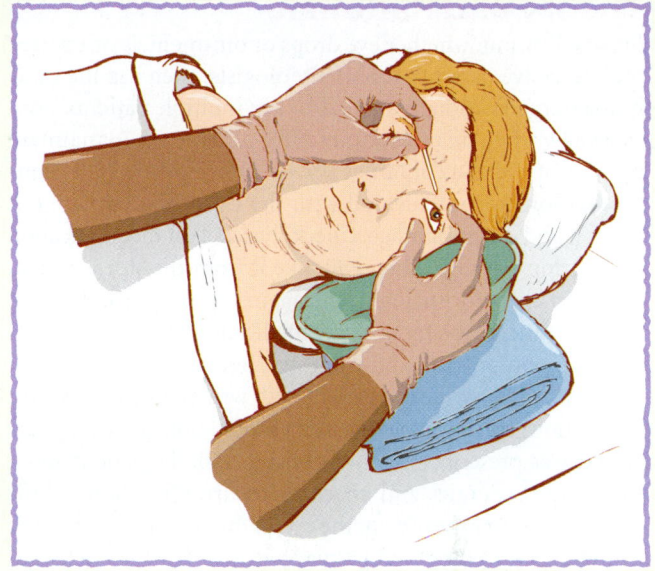

Figure 37-14 ◆ Irrigation of the eye.

16. Wash your hands.
17. Document the patient's tolerance of the procedure, the amount and kind of irrigating solution, and the eye irrigated.

Patient Education

Describe the procedure completely to ensure the patient's cooperation. For safety reasons, the patient will need to remain very still. Tell the patient that eye irrigation will ease the discomfort and help the eye heal faster. Schedule a followup visit.

Charting Example

07/15/XX 2:45 p.m. Fussy 8-year-old pt presents with sand in both eyes from a sibling scuffle in the family's sandbox. Per physician's order, each eye was irrigated per procedure with 180 cc normal saline with holding assistance from mother. Both right and left conjunctival sacs and cornea are clear after irrigation. Child stated that both eyes now feel better. Ann Maynard, CMA (AAMA)

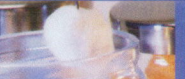

PROCEDURE 37-4 Perform Instillation of Eye Medication

Theory and Rationale

Eye medication, whether eye drops or ointment, is often used for successive patients. Ophthalmologists often use the same bottle of medication to instill drops in multiple patients' eyes, especially when dilating pupils or for anesthesia. To maintain the sterility of the container tip and prevent microbial contamination, keep it covered with the cap when you are not using it and during storage. Check the label on the medication or solution package when you take it from the storage shelf, immediately before using it, and against the physician's order.

A patient who requires eye medication often has not only a medication prescribed for one eye, but another medication for both eyes. Provide the patient with written as well as verbal instructions concerning the correct medication and dosage for each eye as prescribed by the physician. Ask the patient about medication allergies and check the chart. Only ophthalmic preparations may be used in the eye, as other preparations have a different concentration that may harm or damage eye tissue.

Materials

- prescription medication (drops or ointment)
- disposable gloves
- tissues
- patient chart

Competency

(**Conditions**) With the necessary materials, (**Task**) you will be able to instill eye medication (**Standards**) safely within 30 minutes.

1. Wash your hands. Gather equipment and supplies.
2. Take the medication from the storage shelf. Check the label against the physician's order.
3. Identify the patient and guide him or her to the treatment area. Check the patient's identification against the physician's order and medication name.
4. Note the medication dosage to be administered.
5. Ask the patient about allergies. Explain the entire procedure.
6. Wash your hands and put on disposable gloves.
7. Ask the patient to lie down or sit with the head tilted back with both eyes open. (It may be necessary to ask the sitting patient to look at the ceiling.) If the patient is wearing an eye patch, remove it.
8. Give the patient a tissue to hold in each hand until after the procedure.
9. With your nondominant hand and a tissue, press on the lower cheekbone and gently pull the lower eyelid down to expose the cornea and conjunctival sac.
10. To administer eye drops, fill the eyedropper with your dominant hand. Hold the dropper approximately 1/2 inch away from the patient's eye, and administer the prescribed dose into the conjunctival sac (Figure 37-15 ◆). To administer the ointment, rest your dominant hand on the

patient's forehead, hold the tube, and lightly squeeze ointment into the conjunctival sac from the inner to outer corner of the patient's eye.

11. Release the patient's lower eyelid and tell the patient to close the eye.
12. Repeat the procedure in the other eye, if ordered by the physician.
13. Instruct the patient to use a separate tissue for each eye to wipe away excess medication.
14. Apply an eye patch, if ordered by the physician.
15. Provide a waste container for the patient to discard the used tissue into.
16. Dispose of the gloves and tissue.
17. Wash your hands.
18. Document the patient's tolerance of the procedure, the amount and kind of medication administered, and the eye(s) treated.

Patient Education

Give the patient verbal and written instructions for administering eye medications at home. If the patient has not done it before, talk him or her through the instillation procedure. If the patient has done it but had a problem, observe how he or she does it. Tactfully discuss how the patient's technique might be improved, if necessary. Give the patient written instructions about each medication, including frequency and amount. Warn the patient to use only ophthalmic preparations in the eye.

Charting Example

02/25/XX 9:00 a.m. One eye gtt of Timoptic solution administered OS as prescribed. Instructions given to pt about the administration of eye drops and the pt demonstrated correctly how to administer one gtt OD as prescribed by physician. Patrick Cooper, RMA (AMT)

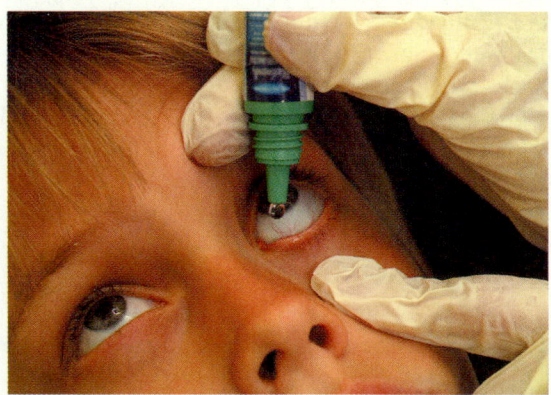

Figure 37-15 ◆ Administer the prescribed dose into the conjunctival sac.

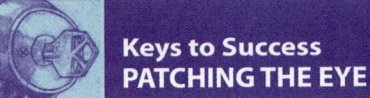
The physician may order that a patient's eye be patched to keep the eyelid from passing back and forth over the cornea as the eyeball moves. The eye patch must apply a gentle pressure on the closed lid to prevent it from opening and closing in the normal process of blinking.

When one eye has a foreign body or abrasion, both eyes are usually patched to limit eye movement and further trauma to the cornea or eyelid, since the eyes move together (Figure 37-16 ◆).

Also, if only one eye is patched, warn the patient that depth perception will be impaired. The patient should use caution when going up and down stairs and when trying to see distant objects. The patient should be advised not to drive.

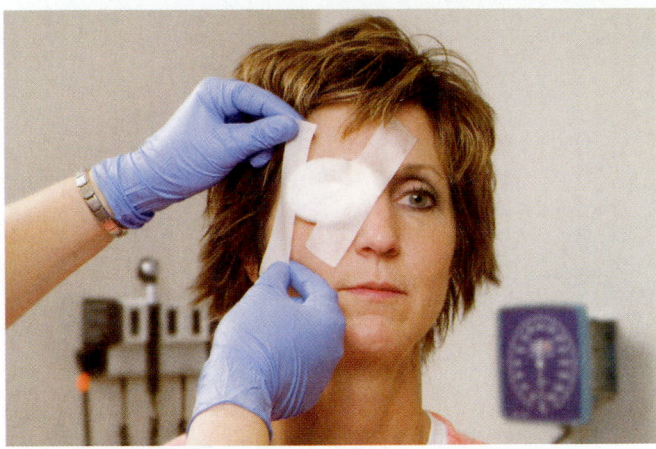

Figure 37-16 ◆ Patching the patient's eye.

The Anatomy and Physiology of the Ear

The ear is the organ for hearing. It is divided into three areas—the external ear, middle ear, and internal ear (Figure 37-17 ◆).

- The external ear comprises the auricle, or pinna, which is the visible portion that projects from the side of the head, and the external auditory canal. The auditory canal is the pathway to the middle ear. It is lined with glands that secrete **cerumen,** or earwax, which protects the canal from infection.
- The tympanic membrane (eardrum) separates the outer or external ear from the middle ear. There are three small bones, called ossicles, in the middle ear: the malleus, incus, and stapes. The oval window connects the middle ear and the inner ear.
- The inner ear, or labyrinth, is made up of three compartments: the cochlea, vestibule, and semicircular canals. Perilymph and endolymph are fluids that transmit vibrations through the canals in the inner ear. The cochlea, a snail-shaped structure, houses the organ of Corti with its sound receptors. The vestibule and semicircular canals assist with equilibrium by transmitting information about the position of the body to the brain via the vestibular nerve.

The process of hearing occurs when sound waves move through the ear. The sound waves:

- enter the auditory canal from the auricle,
- then vibrate the tympanic membrane (eardrum),
- move the three tiny ossicles in the middle ear (malleus, incus, and stapes),
- pass through the oval window,
- continue into the inner ear or labyrinth, which contains the cochlea,
- enter the cochlea, where the fluids perilymph and endolymph allow the sound waves to continue to the auditory receptors in the organ of Corti,
- move to the tiny hairs in the receptors to be relayed on the auditory nerve fibers,
- are sent to the auditory center in the cerebral area of the cortex. These impulses are interpreted as sound by the brain.

An additional function of the ear is balance. Three organs in the inner ear maintain equilibrium: the semicircular canals, saccule, and utricle. Endolymph and tiny, sensitive hair cells move with the movement of the head to help maintain the body's balance.

Diseases and Disorders of the Ear

In conduction disorders, hearing loss may result when sounds are blocked from reaching the auditory nerve by one of a number of factors.

- Cerumen may block the passage of sound waves to the middle ear.
- Inflammatory and infectious disorders may cause edema and block the passage of sound waves to the inner ear.
- Otosclerosis prevents the ossicles from vibrating and sending the sound waves on.

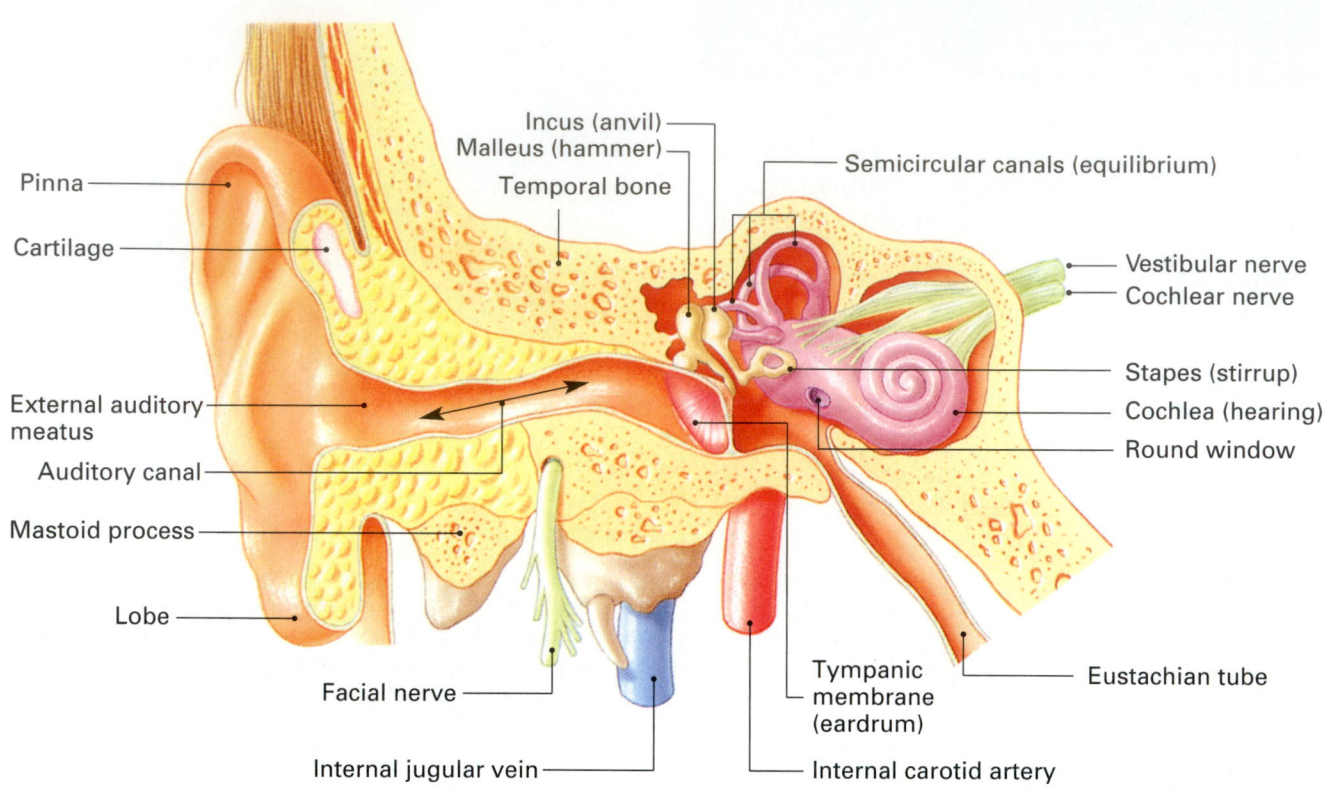

Figure 37-17 ◆ Anatomy of the ear.

Infectious disorders of the ear include otitis externa, otitis media, and labrynthitis (otitis interna). Injury to the ear may take the form of nerve trauma or a foreign body in the ear.

Table 37-2 summarizes common disorders and diseases of the ear.

Diagnostic Procedures

Instruments used in otic examinations include:

- Otoscope: a handheld device that beams light into the ear canal (Figure 37-18 ◆)
- Vienna speculum: a device used to examine the external auditory canal and eardrum (Figure 37-19 ◆)
- Zeiss microscope: magnifies the tympanic membrane

Hearing tests include audiometry and tuning fork testing.

Simple Audiometry

Simple audiometry testing helps determine a patient's hearing level in each ear and can also be used to confirm the presence of underlying disease. The audiometer measures the patient's response to acoustic stimuli of specific frequencies. Employers often order an audiometry exam to establish baseline information for new hires and monitor the hearing status of long-term

employees. The MA will need additional training from an **audiologist** or physician to perform this procedure.

Ear Treatments

Irrigating the ear clears the external auditory canal of cerumen or other foreign material. The physician may order an ear irrigation to make the tympanic membrane easier to see (Figure 37-20 ◆).

Drugs instilled in the ear include antibiotics, topical anesthetics, and solutions or oils that soften cerumen. These drugs must be labeled for use in the ear.

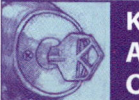

Keys to Success
ASSISTING THE HEARING OR VISUALLY IMPAIRED

The visually impaired patient may require assistance when completing office forms. To provide privacy and prevent embarrassment, politely and discreetly escort the patient to a private area and offer your assistance. Do not assume the visually impaired patient has hearing problems and speak loudly.

The hearing-impaired patient may require written instructions to complete medical forms. Face the patient directly and speak in normal tones.

TABLE 37-2 DISEASES AND DISORDERS OF THE EAR

Disorder	Symptoms	Diagnosis	Treatment
Impacted cerumen ■ Conducted disorder ■ Earwax becomes hardened ■ May result from using cotton swabs to clean the ear	■ Impaired hearing ■ Tinnitus (ringing in the ears) ■ Plugged or stuffed feeling in outer ear	■ Patient presenting symptoms ■ **Otic** examination	■ Irrigation to soften or loosen plug ■ Cryotherapy
Labyrynthitis ■ Inflammation and infection of labyrinth or semicircular canals of the inner ear ■ Cause may be bacterial or viral infection	■ Impaired hearing ■ Vertigo ■ Nausea ■ Vomiting ■ Tinnitus	■ Patient presenting symptoms	■ Antibiotics for bacterial infection ■ Corticosteroids for viral infection
Ménière's disease ■ Conduction disorder characterized by sudden onset of symptoms ■ Abnormality caused by change in volume of endolymph fluid, edema, or rupture of membranous labyrinth ■ No cure	■ Pressure or pain in ear ■ Impaired hearing ■ Vertigo (dizziness) ■ Tinnitus	■ Hearing tests ■ Balance tests ■ Physical examination	■ Drug therapy to control symptoms ■ Surgery—either cutting of vestibular nerve or labyrinthectomy (portion of inner ear is removed, resulting in total hearing loss)
Nerve trauma ■ Injury caused by extended exposure to high noise levels (loud music, loud radio, jackhammers, sirens, machinery, gunshots, Jet engines)	■ Impaired hearing	■ Hearing tests	Prevention (damage is not reversible)
Otitis externa ■ Inflammation of outer ear, also called swimmer's ear (often occurs after swimming); other ear also inflamed and reddened	■ Impaired hearing ■ Pain ■ Fever	■ Visual inspection of outer ear	■ Antibiotic drops for infection ■ Steroid drops ■ Keeping ear dry
Otitis media ■ Inflammation or bacterial infection of middle ear, usually with fluid that cannot drain ■ Eardrum bulges and may be reddened ■ Often comes before or just after upper respiratory or a cold ■ Two forms: serous and purulent	■ Pain ■ Fever ■ Discharge ■ Impaired hearing ■ Young children cry, pull at their ears, or sit with head held to one side	■ Audiology testing ■ Balance tests ■ Physical examination	■ Antibiotics to treat the infection
Otosclerosis ■ Conductive disorder caused by fusion of three main bones of middle ear ■ Movement of stapes is restricted, so sound waves cannot be sent to inner ear	■ Progressive hearing impairment	■ Hearing tests ■ Physical examination	■ Surgery to replace stapes with a metal or plastic prosthesis

continued

TABLE 37-2 DISEASES AND DISORDERS OF THE EAR (CONTINUED)

Disorder	Symptoms	Diagnosis	Treatment
Ruptured tympanic membrane ■ Conductive disorder caused by injury or infectious process of otitis media. ■ Scarring and impaired hearing may remain after membrane heals	■ Impaired hearing	■ Otic examination	■ Antibiotics for otitis media
Foreign bodies ■ Injury caused by object placed in ear or by insect flying or crawling into ear ■ Children often place peas, beans, or other small foods into ear that absorb moisture in ear and swell, further obstructing canal	■ Impaired hearing	■ Physical examination	■ Earwax spoon to remove object ■ Gentle suction ■ Gentle irrigation ■ For insect: in a dark room, shining a light into ear (insect often moves toward light and out of ear)

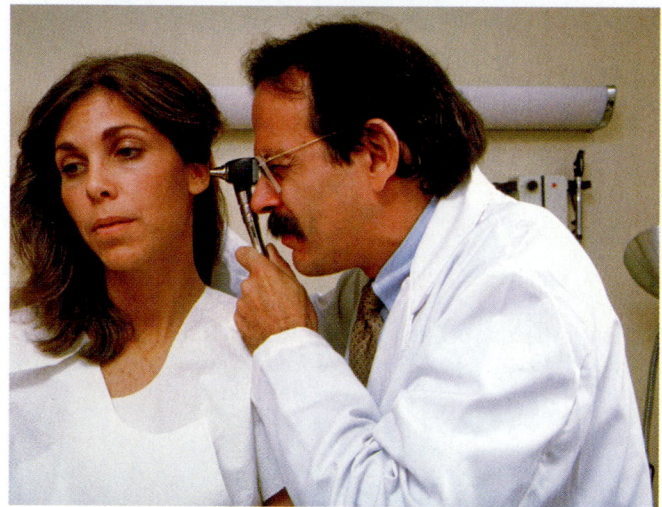

Figure 37-18 ◆ Examination of the ear using an otoscope.
Source: Michal Heron Photography.

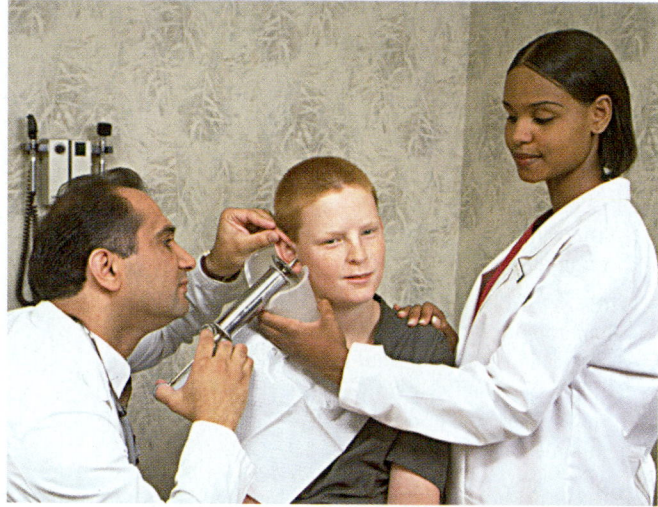

Figure 37-20 ◆ Ear irrigation.

In Practice

David Henson presents to the office complaining that he is having a hard time hearing people. He states that other people's voices sound muffled. After performing a thorough examination, the physician diagnoses the patient with cerumen impaction. The patient seems worried and asks the medical assistant if he is going to lose his hearing. What is cerumen? What should you as the medical assistant tell the patient?

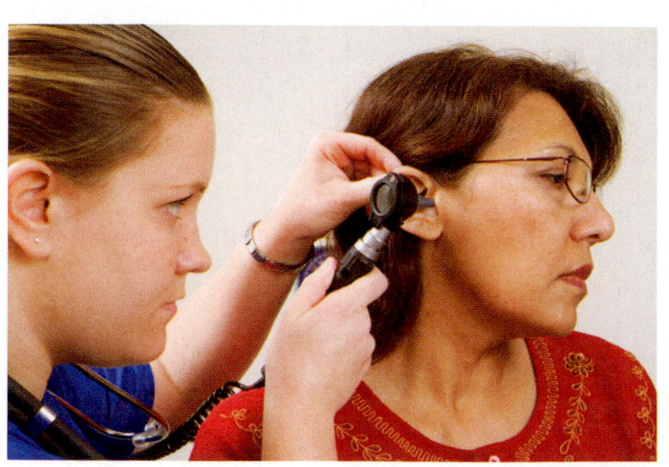

Figure 37-19 ◆ A patient being examined with Vienna speculum.

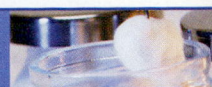

PROCEDURE 37-5 Perform Simple Audiometry

Theory and Rationale

Audiometry provides information about sound frequencies the patient is able and unable to hear. The test is performed in a quiet room or soundproof booth because outside noises affect the accuracy of the results. You should begin testing tones on the ear with better hearing, if known. Earphones are marked for the right or left ear. It is important that earphones are placed correctly for tones to be delivered to the correct ear and results to be accurate.

Make sure the tones do not follow a rhythm, as the patient may guess correctly when the next increasing tones are done. If the patient finds the test too long or the results are inconsistent, inform the physician and reschedule the test. Before performing the rescheduled test, try to correct or improve on the failed first test.

Materials

- audiometer
- earphones
- audiometric test report form
- patient chart

Competency

(**Conditions**) With the necessary materials, (**Task**) you will be able to perform bilateral audiology testing (**Standards**) correctly within 30 minutes.

1. Wash your hands. Gather equipment and supplies.
2. Prepare the testing area to ensure quiet during the procedure.
3. Identify the patient and guide him or her to the testing area.
4. Inform the patient that only one ear at a time will be tested. Instruct the patient to raise one finger or nod when he or she first hears the sound, no matter how soft.
5. Place earphones on the patient.
6. Administer low-frequency sounds to one ear to determine the patient's baseline hearing measurements and ability to follow test instructions (Figure 37-21 ◆).

7. Plot the results from each tone on the graph immediately.
8. Continue raising the tone frequency by 10 **dB** (**decibels**) and recording the results until the patient can no longer hear in the first ear.
9. Lower the tone by 5 dB until the patient signals, to confirm the lowest frequency the patient can hear in that ear.
10. Repeat the procedure with the other ear.
11. Give the audiometric test results to the physician.
12. Prepare the audiometric equipment and room for next the patient.

Patient Education

It is important that the patient understand the testing instructions to obtain the most accurate results. Always ask the patient to repeat the instructions back to you before testing.

Charting Example

09/26/XX 1:30 p.m. Pt demonstrated understanding of audiometry test instructions before the procedure. Results given to physician for discussion with pt. Lauren Willis, RMA (AMT)

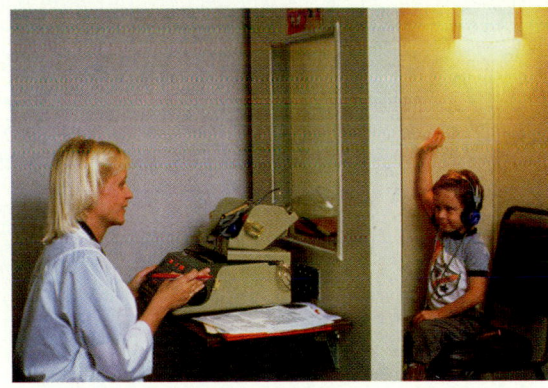

Figure 37-21 ◆ Hearing test.
Source: Phototake, NYC.

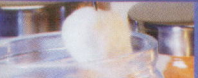

PROCEDURE 37-6 Perform Ear Irrigation

Theory and Rationale

Check the condition of the external auditory canal with an otoscope before and after the procedure to observe any changes. Additional otoscopic examination may be required during the procedure if the patient complains of pain.

The patient's head is tilted toward the affected ear to allow fluid to enter the canal. If it is expected that the earwax will be difficult to remove, the physician may order that a couple of drops of hydrogen peroxide or oil be placed on the surface of the ear canal. As the hydrogen peroxide or oil slides toward the tympanic membrane, the earwax is softened.

For a child 3 years old or an adult, the auricle is pulled back and up to position the ear canal. For a child under 3, whose external auditory canal is narrower, the auricle is pulled back and down.

When you are ready to begin, instruct the patient or other office staff to hold the basin under the ear and next to the neck. Place a towel under the basin to protect the patient's clothing. Place the solution-filled syringe at the opening of the external auditory canal and direct the tip toward the side or top.

Severe pain, and possibly the rupture of the tympanic membrane, will result if you irrigate with the tip aimed straight at the canal because of the force of the irrigating fluid moving directly through the canal.

When you have completed the procedure, examine the auditory canal with the otoscope. Help the patient lie down on the side of the irrigated ear to allow complete drainage. Some physicians also perform a final otoscopic examination to check the ear canal and tympanic membrane.

Note: Store the solution at room temperature to maintain the correct temperature for irrigation.

Materials

- irrigating solution
- sterile basin
- irrigating syringe
- towels
- cotton ball(s)
- patient chart

Competency

(**Conditions**) With the necessary materials, (**Tasks**) you will be able to irrigate the patient's ear (**Standards**) safely and correctly within 30 minutes.

1. Wash your hands. Gather equipment and supplies.
2. Identify the patient and guide him or her to the treatment area. Explain the entire procedure.
3. Check the label of the irrigating solution when you take it from the shelf and against the physician's order.
4. Position the patient in a sitting position and instruct him or her to lean the head toward the side to be irrigated.
5. Check the condition of the external auditory canal with the otoscope.
6. Drape a towel across the patient's shoulder, under the ear.
7. Fill the irrigating syringe with prescribed solution.
8. Place the basin under the ear and against the skin. Instruct the patient or other office personnel to hold the basin in place.
9. For a child under 3 years, gently pull the auricle down and back (Figure 37-22 ◆). For a child over 3 years or an adult, gently pull the auricle ear up and back (Figure 37-23 ◆).
10. Gently place the tip of the irrigating syringe into the external auditory canal and point to the side or top. Do *not* point directly toward the tympanic membrane.
11. Instill the irrigating solution with gentle pressure on the plunger of the syringe.
12. Place the irrigation basin aside.
13. Use the otoscope to determine if more irrigation is needed.
14. Repeat the procedure until the desired results are obtained. If the patient experiences discomfort or other difficulties, report to the physician.

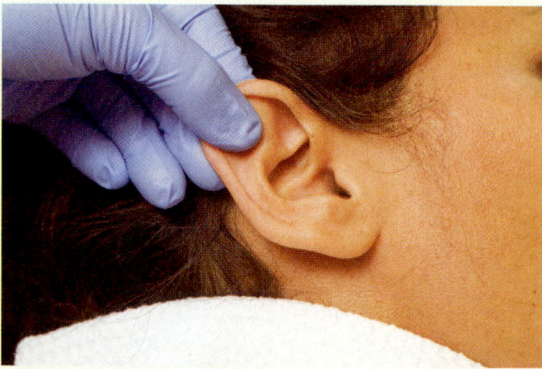

Figure 37-22 ◆ Proper holding position of the ear lobe for children.

Figure 37-23 ◆ Proper holding position of the outer ear for adults.

PROCEDURE 37-6 **Perform Ear Irrigation** (continued)

15. After irrigation, instruct and/or assist the patient to lie down with the head tilted toward the irrigated ear.
16. Place a towel under the head to catch the drainage.
17. Help the patient to a sitting, then standing position. Assess the patient for light-headedness or dizziness. Escort the patient to the waiting room.
18. Clean the treatment area and remove reusable equipment to the utility cleaning area.
19. Wash your hands.
20. Document the patient's tolerance and the results of the procedure.

Patient Education

Explain the procedure before and during the irrigation, including the normal feeling of fullness and flushing discomfort. Instruct the patient to report any new or increased pain.

Charting Example

10/09/XX 9:30 a.m. Otoscope showed moderate amount of cerumen present in the rt external auditory canal. Ear irrigation was done. Pt stated no additional discomfort. Post-otoscopic examination shows clear auditory canal with pearly gray membrane visible. Pt states she can hear better with the rt ear. Liam Marks, RMA (AMT)

PROCEDURE 37-7 **Perform Instillation of Ear Medication**

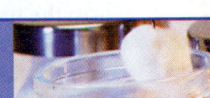

Theory and Rationale

Ear medication is generally prescribed for the patient in multiple doses, and it is important to keep the dropper or bottle tip sterile. This is done by storing it in the bottle when it is not in use and avoiding contact with any surface other than the medication in the bottle.

Ear medication should be at room temperature as the internal ear is sensitive to temperature extremes. If the medication is cold, the patient may experience nausea and/or vertigo.

Check the label when removing the medication from the storage shelf, immediately before using, and against the physician's order. Check the written instructions to verify the correct medication and dosage for each ear as prescribed by the physician. Ask the patient about medication allergies and check the chart as well. After administering the medication, instruct the patient to lie still for approximately 10 minutes to allow the medication to coat the external auditory canal and eardrum.

Materials

- medication
- disposable gloves
- cotton balls
- patient chart

Competency

(**Conditions**) With the necessary materials, (**Task**) you will be able to instill medication into the patient's ear (**Standards**) safely and correctly within 30 minutes.

1. Wash your hands. Gather equipment and supplies.
2. Check the label when removing the medication from the shelf and against the physician's order. Do *not* administer the medication unless it is at room temperature.
3. Identify the patient and guide him or her to the treatment area. Check the patient name against the physician's order and against the medication.
4. Explain the entire procedure to the patient. Ask about any allergies.
5. Instruct the patient to lie on the side opposite the ear to be treated.
6. Position the auricle as in Procedure 37-6.
7. Hold the ear dropper or bottle tip about 1/2 inch above the external auditory canal and gently squeeze the bulb to administer the prescribed number of drops (Figure 37-24 ◆).
8. Instruct the patient to lie still for 10 minutes.
9. Loosely place a small cotton ball, if the physician orders it, at the opening to the canal.
10. Repeat the procedure for the other ear, if ordered.

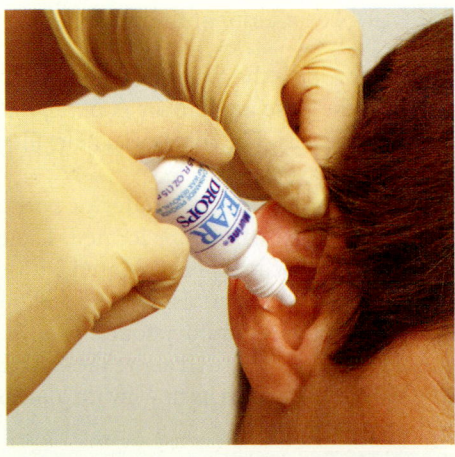

Figure 37-24 ◆ Instilling medication drops in the patient's ear.

continued

PROCEDURE 37-7 Perform Instillation of Ear Medication *(continued)*

11. Recap the medication bottle and dispose of waste materials.
12. Remove and dispose of the gloves. Wash your hands.
13. Escort the patient back to the waiting room.
14. Document the patient's tolerance of the procedure, the medication, the dosage administered, and which ear received treatment.

Patient Education

Provide verbal and written instructions for administering ear medications at home, including frequency and dosage. If the patient is new to instillation, talk him or her through the procedure. If the patient is physically unable or too young to perform the procedure, give the instructions to a significant other.

Charting Example

03/08/XX 9:00 a.m. Auraglan five gtts instilled into each ear per procedure and physician's order. Cotton ball loosely placed at opening to each ear canal. Pt demonstrated ability to instill medication correctly in right ear after demonstration and instilling by undersigned. Pt did not complain of any side effects. Pt said he understood how to instill eardrops at room temperature for seven days, twice daily. Jill Franklin, CMA (AAMA)

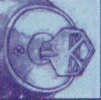

Keys to Success
TYMPANOMETRY

Tympanometry is a process that measures the flexibility of the patient's tympanic membrane when sound waves and pressure are applied. A tympanometer (Figure 37-25 ◆) has an earpiece that is positioned against the ear canal. If fluid is present behind the tympanic membrane (as in otitis media), the machine will record the absence of tympanic membrane movement.

The Anatomy and Physiology of the Nose

The nose and throat comprise the upper airway (Figure 37-26 ◆). The two sides of the interior nose are separated by the **nasal septum** (dividing wall). The interior of the nose has three zones:

- The vestibular zone is the outermost opening of the nose. The holes in the nose are known as *nares;* the anterior nares are the nostrils. The cilia (nasal hair) filter inhaled air by trapping particles.
- The olfactory zone is the most interior portion of the nose where the sense of smell is located. The chonchae (nasal bones) are located here, covered with membranous tissue. The entering air is warmed and humidified before it reaches the respiratory zone.
- The respiratory zone is located above the soft palate. This is where the airflow begins its downward journey toward the oral cavity.

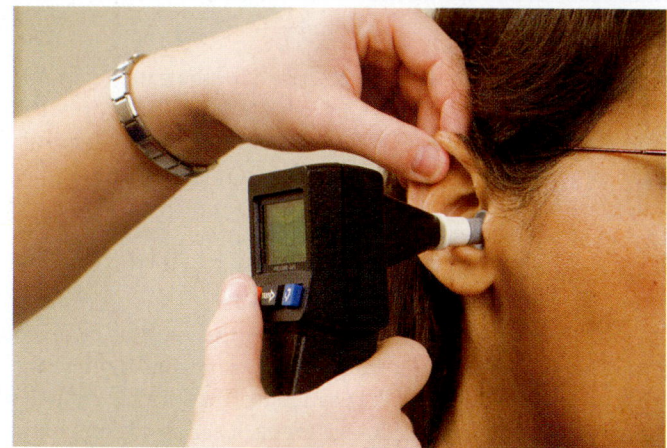

Figure 37-25 ◆ Tympanometer.

Surrounding the nose in the skull are the sinuses. The functions of the sinuses are believed to include lightening the weight of the skull and enhancing phonation (the production of vocal sounds).

Diseases and Disorders of the Nose and Nasal Passages

Disorders of the nose or nasal passages include the inflammatory conditions of rhinitis and paranasal sinusitis, structural conditions of the septum, nasal polyps, epistaxis, traumatic insult, the common cold, and foreign bodies (Table 37-3). An allergic response may be the cause of both rhinitis

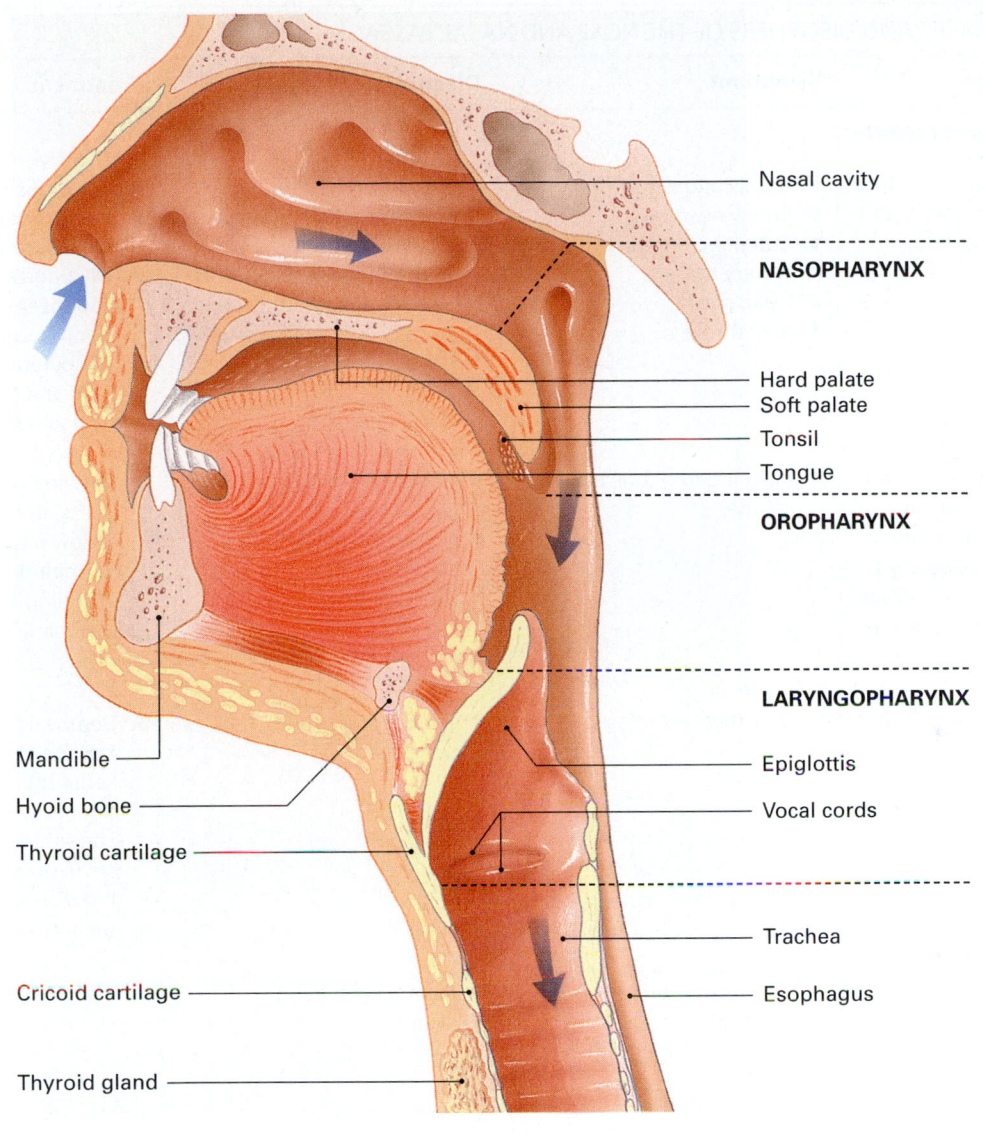

Figure 37-26 ◆ Anatomy of the upper airway.

and sinusitis. Hay fever is typically an allergic response. Therefore, patients who experience chronic or recurrent episode of both upper respiratory conditions may be referred to an allergy specialist.

Diagnosis and Treatment

There are several instruments that facilitate the examination of the nasal passages.

- The otoscope is used to examine not only the ear, but also the nasal cavities. A speculum with a larger opening is usually placed on the scope. The light source enables the examiner to see the mucous membranes lining the nasal cavities.
- The Vienna speculum is used to open the nares and see the nasal membranes. An outside light source is required as well.
- A pharyngeal mirror helps the examiner see into the posterior part of the nasal cavity, or nasopharynx, with an external light source (Figure 37-27 ◆).

Decongestants and steroid-containing nasal sprays are among the drugs used in the care of nose-related conditions.

 Critical Thinking Question 37-3

What items should Stacy lay out for the physician so that he can remove the toy from the child's nose?

The Anatomy and Physiology of the Throat

The pharynx is where the nasal, oral, and laryngeal cavities meet. The pharynx has three regions:

- The nasopharynx is just above the soft palate. It includes the pharyngeal tonsils (adenoids) and the eustachian tubes. Each eustachian tube connects the nasopharynx to the middle ear and maintains equal pressure between these two areas.

TABLE 37-3 DISEASES AND DISORDERS OF THE NOSE AND NASAL PASSAGES

Disease or Disorder	Symptoms	Diagnosis	Treatment
Common cold/Upper respiratory tract infection ■ Inflammatory process affecting upper respiratory tract ■ Caused by viruses	■ Nasal congestion ■ Runny nose ■ Coughing, sneezing ■ Watery eyes ■ Hoarseness ■ Sore throat	■ Patient presenting symptoms and patient history ■ Cultures of nasal discharge and sputum may be necessary to rule out other conditions or to confirm diagnosis of viral cause	■ Condition is usually self-limiting to less than ten days' duration ■ Decongestants and steam vaporizer for nasal congestion, cough syrup for cough, antipyretic agents for fever; mild analgesics ■ Rest and fluids
Epistaxis (nosebleed) ■ Nasal hemorrhage that may occur spontaneously or as result of traumatic injury ■ Often caused by upper respiratory infections or may be recurrent and secondary to other diseases	■ Bleeding from one or both nostrils	■ Patient presenting symptoms ■ Physical examination	■ Blowing nose, then compressing soft tissues just below nasal bones for 5 to 10 minutes (usually stops bleeding, except in case of traumatic injury)
Foreign bodies ■ Objects inserted, usually accidentally, in nares, where they absorb moisture from nasal mucosa (children often insert small objects such as dried peas or grapes into nose)	■ Difficulty breathing	■ Patient presenting symptoms	■ Removal by physician (child may have to be mildly sedated) ■ Squeezing nose if object is something like cereal or small grape; child can then blow object out after it has been crushed
Nasal polyps ■ Masses develop from nasal mucosa and hang down in nasal cavity	■ Difficulty breathing ■ Sinusitis	■ Patient presenting symptoms	■ Surgery to improve airway
Rhinitis ■ Inflammation and/or infection of nasal mucosa ■ Usually caused by virus; part of common cold ■ Causes nasal congestion and rhinorrhea (sneezing and/or itching of nose) ■ Inflammation results in increased mucus secretion and runny nose	■ Runny nose ■ Fever ■ Congestion ■ "Stuffy" head	■ Patient presenting symptoms	■ Liquids ■ Vaporizer to humidify room ■ Over-the-counter (OTC) medications to relieve symptoms—antipyretics for fever and analgesics for discomfort ■ Rest ■ Decongestant sprays (continued use is not recommended)
Septal defects ■ Septum is deviated ■ May be congenital or result of physical injury	■ Sinusitis and nosebleed when there is nasal obstruction	■ Patient presenting symptoms	■ Surgery to improve airway
Sinusitis ■ Inflammation and/or infection of paranasal sinuses ■ Often the forerunner of a cold ■ May be caused by bacteria or virus ■ Acute sinusitis may become chronic	■ Pain and tenderness in cheeks and forehead above eyes	■ Patient presenting symptoms ■ Sinus X-ray	■ Antibiotics and decongestants for bacterial sinusitis ■ OTC medications—antipyretics for fever and analgesics for discomfort ■ Decongestant sprays (continued use is not recommended)

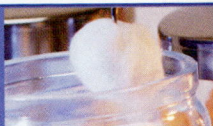

PROCEDURE 37-8   Assist with the Nasal Examination and Obtain Nasopharyngeal Specimen

Theory and Rationale

Examination of the nose and throat is a part of a physical examination and is considered routine in most offices. You may be asked to assist with the examination of the nasal mucosa and the throat. The nasal cavity is examined to inspect the mucous membranes of the nostrils. Typically, the common cold and allergies are the main causes of changes in the mucosa. The physician may use a nasal speculum to inspect the mucous lining of the nose and examine the nasal sinuses by palpation and transillumination. He may note any discharges, lesions, swelling, obstructions, or inflammation. A specimen may be collected to evaluate nasopharyngeal secretions for the presence of pathogenic organisms.

Materials

- penlight
- tongue blade
- sterile swab and transport device
- specimen label
- personal protective equipement
- patient chart
- waste container

Competency

(Conditions) With the necessary materials, you will be able to **(Task)** perform collection of a nasopharyngeal specimen and prepare it **(Standards)** correctly for transport and processing within 15 minutes.

1. Wash your hands.
2. Gather equipment and supplies.
3. Identify and greet the patient, then escort her to the examination room. Explain the process collection.
4. Wash your hands and put on your personal protective equipment.

5. Nasopharyngeal specimen collection:
   - Position the patient with her head tilted back.
   - Using a tongue blade and penlight, examine the nasopharyngeal area and make note of any discharge, lesions, swelling, obstructions, or redness.
   - Gently pass the swab through the nostril and into the nasopharynx. Rotate the swab quickly, then remove it and place in the transport container and medium, if used.
6. Label the container with the patient's name (first and last), date and time of collection, and source of specimen.
7. Dispose of any waste materials in the appropriate container(s).
8. Transport the specimen to the testing area.
9. Wash hands and remove PPE.
10. Perform the required charting or laboratory documentation relating to specimen collection.

Patient Education

Ask the patient to verbalize her understanding of why the test was performed. Usually, the physician prescribes an antibiotic based on clinical symptoms and the usual microorganisms present in the nasopharyngeal infection. If so, reinforce medication instructions. If a C & S is performed, inform the patient that the results usually take three days, but this can vary depending upon the type of pathogen present. The test results will determine if the patient will remain on the same antibiotic or receive another prescription for a more effective medication.

Charting Example

10/15/xx 10:15 a.m. Nasopharyngeal specimen obtained per office procedure. Specimen placed in culturette tube and transported to the laboratory immediately. Pt. Medication instructions received. Daniel Brown, CMA (AAMA)

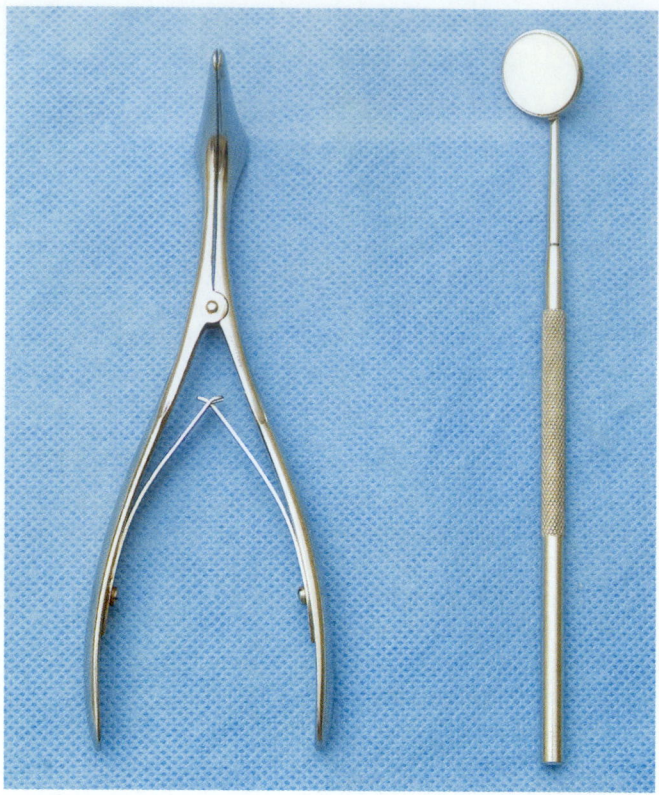

Figure 37-27 ◆ Nasal speculum and pharyngeal mirror.

- The oropharynx is the region you see when you look into a patient's mouth. The palatine tonsils flank either side of this region and the tongue. This region, also called the oral cavity, contains the teeth, the tongue and its taste buds, the inner portion of the cheeks (buccal membranes), and the salivary glands.
- The laryngopharynx is just above the vocal cords. The lingual tonsils (at the base of the tongue), and the epiglottis are located here. The epiglottis is the cartilage (elastic tissue) that covers the trachea (windpipe) during swallowing. The epiglottis prevents food or liquids from entering into the airway.

The vocal cords are housed in the larynx and mark the beginning of the lower airway (Figure 37-28 ◆). They vibrate during exhalation, which creates the sound of the voice.

Diseases of the Mouth and Throat

Common infectious conditions of the throat include pharyngitis, laryngitis, and strep throat. Tonsillitis and adenoiditis are the inflammation and usually infection of the tonsils and adenoids. Thrush is a fungal infection usually affecting infants. Oral cancer may occur in a number of locations in the mouth, lips, and tongue (Table 37-4).

Diagnosis and Treatment

Structures in the oral cavity and pharynx are viewed with the following instruments:

- External light source and tongue depressor
- Laryngeal mirror and external light source—mirror is usually warmed under warm running water to prevent fogging by the patient's breath
- Laryngoscope—requires sedation of the patient and application of a topical anesthetic

Drug therapy includes lozenges, gargles, throat sprays, and antibiotics.

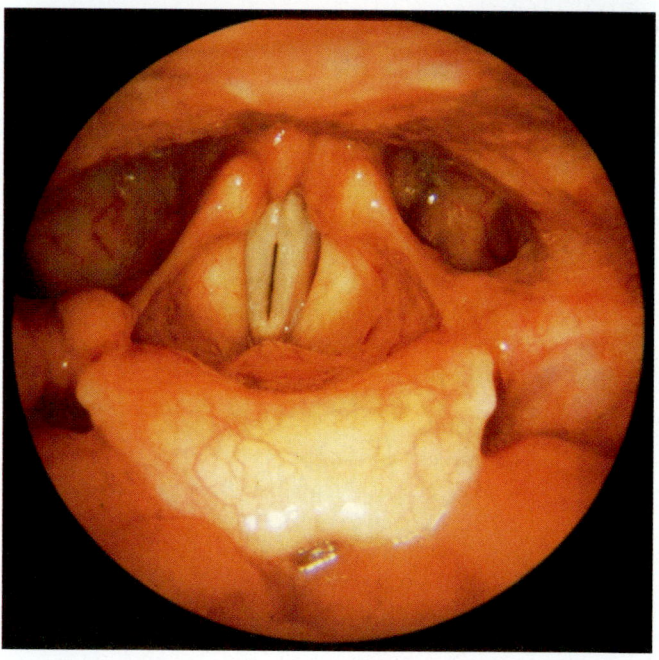

Figure 37-28 ◆ Vocal cords.
Source: Phototake NYC.

TABLE 37-4 INFECTIOUS CONDITIONS OF THE MOUTH AND THROAT

Disease	Symptoms	Diagnosis	Treatment
Laryngitis ■ Inflammation and/or infection of larynx ■ Inflammation of vocal cords makes it difficult to speak ■ May be bacterial or viral in origin ■ May be caused by irritation of respiratory passage or excessive use of the voice	■ Difficulty speaking ■ Sore throat ■ Fever ■ Chills	■ Patient presenting symptoms ■ Visual examination with laryngeal mirror	■ Voice rest ■ Drinking liquids ■ Humidified air ■ Antibiotics for bacterial infections ■ Removing the cause
Oral cancer ■ Cancer on the lips, buccal mucosa, anterior tongue, hard palate, floor of the mouth, or lower gingivia ■ May be in the form of squamous cell carcinoma or adenocarcinoma	■ White patchy lesions in the mouth that do not heal ■ Ulcers on lips and tongue are or become painful ■ Possible difficulty eating, chewing, or swallowing ■ Reduced appetite ■ Possible weight loss	■ If not painful, lesions often discovered on a dental visit ■ Patient history and exam	■ Depends on extent and location of lesion ■ Radiation and surgery (surgery may have to be extensive to remove diseased tissue)
Pharyngitis (sore throat) ■ Inflammation and/or infection of pharynx ■ Caused by bacteria or virus, sometimes smoke or foreign objects ■ May precede a cold or sinusitis or be secondary to a virus	■ Dry or burning sensation in throat ■ Fever ■ Chills ■ Difficulty swallowing and speaking ■ Enlarged cervical lymph nodes ■ Red or swollen membranes	■ Patient presenting symptoms ■ Visual examination	■ Antipyretics and analgesics for bacterial infections ■ Saltwater gargles and throat lozenges to ease discomfort ■ Tonsil removal for chronic pharyngitis that may be result of tonsillitis ■ Rhinitis and sinusitis treatment when these conditions are present
Thrush ■ Fungal infection in mouth caused by *Candidiasis albicans* ■ Occurs most often in infants and young children, but the elderly and immunodeficient individuals also susceptible	■ Usually noticed in infants as slightly raised yellow patchy areas in mouth on inner aspects of cheeks, tongue, and upper palate, and on mucous membrane of inner lip ■ Burning sensation	■ Patient history, oral examination, and laboratory examination of tissue samples	■ Antifungal medications ■ Antifungal mouthwash
Tonsillitis and adenoiditis ■ Inflammation and infection of tonsils and adenoids ■ Patient may refer to this condition as sore throat ■ Most common in children ages 5 to 10; may lead to rheumatic heart disease ■ Non-streptococcal tonsillitis resolves in a few days	■ Pain ■ Difficulty swallowing ■ Fever ■ Chills ■ Earache ■ Muscle aches ■ General malaise ■ Cervical lymph nodes swollen and tender to touch	■ Patient presenting symptoms ■ Visual examination	■ Strep screen or a culture to identify infection ■ Antibiotics ■ Tonsillectomy for patients, especially children, who have more than four sore throats in a year (removal of adenoids in children is common during this procedure)

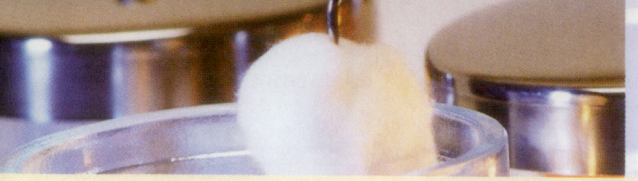

Chapter Summary

- Eye specialists include:
  - *ophthalmologists*—diagnose and treat eye diseases and conditions
  - *optometrists*—examine eyes, test visual acuity, and prescribe adaptive lenses
  - *opticians*—grind lenses, insert lens into frames, and fit patient glasses
- Ear, nose, and throat specialists include:
  - *otorhinolaryngologists*—ear, nose, and throat diseases and conditions
  - *otolaryngologists*—ear and throat diseases and conditions
  - *laryngologists*—throat diseases and disorders
  - *rhinologists*—nose diseases and disorders
- Medical assistants may take vital signs, record patient histories, and perform visual acuity testing, simple audiometry, and irrigation and instillation of the eyes and ears.
- Refractive errors of the eye cause myopia, hyperopia, astigmatism, and presbyopia.
- Infectious disorders of the eye include conjunctivitis, keratitis, blepharitis, and styes. Conjunctivitis is an inflammation and infection of the conjunctiva, the mucous membrane covering the eyeball and lining the eyelid. Keratitis is an inflammation and ulceration of the surface of the cornea. Blepharitis is an inflammation and infection of the hair follicles and glands of the eyelid margins. A stye is an inflammatory and infectious process of an eyelid sebaceous gland.
- Degenerative disorders of the eye include cataracts, diabetic retinopathy, macular degeneration, and glaucoma. Visual acuity typically becomes impaired with aging. Retinal detachment may be the result of a degenerative process or of a traumatic insult.
- Foreign bodies in the eye cause tearing, pain, and occasionally impaired visual acuity or photophobia.
- Visual acuity testing and eye irrigations and instillations are the assessments and diagnostic procedures commonly performed by an MA. Instruments used in eye care include the ophthalmoscope, slit lamp, eye spud, and tonometer.
- Ear disorders include impacted earwax; inflammatory and infectious disorders such as Ménière's disease, otitis externa, otitis media, and otitis interna (labyrinthitis); otosclerosis, a fusion of three main ear bones (ossicles); ruptured tympanic membrane; nerve trauma; and foreign bodies. Diagnostic procedures and hearing assessments performed by an MA include simple audiometry and ear irrigations and instillations. Instruments used in ear care include the otoscope, Vienna speculum, and Zeiss microscope.
- Nose or nasal passage disorders include the inflammatory conditions of rhinitis and sinusitis, structural conditions of the septum, nasal polyps, epistaxis (nosebleed), traumatic insult, and foreign bodies. Instruments used in nose care include the otoscope, Vienna speculum, and pharyngeal mirror.
- Common throat disorders include pharyngitis, laryngitis, strep throat, tonsillitis, adenoiditis, and thrush. Oral cancer may affect a number of locations. Instruments used in throat care include the tongue depressor, laryngeal mirror, and laryngoscope.

Chapter Review

Multiple Choice

1. A patient being tested for visual acuity must keep both eyes open, because
   a. it prevents squinting.
   b. it is easier to see through the spatula.
   c. the patient is standing 20 feet away from the chart.
   d. it helps the patient keep his or her balance.

2. Which of the following specialists is trained to grind lenses?
   a. Ophthalmologist
   b. Optometrist
   c. Optician
   d. Otolaryngologist

3. Myopia is a/an
   a. infection.
   b. refractive disorder.
   c. foreign body.
   d. inflammation.

4. When you irrigate a patient's eye, the patient should
   a. lie flat on his or her back.
   b. sit and look straight at you.
   c. turn the head away from the eye being irrigated.
   d. turn the head in the direction of the eye being irrigated.

5. Ear medication must be administered at
   a. room temperature.
   b. 35°F.
   c. 40°F.
   d. 45°F.

6. A child with otitis media often
   a. smiles and laughs.
   b. falls asleep easily.
   c. pulls at the ear.
   d. keeps the head totally straight.

Chapter Review (continued)

7. The sense of smell is located in the
   a. vestibular zone.
   b. respiratory zone.
   c. nasopharyngeal zone.
   d. olfactory zone.

8. Which of the following is a function of the sinuses?
   a. Sinusitis
   b. Phonation
   c. Balance
   d. Filtration

9. Which of the following is a function of the Eustachian tube?
   a. Phonation
   b. Filtration
   c. Balance
   d. Sinusitis

10. A tonsillectomy is usually recommended if a patient has more than how many sore throats in a year?
    a. Four
    b. One
    c. Two
    d. Three

True/False

T F 1. The mucous membrane covering the eyeball and lining the eyelid is conjunctivitis.

T F 2. The iris is responsible for regulating the amount of light that enters the eye.

T F 3. The superior rectus muscle moves the eye to look down.

T F 4. The ophthalmoscope is used to examine the ear.

T F 5. A tonometer is used to test the pressure within the eye.

Short Answer

1. What does the top number or first number recorded on a Snellen measurement indicate?

2. What does the second or bottom number on a Snellen measurement indicate?

3. Which medications cause the pupils to constrict?

4. What is the purpose of simple audiometry testing?

5. Name the three zones of the interior of the nose.

Research

1. Is there a low-cost clinic for patients in your community who need hearing aids?

2. Optometrists' services offered in "superstores" such as Wal-mart are gaining in popularity. What are some of the pros and cons of these practices?

Externship Application Experience

The medical assistant has prepared to irrigate the eyes of a 5-year-old patient who has sand in her eyes from playing in a sandbox. The MA has explained the procedure to the patient and her mother. When the MA begins the procedure, the patient begins screaming and squirming. What should the medical assistant do?

Resource Guide

American Academy of Ophthalmology
655 Beach Street
San Francisco, CA 94109-7424
(415) 561-8500
www.aao.org

American Optometric Association
243 Lindbergh Boulevard
St. Louis, MO 63141
(314) 991-4100
www.aoanet.org

American Diabetes Association
1701 N. Beauregard Street
Alexandria, VA 22311
(703) 549-1500
1-800-342-2383
www.diabetes.org

Juvenile Diabetes Foundation International
432 Park Avenue South
New York, NY 10016
(212) 889-7575
www.jdfcare.com

National Diabetes Information Clearinghouse
National Institute of Diabetes and Digestive and Kidney Diseases
1 Information Way
Bethesda, MD 20892-3560
(301) 654-3327
www.niddk.nih.gov

National Eye Institute
2020 Vision Place
Bethesda, MD 20892-3655
(301) 496-5248
www.nei.nih.gov

Resource Guide (continued)

Prevent Blindness America
500 East Remington Road
Schaumburg, IL 60173
1-800-331-2020
(847) 843-2020
www.preventblindness.org

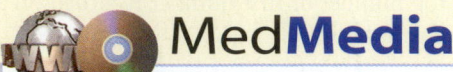 Med**Media**

http://www.MyMAKit.com

More on this chapter, including interactive resources, can be found on the Student CD-ROM accompanying this textbook and on http://www.MyMAKit.com.

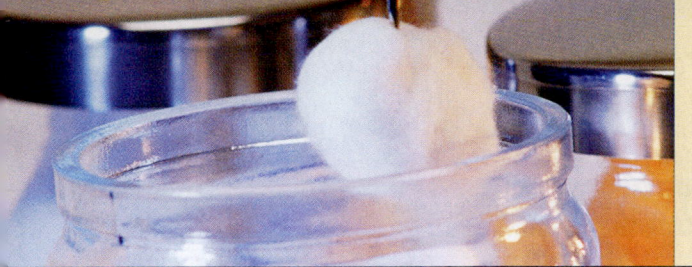

Objectives

After completing this chapter, you should be able to:

- Define and spell the key terminology in this chapter.
- Define the medical assistant's role in the immunology office.
- Discuss the anatomy and physiology of the immune system.
- List and describe immunodeficiency diseases.
- List and describe common autoimmune disorders.
- Explain hypersensitivity and allergic reactions.

Immunology and Allergies

Case Study

Eric is assisting an AIDS patient who has come in for an assessment of a rash on his left and right flanks that wraps around to his back. The rash itself is not itchy, but the area is very painful and nothing seems to be helping. After Eric checks in the patient, he will assist the doctor in performing a prick skin test on another patient to determine if she can have a new puppy for her eighth birthday. The child's mother is concerned because she has other allergies, and she wants to make certain they won't bring a puppy home only to have to return it a few days later.

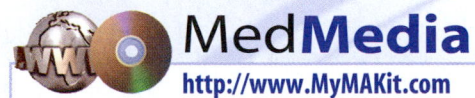

MedMedia
http://www.MyMAKit.com

Additional interactive resources and activities for this chapter can be found on http://www.MyMAKit.com. For a video, tips, audio glossary, legal and ethical scenarios, job scenarios, quizzes, and games related to the content of this chapter, please access the accompanying CD-ROM in this book.

Video
Audio Glossary
Legal and Ethical Scenario: *Immunology and Allergies*
On the Job Scenario: *Immunology and Allergies*
A & P Quiz: The Immune System
Multiple Choice Quiz
Games: Crossword, Strikeout, and Spelling Bee
Tips
HIPPA Quiz

Key Terminology

allergen—substance that is not necessarily harmful, such as dust or eggs, but that produces a hypersensitive reaction in some individuals

ankylosis—condition of joint immobility

antibody—substance produced by the body in response to a specific antigen

antigen—foreign substance that stimulates the production of antibodies against it when it is introduced into the body

antipyretic—fever reducing

autoimmunity—body's negative reaction to its own cells

carditis—inflammation of the heart

dysfunction—abnormal or impaired function

dysphagia—difficulty swallowing

dysphasia—difficulty speaking

ecchymosis—bruise; area of bleeding under the skin

electromyography—procedure in which a needle is inserted into muscle tissue to record electrical activity

hematopoietic—pertaining to normal blood cell development in the bone marrow

hemolytic—pertaining to the breakdown of RBCs

immunodeficiency—inability of the immune system to function normally to protect the body from infection

interphalangeal—between the joints of the fingers or toes

intrinsic factor—substance secreted by the gastric mucosa that is necessary for the absorption of vitamin B_{12} and the development of RBCs

megakaryocytes—large bone marrow cells that play an important role in the production of platelets in the bone marrow

neuritis—inflammation of a nerve or nerves

petechiae—small hemorrhages under the skin

reactive—able to respond to a stimulus

subcutaneous—under the epidermal and dermal layers of the skin

⊕ MEDICAL ASSISTING STANDARDS

CAAHEP ENTRY-LEVEL STANDARDS	ABHES ENTRY-LEVEL COMPETENCIES
■ Perform within scope of practice (psychomotor) ■ Apply ethical behaviors, including honesty/integrity in performance of medical assisting practice (affective) ■ Explain the rationale for performance of a procedure to the patient (affective) ■ Use language/verbal skills that enable patients' understanding (affective) ■ Describe the normal function of each body system (cognitive) ■ Identify common pathology related to each body system (cognitive) ■ Analyze pathology as it relates to the interaction of body systems (cognitive) ■ Discuss implications for disease and disability when homeostasis is not maintained (cognitive) ■ Describe implications for treatment related to pathology (cognitive) ■ Explore issue of confidentiality as it applies to the medical assistant (cognitive)	■ Project a positive attitude. ■ Maintain confidentiality at all times. ■ Be a "team player." ■ Be cognizant of ethical boundaries. ■ Exhibit initiative. ■ Adapt to change. ■ Evidence a responsible attitude. ■ Be courteous and diplomatic. ■ Conduct work within scope of education, training, and ability. ■ Be impartial and show empathy when dealing with patients. ■ Adapt what is said to the recipient's level of comprehension. ■ Serve as a liaison between the physician and others. ■ Interview effectively. ■ Use appropriate terminology. ■ Recognize and respond to verbal and nonverbal communication. ■ Adaptation to individualized needs. ■ Apply principles of aseptic techniques and infection control. ■ Take vital signs. ■ Recognize emergencies. ■ Prepare and maintain examination and treatment areas. ■ Collect and process specimens. ■ Prepare and administer oral and parenteral medications as directed by the physician. ■ Maintain medication and immunization records.

Introduction

An immunologist is a physician who specializes in the immune system and its functions. An allergist is a physician who specializes in diagnosing and treating allergies. Immunology and allergy are often combined within one practice, where allergy testing, allergy desensitization, and laboratory testing are performed.

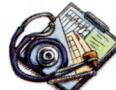

The Medical Assistant's Role in Immunology and Allergy

The medical assistant in an immunology and allergy medical office will:

- Obtain the patient's medical history.
- Take vital signs.
- Instruct the patient about removing clothing, provide a gown and drape, and help the patient, if necessary.

Abbreviations

AIDS—acquired immunodeficiency syndrome

CSF—cerebral spinal fluid

EMG—electromyography

MS—multiple sclerosis

N & V—nausea and vomiting

RA—rheumatoid arthritis

SCID—severe combined immunodeficiency disease

SLE—systemic lupus erythematosus

- Assist the immunologist or allergist, as necessary, with the examination and procedures.
- Watch for signs of allergic reaction when allergy desensitization injections are given.
- Instruct the patient about medication orders, written pre- or postprocedure instructions, and any other written instructions.
- Stress the importance of keeping follow-up appointments.

The Anatomy and Physiology of the Immune System

The immune system provides physical and chemical barriers to bacterial and viral infection and foreign bodies. Barriers include intact skin, secretions, the mucous membranes of organs, the actions of coughing and sneezing, and the acidity of body fluids such as urine and gastric juices.

Allergens are substances that are capable of producing a hypersensitive allergic reaction but may not be harmful to the organism. **Antigens** are foreign substances, usually proteins, that can evoke an allergic response. When an antigen enters the body, the immune system reacts to deactivate, neutralize, or kill it.

There are four components to the body's immune response.

- The *cell-mediated response* is responsible for the production of T-cell lymphocytes. It is part of the response to some infections, malignancies, and delayed hypersensitivity reactions. It is also responsible for tissue transplant rejection.
- The *humoral immune response* is responsible for the production of B-cell lymphocytes with antigen exposure and the resulting **antibody** development. This process renders the patient immune or hypersensitive to the specific antigen.
- Body tissues respond to injury with inflammation, also known as a *nonspecific immune response.* The inflammatory response involves chemical, vascular, and leukocyte activities. Signs of inflammation include redness, swelling, pain, and warmth.
- The *specific immune response* activates when the inflammatory response is not adequate to manage the infectious or inflammatory process. This response is controlled by the T- and B-cells of the cell-mediated and humoral immunity processes, respectively.

The lymphatic vessel system filters infectious microorganisms from the lymph system and uses substances within the plasma portion of the blood to activate the inflammatory response. When blood, tissue, or organs are transplanted, a transfusion reaction or tissue rejection may result in response to the presence of foreign, or non-self, cells, tissue, or fluid. Suppression of the inflammatory response to prevent tissue rejection is accomplished with medication for the remainder of the recipient's life. Blood transfusion reactions are temporary, are often prevented by administering medications during the procedure, or are treated at the onset of symptoms.

The immune system (Figure 38-1 ◆) is made up of:

- A primary set of organs, the thymus gland and bone marrow, that are responsible for the development of lymphocytes.
- A secondary set of organs—the lymph glands and vessels, tonsils, liver, and spleen—that filter substances and stimulate the production of lymphocytes.
- **reactive** leukocytes.

There are five kinds of leukocytes.

- Polymorphonuclear leukocytes (PMNs), also known as polys or neutrophils, react to infection threatening the health of body cells and protect cells from damage.
- Monocytes, which mature into macrophages, are the first line of defense in phagocytosis, a process in which specific cells ingest foreign agents and substances. Other phagocytes include Kupffer's cells of the liver and lymph node reticular cells (Figure 38-2 ◆).
- Eosinophils are attracted to cells and parasites coated with C3B substance, such as helminths. The eosinophils then secrete chemicals to erode the walls of the invading organism.
- Basophils are important in hypersensitivity reactions in the allergic response.
- Lymphocytes (B-cells and T-cells) are responsible for the antigen–antibody response and sensitization, or memory, of cells to previous antigen exposure.

All lymphocytes form in the bone marrow. B-lymphocytes (also called B-cells) mature in the bone marrow, whereas T-lymphocytes (T-cells) migrate and mature in the thymus

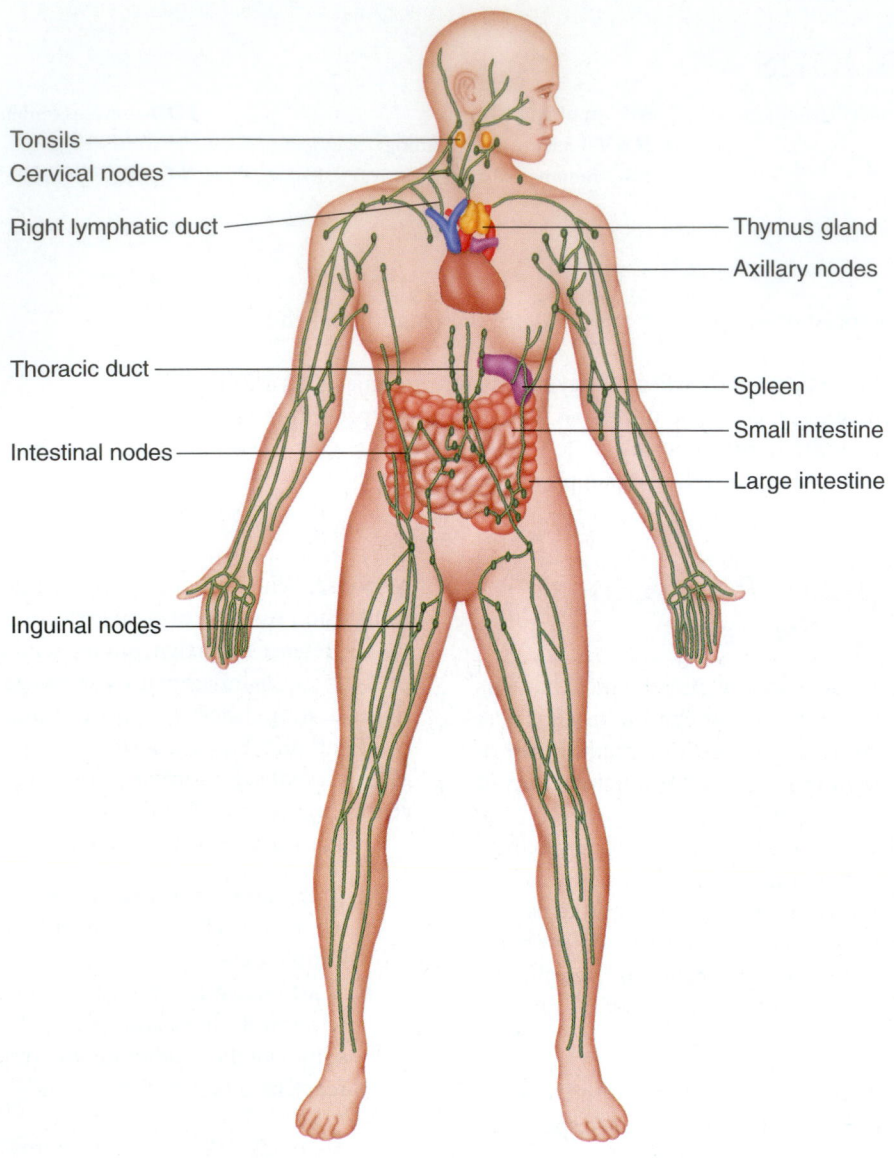

Tonsils

Cervical nodes

Right lymphatic duct

Thymus gland

Axillary nodes

Thoracic duct

Spleen

Small intestine

Intestinal nodes

Large intestine

Inguinal nodes

Figure 38-1 ◆ The lymphatic system.

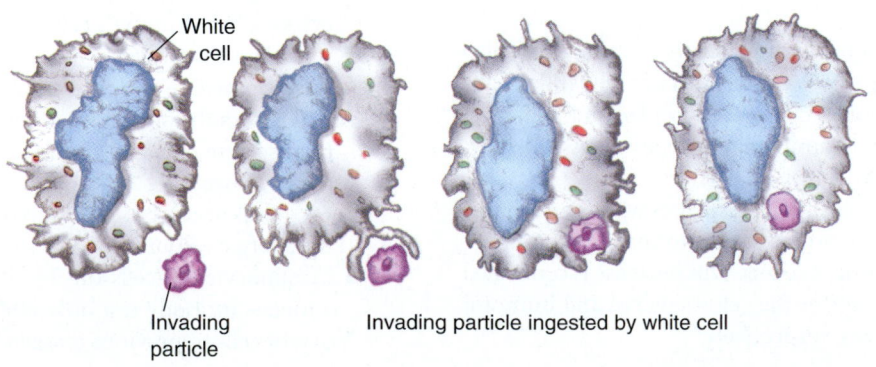

White cell

Invading particle

Invading particle ingested by white cell

Figure 38-2 ◆ Phagocytosis.

gland. Macrophages absorb the foreign substance or infection after T-cells and B-cells destroy it. This process is called cell-mediated immunity when only T-cells are involved, and humoral or antibody-mediated immunity when T- and B-cells are involved.

Immunity is the ability to resist a particular disease or condition. *Natural immunity* is inherited. *Acquired immunity* results from being exposed to the disease or being immunized. Natural immunity and immunity acquired by exposure stimulate the development of antibodies to create active immunity.

Active immunity is long-term and often lifelong. For example, a patient who has had chickenpox is immune for life and will never need a chickenpox vaccination. Immunizations (administered vaccines) also lead to active immunity. *Passive immunity,* on the other hand, is short-term and involves the administration of already formed antibodies. Further vaccination is required to acquire immunity. For example, newborns, because of the placental transfer of the mother's antibodies, have passive immunity to some diseases for a short time after birth. Breast-fed babies keep this immunity even longer because of the transfer of antibodies in breast milk. However, the child requires vaccinations when the antibody protection wears off. (See ∞ Chapter 45 for more information on childhood immunizations.)

Diseases and Disorders of the Immune System

Diseases and disorders of the immune system fall into three general categories: immunodeficiency diseases, autoimmune disorders, and hypersensitivity and allergy reactions. Immunodeficiency diseases occur when the immune system is unable to fight the disease and protect the body. In autoimmune conditions, the body fails to recognize its own cells as self and develops self-antigens, which leads to the destruction of the perceived foreign cells. Hypersensitivity and allergy reactions result from the entry of a foreign body or substance into the system with resulting inflammation and organ **dysfunction.**

Immunodeficiency Diseases

Immunodeficiency diseases result when the immune system is unable or becomes unable to fight and protect the body from disease (Table 38-1). Some immunodeficiency diseases are caused by hereditary, or genetic, patterns. More commonly, however, the immune system is weakened by chemotherapy or radiation, immunosuppressive drugs for organ/tissue transplants, or disease. Treatments such as chemotherapy, radiation, or immunosuppressive drugs decrease the ability of white blood cells to fight infection or foreign substances. The patient may

TABLE 38-1 IMMUNODEFICIENCY DISEASES

Disease	Symptoms	Diagnosis	Treatment
Acquired Immunodeficiency Syndrome (AIDS) ■ Caused by human **immunodeficiency** virus (HIV) ■ Virus is easily killed outside body with diluted bleach or other solutions ■ Virus destroys lymphocytes, particularly T-cells and macrophages, leaving immune system defenseless against all infections ■ Inability to fight infections, even with antibiotic treatment, results in death	■ Influenza ■ Kaposi's sarcoma ■ Pneumocystis carinii pneumonia (PCP) ■ Candida albicans ■ Tuberculosis ■ Herpes zoster (shingles)	■ Patient presenting symptoms ■ Serologic studies ■ ELISA test detects HIV antibodies ■ Western blot test confirms AIDS diagnosis ■ T-cell count, in addition to clinical symptoms, defines early, late, or advanced stages of HIV infection	■ Antibiotics for infections ■ Antiviral medications for viruses ■ AIDS drugs—various drugs in most effective combination for patient ■ Rebuilding lymphocytes to increase patient's immunity; T-cells especially important ■ Support and counsel
Severe Combined Immuno-deficiency Disease (SCID) ■ Inherited condition that puts infant in danger of severe infection ■ No T-cell mediated or B-cell antibody-mediated immunity ■ Most infants die within the first year	■ Failure to thrive (grow and gain weight) ■ Various infections such as pulmonary, ear, and systemic infections	■ Difficult to diagnose before 6 months to 1 year of age ■ Serologic tests	■ Bone marrow transplant to increase healthy T- and B-cells ■ Sterile environment to prevent exposure to any infection

TABLE 38-2 OPPORTUNISTIC CONDITIONS COMMON TO AIDS

Malignancies	Gastrointestinal Symptoms
■ Kaposi's sarcoma	■ Nausea and vomiting
■ Lymphomas	**(N & V)**
Infections	■ Diarrhea
■ Pneumocystis carinii pneumonia	■ Lack of appetite
■ Candida albicans	**Neurological Symptoms**
■ Herpes zoster (shingles)	■ Confusion and memory loss
■ Tuberculosis	■ Headache and visual changes
■ Toxoplasmosis	
■ Herpes simplex	

suffer severe or recurrent opportunistic infections, and it is often these complications that prove life-threatening or fatal (Table 38-2).

? — Critical Thinking Question 38-1-
What precautions should Eric take when setting up the patient with AIDS for examination by the physician?

HIV/AIDS Transmission Prevention Strategies

HIV/AIDS is transmitted by person-to-person contact. The following are suggestions for avoiding direct contact with the transmission source while still living as normal a life as possible.

- Avoid sex with multiple partners. Maintain a monogamous relationship.
- Use condoms and spermicides to prevent the transmission of body fluids during sex.
- Do not use intravenous (IV) drugs or share used needles of any kind with another person.
- Make sure that people providing tattoo and body piercing services use new needles.
- Control your behavior. Avoid using drugs or overindulging in alcohol, both of which lower your guard in social situations and place you at risk for unprotected sex.

In Practice

David Robinson, 25 years old, has recently been diagnosed with HIV. He states that he is taking his medications as prescribed and has enrolled in a support group for HIV-positive men. The patient has learned that there are several opportunistic conditions that are common to AIDS. He wants to know what the opportunistic conditions are. What information will you as the medical assistant provide to this patient?

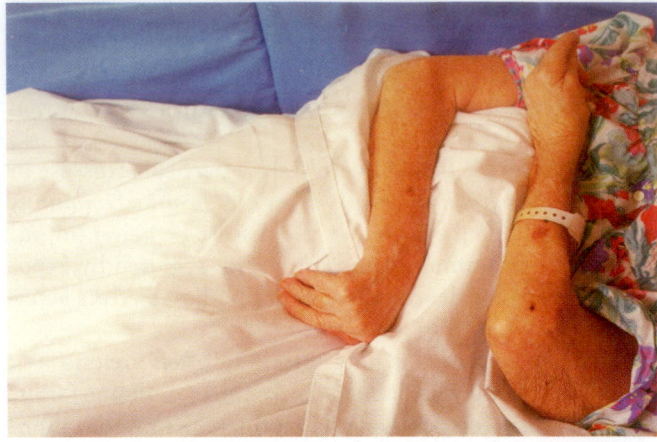

Figure 38-3 ◆ A patient with rheumatoid arthritis in the hands.

Autoimmune Diseases

Autoimmune diseases result from antigens that develop from aggressive activity by the body's immune system against itself (Figures 38-3 ◆ and 38-4 ◆). This type of disorder can affect any body area, including collagen (protein found in connective joints), **hematopoietic** tissue, cardiovascular system tissue, and nervous system tissue (Table 38-3). For example, in hemolytic anemia, the body fails to recognize its own blood cells and destroys RBCs and lymphocytes that have been produced in its own hematopoietic system. Autoimmune disorders may result from unknown causes, but may also be awakened by genetic weaknesses or in combination with other disease complications.

Autoimmune disorders may also affect other systems of the body:

- Gastrointestinal system: ulcerative colitis (a colon disease), atrophic gastritis (a stomach disease)
- Endocrine system: Hashimoto's thyroiditis (a thyroid gland disease), thyrotoxicosis (a thyroid gland disease)

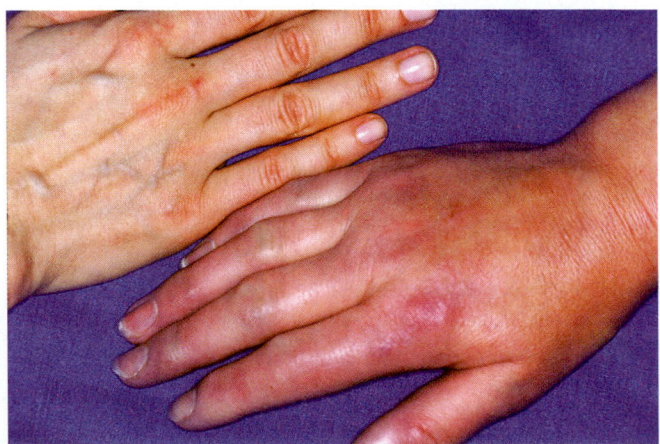

Figure 38-4 ◆ Systemic scleroderma of the hand.
Source: Phototake NYC.

TABLE 38-3 AUTOIMMUNE DISEASES

Disease	Symptoms	Diagnosis	Treatment
Autoimmune hemolytic anemia ■ RBCs are not recognized and are destroyed by B-cells ■ Decreased numbers of RBCs, platelets, hemoglobin, and hematocrit ■ Destroys lymphocytes, particularly T-cells and macrophages, leaving immune system defenseless against all infections	■ Weakness ■ Fever ■ Chills ■ Dyspnea ■ Bruising ■ Skin color pale and jaundiced	■ Patient presenting symptoms ■ Serologic studies ■ Coombs' test for presence of antibodies	■ Immunosuppressive drugs to suppress antigen–antibody response ■ Antiviral medications for viruses ■ Transfusions of washed RBCs, platelets, and plasma in some cases ■ Splenectomy to halve RBC destruction; can increase patient's immunity; T-cells especially important
Idiopathic thrombocytopenic purpura ■ Bleeding into skin and other organs ■ Results when platelets are destroyed by body's own immune response ■ Hematopoietic conditions may result after some viral infections ■ Decreased platelet count and longer bleeding time ■ **Megakaryocytes** in bone marrow	■ **Petechiae** ■ **Ecchymosis** ■ Epistaxis ■ Hematuria ■ Gastrointestinal bleeding	■ Serologic tests	■ Blood transfusions to increase platelet count ■ Vitamin K to stop prolonged bleeding ■ Steroids to stop capillary bleeding ■ Plasma exchange and splenectomy to increase circulating platelets
Multiple sclerosis (MS) ■ Chronic and progressive neurological disorder affecting myelin sheath (covering that insulates and protects some nervous system cells) ■ May be autoimmune disorder but may also result from genetic tendency or viral infections	■ Double vision ■ Muscle weakness ■ Lack of coordination, progressing to paralysis ■ Numbness ■ Prickling ■ Tingling ■ **Dysphasia** ■ Incontinence ■ Mood swings from depression to euphoria	■ Patient presenting symptoms ■ Medical history ■ MRI ■ Cerebrospinal fluid **(CSF)** analysis	■ Physical therapy to increase muscle strength ■ Muscle relaxants for muscle spasms ■ Antidepressants for depression ■ Steroids to suppress autoimmune process ■ Psychological support for patient and significant others
Myasthenia gravis ■ Neuromuscular disease that results in chronically sporadic and progressive periods of weakened muscles ■ Muscle weakness usually occurs after strenuous activity or during afternoon/evening ■ Progresses to complete muscular and respiratory paralysis	■ Fatigue ■ Muscle weakness ■ Double vision ■ Ptosis (drooping eyelids) ■ Difficulty swallowing ■ Backward flow of fluids through nose ■ Other symptoms of cranial nerve dysfunction (see ∞ Chapter 46)	■ Patient presenting symptoms ■ **Electromyography (EMG)** ■ Neostigmine injection	■ Anticholinesterase drugs to reduce muscle weakness ■ Corticosteroid and immunosuppressive drugs to suppress autoimmune process ■ Thymectomy for a select number of patients ■ Psychological support for patient and significant others

continued

TABLE 38-3 AUTOIMMUNE DISEASES (CONTINUED)

Disease	Symptoms	Diagnosis	Treatment
Pernicious anemia ■ May be inherited or autoimmune blood cell production disorder ■ Results from deficiency of **intrinsic factor** ■ Macrocytic (abnormally large) RBCs develop when B_{12} is deficient ■ Patient's life will be normal	■ Weakness ■ Fatigue ■ Pallor ■ Light-headedness ■ Tachycardia and/or palpitations ■ Nausea and/or vomiting ■ **Neuritis** ■ Numbing and tingling of extremities	■ Patient presenting symptoms ■ Medical history ■ Laboratory studies ■ CBC ■ B_{12} serum levels ■ Schilling test to assess gastrointestinal absorption of B_{12} ■ Gastric analysis ■ Bone marrow test	■ **Subcutaneous** injections of cyanacobalamin on a weekly, biweekly, or monthly basis
Rheumatoid arthritis (RA) and juvenile rheumatoid arthritis ■ Chronic disease causing inflammation and destruction of synovial membranes of multiple joints; cartilage and bone erode and joints become deformed ■ May be hereditary; generally thought to be autoimmune disorder ■ **Ankylosis** can cause joint immobility ■ Edema may be present in **interphalangeal** joint areas in severely affected patients ■ Rheumatoid arthritis in children is also called Still's disease	In adults: ■ Joint pain ■ Mild or low-grade fever ■ Fatigue ■ Malaise ■ Weight loss In children: ■ Joint pain ■ Weight loss ■ High fever in the evening ■ Red rash over trunk and limbs ■ Swollen neck and axillary area lymph glands ■ Acute pericarditis ■ Growth may be affected	■ Patient presenting symptoms ■ Serologic test	■ Balanced activity and rest to control pain and inflammation ■ Salicyclates (e.g., aspirin) to control pain and inflammation ■ Ibuprofen or other enteric coated anti-inflammatory drugs for patients with gastric irritation or gastric ulcers to reduce pain and inflammation (medication dosages for children based on weight) ■ Physical therapy, paraffin wax therapy, and braces to improve mobility ■ Surgery—complete joint replacement for severe cases
Rheumatic fever and rheumatic heart disease ■ Rheumatic fever is caused by development of hypersensitive antibodies to group A hemolytic streptococci; reaction causes lesions to grow at cardiac tissue (myocarditis) and joints (arthritis) ■ Characterized by elevated WBCs, cardiac enzymes, ESR	■ Strep throat (about four weeks before fever) ■ Malaise ■ Fever ■ Joint pain	■ Patient presenting symptoms ■ Medical history ■ Laboratory tests such as ESR	■ Antibiotics for strep throat to prevent it from progressing to rheumatic heart disease ■ Analgesics, cardiac medications, and rest to prevent heart damage ■ Surgery to replace damaged heart valves
Scleroderma (systemic sclerosis) ■ Chronic disorder involving skin and connective tissue ■ Ranges in severity from mild (only skin or part of skin involved) to severe (skin and internal organs involved) ■ Collagen production leads to hardening and thickening of tissue, with decrease in function	■ Pain ■ Stiffness ■ Joint swelling ■ Leathery, shiny, tightly stretched skin ■ Raynaud's phenomenon (small artery and arteriole disease) ■ Difficulty eating	■ Patient presenting symptoms ■ Skin biopsy ■ Urinalysis	■ Analgesics for pain ■ Anti-inflammatories for inflammation ■ Immunosuppressive drugs to control or slow autoimmune process ■ Vasodilator and/or antihypertensive drugs to treat Raynaud's phenomenon

TABLE 38-3 AUTOIMMUNE DISEASES (CONTINUED)

Disease	Symptoms	Diagnosis	Treatment
Scleroderma (systemic sclerosis) (*cont.*) ■ Usually slowly progressive disease, but sometimes can progress rapidly toward death	■ Gastric symptoms: efflux heartburn, **dysphagia, diarrhea, constipation**		
Systemic lupus erythematosus (SLE) ■ Chronic systemic disorder affecting any part of connective tissue throughout the body ■ Prognosis is grave; high mortality rate within five years of onset	■ Butterfly rash on face ■ Fever ■ Malaise ■ Weakness ■ Weight loss ■ Photosensitivity ■ Joint symptoms ■ Raynaud's phenomenon ■ Pleuritis (inflammation of pleural membranes) ■ **Carditis** ■ Spotty alopecia (hair loss) ■ Ulcerations in nose, pharynx, oral cavity	■ Patient presenting symptoms ■ Patient history ■ Serologic tests, including CBC, ESR, anti-DNA, LE, and bone marrow	■ Aspirin to relieve inflammation ■ Corticosteroids to relieve inflammation ■ Clothing protection (hats, long sleeves, and long pants) for patients with photosensitivity

■ Renal system: Goodpasture's syndrome (a kidney disease)
■ Circulatory system: vasculitis (a blood vessel disease)

A Coombs' test assesses the development of antibodies to **hemolytic** diseases. Antinuclear antibody testing can be performed to assist in the diagnosis of SLE or RA. Treatment focuses on steroids and immunosuppressive drugs to reduce the self-antigen/antibody response. Support treatment prevents possible further harm to the organ system(s) affected. Analgesics are prescribed for pain as necessary. Psychological support and therapy may be needed for these progressive and physically debilitating diseases.

Hypersensitivity and Allergic Reactions

An allergy is an immune system response to a foreign body that results in inflammation and organ dysfunction. Hypersensitivity, an abnormal condition, is an exaggerated response of the immune system. Allergies develop after repeated exposure to an antigen (Table 38-4). Allergic reactions include the following.

■ Hay fever is a respiratory reaction to allergens such as pollen. It is usually seasonal.
■ Asthma is a more serious respiratory reaction. It can be life-threatening if the person experiences status asthmaticus (severe and prolonged asthma attack).
■ Urticaria, also known as hives, is characterized by a spreading area of reddened and elevated lesions (Figure 38-5 ◆). Causes include insect bites, stress, drugs, and food.
■ Food allergies can be severe and life-threatening. For example, people who are allergic to peanuts cannot eat them or touch anything that has been touched by peanuts.

TABLE 38-4 COMMON ALLERGENS

Environment	
dust	animal dander
plant pollen	insect stings
mold	medications
latex	chemicals
cockroaches	strong aerosol odors
hair	cigarette smoke
Food	
peanuts and peanut products	nuts
	eggs
shellfish	milk
fish	

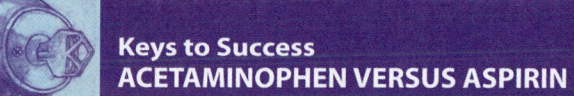

Keys to Success
ACETAMINOPHEN VERSUS ASPIRIN

Aspirin has **antipyretic,** analgesic, and anti-inflammatory properties. Acetaminophen has only antipyretic and analgesic properties. It is not used to treat inflammatory disease conditions except to enhance the pain-relieving properties of another medication.

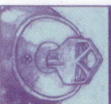

**Keys to Success
AGING AND IMMUNITY**

The thymus gland, which aids in the maturing of T-cells during childhood, gradually decreases in size and function from puberty on. T-cells in the shrinking thymus gland also decrease the immune system's fighting ability. B-cell antibody function decreases as the body ages, too. It is thought that the decline in function of the immune system leads to a higher risk of disease development in the elderly. But there are other factors, such as general health, medications, nutrition, psychological stresses, and lack of social activity, that may raise their vulnerability to disease.

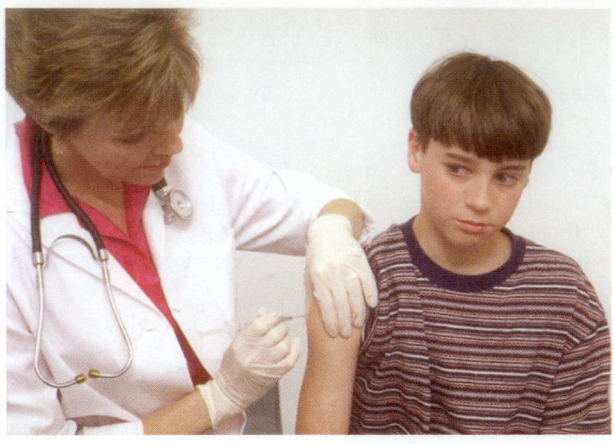

Figure 38-6 ◆ Diagnostic allergy testing: intradermal injection.

■ Anaphylactic reactions are increasingly severe antigen–antibody reactions to repeated exposure to an allergen. They can be mild or life-threatening. If symptoms progress toward swelling of airway passages and increasingly severe shortness of breath, emergency treatment is necessary. Anaphylactic reactions can occur after unexpected exposure to allergens or planned exposure to weakened allergens used in allergy desensitization injections (explained later in the chapter).

Diagnostic Procedures and Treatments

There are four methods of diagnostic allergy testing:

■ Intradermal: injecting a small amount of potential antigen under the skin (Figure 38-6 ◆).
■ Skin patch: putting a patch soaked with potential antigen on the skin.
■ Scratch testing: putting the potential antigen into a scratch made on the skin (Figure 38-7 ◆).

■ CBC for RBCs, platelets, and WBCs, including B and T lymphocytes.

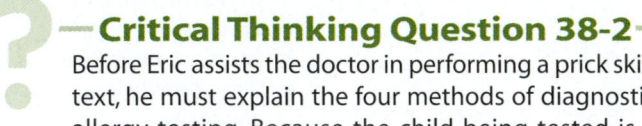

? — Critical Thinking Question 38-2 —
Before Eric assists the doctor in performing a prick skin text, he must explain the four methods of diagnostic allergy testing. Because the child being tested is a minor, what else does Eric need to do?

Treatment of allergic reactions involves first trying to identify the cause. If possible, the allergen is removed from the patient's environment. Antihistamines are prescribed to treat symptoms and halt their progression. Allergy injections may be recommended to desensitize the patient to certain allergens. If the patient cannot be removed from environmental exposure to the allergen, a special serum may be prescribed. Each prescription is specially formulated to introduce very weak concentrations of the allergen and stimulate the patient's body to produce immunity to the allergen.

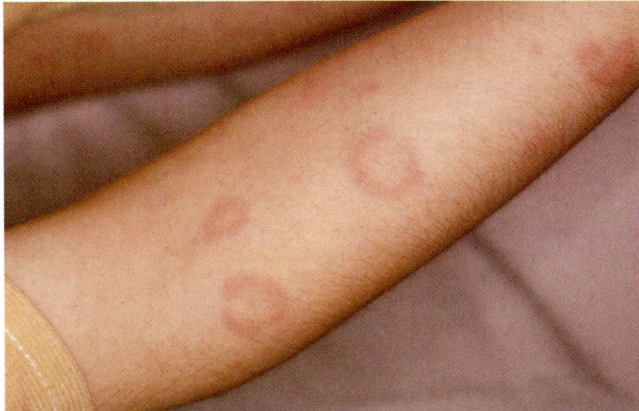

Figure 38-5 ◆ Urticaria is characterized by a spreading area of reddened and elevated lesions

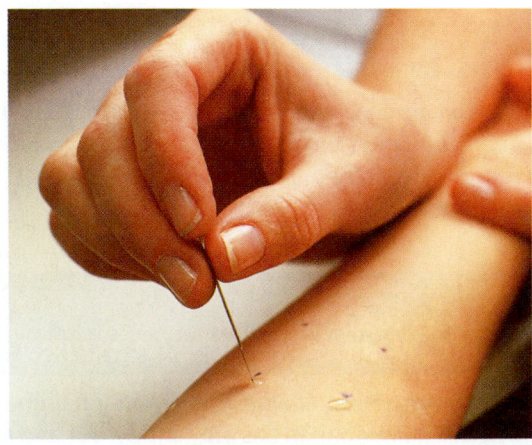

Figure 38-7 ◆ Diagnostic allergy testing: performing a scratch test on a patient.

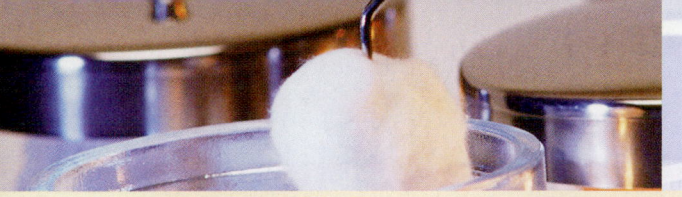

REVIEW

Chapter Summary

- Obtaining the medical history and routine vital signs and assisting patients and the physician are key functions of the MA in an immunology and allergy practice.
- Procedures performed in an immunology and allergy office are allergy testing, allergy desensitization, electromyography, and laboratory testing.
- The immune system provides a physical and chemical barrier to bacterial and viral infection and foreign bodies. It has a primary set of organs, a secondary set of organs, and reactive leukocytes.
- All lymphocytes form in the bone marrow, but B-cells mature in the bone marrow and T-cells migrate and mature in the thymus gland. T-cells defend the body with a cell-mediated response. B-cells defend the body with an antibody-mediated response.
- When the immune system malfunctions, a patient can become immunodeficient, autoimmune, and/or hypersensitive to allergens. A patient who receives a transplant may experience a transfusion reaction or tissue rejection.
- Immunodeficiency diseases result when the immune system no longer functions to protect the body against disease. Some

immunodeficiency diseases are caused by hereditary, or genetic, patterns, but generally the immune system is weakened by chemotherapy or radiation, immunosuppressive drugs for organ/tissue transplants, or disease. Examples of immunodeficiency diseases are AIDS and SCID.
- Autoimmune diseases result from developed self-antigens that stimulate aggressive activity by the immune system against itself. This disorder can affect any body area. Examples of autoimmune diseases are RA and MS.
- Allergy responses are hypersensitive reactions of the immune system to allergen and antigens. Reactions include hay fever, asthma, urticaria, and life-threatening anaphylaxis. Common allergens include pet dander, house dust, mold, plant pollen, medications, foods, and household solutions that come in contact with the skin.
- The four methods of diagnostic allergy testing are intradermal, skin patch, scratch testing, and CBCs. Treatment of allergic reactions involves identifying the cause, removing the patient from the environment, if possible, and prescribing antihistamines. Allergy injections may be recommended to desensitize the patient to certain allergens.

Chapter Review

Multiple Choice

1. Which of the following organs is responsible for producing lymphocytes?
   a. Spleen
   b. Liver
   c. Thymus gland
   d. Heart

2. Which of the following organs filters and removes foreign substances?
   a. Spleen
   b. Thymus gland
   c. Bone marrow
   d. Heart

3. Active immunity is
   a. an outcome of breastfeeding a child longer than is recommended.
   b. short-term, with the need for further vaccination.
   c. long-term and results from being exposed to and having the disease.
   d. an outcome of placental transfer of the mother's antibodies to the child.

4. AIDS can be transmitted by
   a. kissing.
   b. shared needles.
   c. hand contact.
   d. drinking alcohol.

5. SCID is a disease that affects
   a. elderly.
   b. teens.
   c. adults.
   d. children.

6. Autoimmune hemolytic anemia is treated by
   a. hysterectomy.
   b. appendectomy.
   c. splenectomy.
   d. lumpectomy.

7. Vitamin K is prescribed for idiopathic thrombocytopenic purpura to
   a. stop prolonged bleeding.
   b. increase platelet count.
   c. increase megakaryocytes.
   d. stop viruses.

8. Which of the following is a symptom of juvenile RA?
   a. Vomiting
   b. Strep throat
   c. Pallor
   d. Acute pericarditis

9. A serious anaphylactic reaction requires
   a. an MRI.
   b. a blood test.
   c. emergency care.
   d. a skin biopsy.

Chapter Review (continued)

10. Which of the following is used to test for allergies?
    a. Schilling test
    b. Intradermal test
    c. Coombs' test
    d. ESR

True/False

T F 1. Immunology and allergy treatment are combined into one practice.

T F 2. Coughing, sneezing, and the acidity of body fluids such as urine and gastric juices are all types of barriers to bacterial and viral infection and foreign bodies.

T F 3. Allergens are foreign substances, usually proteins.

T F 4. Antigens are substances capable of producing a hypersensitive allergic reaction.

T F 5. All lymphocytes are formed in the bone marrow.

Short Answer

1. What is another term for *inflammation?*
2. List the organs that make up the immune system.
3. What are the five kinds of leukocytes?
4. What is the difference between active and passive immunity?
5. Name the four methods of diagnostic allergy testing.

Research

1. How many AIDS cases were reported in your state last year?
2. Are there any AIDS/HIV support groups or activity centers in your community?

Externship Application Experience

An adult patient presents with redness, swelling, fluid-filled vesicles, and itching on the hands and lower arms. The patient states he has no history of allergies. What questions should you ask this patient?

Resource Guide

American Lupus Society
260 Maple Court, Suite 123
Ventura, CA 93003
1-800-331-1802

Arthritis Foundation
3400 Peachtree Rd. NE
P.O. Box 7669
Atlanta, GA 30357-0669
1-800-283-7800
www.arthritis.org

Lupus Foundation of America
2000 L Street NW, Suite 710
Washington, DC 20063
800-558-0121
www.lupus.org

National AIDS Hotline
P.O. Box 13827
RTP, NC 27709
1-800-342-AIDS, 24 hours a day
www.ashastd.org/nah
www.hivmail@cdc.gov

National Multiple Sclerosis Society
733 Third Ave.
New York, NY 10077
1-800-344-4867 (FIGHT-MS)
www.nmss.org

Primary Immunodeficiency Association, United Kingdom
+44(0)20-7976-7640
www.pia.org.uk

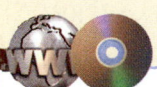

MedMedia

http://www.MyMAKit.com

More on this chapter, including interactive resources, can be found on the Student CD-ROM accompanying this textbook and on http://www.MyMAKit.com.

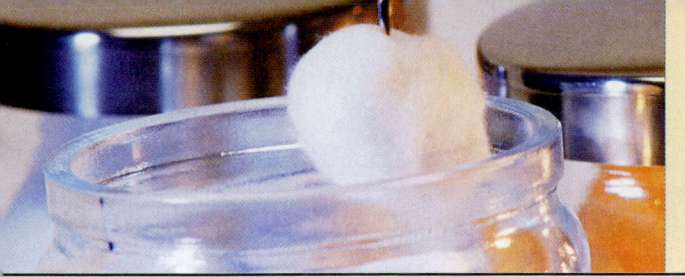

Objectives

After completing this chapter, you should be able to:

- Define and spell the key terminology in this chapter.
- Define the medical assistant's role in the dermatology office.
- List and describe common types of dermatitis.
- List and describe common types of congenital skin disorders.
- List and describe common types of infectious skin disorders.
- List and describe common types of fungal skin diseases.
- List and describe common types of parasitic skin diseases.
- List and describe common types of pigmentation disorders.
- List and describe common types of benign skin disorders.
- List and describe the three types of skin cancer.

Dermatology

Case Study

Manny is busy rooming patients at the dermatology office where he works and notices that he has two walk-in patients today. The first is a teenage girl who has come with her mother to check on what she describes as a "suspicious mole" she found while sunbathing. In the next room, a mother has brought in her four children after being notified of a lice outbreak at school.

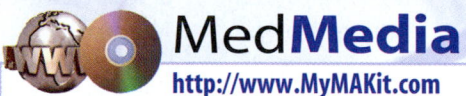

MedMedia
http://www.MyMAKit.com

Additional interactive resources and activities for this chapter can be found on http://www.MyMAKit.com. For a video, tips, audio glossary, legal and ethical scenarios, job scenarios, quizzes, games, and activities related to the content of this chapter, please access the accompanying CD-ROM in this book.

Video
Audio Glossary
Legal and Ethical Scenario: *Dermatology*
On the Job Scenario: *Dermatology*
A & P Quiz: The Integumentary System
Multiple Choice Quiz
Games: Crossword, Strikeout, and Spelling Bee
Drag and Drop: Integumentary System: Anterior View of the Body; Integumentary System: Posterior View of the Body; Integumentary System: Hair Follicle; Integumentary System: Layers of the Skin; Integumentary System: Features of the Integumentary System
Tips
HIPAA Quiz

Key Terminology

appendage—anything attached to a larger or major body part

cauterization—destruction of tissue with a caustic, electric current, hot iron, or by freezing

collagen—fibrous connective tissue

cryosurgery—freezing lesions with nitrous oxide

dermatitis—skin inflammation

dermatologist—physician who specializes in the treatment of skin diseases and conditions

dermatology—study and treatment of integumentary system diseases and conditions

dermatophytoses—superficial fungal infections of the skin and its appendages

integumentary system—the skin and its supporting structures (nails, hair, and sebaceous and sweat glands)

keratin—tough protein substance found in hair, nails, and horny tissue

lesion—tissue abnormality that may be hard or soft, small or large, flat or raised, crusted or filled with fluid or pus, and, when associated with skin, on or within the skin tissue

melanin—pigment (color) in the skin and hair

melanocytes—cells that produce melanin

neuralgia—sharp, stabbing, or burning pain that occurs along the course of a nerve

sebaceous glands—small glands in the dermis that secrete sebum, usually through ducts that empty into the hair follicles

Abbreviations

AK—actinic keratosis

BCC—basal cell carcinoma

SCC—squamous cell carcinoma

UV—ultraviolet

MEDICAL ASSISTING STANDARDS

CAAHEP ENTRY-LEVEL STANDARDS	ABHES ENTRY-LEVEL COMPETENCIES
■ Perform within scope of practice (psychomotor) ■ Apply ethical behaviors, including honesty/integrity in performance of medical assisting practice (affective) ■ Explain the rationale for performance of a procedure to the patient (affective) ■ Use language/verbal skills that enable patients' understanding (affective) ■ Describe the normal function of each body system (cognitive) ■ Identify common pathology related to each body system (cognitive) ■ Analyze pathology as it relates to the interaction of body systems (cognitive) ■ Discuss implications for disease and disability when homeostasis is not maintained (cognitive) ■ Describe implications for treatment related to pathology (cognitive)	■ Project a positive attitude. ■ Maintain confidentiality at all times. ■ Be a "team player." ■ Be cognizant of ethical boundaries. ■ Exhibit initiative. ■ Adapt to change. ■ Evidence a responsible attitude. ■ Be courteous and diplomatic. ■ Conduct work within scope of education, training, and ability. ■ Practice Standard Precautions. ■ Use quality control. ■ Dispose of biohazardous materials.

Introduction

A **dermatologist** is a physician who specializes in treating skin diseases and conditions. Procedures performed in the **dermatology** office include biopsies, **cryosurgery,** and the surgical removal of lesions. Suture removal and dressing application may be the responsibilities of the MA.

The Medical Assistant's Role in Dermatology

The MA in a dermatology office will:

- Obtain the patient's medical history.
- Take vital signs.
- Instruct the patient about removing clothing, provide a gown and drape, and help the patient as necessary.
- Assist the dermatologist, as necessary, with the examination and procedures.
- Instruct the patient about medication orders, written pre- or post-procedure instructions, and any other written instructions.
- Stress the importance of keeping follow-up appointments.

The Anatomy and Physiology of the Skin

The **integumentary system** is the largest organ of the body. The other structures of the integumentary system are the nails, hair, and sweat and **sebaceous glands.** The skin serves several bodily functions, including the following:

- Barrier to prevent microorganisms and other foreign bodies from entering.
- Temperature regulator.
- Protection against dehydration.
- Environmental sensor, including pain, temperature, and touch.
- Synthesizing vitamin D from sunlight.
- Excreting toxins in perspiration.

Skin is composed of three layers (Figure 39-1 ◆):

- Epidermis.
- Dermis.
- Subcutaneous tissue.

Skin cells originate in the basal layer of the epidermis (just above the dermis) and progress upward. As they move toward the surface, the cells die and are eventually sloughed off, or shed. The life cycle of epidermal cells lasts approximately four weeks. They are made up largely of **keratin,** a protein found also in hair and nails. **Melanin,** also produced in the epidermis, is the pigment that colors the skin, hair, and iris of the eye. It also serves to protect the skin from harmful ultraviolet (**UV**) rays.

The dermis contains blood and lymph vessels, nerve cell endings, and skin support organs—nails, hair follicles, and sweat and sebaceous glands. The elasticity of the skin depends on the connective cells and **collagen** within the dermis. The nerve cell endings in the dermis sense touch, pain, and temperature.

The innermost layer, the subcutaneous tissue, is made up of connective tissue and fat cells. This layer acts as insulation for the body. It provides protection against extreme heat and cold and against heat loss. The layers of fat cells cushion and protect underlying structures.

The **appendages** of the skin are the following:

- Hair, which covers most of the body surface.
- Nails, which protect the finger and toe tips.
- Sweat glands, which regulate body temperature.
- Sebaceous glands, which prevent the skin and hair from drying.

Hair is a nonliving keratin tissue. Each hair is formed within a sheath-like follicle and extends upward to the skin surface (Figure 39-2 ◆). Nails, also nonliving keratin, grow from the nail root (Figure 39-3 ◆). The condition of the nails can reflect a person's overall health. Sweat glands are located in the dermis and subcutaneous tissue (Figure 39-4 ◆). They have excretory tubes extending to the surface of the skin, where they open as sweat pores. Sweat evaporating from the pores cools the body. The sebaceous glands open into the hair follicles and secrete an oily substance, sebum, that lubricates the skin and hair (Figure 39-5 ◆).

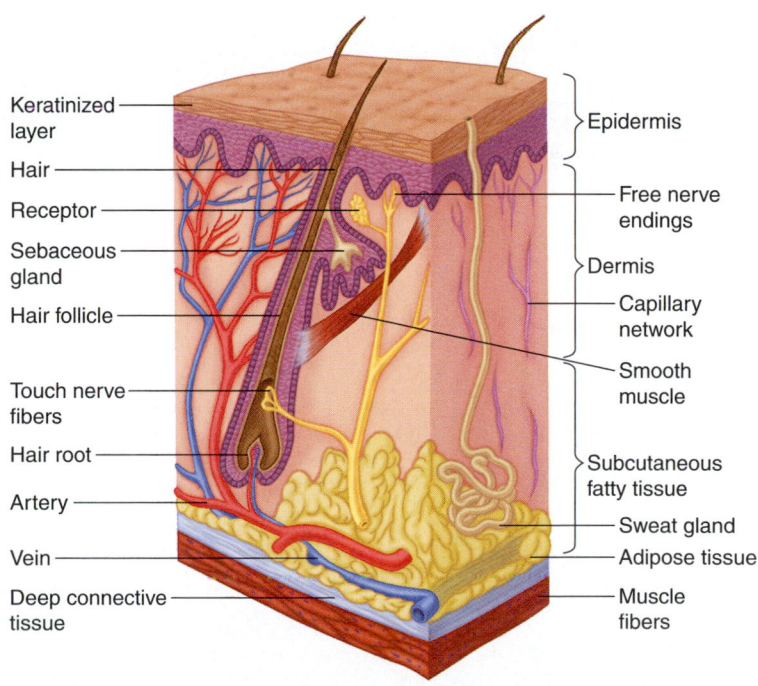

Figure 39-1 ◆ Structure of the skin.

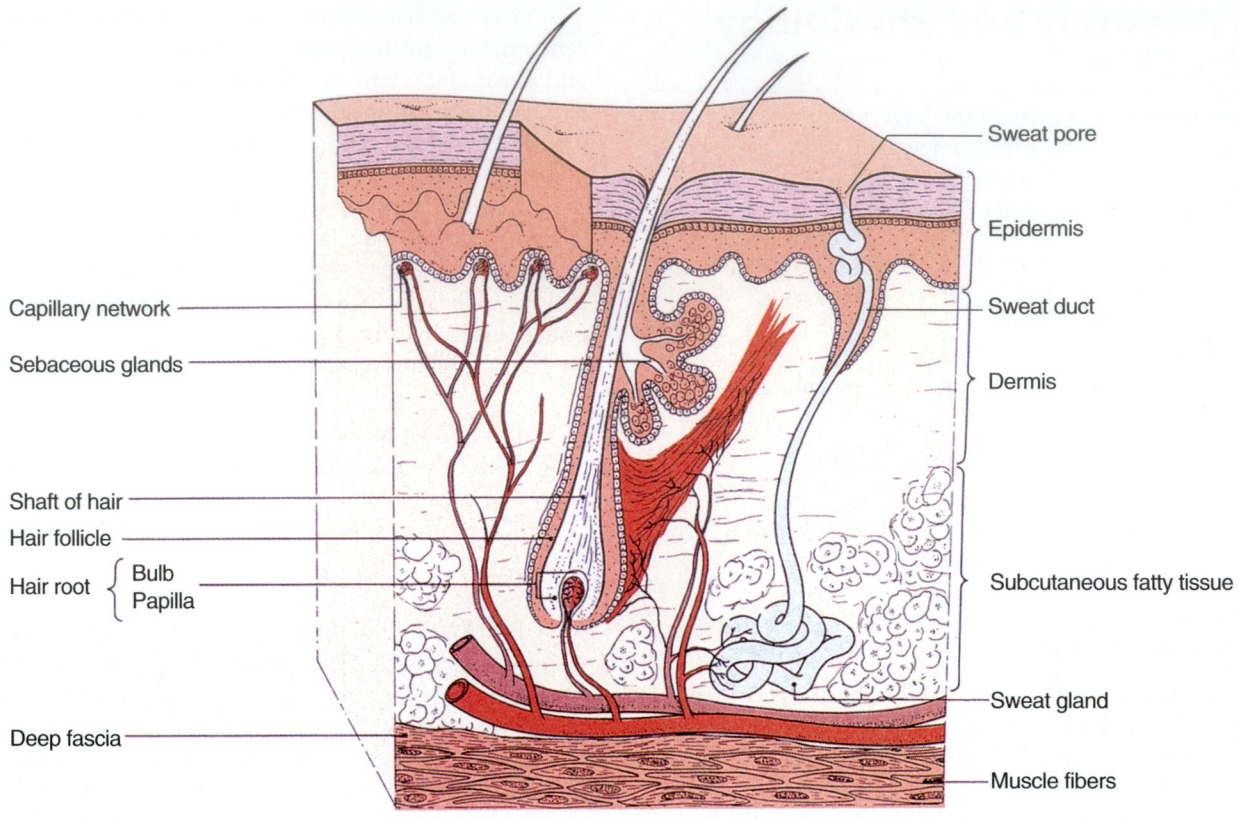

Figure 39-2 ◆ Hair follicle/skin structures.

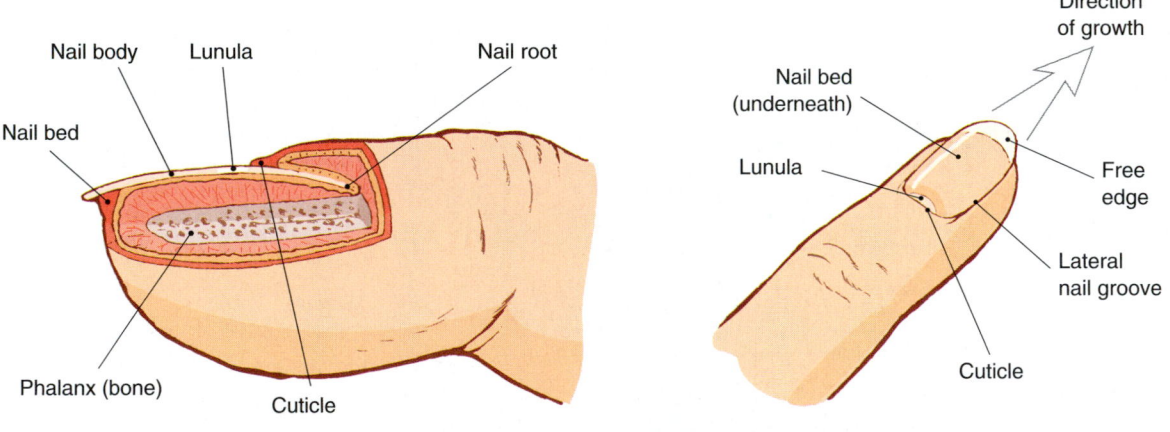

Figure 39-3 ◆ Nail bed and structure.

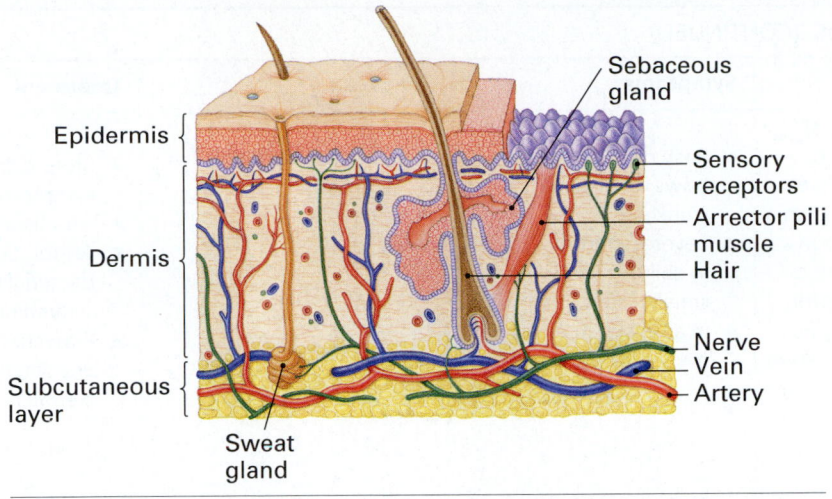

Figure 39-4 ◆ The sweat glands are located in the dermis and subcutaneous tissue.

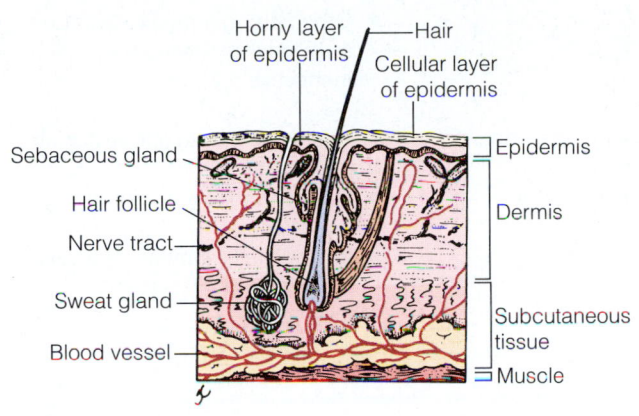

Figure 39-5 ◆ The sebaceous glands open in the hair follicles and secrete sebum.

Diseases and Disorders of the Skin

As the largest organ of the body, the integumentary system has a large exposed surface and is the site of many diseases and disorders. A break in this defense system of the body may result in generalized illness as well as localized irritations or **lesions.** Insults or injuries to the skin may disrupt any of several bodily functions involved with the skin.

Dermatitis

Dermatitis is an inflammatory condition that occurs on or in the layers of the skin. It may be chronic or acute. There are several types of dermatitis: seborrheic dermatitis, allergic contact dermatitis, contact dermatitis, eczema, and urticaria (hives) (Table 39-1; Figures 39-6 ◆ through 39-9 ◆).

TABLE 39-1 DERMATITIS

Type of Dermatitis	Symptoms	Diagnosis	Treatment
Allergic contact dermatitis ■ Skin condition resulting from contact with an allergen ■ Common allergens are plants (poison oak, poison ivy, sumac), latex, preservatives, laundry products, detergents, dyes, drugs, furs, fragrances, and cosmetics; sometimes radiation from sun or tanning beds	■ Skin redness ■ Swelling ■ Oozing small vesicles that may burn, itch, and sting	■ Patient presenting symptoms ■ Patient history	■ Removing the source when possible; irritation continues to spread as long as skin is in contact with source ■ Cleansing skin to remove irritant from skin surface ■ Steroid cream to ease irritation and help healing ■ Oral steroids at decreasing dosages for more involved cases to reverse reaction and for healing
Contact dermatitis ■ Skin irritation caused by contact with a chemical substance on skin's surface ■ Common chemicals are latex, fragrances, dyes, detergents, laundry products, acids, and cleaning products	■ Skin redness ■ Swelling ■ Small, oozing vesicles that may burn, itch, and sting	■ Patient presenting symptoms ■ Patient history	■ See "Allergic contact dermatitis"

continued

TABLE 39-1 DERMATITIS (CONTINUED)

Type of Dermatitis	Symptoms	Diagnosis	Treatment
Eczema (atopic dermatitis) ■ Inflammation of the skin ■ Generally found in people with family history of eczema or other allergic conditions ■ May be triggered by stress and sudden, severe weather changes; in infants, may be triggered by milk and orange juice ■ No known cure, but heals in time	■ Rash on face, neck, elbows, knees, and upper trunk ■ Severe itching ■ In children: rash with small blisters and oozing ■ In adults: rash with small, dry, leathery blisters	■ Patient presenting symptoms ■ Patient history	■ Steroid cream to control symptoms ■ Antihistamines to relieve itching ■ Antibiotics when necessary for bacterial infection due to scratching ■ Pimecrolimus cream (steroid-free anti-inflammatory) in place of steroids
Seborrheic dermatitis ■ Chronic, inflammatory, and noncancerous ■ Caused by increased secretion by sebaceous glands ■ Called cradle cap in infants and toddlers	■ Skin redness ■ Itching ■ Yellow-tinged and greasy-looking scales	■ Patient presenting symptoms	■ Hydrocortisone or low-strength cortisone cream for topical application ■ Other, stronger medications prescribed when creams are ineffective
Urticaria (hives) ■ Acute allergic response to allergen contact ■ Life-threatening when respiratory system is involved because of sudden and acute edema of airway tissue ■ Contact with allergen may be through dermal contact, ingestion, injection (for example, bee stings), or inhalation	■ Eruptions on body, skin surfaces, or mucous membranes ■ Local swelling ■ Skin redness	■ Patient presenting symptoms ■ Patient history	■ Antihistamines to relieve itching and allergy ■ Epinephrine to reduce swelling and edema ■ Immediate treatment necessary when respiratory system is involved

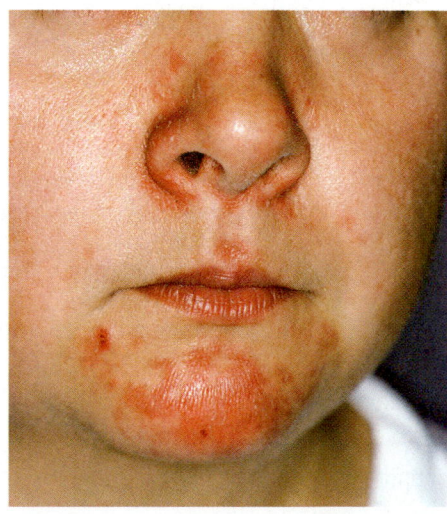

Figure 39-6 ◆ Acute facial seborrheic dermatitis.
Source: Phototake NYC

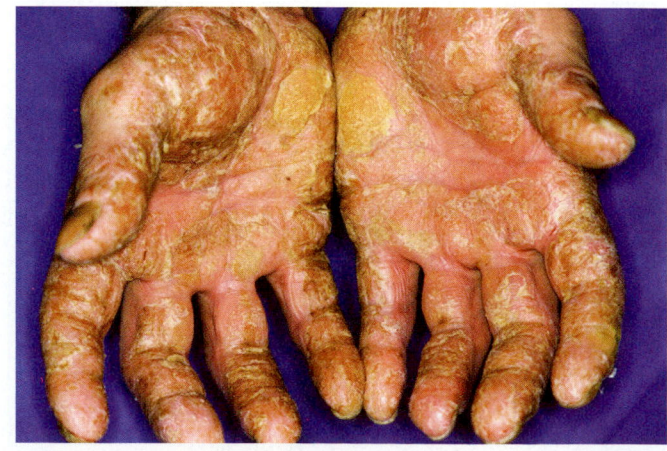

Figure 39-7 ◆ Contact dermatitis on the hands.
Source: Phototake NYC

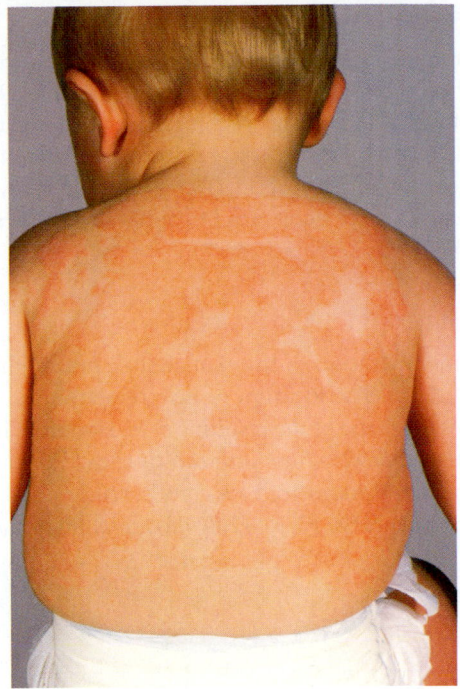

Figure 39-8 ◆ An infant afflicted by atopic eczema.
Source: Phototake NYC

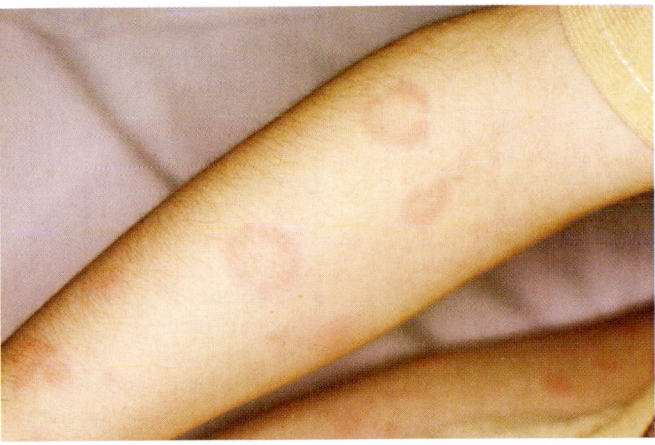

Figure 39-9 ◆ Urticaria.
Source: CNRI/Phototake NYC

In Practice

The medical assistant is working in a busy pediatric office and the receptionist informs the MA that there is a patient who has just arrived and is complaining of a rash that is "itching." The receptionist is concerned that the patient may be contagious. What should the medical assistant do?

Infectious Skin Disorders

Infectious skin disorders include herpes zoster (shingles), herpes simplex, acne, furuncles/carbuncles, and impetigo (Figures 39-10 ◆ through 39-13 ◆). See also Table 39-2.

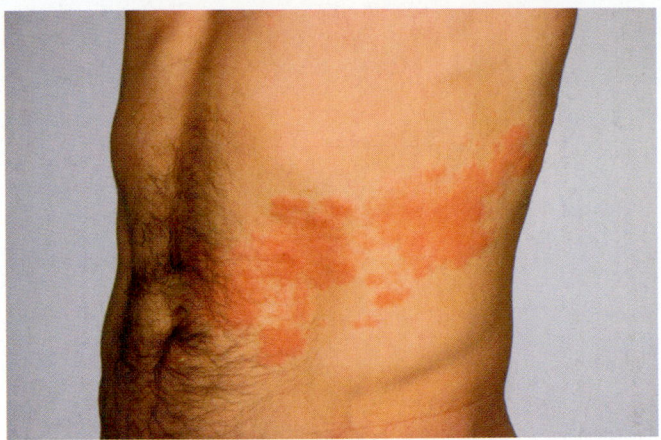

Figure 39-10 ◆ Shingles on the torso.
Source: Phototake NYC

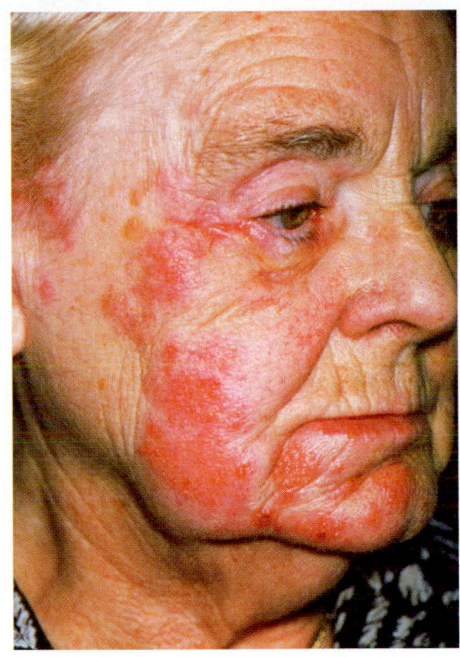

Figure 39-11 ◆ Shingles on the face.
Source: Photo Researchers, Inc.

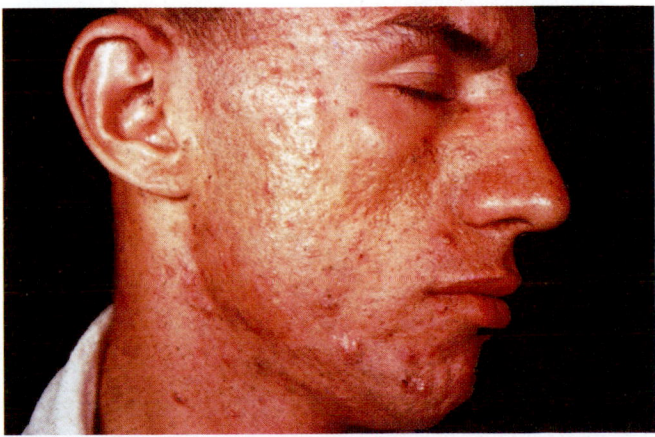

Figure 39-12 ◆ A patient with acne.
Source: Custom Medical Stock Photo

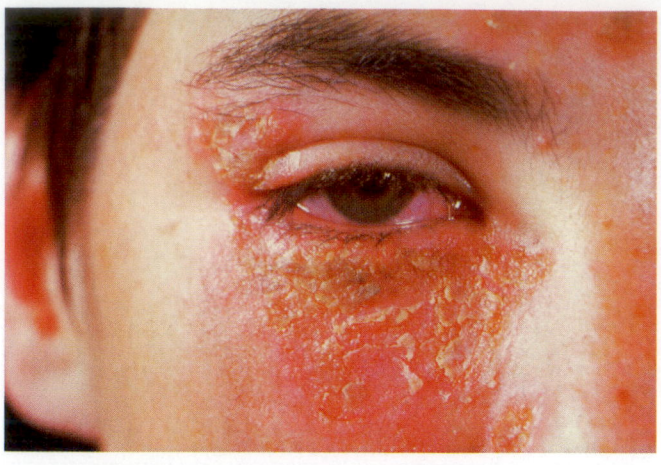

Figure 39-13 ◆ Impetigo.
Courtesy of Charles Stewart, M.D. and Associates.

Fungal Skin Conditions

Dermatophytoses—superficial skin conditions caused by fungi—affect the epidermal layer of the skin (Table 39-3). General symptoms include blisters, itching, scales, and swelling. These conditions thrive on moist, close skin surfaces. Tinea, or ringworm, occurs on the scalp, body, feet, groin, and nails, and each type is named for the body area of habitation (Figures 39-14 ◆ through 39-16 ◆).

Parasitic Skin Conditions

Two common parasites of the skin are itch mites, which cause scabies, and lice. The location of lice infestation on the body determines the name of the resulting skin condition. In school-age children, *Pediculus humanus capitis* (head lice) are spread easily through the sharing of hats, combs, brushes, and common coat rooms (Figure 39-17 ◆). *Pediculus humanus corporis* (body

---

TABLE 39-2 INFECTIOUS SKIN DISORDERS

Disease	Symptoms	Diagnosis	Treatment
Acne vulgaris (commonly called acne) ■ Condition of plugged pores, pimples, and cysts involving sebaceous glands and hair follicles ■ Appears on face, neck, arms, and upper back ■ Onset usually begins with puberty and increased levels of testosterone (sex hormone) ■ Pore becomes plugged with dead cells and sebum that does not reach skin surface, allowing bacterial growth; pore becomes inflamed and wall breaks, spilling sebum, dead cells, and bacteria into skin	■ Pimples ■ Pustules ■ Tender, reddened areas ■ Skin redness ■ White pustules	■ Patient presenting symptoms	■ Avoiding picking or squeezing pimples to avoid spread of bacteria, damage to skin, and scarring ■ Vitamin A acid cream or lotion for topical treatment to reduce bacteria and unblock pores ■ Antibiotic for topical treatment to reduce bacteria and help healing ■ Oral antibiotics for more involved cases when topical treatments fail ■ Female hormones to counteract testosterone
Furuncles and carbuncles ■ Furuncle: localized infection or abscess involving entire hair follicle and surrounding subcutaneous tissue ■ Carbuncle: very large furuncle or multiple furuncles in surrounding tissue often connected by several drainage canals ■ Usually caused by bacterial infection; *S. aureus* is common causative microbe	■ Reddened tissue ■ Swelling around hair follicle/follicles ■ Pain ■ Discharge or drainage through the skin or internally ■ Carbuncles are larger	■ Patient presenting symptoms ■ Culture to identify causative agent	■ Hot compresses ■ Surgical incision and drainage ■ Antibiotics

TABLE 39-2 INFECTIOUS SKIN DISORDERS (CONTINUED)

Disease	Symptoms	Diagnosis	Treatment
Herpes simplex ■ Systemic disorder resulting from previous infection with herpes simplex virus; virus moves to nerve root, where it is dormant until triggered by stress	■ Severe pain on lips and in mouth ■ Possible fever ■ Possible headache ■ Malaise ■ Blisters within hours to 1 day, lasting 4–5 days, eventually turning to scabs	■ Patient presenting symptoms	■ Cool compresses to ease pain ■ Antiviral drugs ■ Corticosteroids ■ Pain medication ■ Antiviral cream for application to lips
Herpes zoster (shingles) ■ Systemic disorder resulting from previous infection with herpes varicella (chickenpox) virus; virus moves to nerve root, where it is dormant until triggered by stress ■ Immunocompromised people at high risk for developing shingles; many suffer from post-herpetic **neuralgia** for weeks or months after blisters have disappeared ■ Repeat cases are rare ■ Not contagious to anyone who has had chickenpox ■ Newborns and adults who have never had chickenpox or have decreased immunity are at risk when exposed to fluid from blisters	■ Severe pain ■ Fever ■ Headache ■ Malaise ■ Rash ■ Blisters within 2 to 3 days, lasting 2 to 3 weeks, followed by pus or dark blood in blister pockets, eventually turning to scabs ■ Trunk of body most often affected, but cranial and spinal nerve dermatomes (bands of skin supplied by one nerve) may also be affected	■ Patient presenting symptoms	■ Cool compresses to ease pain ■ Antiviral drugs ■ Corticosteroid drugs ■ Pain medications
Impetigo ■ Contagious skin infection caused by *Streptococcus* or *Staphylococcus aureus* ■ Found around nose, mouth, cheeks, and extremities ■ Fluid from pustules can spread infection to nearby skin areas	■ Lesions that are yellow or red, weeping, crusted, pustular, and swelling	■ Patient presenting symptoms	■ Antibiotics for topical treatment to reduce bacteria and help healing

TABLE 39-3 FUNGAL SKIN CONDITIONS

Disease	Symptoms	Diagnosis	Treatment
Tinea capitis (scalp ringworm) ■ Affects scalp	■ Lesions: round, scaly, itchy	■ Patient presenting symptoms	■ Antifungal cream to reduce fungus and help healing ■ Oral antifungal drugs when antifungal creams are not recommended

continued

TABLE 39-3 FUNGAL SKIN CONDITIONS (CONTINUED)

Disease	Symptoms	Diagnosis	Treatment
Tinea corporis (body ringworm) ■ Affects hairless body skin ■ May be transmitted by infected animals, including cats.	■ Red scaly patches (center of patch clears, leaving a ring) ■ Vesicles ■ Itching	■ Patient presenting symptoms	See "Tinea Capitis"
Tinea cruris (jock itch) ■ Affects groin area	■ Patches on groin area and inner part of upper thigh ■ Redness ■ Vesicles ■ Itching	■ Patient presenting symptoms	■ Antifungal cream to reduce fungus and help healing. ■ Oral antifungal drugs when antifungal creams are not recommended
Tinea pedis (athlete's foot) ■ Affects the feet ■ Commonly found in athlets	■ Cracks and blisters between toes and on soles ■ Burning ■ Itching	■ Patient presenting symptoms	■ Antifungal cream to reduce fungus, itching, and burning and help healing
Tinea unguium (yellow nail) ■ Affects fingernails and toenails	■ Nails: thickened, hardened, brittle, yellow-tinged (usually toenails)	■ Patient presenting symptoms	■ Antifungal cream for application to nail and nail bed

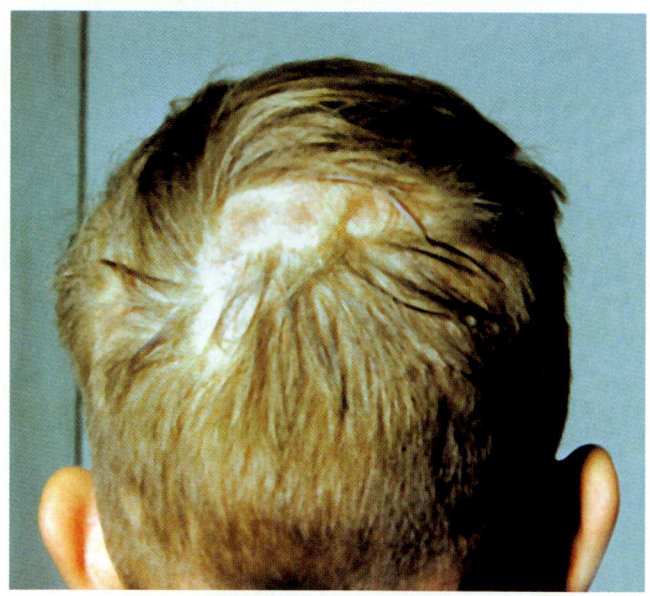

Figure 39-14 ◆ Scalp ringworm.
Source: Courtesy of the CDC, 1959.

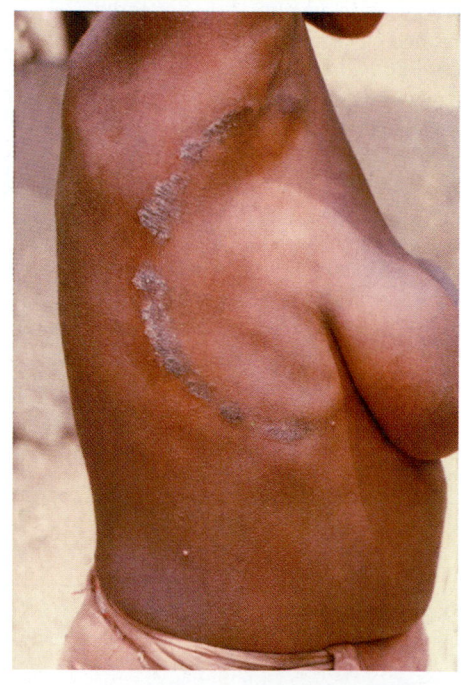

Figure 39-15 ◆ Body ringworm.
Source: Courtesy of the CDC/Lucille K. Georg, 1964.

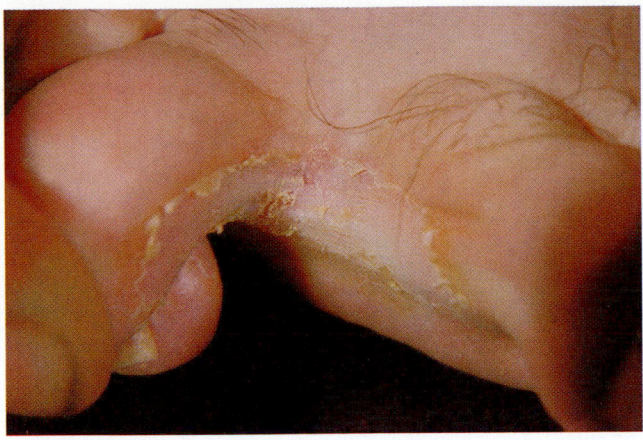

Figure 39-16 ◆ Athlete's foot.
Source: Courtesy of the CDC/Dr. Lucille K. Georg, 1964.

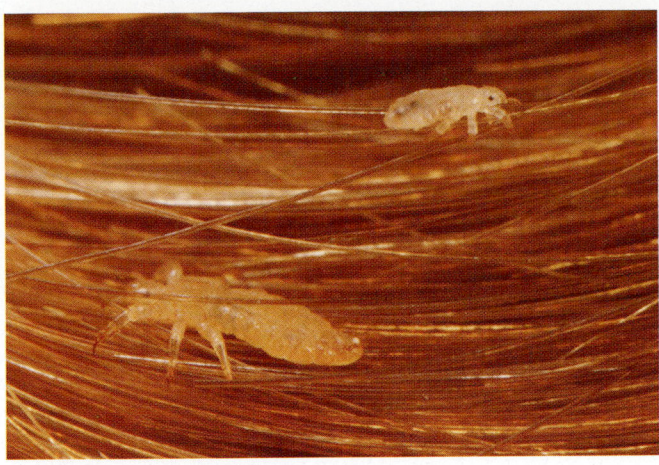

Figure 39-17 ◆ Head lice.
Source: National Geographic Image Collection.

lice) and itch mites are frequently spread by poor hygiene and close body contact or the sharing of clothing or bedding (Figures 39-18 ◆ and 39-19 ◆). *Pediculus humanus pubis* (pubic lice) are spread through sexual contact. Table 39-4 describes various common parasitic conditions.

?─Critical Thinking Question 39-1─
The mother is very concerned that her children may have lice and is under the impression that they will be labeled "dirty" or that she will be seen as an unfit mother. In addition, she has assumed that all lice are the same and attach to all types of hair. What should Manny tell her about the different kinds of head lice and how they're transmitted?

Pigmentation Disorders

Pigmentation refers to the natural coloring of the skin and hair. Pigmentation disorders include albinism, vitiligo, and chloasma (Table 39-5; Figures 39-20 ◆ through 39-22 ◆).

Benign Neoplasms

Benign neoplasms are lesions or localized growths that do not invade surrounding tissue. They do not metastasize, or spread, to distant sites in the body, although they may affect tissue function and cause physical symptoms. Malignant neoplasms are invasive and metastasize to distant sites. Benign skin disorders include actinic keratosis (**AK**), seborrheic keratosis, moles, warts, keloids, sebaceous cysts, and skin tags (Table 39-6; Figures 39-23 ◆ through 39-29 ◆).

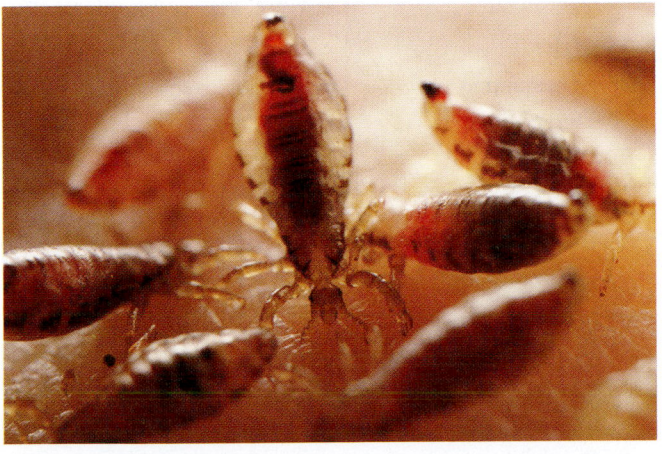

Figure 39-18 ◆ Body lice.
Source: National Geographic Image Collection.

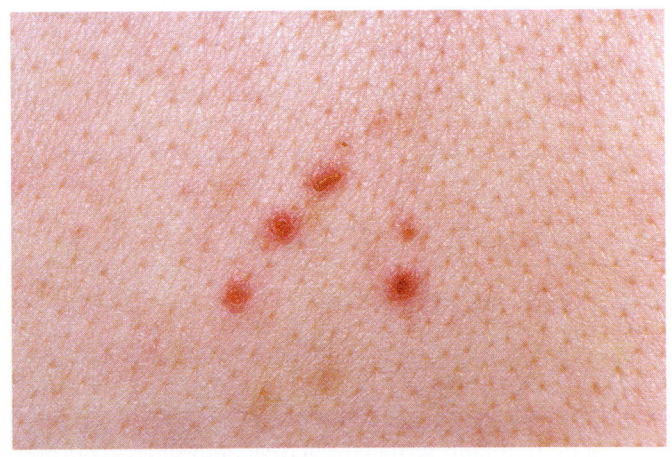

Figure 39-19 ◆ Itch mites.
Source: Phototake NYC.

TABLE 39-4 PARASITIC SKIN CONDITIONS

Parasite	Symptoms	Diagnosis	Treatment
Pediculus humanus capitis/Pediculosis capitus (head lice) ■ Highly contagious ■ Affects the head ■ Commonly found among school-age children	■ Rash ■ Itching ■ Presence of lice and nits on hair shafts on head	■ Patient presenting symptoms	■ Special shampoo, cream, and sulfur preparation to thoroughly wash hair and body ■ Washing all contaminated clothing and bedding in hot water with bleach, then drying in dryer ■ Patient education to prevent re-exposure ■ Special hair combing to remove lice and nits
Pediculus humanis corporis/Pediculosis corporis (body lice) ■ Highly contagious ■ Affects the body	■ Rash ■ Itching ■ Presence of lice and nits on body and clothing	■ Patient presenting symptoms	■ Special shampoo, cream, and sulfur preparation to thoroughly wash hair and body ■ Washing all contaminated clothing and bedding in hot water with bleach, then drying in dryer ■ Patient education to prevent re-exposure
Pediculus humanus pubis/Pediculosis pubis (pubic lice or crabs) ■ Highly contagious ■ Transmitted sexually	■ Presence of lice and nits on pubic, groin, and armpit hair ■ Intense itching, especially at night ■ Brown-red dust in underwear ■ Blue-gray flat rash on trunk, thighs, or armpit	■ Patient presenting symptoms	■ See "Pediculus humanus corporis"
Scabies ■ Highly contagious ■ Caused by itch mites ■ Affects entire body	■ Rash ■ Intense itching ■ Feeling of something crawling on the body ■ Presence of scabies on the body and on clothing	■ Patient presenting symptoms	■ See "Pediculus humanus corporis"

Cancerous Skin Disorders

Many skin conditions seen in the dermatology office are benign and, while troublesome, are not life-threatening. Basal cell carcinoma (**BCC**), squamous cell carcinoma (**SCC**), and malignant melanoma are cancerous conditions affecting the skin (Figures 39-30 ◆ through 39-32 ◆). Skin cancers are the most common type of cancer as well as the most curable when diagnosed early (Table 39-7).

Skin cancers are initially diagnosed according to their appearance. Malignant melanoma is often identified by the "ABCD rule":

A = Asymmetry (the shape of one half is different from the shape of the other half)
B = Border (the edges of the lesion appear irregular and ill-defined, ragged, and uneven)

TABLE 39-5 PIGMENTATION DISORDERS

Disorder	Symptoms	Diagnosis	Treatment
Albinism ■ Genetic disorder resulting in partial or total lack of skin color ■ No known cure	■ Very pale skin ■ Light or white hair ■ Eye color varies, but extreme is light or red irises ■ Visual difficulties: nystagmus (irregular or rapid eye movement), strabismus (eye muscle imbalance), astigmatism (distorted viewed image), photophobia (sensitivity to bright light)	■ Patient presenting symptoms	■ Sunscreen used outdoors ■ Treatment for specific vision difficulties
Chloasma (also called melasma) ■ Skin disorder characterized by tan to brown patches ■ More common in women than men ■ Chloasma gravidarum is called mask of pregnancy but can also affect women using hormonal contraceptives ■ Also occurs in patients with underlying liver disease ■ No cure	■ Tan and brown patches found on forehead, temples, cheeks, and upper lip	■ Patient presenting symptoms	■ Sunscreen used outdoors ■ Makeup to cover patches
Vitiligo ■ Characterized by large white patches of skin ■ Cause unknown ■ No known cure	■ Large white patches of skin, commonly on hands and face	■ Patient presenting symptoms	■ Sunscreen used outdoors ■ Makeup to cover patches

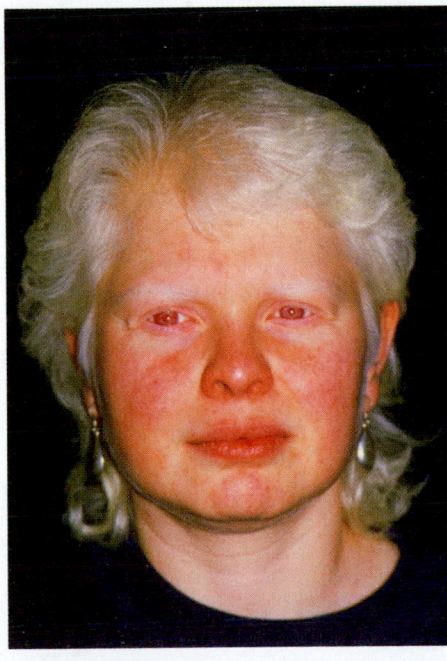

Figure 39-20 ◆ Albinism.
Source: Photo Researchers, Inc.

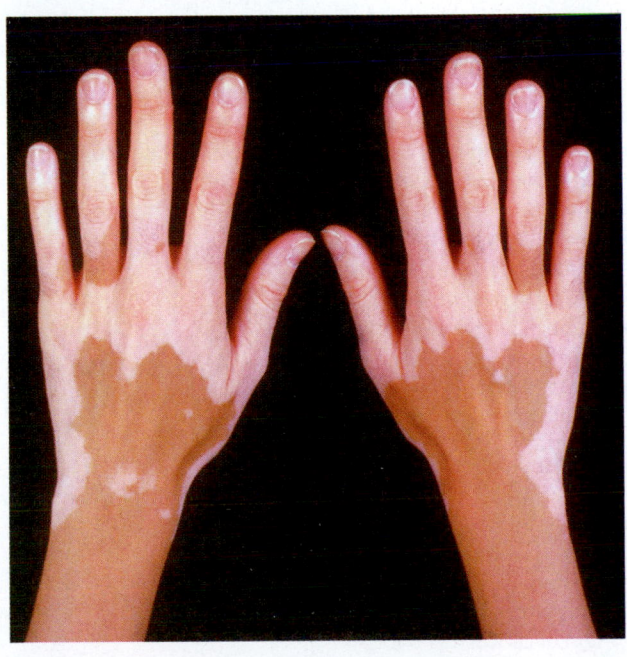

Figure 39-21 ◆ Vitiligo.
Source: Custom Medical Stock Photo

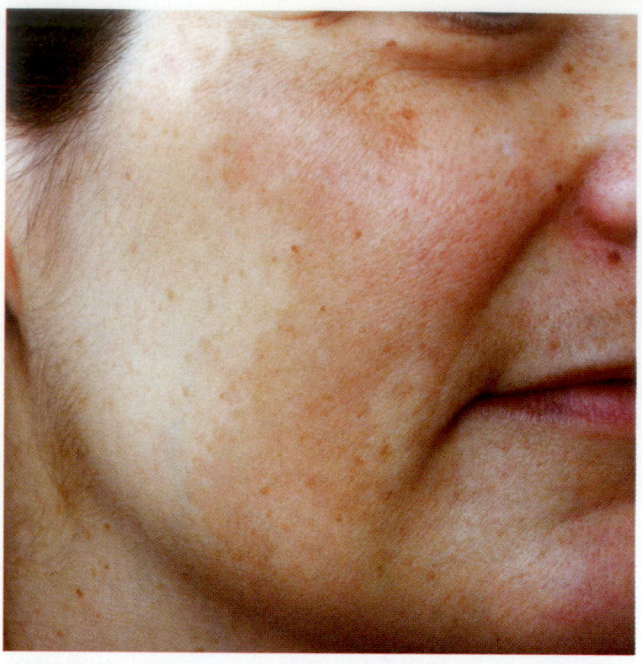

Figure 39-22 ◆ Chloasma.

C = Color (commonly a mix of tan, black, and brown, but can also include blue, red, and white)

D = Diameter (lesions can be larger than 6 millimeters in diameter, or bigger than a pencil eraser)

Exposure to the sun is considered the main risk factor for skin cancer. Certain common-sense guidelines may be followed to reduce harmful exposure.

1. Avoid sun exposure when UV rays are strongest, from 10 am to 3 pm.
2. Apply sunscreen with UV protection greater than SP15, following product instructions.
3. Wear protective clothing outdoors, including a hat and clothing with sleeves and pant legs.
4. Plan outside activities for the periods of weaker UV rays.

?— Critical Thinking Question 39-2

The teenage girl with the mole admits to sunbathing regularly in the summer at the lake and describes her mole only as "suspicious." What questions should Manny ask her regarding this condition? What advice should he give?

TABLE 39-6 BENIGN SKIN DISORDERS

Disorder	Symptoms	Diagnosis	Treatment
Actinic keratosis (AK, also called solar keratosis) ■ Benign skin disorder, but can also be precancerous (squamous cell cancer) ■ Usually caused by exposure over time to solar or artificial UV rays ■ Biopsy of tissue is recommended after removal	■ Scaly, bumpy, crusty areas on face, ears, neck ■ Affected area may be flesh-colored, light or dark tan, pink, red, or combination ■ Itch ■ Tenderness	■ Patient presenting symptoms	■ Immediate examination by physician ■ Topical medication ■ Cryosurgery, curettage (scraping), electrosurgery, minor surgery, or laser surgery for removal ■ Routine examinations to track changes
Keloids (hypertrophic scars) ■ Benign overgrowths of collagenous scar tissue, often raised and hard ■ Secondary to surgical process or traumatic injury and form over incision scar ■ Surgery can cause further scarring ■ Some disappear by themselves	■ Flesh- or light-colored growths	■ Patient presenting symptoms	■ Cryotherapy for small keloids ■ Surgery followed by X-ray treatment or steroid injection at site as necessary
Moles (nevi) ■ Usually benign ■ Cause unknown ■ Should be monitored for changes in color or size; itching, pain, or bleeding may be sign of cancer ■ Almost everyone has moles, often developed in childhood	■ May be flesh-colored, brown, black, or blue	■ Patient presenting symptoms	■ Routine examinations to track any changes in people who have had extensive exposure to UV rays ■ Surgery only for cosmetic purposes

TABLE 39-6 BENIGN SKIN DISORDERS (CONTINUED)

Disorder	Symptoms	Diagnosis	Treatment
Sebaceous cysts ■ Growths arising from epidermal tissue ■ Result of blocked sebaceous gland duct	■ Soft, smooth lump	■ Patient presenting symptoms	■ Incision and drainage (I & D) to drain cyst ■ Antibiotics as needed
Seborrheic keratosis ■ Benign skin disorder on outer ■ Cause unknown ■ Looks like waxy growth stuck onto skin surface ■ Lesions appear as individual ages and grow larger over time	■ Single or in clusters ■ Very light to very dark brown ■ Minute to over 2 inches in diameter	■ Patient presenting symptoms ■ Any lesion removed is sent to pathology lab to identify any malignant condition	■ Cryosurgery, curettage, or electrosurgery when growth becomes unsightly or irritated by clothing
Skin tags (acrochordons) ■ Small, skin-colored, benign outgrowths of skin tissue ■ Become more common after midlife	■ Small overgrowths of skin attached by narrow stalk	■ Patient presenting symptoms	■ Cryotherapy, electrical burning, or minor surgery for removal
Warts (verrucae) ■ Small, contagious growths on skin ■ Often caused by a virus ■ Most occur on hands and feet	■ Small ■ Hard ■ May be flesh-colored, white, or pink ■ Painful if on bottom of foot	■ Patient presenting symptoms	■ Over-the-counter (OTC) medication to remove warts ■ Cryosurgery, electrical burning, minor surgery, or laser surgery for removal

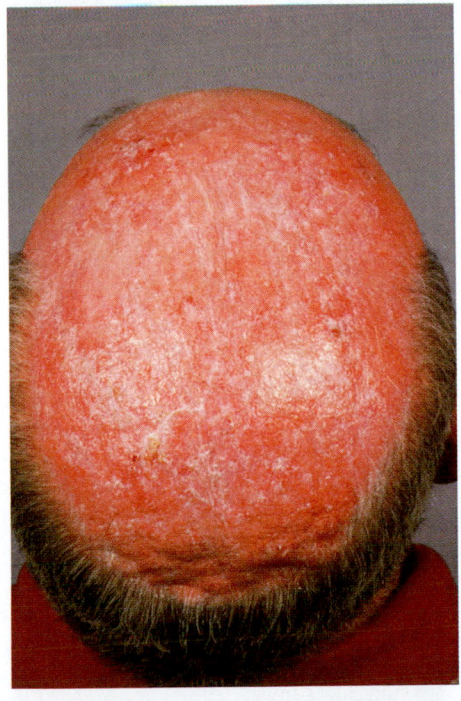

Figure 39-23 ◆ Actinic keratoses.
Source: Phototake NYC.

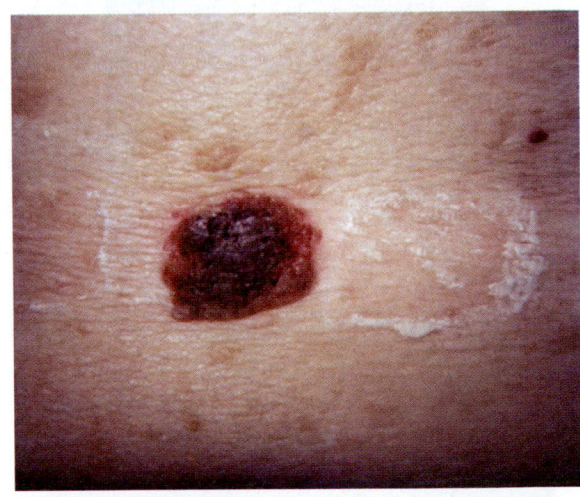

Figure 39-24 ◆ Seborrheic keratoses.
Source: Courtesy of the CDC/Dr. Steve Kraus, 1981.

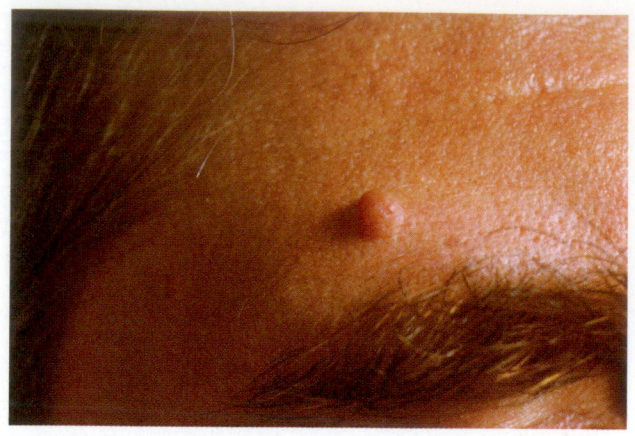

Figure 39-25 ◆ Raised mole.
Source: Custom Medical Stock Photo

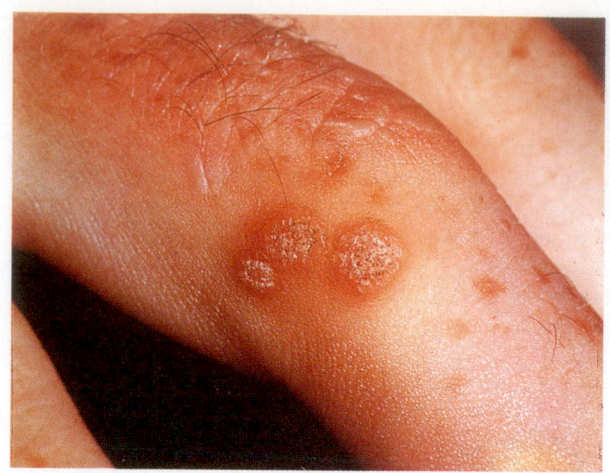

Figure 39-26 ◆ Warts.

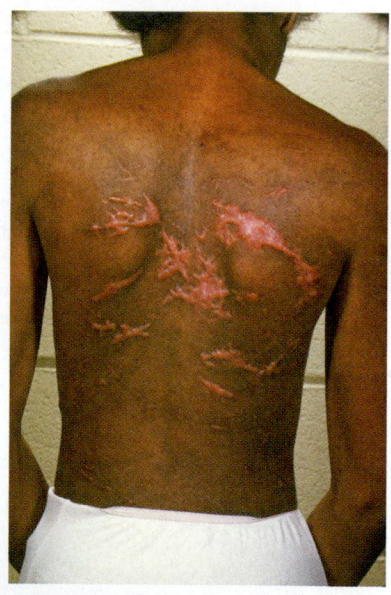

Figure 39-27 ◆ Keloids.
Source: Phototake NYC

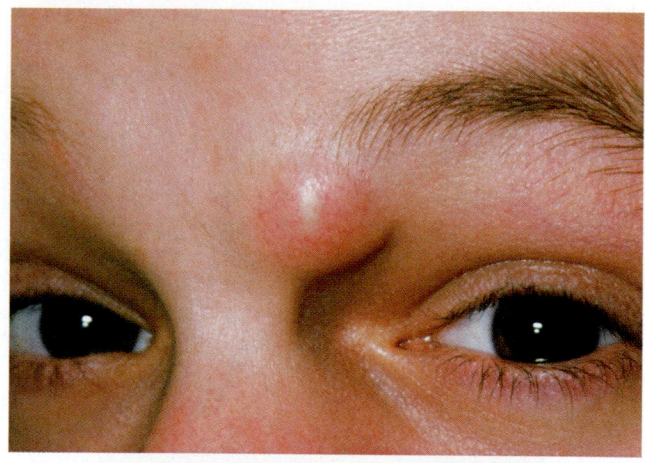

Figure 39-28 ◆ Sebaceous cyst.
Source: Photo Researchers, Inc.

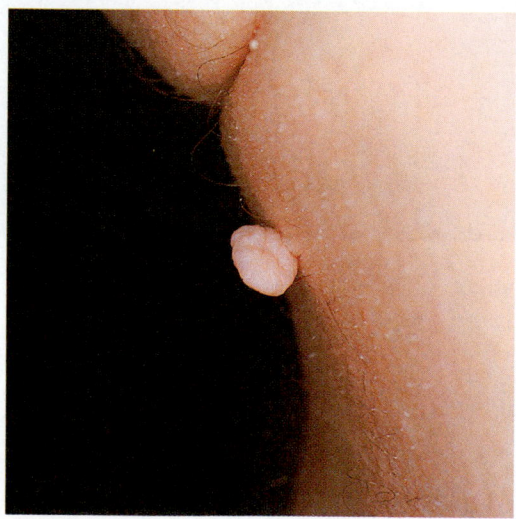

Figure 39-29 ◆ Skin tag.
Source: Peter Arnold, Inc.

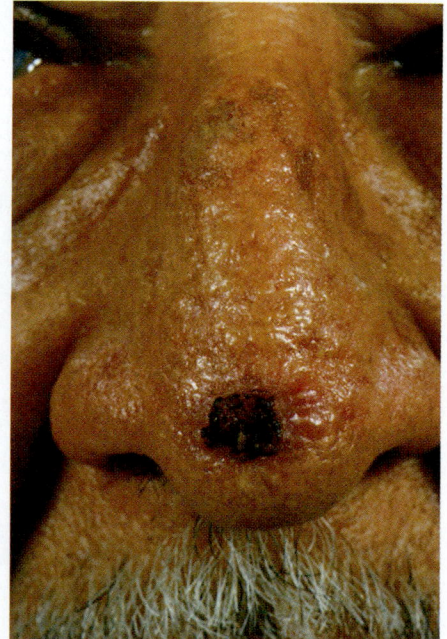

Figure 39-30 ◆ Basal cell carcinoma.
© *Caliendo/Custom Medical Stock Photo*

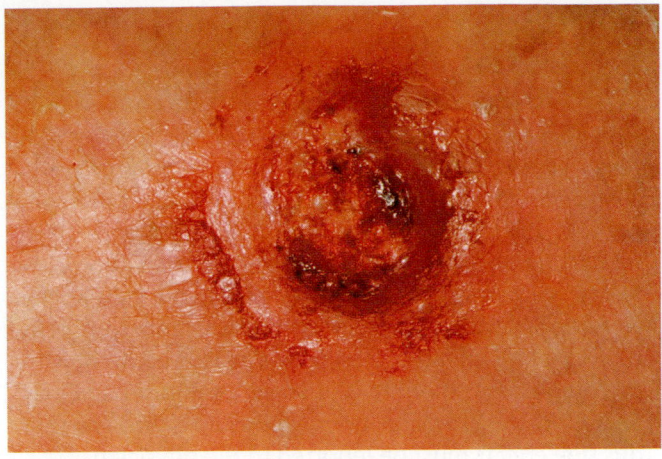

Figure 39-31 ◆ Squamous cell carcinoma.
Source: Photo Researchers, Inc.

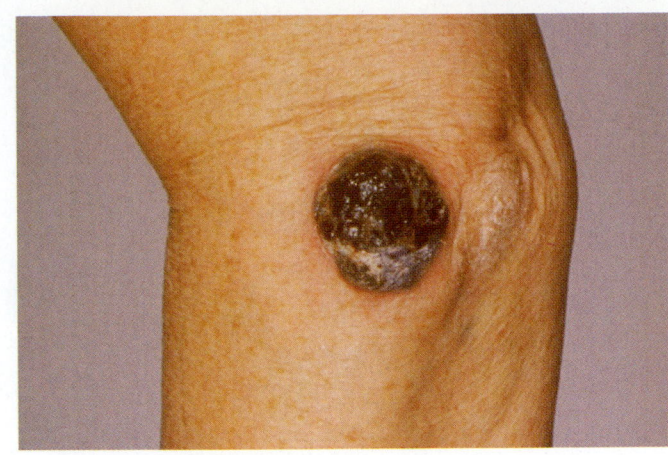

Figure 39-32 ◆ Malignant melanoma.
Source: BioPhoto Associates/Science Source/Photo Researchers, Inc.

Miscellaneous Integumentary Conditions

In addition to the common disease conditions described above, the following may also be encountered in the medical office setting.

- Psoriasis is a chronic, noninfectious, and inflammatory skin disorder with an unknown cause and no known cure (Figure 39-33 ◆). It is characterized by plaques (patches) of various sizes that are thick, flaky, red, and dry, with silvery scales. Patches are usually found on the patient's scalp, knees, elbows, and trunk. Other symptoms include itching, soreness, and pustules. Treatment is palliative because the disease has no cure.
- Cellulitis is a condition of inflammation and infection of the skin and subcutaneous tissue. *Staphylococcus* is usually the cause. IV antibiotics are generally prescribed, along with pain medication, elevation of the extremity,

TABLE 39-7 CANCEROUS SKIN DISORDERS

Disorder	Symptoms	Diagnosis	Treatment
Basal cell carcinoma (BCC) ■ Slow-growing malignancy in basal cell layer of epidermis ■ Most common skin cancer ■ Lesions do not heal but are not likely to spread ■ Treatment based on depth and location of the lesions	■ Pearly nodule with a rolled edge when found on face, ears, or neck ■ Flat, flesh-colored, or brown scar-like lesion when found on chest or back ■ Itching ■ Bleeding	■ Patient presenting symptoms ■ Skin biopsy	■ X-ray radiation ■ Scraping and **cauterization,** surgical excision, cryosurgery, or Mohs' surgery (controlled shaved excisions) for removal ■ Sunscreen used outdoors
Squamous cell carcinoma ■ Malignant tumor in squamous cells of middle portion of epidermis ■ Can metastasize to other organs, such as lymph nodes ■ May start as a precancerous tumor	■ Firm red nodules that crust and bleed ■ May appear on face, ears, neck, hands, arms ■ Pain (later)	■ Patient presenting symptoms ■ Skin biopsy	■ X-ray radiation ■ Surgical excision for removal ■ Mohs' surgery for removal if cancer returns ■ Sunscreen used outdoors
Malignant melanoma ■ Deadliest form of skin cancer ■ Metastasizes rapidly ■ Commonly occurs on normal skin, but some arise from a mole ■ Begins in **melanocytes**	■ Lesions of various colors and with irregular edges ■ Mole with color change, size change, itch, or soreness	■ Patient presenting symptoms ■ Skin biopsy	■ Surgical excision for removal; surrounding normal skin or lymph nodes also usually removed to stop spread

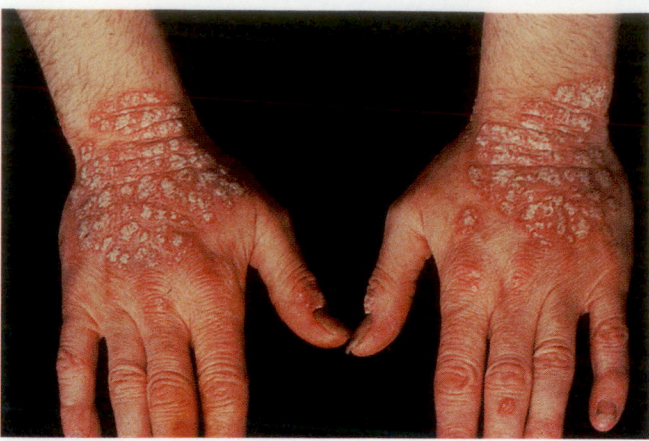

Figure 39-33 ◆ Psoriasis lesions.

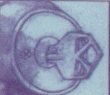
and/or heat treatment to address the impaired circulation of the swollen tissue.

■ Folliculitis is the inflammation and infection of a hair follicle, usually caused by *Staphyloccus*. This condition is characterized by small pustules at the hair follicle and is usually treated by daily cleansing with antiseptic cleanser. Oral antibiotics may be required as well.

■ Alopecia is a condition of partial or complete hair loss. Causative factors include heredity, aging, iron deficiency, thyroid disease, skin infection of the scalp, chemotherapy, and radiation. Some hair loss is temporary if the causative factor is addressed or removed.

■ Hirsutism is a condition of excessive hair growth. Polycystic ovaries or tumors of the adrenal glands and ovaries may be the cause. Treatment varies but may include medications to suppress production of the hormone causing the condition or removal of tissue or organs causing the hormonal imbalance.

■ Lyme disease is transmitted by ticks found on deer and other outdoor animals. It affects multiple systems of the body and is first recognized by a red ringed area with a white or faded center around the bite. If the disease is not diagnosed shortly after the tick bite, a range of mild flu-like symptoms and joint and muscle pains can progress to severe neurologic involvement. Complete recovery can occur over time with antibiotic treatment.

■ Rosacea often occurs in middle-aged and elderly individuals, and the cause is unknown. Signs of rosacea include varying degrees of pustules (elevated and pus-filled skin lesions), papules (small, red, elevated skin lesions), and rhinopyema (hyperplasia, or overgrowth of nasal soft tissue). Rosacea is treated with medications, including antibiotics.

Cosmetic Treatment for Skin Conditions

In addition to traditional medical treatment for skin diseases and disorders, many patients are interested in removing residual effects, such as scarring or color changes, and in improving the skin's cosmetic appearance. Treatments include dermabrasion, chemical peel, and laser resurfacing. Dermabrasion involves a controlled scraping of the skin that gives it a smoother surface. The procedure removes or softens scars from acne, surgery, or accidents; smooths facial wrinkles; and removes some precancerous karatoses. A chemical peel removes the damaged outer layers of the skin, including blemishes, wrinkles, uneven skin coloration, and some precancerous skin growths. Laser resurfacing, also called laser peel, uses a carbon dioxide laser to remove wrinkles, scars, and uneven skin coloration.

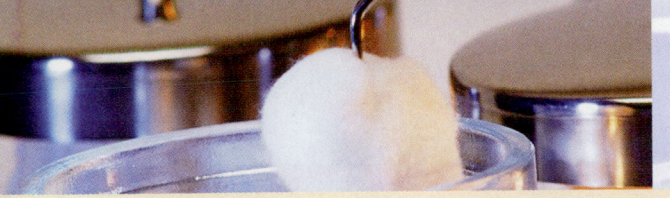

REVIEW

Chapter Summary

- A dermatologist is a physician who specializes in treating skin diseases and conditions. Procedures performed in the dermatology office include biopsies, cryosurgery, and surgical removal of lesions.
- The integumentary system is the largest organ of the body. Its functions include barrier protection, temperature regulation, and toxin excretion. Other structures of the integumentary system are the nails, hair, and sweat and sebaceous glands.
- Skin is composed of three layers: the epidermis, dermis, and subcutaneous tissue. The epidermis is the outermost layer. Melanin (the pigment in the skin, hair, and iris) and keratin (a protein that makes up epidermal cells) are produced in the epidermis. Melanin protects the skin from harmful ultraviolet (UV) rays. The dermis, the middle layer, contains blood and lymph vessels, nerve cell endings, sweat and sebaceous glands, and hair follicles. The innermost layer, or subcutaneous tissue, is composed of connective tissue and fat cells and acts as insulation for the body.
- There are several types of dermatitis, including seborrheic dermatitis, allergic contact dermatitis, contact dermatitis, eczema, and hives (urticaria).
- Psoriasis is considered a chronic, inflammatory skin disorder. It is characterized by thick and flaky red patches covered with white, silvery scales. This condition is noninfectious, and its cause is unknown.
- Infectious skin disorders include shingles (herpes zoster), acne, and impetigo.
- Fungal skin conditions or dermatophytoses affect the epidermal layer of the skin. General symptoms include blisters, itching, scales, and swelling. Ringworm and athlete's foot are common fungal conditions.
- Common parasites of the skin include itch mites and lice.
- Pigmentation refers to the natural coloring of the skin and hair. Pigmentation disorders include albinism, vitiligo, and chloasma.
- Seborrheic keratosis, actinic keratosis, moles, warts, keloids, sebaceous cysts, and skin tags are all benign (noncancerous) skin disorders.
- Basal cell carcinoma (BCC), squamous cell carcinoma (SCC), and malignant melanoma are cancerous skin conditions.

Chapter Review

Multiple Choice

1. Which of the following is a function of the integumentary system?
   a. Blood sensor
   b. Environmental sensor
   c. Kidney regulator
   d. Growth regulator

2. The dermis is the layer that
   a. is made up of connective tissue and fat cells.
   b. sloughs skin cells.
   c. is considered an appendage of the skin.
   d. contains nerve cell endings.

3. The epidermis is the layer that
   a. sloughs skin cells.
   b. is made up of connective tissue and fat cells.
   c. contains nerve cell endings.
   d. is considered an appendage of the skin.

4. The subcutaneous tissue is the layer that
   a. contains nerve cell endings.
   b. sloughs skin cells.
   c. is made up of connective tissue and fat cells.
   d. is considered an appendage of the skin.

5. Psoriasis is
   a. curable.
   b. not curable.
   c. not congenital.
   d. contagious.

6. Which of the following is a pigmentation disorder?
   a. Albinism
   b. Actinic keratosis
   c. Scabies
   d. Impetigo

7. A skin tag is a
   a. fungal infection.
   b. red surface bump.
   c. flat lesion.
   d. benign tumor.

8. Which of the following is a leading cause of skin cancer?
   a. Unprotected sun exposure
   b. Contact with chemicals
   c. Contact with allergens
   d. Untreated fungal skin infections

9. Actinic keratosis can develop into
   a. melanoma.
   b. moles.
   c. birthmarks.
   d. squamous cell cancer.

10. Melanoma is a(n)
    a. infection.
    b. precancerous condition.
    c. highly cancerous disease.
    d. fungal condition.

Chapter Review (continued)

True/False

T F 1. Biopsies, cryosurgery, and lesion removal can all be performed in a dermatology office.

T F 2. Suture removal and dressing application may be the responsibility of the medical assistant.

T F 3. Structures of the integumentary system include nails, hair, and sweat glands but not nerves or sebaceous glands.

T F 4. The skin synthesizes vitamin D from sunlight.

T F 5. Skin cells originate in the basal layer of the dermis, above the epidermis.

Short Answer

1. How long is the life cycle of epidermal cells?

2. What are the functions of subcutaneous tissue?

3. What is melanin?

4. List four symptoms of psoriasis.

5. Which parasite causes scabies?

Research

1. Research leprosy and find out if there are still any leper colonies in the United States.

2. Find the most recent report on head lice outbreaks in schools in your community. How many children were affected?

Externship Application Experience

You are assisting a male dermatologist as he examines a 65-year-old female patient. He has discovered what he thinks are several malignant melanoma lesions on her face, neck, arms, and legs. A visual examination of her entire body is required, and she is asked to disrobe. He steps out of the room. The patient holds her clothing tightly and refuses to disrobe. What should you do?

Resource Guide

American Academy of Dermatology
930 N Meacham Road
P.O. Box 4014
Schamburg, IL 60168-4014
1-888-462-DERMx22
www.aad.org

American Cancer Society
1-800-ACS-2345
www.cancer.org

Melanoma Research Foundation
P.O. Box 747
San Leandro, CA 94577
1-800-MRF-1290
MRFI@melanoma.org

National Pediculosis Association
P.O. Box 610189
Newton, MA 02161
781-449-NITS (6487)
www.headlice.org

National Psoriasis Foundation
6600 SW 92nd Ave, Ste 300
Portland, OR 97223
503-244-7404
www.psoriasis.org

National Skin Cancer Prevention Education Program
1-888-842-6355
www.cdc.gov/cancer/nscpep

Skin Cancer Foundation
245 5th Ave, Suite #1403
New York, NY 10016
1-800-SKIN-490
www.skincancer.org

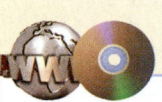

MedMedia

http://www.MyMAKit.com

More on this chapter, including interactive resources, can be found on the Student CD-ROM accompanying this textbook and on http://www.MyMAKit.com.

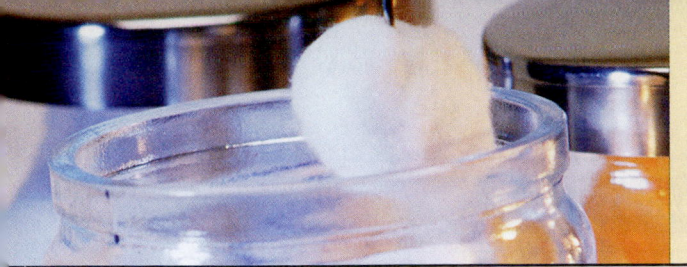

Objectives

After completing this chapter, you should be able to:

- Define and spell the key terminology in this chapter.
- Define the medical assistant's role in the endocrinology office.
- Label the structures of the endocrine system.
- Discuss the physiology of the endocrine system.
- Identify and discuss pituitary gland disorders.
- Identify and discuss thyroid disorders.
- Identify and discuss parathyroid disorders.
- Identify and discuss glucose metabolism disorders.
- Identify and discuss adrenal gland disorders.

Endocrinology

Case Study

Dr. Cabe has asked her CMA, Charles, to provide instructions to her patient, Mr. Wiat, who was recently diagnosed with adult Type 2 diabetes. The patient is more than 50 pounds overweight, does not participate in any type of exercise, and continues to eat a high-carbohydrate, high-fat diet. Reviewing Mr. Wiat's three-day diet journal, Charles notes that he consumes more than 2 liters of soda per day and regularly consumes fast food. When Charles mentions the danger of continuing this lifestyle, Mr. Wiat responds that he has lived this long with these lifestyle habits and isn't about to change. "It's not like it's going to kill me," he says.

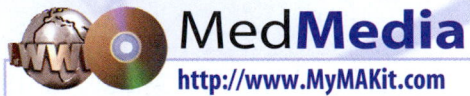

Med**Media**

http://www.MyMAKit.com

Additional interactive resources and activities for this chapter can be found on http://www.MyMAKit.com. For a video, tips, audio glossary, legal and ethical scenarios, job scenarios, quizzes, games, virtual tours, and activities related to the content of this chapter, please access the accompanying CD-ROM in this book.

Video
Audio Glossary
Legal and Ethical Scenario: *Endocrinology*
On the Job Scenario: *Endocrinology*
A & P Quiz: The Endocrine System
Multiple Choice Quiz
Games: Crossword, Strikeout, and Spelling Bee
3D Virtual Tour: Endocrine System: The Endocrine System; The Lymphatic System: The Lymphatic System
Drag & Drop: The Lymphatic System
Tips
HIPAA Quiz

Key Terminology

endocrine glands—glands that secrete and release hormones directly into the bloodstream; also known as ductless glands

exocrine glands—glands that secrete substances through ducts, such as sweat glands

gluconeogenesis—conversion of noncarbohydrate sources stored in the liver into glucose

hormones—chemical messengers secreted by the endocrine glands

hypothalamus—very small structure in the midbrain, below the thalamus, that controls many body functions and endocrine processes

Abbreviations

ACTH—adrenocorticotropic hormone

ADH—antidiuretic hormone

FBS—fasting blood sugar

FSH—follicle-stimulating hormone

GHB A1c—glycohemoglobin/ glycosylated hemoglobin

GH—growth hormone

IDDM (type I)—insulin-dependent diabetes mellitus

LH—luteiniziing hormone

MSH—melanocyte-stimulating hormone

NIDDM (type II)—non-insulin-dependent diabetes mellitus

PTH—parathyroid hormone

T₃—triiodothyronine

T₄—thyroxine

TSH—thyroid-stimulating hormone

✚ MEDICAL ASSISTING STANDARDS

CAAHEP ENTRY-LEVEL STANDARDS	ABHES ENTRY-LEVEL COMPETENCIES
■ Perform within scope of practice (psychomotor) ■ Apply ethical behaviors, including honesty/integrity in performance of medical assisting practice (affective) ■ Explain the rationale for performance of a procedure to the patient (affective) ■ Use language/verbal skills that enable patients' understanding (affective) ■ Describe the normal function of each body system (cognitive) ■ Identify common pathology related to each body system (cognitive) ■ Analyze pathology as it relates to the interaction of body systems (cognitive) ■ Discuss implications for disease and disability when homeostasis is not maintained (cognitive) ■ Describe implications for treatment related to pathology (cognitive)	■ Apply principles of aseptic techniques and infection control. ■ Prepare and maintain examination and treatment areas. ■ Prepare patients for procedures. ■ Assist physician with examinations and treatments. ■ Maintain medication records. ■ Interview effectively. ■ Recognize and respond to verbal and nonverbal communication. ■ Maintain confidentially at all times. ■ Use appropriate medical terminology. ■ Document accurately. ■ Adapt what is said to the recipient's level of comprehension. ■ Instruct patients with special needs. ■ Teach patients methods of health promotion and disease prevention. ■ Locate resources and information for patients and employers.

Introduction

The endocrine system consists of ductless glands that affect the functions of targeted organs in the body by secreting hormones. Disorders of the endocrine system usually involve the overactivity or underactivity of these glands. An endocrinologist diagnoses and treats disorders of the endocrine system such as diabetes and thyroid dysfunction.

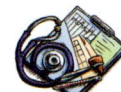

The Medical Assistant's Role in the Endocrinology Office

In an endocrinology office the MA may perform a variety of assessment and other tasks, including the following:

- Obtaining and recording vital signs, history information, and reason for current visit, as requested by the physician.
- Obtaining blood and urine specimens for laboratory analysis (as discussed in ∞ Chapters 32 and 33).
- Performing blood glucose tests with a glucometer (∞ discussed in Chapter 30).
- Discussing with the patient written instructions concerning diet, diabetic foot care, the use and care of glucose self-monitoring equipment, or preparation for diagnostic testing.

Anatomy and Physiology of the Endocrine System

There are two control systems in the body: the nervous system and the endocrine system.

- The nervous system, including the autonomic system, exerts control over body functions in a way similar to an electrical system. Impulses travel through the nerves at an extremely rapid speed and elicit an immediate response.
- The endocrine system is slightly slower in its elicited response, which is chemically mediated by **hormones.** The endocrine system is composed of **endocrine glands** that secrete and release hormones directly into the bloodstream (Figure 40-1 ◆). These glands include the pituitary gland, thyroid gland, parathyroid gland, pancreas, adrenal glands, gonads (testicles and ovaries), pineal gland, and thymus gland. (Refer to ∞ Chapter 33, Urology and Nephrology, and ∞ Chapter 44, Obstetrics and Gynecology, for a discussion of the sex hormones.)

Endocrine disorders are the result of too much or too little of a particular hormone being stimulated or released. Therefore, most endocrine disorders are referred to as either the hyper- or hypoactivity of the gland.

Hormones are chemical substances that influence and control body functions such as growth and development, sexual maturity, and metabolism. Hormones send messages to other glands and target organs (Figure 40-2 ◆). Regulation of this system is accomplished by a positive–negative feedback process. Negative feedback originates when blood hormone levels are elevated and a message is sent slowing or stopping of the gland's activity, thereby ceasing or reducing the production of the hormone. In this manner, blood levels of various hormones control the secretion of other hormones and their resulting blood levels.

The Endocrine Glands

The *pituitary gland* is a minute structure located in the midbrain, in the middle of the skull (Figure 40-3 ◆). It consists of two lobes, the anterior lobe and the posterior lobe. This gland

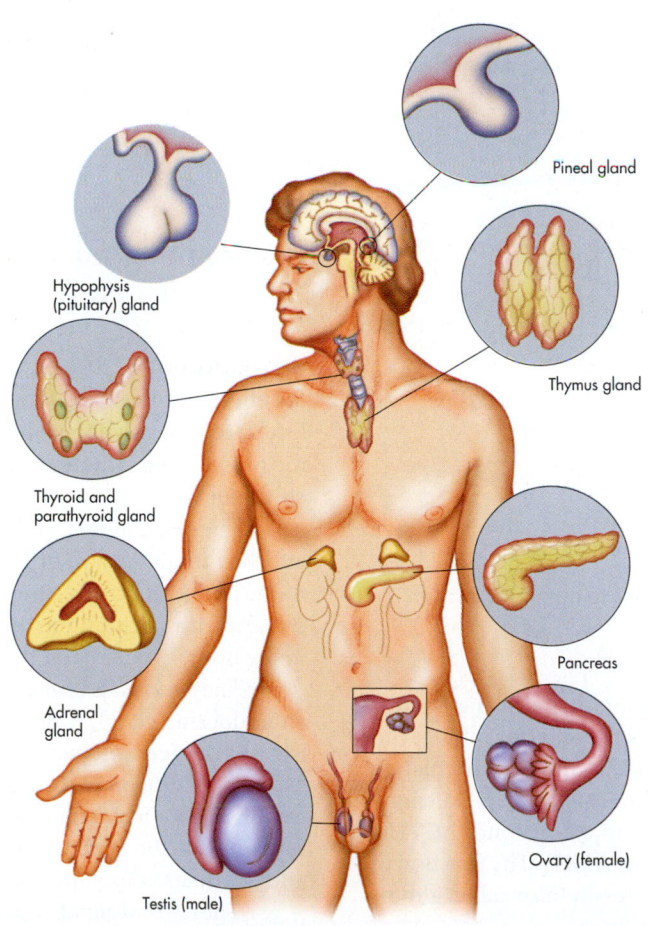

Figure 40-1 ◆ Endocrine glands scattered throughout the body.

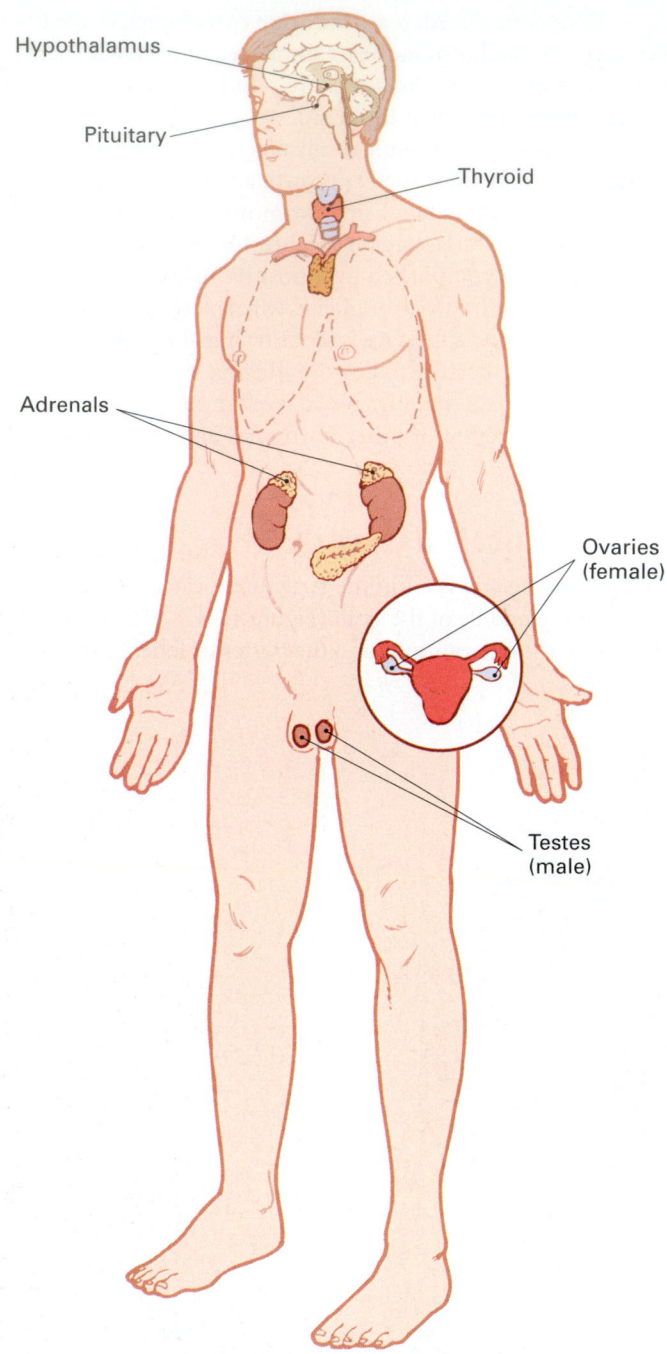

Figure 40-2 ◆ Hormones send messages to other glands and target organs.

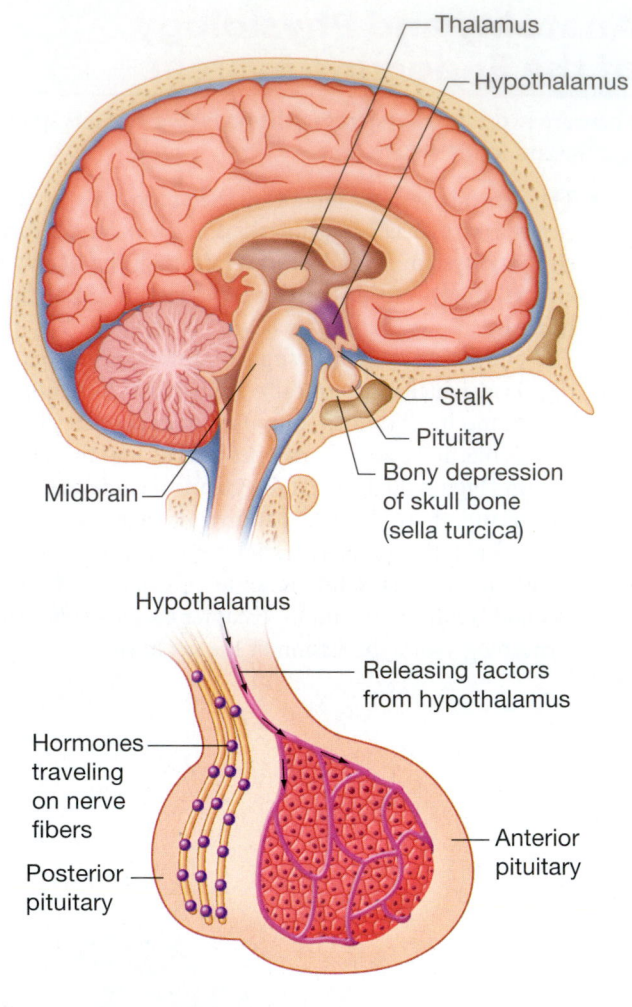

Figure 40-3 ◆ The pituitary gland and its relation to the brain.

is controlled by the **hypothalamus** and its releasing factors. Hypothalamic releasing factor causes the anterior pituitary to release growth hormone (**GH**), prolactin, follicle-stimulating hormone (**FSH**), thyroid-stimulating hormone (**TSH**), luteinizing hormone (**LH**), adrenocorticotropic hormone (**ACTH**), and melanocyte-stimulating hormone (**MSH**). The function of the posterior lobe is to secrete vasopressin (also called antidiuretic hormone, or **ADH**) and oxytocin.

The *thyroid gland,* also composed of two lobes, is located in the neck on either side of the trachea. It secretes triiodothyronine (T_3), thyroxine (T_4), and calcitonin. T_3 and T_4 are under the control of TSH, stimulate cell metabolism, and are essential for energy and cell building and repair. When blood calcium levels are high, calcitonin stimulates some of the calcium to exit the blood and go into the bones, returning blood calcium levels to normal.

The *parathyroid glands,* usually four in number, are attached to the surface of the thyroid gland. Parathyroid hormone (**PTH**) affects calcium levels in the blood. It functions in concert with calcitonin to maintain appropriate calcium levels in the body.

The *pancreas* is both an endocrine and **exocrine gland.** As an endocrine gland, it produces insulin and glucagon in the islets of Langerhans. Insulin is produced in the beta cells of the islets and glucagon in the alpha cells. These two hormones are responsible for maintaining glucose levels in the blood. Exocrine functions of the pancreas are related to the digestive process, and the ducts empty into the GI tract.

The *adrenal glands* are two small glands on the upper surface of each kidney. Each gland has two portions.

■ The *adrenal medulla,* or inner portion, works in concert with the sympathetic nervous system during activation of the sympathetic response, producing epinephrine (adrenaline) and norepinephrine (noradrenaline)

- The *adrenal cortex,* or outer portion, produces hormones called corticosteroids (steroids), including mineralcorticoids, glucocorticoids, androgens, estrogens, and progestins.

The *thymus gland* functions early in life, helping to develop the immune system. It is located in the mediastinum and is composed of lymphoid-type tissue. The thymus usually shrinks or atrophies during adolescence.

The *pineal gland* is located in the central portion of the brain. This gland is believed to secrete melatonin. It has a tendency to calcify during the aging process.

Table 40-1 summarizes the endocrine glands, the hormones they secrete, and the functions the various hormones perform.

TABLE 40-1 THE ENDOCRINE GLANDS		
Gland	**Location**	**Hormone(s) Secreted**
Pituitary, anterior lobe	Cranial cavity, brain	■ Growth hormone: stimulates growth, protein synthesis, and lipid mobilization and catabolism ■ Thyroid-stimulating hormone: stimulates secretion of thyroid hormones ■ Adrenocorticotropic hormone: glucocorticocoid secretion ■ Follicle-stimulating hormone: stimulates estrogen secretion and follicle development (female) and sperm maturation (male) ■ Luteinizing hormone: stimulates ovulation, corpus luteum development, secretion of progesterone
Pituitary, posterior lobe	Cranial cavity, brain	■ Antidiuretic hormone: absorbs H_2O, elevates blood pressure and volume ■ Oxytocin: stimulates uterine contractions and milk ejection (female), and contractions of the prostate (male)
Thyroid	Neck	■ Triiodothyronine (T_3): increases metabolic rate ■ Thyroxine (T_4): increases metabolic rate ■ Calcitonin: increases calcium storage in bones
Parathyroid	Neck, attached to thyroid	■ Parathormone (PTH): increases calcium removal from the bones
Adrenal cortex	Retroperitoneal (above kidneys)	■ Mineralocorticoids (aldosterone): stimulate reabsorption of sodium in kidney tubules, accelerate loss of potassium ions from urine ■ Glucocorticoids (cortisol, corticosterone, cortisone): influence metabolism of food, exhibit anti-inflammatory effect ■ Gonadocorticoids (androgens, estrogens, progestins): possible support of sexual function
Adrenal medulla	Retroperitoneal (above kidneys)	■ Catecholamines, epinephrine, norepinephrine: enhance and prolong effects of sympathetic nervous system
Pancreas islets	Abdomen	■ Insulin: promotes movement of glucose across cell membranes ■ Glucagon: promotes movement of glucose from storage into the blood
Thymus	Mediastnum	■ Thymosin: involved with immune response, essential for maturation of T cells
Pineal gland	Cranial cavity, brain	■ Melatonin: may affect circadian rhythms

continued

TABLE 40-1 THE ENDOCRINE GLANDS (CONTINUED)

Gland	Location	Hormone(s) Secreted
Ovaries	Pelvic cavity	■ Estrogens: develop and maintain female sex characteristics and female reproductive cycle ■ Progesterone: maintains lining of uterus during pregnancy
Testes	Scrotum	■ Testosterone: develops and maintains male sex characteristics and sperm production

Endocrine Disorders

Most endocrine disorders are the result of either hyposecretion (diminished activity) or hypersecretion (increased activity) of the gland. For example, hypersecretion of the pituitary gland during the years of growth results in gigantism and, during post-growth years, in acromegaly. Hypopituitarism in children results in a condition called dwarfism (Figure 40-4 ◆). Table 40-2 lists a few of the disorders caused by hyper- and hyposecretion.

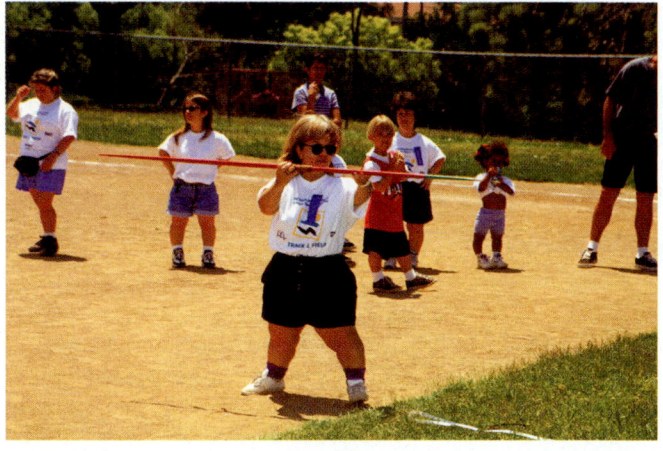

Figure 40-4 ◆ Dwarfism.
Source: Photoedit, Inc.

Pituitary Gland Disorders

The pituitary gland is often referred to as the master gland. The hypothalamus controls the activity of the gland by releasing factors to the anterior pituitary gland. Releasing factors, peptides produced by the hypothalamus, are secreted directly into the anterior pituitary gland to stimulate the secretion of specific tropic hormones. Tropic hormones control or stimulate the activities of other glands. Growth hormone (GH) secreted by the pituitary gland reaches all body tissues. Hypersecretion causes excessive growth, and hyposecretion retards growth. The overstimulation of bone and other tissue by GH results in abnormal growth during the growth period and gigantism. If overstimulation occurs after the growth period has ended, the result is acromegaly—overgrowth of the bones of the hands, feet, and face. In both conditions, the usual cause is a pituitary tumor. Although the overproduction of growth hormone can be controlled, excessive growth cannot be reversed.

Hypopituitarism is a reduction in the excretion of any of the pituitary hormones. This complex condition may involve retarded growth, retarded or delayed sexual maturation, or metabolic dysfunction. Growth retardation in children results in dwarfism, and growth hormone is administered to encourage growth.

Diminished release of vasopressin, or antidiuretic hormone, by the posterior lobe of the pituitary gland causes excessive amounts of very dilute urine to be secreted by the kidneys. This condition is known as diabetes insipidus. Individuals with this condition may secrete as much as 3 to 6 liters of dilute urine in a 24-hour period. Injections of vasopressin or the use of nasal spray containing vasopressin help to replace the diminished supply and slow the excessive output of urine.

TABLE 40-2 EXAMPLES OF ENDOCRINE DISORDERS CAUSED BY HYPERSECRETION AND HYPOSECRETION

Gland	Hypersecretion	Hyposecretion
Pituitary gland	Growth hormone: gigantism in childhood, acromegaly in adulthood	Growth hormone: dwarfism in childhood, hypopituitarism in adulthood
Thyroid gland	Thyroid hormones: Graves' disease	Thyroid hormones: simple goiter or hyperplasia of thyroid gland
Parathyroid gland	Parathyroid hormone: hypercalcemia	Parathyroid hormone: hypocalcemia
Pancreas	Insulin: hypoglycemia, or insulin shock	Insulin: hyperglycemia, or diabetic coma
Adrenal glands	Glucocorticoids: Cushing's syndrome	Adrenocortical hormones: Addison's disease

Thyroid Gland Disorders

Iodine must be supplied in the diet to assure the proper functioning of the thyroid gland. Hyperplasia or enlargement of the thyroid gland, also known as simple goiter, results from inadequate iodine intake and the inability of the gland to secrete thyroid hormones. The hyperplasia must be halted before it compromises the airway. Treatment options include iodine supplements, drug therapy to provide required amounts of T_3 and T_4, and surgical intervention to remove the overgrowth of tissue.

Hypothyroidism, the result of underproduction and undersecretion of thyroid hormones, is a common condition that is treated with hormone replacement therapy that must continue for life. Signs of hypothyroidism include a slowed metabolic rate, low levels of T_3 and T_4, pale, cool skin, slow heart rate, lethargy, decreased appetite, weight gain, intolerance to cold, and possible goiter.

Several conditions are related to hypothyroidism.

- Hashimoto's disease, also known as chronic thyroiditis, is a form of hypothyroidism and occurs as an autoimmune reaction.
- Myxedema is a severe or acute hypothyroid state in adults that may lead to hypoglycemia, hypotension, hypothermia, reduced levels of consciousness, and, when untreated, to death.
- Cretinism is a congenital condition of hypothyroidism resulting from iodine deficiency during fetal development or during early life development. This condition is characterized by mental retardation and impaired growth patterns.

Hyperthyroidism, an oversecretion of thyroid hormones, is also known as Graves' disease. This condition is often accompanied by an outward protrusion of the eyes, called exophthalmos. Other symptoms include a feeling of unusual nervousness, excessive perspiration, insomnia, palpitations and rapid heart rate, and intolerance to heat. Individuals may also experience weight loss, excessive thirst, muscle weakness, and fatigue. Treatment involves drug therapy with antithyroid drugs (propylthiouracil and methimazole) to slow the production of thyroid hormones, and cardiac drugs, including beta-blockers, to treat the cardiac arrhythmias. When drug therapy does not bring about a sufficient response, radioactive iodine or surgical removal of a portion of the thyroid gland may be necessary.

In Practice

Camille Banks, 40 years old, is seen in the office for a complaint of weight gain, decreased appetite, and being tired all of the time. After the physical examination, she asks the medical assistant why the physician felt the front of her neck. How should the MA respond? What gland is located there? What tests do you think the physician will request?

Parathyroid Disorders

Parathyroid disorders include hypoparathyroidism and hyperparathyroidism. Hypoparathyroidism causes low serum calcium levels, or hypocalcemia. Two consequences of hypocalcemia are increased nerve excitability (spontaneous muscle contractions or twitching), also known as tetany, and weak cardiac muscle contractions. Treatment involves lifelong calcium replacement therapy along with vitamin D supplements.

Excessive production and secretion of parathyroid hormone causes an elevation in blood calcium levels, or hypercalcemia, as calcium migrates from bone tissue into the blood serum. Symptoms of this condition include joint pain, kidney stones, CNS and gastrointestinal disturbances, and brittle bones. Treatment varies depending on the cause and includes partial resection of the parathyroid glands, hydration of the patient, and drug therapy to inhibit reabsorption of calcium from bone tissue.

Disorders of the Pancreas

The pancreas is both an endocrine gland and an exocrine gland. As an exocrine gland it secretes enzymes necessary for the digestive process that are released into the GI tract through the pancreatic duct. Endocrine activity occurs in the alpha and beta cells of the islets of Langerhans. In response to low blood glucose levels, the alpha cells secrete glucagon. Glucagon increases blood glucose levels by stimulating the liver to convert stored noncarbohydrate substances into glucose, a process called **gluconeogenesis.**

Insulin is produced in and secreted by the beta islet cells. Insulin is necessary for the transport of glucose across cell membranes into cells for cellular metabolism. When insulin is not available to assist in this transport, blood levels of glucose increase. The condition that results from the continued decrease of available insulin and the increase in blood glucose levels is diabetes mellitus. Normal blood glucose levels generally range between 60 and 120 mg/dl, although a 10 percent variable is considered within normal range.

Diabetes mellitus is classified into two different forms, insulin-dependent diabetes mellitus (**IDDM, type I**) and non-insulin-dependent diabetes mellitus (**NIDDM, type II**).

- IDDM often has an abrupt onset, usually appears before the age of 30, and is sometimes called juvenile-onset diabetes. In this condition, the pancreas does not secrete insulin. Treatment consists of insulin administration by injection or parenteral insulin pump.
- NIDDM often has a gradual onset, usually appearing in adults over the age of 40, and is often referred to as adult-onset diabetes. The pancreas still secretes some insulin, and it is possible to stimulate it to secrete more.

?—Critical Thinking Question 40-1-

Mr. Wiat is apparently unaware of how adult-onset diabetes occurs and what the treatment options are. How should Charles educate him?

Two serious glucose metabolism disorders, hypoglycemia and hyperglycemia, are complications of diabetes mellitus. Too much insulin, whether by injection or beta cell production stimulation, results in a dramatic drop in blood glucose levels, or hypoglycemia, also referred to as insulin shock. Other causes are inadequate food intake, excessive exercise, or other underlying illnesses. Hypoglycemia is a life-threatening condition that requires immediate intervention. The individual experiences a feeling of weakness, shakiness, light-headedness, and sweating. Without immediate intervention—ingestion or infusion of glucose—an altered level of consciousness follows and the individual may become agitated and uncooperative. ∞ This condition constitutes a true medical emergency, as described in Chapter 41, Emergency Care.

The opposite of hypoglycemia or insulin shock is hyperglycemia, or diabetic coma. The glucose level of the blood rises well above 120 mg/dl, the upper end of the normal range. As this condition evolves, the blood pH level drops, creating a condition of metabolic acidosis. As the body tries to rid itself of the excess glucose in the blood, more urine is produced and the respiratory system excretes acetones (ketones). Skipping or delaying an insulin injection, illness, and ingestion of too much food, especially food high in sugar content, can cause this complication. Symptoms include a fruity odor to the breath, intense thirst, lethargy, dry skin, occasionally abdominal pain, and possible coma. Intervention consists of hydration and the administration of insulin.

Critical Thinking Question 40-2

Mr. Wiat seems to be in denial about his condition and how his lifestyle may cause additional health problems and even death. How should Charles proceed in educating him?

Gestational diabetes mellitus is a form of diabetes that has its onset during pregnancy. The inability to produce adequate amounts of insulin or to utilize it effectively is usually first noticed during the second or third trimester. Many physicians routinely order glucose tolerance tests or two-hour postprandial glucose during the last half of the pregnancy as a screening for gestational diabetes. Management of this disease is similar to the usual management of diabetes mellitus. It involves the monitoring of blood glucose levels and the administration of oral hypoglycemic agents and, on occasion, insulin.

The signs, symptoms, and treatment of hypoglycemia and hyperglycemia are summarized in Table 40-3.

Drug therapy for diabetes mellitus includes insulin replacement. Research is currently being conducted on new methods of insulin administration in addition to the current methods—injection or, in an emergency, IV. Oral hypoglycemic agents work in various ways to stimulate the pancreas to secrete more insulin by blocking gluconeogenesis, increasing insulin sensitivity, reducing insulin resistance and allowing better utilization of available insulin, and slowing absorption of dietary glucose in the gut.

In addition to daily "finger sticks" for glucose monitoring, the physician may order laboratory blood tests on a regular basis. A fasting blood sugar (**FBS**) drawn first thing in the morning is an accurate determination of blood glucose levels. A second blood test, also a fasting test, is the glycohemoglobin or glycosylated hemoglobin (**GHB A1c**) test. This test indicates an average of blood glucose levels over the previous 120 days as an indication of how well blood glucose has been controlled in that time frame.

The medical assistant may play one or more roles in dealing with the diabetic patient, including the following:

- Teaching the patient about insulin administration (depending on state practice acts and physician direction).
- Instructing the patient in how to use a glucometer and record the information in a "diabetic diary," if the glucometer is not equipped with an internal memory.

TABLE 40-3 HYPOGLYCEMIA VERSUS HYPERGLYCEMIA		
	Hypoglycemia, Insulin Reaction	**Hyperglycemia, Diabetic Coma**
Signs and Symptoms	Rapid, abrupt onset Patient complains of hunger Cool, moist skin and profuse perspiration (diaphoresis) Pale, clammy skin Blood glucose level below 70 mg/dl Rapid onset of decreased level of consciousness	Slow, insidious onset Patient complains of intense thirst and dry mouth Dry, warm skin Flushed skin Blood glucose level elevated above normal Increased urine output Rapid and deep respirations Abdominal pain and vomiting Slow onset of decreased level of consciousness Acetone-smelling breath
Treatment	Give patient a simple sugar source such as hard candy, soda, or orange juice. If patient is unable to swallow or is comatose, give dextrose or glucagon by intravenous route.	Give patient insulin by subcutaneous injection, plus fluids and sodium (such as salt) by mouth. If patient is unable to swallow or is comatose, give insulin, fluids, and sodium by intravenous route.

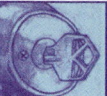

Keys to Success
HELPING PATIENTS WITH THE COST OF DIABETIC SUPPLIES

The treatment of disease conditions usually involves medication or a specific therapy for a certain amount of time. But the diabetic patient needs medical supplies for a lifetime: a glucometer, glucometer strips, insulin syringes, insulin, lancets, lancet holders, syringe waste disposal, and healthier food. Patients may not understand the importance of preventive health maintenance and may risk hospitalization and other complications when their budgets are limited. The medical assistant can help patients by researching pharmaceutical companies that provide free or low-cost insulin and medical supplies. The MA should also know how to help patients contact the local trustee office or welfare office and provide assistance with filing insurance claims for Medicaid, Medicare, and other third-party payers.

- Discussing the importance of foot care.
- Encouraging the patient to follow dietary plans, glucose monitoring, and medication instructions and to keep follow-up appointments as scheduled. (∞ Refer to Chapter 30 for glucose monitoring information and Chapter 42 for dietary information.)

- Encouraging patients to discuss possible side effects of drugs with their physician or pharmacist and to immediately report to the physician any side effects that do occur.

Adrenal Gland Disorders

There are two major adrenal gland disorders.

- Cushing's syndrome is caused by hypersecretion of glucocorticoids. The individual takes on an appearance typical of obesity, with the characteristic round or moon face. There is a wasting away of muscle tissue as well as the development of a thick trunk and a "buffalo hump" at the back of the neck. These individuals are at high risk for infection and have a poor stress response. They experience fatigue, weakness, hypertension, glucose intolerance, and delayed healing. Drug therapy, radiation, and surgery are intervention options for this disorder.
- Addison's disease is caused by the hyposecretion of adrenocortical secretions. Possible causes are autoimmune response and infectious processes. The individual experiences weight loss, fatigue, frequent infection, anorexia, nausea and vomiting, syncope, and poor stress response. Replacement of the deficient hormones and dietary and electrolyte balance are the usual forms of treatment.

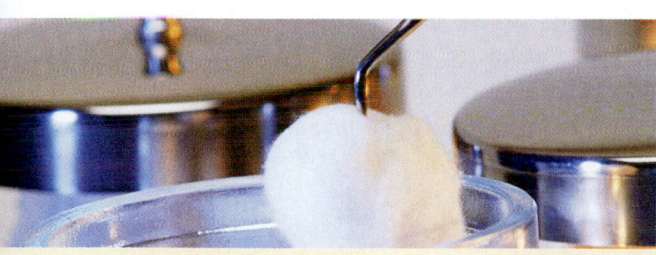

REVIEW

Chapter Summary

- The MA in an endocrinology office may perform typical assessment tasks, such as obtaining and recording vital signs and history information, as well as obtaining blood and urine specimens and performing blood glucose tests. The MA may also discuss dietary instructions, diabetic foot care, and glucose self-monitoring equipment with the patient.
- The nervous and endocrine systems are the two control systems in the body. The endocrine system is composed of glands that secrete and release hormones directly into the bloodstream. They include the pituitary gland, thyroid gland, parathyroid gland, pancreas, adrenal glands, gonads, thymus gland, and pineal gland. Hormones are chemical messengers that influence and control body functions.
- Endocrine disorders are the result of too much hormone being stimulated or released (hyperactivity) or too little (hypoactivity).

- The pituitary gland is controlled by the hypothalamus and its releasing factors. The anterior pituitary lobe releases growth-stimulating hormone, prolactin, follicle-stimulating hormone, thyroid-stimulating hormone, luteinizing hormone, adrenocorticotropic hormone, and melanocyte-stimulating hormone. The posterior lobe's function is to secrete vasopressin and oxytocin. Hyperfunctioning of the pituitary gland results in gigantism or acromegaly. Hypopituitarism in children causes dwarfism. Decreased secretion of the posterior lobe results in diabetes insipidus.
- The two lobes of the thyroid gland are located in the neck on either side of the trachea. The thyroid gland secretes triiodothyronine (T_3), thyroxine (T_4), and thyrocalcitonin (TCT). T_3 and T_4 stimulate cell metabolism and are essential for energy, cell building, and repair and are under the control of TSH. TCT or calcitonin serves to maintain normal blood

Chapter Summary (continued)

calcium levels. Iodine deficiency causes simple goiter, or enlargement of the thyroid gland. Hypothyroid conditions include Hashimoto's disease, myxedema, and, in children, cretinism. Graves' disease is a hyperthyroid condition. Hypothyroidism is treated with lifetime hormone replacement therapy. Treatment options for hyperthyroidism include iodine supplements, drug therapy to replace required amounts of T_3 and T_4, or surgical intervention to remove the over-growth of tissue.

■ Parathyroid hormone (PTH) affects calcium levels in the bone. With calcitonin it maintains appropriate calcium levels in the body. Hypoparathyroidism causes low serum calcium levels, or hypocalcemia. Hyperparathyroidism causes elevated blood calcium levels, or hypercalcemia.

■ The pancreas produces insulin and glucagon in the islets of Langerhans and is responsible for maintaining glucose levels in the blood. Glucose metabolism disorders include diabetes mellitus and hypoglycemia. There are two forms of diabetes mellitus: insulin-dependent diabetes mellitus (IDDM, type I)

and non-insulin-dependent diabetes mellitus (NIDDM, type II). Drug therapy for diabetes mellitus includes insulin replacement. Hypoglycemia, or insulin shock, is a life-threatening condition resulting from too much insulin and requiring immediate intervention. In hyperglycemia, or diabetic coma, blood glucose levels rise well above normal. Intervention includes hydration and insulin administration.

■ The adrenal glands are two small glands on the kidneys. They produce epinephrine (adrenaline), norepinephrine (noradrenaline), and corticosteroids (steroids). Cushing's syndrome is caused by hypersecretion of glucocorticoids. Drug therapy, radiation, or surgery are treatment options for this disorder. Addison's disease is caused by hyposecretion of adrenocortical secretions and is treated with replacement of the deficient hormones and dietary and electrolyte balance.

■ The thymus gland helps to develop the immune system. It is located in the mediastinum and usually shrinks or atrophies during adolescence. The pineal gland, located in the brain, is believed to secrete melatonin.

Chapter Review

Multiple Choice

1. The conversion of noncarbohydrates stored in the liver into glucose is known as
   a. gluconeogenesis.
   b. absorption.
   c. endocrine release.
   d. hypothalamus conversion.

2. Which of the following is not part of the endocrine gland system?
   a. Ovaries
   b. Testicles
   c. Mammary glands
   d. Thymus

3. The pituitary gland is controlled by the
   a. pineal gland.
   b. parathyroid.
   c. adrenal gland.
   d. hypothalamus.

4. Which of the following is *not* released by the anterior pituitary?
   a. LH
   b. ADH
   c. MSH
   d. TSH

5. How many parathyroid glands are there?
   a. 5
   b. 3
   c. 2
   d. 4

6. The two small glands on the upper surface of each kidney are
   a. adrenal medulla glands.
   b. adrenal glands.
   c. adrenal cortex glands.
   d. thymus glands.

7. The gland in the central portion of the brain that is believed to secrete melatonin is the
   a. pineal gland.
   b. thymus gland.
   c. adrenal gland.
   d. parathyroid gland.

8. Which hormone is *not* secreted by the anterior lobe of the pituitary gland?
   a. Follicle-stimulating hormone
   b. Luteinizing hormone
   c. Antidiuretic hormone
   d. Thyroid-stimulating hormone

9. Which of these is *not* secreted by the adrenal cortex?
   a. Mineralocorticoids
   b. Parathormone (PTH)
   c. Glucocorticoids
   d. Gonadocorticoids

10. Which of these hormones is *not* secreted by the thyroid?
    a. Thymosin
    b. Thyroxine
    c. Triiodothyronine
    d. Calcitonin

Chapter Review (continued)

True/False

T F 1. Most endrocrine disorders are the result of hyposecretion.

T F 2. Hypopituitarism in children results in a condition called *dwarfism.*

T F 3. The hypothalamus is often referred to as the "master gland."

T F 4. Hypopituitarism is a reduction in the excretion of a single pituitary hormone.

T F 5. An excessive urinary output may be caused by a diminished release of vasopressin.

T F 6. Hashimoto's disease is a form of hypothyroidism and can occur as an autoimmune reaction.

T F 7. Elevation of blood calcium levels is a reaction to excessive secretion from the thyroid gland.

T F 8. The pancreas is both an endocrine and an exocrine gland.

T F 9. Hyperglycemia is a life-threatening disorder in which skin appears cool and moist.

T F 10. Hypoglycemia is known as *insulin shock* and can cause a diabetic coma.

Short Answer

1. What is the range of normal blood glucose levels?

2. Which form of DM has its onset during pregnancy?

3. What is the difference between hypoglycemia and hyperglycemia?

Research

1. Does the hospital or other facility in your community run patient education programs for diabetic patients?

2. If you were to help your local clinic create a patient education brochure about endocrine disorders, which diseases, symptoms, and organs would you include? What would you leave out and why? What additional information would your brochure include?

Externship Application Experience

A patient is waiting in the reception area to be seen by the physician for nausea and vomiting. You notice that the patient is pale and very diaphoretic. Her spouse approaches you and says that the patient has had insulin but nothing to eat. The patient is conscious at present. What do you do?

Resource Guide

American Diabetes Association
1701 North Beauregard St.
Alexandria, VA 22311
1-800-DIABETES, 1-800-342-2383
www.diabetes.org

American Thyroid Association
6066 Leesburg Pike, Suite 650
Falls Church, VA 22041
703-998-8890; patients 1-800-THYROID
www.thyroid.org

Endocrine Society
8401 Connecticut Ave., Suite 900
Chevy Chase, MD 20815-5817
301-941-0200
www.endo-society.org

National Diabetes Information Clearinghouse (NDIC)
1 Information Way
Bethesda, MD 20892
1-800-860-8747
diabetes.niddk.nih.gov

National Institute of Diabetes and Digestive and Kidney Diseases
NIH – Building 31, Room 9A04
31 Center Drive, MSC 2560
Bethesda, MD 20892-2560
www.niddk.nih.gov

Med**Media**

http://www.MyMAKit.com

More on this chapter, including interactive resources, can be found on the Student CD-ROM accompanying this textbook and on http://www.MyMAKit.com.

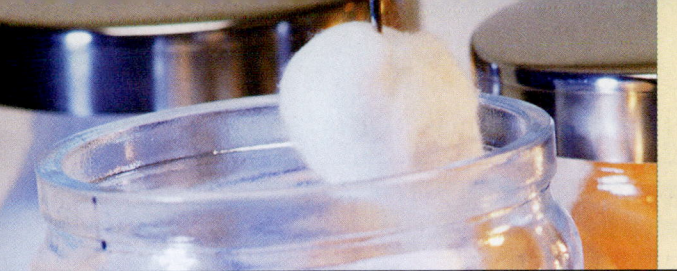

Objectives

After completing this chapter, you should be able to:

- Define and spell the key terminology in this chapter.
- Define the medical assistant's role in emergency care.
- Describe the role of the EMS.
- List the equipment and supplies maintained for emergencies in a medical office.
- Explain the principles of early intervention with CPR and AED.
- Discuss how chest pain emergencies are handled in the medical office.
- Describe the types of respiratory distress and appropriate interventions.
- Identify the different types of shock.
- Compare the different types of bleeding.
- Compare open and closed wounds and their treatment.
- Describe burns, frostbite, and other thermal insults and their appropriate treatment.
- Discuss the appropriate interventions for musculoskeletal injuries.
- Explain allergic reactions and appropriate interventions.
- Describe neurological emergencies and interventions.
- Discuss interventions for acute abdominal pain, diabetic crises, poisoning, and foreign bodies in the eyes, ears, and nose.
- Describe appropriate interventions for psychosocial emergencies.
- Know how to respond in the event of a manmade or natural disaster.

Emergency Care

Case Study

Ariko, a medical assistant, receives a phone call from a young mother, Brenna, who is frantic and crying. Brenna explains that her 2-year-old was playing in the living room while she was doing dishes in the kitchen, one room away. Brenna reports hearing a loud thud against what she believes was the hardwood floor. When she rushed in, she found her daughter curled in a fetal position between a chair and an ottoman.

Brenna says her daughter did not say anything or explain what had happened. The child appears normal, with no bump or bruising and no bleeding that Brenna can see.

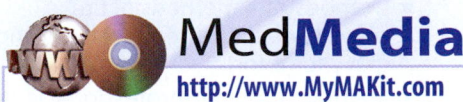

MedMedia

http://www.MyMAKit.com

Additional interactive resources and activities for this chapter can be found on http://www.MyMAKit.com. For a video, tips, audio glossary, legal and ethical scenarios, job scenarios, quizzes, and games related to the content of this chapter, please access the accompanying CD-ROM in this book.

Audio Glossary
Legal and Ethical Scenario: *Emergency Care*
On the Job Scenario: *Emergency Care*
Tips
Video: *Facing Emergencies*
Multiple Choice Quiz
HIPAA Quiz
Games: Crossword, Strikeout, and Spelling Bee

Key Terminology

abrasion—open wound in which the outer layer of skin is scraped away, leaving underlying tissue exposed

Ambu bag—bag-valve-mask unit used to provide ventilation to a nonbreathing patient or to assist ventilations for a patient whose breathing (respiratory effort) is inadequate to support life

anaphylaxis—severe allergic reaction

avulsion—open wound in which skin or tissue is torn loose or pulled completely from underlying tissue

cyanosis—bluish tint in skin or mucous membrane, usually appearing in fingernail beds, oral mucous membranes, and circum-oral tissue (tissue surrounding the mouth) and indicating excessive deoxygenated hemoglobin or reduced hemoglobin in the blood

epistaxis—nosebleed

hyperglycemia—condition in which blood glucose is elevated above normal

hypertension—continued elevation of blood pressure above normal

hyperthermia—condition in which body temperature is much higher than normal for a prolonged period of time

hypoglycemia—condition in which blood glucose is below normal

hypothermia—condition in which body temperature is below normal for a prolonged period of time

incision—open wound with smooth edges made with a knife or other sharp object

laceration—open wound in which the skin and underlying tissue are torn and skin integrity is broken

patent—open

sepsis—febrile state characterized by pathogens in the bloodstream

status epilepticus—continuous seizure activity

venous—pertaining to blood vessels that carry blood toward the heart

✚ MEDICAL ASSISTING STANDARDS

CAAHEP ENTRY-LEVEL STANDARDS	ABHES ENTRY-LEVEL COMPETENCIES
■ Perform within scope of practice (psychomotor)	■ Project a positive attitude.
■ Apply ethical behaviors, including honesty/integrity in performance of medical assisting practice (affective)	■ Maintain confidentiality at all times.
■ Practice Standard Precautions (psychomotor)	■ Be a "team player."
■ Identify safety techniques that can be used to prevent accidents and maintain a safe work environment (cognitive)	■ Be cognizant of ethical boundaries.
■ State principles and steps of professional/provider CPR (cognitive)	■ Exhibit initiative.
■ Describe basic principles of first aid (cognitive)	■ Adapt to change.
■ Describe fundamental principles for evacuation of a healthcare setting (cognitive)	■ Evidence a responsible attitude.
■ Discuss fire safety issues in a healthcare environment (cognitive)	■ Be courteous and diplomatic.
■ Discuss critical elements of an emergency plan for response to a natural disaster or other emergency (cognitive)	■ Conduct work within scope of education, training, and ability.
■ Identify emergency preparedness plans in your community (cognitive)	■ Practice Standard Precautions.
■ Discuss potential role(s) of the medical assistant in emergency preparedness (cognitive)	■ Recognize emergencies.
■ Develop a personal (patient and employee) safety plan (psychomotor)	
■ Develop an environmental safety plan (psychomotor)	
■ Participate in a mock environmental exposure event with documentation of steps taken (psychomotor)	
■ Explain an evacuation plan for a physician's office (psychomotor)	
■ Demonstrate methods of fire prevention in the healthcare setting (psychomotor)	
■ Maintain provider/professional level CPR certification (psychomotor)	
■ Perform first aid procedures (psychomotor)	
■ Maintain a current list of community resources (psychomotor)	
■ Recognize the effects of stress on all persons involved in emergency situations (affective)	
■ Demonstrate self awareness in responding to emergency situations (affective)	

Abbreviations

ABCD—airway, breathing, circulation, defibrillation
AED—automatic external defibrillator
AHA—American Heart Association
ARC—American Red Cross
CPR—cardiopulmonary resuscitation

CVA—cerebrovascular accident/stroke
ED—emergency department
ETA—estimated time of arrival
FEMA—Federal Emergency Management Agency

LOC—level of consciousness
NS—normal saline
SOB—shortness of breath
TIA—transient ischemic attack

✓ COMPETENCY SKILLS PERFORMANCE

Training in cardiopulmonary resuscitation (CPR), clearing an obstructed airway, and using an automated external defibrillator (AED) must be supervised by an instructor certified by the American Red Cross (ARC) or the American Heart Association (AHA). Because it is an educational requirement for medical assistants, certification training must be at the same level as that required for all healthcare employees. The general information presented in this chapter for CPR, obstructed airway, AED use, and first aid skills is superseded by AHA or ARC skill training and certification. For this chapter, you will be responsible for learning the following emergency procedures:

1. Perform adult rescue breathing and one-rescuer CPR.
2. Use an automated external defibrillator (AED).
3. Respond to an adult with an obstructed airway.
4. Administer oxygen.
5. Respond to a patient who has fainted.
6. Demonstrate the application of a pressure bandage.
7. Demonstrate the application of triangular, figure 8, and tubular bandages.
8. Demonstrate the application of a splint.
9. Develop an environmental exposure plan.

Introduction

A positive outcome for a medical office emergency depends on prompt and effective assessment and intervention by the medical team members. Medical emergencies in the office can range from a nosebleed or simple laceration to shortness of breath, chest pain, and full cardiac arrest. They can occur on site or over the phone. It is the responsibility of each team member to know his or her role in any medical emergency. At all times, Universal Precautions and office protocol for emergency situations must be followed.

The Medical Assistant's Role in Emergencies

Medical assistants and other staff members must stay up to date on the emergency plans of the office, facility, and community. These plans should be reviewed on a regularly scheduled basis. For major or catastrophic events, the disaster plan of the American Red Cross (**ARC**) should be considered. Local law enforcement and emergency management agencies direct rescue, treatment, and transportation efforts after catastrophic events. The standard policy is to treat the least seriously injured, also called the walking wounded, as soon as possible so they can assist in any rescue attempts.

After the appropriate training, the MA will be expected to render emergency care as directed. The MA's role will include:

■ Applying CPR, AED, and the Heimlich maneuver.
■ Bandaging and manipulating pressure points.
■ Immobilizing head, neck, and limbs.

More advanced responsibilities will be determined by the physician and the clinical specialty.

Emergency Resources

Those seeking medical care in an emergency have several options.

- During normal office hours, minor emergencies may be handled in a medical office. Some physician group practices may have an emergency clinic where emergency service is provided both during and after office hours.
- Freestanding clinics or urgent care centers provide emergency care during and after hours until late in the evening and often on weekends. However, many of these facilities do not offer critical care intervention.
- Hospitals usually have 24-hour emergency departments (**EDs**) that are open seven days a week. These "24-7 EDs" can usually handle most emergencies and transport patients to critical care trauma centers.
- Critical care centers, such as cardiac, burn, and surgical centers, have specialty trained physicians, surgeons, anesthesiologists, and other critical care staff on duty at all times.

The MA should be aware of the emergency care options available in his or her community.

EMS

The Emergency Medical System (EMS) was established to provide prehospital care and safe and prompt transportation to an emergency facility. Guidelines have been established for consistency in care and for ongoing evaluation of the system services. The role of the EMS is to:

- Provide on-the-scene intervention and treatment.
- Prepare the victim with injuries, trauma, or illness for transport.
- Transport the victim to the emergency facility.

Emergency transportation is accomplished by ambulance, helicopter, or fixed-wing aircraft (Figure 41-1 ◆). Once the patient is safely delivered to the receiving facility, the patient's care is passed to medical personnel at that facility.

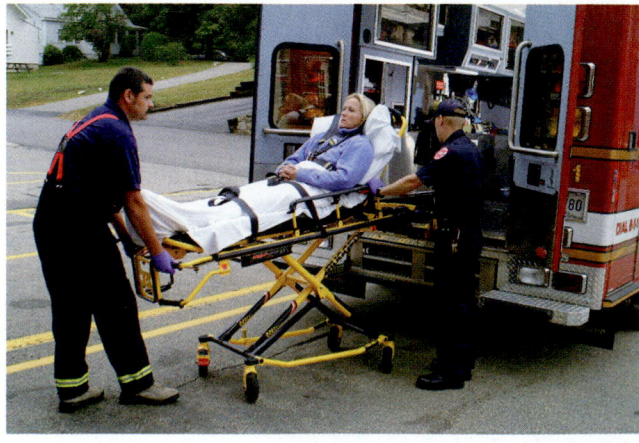

Figure 41-1 ◆ Ambulance transport.

Good Samaritan Laws

A healthcare professional who volunteers in an emergency situation is generally protected by various state laws that hold the medical professional *not* legally liable when rendering first aid. These laws are often referred to as Good Samaritan laws. A healthcare professional has a commitment to render care to a victim(s) according to the scope of his or her license, certification, or training. He or she must remain with the victim until relieved by another healthcare professional with an equal or higher level of training. It is important that every healthcare professional be aware of the laws in his or her own state and remember that the standard of care must be met within his or her license, certification, or training.

Medical Office Preparedness

Most offices keep supplies specifically for emergencies. The office specialty often determines the choice of supplies.

Emergency Equipment and Supplies

Most offices have a crash cart fitted with equipment and supplies appropriate for the office specialty (Figure 41-2 ◆). For example, an allergy office has medications and injections to treat allergic responses.

Crash Cart and Emergency Medical Box

The crash cart is usually kept in an emergency area with easy access from other areas of the office. It is mounted on wheels for easy transport of the equipment and various supplies to any

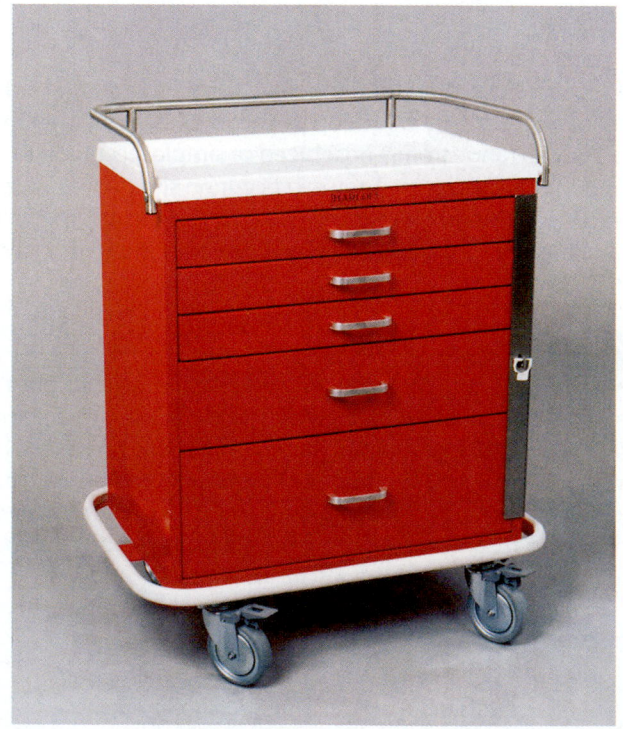

Figure 41-2 ◆ Crash cart.

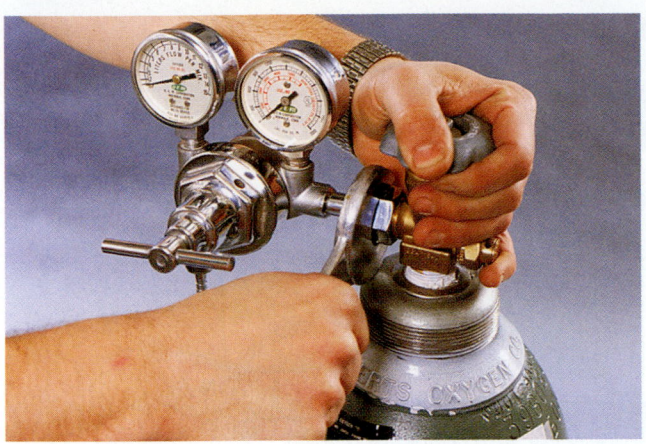

Figure 41-3 ◆ Oxygen tank with flow meter and wrench.

TABLE 41-1 DRUGS COMMONLY STOCKED IN AN EMERGENCY MEDICAL BOX	
■ Activated charcoal	■ Nitroglycerin
■ Atropine	■ Normal saline
■ Diphenhydramine	■ Phenobarbital and
■ Epinephrine	diazepam
■ Furosemide	■ Sodium bicarbonate
■ Instant glucose	■ Solu-Cortef™
■ Insulin	■ Spirits of ammonia
■ Lidocaine	■ Syrup of ipecac
■ Local anesthetics	■ Verapamil

part of the office. Respiratory aids on the cart should include the following:

- Oxygen tank with flow meter and wrench for opening the tank (Figure 41-3 ◆)
- Airways of all sizes, both nasal and oral
- Tubing
- Nasal cannula
- Oxygen masks, both adult and pediatric
- Ambu bags
- Resuscitation masks in a variety of sizes
- Bulb syringe for suctioning

The following IV supplies are also kept on the crash cart:

- IV fluids, including D5W, **NS,** D10W, and Ringer's lactate in 500 ml bags
- At least three butterflies of each size (#19, #21, #23, #25)
- At least three angiocaths of each size (#16, #18, #20, #22)
- Hemostats
- Tourniquets
- Iodine

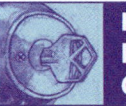

Keys to Success
LEGAL ISSUES CONCERNING CRASH CARTS

Offices with crash carts, AEDs, and emergency drug boxes face certain liability concerns. During office hours, office personnel trained in the use of emergency equipment and the administration of medications must be present. A physician must also be present during office hours to supervise the emergency and administer emergency medication (or supervise administration by qualified staff). Many offices choose to rely on EMS to provide advanced emergency care. The type of office, its location (proximity to a major medical center), and the availability of trained staff are decisive factors in determining what supplies and equipment to keep on hand.

- Alcohol preps
- IV tubing
- A collapsible IV pole

The emergency medical or drug box is kept on or close to the crash cart. Table 41-1 lists some of the drugs that may be stocked in an emergency medical box. Each office determines which drugs are appropriate for its practice, as established by emergency algorithms (Figure 41-4 ◆).

Other supplies usually stocked on a crash cart include alcohol prep pads, blood pressure cuffs (in standard, pediatric, and large sizes), a sphygmomanometer, a stethoscope, scissors, sterile 4 × 4s, sterile Kling™ gauze, pressure bandages in various sizes, sterile and examination gloves, prepackaged needles and syringes in assorted sizes, hypoallergenic tape, nasogastric tubes, a catheter tip syringe, water-soluble lubricant, a pen light, batteries, hot/cold packs, and a pen and note paper.

Emergency Intervention

Emergency intervention is called for in any situation that may be life-threatening (Table 41-2). The responder provides appropriate intervention and stays with the injured or ill person until more advanced care can be provided. Triage of emergency patients is a critical care issue.

Emergency Assessment

In any emergency, even if you are familiar with your office surroundings, the first step is to survey the scene. *Never* put yourself in harm's way. You could become injured or incapacitated. If the scene is safe, the next step is to conduct a primary survey of the injured or ill person, evaluating the airway, breathing, and circulation. If EMS services are required, call or designate an individual to call 911.

Do not move the victim of a fall or injury involving a sudden stop or acceleration, such as in a car. If the victim is conscious, tell him or her not to move, then introduce yourself and ask permission to render care. Ask the victim his or her name and use it. If you are given permission to proceed or if the victim is unconscious, immobilize the neck and possibly the spine. The victim must be log-rolled (moving the head, spine, and legs as a single unit to prevent additional spinal injury), or the

PATIENT ASSESSMENT

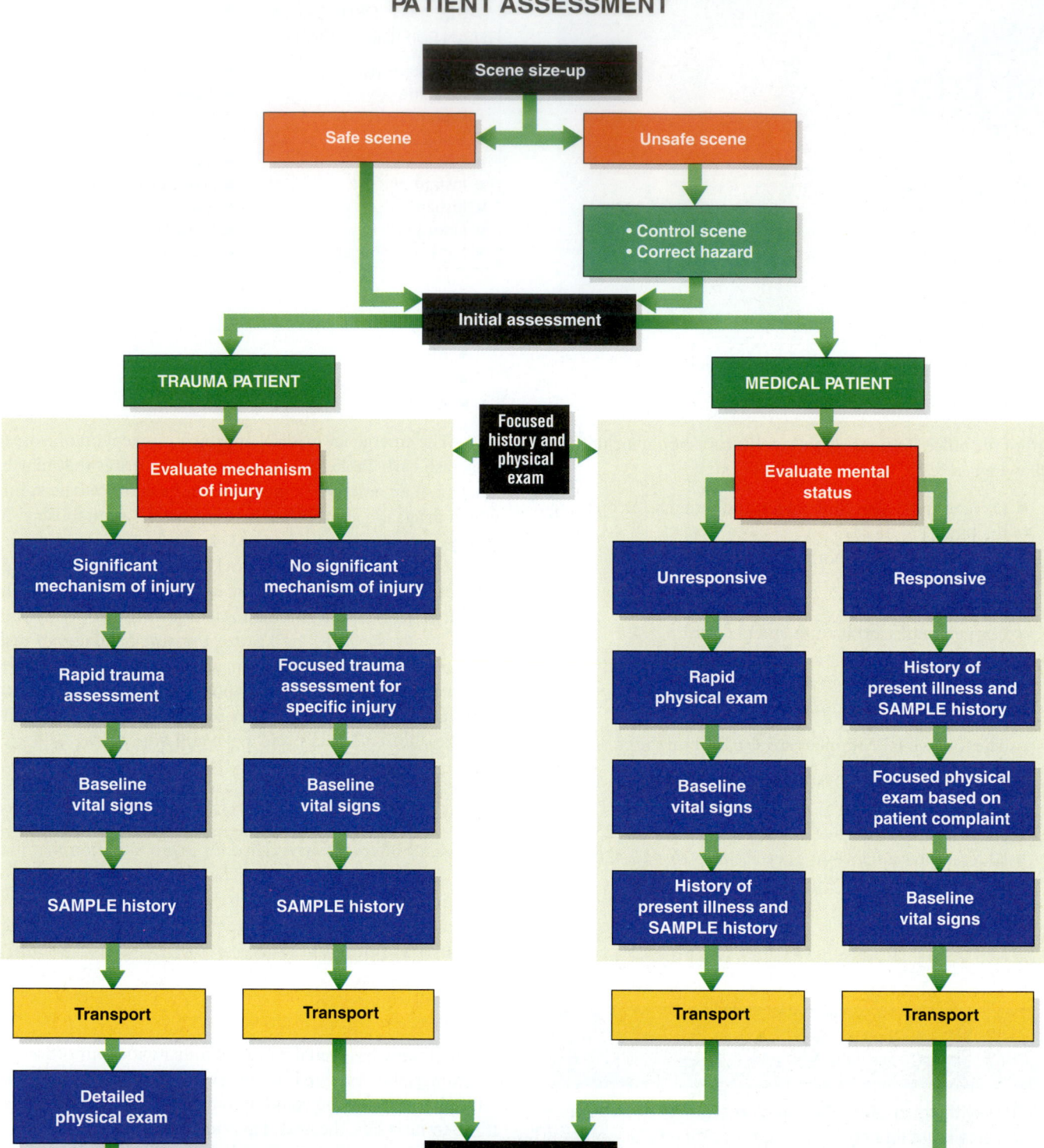

Figure 41-4 ◆ Example of emergency algorithm.

Source: Limmer, Daniel; O'Keefe, Michael F.; Dickinson, Edward V.; Grant, Harvey; Murray, Bob; Bergeron, David J., Emergency Care, *10th Edition, © 2005. Reprinted by permission of Pearson Education, Inc. Upper Saddle River, NJ.*

TABLE 41-2 EMERGENCY INTERVENTION

Life-Threatening Condition	Not Life-Threatening: Immediate Intervention	Not-Life Threatening: Intervention as Soon as Possible
■ extreme **SOB** (airway or breathing problems) ■ cardiac arrest ■ severe, uncontrolled bleeding ■ head injuries ■ poisoning ■ open chest or abdominal wounds ■ shock ■ severe burns, including face, hands, feet, and genitals ■ potential neck injuries	■ decreased levels of consciousness ■ chest pain ■ seizures ■ major or multiple fractures ■ neck injuries ■ severe eye injuries ■ burns not on face, hands, feet, or genitals	■ severe vomiting and diarrhea, especially in the very young and the elderly ■ minor injuries ■ sprains ■ strains ■ simple fractures

spine must be immobilized and splinted. Ask the victim what happened and for medical information, including:

- The presence and location of pain.
- Any history of medical problems, such as diabetes or seizures.
- Last time the patient ate or drank.
- What medications were taken and when.
- Allergies.

Determine the cause of the injury, perform a rapid, focused trauma assessment and baseline vital signs, and plan for the victim's transport, if necessary.

?—Critical Thinking Question 41-1—
What questions should Ariko ask Brenna regarding the accident and the child's behavior?

Primary and secondary surveys follow. Check or recheck vital signs, including pulse, respirations, and blood pressure. Assess the skin for color, moisture, and temperature. Check for cuts, bruises, and any other signs of injury while assessing the victim from head to toe. Examine the pupils of the eyes for reactivity and equality of size, then the ears, nose, and mouth for fluid drainage. Palpate the sides of the victim's neck for pain, tenderness, or injury, then the shoulders, collarbones, rib cage, and chest. Feel the patient's abdomen in all quadrants for any signs of tenderness or rigidity. Check the arms, hips, legs, and feet.

In the event of sudden illness, acute pain, bleeding, or reduced level of consciousness in the medical office, move or assist the patient to an examination room where an assessment can be made. As with a trauma victim, the severely ill person should be assessed following established office guidelines. Evaluate the person's mental status. If the patient is responsive, obtain a rapid medical history. If the victim is unresponsive, quickly do a physical assessment and take vital signs. If the physician is unavailable to provide direction and orders, call EMS, then prepare the victim for transport to an emergency facility.

As a rescuer, remain calm and in control of the situation. Office personnel not involved in the emergency response should return to work. One person should be designated to keep family members informed of the situation. Both the patient and the family need emotional support. If necessary, maintain crowd control. Another person should be designated to document or take notes about all the events. Record vital signs, times, symptoms and signs elicited, and any action or intervention, then complete an incident report.

OSHA Guidelines

OSHA guidelines apply to emergency as well as routine medical office procedures.

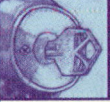

**Keys to Success
EYEWASH STATIONS**

Emergency eyewash stations are essential tools that are used when chemicals or small particles come into contact with the eye. Perform the following steps in the case of such an emergency:

1. Immediately remove contact lenses if a chemical or other substance enters the eye. If not removed, the lenses can hold the substance in the eye and cause serious damage.
2. Gently hold your eyes open and place them on the designated spot on the eyewash station.
3. The eyewash station is designed to deliver a continuous flush of water to ensure that substances are moved from the eye. While holding your eyes open, have another individual turn on the water. Irrigation should last for at least 15 minutes.
4. Never rub your eyes if dust or debris is thought to be inside as this can further irritate and possibly damage the eye.
5. Emergency response units should be called. Request that a co-worker make the call for EMS while you continue to irrigate your eyes. Again, be sure to irrigate for at least 15 minutes, even after the emergency response team arrives.

- Wear examination gloves when handling body fluids and infectious materials and when hands come in contact with mucous membranes, non-intact skin, or contaminated instruments or equipment.
- Dispose of any biohazardous materials in an appropriate waste receptacle.
- Wash your hands immediately after removing gloves and before caring for another patient.
- Wear additional PPE, such as a face shield or mask, whenever there is a risk of exposure.
- If you perform **CPR,** use a face mask barrier device.
- If your hands, arms, or any uncovered skin come into contact with blood or body fluids, wash with soap and water immediately. Flush mucous membranes, such as those in the mouth, eyes, and nose, immediately with water.
- To prevent accidental or careless exposure, *do not* eat, drink, or touch your face during emergencies without first washing your hands.
- Follow sharps precautions when using syringes and needles, and handle accidents involving glass carefully and without direct contact to avoid injury.
- Follow the correct sanitization, disinfection, and sterilization procedures when cleaning surfaces and instruments.

CPR, AED, and Obstructed Airway

Respiratory and cardiac arrest may be caused by an occluded airway, electrocution, shock, drowning, heart attack, trauma, **anaphylaxis,** drugs, poisoning, or traumatic head or chest injury. Intervention must be immediate if resuscitation is to be successful. For individuals experiencing acute chest pain, loss of consciousness, or respiratory arrest, follow CPR protocol.

Guidelines are similar for respiratory arrest, cardiac arrest, and obstructed airway but vary somewhat according to age group. Table 41-3 lists the major differences in the performance of CPR-related skills as defined by the **AHA.** Early access to EMS is important. Access for the adult victim is initiated by calling 911 as soon as it has been determined that the victim is unconscious and not breathing. In general, "phone first" for an unresponsive adult. With children and infants, EMS access is made after 2 minutes of CPR. In general, perform "CPR first" for unresponsive children and infants. The sequence normally followed is airway, breathing, circulation, and defibrillation (**ABCD**).

Airway

First, roll the victim onto his or her back, using the log-roll technique. Next, assess the unconscious victim for responsiveness. With an adult or child, shake the shoulders and ask, "Are you

TABLE 41-3 ADULT, CHILD, AND INFANT CPR SKILLS

CPR Skill	Adult: 8+ years	Child: 1 year–puberty (approximately 12–14 years)	Infant: under 1 year
EMS access by calling 911 and giving emergency information	If sudden collapse is witnessed, immediately activate EMS and get AED. If asphyxiation (e.g., drowning, injury, overdose) suspected, first perform 2 minutes of CPR (or 5 cycles), then activate EMS.	If sudden collapse is witnessed, immediately activate EMS and get AED. Otherwise perform 2 minutes of CPR (5 cycles), then activate EMS.	If sudden collapse is witnessed, immediately activate EMS. Otherwise, perform 2 minutes of CPR (5 cycles), then activate EMS.
Assessment of unresponsiveness	Shake the shoulders.	Shake the shoulders.	Snap or poke the feet. Do *not* shake the shoulders.
Rescue breathing rate of 1 second long, normal breath until chest rises	10–12 breaths per minute or one breath every 5–6 seconds	12–20 breaths per minute or one breath every 3–5 seconds	12–20 breaths per minute or one breath every 3–5 seconds
Obstructed airway foreign body	Abdominal thrusts	Abdominal thrusts	Back slaps and chest thrusts
Pulse check location	Carotid	Carotid	Brachial or femoral
Compression technique	One hand linked over second hand, with heel of second hand on sternum	Heel of one hand on sternum	Single rescuer: two fingertips on sternum Two rescuers: two thumbs touching on sternum and hand encircling chest and back technique
Compression landmarks	Center of chest, between nipples	Center of chest between nipples	Center of chest, just below nipple line
Compression depth	1-1/2—2"	1/2 to 1/3 depth of chest	1/2 to 1/3 depth of chest
Compression rate	100 per minute	100 per minute	100 per minute
Compression ratio to rescue breathing	Single rescuer: 30:2 Two rescuers: 30:2	Single rescuer: 30:2 Two rescuers: 15:2	Single rescuer: 30:2 Two rescuers: 15:2

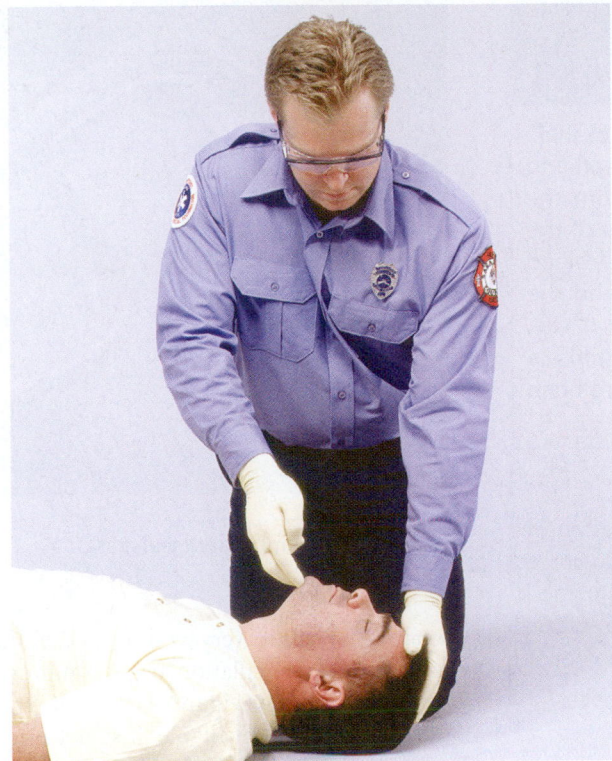
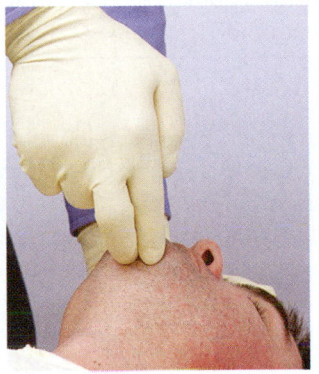

Figure 41-5 ◆ Head-tilt, chin-lift maneuver.

choking?" With an infant, poke or snap the feet. Do not shake the shoulders, as shaking may cause Shaken Baby Syndrome.

If the victim does not respond, check the airway. With an adult, child, or infant, place the palm of one hand on the forehead and two or three fingers under the lower jawbone to gently tilt the head backward (Figure 41-5 ◆). If cervical or other spinal injuries are suspected, a jaw-thrust maneuver must be used to open the airway (Figure 41-6 ◆). When the airway is opened, the victim may begin spontaneous breathing because the tongue is lifted from covering the trachea. While keeping close to the

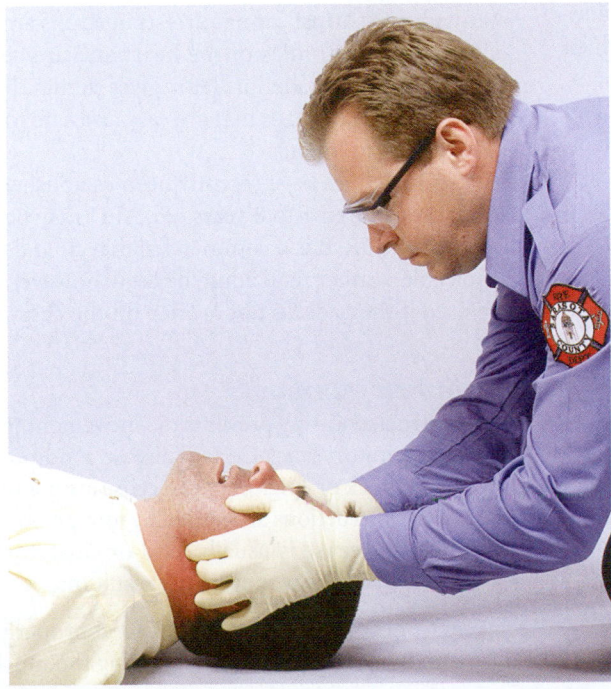
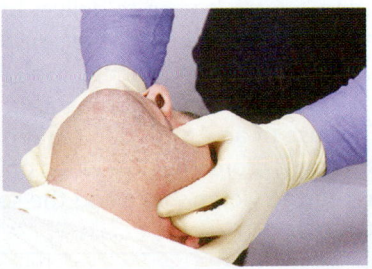

Figure 41-6 ◆ Jaw-thrust maneuver.

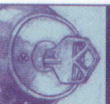
victim's mouth, listen for air movement, look for chest movement, and feel for air movement on your cheek. If you do not feel air on your cheek, remove any clothing from the victim's neck. It is possible the victim has a tracheotomy, a surgically created opening for breathing, which may be the reason you do not feel air movement.

Breathing

If you have looked, listened, and felt for breathing and found none, pinch the patient's nose shut, seal your lips tightly around the patient's mouth, and deliver two breaths, each lasting 1 second. You will know the artificial ventilation is effective if the victim's chest rises with each delivered breath. For a victim with a tracheotomy, it may be necessary to close the mouth and nose and administer breaths to the tracheotomy.

Circulation

According to the most recent AHA Basic Life Support guidelines, the rescuer should check for signs of circulation, defined as pulse, color and warmth of skin, and victim movement. After you deliver breaths to the victim, check the pulse. In an adult or child, feel the carotid pulse in the neck. In an infant, feel the brachial pulse. Count the pulse for at least 5 to 10 seconds (no more than 10 seconds) because it may be erratic and

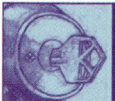

Keys to Success
USING A MASK

In the medical setting, a mask is used to deliver breaths and serves as a barrier device to prevent transmission of infectious disease. The mask is often attached to an **Ambu bag** for delivery of artificial ventilations and oxygen (Figure 41-7 ◆). (The use of an Ambu bag requires CPR training.) The Ambu bag is more effective when one person holds the mask to the victim's face and the second person squeezes the bag.

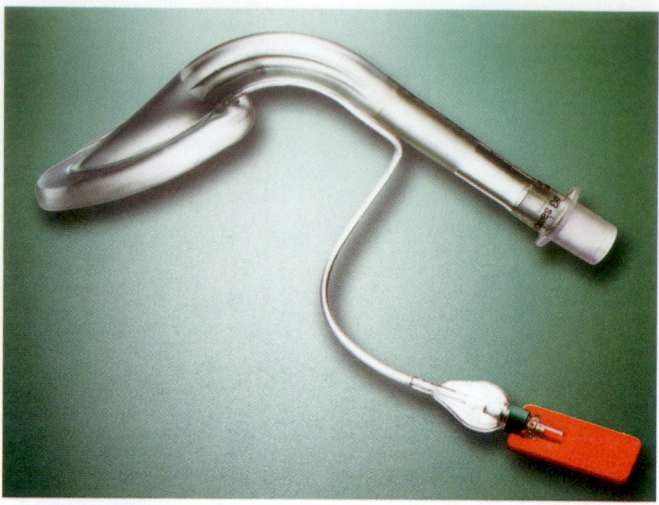

Figure 41-7 ◆ Ambu laryngeal mask.
Ambu Inc., Baltimore, MD

weak. If the pulse is very weak, erratic, or nonexistent and there are no signs of circulation, begin compressions as appropriate to the victim's age (Figures 41-8 ◆, 41-9 ◆, and 41-10 ◆). If a second rescuer is available, instruct him or her to monitor compression quality by checking the carotid, brachial, or femoral pulse. If your compressions are effective, a pulse will be felt. If the compressions do not generate a palpable pulse, the second rescuer should take over the compressions in two-man CPR or the entire sequence in one-man CPR. The one-man sequence allows the original rescuer to rest or get help.

Defibrillation

Automated external defibrillation (**AED**) is highly effective when provided immediately after or within minutes of an adult cardiac arrest. Most cardiac arrests in adults are related to fatal electrical arrhythmias of the heart and are correctable with defibrillators. The defibrillator gives verbal directions to the rescuer or rescue team that are easy and safe to follow. AED is not applied to infants.

Guidelines have recently been established for the use of AED on children 1 to 8 years old. AED may be used after one minute of CPR. It is recommended that child defibrillator pads and cables, rather than adult, be used; however, adult pads can be used if the pads do not overlap on the chest.

Heimlich Maneuver

An obstructed airway prevents the movement of air into or out of the respiratory tract. Certain disease conditions, such as anaphylactic shock or epiglotitis, can cause an anatomical blockage, but most obstructions are caused by foreign objects. With small children, the cause is usually food or small toys. With adults, an obstructed airway may be the result of:

■ Not chewing large pieces of food properly.
■ Talking too excitedly or laughing too much while eating.

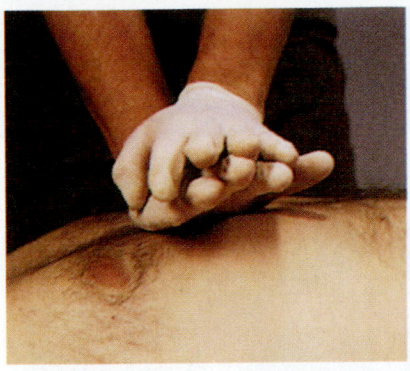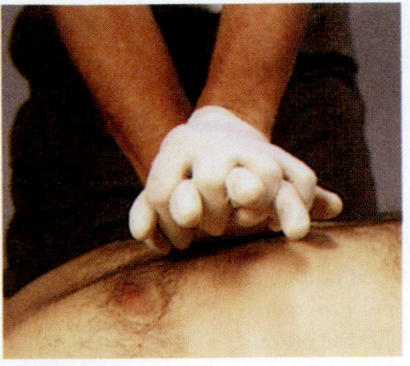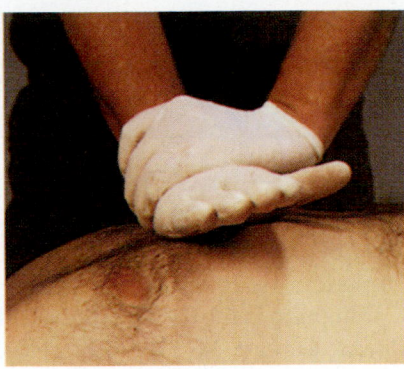

Figure 41-8 ◆ Location and position of hand during chest compressions for adult.

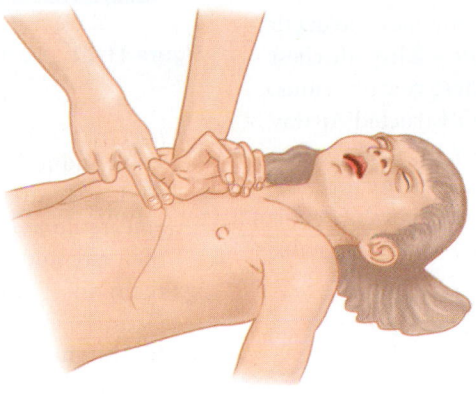

Figure 41-9 ◆ Compressions for a child.

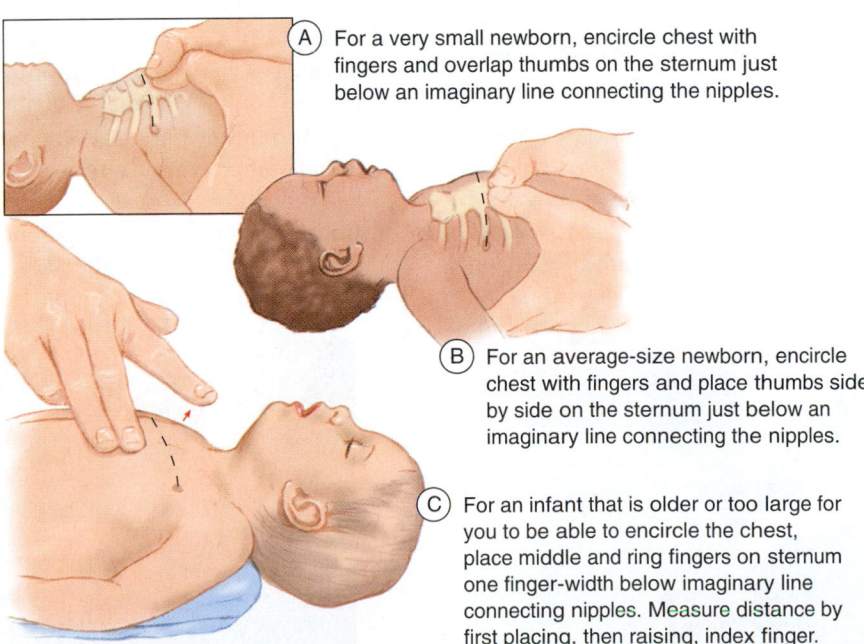

(A) For a very small newborn, encircle chest with fingers and overlap thumbs on the sternum just below an imaginary line connecting the nipples.

(B) For an average-size newborn, encircle chest with fingers and place thumbs side by side on the sternum just below an imaginary line connecting the nipples.

(C) For an infant that is older or too large for you to be able to encircle the chest, place middle and ring fingers on sternum one finger-width below imaginary line connecting nipples. Measure distance by first placing, then raising, index finger.

Figure 41-10 ◆ Compressions for an infant.

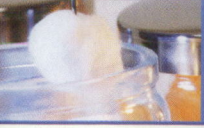

PROCEDURE 41-1 Perform Adult Rescue Breathing and One-Rescuer CPR

Theory and Rationale

Chest compressions and rescue breathing are performed in adults with an absence of respiratory and cardiac function. The American Heart Association recently revised guidelines for Cardiopulmonary Resuscitation (CPR) and Emergency Cardiovascular Care (ECC) in an effort to simplify the process. The new guidelines require healthcare providers to increase the number and quality of uninterrupted compressions delivered. Revised guidelines recommend a universal compression-to-ventilation of 30 to 2 for lone rescuers for victims of all ages (except newborns). Rescuers must provide compressions of adequate rate (approximately 100 beats/minute) and depth (1 1/2 to 2 inches) for adult victims and allow adequate chest recoil with minimal interruptions in chest compressions. Additionally, actions for Foreign Body Obstructed Airway (FBOA) were simplified. The tongue-jaw lift is no longer taught, and blind finger sweep should not be performed.

   Using a mouth guard with a one-way valve prevents vomit or other body fluids from contaminating the rescuer's mouth.

Materials

■ approved mannequin
■ gloves
■ ventilator mask
■ mouth guard

Competency

(**Conditions**) With the necessary materials, (**Task**) you will be able to administer rescue breathing for an adult and one-rescuer CPR for an adult (**Standards**) correctly, within the time frame designated by the instructor.

1. Assess the victim and determine if help is needed. Shout "Are you OK?" while gently shaking the victim's shoulders.
2. If the adult victim is determined to be unresponsive, activate EMS immediately by calling 911 and get an AED if available.
3. Assess the ABCs. Airway: Perform a head-tilt chin lift, or, if a neck injury is suspected, a jaw thrust (Figure 41-11 ◆).

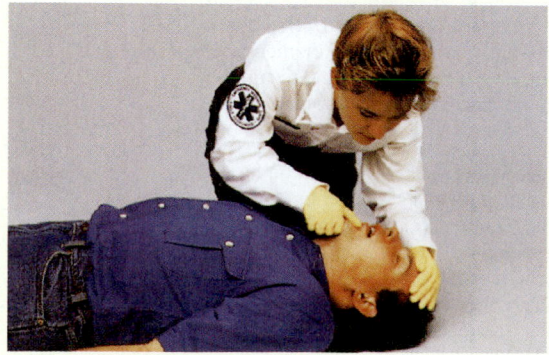

Figure 41-11 ◆ Establish an open airway.

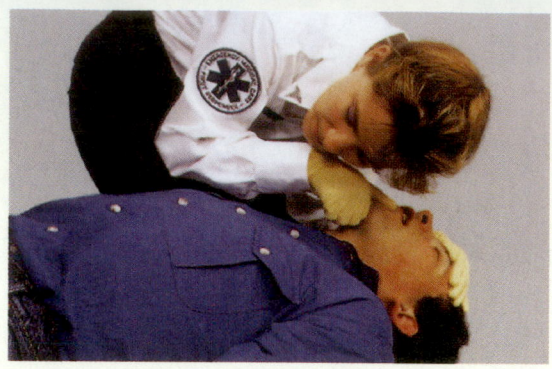

Figure 41-12 ◆ Look and feel for breath and chest movements.

Look and feel for breath and chest movements (Figure 41-12 ◆). Attempt to get another person to call 911. If you are alone, begin the rescue sequence for 1 minute and then attempt to call yourself. If gloves are available, put them on. If you have a ventilator mask, place it on the victim.

4. If breathing is absent, put on a mouth guard and administer two rescue breaths (Figure 41-13 ◆). If your breaths do not cause the chest to rise, look in the victim's mouth and remove an object if one is seen. If no object is seen, make a second attempt to administer a rescue breath. If the breath still does not enter the chest, proceed to abdominal thrusts for unconscious victims.
5. If the breaths cause the chest to rise, assess the patient's circulation by feeling for a pulse at the carotid artery (Figure 41-14 ◆). If you feel a pulse, begin rescue breathing. Administer 1 breath every 5 seconds, or 10–12 every minute. After 1 minute, reassess the victim for breathing and pulse.
6. If you do not feel a pulse, begin chest compressions. Kneel at the victim's side. Find the sternum and place the heel of one hand just below the nipple line.

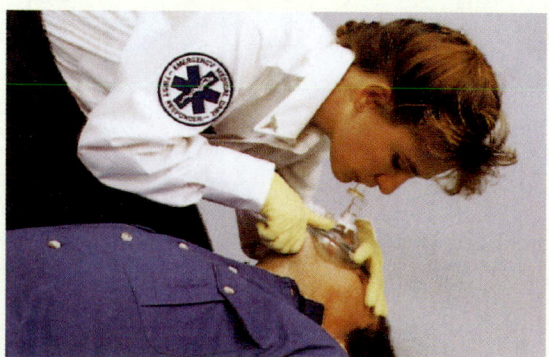

Figure 41-13 ◆ Administer two rescue breaths.

PROCEDURE 41-1 Perform Adult Rescue Breathing and One-Rescuer CPR (continued)

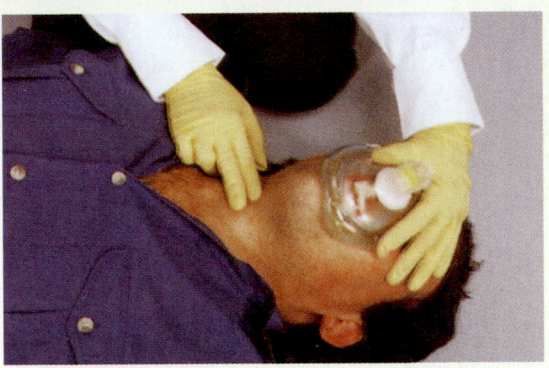

Figure 41-14 ◆ Assess the patient's circulation by feeling for a pulse at the carotid artery.

7. Place your other hand on top of the first hand, making sure to lift your fingers off the chest, using only the heels of your hands to administer compressions.
8. Keeping your shoulders directly over your hands, compress the chest 1-1/2 to 2 inches, then allow the sternum to relax (Refer to Figure 41-8). Do not lift your hands off the chest.

9. Continue to compress the chest a total of 30 times, then administer 2 breaths.
10. Repeat this sequence for 4 total cycles. Reassess the victim.
11. If necessary, continue CPR until pulse and breathing return or you are relieved by more advanced medical personnel.

Patient Education
Advise the patient to follow up with his or her personal physician after release from the EMS.

Charting Example
08/05/XX 7:30 PM Patient found collapsed in bathroom and unresponsive. 911 call placed and CPR started. EMS arrived in approximately 10 minutes and took over care. Patient was transferred to Deaconess Medical Center. Vivian Nagle, RMA (AMI)

PROCEDURE 41-2 Use an Automated External Defibrillator (AED)

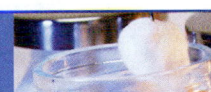

Theory and Rationale
The use of AEDs as lifesaving devices is becoming more and more common. AEDs are now found in doctors' offices, malls, airplanes, and private residences (Figure 41-15 ◆). An AED works by sending an electrical current through the myocardium of the heart, briefly causing the heart to stop and allowing the heart's natural pacemaker to take over. The goal is for the heart to resume function. All AEDs function in the same manner.

The AED is brought by a second- or third-party rescuer after the initial chest compressions and rescue breathing have begun.

Materials
■ AED machine
■ patient chart

Competency
(**Conditions**) With the necessary materials, (**Task**) you will use an AED (**Standards**) correctly within the time frame designated by the instructor.

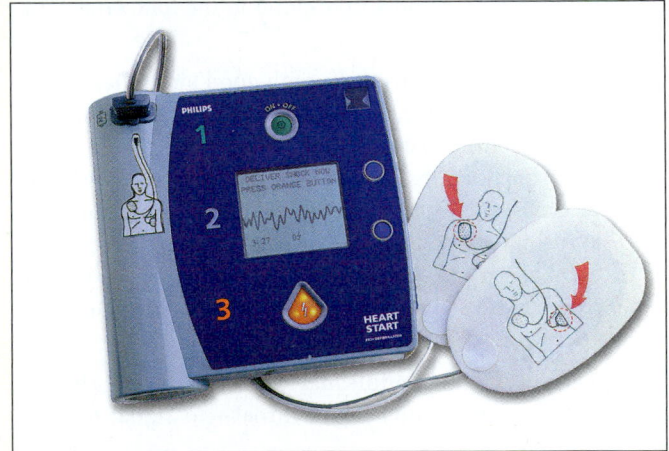

Figure 41-15 ◆ Philips Medical Systems SMART Biphasic Automated External Defibrillator, Model Heart Start FR2+.
Reprinted by permission of Philips Medical Systems.

continued

PROCEDURE 41-2 **Use an Automated External Defibrillator (AED)** (continued)

1. Place the AED next to the victim's left ear. This position allows the rescuers clear access to the chest and airway for continued rescue measures.
2. Turn the AED on and follow the voice prompts.
3. You will be prompted to attach the electrode pads to the patient's chest, on the sternum and at the apex of the heart, following the diagram for correct placement.
4. Next, you will be directed to allow the machine to analyze the heart rhythm to determine if it is a shockable rhythm. CPR should cease while the machine is analyzing.
5. The machine will begin a charging sequence prior to shocking and warn rescuers to stand back. The voice prompt will then tell you to press the "shock" button to administer the electrical current to the patient.
6. If the machine indicates "No shock is advised," assess the patient for breathing and circulation. Continue CPR as needed until advanced medical personnel arrive.

Patient Education

If a friend or family member of the patient is present at the time of rescue, you will need to help that person remain calm and out of the way so that advanced rescue personnel can treat the victim. It is also helpful if you can explain to friends or family members what is happening and to what hospital the victim will be transported. Be careful not to make comforting statements that may not be accurate, such as "He'll be all right" or "She's going to be just fine."

Charting Example

11/25/XX 3:30 PM Patient found in stairwell, unresponsive, with absence of pulse and respirations. 911 protocol initiated with 2 rescuer CPR. Third rescuer initiated AED response and patient was analyzed for shockable rhythm. CPR and AED shocks administered a total of 8 cycles prior to advanced medical support arriving. Patient released to EMS care and transferred to Sacred Heart Medical Center. Martin Cowan, CMA (AAMA)

- Drinking alcohol before and during eating.
- Choking on body or extraneous fluids, such as vomit or blood.

The MA should know how to respond to the following choking scenarios:

1. Partial airway obstruction with good air exchange: The victim is conscious, is capable of speaking, and is making a strong effort to cough.
2. Partial airway obstruction with poor air exchange: The victim is conscious but is weakening in clinical condition and ability to cough.
3. Total obstructed airway: The victim is unconscious, and there are no signs of breathing or the victim is unable to vocalize.

The conscious choking adult may use the universal choking sign—crossing the hands at the throat—to signal for help (Figure 41-16 ◆).

A partial airway obstruction may allow some air into the respiratory tract and is characterized by a high-pitched noise from the victim. The victim may be able to cough and expel the foreign object. *Do not* pat the victim on the back—it may lodge the object in the airway. If a phone call comes in to the medical office and the caller states, "My child is not breathing" and you hear the child crying in the background, the airway is

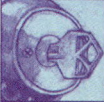

Keys to Success
EFFECTIVE ABCD

Breaths that are not successfully delivered do not help the victim. If you do not see the chest rise and fall with the first delivery of artificial ventilation, reposition the head and neck and attempt ventilation again. If it is still unsuccessful, change the ABCD sequence to obstructed airway. Call for help, reposition the head, and apply 6 to 10 abdominal thrusts to the patient's abdomen. If the obstruction is not cleared, look for an object in the victim's mouth and remove it if visible. A blind finger sweep is no longer recommended and should not be performed. It does not help to proceed from artificial ventilation to a pulse check and compressions if the airway is not partially or totally open and oxygen cannot be delivered to the lungs and bloodstream. *Do not* proceed with the ABCD sequence unless you have restored an open airway to deliver artificial ventilations.

If you find a pulse, provide breaths only. Monitor the victim's pulse every few minutes. If you can still feel the pulse, continue to provide only breaths. If the pulse ceases, continue breaths and begin compressions.

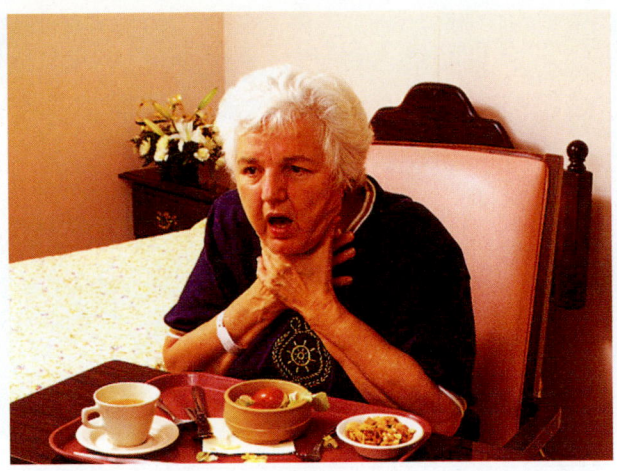

Figure 41-16 ◆ The universal choking sign.

not obstructed. Anytime the victim can speak or cry, air is moving in and out of the airway.

As a rescuer, ask the victim, "Can you speak?" If the victim responds by shaking the head, the airway is obstructed and immediate intervention is required. Request permission to assist the victim and perform the Heimlich maneuver for the adult or child (or abdominal thrusts for the supine victim) and back blows and chest thrusts for the infant (Figure 41-17 ◆). You should also use the Heimlich maneuver if the victim's coughing weakens or if the victim cannot speak.

To perform the Heimlich maneuver, stand behind the victim and put your arms around his or her chest halfway between the xiphoid process of the sternum and the umbilicus. Make a fist with one hand, with the thumb turned into the fist. Wrap your other hand around the fisted hand and pull the fisted hand in and up toward the diaphragm. This force against

the diaphragm is usually sufficient to loosen the foreign object and propel it out of the mouth. If the victim becomes unconscious, ease him or her to the floor to prevent any additional injuries, and proceed with the technique described below for unconscious obstructed airway. The Heimlich (or abdominal thrusts in the supine victim) is adjusted for infants, very obese people, and visibly pregnant women to chest thrusts that are identical to the chest compressions of CPR.

If the victim is unconscious, you will need to add artificial ventilations to the obstructed airway procedure. If the obstruction is loosened during the procedure, it may be possible to get oxygen around the object and into the bloodstream. Reposition the airway each time ventilations are attempted.

For an unresponsive, nonbreathing adult with an obstructed airway, the sequence is:

- Attempt ventilation
- Perform chest compressions
- Reattempt ventilations.
- Return to chest compressions.

Chest Pain

Heart attacks are the leading cause of death for both men and women. The patient experiencing chest pain may display various symptoms. The primary complaint will be pain in the middle or left side of the chest, described as sharp, stabbing, crushing, squeezing, or aching. The pain may radiate to the left arm, to the back, or up the neck. Sometimes the pain is brought on by exertion, but other times onset is sudden and unexplained. Other symptoms are nausea, weakness, SOB, apprehension, and the feeling of impending doom. The skin may be clammy, moist, pale, or cyanotic. Denial is common, as the individual tries to explain the pain as heartburn or indigestion.

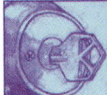

Keys to Success
SAVING CHILDREN AND INFANTS

Blind sweeps of the mouth are *never* attempted on children and infants. A child's or infant's airway is narrow, and it is possible to push the foreign object farther into the respiratory tract. You can look in the mouth of a child or infant for an object that can be removed.

Use chest thrusts followed by back blows for obstructed airways in infants and in children in an upright position (Figure 41-18 ◆). Attempt ventilations, reattempt ventilations, then return to chest thrusts and back blows. For children in a supine position, use a similar sequence, but use abdominal thrusts only.

Abdominal thrusts are done by placing the child on a flat surface. Place the middle and index fingers of both hands below the rib cage and above the navel. Make a quick upward thrust. *Do not* squeeze. Repeat until the object is expelled.

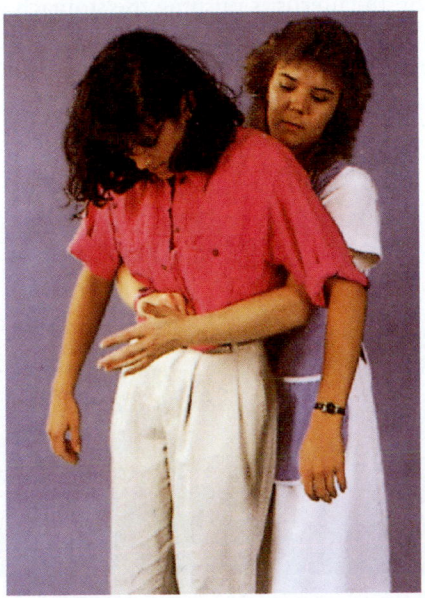

Figure 41-17 ◆ Heimlich maneuver.

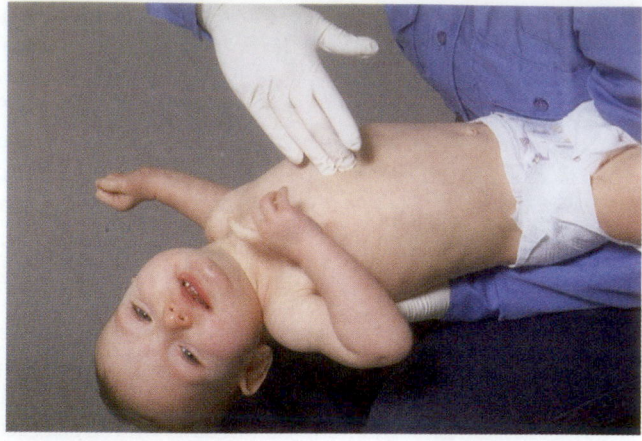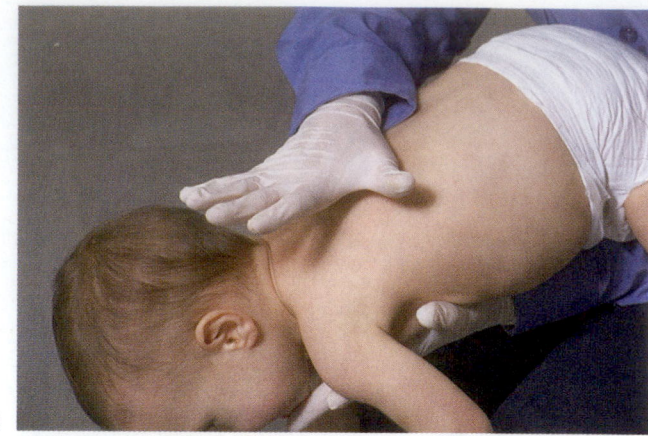

Figure 41-18 ◆ (A) Use chest thrusts followed by (B) back blows.

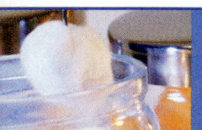

PROCEDURE 41-3 Respond to an Adult with an Obstructed Airway

Theory and Rationale

A bolus of food is the most common object adults choke on. When the food is lodged in the upper airway, the person may put his or her hands around the throat, the universal sign of choking, to let bystanders know he or she cannot breathe properly. If the person can wheeze, make a high-pitched sound, cough, or speak, do not take any action. Instead call 911 and encourage the person to continue to cough forcefully to try to dislodge the object. If the person is unable to speak or cough, he or she is in immediate danger and action must be taken.

It is important that the rescuer call 911 even if the victim's airway is not completely blocked or the Heimlich maneuver was successful. Once the object has been expelled, the throat is likely to continue to swell as a result of the irritant, so the victim should be assessed in an emergency room.

Materials

- approved mannequin
- gloves
- ventilation mask with one-way valve for unconscious victim

Competency

(**Conditions**) With the necessary materials, (**Task**) you will administer the Heimlich maneuver to an adult (**Standards**) correctly within the time frame designated by the instructor.

1. Once it has been established that the victim is choking, with no air exchange, direct someone to call 911 and shout, "Are you choking?" or "Can you speak?" If the answer is no—as indicated by a head shake—tell the victim you are going to begin emergency treatment.

2. Stand behind the victim with your feet slightly apart, placing one foot between the victim's feet and one to the outside. This stance will give you greater stability, and if the victim should pass out, you can safely guide him or her to the ground by sliding him or her down your thigh.

3. Place the index finger of one hand at the person's navel or belt buckle. If the victim is a pregnant woman, place your finger above the enlarged uterus.

4. Make a fist with your other hand and place it, thumb side to victim, above your other hand. If the person is very pregnant, the uterus is pushing the stomach and other internal organs under the rib cage and you may have to do chest compressions.

5. Place your marking hand over your curled fist and begin to give quick inward and upward thrusts (Figure 41-19 ◆).

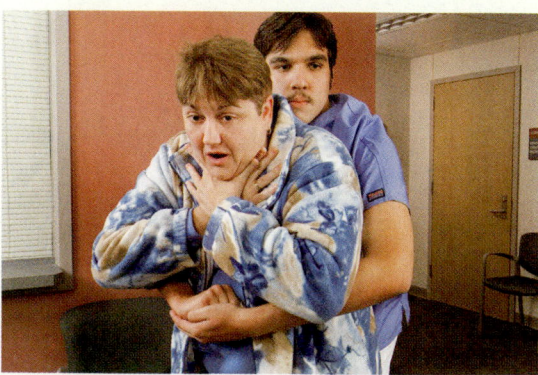

Figure 41-19 ◆ Deliver a firm thrust into the patient's abdomen in an upward direction toward you.

PROCEDURE 41-3 Respond to an Adult with an Obstructed Airway *(continued)*

6. There is no set number of thrusts to give to an adult who remains conscious. Continue to give thrusts until the object is removed *or* the victim becomes unconscious.
7. If the victim becomes unconscious, gently lower him or her to the ground.
8. Activate EMS and put on gloves.
9. Immediately begin CPR with 30 chest compressions and 2 rescue breaths.
10. Before administering the rescue breaths, open the airway with the head-tilt chin lift and look for a foreign body in the victim's mouth and remove if visible. Blind finger sweeps are no longer recommended and should not be performed.
11. Continue with cycles of 30 compressions and 2 rescue breaths until the foreign body is expelled or advance medical personal arrive to relieve you.

Patient Education

If the object has been successfully removed and the patient did not lose consciousness, the patient may feel he or she no longer needs medical treatment. As a rescuer you must insist that the victim seek medical attention anyway. The lodged object may have caused swelling in the lining of the esophagus, constricting the throat and impairing the breathing.

Charting Example

10/25/XX 11:30 AM Jason Jones, CMA, exhibited signs of choking at lunch. Jason grabbed his throat and was unable to cough or make noise. Tina Muller, RMA, (AMT) alerted the physician and placed a call to 911. Chest compressions and rescue breaths were given until the piece of apple was expelled. EMS arrived and checked Jason for signs of throat irritation and swelling. Janice Walker, CMA (AAMA)

The first intervention is to have the individual stop what he or she is doing and sit down, with the feet elevated if possible. Request help and/or call EMS, and inform the physician. If oxygen is available, administer it according to office protocol by nasal cannula at 6 to 8 liters per minute until the physician or emergency personnel arrive.

If the victim has previously been diagnosed with angina and has nitroglycerin tablets, insert one tablet under the tongue.

Administering Nitroglycerin

Nitroglycerin is a vasodilator. Wear gloves when handling a patient's nitroglycerin tabs to prevent your own blood vessels from suddenly dilating (Figure 41-20 ◆). Be sure to check the expiration date on the bottle. If gloves are not readily available, put a tablet into the cap of the bottle. Ask the patient to place the tablet under his or her tongue or to raise the tongue so you can drop the tablet there (Figure 41-21 ◆). Ask the patient if the tablet is "fizzling" under the tongue. A fizzle indicates the tablet is dissolving. Tablets may be administered every 5 minutes up to three doses. If the pain is not relieved, inform the physician and/or EMS on the scene.

If a patient calls complaining of chest pain:

■ Keep the caller on the line while asking for help from another office staff member.
■ Write down the caller's name and location (if someone is calling for the victim, ask the caller for the victim's name and location).

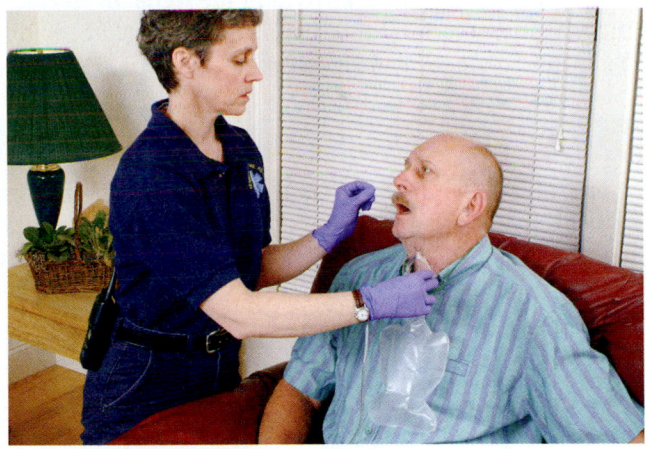

Figure 41-20 ◆ Administering nitroglycerin tablets.

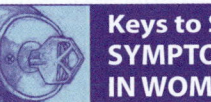

Keys to Success
SYMPTOMS OF HEART ATTACK IN WOMEN

A heart attack in a woman is usually more difficult to diagnose because typical chest pain is not described. A burning sensation in the chest is often dismissed as heartburn. Flu-like symptoms of nausea, clamminess, cold sweats, and vomiting are common. Unexplained fatigue, weakness, or dizziness may also occur. A woman is therefore more likely to ignore the symptoms. It is important to monitor symptoms and check the patient's history for hereditary heart disease.

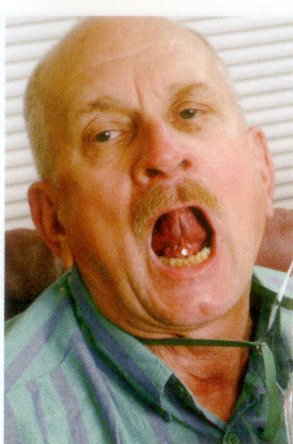

Figure 41-21 ◆ Self-administration of nitroglycerin tablets.

- Advise the caller that you are calling EMS.
- Instruct the caller to stay on the line with you.

The other staff member contacts EMS to relay the information and to enter the victim's name into the EMS system. Remain calm and assure the caller that help is on the way. The EMS dispatcher will keep you advised of the location of the EMS unit dispatched and an estimated time of arrival (**ETA**). End the phone conversation with EMS *only* when directed to do so or when EMS personnel have arrived on the scene. In all emergency situations, record times and interventions and add this documentation to the patient's chart.

In Practice

When Courtney Molino enters the medical office for her physical exam, she says she feels unwell after choosing the stairs over the elevator. In fact, she says she is having chest pain and extreme dizziness. What should the medical assistant do?

Another cardiac emergency is congestive heart failure (CHF). The patient complains of SOB, swelling in the feet and hands, palpitations, and rapid heartbeat. He or she may appear anxious, cyanotic, diaphoretic, and slightly confused. Inform the physician immediately. Take the patient to an examination room and seat him or her on the examination table. If oxygen is available and the physician orders it, administer oxygen according to orders. Usually, EMS is called to transport the patient to an emergency facility. Monitor and record vital signs, any medication administered, and treatment performed.

Respiratory Distress

Respiratory distress may be a reaction to a long-term debilitating disease, such as chronic pulmonary obstructive disease (COPD), or to an emergency situation, such as anaphylactic response to medication. It can also be the result of other disease processes, including obstructive conditions, such as asthma, chronic bronchitis, and emphysema, pneumonia, and acute pulmonary edema. Conscious control is usually not a factor in respiratory distress. Being unable to get enough oxygen causes extreme anxiety, and medical staff should be prepared to give the patient emotional support.

Signs and symptoms vary, depending on the cause. One of the most serious is an occluded airway that causes the patient to grasp at the neck and attempt to cough. Unconsciousness soon follows, then cardiac arrest. Other conditions of respiratory distress may cause symptoms such as:

- Acute anxiety with gasping breaths
- Bradypnea, abnormally slow breathing (fewer than eight breaths a minute)
- **Cyanosis**
- Failure of the chest to rise and fall
- Nasal flaring
- Pursing of the lips
- Noisy breathing (snoring, gurgling, wheezing, rattling, sternal retraction, stridor)
- Tachypnea, abnormally rapid breathing (more than 24 breaths per minute)

If respiratory distress is the result of a known diagnosis, the patient will need medical followup with an emergency facility and/or physician, depending on the severity or change in the condition. If respiratory distress is caused by an obstructed airway, the appropriate sequence for obstructed airway should be initiated.

Shortness of Breath (SOB)

Any individual experiencing SOB needs immediate intervention. A **patent** airway is necessary to support life. If the person can speak, air is moving in and out. Ask the patient about the onset for difficult breathing and what activity caused it. This information helps to identify the problem.

The patient experiencing SOB may be gasping for air, pale or cyanotic, and may exhibit nasal flaring and extreme anxiety (Figure 41-22 ◆). Usually the patient sits in an upright position and may be quite weak. If the airway is partially obstructed, the patient may cough in an attempt to clear the passages. It the patient is not in a sitting position, help him or her to a sitting position with support to the back. Call out for assistance.

Hyperventilation

Hyperventilation is quick, shallow breathing or rapid, deep breathing that results in decreasing carbon dioxide in the blood, dilation of blood vessels, and lowered blood pressure. The patient feels faint or light-headed and may experience:

- Chest tightness
- Cardiac palpitations
- Rapid pulse
- Deep sighing breaths

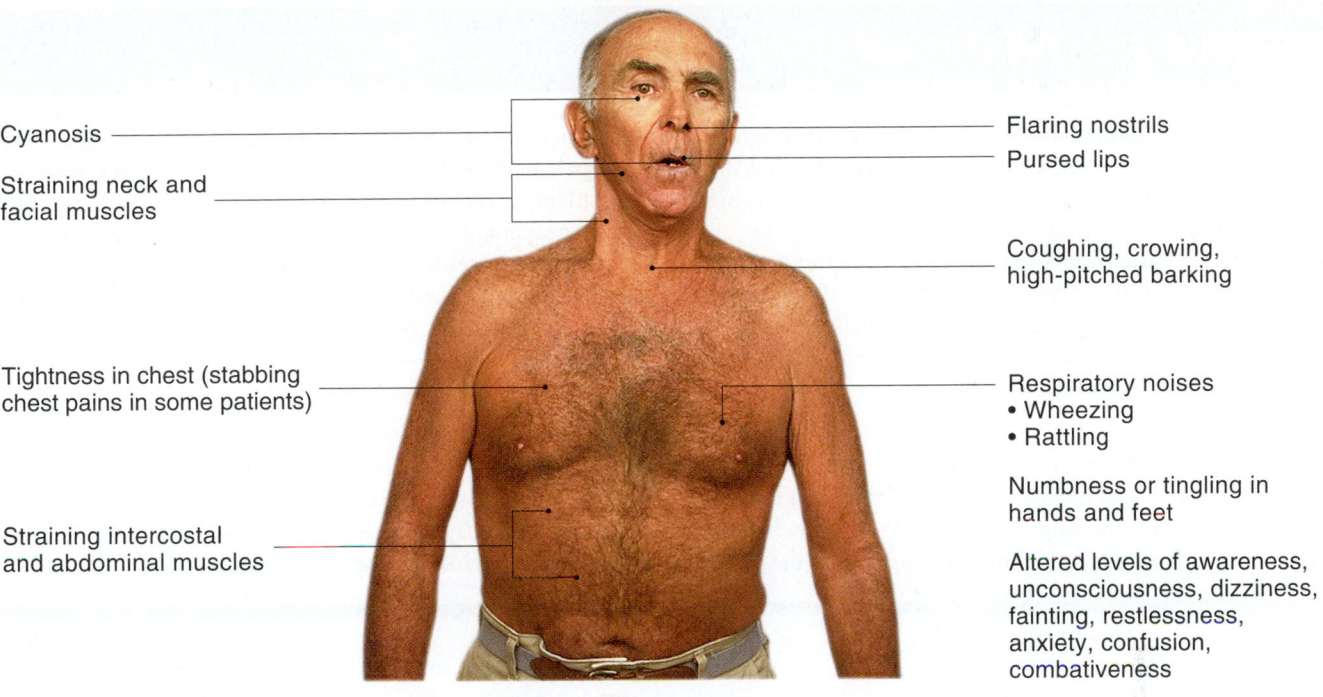

Cyanosis

Straining neck and facial muscles

Tightness in chest (stabbing chest pains in some patients)

Straining intercostal and abdominal muscles

Flaring nostrils

Pursed lips

Coughing, crowing, high-pitched barking

Respiratory noises
• Wheezing
• Rattling

Numbness or tingling in hands and feet

Altered levels of awareness, unconsciousness, dizziness, fainting, restlessness, anxiety, confusion, combativeness

Figure 41-22 ◆ Signs and symptoms of breathing difficulty.

PROCEDURE 41-4 Administer Oxygen

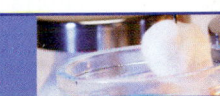

Theory and Rationale

Patients with chronic lung conditions often require oxygen therapy to breathe more easily. The delivery of oxygen helps improve the status of most patients' breathing. However, patients with severe lung conditions such as emphysema, COPD, and lung cancer should be transferred to a hospital immediately.

Materials

■ portable oxygen tank
■ pressure regulator
■ oxygen flow meter
■ sterile, prepackaged, disposable nasal cannula with tubing
■ gloves
■ oximeter
■ patient chart

Competency

(**Conditions**) With the necessary materials, (**Task**) you will be able to administer oxygen therapy to an adult (**Standards**) correctly within the time frame designated by the instructor.

1. Gather all needed equipment.
2. Wash your hands.
3. Identify the patient and confirm the physician's order for oxygen therapy.
4. Check the pressure reading on the oxygen tank to make sure it has enough oxygen in it.
5. Start the flow of oxygen by opening the cylinder.

6. Attach the cannula tubing to the flow meter. Adjust the oxygen flow to the physician's order.
7. Hold the cannula tips over the inside of your wrist, without touching the skin, to determine if the oxygen is flowing.
8. Don gloves, if necessary. You may prefer to wear gloves with patients who demonstrate a chronic cough, nasal drip, or other situation of potential exposure.
9. Place the tips of the nasal cannula into the patient's nostrils. Wrap the tubing behind the patient's ears (Figure 41-23 ◆).

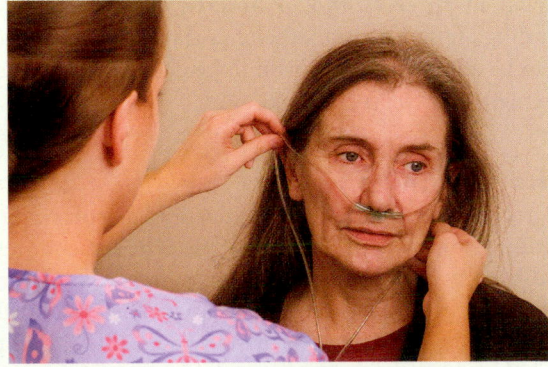

Figure 41-23 ◆ Adjust the tubing around the back of the patient's ears.

continued

PROCEDURE 41-4 Administer Oxygen (continued)

10. Instruct the patient to breathe normally through the mouth and nose. Some patients instinctively hold their breath or avoid breathing through the nose when an object is placed in the nostrils.
11. Check the patient's oxygen level with an oximeter. Place the probe over the index finger and record the reading. If necessary, have the patient take a short walk to verify that the oxygen flow rate is sufficient for activity.
12. Document the procedure in the patient's chart.

Patient Education

Instruct the patient on the safety protocol for oxygen use, such as refraining from smoking, not laying the oxygen container on its side, and other manufacturer instructions. If the oxygen will be required on a continuous basis, you will need to set the patient up with a portable oxygen unit for home use. Once a patient account has been established with a home health-care company, per the physician's instructions, the respiratory therapy representative will explain different models and mobile units available to the patient for home use, as well as the necessary safety precautions.

Charting Example

10/25/XX 11:30 AM Patient evaluated for oxygen use. Patient tested on 2 lpm [liters per minute] continuous flow while at rest. 4 lpm needed for activity to maintain 90% blood oxygen saturation. Order for O$_2$ two lpm rest / four lpm with exertion faxed to Apria Home Health Care. Connie Hughes, CMA (AAMA)

■ Anxiety
■ Tetany

Inform the physician and encourage the patient to breathe slowly. Have the patient breathe into an oxygen mask (not connected to any oxygen), block one nostril, or breathe into a brown paper bag. One of these methods is usually effective. This condition can generally be resolved quickly and without further intervention.

Chronic Obstructive Pulmonary Disease (COPD)

Asthma, chronic bronchitis, and emphysema are considered chronic obstructive pulmonary diseases. Air is trapped in the lungs and the patient is unable to expel all the carbon dioxide from the alveoli. Although each condition has specific signs and symptoms, they share many of the same problems. A person with COPD has SOB and a rapid heart rate and experiences weakness. Asthma may also be characterized by audible wheezes, diaphoresis, and tightness in the chest. Inform the physician in all cases and, if ordered, administer oxygen. Depending on the situation, the physician may order medications to be administered, oxygen to be delivered, or transport to an emergency facility by EMS.

Pulmonary Edema

Fluid accumulation in the lung tissue and alveoli result in a condition known as pulmonary edema. The patient presents with difficulty breathing, wheezing sounds, cyanosis, rapid heartbeat, distended neck veins, extreme anxiety, and orthopnea. Inform the physician. Place the patient in a sitting position with feet and legs up on a bed or cart. Administer supplemental oxygen if ordered and available. Call EMS for transport to an emergency facility.

Shock and Anaphylactic Shock

Shock, the collapse of the cardiovascular system, is caused by insufficient cardiac output. Blood supply and nourishment (oxygen and nutrients, including glucose) to the tissue and perfusion to the organs are inadequate. Untreated shock can progress very rapidly to death. Shock may be the result of many insults to the body, including anaphylaxis, cardiac failure, hemorrhage, extreme emotional upset, respiratory distress, neurological collapse, severe metabolic insult, and **sepsis.** The types and causes of shock are summarized in Table 41-4. Some of the symptoms that may occur after the initial crisis are listed in Table 41-5.

Regardless of the cause, immediate, aggressive intervention is required to stop the progression of the condition and the possible death of the patient. Have the patient lie down, keep him or her warm, maintain a patent airway, control all bleeding, monitor vital signs, and provide emotional support. Inform the physician and call EMS for further assessment and transport. Oxygen may be administered, if ordered and available, by trained personnel.

TABLE 41-4 CLASSIFICATIONS OF SHOCK

Type of Shock	Cause
anaphylactic shock	heart failure
cardiogenic shock	blood loss
hemorrhagic shock	loss of body fluids and
metabolic shock	electrolytes
neurogenic shock	nervous system failure
psychogenic shock	dilated blood vessels
respiratory shock	respiratory failure
septic shock	infection in bloodstream
severe allergic reaction	

TABLE 41-5 SYMPTOMS OF SHOCK FOLLOWING A CRISIS SITUATION

■ Weakness	■ Cool skin
■ Rapid heartbeat	■ Clammy skin
■ Thirst	■ Cyanosis
■ Nausea	■ Confusion
■ Dizziness	■ Disorientation
■ Restlessness	■ Unresponsiveness
■ Pallor	■ Shallow breathing

Anaphylactic Shock

Anaphylactic shock is a severe allergic reaction to a foreign substance, characterized by antigen formation and physiological reaction. See Table 41-6 for symptoms. Examples of foreign substances include medications, bug bites, and latex gloves. Inform the physician immediately. Call EMS. The physician may order epinephrine and/or an antihistamine. An IV may also be started.

Prevention is the most important factor in anaphylactic shock. Always ask the patient about allergies to any medication before administering it and record this information on the front of the chart in red. After administering medication, ask the patient to wait 20 minutes before leaving the office and observe for any potential reactions. In offices where antibiotics and allergy injections are given on a regular basis, you must be alert to possible reactions and be prepared with an emergency drug box for rapid intervention.

Assisting Patients in Shock

Patients go into shock for varied reasons, including blood loss, infection, and pain. The most common signs of shock include pale, gray, or bluish skin; moist, cool skin; dilated pupils; a weak, rapid pulse; shallow, rapid respirations; and extreme thirst. When patients exhibit signs of shock, medical assistants should ensure that those patients have an open airway and proper circulation. Assistants should encourage patients to lie down with their legs elevated to return blood to the vital organs. Next, assistants should cover patients with blankets for warmth and keep them calm until emergency personnel arrive. Most emergency treatments for shock patients will need to be administered by a physician or emergency personnel.

TABLE 41-6 SYMPTOMS OF ANAPHYLACTIC SHOCK

■ sudden onset of anxiety	■ cardiac arrhythmias
■ sneezing	■ respiratory arrest
■ difficulty breathing	■ cardiac arrest
■ hives	■ cyanosis
■ itching and rash	■ weakness
■ nasal congestion	■ weak rapid pulse
■ swelling of the lips and tongue	■ hypotension
■ flushed or dry skin	■ altered levels of consciousness

TABLE 41-7 TREATMENT FOR SHOCK IN THE MEDICAL OFFICE

Cause	Treatment
Anaphylactic shock	Epinephrine
Cardiogenic shock	IV dopamine, immediate transport to the emergency room
Hemorrhagic shock	Stop bleeding, replace volume, immediate transport to the emergency room
Hypovolemic shock	Replace volume
Insulin shock	Sugar given to the patient by any means tolerated
Neurogenic shock	IV dopamine, immediate transport to the emergency room
Poisoning	Consult the poison center for treatment specific to the poison
Respiratory shock	Intubation and immediate transport to the emergency room
Sepsis	Fluids, IV dopamine, and immediate transport to the emergency room

Source: Beaman, N. and Fleming, L. Pearson's Comprehensive Medical Assisting, © 2007. Reprinted by permission of Pearson Education, Upper Saddle River, NJ.

Table 41-7 outlines the cause and treatment of different types of shock.

Bleeding

Bleeding can be either external or internal. External bleeding occurs when the skin is broken. Internal bleeding occurs with tissue damage, while the skin remains intact. Bleeding can originate from any of the three types of blood vessels—arteries, veins, and capillaries.

Arterial bleeding is usually copious, rapid, and bright red. The blood often spurts, echoing the heartbeat. Arterial bleeding must be brought under control as soon as possible. Pressure applied directly over the exit wound may halt the flow of blood. If this is not successful, external pressure on the pressure points may be. Elevating the injured part higher than the heart may also slow the blood flow.

Venous blood flows more slowly, is darker in color, and can usually be controlled by direct pressure. Blood from capillaries oozes rather than flows and can also be halted with direct pressure. Bleeding from the scalp or face is often copious because of the many circulatory vessels in the area. Caution must be exercised if a fracture in the area is suspected.

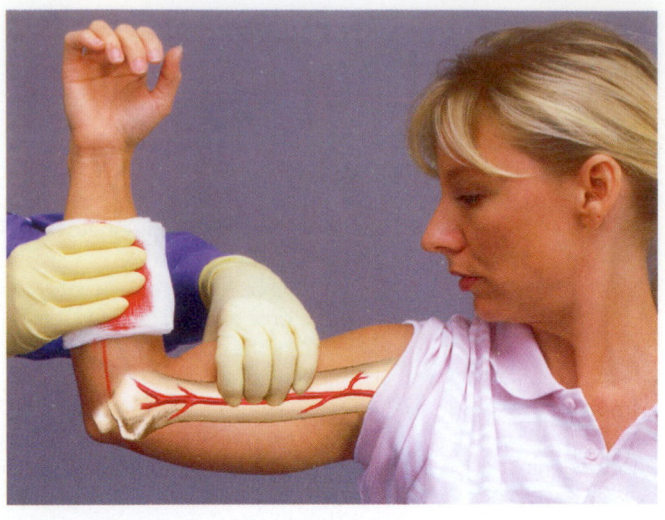

Figure 41-24 ◆ Apply direct pressure to the patient's wound.

Direct pressure is applied by placing a sterile dressing over the wound and holding it in place (Figure 41-24 ◆). A pressure bandage may be wrapped around the injured part to maintain pressure on the site. If blood seeps through, reinforce the bandage by applying more dressings and bandages over it. Do *not* remove the original dressing.

Pressure Points

Pressure points may be used to help control external bleeding (Figure 41-25 ◆). Pressure is applied to the artery where it lies close to the skin and can be compressed against an underlying bone. These arteries include the temporal, carotid, facial, brachial, radial-ulnar, subclavian, femoral, and dorsalis pedis (Table 41-8). It is possible to control external bleeding in regions distal to the pressure point.

Application of Direct Pressure

When direct pressure alone is not effective, direct pressure and bandaging must be applied while the EMS system is activated.

Internal Bleeding

Internal bleeding may be obvious or insidious. Bruising or discoloration of the skin may be an indication of bleeding in

---

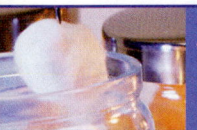

PROCEDURE 41-5 Respond to a Patient Who Has Fainted

Theory and Rationale

Patients who are ill, pregnant, or who have just received upsetting news may faint. Medical assistants must be properly trained to respond to these patients, since patients may injure themselves if they lose consciousness and fall in the medical office.

Materials

- blanket
- footstool or box

Competency

(**Conditions**) With the necessary materials, you will be able to (**Task**) care for a patient who has fainted (**Standards**) correctly within the time limit set by the instructor.

1. If the patient communicates a faint feeling, help the patient sit, bend forward, and place the head on the knees. If the patient collapses with no warning, do not move the patient. The patient may have sustained a neck or back injury.
2. Notify the physician.
3. Loosen any tight clothing, and cover the patient with the blanket for warmth.
4. If the physician directs, use the footstool to support the patient's legs in a raised position.
5. If the physician directs, call for emergency services.
6. Once the emergency passes, document all activities in the patient's medical record.

Patient Education

Observe the patient carefully, monitoring breathing and level of consciousness. Allow the patient to rest 10 minutes after she regains full consciousness. If the patient's vital signs are unstable or the patient does not respond quickly, notify the physician and be prepared to activate the emergency medical system.

Charting Example

6/8/XX 10:45 AM Patient in exam room states that she feels faint. Patient instructed to lower her head to her knees. Instructed to and assisted with loosening of clothing. Physician notified. BP 116/62, P-82 and regular, R-20. Patient remained in position for 3 minutes until symptoms subsided. Patient transferred to exam room and physician notified and evaluated patient. Maria Jimenez, RMA (AMI)

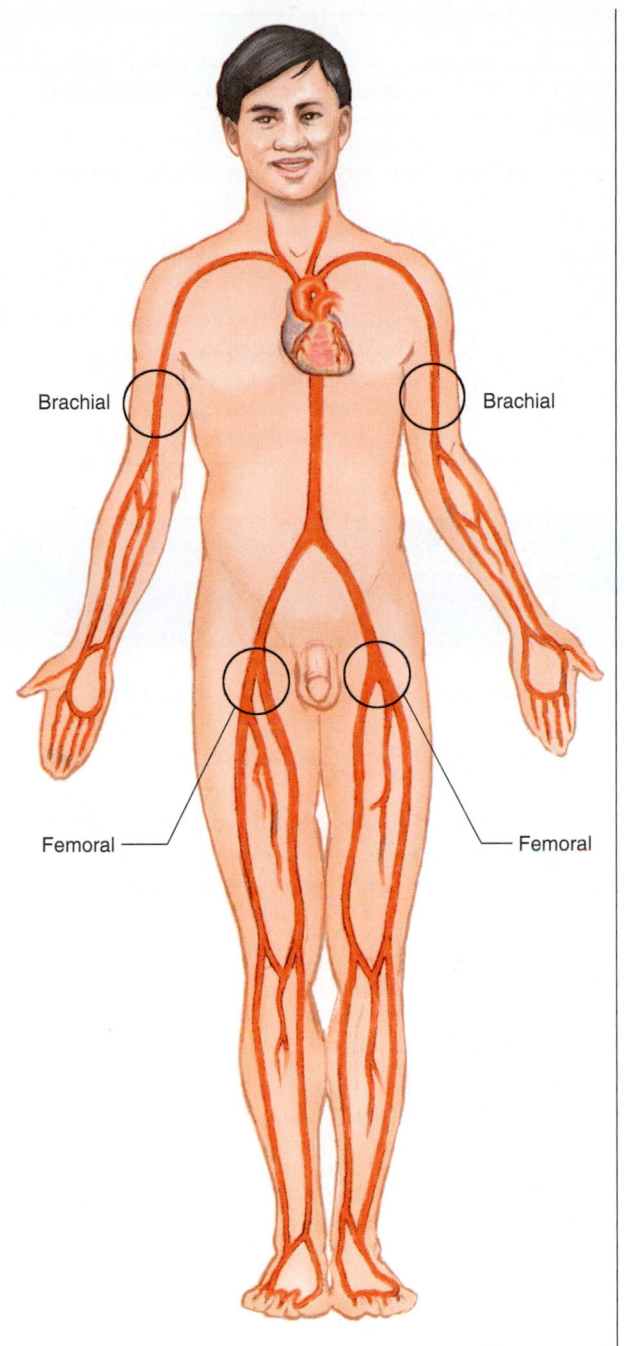

Figure 41-25 ◆ Brachial and femoral pressure points.

pulse, cold, clammy and pale skin, nausea and vomiting, extreme thirst, anxiety, a drop in blood pressure, and possibly a decreased level of consciousness. Inform the physician of the signs and symptoms of internal bleeding. Call EMS for transport.

Until advanced intervention is available, try to prevent or slow the onset of shock. Keep the victim quiet, warm, and lying down with the feet slightly elevated.

Epistaxis

Epistaxis is the medical term for nosebleed. As an external form of bleeding, epistaxis can occur spontaneously or following a blow to the nose. Spontaneous forms may be the result of upper respiratory infection, low humidity in the environment, **hypertension,** strenuous activity, or exposure to high altitudes. While most nosebleeds are only a nuisance, those caused by hypertension are a signal of a more serious underlying problem.

Intervention begins with the patient sitting in a chair and the head tilted forward. Ask the patient to apply direct pressure by pinching and holding the sides of the nose together. It may take up to 15 minutes for the blood to clot and bleeding to be controlled. Apply an ice or cold pack after bleeding is controlled. An additional measure is to apply pressure to the upper lip just below the nose. Instruct the patient not to blow the nose for several hours after the bleeding is controlled to prevent the nosebleed from recurring. If the bleeding cannot be controlled, alert the physician and EMS.

Open Wounds

With an open wound, the integrity of the skin and its defenses are compromised. Open wounds include abrasions, avulsions, amputations, lacerations, incisions, and punctures. The area must be cleansed, and most wounds require some type of dressing to promote healing and prevent infection. Tetanus prophylaxis should be administered if appropriate. The size, length, depth, location and condition of the wound should be noted and recorded on the chart.

Tetanus, also referred to as *lockjaw,* is an infection caused by an anaerobic bacillus, *Clostridium tetani.* This bacillus may be introduced into the body through an open wound or a burn. It affects the central nervous system and causes muscle spasms. If not promptly diagnosed and treated, tetanus can be fatal. Tetanus can be prevented with prophylactic immunizations. In the event of an insult to the skin or tissue, it is recommended that the previously immunized person be given a booster injection of tetanus toxoid. If the patient has never been immunized or immunization cannot be confirmed, an injection of tetanus immune globulin is administered, followed by a series of tetanus toxoid injections.

the underlying tissues. Be alert for signs and symptoms of internal bleeding and initiate intervention before the condition becomes grave. Observe the injured person for bruising, tenderness, and swelling at the site of injury. He or she may complain of pain in the area of injury. The systemic signs that are precursors to shock include a rapid

TABLE 41-8 MAJOR ARTERIES AND PRESSURE POINT SITES

Arteries	Location	Area in Which Bleeding Is Controlled
Temporal arteries	Temples in front of ears	Temporal region of scalp
Carotid arteries	Front of neck on either side of trachea, face, ears, scalp	Face, ears, scalp area above pressure point
Facial arteries	Under mandible	Nose and mouth
Brachial arteries	Just above the hand, arm, elbow	Inner aspect of elbow below pressure point
Radial-ulnar arteries	Just above or at wrists	Hands and fingers below pressure point
Subclavian arteries	Just above clavicles	Hand, arm, shoulder, and portion of anterior chest wall
Femoral arteries	Anterior aspect midthigh	Leg below pressure point
Dorsalis pedis arteries	Anterior aspect of the foot	Toes and foot below pressure point

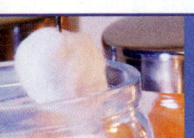

PROCEDURE 41-6 Demonstrate the Application of a Pressure Bandage

Theory and Rationale

In the medical office setting, wear gloves and any other PPE necessary and available to prevent contact with blood and body fluids. Direct pressure is applied with a dressing. If clean or sterile dressings are not available, handkerchiefs, washcloths, sanitary napkins, socks, or other cloth material may be used. Do *not* remove the original pressure dressing but add dressings as needed to help form clots and slow the bleeding. Removing the original dressing would remove any clot formation and start fresh bleeding. If possible, elevate the bleeding area. If bleeding continues with pressure dressing, apply pressure at the pressure point above the injury.

It is important to be cautious when working with bleeding injuries because of the possibility of fractures or internal injuries. Apply only mild pressure if, for example, you see or suspect a fracture.

Materials

- dressing supplies or makeshift materials
- gloves and/or other PPE available

Competency

(**Conditions**) With the necessary materials, (**Task**) you will be able to demonstrate the application of a pressure dressing (**Standards**) correctly.

1. Escort the patient immediately to an examination room.
2. Wash your hands.
3. Put on disposable gloves.
4. Under physician's supervision, apply direct pressure with a dressing placed on the open wound. If possible, elevate the affected part.
5. After assessment, the physician will decide EMS should be activated.
6. Apply additional dressings as needed. Do *not* remove the original dressing.
7. Apply pressure to pressure points as necessary and with the physician's supervision.
8. If bleeding is controlled, anchor the dressing to maintain pressure.
9. Prepare the patient for transport to an emergency care facility.
10. Dispose of waste in a biohazardous container.
11. Remove your gloves and discard.
12. Wash your hands.
13. Document the procedure.

Patient Education

The patient will be anxious. Explain the basic procedure in a calm, quiet, authoritative manner. The physician will answer patient questions based on the patient's ability to deal with information. Engage the patient in general conversation as a focused distraction. This may help maintain the patient's consciousness, as the patient may be prone to fainting.

Charting Example

08/31/xx 8:00 a.m. Pt came to office with 6" laceration to right forearm. Injury occurred from fight with 7-year-old brother when older brother fell into glass patio door. Bleeding profusely. Physician called to examination room. B/P 96/60 P 100, regular but weak. R 26. Pt appears very nervous. Pt transported to Emergency to further control bleeding and take to surgery. Pt is alert and talking to parents. Stephen Porter, CMA (AAMA)

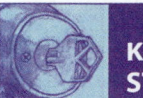

Keys to Success
STOPPING A NOSEBLEED

Some practitioners prefer to have the patient blow the nose before applying pressure to the outside of the nose. This step removes any clots that may be in the nasal passages.

Anyone with soft tissue trauma, especially a puncture wound, should be asked about his or her tetanus immunization status.

Abrasions

An **abrasion** occurs when the outer layer of skin is scraped away, leaving the underlying tissue exposed (Figure 41-26 ◆). Common terms for abrasions include friction burns, rug burns, road rashes, and scrapes. Bleeding is usually in the form of oozing and the injury is quite painful because nerve endings are exposed and/or damaged. As with all open wounds, the area is cleansed and any debris removed. Depending on the physician's choice, antibacterial ointment may be applied to the area and covered with a sterile dressing. Large areas of abraded tissue may require burn treatment.

Avulsions and Amputations

An **avulsion** is the tearing away of skin or tissue (Figure 41-27 ◆). Avulsions usually occur on limbs and appendages, including fingers, toes, hands, arms, feet, legs, nose, and penis. The body part may become entangled in machinery or be injured in a motor vehicle accident or a confrontation with an animal. Cleanse minor avulsion wounds with soap and water and return any skin flap to its normal position. Apply direct pressure, then apply a dressing when bleeding is controlled.

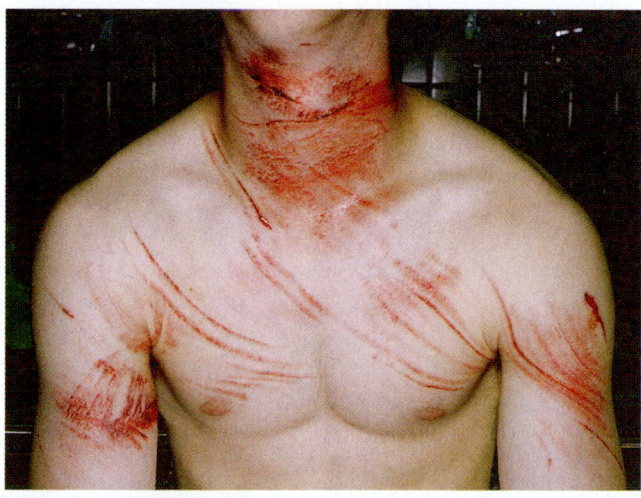

Figure 41-26 ◆ Abrasion.
Courtesy of Charles Stewart, M.D. and Associates

If the body part has been amputated and recovered, cleanse the dismembered part with sterile saline. Wrap it with moist, sterile gauze, seal it in a plastic bag, and place the plastic bag in a container on ice. Prompt medical attention and preservation of the body part enhance the chances for successful reattachment. Cover the wound or stump with a sterile dressing until advanced treatment is available.

Lacerations and Incisions

A **laceration** is an open wound in which the skin and underlying tissue are torn (Figure 41-28 ◆). It usually has jagged edges that may interfere with the healing process. When vessels are torn, bleeding results and must be controlled by direct pressure, pressure on pressure points, or eventual suturing or application of Steri-strips™. Cleanse the laceration with soap and water or an antiseptic solution, removing all debris and foreign matter. If bleeding is severe, a physician should direct the cleansing process.

On minor lacerations, after cleansing, the edges are approximated and then held together with a small dressing, such as a Band-aid™, Steri-strip™ or sterile butterfly. Lacerations over

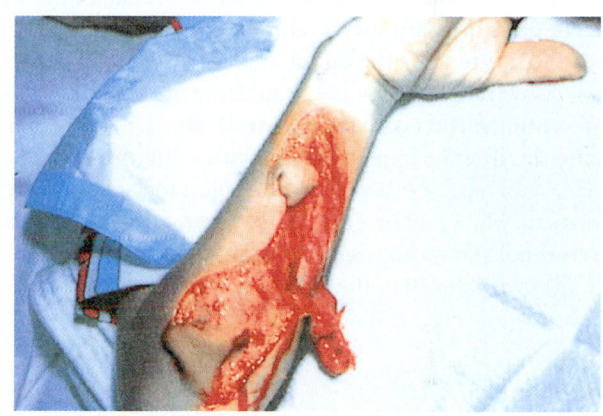

Figure 41-27 ◆ Avulsion.
Courtesy of Edward T. Dickinson.

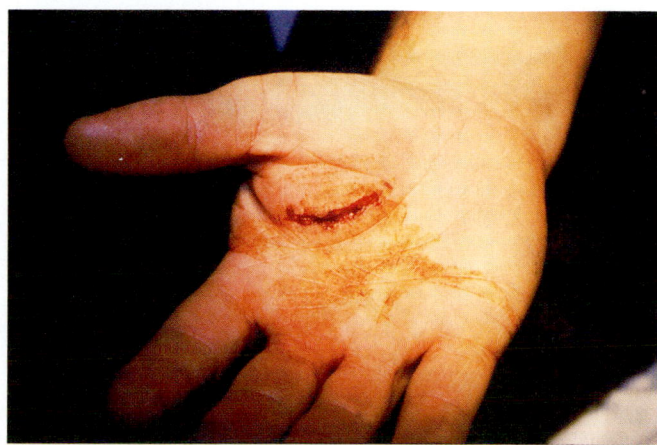

Figure 41-28 ◆ Laceration.

a joint may require joint immobilization for a few days as healing progresses.

An **incision** is a cut with smooth edges made with a knife or other sharp object. It is treated in the same manner as any laceration. If the wound is deep or extensive, the physician usually performs a surgical intervention consisting of debridement, hemostasis, and trimming away of the jagged wound edges. If there is damage to underlying tissue, such as a tendon or ligament, further surgical intervention is required.

Puncture Wounds

A puncture wound results from a pointed foreign body penetrating the skin and tissue (Figure 41-29 ◆). Often the wound edges close, trapping pathogens and debris in the tissue. Depending on the nature of the pointed object, cleansing may consist of simply soaking the area or may require invasive irrigation. After cleansing, a dressing is applied. Bleeding from a puncture wound is usually minimal.

Impaled Objects

A patient who has been impaled by an object such as a large piece of glass or sharp metal requires special treatment. The general rule is to leave the object in place until it can be safely removed by trained personnel. Stabilizing the object is critical to preventing further damage (Figure 41-30 ◆). Control bleeding and stabilize the impaled object with a bulky dressing held in place with tape or other bandages. Splint the area to prevent movement. For a small penetrating object, a small paper cup may be used. Make a hole in the bottom of the cup, place it over the object with the lip of the cup against the skin, and secure it with bandages (Figure 41-31 ◆).

Soft-Tissue Injuries

Soft-tissue trauma involves both the skin and underlying tissue. Abrasions, incisions, lacerations, and puncture wounds are easily identified as open-wound skin injuries. Avulsions, amputations, and thermal insults are considered soft-tissue injuries because tissue as well as skin is involved.

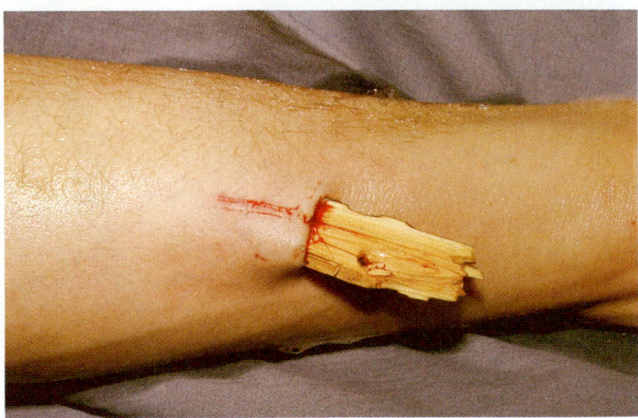

Figure 41-29 ◆ Puncture wound.
Courtesy of Charles Stewart, M.D. and Associates.

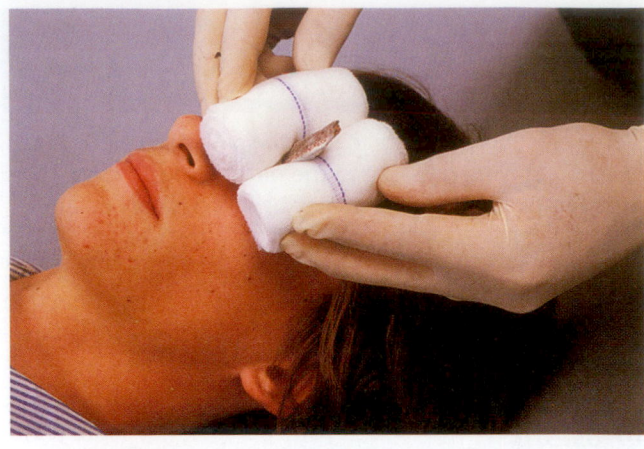

Figure 41-30 ◆ Stabilizing an impaled object.

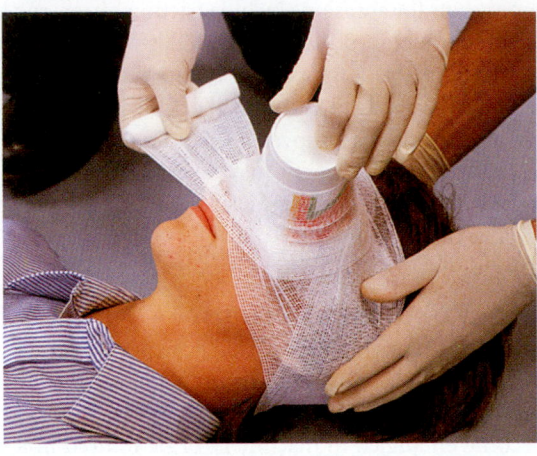

Figure 41-31 ◆ Securing a small penetrating object with a paper cup.

Contusions are closed wounds in which the skin is not broken. Damage to the underlying tissue may involve blood vessels, nerves, muscles, and subcutaneous tissue. The tearing of minute to larger blood vessels results in bleeding into the tissue and discoloration of the area. Swelling may exert pressure on nerve endings, creating pain.

Crush injuries result when force is applied to the tissue. Depending on the area involved, the crush may be similar to pinching of tissue or it may be so severe as to involve organs and bones.

Elevating the body part above the heart and applying cold are often the only intervention needed. With a more severe injury, the body part should be immobilized. Monitoring vital signs and observing skin color, temperature, and moisture are essential to deciding whether more extensive intervention is needed.

Traumatic Injury Emergencies

Traumatic insults to the body may result in minor to very severe injuries. These injuries may be classified as soft-tissue injuries and musculoskeletal injuries. Soft-tissue injuries involve the skin and underlying tissue, including subcutaneous tissue,

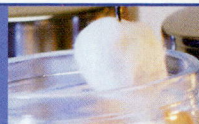

PROCEDURE 41-7 **Demonstrate the Application of Triangular, Figure 8, and Tubular Bandages**

Theory and Rationale

Bandage application varies according to whether an open wound, surgical incision, or intact skin is being bandaged. For an open wound or surgical wound, a sterile dressing must be applied before the bandage. For application to intact skin, medical asepsis must be practiced for the entire procedure.

If necessary, clean and dry the area to be bandaged. If the skin integrity were to be broken under a dirty bandage, the new wound would be easily contaminated. As bandages are applied, avoid skin-to-skin contact. Microbial growth can occur when skin touches other skin and moisture develops. Protect bony prominences from rubbing, irritation, and potential skin breakdown by padding before wrapping with bandages. Position any extremities in a slightly flexed position before bandaging for additional comfort and protection from injury.

To help venous blood flow return to the heart, always apply bandages distally to, proximally, or far to near. Leave as much of the fingers and toes exposed as possible to monitor circulation (Figure 41-32 ◆). Ask the patient if the bandage is snug but not too tight. A tight dressing impairs circulation and predisposes the patient to complications. Check beneath the distal end of the bandage for signs of impaired circulation. Loosen the bandage and inform the physician if signs of impaired circulation occur.

Bandages come packaged in rolls and are often easy to drop. If you drop a bandage on a clean surface, you may use it again. A bandage dropped on a dirty surface should not be used.

In the medical office, three basic types of bandages are used:

■ Elastic—often known by name brand, such as Ace™; washable for repeat use; secures bandages for comfort and support; if applied too tightly, can impair circulation

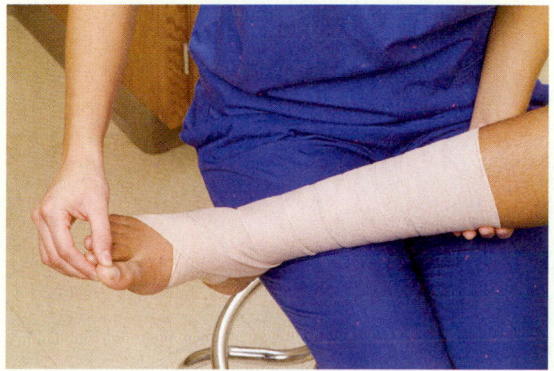

Figure 41-32 ◆ Bandage the patient's foot with toes exposed for monitoring circulation.

■ Roller—made of sterilized gauze; molds to extremities or body parts
■ Kling™—made of sterilized gauze; stretches to mold easily; layers cling together to stay in place

Different turns are used to apply bandages smoothly and to fit the body parts. They include figure 8, spiral and spiral reverse turn, circular turn, and recurrent turn. A tubular gauze bandage is applied to extremities with an applicator. A triangular bandage supports and immobilizes the arm. Regardless of type of bandage material, remember to choose the appropriate width for proper fit and patient comfort.

Materials

■ elastic bandage
■ roller bandage
■ Kling™ bandage
■ tubular gauze and applicator
■ triangular bandage
■ tape
■ scissors

Competency

(**Conditions**) With the necessary materials, (**Task**) you will be able to apply triangular, figure 8, and tubular bandaging (**Standards**) correctly.

1. Escort the patient immediately to an examination room. You may need to assist the patient, depending on the severity, location, and type of injury.
2. Explain the procedure to the patient.
3. Wash your hands.
4. Gather necessary supplies.
5. Apply the bandage as follows.
   Triangular bandage
   • Keep the injured arm as immobile as possible.
   • Carefully slide the triangular bandage under the area to be held. The two shorter sides of the triangle should be pointing toward the elbow, and the remaining longer edge should be parallel to the opposite body side.
   • Bring the lowest side of the triangle up and over the arm.
   • Tie the ends of the bandage behind and slightly to the side of the neck. Tuck the peak of the bandage in toward the elbow point of the bandage.
   • The triangular bandage may also be wrapped around the head as a turban to anchor dressings onto the head.
   Figure 8 bandage
   • Place the thumb of one hand on one end of the bandage to hold it in place.

continued

PROCEDURE 41-7 Demonstrate the Application of Triangular, Figure 8, and Tubular Bandages *(continued)*

- Anchor the bandage with your other hand, then complete one circle around the extremity or body part (Figure 41-33 ◆).
- Continue to alternate wrapping above and below the body joint or dressing and circling behind the joint or dressing area until the injured area is covered adequately (Figure 41-34 ◆).

Tubular bandage

- Choose an applicator that is larger than the extremity to be bandaged.
- Cut an approximate amount of tubular gauze bandage and slide the gathered bandage onto the applicator (Figure 41-35 ◆).
- Slide the applicator over the extremity (Figure 41-36 ◆).

- Hold the bandage against the proximal end of the extremity and pull the applicator approximately 1 inch past the distal end (Figure 41-37 ◆).
- Twist the bandage gauze one complete turn.
- Next, slide the applicator toward the proximal end of the injury (Figure 41-38 ◆).
- Hold the proximal end of the tubular bandage gauze in place, and pull the applicator toward the distal end.
- After pulling past the distal end, complete one twist.
- Slide back and forth and twist the distal end of the dressing until the injured area is adequately covered.
- Cut excess dressing, but remember to anchor the bandage at the proximal end.

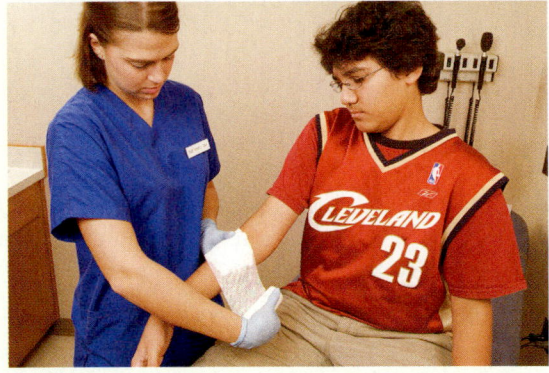

Figure 41-33 ◆ Complete one circle around the extremity or body part.

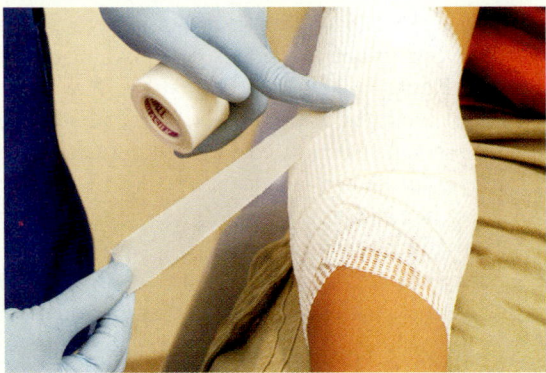

Figure 41-34 ◆ Wrap above and below the body joint or dressing.

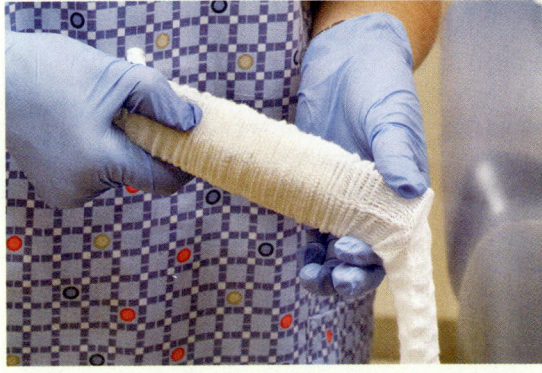

Figure 41-35 ◆ Gather the gauze bandage onto a tubular gauze applicator.

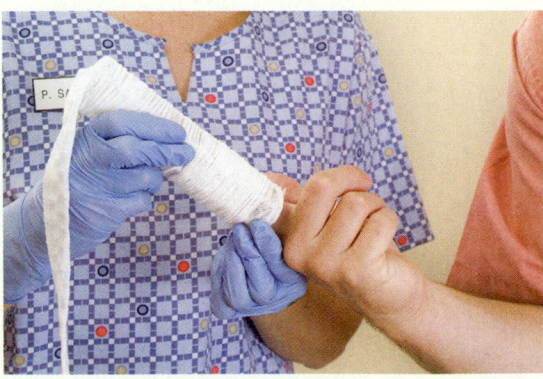

Figure 41-36 ◆ Slide the applicator on the body part.

PROCEDURE 41-7 **Demonstrate the Application of Triangular, Figure 8, and Tubular Bandages** (continued)

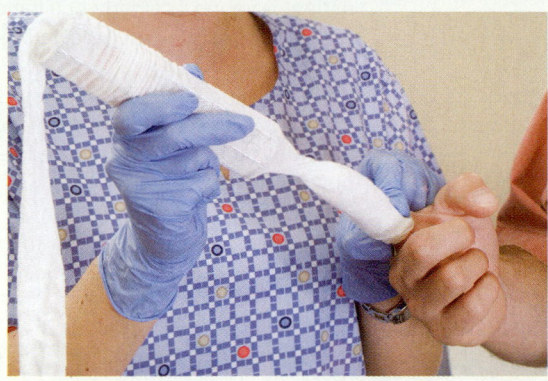

Figure 41-37 ◆ Position the applicator one inch past the distal end.

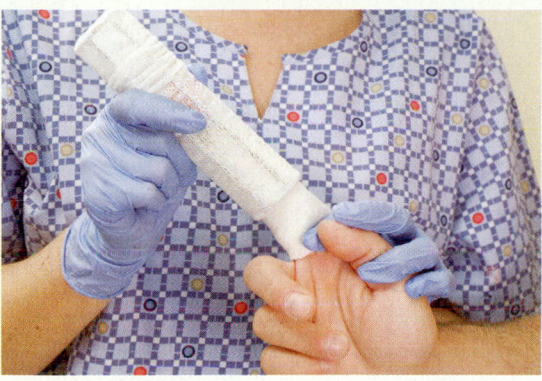

Figure 41-38 ◆ Slide the applicator toward the proximal end of the injury.

6. Instruct the patient to watch for signs of circulation impairment (Table 41-9).
7. Wash your hands.
8. Document the procedure and patient teaching.

Patient Education

Instruct the patient to watch for increasing pain, numbness, skin tightness, pale skin color, swelling, cold fingers and toes, and blue nail beds. Explain that some swelling, pain, numbness, and color changes may be expected for a short period, but to check with the physician for more specific information.

Charting Example

07/22/xx 9:30 a.m. Figure 8 bandage applied to arm as instructed by physician. Pt stated that arm feels supported and less painful. Pt stated awareness of return appointment and that he will call if pain and swelling become worse. Monica Mason, RMA (AMT)

TABLE 41-9 SIGNS OF IMPAIRED CIRCULATION	
■ Pain, numbness	■ Swelling
■ Tight skin	■ Cold fingers, toes
■ Pale skin color	■ Cyanotic fingernails and/or toenails

nerves, blood vessels, fat, muscles, fibrous tissues, membranes, and glands. Musculoskeletal injuries involve bones, joints, cartilage, ligaments, tendons, and muscles.

Pressure Bandages

Bandages anchor dressings in place, prevent contamination of a recent wound or surgical site, support and immobilize injured extremities, and may be used to apply pressure to slow and/or stop bleeding.

Thermal Injuries: Integumentary and Systemic

Thermal insults are integumentary or systemic injuries caused by extremes of heat or cold. Integumentary system injuries include burns and frostbite. Systemic injuries include heat exhaustion, **hyperthermia,** and **hypothermia.**

Integumentary Insults: Burns

Burns may be the result of thermal, chemical, electrical, light, or radiation insults to the skin and underlying tissue. Physical contact with heat sources, such as flames or fire, radiation, steam, hot liquids, or hot objects, can cause a thermal burn. Acids, bases, and caustics can cause chemical burns. Electrical current, including lightning, enters the body, causing burns at the point of entry, the traveled pathway, and the point of exit. Intense light can cause radiation burns to the skin and/or eyes. Radiation from nuclear sources is also capable of causing burns.

TABLE 41-10 BURNS ACCORDING TO DEGREE OF INJURY, SYMPTOMS, AND TREATMENT

Burn Type	Symptoms	Treatment
First degree: superficial burns; heal without scarring	Reddened skin; no blisters; painful	Submerge in cool water 2 to 5 minutes. If patient is young or elderly, or if hands, face, feet, or genitals are involved, see physician.
Second degree: partial-thickness burns; heal with very little scarring	Reddened skin; fluid-filled blisters within 48 hours; very painful; white spots possible	Stop the burning. Do not break blisters. If patient is young or elderly, or if hands, face, feet, or genitals are involved, see physician.
Third degree: full-thickness burns; scarring is likely	Gray, black, or charred skin; underlying tissue involved; extremely painful or no pain if nerve endings are damaged	Call EMS. Treat for shock. Physician evaluation is necessary for treatment. Skin grafting may be necessary.

Without endangering yourself, your first priority is to remove the victim from the source.

Burns are classified by depth, area involved, and source of burn (Table 41-10). Classifications by depth are:

- Superficial or first-degree burns, involving the epidermis (Figure 41-39 ◆)
- Partial-thickness or second-degree burns, involving the epidermis and dermis (Figure 41-40 ◆)
- Full-thickness or third-degree burns, extending through all the layers of the skin to the underlying tissue, including muscle, fat, blood vessels, nerves, and bone (Figure 41-41 ◆)

Age also plays an important part in the outcome of burns. Adults over the age of 55, children under the age of 5, and infants are all at greater risk for unfavorable outcomes and complications.

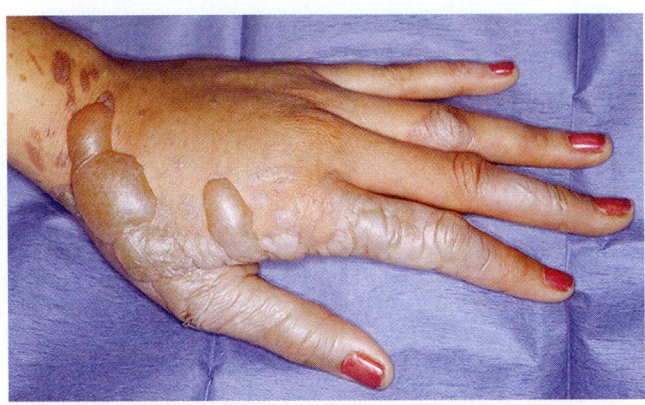

Figure 41-40 ◆ Second-degree burn.
Courtesy of Charles Stewart, M.D. and Associates.

The Rule of Nines is a common way to calculate the extent of the burn area. Specialty burn treatment centers make a more detailed calculation. On the Rule of Nines chart, anterior and posterior outlines of the body are shaded to indicate the burned surface areas (Figure 41-42 ◆). Note if the face, hands, feet, or genitals are involved. While these areas do not comprise a large percentage of the body's surface, they require special attention to promote healing and future functioning.

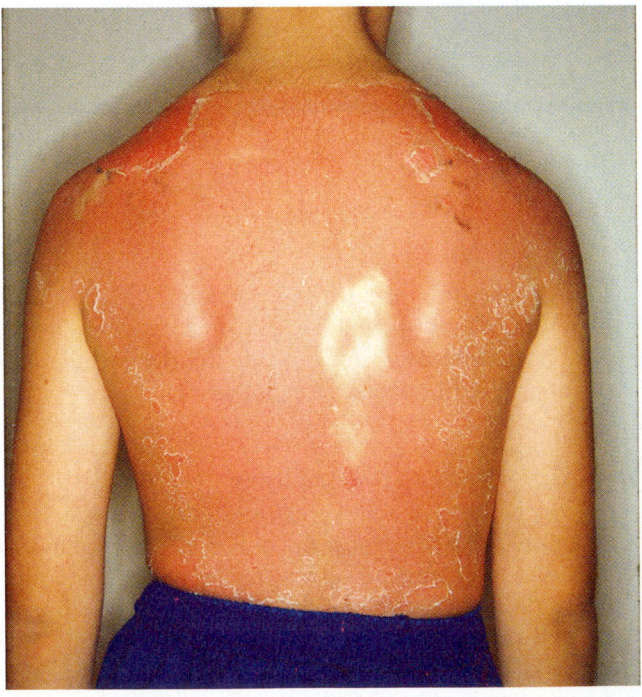

Figure 41-39 ◆ First-degree burn.
Courtesy of Charles Stewart, M.D. and Associates.

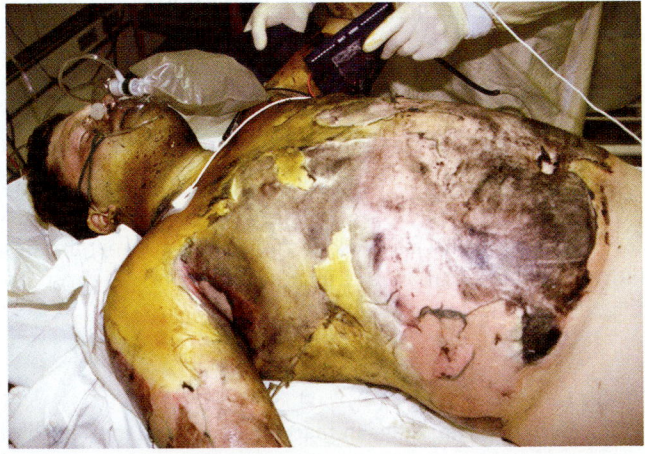

Figure 41-41 ◆ Third-degree burn.
Courtesy of Edward T. Dickinson

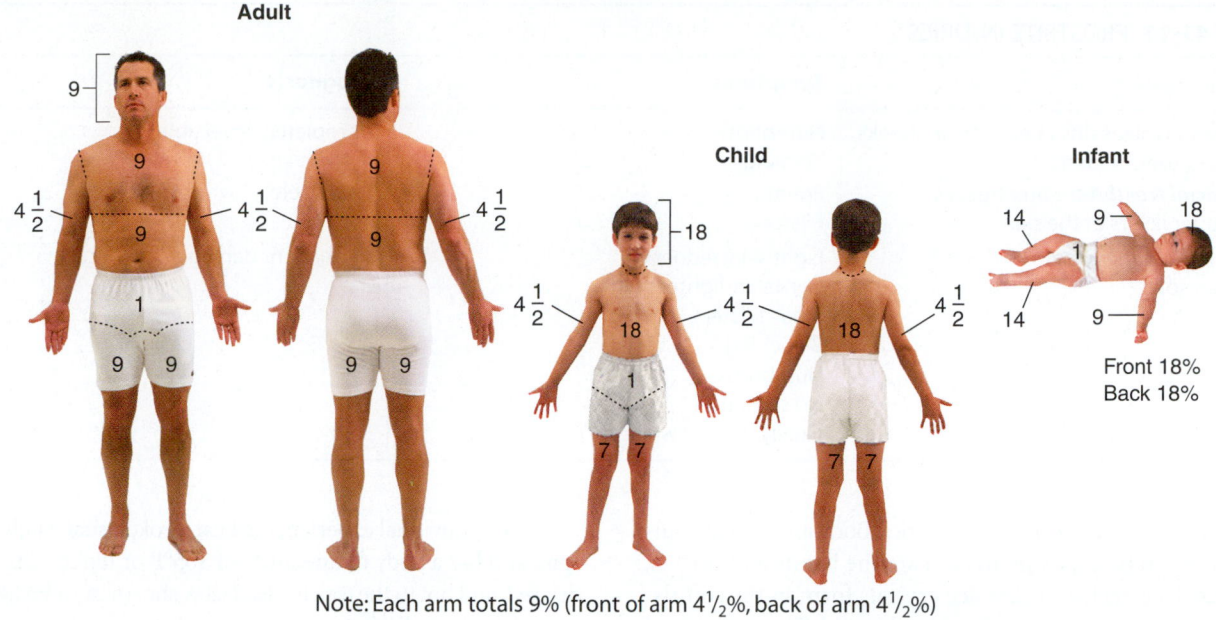

Adult

9

9

4 1/2   4 1/2   4 1/2

9   9

1

9   9   9   9

Child

18

4 1/2   4 1/2   4 1/2

18   18

1

7   7   7   7

Infant

14   9   18

1

14   9

Front 18%
Back 18%

Note: Each arm totals 9% (front of arm 4¹/₂%, back of arm 4¹/₂%)

Figure 41-42 ◆ Rule of nines.

Burns from flames and intense heat may involve areas other than the skin. The respiratory system is often affected. As you assess a burn victim, note any singeing of the eyebrows, nasal hair, or facial hair, as well as any charring or soot. These signs indicate respiratory involvement and possible airway compromise.

Halt the burning process by immersing the injured part in cool water, if possible. If not, soak sterile gauze with cool normal saline and place it over the burned area. When the area has cooled, cover it with dry sterile towels or gauze until the burn can be assessed and treatment prescribed by the physician. Full-thickness burns are left untouched, covered with sterile dressings, and the victim is transported to an emergency facility, usually by EMS. Keep the patient warm to prevent shock.

If a liquid chemical is the cause of a burn, remove it from the skin by flushing with copious amounts of water. A dry or powdery chemical should be carefully wiped from the victim while avoiding exposure to yourself or bystanders. After all the powder has been brushed away, flush the area with a copious but gentle stream of water.

When an electrical burn is involved, the entry and exit points of the electrical current are evident, but the internal damage is difficult to assess. Therefore, first aid consists of covering the wounds with sterile material and transporting the victim to an emergency facility. If the victim is still touching the electrical source, *do not* attempt to remove him or her until the power has been disconnected. You could be electrocuted. If the electrical impact has thrown the victim, assess respiratory status. If cardiac arrest occurs, start CPR. Other considerations include musculoskeletal involvement.

Exposure to lightning also causes burns. If the victim is hit directly by lightning, the electrical charge usually travels through the body in a forceful or violent manner. Treat the entry and exit wounds the same way you would electrical burns. If respiratory arrest has occurred, start rescue breathing. Often cardiac arrest rapidly follows the cessation of breathing. CPR with AED must

follow if the victim is to survive. Most lightning strike survivors are transported to an emergency facility. Cardiac and respiratory functions are monitored and the victim is observed for shock and blood pressure fluctuations. Other possible effects include ruptured tympanic membranes, caused by the shock of the impact, and damage to the eyes, such as eventual cataract development from the intense brightness of the lightning.

Radiation burn treatment is similar to thermal burn treatment after the victim is removed from the source. Radiation burns can include overexposure to the ultraviolet rays of the sun and tanning booths, X-rays, and radiation therapy for cancer.

Frostbite

Extreme cold can cause local injuries as severe as frozen soft tissue, or frostbite (Figure 41-43 ◆). Cold air, moisture, water,

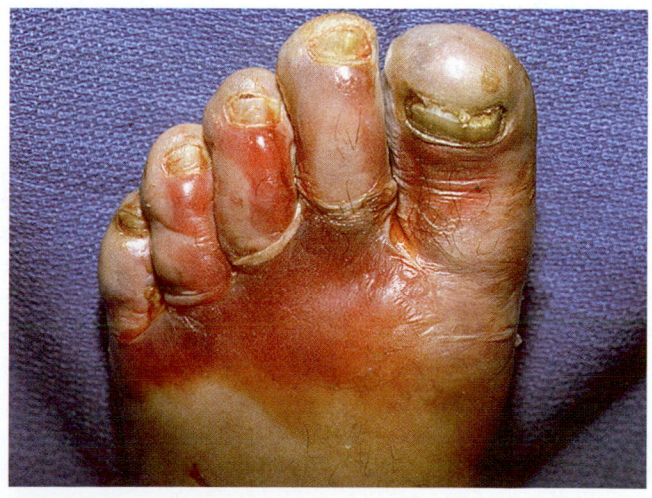

Figure 41-43 ◆ Frostbite.
Courtesy of Charles Stewart, M.D. and Associates.

TABLE 41-11 FROSTBITE INJURIES

Injury	Symptoms	Prognosis
Frostnip: involves tips of ears, nose, cheeks, fingers, toes, or chin	Numbness Tingling	Completely reversible
Superficial frostbite: water freezes in upper layers of the skin	Edema Blisters	Reversible
Frostbite: tissue beneath skin is frozen solid	Light skin: redness Dark skin: lightening Small blisters Blanching Numbness No sensation Finally, area all white	Permanent damage may occur

and wind may all be contributing factors. Body areas most commonly affected by exposure to cold are the hands and fingers, ears, nose, face, feet, and toes. Ice crystals form in the soft tissue as circulation is compromised by the cold. The first sign of frostbite is a developing redness to the skin in a light-skinned individual and a lightening of the skin of a darker-skinned person. This is followed by blanching of the skin. The skin and underlying tissue become numb, all sensation ceases, and the area turns white. Tissue death and loss of the affected body part are possible outcomes (Table 41-11).

Move the victim from the cold to a warmer environment so the tissue can be gently warmed. A person with early frostbite may start the warming process by gently blowing on the area. If the fingers are involved, placing the hands under the armpits or immersing the affected part in tepid water often starts the warming process.

If the tissue has been frozen and is hard to the touch, call EMS or the physician. *Never* rub, squeeze, or massage frozen tissue. Wrap it in sterile gauze, if available, and clean towels in preparation for transport to an emergency facility or until the physician can intervene.

Heat Exhaustion

Heat exhaustion occurs as the result of sodium and water depletion from the body. Strenuous activity often precedes heat exhaustion, as the individual becomes overheated and perspires profusely. The skin is moist, pale, and cool, and body temperature is normal. The individual may complain of headache, muscle cramps, weakness, dizziness, and nausea. He or she should be moved to a cooler environment and encouraged to lie down. Apply cool compresses and give sips of water if the individual is conscious. Heat exhaustion can usually be prevented by taking salt pills and drinking lots of water before, during, and after strenuous activities in a warm environment.

Hyperthermia

Prolonged exposure to extremely hot temperatures often results in hyperthermia. The loss of water and salt through perspiration leads to a state of mild shock. If the body's cooling mechanisms fail, heat exhaustion can progress into heat stroke.

An individual experiencing heat stroke usually fails to perspire and has a body temperature of 105°F or higher. The skin is dry, red, and hot to the touch. Headache, shortness of breath, nausea or vomiting, dizziness, weakness, and dry mouth are common symptoms. At the onset the pulse is rapid, but it gradually slows and becomes weak, and the blood pressure begins to drop. Mental confusion may appear, possibly accompanied by irritability and hysterical behavior. In some cases the victim collapses. If he or she remains exposed to heat, brain cells begin to die and permanent brain damage or even death may eventually result.

The victim must be removed from the environment immediately. Loosen the clothing and cool the body down as quickly as possible by pouring cool water over the victim or sponging with a cool, wet cloth. If heat stroke is suspected, EMS should be contacted after the initial emergency treatment to transport the victim to an emergency facility where vital signs and cardiac status can be monitored. The victim should not be left alone and should be assessed by a physician as promptly as possible.

Hypothermia

The victim of hypothermia is also at great risk. Prolonged exposure to cold or cold water can cause the core temperature to drop below 95°F. The victim shivers and experiences a numbness and tingling over the body. The skin becomes very cool to the touch and is pale with a blue or ashy tinge. Respirations are slow and shallow, and the victim becomes disoriented and eventually unconscious as body functions and organs slow down to the point of complete shutdown.

Treatment involves removing any cold, wet clothing and wrapping the victim in warm blankets. Heat packs may be used, but not directly on the skin. Once the victim is conscious, offer sips of warm liquid. When possible, the victim should be transported to a treatment facility for assessment by a physician.

Table 41-12 summarizes the symptoms, causes, and treatment of thermal insults.

Musculoskeletal Injuries

Musculoskeletal injuries involve bones, muscles, tendons, and ligaments and include fractures, dislocations, sprains, and strains. Definitive diagnosis is made by X-ray, but these injuries

TABLE 41-12 THERMAL INSULTS

Insult	Causes	Symptoms	Treatment
Heat stroke	Continued exposure to extremely hot temperatures Failure of the body to cope with excessive heat	Body temperature >105°F Dry, hot, red skin Dry mouth Nausea Vomiting Dizziness Weakness SOB Rapid pulse Decreasing BP Anxiety, confusion Possible seizures	Cool the body rapidly. Pour cool water over the body to bring the core temperature down below 100°F. Transport to an emergency facility.
Heat exhaustion	Continued exposure to extremely hot temperatures Depletion of salt or water in the body	Normal or below normal body temperature Profuse sweating Skin: moist, cool, pale Headache Dizziness Fatigue Nausea Muscle cramps Pulse: weak, rapid Dilated pupils	Move to a cool place. Apply cool compresses. Elevate the feet. If conscious, give small amounts of liquid.
Hypothermia	Continued exposure to wind, cold, or cold water	Numbness or cold feeling Fatigue Core body temperature < 95°F Skin: blue, puffy Pulse: weak, slow Confusion Decreased level of consciousness	Remove wet clothing. Warm the patient by wrapping in warm blankets. Transport to an emergency facility.

must be considered fractured bones until determined to be otherwise. Therefore, the affected part must be immobilized.

Fractures

In a closed or simple fracture, the bone is broken but does not penetrate the skin (Figure 41-44 ◆). In an open or compound fracture, the bone pierces the skin, or the skin is torn open by the bone or by an external force (Figure 41-45 ◆). Fractures may also be single or multiple breaks in the bone (Figure 41-46 ◆). Bone breaks can be complete, twisted, or splintered. The affected part is immobilized and examined for impaired circulation to the distal aspect. The location of

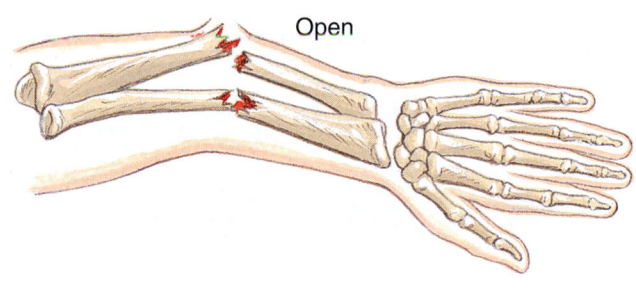

Open

Figure 41-45 ◆ An open fracture.

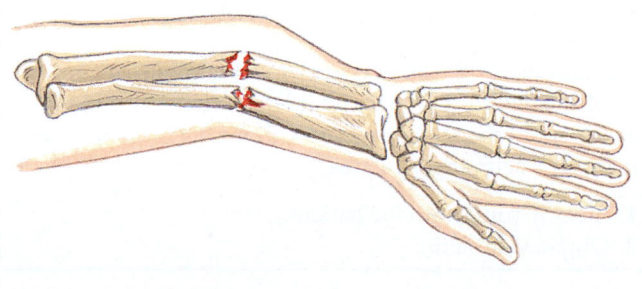

Figure 41-44 ◆ A closed fracture.

the fracture and the possible presence of heavy bleeding or bruising are also determined. Knowing the cause of the injury is very helpful in this assessment.

A fracture may occur in any bone. Special precautions must be taken for suspected fractures of the spinal column or skull. For any injury caused by sudden acceleration and deceleration, the cervical spine must be immobilized. Other injuries to the spinal column require extreme caution when moving the victim. The best response is to call 911. Allow EMT professionals to immobilize the cervical spine with a cervical collar and log-roll the victim onto a spine board for transport to a facility where X-rays can be taken to determine the extent of

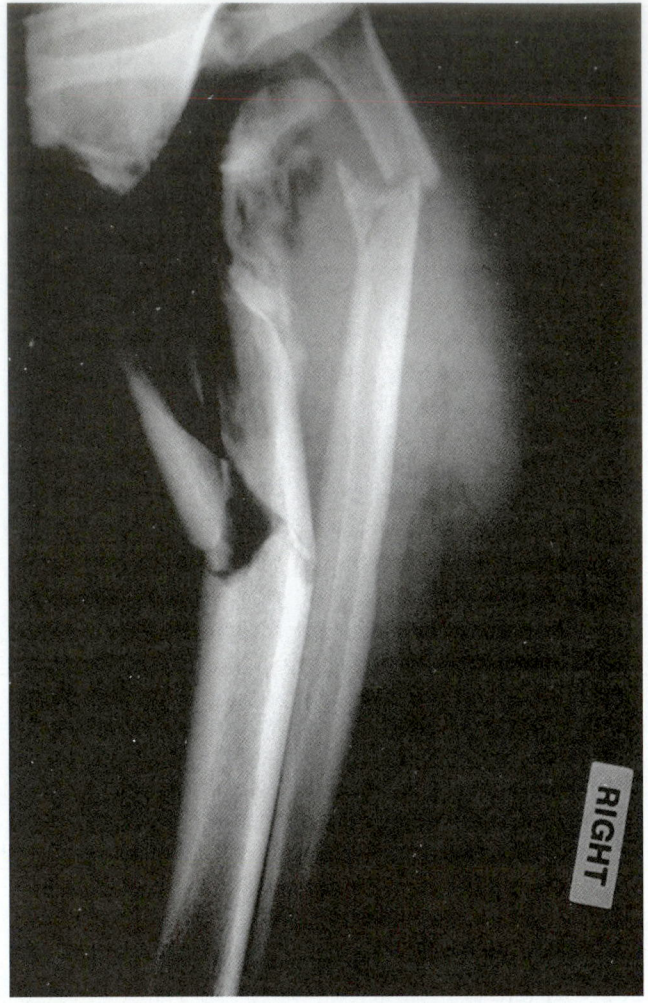

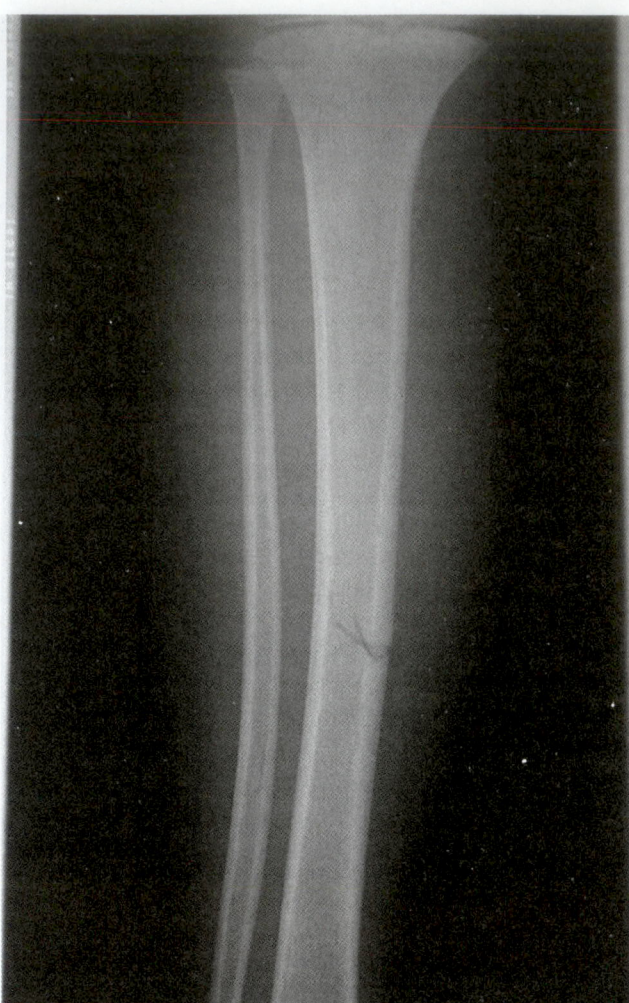

Figure 41-46 ◆ Fractures may be single or multiple breaks in the bone. (A) Severe fracture. (B) Subtle fracture; difficult to detect without an X-ray.

Courtesy of Charles Stewart, M.D. and Associates.

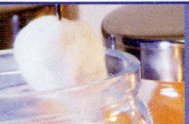

PROCEDURE 41-8 Demonstrate the Application of a Splint

Theory and Rationale

Manufactured splints may be available in the medical office. However, it may sometimes be necessary to improvise a splint using materials at hand, such as narrow boards, before a physician examines the victim. Rolled-up newspapers, magazines, a pillow, a folded blanket, or a rigid object may also be used. Pad the splint with a towel or other soft material before placing it under or beside the injured limb. The secured splint should be snug, but not so tight as to impair circulation or neurological status. If possible, leave a "window" or open area in the splint to allow observation of the extremity. Elevating the limb, especially a lower limb, is helpful in preventing pain and swelling.

Materials

- makeshift or sterile dressing supplies
- stiff or solid materials to immobilize the extremity
- bandages or strips of material to secure splint materials

Competency

(**Conditions**) With the necessary materials, (**Task**) you will be able to apply a splint (**Standards**) correctly with minimal movement to the extremity and without impairment to circulation or neurological status.

1. Identify yourself to the patient.
2. Obtain vital signs.

PROCEDURE 41-8 Demonstrate the Application of a Splint (continued)

3. Ask the patient, if conscious, to speak his or her name.
4. Ask about medical allergies and medications and whether the patient has a medical history.
5. Assess the area of suspected fracture for bruising, bleeding, and open areas or protruding bones.
6. Moving the limb as little as possible and with gentle traction on the distal side, place the splint with padding under the limb or alongside the limb. You may have to ask other clinical staff for help to ensure the least amount of discomfort for the least amount of time.
7. Place sterile dressings or clean makeshift dressings gently over open areas.
8. Secure the splint by wrapping bandages or strips of material around the splint and the limb. The ties must be above and below the joints on both sides of the suspected fracture.
9. Add additional ties as necessary along the length of the splint.
10. If possible, leave an exposed area, such as toes or fingers, so that circulation can be monitored.
11. The splint should be snug enough to immobilize the limb, but not tight.

Patient Education

If the patient is conscious or significant others are present, instruct them to watch for increased pain, numbness, discoloration, and swelling. Emphasize the importance of immobilization and the need for physician and X-ray followup for additional diagnosis and care.

If the patient is unconscious, give the family or friends basic information and make EMS transport arrangements immediately.

Charting Example

12/23/xx 8:30 a.m. Pt came to office with splint applied to lower leg and foot. Pt states that brakes failed on bike, he swerved to miss a dog, and was thrown from bike when it ran into a tree. A passerby called his wife, who splinted the lower leg. Pt complains of severe pain and has pliable cold pack applied to area of leg pain. Pt is able to move toes and toes are pink and warm. William Hughley, CMA (AAMA)

---

the injury. Suspected fractures of the thigh (femur) and pelvis also require immobilization and transport and are best handled by the EMS.

In open or compound fractures, the soft-tissue injury must be tended. Cover the open wound with a sterile, saline-moistened dressing, then place a sterile occlusive dressing over that. Generally, the tissue must be surgically cleaned and debrided.

∞ Descriptions of specific fractures and their treatment are given in Chapter 43.

Splint Application

Fractures of long bones require immobilization by splinting to prevent joint movement above and below the fracture. In addition to preventing additional damage to the bone and surrounding soft tissue, the splint helps to relieve pain and allows safe movement of the injured part. Another comfort measure is the application of cold, usually after splinting, to prevent swelling.

Sprains, Strains, and Dislocations

A sprain occurs when muscles, tendons, or ligaments are torn. It may be the result of trauma or cumulative overuse of the joint.

A strain, often called a pulled muscle, occurs when a muscle or tendon is overextended by stretching. The patient complains of pain and may be unable to use the joint. In the lower extremities, weight-bearing is painful and sometimes impossible.

In a dislocation, the bone is actually pulled away from the joint, stretching or tearing the ligaments and tendons. A deformity is generally noted. Dislocations must be reduced and the bone reinserted into the joint.

The injured body parts should be immobilized to prevent additional damage and reduce pain. Applications of cold also help with the pain and slow edema. The physician assesses the injury and usually orders radiographs to eliminate the possibility of fracture and diagnose sprain, strain, or dislocation.

Allergic Reactions

Allergic reactions can range from possibly catastrophic anaphylaxis to the troublesome itching of hives. Respiratory reactions may be triggered by such common factors as perfume, hair spray, insect repellents, and other airborne irritants. Symptoms may range from hives, welts, wheezing, and anxiety, to airway constriction, respiratory arrest, vascular collapse, and cardiac arrest.

Each exposure to the same allergen may cause more intense symptoms. Many individuals with known allergic conditions wear identification, such as a bracelet, charm, or necklace, to alert healthcare providers or emergency responders to the allergy.

Treatment consists of removing the allergen or removing the victim from the environment causing the reaction. In the medical office setting, if a physician is available, antihistamines or steroids may be ordered and administered to neutralize, slow, or stop the histamine-induced reaction. Cold-water compresses may be helpful in relieving the itching.

Neurological Emergencies

Neurological emergencies include head trauma, seizures, **status epilepticus,** sudden onset of paralysis or hemiparesis, spinal cord involvement, and altered level of consciousness. An insult to the brain or spinal cord can be either internal or external. External insults with open wounds require additional attention.

Many neurological emergencies require more intense intervention, monitoring, and treatment than is possible in a physician's office. Usually the best course of action is to place the victim in a supine or semi-Fowler's position (at a 45-degree angle), inform the physician, complete a rapid assessment, and stay with the patient. Have another person call 911 to transport the patient to an emergency facility. Take and record vital signs, note the level of consciousness (**LOC**), and implement shock prevention measures. Evaluate pupil reaction, if possible (Figure 41-47 ◆). Keep the patient quiet and remain calm.

The basic neurological assessment includes level of consciousness, pupil reaction, motor and sensory skills, and

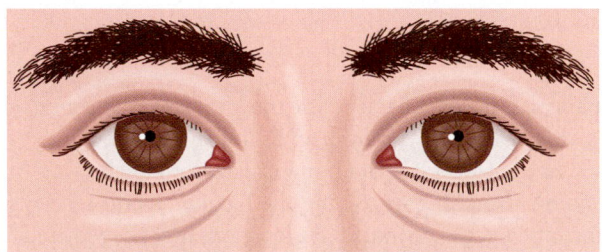
Constricted pupils

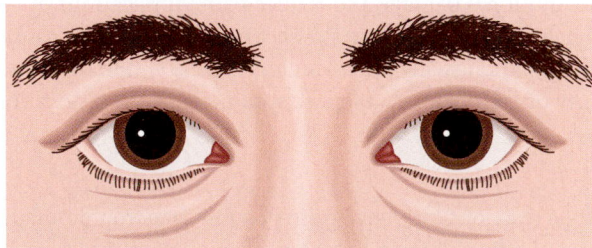
Dilated pupils

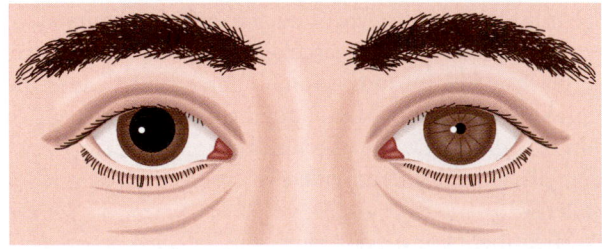
Unequal pupils

Figure 41-47 ◆ Evaluate pupil reaction.

Keys to Success
GLASGOW COMA SCALE

Eye opening	Spontaneous	4	_____
	To voice	3	_____
	To pain	2	_____
	None	1	_____
Verbal response	Oriented	5	_____
	Confused	4	_____
	Inappropriate words	3	_____
	Incomprehensible sounds	2	_____
	None	1	_____
Motor response	Obeys commands	6	_____
	Localizes pain	5	_____
	Withdrawal (pain)	4	_____
	Flexion (pain)	3	_____
	Extension (pain)	2	_____
	None	1	_____
Glasgow Coma Score total			_____

Total Glasgow Coma Scale Points (conversion = approximately one-third total value):

14–15 = 5	5–7 = 2
11–13 = 4	3–4 = 1
8–10 = 3	

Neurological Assessment _____

ability to cooperate. Emergency medical personnel may use the Glasgow Coma Scale to establish a baseline assessment of a head injury patient. The lower the score, the greater the chance of a negative outcome. Throughout the course of treatment, comparing scores may provide an indication of trauma progression or condition improvement.

A more complete and thorough examination is conducted by the physician and includes six components:

1. Cerebral function (mental status)
2. Cranial nerve function
3. Cerebellar function
4. Motor function
5. Sensory function
6. Deep tendon reflexes (DTRs)

It is important to note and compare the functions on the right and left sides of the body. If the findings are not symmetrical, that is usually an indication of an abnormal condition.

Decreased Level of Consciousness

Decreased levels of consciousness range from dizziness and light-headedness to complete loss of consciousness. As the patient's level of consciousness drops, he or she may fall to the ground or floor, possibly sustaining an injury. If a patient complains of light-headedness or feeling faint, assist him or her to a sitting position, with the head between the knees. Or help lower the patient to a lying position and slightly elevate the feet and legs about 12 inches. Observe the airway to ensure that it remains open. Check and record vital signs and inform the physician. Light-headedness often passes quickly once sufficient blood flow has been reestablished to the brain.

If the patient is completely unresponsive, immediately have someone notify the physician, remain with the patient, contact EMS for transport, assess vital signs, administer oxygen if available, and follow office procedure.

?—Critical Thinking Question 41-2

After Ariko has collected all the information on the accident as reported by Brenna, how should she advise Brenna?

Seizures

Seizures are involuntary muscular contractions or a series of muscular contractions that result from abnormal cerebral stimulation. Since the primary concern with a person experiencing a seizure is to prevent injury, you should do the following.

- If the person is in an upright position when the seizure begins, ease him or her to the floor. Move furniture and other objects out of the way to minimize the risk of injury to the patient (Figure 41-48 ◆).
- Do *not* attempt to force open the mouth to hold the tongue from blocking the airway. Forcing the mouth open will break teeth and cause mouth injuries.
- Stay with the person and provide privacy.
- Loosen any constricting clothing.
- Ensure the airway is patent when the seizure stops.
- If the victim is not breathing, open the airway with the head-tilt or jaw-thrust maneuver. These maneuvers lift the tongue away from the airway (the tongue is never

swallowed but only relaxes against the airway), and spontaneous breathing usually returns.

- If mucus and saliva are present in the person's mouth, turn the head to the side to drain the fluids and prevent aspiration.
- Note the length of the seizure, the part of the body involved, and any other pertinent information.
- Ask a family member to assist the person home after the seizure because the person may experience a postictal period during which he or she is responsive but disoriented. Do *not* allow the individual to drive or be alone.

Status epilepticus, a condition of continuous seizure activity, is considered a life-threatening emergency. Respiratory activity may be compromised and the seizures must be brought under control. Activate EMS and inform the physician immediately. The victim will need oxygen, and anti-seizure medication must be administered intravenously. If the physician is not available, the patient must be transported to an emergency facility for treatment and observation.

Cerebrovascular Accidents and Transient Ischemic Attacks

Cerebrovascular accidents (**CVA** or stroke) occur when circulation to the cerebral tissue in the brain is compromised, resulting in an interruption of neurological functioning. A plaque-narrowed artery may be occluded by a cerebral thrombosis or an embolism. Hemorrhage may also occur in an artery, causing bleeding into the tissue, pressure on other vessels, and the interruption of blood circulation in the area.

The onset of an occlusion is usually very sudden. Signs and symptoms are unilateral paralysis, impaired or slurred speech, confusion, dizziness, facial droop, arm drift, loss of balance and coordination, visual difficulties, and/or loss of consciousness (Figure 41-49 ◆). The patient with cerebral hemorrhage may experience a slower onset over a few minutes, and a headache may be one of the symptoms.

A transient ischemic attack (**TIA**) is temporary in nature but similar to a CVA. Usually, the symptoms are less severe, do not involve a loss of consciousness, and resolve within 24 hours.

Since it is not possible to determine the seriousness of the attack, emergency treatment for both CVA and TIA victims is the same. In the medical office, take the patient to an examination room and assist him or her onto an examination table. The patient is usually more comfortable in a semi-sitting position. Do not leave the patient alone. Inform the physician and, if it is available and ordered, administer oxygen. Call EMS for transport to an emergency facility. Monitor and record vital signs.

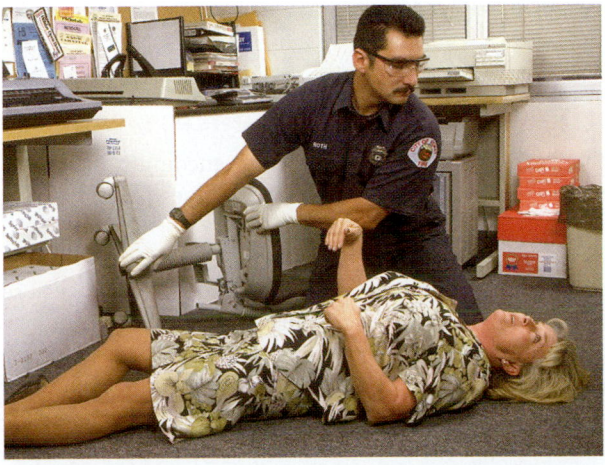

Figure 41-48 ◆ Emergency personnel protecting the seizure patient from injury.

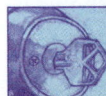

Keys to Success
ASPIRIN AND STROKES

At the first sign of an impending stroke, the patient should chew one 5-grain aspirin tablet. Patients should consult a physician before adding aspirin to their treatment regimen.

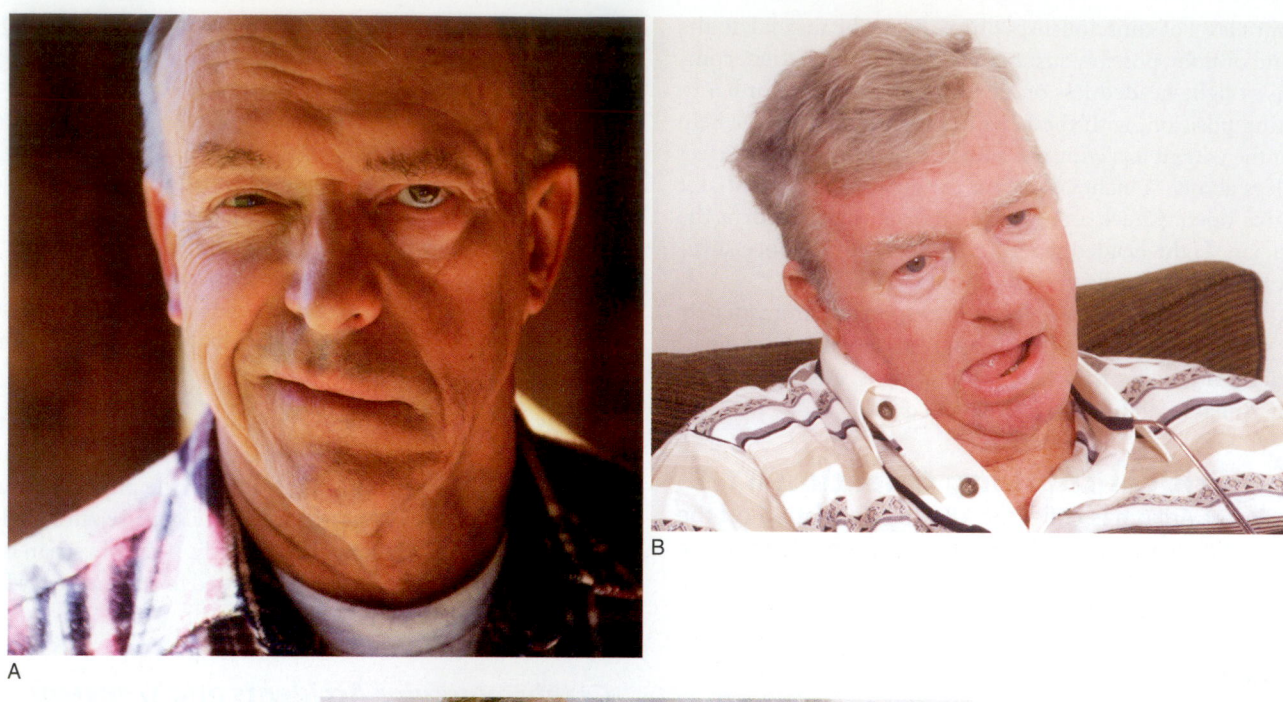

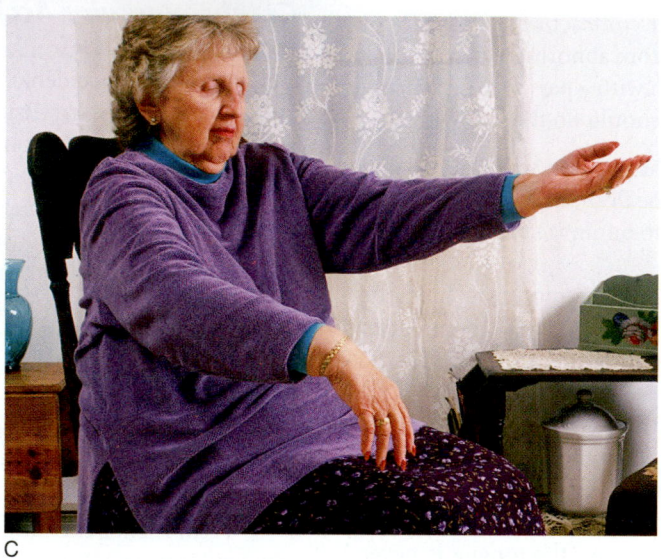

Figure 41-49 ◆ Stroke symptoms: (A) Facial droop. (B) Speech difficulties. (C) Arm drift.
Source: Photo A) Michal Heron.

Head Injuries

The severity of trauma to the head depends on what caused the injury, the force of the offending object, and the location of the trauma. Injuries may be open or closed and involve a fracture of the skull and soft-tissue damage (Figure 41-50 ◆). Most severe head and facial injuries, including open skull fractures, require advanced medical treatment, and the patient should be transported to an emergency facility. If severe bleeding is present, gently apply an absorbent dressing.

A neurological assessment is helpful to EMS and the physician. If the victim is conscious, attempt to keep him or her quiet and ask what happened.

Other Medical Emergencies

Other medical emergencies you may encounter include sudden onset of abdominal pain, diabetic crises, and poisoning.

Acute Abdominal Pain

Acute abdominal pain with a sudden onset often signals a serious underlying condition and must be assessed by the physician to determine the cause. Assessment is done in quadrants. Palpation begins in the upper right quadrant and moves clockwise around the abdomen, terminating in the lower right quadrant. While not definitive in a diagnosis, pain located in certain quadrant(s) signals possible acute conditions:

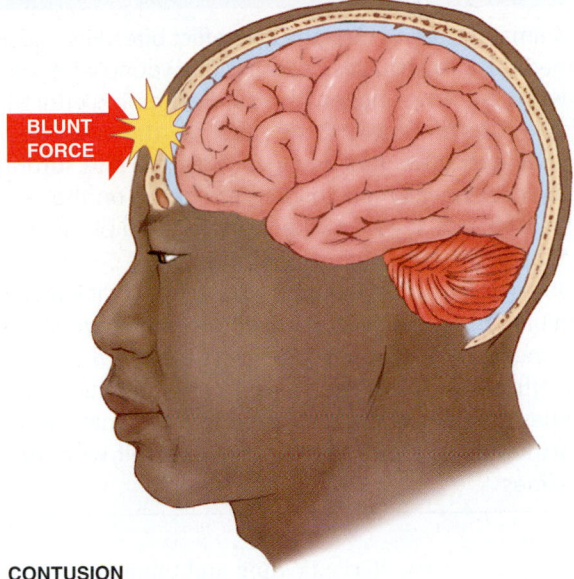

CONCUSSION
- Mild injury, usually with no detectable brain damage
- May have brief loss of consciousness
- Headache, grogginess, and short-term memory loss common

BLUNT FORCE

CONTUSION
- Unconsciousness or decreased level of responsiveness
- Bruising of brain tissue

Figure 41-50 ◆ Closed head injuries.

- Upper right quadrant—gallbladder disorders
- Lower right quadrant—appendicitis
- Back or flank region (retroperitoneal)—kidney disorders
- Pelvis—urinary infection, pelvic infection, or problem in lower GI tract; patient may guard the abdomen and sit with the knees drawn up

In the medical office, make the patient as comfortable as possible, preferably sitting with the knees drawn up on an examination table. Keep the patient warm, and take and record vital signs. Do not allow the patient to eat or drink or take pain medication unless you have the physician's permission. If the patient becomes unconscious and vomits, there is a risk of aspiration and further complications. If an undiagnosed condition is found, the patient may have to have surgery. Keep the patient NPO if there is the potential need for general anesthesia and until the physician gives orders to provide food and fluids.

For acute abdominal, flank, or pelvic pain, the patient must be examined by a physician. Laboratory and radiographic studies along with the examination and history assist the physician in a diagnosis and subsequent orders for treatment.

Diabetic Coma or Insulin Shock

A patient with diabetes may exhibit signs of either **hypoglycemia** or **hyperglycemia.** Both conditions may cause the rapid onset of altered levels of consciousness. The greatest risk for a patient is hypoglycemia.

Hypoglycemia, in which blood sugar falls below 70 mg per deciliter, may be the result of a skipped meal, vomiting after

taking diabetic medications, excessive exercise, or an unknown reason. A patient may appear to be intoxicated (slurred speech, balance disturbances, and uncharacteristic behavior), have cold clammy skin, and be anxious or combative. Intervention must be immediate and consists of some form of glucose administration. If the patient is conscious, ask about the last intake of food and diabetic medication. If the patient is able to swallow, glucose paste may be placed inside the mouth behind the lip and along the cheek, or the patient may drink orange juice with added sugar. If the patient is unconscious, IV glucose is administered. The person experiencing hypoglycemia is in grave danger when the blood glucose drops below 40. The brain requires glucose to survive, and brain cells begin dying unless glucose is administered promptly. If possible, blood glucose levels should be checked with a blood glucose monitor. Contact EMS if a physician is not available to administer IV glucose.

If there is doubt about whether the patient is hypoglycemic or hyperglycemic, glucose may be administered. It will raise the glucose 25 to 50 points, but this rise can be reversed with an insulin injection as soon as an elevated glucose is diagnosed.

The hyperglycemic individual may experience acidosis. As this condition progresses the patient's breath develops a sweet, fruity odor, indicating the presence of ketones. The patient may progress to an unconscious state, reversible with insulin. The physician orders the amount and route of the insulin.

Whether the patient is hypoglycemic or hyperglycemic, keep him or her as warm and comfortable as possible on an examination table until the physician arrives.

∞ Table 40-3 (p. 862) compares hypoglycemic and hyperglycemic reactions.

Poisoning and Overdose

Poisoning and overdoses may be accidental or intentional. The poison and its means of entry must be identified before appropriate treatment can begin. Poisons can be introduced into the body in four ways.

- Ingestion (swallowing): Ingested poisons include drugs, cleaning materials, food toxins, poisonous plants, and petroleum products. Depending on the substance, the patient drinks water or milk, or vomiting is induced. Vomiting is never induced when petroleum products or caustic substances have been ingested or when the patient is unconscious. Activated charcoal is often administered after emesis has been successfully induced to absorb any poison left in the GI tract.
- Injection: Injected poisons include drugs and any other poisonous substance delivered by insect sting, bite, sharp or piercing object, or needle. A patient who has been injected with a poison usually requires an antidote to counteract it.
- Absorption: Some poisons, such as insecticides, may be absorbed through the skin. The process of absorption

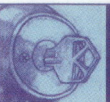

Keys to Success
TREATING INSECT STINGS

Insect stings may be insignificant or life-threatening. Some are quite painful, while others cause no pain and the victim is unaware of the sting until itching, redness, or a reaction develop. Help the victim by following these steps.

1. Remove the stinger by scraping across the affected area with a credit card or other rigid object. This is usually the only treatment necessary to remove the stinger.
2. Apply a paste of baking soda and water to the area.
3. If the victim is allergic to certain types of insect stings (bees, wasps, hornets), administer antihistamine or epinephrine, as ordered by the physician.

can be slowed if the area is cleansed immediately with copious amounts of water.

- Inhalation: Inhaled poisons such as carbon monoxide enter the body through the respiratory tract. The patient must be given respiratory support—usually supplemental oxygen—and an antidote, if applicable.

Poison Control Centers

Poison Control Centers have been established in most areas of the United States. The American Association of Poison Control Centers and Rocky Mountain Poison Control Centers offer telephone contact information for local centers. Telephone books usually list toll-free numbers as well.

Poison Control Centers offer emergency advice concerning accidental poisoning and overdose. In most cases there is no charge for this service. Registered nurses, pharmacists, and often physicians are available 24 hours a day, seven days a week, to provide emergency treatment instructions. The caller's name and phone number are recorded for followup contact within 24 hours after the initial patient contact and instructions. After followup, the caller's identity is discarded and the remaining information is used for statistics and for events reportable to the CDC. The caller provides the following information: sex, age, and weight of the poisoning victim; the substance ingested, including amount and any information on container; the time of occurrence; any other pertinent information; and any intervention made. Instructions are then given for the appropriate intervention.

Foreign Bodies in the Eye, Ear, and Nose

Foreign bodies present a unique challenge in the medical office. They include dirt, rust particles, metal, insects, and other small objects.

A foreign body in the eye requires immediate attention to prevent further damage. Sterile eyewash may be used in some cases. Have the victim turn the head toward the affected side. Apply sterile wash across the eye from the inner cannula outward, gently letting it flow across the eye. If sterile eyewash is not

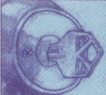

Keys to Success
ANIMAL BITES

Any animal, including humans, can inflict bites. First aid in the medical office involves cleansing the wound with soap and water and covering it with a sterile dressing until the physician assesses it and decides on the next step. Depending on the extent and location of the bite, sutures may be necessary. When children are bitten on the face, arms, and hands, they are often referred to a plastic surgeon for repair with minimal scarring.

Obtain information regarding the animal that inflicted the injury. Contact your local law enforcement agency for the name of the appropriate agency to call. A law enforcement officer may notify the agency for you. In many communities, animal bites are reported to an animal control department. You should familiarize yourself with local guidelines.

available, you may use sterile IV fluid and tubing to wash the eye. As a last resort, have the victim place his or her head under water running in a slow stream, also from the inner cannula out. If both eyes are affected, irrigate one eye, then the other.

Impaled objects must be secured. Both eyes are closed and patched to prevent further damage, as the eyes are sympathetic and move together. The good eye is patched first to limit movement of the injured eye. Rust in the eye causes a rust ring residue that must be removed by a physician. Patients are often referred to an ophthalmologist for additional treatment. Surgery may be required to remove the impaled object.

An insect in the ear is easily removed by placing the patient in a dark room and shining a flashlight into the ear. If the insect is alive, it will migrate to the light source and come out of the ear on its own accord. If the insect is dead, gentle irrigation of the outer ear canal with a solution of 50 percent hydrogen peroxide and 50 percent warm water will wash it out.

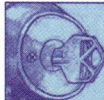

Keys to Success
TEACHING CHILDREN ABOUT POISONS

Mr. Yuk and Officer Ugg are two television characters who teach children how to identify potential poisons and containers containing poisonous materials.

Mr. Yuk was developed by the Children's Hospital of Pittsburgh to promote awareness of poisons among children by telling them never to touch anything with the picture of Mr. Yuk on it. Mr. Yuk has a green face and is sticking out his tongue. Stickers with Poison Control Center telephone number and a picture of Mr. Yuk are available to place on telephones.

Officer Ugg is used by Rocky Mountain Poison Control Centers as a symbol to warn children about poisonous substances. Officer Ugg wears a blue uniform and has a green face with white hands across the mouth.

Children sometimes push small objects up their noses. If the object is a dry item, such as a bean or dried pea, it will absorb moisture from the nasal mucosa and swell, blocking air passage through that nostril. Encourage the patient to blow the nose. If the object does not come out, a physician will have to remove the object, usually with instruments.

Psychosocial Emergencies

Psychosocial emergencies presenting on the phone or in person require prompt attention. They include child abuse, domestic violence, elder abuse, rape or sexual abuse, drug abuse, threatened suicide, depression, alcoholic intoxication, rage, and psychotic behavior.

Child and elder abuse are often detected during a routine office visit, or the victim may be seeking treatment for injuries resulting from abuse. By law these incidents are considered mandatory reportable incidents. Record all the information the victim or a family member provides. Reassure the victim that he or she does not deserve to be abused and is not responsible for the abuser's action. Treat any injuries and provide emotional support as required.

Domestic Violence

A victim of domestic violence may be reluctant to reveal any information, and according to state law that wish must be respected. If the victim chooses to share information about the abuse, listen in a calm, nonjudgmental manner, and inform the physician, who will determine the course of action. In most states, reporting is mandatory only in cases of child or elder abuse. Familiarize yourself with state and local statutes pertaining to abuse.

Sexual Abuse and Rape

Most states have statutes regarding rape and sexual abuse victims, and medical office protocol is designed accordingly. A calm and understanding approach helps the victim feel comfortable and secure. Assure her that she did not ask for this treatment and did not deserve to be sexually abused or raped. If the victim requests that no law enforcement agency be contacted, her wishes should be honored unless state law dictates otherwise.

Depression

Severely depressed persons look sad, may be tearful, and avoid eye contact. They require understanding and someone to listen to their problems. In an emergency situation, the physician must be notified as soon as possible, and the patient should not be left alone. Depression is a complex disorder that is further discussed in ∞ Chapter 47, Mental Health.

Suicide

The patient or individual who voices the intent to commit suicide on the phone or in the office should be taken seriously. Note if the person refers to the future or to details of the planned suicide. If the suicide threat is made over the phone, ask the following specific questions:

- "What is your name?"
- "How old are you?" or "When were you born?"
- "Where are you right now?"

- "Do you have an address?"
- "What is the telephone or cell phone number from where you are calling?"
- "Are you alone?"
- "Have you ever felt this way before?"
- "Do you have access to any weapons, pills, or other means of suicide?"

These questions demonstrate your concern while providing you with the necessary information to get help. If the person is in the office, ask why he or she feels this way and if he or she has attempted suicide before.

When dealing with any potential suicide victim, help him or her identify reasons to go on living. Ask who will take care of the children, pets, home, and so on. Ask how you can help. Make the physician aware of the situation as soon as possible. Individuals at risk for suicide are often referred to a mental health facility for further intervention and treatment. Document any information you obtain and any action taken.

Rage

If the patient or other individual is agitated or hostile, the primary intervention is to defuse the situation. It is important to remain calm and speak in a quiet voice, which may help convince the person to accept assistance. Address the person by name. Do *not* interrupt, and do not respond in anger. Listen and try to understand the person's feelings. Sometimes an angry person just wants to air his or her frustration. Take notes so the person feels you are taking him or her seriously and repeat back the information.

If the individual has been diagnosed with psychotic behavior, recognize that you may need help. Attempt to redirect the rage to an inanimate object or to something outside the office environment. If you cannot defuse the situation, follow office protocol for contacting local law enforcement for assistance. An agitated psychotic individual is a danger to him- or herself and to everyone else in the building. Keep in mind that the leading cause of death in the workplace is homicide.

Alcohol Intoxication

The intoxicated patient may be unruly and uncooperative or very subdued. The odor of alcohol is usually noticeable. The patient should not be left alone; help should be requested and the physician notified for orders. It is best not to confront the alcohol-intoxicated patient until the physician is present to direct treatment and assist in handling the situation.

Psychotic Behavior

Psychotic behavior is discussed in ∞ Chapter 47, Mental Health. It is best to be cordial to a patient exhibiting psychotic behavior and to request help from other staff. Ask the patient to sit down so you can talk quietly together. During a psychotic episode a patient may experience hallucinations (auditory or visual) and will require immediate intervention by a physician. Have someone advise the physician that his or her presence is required immediately.

Emergency Preparedness

The medical assistant should be knowledgeable in the area of emergency preparedness. This includes knowing how to respond in the event of a manmade disaster, such as a terrorist event, and to a natural disaster, such as a hurricane.

Earthquakes

Because earthquakes can happen at any time, and without any warning, the medical assistant should know how to respond to this type of emergency. One of the first steps to preventing injury during an earthquake is to prepare before an earthquake happens. Advance preparation may save lives as well as prevent injuries.

According to the Federal Emergency Management Agency (**FEMA**), there are six steps involved in planning ahead for an earthquake. These steps are:

1. Check for hazards around the facility.
   - Make sure shelves are fastened securely to walls.
   - Do not place large or heavy objects on higher shelves.
   - Store any breakable items in low, closed cabinets equipped with locks.
   - Heavy items should not be hung on walls above where patients will sit or lie.
   - Overhead light fixtures should be secured.
   - Any defective electrical wiring or leaky gas connections should be repaired.
   - Water heaters should be strapped to wall studs and bolted to the floor.
   - Any deep cracks in ceilings or foundations should be repaired.
   - All flammable products should be stored in closed cabinets with locks, on the bottom shelf.
2. Identify safe places both indoors and outdoors.
   - Under study furniture.
   - Against an inside wall.
   - Away from glass that could shatter.
   - Away from bookcases or furniture that could fall over.
   - In the open, away from buildings, trees, telephone or electrical lines, overpasses, or elevated expressways.
3. Educate yourself and your co-workers.
   - Contact the local emergency management office or the American Red Cross chapter for information.
   - Teach all staff members how and when to turn off gas, electricity, and water.
4. Have disaster supplies on hand.
   - Flashlight and extra batteries.
   - Portable battery-operated radio and extra batteries.
   - First aid kit and manual.
   - Emergency food and water.
   - Nonelectric can opener.
   - Sturdy shoes.
5. Develop an emergency communication plan.
   - In case staff members are separated from one another during an earthquake, develop a plan for reuniting after the disaster.
   - Define the expectations of each staff member: Who will escort patients from the building? Who will check the treatment rooms?
6. Help your community get ready.
   - Provide literature for patients on how to prepare for an earthquake.

Fire

Because more than 4,000 Americans die and more than 25,000 are injured in fires each year, the medical assistant should be prepared to respond to this type of disaster. Fire spreads quickly, and there is typically no time to gather belongings or make a telephone call. In just 2 minutes, a fire can become life-threatening, and in 5 minutes a fire can engulf a building. Heat and smoke from fire are often more dangerous than the flames.

The medical office should be equipped with properly working smoke alarms. These should be placed on every level of the building on the ceiling or high on the walls. Every room of the office should be equipped with a smoke detector, and each should be tested and cleaned once per month. The batteries should be replaced at least once per year and every smoke alarm should be replaced once every ten years.

The medical assistant should know the escape routes to use in the event of a fire. Staff members should practice those escape routes. If the office is located above the first level, escape ladders may be used.

Any flammable items must be stored in well-ventilated areas, and care must be taken in placing any items near a heat source or heating vent. Any defective wiring must be repaired to avoid a fire hazard. Fire extinguishers should be located throughout the office and staff should be trained in their use.

During a fire, the medical assistant should be aware that if a person's clothes are on fire, that person should stop, drop, and roll until the fire is extinguished. Running makes the fire burn faster.

In order to escape a fire, the medical assistant should check closed doors for heat before opening. This is done by using the back of the hand to feel the top of the door, the doorknob, and the crack between the door and the door frame before opening the door. If the door is hot, it should not be opened, and another route of escape should be sought. If the door is cool, it should be opened slowly.

When escaping a fire, the medical assistant should crawl low under any smoke on the way to the exit and close doors as they are passed through to delay the spread of fire. Once out of the building, the medical assistant should not attempt to reenter until or unless the fire department declares that action to be safe.

Floods

FEMA declares floods to be the most common hazard in the United States. Some floods can develop over days of rainy weather; others may be in the form of flash floods and may come on very quickly. The medical assistant should be aware of the flood dangers that exist in his or her local area.

During a flood, the medical assistant should listen to the radio for information. In the event of a flash flood, the MA should move to higher ground. If there is time before evacuating, the medical assistant should be sure to disconnect any electrical equipment and shut off utilities at their main valve.

When evacuating, the medical assistant should be careful not to walk through moving water. Only six inches of moving water can make a person fall.

Hurricanes

Hurricanes can strike with little warning, although most will allow for some advance warning, giving the medical office staff time to prepare. If the office is in the path of the hurricane, the windows may need to be secured. This can be done using plywood. Trees and shrubs around the office should be well trimmed.

If the medical office is to be evacuated before a hurricane, the medical assistant should listen to the radio or television for information provided by local emergency management personnel.

During the hurricane, the medical assistant should listen to the radio or television for information and prepare for high winds and possible flooding.

Terrorism

In the event of a terrorist attack, the medical assistant should be aware of the steps to take in each of the following types of emergencies.

Explosions

In the event of a bomb threat, the medical assistant should try to obtain as much information from the caller as possible. The following questions should be asked.

1. When is the bomb going to explode?
2. Where is the bomb right now?
3. What does it look like?
4. What kind of bomb is it?
5. What will cause it to explode?

This information should be immediately provided to the police, and their directions should be followed. If an explosion has occurred, the medical assistant should respond by following the steps as if an earthquake and/or fire has happened.

Biological Threats

There are four methods of delivery of a biological agent:

1. Aerosols—agents are dispersed into the air, forming a mist that may drift for miles.
2. Animals—some diseases are spread by insects or animals.
3. Food and water contamination—some agents are placed in the food or water supply.
4. Person-to-person—some spread of agents is possible via direct contact between people.

In order to prepare for a biological attack, the medical facility may have a high efficiency particulate air (HEPA) filter installed.

In the event of a biological attack, the medical assistant should be prepared to move away quickly, wash with soap and water, contact authorities, listen to the radio for instructions, and remove and bag clothing if contaminated.

Nuclear Blast

In the event of a nuclear attack, the medical assistant should take cover as quickly as possible, below ground if the building has a basement. The medical assistant should remain in a safe location, listening to the radio for instructions. The medical assistant should not look at the flash or fireball, lie flat on the ground with the head covered, and seek shelter as quickly as possible.

Mock-Environmental Exposures

Medical assistants can play a vital role in the event of an environmental emergency. It is helpful to be prepared for such events by understanding how to help victims and providing assistance to other healthcare providers.

Organizations within the community, colleges, and hospitals may offer mock-environmental exposure events. These events provide real-life scenarios and situations that may arise during times of disaster. Scenarios of mock-environmental events may include a tornado site with injured victims, an exposure to a biological chemical, or treating injured victims of flash floods or hurricanes. The role of the medical assistant will vary in every situation; however, overall, MAs may be able to provide assistance by:

- Aiding in evacuation plans
- Triaging patients to determine which patients require immediate attention
- Assisting in first-aid response for wounded individuals
- Administering tetanus and other vaccines under the direction of a physician
- Facilitating order and organization in the midst of chaos
- Implementing and following through on an environmental safety plan

PROCEDURE 41-9 Develop an Environmental Exposure Plan

Theory and Rationale

Medical assistants are playing an increasing role in emergency preparedness. Emergencies include not only medical emergencies, but also natural disasters and man-made disasters. The most important rule to follow is to always be prepared for any situation that may arise. By adequate preparedness we not only help ourselves and our patients, but also the community that surrounds us.

Materials

- pen
- paper
- computer
- copy machine
- various emergency supplies
- waterproof containers

Competency

(**Condition**) With the necessary materials, you will be able to (**Task**) develop an environmental exposure plan (**Standards**) with correct items in the time designated by the instructor.

1. Create an emergency kit that can be used by your office in the event of an environmental emergency. Supplies may include:
   - flashlights
   - batteries
   - bottles of water
   - nonperishable food
   - bandages
   - alcohol and hydrogen peroxide
   - blankets
   - vinyl or latex gloves
   - tweezers, scissors
   - medication—ibuprofen, acetimetophen, antihistamines, antibiotic ointment, tetanus vaccines, etc.
   - self-powered radio
2. Enclose the kit in a waterproof container.
3. Place the kit in a safe area, such as a medicine closet or storage closet.
4. Create evacuation plans and make sure that every room in the medical office shows a detailed exit route.
5. Create a delineation chart that outlines responsibilities of office staff members in the event of an emergency.
6. Create a list of "safety zones" that can be used in the event of an emergency. For instance:
   - a safety zone in the event of a tornado
   - an outdoor safety zone in the event of a fire
   - a safety zone in the event of a flood
7. Make photocopies of the safety zone list, evacuation plan, and delineation chart for everyone in the office. Laminate and hang copies in the employee break room.
8. Train all office staff on the environmental exposure plan within ten days of hire.

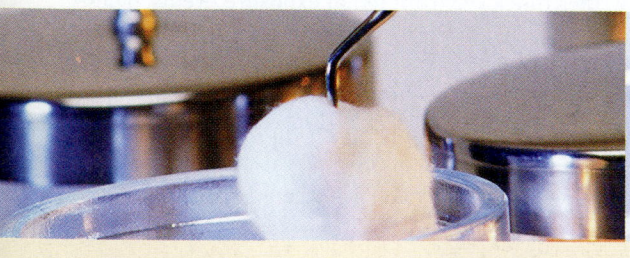

REVIEW

Chapter Summary

- Each team member must know what procedures to follow in a medical emergency. As an MA, you will need advanced training in CPR, AED, and treating specialty office emergencies, such as allergic reactions.
- Patients may experience fainting, seizures, anaphylactic shock, and other conditions when visiting the medical office for other health reasons. Contacting the physician and EMS, if necessary, is part of office protocol. Good Samaritan laws were established to encourage healthcare professionals to volunteer in emergencies without fear of financial liability.

It is important that you and other healthcare professionals render emergency care according to scope of license, certification, or training until relieved by another health professional.

- EMS may be called for on-the-scene care, stabilization of the victim, and transport to the appropriate emergency room for further assessment and treatment.
- Equipment is kept for medical emergencies in the medical office. The amount and type of equipment vary according to the types of patients seen and proximity to advanced

Chapter Summary (continued)

emergency care. Examples of emergency equipment are the crash cart, oxygen supplies, emergency drugs, and intravenous supplies.

■ In an emergency, you must first determine if the scene is safe to enter. If it is not safe, wait for emergency assistance. If it is safe, a primary survey determines the care for life-threatening conditions, followed by a secondary survey to assess and set priorities for additional care.

■ For individuals experiencing acute chest pain, loss of consciousness, or respiratory arrest, CPR protocol is followed. First, establish whether the individual is unconscious. If the patient is conscious, there is no need to proceed with CPR. If the patient is unconscious, you will need to open the airway. If it is obstructed, determine whether the obstruction is total, partial with good air exchange, or partial with poor air exchange. If the breathing is obstructed, reposition the airway and attempt to ventilate. If you cannot ventilate the victim, proceed with the obstructed airway sequence until the obstruction is removed. When the airway is functioning, the third step is to check the pulse—carotid in the adult and child and brachial in the infant. If there is no pulse, begin compressions. Use AED on adults, but not on children or infants. If CPR is not needed, keep the victim comfortable, warm, and in the recovery position until EMS help arrives.

■ Other cardiac and respiratory emergencies include chest pain, respiratory distress, SOB, hyperventilation, congestive heart failure, chronic obstructive pulmonary disease, and pulmonary edema. Chest pain may require emergency treatment with oxygen and/or nitroglycerin. If a patient with chest pain calls the medical office, keep the caller on the line and arrange for EMS to transport the patient to an emergency facility for evaluation and treatment.

■ Shock is the collapse of the cardiovascular system and may occur in any of several forms, including anaphylactic, cardiogenic, hemorrhagic, metabolic, neurogenic, psychogenic, respiratory, and septic. Shock may be life-threatening and require emergency treatment.

■ Vascular and soft tissue emergencies include bleeding, open wounds, and closed wounds. Pressure bandages on the bleeding site and direct pressure on pressure points are part of the treatment. You should be aware of and monitor the signs and symptoms of internal bleeding, bruising, tenderness, swelling, and pain at the site of the injury. Treatment varies according to type and extent of injury but includes elevation and ice, cleansing and bandages, and pain medication.

■ Thermal injuries to the skin and body systems caused by cold or heat may be considered medical emergencies. Burns and frostbite are integumentary insults. Treatment varies according to the depth of the injury. Systemic insults are often life-threatening and include hyperthermia and hypothermia.

■ Musculoskeletal injuries include fractures, dislocations, sprains, and strains. Fractures may be closed or open, simple or compound, and may lead to circulatory and neurological complications. The injured body part should be immobilized and observed for pain, numbness, swelling, bruising, bleeding, and circulation. If there is a skin break, dressings should be applied to prevent infection.

■ Allergic reactions can be life-threatening if they progress to anaphylactic shock, but can be treated in the office with followup evaluation, additional treatment, and patient education. Neurological emergencies, such as seizures and head trauma, require advanced evaluation and treatment in an acute-care hospital setting. Medical emergencies include sudden acute pain, diabetic coma or insulin shock, and poisoning. The physician assesses the patient, provides initial treatment, and refers the patient to an acute-care facility. Foreign bodies in the eyes, ears, and nose may be removed in the medical office or an emergency care facility, depending on the extent of the injury. If an object is impaled in the eye, it is necessary to cover the good eye first before the affected eye.

■ When handling psychosocial emergencies—rape, domestic violence, drug abuse, depression, psychotic behavior, suicide attempts, and other situations—it is important to know the laws that apply to treatment in the medical office. Encourage the patient to talk, ask questions, and take notes.

■ The medical assistant should be knowledgeable in the area of emergency preparedness, and understand how to respond in the event of a manmade disaster or a natural disaster.

Chapter Review

Multiple Choice

1. Which of the following is a life-threatening medical emergency requiring immediate intervention?
   a. Open chest wound
   b. Seizure
   c. Severe vomiting
   d. Major fracture

2. The victim of a sudden stop in a vehicle should
   a. receive pain medication before the primary survey.
   b. be moved immediately before splinting.
   c. be treated even if he or she refuses.
   d. have his or her neck and possibly spine immobilized.

Chapter Review (continued)

3. The Heimlich maneuver on a child is performed by
   a. using abdominal thrusts.
   b. using chest thrusts.
   c. strongly shaking the child.
   d. strongly squeezing the child.

4. Which of the following should you do when administering nitroglycerin?
   a. Ask the patient to swallow the tablet immediately.
   b. Put the patient's tablet directly on his or her tongue.
   c. Wear disposable gloves before handling the patient's tablet.
   d. Call EMS and wait before administering the nitro- glycerin.

5. If a patient has a partial airway obstruction, you should
   a. help the patient lie down.
   b. assist the patient to a sitting position.
   c. start CPR.
   d. perform the Heimlich maneuver.

6. Septic shock is caused by
   a. infection in the bloodstream.
   b. heart failure.
   c. loss of body fluids and electrolytes.
   d. an allergic reaction to a substance.

7. Blood from capillaries
   a. flows rapidly, echoing the heartbeat.
   b. flows rapidly and copiously.
   c. flows slowly and is darker in color.
   d. oozes slowly.

8. Which of the following steps should you perform when applying a pressure bandage?
   a. Add dressings every 10 minutes.
   b. Add dressings every 5 minutes.
   c. Keep the original dressing in place.
   d. Remove the original dressing and add a new dressing.

9. Which of the following procedures should be used in the treatment of a full-thickness burn?
   a. Immerse the burn in cool water.
   b. Leave it untouched and cover with a sterile dressing.
   c. Soak sterile gauze and apply it to the burn.
   d. Apply burn ointment immediately.

10. When a patient in the medical office experiences a seizure, you should
    a. never force open the mouth.
    b. force open the mouth.
    c. keep the patient in an upright position by holding him or her in place.
    d. keep the patient's head straight, even if saliva has formed in his or her mouth.

True/False

T F   1. A laceration is an open wound in which the outer layer of skin is scraped away.

T F   2. Hypoglycemia is a condition in which blood glucose is below normal.

T F   3. EMS technicians provide on-the-scene intervention and treatment but do not transfer patients.

T F   4. Since its introduction in 1968, the 911 emergency access number has been so successful that it is used in every single U.S. state.

T F   5. Decreased levels of consciousness are not a life-threat- ening condition.

T F   6. The first step in any emergency is to check if the vic- tim is alert.

T F   7. You should not move a victim or help a victim move after a fall or sudden stop, such as a car accident, unless the victim is conscious.

T F   8. Cardiac arrest and heart attack have exactly the same symptoms from onset to death.

T F   9. AED can be used on children 1 year old or younger as long as the rescuer uses pediatric-size pads.

T F 10. If a child is choking on an object but can still move air past the object, a sharp, quick blow to the back between the shoulder blades may help move the item out of the airway.

Short Answer

1. When is the Heimlich maneuver used?

2. Blind finger sweeps can be performed on patients of what age?

3. What is the leading cause of death in both men and women?

Research

1. In your community, is Healthcare Providers CPR and First Aid required for medical assistant certification?

2. Is there a Good Samaritan Law in your community?

Externship Application Experience

While waiting for a scheduled appointment for a pre-employment physical, a 36-year-old female comes to the receptionist's window and states that she does not feel well. You observe that her face is pale and ashen. You check her pulse and note that it is fast and thready. She drops to the floor. What do you do next?

Resource Guide

American Heart Association (AHA)
American Heart Association National Center
7272 Greenville Ave.
Dallas, TX 75231
1-800-AHA-USA1
1-888-4STROKE
www.americanheart.org

American Red Cross
www.redcross.org

Federal Emergency Management Association (FEMA)
500 C Street SW
Washington, DC 20472
Disaster Assistance (800) 621-FEMA
www.fema.gov

National Highway Traffic Safety Administration
1-888-327-4236
www.nhtsa.dot.org

U.S. Department of Transportation (USDOT)
400 7th St. SW
Washington, DC 20590
www.dot.gov

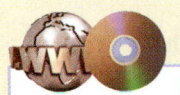

Med**Media**

http://www.MyMAKit.com

More on this chapter, including interactive resources, can be found on the Student CD-ROM accompanying this textbook and on http://www.MyMAKit.com.

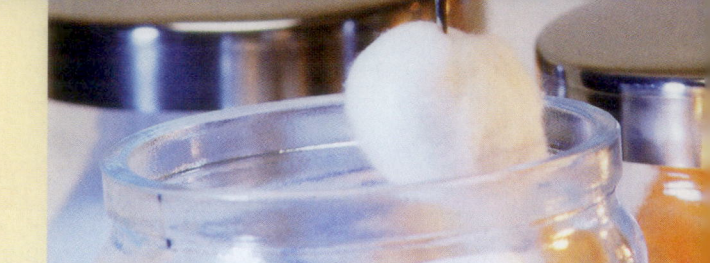

CHAPTER 42

Gastroenterology and Nutrition

Case Study

Reggie, an MA, is rooming a teenage patient, Serena, when her mother asks to speak to him regarding her care. Reggie takes the appropriate measures and makes sure he has the patient's permission to discuss her care with a family member. During the conversation, Serena's mother mentions that her daughter has decided with some of her friends at school to become a vegetarian. The mother is concerned that she is not going to get enough protein and will become anemic.

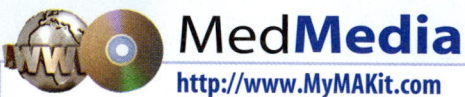

Med**Media**

http://www.MyMAKit.com

Additional interactive resources and activities for this chapter can be found on http://www.MyMAKit.com. For a video, audio glossary, tips, legal and ethical scenarios, job scenarios, quizzes, games, virtual tours and activities related to the content of this chapter, please access the accompanying CD-ROM in this book.

Video
Audio Glossary
Legal and Ethical Scenario: *Gastroenterology and Nutrition*
On the Job Scenario: *Gastroenterology and Nutrition*
A & P Quiz: The Digestive System
Multiple Choice Quiz
Games: Crossword, Strikeout, and Spelling Bee
3D Virtual Tour: Digestive System: The Digestive System
Drag and Drop: Digestive System: The Intestinal Wall
Tips
HIPPA Quiz

Objectives

After completing this chapter, you should be able to:

- Define and spell the key terminology in this chapter.
- Define the role of the medical assistant in the GI medical office.
- Describe the basic anatomy and physiology of the gastrointestinal system and accessory organs.
- Identify disease and disorders of the gastrointestinal system and accessory organs.
- List and describe the basic food components: proteins, carbohydrates, fiber, lipids, vitamins, minerals, and water.
- Explain how the Food Guide Pyramid/MyPyramid is used for healthy meal planning.
- Describe how individual health is affected by nutritional status.
- Discuss the factors that may affect caloric intake.
- Explain the effects of alcohol on nutritional status.
- Describe the relationship between aging and nutrition.
- List and describe the types of disorders associated with altered nutritional status.
- List some common food allergies and how they are diagnosed.
- Name the anatomical divisions and clinical quadrants of the body.
- List the diagnostic procedures performed for GI disorders.
- List and describe special and therapeutic diets commonly prescribed for GI patients.

✚ MEDICAL ASSISTING STANDARDS

CAAHEP ENTRY-LEVEL STANDARDS	ABHES ENTRY-LEVEL COMPETENCIES
■ Perform within scope of practice (psychomotor) ■ Explore issue of confidentiality as it applies to the medical assistant (cognitive) ■ Apply ethical behaviors, including honesty/integrity in performance of medical assisting practice (affective) ■ Explain the rationale for performance of a procedure to the patient (affective) ■ Use language/verbal skills that enable patients' understanding (affective) ■ Describe the normal function of each body system (cognitive) ■ Identify common pathology related to each body system (cognitive) ■ Analyze pathology as it relates to the interaction of body systems (cognitive) ■ Discuss implications for disease and disability when homeostasis is not maintained (cognitive) ■ Describe implications for treatment related to pathology (cognitive) ■ Apply critical thinking skills in performing patient assessment and care (affective) ■ Prepare a patient for procedures and/or treatments (psychomotor) ■ Perform handwashing (psychomotor) ■ Screen test results (psychomotor) ■ Administer parenteral medications (psychomotor) ■ Document patient care (psychomotor)	■ Project a positive attitude ■ Maintain confidentiality at all times ■ Be a "team player." ■ Be cognizant of ethical boundaries. ■ Exhibit initiative. ■ Adapt to change. ■ Evidence a responsible attitude. ■ Be courteous and diplomatic. ■ Conduct work within scope of education, training, and ability. ■ Provide patient education for postprocedural care. ■ Prepare patients for procedures. ■ Apply principles of aseptic techniques and infection control. ■ Prepare and maintain examination and treatment area. ■ Collect and process specimens. ■ Perform selected CLIA waived tests that assist with diagnosis and treatment. ■ Dispose of biohazardous materials. ■ Practice standard precautions. ■ Inform patients of dietary needs and treatment options.

✔ COMPETENCY SKILLS PERFORMANCE

1. Assist with a colon endoscopic/colonoscopy exam.
2. Assist with a sigmoidoscopy.
3. Insert a rectal suppository.

Introduction

The gastrointestinal system is responsible primarily for the nourishment of the body. Salivation, mastication, and the process of **digestion** break food down into nutritional substances. Further processes of **metabolism** and **absorption** convert the products of digestion into fuel and nutrients for cellular functions.

Good nutritional habits help the body maintain a strong immune system and maintain healthy energy levels and mental alertness. During times of impaired health, a healthy nutritional status can speed recovery. For example, when nutritional supplements are given to hospitalized or nonhospitalized patients during the recovery process from surgery, wounds heal faster.

Key Terminology

absorption—passage of digested food products through the wall of the intestine into the bloodstream

alimentary canal—tubelike structure of the gastrointestinal system that originates in the mouth and terminates at the anus

alimentation—entire process of providing nourishment to the body that includes mastication, swallowing, digestion, and absorption

amino acids—chief components of protein, synthesized in the body and obtained from the diet

anastomosis—surgical joining of two tubular structures

anorexia—diminished desire to eat or diminished appetite

anus—terminal aspect of the gastrointestinal tract through which dietary waste is expelled

bolus—mass of masticated food that is swallowed

calorie (also called small calorie)—energy released from the metabolism of proteins, fats, and carbohydrates; amount of heat required to raise 1 gram of water 1 degree Celsius

carbohydrates—simple and compound sugars that are the primary source of energy for metabolism

cholesterol—steroid alcohol formed in the liver and also found in plant and animal fats; may be responsible for fatty deposits of plaque in blood vessels

chyme—mixture of partially digested food and enzymes that enters the small intestines

colonoscopy—visual examination of the colon using a colonoscope

colostomy—surgically created opening connecting the colon to the abdominal surface for fecal evacuation

complete protein—protein containing all the essential amino acids

digestion—physical and chemical conversion of food into substances that can be used by the body

dyspepsia—painful digestion

dysphagia—difficulty swallowing

electrolytes—substances present in the bloodstream, cells, and tissues that are involved in homeostatic changes in acid-base balance, movement of tissue fluid, and activities of the cells and cellular walls

elimination—expulsion of waste products from the body

Key Terminology *(continued)*

emesis—regurgitation of partially digested food from the stomach; vomit

emulsification—transformation of ingested particles of fat into small globules with bile

fat—food component that is a source of energy and aids in growth and development by providing fatty acids

feces—waste product of digestion that is expelled through the rectum and anus

fiber—nondigestible substances found in food, such as cellulose and pectin, that provide bulk and roughage for the evacuation of fecal waste

flatulence—excessive gas or air generated in the stomach or intestinal tract

gastric—pertaining to the stomach

gastroenterology—the study of diseases affecting the gastrointestinal tract

gastroscopy—visual examination of the stomach using a gastroscope

hematemesis—vomiting of blood, an indication of bleeding in upper GI tract

hepatomegaly—enlargement of the liver

ileostomy—surgical opening of the ileum onto the surface of the abdomen for the elimination of fecal material

incomplete protein—protein lacking one or more of the essential amino acids

intrinsic factor—A glycoprotein secreted by the parietal cells of the gastric mucosa

jaundice—yellowing of skin and mucous membranes resulting from deposit of bile pigment; usually a symptom of a biliary disease process

kilocalorie—1000 small calories; amount of heat required to raise 1 kilogram of water 1 degree Celsius

large intestine—extending from the ileum to the anus and is approximately 5 ft. in length; includes the cecum and colon.

lipids—fat-related substances not soluble in water (triglycerides, fats, oils, phospholipids, sterols)

malnutrition—condition of excess or deficient nutrient and caloric intake

melena—black, tarry stools

metabolism—process of changing nutrients from food into substances for anabolic or catabolic activity

minerals—elements essential to every cell, naturally occurring in nature, and used by the body in the processes of blood clotting, muscle contraction, and nervous system impulse conduction

obesity—excess body weight 20 to 30 percent above average for gender, age, and height, with abnormal amounts of body fat

overweight—general term for early stage of excess body weight above standard for gender, age, and height

peristalsis—rhythmic, involuntary, wave-like motion in the hollow tubes of

the body that assists the passage of contents

polyps—fingerlike growths on the mucous membranes throughout the body

portal hypertension—condition of increased blood flow pressure through the blood vessels of the liver (portal circulation), often caused by cirrhosis of the liver or compression of the hepatic blood vessels

proctology—medical practice specializing in disorders of the rectum and anus

protein—food component composed of amino acids; provides a source of energy and assists in building and renewing body tissues

saturated fats—fats derived from animal sources that are solid at room temperature

small intestine—starting from the duodenum to the large intestine; includes the jejunum and ileum.

total parenteral nutrition—nutrition ingested by means other than oral intake

triglycerides—chief form of fat found in foods

unsaturated fats—fats derived from plant sources that are liquid at room temperature

upper gastrointestinal tract—oral cavity (mouth), pharynx, esophagus, duodenum, and stomach

vitamins—components required for metabolism, growth, and development

Abbreviations

BMI—body mass index

DGA—Dietary Guidelines for Americans

DHHS—Department of Health and Human Services

ERCP—endoscopic retrograde cholangiopancreatography

FNB—Food Nutrition Board

GI—gastrointestinal

HDL—high-density lipoproteins

LDL—low-density lipoproteins

LGI—lower gastrointestinal

LLQ—left lower quadrant

LUQ—left upper quadrant

N & V—nausea and vomiting

RDA—recommended dietary allowance

RLQ—right lower quadrant

RUQ—right upper quadrant

S & S—signs and symptoms

TPN—total parenteral nutrition

UGI—upper gastrointestinal

USDA—U.S. Department of Agriculture

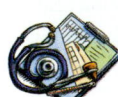

The Medical Assistant's Role in the Gastroenterology Office

Obtaining and recording the patient's medical history and vital signs are routine and essential functions of the medical assistant in the **gastroenterology** or **proctology** medical office. The MA will need to be familiar with the anatomy of the GI tract as well as the regions of the abdomen. Medical assistants will record specific symptoms as reported by the patient. Assisting the physician as necessary during examinations and procedures is a routine function, along with instructing the patient in the removal of necessary clothing and providing a gown and drape. The MA will also arrange appointments for diagnostic tests and procedures and provide patient instruction concerning dietary guidelines and the collection of specimens. MAs should be aware of community resources for gastroenterology patients such as cancer screening, food pantries, and **colostomy** support.

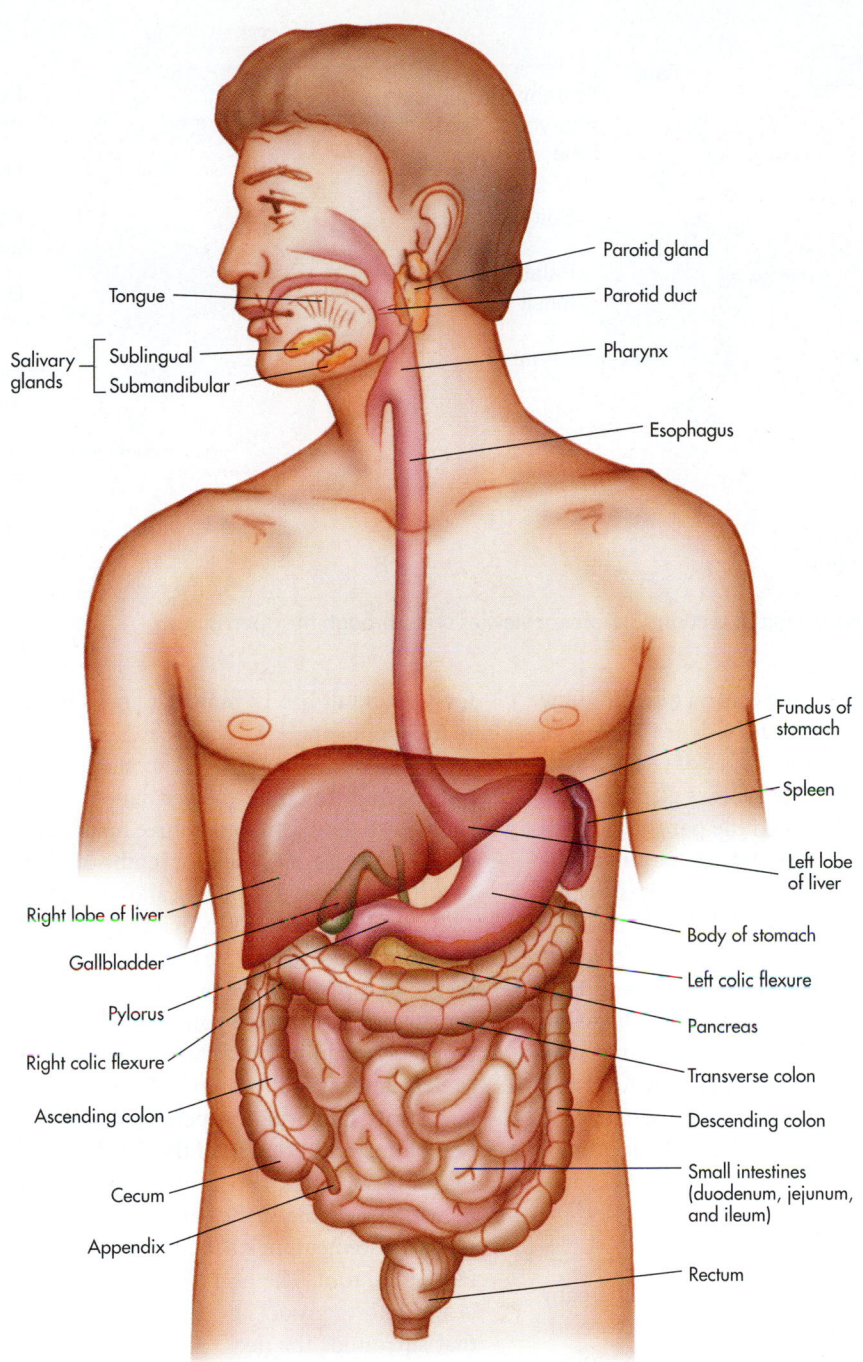

Figure 42-1 ◆ The digestive system.

The Anatomy and Physiology of the Gastrointestinal System

The gastrointestinal (**GI**) system, or digestive tract, is composed of the **alimentary canal** and accessory organs (Figure 42-1 ◆). The alimentary canal, a tubelike structure, begins with the **upper gastrointestinal tract (UGI),** or upper digestive tract.

The Upper Gastrointestinal Tract (UGI)

The UGI includes the mouth, pharynx, esophagus, stomach, and duodenum.

Mouth

The mouth is the cavity formed by the palate (roof), the lips and cheeks on the sides, and the tongue on the floor (see Figure 42-2 ◆). The oral cavity (the mouth) contains the teeth and the salivary glands. The cheeks form the lateral walls and are continuous with the lips. The vestibule includes the space between the cheeks and the teeth. The gingivae (gums) surround the neck of the teeth, helping to hold the teeth in place. The hard and soft palates form a roof for the oral cavity, and the tongue is connected to the floor of the mouth by the lingual frenulum. The tongue is made of skeletal muscle and is covered with mucous membrane. The tongue can be divided

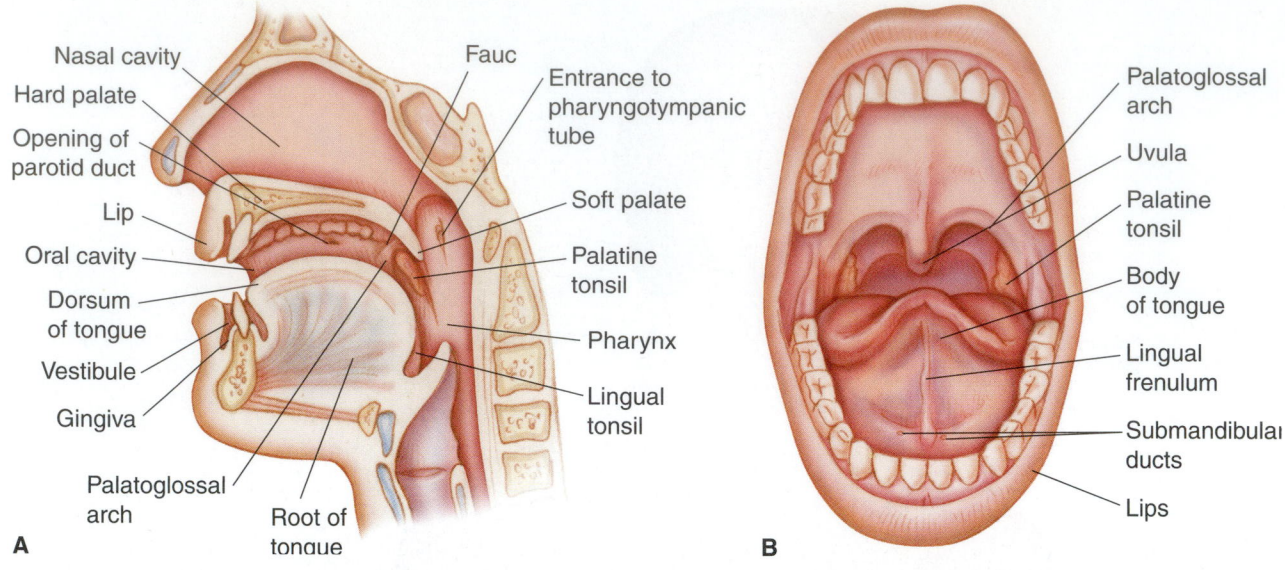

Figure 42-2 ◆ The oral cavity: (A) Sagittal section. (B) Anterior view as seen through the open mouth.

into the rear portion called the root, the central body, and the pointed tip. Papillae (elevations) and taste buds are located on the surface of the tongue. There are four types of taste buds—sweet, salt, sour, and bitter. Three pairs of salivary glands secrete saliva into the oral cavity. They are called the parotid, sublingual, and submandibular glands. The posterior margins of the soft palate support the muscular pharyngeal arches, which function in swallowing and phonation, and the uvula—the dangling tissue hanging down from the center of the pharyngeal arches. The line formed by the pharyngeal arches and the uvula separates the oral cavity from the pharynx. Digestion begins in the mouth with the process of mastication (chewing) and the secretion of saliva, which moistens the food and starts the chemical breakdown of food. The combination of the chewing action and the saliva helps to form the food into a **bolus** (ball) for swallowing.

Teeth

Humans have two sets of teeth: 28 deciduous teeth (the baby teeth) and 32 permanent teeth (see Figure 42-3 ◆). The 28 deciduous teeth include 8 incisors, 4 canines (cuspids), and 8 molars. The permanent teeth include 8 incisors, 4 canines, 8 premolars, and 12 molars. The incisors are so named because of their sharp, cutting edge used for biting food. The incisors are the four front teeth of the dental arch. The upper incisors are larger and stronger than the lower ones.

The canine teeth are also known as the cuspids. These teeth have their roots stuck deeply into the bones of the jaw. The upper canines are also known as the "eye teeth" and are larger than the lower canines. The lower canines are also known as the "stomach teeth."

The premolar teeth are situated lateral to, and behind, the canine teeth. They are also known as the bicuspid teeth and are smaller and shorter than the canine teeth. There are four premolars in each arch. The molar teeth are the largest teeth in the permanent set and are adapted to grinding and pounding

food. An adult has 12 molars, 6 in each arch, placed posterior to the premolars.

The deciduous teeth are smaller than the permanent teeth, but generally resemble the permanent teeth on a smaller scale.

Each tooth consists of three main portions: the crown (the part above the gum); the root (embedded in the gums); and the neck, the part between the root and the crown (see Figure 42-4 ◆). The root of each tooth sits in a bony socket called the alveolus. Collagen fibers of the periodontal ligament extend from the dentin of the root to the bone of the alveolus, creating a strong articulation known as a gomphosis (that binds the teeth to the bony sockets in the maxillary bone and mandible). A layer of cementum covers the dentin of the root, providing protection and firmly anchoring the periodontal ligament. The solid portion of the tooth consists of the dentin, which forms the bulk of the tooth, and the enamel, which covers the exposed part of the crown. The enamel is the hardest and most compact part of the tooth. The cementum is a thin layer of bone, deposited on the surface of the root. The neck of the tooth is the part between the crown and the root. The gingiva is the soft tissue of the gum that surrounds the neck. A shallow groove called the gingival sulcus surrounds the neck of each tooth.

Teeth erupt from the gums when there is sufficient calcification for the tooth to be able to tolerate the stress that it will be subjected to later on. Deciduous teeth erupt from the gums starting at about 7 months and finishing at about age 2 1/2. The permanent teeth erupt at about the following ages:

First molars	6th to 7th year
Two central incisors	7th to 8th year
Two lateral incisors	8th to 9th year
First premolars	10th to 11th year
Second premolars	10th to 12th year
Canines	11th to 12th year
Second molars	12th to 13th year
Third molars	17th to 21st year

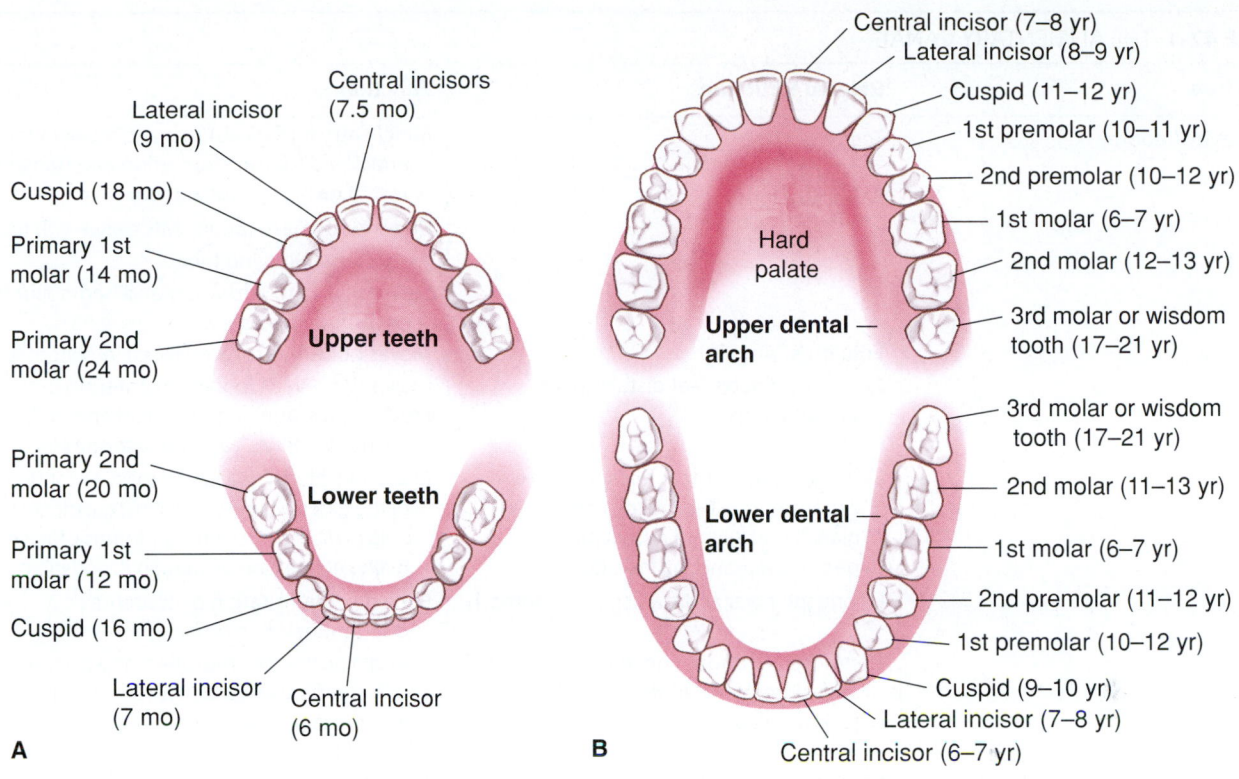

Figure 42-3 ◆ Deciduous and permanent teeth: (A) Deciduous teeth, with the age at eruption given in months. (B) Permanent teeth, with the age at eruption given in years.

Pharynx

The pharynx lies posterior to the mouth and is the beginning of the tube leading to the stomach. The pharynx is used by both the respiratory system and the digestive system. Both the larynx and the esophagus begin in the pharynx. Anything that is swallowed passes through the pharynx into the esophagus reflexively. Muscular constructions move the ball of food into the esophagus while closing the trachea to prevent food from entering the trachea.

Esophagus

The esophagus is a collapsible tube, about 10 inches long, that starts at the pharynx and ends at the stomach. Food is carried down the esophagus by a series of muscular contractions called

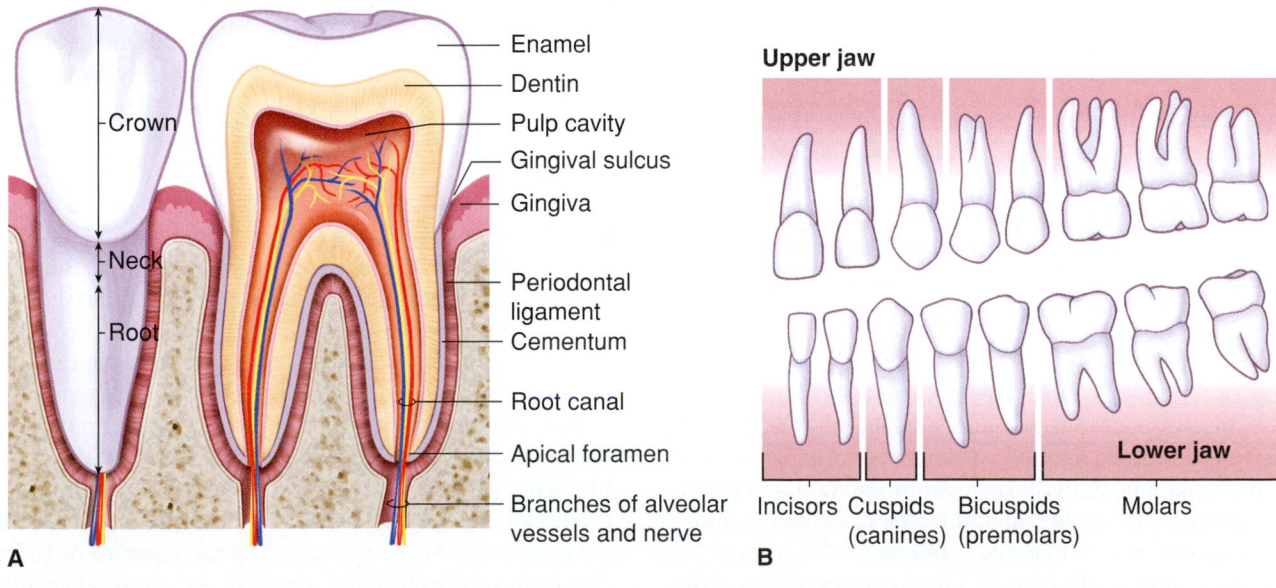

Figure 42-4 ◆ Teeth: (A) A diagrammatic section through a typical adult tooth. (B) The adult teeth.

TABLE 42-1 THE ALIMENTARY CANAL

Structure	Related Structures	Function
Oral cavity (mouth)	Teeth Tongue Salivary glands	Initial entry into digestive tract; receives food and liquid for transformation and transport to rest of gastrointestinal tract. Chew food (mastication). Mix saliva with food. Assists in swallowing food. Secrete saliva to add water and begin digestion of carbohydrates.
Esophagus	Epiglottis Cardiac sphincter—at distal aspect of esophagus	Moves bolus (masticated food) into stomach. Closes to prevent food from entering bronchi. Prevents passage of gastric acid and other gastric contents back into esophagus.
Stomach	Muscular walls contain folds (rugae) for expansion; gastric mucosa contains glands that secrete hydrochloric acid, pepsinogen, and intrinsic factor Pyloric sphincter at distal aspect of stomach	Mixes and dilutes swallowed mass as continuation of the digestive process. Acidic gastric secretions help in digestion of protein. Intrinsic factor makes absorption of Vitamin B_{12} possible. Prevents regurgitation of contents of duodenum into stomach.
Small intestine	Composed of duodenum (which contains ampulla of Vater at proximal junction), jejunum, ileum	Absorbs nutrients. Emulsifies fat with the help of bile and digests carbohydrates, fat (lipids), and protein with the help of pancreatic enzymes.
Large intestine (also known as colon)	Composed of cecum, ascending colon, transverse colon, descending colon, sigmoid colon	Absorbs water and electrolytes.
Rectum	Terminates at anus at body surface	Stores waste for defecation.

peristalsis. These wave-like contractions will move the bolus of food along through the entire digestive system.

Stomach

The stomach is a large sac-like organ that holds food for the beginning of the digestive process. The stomach holds about 1 to 1.5 liters of food and fluid at a time. The stomach secretes hydrochloric acid and gastric juices to convert food into a semiliquid state to be passed into the small intestine for further digestion.

Duodenum

The first 12 inches of the small intestine is the duodenum. It is the first part of the small intestine, and it connects the stomach to the second 8 feet of small intestine, the jejunum. The duodenum is where most chemical digestion takes place, and it is largely responsible for the breakdown of food in the small intestine.

The Lower Gastrointestinal Tract (LGI)

The next portion, called the lower gastrointestinal tract (**LGI**) or lower digestive tract, includes the small intestine, large intestine, cecum, appendix, sigmoid portion, rectum, and **anus.** The **small intestine** consists of the duodenum, jejunum, and ileum. The **large intestine** is made up of the cecum, ascending colon, transverse colon, descending colon, and sigmoid regions of the colon, terminating in the rectum. The accessory organs of the GI system are the pancreas, liver, gallbladder, and connecting

ducts. The structures of the GI system and their functions are summarized in Table 42-1.

The alimentary canal is composed of four layers: the mucosa, submucosa (containing the main blood vessels of the GI tract), mucularis, and serosa (Figure 42-5 ◆). The outer surface of the stomach and intestines is covered and protected by a serosal-type surface called the parietal peritoneum. The peritoneal surface next to the GI organs is referred to as the visceral peritoneum. Blood is supplied to the GI system by the upper and lower mesenteric arteries and is drained away by the portal system.

The liver performs several functions. One primary function is assisting in the metabolism of proteins, fats, and carbohydrates. The liver removes nutrients from the blood, and during a process called glycogenesis, it stores glucose as glycogen and converts glycogen as needed into glucose. In another process called glyconeogenesis, the liver stores fat and protein for conversion into glucose. The liver also helps in the formation of clotting factors and blood plasma proteins as well as in the detoxification of drugs and some toxic substances.

The biliary tract comprises the organs and ducts involved in the secretion, storage, and transport of bile and digestive enzymes to the duodenum (Figure 42-6 ◆). The liver secretes bile, which functions in the emulsification of fats (lipids). The bile leaves the liver via the common hepatic duct to be stored in the gallbladder. When stimulated by the presence of fat in the duodenum, the gallbladder contracts and releases bile into the cystic duct. The cystic duct and the hepatic duct join to form

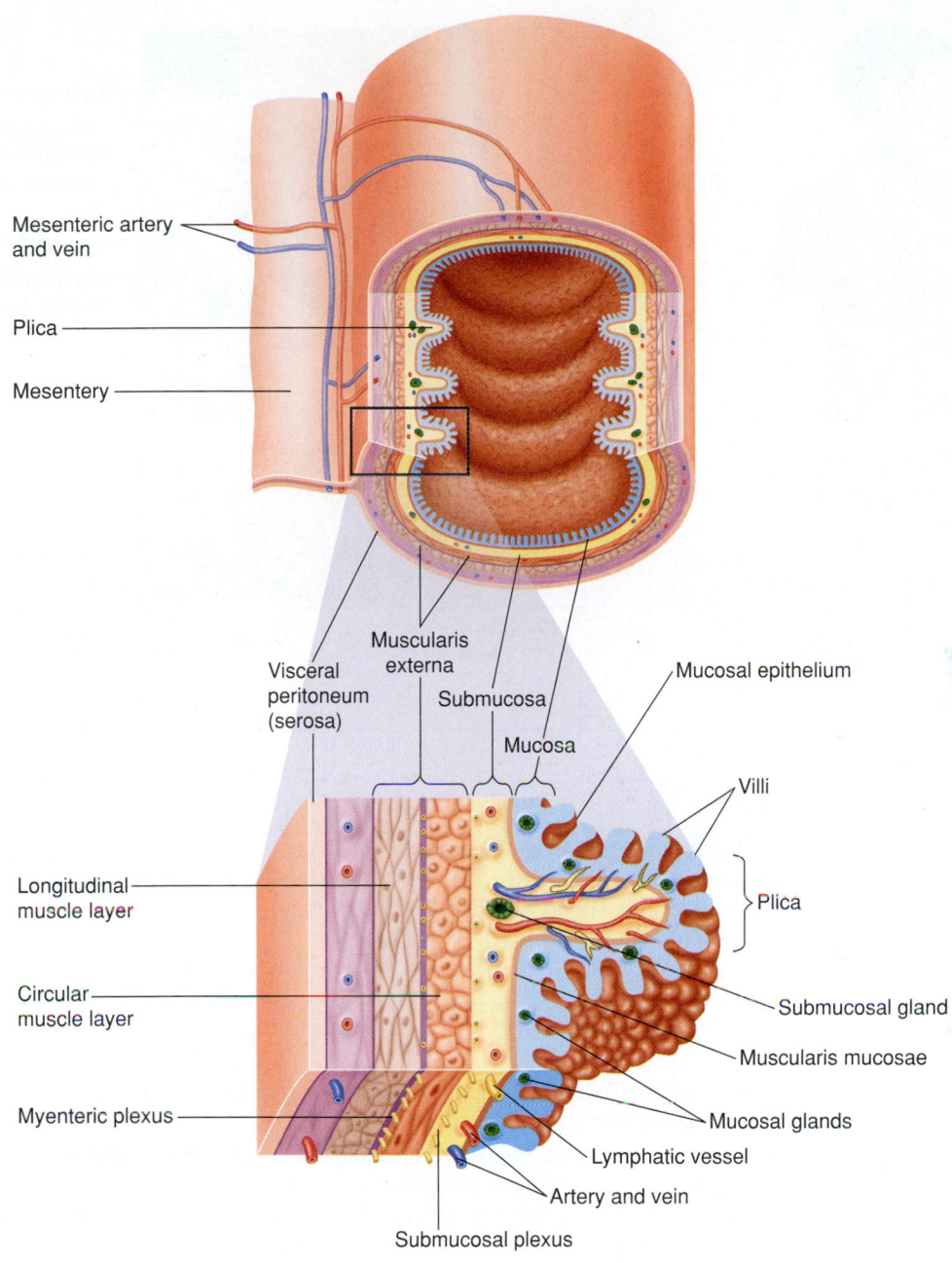

Figure 42-5 ◆ Mucosal surface of the small intestine.

the common bile duct, which empties into the duodenum. Pancreatic enzymes are also released through the common bile duct into the duodenum at an opening called the ampulla of Vater. The components of the biliary tract and their functions are listed in Table 42-2.

The Functions of the Gastrointestinal System

The major functions of the GI system are digestion and **alimentation,** which provide nourishment for the body, and the **elimination** of the waste products of digestion. This process is divided into the following steps:

- Ingestion: Food is taken through the mouth.

- Mastication (chewing): The initial, mechanical breaking up of food starts in the mouth with the teeth, mandible, maxilla, cheeks, tongue, and salivary glands. The resulting food mass is called a bolus.
- Deglutition (swallowing): This process involves the tongue, pharynx, and esophagus. Peristalsis begins in the esophagus.
- Digestion: Mastication or chewing is the first step of digestion and is the process by which food is crushed and ground by teeth. As chewing continues, the food is chemically broken down into substances that can be absorbed into the bloodstream. This process begins in the mouth when the salivary glands release amylase, which begins the digestion of starches, and progresses to the stomach,

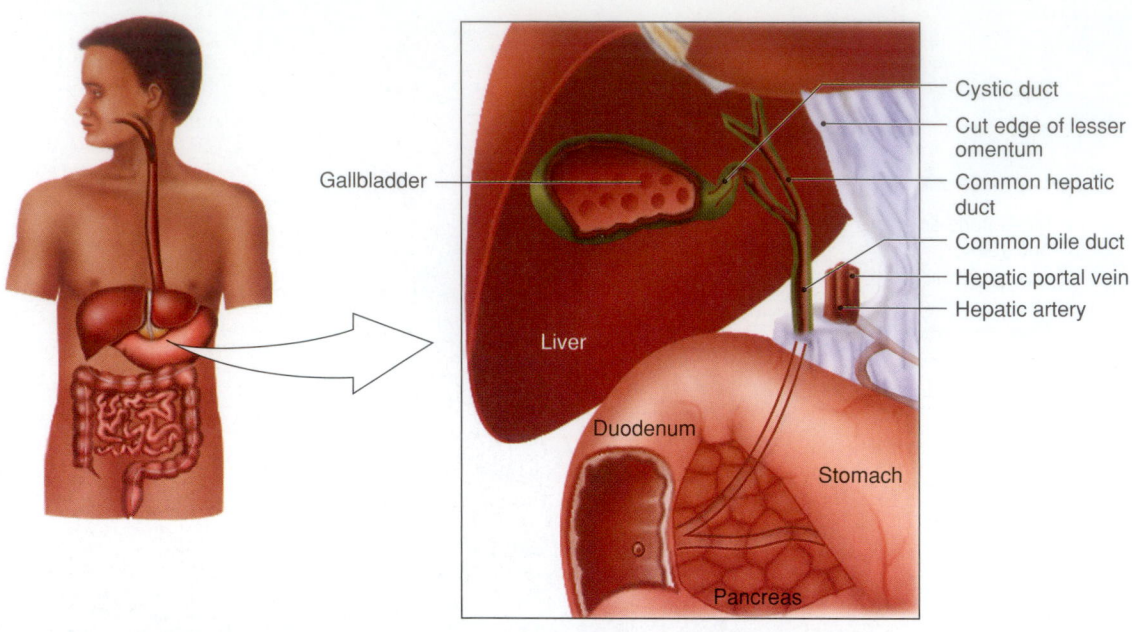

Figure 42-6 ◆ The gallbladder.

TABLE 42-2 THE BILIARY TRACT	
Accessory Organ	**Function**
Liver	■ Manufactures bile for emulsification of fat (lipids) ■ Stores glucose as glycogen and converts glycogen as needed into glucose (glycogenesis) ■ Stores fat and protein for conversion into glucose (glyconeogenesis) ■ Detoxifies drugs and some toxic substances ■ Helps in the formation of clotting factors and blood plasma proteins
Common hepatic duct	Joins with the common cystic duct to form the common bile duct; carries bile from the liver to the common hepatic duct
Gallbladder	Stores bile from the liver
Common bile duct	Exits from the gallbladder and joins the pancreatic duct to deliver bile and pancreatic enzymes to the duodenum
Pancreas	■ Manufactures amylase for carbohydrate digestion, lipase for fat (lipids) digestion, trypsinogen, chymotripsinogen to digest proteins ■ Produces insulin, which transports glucose from the bloodstream into body cells for metabolism
Ampulla of Vater	Hepatopancreatic duct opening into the duodenum; releases bile and pancreatic enzymes from common bile duct into duodenum

where hydrochloric acid and **gastric** enzymes (pepsin, gastrin, **intrinsic factor**) enter the digestive process. The end product of this process is called **chyme.** In the duodenum, bile for the **emulsification** of **fats** is joined by pancreatic enzymes (lipase and protease) and intestinal enzymes (enterokinase, cholecystokinin, and secretin) to break down **carbohydrates, lipids,** and **proteins.**

■ Absorption: In the small intestine, nutrients from the chemically digested food are absorbed into the bloodstream for transport to body cells. Water, fluids, and **electrolytes** are absorbed mainly in the large intestine.

■ Excretion: Food that has not been digested, miscellaneous secretions, and the excretory products of metabolism are

eliminated from the body through the rectum and anus. This final waste product of digestion is termed **feces.**

Diseases and Disorders of the GI Tract

Diseases of the GI system include inflammatory conditions, obstructive conditions, infectious disorders, disorders due to increased or decreased peristalsis, circulatory and hemorrhagic disorders, congenital disorders, functional disorders, neoplasms, parasitic invasion, and food poisoning (Tables 42-3 and 42-4).

(*text continues on p. 927*)

TABLE 42-3 DISORDERS AND CONDITIONS OF THE GASTROINTESTINAL TRACT

Condition or Disorder	Signs/Symptoms	Area Affected	Diagnosis	Treatment
Abnormal Function				
Constipation	Inability to move bowels, distension of abdomen, abdominal cramping	Small intestine, colon, rectum	Palpation of abdomen, auscultation of abdomen, imaging studies	Laxatives, colonic irrigations, dietary changes
Diarrhea	Loose, watery stools, abdominal cramping	Colon, rectum	Reports of loose, watery stools	Antidiarrheal medications and dietary changes
Paralytic obstruction, also called paralytic ileus	Vomiting, abdominal distension, no bowel movements, severe abdominal pain	Esophagus, stomach, small intestine, colon, rectum	Palpation of abdomen, auscultation of abdomen, imaging studies	Drug therapy, surgical intervention
Vomiting	Expulsion of gastric contents through the mouth	Esophagus, stomach, small intestine	Visual exam, palpation, auscultation, imaging studies	Drug therapy, surgical intervention
Anatomical and Congenital Abnormalities				
Diverticulosis	Abdominal pain, abdominal distension, flatulence, difficulty and pain in defecation; small outpouching of intestinal lining that makes little pockets	Colon	Palpation, auscultation, imaging studies	Dietary changes, increase in roughage and fluids, avoiding seeds, nuts, and foods with skins
Gastroesophageal reflux disease (GERD)	Regurgitation of stomach and duodenal contents up into the esophagus. Usually occurs at night or when patient lies down	Esophagus, stomach, duodenum	Palpation, auscultation, imaging studies	Drug therapy, avoiding lying down for at least one hour after eating, elevating head of bed
Hiatal hernia	Portion of stomach slips up above the diaphragm into thoracic cavity	Esophagus, stomach, diaphragm	Imaging studies	Drug therapy, avoiding lying down for at least one hour after eating, elevating head of bed
Organic obstructions	Mechanical obstructions anywhere in GI tract. May be caused by tumors, strictures, foreign bodies, fecal impactions, adhesions, strangulated hernias	Esophagus, stomach, small intestine, colon, rectum	Visual exam, palpation, auscultation, imaging	Usually surgical intervention to relieve obstruction; fecal impaction may be removed digitally through rectum
Abdominal hernia	Lump appears in abdominal wall that can be painful or painless	Organ or part of an organ (usually the bowel) breaks through weak portion of muscles and membranes of a wall	Visual exam, palpation, auscultation, imaging studies	Surgical intervention usually the only way to resolve a hernia
Infections				
Gastroenteritis	Abdominal pain and cramping with or without vomiting and/or diarrhea	Stomach, small intestines, colon; commonly caused by rotavirus and Norwalk virus	Visual examination of individual, palpation and auscultation of abdomen	Drug therapy, hydration, diet modifications until condition improves

continued

TABLE 42-3 DISORDERS AND CONDITIONS OF THE GASTROINTESTINAL TRACT (CONTINUED)

Condition or Disorder	Signs/Symptoms	Area Affected	Diagnosis	Treatment
Infections (*cont.*)				
Enteritis	**N & V,** diarrhea, abdominal cramping, fever, malaise	Caused by invasion of protozoa or bacteria	Patient history, blood and stool cultures	Fluid and electrolyte replacement by mouth or IV therapy; nutritional support; antimicrobial, antinausea, and antiemetic medication; bed rest
Acute appendicitis	Sudden onset of acute pain in lower right quadrant of abdomen	Infection in appendix, causing inflammation, usually caused by bacteria	Palpation of abdomen, positive reaction to pressure on McBurney's point	Surgical excision of appendix to prevent rupture and peritonitis, accompanied by antibiotic therapy
Food Poisoning				
Salmonellosis	Abdominal pain, diarrhea, vomiting, abdominal cramping, fever	Stomach and intestines	Presence of salmonella in stool specimen	Usually resolves within a week; IV therapy may be required
Clostridium botulinum	Initial vomiting or diarrhea, later neurological complications, blurred vision, slurred speech, difficulty swallowing, paralysis, and respiratory failure	GI tract and nervous system	Presence of toxin in blood or stool	Antitoxin and support of systems when necessary
Escherichia coli	Abdominal cramping, vomiting, watery diarrhea possibly containing blood and mucus	GI tract	Presence of *E. coli* in stool specimens	Usually resolves without antibiotic intervention; supportive therapy may be required
Staphylococcus aureus	Severe nausea and vomiting, abdominal cramping, hypotension, reduced body temperature	Upper GI tract	Presence of *S. aureus* in suspected food	Usually resolves but supportive therapy may be required
Inflammation				
Esophagitis	Difficult and/or painful swallowing, heartburn, mouth sores.	Irritation of mucosa caused by chemical sources, infections, or reflux of gastric contents	Visual exam of esophagus, often with a gastroscope	Drug therapy and dietary modification
Gastritis	Pain, vomiting, eructation (belching). Acute: shallow lesions or erosions of gastric lining. Chronic: atrophy of gastric mucosa, mild and chronic inflammation.	Irritation of mucosa lining the stomach, caused by chemical or bacterial sources.	Symptoms aid in diagnosis. Visual exam, palpation, auscultation, imaging studies, often including gastroscopic exam	Drug therapy and dietary modification. Acute gastritis usually self-limiting
Peritonitis	Sudden, severe, general abdominal pain localizing at causal site; cool, clammy skin; possibly N & V and rigidity of abdomen	Inflammation of peritoneum caused by infection or foreign substance entering peritoneal cavity	Auscultation of bowel sounds, abdominal and chest X-rays, blood studies	NPO and nasogastric tube to keep GI tract empty; fluids and electrolytes by IV therapy; aggressive antibiotic therapy; surgery if perforation of GI tract occurs

TABLE 42-3 DISORDERS AND CONDITIONS OF THE GASTROINTESTINAL TRACT (CONTINUED)

Condition or Disorder	Signs/Symptoms	Area Affected	Diagnosis	Treatment
Inflammation (*cont.*)				
Gastric/duodenal ulcer	Abdominal pain, possible bloody emesis or occult blood in the stool, abdominal distension and tenderness	Erosion of gastric or duodenal mucosa with or without bleeding, *H. pylori*	Visual exam, palpation, auscultation, imaging studies, including endoscopic examination (gastroscopy)	Drug therapy, diet modification, stress reduction, surgical intervention if other treatments unsuccessful
Stomatitis	Pain, swelling and redness of the oral mucosa.	Inflammation of tissue in the mouth; may be caused by bacteria, virus or fungus.	Visualization of oral cavity, microbiological smear or culture	Warm water mouth rinses, topical anesthetic for pain, bland or liquid diet; antiseptic mouth washes further irritate condition and should not be used
Proctitis	Feeling of rectal fullness, constant urge to defecate, abdominal cramps, constipation, involuntary straining; pain; blood and mucus in stool	Inflammation of mucosa lining the rectum	Patient history, sigmoidoscopy, biopsy, microbiological smear or culture	Tranquilizers for emotional stress; elimination of laxatives; soothing enemas or suppositories to counteract effects of radiation
Diverticulitis	Abdominal pain, abdominal distension, flatulence, difficulty and pain in defecation	Colon inflammation in small outpouching of intestinal lining, occasionally infection of area	Palpation, auscultation, imaging studies	Dietary changes, increase in roughage and fluids, avoiding seeds, nuts, foods with skins; hydration and antibiotics if infection is present
Regional enteritis (Crohn's disease)	Abdominal pain, abdominal distension, flatulence, watery stools often containing blood, anorexia, weight loss, anemia, fatigue	Usually small intestine and ascending colon of large intestine, with inflammation of mucosa	Patient history, symptoms	There is no cure; antibiotics, corticosteroids, and surgical removal of the affected part
Chronic ulcerative colitis	Abdominal pain, abdominal distension, flatulence, watery stools often containing blood	Usually large intestine with inflammation of mucosa	Symptoms, patient history, colonoscopy	Antibiotics, corticosteroids, pain medication, possible surgical removal of affected area
Malignancies				
Carcinoma of the lip and tongue	Lesion on tongue or lip that does not heal; may be painful or painless	Tongue, lip, or mucosa inside mouth	Visual examination and biopsy	Surgical removal, possible radiation
Cancer of the esophagus	Lesion on esophagus that causes difficulty swallowing, spitting up of blood; may be asymptomatic	Esophagus may become obstructed, causing inability to swallow	Visual examination with endoscope, biopsy	Surgical removal, possible radiation and chemotherapy
Stomach cancer	Lesion in stomach that may cause pain or be painless, vomiting with mucus and blood	Usually on lesser curve of stomach; may cause obstruction in addition to pain	Tenderness in upper abdomen, possible pain, auscultation and palpation of upper abdomen, endoscopic exam with biopsy, ultrasound of stomach	Surgical removal, possible chemotherapy and radiation

continued

TABLE 42-3 DISORDERS AND CONDITIONS OF THE GASTROINTESTINAL TRACT (CONTINUED)

Condition or Disorder	Signs/Symptoms	Area Affected	Diagnosis	Treatment
Malignancies (*cont.*)				
Colon cancer	Weight loss, presence of blood in stool or melena, changes in character of stool, fatigue	Colon	Discovery of polyps during colonoscopy, occult blood in stool, imaging studies, confirmation by biopsy	Surgical removal of involved area, possible chemotherapy and radiation, possible colostomy
Rectal cancer	Weight loss, presence of blood in stool or melena, changes in character of stool, fatigue	Rectum	Proctoscopic exam, sigmoidoscopy, imaging studies, biopsy	Surgical removal, possible chemotherapy and radiation, possible colostomy
Vascular-Related Conditions				
Esophageal varices	Abdominal pain and distension; in emergency conditions, presence of bloody emesis	Blood vessels of esophagus, often resulting from **portal hypertension**	Endoscopic examination	Ice water lavage and epigastric tamponade with NN tube anchored by esophageal balloon
Hemorrhoids	Rectal and lower back pain, bloody stools	May be internal or external (protruding)	May be result of obesity, pregnancy, straining at stools, hard dry stools	Stool softeners, drug therapy, surgical excision

Imaging studies can include MRI, ultrasound, CT, PET, or X-ray, depending on the needs of the physician. The physician will order the study based on patient symptoms, suspected diagnosis, and location. Other factors may include patient allergies, claustrophobia, and availability. MRI is used to view alterations of living tissues, such as tumors or structural abnormalities in locations such as the lungs or brain. MRI gives multiple views or "cuts" as it passes over the body. The images produced by an MRI can be thought of as slices in a loaf of bread, with the entire body being the loaf of bread and each slice being a single MRI image. Ultrasound is commonly used during pregnancy to obtain an image of the fetus and its internal structures. Ultrasound is also used to view the structure, size, and location of internal organs, muscles, and tendons. Positron emission tomography (PET) scans are used to create a 3D image of the body, including the organs and other structures. PET scans allow physicians to see anatomic blood flow, or lack thereof, to different organs. X-rays are most commonly used to view the bony structures of the body but can also be useful in identifying abnormal conditions in soft tissues. Some organs such as the gallbladder create stones that can be identified by X-ray because the gallbladder is normally radiolucent and the gallstones appear radiopaque.

TABLE 42-4 DISEASES AND CONDITIONS OF THE DIGESTIVE ACCESSORY ORGANS

Condition or Disorder	Signs/Symptoms	Area Affected	Diagnosis	Treatment
Abnormal Function Cholelithiasis (gallstones)	Pain in right upper quadrant radiating to right shoulder blade, nausea and vomiting, bile-colored emesis and stool, **jaundice**	Stones may be present in gallbladder and/or in common bile duct	**S & S,** physical exam, tenderness in right upper quadrant, imaging studies including cholecystogram and ultrasound of gallbladder	Pain medication, surgical intervention (laparoscopy or endoscopy) to remove stones
Infections Hepatitis A (infectious)	Jaundice, anorexia, fatigue, weakness, fever, joint pain, enlarged liver, lymph node involvement	Liver and blood	Virus or antibodies in the blood identified; liver function tests, possible liver biopsy	Immune globulin vaccination upon exposure; bed rest, low-carbohydrate diet; individual symptoms treated
Hepatitis B (serum)	Jaundice, anorexia, nausea and vomiting, general malaise, pruritic rash, enlarged liver, dark-colored urine, swollen joints	Liver and blood, body fluids	Virus or antibodies in the blood identified; liver function tests, possible liver biopsy	Prevention by vaccination is primary goal; bed rest, supportive treatment of symptoms

TABLE 42-4 DISEASES AND CONDITIONS OF THE DIGESTIVE ACCESSORY ORGANS (CONTINUED)

Condition or Disorder	Signs/Symptoms	Area Affected	Diagnosis	Treatment
Infections (*cont.*)				
Hepatitis C (non A, non B)	Acute onset consisting of fever, chills, nausea and vomiting, malaise	Liver and blood	Virus or antibodies in the blood identified; liver function tests, possible liver biopsy	There is no cure; rest, well-balanced diet; interferon alpha to treat symptoms; additional symptom treatment
Inflammation				
Acute pancreatitis	Severe pain and tenderness in epigastric region and over pancreas, nausea and vomiting	Pancreas, ampulla of Vater, common bile duct, duodenum	S & S, physical exam, upper abdominal tenderness, imaging studies, ultrasound of pancreas	Pain medication, antibiotics, hydration, supportive therapy
Cholecystitis	Inflammation of gallbladder caused by gallbladder disease or gallstones	Gallbladder	S & S, physical exam, ultrasound or CT scan, stool test for fat	Surgery
Cirrhosis	Anorexia, weight loss, nausea and vomiting, indigestion, abdominal distention, dependent edema (edema of any body part lower than the heart regardless of vertical or horizontal body position) and ascites, jaundiced skin, greater tendency to bleed (including nosebleeds and bruising); untreated advanced cirrhosis leads to hepatic failure and death	Liver, usually caused by alcoholism; may also be caused by some forms of hepatitis, malnutrition parasites, toxic chemicals	Hard, palpable, enlarged liver, elevated liver enzymes and bilirubin levels; liver scan and biopsy for confirmation	Prevention of further damage by treating cause; rest, vitamins, minerals, diuretics, transplant in some cases
Liver cancer	Weight loss, anemia, **hepatomegaly,** pain, jaundice	Liver, usually metastatic from another site	Physical exam, liver scan, biopsy	Surgical removal of as much affected portion as possible, chemotherapy, radiation therapy
Pancreatic cancer	Weight loss, anemia, enlargement of pancreas, pain, nausea and vomiting	Pancreas may be primary site	Physical exam, ultrasonic examination and other imaging studies, biopsy	Surgical removal of as much affected portion as possible, chemotherapy, radiation therapy

Nutrition

Food is required for the growth and repair of body tissues, provides nutrients that regulate body processes, and serves as the fuel for heat production. The basic components of food are carbohydrates, proteins, fats, **minerals, vitamins, fiber,** and water (Table 42-5).

■ Carbohydrates are the body's primary source of energy and are found primarily in breads and cereals, pasta products, rice, fruit, and potatoes.

■ Proteins assist in the building and renewing of body tissues. **Amino acids** are the building blocks of protein. There are eight *essential* amino acids, which cannot be manufactured by the body and must be supplied in the diet. The other eleven amino acids are *nonessential,* which means they can be manufactured internally by the body. A **complete protein** is one that supplies all the essential amino acids; meat, fish, eggs, and other animal products are a common source. Nuts, legumes, whole grains, and other vegetable sources provide **incomplete proteins.**

TABLE 42-5 FOOD CATEGORIES AND FOOD SOURCES

Category	Functions	Sources
Carbohydrates (CHO) ■ Simple sugars ■ Complex carbohydrates (starch) ■ Dietary fiber	■ Supply fuel for energy, metabolism, and all cellular activities ■ Metabolize at a rate of 4 kcal/g ■ Converted by the body for use as glucose ■ Fiber/roughage provides bulk for elimination of intestinal wastes	■ Simple sugars: table sugar, corn and maple syrup, honey, candy, molasses, milk, fruits, sweets (cakes, cookies, pastries) ■ Complex carbohydrates: legumes, potatoes, seeds, vegetables, grain and grain products, cereal, whole-grain breads, pasta, corn, barley, rice ■ Fiber: bran, fruits, vegetables, dried fruits, beans, oatmeal, seeds, whole-grain breads and cereals
Fats (lipids)	■ Concentrated form of fuel; secondary energy source ■ Metabolize at the rate of 9 kcal/g ■ Necessary for essential fatty acids and absorption of fat-soluble vitamins ■ As adipose tissue, provides protection, insulates body, regulates temperature, and supports body organs	■ Saturated fats: animal sources (dairy products, eggs, fish, meat), coconut and palm oils ■ Unsaturated fats: polyunsaturated fats (fish, walnuts, corn, soybeans, sunflower seeds, safflower oil) and monounsaturated fats (fowl, almonds, pecans, cashews, peanuts, olive oil, avocados)
Protein	■ Builds and repairs tissues ■ Aids in body's defense against disease ■ Provides energy and regulates body secretions and fluids ■ Metabolizes at the rate of 4 kcal/g	■ Complete proteins: beef, chicken, poultry, fish, eggs, dairy products ■ Incomplete proteins: rice, whole grains, legumes, soybeans, nuts, soy flour
Vitamins: ■ Water soluble: B_1, B_2, B_6, B_{12}, niacin, folic acid, biotin, C ■ Fat soluble: A, D, E, K	■ Regulate the formation of body tissues ■ Aid in food metabolism ■ Prevent diseases resulting from nutritional deficiency	See Table 42-6
Minerals: ■ Calcium ■ Chlorine ■ Magnesium ■ Phosphorus ■ Potassium ■ Sodium Trace elements: ■ Iron ■ Copper ■ Chromium ■ Iodine ■ Fluorine ■ Manganese ■ Zinc ■ Selenium ■ Cobalt	■ Required in small amounts for electrolytes, water, and acid-base balance ■ Essential component of enzymes ■ Involved in regulation of heart rhythm, blood clotting, neuromuscular activities, and the building and maintenance of bones, muscles, and teeth	See Table 42-6
Water	■ Transport vehicle for nutrients, hormones, antibodies, and metabolic waste ■ Helps regulate body temperature ■ Solvent for most biochemical reactions ■ Lubricant for joints and mucous membranes	■ Healthy diet, eight glasses of water daily

Strict vegetarians, or vegans, must combine certain foods—such as beans and rice—to ensure an adequate intake of complete proteins.

■ Fats are also a source of energy, and fatty acids aid in growth and development. Saturated, unsaturated, and polyunsaturated fatty acids are components of **triglycerides.** The amount of hydrogen holding the fatty acids together determines the degree of saturation. **Saturated fats** such as butter, with the greatest hydrogen hold, are solid and are usually derived from animal sources.

Unsaturated fats, with the lowest hydrogen hold, are softer or liquid and usually come from plant sources. Polyunsaturated fats from such sources as fish and corn, soybean, and safflower oils contain two or more unfilled hydrogen bonds. Monounsaturated fats in avocados, peanuts, and olive oil contain one unfilled hydrogen bond. Maintaining a diet lower in saturated fats and higher in unsaturated fats is one way to lower the risk of heart disease.

Lipoproteins are simple proteins that combine with lipid components, including **cholesterol,** phospholipids, and triglycerides. High-density lipoprotein (**HDL**) and low-density lipoprotein (**LDL**) are transport media that carry fats in the bloodstream. LDLs transport fats manufactured in the liver to body cells, while HDLs transport fats from body cells to the liver for disposal. A diagnostic test called a lipid profile provides information concerning LDL and HDL ratios as an assessment for possible heart and vascular disease.

■ Water, an element in almost every body process, is essential to life. The body can sustain life longer without food than without water. The body is composed of approximately 70% water. Water regulates body temperature, lubricates the joints, carries nutrition to and waste materials from body cells, and aids in other body processes. A healthy body maintains a normal balance of intake and excretion of water through the function of the circulatory, renal, and endocrine systems. Water is excreted from the body by urination, perspiration, respiration, and through the GI tract. When excessive water is lost through vomiting, diarrhea, bleeding, or burns, electrolyte imbalances may occur to a life-threatening degree. When body systems do not function properly and retain fluids, edema and possibly pulmonary congestion result. Other than plain water, sources of water include liquids such as juice, milk, coffee, tea, fruits, vegetables, broths, and soups. Drinking six to eight glasses of water daily is recommended to maintain water balance.

■ Vitamins are organic compounds required in small amounts for metabolism, growth, and development (Table 42-6). They

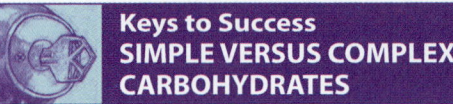

Keys to Success
SIMPLE VERSUS COMPLEX CARBOHYDRATES

Simple carbohydrates are sugars found in natural sources such as fruit and honey as well as in candy and other sweets. Complex carbohydrates are the starches in foods such as bread, potatoes, and whole grains. Ultimately, all carbohydrates are digested into simple sugars that are used by the body for cellular energy and as fuel for body activities. Digesting complex carbohydrates into glucose takes longer than digesting simple carbohydrates. Eating simple carbohydrates can give you a quick "energy boost" but can also lead to a rapid drop in blood glucose levels when the energy has been "spent." Ingestion of simple carbohydrates without complex carbohydrates can result in fluctuating blood glucose and energy levels. For diabetic patients, it is sometimes necessary to ingest simple carbohydrates to raise blood glucose levels quickly, but a combination of simple and complex carbohydrates not only allows levels to rise to normal quickly but also supplies a developing and longer-term source of glucose.

are classified as fat-soluble (A, D, E, and K) and water-soluble (B complex and C). Antioxidants such as lycopene, lutein, beta carotene (a form of Vitamin A), and vitamins A, C, and E are substances believed to prevent cellular damage that may lead to cancer, atherosclerosis, and other conditions.

■ Minerals play an important role in specific regulatory processes and in tissue development and repair. They are essential to every cell, occur naturally in nature, and are used by the body in the processes of blood clotting, muscle contraction, and nervous system impulse conduction. The term *trace element* is applied to any mineral required in very small amounts.

■ Dietary fiber—carbohydrates that the body does not digest—promotes intestinal health and helps to prevent

TABLE 42-6 VITAMINS AND MINERALS

Vitamins/Nutrient	Source	Functional Deficiency	Toxicity	Recommended Dietary Allowances (RDA)[a]
Vitamin A (carotene): necessary for formation and maintenance of skin, mucous membranes, teeth and hair, and normal vision	Egg yolk, fish-liver oils, liver, green leafy or yellow vegetables, yellow and orange fruits, dairy products	Night blindness, fatigue, scaly skin	Headache, skin peeling, bone thickening, liver and spleen enlargement	5000 IU/day
Vitamin B₁ (thiamine): carbohydrate metabolism, nerve cell function, heart muscle function	Dried yeast, whole grains, meat (liver and pork), nuts, enriched cereals, potatoes, legumes	Beriberi, fatigue, mental confusion		1.5 mg/day

continued

TABLE 42-6 VITAMINS AND MINERALS (CONTINUED)

Vitamins/Nutrient	Source	Functional Deficiency	Toxicity	Recommended Dietary Allowances (RDA)[a]
Vitamin B$_2$ (riboflavin): releases energy during protein metabolism	Milk, cheese, eggs, liver, enriched cereals, almonds	Anemia, dermatosis, skin cracks		1.2 mg/day
Vitamin B$_6$ (group): nitrogen and protein metabolism, assists in building body tissue	Dried yeast, liver, whole grain cereals, fish, legumes, bananas, avocados	Anemia, seborrheic dermatitis, nervous system disorders, convulsions, skin cracks	Nerve damage	2 mg/day
Vitamin B$_{12}$ (cyanocobalamin): nervous system function, fat and protein metabolism	Milk products, seafood, meat, liver, cheese	Pernicious anemia, fatigue, nervousness		6 mcg/day
Niacin (nicotinic acid): carbohydrate, fat, and protein metabolism	Dried yeast, fish, liver, meat, legumes, enriched cereals, eggs, peanuts, and poultry	Pellagra, dermatosis, glossitis, CNS dysfunction, fatigue		20 mg/day
Vitamin C (ascorbic acid): needed to build bones, muscles, blood vessels, and connective tissue; aids in iron absorption	Citrus fruits, tomatoes, broccoli, potatoes, cabbage, green peppers, berries, and strawberries	Scurvy, loose teeth, hemorrhoids, gingivitis, fatigue	Nausea and diarrhea	60 mg/day
Vitamin D: necessary for calcium and phosphorus absorption, bone and tooth development and maintenance; helps maintain nervous system and heart muscle action	Fortified milk, butter, margarine, eggs, fish-liver oils, liver, sunlight	Rickets, tetany, loss of bone calcium	Diarrhea, weight loss, renal failure	400 IU/day
Vitamin E: protects blood cell membranes, body tissues and fatty acids from destruction	Vegetable oil, wheat germ, margarine, egg yolks, leafy vegetables, legumes, cereals	Anemia, nerve damage, RBC hemolysis, muscle damage		30 IU/day
Vitamin K: normal blood coagulation, prothrombin formation	Leafy vegetables, liver, pork, vegetable oils, fruit, dairy	Hemorrhage in newborn and in person taking blood thinner		No RDA for Vitamin A
Biotin: metabolism of protein, carbohydrates, and fats	Yeast, liver, kidney, egg yolks, nuts, legumes, cauliflower	Dermatitis, glossitis		0.5 mg/day
Folic acid: RBC production	Dried legumes, green leafy vegetables, organ meats	Anemia, GI disorders, mouth cracks		0.4 mg/day
Pantothenic acid: aids in energy release from carbohydrates and fats	Whole grains, meats, vegetables, fruits, legumes	Muscle cramps, fatigue, vomiting		10 mg/day
Calcium: bone and tooth formation, muscle contractility, blood coagulation, myocardial conduction, neuromuscular function	Milk and milk products, meat, fish, eggs, beans, cereals, fruits, vegetables, tofu, fortified orange juice	Hypocalcemia, tetany, neuromuscular excitability, osteoporosis	Hypercalcemia, kidney stones, renal failure	800 mg/day

TABLE 42-6 VITAMINS AND MINERALS (CONTINUED)

Vitamins/Nutrient	Source	Functional Deficiency	Toxicity	Recommended Dietary Allowances (RDA)[a]
Chromium: part of glucose tolerance factor (CTF)	Brewer's yeast and widely distributed in other foods	Impaired glucose tolerance in malnour- ished children and diabetics		No RDA
Cobalt: part of vitamin B_{12} molecule	Green leafy vegetables	Anemia in children		20 mg/day
Copper: enzyme component	Oysters, organ meats, nuts, dried legumes, whole grain cereals	Anemia in malnourished children		0.3 mg/kg per day
Fluorine: bone and tooth formation	Coffee, tea, fluoridated water	Dental caries	Mottling and pitting of permanent teeth	No RDA
Iodine: thyroxine (T_4) and triiodothyronine (T_3) formation, necessary for energy formation	Seafood, iodized salt, dairy products	Goiter, cretinism	Myxedema	150 mcg/day
Iron: hemoglobin, enzymes	Soybean flour, kidney, beef, liver, beans, peaches	Anemia		30 mg/day
Magnesium: bone and tooth formation, nerve conduction, muscle contractility, enzyme activity	Green leafy vegetables, cereals, nuts, wheat bran, grains, seafood, chocolate	Neuromuscular irritability, weakness	Hypotension, respiratory failure, cardiac disturbances	280 mg/day
Phosphorus: bone and tooth formation, acid–base formation	Milk, cheese, meat, fish, poultry, cereals, nuts, legumes	Irritability, weakness, blood cell disorders		300 mg/day
Potassium: muscle activity, nerve transmission, intracellular acid–base balance, water retention	Milk, bananas, kiwi, raisins, vegetables	Hypokalemia, paralysis, cardiac arrhythmia (irregular heartbeat)	Hyperkalemia, paralysis, cardiac arrhythmia	2000 mg/day
Sodium: maintain acid–base balance, muscle contractility, nerve transmission	Meat (beef, pork), cheese sardines, olives, potato chips, table salt	Hyponatremia, muscle cramping	Hypernatremia, coma, confusion, high blood pressure	500 mg/day
Zinc: growth, wound healing component of insulin and enzyme	Vegetables	Growth retardation		30 mg/day

[a]*IU, international units; mg, milligrams; mcg, micrograms.*
Source: Beaman, Nina; Fleming–McPhillips, Lorraine. Pearson's Comprehensive Medical Assisting, *1st Edition, © 2007. Reprinted by permission of Pearson Education, Inc.*

intestinal disease. Fiber is found in food plants, including fruits, vegetables, grains, and legumes. Good sources of dietary fiber include whole-grain products (wheat, barley, oats, brown rice, bran), apples, pears, berries, avocados, carrots, celery, nuts, seeds, and legumes (dried peas, beans, and lentils).

Energy released from the metabolism of proteins, fats, and carbohydrates is measured in units called **kilocalories** (kcal). One kilocalorie is equal to 1,000 small calories (calories as counted in food intake). The amount of energy released through metabolism is 4 kcal per gram of carbohydrate, 4 kcal per gram of protein, and 9 kcal per gram of fat.

The Food Guide Pyramid/MyPyramid Food Guidance System

"We are what we eat" is a statement often made by nutritionists and healthcare providers. How do we decide what makes a nutritious diet? Guidelines have been established by various agencies and organizations, including the American Dietetic Association, the U.S. Department of Agriculture (**USDA**), and the American Home Economics Association.

The Food Guide Pyramid was an educational tool developed by the USDA to help healthy Americans maintain good eating habits. The pyramid recommended eating a specified number of servings of different food groups to meet daily

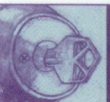

Keys to Success
CONSEQUENCES OF DEHYDRATION

One consequence of dehydration is decreased blood volume. The felt pulse is weaker and described as "thready," and the person is susceptible to hypotension and therefore fainting or falls. The individual may also experience hypotension when sitting or standing abruptly. To compensate, the heart beats faster to circulate blood around the body. Dehydration may also affect kidney function, as the filtering of waste products and production of urine are decreased. Dehydration can be gradual and limited or sudden and severe. Severe dehydration can lead to hypovolemic shock and possibly death.

TABLE 42-7 RELIGIOUS AND PERSONAL DIETARY RESTRICTIONS

Buddhist	See Vegetarian.
Greek Orthodox	Avoid meat on fast days.
Hindu	See Vegetarian.
Mormon	Avoid alcohol and caffeine-containing products, including coffee and tea.
Muslim	Abstain from pork, pork products, and alcohol.
Orthodox Jewish	■ Abstain from pork, shellfish, and nonkosher meats. ■ Abstain from leavened bread during Passover. ■ Observe fasting days. ■ Do not serve milk and meat products together.
Roman Catholic	■ Avoid meat before Communion, Ash Wednesday, and Good Friday. ■ Observe religious fasting days.
Seventh-Day Adventist	■ Primarily vegetarian. ■ Do not eat meat from cloven-hoofed animals, such as cows, pigs, sheep. ■ Do not eat shellfish and other scavenger sea animals. ■ Discourage intake of caffeine-containing products.
Vegetarian	■ Diet consists mainly of vegetables, fruit, and grains. ■ Some may eat dairy product.

nutritional needs. Since the creation of the first food pyramid, other versions have been developed for specific groups such as Asians, Latinos, vegetarians, the elderly, and children aged 2 through 6. Persons with medical needs require the assistance of professional dieticians and physicians to maintain healthful eating habits within the constraints of their particular situations.

In April 2005, the USDA replaced the Food Guide Pyramid with MyPyramid Plan, establishing a new nutritional attitude: "One size does not fit all." MyPyramid is suitable for all individuals of normal health over the age of 2. It can be found online at www.MyPyramid.gov and can be tailored to each individual based on eating habits, exercise levels, and nutritional requirements (see ∞ Chapter 6).

The USDA bases its recommendations on scientific information and consensus from a variety of sources and experts. Since 1985, Dietary Guidelines for Americans (**DGA**) have been developed and published jointly by the USDA and the Department of Health and Human Services (**DHHS**). The DGA serves as the basis for federal policy regarding federal nutritional programs, including school lunches.

In general, the DGA recommends a variety of foods for energy, essential nutrients, and a healthy physical and emotional state. Another recommendation is to limit intake of alcohol, sugar, salt or sodium, fat, saturated fat, and cholesterol. Eating a variety of whole-grain products, fruits, and vegetables provides complex carbohydrates, vitamins, minerals, and fiber and helps to decrease fat intake. Maintaining a healthy body weight by balancing caloric intake with an exercise program is also recommended.

The Food and Nutrition Board (**FNB**), which helps develop the DGA, also provides criteria for setting Recommended Daily Allowances (**RDA**). RDAs represent the amount of nutrients required to meet the daily nutritional needs of most healthy people. These recommendations cover caloric, vitamin, mineral, and water intake.

There are many variables in nutritional guidelines, such as cultural and religious background, age, social status, physical status, and availability of dietary components. Table 42-7 lists some typical religious and other restrictions.

How to Read a Food Label

Reading a food label is an important tool in maintaining a healthy lifestyle (Figure 42-7 ◆). In 1994 the federal government made reading food labels easier with the Nutrition Labeling and Education Act. Under this law, any special health claims on a product label must be stated using specific terms, and the nutritional content must meet USDA standard definitions for those terms. For example, if the label contains the term "reduced fat" or "low fat," that food must contain a minimum of 25% less fat per serving than the regular offered product. Any food that has the words "low fat" on the label must contain no more than 3 grams of fat per serving. A "fat-free" food must contain no more than 0.5 gram of fat per serving. Foods labeled "lite" or "light" must have a minimum of 1/3 fewer calories than the regular product or at least 50% less fat. Food manufacturers are allowed to use words that are not federally regulated, such as "right," "smart choice," or "natural," at their own discretion.

It is important to note that the percentages on a nutrition label are based on a 2,000-calorie-per-day diet, so if you eat more or less than 2,000 calories per day, you will need to adjust the nutritional values accordingly.

Another important component of the food label is the ingredients list. All manufacturers must list ingredients in descending order of predominance and weight. For example, if the first ingredient is sugar, then sugar makes up the majority of the product. Food manufacturers are allowed to list similar ingredients as separate compounds, a fact consumers should be aware of. In ketchup,

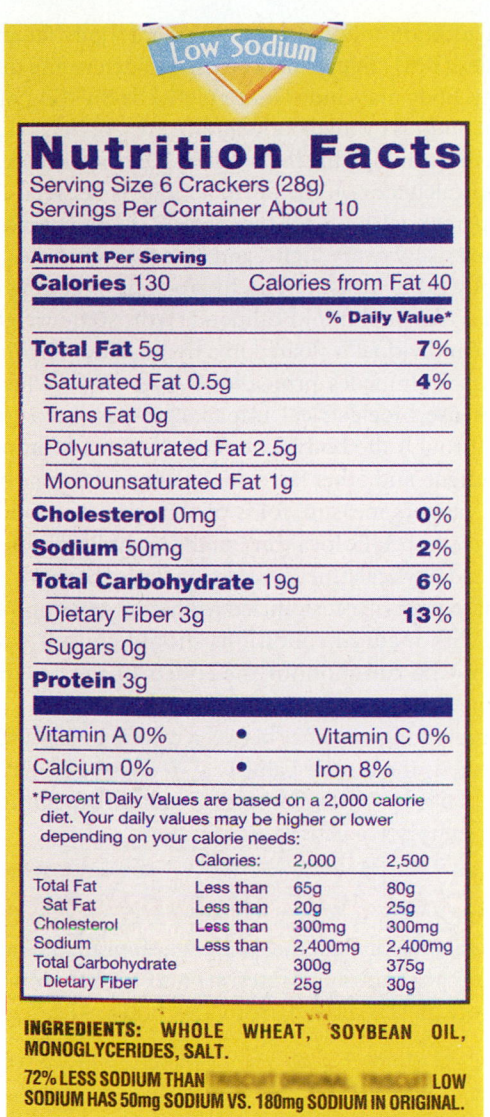

Figure 42-7 ◆ Food label listing nutritional information.

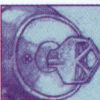

Keys to Success
READING FOOD PRODUCT LABELS

Consumers can obtain important nutritional information by reading labels on food products. Since the early 1990s, under USDA regulations, all food products must carry a label listing nutritional information, including:

- the serving size for each product, in both household and metric measurements
- the number of servings per container
- total **calories** per serving and calories from fat
- grams of total fat, saturated fat, cholesterol, total carbohydrates, protein, and sodium by serving size
- a breakdown of total carbohydrates into dietary fiber and sugars
- a list of ingredients in the order of importance
- daily percentage of RDA for vitamins A, B complex, C, iron, and calcium
- any special health claim
- artificial color(s)

Busy lifestyles can contribute to poor eating habits and a deterioration in health. Individuals with existing health problems often have poor eating habits. Dental health is another contributing factor to nutritional status. Proper chewing is the essential first step in the breakdown and digestion of foods for maximum absorption of nutrients. Persons with poor dental health, missing teeth, or dentures cannot chew fiber and other foods thoroughly, which contributes to decreased motility of the GI system and may result in constipation or diarrhea. Persons with painful or malodorous mouth conditions also may not eat well.

Healthy habits include good oral hygiene; eating nutritious foods, including fiber to assist in peristalsis and evacuation; and exercising regularly. These basic practices help prevent disease as well as a declining nutritional status resulting from disease or illness. They also help prevent the additive effects of poor nutritional status on a disease condition.

The physician will evaluate if a patient is able to manage his or her own nutritional needs or if a regimen of diet, exercise, medications, or other treatments is required. If a patient cannot take nutrients orally, the physician will prescribe **total parenteral nutrition** (**TPN**) by tube feedings directly into the stomach or by IV therapy.

for example, sugar, high-fructose corn syrup, and sucrose may be listed as separate ingredients, but they are all forms of sugar.

Critical Thinking Question 42-1

What questions should Reggie ask Serena about her newfound interest in vegetarianism so that he can more accurately assess her nutritional needs?

Nutrition and Health

Nutritional status has single, seesaw, or cascading effects on an individual's health. Single problems are caused by single deficiencies. Seesaw effects occur when the body overcompensates for a deficiency in nutrients, resulting in breakdown of tissue or other problems. Cascading occurs when a deficiency in one nutrient causes deficiencies in other nutrients because of impaired ability to transport, create, or absorb the other nutrients.

Critical Thinking Question 42-2

Once Reggie has established what type of vegetarian Serena would like to become, how should he proceed to help her reach her nutritional as well as lifestyle goals?

Factors That May Affect Caloric Intake

Caloric intake is affected by many potentially harmful cultural, economic, and lifestyle factors.

- Economic: People with low incomes tend to buy more high-carbohydrate foods in an effort to get more food on a limited budget.
- Culture: In some cultures social gatherings are often centered around large meals, and it is an insult to decline the offer of food.
- Lifestyle: As people's lives become busier, they tend to eat more fast food and exercise less.

Education and individual motivation are the best tools for counteracting these harmful influences. Most people need to eat higher-quality food in smaller quantities. The money "saved" from buying foods high in simple carbohydrates is actually money wasted, as **obesity** and other medical conditions lead to poor health. The influence of culture on dietary habits is a bigger challenge, but higher caloric intake can be balanced with more exercise, and modest daily intake can allow for family feasts. Lifestyle changes are also a challenge, and short-term and long-term individual goals must be established to achieve lasting benefits.

Obesity

Excess ingested food is metabolized, converted, and stored as fat. Obesity, a symptom of caloric intake greater than the body requires, is both a cause and a result of medical conditions. It is often directly linked to diabetes, cardiovascular disease, hypertension, and many other disease conditions. Obesity may also be a residual effect of disease conditions that may cause a decrease in activity, such as myocardial infarction and congestive heart failure.

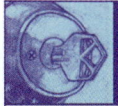

Keys to Success
FAD DIETS, AT BEST, ARE TEMPORARY MEASURES

Americans spend over $30 million a year on weight loss programs and products. Fad diets promising rapid weight loss and beautiful figures contribute to this big business. Some examples are the Atkins Diet, the Cabbage Soup Diet, the Grapefruit Diet, and the Zone Diet. Fad diets have a common theme: restricting a particular food or food group and promoting high intake of another food or food group. For example, the Atkins Diet promotes restriction of carbohydrates in favor of proteins and fats. The Cabbage Soup Diet promotes a steady regimen of cabbage-based soups and restriction of other food groups. The Grapefruit Diet promotes an excess of grapefruits. The Zone Diet promotes a slightly higher intake of carbohydrates and dividing the remaining calories equally between protein and fat. The advantage to following a fad diet is usually rapid weight loss. The disadvantages are rebound weight gain, compromised self-image because of weight loss failure, and the absence of healthy, permanent lifestyle changes. Studies continue to prove that maintaining a balance between caloric intake and exercise is the only way to effectively manage weight.

In addition to weight measurement, body fat and body mass index (**BMI**) figures may be used to determine the extent of obesity. Body mass index is calculated by dividing a person's weight in pounds by total body surface area, or height in inches squared, then multiplying the result by 703. (Several online sites have BMI calculators.) The normal range is between 18.5 and 24.9. A person with a BMI below 18.5 is considered underweight, over 24.9 **overweight,** and 30 or above obese.

Body fat is measured by hydrostatic weighing or with body fat scales or skinfold calipers. Hydrostatic weighing, in which the individual is floated in a hydrostatic weighing tank, is based on Archimedes' principle of water displacement. Body fat scales use bioelectrical impedance, passing a low-level current through the body. The measurement of impedance, height, weight, and other factors is used to determine body fat. Skinfold calipers measure folds of skin and their underlying layers of fat at specific locations on the body. Physicians, nutritionists, and physical fitness professionals use the body fat measurement to prescribe customized regimens of diet and exercise. Patients with medical conditions should consult with their physician, who can monitor the effects of the program and change the treatment plan if necessary.

Maintaining a balance between caloric intake and caloric expenditure is the most reliable way to control weight (Figure 42-8 ◆). Table 42-8 lists examples of caloric expenditure during different types of activity or exercise.

The Effects of Alcohol on Nutrition

Alcohol is a non-nutrient that yields 7 kcal/gram. It is absorbed by the stomach and small intestine and broken down by the liver before it is excreted from the body. Although small

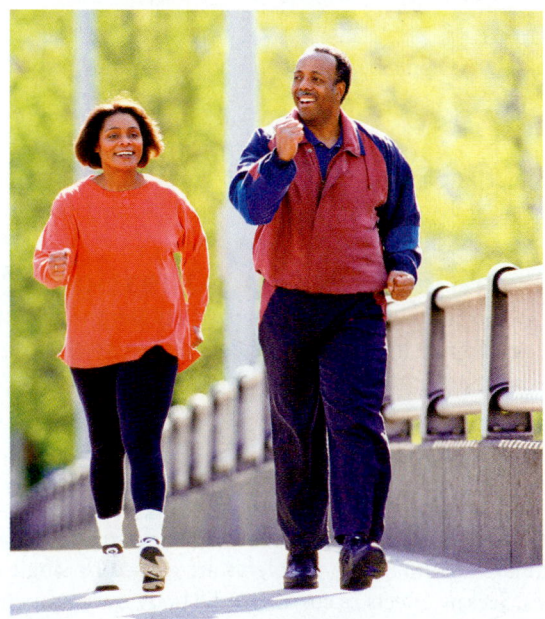

Figure 42-8 ◆ Maintaining a balance between caloric intake and caloric expenditure is the most reliable way to control weight.
Source: Jim Cummins/Getty Images, Inc.

TABLE 42-8 CALORIC EXPENDITURE DURING SELECTED ACTIVITIES OR EXERCISE

Activity	Caloric Expenditure per Hour
Sitting	80 calories
Weight lifting	215 calories
Walking (4 mph)	325 calories
Aerobics (high impact)	505 calories
Tennis	505 calories
Bicycling (15 mph)	720 calories
Running (10 minutes/mile)	720 calories
Swimming (crawl stroke)	790 calories

amounts have some therapeutic benefits, in general, alcohol interferes with metabolism and contributes to the development of liver and other medical conditions.

- When too much alcohol is delivered to the liver, it accumulates as fat and may eventually cause cirrhosis.
- The metabolism of alcohol prevents enzyme use for other necessary nutritional reactions.
- Long-term use leads to other medical disorders, including **malnutrition,** obesity, ulcers, cancer, hypertension, and diabetes mellitus.
- Pregnant women are advised against taking *any* alcohol because of its devastating effects on the fetus, a condition known as fetal alcohol syndrome.

Recent studies suggest that one drink per day for women and two drinks per day for men may be beneficial for overall health status. A drink unit is 1.5 ounces of liquor, 5 ounces of wine, or 12 ounces of beer. Research is inconclusive as to whether beer or wine offers more health benefits. At this time, however, this finding is not generally accepted in medical practice.

The Effects of Aging on Nutritional Status

The physiological functioning of the gastrointestinal system becomes less efficient as an individual ages. Teeth, so important in the initial breakdown of food, often are absent or have been replaced by less effective false teeth. The sense of taste and sense of smell become dull, and the declining function of the nervous system results in slower peristalsis of the esophagus, stomach, and small and large intestines. The metabolism slows and, in general, activity levels decrease. Elderly persons also tend to lose the capacity or desire to shop and/or cook. Medications may affect digestion and food absorption. These conditions heighten the challenge of maintaining a balanced diet as a person ages.

Social interaction aids in the digestion process in people of all ages. Among the elderly, social interaction often decreases, leading to isolation from family and friends. One common reason for growing isolation is the loss of spouse. Elderly individuals also often become depressed as they fail to cope with the effects of aging.

The nutritional status of the elderly is the result of lifestyle habits and choices made during their younger years. The individual who establishes wellness habits early in life avoids inactivity, malnutrition, obesity, and the development or advancement of medical and dental conditions later. As an individual ages, nutritional status can affect or cause medical conditions. For example, obesity contributes to the development or advancement of hypertension, diabetes, arthritis, and other conditions. The loss of teeth affects the chewing, swallowing, and digestion of food. A person who cannot chew, lacks roughage in the diet, and is not active has slower GI motility and becomes constipated more easily.

Under the direction of dieticians and physicians, you should encourage elderly patients to eat nutritious foods and maintain or increase physical activity. Regular activity increases appetite, mobility, physical endurance, and immune response.

Diseases and Disorders Involving Nutrition

Disease conditions result from and are the cause of altered nutritional states.

- Heart disease, hypertension, and atherosclerosis often result from dietary intake of foods high in lipids (fats) and cholesterol (hyperlipedimia, hypercholesteremia).
- Prolonged nausea and vomiting, with the resulting loss of fluids, often lead to electrolyte imbalances.
- Parasitic infestation and infections caused by contaminated food and/or water, malabsorption syndrome, irritable bowel syndrome, gastric bypass surgery, cancer of the colon and other organs in the digestive tract, starvation (self-induced or otherwise), and starvation-related conditions including **anorexia,** bulimia, and binge eating are other factors in compromised nutritional status.
- Gastrointestinal obstructions, which can occur at any point along the GI tract, cause an interruption in the absorption of nutrients.
- Constipation and diarrhea are symptoms of altered gastrointestinal mobility.
- Inborn errors of metabolism negatively affect the normal absorption of nutrients by altering the metabolic process involved in digestion.
- Eating disorders include anorexia nervosa and bulimia.

Food Allergies and Food Intolerances

Food allergies and food intolerances occur in both children and adults (Table 42-9). Food intolerances are unpleasant reactions to certain foods, but they do not cause severe or life-threatening medical emergencies. Food allergies result from a hypersensitivity of the immune system to certain foods. Persons with food allergies often have a genetic predisposition and a history of other allergies. Children often outgrow allergies, but adults have their allergies for life. The frequency of particular allergies may be enhanced by geographic location; an example is the high rate of rice allergies in Japan.

TABLE 42-9 COMMON FOOD ALLERGIES AND INTOLERANCES

Food Allergies: Adults	Food Allergies: Children
■ Shellfish: crab, crayfish, lobster, shrimp ■ Legumes: peanuts ■ Tree nuts: walnuts, Brazil nuts ■ Fish ■ Eggs ■ Cantaloupe and other fruit	■ Eggs ■ Milk ■ Legumes: peanuts, soy products ■ Fish ■ Shrimp ■ Fruit juices

Food Intolerances: Adults and Children

■ Lactose-containing products
■ Sulfites
■ Monosodium glutamate (MSG)
■ Yellow dye #5
■ Red dye

Food allergies are similar to other allergies, such as drug allergies, in the way they develop. When a person with a genetic predisposition eats an allergy-causing food, the body's immune system produces immunoglobulin E (IgE), a protein antibody that circulates in the bloodstream. IgE attaches to mast cells that may be present in all body tissues but mostly in the nose, throat, lungs, gastrointestinal tract, and skin. After a person has been exposed to the food and initiated IgE production and mast cell attachment, histamine is released. The area of histamine release directly relates to the symptoms. If it is released in the nasopharyngeal region, itching, difficulty swallowing, and difficulty breathing may develop. If histamine is released in the gastrointestinal system, symptoms may be diarrhea and/or pain, and when released in the skin, hives.

It is important to differentiate between a food allergy and food intolerance to prevent serious illness and fatality. After clinical assessment and intervention, food allergy percentages in the adult population decrease to 1 percent and in the pediatric population to 3 percent. To confirm a diagnosis of food allergy, the physician first rules out other possibilities.

- The reaction may be caused by the toxins in contaminated food.
- Some foods have a naturally high histamine content, such as mackerel, tuna, some wines, and cheeses.
- Lactase deficiency and food additives (MSG, sulfites) may cause food intolerances that are mistaken for food allergies.
- The symptoms of other medical conditions, such as ulcers and gastrointestinal cancers, can mimic those of food allergy.
- Psychological triggers may mimic food allergy symptoms.

When considering a diagnosis of food allergy, the physician performs a detailed health history. Often the patient is asked to keep a detailed food diary. Elimination diets are often used to determine if the absence of a food is related to the absence of symptoms. Skin and patch testing may be performed, but is not preferred if the person has experienced a severe anaphylactic reaction. Blood tests such as RAST and ELISA are performed to measure the presence of IgE.

The first step in treating a food allergy is avoiding the offending food. The patient must learn to read all food labels. Even then, however, anaphylactic reactions are possible, and the patient must be prepared to react quickly. The patient should wear an allergy bracelet, carry an emergency kit with adrenaline (epinephrine), and get help immediately. Emergency medication may also include antihistamines and bronchodilators, among others. It is important to communicate to the patient that cross reactivity may result, in which the patient may become allergic to similar foods. The patient should also be made aware of the possibility of exercise-induced food allergy, when a certain food eaten before exercise causes symptoms that range from light-headedness and itching to anaphylaxis and death.

Diagnosis and Treatment of GI Disorders

The location of patient signs and symptoms can be significant in guiding the physician to a diagnosis of conditions and disorders (Table 42-10). There are two methods for describing the location of the abdominopelvic regions: by the nine anatomical divisions or by the four clinical quadrants (Figures 42-9 ◆ and 42-10 ◆). The MA and other clinical staff assist the physician by listening to the patient's description and accurately documenting symptom location.

Warning signs of GI problems include:

- Nausea: motion sickness, pregnancy, emotional distress, gallbladder disease, intestinal obstruction, food poisoning, enteroviruses
- Vomiting, especially **emesis** containing blood (**hematemesis**): food poisoning, intestinal obstruction, esophageal varices, ulcers, early pregnancy
- Coffee-ground emesis: bleeding in GI tract from ulcers, esophageal varices
- Diarrhea: enteroviruses, food poisoning, gallbladder disease
- Constipation: intestinal obstruction, lack of fiber and fluids in diet, constipating foods
- Bright red blood in stools: hemorrhoids, rectal polyps, cancer of rectum or lower GI tract
- Black stools (**melena**): bleeding in GI tract, usually in stomach, upper GI tract, or upper portion of large intestine
- Abdominal pain: intestinal obstruction, food poisoning, enteroviruses, flatus, constipation, appendicitis, many other conditions
- Abdominal distension: intestinal obstruction, constipation, food poisoning, many other conditions
- **Dyspepsia:** Difficulty in digestion.
- Anorexia: Loss of appetite, not to be confused with Anorexia Nervosa, the mental condition in which an individual refuses to eat due to poor self-image.
- **Flatulence:** Excessive gas in the stomach and intestines.
- **Dysphagia:** Difficulty in swallowing

TABLE 42-10 ABDOMINAL REGIONS AND DISORDERS

Structures	Possible Disorders
Right Upper Quadrant (RUQ)	
Liver	Cancer of the liver, cirrhosis, hepatitis: A (infectious), B (serum), C (non A, non B), D (delta virus), E, G
Gallbladder	Cholecystitis, cholelithiasis, obstruction of bile ducts
Duodenum	Duodenal cancer, duodenal ulcer
Head of pancreas	Pancreatitis, cancer of pancreas
Right kidney and adrenal glands	Pyelitis, pyelonephritis, renal calculi, adrenal disorders
Hepatic flexure of the colon	Obstruction, cancer of colon
Portion of ascending and transverse colon	Obstruction, cancer of colon
Right Lower Quadrant (RLQ)	
Cecum	Obstruction, cancer of colon
Appendix	Appendicitis
Right ovary and fallopian tube	Cancer of ovary, ovarian cyst, ectopic pregnancy, endometriosis, PID
Right ureter	Renal calculi, UTI
Left Upper Quadrant (LUQ)	
Stomach	Gastric ulcer, gastric cancer, hiatal hernia
Spleen	Traumatic injury to spleen, enlarged spleen due to disease
Left lobe of liver	Cancer of liver, cirrhosis, hepatitis: A (infectious), B (serum), C (non A, non B), D (delta virus), E, G
Body of pancreas	Pancreatitis, cancer of pancreas
Left kidney and adrenal gland	Pyelitis, pyelonephritis, renal calculi, adrenal disorders
Splenic flexure of colon	Splenic flexure syndrome
Portion of transverse and descending colon	Obstruction, cancer of colon, diverticulosis, diverticulitis
Left Lower Quadrant (LLQ)	
Portion of descending colon	Obstruction, cancer of colon, diverticulosis, diverticulitis
Sigmoid colon	Obstruction, cancer of colon, diverticulosis, diverticulitis
Left ovary and fallopian tube	Cancer of ovary, ovarian cyst, ectopic pregnancy, endometriosis, PID
Left ureter	Renal calculi, UTI
Middle of Abdomen, Midline	
Aorta	Dissecting aorta
Abdominal wall	Umbilical hernia
Uterus (when enlarged)	Pregnancy, fibroid tumors, cancerous tumors
Bladder (when distended)	Urinary retention

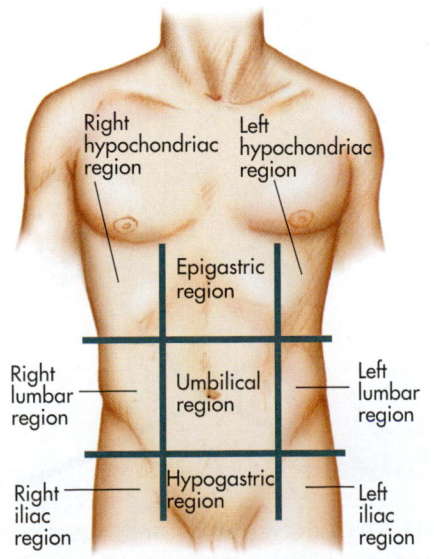

Figure 42-9 ◆ Anatomical divisions of the abdomen.

Diagnostic Procedures

Various diagnostic procedures may be ordered for GI disorders, some of which are performed in the office setting. Procedures include but are not limited to:

- Palpation, auscultation, and visualization of the abdomen
- Upper GI series
- Lower GI series (barium enema, air contrast study)
- Gallbladder series (cholecystography)
- Endoscopic examination (**gastroscopy, ERCP, colonoscopy**)
- Stool specimen studies for ova/parasites (refer to ∞ Chapter 31)
- Occult fecal blood specimen tests (∞ refer to Chapter 31)
- Blood tests (CBC, bilirubin studies)
- Ultrasound studies of abdomen and abdominal organs
- MRI of abdomen

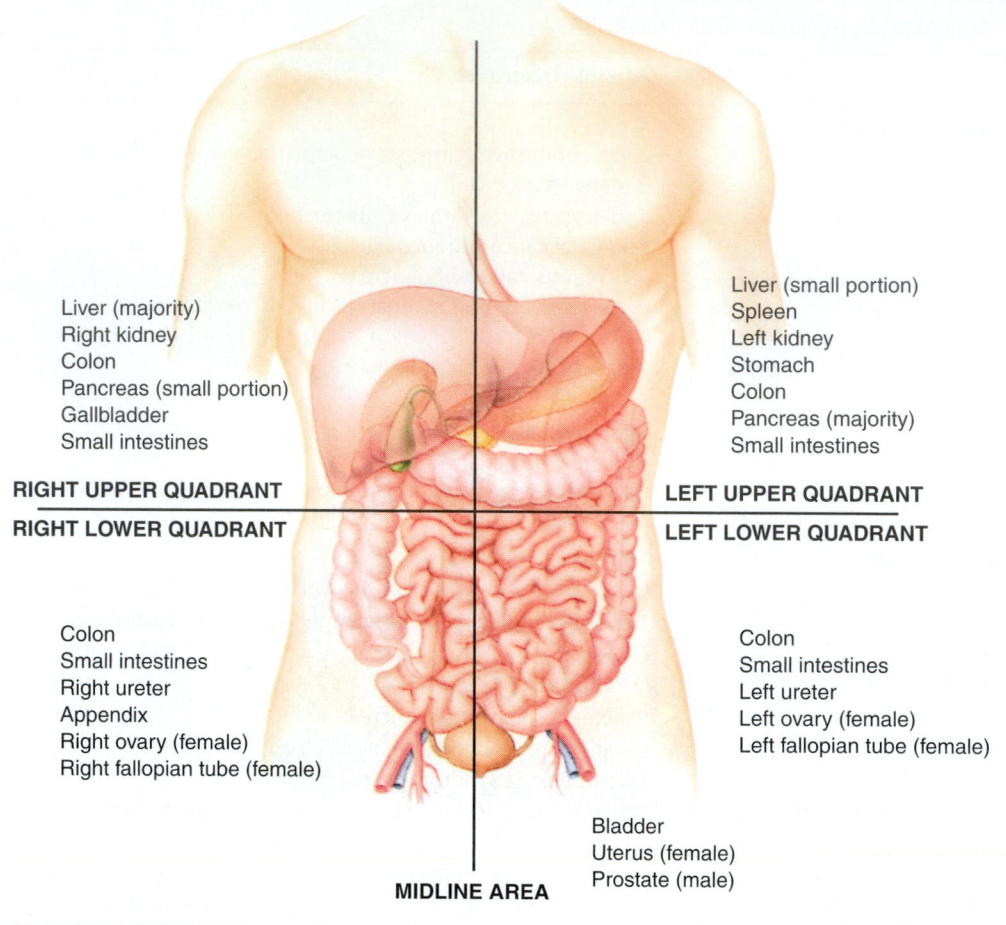

Liver (majority)
Right kidney
Colon
Pancreas (small portion)
Gallbladder
Small intestines

Liver (small portion)
Spleen
Left kidney
Stomach
Colon
Pancreas (majority)
Small intestines

RIGHT UPPER QUADRANT

LEFT UPPER QUADRANT

RIGHT LOWER QUADRANT

LEFT LOWER QUADRANT

Colon
Small intestines
Right ureter
Appendix
Right ovary (female)
Right fallopian tube (female)

Colon
Small intestines
Left ureter
Left ovary (female)
Left fallopian tube (female)

Bladder
Uterus (female)
Prostate (male)

MIDLINE AREA

Figure 42-10 ◆ Clinical divisions of the abdomen.

Obstructive conditions of the colon may require surgical intervention, including colostomy, either temporary or permanent, or resection (surgical removal) of the affected length of the colon. In resection, the ends of the remaining sections of the colon are sutured together in a procedure known **anastomosis.** Temporary colostomies are reversed, also by anastomosis, after the patient has healed and recovered from the causative factor.

Obstructive conditions involving the small intestine, including the ileum, are often treated with an **ileostomy.** During this procedure, the involved structure may be removed and an opening created through the wall of the abdomen for the expulsion of waste products. This procedure may also be reversed, or it may be permanent.

Colonoscopy

A colonoscopy is performed to assess healthy or disease states of the colon (Figure 42-11 ◆). The American Cancer Society recommends that all individuals over the age of 50 have a colonoscopy to screen for cancer. The procedure is also done to check for hemorrhoids, polyps, fistulas, and abscesses within the colon.

To properly view the entire length of the large intestine, the physician performs the colonoscopy in a hospital setting, where sedation is available for the patient's comfort. There are

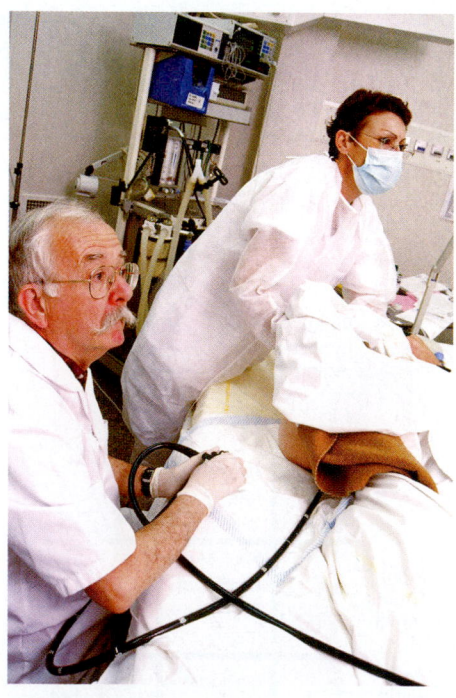

Figure 42-11 ◆ A gastroenterologist and enterological surgeon with staff performing a colonoscopy.
Source: Phototake NYC.

several types of flexible colon fiberscopes that allow the physician to view the colon, rectum, anus, sigmoid colon, and descending, transverse, and ascending colon sections as an in-office procedure.

The procedure serves to:

- Obtain baseline information during a healthy state when the patient has a family history of colon cancer or **polyps.**
- Evaluate symptoms such as abdominal pain, persistent diarrhea, or unexplained blood in the stool.
- Evaluate the type and extent of an inflammatory bowel condition such as Crohn's disease or ulcerative colitis.

The physician explains to the patient why a colonoscopy is necessary and what the risks are. Risks include possible bowel perforation, which requires surgical repair, bleeding from tissue biopsy or polypectomy (removal of polyps) performed during the procedure, reactions to sedative or anesthetic medications, possible infections, and GI symptoms relating to preparation for the procedure.

Many patients are apprehensive about having a rectal exam. To ease their apprehension, the MA should carefully explain the procedure, what it will feel like, sedation methods (if used), recovery time, and how to prepare the colon, if necessary.

In Practice

As the medical assistant for a busy gastroenterology office, you are often required to prepare patients for colonoscopy exams. Ms. Jones calls the office to verify her appointment scheduled for later in the day; however, she admits that she has not been able to follow the clear-liquids-only diet. What should you do? What patient preparation information should be given to all patients before they have a colonoscopy procedure performed?

PROCEDURE 42-1 Assist with a Colon Endoscopic/Colonoscopy Exam

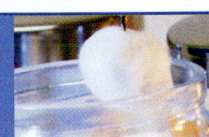

Theory and Rationale

Because of the personal nature of this invasive test, the patient may need your encouragement to discuss any concerns with the physician. You may prepare the Informed Consent form, and the physician or nurse secures the patient signature after discussing the procedure and risks. You will also give the patient pre-colonoscopy preparation instructions and post-colonoscopy care instructions.

Before the colonoscopy:
- The physician will order a cathartic to be administered at different intervals during the day before the procedure.
- The physician will order a high intake of fluids to prevent dehydration, unless there is a medical contraindication.
- The physician will order a clear-liquids-only diet for the day before the procedure.
- The following are *prohibited* from the beginning of the preparation day until after the colonoscopy:
  - milk, dairy products, and solid food
  - fruit juices with pulp
  - any liquids that are red or purple

After the colonoscopy:
- The physician will provide additional information relating to the procedure(s) performed during the colonoscopy.
- If specimens are taken for analysis, the physician will inform you when to expect the biopsy results. The physician may discuss diagnosis during the recovery period or during a later office visit.
- The physician will discuss postoperative care that may include the following:

1. During the first 12–24 hours, restrict activities and driving until the effects of the sedative or anesthetic have worn off, restrict weight lifting, and take plenty of fluids, a soft diet, and pain control if needed.
2. During days 2–14, expect some very minor bleeding in the stool, shift to a high-fiber diet, and take Metamucil or Citrucel if necessary to promote regular bowel movements. Take Milk of Magnesia if you do not have a bowel movement within 72 hours, and drink plenty of fluids.
- Recommendations will be given for a repeat colonoscopy or Hemoccult stool test.

Materials
- two pairs of nonsterile gloves
- instrument for viewing, depending on procedure being performed
- water-soluble lubricant
- patient drapes and gown
- sterile cotton-tipped applicators, for collection of fecal samples
- suction device
- sterile biopsy forceps
- disposable or sterile rectal speculum
- specimen containers with lab requisition form, as needed
- disposable tissue
- biohazard container
- patient chart

continued

PROCEDURE 42-1 Assist with a Colon Endoscopic/Colonoscopy Exam *(continued)*

Competency

(**Conditions**) With the necessary materials, (**Task**) you will be able to set up an exam room and assist the physician with a colon endoscopic procedure (**Standards**) within the time frame designated by the instructor.

1. Gather all needed supplies.
2. Identify the patient and explain the procedure. Verify that the patient has followed pre-exam instructions regarding foods, medications, and activities to avoid, such as enemas. The patient should be asked to empty the bladder prior to the exam.
3. Give the patient drapes and a gown and instructions on proper gown opening placement.
4. Take the patient's vital signs.
5. Assist the patient to the table and position him or her for the exam.
6. Wash your hands and put on gloves.
7. Assist the physician by handing him or her supplies as requested. To ease equipment entry into the anal canal, the physician will use an anal speculum. A suction device may be required to remove any fecal matter that obstructs the physician's view. If polyp tissue samples are needed, the physician will use sterile biopsy forceps.
8. To ease any discomfort, instruct the patient to breathe slowly and deeply. Observe the patient for any change in vitals, increased pain level, or other undue reactions.
9. After the physician has collected the necessary samples, you will place them in sterile specimen containers.
10. When the physician has completed the examination, cleanse the patient's anal area with tissues.
11. Remove the gloves, wash your hands, and assist the patient into a recovery position.
12. While the patient is resting, recheck vital signs. Invasive procedures often cause a drop in blood pressure.
13. Once the blood pressure is stable, allow the patient to get off the exam table and get dressed.
14. Complete laboratory forms. Seal the specimen containers in an appropriate biohazard-labeled transport bag.
15. When the patient has been released from the room, wash your hands, put on new gloves, and disinfect the area. A disposable speculum should be discarded into a biohazardous container; a stainless steel speculum should be prepared for autoclaving.
16. Document the procedure in the patient's chart.

Patient Education

Give the patient verbal and written instructions for care after this invasive procedure. The patient should report any undue effects, such as fainting, dizziness, loss of appetite, or rectal bleeding. Advise the patient to refrain from intense physical activity until directed by a physician.

Charting Example

08/05/XX 7:30 PM Assisted in colon endoscopic procedure. Patient vital signs monitored and remained stable. Patient reported no feelings of faintness, dizziness, or discomfort following the procedure. Specimens collected and sent to laboratory. Anita Estrada, RMA (AMI)

Sigmoidoscopy

To correctly evaluate suspected lower gastrointestinal disorders, tumors, positive fecal occult blood tests, bleeding, polyps, or suspected cancer, the physician must examine the lower gastrointestinal system. A sigmoidoscopy allows the physician to visualize the anus, rectum, large intestine, and appendix.

A sigmoidoscopy is performed with a sigmoidoscope, which can be rigid (metal) or flexible (plastic). All sigmoidoscopes are equipped with a light source and a magnifying lens that gives the physician a clear view of the sigmoid structure. To provide better access to the sigmoid colon, an obturator, a firm plastic device, is attached within the hollow tubing of the sigmoidoscope. A few inches of the tapered end of the obturator extend beyond the tube, facilitating entry past the anal sphincter. Both instruments are lubricated and threaded into the rectum. The obturator is then removed by pulling it straight out of the opposite end of the sigmoidoscope. The sigmoidoscope is left in place, providing a clear view of the sigmoid colon.

Rectal Suppositories

If rapid absorption of a medication without the risk of GI upset is an issue, suppositories are a good option. The rectal mucosa are ideal for absorption due to the high vascularity of the membranes. When medication is introduced via the rectum, it is also not altered, as it would be by gastric juices. The ideal time to insert a rectal suppository is immediately after a bowel movement and when the patient can remain lying down in a supine position for at least 20 minutes.

Patient Instruction in Nutrition

Medical assistants may be responsible for providing patients with information about special diets. Many offices have printed dietary plans available for distribution to patients. The MA should be familiar with the various dietary options and review the prescribed diet with the patient. Some common diets are described in Table 42-11.

TABLE 42-11 SPECIAL DIETS

Name or Type of Diet	Reason for Diet	Dietary Concepts
Clear liquid diet	May be prescribed as a preoperative diet, postoperative diet, prep diet for certain diagnostic tests, or to treat GI upsets	Broth, tea, Jell-O; apple juice and cranberry juice occasionally allowed
Liquid diet (full liquid diet)	May be prescribed as a preoperative diet, postoperative diet, prep diet for certain diagnostic tests, or to treat GI upsets	Clear liquids, milk, custards, ice cream, fruit juices, eggnog, milkshakes
Soft diet	May be prescribed postoperatively to reduce strain on GI system or for certain gastrointestinal disorders	Foods containing very little roughage, no raw fruits or vegetables, no gas-forming foods, and reduced or no spices
Mechanical soft diet	Prescribed when mastication is difficult or impossible.	Pureed, chopped, or ground foods
High-fiber diet	Provides bulk in GI tract as an aid to elimination	Fruits, vegetables, whole-grain cereals, green leafy vegetables, deep yellow fruits and vegetables, members of cabbage family, and decreased fat and salt intake
Low-fiber diet	Elimination of high-fiber foods that may irritate intestinal mucosa and diverticulosis	No nuts, seeds, fruits or vegetables with skins (peas, corn, plums) or a high fiber content (whole grains, cabbage, celery)
Bland diet	Elimination of foods that may irritate gastric mucosa	No spices, fried foods, substances containing caffeine, pepper, chili, alcohol, and high-fiber foods
Elimination diet	Determination of food substances that may be causing an allergic response	One or two foods eliminated for a period of time to see if allergic response abates
Diabetic diet	Control of blood glucose levels in the diabetic patient; usually includes controlling caloric intake and reducing simple sugars	Balanced diet containing complex carbohydrates, monounsaturated fats, five servings of dark-colored vegetables or fruits daily, six servings of whole grains daily, two weekly servings of fish, reduced salt intake, avoidance of saturated fats
Low-fat or low-cholesterol diet	Reduction of blood levels of lipids and cholesterol	Reduced intake of foods high in cholesterol and saturated fats
Reduced-calorie diet	Weight loss	Reduced calories while maintaining nutritional status
Low-sodium diet	Hypertension, heart problems, kidney disorders	Additional salt withheld from diet
Infant and pediatric diets	Provision of nutrients necessary for growth	High protein, vitamins, minerals, other nutrients
Diet for pregnancy and lactation	Provision of adequate calories and nutrients to support growing fetus and nursing infant	High protein, additional calcium and iron
Geriatric diet	Dentition, activity, and medication needs of geriatric patients	Softer or pureed food, fewer calories for less active patients, lower carbohydrates for diabetic patients, low-sodium diet for patients with CHF
High-energy diet	Prevention of fluctuating levels of blood sugar	Higher intake of raw or lightly cooked vegetables, fresh fruit, beans, nuts, whole grains, fish, free-range chicken, herb teas; exclusion of coffee, tea, alcohol, most meats; three regularly spaced meals and two snacks

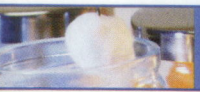

PROCEDURE 42-2 Assist with a Sigmoidoscopy

Theory and Rationale

During a sigmoidoscopy, the physician may occasionally need to distend the walls of the colon for easier viewing by introducing air into the colon via an inflation bulb, or insufflator, attached to the scope. This part of a sigmoidoscopy is uncomfortable and sometimes painful. To help ease discomfort, coach the patient to take slow, deep breaths.

Sigmoidoscopies can be performed with disposable or sterile equipment.

Materials

- sigmoidoscope
- insufflator
- water-soluble lubricant
- patient drapes and gown
- sterile cotton-tipped applicators
- suction device
- sterile biopsy forceps, as directed by physician
- disposable or sterile rectal speculum
- specimen containers with lab requisition form, as needed
- disposable tissue
- chucks pads
- water basin
- 500 ml of warmed water
- gloves
- biohazard container
- patient chart

Competency

(**Conditions**) With the necessary materials, (**Task**) you will be able to set up an exam room and assist the physician with a sigmoidoscopy procedure (**Standards**) within the time frame designated by the instructor.

1. Gather all needed supplies.
2. Identify the patient and explain the procedure. Verify that the patient has followed pre-exam instructions regarding foods, medications, and activities to avoid and performed an enema. The patient should be asked to empty the bladder prior to the exam for greater comfort.
3. Give the patient drapes and a gown and instructions on proper gown opening placement.
4. Take the patient's vital signs.

5. Assist the patient to the table and position for the exam.
6. Place a chucks pad, examination pad, or other absorbent material under the patient's perineal area.
7. Wash your hands and put on gloves.
8. Assist the physician as needed.
9. Attach the light source and insufflator to the sigmoidoscope, but do not turn on the light until the physician is ready to use it. The light generates heat the longer it is on and can potentially burn the patient.
10. To ease the patient's discomfort, instruct him or her to breathe slowly and deeply. Observe the patient for any change in vitals, increased pain level, or other undue reactions.
11. When the physician has completed the examination, cleanse the patient's anal area with tissues.
12. Remove the gloves, wash your hands, and assist the patient into a recovery position.
13. While the patient is resting, recheck vital signs. Invasive procedures often cause a drop in blood pressure.
14. Once the blood pressure is stable, allow the patient to get off the exam table and get dressed.
15. Complete the laboratory forms and send samples to be examined.
16. When the patient has been released from the room, wash your hands, put on new gloves, and disinfect the area.
17. Document the procedure in the patient chart.

Patient Education

When air is introduced into the gastrointestinal tract, it can cause mild discomfort or even pain for some patients. After the procedure, instruct the patient to lie in the supine position to relieve this discomfort. Placing a pillow across the abdomen or between the knees can also help relieve gastric pressure. Encourage the patient to find the most comfortable position that will allow the passing of excess gas. Do not recommend that the patient take any gas-relief medication.

Charting Example

08/05/XX 7:30 PM Assisted in sigmoidoscopy procedure. Patient vital signs monitored and remained stable. Patient reported no feelings of faintness, dizziness, or discomfort following the procedure. Specimens collected and sent to laboratory. Lisa Kim, RMA (AMI)

PROCEDURE 42-3   Insert a Rectal Suppository

Theory and Rationale

For patients who are experiencing extreme nausea or are unable to tolerate GI medications, rectal suppositories are often prescribed for medication administration.

Materials

- physician-prescribed rectal suppository
- water-soluble lubricant
- tissues
- biohazardous container
- disposable gloves
- patient instructions
- patient chart

Competency

(Conditions) With the necessary materials, **(Task)** you will be able to correctly administer a rectal suppository **(Standards)** within the time allotted by the instructor.

1. Verify the patient's identification and check for allergies.
2. Verify the physician's medication order.
3. Collect all necessary supplies.
4. Explain the procedure to the patient.
5. Wash your hands and put on gloves.
6. Ask the patient to remove all clothing from the waist area down.
7. Assist the patient into a Sims position and provide proper drapes (Figure 42-12 ◆).
8. Take the protective foil wrap from the suppository and carefully smooth any rough or jagged edges. Lubricate the suppository with the water-soluble lubricant.
9. Expose the patient's buttocks.
10. Holding the suppository in one hand, lift the upper buttock with your other hand, exposing the anus (Figure 42-13 ◆).
11. Firmly guide the suppository into the anus with your index finger, past any fecal masses and the internal sphincter. This will prevent it from being expelled (Figure 42-14 ◆).

12. With a tissue, apply firm pressure on the anus for 1–2 minutes to allow the medication to be retained. Discard the tissue into the biohazardous container.
13. With another tissue, wipe away any excess lubricant or fecal matter from the anus and discard the tissue into the biohazardous container.

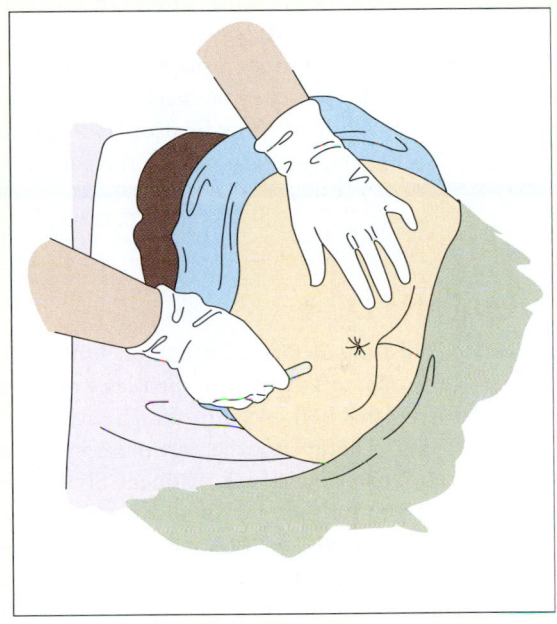

Figure 42-13 ◆ Lift the upper buttock, exposing the anus.

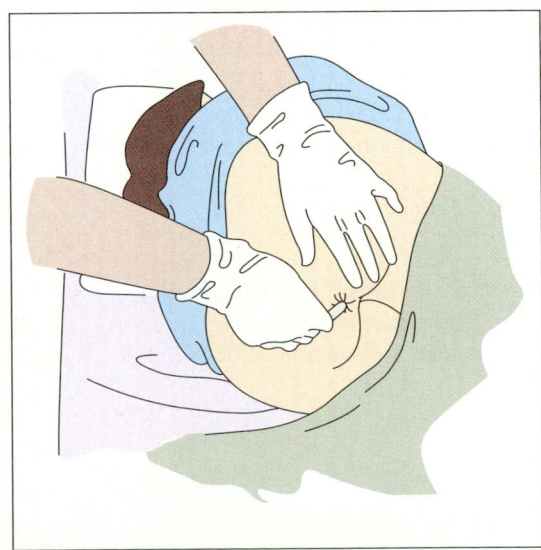

Figure 42-14 ◆ Insert the suppository.

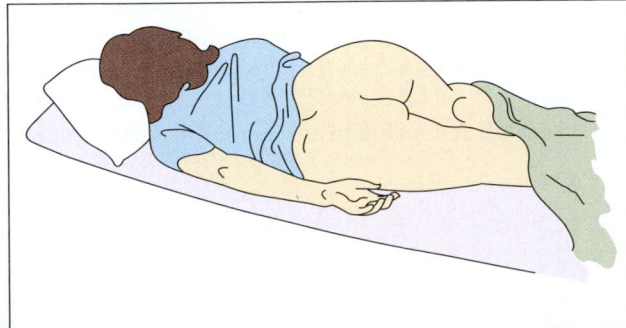

Figure 42-12 ◆ Assist patient into Sims position.

continued

PROCEDURE 42-3 **Insert a Rectal Suppository** (continued)

14. Instruct the patient to get into a comfortable position and rest for 30 minutes as the medication is absorbed.
15. Clean the area, providing a new drape if necessary, and dispose of all materials in the biohazardous container.
16. Remove the gloves and wash your hands.
17. Document the procedure in the patient chart.

Patient Education

Inform the patient of the time frame in which the medication takes effect. The patient may need to rest in a comfortable position while the medication is absorbed, as directed by office protocol. Also inform the patient of any side effects that may be experienced, such as flatulence or anal leakage. Some medications may also cause dizziness. Patients taking medication known to cause excessive sleepiness or dizziness should be monitored carefully and assisted when moving off the exam table. These patients will also require someone to drive them home, as it would be unsafe for them to operate a motor vehicle.

Charting Example

08/05/XX 7:30 PM Dulcolax 15 mg rectal suppository administered for relief of constipation. Patient advised to call office in 24 hours to report effectiveness. Alex Rodriguez, RMA (AMT)

Therapeutic Diets

In addition to providing dietary information, it may be necessary to refer the patient to a dietitian. A dietitian works with the patient to plan a diet that both meets medical needs and appeals to the patient's taste. Therapeutic diets are prescribed to alleviate symptoms and manage medical treatment. Some disorders that may benefit from a therapeutic diet are hypertension, hypercholesteremia, diabetes mellitus, and some gastrointestinal disorders. For example, eliminating foods high in sodium controls fluid retention that may be responsible for a patient's hypertension. Reducing foods high in cholesterol or cholesterol-forming agents may lower blood cholesterol and slow the progression of atherosclerosis. The American Heart Association, American Cancer Society, and American Diabetic Association all offer dietary recommendations for these medical conditions and for overall healthier eating habits. The guidelines of two of the groups are listed in Table 42-12.

Another area in which you can be helpful to patients concerns simple, common-sense treatments for common digestive problems:

Nausea

- Eat crackers slowly, in small amounts
- Keep the eyes open.
- Avoid head movements.

- Avoid milk and milk products.
- Avoid high-fat foods.
- Drink flat carbonated water or soft drinks (soda).

Vomiting

- Avoid food or fluids for one hour after emesis.
- Freshen the mouth by rinsing with water.
- Sip a soft drink in small amounts after one hour.
- When able to resume eating, start with bland foods.

Diarrhea

- Drink clear liquids.
- Use sports drinks to replace glucose and electrolytes.
- Avoid alcohol.
- Eat cultured yogurts.

Constipation

- Increase fluid intake.
- Increase fiber in the diet.
- Avoid milk, cheese, and other dairy products.
- Increase your level of exercise, including walking.
- *Do not* ignore the urge to defecate. Respond in a timely manner.
- Establish and maintain a daily routine for defecation.

TABLE 42-12 THERAPEUTIC DIETS

Heart-Healthy Dietary Guidelines (AHA)
- Maintain a daily fat intake of 30% of total calories or less, distributed as follows:
  - Saturated fatty acids (the "bad" type) less than 10% of total calories
  - Polyunsaturated fats (the "good" type) less than 10% of total calories
  - Monounsaturated fats (the "good" type) less than 15% of total calories
- Avoid products made with white flour. Substitute whole-grain products.
- Replace granola and other cereals made with coconut or palm oil with whole-grain cereals low in fat and sugar but high in fiber.
- Avoid deep-fried vegetables. Eat steamed or baked dark-green leafy vegetables.
- Avoid cream, butter, margarine, lard, mayonnaise, and salad dressings.
- Substitute skim, low-fat, or 1% milk products for whole milk, condensed milk, and evaporated milk.
- Avoid whole-milk cheeses, processed cheeses, cheese spreads, and cream cheese. Substitute low- or nonfat hard cheese, low-fat cottage cheese, and part-skim ricotta cheese.
- Avoid coconuts, coconut products, and dried fruits with sodium preservatives. Substitute fresh and frozen fruit without added sugar.
- Instead of goose and duck, organ meats, or fried and processed meats, choose lean beef, veal, pork, and lamb.
- Avoid smoked, fried, or salted fish, tuna packed in oil, sardines, anchovies, oysters, and crab. Substitute fresh or frozen fish, clams, scallops, and lobster.

American Cancer Society Dietary Guidelines
- Include more high-fiber foods in the diet (fruits, vegetables, and whole-grain products).
- Increase your intake of dark-green and yellow fruits and vegetables, broccoli, cabbage, brussel sprouts, kohlrabi, and cauliflower.
- Limit your intake of processed, salt-cured, smoked, and nitrite-cured foods (bacon and smoked sausage).
- Reduce total fat intake, especially animal fats.
- Maintain a healthy weight.
- Limit your intake of alcoholic beverages.

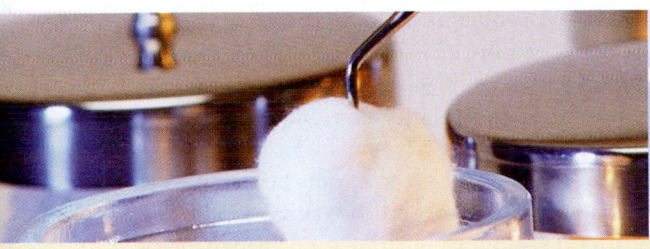

REVIEW

Chapter Summary

- The gastrointestinal system is primarily responsible for nourishing the body. Salivation, mastication, and the process of digestion break food down into nutritional substances. Habits of good nutrition help the body maintain a strong immune system, healthy energy levels, and mental alertness. During times of altered health, a healthy nutritional status can speed recovery.
- Obtaining and recording the medical history and vital signs are an MA's routine functions in a gastroenterology or proctology medical office. The MA records specific symptoms, assists the physician in examinations and procedures, arranges appointments for diagnostic tests and procedures, and provides patient instruction.
- The gastrointestinal system or digestive tract is composed of the alimentary canal and accessory organs. The upper digestive tract begins at the mouth and goes on to the pharynx, esophagus, stomach, and duodenum. The lower digestive tract includes the small intestine and large intestine, cecum, appendix, sigmoid portion, rectum, and anus. The small intestine is made up of the duodenum, jejunum, and ileum. The large intestine comprises the cecum, ascending colon, transverse colon, descending colon, and sigmoid regions of the colon, terminating at the rectum. The accessory organs are the pancreas, liver, gallbladder, and connecting ducts.

- The major functions of the GI system are digestion, alimentation, and elimination. The digestion process is divided into ingestion, mastication, deglutination, digestion, and absorption. Elimination is the process of excretion.

- Healthy living habits help prevent disease as well as the additive effects of poor nutritional status upon a disease condition.

- Food is required for the growth and repair of body tissues, for the regulation of different body processes, and for heat production. Individuals fulfill their dietary needs based on such

Chapter Summary (continued)

factors as cultural and religious background, financial resources, and appetite.

■ The basic components of nutrition are carbohydrates, proteins, fats, minerals, vitamins, fiber, and water. Carbohydrates are the primary source of energy and are primarily found in fruit, breads and cereals, pasta products, rice, and potatoes. Fats and proteins are also a source of energy. Fats aid in growth and development by providing fatty acids, and proteins build and renew body tissues.

■ Vitamins are required components for metabolism and growth and development. Minerals help in specific regulatory processes, tissue development and repair, blood clotting, muscle contractions, and nervous system impulse conduction. Fiber is important to intestinal health and the prevention of intestinal diseases. Water regulates body temperature, lubricates joints, carries nutrition to and waste materials from body cells, and aids in other body processes.

■ Weight management is best achieved by maintaining a balance between caloric intake and caloric expenditure. Obesity, a symptom of caloric intake greater than required caloric needs, is both a cause and a result of medical conditions.

■ The MyPyramid is an educational tool developed by the USDA to assist healthy Americans over 2 years of age to maintain good eating habits.

■ The pyramid lists the recommended servings of different food groups to meet daily nutritional needs. Alternate versions of the Food Pyramid address specific groups such as Asian, Latin, Mediterranean, vegetarian, the elderly, and children ages 2 through 6. Persons with medical needs require the professional assistance of dietitians and physicians to design optimum diets.

■ The physiological functioning of the gastrointestinal system decreases as an individual ages. Functioning is also affected by past and present medical conditions, medications, and social interaction. Establishing wellness habits early in life prevents malnutrition, obesity, inactivity, and the advancement or development of medical and dental conditions later. The nutritional status of an individual as he or she ages can affect or cause medical conditions. The elderly should be encouraged to eat high-nutrition foods and maintain or increase physical activity, which in turn increases appetite, mobility, physical endurance and immune response.

■ Food allergies and food intolerances occur in both children and adults. Food allergy reactions result from a hypersensitivity of the immune system to certain kinds of food substances. Persons with food allergies often have a genetic predisposition and a history of other allergies.

■ Diseases of the GI system include inflammatory conditions, obstructive conditions, infectious disorders, disorders due to increased or decreased peristalsis, circulatory or hemorrhagic disorders, congenital disorders, functional disorders, neoplasms, parasitic invasion, and food poisoning. Various diagnostic procedures may be ordered, some of which are performed in the office setting, including palpation, auscultation, visualization of the abdomen, blood tests, upper and lower GI series, stool specimen studies, and others.

■ Disease conditions result from and are the cause of altered nutritional states. For example, heart disease, hypertension, and atherosclerosis often result from dietary intake of foods high in fats and cholesterol. Prolonged nausea and vomiting are often responsible for electrolyte imbalances due to excessive loss of fluids. Parasitic infestation and infections result from the ingestion of contaminated food and/or water.

■ Colonoscopies are performed to assess healthy or disease states of the colon.

■ Warning signs of GI problems include nausea, vomiting, hematemesis, coffee ground emesis, diarrhea, constipation, bright red blood in stools, black stools, abdominal pain and distension, dyspepsia, anorexia, flatulence, and dysphagia.

■ Disorders or conditions of the GI tract may be classified as abnormal function, anatomical and congenital abnormalities, infections, food poisoning, inflammation, malignancies, vascular-related conditions, and conditions of the accessory digestive organs.

■ The medical assistant provides patients with information regarding special diets. It is customary for offices to have printed diets available for distribution to patients.

Chapter Review

Multiple Choice

1. Which of the following terms means "difficulty swallowing"?
   a. Hematemesis
   b. Dyspepsia
   c. Dysphagia
   d. Hepatomegaly

2. The lower GI tract includes all of the following except the
   a. duodenum.
   b. small intestine.
   c. large intestine.
   d. sigmoid.

Chapter Review (continued)

3. The upper GI tract includes all of the following except the
   a. pharynx.
   b. cecum.
   c. esophagus.
   d. duodenum.

4. The alimentary canal is composed of how many layers?
   a. 2
   b. 3
   c. 0
   d. 4

5. The parietal peritoneum covers which two organs?
   a. Upper and lower intestines
   b. Stomach and intestines
   c. Esophagus and small intestine
   d. Rectum and esophagus

6. The duct opening into the duodenum that releases bile and pancreatic enzymes is the
   a. ampulla of Vater.
   b. pancreatic duct.
   c. common hepatic duct.
   d. common bile duct.

7. *Mastication* means
   a. swallowing.
   b. elimination.
   c. chewing.
   d. ingestion.

8. Which of the following is *not* involved in the initial breakdown of food?
   a. Teeth
   b. Cheeks
   c. Tongue
   d. Esophagus

9. How many essential amino acids are there?
   a. 11
   b. 8
   c. 10
   d. 4

10. How many amino acids can be produced by the body?
    a. 11
    b. 8
    c. 6
    d. 4

True/False

T F 1. LDLs transport fats manufactured in the liver to body cells.
T F 2. HDLs transport fats from body cells to the liver.
T F 3. Lipoproteins contain cholesterol.
T F 4. Dietary fiber is a carbohydrate that takes the longest to digest, making a person feel full longer.
T F 5. Complex carbohydrates are sugars found in natural sources such as fruit and honey.

Short Answer

1. What is a calorie?
2. How much energy is released through the metabolism of 1 gram of carbohydrate, 1 gram of protein, and 1 gram of fat?
3. According to the American Cancer Society, who should have colonoscopies for cancer screening?
4. Which procedure is often used to treat obstructive conditions involving the small intestine?
5. What is the function of the organs and ducts of the biliary tract?

Research

1. Research the different types of vegetarian diets, such as full vegan.
2. Research the top five diet trends of the year. How are they similar? How are they different? What is the main "promise" of each?

Externship Application Experience

A patient sitting in the exam room states that he is feeling nauseous and very uncomfortable. What should you do?

Resource Guide

American College of Gastroenterology (ACG)
P.O. Box 3099
Alexandria, VA 22302
www.acg.gi.org

American Dental Association
211 E Chicago Ave.
Chicago, IL 60611-2678
www.ada.org

American Dietetic Association
216 W. Jackson Blvd.
Chicago, IL 60606-6995
800-877-1600
www.eatright.org

American Dietetic Association Foundation
120 South Riverside Plaza, Suite 2000
Chicago, IL 60606
1-800-877-1600
www.adaf.org

American Gastroenterology Association
493 Del Ray Ave.
Bethesda, MD 20814
301-654-2055
www.gastro.org

Food Allergy and Anaphylaxis Network
10400 Eaton Place, Suite 107
Fairfax, VA 22030
800-929-4040
www.foodallergy.org

National Institute of Allergy and Infectious Diseases
National Institutes of Health
U.S. Department of Health and Human Services
Bethesda, MD 20892
www.niaid.nih.gov

U.S. National Library of Medicine
National Institutes of Health
www.nlm.nih.gov

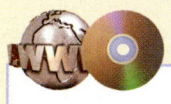

Med**Media**

http://www.MyMAKit.com

More on this chapter, including interactive resources, can be found on the Student CD-ROM accompanying this textbook and on http://www.MyMAKit.com.

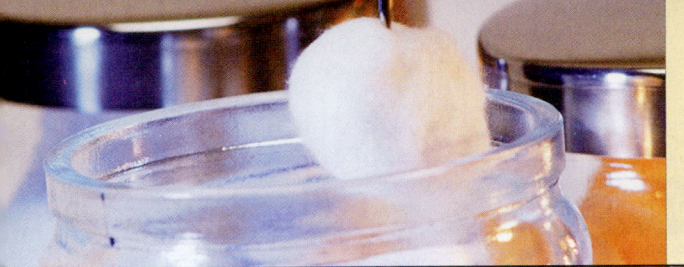

Objectives

After completing this chapter, you should be able to:

- Define and spell the key terminology in the chapter.
- Define the role of the medical assistant in the orthopedic office.
- Describe the anatomy and physiology of the bones and skeleton.
- Describe the anatomy and physiology of muscles.
- Discuss congenital, degenerative, infectious, malignant, and traumatic musculoskeletal conditions.
- List and describe diagnostic procedures for musculoskeletal conditions.
- Explain how splints and braces are used.
- Describe different types of casts and cast application.
- Describe major physical therapy modalities, including thermodynamics.
- Discuss ambulation modalities, including walking with crutches, a cane, and a walker.
- Explain the use of prostheses in orthopedics.
- Discuss proper body mechanics.

Orthopedics and Physical Therapy

Case Study

Xavier is restocking the exam rooms at the urgent care center where he works after a midafternoon rush of patients. Just as he is finishing, Jorge Ramirez hops in, assisted by two of his friends. Jorge explains that he was playing a game of touch football with his friends when he was tackled and twisted his ankle. It started swelling immediately, is very painful to move, and cannot bear any weight. Xavier directs Jorge's friends to assist him onto the X-ray table so the ankle can be checked for a fracture.

After the initial exam and X-ray by the physician, Jorge is told a fracture cannot be ruled out due to the swelling. The doctor says he will refer Jorge to an orthopedic specialist. In the meantime, prior to the appointment, Jorge is to wear an air brace for support and use crutches. It is Xavier's responsibility to teach him the proper technique for crutch use.

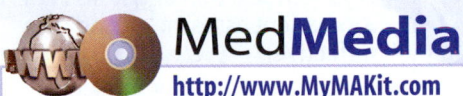

MedMedia

http://www.MyMAKit.com

Additional interactive resources and activities for this chapter can be found on http://www.MyMAKit.com. For videos, tips, audio glossary, legal and ethical scenarios, job scenarios, quizzes, games, virtual tours, and activities related to the content of this chapter, please access the accompanying CD-ROM in this book.

Audio Glossary
Legal and Ethical Scenario: *Orthopedics and Physical Therapy*
On the Job Scenario: *Orthopedics and Physical Therapy*
Video: Crutch Instruction
Multiple Choice Quiz
Games: Crossword, Strikeout, and Spelling Bee
3D Virtual Tour: Muscular System: Head & Neck; Muscular System: Hip & Thigh; Muscular System: Leg & Foot; Muscular System: Lower Limb; Muscular System: Pelvis (Female); Muscular System: Arm & Shoulder; Muscular System: Trunk & Abdomen; Muscular System: Upper Limb
Drag and Drop: Muscular System: Muscle Structures, Muscles of the Anterior, Muscles of the Posterior
Tips
HIPAA Quiz

Key Terminology

amphiarthrosis—condition of slight joint movement in all directions

arthritis—inflammation of a joint

articular—pertaining to a joint

atony—lack of normal tone or strength in a muscle

atrophy—decrease in size of normal muscle mass

axillary—pertaining to the axilla (armpit)

body mechanics—procedures for standing and efficient body movement, including lifting, pushing, or pulling, that prevent injury and maintain required energy levels for long employment

bursa (plural: bursae)—a sac filled with synovial fluid that reduces friction and provides ease of movement between tendons and ligaments, ligaments and bone, and other tissues

bursitis—inflammation of bursa(e)

cartilage—smooth, elastic connective tissue that covers the ends of the bones

cast—a plaster or fiberglass device used to immobilize a body part

compress—folded piece of material used to apply dry or moist heat or cold therapeutic applications

cryotherapy—the use of cold applications to prevent or reduce swelling and pain

diarthrosis—condition of bone joints moving freely

endosteum—membrane lining the inner portion and marrow cavity of the bone

hematopoiesis—formation of blood cells

ligament—a tough, elastic tissue that connects ends of bones

neoplasia—abnormal cell development

orthopedics—the study and treatment of diseases and disorders of the musculoskeletal system

osteoblast—a precursor cell in bone formation

periosteum—a fibrous membrane covering the outside of bone tissue

prosthesis (plural: prostheses)—artificial replacement for a body part

range of motion—the full extent of any joint potential for movement, including actions such as flexion, extension, circumduction, adduction, and abduction

✚ MEDICAL ASSISTING STANDARDS

CAAHEP ENTRY-LEVEL STANDARDS	ABHES ENTRY-LEVEL COMPETENCIES
■ Perform within scope of practice (psychomotor) ■ Explore issue of confidentiality as it applies to the medical assistant (cognitive) ■ Apply ethical behaviors, including honesty/integrity in performance of medical assisting practice (affective) ■ Apply local, state and federal health care legislation and regulation appropriate to the medical assisting practice setting (psychomotor) ■ Recognize the importance of local, state and federal legislation and regulations in the practice setting (affective) ■ Explain the rationale for performance of a procedure to the patient (affective) ■ Use language/verbal skills that enable patients' understanding (affective) ■ Describe the normal function of each body system (cognitive) ■ Identify common pathology related to each body system (cognitive) ■ Analyze pathology as it relates to the interaction of body systems (cognitive) ■ Discuss implications for disease and disability when homeostasis is not maintained (cognitive) ■ Describe implications for treatment related to pathology (cognitive) ■ Apply critical thinking skills in performing patient assessment and care (affective) ■ Prepare a patient for procedures and/or treatments (psychomotor) ■ Assist physician with patient care (psychomotor) ■ Document accurately in the patient record (psychomotor) ■ Practice Standard Precautions (psychomotor) ■ Show awareness of patients' concerns regarding their perceptions related to the procedure being performed (affective)	■ Project a positive attitude. ■ Maintain confidentiality at all times. ■ Be a "team player." ■ Be cognizant of ethical boundaries. ■ Exhibit initiative. ■ Adapt to change. ■ Evidence a responsible attitude. ■ Be courteous and diplomatic. ■ Conduct work within scope of education, training, and ability. ■ Interview and take a patient history. ■ Prepare patients for and assist physician with routine and specialty examinations and treatments and minor office surgery. ■ Apply principles of aseptic techniques and infection control. ■ Prepare and maintain examination and treatment area. ■ Collect and process specimens. ■ Dispose of biohazardous materials. ■ Practice Standard Precautions. ■ Prepare and administer oral and parenteral medications as directed by the physician. ■ Maintain medication and immunization records.

Key Terminology *(continued)*

reduction—the process of open or closed manipulation that returns bony ends to correct anatomical position before healing

soak—procedure in which the total body or body part is immersed in water for heat or cold therapeutic applications

splint—a temporary orthopedic device used to immobilize, restrain, and support any extremity of the body

synarthrosis—condition of absent joint movement

tendon—tough, elastic tissue that connects muscle to bone

tetany—painful, intense, spasmodic muscle contractions

thermodynamics—the use of cryotherapy or thermotherapy for therapeutic treatment

thermotherapy—the use of heat application to increase circulation to an area and promote healing

Abbreviations

AKA—above knee amputation

BEA—below elbow amputation

BKA—below knee amputation

C1—cervical vertebra number 1 (number identifies 1-7 of cervical vertebrae)

Ca—calcium

DJD—degenerative joint disease

Fx—fracture

L1—lumbar vertebra number 1 (number identifies 1-5 of lumbar vertebrae)

LLE—left lower extremity

LLL—left lower leg

LS—lumbosacral

LUE—left upper extremity

PT—physical therapy

RA—rheumatoid arthritis

RLE—right lower extremity

RLL—right lower leg

ROM—range of motion

RUE—right upper extremity

T1—thoracic vertebra number 1 (number identifies 1-12 of thoracic vertebrae)

✔ COMPETENCY SKILLS PERFORMANCE

1. Assist with fiberglass cast application.
2. Assist with cast removal.
3. Assist the patient with cold application/cold compress.
4. Assist the patient with hot moist application/hot compress.
5. Assist with therapeutic ultrasonography.
6. Demonstrate measuring for axillary crutches.
7. Assist a patient with crutch walking.
8. Assist a patient in using a cane.
9. Assist a patient in using a walker.
10. Assist a patient in a wheelchair to and from an exam table.

Introduction

Orthopedics is the study of the musculoskeletal system: the bones, muscles, joints, ligaments, tendons, and nerves. The bones of the skeletal system give the body its shape and support and also protect internal organs. The muscles cover the skeleton and move the different parts of the body. All parts of the musculoskeletal system are subject to disease and trauma.

An orthopedic surgeon is a surgical physician who specializes in the diagnosis and treatment of musculoskeletal conditions. Physicians in this practice are often called orthopedists or orthopods.

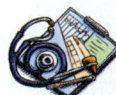

The Medical Assistant's Role in the Orthopedic Office

The medical assistant in an orthopedic office should be familiar with the anatomy, terminology, and disorders and diseases of the musculoskeletal system. The MA will have a variety of tasks, depending on the area of the medical office to which he or she is assigned:

- Obtaining and recording medical history, vital signs, and specific symptoms as reported by the patient
- Assisting the physician in examinations and procedures
- Placing X-ray films on the radiograph viewbox for the physician
- Instructing the patient about undressing, and providing a gown and drape
- Assisting the patient in ambulating or moving to and from the examination table
- Arranging appointments for diagnostic tests and procedures
- Providing patients with supportive and ambulation devices, including crutches, canes, and wheelchairs
- Instructing patients and family members in proper **body mechanics** and **thermodynamic** treatments
- Providing information on community resources for orthopedic patients such as rehabilitation, transportation, and mobility services, and physical therapy

The Anatomy and Physiology of the Musculoskeletal System

The musculoskeletal system is composed of bones and muscles. The skeleton provides the framework for the body, allowing the individual to stand erect, and protects the internal organs. Muscles facilitate the movement of the various bones and joints of the skeleton.

Bones

The skeleton can be divided into axial and appendicular sections (Figure 43-1 ◆). The axial skeleton consists of bones in the head and trunk, such as the cranial, facial, and ear bones; the vertebrae of the spinal column; the sternum; and the ribs. The spinal column consists of cervical, thoracic, lumbar, sacral, and coccygeal sections. It serves as an anchor for the head and extremities and provides structure for the positions of sitting, standing, and lying.

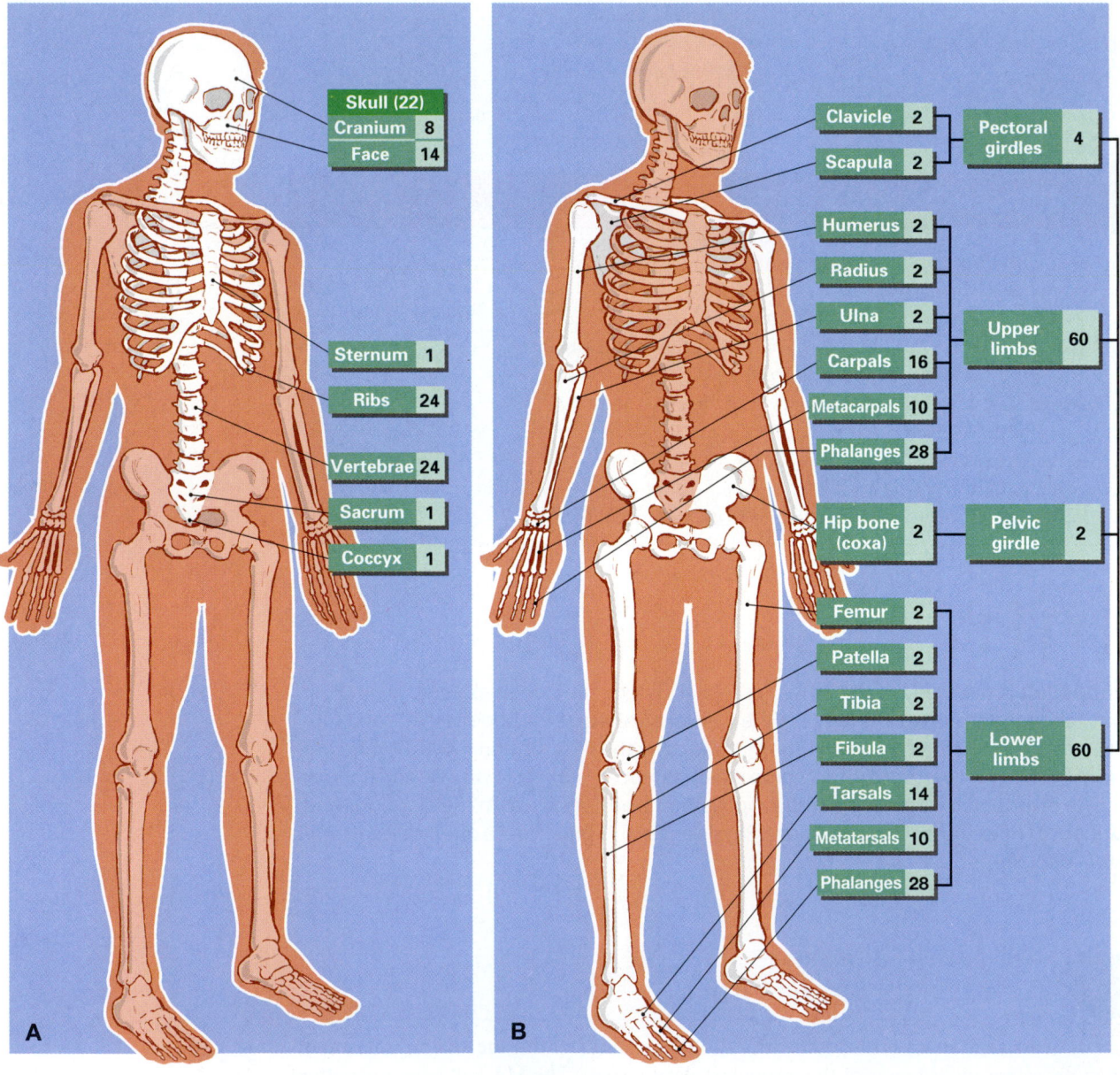

Figure 43-1 ◆ (A) The axial skeleton. (B) The appendicular skeleton.

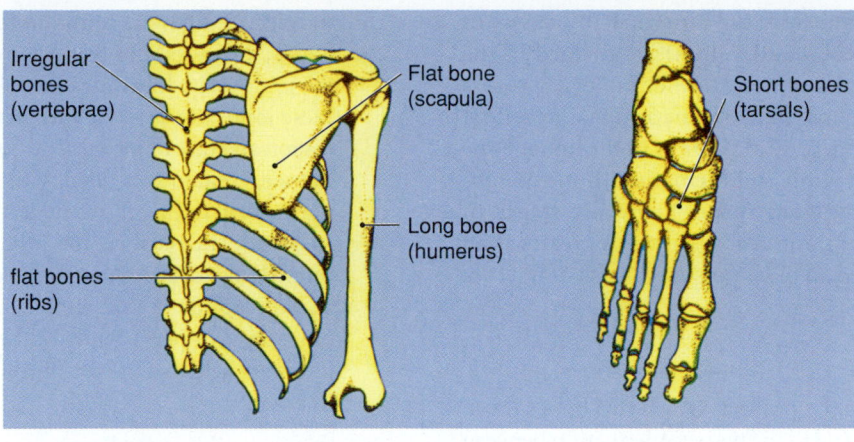

Figure 43-2 ◆ Classification of bones.

The appendicular section of the skeleton consists of the extremities and the shoulder and hip framework to which the extremities are attached. Examples of upper-division appendicular skeleton bones are the clavicle, scapula, humerus, radius, ulna, carpals, metacarpals, and phalanges of the fingers. The lower-division appendicular skeleton contains the pelvic bones, femur, patella, fibula, tibula, tarsals, metatarsals, and phalanges of the toes.

The skeleton is composed of 206 bones. These bones are classified according to structure (Figure 43-2 ◆).

- Long bones are located in the thigh, lower leg, upper arm, lower arm, and digits.
- The wrists and ankles consist of short bones that enable more specific movement.
- Flat bones include the shoulder bones (scapulae), ribs, and pelvic bones.

- Sesamoid bones, which are formed within **tendons** or joint capsules, include the patella, also known as the kneecap.

The bones come together to form joints and serve as points of attachment for muscles, thereby making movement possible. Bone tissue also serves as a repository for calcium (**Ca**) and other mineral reserves. When calcium blood levels are low, such as during low dietary supply, bone tissue releases calcium into the blood.

The outside layer of bone is covered with a membrane called **periosteum** (Figure 43-3 ◆). **Cartilage,** a strong and flexible connective tissue, helps to reduce friction between the moving bones and serves as a shock absorber. Cartilage is also found in the tip of the nose, the pinna (outer ear), and the larynx and trachea. The periosteum layer contains **osteoblasts** for bone tissue formation, blood and lymphatic vessels, and nerve fibers.

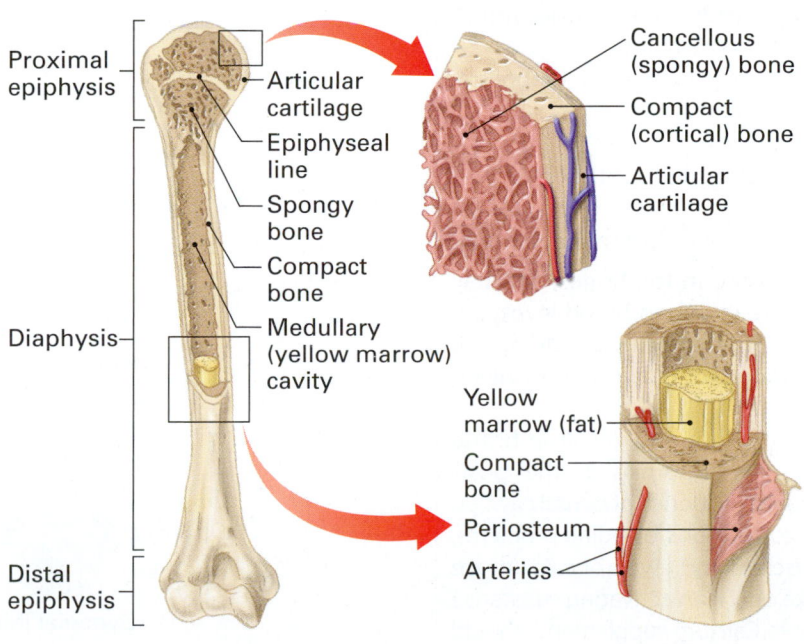

Figure 43-3 ◆ Bone and its anatomy.

The **endosteum** membrane lines the inner marrow cavity of the bone. Blood cells (RBCs and WBCs) are formed in the ends of long bones and the center of other bones, a process called **hematopoiesis.** Yellow marrow, made up largely of fat tissue, is found in the long, central portion of the bone. Bone tissue undergoes reabsorption and formation (bone metabolism) as the body progresses through the life stages of growth and aging. When bone reabsorption is greater than bone formation, such as in an older person, the risk of fracture increases.

Joints

A joint, or articulation, is the point at which two bones meet. Joints are classified according to the tissue construction between the bones and the amount of movement allowed by each joint.

- Cartilaginous joints are slightly movable because of the cartilage between the bones. They exhibit a type of movement called **amphiarthrosis.** There is no joint cavity. An example of a cartilaginous joint is the pubic symphysis between the pelvic bones; there are also cartilaginous joints between the vertebrae bodies of the spine.
- Fibrous joints, such as the sutures of the skull, are made of fibrous tissue. These joints exhibit **synarthrosis,** or no movement, because of the connective tissue between the bones. There is no joint cavity.
- Synovial joints are freely movable (**diarthrosis**) and have a joint cavity with anatomical structures to support full

movement. They are found in the neck, shoulders, arms, hands, hips, legs, and feet. Synovial fluid secreted within the joint cavity lubricates the joint. The bone surfaces of these joints are covered with **articular** cartilage for protection and ease of movement. Some synovial joints, called **bursae,** contain sacs filled with synovial fluid. In health, bursae help to ease movement of the often stressed joint. In disease, bursae become inflamed, a condition called **bursitis.** Synovial joints are also covered and protected by a joint capsule of connective tissue that joins with the outer layer, or periosteum, of the bone. Bones of synovial joints are held together by fibrous connective tissue called **ligaments.**

There are several types of synovial joints (Figure 43-4 ◆). They are capable of many different types of movement (Table 43-1 and Figure 43-5 ◆).

- The ball-and-socket joint allows free movement in many directions from its central point. It is found in the shoulders and hips where they connect to the axial skeleton.
- The condyloid joint allows for two-way movement. It is found at the junction of the skull occipital bone and the first cervical bone, and at the junction of the metacarpal joint and the first phalanx of each finger.
- The gliding joint allows for the gliding of one bone over the surface of another. The wrist and ankle are gliding joints.
- The hinge joint allows for extension or flexion of joints in the knee, elbow, fingers, and toes.
- The pivot joint facilitates internal or external rotation. This joint is found between the first and second cervical vertebrae and at the proximal ends of the radius and ulna in the arm.

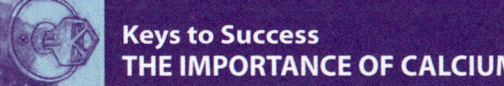

Keys to Success
THE IMPORTANCE OF CALCIUM

Calcium is essential to many body functions:

- It is important for blood clotting (coagulation).
- It helps nerves and muscles to function normally, including the myocardial muscle of the heart.
- It is essential for healthy bone growth and metabolism.
- It provides rigidity in bones and teeth.
- It is necessary for lactation.
- It serves as an activating enzyme for other chemical reactions in the body.
- It maintains the permeability of cellular membrane.

Calcium deposits are stored in the bones, but may be released to the bloodstream when blood levels are low. The parathyroid glands (behind the thyroid gland) are responsible for regulating blood levels of dissolved calcium.

A deficiency of blood calcium may result in brittle bones and teeth, rickets, osteoporosis in the postmenopausal female, increased incidence of dental cavities, **tetany,** muscle twitching, convulsions, bleeding problems, or **atony** of the heart muscle. Blood levels of calcium are increased by dietary intake only if an activating substance such as vitamin D is available. Calcium supplements should therefore be accompanied by sources of vitamin D.

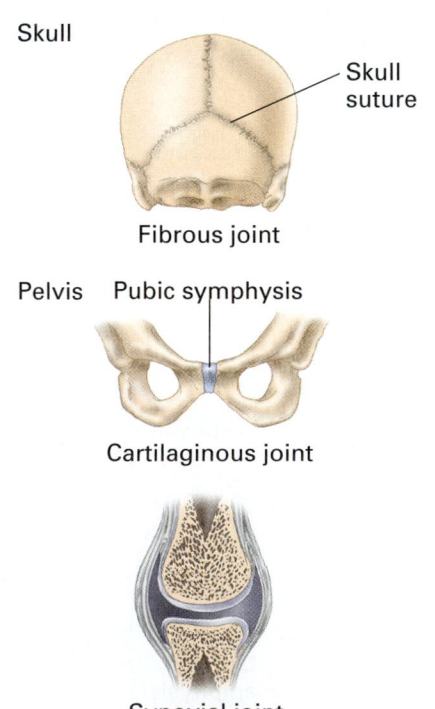

Figure 43-4 ◆ Types of joints found in the body.

TABLE 43-1 SYNOVIAL JOINT MOVEMENTS

Name of Movement	Description	Examples
Flexion	Decreasing the angle of the joint	Bending the lower arm toward the shoulder or making a fist by bending the fingers in toward the palm of the hand
Extension	Opposite of flexion; increasing the angle of the joint	Opening a closed fist to straighten the fingers or unfolding a bent elbow to straighten an arm
Adduction	Bringing the joint toward the body's midline	Moving an arm toward the body
Abduction	Moving the joint away from the body's midline	Moving an arm away from the body
Circumduction	Combination of flexion, extension, adduction, and abduction, accomplished by drawing a circle with an extremity	Rotating the distal portion of the arm while the proximal end remains fixed
Rotation	Turning the bone joint upon its own axis	Turning the head upon the first cervical vertebra
Supination	Describes movements of the hand, spine, and foot, referring to the spine or bony portion of the hand, spine, or foot in the dominant position (it is helpful to remember "supine on spine")	Having the palm facing upward when it is extended away from the body
Pronation	Describes movements of the hand, spine, and foot, referring to the soft tissue of the hand, palm, or abdomen in the dominant position	Having the palm facing downward when it is extended away from the body
Inversion	Turning inward	Turning the foot inward
Eversion	Turning outward	Turning the foot outward
Plantar flexion	Flexing of the foot with toes pointed downward and arch exaggerated	Ballet dancing on the toes

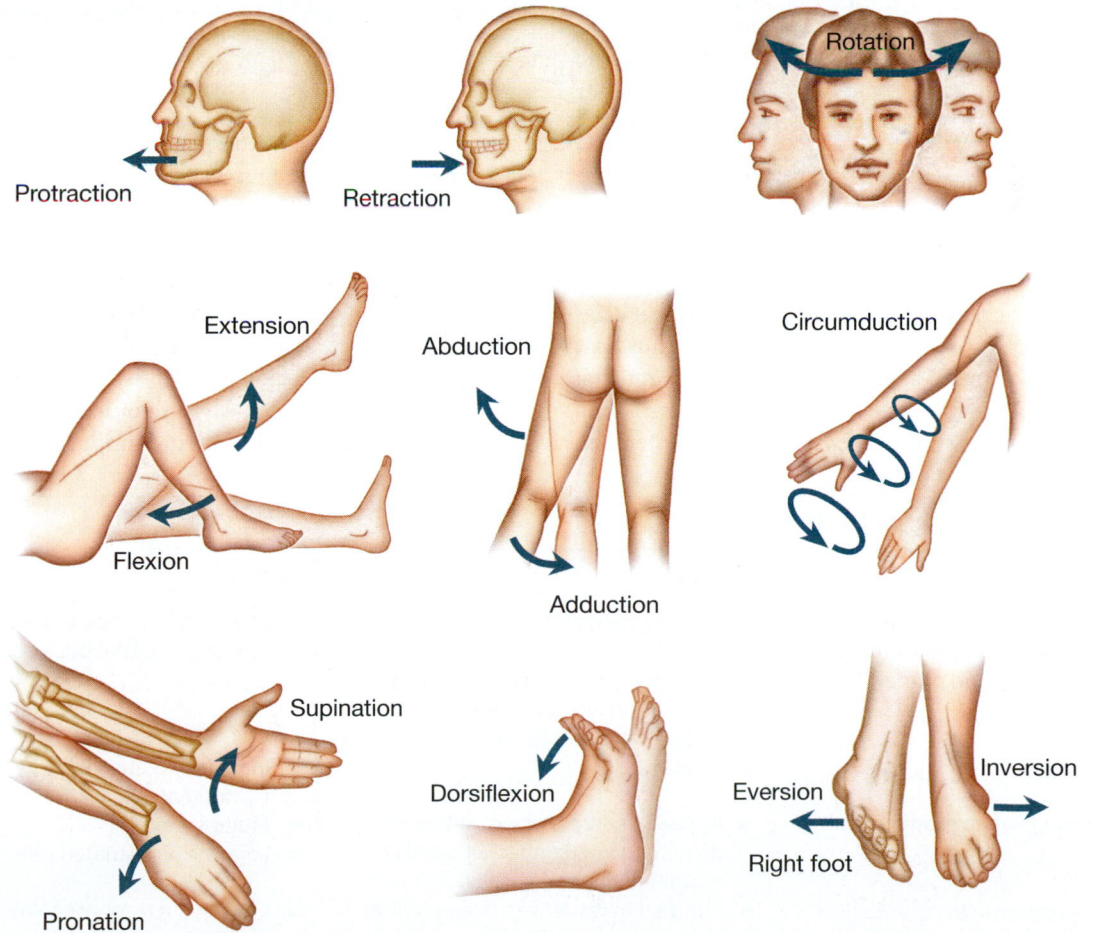

Figure 43-5 ◆ Range of motion exercises.

■ The saddle joint allows for two-way joint movement like the condyloid joint, but with deeper articulating movement between surfaces. An example of this type of joint is found between the metacarpal bone of the thumb and the wrist.

Range of motion (ROM) is the full degree of movement a joint is capable of (Figure 43-5). When a patient is immobile for any length of time, joint range of motion and muscle strength diminish. Range-of-motion exercises are prescribed to maintain joint flexibility and muscle strength. Active range of motion is performed by the patient without any help. Passive range of motion is performed by another person for the patient. Joint contractures and muscle **atrophy** may result when ROM is not prescribed and performed for patients who are immobile for extended periods of time.

Muscles

A muscle is tissue composed of fibers that have the ability to contract and relax, facilitating the movement of body parts and organs. There are three kinds of muscle tissue in the body: skeletal, smooth, and cardiac. This chapter addresses the functions, disorders, and/or insults to skeletal muscle. Muscles are attached to bones by connective tissue known as tendons and contract when they are stimulated by the nervous system.

Muscles help to maintain an upright posture and generate heat by shivering when the body responds to cold. Other functions include a wide range of movements, from opening and closing the eyes to running and throwing a ball, from digesting food to enlarging the thoracic cavity. Muscle tissue is stimulated by voluntary or involuntary muscle control. Smooth and cardiac muscle tissue are classified as involuntary, and skeletal muscle is classified as voluntary (Figure 43-6 ◆ and Table 43-2).

Involuntary muscles are controlled by the autonomic nervous system. Individuals cannot control involuntary responses such as the ongoing process of peristalsis or the beating of the heart. Cardiac muscle usually responds to a stimulus that originates at the sinoatrial (SA) node. The path of neuromuscular conduction spreads through and down the normal channel of electrical conduction to stimulate cardiac muscle contraction and relaxation. Different stimuli such as trauma, excitement,

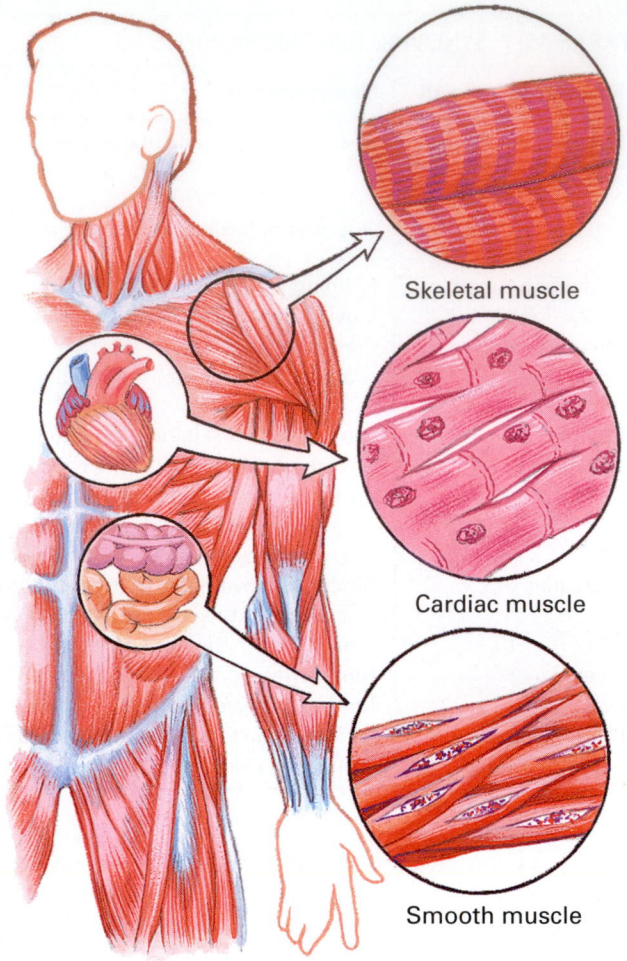

Figure 43-6 ◆ Types of muscles.

or a medical condition can affect whether the impulse originates in the SA node or in any of the other individual cardiac muscle cells of the atria, nodal region, or ventricles. The property of automaticity, belonging only to the cardiac cells, explains why the heart can beat slowly, fast, or irregularly, according to the location of the initiated cardiac impulse.

TABLE 43-2 SMOOTH, CARDIAC, AND SKELETAL MUSCLES

Smooth	Cardiac	Skeletal
■ Line the walls of blood vessels, respiratory tree, and hollow organs	■ Line the walls of the heart	■ Attached to bones and responsible for movement of the body and extremities
■ Move involuntarily and produce peristalsis	■ Involuntary reaction to nervous system stimulation results in pumping of heart and pulsation of vessels	
■ Single nucleus	■ Single nucleus	■ Movements are voluntary (consciously controlled)
■ Appear smooth when examined microscopically	■ Appear striated (striped) and have branching interconnections when examined microscopically	■ Multiple nuclei ■ Long, heavily striated cells
■ Contract in response to neurological electrical impulse, hormonal influence, exercise, medications	■ Contract in response to neurological electrical impulse, hormonal influence, exercise, medications	■ Contract in response to neurological electrical impulse, hormonal influence, exercise, medications

Voluntary muscles respond to individual control as well as autonomic nervous system control. The action of skeletal muscles under voluntary control can be changed. For example, a person walking can decide to run. Skeletal muscles can also respond involuntarily—for instance, the action of jerking the hand back after touching a hot pan.

The Contraction of Muscle Cells

A nerve cell contacts the muscle cell at the neuromuscular junction. Between the nerve cell and muscle cell is a small space called a synaptic gap (Figure 43-7 ◆). A stimulus causes the release from the neuron of neurotransmitters that excite and prompt a response from the muscle fiber, or cell. Neurotransmitters, including acetylcholine and others, are stored in nerve-ending vesicles until stimulated to release and carry the electrical impulse across the synaptic gap. The neurotransmitter chemicals attach to receptors of the muscle cell that spread the electrical impulse along the entire muscle cell.

When all elements of the neuromuscular system are healthy and functioning properly, the transmission of the nervous impulse results in contraction. In certain disease conditions, degeneration of the neuromuscular systems occurs. For example, Parkinson's disease results from a deficiency of the neurotransmitter dopamine, muscular dystrophy from the death of muscle fibers, and multiple sclerosis from demyelination (destruction of the myelin sheath present on some neurons) (see ∞ Chapter 46 for information on neuromuscular disorders).

Good health can prevent or inhibit the progression of neuromuscular diseases. A well-balanced diet provides vitamins

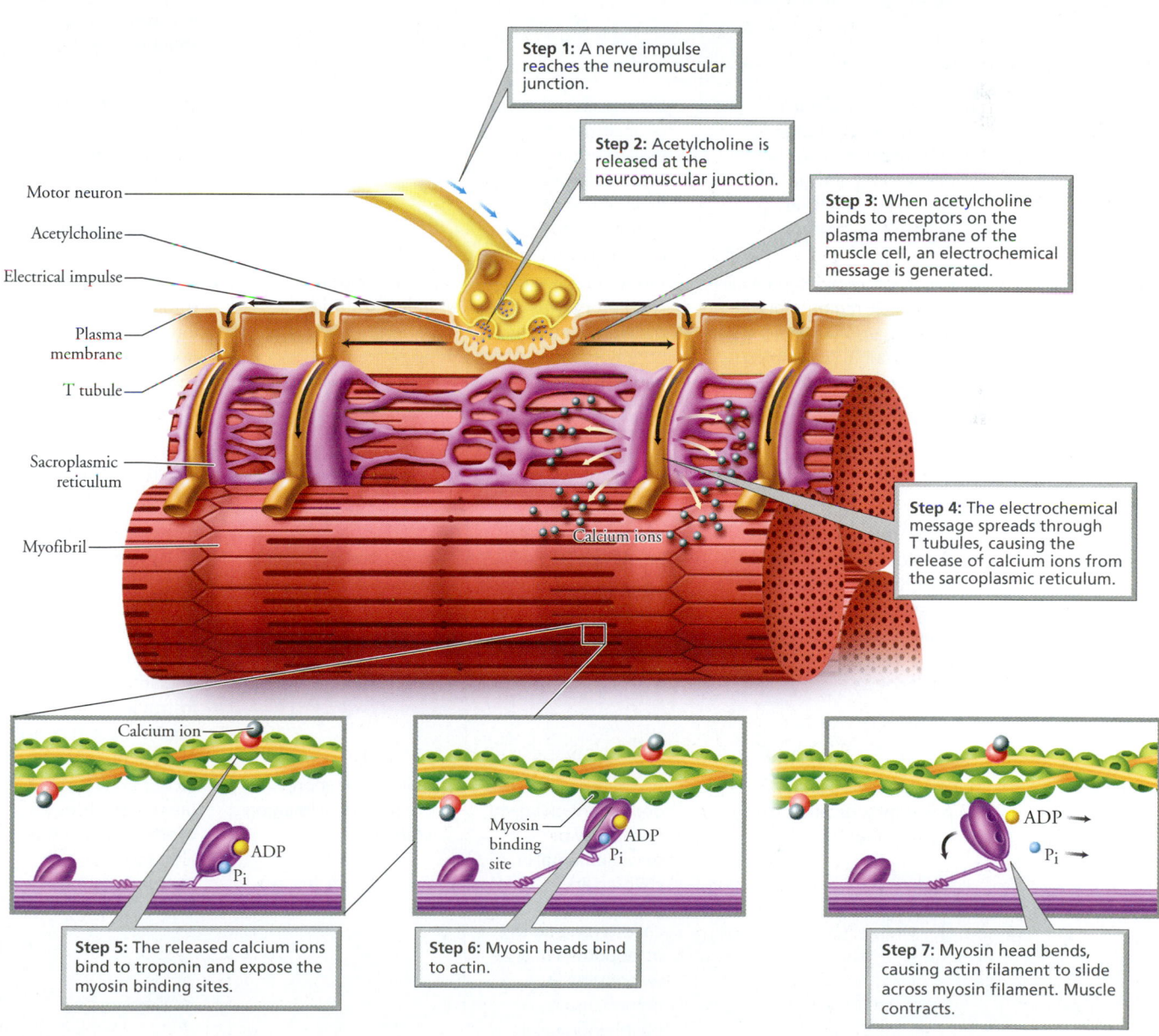

Step 1: A nerve impulse reaches the neuromuscular junction.

Step 2: Acetylcholine is released at the neuromuscular junction.

Step 3: When acetylcholine binds to receptors on the plasma membrane of the muscle cell, an electrochemical message is generated.

Motor neuron

Acetylcholine

Electrical impulse

Plasma membrane

T tubule

Sacroplasmic reticulum

Myofibril

Calcium ions

Step 4: The electrochemical message spreads through T tubules, causing the release of calcium ions from the sarcoplasmic reticulum.

Calcium ion

ADP
Pᵢ

Step 5: The released calcium ions bind to troponin and expose the myosin binding sites.

Myosin binding site

ADP
Pᵢ

Step 6: Myosin heads bind to actin.

ADP →
Pᵢ →

Step 7: Myosin head bends, causing actin filament to slide across myosin filament. Muscle contracts.

Figure 43-7 ◆ Neuromuscular junction.

and other nutrients that promote proper growth and development and help protect the neuromuscular system. Exercise enhances the circulation and transport of nutrition and oxygen to the cells and waste materials from the cells. It improves muscle tone and prevents muscles from atrophying. Exercise also strengthens bone tissue, thereby lowering the risk of fractures. Additionally, medical checkups, for health maintenance or management of neuromuscular symptoms, promote optimal health.

Common Musculoskeletal Diseases and Disorders

Conditions encountered in the orthopedic office can be classified as congenital, degenerative, infectious, and malignant or traumatic (Tables 43-3, 43-4, and 43-5). Another way to classify them is by the anatomical structure affected: bones, joints, or muscles.

TABLE 43-3 CONGENITAL AND DEVELOPMENTAL MUSCULOSKELETAL CONDITIONS

Condition	Signs and Symptoms	Cause	Diagnosis	Treatment
Clubfoot	Anterior aspect of foot of newborn is adducted and inverted, and potential for standing with foot flat is nil	Unknown; possibly congenital	Visual examination, manipulation, radiographs	Splinting in early months of life; if unsuccessful, surgical intervention may be required to straighten ankles and feet
Congenital hip dysplasia	Hip joint unstable due to abnormal development; folds of thigh in newborn uneven and one femur appears shorter during visual examination	Cause usually unknown or uncertain; possibly fetal position such as in breech presentation or softening of ligaments due to maternal hormones	Visual examination after birth, confirmed by imaging studies	Application of device to stabilize joint in proper position; if unsuccessful, surgical intervention may be required
Kyphosis	Outward curve of spine, usually in thoracic region; "hump" noted in upper spine, sometimes accompanied by pain and decreased mobility of spine	Etiology unknown in children; may be developmental, result of tumors, tuberculosis of the spine, or ankylosing spondylitis; in postmenopausal females, cause is frequently osteoporosis	Visual examination, imaging studies	Exercises, braces, and eventually surgical intervention for nonresponsive cases
Scoliosis	Lateral curve to spine, with one shoulder or hip higher than the other; often insidious onset; pain, occasional shortness of breath; occurs more frequently in adolescents	Etiology in some cases unknown; in others, cause may be uneven leg lengths, muscle degeneration, or vertebral deformity	Visual diagnosis, confirmed by imaging studies	Exercises, muscle electrostimulation, and braces; if unsuccessful, surgical intervention, fusion of vertebrae, possible implantation of instrumentation to secure spine in proper alignment
Lordosis (swayback)	Increased inward (anterior-posterior) curvature to the lower spine	Cause may be dependent on age of onset; may be developmental in children and degenerative in older children and adults; osteoporosis may be responsible in menopausal and postmenopausal females	Visual examination, confirmed by imaging studies	Exercises and braces; if unsuccessful, fusion of affected vertebrae along with instrumentation

TABLE 43-3 CONGENITAL AND DEVELOPMENTAL MUSCULOSKELETAL CONDITIONS (CONTINUED)

Condition	Signs and Symptoms	Cause	Diagnosis	Treatment
Muscular dystrophy	Progressive, degenerative weakening of muscles; onset in childhood; deterioration of muscle tissue is followed by eventual immobility and contractures	Generally considered genetic	Extensive family medical history; muscle biopsy and EMGs help confirm diagnosis	No cure at present, but exercise, PT, braces, and surgery help maintain child's ability to walk and move limbs; most children succumb before adulthood
Myasthenia gravis	Chronic weakness of muscles; initial onset usually in facial muscles, progressing to other muscles; droopy eyelids, difficulty swallowing often first symptoms; eventually progresses to paralysis	Possibly autoimmune disorder	Physical examination EMG; Tensilon test confirms involvement of acetylcholine receptors	Drug therapy including anticholinesterase medications, possibly corticosteroids; remissions are possible

TABLE 43-4 DEGENERATIVE AND INFLAMMATORY MUSCULOSKELETAL CONDITIONS

Condition	Signs and Symptoms	Cause	Diagnosis	Treatment
Osteoarthritis	Gradual onset of joint pain with edema and limited range of motion; muscles around affected joint become weak; bone spurs may be observed with imaging studies	Cause unknown; may be connected to aging process or follow insult to joint area	Physical examination, history, imaging studies	Drug therapy, including NSAIDs and steroids; exercise, heat applications provide pain relief
Rheumatoid arthritis	Deformed, painful joints; may become systemic, affecting many joints throughout body	Cause unknown at present; may be autoimmune response	Physical examination, history, imaging studies	Drug therapy, including NSAIDs and steroids; exercise, heat applications provide pain relief
Gout	Form of arthritis that normally affects great toe or fingers; pain and swelling in affected joints and possible limited movement	Deposits of uric acid crystals in joint spaces because of failure to fully metabolize purines in foods	Physical examination of joints, imaging studies; confirmed by urate crystals in joint fluid aspirate; elevated blood levels of uric acid may be indicator	Drug therapy including NSAIDs; rest to affected joint to relieve pain; avoidance of foods high in purine content
Bursitis	Inflammation of bursae in synovial tissue of joint; pain in joint area accompanied by limited range of motion	Repetitive motion to joint, friction in bursal space, or systemic disorders may lead to inflammatory condition	Imaging studies, physical examination	Resting affected joint, moist heat applications alternating with cold applications; drug therapy, including corticosteroids or NSAIDs
Osteoporosis	Usually asymptomatic until fracture occurs in older age, particularly to females; loss of height possible	Loss of calcium in bones, often after menopause as estrogen levels decrease	Blood serum studies, CT scan, bone scan, DEXA scans	Exercise helps to slow progress; drug therapy options are calcium and Vitamin D, hormone replacement therapy, or drugs such as Fosamax, Actonel, or Boniva.

continued

TABLE 43-4 DEGENERATIVE AND INFLAMMATORY MUSCULOSKELETAL CONDITIONS (CONTINUED)

Condition	Signs and Symptoms	Cause	Diagnosis	Treatment
Osteomalacia, rickets, softening of bone	Soft bones that deform during growth, bend easily or are brittle and painful; weakness	Vitamin D deficiency and loss of calcium; lack of sunlight	Bone scans and other imaging studies; blood tests including serum levels of calcium, alkaline phosphatase and Vitamin D; bone biopsy	Supplemental Vitamin D, calcium and phosphorus; exposure to sunlight for synthesis of natural Vitamin D.
Fibromyalgia	Chronic muscle pain, often accompanied by joint stiffness and tenderness; associated symptoms include fatigue, sleep disturbances, concentration problems, depression	Cause unknown at present; smoking tends to aggravate symptoms	Physical examination and tests to rule out other musculoskeletal conditions; tenderness in 11 of 18 specific trigger points indicates fibromyalgia	Improvement in sleep patterns, often with drug therapy; NSAIDs and muscle relaxants; exercise and relaxation techniques to relieve pain; no known cure at present.
Carpal tunnel syndrome	Chronic burning or aching pain in muscles and joint soft tissue	Cause unknown at present often trauma, infection; or emotional stress may precede onset	Pain in hand and wrist when median nerve is tapped indicates presence of trapped nerve; history and physical examination	Surgical release of compression on median nerve
Herniated disk	Severe pain in back area where disk is located; pain usually has sudden onset and is often sharp, radiating down to buttocks and thighs; possible muscle weakness of leg	Repetitive trauma or sudden impact; often caused by incorrect body mechanics when lifting heavy objects	Patient history and physical examination; MRI or radiographs confirm disk is protruding from normal area of spinal column and pressing on spinal cord and nerves	Rest and anti-inflammatory medication; surgical intervention to either trim bulging portion or remove entire disk
Tendonitis	Nonspecific pain along pathway of tendon or at its attachment	Injury to tendon or repetitive movement of tendon and joint	History and physical examination	Rest, drug therapy with NSAIDs or other anti-inflammatory drugs, cold therapy

TABLE 43-5 INFECTIOUS MUSCULOSKELETAL CONDITIONS

Condition	Signs and Symptoms	Cause	Diagnosis	Treatment
Lyme disease	Fever, chills, fatigue, headache, joint and muscle pain; characteristic itchy rash surrounding a red circle in early stages; untreated infection leads to arthritis-type pain, possible abnormalities in nervous system and/or cardiac arrhythmias	Infection spread by bite of a deer tick infected with the spirochete *Borrelia burgdorferi*	Patient history, physical examination revealing typical target lesion; skin biopsy revealing presence of spirochete confirms condition	Prompt removal of offending tick is essential; oral antibiotics in initial or early stages and IV in advanced stages; antipyretics to relieve fever
Osteomyelitis	Pain and tenderness in bone; fever; patient tends to guard against movement of the bone; possible bone trauma or a surgical procedure preceding infection	Bacterial invasion of bone tissue or bone marrow may result from insult to bone tissue during surgical or traumatic event. Usual causative organism is staphylococci	Blood cultures and culture of aspirate or drainage confirms presence of offending microorganism	Antibiotic therapy; extensive infections may require surgical removal of infected tissue

Common musculoskeletal diseases may involve muscles and bones of the body as a whole, the spine, the joints, or other connective tissue such as ligaments and cartilage. Others arise as the result of genetic predisposition.

Congenital conditions such as clubfoot and congenital hip dysplasia are present at birth. During development and throughout the growth periods, kyphosis, lordosis, and scoliosis, called developmental conditions, may occur. Some people have predispositions to certain conditions that are not observable at birth but are still present in underlying tendencies. Muscular dystrophy is a genetically transmitted disease. This progressive atrophy of skeletal muscles, with insidious loss of muscle strength, has no cure and leads to eventual death. Myasthenia gravis has an onset later in life as the individual experiences loss of muscle strength and function.

Degeneration of different areas of the musculoskeletal system occurs at various stages in life and affects numerous structures. **Arthritis** is the inflammation and degeneration of joint structures and appears as osteoarthritis or rheumatoid arthritis. Another form is gouty arthritis, which results from the improper metabolism of uric acid and the deposit of urate crystals in the joint spaces. Bursitis is an inflammatory process in the bursae or tissue surrounding the joints. In osteoporosis, bone loses density, predisposing the patient to a higher risk of fracture as the bones become porous. Osteomalacia literally means the softening of bone, with deformities and increased flexibility of the bone tissue. Carpal tunnel syndrome and other related conditions are the result of repetitive trauma. Fibromyalgia—muscle pain accompanied by sleep disturbances—has no known etiology and no known cure and is difficult to diagnose.

Infectious musculoskeletal conditions include Lyme disease and osteomyelitis. Lyme disease is a bacterial infection that develops from the bite of an infected deer tick. Osteomyelitis is an inflammation of bone tissue, caused by bacteria and usually following a traumatic insult or a surgical procedure.

Neoplasia

Neoplasia and/or malignant musculoskeletal conditions may involve any of the structures of the system—bone, cartilage or muscle—and usually take the form of tumors. Not all abnormal tissue growths (neoplasia) are malignant; some may be benign. Benign bone tumors are called osteomas.

Pain is a common factor in both benign and malignant tumors, often accompanied by swelling or growth. When a joint is affected, range of motion may be reduced. Diagnosis is often achieved through imaging studies; biopsy is required for positive differentiation of tumor origin and composition.

Malignant bone tumors usually occur in young people and affect the ends of the bones. Chemotherapy is administered to shrink a tumor prior to surgical removal. Primary carcinomas of the bone are called osteogenic sarcomas. Secondary or other forms of bone malignancy are the result of metastasis from primary malignancy sites. The bone destruction from metastatic carcinoma is quite painful, and fractures of the involved bone are frequent.

Rhabdomyosarcomas are rare, highly malignant tumors of muscle tissue. Early surgical removal is recommended. Many tumors metastasize before they are discovered and prognosis is not favorable.

Traumatic Musculoskeletal Conditions

Trauma to the musculoskeletal system includes insults to the bones in the form of fractures, soft-tissue insults to ligaments and tendons, and insults to the muscles. Sports injuries and motor vehicle accidents account for many traumatic musculoskeletal insults. Fractures resulting from falls are fairly common among the elderly.

Fractures

Fractures result from traumatic insult and challenge to the integrity of the bone structure. They take many forms, depending on the location of the traumatic insult, the type of insult, and the health status of the individual (Table 43-6).

Other Traumatic Conditions

Sprains, strains, dislocations, severed tendons, and torn meniscus in the knee are some of the soft-tissue injuries that involve the musculoskeletal system.

TABLE 43-6 TYPES OF FRACTURE

Name	Description	Usual Sites Affected
Avulsion	Fragment of a fractured bone is torn away with the muscle or ligament	Appendages; often occurs when clothing or a digit are entangled during the traumatic event
Comminuted fracture	Crushing or splintering of the bone	Long bones and any other bone vulnerable to crushing
Compound fracture	Open wound over the ends of the fractured bones; often an end of the bone is visible	Long bones
Compression	Collapse of the bone due to pressure exerted on it	Spinal vertebrae
Depression	Fragments or portions of bone pressed down in the skull and into the brain and surrounding tissue	Head, usually the result of acceleration-deceleration insult
Displaced fracture	Bone ends out of alignment	Long bones
Greenstick fracture	Bone partially bent and partially broken, like a twig or branch of a tree	Long bones, usually the arms; often occurs in children

continued

TABLE 43-6 TYPES OF FRACTURE (CONTINUED)

Name	Description	Usual Sites Affected
Impacted fracture	One end of a fractured bone driven or wedged into the other end of the same bone	Long bones and bones of wrists, elbows, shoulders, ankles, knees and hips
Longitudinal fracture	Fracture parallel with the long axis of the bone, usually running along part of the length of the bone	Long bones
Nondisplaced fracture	Bone ends remain in alignment	Any bone
Oblique fracture	Fracture runs obliquely across the bone	Long bones
Pathological fracture	Result of insult to diseased or weakened bone that normally would not cause a fracture in healthy bone tissue	Any bone, particularly of the spine and hips
Simple fracture	Skin intact over the fracture	Any bone
Spiral fracture	Fracture follows a helical pattern, twisting around the axis of the bone	Long bones
Transverse fracture	Fracture crosses the bone at a 90° angle to the bone's axis	Long bones

- A sprain, or acute partial tear of a ligament, occurs as the result of a traumatic insult to the muscle, tendon, or ligament surrounding a joint. Careful questioning of the patient helps to ascertain the mechanism of injury, often a twisting action from a fall or partial fall. Severe pain is usually felt immediately, followed by swelling and discoloration. If a leg, ankle, or foot is injured, it is usually very difficult, if not impossible, to bear weight on it. Sprains to the upper appendages are usually characterized by limited range of motion or restricted movement. Imaging studies verify a sprain and rule out fracture. Treatment consists of immobilizing the joint.

- A strain, or the overstretching of a muscle, tendon, or ligament, also occurs when a muscle is used or stretched beyond its normal capacity. In addition to pain, the individual may experience numbness or loss of feeling in the affected area, weakness, and reduced function. Edema is common. Cool therapy, usually with ice, helps to reduce swelling and relieve pain.

- A dislocation involves a bone being displaced or separated from a joint and is usually the result of a traumatic insult. A subluxation is an incomplete or partial dislocation. A dislocation is painful, the joint appears deformed, and the range of motion is limited, if not absent. Dislocation can affect the shoulders, elbows, hand and finger joints, hips, knees, ankles, and toes. A serious dislocation of the vertebrae may cause damage to the spinal cord. Blood vessels and nerves may be injured, edema is spontaneous, and tissue is damaged. Imaging studies confirm the diagnosis. Dislocations must be reduced by manipulation or by surgical intervention. Depending on the joint involved, immobilization is generally required.

- A severed tendon generally also involves a laceration or acute tear to the surrounding tissue. Since tendons connect bone to muscle, severing renders the connected part unable to move. The tendons usually affected are those in the hands, fingers, forearms, feet, toes, and calves of the legs. Occasionally, the tendon is torn rather than severed with a sharp object.

- A torn meniscus (cartilage in the knees and other joints) often results from a fall, but could also result from a twisting motion or a sports injury. The patient experiences pain, edema, limited range of motion, and a limited ability to bear weight. Arthroscopy is performed as an outpatient procedure to examine and often repair the damage. Upon discharge, the patient ambulates with the aid of crutches. The patient receives a prescription for pain medication along with instructions to elevate the extremity and apply ice intermittently.

In Practice

A youth baseball player is seen in the office after twisting his ankle during a game. He states that he began to experience pain and swelling almost immediately after the injury. The physician diagnoses the patient with an ankle sprain. After the physical examination, the patient asks the medical assistant what the difference is between a strain and a sprain. How are each of these musculoskeletal conditions treated?

Amputation

Amputation—the total or partial removal of a limb or digit—may be the result of trauma or of disease process. An accidental amputation may be complete, or a surgical procedure may be required to completely sever the body part or revise the remaining stump and close the wound. Often a traumatic amputation is the result of a crushing, tearing, or incising event. Impaired circulation resulting from compromised arteries, peripheral vascular disease, tumors, infection or other disease processes leads to ischemia to the tissue and necrosis, making amputation necessary.

After an amputation, the individual may feel pain or other sensations in the area where the amputated part had been, as if it were still attached. This feeling is referred to as phantom limb or phantom pain. Damage to the sensory nerves during amputation is difficult to treat but may diminish with time.

After the stump has healed, rehabilitation of the affected limb, with a **prosthesis** and patient training, is recommended.

Diagnostic Procedures

In conjunction with the physical examination and the patient's description of symptoms, diagnostic procedures are performed to rule out or confirm diagnoses of musculoskeletal conditions (Table 43-7). Noninvasive diagnostic screening includes radiographs and most bone scans and CT scans. (When ordered by the physician, bone scans and CT scans can become invasive with the injection of contrast medium.) Arthrograms, myelograms, electromyograms, biopsies, and blood studies are invasive diagnostic procedures.

While most major fractures receive treatment at emergency facilities, many may be treated in the orthopedic office. Displaced, compound, avulsed, and other types of fractures usually receive surgical intervention at an emergency or urgent care center, and the patient has been referred to the orthopedic office for followup care. Radiographs and imaging studies are usually required to make a diagnosis. Most orthopedic clinics and offices have an imaging department on site.

Treatment of Musculoskeletal Conditions in the Orthopedic Office

The correction of a fracture, in which the bone fragments are realigned, is called **reduction.** A closed reduction is performed by external manipulation, and an open reduction is done through surgery.

Fractures are generally immobilized with **splints,** braces, or **casts.** Ambulation or mobility devices such as crutches and canes are prescribed as well. The MA often assists with procedures and patient education in these treatments as well as in physical therapy, particularly heat and cold treatments. Sutures or staples sometimes have to be removed and dressings inspected and replaced.

Splints and Braces

Splints are temporary devices used post-trauma primarily to prevent movement of the affected extremity(ies), including bones and joints, and to prevent further insult until the physician has assessed the extent of the injury (Figure 43-8 ◆). Sometimes a splint is used for post-reduction in place of a cast.

A brace is usually a more permanent device that provides support for a weak muscle or joint and allows it to function normally. With specialized padding, braces can provide corrective alignment for patients with scoliosis, congenital hip dysplasia, and other conditions. Braces can often be removed temporarily to allow observation of the affected area and hygiene care.

? Critical Thinking Question 43-1

Xavier must give information and instructions to the patient, Jorge, who is in pain and will probably not remember most of their conversation in the morning.

TABLE 43-7 DIAGNOSTIC PROCEDURES FOR MUSCULOSKELETAL DISORDERS

Radiograph	X-ray image of various body structures, used to detect fractures or other abnormalities based on the density of tissues
CT scan (Computed Axial Tomography)	Cross-sectional images in fine detail that assist in diagnosis of tumors, lesions, and other soft-tissue anatomical abnormalities
Arthrogram	Fluoroscopic examination of the internal aspects of the joint, accomplished by injecting contrasting medium into the joint capsule
Myelogram	Injection of a contrast medium into the spinal canal to diagnose/confirm intervertebral disc disorders
Bone scan	Imaging technique to evaluate bone density, bone growth, bone tumors, and other bone disease patterns
Electromyogram (EMG) and nerve conduction velocity studies	Diagnostic test to measure muscle contraction as a result of electrical stimulation (nerve conduction); evaluates the passage of nervous system impulses to and through the muscle and the muscular response
Bone and muscle biopsy	Removal of tissue samples to identify cancerous and benign neoplasms and other pathogenic conditions
Serum calcium (blood levels of calcium), serum phosphorus, serum alkaline phosphatase	Test for increased or decreased levels of blood calcium, phosphorus, or alkaline phosphatase to diagnose various bone and muscle diseases

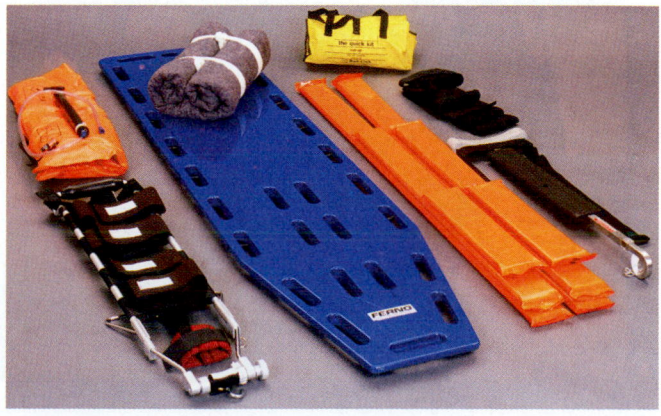

Figure 43-8 ◆ Splints and accessories for musculoskeletal injuries.

What is the best approach Xavier can take to make certain Jorge understands his instructions for ankle care, using the brace, and his orthopedic appointment?

Casts

Casts are solid, rigid, cylindrical casings that immobilize joints or body parts and facilitate the healing of fractures, of joints with or without surgery, and of anatomical deformities without surgery. There are two basic types of casting materials (Figure 43-9 ◆). Traditionally, casts have been made of plaster. Today newer synthetic casts made of fiberglass, polyester, or cotton are more commonly used. Both types have benefits and drawbacks.

- Plaster casts are heavier, may soften or crumble with moisture, and can crack or break. Plaster casts are more easily molded to the body part, so immobilization is more effective.
- Synthetic casts are lighter in weight, are not affected by moisture, and usually do not crack or break. They dry more quickly than plaster casts and are less likely to dent and create a pressure area. However, synthetic casts are not flexible and do not mold to the body part, they are more expensive, and the rougher surface can tear clothing and scratch the skin.

Cast Application

Casts are applied and removed by the orthopedist with the help of the medical assistant or specially trained technician. The MA prepares the treatment room with equipment and supplies, assists the physician as instructed and trained, provides printed instructional materials to the patient, and schedules appointments and referrals.

Before the cast is applied, X-rays are taken to assess the extent of the fracture. The physician performs reduction on the fracture and realigns the bone(s). The physician inspects the skin for lesions, redness, and bruises. The skin must be clean and dry for cast application. Either the physician or the MA does the cleansing.

TABLE 43-8 PATIENT INSTRUCTIONS: CAST CARE
Immediate Care Instructions
■ Elevate the casted limb above heart level for the first 24-48 hours to prevent swelling and reduce pain.
■ Move the toes or fingers frequently to maintain joint and muscle mobility.
■ Cold dry therapy in the form of ice bags may be applied at the local area of injury for 20 minutes per hour to reduce swelling. The cast should be protected from water damage.
■ With a plaster cast, avoid weight-bearing activity for 24 hours. With a synthetic cast, avoid activity for one hour.
General Care Instructions
■ To avoid injuring the skin, do not force anything under the cast.
■ Keep the cast dry. If the synthetic cast becomes wet, blot it dry, then sweep a blow-dryer on low or cool setting back and forth across the area.
■ Check the skin around the cast for signs of redness, sores, or swelling. Report any such findings to the physician.
■ Do not trim or break the cast. Notify the physician about any broken or loose areas.
■ Follow the exercise instructions prescribed by the physician or physical therapist to maintain muscle tone while the extremity is immobilized.
■ Follow the schedule for return appointments.
■ Report the following symptoms:
● Numbness or tingling in the fingers or toes.
● Blue, pale, or cold fingers or toes.
● Increased pain or swelling that is not helped with elevation or rest.
● Pain or burning under the cast.
● Drainage or foul odor coming from the cast.
● Sores around the edge of the cast.
● Fever, chills, nausea, or vomiting.

After the cast has been applied, radiograph films are taken again to confirm that the ends of the bone are correctly aligned. Observe exposed areas for circulation, sensation, and movement. The instructions in Table 43-8 help patients care for their casted limbs at home.

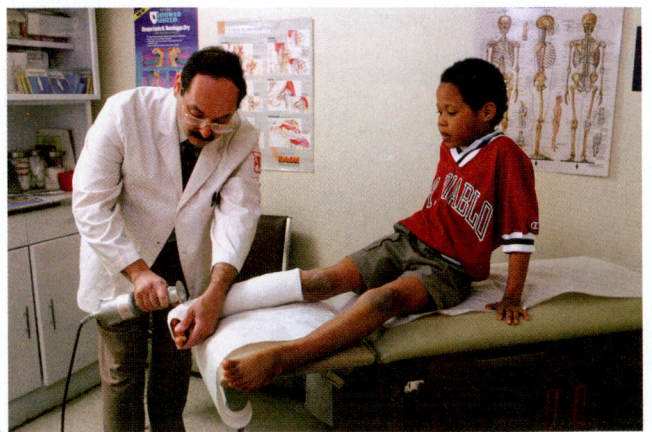

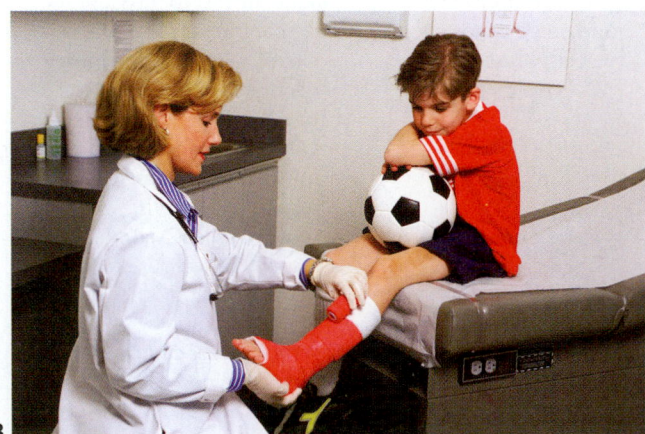

Figure 43-9 ◆ (A) Plaster cast; (B) Synthetic cast.
Source: Michal Heron Photography.

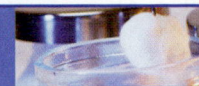

PROCEDURE 43-1   Assist with Fiberglass Cast Application

Theory and Rationale

There are many types of casts and many reasons for application. The physician will determine which is the most suitable for the patient's needs. Casts can be made from plaster of Paris, fiberglass, plastics, other synthetic materials, or fabric. If the cast must remain in place 24 hours a day for an extended period of time, fiberglass is generally used. Fiberglass is strong, lightweight, and waterproof. However, if the patient needs to wear the cast only when using the limb, the physician may choose to make a removable cast from synthetic materials that can be attached to the limb with Velcro straps. Air casts are fabric sleeves that fit over the injured limb and are inflated with air to immobilize the area. They can be used for a short time, depending on how much the limb is used.

Materials

- rolls of fiberglass casting material
- stockinette
- padding
- tape
- blunt/sharp nose scissors (for cutting material)
- warm tap water
- basin (2–4 liter)
- bandage
- gloves
- stool or low chair for support (if casting a foot or lower leg)
- patient drapes

Competency

(**Conditions**) With the necessary materials, you will be able to (**Task**) assist with the application of a fiberglass cast (**Standards**) correctly within the time frame designated by the instructor.

1. Assist the patient to the exam room and into a comfortable position. Explain that the patient should be comfortable to avoid having to shift the body weight during the lengthy casting process.
2. Identify the patient and verify the physician's orders.
3. Explain the procedure.
4. Wash your hands and put on gloves.
5. Cleanse and inspect the area to which the cast will be applied. Note any open wounds, bruising, or excessive swelling and report these to the physician.
6. Drape the patient to protect clothing.
7. Open one package of fiberglass material. Do not open the other packages until they are needed, to prevent waste.
8. Hand the physician the materials requested. If your clinic allows medical assistants to perform casting, cut the stockinette to fit the area.
9. Cover the affected body part with the stockinette, making sure it is smooth against the patient's skin and extends 1–2 inches beyond where the cast will end (Figure 43-10 ◆). If the stockinette is allowed to wrinkle or become bulky, it may cause a pressure sore on the patient's skin.
10. If you are casting the ankle, cut away excess wrinkled stockinette from the bend in the front of the ankle (Figure 43-11 ◆).
11. Use a spiral bandage turn to cover the casting area with padding (Figure 43-12 ◆). Apply extra padding to any bony areas.
12. Soak the inner layer of fiberglass tape in the basin of warm water (Figure 43-13 ◆). The tape material will be activated on contact with the water, so only wet as much as you need at a time.
13. The physician will roll and form the cast to the patient.
14. Roll the excess stockinette over the edges of the casting material to form a smooth edge.
15. Open the package of outer fiberglass tape for the physician (Figure 43-14 ◆).
16. The physician will shape and smooth the cast or may direct you to do so (Figure 43-15 ◆).
17. Clean up the work station.

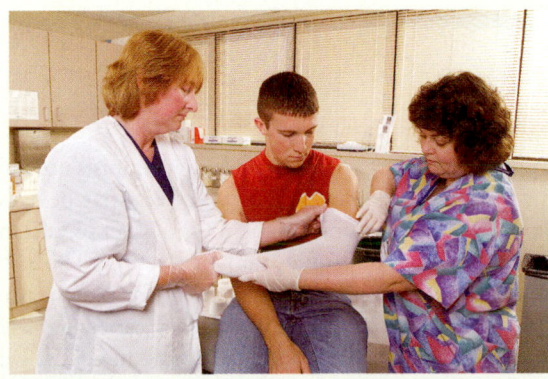

Figure 43-10 ◆ Apply stockinette to area that cast will cover.

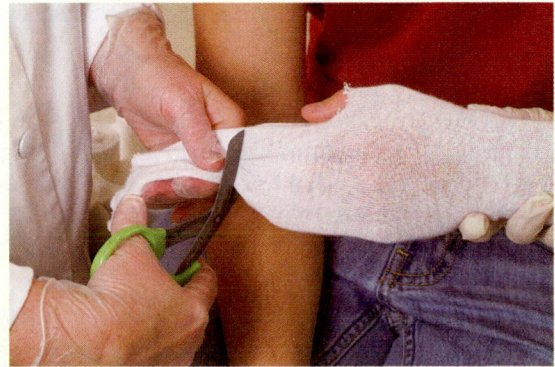

Figure 43-11 ◆ Cut away excess stockinette.

continued

PROCEDURE 43-1   Assist with Fiberglass Cast Application *(continued)*

18. Remove the gloves and wash your hands.
19. Document the procedure in the patient chart.

Patient Education

Provide the patient with verbal and written cast care instructions to help ensure compliance. Make appointments or referrals for followup care.

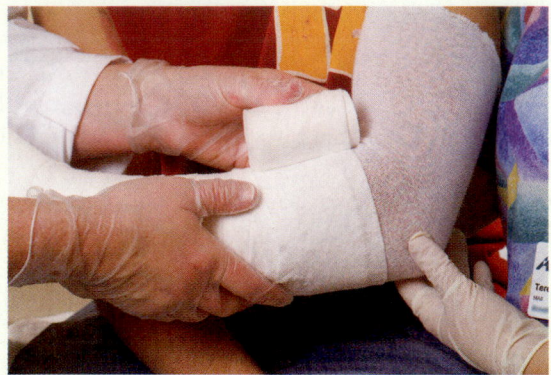

Figure 43-12 ◆ Use a spiral bandage turn to cover the casting area with padding.

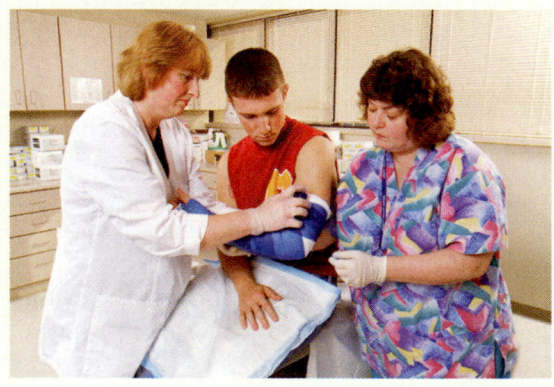

Figure 43-14 ◆ Open and apply an outer layer of fiberglass tape.

Charting Example

01/26/XX 8:00 am Application of fiberglass cast to patient's left forearm. Fingertips checked for capillary refill, movement, and circulation. Patient sent to X-ray to verify correct bone alignment. Stacy Robbins, CMA (AAMA)

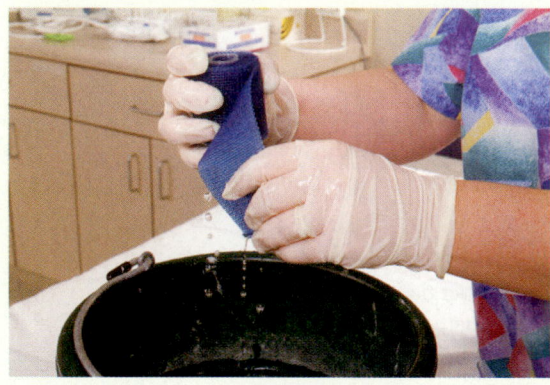

Figure 43-13 ◆ Soak the inner layer of fiberglass tape in the basin of warm water.

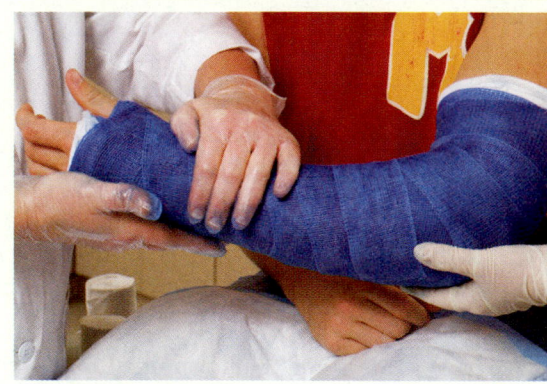

Figure 43-15 ◆ Assist in shaping the cast, as directed by the physician.

? Critical Thinking Question 43-2

What signs and symptoms should Xavier tell Jorge to watch for as his ankle heals? What can Jorge do to relieve some of the pain of his injury?

Cast Removal

When the normal healing period has passed, the physician orders a radiograph to confirm that the cast may be removed. The physician usually performs the cast removal but occasionally delegates the task to a specially trained clinical staff person.

Physical Therapy Modalities

Many physicians refer patients to physical therapists not only for therapy but for instruction in the use of assistive devices and thermodynamic applications (Table 43-9). Other physicians ask the medical assistant to provide patient teaching. The MA may be required to measure and fit the patient for crutches and/or to instruct the patient in the use of crutches, canes, and walkers. Other assignments may include instructing the patient in the therapeutic use of heat and cold, assisting in the evaluation of the patient's range of motion, and explaining proper body mechanics.

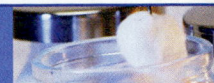

PROCEDURE 43-2 Assist with Cast Removal

Theory and Rationale

A cast cutter is used in a procedure known as *bivalving the cast.* Cuts are made on two sides, and the cast is then pried apart with a cast spreader (Figure 43-16 ◆). The cast padding and stockinette are cut away with bandage scissors. Occasionally, bivalving is done within the first few days after cast application to reduce pressure and pain on traumatized tissue. In this case, the cast may need to be replaced.

Materials

- cast-cutting device
- cast spreader
- bandage scissors
- heavy-duty bag in which to discard cast materials
- patient drape
- 500 ml basin
- 500 ml of warm water
- hypoallergenic soap
- towel
- hypoallergenic lotion

Competency

(**Conditions**) With the necessary materials, you will be able to (**Task**) assist in the removal of a cast (**Standards**) correctly within the time frame designated by the instructor.

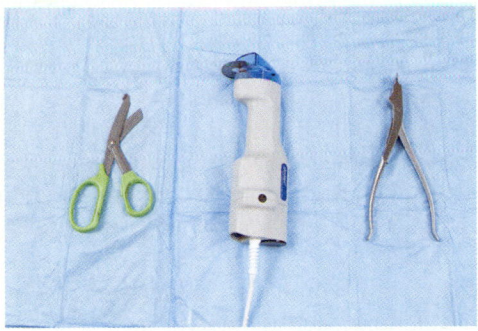

Figure 43-16 ◆ Cast cutter and cast spreader.

1. Making certain that the limb is properly supported, make two cuts along the medial and lateral side of the long axis of the cast (Figure 43-17 ◆).
2. Pry the cast apart with a cast spreader.
3. Carefully remove the two halves of the cast.
4. Cut away the stockinette and padding with the large bandage scissors.
5. Wash the previously casted area with hypoallergenic soap.
6. Dry the skin and apply a gentle skin lotion.
7. Provide the patient with written and verbal instructions for care of the limb.
8. Make an appointment for physical therapy as directed by physician.

Patient Education

The patient may be apprehensive about the cast-cutting device. Explain that the cutter blade vibrates but does not spin. The patient will feel some pressure and warmth as the cutter vibrates. The patient should also be advised that the skin under the cast will appear lighter in color and possibly wrinkled, and muscle tone may be noticeably decreased. Reassure the patient that physical therapy will help in regaining lost muscle tone and strength and that skin color and appearance will gradually return to normal with exposure to air and sunlight.

Charting Example

01/26/XX 8:00 am Patient came in for removal of left arm cast. Successful removal performed. Patient reports weakness in limb but no adverse effects. Appointment for physical therapy initiated. Lawrence Graham, RMA (AMI)

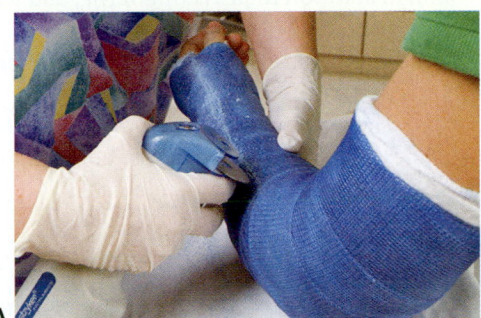
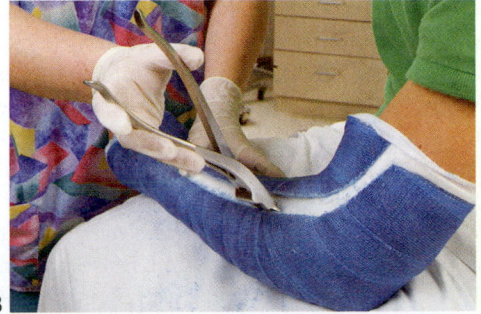

Figure 43-17 ◆ (A) Cut the medial and lateral side of the long axis of the cast. (B) Spread the cast.

TABLE 43-9 PHYSICAL THERAPY MODALITIES

Therapy	Description and Purpose
Cryotherapy	■ Also known as cold therapy ■ Constricts blood vessels; slows circulation to affected area; reduces swelling, inflammation, and pain; decreases body temperature ■ Dry cryotherapy: ice collars, ice-filled gloves, or other forms of commercial or improvised ice bags ■ Moist cryotherapy: cold compresses
Exercise therapy	■ Improves joint flexibility, muscle tone, strength, and mobility ■ Should be monitored by a physician or physical therapist
Hydrotherapy	■ Affected part is immersed in a whirlpool or container of water ■ Water exercise takes place in swimming pools or spas, directed by a physical therapist trained in hydrotherapy
Massage	■ Stimulates circulation and promotes healing ■ Helps to relieve muscle spasms, soreness, and tightness, and to restore motion and function to the body part
Range of motion (ROM) exercises	■ Prescribed by the physician and defined by the physical therapist ■ Improve flexibility and mobility ■ Active ROM exercises are performed by the patient without assistance; passive ROM exercises are performed by the patient with assistance from another person
Thermotherapy	■ Increases circulation to the area for greater comfort and healing ■ Moist thermotherapy: hot soaks or compresses ■ Dry thermotherapy: heat lights, infrared lights, light bulbs, and heating pads
Ultrasound	■ Vibrates tissues, generates heat, promotes circulation

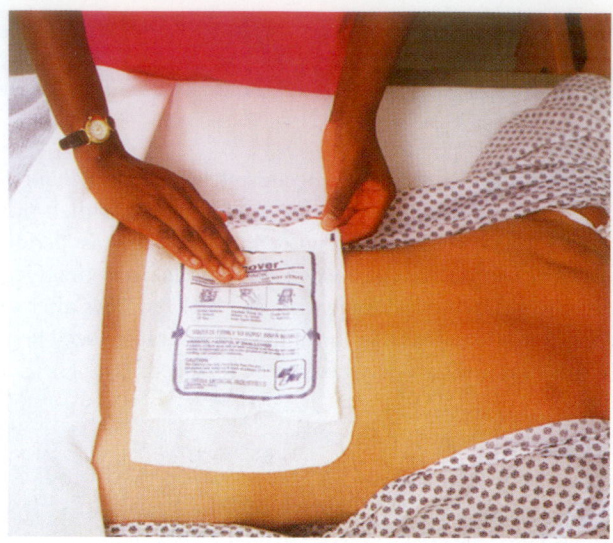

Figure 43-18 ◆ Applying heat and ice.

Thermodynamics

Thermodynamics consists of heat (**thermotherapy**) or cold (**cryotherapy**) applications that promote healing and prevent further tissue injury to areas affected by trauma, infection, and inflammation (Figure 43-18 ◆). The physician prescribes the appropriate treatment. The MA will be responsible for application in the medical office and patient instruction for self-care at home.

Heat dilates blood vessels and increases circulation. It can also speed up the localized formation of pus, also known as suppuration. The rate of healing is improved by increased oxygen and nutrition to the cells and the removal of the waste products of metabolism and inflammation. Heat relaxes the muscles and can reduce pain.

Cold constricts blood vessels, reducing blood flow and the leakage of fluid into tissues. By reducing swelling and stimulating nerve receptors, cold also acts as a temporary anesthetic, reducing discomfort and pain. In the early stages of infection, cold application can inhibit microbial growth and activity. For traumatic injury, with some exceptions, cold is usually applied for the first 24 to 48 hours to decrease swelling and pain, and heat is usually applied thereafter to increase circulation and healing.

In moist applications, water-immersed material is held against the skin. Thermodynamic treatments are applied for short, intermittent intervals (15 to 30 minutes) to prevent the reversal of the intended therapeutic effects. Covering the pack or other application prevents discomfort and pressure that might cause tissue damage and a breakdown in skin integrity.

Patients with neurological impairment due to aging or a medical condition, such as diabetes, may be more susceptible to harm from a thermodynamic treatment because they may not be aware that it is too hot or too cold and injuring the skin. In addition to providing verbal and written instructions to the patient, the MA may need to advise a family member or friend regarding potential complications from heat and cold applications.

The most common types of heat and cold application are the heating pad, hot **compress,** hot **soak,** ice bag, cold compress, and chemical hot or cold pack.

- In a heating pad, wires conduct electrical energy that is converted into heat.
- A hot compress increases circulation, suppuration, and infectious drainage. If a compress is used on an open

TABLE 43-10 PATIENT INSTRUCTION: MOIST AND DRY, HEAT AND COLD APPLICATIONS

Dry Heat Application: Heating Pad

- A heating pad uses electrical current to produce dry heat. Safety precautions must be followed to avoid overheating or electric shock. Inspect the heating pad for broken wires, do not use safety pins to hold the ends together or to attach the pad to bed linens, and inspect the cord for integrity.
- Cover the pad with a protective covering. Set the temperature as prescribed by the physician and place the pad on the area to be treated. The pad should feel warm but not uncomfortable.
- Do *not* turn the heating pad control to a higher temperature for more warmth. Doing so could cause serious burns.
- Call the physician if you notice increased swelling and redness or if pain increases.

Moist Heat Application: Hot Soak

- Wash and dry your hands before and after the treatment.
- Assemble a basin of very warm water or prescribed solution. The temperature should be between 105 and 110 degrees Fahrenheit (41–44 degrees Celsius).
- Immerse the body part gradually in the water or solution. To maintain the temperature of the soak, remove some water/solution and replace it with hotter water/solution every few minutes. Add the liquid toward the edge of the basin, away from rather than close to the immersed body part.
- Immerse the part for approximately 20 minutes.
- Call the physician if you notice increased swelling and redness or if pain increases.
- Clean and air-dry the basin for the next treatment.

Dry Cold Application: Ice Bag

- Fill an ice bag 1/2 to 2/3 full with small pieces of ice. Expel enough air to make the ice bag flexible.
- Cover the ice bag and lightly mold it to the treatment area. It may be slightly uncomfortable for a short time until skin sensitivity has adjusted.
- Remove the ice bag after 20 to 30 minutes. The skin may feel numb.
- Call the physician if the skin is pale, mottled blue, or very numb; if the pain becomes more intense; or if swelling or redness increases.
- Refill the ice bag and change the protective covering as necessary. Repeat the procedure as directed by the physician.
- If you do not have an ice bag, you may substitute a covered bag of frozen vegetables.

Dry Heat or Cold Application: Chemical Pack

- Follow the directions on the chemical pack to activate it. Generally this involves shaking the chemical crystals to the bottom of the bag, firmly squeezing and breaking the smaller inner bag of water, and shaking the bag to thoroughly mix the contents.
- Cover the pack with a protective cover and place it on the affected area for the prescribed period of time.
- Dispose of the pack as recommended by the manufacturer.

wound, sterile technique and supplies must be used to prevent the introduction of pathogens.

- Hot soaks serve the same purposes as compresses. The affected body area is immersed in water or a medicated solution.
- Ice bags are used initially to treat pain and swelling.
- Cold compresses are used in the same ways as ice bags but conform more easily to the area being treated. They are also effective for treating eye injuries, headaches, and the jaws after dental extraction.
- Chemical cold or hot packs do not require cleaning, require very little storage space, and are flexible, easily activated, and disposable.

Patient instructions for the safe use of thermodynamic devices are listed in Table 43-10.

Ultrasonography

Ultrasound therapy is performed by a trained therapist with an ultrasound machine, a special gel that allows ultrasound waves to be conducted through the skin, and an applicator. Ultrasound waves, with frequencies that cannot be heard by the human ear, penetrate deep into muscle tissue and are converted to heat.

Ultrasound therapy can be used to treat chronic pain or acute muscle injuries, such as sprains or strains. It relaxes the muscles and increases the elasticity of tendons and ligaments. Ultrasound also increases circulation, which speeds the healing process.

Assistive Aids for Ambulation

Assistive aids for ambulation include **axillary** crutches and forearm crutches (also known as Lofstrand crutches); standard and legged canes; and standard and rolling walkers. The decision to use crutches, a cane, or a walker depends on various factors, including the patient's muscular coordination and weight-bearing capability and the type and severity of the physical impairment.

Crutches

Crutches remove or reduce weight bearing from one or both legs and transfer it to the arms and upper chest. The typical

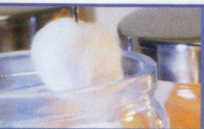

PROCEDURE 43-3 Assist the Patient with Cold Application/Cold Compress

Theory and Rationale

Cold applications cause the contraction of involuntary muscles, act as a vasoconstrictor, numb sensory nerve endings, and slow the inflammatory process. Inform the patient that although the cold application will prevent further swelling, it will not reduce swelling that is already present, which must be treated later with heat therapy. Cold compresses are generally ordered for application in 3- to 5-minute increments, with short breaks for tissue recovery. The skin should be monitored for redness and increased pain.

Materials

- water
- 4 × 4 gauze pads or other absorbent material, or washcloths
- waterproof pad
- waterproof wrap (plastic bag or plastic wrap)
- basin
- ice cubes

Competency

(**Conditions**) With the necessary materials, you will be able to (**Task**) apply a cold compress (**Standards**) correctly within the time frame designated by the instructor.

1. Wash your hands.
2. Identify the patient and verify the physician's order.
3. Explain the procedure to the patient.
4. Fill the basin with ice and water and soak the gauze pads or washcloths.

5. Wring out the compress so it is damp but not dripping.
6. Place the compress on the patient's injured body part and wrap it with plastic wrap to protect the patient's clothing.
7. Check the compress every 3–5 minutes, replacing it with a colder compress as needed. Remove water as necessary from the basin and add more ice to keep the water cold.
8. After applying compresses for the time specified by the physician, remove them and dry the affected area. Call the physician if you notice increased swelling and redness, or if the pain intensifies.
9. Launder the linens or place them in the appropriate laundry hamper, according to office protocol, and clean the room.
10. Wash your hands and document the procedure.

Patient Education

Physicians often prescribe cold compresses to be administered at home. Instruct the patient on the duration and frequency of application to avoid further injury or irritation to the skin.

Charting Example

01/26/XX 8:00 am Application of cold compress to left wrist for 20 minutes. Patient reports decrease in pain and swelling post application. Patient has been given written and verbal instructions for continued cold application at home. Tammy Lee, CMA (AAMA)

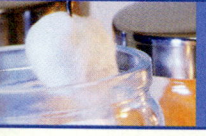

PROCEDURE 43-4 Assist the Patient with Hot Moist Application/Hot Compress

Theory and Rationale

Heat therapy increases circulation in the area to which it is applied, causes the muscles to relax, and helps tissues begin repair. Heat applications are often used to relieve tissue congestion or shorten the healing time of a sprained joint. Be sure to give clear written and verbal instructions to the patient, as heat can also be harmful. Prolonged exposure to heat can reduce the skin's resistance to injury. Extreme heat can cause severe nerve damage and burns.

Materials

- water
- digital or disposable strip thermometer
- 4 × 4 gauze pads or other absorbent material, or washcloths
- waterproof pad
- waterproof wrap (plastic bag or plastic wrap can be used)
- basin

Competency

(**Conditions**) With the necessary materials, you will be able to (**Task**) apply a cold compress (**Standards**) correctly within the time frame designated by the instructor.

1. Wash your hands.
2. Identify the patient and verify the physician's order.
3. Explain the procedure to the patient.
4. Fill the basin with water heated to 105 to 110 degrees F, as verified with the thermometer, and soak the gauze pads.
5. Wring out the pads or washcloths until damp but not dripping.
6. Place the waterproof pad under the injured body part. Apply the compress to the patient's injured body part and wrap with plastic wrap to protect clothing. Ask the patient to confirm that the temperature is comfortable but not burning (Figure 43-19 ◆).
7. Check the compress every 3–5 minutes, replacing it with a warmer compress as needed. Call the physician if you notice increased swelling and redness, or if pain increases.
8. After applying the compress for the time specified by the physician, remove it and dry the affected area.
9. Launder the linens or place them in the appropriate laundry hamper, according to office protocol, and clean the room.
10. Wash your hands and document the procedure.

PROCEDURE 43-4   Assist the Patient with Hot Moist Application/ Hot Compress *(continued)*

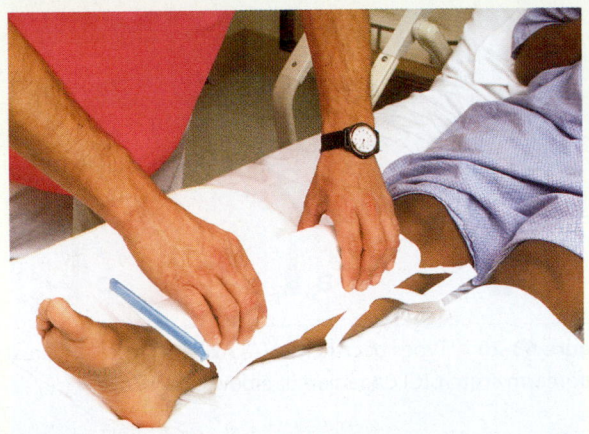

Figure 43-19 ◆ Apply a hot compress to the patient's leg.

Patient Education

Physicians often prescribe hot compresses to be administered at home. Instruct the patient on the duration and frequency of application to avoid further injury or irritation to the skin.

Charting Example

11/16/XX 4:00 pm Application of hot compress to right ankle for 20 minutes. Patient reports decrease in pain and swelling post application. Patient has been given written and verbal instructions for continued hot application at home. Bonnie Barkley, CMA (AAMA)

PROCEDURE 43-5   Assist with Therapeutic Ultrasonography

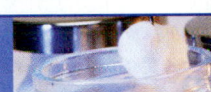

Theory and Rationale

The ultrasound machine creates a steady vibration when placed in contact with the skin and a coupling agent. The ultrasonic waves vibrate the muscles and tissue, increasing blood flow and speeding recovery. Ultrasonic waves travel best through water, so they penetrate muscles and tissues more deeply than bone, which has almost no water content. Extra care must be taken when passing the machine over bony structures.

Materials

- ultrasound gel (coupling agent)
- ultrasound machine
- tissue
- patient chart

Competency

(Conditions) With the necessary materials, you will be able to **(Task)** assist with therapeutic ultrasonography **(Standards)** correctly within the time frame designated by the instructor.

1. Prepare the equipment and identify the patient.
2. Verify the physician's orders for duration and frequency of treatment.
3. Explain the procedure and encourage the patient to inform you of any pain or discomfort.
4. Have the patient remove clothing from the area to be treated.
5. Apply warmed ultrasonic gel to the area to be treated and to the applicator head.
6. Set the machine at the lowest treatment setting and increase gradually as needed. Set the timer to the specified treatment time.

7. Place the applicator head firmly against the patient's skin and move the applicator in a circular motion at a speed of 2 inches per second. Keep the applicator head in contact with the patient's skin and moving at all times when the machine is running.
8. When the set time has expired, the machine will shut off automatically.
9. Return the intensity control back to zero.
10. Wipe the ultrasonic gel from the patient's skin and assist with dressing if necessary.
11. Wash your hands and document the procedure in the patient's chart.

Patient Education

Ultrasound therapy should be soothing and relaxing. The patient should not feel any burning, pressure, or other discomfort. Any adverse reactions should be reported immediately. The patient should also be advised to avoid heavy lifting or quick movement with the treated muscles until advised by a physician, because they are more susceptible to injury immediately following therapy.

Charting Example

10/04/XX 6:00 pm Ultrasonic treatment of left levator scapula area on setting of 3 intensity for 12 minutes. Patient is instructed to return for treatment three times per week for the next three weeks. Patient tolerates treatment well and reports pain relief and decreased muscle spasm. Leslie Miller, RMA (AMT)

crutch is made of aluminum or wood and can be adjusted for hand placement and axillary height (Figure 43-20 ◆). Crutches are equipped with padded armrests, hand grips, and rubber tips to prevent sliding. Lofstrand crutches are used primarily by patients with cerebral palsy or paraplegia.

Axillary crutches that fit the patient properly are very important for his or her safety, comfort, and recovery. Crutches that are too short or too long will create balance problems and unsafe conditions that may further injure the patient, who may then avoid ambulation altogether. The physician may instruct the patient to see a physical therapist or convalescent aid provider for crutch fitting and instruction, or an MA may perform both functions.

Patients who use crutches should be taught the safest and most efficient way to walk with them. There are several different gaits, or step patterns, a patient can use, depending on his or her condition (Table 43-11).

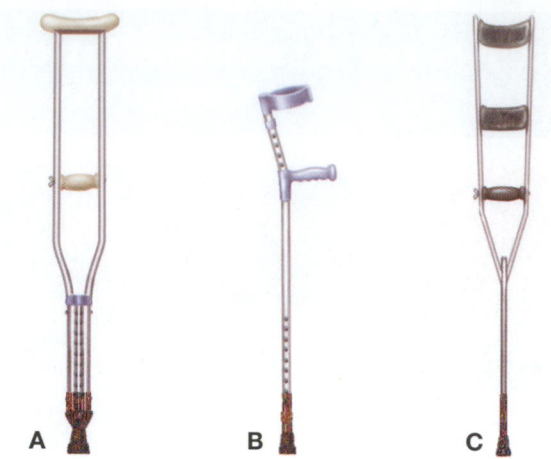

Figure 43-20 ◆ Types of crutches: (A) Axillary crutch. (B) Lofstrand or forearm crutch. (C) Canadian or elbow crutch.

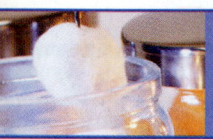

PROCEDURE 43-6 Demonstrate Measuring for Axillary Crutches

Theory and Rationale

The goal of measuring for axillary crutches is to ensure the correct length and hand grip placement. Crutches that are too long are difficult to use because the patient cannot use shoulder force to push the body off the ground. The patient may experience axillary pain and subsequent crutch palsy, a sign of neurological damage characterized by muscular weakness of the lower arm, wrist, and hand. With crutches that are too short, the patient is bent forward, raising the risk of back pain.

The first step in proper measurement is to assist the patient to a standing position. The crutch tip should be placed 2 inches in front of the foot and 4 to 6 inches from the lateral aspect. The height of wooden crutches is adjusted by removing a bolt and wing nut from a lower central piece and sliding the central piece up or down. When the correct height is established, the bolt and wing nut are replaced and tightened. Aluminum crutches are adjusted by pushing in a spring button to allow sliding and, at the correct height, popping the button into a locked position. The last step is to place the hand grip so the patient's hand is flexed 30 degrees. The bolt and wing nut for the hand grip are removed, the grip is slid to the correct position, and then the bolt and wing nut are replaced and tightened. The patient should wear the same shoes (with nonskid soles) when being measured for the crutches and when using them.

Instruct the patient to observe for signs that crutch height may need to be adjusted. Back pain; weakness in the lower arm, wrist, and hand; inability to keep the back straight and avoid leaning forward; or general awkwardness in using the crutches are all signs that the handgrip and/or central strut should be adjusted.

Materials

- patient chart
- order for axillary crutches
- adjustable axillary crutches

Competency

(**Conditions**) With the necessary materials, you will be able to (**Task**) measure for axillary crutches (**Standards**) correctly within 20 minutes.

1. Wash your hands and gather the necessary materials.
2. Identify the patient and escort him or her to the treatment area.
3. Assist the patient, with shoes on, to a standing position. With the crutch armrests under the patient's axillae, adjust the crutches first for height and then for hand position, using the following criteria: (a) a space of two fingerwidths between the axilla and the crutch armrest; (b) body weight supported by the hands on the hand grips; and (c) crutch tip placement approximately 2 inches in front of the foot and 4 to 6 inches from the lateral aspect.
4. After the crutches have been correctly measured and fitted to the patient, provide verbal and written instruction about general guidelines, crutch gait, and symptoms of improper fit.
5. Document the procedure and prepare the treatment area for the next patient.

Patient Education

See patient instructions in Table 43-11.

PROCEDURE 43-6   Demonstrate Measuring for Axillary Crutches (continued)

Charting Example

08/23/XX 10:45 A.M. 23-year-old male seen for severely sprained Lt ankle. Physician splinted and ordered crutch walking with followup appointment in two weeks. Pt fitted for crutches with two-fingerwidth space between axilla and armrest, body support on wrists, and crutches approx 5 inches from the foot. Patient instructed on symptoms of improper crutch fitting, and instruction given on the three-point gait. Appointment scheduled for two-week return visit. John Young, CMA (AAMA)

TABLE 43-11   PATIENT INSTRUCTION: GUIDELINES FOR WALKING WITH CRUTCHES

General Guidelines

- Practice arm strengthening exercises regularly before and during the early stages of crutch walking.
- Practice the crutch gait prescribed by the physician before leaving the medical office, physical therapy department, outpatient treatment center, or convalescent aid supplier.
- Keep the back straight to maintain correct body posture, prevent back strain, and maintain balance.
- Look ahead when walking. Do *not* look at your feet.
- Nonskid shoes will provide stability when crutch walking.
- When crutch walking, body weight should be on the hand grips, and the armrests should be against the sides of the rib cage.
- Be aware of your environment and enlist the support of others to remove obstacles that might cause falls, including dark areas, throw rugs, and wet floors.
- Extra padding may be applied to the hand grips and shoulder rests, although the crutches may then need to be adjusted for height and hand placement.
- Dry crutch tips can become wet. Replace crutch tips that become smooth.
- Check the bolts and wing nuts frequently to make sure they are tight.
- Report symptoms of numbness, tingling, and weakness in the arms, wrists, or hands.

Four-Point Gait (Figure 43-21 ◆)
Start in the tripod position (crutch 4 to 6 inches in front of the foot and 4 to 6 inches to the lateral aspect) with your feet approximately a foot apart for balance (you may widen the base distance if you have a large frame). The sequence of steps is:

- Right crutch forward.
- Left foot forward.
- Left crutch forward.
- Right foot forward.
- Repeat.

Three-Point Gait (Figure 43-22 ◆)
Start in the tripod position with the feet base distance apart. The sequence of steps is

- Move the affected leg forward with the crutches.
- Balancing on the crutches, move the unaffected leg forward.
- Repeat.

Two-Point Gait (Figure 43-23 ◆)
Start in the tripod position with the feet base distance apart. The sequence of steps is:

- Move the left crutch and right foot forward at the same time.
- Move the right crutch and left foot forward at the same time.
- Repeat.

Swing Gait (Figure 43-24 ◆)
Start in the tripod position with the feet base distance apart. The sequence of steps for the swing-to gait is:

- Move both crutches forward.
- Lift and swing the extremities to the crutches.
- Repeat.

For the swing-through gait:

- Move both crutches forward.
- Lift and swing the extremities to and past the crutches.
- Repeat.

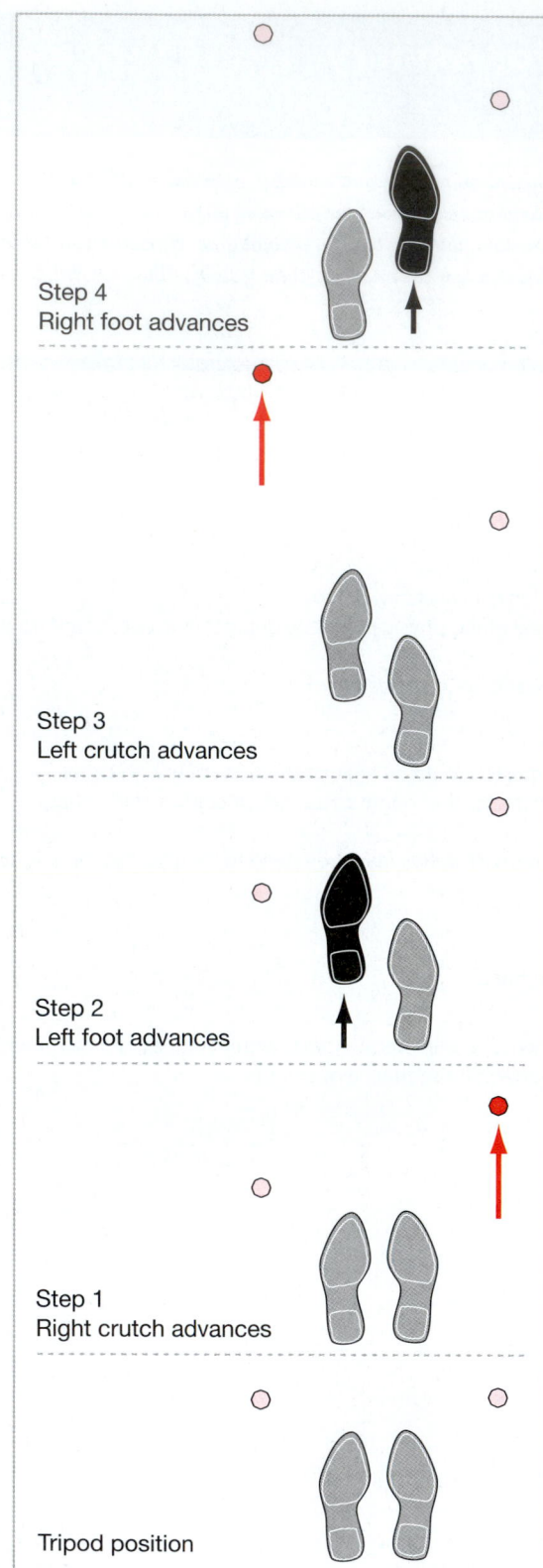

Step 4
Right foot advances

Step 3
Left crutch advances

Step 2
Left foot advances

Step 1
Right crutch advances

Tripod position

Figure 43-21 ◆ Four-point gait.

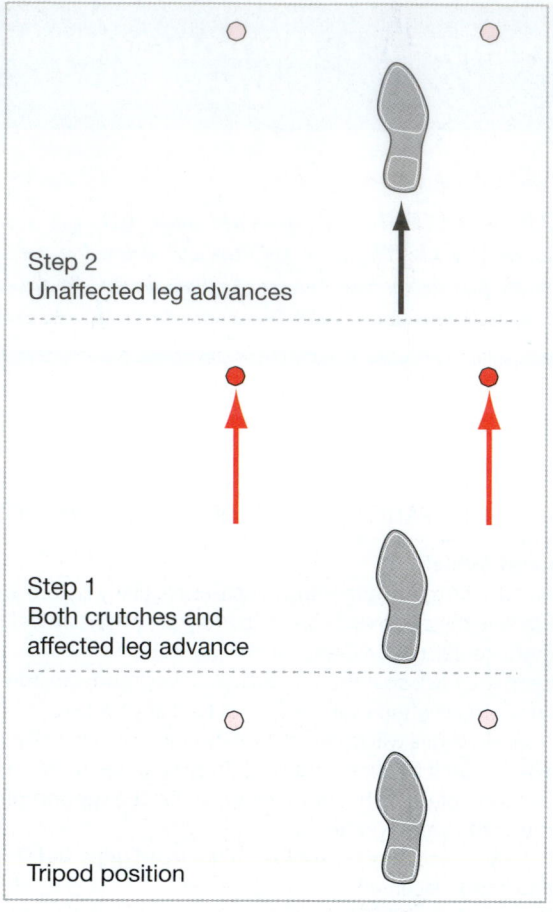

Step 2
Unaffected leg advances

Step 1
Both crutches and
affected leg advance

Tripod position

Figure 43-22 ◆ Three-point gait.

■ Patients with degenerative joint disease, impaired muscle coordination, muscle spasticity, or muscle weakness may be taught the four-point gait, the most stable gait.

■ The three-point gait is for patients who can bear weight on only one leg, such as patients with fractures, sprains, amputations, or lower leg inflammations, or during post-surgical healing. Good upper arm strength and muscular coordination are required.

■ The two-point gait is similar to the four-point gait, but with fewer steps. It is used by patients with better balance and muscular coordination who can bear more weight.

■ Swing-to and swing-through gaits are used by those with lower extremity injuries or disabilities. These gaits require very strong arms and good muscular coordination.

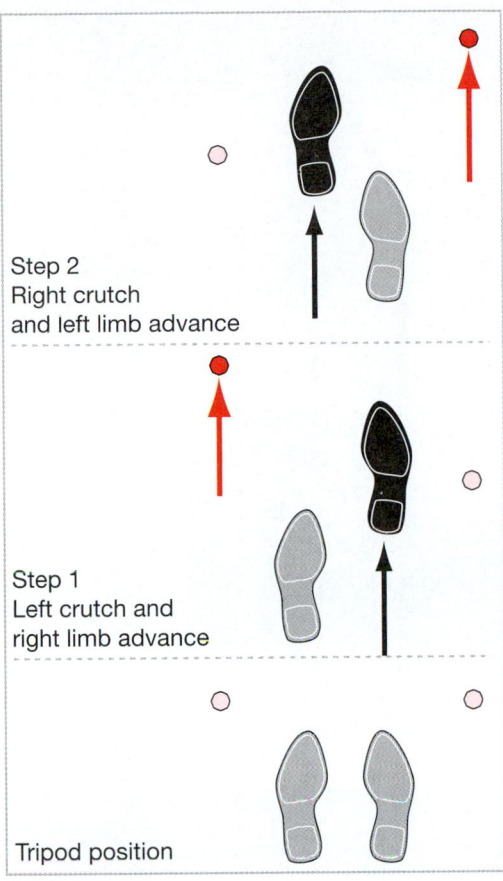

Figure 43-23 ◆ Two-point gait.

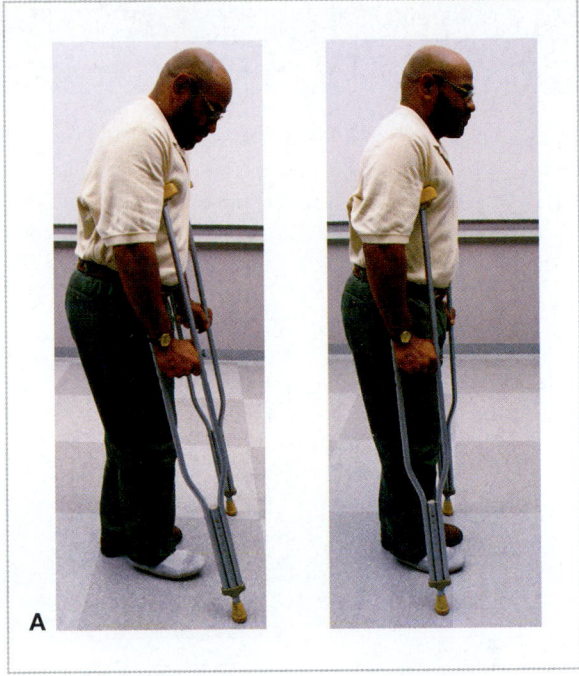

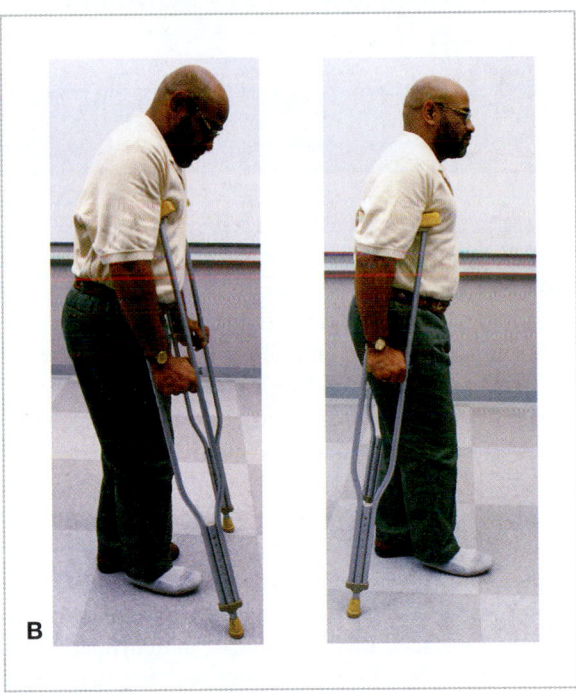

Figure 43-24 ◆ Swing gaits: (A) Swing-to gait. (B) Swing-through gait.

Patients using assistive ambulation aids should be made aware of certain safety considerations. The patient or caregiver should monitor the rubber safety tips for replacement needs. All screws or connections should be regularly checked. Patients and their caregivers should be observant of the surrounding environment to avoid falls and injury. Two common hazards are throw rugs and dim lighting.

Canes

Canes are also commonly used as assistive ambulation devices by patients with one-sided weakness, such as hemiparesis, joint impairment, or other neuromuscular conditions. All canes consist of a grip handle, a pole portion, and rubber-tipped footing or legs (Figure 43-25 ◆). The standard cane has one rubber-tipped leg and is used by patients who require very little support for walking. The three-footed tripod cane and four-footed quad cane provide additional walking stability and support. Tripod and quad canes can stand alone as patients momentarily remove the hand to manage other activities, such as opening a door. However, tripod and quad canes are considered bulkier and harder to move because of their extra feet.

Walkers

Walkers are another common assistive device. They are used by patients who need more support, have symptoms of poor balance and weakness, or have had hip or knee replacement

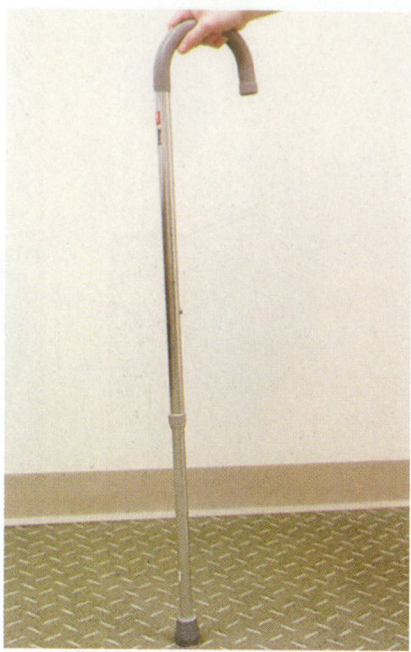
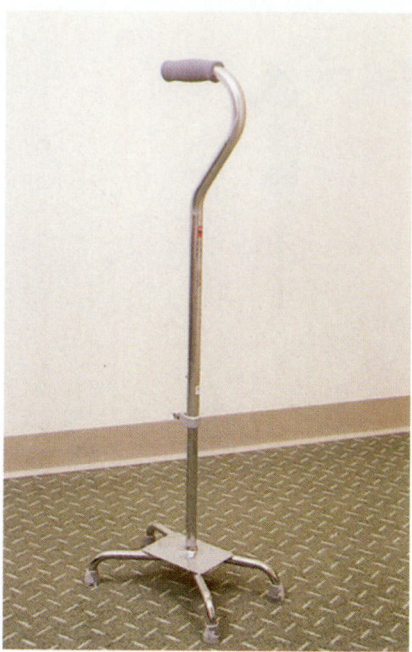

Figure 43-25 ◆ Two types of canes.

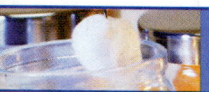

PROCEDURE 43-7 Assist a Patient with Crutch Walking

Theory and Rationale

The goal of proper patient instruction in the use of crutches is to reduce the risk of injury and accident in the patient's home and during day-to-day activities. Crutches provide support for greater mobility and allow for a wide range of gait patterns and speed. Several types of crutches are available: platform, forearm (or Lofstrand), and axillary. The type of crutches prescribed depends on the injury and the patient's ability and physical limitations.

Axillary crutches are the most commonly prescribed crutches. They are ideal for physically strong patients who need them only for a short time. Axillary crutches are easily transported, stored, and adjusted. They are easy to maneuver on unstable surfaces, such as stairs, or in tight spaces.

Forearm crutches are prescribed for patients who require crutches permanently or for a long period of time. They are built with a hard plastic or metal sleeve that fits around the patient's forearm. The patient's body weight is supported on the hand grips below the arm cuffs. Forearm crutches are shorter and provide less stability than axillary crutches and require a longer training session.

The platform crutch is most often recommended for elderly patients who cannot grip the handgrips of forearm crutches or support their weight on their hands or wrists with axillary crutches. The platform crutch has a platform attached to the top with a handgrip. The crutch is adjusted so that the patient's forearm rests on the platform, with the arm bent at a 45-degree angle. The forearm bears all the weight but does not provide much stability. Platform crutches require strength and coordination, and it may be difficult for some patients to learn proper technique.

Materials

■ crutches correctly fitted to the patient

Competency

(**Conditions**) With the necessary materials, you will be able to (**Task**) assist a patient with crutch walking (**Standards**) correctly within 20 minutes.

1. Inspect the crutches for correctly fitted arm pads, tight wing nuts, and comfortable handgrips.
2. Instruct the patient to relax the injured knee and keep it slightly bent to avoid touching the foot to the ground.
3. Instruct the patient in the crutch-walking gait ordered by the physician (see Table 43-11).
4. Have the patient practice taking several steps to ensure correct technique.

Patient Education

See patient instructions in Table 43-11.

Charting Example

08/23/XX 10:45 A.M. Patient instructed on proper crutch walking and how to inspect the crutches for wear and tear. Patient correctly demonstrated knowledge of crutch use. Maurice Ellis, RMA (AMT)

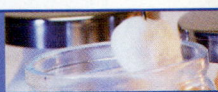

PROCEDURE 43-8 Assist a Patient in Using a Cane

Theory and Rationale

To measure for the correct cane height, instruct the patient to stand upright without leaning and to flex the elbow approximately 30 degrees. The grip handle of the cane should be located at the greater trochanter of the femur neck to maximize stability and support.

Materials

- single-tipped cane as ordered by physician
- gait belt

Competency

(**Conditions**) With the necessary materials, you will be able to (**Task**) instruct a patient on correct cane use (**Standards**) within the time frame allowed by the instructor.

1. Identify the patient and explain why instruction in cane use is necessary.
2. Wash your hands.
3. Verify the type of cane the patient and physician have agreed on and assemble equipment.
4. Make sure the suction tip on the cane is in good condition.
5. Place the gait belt snugly around the patient's waist, tucking any excess length into the belt.
6. Place the cane tip 4 to 6 inches to the side of the patient's foot, on the patient's stronger, unaffected side. Adjust the cane so that the handle grip is level with the patient's hip and the patient's elbow is flexed at a 20- to 30-degree angle.
7. Stand on the patient's weaker side with a firm underhand grip on the gait belt.
8. Instruct the patient to move the injured leg and cane forward simultaneously (Figure 43-26 ◆).
9. The patient should then advance the stronger leg and rest it slightly in front of the injured leg. Repeat this process.
10. Going up stairs:
    - Instruct the patient to use hand rails whenever possible.
    - The patient moves the stronger leg forward to the next step while the injured leg and cane rest on the lower step.
    - With a firm grip on the cane and the handrail, the patient moves the injured leg up to the same step as the uninjured leg.
    - Repeat as needed.

11. Going down stairs:
    - The patient steps down with the uninjured leg and the cane.
    - The injured leg follows to the same step.

Patient Education

During the early stages of using the cane, the patient may have to think through the sequence, but practice will make it second nature. The patient should be careful not to attempt too much at first, especially on stairs, in unfamiliar conditions, or when he or she is home alone.

Charting Example

05/23/XX 10:45 A.M. Patient arrived for cane adjustments and walking instructions post knee replacement surgery. Single-tip cane was adjusted to patient's hip joint. Patient was instructed on ambulating on flat surfaces and going up and down stairs. Patient successfully demonstrated understanding of instructions. Dawn Maynard, CMA (AAMA)

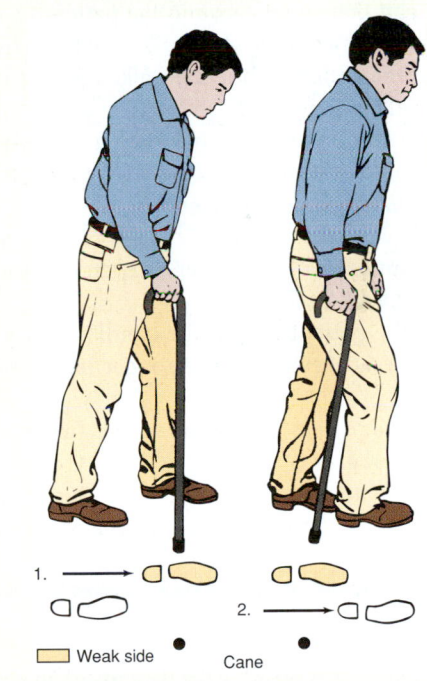

1. → ⬜ 2. → ⬜

⬜ Weak side ● Cane

Figure 43-26 ◆ Instruct the patient to move the injured leg and cane forward simultaneously.

surgery. Because the walker provides a larger base of support than the cane or crutch, patients generally feel more secure during walking. However, the walker can slow ambulation and is more cumbersome to maneuver in some situations. Correct walker height is slightly below the patient's waistline.

Prostheses

Prostheses replace not only extremities and joints but also diseased tissues and organs, often temporarily. Today there are prostheses for the heart, breasts, kidney, skin, blood vessels, blood, and teeth. Lighter-weight, stronger, more durable materials have

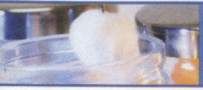

PROCEDURE 43-9 Assist a Patient in Using a Walker

Theory and Rationale

Patients who have the strength to support their body weight but have difficulty keeping their balance may use a walker to get around and maintain their independence. The patient should wear good, supportive walking shoes and loose-fitting, comfortable clothing.

Materials

- walker
- gait belt

Competency

(**Conditions**) With the necessary materials, you will be able to (**Task**) teach a patient how to use a walker (**Standards**) correctly within the time frame allowed by the instructor.

1. Identify the patient and explain why instruction in using a walker is necessary.
2. Wash your hands.
3. Place a gait belt snugly around the patient's waist. Tuck any excess belt length under the belt near the hip.
4. Position the patient inside the walker. Adjust the height of the walker as needed. The patient's arms should be flexed at a 30-degree angle when resting on the hand grips.
5. Stand behind and slightly to the side of the patient, with an underhand grip on the gait belt.
6. Instruct the patient to move the walker directly ahead until the back supports of the walker are even with the patient's toes (Figure 43-27 ◆).
7. Instruct the patient to grip the handles firmly and step toward the walker with the stronger leg first, then the other leg.
8. Repeat: The patient moves the walker first, then moves toward the walker.
9. Watch the patient for signs of fatigue. Some walkers are equipped with platforms on which the patient can sit to rest.

Patient Education

At first the patient may have to think the sequence through, but practice will make it second nature. For stability and support, remind the patient to move the feet when the walker is stationary and to move the walker when the feet are stationary. The family can help the patient adjust to using the walker by rearranging furniture as necessary and removing loose carpets, cords, or other hazards from the patient's home.

Charting Example

08/23/XX 10:45 A.M. Patient assisted with use of her new walker. Patient practiced ambulating around the clinic. Patient states she is "comfortable" using the walker on her own. Steve Sanders, RMA (AMI)

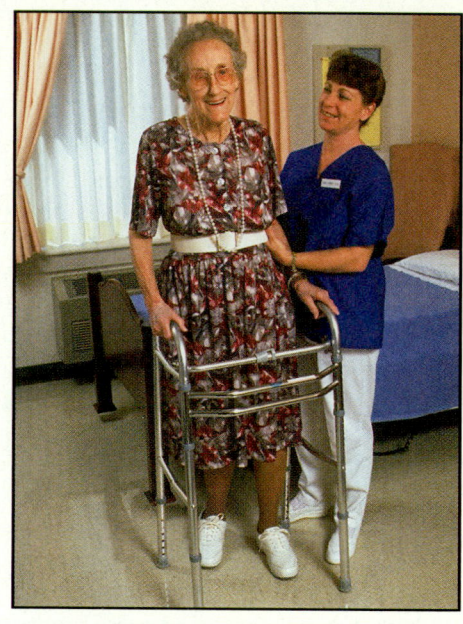

Figure 43-27 ◆ Using a walker for support.

---

made joint replacement possible for patients of all ages. Artificial limbs look more natural. Surgical techniques have been modified so they are less traumatic for the patient. As an example, a lateral approach for knee replacement, rather than the traditional frontal approach, has eliminated incising major muscles, thereby reducing pain and recovery time.

Body Mechanics

The principles of body mechanics should be followed when transferring patients from a chair or wheelchair to an examination table and vice versa, when assisting a patient to a sitting or standing position, and when assisting the physician with procedures. Using

proper body mechanics can prevent injury to yourself and to the patient. Follow these guidelines during a wheelchair transfer.

- Know the patient's level of functioning, both physical and mental, before transferring to an examination table, or vice versa. You may need to call on another staff member if the patient is unable to help.
- Keep the wheelchair brakes on during the transfer to keep it from rolling.
- If possible, remove armrests or leg attachments, which may act as obstacles in the transfer.
- Help the patient to stand. Holding him or her close to your center of gravity, pivot or guide the patient into position for

PROCEDURE 43-10 Assist a Patient in a Wheelchair to and from an Exam Table

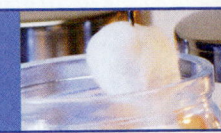

Theory and Rationale

Patients may present to the office in a wheelchair and not have the strength or mobility to move themselves to an examination table. You should be able to physically transfer these patients in a way that is effective and safe for both you and the patient.

Materials

- gait belt
- long-handled stool (if exam table is not equipped with pull-out step)

Competency

(**Conditions**) With the necessary materials, you will be able to (**Task**) transfer a patient from a wheelchair to an examination table and from an examination table to a wheelchair (**Standards**) correctly within the time frame allowed by the instructor.

To transfer the patient from a wheelchair to an exam table:

1. Identify the patient and explain what you are going to do.
2. Wash your hands.
3. Position the wheelchair so that the patient is sitting with his or her strongest side next to the examination table.
4. Lock the wheelchair brakes.
5. Place the gait belt snugly around the patient's waist, making certain the belt is tight enough that it will not slip and put unnecessary pressure on the ribs. Tuck any excess belt length under the belt.
6. If the wheelchair allows, remove the foot rests. If not, move them as far out as possible to avoid hitting your shins against them during the transfer.
7. Standing directly in front of and as close to the patient as possible, grip the gait belt with both hands in an underhand grip. Bend at the knees and hips to avoid back strain.
8. If the patient is able, have him or her grip the arm rests and push off at the same time that you lift, for added leverage. If possible, the patient can also assist by pushing upward with his or her legs (Figure 43-28 ◆).
9. With the patient now standing, have him or her place the stronger leg on the stool or exam table step, and together you will lift as the patient steps up.
10. Have the patient place one hand on the table and guide him or her to a sitting position.
11. Move the wheelchair out of the way.

To transfer the patient back to the wheelchair:

1. After identifying the patient, explaining the procedure, and washing your hands, place the stool (if the exam table does not have a step) next to the exam table.
2. Place the wheelchair next to the exam table with the brakes locked.
3. With a firm underhand grip on the gait belt, assist the patient to a standing position. If the patient is able, have him or her push off with the legs and arms.
4. Once the patient is steady on the step or stool, have him or her step to the floor with the stronger leg.
5. Have the patient take small steps backward until the backs of the knees touch the wheelchair.
6. Ask the patient to reach back and place the hands on the wheelchair armrests for support. Bending at the hips and knees, slowly lower the patient to the chair.
7. Help the patient adjust to a comfortable position in the wheelchair.
8. Replace the foot rests.

Patient Education

Make sure the patient understands the importance of moving with you as you lift and turn him or her, to avoid injury.

Charting Example

02/10/XX 3:15 P.M. Patient arrived for yearly physical and was successfully transferred to the exam table using a single-person transfer method and gait belt. Heather Brown, RMA (AMT)

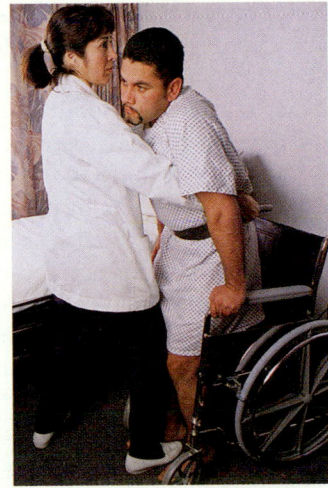

Figure 43-28 ◆ Using a transfer (gait) belt.

sitting in the wheelchair or on the examination table. Some employers require the use of safety belts when lifting or transferring patients to help prevent back injury to the employee.

Although proper body mechanics are emphasized for employee health and safety, they also prevent injury to other workers and patients. (Body mechanics are more fully discussed in ∞ Chapter 23.)

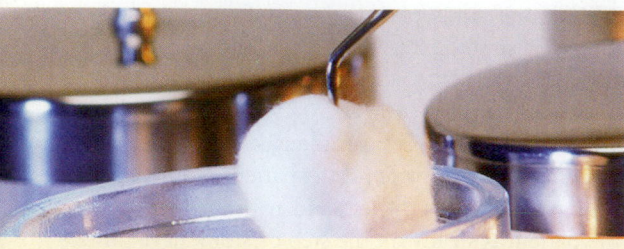

REVIEW

Chapter Summary

- Orthopedics is the study of the musculoskeletal system: bones, muscles, joints, ligaments, tendons, and nerves. An orthopedic surgeon specializes in the diagnosis and treatment of musculoskeletal conditions.
- The MA obtains and records medical history and vital signs, notes any obvious deformities, assists the physician in examinations and procedures, and instructs and assists the patient as necessary. The MA may also provide patients with ambulation devices, including crutches, canes, and wheelchairs, and provide instruction about proper body mechanics and thermodynamic treatments.
- The bones and muscles provide a framework for the body, help the individual to stand erect, protect internal organs, and make movement possible. Bone tissue serves as a repository for calcium reserves. Cartilage, a connective tissue, helps reduce friction between moving bone surfaces. The outside layer of bone is covered with a membrane called periosteum, which contains osteoblasts for bone tissue formation, blood and lymphatic vessels, and nerve fibers. The inner marrow cavity of the bone is lined with endosteum.
- Red bone marrow contains hematopoietic tissue in which precursor blood cells are manufactured. Yellow marrow is found in the long central portion of the bone. Bone tissue undergoes reabsorption and formation throughout life. When bone reabsorption is greater than bone formation, such as in an aging person, the risk of fractures rises.
- The skeleton consists of the axial skeleton (bones in the head and trunk) and appendicular skeleton (extremities and shoulder and hip framework for the attachment of the extremities). Bones are classified according to structure: long bones (thigh, lower leg, upper arm, lower arm, digits), short bones (wrists and ankles), flat bones (scapula, ribs, pelvic bones), and sesamoid bones (patella).
- Range of motion (ROM) is the total degree of movement a joint is capable of. When a patient is immobile for any length of time, joint range of motion and muscle strength diminish. Range-of-motion exercises maintain joint flexibility and muscle strength.

- Muscles are attached to bones by connective tissue called tendons and contract in response to nervous system stimulation.
- Musculoskeletal conditions seen in the orthopedic office are congenital, degenerative, infectious, malignant, or traumatic. They may also be classified by the anatomical structure affected: bones, joints, or muscles. Common musculoskeletal diseases involve the body as a whole, the spine, the joints, or the collagen. Some diseases are characterized by genetic predisposition.
- Congenital conditions are present at birth (for example, clubfoot and congenital hip dysplasia). Developmental conditions occur as the individual progresses into adulthood, such as kyphosis, lordosis, and scoliosis. Muscular dystrophy is the result of genetically transmitted disease. Myasthenia gravis may be an autoimmune disorder.
- Degeneration of different areas of the musculoskeletal system comprises another group of conditions. Arthritis is inflammation and degeneration of the joint structures. Three types are osteoarthritis, rheumatoid arthritis, and gouty arthritis. Bursitis is an inflammatory process in the bursae, or tissue surrounding the joints. Osteoporosis occurs as bone density diminishes and the bones become porous and susceptible to fracture. Osteomalacia is the softening of bone tissue, with deformities and increased flexibility. Carpal tunnel syndrome is the result of repetitive trauma. Fibromyalgia, with symptoms of muscle pain and sleep disturbance, has an unknown etiology and no known cure.
- Infectious musculoskeletal conditions include Lyme disease, the result of the bite of an infected deer tick, and osteomyelitis, inflammation of the bone tissue.
- Fractures result from traumatic insult and take many forms, depending on type and location and the individual's health status. Types of fractures include comminuted, compound, simple, compression, depression, displaced, nondisplaced, greenstick, impacted, longitudinal, oblique, transverse, spiral, and pathological fractures, as well as avulsions. Insults to joints, tendons, ligaments, and muscle tissue are other types of trauma.
- Neoplasia and/or malignant musculoskeletal conditions may affect any of the structures of the system, usually in the form

Chapter Summary (continued)

of tumors. Not all abnormal tissue growths in the system are malignant. Pain, swelling, growth, and reduced range of motion are some symptoms. Chemotherapy is administered to shrink tumors prior to surgical removal. Rhabdomyosarcomas are rare malignant tumors of muscle tissue that should be surgically removed as early as possible.

■ Sprains occur as the result of traumatic insult to the muscle, tendon, or ligament surrounding a joint. Strains result from the overuse or overstretching of a muscle. Dislocations involve a bone being displaced or separated from the joint and are usually the result of a traumatic insult. A severed tendon leaves the connected part unable to move. A torn meniscus may result from a fall, a twisting motion, or a sports injury.

■ Many physicians refer patients to physical therapists for therapy and instruction in the use of assistive devices and thermodynamics, but sometimes the MA may provide patient instruction. The MA may measure and fit the patient for crutches, instruct the patient about the therapeutic use of heat and cold, assist in evaluating the patient's range of motion, or explain proper body mechanics.

■ Thermodynamics involves the use of heat (thermotherapy) or cold (cryotherapy) applications to promote healing and prevent further tissue injury in areas affected by trauma, infection, and inflammation. Heat, by virtue of increasing circulation, increases nutrition to cells and carries away waste products. Cold constricts blood vessels, reduces leakage of fluid into tissues, acts as a temporary anesthetic, and reduces the number of pathogens in the area. Devices used in heat or cold therapy include heating pads, chemical hot or cold packs, ice bags, and cold or hot moist soaks or compresses.

■ Assistive aids for ambulation include axillary crutches and forearm crutches (Lofstrand crutches); standard, tripod, and quad canes; and standard and rolling walkers. Special safety guidelines must be followed when assistive aids are used.

■ To prevent musculoskeletal injury and maintain health and safety, health care team members must practice proper body mechanics such as keeping the back straight when sitting, standing, and walking; bending at the hips and knees and keeping objects close to the body when lifting and lowering them; and maintaining the center of gravity within the body.

Chapter Review

Multiple Choice

1. Which of the following terms means "decrease in the size of normal muscle mass"?
   a. Atony
   b. Atrophy
   c. Axillary
   d. Articular

2. Which of the following is *not* part of the axial skeleton?
   a. Clavicle
   b. Sternum
   c. Cranium
   d. Ribs

3. Which of the following is *not* part of the appendicular section of the skeleton?
   a. Scapula
   b. Femur
   c. Ulna
   d. Facial bones

4. The type of membrane covering the outside layer of bone is
   a. cartilage.
   b. osteoblast.
   c. periosteum.
   d. endosteum.

5. Which of the following means "no movement of a joint"?
   a. Bursae
   b. Diarthrosis
   c. Amphiarthrosis
   d. Synarthrosis

6. The type of fracture that results in the crushing or splintering of the bone is the
   a. compression fracture.
   b. compound fracture.
   c. comminuted fracture.
   d. depression fracture.

7. A fractured bone that is partially bent and partially fractured is called
   a. greenstick.
   b. displaced.
   c. comminuted.
   d. impacted.

8. Which of the following is *not* a soft-tissue knee injury?
   a. Sprain
   b. Avulsion
   c. Torn meniscus
   d. Severed tendon

9. Which of the following terms means "overstretching of a muscle, tendon, or ligament"?
   a. Severed
   b. Sprain
   c. Dislocation
   d. Strain

10. An imaging technique used to evaluate bone density is the
    a. myelogram.
    b. bone scan.
    c. arthrogram.
    d. radiograph.

Chapter Review (continued)

True/False

T F 1. The correction of a fracture is called *reduction*.

T F 2. Surgical intervention is not necessary for compound, avulsed, or displaced fractures.

T F 3. Cotton is a common material that can be used to make a cast.

T F 4. Thermotherapy includes both moist and dry applications.

T F 5. Heat can be used to speed up the localized formation of pus.

Short Answer

1. What is a compression fracture?

2. Which physical therapy modality vibrates tissue, generates heat, and promotes circulation?

3. What are the two types of thermodynamic applications?

4. The correct placement of the crutch pad is how many inches below the armpit?

5. What is the best gait for patients who need crutches but can bear weight on only one leg?

Research

1. In your local area, are there orthopedic physicians who specialize in pediatrics as well as geriatrics?

2. Are there physical therapists in your community who specialize in sports-related injuries and rehabilitation?

Externship Application Experience

As an extern, you have been sent into a room to prepare a 10-year-old boy for the removal of an arm cast. You prepare the materials and equipment with the mother and child present. When the patient sees the cast saw and orthopedic vacuum, he screams, "Don't cut off my arm!" How will you prepare the patient and mother for the cast removal?

Resource Guide

American Academy of Orthopedic Surgeons
6300 N. River Rd.
Rosemont, IL 60018-4262
1-800-346-AAOS
www.aos.org

American Lyme Disease Foundation
Mill Pond Offices
293 Route 100
Somers, NY 10389
1-914-277-6970
www.aldf.com

American Physical Therapy Association
1111 N. Fairfax St.
Alexandria, VA 22314-1488
1-800-999-2782
www.apta.org

Arthritis Foundation
PO Box 7669
Atlanta, GA 30357-0669
1-800-283-7800
www.arthritis.org

Muscular Dystrophy Association
3300 E. Sunrise Drive
Tucson, AZ 85718
1-800-572-1717
www.mdausa.org

National Osteoporosis Foundation
1232 22nd Street, NW
Washington, DC 20037-1292
1-202-223-2226
www.nof.org

National Rehabilitation Information Center
4200 Forbes Blvd.
Lamham, MD 20706
1-800-346-2742
www.naric.com

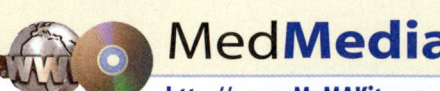

MedMedia

http://www.MyMAKit.com

More on this chapter, including interactive resources, can be found on the Student CD-ROM accompanying this textbook and on http://www.MyMAKit.com.

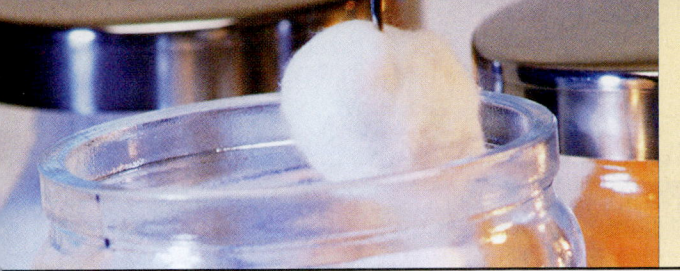

Objectives

After completing this chapter, you should be able to:

- Define and spell the key terminology in this chapter.
- Define the medical assistant's role in the obstetric/gynecology medical office.
- Discuss the anatomy and physiology of the female reproductive system.
- Explain the menstrual cycle and menopause.
- Describe common disorders and conditions related to the menstrual cycle.
- List and describe the different methods of contraception.
- Explain some of the causes of female infertility.
- Discuss the processes of pregnancy and childbirth.
- List the information required for a complete obstetrical history.
- Explain common complications of pregnancy.
- Discuss the benefits and drawbacks of breastfeeding and formula feeding.
- List and describe disease conditions related to the female reproductive system.
- Explain how to assess vaginal bleeding.
- List and describe sexually transmitted diseases affecting women.
- Discuss disorders and conditions that affect the breasts.
- Discuss patient assessment in the OB/GYN office.
- Describe the various diagnostic procedures performed in the OB/GYN office.
- List and explain different treatment modalities for OB/GYN patients.
- Discuss psychological interventions for various OB/GYN conditions.

Obstetrics and Gynecology

Case Study

Sydney Jackson, RMA (AMT) is taking phone calls one afternoon when she receives a frantic message from Tina Blakely, a 72-year-old patient. Mrs. Blakely is concerned about recent news reports linking hormone replacement therapy to breast cancer and has stopped her medication. Now she is experiencing multiple symptoms and would like to know if there are any nonpharmaceutical therapies she can take.

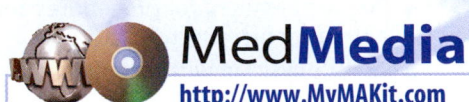

MedMedia
http://www.MyMAKit.com

Additional interactive resources and activities for this chapter can be found on http://www.MyMAKit.com. For videos, tips, audio glossary, legal and ethical scenarios, job scenarios, quizzes, games, virtual tours, and activities related to the content of this chapter, please access the accompanying CD-ROM in this book.

Audio Glossary
Legal and Ethical Scenario: *Obstetrics and Gynecology*
On the Job Scenario: *Obstetrics and Gynecology*
Video: Assisting with the Gynecological Exam
A & P Quiz : The Reproductive System
Multiple Choice Quiz
Games: Crossword, Strikeout, and Spelling Bee
3D Virtual Tour: Reproductive System: Female Reproductive System
Drag & Drop: Reproductive System: Ovulation; Reproductive System: Female Reproductive System
Tips
HIPAA Quiz

Key Terminology

abortus—an aborted fetus

amniocentesis—procedure in which a needle is inserted into the amniotic sac to withdraw amniotic fluid for testing; used to identify genetic abnormalities, often neural tube deficits and Down syndrome, in the fetus; also used to determine the sex of the fetus

cervix—entrance to the uterus

colostrum—fluid secreted by the breasts after delivery, before milk production, that contains antibodies and provides the infant with immunological protection

effacement—thinning of the cervix during the labor process

embryo—initial physical stage of human development following fertilization of the ovum until the end of the seventh or eighth week

endometrium—lining of the uterus

fetus—human child in utero from embryonic stage until birth

fundal height—height of the fundus from the top of the symphysis pubis to the highest point at the top of the uterus; used to estimate the size of the fetus

gravida—combining form meaning a pregnant female or pregnancy

gynecology—branch of medicine pertaining to the female reproductive system, diseases, and disorders

gynecologist—physician specializing in the medical care of the female reproductive system, diseases, and disorders

menarche—onset of menses or menstrual cycle during adolescence

menopause—cessation of menses

menses—cyclic shedding of the uterine lining (endometrium) when fertilization of the ovum does not occur

obstetrician—physician specializing in the medical care of women during pregnancy, including prenatal, delivery, and postnatal care

obstetrics—branch of medicine pertaining to the medical care of women during pregnancy, including prenatal, delivery, and postnatal care

ovum (plural: ova)—human gamete (egg)

 MEDICAL ASSISTING STANDARDS

CAAHEP ENTRY-LEVEL STANDARDS	ABHES ENTRY-LEVEL COMPETENCIES
■ Perform within scope of practice (psychomotor) ■ Explore issue of confidentiality as it applies to the medical assistant (cognitive) ■ Apply ethical behaviors, including honesty/integrity in performance of medical assisting practice (affective) ■ Apply local, state and federal health care legislation and regulation appropriate to the medical assisting practice setting (psychomotor) ■ Recognize the importance of local, state and federal legislation and regulations in the practice setting (affective) ■ Explain the rationale for performance of a procedure to the patient (affective) ■ Use language/verbal skills that enable patients' understanding (affective) ■ Describe the normal function of each body system (cognitive) ■ Identify common pathology related to each body system (cognitive) ■ Analyze pathology as it relates to the interaction of body systems (cognitive) ■ Discuss implications for disease and disability when homeostasis is not maintained (cognitive) ■ Describe implications for treatment related to pathology (cognitive) ■ Apply critical thinking skills in performing patient assessment and care (affective) ■ Prepare a patient for procedures and/or treatments (psychomotor) ■ Assist physician with patient care (psychomotor) ■ Screen test results (psychomotor) ■ Document accurately in the patient record (psychomotor) ■ Practice Standard Precautions (psychomotor) ■ Show awareness of patients' concerns regarding their perceptions related to the procedure being performed (affective)	■ Interview and record patient history. ■ Prepare patients for procedures. ■ Apply principles of aseptic techniques and infection control. ■ Take vital signs. ■ Prepare and maintain examination and treatment area. ■ Prepare patient for and assist physician with routine and specialty examinations and treatments and minor office surgeries. ■ Use quality control. ■ Collect and process specimens. ■ Screen and follow up patient test results. ■ Prepare and administer oral and parenteral medications as directed by physician. ■ Maintain medication and immunization records. ■ Dispose of biohazardous materials. ■ Practice Standard Precautions. ■ Perform electrocardiograms. ■ Perform respiratory testing. ■ Perform telephone and in-person screening.

✔ **COMPETENCY SKILLS PERFORMANCE**

1. Assist with a prenatal exam.

2. Instruct the patient in breast self-examination.

3. Assist the physician in the performance of a pelvic examination and Pap test.

4. Perform a urine pregnancy test.

5. Assist with cryosurgery.

Key Terminology *(continued)*

Pap Smear (Papanicolaou test)—A screening test to aid in the detection of cervical/uterine cancer and cancer precursors.

para—combining form signifying the number of deliveries after the 20th week of gestation

perineum—area between the vaginal orifice and the anus

postnatal/postpartum—after childbirth

prenatal—prior to birth

zygote—the fertilized ovum created by the union of the male and female sex cells (sperm and ovum)

Abbreviations

AFP—alpha-fetoprotein

BSE—breast self-exam

C-section—cesarean section

EDC—estimated date of confinement

EDD—expected date of delivery

FHT—fetal heart tones

g—gravida (followed by number for each pregnancy experienced)

L & D—labor and delivery

LH—luteinizing hormone

LMP—last menstrual period

OB/GYN—obstetrics and gynecology

PMS—premenstrual syndrome

PP—postpartum

p—para (followed by number for each birth of a fetus over 20 weeks gestation)

UCG—urine chorionic gonadotropin

Introduction

The **OB/GYN** practice focuses on the female reproductive system. **Obstetrics** focuses specifically on pregnancy and childbirth. Many pregnancies progress without complications and the infant is delivered spontaneously, without difficulty. The expectant mother and developing **fetus** are monitored throughout the pregnancy during routine **prenatal** visits. The expectant parents are provided with information regarding pregnancy, labor and delivery **(L & D), postnatal** or **postpartum (PP)** care, and parenting. The **obstetrician** assists the mother during a normal vaginal delivery and with any surgical intervention that may be required if complications arise.

The **gynecology** practice addresses diseases and disorders of the female reproductive system. These conditions include ovarian, tubal, uterine, and vaginal disorders. Sexual dysfunction and sexually transmitted diseases are also treated. Fertility problems may be addressed by either the obstetrician or the **gynecologist.** Assisting women in dealing with normal life cycle changes is another goal of the OB/GYN practice.

The Medical Assistant's Role in the OB/GYN Office

The medical assistant in an OB/GYN office assists with obtaining the patient history, paying special attention to OB/GYN-related information. The MA will obtain vital signs according to office protocol and assist the physician with physical examinations, including pelvic exams, and obtaining **Pap smears** and other specimens. The MA may also assist with other procedures the physician may perform.

Normal prenatal visits include obtaining and recording the patient's weight and blood pressure and checking a urine specimen for protein and sugar. Urine pregnancy tests (**UCG**) are done on the initial visit and any visit when the patient reports vaginal bleeding.

Patient teaching involving the breast self-exam (**BSE**) is often delegated to the medical assistant. The MA may also be expected to give the patient information regarding nutritional requirements during pregnancy and lactation and to discuss breast and formula feeding options. Other important information for the patient and her partner addresses labor and delivery, prenatal classes, and caring for the newborn infant.

The Anatomy and Physiology of the Female Reproductive System

The female reproductive system consists of the following structures (Figure 44-1 ◆).

- Ovaries: The two ovaries are small almond-shaped structures located bilaterally in the lower aspect of the pelvis, beside the uterus, in a fold of the broad ligament. The process of ovulation occurs when the ovaries produce and release an egg, or **ovum,** in response to stimulation by the

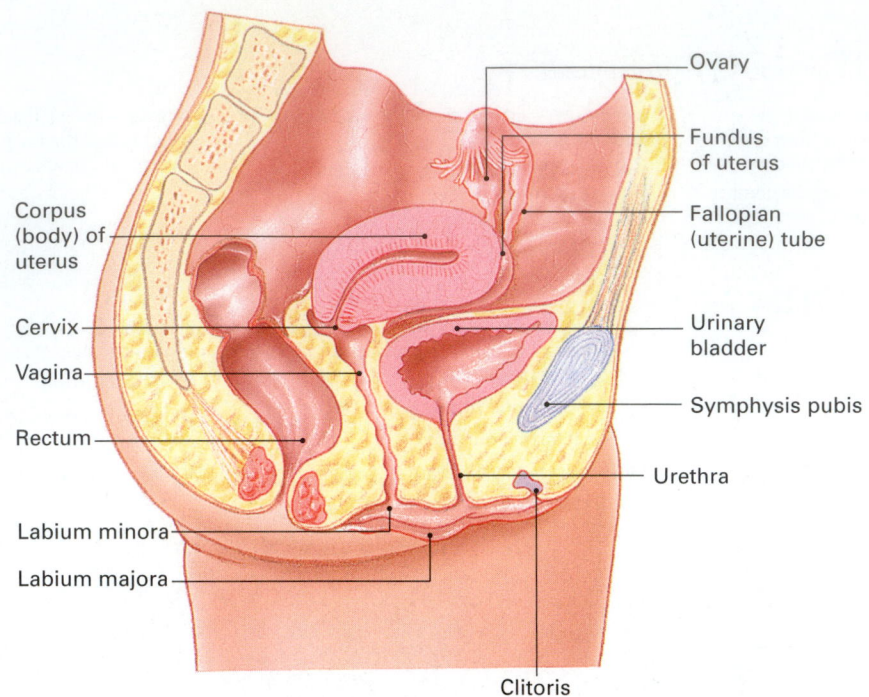

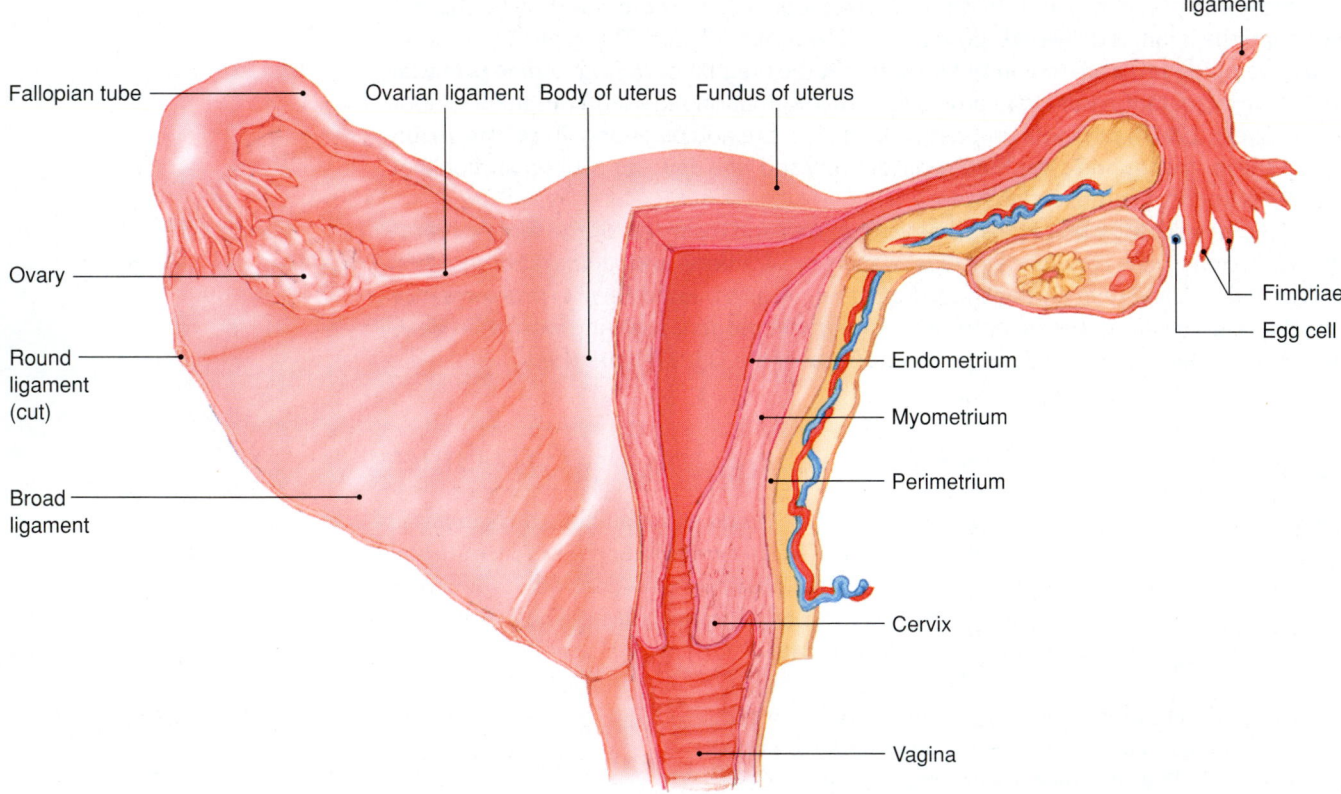

Figure 44-1 ◆ Female organs of reproduction.

follicle-stimulating hormone. Hormones produced by the ovary control the entire reproductive process: the menstrual cycle, its onset (**menarche**), the fertility cycle and **menses,** and the cessation of menses (**menopause**). At the moment of birth, the ovaries contain all the eggs that will be needed throughout a woman's child-bearing years.

■ Fallopian tubes: Two fallopian tubes are also bilaterally located in the pelvis. Their distal aspect is close to the ovaries, and at their dorsal aspect they connect to the uterus. The ova travel through the fallopian tubes from the ovaries to the uterus. The fallopian tubes are also the route the sperm travels to meet the ovum and fertilize it.

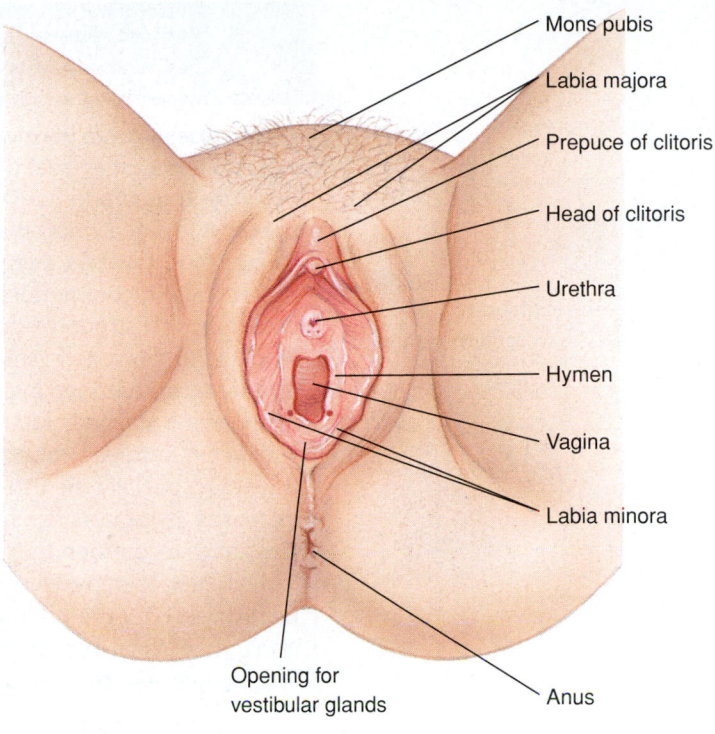

Mons pubis

Labia majora

Prepuce of clitoris

Head of clitoris

Urethra

Hymen

Vagina

Labia minora

Opening for vestibular glands

Anus

Figure 44-2 ◆ The female external genitalia.

The distal portions of the fallopian tubes have fingerlike projections called *fimbriae* that move to capture the egg and direct it into the tube for its journey to the uterus.

- Uterus: A hollow pear-shaped organ centered in the pelvis, the uterus is the internal female organ of reproduction. It is composed of three layers: the **endometrium,** or internal lining; the myometrium, the middle muscular layer; and the perimetrium, the outermost layer, composed of serous connective tissue. The endometrium is sensitive to hormonal influence and is where the fertilized egg is implanted for growth and development. When pregnancy does not occur, the endometrium is shed and menses begin.
- Vagina: The vagina is the tubelike portion of the reproductive tract extending from the outer opening (vaginal orifice) to the **cervix.** During the process of natural birth, the fetus must pass through this birth canal, often referred to as the vaginal vault.
- Cul-de-sac: The cul-de-sac is located directly behind the cervix and is a highly sensitive area.

Other structures associated with the female reproductive system comprise the external genitalia (Figure 44-2 ◆). *Vulva* is the collective term for these external structures.

- Labia majora: the outer lips of the vagina
- Labia minora: the smaller inner structures of the vagina
- Bartholin's glands: glands on either side of the vaginal orifice that produce mucus to lubricate the vagina
- Clitoris: erectile tissue anterior to the vaginal orifice and in front of the urethral meatus
- **Perineum:** area between the vaginal orifice and the anus

Anatomy and Physiology of the Female Breast

The female breasts, also known as mammary glands, develop during puberty but remain nonfunctional until the end of a pregnancy. Following birth, **colostrum** and the milk that follows serve as the source of the newborn's nutrition and passive immunity. Breastfeeding also establishes an emotional bond between mother and child.

Each mammary gland is composed of lobes containing fatty and glandular tissue and lactiferous (milk) ducts (Figure 44-3 ◆). On the exterior of each breast, in the center of the areola, the nipple is the convergence of the lactiferous ducts. With the birth of the child, a hormone called prolactin is secreted, thereby causing the glandular tissue to secrete colostrum, then breast milk, into the lactiferous ducts. The infant's sucking stimulates the release of oxytocin, a hormone that causes the lactiferous ducts to contract and release the milk, a process known as *milk letdown* or the *letdown reflex*. Breast milk production can be maintained for several months by continuous breastfeeding or by breast pumping.

The Menstrual Cycle

As the young female develops physically and approaches adolescence, hormonal changes stimulate the onset of menses and the menstrual cycle. Menarche signals the beginning of the female's reproductive capability. Hormones control the development, maturation, and release of ova for fertilization and implantation. If the ovum is not fertilized or the zygote is not implanted, the endometrial lining is shed as menstrual flow to prepare the uterus for the next potential pregnancy.

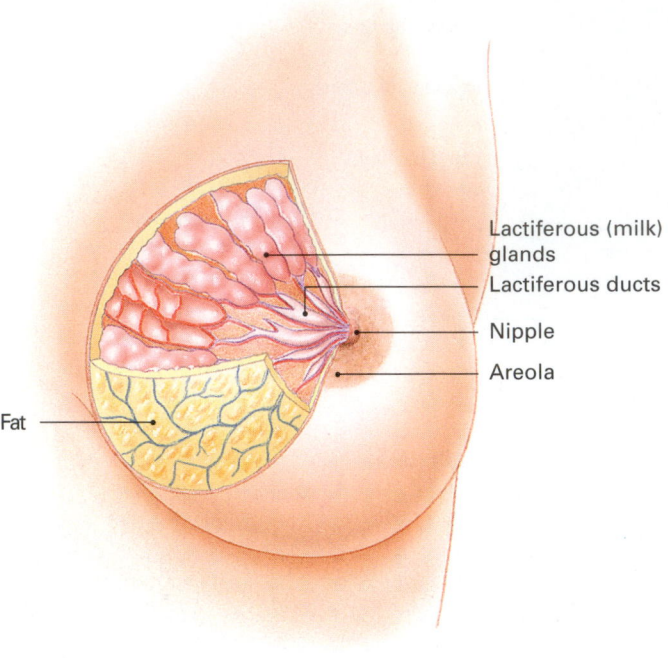

Fat
Lactiferous (milk) glands
Lactiferous ducts
Nipple
Areola

Figure 44-3 ◆ The female breast.

Normal menstruation is based on a 28-day cycle, also referred to as a lunar month. The onset of a menstrual period, or menses, is considered the first day of the cycle (Figure 44-4 ◆). The menstrual period normally lasts around five days, during which the disintegrated cells of the endometrium are shed in a bloody fluid with glandular secretions and blood cells. This process is usually followed by the repair of the endometrium, the release of estrogen by the maturing graafian follicles, also known as ovarian follicles, and the maturation of another ovum during days 6 to 13 of the cycle. Just before ovulation, or the release of the egg, on approximately the fourteenth day, secretion of luteinizing hormone (**LH**) sharply increases. The ovarian follicle ruptures (ovulation), and the follicle is transformed into a corpus luteum. The corpus luteum is responsible for producing some estrogen and large amounts of progesterone, which causes the endometrium and uterine blood vessels to thicken in anticipation of a potential pregnancy. As ovulation occurs and the ovum is released, waving fimbriae at the distal end of each fallopian tube assist in moving the ovum through peritoneal fluid toward the mouth of the fallopian tube. The journey of the ovum from fallopian tube to uterus takes about five days and would not occur without the propelling movement of cilia within the tube. If fertilization does not occur, the corpus luteum deteriorates, and levels of estrogen and progesterone decrease. This drop in hormone levels is a signal to the body to begin the menses and prepare for the next cycle.

Menopause, or the cessation of the menses, usually occurs between the ages of 45 and 55. This expected, normal condition occurs because of aging and the decline of ovarian function. Menopause also occurs after a surgical procedure called a hysterectomy. Hormone replacement therapy (HRT) is one possible treatment for the symptoms of menopause. The physician should

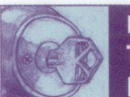

**Keys to Success
THE DEBATE OVER HORMONE REPLACEMENT THERAPY**

Recent research into hormone replacement therapy (HRT) has created a great deal of controversy. HRT had previously been recommended for postmenopausal women to help alleviate symptoms such as vaginal dryness, hot flashes, mood swings, sleep problems, and panic attacks. HRT was also recommended to prevent heart attacks and osteoporosis. Estrogen alone was prescribed for women who had undergone hysterectomies; progestin (progesterone) was prescribed in combination with estrogen for women who still had a uterus.

Recent studies suggest that hormone replacement therapy, especially the estrogen-progestin combination, increases a woman's risk for breast cancer. Many physicians have recommended that their patients discontinue combination therapy. Any decisions regarding HRT should be discussed by the patient, her partner, and the physician before a final decision is made. This discussion should include information regarding risks and benefits.

discuss the benefits and risks of HRT and other treatments with the menopausal patient and allow her to make an informed decision about whether to treat the symptoms. It is common for women undergoing the physical changes of menopause to feel too embarrassed to discuss their condition. Provide emotional support and reassurance that this is a normal condition.

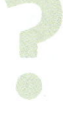

Critical Thinking Question 44-1

How should Sydney handle the phone call from Mrs. Blakely? How can she reassure her and offer support until Mrs. Blakely can speak to the physician? Should Sydney offer suggestions for nonpharmaceutical therapy?

Menstrual Disorders

Disorders relating to the menstrual cycle include dysmenorrhea, amenorrhea, menorrhagia, metrorrhagia, mittelschmertz, and premenstrual syndrome (**PMS**) (Table 44-1). Causes are varied, as are the treatments.

Contraception

The OB/GYN office provides information on contraception as well as prescriptions for contraceptive drugs and devices. Contraception, or birth control, may be achieved by various methods, including barriers, chemical contact, hormonal control, intrauterine devices, surgical sterilization, and periodic sexual abstinence. The use of contraception does not guarantee prevention of pregnancy. Although various contraceptive methods have established effectiveness rates, human factors, such as the consistency of correct use, and hormonal factors, such as those relating to breastfeeding, may affect the results and lead to unintended pregnancies.

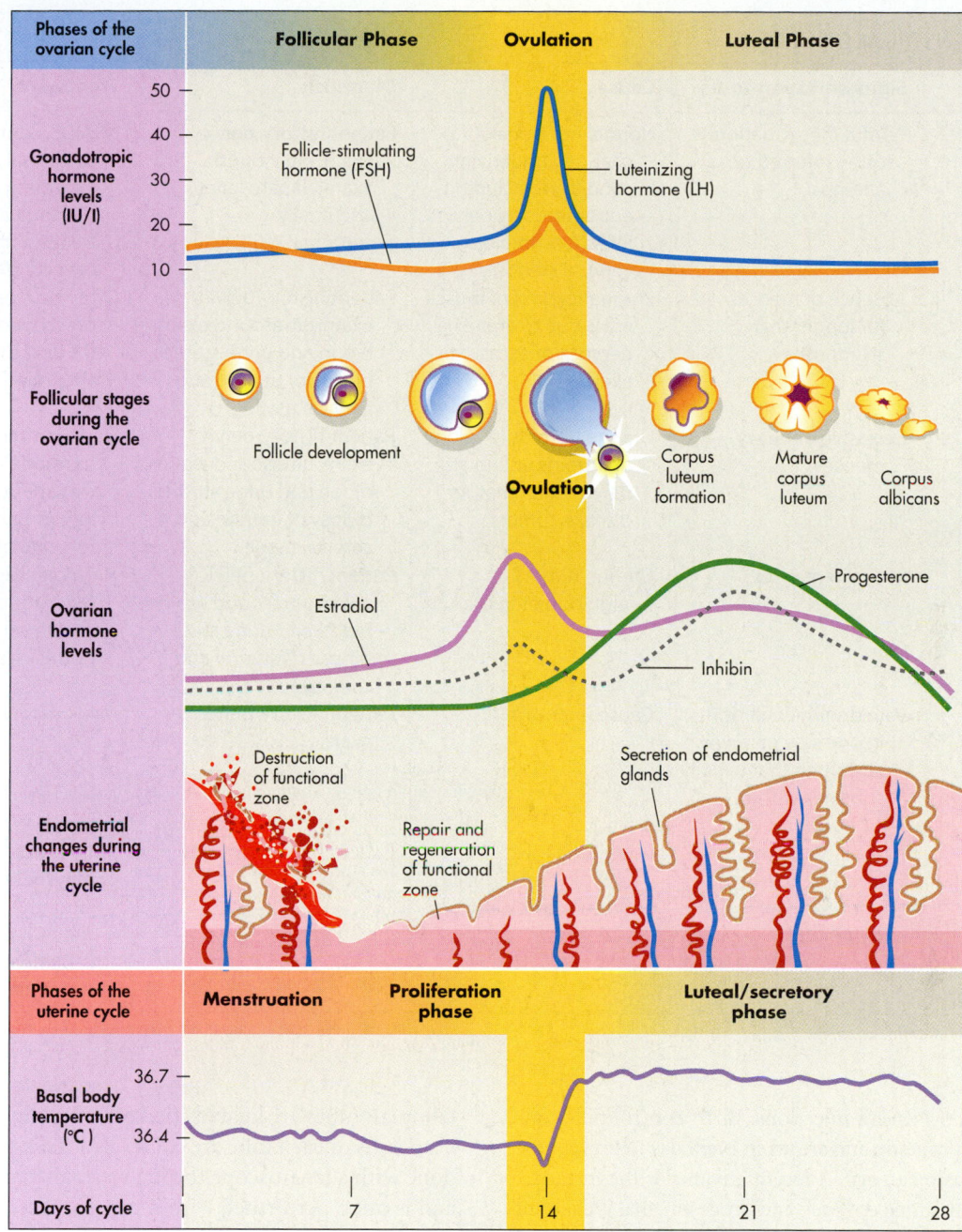

Figure 44-4 ◆ The menstrual cycle.

Barrier methods of birth control are designed to prevent the sperm from entering the cervix, traveling through the uterus to the fallopian tube, and fertilizing the ovum. Barriers include condoms, diaphragms, and cervical caps, which are usually made of latex. In addition to blocking fertilization, condoms also help to protect against the spread of STDs by preventing contact between the causative organism and the mucous membrane of the vagina. Barriers are usually the least expensive method of contraception. One drawback, however, is the inconvenience of inserting the diaphragm into the vagina, positioning the cervical cap on the cervix, or placing the condom on the penis before sexual intercourse.

Contraception may be achieved by contact between sperm and a chemical spermicide. Spermicides are available in foam, jelly, or cream form and may be purchased in drugstores or other stores without a prescription. They are recommended for use with diaphragms and cervical caps to make these devices more effective, but they may also be used alone, inserted into the vagina following sexual intercourse for moderate efficacy.

Another chemical intervention is vaginal irrigation or douching with solutions that create unfavorable conditions for the survival of sperm. Douching also washes out many sperm remaining in the vagina following intercourse.

Hormonal contraception includes the oral form (birth control pills), hormonal implants, intradermal patches, Norplant,

TABLE 44-1 MENSTRUAL DISORDERS

Condition	Signs and Symptoms	Cause	Diagnosis	Treatment
Dysmenorrhea	Painful menstruation, often referred to as "cramps"	Normal hormonal changes, underlying conditions including endometriosis, pelvic infection, fibroids, cervical stenosis	Patient history, pelvic exam, ultrasound exams, laparoscopy, and finally surgery (D&C)	NSAIDS, contraceptives (oral or dermal patches), treatment of endometriosis, surgical approach to treating fibroids and cervical stenosis
Amenorrhea	Absence of menses for longer than six months	Pregnancy; loss of muscle mass due to anorexia nervosa or excessive exercise	Patient history, pelvic exam, ultrasound exams, blood and urine studies, biopsy of uterine and cervical tissue	Often no treatment prescribed; hormone therapy may be used after ruled out pregnancy
Menorrhagia	Excessive or heavy menses	Uterine fibroids (etiology of fibroids unknown), pelvic inflammatory disease, tumors	Patient history, pelvic exam, ultrasound exams, blood and urine studies, biopsy of uterine and cervical tissue	Depending on cause: hormone replacement, treatment of pelvic inflammatory disease, removal of tumors
Metrorrhagia	Irregular menses	Uterine tumors or foreign bodies in uterus	Patient history, pelvic exam, ultrasound exams, blood and urine studies, biopsy of uterine and cervical tissue	Hormone replacement, D & C to restore endometrium to normal status
Mittelschmertz	Pain during ovulation in one side of lower abdomen that usually subsides within 12 hours	Cause unknown	Patient history, pelvic exam	Mild analgesics
Premenstrual syndrome (PMS)	Irritability, depression, breast tenderness prior to onset of period	Cause unknown; may be due to cyclic hormone deviation	Patient history, physical exam	Individualized treatment may include dietary alterations (reduction of salt, sugar, alcohol, and caffeine intake), exercise, stress management

Nuvaring, or Depo-Provera injections. Birth control pills contain estrogen and progestin and are taken every day to prevent the ovaries from releasing an egg. A recent advance is the intradermal patch, also containing estrogen and progestin, that is changed every week. The Norplant concept involves the placement of progestin rods under the skin of the upper arm. These rods release progestin slowly and last for two or five years depending on the number of rods implanted. The NuvaRing is a flexible contraceptive ring that is used to prevent pregnancy. It is about two inches in diameter and is inserted into the vagina once a month. It is kept in place for three weeks, during which the ring releases a synthetic estrogen to protect against pregnancy for one month. Depo-Provera is a form of progestin that is injected intramuscularly every three months.

Another form of contraception is the intrauterine device (IUD). The physician inserts the IUD through the cervix into the uterus, where it prevents the fertilized egg from implanting in the uterine wall. IUDs may remain in place for up to ten years and require removal by a physician.

Contraception by surgical sterilization is usually permanent. Tubal ligation is a surgical procedure in which both fallopian tubes are ligated (tied off), usually with a laser, and both ends of each tube are cauterized. This procedure can be done with a laparoscope through a small abdominal incision and is often performed within two days after delivery. Tubal ligation prevents the egg from traveling through the fallopian tube and the sperm from traveling up the fallopian tube to meet the egg. In the male, a vasectomy, or ligation of the vas deferens, permanently prevents the sperm transfer during ejaculation. Surgical reversals to reestablish a fertilization pathway in the male or female are usually only minimally successful.

Periodic sexual abstinence involves avoiding sexual intercourse during the probable fertile period of the menstrual cycle. The fertile period can be determined by monitoring the menstrual cycle; taking the female's body temperature, which rises slightly with ovulation; and interpreting the vaginal mucus, which is clear, slick, and stretchy during ovulation. Abstinence is the most reliable method of birth control. In some religions, however, it is the only acceptable method. Be careful not to impose your religious beliefs or feelings about birth control on the patient.

Infertility

An area of the OB/GYN practice that closely parallels contraception is fertility concerns, specifically the inability of the female to conceive. Obstetricians and gynecologists are both qualified to address fertility problems, but some choose to specialize in fertility.

The term *infertility* is used to describe partners who are under the age of 35 and have actively tried to conceive, without medical assistance, for one year without a resulting pregnancy. For couples over the age of 35, the time frame is shortened to six months. The term primary infertility refers to couples who have never achieved a pregnancy, while secondary infertility refers to infertility that affects couples after one or both have achieved a viable pregnancy.

Fertility issues are broken down into percentages of which partner is the most likely result of the inability to conceive. Currently fertility issues are 40% female factor, 40% male factor, 10% combined factor, and 10% unknown origin.

Some OB/GYN practitioners choose to only treat female issues, while others will run the necessary tests on both partners.

If neither partner has no previous successful pregnancies or caused a pregnancy, and there is no medical reason to suspect either partner, the male factors are the first to be tested and ruled out due to the simplicity and noninvasive testing approaches. The testing for male factors is a simple blood test to check hormone levels and a semen analysis through a donated sperm sample. By microscopically examining the semen, the physician can verify if there is sufficient sperm, the sperm are mobile (no double tails, missing tails, double heads, etc.), the ejaculate is the correct viscosity, checking the total morphology and motility. If male factor is diagnosed, there are multiple treatment options or even the possibility for the couple to explore donor sperm options.

Donor sperm options are also an option for women wishing to become single parents or for same sex couples to achieve a pregnancy.

Testing for female fertility issues are much more complex and costly. Multiple issues can arise in the female anatomy: Are the ovaries producing enough estrogen and progesterone? Is an egg being produced? Is the uterine lining adequate to support a fertilized egg? Can the uterus and cervix support a pregnancy? Can the ovum travel through the fallopian tubes? Is the cervical mucus thin enough to allow sperm passage into the uterus? Women can suffer from one or more fertility issues. To test female issues, the physician may choose to start with a complete blood analysis to determine if hormonal levels are normal. Specifically, a blood analysis can test for LH, FSH, progesterone, TSH, and prolactin as well as a variety of STDs that may have been contracted without showing symptoms. LH stands for luteinizing hormone, which aids in triggering the female body to ovulate or the male to produce testosterone. FSH is follicle-stimulating hormone. High levels may indicate a low egg reserve, especially in older women, while a low FSH level may indicate the woman is not ovulating at all. Low progesterone levels may indicate the body cannot ovulate. The thyroid functioning is checked with the TSH testing, to determine if it is over- or underfunctioning.

Either may affect the menstrual cycle and ability to ovulate. Prolactin is a by-product of the pituitary gland that can also affect the woman's ability to ovulate.

Once it is determined that the woman is ovulating and there are no male factors, the practitioner must determine if there are structural abnormalities. This can be done through a variety of tests such as an ultrasound of the pelvis to determine if follicle development is normal or a hysterosalpingogram in which a contrast dye is injected via the vagina to check that the cervix opens and the uterus and fallopian tubes are free of damage or structural problems. A much more invasive test is a laparoscopy, in which the uterus and fallopian tubes are viewed from surgical incisions in the abdomen. The laparoscopy can determine if there is scarring from pelvic inflammatory disease, endometriosis, or uterine fibroids. If those conditions are present, the practitioner can remove them during the viewing procedure.

If fertility issues are present, there are multiple medical advancements to help with these family-building challenges. Patients should be aware that most testing and infertility treatments are not covered by insurance. The patient should verify all financial responsibilities with their insurance carrier and practitioner prior to treatment.

Some religions and cultures regard the treatment of fertility problems as improper. Again, the patient's feelings and beliefs must be respected.

Pregnancy and the Birth Process

The release of an ovum from the ovary is the first step in the female reproductive process. If the ovum is fertilized by a sperm in the fallopian tube, a **zygote** is formed. As it divides

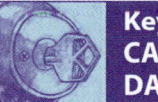

Keys to Success
CALCULATING THE EXPECTED DATE OF DELIVERY

The normal gestational period is 266 days, or 38 weeks, from the date of conception. The expected date of delivery (**EDD**), also called the estimated date of confinement (**EDC**), can be estimated using Nagele's Rule or the lunar method. To use Nagele's Rule, take the date of onset of the last period, subtract 3 months, then add 1 year and 7 days. If the date of onset is June 5, 2007, for example, the EDD would be March 12, 2008. To calculate EDD with the lunar method, add 9 months to the date of onset of last period, then add 7 days to that new date. Again, for a date of onset of June 5, 2007, the EDD would be March 12, 2008. Both methods yield the same result; preference depends on which is easier for the user.

Many wheel-type charts are available for calculating EDD and are used in the OB office. If the exact date of fertilization is known, 38 weeks are added to that date. Ultrasounds of the pelvis and developing fetus are also fairly accurate in establishing the age of the fetus. (This method is not available in all locations, however, and may be too expensive for some patients.)

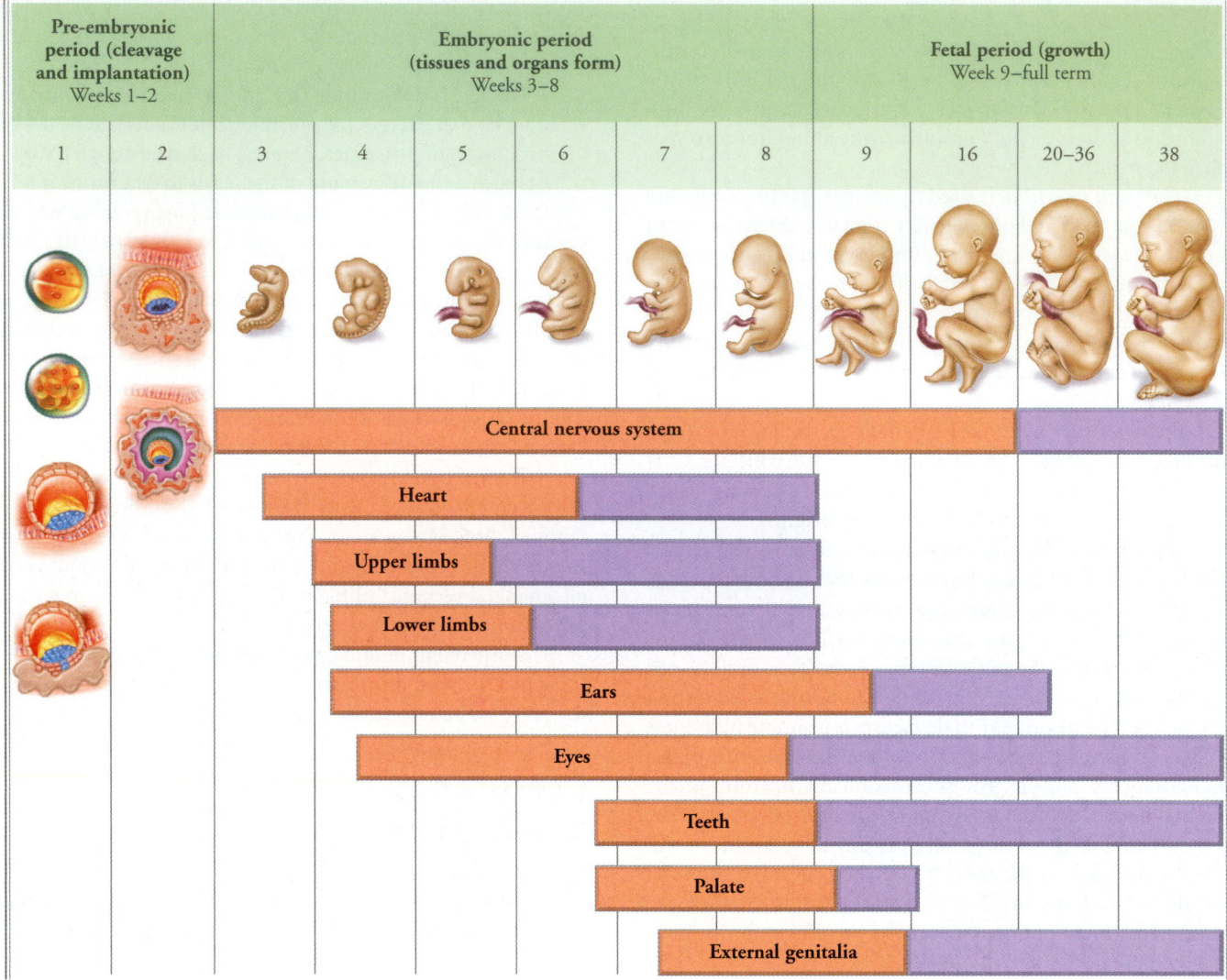

Figure 44-5 ◆ Stages of development.

and grows, it is transformed into an **embryo.** The embryo completes the journey through the fallopian tube to the uterus, where it implants itself in the endometrium. If conditions are favorable, the implanted embryo develops and grows into a fetus. It normally takes 38 to 40 weeks for the fetus to mature (Figure 44-5 ◆).

Delivery

In a normal delivery, the **cervix,** or mouth of the uterus, dilates and begins **effacement,** and uterine contractions propel the fetus through the vagina and into the external environment (Figure 44-6 ◆). Many of the movements the fetus makes as it travels down the birth canal stimulate its breathing after delivery. If the fetus is not in a head-down (cephalic) presentation, or if it shows signs of distress during labor, the physician may elect to perform a **C-section** to prevent fetal death. In this procedure, a surgical incision is made either midline in the abdomen or lower on the abdomen and into the uterus to deliver the baby.

Obstetrical History

Routine prenatal visits are usually scheduled once a month until the seventh month. If the physician feels the patient should be seen more often because of emerging problems for the mother or fetus, visits may be more frequent. After the seventh month, the expectant mother is seen every two or three weeks, then every week in the final month. A nurse practitioner often manages routine visits.

The routine prenatal visit includes measuring the patient's weight and blood pressure and checking a urine specimen for protein and glucose. Fetal heart tones (**FHT**) and the fetal position are also assessed, and the physician measures **fundal height.** Other areas that may be addressed, depending on the clinical progression of the pregnancy and the condition of the mother, include dietary modifications as well as instruction on labor and delivery, breastfeeding, and postpartum visits.

During the initial visit, you will obtain an obstetrical history of the patient. Important information includes the following:

- Date of the last menstrual period (**LMP**)
- Age at the onset of menses (menarche)

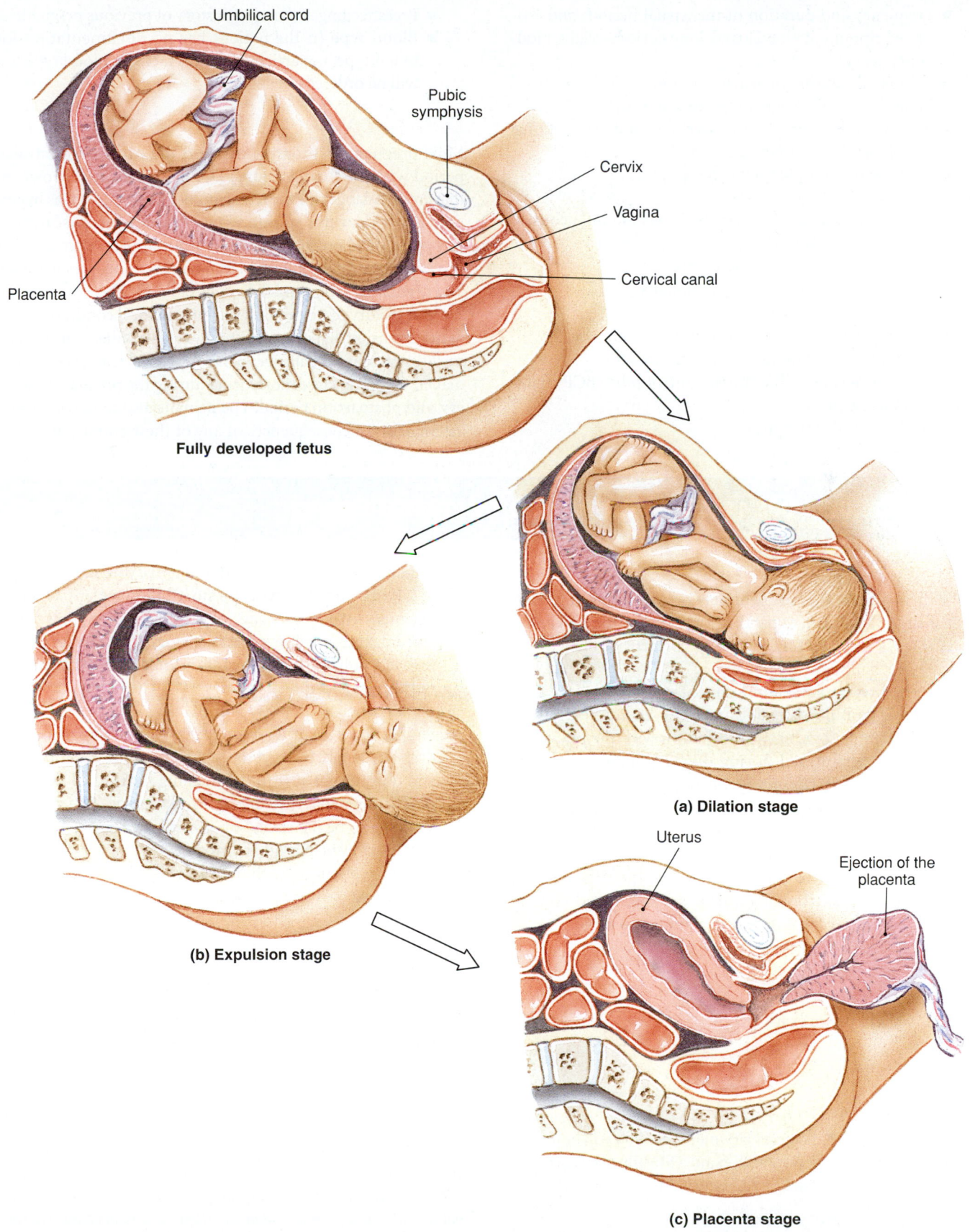

Figure 44-6 ◆ Stages of delivery.

- Frequency and duration of menstrual periods and estimated amount of blood loss during periods (slight, moderate, heavy)
- Pain, if any, during menstrual period
- Total number of pregnancies (**gravida** [**g**])
- Number of live births (fetus born alive and of gestational age of viability, or **para** [**p**])
- Number of multiple pregnancies
- Number of stillbirths
- Number of miscarriages or abortions (spontaneous or induced) (**abortus** [**a**])
- Infants born with congenital defects
- Age at cessation of menses (menopause)
- Surgical procedures, if any
- History of any sexually transmitted disease
- Dates of last mammogram and Pap smear
- Medications, including birth control pills (BCP), vitamins and aspirin
- Method of contraception

- Breastfeeding, if there is a history of previous pregnancies
- Blood type (if the patient has no documentation for blood type, in particular the Rh factor, a blood type test will be ordered)

Complications of Pregnancy

Most pregnancies progress through the normal gestational period without complications. Difficulties do arise, however, that create a danger for the fetus, mother, or both, such as hyperemesis gravidarum; spontaneous abortion or miscarriage; ectopic or tubal pregnancy; hydatidiform mole; toxemia, either pre-eclampsia or eclampsia; placenta previa; abruptio placenta; and premature labor and delivery (Table 44-2).

A history of previous or current medical conditions such as hypertension, hypothyroidism, hyperthyroidism, or diabetes mellitus presents a challenge to the obstetrical team. Gestational diabetes requires close monitoring during the pregnancy, delivery, and postpartum period. The neonate also requires prompt assessment for consequences of any of these conditions.

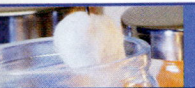

PROCEDURE 44-1 Assist with a Prenatal Exam

Theory and Rationale

The first prenatal appointment may be an exciting or terrifying visit for a woman, depending on whether the pregnancy was intentional. The physician will confirm or deny a suspected pregnancy during this visit.

The first prenatal appointment takes more time than subsequent routine visits and includes several blood tests, manual examinations, and consultation with the physician. Information established during this visit includes how far along the pregnancy has progressed, onset of menses, duration and amount of flow, any cycle problems, previous pregnancies or complications, previous births or complications, and all other obstetrical history. It is important to offer the patient guidelines for a healthy pregnancy, such as the safest amount of weight gain, nutritional guidelines, vitamin and mineral requirements, and substances and activities to avoid.

Materials

- EDD calculator
- full Pap and pelvic exam setup
- gloves
- patient's chart

Competency

(**Conditions**) With the necessary materials, you will be able to (**Task**) assist with a prenatal exam (**Standards**) correctly within the time limit set by the instructor.

1. Verify the patient's identification.
2. Explain the tests that will be done as a baseline to compare to in the later stages of pregnancy.
3. Measure the patient's height and weight.

4. Depending on your office requirements, you may be asked to take a complete physical history of the patient. Obtain her menstrual history (age of onset, duration, flow rate, and intervals) and pregnancy history (number of pregnancies, number of live births, number of miscarriages, number of abortions).
5. Obtain a urine sample to run a UA.
6. Supply the patient with a paper gown and appropriate drape materials. Instruct the patient to undress completely and don the gown with the opening in front so that the practitioner may perform a breast exam. The patient should also be instructed on how to appropriately cover herself with the provided drape.
7. Assist the physician with the Pap and pelvic examination as required by office protocol.

Patient Education

It is important that the patient understand the importance of proper nutrition and which foods to avoid. If the patient qualifies, there are government programs that provide assistance to ensure a healthy pregnancy and delivery.

Charting Example

04/28/XX 9:41 AM Patient came in for confirmation of pregnancy and baseline testing. Pregnancy confirmed and patient was given prenatal package containing information about HIV and STD testing, Quad-screen testing for genetic disorders, and a prescription for prenatal vitamins. Copy placed in chart. Patient was asked about hospital preference and is undecided. Patient received paperwork for Lamaze class and nutritional guidelines. Payton Ferraro, CMA (AAMA)

TABLE 44-2 COMPLICATIONS OF PREGNANCY

Condition	Signs and Symptoms	Cause	Diagnosis	Treatment
Hyperemesis gravidarum ("morning sickness")	Often first sign of pregnancy; nausea and/or vomiting; generally resolves as pregnancy progresses	Changes in hormone levels	Patient history of vomiting in the morning early in pregnancy	IV replacement of fluids and electrolytes in case of severe vomiting
Spontaneous abortion or miscarriage	Vaginal bleeding during early phases that results in termination of pregnancy	Etiology unknown; suggested causes include genetic fetal abnormality, hormonal imbalances, incompetent cervix, infection, immunological responses	Uterine bleeding, cramping, expulsion of products of conception from uterus	D&C if bleeding is severe to remove all products of conception from uterus
Ectopic or tubal pregnancy	Severe pain in pelvic area, usually vaginal bleeding, signs of shock	Zygote implants in area other than endometrium (usually fallopian tube but also ovary, outer wall of uterus, intestine, vaginal vault); in fallopian tube grows into embryo and causes tube to rupture	Patient history, pelvic exam, signs of shock	Immediate intervention: surgical termination of pregnancy, treatment of shock, replacement of lost fluids
Hydatidiform mole	Growth of abdomen but no fetal heart tones; bright vaginal bleeding during third month after cessation of menses	Error in conception involving chorionic villi; mass of vesicles develops and mimics early stages of pregnancy	Ultrasound	Mole may be expelled spontaneously, otherwise surgical removal; patient at risk for choriocarcinoma
Toxemia: preeclampsia is milder form, with no convulsions; can progress to more severe form, eclampsia, when convulsions occur	Sudden changes in blood pressure, weight, nausea, vomiting, headache, dizziness or spots before the eyes, edema in face, hands, and feet; usually affects primaparas under 18 or over 35; onset of convulsions (eclampsia) may trigger abruptio placentae	Sudden hypertension in last trimester	Routine urine testing and blood pressure monitoring	Dietary changes in early stages (low sodium, adequate protein); hospitalization if condition cannot be controlled and to avoid convulsions; delivery usually resolves condition quickly. Termination of pregnancy by induction or surgical intervention is the only cure. Preeclampsia requires close monitoring and often hospitalization; eclampsia is serious and requires constant monitoring.
Abruptio placentae	Sudden onset of abdominal pain, bright vaginal bleeding that may be copious; signs of shock, rigid and tight abdomen, fetal distress	Placenta prematurely separates from wall of uterus	Patient history, exam, ultrasound studies indicating location of placenta, vaginal bleeding	C-section to save mother's life and possibly child's life
Placenta previa	Painless vaginal bleeding during second and third trimester	Placenta implanted across cervical os or low in uterus close to cervical os	Patient history, exam, ultrasound studies showing location of placenta and vaginal bleeding	Bed rest often allows mother to carry baby to term; delivery by C-section

continued

TABLE 44-2 COMPLICATIONS OF PREGNANCY (CONTINUED)

Condition	Signs and Symptoms	Cause	Diagnosis	Treatment
Premature labor	Labor before gestational period of 36 weeks; contractions, rupture of amniotic sac, vaginal bleeding or spotting, cervical effacement and dilation	Etiology often unknown; causes may include maternal infection, illness, injury, surgical procedures, incompetent cervix, placenta previa, placenta abruptio, toxemia, or presence of multiple fetuses.	Patient history, examination, fetal and uterine monitoring, observation of contractions by watching fundus	Restricted activities or bed rest; medications to slow or stop contractions; delivery if amniotic sac breaks to prevent infection; neonatal team present to care for high-risk premature infant

Breastfeeding

Breastfeeding is a matter of personal choice. Both breast-feeding and formula feeding have their advantages. Breast milk provides the infant with immunity to certain diseases and a readily available supply of nutrition that is always the correct temperature. The baby's suckling stimulates further milk production, and with continued breastfeeding the mother can usually produce adequate milk indefinitely. The APA (American Pediatric Association) recommends twelve months at minimum. For optimum milk production, the mother requires good nutrition and adequate fluid intake. A drawback to breastfeeding is that the mother must be available to nurse the baby on a regular basis or pump her breasts to obtain milk for the infant to be fed with a bottle. It takes some new mothers a while to develop the breastfeeding technique. Patient instruction is important in this area. The mother should never feel pressured into doing something she does not feel comfortable doing.

Formula feeding allows the mother more freedom to leave her infant in someone else's care. Bottle feeding provides a way to measure the calories and amount of liquid the infant is taking in. However, formula is expensive and requires preparation, while breast milk is essentially free and immediately available.

Gynecological Diseases and Disorders

The female reproductive system is prone to several diseases or conditions. Any structure in the system may be affected. For example, the ovaries may develop cysts or carcinoma. The fallopian tubes may be the site of an infectious process, scarring, and subsequent obstruction. The uterus is vulnerable to endometriosis, pelvic inflammatory disease, fibroids, and endometrial cancer. The cervix may be affected by infection, carcinoma, or dysplasia. The vagina is susceptible to vaginitis and uterine prolapse. Cystoceles and rectoceles also occur in the vaginal area.

Table 44-3 describes some of the common conditions of the female reproductive system that you the MA is likely to encounter in the OB/GYN office. Table 44-4 lists risk factors and points of instruction for the patient concerning cervical and uterine cancer.

Assessing Vaginal Bleeding

A primary symptom of problems in the female reproductive tract is vaginal bleeding other than during the regular menstrual period. Abnormal bleeding can occur at any age. In the very young female, from infancy until puberty and menarche, vaginal bleeding may be an indication of sexual abuse. (Bleeding in the sexually and physically mature child-bearing adult or elderly female may also result from sexual abuse.)

Vaginal bleeding other than normal menses in the female who has passed menarche may indicate a hormonal imbalance or a pathology in the reproductive tract. During pregnancy vaginal bleeding is an abnormal occurrence and requires prompt assessment for the cause.

When a patient reports abnormal vaginal bleeding, even an unusually heavy menstrual flow, the actual amount lost, as well as its color, must be determined. The MA may need to ask the patient questions such as these:

- Describe the flow. Is it spotty or continuous?
- What type of pad or sanitary napkin are you using—a mini-pad or maxi-pad? Do you use tampons?
- How much blood is present? Is the pad spotted or saturated? How much of the pad is covered?
- How long does it take to saturate the pad? How frequently does it need to be changed?
- Describe the color of the blood. Is it dark, light pink and watery, or bright red?

The MA will document on the chart the patient's description of the type and amount of blood flow. This information enables the physician to estimate the amount of blood lost.

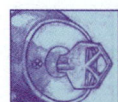

Keys to Success
CULTURAL CONSIDERATIONS ABOUT BREASTFEEDING

In many cultures, new mothers are expected to breastfeed their infants. Other societal pressures may also affect a new mother's decision whether to breastfeed. Some mothers are unable to breastfeed because of various health and emotional problems. As a medical assistant, you should accept the patient's decision in a nonjudgmental way.

TABLE 44-3 DISEASES AND DISORDERS OF THE FEMALE REPRODUCTIVE SYSTEM

Condition	Signs and Symptoms	Cause	Diagnosis	Treatment
Ovarian cyst	Pain in one side of lower abdomen, possible vaginal bleeding; may be cyclic or may enlarge and rupture unless surgically removed	Often no known etiology; some caused by normal functioning of ovary from ovarian follicle or corpus luteum; some may be result of infectious process; others may be malignant	Patient history, exam, ultrasound, laparoscopy	Some resolve on their own; others require surgical removal
Pelvic inflammatory disease (PID)	Fever, chills, foul-smelling vaginal discharge, severe pelvic pain, backache, tender abdomen	Bacterial invasion of vagina and pelvic cavity, often caused by STDs	Patient history, exam, elevated white blood cell count, tender abdomen	Antibiotics; scarring often irreversible
Endometriosis	Pain caused by microscopic bleeding of displaced endometrial tissue; most attacks subside after menopause	Endometrial tissue displaced to other tissue in reproductive system or into abdominal cavity, where it implants, grows, and continues to respond to hormonal changes	Patient history, exam, laparoscopy	Hormones, surgical removal of ovaries, D&C
Uterine fibroids	Vaginal bleeding, heavy menstrual periods, pelvic pain and pressure	Benign fibrous growths or tumors of myometrium	Patient history, exam, ultrasound studies, laparoscopy, D&C	Surgical removal of fibroids (for women still planning to become pregnant), hysterectomy (for women no longer desiring children)
Vaginitis	Vaginal discharge, often yellow and foul-smelling	Inflammation of vagina, usually caused by *Trichomonas* infection	Patient history, exam, positive culture of vaginal smears	Antibiotics, antifungal medications, steroid creams
Uterine prolapse	Pressure in pelvic region, difficulty urinating	Uterus drops from normal suspension in pelvis into vagina; may protrude from vaginal orifice; caused by weakened pelvic muscles and ligaments	Patient history, pelvic exam, visualization of uterus protruding from vaginal canal	Minor prolapse helped by exercises that strengthen muscles of pelvic floor, weight loss; surgical repair
Cystocele	Frequent urination, urgency, incontinence, pressure	Downward displacement of urinary bladder into vagina; caused by weakened muscles in pelvic floor, often result of childbearing and aging	Patient history, pelvic exam	Exercises to strengthen pelvic floor muscles, surgical repair
Rectocele	Incontinence of flatus and stool	Downward displacement of rectum into vagina; caused by weakened muscles in pelvic floor, often result of childbearing and aging	Patient history, pelvic exam	Surgical repair
Ovarian cancer	Symptoms not specific for ovarian cancer: lower back pain, constipation, lower abdominal discomfort, irregular menstrual periods	Etiology unknown	History, exam revealing pelvic adnexal mass, laparoscopic exam, elevated tumor markers	Surgical removal if possible, chemotherapy

continued

TABLE 44-3 DISEASES AND DISORDERS OF THE FEMALE REPRODUCTIVE SYSTEM (CONTINUED)

Condition	Signs and Symptoms	Cause	Diagnosis	Treatment
Uterine or endometrial cancer	Vaginal "spotting" or bleeding in early stages, pain later	Etiology unknown; possibly caused by overexposure to estrogen, including postmenopausal HRT	Biopsy and staging with imaging procedures to determine extent of metastasis	Surgical excision and radiation
Cervical cancer	Often asymptomatic; bloody vaginal discharge and bleeding between menstrual periods; cervical lesions may be noted during visual pelvic exam	Possibly exposure to human papillomavirus; other causes not yet identified	Pelvic exam, Pap smear, biopsy	Surgical excision of lesion, followup chemotherapy and/or radiation (Note: vaccine for HPV is now available)
Labial cancer	Nodule or ulcer on labia, pruritis, burning, dysuria, possible enlarged lymph nodes	Unknown cause; occurs more often in females over age 60; history of herpes virus, multiple sexual partners, cigarette smoking; prior history of reproductive system cancers	Biopsy and evaluation for metastasis	Surgical excision of lesion and surrounding tissue; chemotherapy for systemic involvement

Sexually Transmitted Diseases

Both OB and GYN offices care for patients with contagious diseases that are transmitted through sexual contact, commonly referred to as sexually transmitted diseases (STDs) or venereal diseases (Table 44-5). STDs may be experienced by either the male or female and are transmitted during sex by blood, semen, and vaginal secretions.

TABLE 44-4 RISK FACTORS AND EDUCATION RELATING TO CERVICAL AND UTERINE CANCER

Risk Factors
- A family history of various cancers, particularly breast, uterine, and cervical.
- Promiscuous sexual behavior.
- Frequent vaginal infections.
- Nonsurgical menopause.

Education
- An annual pelvic exam and Pap test are recommended after age 18 or when sexual activity has begun, whichever is earlier.
- The patient should report a family history of ALL cancers to the physician, particularly breast, uterine, and cervical.
- The patient should not douche or engage in sexual relations within 48 hours of the Pap test.
- Further examinations are required when abnormal symptoms are present, including pelvic or vaginal pain; vaginal discharge other than bleeding; abnormal bleeding such as heavy, scanty, or spotting, or at times other than during the monthly menstrual period; changes in the breasts such as a new lump or mass; or lack of pregnancy without contraceptives during the childbearing years.

In Practice

Melanie Forbes, 23 years old, is diagnosed with genital warts. She wants to know if the doctor will give her a shot or a prescription to treat the condition. She also wants to know if her condition is contagious. How should the medical assistant respond? What organism causes genital warts?

Breast Disorders and Conditions

The female breast is prone to a number of conditions that may be seen in the OB/GYN office. Fibrocystic changes, mastitis, carcinoma, diminutive size, and massive size are examples. Some patients may wish to discuss the necessity of monthly breast self-exams and regular mammogram screenings. Those anticipating either breast reduction or augmentation procedures may seek additional information or reassurance.

Many females connect the size and shape of their breasts with their sexuality. For other women, the ability to bear children is essential to their self-esteem and femininity. Encouraging the female patient to vocalize her concerns and listening in a nonjudgmental way promotes a more positive outlook.

Hormonal changes during the menstrual cycle can cause changes in breast tissue. Fibrocystic changes are usually responses to hormone stimulation. Progesterone may cause an increase in fluid in the breast tissue, creating tenderness and an uncomfortable feeling. Fibrous tissue and cysts develop, and lumps may be felt upon palpation. Manual examination of the breasts, accompanied by a mammogram, is helpful in ruling out carcinoma. Caffeine is thought to aggravate the cystic condition, and avoiding or limiting caffeine intake is encouraged. A firm, supporting

TABLE 44-5 SEXUALLY TRANSMITTED DISEASES

Condition	Signs and Symptoms	Causative Agent	Diagnosis	Treatment
Candidiasis	Irritation, itching, thick white vaginal discharge; often occurs in immunocompromised patients or following antibiotic therapy	*Candida albicans*	Microscopic examination	Antifungal creams or suppositories, including myconazole, clotrimazole, nystatin
Chlamydia	Usually asymptomatic before complications	*Chlamydia trachomatis*	Swab cultures, Giemsa stain, serologic testing for antibodies	Oral antibiotics, including doxycycline and erythromycin
Genital herpes	Painful, blister-like lesions in genital region; systemic influenza symptoms, including fever, headache, swollen glands; possible painful urination	Herpes simplex virus type 2 (HSV 2)	Observation of lesions, tissue culture	No cure; symptom relief with antiviral medications such as acyclovir, famcyclovir, and valacyclovir
Genital warts (condylomata acuminata)	Warts on genitalia; burning, itching lesions	Human papillomavirus (HPV)	Observation of warts, potential biopsy to rule out cancer/carcinoma	Chemical or surgical removal
Gonorrhea	Purulent discharge from GU tract; painful urination; occasionally asymptomatic	*Neisseria gonorrhoeae*	Gram stain of discharge	Antibiotics (penicillin, tetracycline, ceftriaxone)
Syphilis	Painless chancre(s) on genitalia	*Treponema pallidum*	Microscopic examination of smear with causative organism	Penicillin G
Trichomoniasis	Mainly asymptomatic; possible profuse green-yellow discharge	*Trichomonas vaginalis*	Wet prep slide and microscopic visualization of causative organism; urinalysis	Anti-infective medications

bra may also afford some relief and comfort. The most important aspect of the condition is ruling out breast cancer.

A small, painless lump in the breast is often the first sign of breast cancer (Table 44-6). The lump may be discovered by the female during a monthly breast self-exam or by the physician during a routine or annual physical. A mammogram is helpful in the diagnosis, but a biopsy is necessary to confirm it. Suggested treatment usually involves excision of the lesion and surrounding tissue by either lumpectomy or mastectomy. Lymph nodes may be removed and examined for the presence of malignant cells. Additional treatment may include chemotherapy and/or radiation.

Breast reduction is done for the female with extremely pendulous breasts that cause pain and discomfort, usually in the shoulders, neck, and back. As a cosmetic procedure, breasts may be reduced to allow the female to wear normal clothes. A reconstructive process for medical purposes may be covered by insurance. Many patients require counseling to adjust to their new image.

The female with small breasts may seek breast augmentation. Implants come in a variety of shapes and types. Implants all come in a form made of Elastomer, which is a rubber-like silicone material. The implant can be filled with gel, saline, silicone/saline combination, PVP-Hydrogel, or even natural plant oil. The shape

TABLE 44-6 RISK FACTORS AND EDUCATION RELATING TO BREAST CANCER

Risk Factors
- Female gender
- Increasing age, particularly over 50
- Ethnicity: non-Hispanic women have the highest incidence, and African American women have the highest mortality rate
- Early onset of menarche
- Later age of first full-term pregnancy (30 and over)
- Later onset of menopause (over 55)
- Personal medical history of abnormal breast changes
- Personal medical history of breast cancer
- Use of birth control pills or HRT (hormone replacement therapy)
- Obesity and physical inactivity
- High alcohol intake
- Family history of breast cancer or other associated cancers
- Radiation exposure, particularly to the chest

Education
- Monthly breast self-examination. Any breast changes such as newly found lumps, swelling, dimpling, skin retraction, or unusual nipple discharge should be evaluated by a physician.
- Routine professional breast examination.
- Routine mammography as determined by the physician based on risk factors and medical/family history.

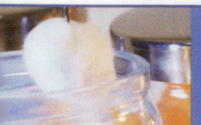

PROCEDURE 44-2 Instruct the Patient in Breast Self-Examination

Theory and Rationale

It is important for women to learn and practice monthly breast self-examination. Breast cancer has a high mortality rate in women with or without risk factors. During their lifetime, 12 percent of women will receive a diagnosis of breast cancer. Over 8 percent will be women without risk factors. Early diagnosis and treatment of malignancies increase survival rates. Patients should be taught how to reduce risk factors and encouraged to follow a preventive and healthier lifestyle.

Women who practice monthly breast self-examinations are more likely to seek medical treatment when they notice breast changes. Changes in appearance and tissue density may be subtle or obvious. Breast lumps may or may not be malignant, but medical management is necessary to monitor and treat the patient for changes that may become malignant later. You will use printed materials, videos, and artificial breast models to educate the patient. It is important to emphasize consistent times and techniques for the monthly exam to ensure that it is performed thoroughly and correctly. Breast inspection is done with the patient standing in front of a mirror, with her arms in different positions, then lying flat or on her side. She should start with the same breast and follow the same palpation search pattern (vertical strip, wedge, or circular) each time, to ensure that all areas are examined. Palpation is done in small, circular motions with the fingertip pads, which are more sensitive to abnormalities or differences in tissue.

Materials

■ patient chart
■ educational materials such as patient brochures or breast models

Competency

(**Conditions**) With the necessary materials, (**Task**) you will be able to instruct the patient in the performance of breast self-examination (**Standards**) correctly within 30 minutes.

1. Wash your hands and gather the necessary supplies.
2. Escort the patient to the patient education area.
3. Emphasize the following habits for the monthly self-exam.
   a. Premenopausal women should perform the examination about one week after the menstrual period, when the breasts are not swollen. Postmenopausal women should select a specific date of the month.
   b. Perform a visual inspection while standing in front of a mirror. With the arms hanging at the sides, above the head, or forward, away from the body, or with the hands positioned on the hips, observe for bilateral similarities or differences, for color or texture changes in the skin and nipples, and for nipple discharge (Figure 44-7 ◆).
   c. Examine each breast in side-lying and flat positions, starting with the same breast each time (Figures 44-8 ◆) For the flat position, place a pillow under the shoulder on each side.
   d. Palpate each breast with the fingertip pads of the opposite hand, using a dime-sized, circular motion (Figure 44-9 ◆).

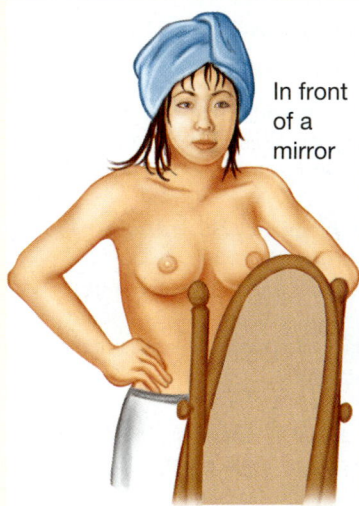

In front of a mirror

Figure 44-7 ◆ Perform a visual inspection while standing in front of a mirror.

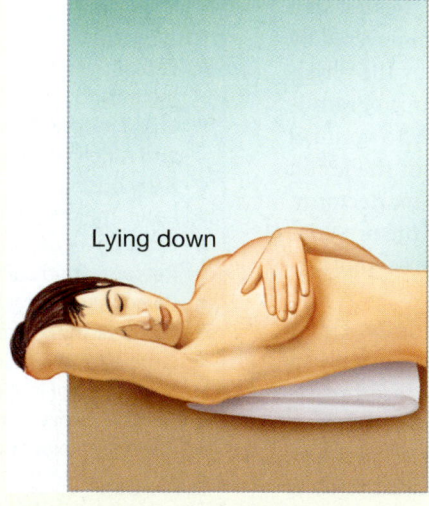

Lying down

Figure 44-8 ◆ Patient in side-lying position for breast self-exam.

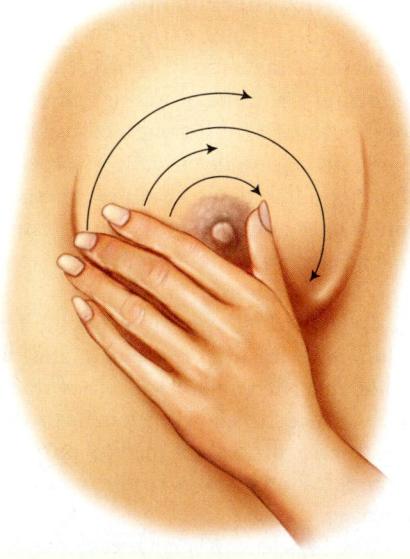

Figure 44-9 ◆ Palpate each breast in a circular motion.

PROCEDURE 44-2 Instruct the Patient in Breast Self-Examination *(continued)*

Use the same search pattern of vertical strip, wedge, or circle search for both breasts.

   e. Finish the breast examination by squeezing for nipple discharge and palpating the breast into the axillary area.

   f. Report any abnormalities or changes to the physician.

4. Document your patient instruction in breast self-examination. Note the patient's level of understanding.

5. Perform any necessary cleaning of teaching models and store for the next patient use.

Patient Education

Reinforce patient education materials with verbal instruction and demonstration. Ask the patient to perform a return demonstration. Encourage questions.

Charting Example

6/7/XX 11:00 AM Patient given written materials, verbal instruction, and demonstration on breast self-examination. Patient gave return demonstration correctly without questions. Edward Lee, RMA (AMT)

---

of the implant can be round or anatomic, also known as teardrop shape. Breast implants have been available since 1976, but it was not until 1992 that they were regulated by the FDA as medical devices. Patients are advised that complications are possible, including pain, capsular contractures, and infection. Any patient who desires a surgical alteration in appearance may benefit from counseling before and after the procedure.

Routine Assessment

Assessment of the female patient in the medical office includes the following:

- Taking a complete history: menstrual, obstetrical, surgical, and drug therapy history.
- Measuring weight and height, blood pressure, and temperature (if infection may be present).
- Performing a UCG for women of child-bearing age and capability.
- Assessing vaginal bleeding.

The pelvic exam and the Pap test are usually performed annually and are routine before oral or dermal forms of birth control are prescribed or prescriptions are renewed. A pelvic exam must be performed when vaginal bleeding, pelvic pain, and/or discharge is present. The MA will assist both the patient and the physician during the exam.

Diagnostic Procedures

Many diagnostic tests are typically performed in the OB/GYN office. The MA may perform certain tests or assist the physician with others.

- Urine tests can be used to determine if a patient is pregnant. Urine specimens from pregnant patients are tested for the presence of protein and glucose (sugar). The presence of protein may indicate impending toxemia of pregnancy; elevated glucose levels may indicate gestational diabetes. These screening procedures are performed along with weight and blood pressure measurement.

PROCEDURE 44-3 Assist the Physician in the Performance of a Pelvic Examination and Pap Test

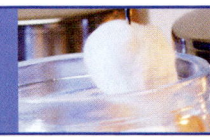

Theory and Rationale

Breast and pelvic exams help to assess the patient's health and diagnose disease conditions. Although both procedures are performed at the annual gynecological examination, specific patient symptoms or presenting complaints may warrant one examination without the other. Your role is to assist the physician as well as to explain the procedure and provide emotional support to the patient.

   The pelvic examination consists of a visual inspection of the external genitalia, bimanual pelvic and rectal-vaginal examinations, and the Pap test. The patient should not douche or engage in sexual intercourse during the 48 hours prior to

the Pap test. Douching alters the vaginal pH, and intercourse may cause inflammatory changes that affect the quality of the specimen and the accuracy of the test results.

   In addition to gathering vital signs and weight, documenting details of the reason for the office visit, and charting allergies, you will ask the patient to void to prevent the discomfort of a full bladder during the examination. A general explanation of the procedure will also alleviate some of the patient's fear and anxiety. Generally, you will instruct the patient to change into a gown and place a cover across the body from the waist down. You will also provide privacy for the patient to change. You may need to stay and

continued

PROCEDURE 44-3 Assist the Physician in the Performance of a Pelvic Examination and Pap Test *(continued)*

offer assistance to some patients during changing or positioning for the procedure.

As the physician performs the Pap test, the bimanual exam, and the rectal-vaginal examination, in that order, you must anticipate his or her needs and have materials prepared ahead of time to ensure that the procedure continues in a professional, efficient manner.

There are two different methods for obtaining specimens during a Pap and pelvic examination: the slide method and the thin-prep method. In the slide method, slides are labeled with the patient's identification and the letters *V* (for vaginal), *C* (cervical), or *E* (endocervical) to indicate where the smear specimen was obtained. Correlating the results of the Pap smear with the location will ensure more accurate and rapid diagnosis and treatment. When completing the laboratory requisition, indicate information that would be helpful to the interpretation of results, such as abnormal bleeding or hormonal, thyroid, steroid, and digitalis medications.

The thin-prep method involves collecting the specimen from the posterior fornix by scraping it with a plastic spatula. When a sufficient sample has been collected on the spatula, the spatula is rinsed by swirling for approximately 10 minutes in a solution specific for the thin-prep procedure. The vial of solution is then closed tightly and sent to the cytology department as soon as possible. Methanol-based solutions preserve the patient cells for approximately three weeks at room temperature.

The physician inserts the vaginal speculum to observe the vagina and cervix and obtain the Pap smears. After withdrawing the speculum, the physician lubricates the index and middle fingers of a gloved hand and inserts the fingers into the vagina while pressing on the lower abdomen with the other hand. This bimanual technique is used to palpate the uterus and ovaries to assess normalcy or changes that might indicate a disease condition (Figure 44-10 ◆). Last, for the rectal-vaginal examination, the physician inserts one gloved finger into the vagina and the gloved finger of the other hand into the rectum to assess for normalcy or disease conditions of the fallopian tubes, ovaries, ligaments of the uterus, and other pelvic organs. Hemorrhoids, fissures, or fistulas may also be diagnosed during the rectal-vaginal examination.

Materials

- patient chart
- examination gloves
- water-soluble lubricant
- physician's gown and eye protection
- vaginal speculum
- gooseneck or other light source
- slide container, glass slides, marker to label slides, and slide fixative for Pap smear
- cervical/spatula scraper
- cotton-tipped applicators
- lab requisition form

Competency

(**Conditions**) With the necessary materials, (**Task**) you will be able to assist the physician during the performance of a pelvic examination and Pap test (**Standards**) correctly within 30 minutes.

1. Wash your hands and assemble the equipment. Label the slide containers with patient information. Label the frosted

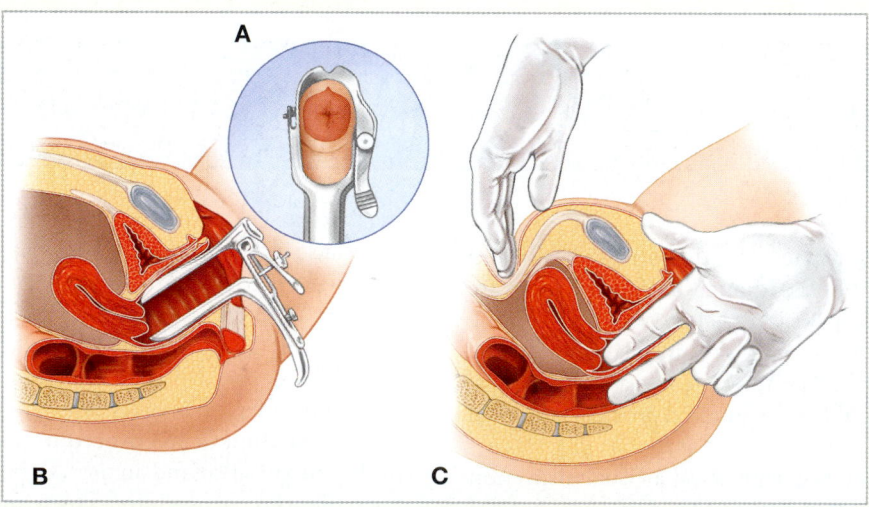

Figure 44-10 ◆ (A) and (B) The physician performs a pelvic examination of a female patient using a vaginal speculum. (C) Bimanual technique.

PROCEDURE 44-3 Assist the Physician in the Performance of a Pelvic Examination and Pap Test (continued)

edge of each slide with patient information and the location from which the specimen was taken.

2. Identify the patient and escort her to the examination room. Obtain the mensuration required by the physician (usually weight, temperature, blood pressure, pulse, and respirations).

3. Interview the patient for the following information:
   a. chief complaint (reason for visit)
   b. medications and known allergies
   c. start date of last menstrual period
   d. date of most recent Pap smear

4. Explain the procedure to the patient.

5. Before the procedure, assist the patient to the bathroom to void.

6. When the patient returns to the examination room, instruct her to remove clothing from the waist down. Assist as necessary. Provide a drape for the body from the waist down. If a breast examination is also to be performed, the patient will need to completely disrobe. Provide a gown cover for the chest area as well. The patient may sit on the examination table or lie comfortably until the physician arrives.

7. When the physician is present, assist the patient into a supine/dorsal recumbent position if a breast exam is to be performed. Slide the patient toward the stirrups and into the lithotomy position for the remainder of the pelvic examination and the Pap test.

8. Observe the patient's tolerance of the procedure and hand the slides, cervical/spatula scraper, and cotton-tipped applicators to the physician for the Pap smear. After the physician has placed the specimen on the slides, immediately

spray or apply ethyl alcohol liquid fixative. Give the physician water-soluble lubricant for the pelvic examination.

9. When the procedure has been completed, assist the patient to a sitting position. Leave the room to allow her to dress in private, or assist if necessary.

10. Remove the used implements to the cleaning area. Dispose of disposable and biohazardous materials in the appropriate containers. Wash your hands.

11. Transport the labeled specimen to the laboratory, or arrange for transport, with the appropriate lab requisitions. Assist the patient with the scheduling of additional procedures, if necessary.

12. Document the patient's response to the procedure, any future appointments, and other patient information, including prescriptions or patient instruction.

Patient Education

If this is the patient's first visit for an annual pelvic examination, instruct her as to office procedure and her responsibility in scheduling subsequent visits. Also instruct her to call the office if any unusual vaginal or lower abdominal problems occur.

Charting Example

03/29/XX 2:30 PM Explained procedure to patient. Patient sent to bathroom to empty bladder. Patient required no assistance during examination. Instructions given to call office in two weeks for results and/or appointment in two weeks. Patient filled out reminder postcard for next year's appointment. Kimberly Rainer, RMA (AMT)

- A colposcopy is a special examination of the vagina and cervix with an optical magnifying instrument. It allows for a microscopic view of the cervix. The physician usually performs the cervical biopsy during this procedure when a Pap smear report indicates cervical dysplasia.
- Patients experiencing heavy or unusual bleeding may have blood tests for hemoglobin and hematocrit.

Keys to Success
CULTURAL CONSIDERATIONS

In some cultures, female patients are prohibited from disrobing in view of others. A woman may not be examined by a male physician, or the husband must be present in the room during any examination or treatment. These customs must be honored. The physician will generally provide guidance in how to handle this situation.

- During the course of the pregnancy, specific diagnostic testing may be ordered. A routine blood test is alpha-fetoprotein (**AFP**) screening for possible neural tube defects, performed between the fifteenth and eighteenth weeks. If results are elevated above acceptable levels, additional testing includes ultrasound examination and **amniocentesis.**
- Glucose tolerance testing is now becoming routine as a part of the prenatal screening process and is useful in the detection of gestational diabetes.
- The use of ultrasound during a pregnancy as well as to assess gynecological conditions is becoming more common. The age and sex of the fetus and possible congenital conditions are often determined during an ultrasonic examination (see ∞ Chapter 34). Ultrasounds are performed prior to and during amniocentesis, to determine the location of the placenta and fetal structures. After the area is anesthetized with local anesthetic, a needle is introduced into the uterus to withdraw a sample of amniotic fluid that is then analyzed in the laboratory.

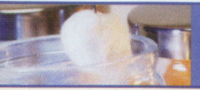

PROCEDURE 44-4 Perform a Urine Pregnancy Test

Theory and Rationale

When a pregnancy occurs, the placenta begins to develop, providing a filter between the mother and fetus for the remainder of the pregnancy. The placenta secretes a hormone called human chorionic gonadotropin (hCG) into the blood serum or urine. In a urine test, it is the presence of this hormone that confirms a pregnancy.

Pregnancy tests are one of the few diagnostic tools that can be purchased over-the-counter for patient use at home. Many pregnancy tests are so sensitive to the hormone hCG that a pregnancy can be detected as early as five days after conception. Any test performed at home should be evaluated by a medical office.

Materials

- gloves
- urine sample
- hCG test
- hCG positive urine control
- hCG negative urine control
- timer
- disinfectant
- patient chart

Competency

(**Conditions**) With the necessary materials, you will be able to (**Task**) test a patient's urine for the presence of hCG (**Standards**) within 5 minutes.

1. Assemble all necessary equipment.
2. Wash your hands and put on gloves.
3. Follow the manufacturer's directions for using the negative control serum.
4. Follow the manufacturer's directions for using the positive control serum.
5. When you are satisfied that the tests are reliable, test the patient's urine sample.

6. Report the results to the physician (Figure 44-11 ◆).
7. Disinfect the work area.
8. Document the test and results in the patient's chart.

Patient Education

Keep in mind that not every pregnancy is a planned or positive event. Be sympathetic to the patient's needs and have appropriate contact numbers available for reference to counselors or other professionals.

Charting Example

04/28/XX 9:41 AM hCG urine test performed. Patient tested positive and was given results by Dr. King. Bryan Gross, RMA (AMI)

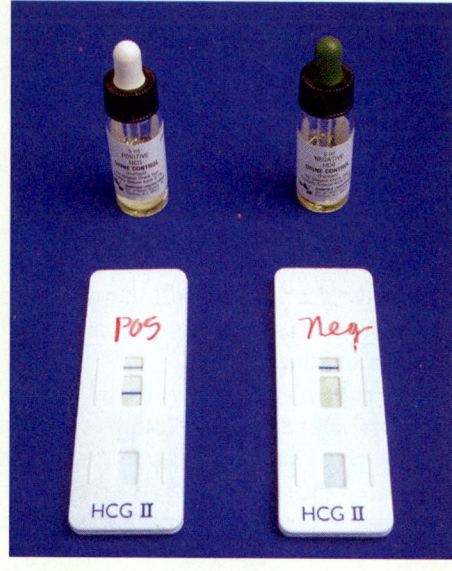

Figure 44-11 ◆ A urine pregnancy control test, positive and negative.

- Pap smears are performed as a screening process for cervical cancer. During a pelvic examination, the physician uses a special, thin wooden cervical spatula and a cervical brush to obtain cells from the cervix and the cervical canal. These cells are sent to a laboratory, where they are examined for the presence of cancer cells. Annual Pap smears help to detect cervical cancer in its early stages.

Treatment Modalities

Dysplasia of the cervix may be treated in a number of ways. Factors influencing the choice of treatment for cervical dysplasia include the extent and severity of the dysplasia, the presence of

the Human Papilloma Virus (HPV) and other gynecological problems, and the availability of equipment. The abnormal tissue can be treated by chemicals (silver nitrate) or freezing, which is known as Cryotherapy. Additional treatment methods include Loop Excision (LEEP), Laser Treatment and Cone Biopsy.

Gynecological surgical procedures are usually done in a clinical or hospital setting and include dilatation and curettage, laparoscopic procedures, tubal ligations and abdominal or vaginal hysterectomies, oophorectomies, and/or salpingectomies. Surgical intervention to suspend a prolapsed uterus or repair a cystocele or rectocele are other gynecological procedures. Obstetrical procedures include episiotomy (incision in the perineum to facilitate delivery of the infant) and C-section (Cesarean section).

- Dilation and curettage (D&C) is a surgical procedure in which the cervix is dilated and the lining of the uterus (endometrium) is scraped with a curette. This procedure is performed to obtain tissue for diagnosis of some uterine diseases, to treat prolonged or painful uterine bleeding, or to empty the uterus of products of conception (usually after a miscarriage).
- Laparoscopic procedures are surgical procedures performed with a laparoscope to view internal body structures with very small incisions. Organs and tissue can be removed or repaired by this method, which does not involve a surgical opening into the abdominal cavity.
- A tubal ligation is a surgical procedure in which both fallopian tubes are ligated, usually with a laser, and both ends of each tube are cauterized. This procedure can be done through a small abdominal incision with a laparoscope and is often performed within two days post delivery. A tubal ligation is a permanent form of contraception, as it prevents the sperm from meeting the egg for fertilization. Reversal is generally not successful, although there are recorded instances of females conceiving after a tubal ligation.
- A hysterectomy is the surgical removal of the uterus. In a total abdominal hysterectomy (or bilateral salpingo-oophorectomy), the surgeon removes the uterus, cervix, both fallopian tubes, and both ovaries. In a vaginal hysterectomy, the uterus is removed through the vagina rather than through an abdominal incision. Some physicians elect to leave a cervical stump intact, and sometimes one ovary or a portion of an ovary is left to produce female hormones. Menses cease with the removal of the uterus.

- An oophorectomy is the surgical removal of one ovary. The remaining ovary continues to ovulate regularly, menses continue, and the female can achieve pregnancy. In a bilateral oophorectomy, often referred to as surgical menopause, both ovaries are removed. The female no longer ovulates, hormones are not produced to stimulate the normal menstrual cycle, and menses cease. Many physicians order hormone replacement therapy to begin while the patient is in the recovery room to prevent or reduce symptoms of surgical menopause.
- A salpingectomy is the surgical removal of one fallopian tube. Bilateral salpingectomy is the removal of both tubes.
- A & P repair (anterior and posterior repair) is a procedure to correct a cystocele and a rectocele.
- A cesarean section (C-section) is a surgical procedure in which an incision is made either midline in the abdomen or lower on the abdomen and into the uterus to deliver the baby. This procedure is performed when the infant is too large to pass through the mother's pelvis, when it is in fetal distress, when the mother's life is in danger and immediate delivery is mandatory, or when the mother has had previous C-sections.
- An episiotomy is an incision made in the perineum to facilitate the delivery of an infant.

Cryosurgery

Cryosurgery is a technique that uses liquid nitrogen, which has an extremely low temperature, to freeze tissue so that it dies and sloughs off, to be replaced eventually by healthy tissue. Cryosurgery is performed to treat cervicitis, cervical erosion, and venereal warts.

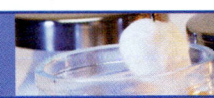

PROCEDURE 44-5 Assist with Cryosurgery

Theory and Rationale

Cryosurgery is performed with the patient in the lithotomy position. It is an uncomfortable procedure, and the patient should be made as comfortable as possible. Offer the patient a pillow for her head and remind her to take slow, deep breaths. Once she is in position, the physician will swab the cervix to remove mucus. The liquid nitrogen probe will be placed against the affected area as the liquid nitrogen flows over the area and freezes the tissue. The patient will feel pain similar to menstrual cramps. She should remain still and continue slow, deep breathing for pain control.

Materials

- gloves
- patient drapes
- light source
- liquid nitrogen
- vaginal speculum

- sterile specimen container (if needed)
- patient chart

Competency

(**Conditions**) With the necessary materials, you will be able to (**Task**) assist with a cryosurgery (**Standards**) within the time limits set by the instructor.

1. Verify the patient's identification.
2. Explain the procedure to the patient.
3. Wash your hands and put on gloves.
4. If necessary, assist the patient in undressing from the waist down. Provide proper patient drapes.
5. When the patient is undressed and draped, assist her into the lithotomy position.
6. Assist the physician as needed.
7. Reassure the patient that as the probe moves over the affected tissue and the liquid nitrogen freezes and kills the tissue, she will feel some discomfort, similar to

continued

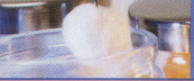

PROCEDURE 44-5 Assist with Cryosurgery *(continued)*

menstrual cramping. The discomfort should not be unbearable, however.

8. After the procedure, assist the patient to a seated position and help her dress as needed.
9. Clean and disinfect the room.

Patient Education

Instruct the patient in post-cryosurgery care:

■ Expect a heavy discharge for up to four weeks. It should have a clear, watery consistency.
■ Cleanse the perineal area often.
■ Use only sanitary napkins, not tampons or other devices that must be inserted, such as silicone cups.

■ Remain on full cervical/pelvic rest for four weeks—no douching, tampon use, or sexual intercourse.
■ Report any signs of infection such as vomiting, foul-smelling discharge, pain, or fever.
■ The next menstrual cycle will be heavier than usual. This is normal.

Charting Example

04/28/XX 9:41 AM Cryosurgery performed for chronic cervicitis. Patient reported slight cramping for 20-30 minutes and was monitored. Vital signs remained stable and patient was released home. Patient received postoperative care instructions, both verbal and written. Diane Edwards, CMA (AAMA)

Psychological Considerations

Many psychologically sensitive issues are addressed in the OB/GYN office. It is important to listen with compassion to patients and their families as they present with various problems. Consider the following examples:

■ Couples attempting to achieve a successful pregnancy or experiencing fertility problems often undergo a severe emotional, physical, and financial drain.
■ Hormonal changes during the menstrual cycle, such as PMS, may disrupt the patient's emotional stability.

Menopause also has a tendency to create emotional turmoil.

■ The diagnosis of cancer of any of the female reproductive structures not only intensifies the fear of death but also stimulates feelings of loss of femininity.
■ Parents who have multiple fetuses or infants from the same pregnancy may face a myriad of stressful problems.
■ The single mother faces many challenges. Understanding and tolerance are crucial when dealing with this patient.

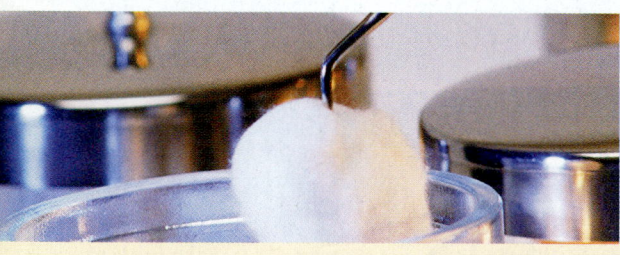

REVIEW

Chapter Summary

■ The OB/GYN practice focuses on the female reproductive system. Obstetrics specifically addresses pregnancy and childbirth. The expectant mother and developing fetus are monitored throughout the pregnancy during routine prenatal visits. The obstetrician assists the mother during a normal vaginal delivery and with any surgical intervention in the course of the delivery. The gynecology practice addresses diseases and disorders of the female reproductive system. Either the obstetrician or the gynecologist may address fertility problems.
■ The medical assistant in the OB/GYN office obtains the patient's OB/GYN history and vital signs, assists the physician with pelvic examinations (including obtaining the Pap smear

and other specimens), and instructs the patient in breast self-examination, nutritional requirements, labor and delivery, breast and formula feeding, and caring for the newborn infant.
■ Mammary glands develop during puberty but remain nonfunctional until the end of a pregnancy. Following birth, colostrum and breast milk are the sources of nutrition and passive immunity for the newborn.
■ As the female approaches adolescence, hormonal changes stimulate the onset of menses (menarche). Hormones influence the development, maturation, and release of an ovum (egg) for fertilization and implantation. If the egg is not fertilized or the fertilized egg is not implanted, menstrual flow

Chapter Summary (continued)

takes place to cleanse, or shed, the endometrial lining and prepare the uterus and body for the next potential pregnancy.

■ Menopause, or the cessation of the menses, usually occurs at 45 to 55 years of age because of aging and the decline of ovarian function. A surgical procedure called a hysterectomy also induces menopause.

■ Disorders relating to the menstrual cycle include dysmenorrhea (painful menstruation), amenorrhea (lack of menstruation), menorrhagia (heavy menses), metrorrhagia (irregular menses), mittelschmertz (pain during ovulation), and premenstrual syndrome (PMS).

■ The OB/GYN office provides contraception information and prescriptions. Contraception, or birth control, may be achieved with barriers, chemical contact, hormonal control, intrauterine devices, surgical sterilization and periodic sexual abstinence.

■ Couples having difficulty conceiving are diagnosed with an infertility problem. Treatment varies but can include hormone treatment for the female to stimulate release of ova, as well as in-vitro fertilization and implantation.

■ During the initial prenatal visit, an obstetrical history is obtained, including such information as age at menarche, frequency and duration of menstrual periods, total number of pregnancies, surgical procedures, sexually transmitted diseases, dates of last mammogram and Pap smear, blood type, medications, and so on.

■ The routine prenatal visit includes measuring blood pressure and weight, checking the urine specimen for protein and glucose, and assessing fetal heart tones (FHT) and fetal position. The physician measures fundal height. Other areas may be addressed as well, depending on the clinical progression of the pregnancy and the mother's condition.

■ Most pregnancies progress without complications. Problems that may arise include hyperemesis gravidarum; spontaneous abortion or miscarriage; ectopic or tubal pregnancy; hydatidiform mole; toxemia, either pre-eclampsia or eclampsia; placenta previa; abruptio placenta; and premature labor and delivery.

■ Conditions affecting the female reproductive system include ovarian, tubal, uterine, or vaginal disorders, as well as sexual dysfunction and sexually transmitted diseases. Any structure in the system may be the site of the disorder.

■ Cancer of the female reproductive system includes ovarian cancer, uterine or endometrial cancer, cervical cancer, labial cancer, and breast cancer. Screening for cervical cancer is routinely done with a Pap smear, breast cancer screening with monthly breast self-examinations and annual mammograms. A physical examination (pelvic or breast) and a biopsy confirm the diagnosis. Some blood tests may indicate the presence of cancer cells. Treatment in most cases includes surgical excision, chemotherapy, and/or radiation.

■ Ovarian cysts, pelvic inflammatory disease, endometriosis, uterine fibroids, uterine prolapse, cystocele, and rectocele are other gynecological diseases and disorders. Sexually transmitted diseases (STDs) or venereal diseases affect both males and females and are transmitted during sex by blood, semen, or vaginal secretions.

■ The female breast is prone to fibrocystic changes, mastitis, carcinoma, diminutive size, and pendulous size. A small painless lump in the breast often is the first sign of breast cancer, which is further diagnosed by mammogram and confirmed by biopsy. Treatment is usually lumpectomy or mastectomy, chemotheraphy, and/or radiation. All women should learn and practice monthly breast self-examination to detect the first signs of breast cancer.

■ Breast reduction is performed on extremely pendulous breasts to relieve pain and discomfort or as a cosmetic procedure. Small breasts may be augmented with implants.

■ Diagnostic procedures include urine tests, colposcopies, fetal ultrasounds, phlebotomy testing, and amniocentesis.

■ Cervical dysplasia may be treated by cautery or cryocauterization. Gynecological surgical procedures in a clinic or hospital setting include D & C, laparoscopic procedures, tubal ligations, abdominal or vaginal hysterectomies, oophorectomies and/or salpingectomies, surgical fixation for suspension of a prolapsed uterus, and repair of cystocele or rectocele. Obstetrical procedures include episiotomy and C-section.

■ Psychological issues are also addressed in the OB/GYN office. It is important to listen to patients and their families and provide emotional support.

Chapter Review

Multiple Choice

1. The lining of the uterus is called a/an
   a. menses.
   b. menarche.
   c. endometrium.
   d. colostrum.

2. The practice of gynecology addresses
   a. STDs.
   b. vaginal disorders.
   c. sexual disorders.
   d. all of the above.

Chapter Review (continued)

3. The internal lining of the uterus is called a/an
   a. endometrium.
   b. myometrium.
   c. perimetrium.
   d. cervimetrium.

4. The projections on the distal portions of the fallopian tubes are called
   a. Bartholin's glands.
   b. fimbriae.
   c. perineum.
   d. myometrium.

5. The glands on either side of the vaginal orifice are known as
   a. lactiferous.
   b. perineum.
   c. Bartholin's glands.
   d. fimbriae.

6. Which of the following hormones is responsible for the secretion of colostrum in the breasts?
   a. Prolactin
   b. Oxytocin
   c. Estrogen
   d. Progesterone

7. The union of male and female sex cells produces a/an
   a. ovum.
   b. zygote.
   c. fetus.
   d. embryo.

8. A woman who has not menstruated for more than six months has a condition called
   a. dysmenorrhea.
   b. mittelschmertz.
   c. metrorrhagia.
   d. amenorrhea.

9. Cervical disorders include
   a. PID.
   b. dysplasia.
   c. endometriosis.
   d. fibroids.

10. Often the first sign of breast cancer is
    a. a small, painless lump.
    b. a small, painful lump.
    c. a large, painless lump.
    d. a large, painful lump.

True/False

T F 1. Fibrocystic disease, mastitis, and cancer are all breast disorders.

T F 2. Breast implants have been available since 1978, but it was not until 1990 that they were regulated by the FDA as medical devices.

T F 3. During their lifetime, 12 percent of women will receive a diagnosis of breast cancer.

T F 4. The pelvic examination consists of a visual inspection of the external genitalia, bimanual pelvic and rectal-vaginal examinations, and the Pap test.

T F 5. Slides prepared during a Pap smear should be labeled with the patient's identification and the letters *V* (for vaginal), *C* (cervical), or *E* (external) to indicate where the smear specimen was obtained.

Short Answer

1. List three ways in which dysplasia of the cervix is treated.

2. What is the medical term for the surgical removal of one ovary?

3. For which two substances are urine specimens from pregnant patients tested?

4. What is a colposcopy?

5. What is the difference between uterine prolapse and cystocele?

Research

1. Where in your local area can pregnant women locate a doula?

2. Are there support groups in your community for women with breast cancer?

3. In your state, at what age can a minor legally obtain birth control without the consent of her parents?

Externship Application Experience

As an extern, you escort a married Muslim woman to the examination room. She is accompanied by her husband. As you attempt to obtain her medical history, her husband answers all your questions. After instructing her to remove her clothing and put on a patient gown, you leave the room. Five minutes later you return and find the woman sitting in a chair completely dressed. You ascertain that her husband will not allow the male physician to examine his wife. What do you do?

Resource Guide

American Cancer Society
1599 Clifton Rd
Atlanta, GA 30329
1-800-ACS-2345
www.cancer.org

American College of Obstetricians and Gynecologists (ACOG)
409 12 St S.W., PO Box 96920
Washington, DC 20090-6920
1-800-673-8444
www.acog.com

Endometriosis Association
8585 N. 76th Place
Milwaukee, WI 53223
1-800-992-3636 or 414-355-2200
www.endometriosisassn.org

Chicago Office
1 Oakbrook Terrace #808
Oakbrook Terrace, IL 60181
1-630-627-9270

National Alliance of Breast Cancer Associations
9 E. 37th St., 10th floor
New York, NY 10016
www.nabco.org

North American Menopause Society
PO Box 94527
Cleveland, OH 44101
216-844-8748
info@menopause.org

Planned Parenthood Federation of America, Inc.
434 W. 33rd St
New York, NY 10001
212-541-7800
www.ppfa.org/ppfa

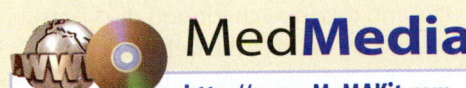

Med**Media**

http://www.MyMAKit.com

More on this chapter, including interactive resources, can be found on the Student CD-ROM accompanying this textbook and on http://www.MyMAKit.com.

CHAPTER 45

Pediatrics

Case Study

Lucas has just finished checking in his first patient of the afternoon, a 6-month-old girl, and is preparing to weigh her. After the mother removes the child's diaper, Lucas observes a thick, raised rash. The mother explains that her daughter has had a diaper rash that "just won't go away" and that when she gave her the prescribed medication, thick white patches appeared in the child's mouth. So the mother stopped giving the medication after the first couple of days.

Objectives

After completing this chapter, you should be able to:

- Define and spell the key terminology in this chapter.
- Define the medical assistant's role in a pediatric specialty office.
- Discuss the physical and developmental factors relating to the age of the child.
- List the procedures that may be performed during a well-child visit.
- Explain the role of growth measurement in the routine or well-child visit.
- List recommended child immunizations and possible side effects.
- Discuss common contagious diseases of childhood.
- List and describe childhood disorders caused by neural tube defects.
- List and describe congenital heart conditions that affect children.
- List and describe common pediatric blood disorders.
- List and describe diagnostic procedures used with pediatric patients.
- Describe different techniques used to position and secure the child for examination and treatment.
- Describe pediatric urine specimen collection.

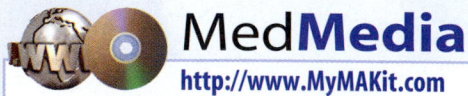

MedMedia

http://www.MyMAKit.com

Additional interactive resources and activities for this chapter can be found on http://www.MyMAKit.com. For videos, audio glossary, legal and ethical scenarios, tips, job scenarios, quizzes, and games related to the content of this chapter, please access the accompanying CD-ROM in this book.

Audio Glossary
Legal and Ethical Scenario: *Pediatrics*
On the Job Scenario: *Pediatrics*
Video: Pediatrics
Multiple Choice Quiz
Games: Crossword, Strikeout, and Spelling Bee
Tips
HIPAA Quiz

MEDICAL ASSISTING STANDARDS

CAAHEP ENTRY-LEVEL STANDARDS	ABHES ENTRY-LEVEL COMPETENCIES
■ Perform within scope of practice (psychomotor) ■ Explore issue of confidentiality as it applies to the medical assistant (cognitive) ■ Apply ethical behaviors, including honesty/integrity in performance of medical assisting practice (affective) ■ Apply local, state and federal health care legislation and regulation appropriate to the medical assisting practice setting (psychomotor) ■ Recognize the importance of local, state and federal legislation and regulations in the practice setting (affective) ■ Use language/verbal skills that enable patients' understanding (affective) ■ Apply critical thinking skills in performing patient assessment and care (affective) ■ Obtain vital signs (psychomotor) ■ Document accurately in the patient record (psychomotor) ■ Demonstrate diversity in approaching patients and families (affective) ■ Maintain growth charts (psychomotor) ■ Compare body structure and function of the human body across the life span (cognitive) ■ Obtain specimens for microbiological testing (psychomotor) ■ Practice Standard Precautions (psychomotor) ■ Show awareness of patients' concerns regarding their perceptions related to the procedure being performed (affective)	■ Project a positive attitude. ■ Maintain confidentiality at all times. ■ Be a "team player." ■ Be cognizant of ethical boundaries. ■ Exhibit initiative. ■ Adapt to change. ■ Evidence a responsible attitude. ■ Be courteous and diplomatic. ■ Conduct work within scope of education, training, and ability. ■ Practice Standard Precautions. ■ Use quality control. ■ Dispose of biohazardous materials. ■ Take vital signs. ■ Prepare patients for procedures. ■ Assist physician with examinations and treatments. ■ Prepare and administer medications as directed by physician. ■ Maintain medication records.

 COMPETENCY SKILLS PERFORMANCE

1. Perform and record measurements of height or length, weight and head and chest circumference.
2. Perform and record pediatric vital signs and vision screening.
3. Perform documentation of immunizations, both stored and administered.
4. Perform urine collection with a pediatric urine collection bag.

Introduction

A **pediatrician** is a physician who specializes in treating children from birth to age 20. A primary care physician may also see pediatric patients. Early care is important for the evaluation of growth and development as well as for disease prevention and diagnosis. A **pediatrics** practice involves wellness and illness, and visits are categorized as well child

Key Terminology

acyanotic—pertaining to an absence of cyanosis

cyanotic—characterized by cyanosis, or a blue tint in the skin, which indicates reduced blood oxygen

fontanelle—"soft spot" on the cranium of a newborn or infant; area of the skull that is not covered by bone at birth but where the cranial bones eventually come together, allowing for the growth of the brain and skull

lavage—washing out of a cavity

pediatrician—physician who specializes in treating children from birth to age 20

pediatrics—medical specialty that focuses on the care and treatment of children from birth through age 20

Abbreviations

FAS—fetal alcohol syndrome

MMR—measles-mumps-rubella vaccine

RSV—respiratory syncytial virus

VIS—vaccination information sheet

or sick child. A well-child visit comprises health maintenance, including routine inoculations. During a sick-child visit, symptoms are assessed and treatment is prescribed. Additional checkups may be required for school, sports, or camp.

The Medical Assistant's Role in Pediatrics

The medical assistant in a pediatric office will:

- Obtain the child's health and developmental history
- Take and record vital signs
- Measure and record growth
- Assist parents in undressing the child if necessary
- Assist the physician during the physical examination and treatment
- Help the parents restrain the child if necessary
- Obtain a urine specimen
- Administer medication injections and immunizations

Children ages zero through 20 go through many changes over time. A child's ability to understand medical care and treatment is based on his or her developmental, mental, and emotional stages. MAs must be sensitive to emotions such as fear, mistrust, and embarrassment, listen to the parent or guardian, and respect his or her instincts and observations. Presenting symptoms may be subtle. A parent's finely tuned understanding of the child can provide vital clues, such as changes in the child's appetite, sleep habits, cry, mental alertness and energy levels, and fussiness. Medical assistants must avoid labeling a seriously concerned and anxious parent or guardian as neurotic or overbearing.

A parent or guardian should be allowed and encouraged to stay with the child unless his or her presence hinders effective care. When necessary, the parent or guardian may be asked to leave or be escorted from the room.

A child should never be taken from the parent. When weighing a child, the MA should ask the parent to place the child on the scales and stand nearby, reassuring the child. If the child can be held to during a portion of the examination, encourage the parent do so. Show the parent how to hold the child during the examination.

The medical assistant should never tell a child "This will not hurt" when a potentially painful procedure is about to be done; the MA should always be truthful and reassure the parent or guardian about the procedure.

The MA should consider how big and threatening he or she may look to a child. Whenever possible, the MA should get down to the child's eye level when conversing. Sitting in a chair while obtaining the history is helpful.

If a child feels uncomfortable and threatened when clothing needs to be removed, the MA should provide covering in the form of a drape, gown, or sheet. The child can keep a security blanket or any other security item he or she has brought along, such as a stuffed animal or doll; it is an excellent source of comfort.

Physical, Developmental, and Emotional Growth of a Child

Every child progresses through a sequence of stages in the growth process (Figures 45-1 ◆ through 45-7 ◆):

- Fetus or embryo: from conception to birth
- Neonate or newborn: birth to 4 weeks
- Infant: 4 weeks to 1 year
- Toddler: 1 to 3 years
- Preschool (early childhood): 3 to 6 years
- School age (late childhood): 6 to 12 years, or puberty
- Adolescence: 12 years or puberty to beginning of adult stage

Factors that influence physical growth include heredity, racial and ethnic characteristics, gender, environment (prenatal and postnatal), and hormonal balance.

Prenatal factors that can cause harm or delays in the normal physical growth of a child include the mother's drug or alcohol use, smoking, physical injury, poor diet, and infection with rubella. Illnesses or injury during childhood may also affect the progression of normal development.

Certain physical, developmental, and emotional growth stages have been found to be common to specific age groups (Table 45-1).

Monitoring Growth Development

Measuring growth and keeping growth records for the pediatric patient is important. The physician uses growth patterns to

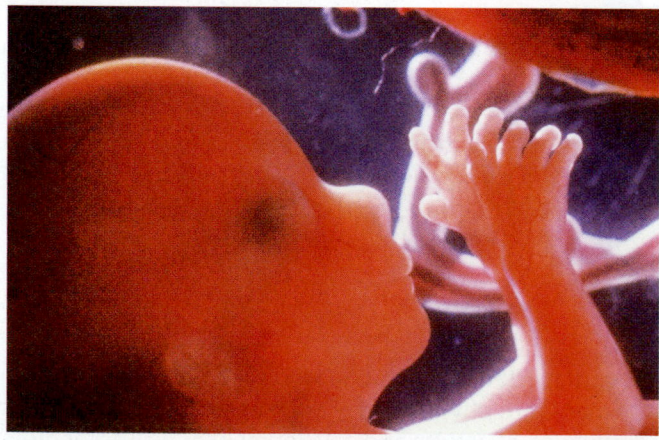

Figure 45-1 ◆ Fetus at four months.
Source: Petit Format/Nestle/Photo Researchers, Inc.

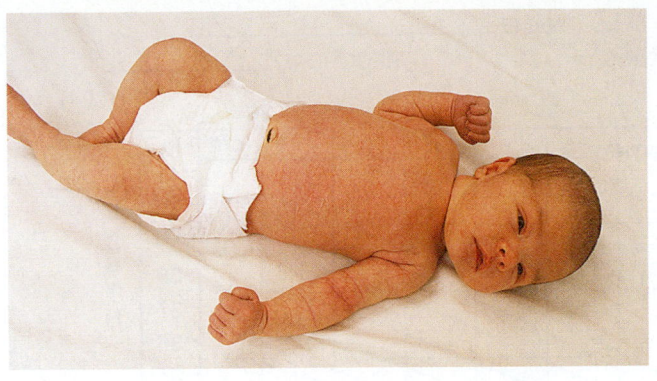

Figure 45-2 ◆ Newborn: birth to 4 weeks.

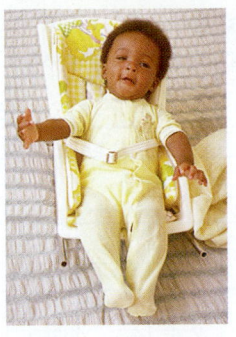

Figure 45-3 ◆ Infant: 4 weeks to 1 year.
Source: Michal Heron Photography

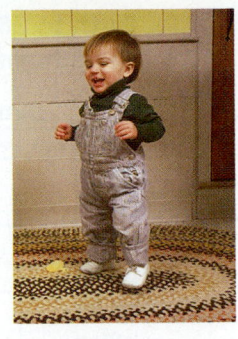

Figure 45-4 ◆ Toddler: 1 to 3 years.
Source: Michal Heron Photography

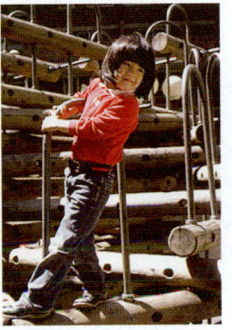

Figure 45-5 ◆ Preschool: 3 to 6 years.
Source: Michal Heron Photography

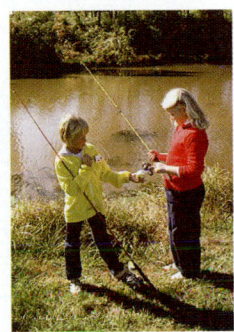

Figure 45-6 ◆ School-age (late childhood): 6 to 12 years, puberty.
Source: Michal Heron Photography

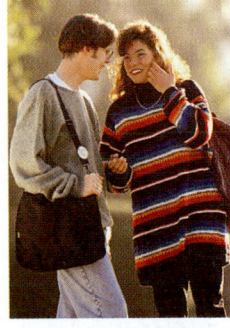

Figure 45-7 ◆ Adolescence: 12 years or puberty to beginning of adult stage.
Source: Michal Heron Photography

TABLE 45-1 NORMAL OR EXPECTED CHILD DEVELOPMENT

Infant:
- Begins to smile at 6 weeks.
- Rolls from stomach to back at 10 weeks.
- Gains strength to raise head from a supine position.
- Begins to recognize sounds and make associations.
- Sits without support at 6 to 8 months.
- Begins to crawl, stand, and take steps at 8 to 12 months.
- Begins to develop language skills with simple words.

Toddler:
- Strength develops to include climbing and running.
- Coordination (including manual dexterity) improves.
- Continues to process information through senses.
- Continues to develop communication and speech skills.
- Begins to develop small motor skills and finger dexterity.
- Begins to develop independence.

Preschooler:
- Begins to mimic older children and adults.
- Becomes more independent.
- Enhances communication techniques.
- Talks in simple, complete sentences.
- Can dress and undress self.

School-age child:
- Eye and body coordination improves.
- Makes choices.
- Feels guilt and shame.
- Can experience emotional withdrawal or shyness.

Preadolescent or teenager:
- Develops secondary sex characteristics.
- Strives for independence.
- Experiences puberty and self-image changes.

Stages of emotional or personality development
- Infancy, birth to 1 year—sense of trust
- Toddler, 1 to 3 years—sense of autonomy
- Preschool, 3 to 6 years—sense of initiative
- School age, 6 to 12 years—sense of industry
- Adolescence, 12 years—sense of identity
- Late adolescence, sense of intimacy

observe normal physical development or diagnose diseases. Growth charts are usually part of a child's medical file and are updated on each visit. Charts for growth record keeping are developed by the National Center for Health Statistics (NCHS) along with the CDC's National Center for Chronic Disease Prevention and Health Promotion. These charts are colored with a blue background for boys and a pink background for girls. They are specific for age groups as well as length-for-age and weight-for-age percentiles; head-circumference-for-age and weight-for-length percentiles; body-mass-index-for-age percentiles and weight-for-stature percentiles (Figure 45-8 ◆ through 45-11 ◆). The age groups are birth to 36 months and two to 20 years.

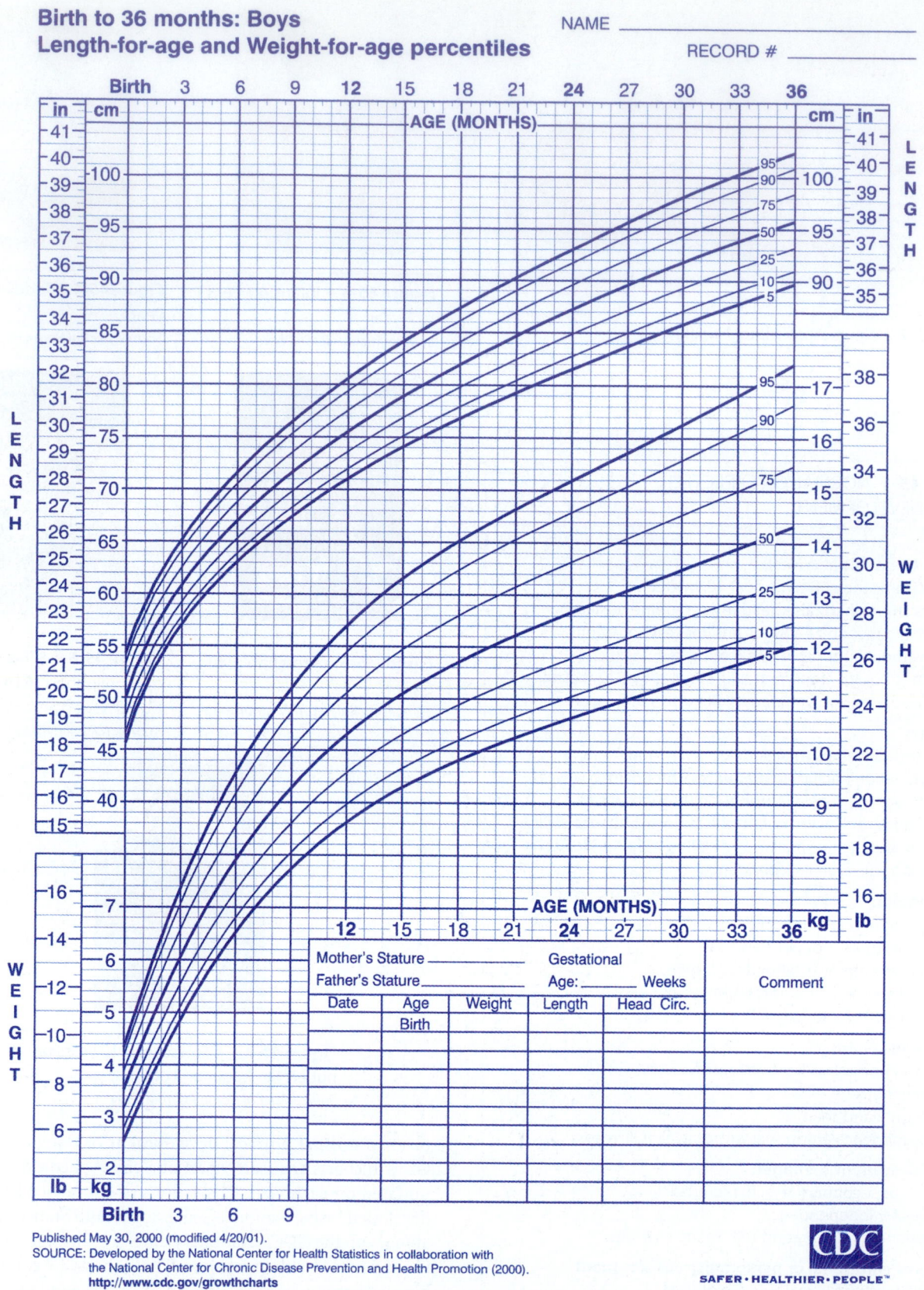

Figure 45-8 ◆ Birth to 36 months: Boys; Length-for-age and Weight-for-age percentiles.

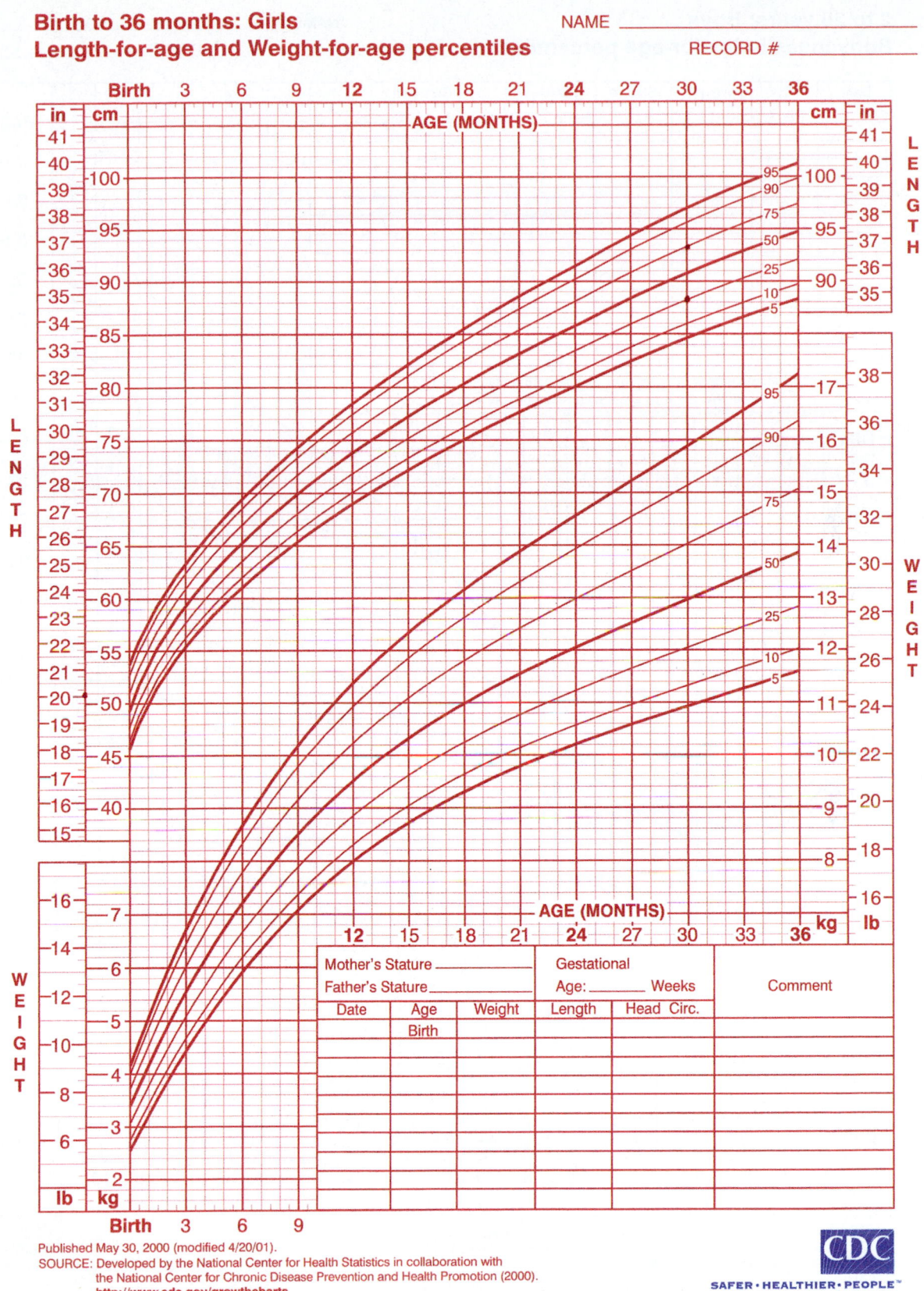

Figure 45-9 ◆ Birth to 36 months: Girls; Length-for-age and Weight-for-age percentiles.

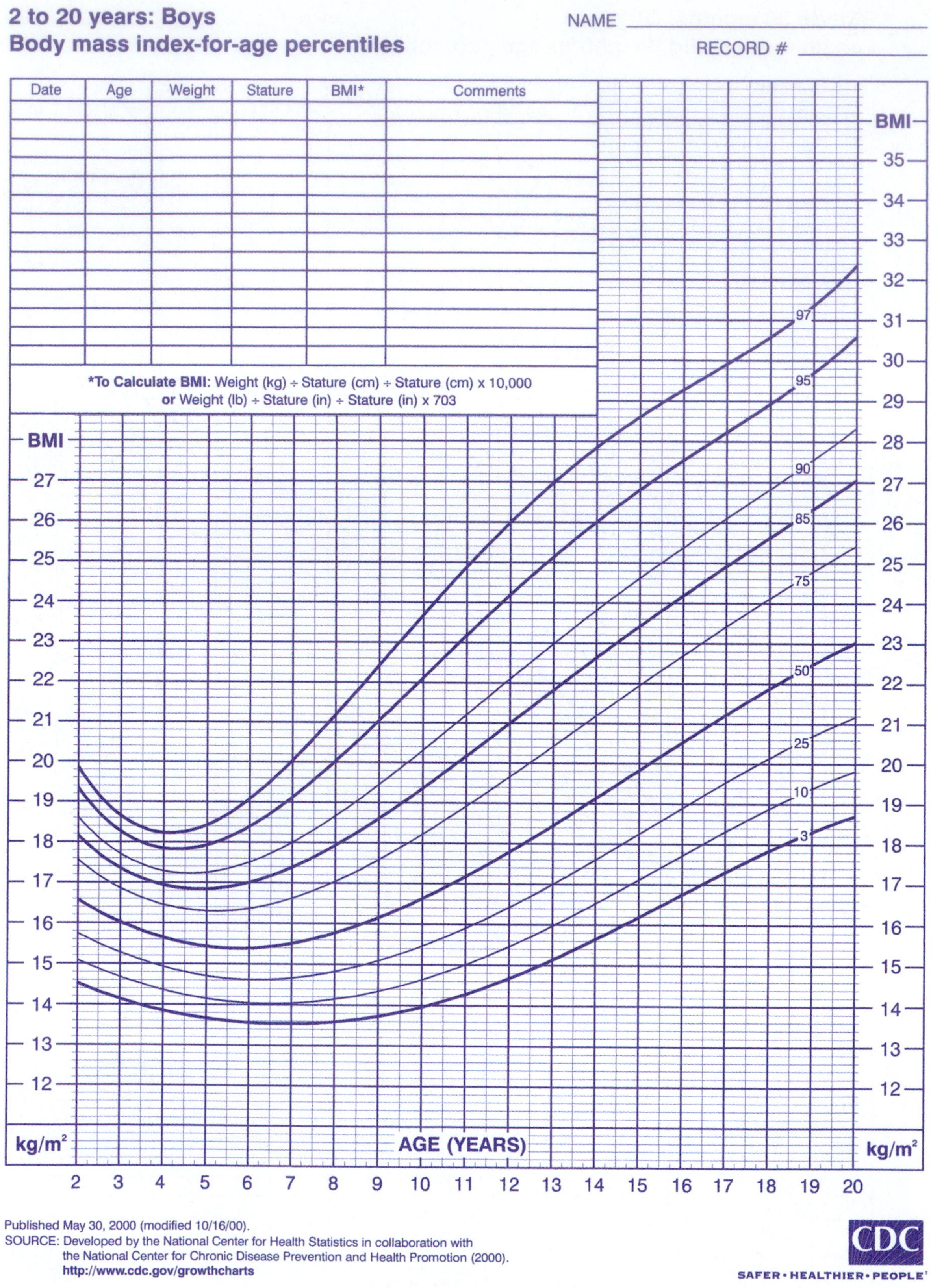
2 to 20 years: Boys
Body mass index-for-age percentiles
NAME
RECORD #
Date
Age
Weight
Stature
BMI*
Comments
*To Calculate BMI: Weight (kg) ÷ Stature (cm) ÷ Stature (cm) x 10,000
or Weight (lb) ÷ Stature (in) ÷ Stature (in) x 703
BMI
35
34
33
32
31
30
29
28
27
26
25
24
23
22
21
20
19
18
17
16
15
14
13
12
97
95
90
85
75
50
25
10
3
kg/m²
AGE (YEARS)
2 3 4 5 6 7 8 9 10 11 12 13 14 15 16 17 18 19 20
Published May 30, 2000 (modified 10/16/00).
SOURCE: Developed by the National Center for Health Statistics in collaboration with
the National Center for Chronic Disease Prevention and Health Promotion (2000).
http://www.cdc.gov/growthcharts
CDC
SAFER • HEALTHIER • PEOPLE

Figure 45-10 ◆ 2 to 20 years: Boys; Body mass index-for-age percentiles.

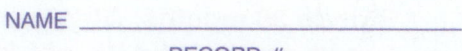

2 to 20 years: Girls
Body mass index-for-age percentiles

NAME _____

RECORD # _____

Date	Age	Weight	Stature	BMI*	Comments

*To Calculate BMI: Weight (kg) ÷ Stature (cm) ÷ Stature (cm) x 10,000
or Weight (lb) ÷ Stature (in) ÷ Stature (in) x 703

BMI

97
95
90
85
75
50
25
10
3

AGE (YEARS)

kg/m²   kg/m²

2 3 4 5 6 7 8 9 10 11 12 13 14 15 16 17 18 19 20

Published May 30, 2000 (modified 10/16/00).
SOURCE: Developed by the National Center for Health Statistics in collaboration with
the National Center for Chronic Disease Prevention and Health Promotion (2000).
http://www.cdc.gov/growthcharts

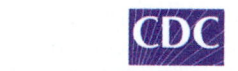

Figure 45-11 ◆ 2 to 20 years: Girls; Body mass index-for-age percentiles.

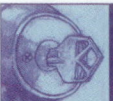

Keys to Success
CIRCUMCISION

A procedure usually performed in the hospital shortly after birth is circumcision, in which the foreskin on an infant boy is surgically removed. The presurgical diagnosis is phimosis (condition in which the foreskin cannot be pushed back over the glans penis). Traditionally a routine procedure on most male babies, circumcision now involves an informed decision by the parents.

The Jewish faith mandates that the male infant be circumcised on the eighth day after birth. A rabbi routinely performs the procedure as part of a religious ceremony and family celebration. The medical office may become involved if an infection or other postoperative complication develops.

Routine Visits (Well-Baby Checks)

Inoculations and well-baby or well-child checks account for many of the visits to the pediatric office (Table 45-2).

Procedures performed during a well-baby visit may include the following:

- Measuring weight and height
- Measuring head and chest circumference
- Taking temperature, pulse, respirations, and in older children, blood pressure
- Testing range of motion (ROM) of limbs, head, and neck
- Testing pupil reaction
- Checking ears, nose, and throat
- Checking cardiac and respiratory status
- Palpating the abdomen

TABLE 45-2 WELL-CHILD VISIT SCHEDULE

First Year of Life	Second Year of Life	After Two Years of Age
2 weeks 1 month 2 months 4 months 6 months 9 months 12 months 　(one year)	15 months 18 months	Annually Preschool check

Depending on the child's age, other assessments include:

- Ambulation (walking or moving about freely)
- Gait
- Scoliosis (curvature of the spine)
- Musculoskeletal abnormalities in the feet and legs
- Dental eruptions

Measuring Growth

Growth is measured to evaluate the child's developmental patterns. A newborn's length, weight, and head circumference are one such measure. When growth patterns are abnormal, further assessment and diagnostic testing are performed to determine the cause.

In Practice

Molly Parks, a 9-month-old girl, is in the office with her father for a well-child checkup. The medical assistant weighs the patient and she weighs 22 pounds. What percentile is this patient according to the growth chart in Figure 45-9? The father asks the medical assistant if the child is growing appropriately. How would the medical assistant explain the percentile to the father of the child?

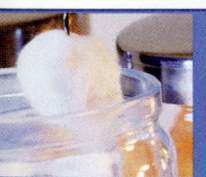

PROCEDURE 45-1 Perform and Record Measurements of Height or Length, Weight, and Head and Chest Circumference

Theory and Rationale

A platform scale is used to weigh an infant. Cover it with a paper protector to prevent cross-contamination between patients. Balance the scale with the protector in place. Set the scale to zero before the weight is taken. Infants are generally weighed without clothing or diaper as standard office policy.

Measuring the infant's length requires the help of the parent or guardian. Some exam tables are equipped with length scales, or the exam table is marked. Ask the parent or guardian to hold the infant's head at the zero mark. With the legs straightened, hold the infant's feet at right angles to the exam table.

Length is measured to approximately 2 years of age. When a child can stand on the stadiometer (device used to

measure height) with minor help from the parent, the exam table is no longer necessary.

Head circumference is measured during the first three years of life. Use a plastic or paper tape measure at the greatest round distance of the head. Do *not* use a cloth measuring tape, because it can stretch and measurements would not be accurate.

Infant chest circumference is not routinely measured, except when respiratory or cardiac abnormalities are suspected.

An infant can move quickly and suddenly. Watch the infant from the periphery of your vision and take the measurements quickly. Keep a hand within reach of the infant to prevent accidental falls when weighing or measuring.

PROCEDURE 45-1 Perform and Record Measurements of Height or Length, Weight, and Head and Chest Circumference *(continued)*

Materials

- plastic or paper tape measure
- infant or platform scale
- stadiometer (if available)
- growth charts
- patient chart

Competency

(**Conditions**) With the necessary materials, (**Task**) you will be able to measure the child's length (height), weight, and head and/or chest circumference (**Standards**) correctly within 15 minutes.

1. Wash your hands and gather equipment and supplies.
2. Identify the parent or guardian with the child and guide them to the treatment area.
3. Remove all clothing except the diaper before weighing.
4. Weigh the child on the platform scale (Figure 45-12 ◆).

5. Record the weight on the growth charts and/or progress notes within the child's chart.
6. Wash your hands.
7. Move or ask the parent or guardian to move the child to the exam table.
8. Measure the length of the child (Figure 45-13 ◆).
9. Record the height on the growth charts and/or progress notes within the child's chart.
10. Measure the child's head circumference (Figure 45-14 ◆).
11. Record the head circumference on the growth charts and/or progress notes within the child's chart.
12. Measure the child's chest circumference, if necessary (Figure 45-15 ◆).
13. Record the chest circumference on the growth charts and/or progress notes within the child's chart.
14. Tell the physician that the child is ready.
15. After the physician has examined the child, tell the parent or guardian to redress the child.
16. Dispose of disposable items.
17. Clean the room.

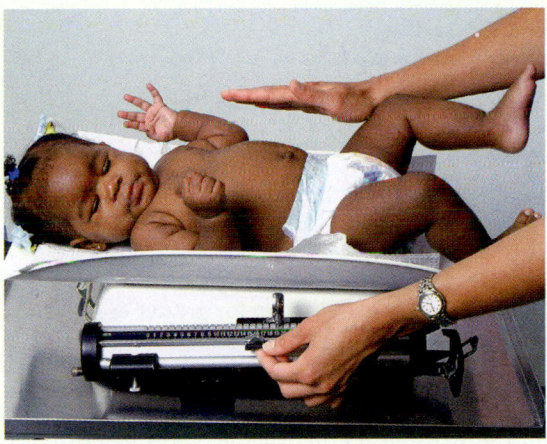

Figure 45-12 ◆ Weigh the infant on the balance baby scale.

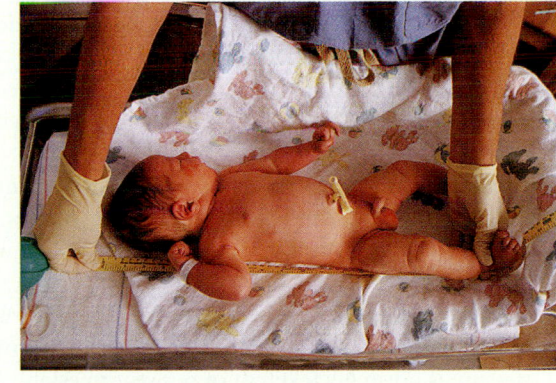

Figure 45-13 ◆ Measure the length of the newborn.

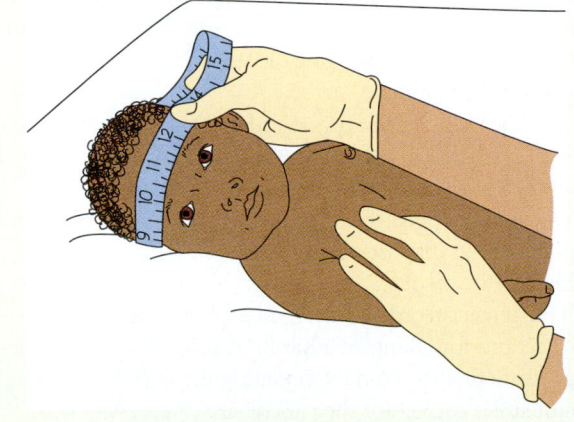

Figure 45-14 ◆ Measure the head circumference of the infant.

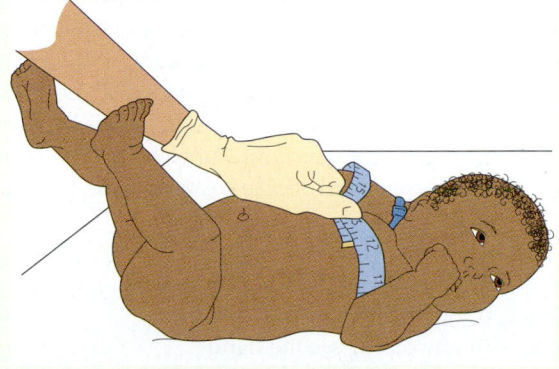

Figure 45-15 ◆ Measure the chest circumference of the infant.

continued

PROCEDURE 45-1 Perform and Record Measurements of Height or Length, Weight, and Head and Chest Circumference *(continued)*

18. Wash your hands.
19. Prepare the room for the next patient.

Patient Education

Tell the parent or guardian the purpose of growth measurements. Encourage questions.

Charting Example

09/23/XX 9:00 a.m. Wt. 15 lbs 9 oz, Ht 26 in., head circumference 42 cm. Results given to physician for evaluation. Vaiden Breen, CMA (AAMA)

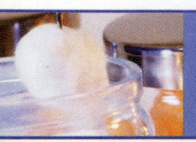

PROCEDURE 45-2 Perform and Record Pediatric Vital Signs and Vision Screening

Theory and Rationale

When taking pediatric vital signs, be sure to have the correct size equipment for the child. Temperature readings on an infant are most accurately obtained anally, although axillary readings may also be taken. If the child is older than 2, an aural temperature may be obtained. For a child is younger than 2, avoid using a tympanic thermometer. The reading may be incorrect by several degrees due to impacted cerumen or chronic ear infections. Oral temperatures are taken only on children age 5 years and older, who can understand directions and will not bite the thermometer.

The pulse of a child is taken at the apex of the heart, without clothing. Although the pulse can be felt at the brachial artery, the apex gives a more reliable pulse rate.

When counting a child's respirations, which are normally irregular, count for one full minute. Count an infant's respirations by watching the rise and fall of the chest as well as the abdomen.

Blood pressure is not normally taken on an infant unless it is specifically requested by the physician. After the age of 3, blood pressure is normally taken once per year to establish a baseline reading.

When children require a vision check to rule out abnormalities, you will use an Allen chart, E chart, or Snellen chart. If the child is old enough to recognize shapes but not directions, use an Allen chart, which features sailboats, hearts, stars, and other easily recognized shapes. For a child old enough to know direction but not the alphabet, you can use the E chart, which is a series of Es pointing in different directions. For children older than 5, most offices use the standard Snellen chart for vision testing.

Materials

- pediatric blood pressure cuff
- Allen, E, or Snellen chart
- watch with a sweeping second hand
- digital thermometer
- patient chart

Competency

(**Conditions**) With the necessary materials, (**Task**) you will be able to measure a child's temperature, pulse, respirations, and blood pressure and perform a vision screening test (**Standards**) correctly within 15 minutes.

Pulse, Respirations, Axillary Temperature, and Blood Pressure

1. Gather equipment and supplies. Wash your hands.
2. Identify the patient and explain the procedure to the parent or guardian.
3. Have the parent disrobe the child down to the diaper or underwear.
4. Place the child in the supine position or allow him or her to remain in the parent's lap for greater compliance.
5. Locate the apex of the heart by feeling for the fifth intercostal space to the left of the sternum on the midclavicular line.
6. Make sure the stethoscope head is warmed and place it on the space, listening for the "lub-dub" of the heart. Count for one minute (each lub-dub equals one beat).
7. Record the results.
8. Place your hand on the child's chest and count inspirations and expirations for one minute. The rise and fall of the chest is counted as one breath.
9. Record the results.
10. Take the temperature probe and apply a disposable sheath.
11. Place the probe in the infant's axillary space, holding the child's arm down close to his or her side.
12. Wait for the beep to indicate the reading has been completed, then dispose of the probe cover.
13. Record the results.
14. If the physician orders that blood pressure be taken, follow the directions for taking an adult BP reading. Palpate the blood pressure first to avoid overinflating the cuff. Make sure the cuff size is correct for the patient size (Figure 45-16 ◆).
15. Record the results.

PROCEDURE 45-2 Perform and Record Pediatric Vital Signs and Vision Screening *(continued)*

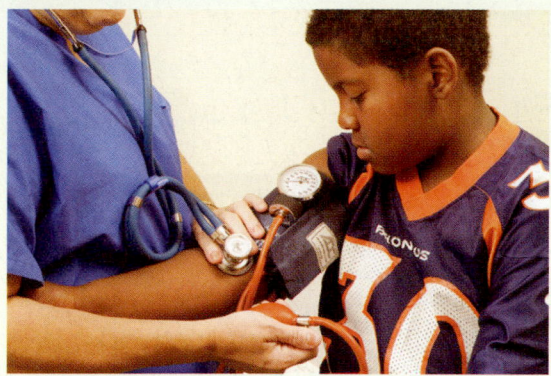

Figure 45-16 ◆ Take the child's blood pressure.

Vision Screening

16. Take the child to the vision screening area, accompanied by the parent. Explain the chart and ask the child to stand at the correct distance from the chart. (Each chart indicates the recommended distance.)
17. Have the child cover one eye and read as many lines as possible (Figure 45-17 ◆). If the child misses two objects, directions, or letters in a single line, stop the test and record the line number. For example, if the child reads line 20/20 correctly with the left eye but misses multiple letters on line 20/15, the vision would be 20/20 in the left eye.
18. Repeat the procedure for the other eye, then both eyes reading together.
19. Record the results in the patient's chart.

Patient Education

Explain to the parent or guardian the purpose of vital signs and vision screening. Encourage questions.

Charting Example

09/23/XX Pediatric vital signs obtained and given to the physician for review. Pediatric E chart vision test administered. Results recorded: 20/15 OD, 20/20 OS, 20/20 OU. Damion Frank, RMA (AMI)

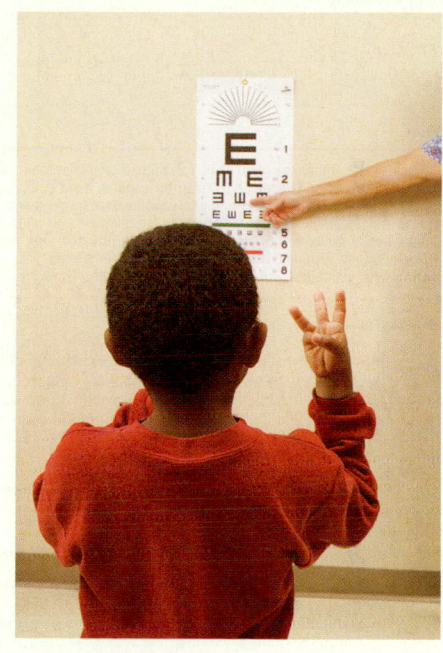

Figure 45-17 ◆ Have the child cover one eye and read as many lines as possible.

Immunizations

Children in the United States are routinely inoculated against such diseases as chickenpox, measles, mumps, and smallpox (Figure 45-18 ◆). Recent additions to routine vaccinations include Hepatitis A, pneumococcal and meningococcal vaccines. Booster injections are recommended by the American Academy of Pediatrics (see Figures 45-19 ◆ and 45-20 ◆ for the CDC Recommended Childhood and Adolescent Immunization Schedules). Epidemics of childhood contagious diseases have a tendency to occur among college students when booster injections are not rigorously scheduled and administered.

Immunizations have dramatically reduced the frequency of many childhood illnesses and the transfer of disease to other children and adults. But it is important to alert parents to potential side effects. Vaccinations commonly cause such reactions as fever, rash, redness, and swelling at the vaccination site.

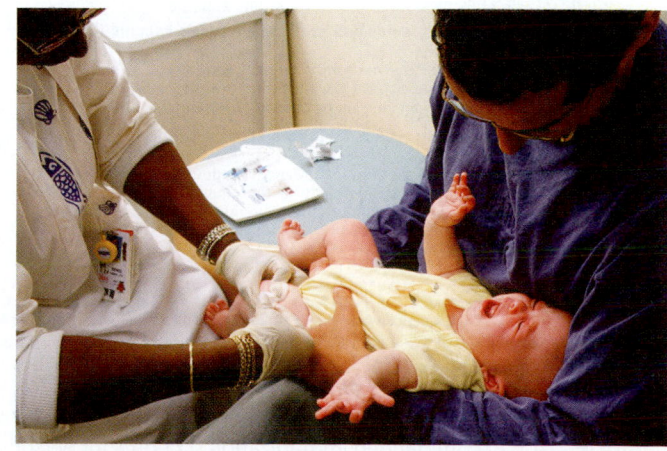

Figure 45-18 ◆ Infant receiving a vaccination.

Recommended Immunization Schedule for Persons Aged 0–6 Years—UNITED STATES • 2008

For those who fall behind or start late, see the catch-up schedule

Vaccine ▼ Age ▶	Birth	1 month	2 months	4 months	6 months	12 months	15 months	18 months	19–23 months	2–3 years	4–6 years
Hepatitis B[1]	HepB	HepB		see footnote 1	HepB						
Rotavirus[2]			Rota	Rota	Rota						
Diphtheria, Tetanus, Pertussis[3]			DTaP	DTaP	DTaP	see footnote 3	DTaP				DTaP
Haemophilus influenzae type b[4]			Hib	Hib	*Hib*[4]	Hib					
Pneumococcal[5]			PCV	PCV	PCV	PCV					PPV
Inactivated Poliovirus			IPV	IPV	IPV						IPV
Influenza[6]					Influenza (Yearly)						
Measles, Mumps, Rubella[7]						MMR					MMR
Varicella[8]						Varicella					Varicella
Hepatitis A[9]						HepA (2 doses)				HepA Series	
Meningococcal[10]										MCV4	

Legend:
- **Range of recommended ages** (yellow)
- **Certain high-risk groups** (purple)

This schedule indicates the recommended ages for routine administration of currently licensed childhood vaccines, as of December 1, 2007, for children aged 0 through 6 years. Additional information is available at **www.cdc.gov/vaccines/recs/schedules**. Any dose not administered at the recommended age should be administered at any subsequent visit, when indicated and feasible. Additional vaccines may be licensed and recommended during the year. Licensed combination vaccines may be used whenever any components of the combination are indicated and other components of the vaccine are not contraindicated and if approved by the Food and Drug Administration for that dose of the series. Providers should consult the respective Advisory Committee on Immunization Practices statement for detailed recommendations, including for **high-risk conditions: http://www.cdc.gov/vaccines/pubs/ACIP-list.htm**. Clinically significant adverse events that follow immunization should be reported to the Vaccine Adverse Event Reporting System (VAERS). Guidance about how to obtain and complete a VAERS form is available at **www.vaers.hhs.gov** or by telephone, **800-822-7967**.

1. Hepatitis B vaccine (HepB). *(Minimum age: birth)*
At birth:
- Administer monovalent HepB to all newborns prior to hospital discharge.
- If mother is hepatitis B surface antigen (HBsAg) positive, administer HepB and 0.5 mL of hepatitis B immune globulin (HBIG) within 12 hours of birth.
- If mother's HBsAg status is unknown, administer HepB within 12 hours of birth. Determine the HBsAg status as soon as possible and if HBsAg positive, administer HBIG (no later than age 1 week).
- If mother is HBsAg negative, the birth dose can be delayed, in rare cases, with a provider's order and a copy of the mother's negative HBsAg laboratory report in the infant's medical record.

After the birth dose:
- The HepB series should be completed with either monovalent HepB or a combination vaccine containing HepB. The second dose should be administered at age 1–2 months. The final dose should be administered no earlier than age 24 weeks. Infants born to HBsAg-positive mothers should be tested for HBsAg and antibody to HBsAg after completion of at least 3 doses of a licensed HepB series, at age 9–18 months (generally at the next well-child visit).

4-month dose:
- It is permissible to administer 4 doses of HepB when combination vaccines are administered after the birth dose. If monovalent HepB is used for doses after the birth dose, a dose at age 4 months is not needed.

2. Rotavirus vaccine (Rota). *(Minimum age: 6 weeks)*
- Administer the first dose at age 6–12 weeks.
- Do not start the series later than age 12 weeks.
- Administer the final dose in the series by age 32 weeks. Do not administer any dose later than age 32 weeks.
- Data on safety and efficacy outside of these age ranges are insufficient.

3. Diphtheria and tetanus toxoids and acellular pertussis vaccine (DTaP). *(Minimum age: 6 weeks)*
- The fourth dose of DTaP may be administered as early as age 12 months, provided 6 months have elapsed since the third dose.
- Administer the final dose in the series at age 4–6 years.

4. *Haemophilus influenzae* type b conjugate vaccine (Hib). *(Minimum age: 6 weeks)*
- If PRP-OMP (PedvaxHIB® or ComVax® [Merck]) is administered at ages 2 and 4 months, a dose at age 6 months is not required.
- TriHIBit® (DTaP/Hib) combination products should not be used for primary immunization but can be used as boosters following any Hib vaccine in children age 12 months or older.

5. Pneumococcal vaccine. *(Minimum age: 6 weeks for pneumococcal conjugate vaccine [PCV]; 2 years for pneumococcal polysaccharide vaccine [PPV])*
- Administer one dose of PCV to all healthy children aged 24–59 months having any incomplete schedule.
- Administer PPV to children aged 2 years and older with underlying medical conditions.

6. Influenza vaccine. *(Minimum age: 6 months for trivalent inactivated influenza vaccine [TIV]; 2 years for live, attenuated influenza vaccine [LAIV])*
- Administer annually to children aged 6–59 months and to all eligible close contacts of children aged 0–59 months.
- Administer annually to children 5 years of age and older with certain risk factors, to other persons (including household members) in close contact with persons in groups at higher risk, and to any child whose parents request vaccination.
- For healthy persons (those who do not have underlying medical conditions that predispose them to influenza complications) ages 2–49 years, either LAIV or TIV may be used.
- Children receiving TIV should receive 0.25 mL if age 6–35 months or 0.5 mL if age 3 years or older.
- Administer 2 doses (separated by 4 weeks or longer) to children younger than 9 years who are receiving influenza vaccine for the first time or who were vaccinated for the first time last season but only received one dose.

7. Measles, mumps, and rubella vaccine (MMR). *(Minimum age: 12 months)*
- Administer the second dose of MMR at age 4–6 years. MMR may be administered before age 4–6 years, provided 4 weeks or more have elapsed since the first dose.

8. Varicella vaccine. *(Minimum age: 12 months)*
- Administer second dose at age 4–6 years; may be administered 3 months or more after first dose.
- Do not repeat second dose if administered 28 days or more after first dose.

9. Hepatitis A vaccine (HepA). *(Minimum age: 12 months)*
- Administer to all children aged 1 year (i.e., aged 12–23 months). Administer the 2 doses in the series at least 6 months apart.
- Children not fully vaccinated by age 2 years can be vaccinated at subsequent visits.
- HepA is recommended for certain other groups of children, including in areas where vaccination programs target older children.

10. Meningococcal vaccine. *(Minimum age: 2 years for meningococcal conjugate vaccine (MCV4) and for meningococcal polysaccharide vaccine (MPSV4))*
- Administer MCV4 to children aged 2–10 years with terminal complement deficiencies or anatomic or functional asplenia and certain other high-risk groups. MPSV4 is also acceptable.
- Administer MCV4 to persons who received MPSV4 3 or more years previously and remain at increased risk for meningococcal disease.

The Recommended Immunization Schedules for Persons Aged 0–18 Years are approved by the Advisory Committee on Immunization Practices (**www.cdc.gov/vaccines/recs/acip**), the American Academy of Pediatrics (**http://www.aap.org**), and the American Academy of Family Physicians (**http://www.aafp.org**).

DEPARTMENT OF HEALTH AND HUMAN SERVICES • CENTERS FOR DISEASE CONTROL AND PREVENTION • SAFER • HEALTHIER • PEOPLE™

CS103164

Figure 45-19 ◆ Recommended immunization schedule for persons aged 0–6 years—United States, 2008.

The Recommended Immunization Schedules for Persons Age 0–18 Years are approved by the Advisory Committee on Immunization Practices (www.cdc.gov/vaccines/recs/acip), the American Academy of Pediatrics (http://www.aap.org), and the American Academy of Family Physicians (http://www.aafp.org).

Recommended Immunization Schedule for Persons Aged 7–18 Years—UNITED STATES • 2008

For those who fall behind or start late, see the green bars and the catch-up schedule

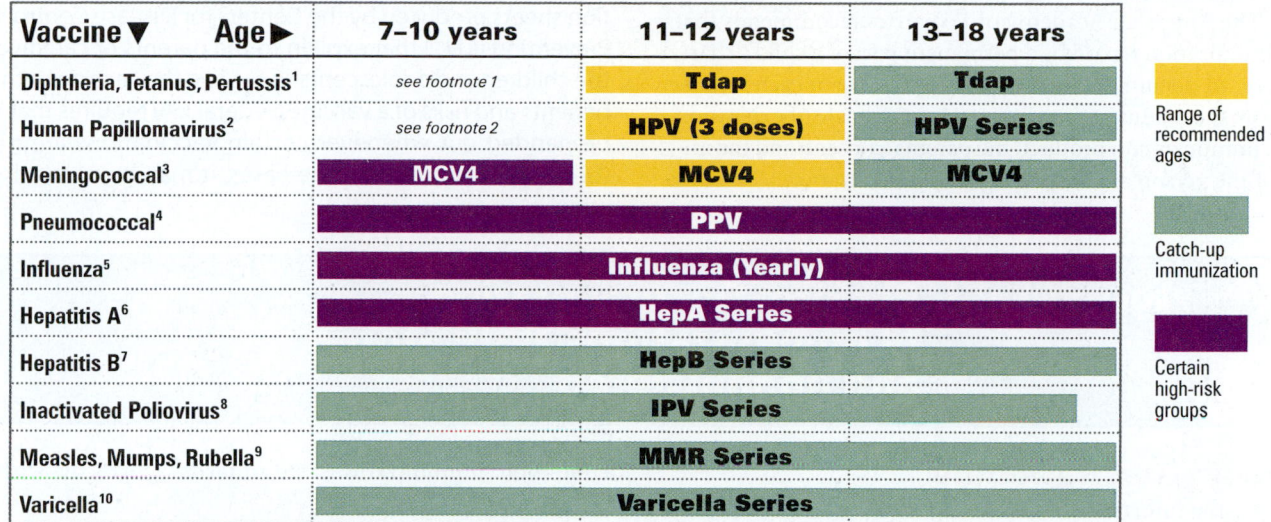

Vaccine ▼ Age ▶	7–10 years	11–12 years	13–18 years
Diphtheria, Tetanus, Pertussis[1]	*see footnote 1*	**Tdap**	**Tdap**
Human Papillomavirus[2]	*see footnote 2*	**HPV (3 doses)**	**HPV Series**
Meningococcal[3]	**MCV4**	**MCV4**	**MCV4**
Pneumococcal[4]	**PPV**		
Influenza[5]	**Influenza (Yearly)**		
Hepatitis A[6]	**HepA Series**		
Hepatitis B[7]	**HepB Series**		
Inactivated Poliovirus[8]	**IPV Series**		
Measles, Mumps, Rubella[9]	**MMR Series**		
Varicella[10]	**Varicella Series**		

Range of recommended ages

Catch-up immunization

Certain high-risk groups

This schedule indicates the recommended ages for routine administration of currently licensed childhood vaccines, as of December 1, 2007, for children aged 7–18 years. Additional information is available at **www.cdc.gov/vaccines/recs/schedules**. Any dose not administered at the recommended age should be administered at any subsequent visit, when indicated and feasible. Additional vaccines may be licensed and recommended during the year. Licensed combination vaccines may be used whenever any components of the combination are indicated and other components of the vaccine are not contraindicated and if approved by the Food and Drug Administration for that dose of the series. Providers should consult the respective Advisory Committee on Immunization Practices statement for detailed recommendations, including for **high risk conditions: http://www.cdc.gov/vaccines/pubs/ACIP-list.htm**. Clinically significant adverse events that follow immunization should be reported to the Vaccine Adverse Event Reporting System (VAERS). Guidance about how to obtain and complete a VAERS form is available at **www.vaers.hhs.gov** or by telephone, **800-822-7967**.

1. Tetanus and diphtheria toxoids and acellular pertussis vaccine (Tdap). *(Minimum age: 10 years for BOOSTRIX® and 11 years for ADACEL™)*
- Administer at age 11–12 years for those who have completed the recommended childhood DTP/DTaP vaccination series and have not received a tetanus and diphtheria toxoids (Td) booster dose.
- 13–18-year-olds who missed the 11–12 year Tdap or received Td only are encouraged to receive one dose of Tdap 5 years after the last Td/DTaP dose.

2. Human papillomavirus vaccine (HPV). *(Minimum age: 9 years)*
- Administer the first dose of the HPV vaccine series to females at age 11–12 years.
- Administer the second dose 2 months after the first dose and the third dose 6 months after the first dose.
- Administer the HPV vaccine series to females at age 13–18 years if not previously vaccinated.

3. Meningococcal vaccine.
- Administer MCV4 at age 11–12 years and at age 13–18 years if not previously vaccinated. MPSV4 is an acceptable alternative.
- Administer MCV4 to previously unvaccinated college freshmen living in dormitories.
- MCV4 is recommended for children aged 2–10 years with terminal complement deficiencies or anatomic or functional asplenia and certain other high-risk groups.
- Persons who received MPSV4 3 or more years previously and remain at increased risk for meningococcal disease should be vaccinated with MCV4.

4. Pneumococcal polysaccharide vaccine (PPV).
- Administer PPV to certain high-risk groups.

5. Influenza vaccine.
- Administer annually to all close contacts of children aged 0–59 months.
- Administer annually to persons with certain risk factors, health-care workers, and other persons (including household members) in close contact with persons in groups at higher risk.

- Administer 2 doses (separated by 4 weeks or longer) to children younger than 9 years who are receiving influenza vaccine for the first time or who were vaccinated for the first time last season but only received one dose.
- For healthy nonpregnant persons (those who do not have underlying medical conditions that predispose them to influenza complications) ages 2–49 years, either LAIV or TIV may be used.

6. Hepatitis A vaccine (HepA).
- Administer the 2 doses in the series at least 6 months apart.
- HepA is recommended for certain other groups of children, including in areas where vaccination programs target older children.

7. Hepatitis B vaccine (HepB).
- Administer the 3-dose series to those who were not previously vaccinated.
- A 2-dose series of Recombivax HB® is licensed for children aged 11–15 years.

8. Inactivated poliovirus vaccine (IPV).
- For children who received an all-IPV or all-oral poliovirus (OPV) series, a fourth dose is not necessary if the third dose was administered at age 4 years or older.
- If both OPV and IPV were administered as part of a series, a total of 4 doses should be administered, regardless of the child's current age.

9. Measles, mumps, and rubella vaccine (MMR).
- If not previously vaccinated, administer 2 doses of MMR during any visit, with 4 or more weeks between the doses.

10. Varicella vaccine.
- Administer 2 doses of varicella vaccine to persons younger than 13 years of age at least 3 months apart. Do not repeat the second dose if administered 28 or more days following the first dose.
- Administer 2 doses of varicella vaccine to persons aged 13 years or older at least 4 weeks apart.

The Recommended Immunization Schedules for Persons Aged 0–18 Years are approved by the Advisory Committee on Immunization Practices (**www.cdc.gov/vaccines/recs/acip**), the American Academy of Pediatrics (**http://www.aap.org**), and the American Academy of Family Physicians (**http://www.aafp.org**).

DEPARTMENT OF HEALTH AND HUMAN SERVICES • CENTERS FOR DISEASE CONTROL AND PREVENTION
SAFER • HEALTHIER • PEOPLE™

CS103164

Figure 45-20 ◆ Recommended immunization schedule for persons aged 7–18 Years—United States, 2008.

The Recommended Immunization Schedules for Persons Age 0–18 Years are approved by the Advisory Committee on Immunization Practices (www.cdc.gov/vaccines/recs/acip), the American Academy of Pediatrics (http://www.aap.org), and the American Academy of Family Physicians (http://www.aafp.org).

Seizures and severe allergic reactions are much rarer side effects. Be sure to forward parents' questions about the benefits and risks of immunizations to the physician.

The American Academy of Pediatrics recommends that an immunization record be a permanent part of a child's chart. This record documents the date, type, and site of each immunization; the manufacturer, lot number, and date of expiration of the immunization product; the parents' consent; and the initials of the person administering the immunization.

Patient Education

Vaccine Information Statements (**VIS**) are written information sheets produced by the Centers for Disease Control and Prevention (CDC) that explain to the parents or caregiver of the children and adolescents to receive the vaccine both the benefits and risks of a vaccine. Federal law requires that VISs be handed out whenever certain vaccinations are given (before each dose). In some cases, it may be necessary to

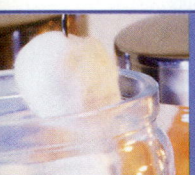

PROCEDURE 45-3 Perform Documentation of Immunizations, Both Stored and Administered

Theory and Rationale

Review the information from the vaccine package insert or from other sources, such as the *Physician's Desk Reference* (*PDR*) or CDC. Know the purpose of the medication, precautions, potential side effects or adverse reactions, correct route for administration, and storage requirements. The National Childhood Vaccine Injury Act of 1988 requires that benefit and risk information about immunizations be given to the parent or legal guardian and that consent to proceed be given by the parent or legal guardian before the child is vaccinated.

Encourage the parent to stay and help when the vaccine is administered. Discourage comments that imply the medical staff is "bad" because they are giving the painful injection. Establishing trust is an important part of the child's visit.

Before any immunization, it is important to obtain the medical history from the parent or guardian. Ask about any known allergies and recent illnesses. The physician will review this information and form an assessment before immunizing. Due to the cost of vaccinations, it is fairly common for a physician to refer patients to the Public Health Department for free or low-cost vaccinations.

After the immunization has been given, record the information. Include in the child's immunization record the date and the initials of the staff member who gave the immunization. The physician's name and number are sometimes recorded as well. In the child's chart, record the date and time of immunization, product name, lot number and expiration date, manufacturer, injection site and/or route given, and the signature of whoever administered the vaccination.

Materials

■ vaccine information sheets (VIS)
■ vaccination dosage
■ sterile gloves
■ patient chart

Competency

(**Conditions**) With the necessary materials, (**Task**) you will be able to provide the parent or guardian instruction and give

childhood immunizations (**Standards**) correctly within 45 minutes.

1. Wash your hands. Gather the equipment and supplies.
2. Identify the parent or guardian with the child and guide them to the treatment area.
3. Ask the parent or guardian about the child's recent health and if there is medical history that would exclude the child temporarily or permanently from any of the immunizations.
4. Provide vaccine information sheets for each immunization to be given.
5. Take and record the child's vital signs.
6. After the physician has seen the patient, wash your hands and put on sterile gloves.
7. Administer the immunizations.
8. Dispose of sharps or biohazardous materials in the appropriate containers.
9. Wash your hands.
10. Document on the child's immunization record for the parent or guardian and on the child's chart.

Patient Education

Educate the parent or guardian about possible side effects of each immunization. The child may be given antipyretics and analgesics as directed by the physician during the first day or two after the immunizations. Instruct the parent or guardian to call the physician during office hours or the emergency room after hours for any symptoms that are worsening or of concern.

Charting Example

08/20/XX 8:00 a.m. Child seen for 12-month well-child visit. Mother stated that insurance has paid maximum benefits for immunizations and she cannot afford immunizations. Physician gave phone number of public health department for free immunizations. Heather Brown, CMA (AAMA)

receive written consent before administering the vaccine. The most current vaccine schedules and information sheets can be found on the Centers for Disease Control and Prevention website (www.cdc.gov).

Storing Vaccines

The potency of vaccines depends on the proper refrigerator or freezer temperature, as stated in the manufacturer's directions. Vaccines are transported inside an insulated cold container with cold packs. The container is placed on the front passenger seat of the vehicle for safety. Upon delivery, immediately move the vaccines to a freezer or refrigerator as required. Refrigerator temperatures must be kept between 35° and 46°F; the safest temperatures are between 41° and 46°F if the refrigerator door is opened frequently. Freezer temperatures should be kept below 5°F. Temperatures should be checked and logged twice daily. It is mandatory that the office keep a month's stock ahead of projected needs and have a back-up plan for emergencies in which power for the refrigerator or freezer may be lost. An emergency generator may be used, or the vaccines may be moved to a hospital, fire station, or other facility.

Common Pediatric Diseases and Conditions

A common complaint during a well-baby checkup is a diaper rash that has not responded to regular treatment. Nonresponsive diaper rash may have a fungal origin and require prescription medications. Frequent diaper changing, gentle cleansing, and gentle handling of the dry, irritated perianal skin are also recommended. After washing, patting the skin dry gently or using a hair dryer *only* on a cool setting will help ease the discomfort of the condition. The medication treats the fungal infection. If oral thrush, an often parallel condition, is also present, a prescription for an oral suspension to coat the white patchy mucous membranes of the mouth is prescribed.

Candida albicans is a fungus that can result from an immunodeficiency-related disease or from overuse of antibiotics. Young, and sometimes older, infants can display signs of oral thrush or a rash of the perianal area that will not resolve without medication.

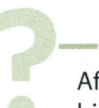

Critical Thinking Question 45-1

After the physician has diagnosed oral thrush combined with a yeast infection, what should Lucas explain to the mother so that the condition is correctly treated?

One of the most common medical conditions that affect infants and toddlers is otitis media (ear inflammation). Fussiness and pulling at the ear or sitting with the head held to one side are often indications of the condition. (Refer to ∞ Chapter 37 for a complete discussion of otitis media.)

The condition responsible for the most lost school time is asthma. Asthma is usually the result of an allergic response. The child experiences shortness of breath (SOB) and usually wheezes. (See ∞ Chapter 36 for a complete discussion of asthma.)

Respiratory conditions are common in children. Two respiratory diseases that are of major concern are respiratory syncytial virus (**RSV**) pneumonia and cystic fibrosis. RSV starts as a mild upper-respiratory infection. As it progresses downward into the lungs, pneumonia develops. Symptoms include fever, coughing, dyspnea, and lethargy. Contact with the respiratory secretions of an infected person is the usual source of the infection. A microscopic exam of a specimen obtained by nasal **lavage** confirms the presence of the virus. Keeping the child hydrated is important, and supplemental oxygen may be required. Fever is treated with antipyretics.

Cystic fibrosis, a genetic metabolic disorder, involves a chronic dysfunction of the exocrine glands. A thick, sticky mucous secretion is produced by the exocrine glands, blocking the ducts. Tissues most frequently affected include the lungs, digestive system (particularly the pancreas), and sweat glands.

Certain contagious diseases are common among children, particularly school-age children. More serious childhood conditions are neural tube defects, congenital heart conditions, and blood disorders. Treatment is required immediately for most of these conditions.

Common Contagious Diseases of Childhood

Thanks to routine preventive inoculations, the common contagious diseases of childhood are far less prevalent now than they were fifty years ago (Table 45-3). These diseases include chickenpox (*herpes varicella*), measles (rubeola), rubella (German measles), mumps (parotitis), whooping cough (pertussis), polio, and diphtheria. Smallpox, once considered extinct globally, is now considered a possible terrorist threat.

Congenital Neurological Disorders/Neural Tube Defects

Neural tube defects are congenital disorders that occur when an embryo's neural tube fails to close during development (Table 45-4). Spinal fusion disorders are spina bifida occulta, meningocele, and myelomeningocele. Cranial fusion disorders are hydrocephalus, microencephaly, and anencephaly.

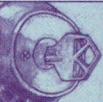

Keys to Success
INFORMATION ON AUTISM

Autism is a mental disorder with symptoms of diminished language, social, and emotional development. The child is described as introverted (withdrawn from reality), often incapable of appropriate social interaction with family and other caregivers. Recent research findings from the University of California suggest that abnormally rapid brain growth during infancy may be a clue for early diagnosis and treatment. Usually, autism is rarely diagnosed before 2 or 3 years of age.

TABLE 45-3 COMMON PREVENTABLE CONTAGIOUS DISEASES

Disease	Symptoms	Diagnosis	Vaccine
Chickenpox ■ Caused by herpes varicella, highly contagious virus ■ Spread by droplets from respiratory tract or direct contact with blisters ■ Virus can be reactivated later in life as herpes zoster (shingles)	■ Blister-like vesicles over body, starting at head and moving downward	■ Patient presenting symptoms	■ Live varicella virus vaccine
Diphtheria ■ Caused by the bacteria *Corynebacterium diphtheriae* ■ Spread by airborne droplets from an infected person's respiratory tract ■ May damage heart or central nervous system (CNS)	■ False membrane develops in throat and interferes with breathing	■ Patient presenting symptoms	■ Diphtheria-pertussis-tetanus (DPT)
Haemophilus influenza type B ■ Occurs mostly in children under age 5 ■ Causes acute respiratory infections ■ Can cause infections of the blood, bones, joints, and head, and bacterial meningitis ■ Can be fatal	■ Fever ■ Nausea and vomiting (N&V) ■ Loss of appetite ■ Irritability ■ Headache ■ Bulging **fontanelles** ■ Stupor ■ Seizures ■ Pneumonia ■ Meningitis ■ Septic arthritis	■ Patient presenting symptoms	■ Haemophilus B conjugate vaccine (HiB)
Hepatitis B ■ Caused by a virus ■ Spread by blood and body fluids ■ May cause death	■ Jaundice ■ Anorexia ■ N&V ■ Joint pain ■ Flulike symptoms ■ Liver damage ■ Liver failure	■ Patient presenting symptoms ■ Blood studies	■ Hepatitis B vaccine (recombinant)
Measles (rubeola) ■ Caused by a virus ■ Spread by airborne droplets	■ Fine rash over the body ■ Fever ■ Malaise ■ Eye problems ■ Otitis ■ Pneumonia ■ Encephalitis	■ Patient presenting symptoms	■ Measles-mumps-rubella (**MMR**) vaccine
Rubella (German measles) ■ Caused by a virus ■ Spread by direct contact with infected persons and nasal or oral secretions ■ Can cause birth defects if pregnant mother contracts the disease	■ Fine rash over body ■ Fever	■ Patient presenting symptoms	■ MMR; immunity confirmed with rubella titer
Mumps (infectious parotitis) ■ Caused by a virus ■ Spread by direct contact with salivary secretions of infected person ■ Male sterility possible if contracted as an adult	■ Swollen parotid glands ■ Fever ■ Diarrhea ■ Malaise ■ Difficulty swallowing	■ Patient presenting symptoms	■ MMR

TABLE 45-3 COMMON PREVENTABLE CONTAGIOUS DISEASES (CONTINUED)

Disease	Symptoms	Diagnosis	Vaccine
Pertussis (whooping cough) ■ Spread by direct contact or airborne droplets ■ Complications include pneumonia, atelectasis, otitis, and convulsions	■ Dry, harsh cough with spasms ■ Fever ■ Dyspnea	■ Patient presenting symptoms	■ DPT injections (series of three)
Poliomyelitis ■ Caused by one of three polio viruses that enter body through the mouth ■ Transmitted in feces of infected individuals ■ Respiratory system affected by paralysis followed by muscle atrophy ■ Post-polio syndrome may occur as late as thirty years post-infection	■ Fever ■ Malaise ■ Headache ■ Paralysis ■ N&V	■ Patient presenting symptoms	■ Trivalent live oral form (Sabin) ■ Inactivated poliovirus vaccine (Salk), given under the skin
Smallpox ■ Caused by a virus ■ Once thought to be completely eradicated worldwide; now may be used as terrorist weapon ■ Usually fatal	■ Pustule-like blisters on the skin	■ Patient presenting symptoms	■ Smallpox vaccine
Tetanus ■ Caused by *Clostridium tetani* entering the body through puncture wound or open skin ■ CNS may become involved, resulting in death if not treated aggressively	■ Headaches ■ Fever ■ Muscle spasms	■ Patient presenting symptoms	■ Tetanus diphtheria (Td) or DPT vaccines ■ Tetanus antitoxin ■ Tetanus toxoid

TABLE 45-4 CONGENITAL NEUROLOGICAL DISORDERS

Disorder	Symptoms	Diagnosis	Treatment
Spina bifida occulta ■ Failure of neural tube to close ■ Usually located in lumbar region with no displacement or insult to the spinal cord	■ Dimpling or depression of skin over affected lumbar region, often with tuft of hair over site	■ Patient presenting symptoms	■ No intervention; close observation for any signs of neurological symptoms
Meningocele ■ Congenital hernia that results in meninges (membranes) protruding through a defect in skull or spinal column ■ Good prognosis if surgery is successful	■ Apparent bulging over spinal column, usually in lumbar region	■ Patient presenting symptoms ■ Imaging studies	■ Surgery to close opening in vertebral column

continued

TABLE 45-4 CONGENITAL NEUROLOGICAL DISORDERS (CONTINUED)

Disorder	Symptoms	Diagnosis	Treatment
Myelomeningocele ■ Form of spina bifida in which a portion of spinal cord and membranes protrude ■ Many patients require intense physical care and often do not survive into teen years	■ Deformity in lumbar region of spinal column ■ Possible paralysis ■ Possible loss of bowel and bladder function	■ Patient presenting symptoms	■ Surgery to protect exposed spinal nerves and cord ■ Supportive care for any paralysis or bowel and bladder dysfunction
Hydrocephalus ■ Accumulation of cerebrospinal fluid (CSF) within brain and skull ■ May be result of developmental error, trauma, infection, or blood clot developing during or shortly after delivery ■ If surgery is performed before permanent neurological damage occurs, child has a good prognosis ■ Requires continual observation for neurological symptoms that signal reduced or impaired functioning of shunt	■ Enlargement of skull, with bulging fontanelles	■ Patient presenting symptoms	■ Surgery to insert shunt to drain excess fluid into circulatory system
Microencephaly ■ Abnormally small brain ■ Most patients die in infancy	■ Small head	■ Patient presenting symptoms ■ Imaging studies	■ Supportive care
Anencephaly ■ Cranial vault missing, and very little cerebral tissue present ■ Most patients are stillborn or die during neonatal period	■ Posterior cranial vault small or absent	■ Patient presenting symptoms ■ Imaging studies	■ Supportive care

Congenital Heart Conditions

Congenital heart conditions are easily identified at birth or before birth by prenatal ultrasound examination (Table 45-5). Some conditions are caused by failure of fetal circulation to convert to normal cardiac circulation after birth. Others are caused by developmental anomalies. There are two classes of congenital heart conditions. **Acyanotic** conditions include ventricular septal defect (VSD), patent ductus arteriosus (PDA), coarctation of the aorta, and atrial septal defect. Tetralogy of Fallot and transposition of the great arteries are **cyanotic** conditions.

Blood Disorders

Disorders affecting the blood that are seen in pediatric patients include anemia, leukemia, and lead poisoning (Table 45-6).

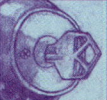

Keys to Success
TAPE TEST FOR WORM/EGG COLLECTION

A classic sign of roundworm and pinworm infestation is scratching of the anus. A microscopic examination of the stool confirms the presence of eggs or worms.

An easy method for collecting the worms is to place clear tape across the rectum when the child goes to bed. The worms have a tendency to migrate to the anus and are trapped on the tape. Examining the tape early the next morning reveals the worms.

Another method of confirming an infestation is to shine a flashlight on the child's anus in the dark. Often the worms can be seen around the anus.

Treatment consists of an antihelminthic regimen for the entire family and laundering all bedding in hot water with bleach, if possible.

TABLE 45-5 CONGENITAL HEART CONDITIONS

Condition	Patient Symptoms	Diagnosis	Treatment
Ventricular septal defect (VSD) ■ Opening in septum between right and left ventricles, resulting in shunting of blood from left to right side of heart	■ Heart murmur ■ Increased heart rate ■ Increased respiratory rate ■ Failure to gain weight ■ Restlessness ■ Irritability	■ Patient presenting symptoms	■ Surgery to repair or patch ventricular septum
Patent ductus arteriosus (PDA) ■ Failure of ductus arteriosus to close after birth, which causes shunting of oxygenated blood to lungs ■ Good prognosis with prompt medication or surgery	■ Heart murmur ■ Retarded growth ■ Signs of heart failure	■ Patient presenting symptoms	■ Antiprostaglandin to inhibit prostaglandin synthesis ■ Surgery to close patent ductus arteriosus
Coarctation of the aorta ■ Portion of aorta is narrowed, restricting blood flow from left ventricle ■ Fair prognosis with prompt surgery	■ Left ventricular failure ■ Pulmonary edema (swelling) ■ Decreased pulse in legs ■ Rapid heart rate ■ Dyspnea	■ Patient presenting symptoms	■ Surgery recommended to remove the coarctation
Atrial septal defect ■ Opening in atrial septal wall ■ Good prognosis with prompt surgery	■ Fatigue ■ SOB ■ Respiratory infections	■ Patient presenting symptoms	■ Surgery to repair wall
Tetralogy of Fallot ■ Combination of ventricular septal defect, pulmonary stenosis, displacement of aorta to the right, and right ventricular hypertrophy ■ Fair prognosis with prompt and successful surgery	■ Cyanosis ("blue baby") ■ Hypoxia ■ Tachycardia ■ Tachypnea ■ Dyspnea ■ Seizures	■ Patient presenting symptoms	■ Immediate surgery to correct defect
Transposition of the great arteries ■ Aorta and pulmonary artery reversed as they exit the heart ■ Variable prognosis with immediate surgery	■ Cyanosis ■ Tachypnea ■ Heart failure ■ Imaging studies	■ Patient presenting symptoms	■ Prostaglandins to keep ductus arteriosus open until surgery ■ Surgery to repair defect

Other Conditions

Some conditions are passed on to the fetus by a mother with a history of substance abuse. A baby with fetal alcohol syndrome (**FAS**) often shows retarded growth in height, weight, and mental capacity. A few days after birth, the baby suffers from alcohol withdrawal. Any neurological damage cannot be reversed, so most treatment involves supportive care. A baby whose mother took crack cocaine during the pregnancy—is very irritable and may also show growth retardation. Many of these children have severe emotional and behavioral problems later in life.

A common digestive disease in children is infestation with helminths, or parasitic intestinal worms. Toxocariasis (roundworm) and enterobiasis (pinworm) infestations are caused by the transfer of larvae by unclean hands and nails to the mouth. In both cases, the larvae are swallowed and hatch in the intestines. Roundworm infestation can cause symptoms of cough, fever, nausea and vomiting, weight loss, or hepatomegaly (enlargement of the liver).

Diagnostic Procedures

Diagnostic procedures that may be performed in the pediatrics office include urinalysis, strep screens, hemoglobin and hematocrit, and culture and sensitivity (C&S). The physician may order blood drawn for a blood lead level and/or theophylline level. Some physicians may perform a lumbar puncture on a child with a fever of unknown origin.

TABLE 45-6 BLOOD DISORDERS

Disorder	Symptoms	Diagnosis	Treatment
Anemia ▪ Several possible causes, but in children commonly caused by iron deficiency and poor diet ▪ Breast milk may have low iron if mother did not take prenatal supplement	▪ Pale skin ▪ Weakness ▪ Fatigue ▪ SOB	▪ Patient presenting symptoms ▪ Physical examination ▪ Hemoglobin (hgb) test ▪ Hematocrit (HCT) test	▪ Fortified formula for infants ▪ Iron supplements for prenatal care ▪ For older children, proper diet with good sources of iron such as egg yolks and fortified cereals ▪ Vitamin and mineral supplements for older children
Leukemia ▪ Abnormal increase in white blood cells ▪ Variable prognosis with treatment	▪ Fatigue ▪ Aching ▪ Infection ▪ Enlarged lymph nodes	▪ Patient presenting symptoms ▪ Blood studies ▪ Lymph biopsy	▪ Chemotherapy ▪ Bone-marrow transplant
Lead Poisoning ▪ Caused by lead in the environment ▪ Can affect physical and mental development ▪ Sources include lead-based paint, water from lead pipes, lead salts in certain foods, ceramic food containers painted with lead-based paint, food grown in contaminated soil, playing in contaminated soil or sand, and older vinyl mini-blinds ▪ Leaded gasoline emissions and seepage are main cause of soil and sand contamination ▪ Neurological damage cannot be reversed	▪ Loss of appetite ▪ Vomiting ▪ Irritability ▪ Difficulty walking ▪ Stumbling ▪ Anemia ▪ Weakness ▪ Colic ▪ Peripheral neuritis ▪ Possible mental retardation ▪ Headache ▪ Stupor ▪ Convulsions ▪ Coma	▪ Patient presenting symptoms ▪ Environmental history ▪ Blood studies ▪ Urine studies	▪ Removing source ▪ Chelating agents to remove lead from blood ▪ Supportive treatment

Positioning and Securing the Child for Examination and Treatment

Medical assistants are responsible for positioning and securing the child for an examination or procedure. When possible, the parent should be involved. The MA will show the parent how to hold and restrain the child and then help the parent to do so.

Position 1: For examining the ears

1. Ask the parent to hold the child upright against his or her body.
2. The child's arms and legs should be tucked in under the parent's arms. The child's head should be turned to the side and held firmly against the parent's chest.
3. Gently turn the child's head and continue holding when the physician examines the other ear.

Position 2: For examining the ears, eyes, nose, and throat

1. Lay the child on the exam table.
2. Ask the parent to hold both of the child's arms against the child's head, grasping the hands together above the head. You may need to gently hold the child's body down on the exam table.
3. Gently turn the child's head from side to side so the physician may examine each ear.

Mummy restraint method: Used when it is not possible for the parent to hold the child but the child must be completely restrained. This method may be adapted to expose an arm or leg.

1. Place the child's arms at his or her sides with the hands open and palms against the body (Figure 45-21 ◆).
2. Wrap the sheet from one side and enclose the arm (Figure 45-22 ◆).

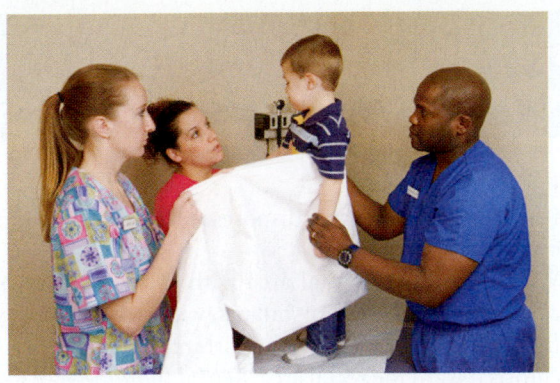

Figure 45-21 ◆ Place the child's arms at sides with palms against the body.

3. Continue wrapping the sheet. Wrap the other end of the sheet around the child and secure it. (Figure 45-23 ◆). The child is now fully restrained, ready for medication.

Papoose board method:

1. Pad the board well (Figure 45-24 ◆).
2. Ask the parent to place the child on the board.
3. Secure the child with the restraining straps and board fasteners (Figure 45-25 ◆).

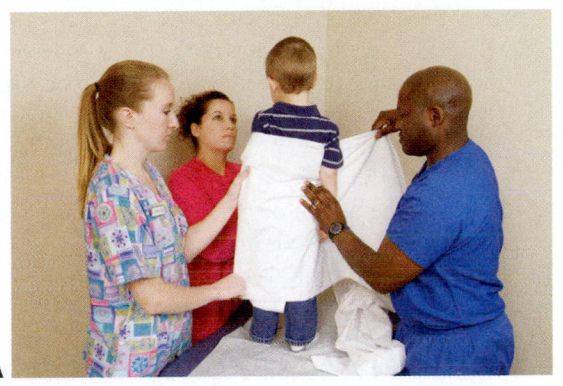

A   B

Figure 45-22 ◆ Wrap the sheet from one side and enclose the arm.

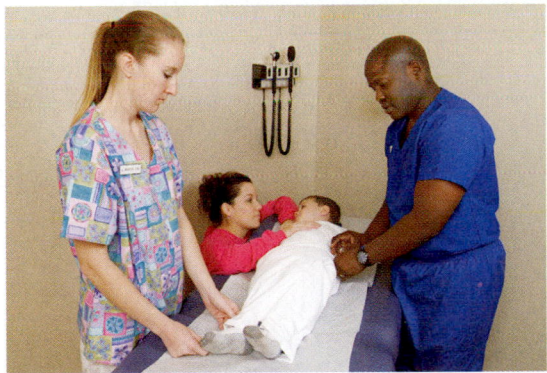

Figure 45-23 ◆ The child is now ready for medication.

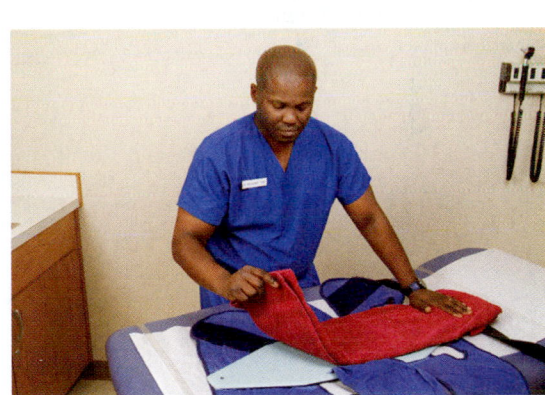

Figure 45-24 ◆ Papoose board method: pad the board well.

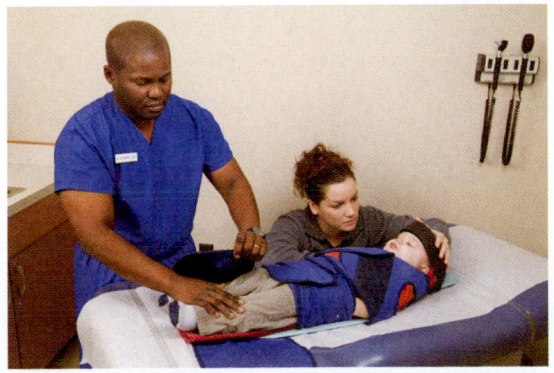

Figure 45-25 ◆ Secure the child.

For extensive procedures, a sedative may be administered to the child.

Pediatric Urine Collection

Urine samples are tested for the presence of blood, glucose, acetone, bilirubin, protein, drugs or hormones, and microorganisms. The specific gravity and pH of the urine may need to be determined. Because the newborn, infant, or toddler cannot physically or mentally follow directions to urinate into a sterile specimen container, the MA may need to attach a urine collection bag, or the physician may perform a catheterization.

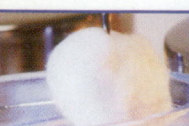

PROCEDURE 45-4 Perform Urine Collection with a Pediatric Urine Collection Bag

Theory and Rationale

It is important that a urine specimen collected with a collection bag be a recent urination. A fresh specimen provides more accurate information for correct diagnosis and treatment. For example, an old specimen may contain bacterial growth above what might have been present at the time of urination. Transport the specimen immediately to the laboratory for proper storage if it is not processed immediately.

Cleansing the skin is also crucial for obtaining accurate information (see ∞ Chapter 33). Microorganisms on the skin may contaminate the urine specimen. To contain the urine specimen in the collection bag, you must create a wrinkle-free seal when you remove the adhesive covers from the tabs and place the bag on the skin. The tight seal is particularly important in the pediatric patient with oliguria (scanty urine production).

Materials

- urine collection bag for newborn or pediatric patient
- sterile gloves
- sterile container with label
- cotton balls
- prepackaged sterile cleansing swabs or towelettes
- laboratory requisition form
- patient chart

Competency

(**Conditions**) With the necessary materials, (**Task**) you will be required to collect a urine specimen in a urine collection bag (**Standards**) correctly within 40 minutes.

1. Wash your hands. Gather the equipment and supplies.
2. Identify the parent or guardian with the child and guide them to the treatment area. Explain the procedure to the parent or guardian.

3. Put on sterile gloves.
4. Remove the diaper and dispose of it in the appropriate container.
5. Wipe the child's genital area with sterile towelettes or cleansing swabs. For boy infants, wipe around and away from the urinary meatus. For girl infants, wipe from the clitoris toward the rectal area. Repeat the wipe with a separate towelette or cleansing swab a second and third time to cleanse the area immediately surrounding the urinary meatus, then cleanse the wider surrounding area.
6. Dry the cleansed area with dry cotton balls.
7. Remove the adhesive tabs of the urine collection bag and apply the bag to the genital area securely, without gaps between the tabs and the skin (Figure 45-26 ◆).
8. Diaper the child.
9. Wash your hands.
10. Instruct the parent or guardian to encourage the infant or toddler to drink or nurse.
11. Recheck the diaper every 20 minutes until a specimen is obtained in the bag.
12. Wash your hands and put on sterile gloves.
13. Remove the urine collection bag. Place the bagged urine specimen in the sterile cup and cover the container tightly.
14. Diaper the child.
15. Remove the gloves and wash your hands.
16. Prepare the container label and laboratory requisition.
17. Transport or arrange for transport of the specimen to the laboratory.
18. Document the procedure in the child's chart.
19. Dispose of biohazardous materials in the proper containers.
20. Clean the area.
21. Wash your hands.

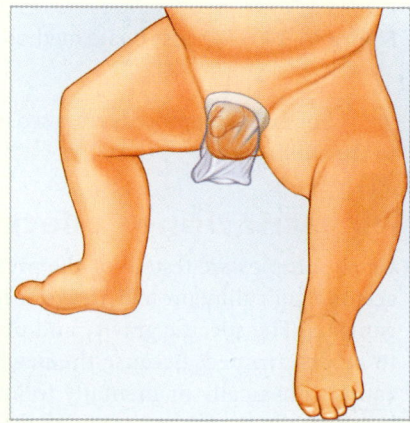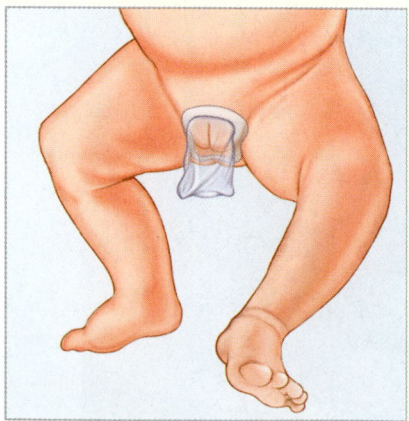

Figure 45-26 ◆ Applying urine collection bags on a male and female infant.

PROCEDURE 45-4 Perform Urine Collection with a Pediatric Urine Collection Bag *(continued)*

Patient Education

Instruct the parent or guardian to increase the child's fluid intake to stimulate urine production. It may be necessary to explain that the urine collection bag is preferred, but the physician may choose to catheterize the child. If the parent or guardian is very anxious, it is often wise to avoid describing too many details. Explain only as much as the parent needs to understand and assist the child through the medical evaluation process.

Charting Example

09/27/XX 2:35 p.m. One-year-old female with history of 101° fever for two days. Mother states child is fussy, not drinking, and urine is darker than normal. Urine collection bag applied per physician order and office procedure. Shane Washington, RMA (AMT)

09/27/XX 3:15 p.m. Urine collection bag removed and placed in sterile urine cantainer. Urine is dark yellow and smells strong. Laboratory requisition sent with labeled urine specimen. Shane Washington, RMA (AMT)

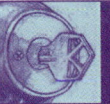

Keys to Success
ADMINISTERING LIQUID MEDICATION

Liquid medications are often prescribed for children. These require special care. A child's body uses and excretes medications differently than an adult's or elderly person's does. Because pediatric dosages are different, medical and other clinical staff must calculate and double-check for accuracy.

It may be tempting for a parent or guardian to use a household teaspoon or tablespoon to measure a liquid medication. Part of your instruction must be the importance of measuring with the spoons or cups supplied by the pharmacist or the manufacturer. For example, it is common to give a child an over-the-counter (OTC) medication, such as acetaminophen. This medication can be administered by drops or liquid. Giving 5 ml of acetaminophen drops on a regular schedule or 150 mg/kg could be toxic for the child, causing liver damage and even death. Instruct parents to read and follow directions carefully.

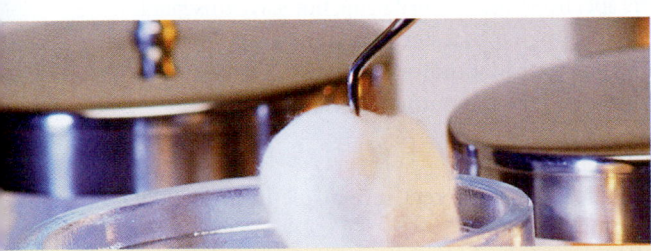

REVIEW

Chapter Summary

■ The pediatric practice offers an MA a variety of tasks: obtaining and recording the child's health, developmental history, and vital signs; measuring and recording growth; assisting the parents or guardian and the physician with the child; obtaining a urine specimen; and administering medications, injections, and immunizations.

■ An important role for the MA is to be aware of the needs and concerns of the parent or guardian and the child. Fear, mistrust, anxiety, and embarrassment are all common emotions. Listening can provide valuable information about the child.

Chapter Summary (continued)

- Growth measurement is usually part of a child's file and is vital information because it can indicate normal and abnormal growth.
- While inoculations and well-baby and child checks are a major part of office visits, diaper rash, thrush, ear inflammation, and asthma are also common.
- Common contagious diseases are more easily controlled today by preventive inoculations. Diseases include chickenpox, measles, German measles, mumps, whooping cough, polio, and diphtheria. Vaccinations for hepatitis B and haemophilus b have been added to routine immunizations.
- Serious respiratory conditions, RSV and cystic fibrosis, require immediate care.

- Neural tube disorders are congenital. They occur when the embryo's neural tube fails to close. There are two categories: spinal and cranial fusion. There is no cure.
- Acyanotic and cyanotic are the two classifications of congenital heart disorders.
- Anemia, leukemia, and lead poisoning are all serious blood disorders.
- Fetal alcohol syndrome and drug-affected babies are more likely to show retarded growth and neurological damage. Often they experience severe emotional and behavioral problems later in life.
- Diagnostic procedures that may be performed include strep screens, urinalysis, hemoglobin and hematocrit, and C&S.

Chapter Review

Multiple Choice

1. Which of the following is an acceptable way to handle an anxious parent?
   a. Ask the parent to leave the room and calm down.
   b. Take the child away from the parent, so you have control of the child.
   c. Show the parent how to hold the child during the exam.
   d. Tell the child and parent "It won't hurt."

2. When you weigh an infant, you must
   a. swab the platform scale before using it.
   b. watch the infant because he or she can move suddenly.
   c. set the platform scale to -.05.
   d. leave the infant's diaper on for comfort.

3. Liquid acetaminophen drops can be administered
   a. only as directed.
   b. in a 5 ml dosage.
   c. in a 6 ml dosage.
   d. in a 7 ml dosage.

4. The "mummy" restraint method involves
   a. the parent holding the child's hands on the child's chest.
   b. using a board.
   c. tucking the infant's arms and legs under the parent's arms.
   d. wrapping a sheet around a child.

5. Which one of the following is a spinal fusion disorder?
   a. Cystic fibrosis
   b. Anencephaly
   c. Meningocele
   d. RSV

6. Hydrocephalus is treated by surgically
   a. closing the opening.
   b. inserting a shunt.
   c. protecting the exposed spinal cord.
   d. repairing the septal wall.

7. Which one of the following is a cyanotic congenital heart condition?
   a. Transposition of the great arteries
   b. Patent ductus arteriosus
   c. Coarctation of the aorta
   d. Atrial septal defect

8. Anemia in an older child is most often caused by
   a. taking supplements.
   b. drinking too much soda.
   c. exercising too little.
   d. eating a poor diet.

9. A urine specimen from a toddler must be
   a. obtained only by catheterization.
   b. recent for an accurate laboratory result.
   c. stored at room temperature.
   d. done as soon as the child wakes in the morning.

10. Immediately after removing the urine collection bag, you must
    a. put the specimen into a sterile cup, but leave unsealed.
    b. put the specimen into a sterile cup and seal.
    c. take the bag to the laboratory sealed.
    d. take the bag to the laboratory unsealed.

True/False

T F 1. The medical assistant can have a role in physically restraining a child.

T F 2. There are two categories of visits to a pediatrician's office: well child or sick child.

T F 3. Children are too young to understand medical procedures, so it is best to tell them "it won't hurt" so that they don't try to wiggle away from you.

T F 4. *Infant* is the term used for a baby from birth to 4 weeks old.

Chapter Review (continued)

T F 5. Each child grows at his or her own individual speed, according to family genetics, so measurements are not important and not done at each visit.

Short Answer

1. What is phimosis?

2. What are the two age groups into which NCHS and CDC charts are divided?

3. Why should you place a paper protector on a platform scale before weighing an infant?

4. At what age can you begin taking a child's temperature orally?

5. Pulling at the ear or sitting with the head held to one side may be indications of what condition in a toddler or infant?

Research

1. Is there a crisis nursery or other organization in your community that provides respite care for children?

2. How many children will be injured or killed this year as a result of poor supervision in the bathtub?

Externship Application Experience

A mother refuses the first immunization series for her child during the first well-child checkup. As a medical assistant, how do you respond?

Resource Guide

American Academy of Allergies, Asthma, and Immunology
611 E. Wells
Milwaukee, WI 53202
1-800-822-ASMA
www.aaaai.org

Cystic Fibrosis Foundation
6931 Arlington Road
Bethesda, MD 20814-5200
1-800 FIGHT-CF
www.cff.org

National Easter Seal Society, Inc.
230 W. Monroe, Ste 1800
Chicago, IL 60606-4802
1-800-221-6872
www.easter-seals.org

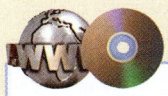

Med**Media**

http://www.MyMAKit.com

More on this chapter, including interactive resources, can be found on the Student CD-ROM accompanying this textbook and on http://www.MyMAKit.com.

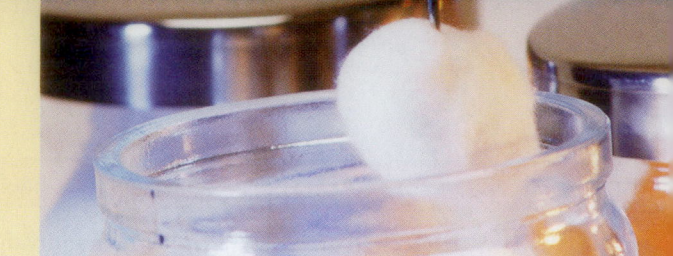

CHAPTER 46

Neurology

Case Study

Dawn Benedict, RMA (AMT), is performing initial questioning with a patient, Milo Stevens, for a consultation regarding back pain. Dawn learns that Milo has recently had what he describes as an allergic reaction that caused a rash on his back, near the axial area on the right side. The patient states that at first he thought the blisters were acne and that his girl-friend helped him "pop" a few. Further questioning reveals that Milo's intense back pain started around the same time Milo had varicella as a child.

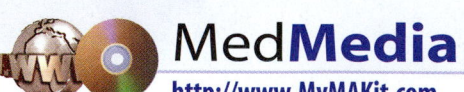

Med**Media**

http://www.MyMAKit.com

Additional interactive resources and activities for this chapter can be found on http://www.MyMAKit.com. For a video, audio glossary, tips, legal and ethical scenarios, job scenarios, quizzes, games, virtual tours, and activities related to the content of this chapter, please access the accompanying CD-ROM in this book.

Video
Audio Glossary
Legal and Ethical Scenario: *Neurology*
On the Job Scenario: *Neurology*
A & P Quiz: The Nervous System
Multiple Choice Quiz
Games: Crossword, Strikeout, and Spelling Bee
3D Virtual Tours: Nervous System: Leg; Nervous System: Arm & Shoulder;
  Nervous System: Spinal Cord; Nervous System: Head
Drag and Drop: Nervous System: Brain & Brainstem
Tips
HIPAA Quiz

Objectives

After completing this chapter, you should be able to:

- Define and spell the key terminology in this chapter.
- Define the medical assistant's role in the neurology/neurosurgery practice.
- Discuss the anatomy and physiology of the central nervous system.
- Discuss the anatomy and physiology of the peripheral nervous system.
- Describe the structures that make up a nerve cell, or neuron.
- Discuss the functions of the various divisions of the nervous system.
- Discuss the various methods of neurological assessment.
- Explain how the Glasgow Coma Scale and lumbar punctures are used in neurological assessment.
- Describe common diseases and disorders of the central nervous system: CVA, TIA, epilepsy, ALS, Parkinson's disease, multiple sclerosis, amyotrophic lateral sclerosis, headache, infectious conditions, head trauma, spinal cord injuries, and disk disorders.
- Describe common diseases and disorders of the peripheral nervous system: Bell's palsy, trigeminal neuralgia, and shingles.

✚ MEDICAL ASSISTING STANDARDS

CAAHEP ENTRY-LEVEL STANDARDS	ABHES ENTRY-LEVEL COMPETENCIES
■ Perform within scope of practice (psychomotor)	■ Project a positive attitude.
■ Explore issue of confidentiality as it applies to the medical assistant (cognitive)	■ Maintain confidentiality at all times.
	■ Be a "team player."
■ Apply ethical behaviors, including honesty/integrity in performance of medical assisting practice (affective)	■ Be cognizant of ethical boundaries.
	■ Exhibit initiative.
	■ Adapt to change.
■ Explain the rationale for performance of a procedure to the patient (affective)	■ Evidence a responsible attitude.
	■ Be courteous and diplomatic.
■ Use language/verbal skills that enable patients' understanding (affective)	■ Conduct work within the scope of education, training, and ability.
■ Describe the normal function of each body system (cognitive)	■ Be impartial and show empathy when dealing with patients.
■ Identify common pathology related to each body system (cognitive)	■ Adapt what is said to the recipient's level of comprehension.
■ Analyze pathology as it relates to the interaction of body systems (cognitive)	■ Serve as a liaison between the physician and others.
■ Discuss implications for disease and disability when homeostasis is not maintained (cognitive)	■ Interview effectively.
	■ Use appropriate terminology.
■ Describe implications for treatment related to pathology (cognitive)	■ Recognize and respond to verbal and nonverbal communication.
■ Apply critical thinking skills in performing patient assessment and care (affective)	■ Adapt to individualized needs.
■ Prepare a patient for procedures and/or treatments (psychomotor)	
■ Assist physician with patient care (psychomotor)	
■ Document accurately in the patient record (psychomotor)	
■ Practice Standard Precautions (psychomotor)	
■ Show awareness of patients' concerns regarding their perceptions related to the procedure being performed (affective)	

✓ COMPETENCY SKILLS PERFORMANCE

1. Assist in a neurological exam.
2. Assist with a lumbar puncture.
3. Prepare a patient for an electroencephalogram.

Key Terminology

affect—emotional expression associated with facial and body behaviors

aura—warning of impending seizure

cephalgia—diffuse acute or chronic pain in any part of the head, commonly known as *headache*

clonic—alternating muscular contraction and relaxation

contrecoup—event on the opposite side, injury in which traumatic impact on the head is strong enough to make the brain strike the opposite side of the cranium and bounce back to strike the impacted side

decerebrate posture—posture characteristic of brain injury in which the patient is rigid, with head retracted and arms and legs extended

decorticate posture— posture characteristic of brain injury in which the patient is rigid, with clenched fists, flexed arms, and extended legs

dermatome—specific area of skin stimulated by a segment of the spinal cord

exacerbation—increasing severity and recurrence of symptoms

hemiparesis—loss of nerve and muscle function on one side of the body

innervate—stimulate

neuralgia—sharp nerve pain

neurology—study of the nervous system

neuron—nerve cell; basic unit of the nervous system

neurotransmitter—chemicals that aid in the transmission of electrical impulses from one neuron, or nerve cell, to the next

nuchal rigidity—severe and painful rigidity of the neck in which the head is bent forward toward the chest

palsy—tremors; temporary or permanent loss of ability to control or make muscle movement

paraplegia—loss of sensation and motor activity (paralysis) of the lower trunk and lower extremities

postictal—pertaining to the period immediately following a seizure

Key Terminology *(continued)*

prodromal—pertaining to symptoms during the period immediately preceding onset of a disease condition

projectile vomiting—vomiting with uncontrollable force

pyogenic—pus-forming

quadriplegia—paralysis of the entire trunk and all four extremities

tonic—pertaining to muscular tension

Abbreviations

ALS—amyotrophic lateral sclerosis

CNS—central nervous system

CSF—cerebrospinal fluid

CVA—cerebrovascular accident

EEG—electroencephalography/ electroencephalogram

LP—lumbar puncture

PNS—peripheral nervous system

TIA—transient ischemic attack

Introduction

Neurology is a branch of medicine that specializes in the diagnosis and treatment of diseases of the nervous system. Conditions affecting the brain, spinal cord, and peripheral nervous system are addressed by neurologists. Neurosurgeons treat neurological conditions requiring surgical intervention, such as traumatic insult to the brain, spinal cord, and peripheral nerves; the presence of a foreign body; tumor or abscess in these structures; and pressure from intracranial hemorrhage. Neurosurgery may also provide pain relief as well as relief from the tremors of parkinsonism.

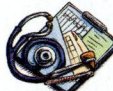

The Medical Assistant's Role in Neurology and Neurosurgery

There are numerous opportunities for the medical assistant in neurology and neurosurgery offices. Many of these opportunities are in the administrative arena; however, clinical positions are generally available as well.

Medical assistants in a neurology office may be responsible for obtaining a preliminary history and information pertaining to the current office visit. The MA will assess and record vital signs, assist the neurologist with the patient examination, assist the patient as required, document the examination on the patient's chart, provide patient instruction, and make and confirm appointments for any additional diagnostic tests.

In a neurosurgical office the MA will have many of the same responsibilities. In addition, when a surgical procedure is to be scheduled, the MA will either obtain precertification and schedule the procedure or coordinate it with the surgical scheduling department. Medical assistants will obtain consent for the procedure according to office policy and instruct the patient and/or family about any presurgical testing or procedures. Following surgical procedures, the MA may remove sutures, staples, or drains and apply appropriate dressings.

The Anatomy and Physiology of the Nervous System

A healthy nervous system coordinates the homeostatic reactions of body systems to internal and external stimuli. As you learned in ∞ Chapter 25, homeostasis is the ability of a living organism to adjust to continually changing internal and external environments for optimum functioning and survival. For example, shivering and diaphoresis are homeostatic reactions to changes in external environment and internal body temperature. When the body senses a cold external environment, the neurological system causes skin blood vessels to constrict and reduce heat loss. Shivering and the resulting voluntary muscle contractions and movement generate heat. Conversely, when the body senses a warm external environment, the neurological system causes skin blood vessels to dilate and allow heat loss and diaphoresis, or sweating. When the nervous system cannot adjust to changing internal and external environments, serious conditions may result, such as hypothermia or hyperthermia in response to temperature changes.

The nervous system has two anatomical divisions (Figure 46-1 ◆):

- Central nervous system (**CNS**)
- Peripheral nervous system (**PNS**)

The Central Nervous System

The central nervous system, consisting of the brain and spinal cord, maintains control of the peripheral nervous system and integrates information between the two divisions. The brain and spinal cord are protected by outer bony structures known as the cranium and vertebral column, respectively. The meninges, extending from the brain to cover the entire length of the spinal cord, form a protective, watertight sheath around the spinal cord known as the cerebrospinal canal. The meninges consist of three protective layers:

- Dura mater: a tough membrane that forms the outer and thickest layer
- Arachnoid meninges: the middle covering, which resembles a spiderweb
- Pia mater: the innermost layer, attached directly to the brain and spinal cord tissues

Cerebrospinal fluid (**CSF**) supports and cushions the brain and spinal cord and protects them from infection and trauma. CSF is produced within the ventricles (spaces within the cerebrum) and circulates through the brain and spinal cord and into the subarachnoid space between the arachnoid and pia mater layers.

The three major areas of the brain are the cerebrum, cerebellum, and brain stem. (The functions of the different areas of the brain are discussed further in ∞ Chapter 47.)

- The outer layer of the cerebrum, or cerebral cortex, consists of six thin layers of gray matter containing many millions of neuron cell bodies. The cerebral interior contains white matter and myelinated axons. The cerebrum controls intelligence, learning and memory, reasoning and judgment, and emotions, and interprets voluntary muscle and sensory activities.
- The cerebellum, also containing an outer layer of gray matter and inner layer of white matter nerve tracts, coordinates the activities of brain structures that control running and walking, maintaining posture and balance, and motor activities such as eating, dressing, writing, riding a bicycle, and tracking movement with the eyes.
- The brain stem, consisting of the midbrain, pons, and medulla oblongata, is composed mainly of white matter and is responsible for regulating vital body functions such as respiration and heart rate.

The Peripheral Nervous System

The peripheral nervous system consists of cranial nerves, spinal nerves, and sympathetic and parasympathetic nerves. Cranial nerves originate from the base of the brain and distribute nervous system impulses mainly to the head and neck. They function in vision, hearing, smelling, the movement of eye muscles and pupil size, facial expression, chewing and tongue movements, and sensations of the head and face. There are twelve pairs of cranial nerves (Table 46-1). The cranial nerve number indicates the order of origination from the base of the brain, and the word name indicates the end distribution of the impulse or function of the nerve.

There are thirty-one pairs of spinal nerves, which originate from the spinal cord. They carry impulses to and from the brain.

The sympathetic and parasympathetic nerves comprise the autonomic nervous system, which is part of the peripheral

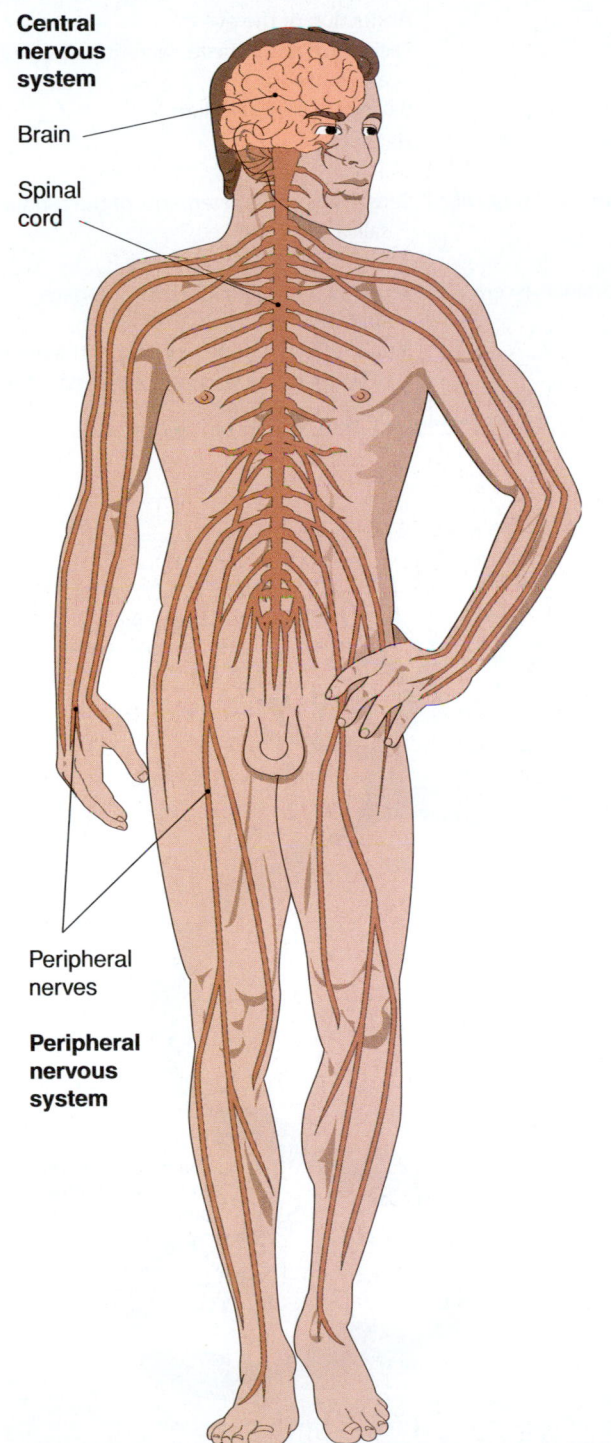

Central nervous system

Brain

Spinal cord

Peripheral nerves

Peripheral nervous system

Figure 46-1 ◆ The nervous system.

TABLE 46-1 THE CRANIAL NERVES

Nerve	Location of Receptors	Function
I. Olfactory	Nasal mucosa	Sense of smell
II. Optic	Retina	Vision
III. Oculomotor	External eye muscles except superior oblique and lateral rectus	Eye movements, regulation of pupil size, accommodation, proprioception
IV. Trochlear	Superior oblique	Eye movements, proprioception
V. Trigeminal	Skin and mucosa of head and teeth	Sensations of head and face, chewing, proprioception
VI. Abducens	Lateral rectus	Abduction of the eye
VII. Facial	Taste buds of anterior two-thirds of the tongue	Facial expression, taste, secretion of saliva and tears
VIII. Vestibulocochlear	■ Vestibular branch: semicircular canals and vestibule	Balance and equilibrium
	■ Cochlear or auditory branch: organ of Corti in the cochlear duct	Hearing
IX. Glossopharyngeal	■ Pharynx: pharynx, taste buds and other receptors of posterior third of tongue	Sensations and movements of the tongue, saliva secretion
	■ Carotid: carotid sinus and carotid body	
X. Vagus	Pharynx, larynx, carotid body, thoracic and abdominal viscera	Sensations and movements of organs supplied
XI. Accessory	Trapezius and sternocleido-mastoid	Shoulder movements, turning of the head, movements of viscera, voice production
XII. Hypoglossal	Tongue muscles	Tongue movements

nervous system. These nerves regulate all involuntary homeostatic functions and responses, including peristalsis, breathing, blinking, and hormonal and chemical activities.

The Neuron

The functional unit of the nervous system is the **neuron,** or nerve cell (Figure 46-2 ◆). Each neuron contains a cell body with a nucleus and other typical cellular components, an axon, and dendrites. Dendrites are fibers that receive impulses from other neurons and carry them to the cell body. The axon, or tail, of the neuron transmits impulses away from the cell body to other neurons, or to neuromuscular junctions. The conduction path of each nervous system impulse travels from the dendrite, through the nerve cell body, continues along the axon, and crosses the synaptic gap to the next dendrite.

Some neurons are protected by a thick, fatty covering called the myelin sheath. Cells with a very thin, almost nonexistent myelin sheath are referred to as unmyelinated. When the conduction path of unmyelinated or myelin fibers is interrupted by disease process, inflammation, or trauma, neurological symptoms include slow or altered gait, altered speech or mental process, or inability to control movements.

The myelinated fiber tissue of dendrites and axons is called white matter because the heavier myelin covering is white. Nerve cell body tissue is called gray matter. Bundles of nerve cell fibers within the central nervous system are known as tracts, and outside the central nervous systems are known as nerves.

Nerve cells are classified by the direction of relayed impulses in relation to the CNS.

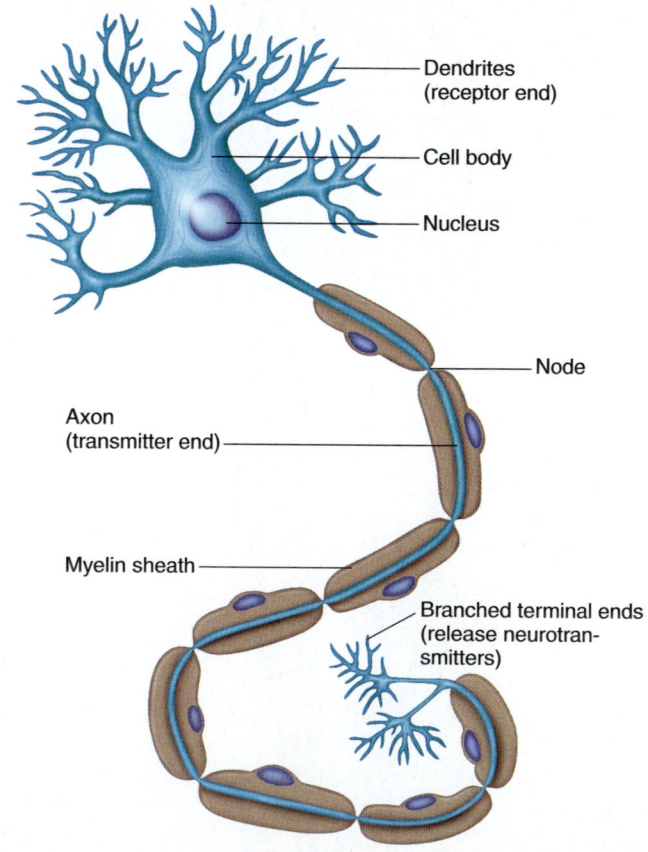

Figure 46-2 ◆ The functional unit of the nervous system is the neuron.

Labels: Dendrites (receptor end); Cell body; Nucleus; Node; Axon (transmitter end); Myelin sheath; Branched terminal ends (release neurotransmitters)

- Afferent, or sensory, neurons carry impulses toward the brain and spinal cord.
- Efferent, or motor, neurons carry impulses away from the CNS to the muscles.
- Interneurons, or central neurons, relay information within the CNS.

Axon branches secrete chemical messengers called **neurotransmitters** that transmit electrical impulses across the synaptic gap. Neurotransmitters function to cause or inhibit reactions of the connected neuron(s). (∞ For a discussion of the role of neurotransmitters in mental disorders, refer to Chapter 47.)

Neuroglia, connective tissue cells of the nervous system, support, protect, and assist in the repair of nerve cells. Neuroglia also act as phagocytes for the nervous system and regulate the fluid composition between cells.

Functions of the Nervous System

The two physiological divisions of the nervous system are:

- Somatic, or voluntary, system: controlled by conscious thought; an example is climbing stairs, which requires conscious thought
- Autonomic, or involuntary, system: responsible for automatic reactions; an example is increased heart and respiratory rates in response to perceived threats

The autonomic nervous system is further divided into sympathetic ("fight-or-flight") and parasympathetic ("brakes") homeostatic nerves (Table 46-2). These two divisions work against each other to control the body's internal functions during normal activity as well as stressful or traumatic periods. Normally, every sympathetic reaction stimulates a physiological response of increased energy and activity, and the body recovers with a slowing or opposing parasympathetic response. The sympathetic nervous system reaction is also known as the "fight-or-flight" response because it engages the nervous system to respond quickly to perceived danger, with increased heart rate, respirations, metabolism, and other physiological reactions. The

TABLE 46-2 EXAMPLES OF SYMPATHETIC AND PARASYMPATHETIC REACTIONS

Sympathetic "Fight-or-Flight"	Parasympathetic "Brakes"
- Faster, stronger heartbeat - Decreased peristalsis of digestive tract - Dilation of pupils - Increased respiratory rate and dilated bronchi - Increased circulation to skeletal muscles and respiratory system - Increased skin perspiration - More glucose released by the liver	- Slower, calmer heartbeat - Increased peristalsis of digestive tract - Constriction of pupils - Decreased respiratory rate and constricted bronchi - Decreased circulation to skeletal muscles and respiratory system - Decreased circulation to skin - Less bladder activity

parasympathetic nervous system later applies the "brakes" to slow and return the body to normal physiological functioning.

In addition to parasympathetic and sympathetic reactions, reflexes also help to protect the body. A reflex is an automatic, rapid neuromuscular reaction to a specific stimulus. Spinal reflexes do not involve coordination with the brain. They include blinking, pulling a hand from a hot pan handle, or reaching out to prevent an off-balance fall. Stretch reflexes, on the other hand, require coordination with the brain. In a stretch reflex, such as the knee-jerk reflex, a muscle is quickly stretched and contracted. Eliciting reflex responses is a simple way to evaluate for neurological disease processes.

Assessing the Neurological System

Assessment of the central neurological system involves different evaluations to locate a deficit in the system. Areas that are assessed are mental status and speech, mood or emotional state, cognitive functioning, level of consciousness, and sensory and motor functions involving the cranial, spinal, and peripheral nerves.

Assessment of mental status usually consists of observation and specific questions such as "What is your name?" "How old are you?" "Do you know where you are?" "What is today's date?" "Who is the president of the United States?" and "Where do you live?" Observation includes noting how long it takes for the patient to respond, the appropriateness of the answers, and whether the patient makes eye contact.

Another assessment area is the individual's mood and behavior. Once again, the presence or absence of eye contact is noted. Does the individual appear sad or happy? Is he or she smiling or frowning? Is the posture straight or slumping? Does the patient have a flat **affect**? Is the patient crying? Does he or she appear angry? Responses that are not typical are noted. If the individual is groggy or unconscious, the Glasgow Coma Scale is used to assess the level of consciousness. A patient who enters the office on his or her own and talks with the staff in an appropriate manner is said to be alert and responding appropriately.

Sensory and motor function assessment is usually performed by the physician or nurse practitioner. A common assessment for motor skills of the hands and fingers is the grip response, in which the patient squeezes the examiner's fingers with both hands (Figure 46-3 ◆). If the grips appear to be unequal, the assessment is documented as "Grips unequal with weakness noted in the right/left side." Assessment of the legs and feet involves having the patient, in the supine or sitting position, push both feet up and down against the examiner's hands. In other common evaluations, the patient is asked to close the eyes and touch the nose with the index finger, walk with the eyes looking straight ahead, and stand on one foot, then the other. A thorough history may indicate another underlying pathology that could cause the patient's inability to perform all the requested tasks.

Sensory abilities are often evaluated by touching the patient's skin in various areas of the body, with a piece of gauze or other item, and asking the patient to close the eyes and state where he or she is being touched. A sterile safety pin may be

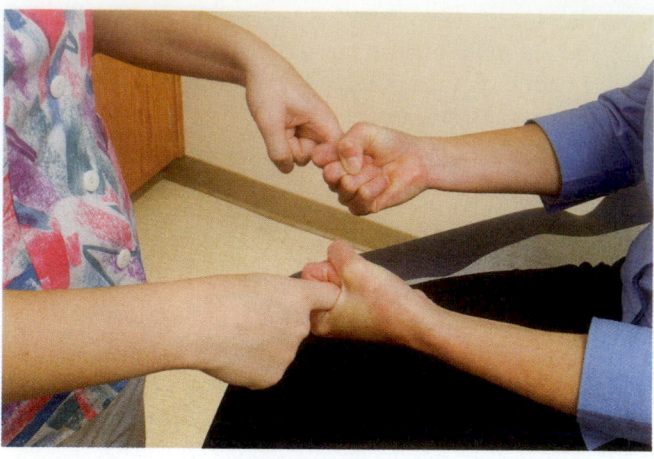

Figure 46-3 ◆ Performing a grip test.

used to prick the skin in this test. Olfactory senses are assessed by asking the patient to identify different odors.

Deep tendon reflexes are assessed by using a rubber reflex hammer to sharply strike a particular tendon at the site of a joint. This action provokes a spinal-mediated jerk response. Absent or diminished reflexes are indicative of nerve insult. Common sites evaluated this way are the elbows, knees, and posterior aspect of the ankles.

Head and facial injuries may affect the motor function of the six muscles controlling eye movement. These muscles and the nerves that **innervate** them are assessed by having the patient hold the head still, then look up, look down, look to the side, and follow the examiner's finger or pen as it moves around the normal field of vision. The innervation of the cranial nerve (III) oculomotor is to the superior rectus muscle that causes the eye to look up, to the inferior rectus muscle

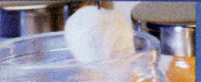

PROCEDURE 46-1 Assist in a Neurological Exam

Theory and Rationale

As a medical assistant, you may be responsible for interviewing patients prior to the physician's physical exam. You will evaluate and record any unusual changes in the patient's behavior—for example, in personal grooming habits and communication skills. As you conduct the interview, pay attention to what the patient is saying and how he or she is saying it. Is the speech slurred? Does the patient fumble for the right words? Is the patient making sense?

When assisting the physician with a neurological exam, you will help the patient assume the correct testing positions and have all instruments ready for use. For example, if the patient is being testing on the Glasgow Coma Scale for damage to the olfactory nerve, you will need to have objects with familiar scents available.

Materials

- reflex hammers
- penlight
- pinwheel
- tongue blade
- tuning fork
- ophthalmoscope
- cold object, as determined by physician
- warm object, as determined by physician
- scent object (coffee grounds, for example), as determined by physician
- patient drapes as determined by office protocol
- patient chart

Competency

(**Conditions**) With the necessary materials, (**Task**) you will be able to assist with a neurological exam (**Standards**) correctly, within the time frame determined by the instructor.

1. Wash your hands and gather equipment and supplies.
2. Interview the patient according to office protocol. Ask standard questions such as:
   A. What is your full name?
   B. Who is the current president of the United States?
   C. What is the date, including the month and year?
3. If your office protocol requires patients to change into cotton shorts and a tank top shirt, assist the patient as necessary.
4. Provide patient drapes as needed.
5. Follow office protocol for assisting the patient into the required positions. If the physician tests reflexes with a hammer first, assist the patient into a seated position on the exam table. Have the patient remove socks and shoes in preparation for testing the Babinski reflex.
6. After the physician has finished reflex testing, assist the patient to dress, as needed. Escort the patient to the gait-and-movement testing area.
7. Document any changes in the patient chart.

Patient Education

Tell the patient what to expect from the tests, any discomfort that may be experienced, and when test results will be ready. Encourage questions.

Charting Example

09/23/XX 2:30 p.m. Patient arrived for neurological testing, appearing disheveled. Patient was unshaven but stated he is not growing a beard. Clothes were wrinkled and unwashed, which is unusual for this patient. Patient was asked several orientation questions and could not identify self or correct time and place. Physician notified of results. Maurice Holmes, CMA (AAMA)

that causes the eye to look down, to the medial rectus muscle that causes the eye to rotate medially, and to the inferior oblique muscle that causes the eye to roll, look up, and look to the side. Cranial nerve VI, the abducens, innervates the lateral rectus muscle and causes the eyes to rotate laterally. Cranial nerve IV, the trochlear nerve, innervates the superior oblique muscle that causes the eye to roll, look down, and look to the side.

Another assessment of neurological function involves cranial nerve function. Areas tested are eye movement, visual acuity, sense of smell, movement of facial muscles on command, taste perception, and hearing.

The Glasgow Coma Scale

The Glasgow Coma Scale (∞ see Chapter 41) is a standardized system for the rapid assessment of brain activity, level of consciousness, possible insults to the brain, and possible outcome. Three responses are assessed: eye response, verbal response, and motor response. Each response is assigned a numerical value, and the three values provide an estimate of the injury.

The best score is noted for each portion of the response scale—for example, E2V2M4. Although it is a dependable rapid evaluation, the Glasgow Coma Scale is only a part of the neurological assessment.

Lumbar Punctures

Lumbar punctures (**LP**) are performed as a diagnostic procedure to evaluate the status of the cerebrospinal fluid and to measure the pressure within the cerebrospinal canal (Figure 46-4 ◆). Pressure is measured with a device called a *manometer,* which is attached to the hub of a needle inserted into the cerebrospinal canal. Laboratory examination and culture and sensitivity of the CSF may reveal the presence of red blood cells, white blood cells, protein, glucose, or microorganisms. Interpreting these test results is helpful in the diagnosis of disorders and diseases of the central nervous system.

Electroencephalography

An electroencephalogram (**EEG**) records electrical impulses in the brain created when brain cells communicate with each other. Electroencephalography is a valuable tool in diagnosing

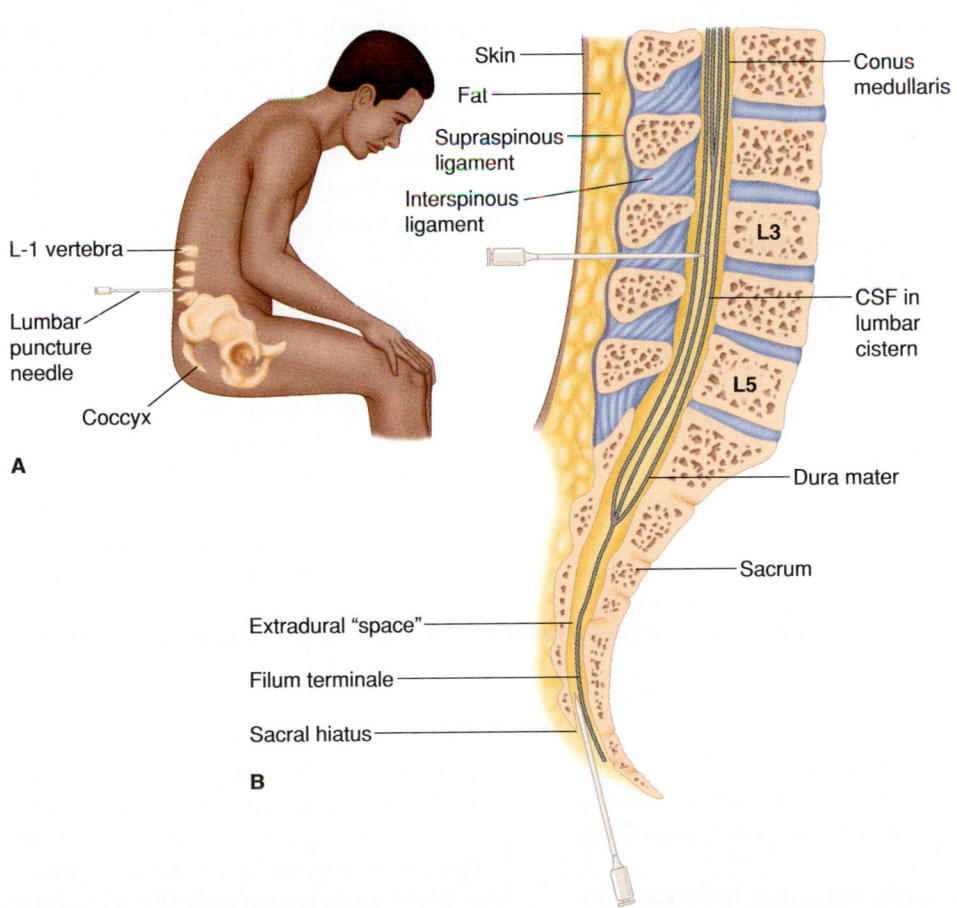

Figure 46-4 ◆ (A) Lumbar puncture (B) Section of the vertebral column showing the spinal cord and membranes.

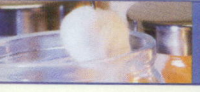

PROCEDURE 46-2 Assist with a Lumbar Puncture

Theory and Rationale

A lumbar puncture is a delicate procedure done under sterile technique in the physician's office. Most offices that perform lumbar punctures set aside a special room for this procedure, which requires that the patient remain at the clinic for several hours. Depending on your office protocol, it may be your responsibility to continuously monitor the patient's vital signs and alert the family of the patient's status. Family members are sometimes allowed to stay with the patient during the postoperative time.

Materials

- lumbar puncture kit: iodine antiseptic, iodine applicator, adhesive bandages, spinal puncture needle, 4 testing tubes
- patient drape
- BP cuff, sized appropriately for the patient
- manometer
- xylocaine 1-2%
- syringe and needle for anesthetic
- sterile gloves
- gauze sponges
- fenestrated drape

Competency

(Conditions) With the necessary materials, **(Task)** you will be able to assist the physician with a lumbar puncture to obtain CSF **(Standards)** correctly within the time determined by the instructor.

1. Identify the patient and explain the procedure. Reinforce the need for postoperative care.
2. Verify that the patient has signed a consent form and that it has been filed in the chart.
3. Have the patient empty his or her bowel and bladder.
4. Obtain the patient's vital signs.
5. Wash your hands, put on gloves, and set up a tray using sterile technique.
6. With the iodine in the kit, disinfect the puncture site (L3 and L4).
7. Have the patient lie on his or her left side and curl into the fetal position. Provide drapes for patient comfort.

8. Assist the physician as necessary in swabbing the patient with antiseptic and placing a fenestrated drape.
9. Assist the physician in aspirating the xylocaine.
10. To avoid potential trauma to the spinal cord, assist the patient in maintaining the fetal position.
11. While the physician is taking a pressure reading, remind the patient to breathe evenly and avoid talking. If the physician requests, assist the patient in straightening his or her legs to get a true pressure reading.
12. Place a gauze pad with firm pressure over the puncture site to absorb any bleeding.
13. After the fluid has been collected, tighten the sample tubes and fill out a lab order form. Correctly label the samples for analysis.
14. Move the patient to the recovery area.
15. Clean and disinfect the treatment area.
16. Remove the gloves and wash your hands.
17. Document the procedure in the patient's chart.

Patient Education

The patient should be instructed to remain in a prone position for 3–4 hours to allow the CSF to be replenished and the puncture site to heal. Make sure the patient understands the importance of not rushing through this vital healing process. The patient should not attempt to sit upright for extended periods, and excessive movement can cause spinal headaches and potential damage. In addition, the patient should increase fluid intake to replace the lost fluid. Any tingling, numbness, paralysis, or severe headaches should be reported immediately.

Charting Example

09/23/XX 9:00 A.M. Lumbar puncture performed by Dr. J. Lee. 3 vials of CSF obtained and sent to laboratory for testing. Patient tolerated procedure well, BP remained stable, checked every 15 minutes for 3 hours postprocedure. Patient was given verbal and written instructions to increase fluid intake, remain flat for 3-4 hours, and report any headaches, fever, bleeding, numbness, paralysis, or tingling. Kathleen Graham, RMA (AMI)

brain death, brain tumors, epilepsy, and other brain conditions. Occasionally, an EEG is ordered to evaluate a sleep disorder, in which case the test is performed in a sleep center, generally in a hospital.

The pattern, height, length, and rate of brain waves are unique to each person, like a brain "fingerprint." The brain-wave activity of the brain is recorded as a written tracing by the EEG machine. The EEG technician attaches electrodes to the scalp and to an amplifier that amplifies the patient's brain waves more than a million times. The technician looks for three distinct types of waves. The occipital alpha wave is an indicator of healthy brain function. This wave comes from the back of the head. Delta waves are normally found in infants and during deep sleep. They are slow, irregular waves that are rarely found in waking adults. A decrease in brain activity shows up as a theta wave, which is a slow, rhythmic wave.

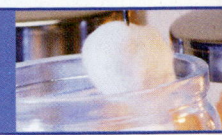

PROCEDURE 46-3 Prepare a Patient for an Electroencephalogram

Theory and Rationale

The EEG technician will ask the patient to remain motionless in a comfortable position, generally lying supine or in a reclining chair, while 16 to 25 electrodes are attached to the scalp. The electrodes are flat metal disks that are applied with a washable paste or adhesive. The placement of electrodes does not require shaving.

There is very little risk involved in performing an EEG. Although the EEG machine records electrical activity in the brain, the patient should be informed that no electricity will pass into the body, and there is no danger of electrocution. The patient should not feel anything during the procedure. If the patient is prone to seizures, which is a common reason for ordering an EEG, the portion of the test involving flashing lights may trigger this response. The EEG technician has been specially trained for this event should it occur.

To ensure an accurate reading, the patient must follow certain pretesting instructions, such as eliminating caffeine, avoiding smoking and other stimulants, and discontinuing certain medications. It may be your job to ensure that the patient has read, understood, and can comply with all pretesting requirements.

Materials

- EEG machine
- electrodes
- approved EEG electrode adhesive

Competency

(**Conditions**) With the necessary materials, (**Task**) you will be able to assist the physician with an EEG (**Standards**) correctly, within the time determined by the instructor.

1. Identify the patient. Explain the procedure and why the physician has ordered it. Try to allay any anxiety the patient might be feeling.
2. Verify that the patient has followed pretesting procedures—avoiding caffeine and other stimulants and eating a well-balanced diet to avoid hypoglycemia.
3. Instruct the patient to remain absolutely motionless during the baseline reading. Even tongue or eyelid movements will alter the baseline.
4. Connect the electrodes to the patient's scalp with the appropriate adhesive.
5. If a sleep EEG has been ordered, the patient should not alter his or her sleeping patterns and avoid using sleep aids.
6. The patient will be shown flickering lights to stimulate the brain. This activity will be recorded by the technician.
7. Remove the electrodes from the patient's scalp. If the patient has been lying supine for the exam, help him or her to a sitting position. The patient should remain seated for a minimum of 1 minute to avoid dizziness caused by orthostatic hypotension.
8. Document the procedure in the patient's chart.

Patient Education

Make sure the patient understands that although the machine records electrical activity within the brain, there is no risk of electrocution. Reinforce that there should be no pain or discomfort during the examination.

Charting Example

06/17/XX 10:00 a.m. EEG performed by Dr. J. Lee. Patient verified she did not use stimulants 48 hours prior to appointment and had a well-balanced meal. Patient tolerated the procedure well and will be given the test results by Dr. Lee. Jason Santos, RMA (AMT)

Disorders and Diseases of the Central Nervous System

CNS diseases and disorders involve the brain and the spinal cord. Cerebral vascular accidents account for a great portion of conditions affecting the brain. Cerebrovascular disease (CVD) is usually a result of atherosclerosis of the cerebral arteries, which deprives the brain of oxygen and is one cause of dementia (∞ see Chapter 35 for a discussion of atherosclerosis). Traumatic insults are another major cause. Other conditions affecting the CNS include epilepsy, multiple sclerosis, Parkinson's disease, and disk disorders.

Cerebrovascular Accidents

Cerebrovascular accidents (**CVA**), also referred to as strokes, may be the result of three vascular conditions in the brain (Figure 46-5 ◆).

- An embolus may lodge in an artery, causing an occlusion and depriving distal brain tissue supplied by that artery of oxygen and nutrition.
- A thrombus may occlude an artery and block distal circulation.
- A vessel rupture, usually from an aneurysm, may hemorrhage into the brain tissue. Malignant hypertension may also cause the rupture.

Regardless of the cause, prompt assessment and intervention are necessary to prevent permanent brain damage or death.

Symptoms of CVA vary, depending on the pathology, location, and extent of the event. Commonly, the person complains of headache and loss of nerve and muscle function on one side of the body (**hemiparesis**). Speech difficulties are typical, and the patient may appear confused. Loss of consciousness is an ominous sign.

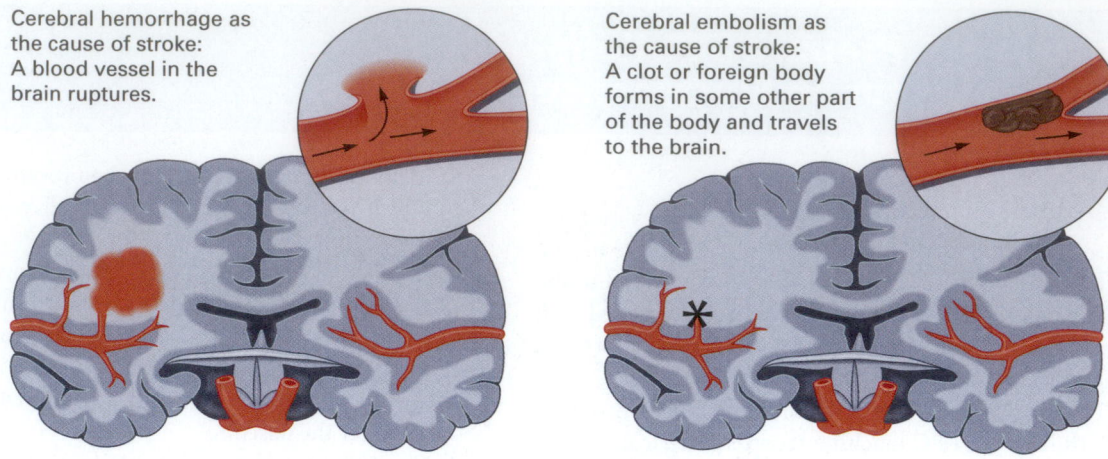

Cerebral hemorrhage as the cause of stroke: A blood vessel in the brain ruptures.

Cerebral embolism as the cause of stroke: A clot or foreign body forms in some other part of the body and travels to the brain.

STROKE

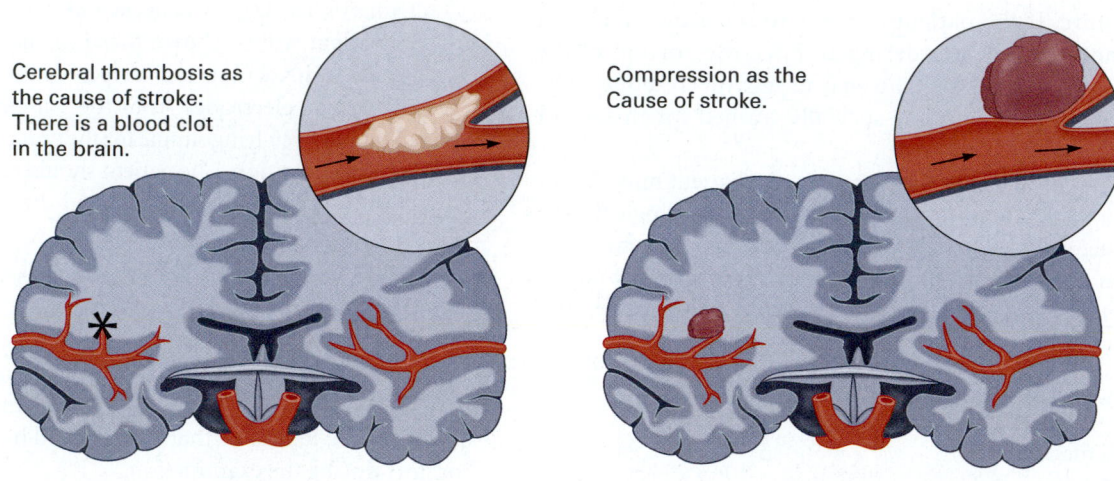

Cerebral thrombosis as the cause of stroke: There is a blood clot in the brain.

Compression as the Cause of stroke.

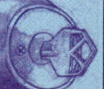

Figure 46-5 ◆ Causes of stroke.

CVAs are considered life threatening. Patients are transported to an emergency facility where anticoagulant and thrombolytic agents are administered to increase blood flow to the affected area. When the insult is the result of a "bleed," surgery may be performed to halt the hemorrhage. Surgery may also be required to reduce pressure on the brain caused by edema. Prognosis is unpredictable and varies according to the type, location, and extent of the insult.

In Practice

Mr. Johanson's son calls the office to schedule an appointment for his father. He states that his father is complaining of a headache and that his left eye is drooping and his speech is slurred. What should the medical assistant tell the patient's son? What are the symptoms and signs associated with cerebrovascular accident (CVA)?

Transient Ischemic Attack

Transient ischemic attacks (**TIA**), caused by brief periods of reduced blood flow to the cerebrum, exhibit symptoms similar to but often less severe than those of a cerebral vascular accident.

Keys to Success
ASPIRIN THERAPY

To reduce the debilitating effects of CVA from thrombus or embolus, the medical community is advocating immediate self-intervention by chewing a single adult-dose aspirin. This is also recommended for anyone displaying the symptoms of a TIA or heart attack.

TIAs usually resolve within 24 hours with little or no residual affects. They are considered a warning sign of possible impending CVA.

Epilepsy

Epilepsy is a chronic disorder characterized by seizure activity in the form of involuntary muscular contractions. The etiology is variable. One possible cause is the electrical disruption of normal brain activity by chemical imbalances, including alcohol withdrawal, poisoning or drug toxicity, eclampsia (severe toxemia of pregnancy), metabolic disease conditions such as diabetes, and the accumulation of waste products in blood when kidneys are not functioning properly. Other causes are CNS infections, CVA, or trauma to the brain.

Seizures occur randomly, as brain impulses are chaotic. Three types of epilepsy seizures are grand mal, petit mal, and status epilepticus.

- The most severe **tonic-clonic** seizures are typical of grand mal epilepsy. Patients frequently experience a warning of impending seizure, called an **aura.** Auras may take the form of distinct odors, special sounds, dizziness, spots before the eyes, tingling in the fingers or toes, and/or loss of consciousness. The seizures are bilaterally symmetrical, involve the entire body, and have no local onset. Following the seizure, the individual is usually unconscious for a brief time and later has no memory of the event. This is called a **postictal** state.
- In petit mal epilepsy, the person, usually a child, experiences brief periods—a few seconds—of unconsciousness. These fleeting periods may go unnoticed as the child blinks or stares briefly into space.
- Status epilepticus is a series of repetitive seizures during which the patient does not regain consciousness. This is a true medical emergency that requires prompt intervention.

Diagnosis of epilepsy is based on a history of recurrent seizure activity, EEG, MRI, and CT scan. Treatment involves anticonvulsant drug therapy, education about the condition, and counseling. For status epilepticus, anticonvulsants are administered to stop the seizures and reduce the possibility of cerebral hypoxia or anoxia and the resulting permanent or fatal damage.

There is no cure for epilepsy. Prognosis is variable, depending on the patient's response to the drug therapy. Compliance is critical to a positive outcome (Figure 46-6 ◆).

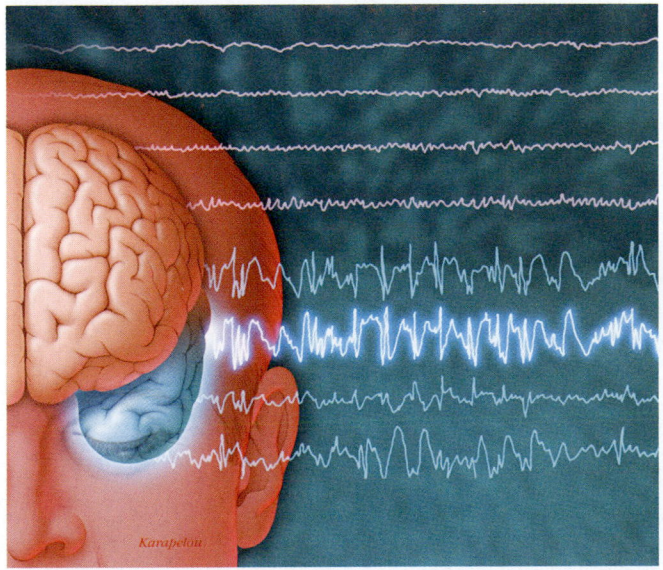

Figure 46-6 ◆ Seizure activity.
Source: Phototake NYC

Amyotrophic Lateral Sclerosis

Amyotrophic lateral sclerosis (**ALS**), also known as Lou Gehrig's disease, is a progressive neuromuscular disease with fatal outcome. The cause is unknown. Muscle weakness and minor involuntary muscular contractions of the arms and hands are early symptoms. The condition progresses to complete loss of neuromuscular function, and the patient requires a ventilator to breathe and tube feedings to compensate for the inability to chew and swallow. But cognitive ability is not affected. Diagnosis is confirmed by EMG and biopsy. Treatment is supportive until death occurs.

Parkinson's Disease

Parkinson's disease is a degenerative condition of the brain characterized by muscular rigidity and **palsy,** or tremors. This slowly progressing chronic condition typically has onset in later life. Fine tremors of the hands are noted, followed by the shaking or nodding of the head. Movements become slower and the facial muscles stiffen. Ambulation becomes a shuffling gait.

The cause of Parkinson's is unknown, but there is a deficiency in the production of the neurotransmitter dopamine. While not a cure, drug therapy with L-dopa and anti-cholinergic drugs helps to replace the missing dopamine. Patients are encouraged to avoid alcohol consumption. Physical therapy is helpful in relieving stiffness and muscle cramps. At present there is no known cure for this debilitating disease.

Multiple Sclerosis

Multiple sclerosis (MS), also a chronic disorder, is characterized by the progressive destruction of the myelin sheath of the nerve and progressive disability. The specific cause is unknown; however, immune, viral, and genetic etiologies have been suggested. Transient motor and sensory disturbances occur and are variable in location, depending on the location of the myelin sheath damage. The vision may become impaired and muscles may weaken. **Exacerbation** is common.

Diagnosis of MS is based on a physical examination, history, CSF analysis, CT scans, and MRIs of the CNS. The goal of treatment is to relieve symptoms and avert exacerbation of the condition. Drug therapy includes the use of adrenocorticotropic hormones. Patients are encouraged to avoid stress and extreme temperatures. There is no known cure for MS and prognosis is variable, depending on the involvement and location of the insulted myelin sheath.

Headache

Headache, also known as **cephalgia,** is diffuse acute or chronic pain occurring in any part of the head. Often the cause is not identifiable; however, the pain results from the irritation of sensory nerve endings in the head or neck. The individual may describe the pain as diffuse, dull, aching, sharp, acute, intense, throbbing, or almost unbearable.

Diagnosis is determined from history and physical examination. Imaging and neurological studies, including EEG, help to identify the underlying pathology and rule out severe pathology. Analgesic drug therapy helps to relieve pain, and stress reduction and massage may be helpful as well.

Migraine headaches are intense, throbbing, and incapacitating. They are thought to be the result of changes in cerebral blood flow—vasoconstriction followed by vasodilation of the arterioles. **Prodromal** symptoms are common, such as photophobia, tinnitus, flashing lights, and cravings for sweets or certain foods. Treatment includes bed rest in a darkened room, analgesics, ergot preparations, and relaxation exercises. Prophylaxis with beta-blockers may be helpful.

Infectious Conditions of the Central Nervous System

Infectious or inflammatory conditions that affect the central nervous system include encephalitis, meningitis, and brain abscess.

Encephalitis

Encephalitis is inflammation of the brain. It can be caused by a virus that is often transmitted to humans from birds or horses via mosquito bite. It may also be a sequela of viral infections such as mumps, measles, chickenpox, influenza, rubella, and mononucleosis. Another form of encephalitis is caused by infection with the herpes simplex virus and has the highest mortality rate when left untreated. Encephalitis caused by the West Nile virus (WNV) occurred only rarely in the United States until recently. Today this form of encephalitis has reached endemic proportions as the virus spreads across the country and into Canada and Mexico.

Symptoms of encephalitis include classic infectious CNS symptoms such as headache, fever, malaise, lethargy, visual disturbances, nausea and vomiting, and decreased level of consciousness. The disease progresses rapidly, causing **nuchal rigidity** (stiff neck), seizures, and loss of consciousness.

Diagnosis is confirmed with a patient history, physical examination, blood tests, and CSF analysis. Treatment involves drug therapy with antiviral agents, steroids, antipyretics, and anticonvulsants, with body system support. Prognosis is variable, depending on the causative agent, the extent and duration of the infection, the age and physical condition of the patient, and the patient's response to treatment.

Eradicating mosquito breeding sites is a primary preventive measure against encephalitis. Mosquito bites can be avoided by installing screens in doors and windows and by using insect repellents and wearing long-sleeved shirts and long pants outdoors.

Meningitis

Meningitis is an inflammation of the meninges, the coverings of the brain and spinal cord. The causative microorganism may be viral or bacterial. Common bacterial agents are *Hemophilus influenzae* type B, *Streptococcus pneumoniae,* and *Neisseria meningitidis.*

As with other CNS disorders, patients with meningitis experience headache, fever, dizziness, blurred vision, and motor problems. A common symptom is nuchal rigidity, indicated when the patient resists any movement of the head. Meningitis is considered a medical emergency and requires prompt diagnosis and aggressive treatment. Vigorous antibiotic therapy and support of systems are the treatments of choice. Prognosis is variable and depends on how quickly diagnosis and treatment are provided.

Brain Abscess

Infectious microorganisms that migrate to the brain from other infections in the body may cause a brain abscess (Figure 46-7 ◆). These **pyogenic** microorganisms may be in encapsulated or free form in the brain tissue. Body infections with a tendency to move

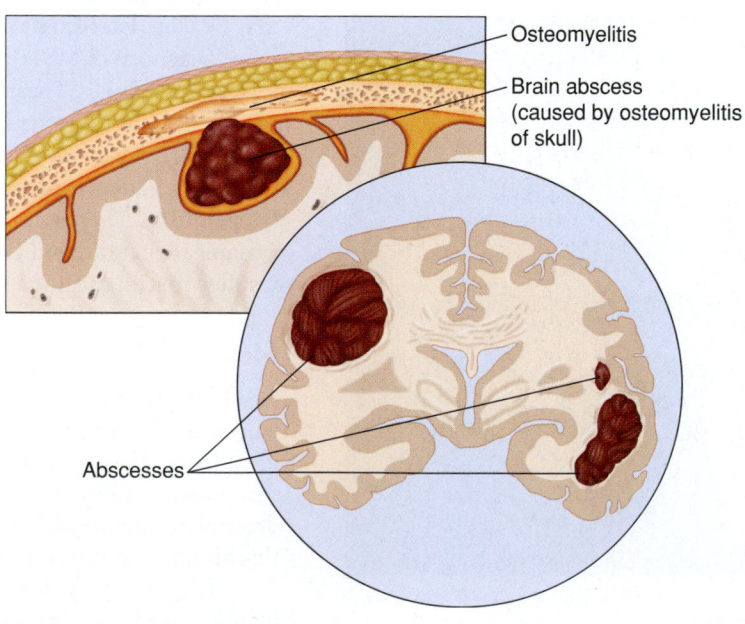

Figure 46-7 ◆ Abscesses of the brain.

to the brain are sinusitis, otitis media, mastoiditis, endocarditis, and pneumonia.

A patient with a brain abscess has a fever and often complains of a headache. Neurological symptoms vary, depending on the location and extent of the abscess. In addition to headache and fever, dizziness, syncope, drowsiness, visual problems, nausea and vomiting, hemiplegia, pallor, and slowed heart rate or respiratory effort are characteristic symptoms. The eyes usually look to the insult.

Imaging studies, including radiographs of the skull, CT scans, and cerebral angiography, are combined with examination of the CSF and measurement of the pressure in the cerebrospinal canal to arrive at a diagnosis. Treatment consists of aggressive antibiotic therapy and support of body systems. Outcome is variable.

Brain Tumors

Tumors of the brain arise from abnormal cell development and are benign or malignant. A malignant tumor may be the primary or secondary metastatic site. As it grows, the tumor exerts pressure on nearby tissues and causes signs and symptoms.

Symptoms include headache, vomiting, and changes in vision, balance and coordination, and muscle strength. Speech, personality, and mental function may also be affected. Diagnostic testing includes MRI, CT scan, EEG, lumbar puncture and examination of CSF, and biopsy of excised tissue. Treatment is primarily surgical to remove the tumor, but can also include chemotherapy and radiation. Other medications are prescribed to reduce or eliminate symptoms created by the pressure or to relieve symptoms associated with chemotherapy, radiation, or the progression of the disease.

Head Trauma

Head injuries are often classified as open or closed. In open head injuries, the skull is fractured and the skin is broken. In closed head injuries, the cranium is not fractured.

Symptoms of head injuries include altered levels of consciousness and mental status, unequal pupils, blood or fluid coming from the ears or nose, severe head pain, alterations in vital signs, dizziness, blurred vision, ringing in the ears, and **projectile vomiting.**

Brain injuries may also have an effect on a patient's posture. It should be noted if the patient displays **decerebrate** or **decorticate posture.**

Direct brain injuries such as lacerations, punctures, and bruises are caused by the fragments or edges of fractured cranial bones. Indirect brain injuries are the result of the impact of the brain on the cranium when force is applied to the skull. Hematomas, concussions, and contusions are indirect brain injuries.

Hematomas are collections of blood that form above or between the meninges (Figures 46-8 ◆ and 46-9 ◆). An epidural or extradural hematoma is above the dura mater, just under the cranial bones. A subdural hematoma lies under the dura mater and above the arachnoid meninges. Some hematomas resolve spontaneously with bed rest, while others may require

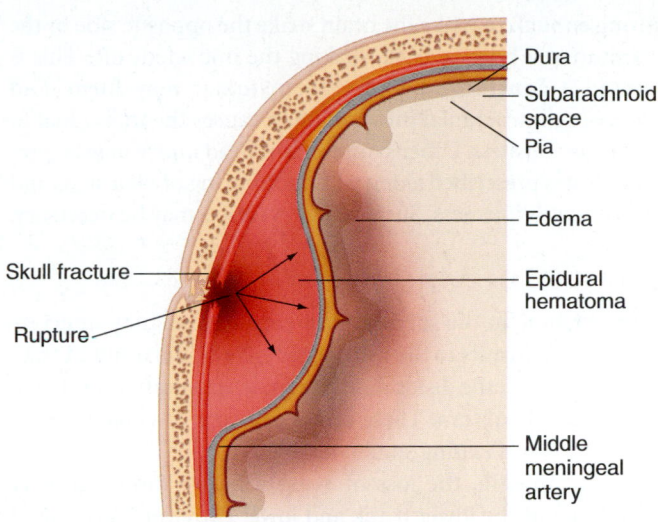

Figure 46-8 ◆ Extradural hematoma.

surgical intervention. The extent and duration of the hematoma as well as its resolution determine whether there are any residual effects.

Concussions and Contusions

A concussion is caused by a blow to the head or an acceleration/deceleration type of injury. The force is transferred through the skull to the brain with no detectable or permanent structural damage. The victim may feel dizzy, often complains of a headache, and may temporarily lose consciousness. Brief, temporary amnesia is not uncommon. The insult usually resolves spontaneously with no residual effects.

A contusion, a more severe form of head injury, is a bruise in the brain where blood vessels are ruptured. The impact is

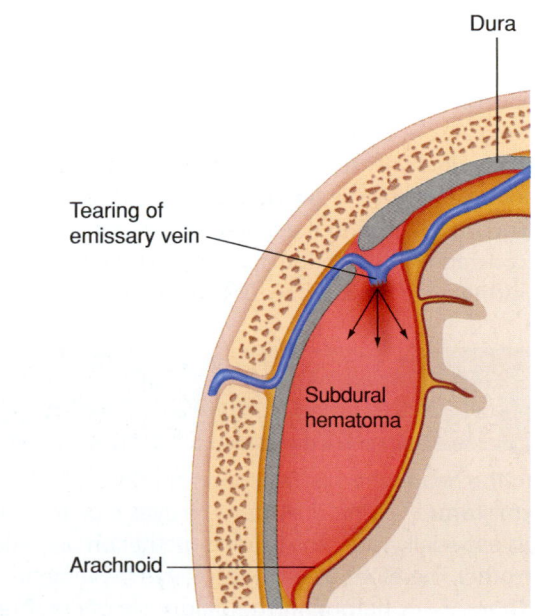

Figure 46-9 ◆ Subdural hematoma.

strong enough to make the brain strike the opposite side of the cranium and bounce back, striking the impacted side. This is termed a **contrecoup** injury. Hematomas may form, and increasing intracranial pressure often causes the individual to lose consciousness. Other symptoms of head injury may be present. Rest is prescribed along with monitoring of vital signs and level of consciousness. Surgical intervention may be necessary.

Spinal Cord Injuries

The vertebrae in the spinal column are separated by intervertebral disks. Insults to the spinal cord may be the result of fractured vertebrae, the dislocation of vertebrae, or other trauma to the vertebral column. These create pressure or edema on the spinal cord and exiting spinal nerves.

Paraplegia, the loss of sensation and motor activity (paralysis) of the lower trunk and lower extremities, is caused by injury to the spinal cord in the thoracic or lumbar region. Ambulatory function may be decreased or completely lost, and control of bowel and bladder function is impaired.

Quadriplegia, the paralysis of the entire trunk and all four extremities, is caused by an insult to the spinal cord in the cervical area. Respiration may be impaired and require mechanical assistance.

Diagnosis of a spinal cord injury is confirmed by observation, physical examination, and history of the insult. Neurological assessment combined with imaging studies helps to identify the location and possible source of the paralysis. Treatment involves reducing pressure on the spinal cord and spinal nerves. Stabilization of fractures and other injuries helps to prevent extension of the insult. Prognosis is variable, but permanent damage to the nerves is possible, as destroyed nerve tissue does not regenerate. Rehabilitation is encouraged.

Impotence is often a side effect for a male patient with a spinal cord injury. Mechanical and drug-based methods for achieving an erection should be explored. Counseling and referrals to a specialist are helpful.

Disk Disorders

Insult to the intervertebral disks from trauma or degenerative disease is one cause of back pain. The cervical and lumbar disks are the most vulnerable, since the cervical and lumbar vertebrae are not held in place by the rib cage as the thoracic vertebrae are. Traumatic insult to the spinal column, whether from a fall, an acceleration-deceleration injury or poor body mechanics when lifting, may squeeze the disk or cause it to bulge or herniate. In a degenerative disease, the disk deteriorates. Regardless of the cause, the damaged disk exerts pressure on the spinal cord and/or the spinal nerves in that region. This pressure causes pain and can lead to loss of function in the area of the body supplied by the compromised nerve.

Imaging studies, patient history, and neurological examination aid in diagnosis. It is not always possible to resolve disk problems. Pain usually dictates the course of treatment. Some bulging disks may resolve spontaneously with rest; others may require surgical intervention. Pain relief may be achieved with rest, drug therapy, physical therapy, or, if necessary, surgery. Prognosis is variable, depending on the cause, location, and extent of the insult.

Sciatica, also known as *spinal stenosis,* is the narrowing of the vertebral canal. The resulting compression of the spinal cord and connecting nerves within the canal cause back and radiating leg pain. Some patients experience numbness in these areas. Increased activity worsens the symptoms. The cause of sciatica may be arthritis or aging. Diagnostic studies include MRI, CT, X-rays, and myelogram. Medications to reduce pain and inflammation are prescribed. A period of bed rest, applications of heat or cold therapy, and massage may help ease the pain. Surgery is performed only in cases of increasing weakness or debilitating pain.

Diseases of the Peripheral Nervous System

Peripheral nervous system disorders include Bell's palsy, trigeminal neuralgia, and shingles. These acute, nonprogressive conditions affect the cranial and spinal nerves.

Bell's Palsy

Bell's palsy is a disorder of the seventh cranial nerve (also called the facial nerve), which is the peripheral nerve supplying the facial muscles. The individual experiences a sudden onset of unilateral facial paralysis, often awakening with one side of the face drooping, in particular the mouth. Sensation on the affected side is diminished or absent.

The etiology of this disorder is unknown, although it may follow a viral infection. Diagnosis is based on observation, physical examination, and history of time of onset and duration of condition. Treatment consists of steroid drug therapy. Resolution may occur spontaneously, or residual effects may remain indefinitely. The patient is warned to use caution when eating and drinking, as sensations of heat and pain are absent. Many physicians recommend patching the eye on the affected side during sleep to prevent corneal abrasions that might otherwise occur because the eye cannot feel pain.

Trigeminal Neuralgia

Like Bell's palsy, trigeminal **neuralgia** (also called *tic douloureux*) has a sudden onset and is generally unilateral. The region of the face affected is supplied by the fifth cranial nerve, the trigeminal nerve. The pain is extremely sharp and can be

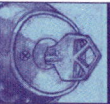

Keys to Success
EYE MOVEMENTS IN HEAD INSULTS

Insults to the head, whether traumatic or infectious, have some symptoms in common. Often the eyes look toward the insult, especially when the insult is greater on one side than the other. Therefore, observation of eye movement—or lack thereof—is helpful in the diagnosis of cerebral insult.

intermittent. One branch or all three branches of the trigeminal nerve may be involved.

The etiology of trigeminal neuralgia is unknown. Diagnosis is based on observation, physical examination, and history. Treatment involves analgesic drug therapy. As a last resort, surgical intervention is performed to cut the nerve and stop the transmission of sensory impulses.

Shingles (Herpes Zoster)

Shingles occurs when the herpes varicella-zoster virus, which remains in a dormant state within the body following a case of chickenpox, is reactivated. Often triggered by emotional or physical stress, this condition is characterized by intense pain and small blisters that follow the affected **dermatome(s)** under the skin. The affected area is often hypersensitive to the touch, and the pain can be burning and tingling. Most incidences are unilateral and do not cross the midline.

The trained clinician recognizes the typical blister-type eruptions and the pattern of distribution along the nerve routes, which, combined with a history of chickenpox infection, confirm the diagnosis. Drug therapy comprises antiviral medications, steroids, analgesics, sedatives, and antipyretics. If the blisters become infected, antibiotics are prescribed. The condition usually resolves in less than a month. Recurrences seldom occur. If the pain persists longer than a month and the blisters have cleared, the condition is termed post-herpetic neuralgia.

Shingles is not contagious to people who have had chickenpox, but those who have never had chickenpox are at risk for developing it after exposure to the herpes varicella-zoster virus. There is no known prevention at this time; however, research is ongoing in the area of preventive vaccines.

? — Critical Thinking Question 46-1 —

What the patient thought was an allergic reaction may in fact be shingles, given the pain level and past history of varicella. What information can Dawn give the patient? How should Dawn handle the information that the patient's girlfriend ruptured some of the blisters?

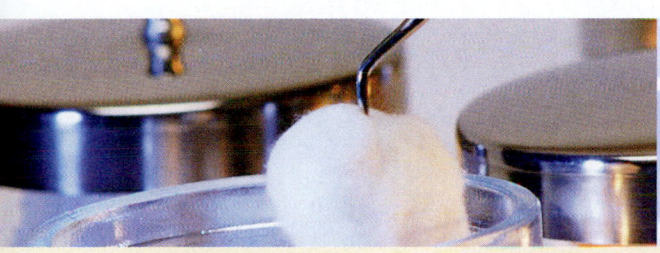

REVIEW

Chapter Summary

- Many opportunities exist for the medical assistant in neurology and neurosurgery offices. Many of these opportunities are in the administrative arena; however, clinical positions are generally available also.
- The central nervous system consists of the brain and spinal cord. The peripheral nervous system consists of cranial nerves, spinal nerves, and the sympathetic and parasympathetic nerves of the autonomic nervous system.
- The neuron is the functional unit of the nervous system. It is made up of a nerve cell body, an axon, and dendrites. Nervous system impulses cross the synaptic gap between neurons via neurotransmitters.
- The nervous system has two physiological divisions: the somatic or voluntary system, controlled by conscious thought, and the autonomic or involuntary system, controlled by homeostatic reactions of the body to sympathetic and parasympathetic stimuli. The sympathetic nervous system prepares the body for the "fight-or-flight" response to perceived dangers. The parasympathetic system applies the "brakes" to return the body to its normal physiological state.
- Neurological assessment utilizes a variety of tools to evaluate mental status, speech, mood or emotional state, cognitive functioning, level of consciousness, and sensory and motor functions. The Glasgow Coma Scale is a standardized system used to rapidly assess brain activity, level of consciousness, possible insults to the brain, and possible outcome based on eye, verbal, and motor responses. Lumbar punctures are a diagnostic procedure involving the analysis of cerebrospinal fluid.
- A CVA, or stroke, may be caused by an embolus, thrombus, or vessel rupture. Symptoms include headache, loss of unilateral nerve and muscle function, speech difficulties and confusion, and possible loss of consciousness.
- Transient ischemic attacks exhibit symptoms similar to those of a CVA. TIAs usually resolve within 24 hours with little or no residual effects.
- Epilepsy is characterized by seizures. Tonic-clonic seizures are observed in grand mal epilepsy. Petit mal seizures are brief periods of unconsciousness. Status epilepticus, repetitive seizures from which the patient does not regain consciousness, is a medical emergency requiring prompt intervention with anticonvulsive drugs.
- Parkinson's disease is a chronic degenerative condition of the brain characterized by muscular rigidity and palsy (tremors). Multiple sclerosis, also a chronic disorder, results

Chapter Summary (continued)

in the progressive destruction of the myelin sheath of the nerve and progressive disability.

■ A headache, or cephalgia, is diffuse acute or chronic pain occurring in any part of the head when sensory nerve endings in the head or neck are irritated. Migraine headaches may be caused by changes in cerebral blood flow.

■ Head trauma can be classified as an open head injury (skull is fractured and skin is broken) or a closed head injury (skull is not fractured). Direct brain injuries (lacerations, punctures, bruises) are caused by fragments or edges of fractured cranial bones. Indirect brain injuries include hematomas, concussion, and contusion. Hematomas are collections of blood above the meninges (epidural) or between the dura mater and arachnoid meninges (subdural).

■ A concussion is the result of a blow to the head or an acceleration/deceleration injury. A contusion is a bruise to the brain in which blood vessels are ruptured.

■ Spinal cord injuries may result in paraplegia or quadriplegia. Injuries may be caused by fractured or dislocated vertebrae or other trauma to the vertebral column.

■ Infectious conditions of the CNS include encephalitis, meningitis, and brain abscess. Encephalitis, inflammation of the brain, is usually caused by a virus or may be a sequela of a viral infection. Meningitis is an inflammation of the meninges caused by a virus or bacteria. Infectious microorganisms that migrate to the brain from other infections in the body may cause brain abscess.

■ Diseases of the peripheral nervous system include Bell's palsy, trigeminal neuralgia, and shingles (herpes zoster). Bell's palsy is characterized by a sudden onset of unilateral facial paralysis. Trigeminal neuralgia also has a sudden onset and is generally unilateral. Shingles occurs when a dormant herpes varicella-zoster virus in the body is reactivated.

Chapter Review

Multiple Choice

1. Which of the following terms means "sharp nerve pain"?
   a. Neuron
   b. Neurodynia
   c. Neuralgia
   d. Nuchal rigidity

2. Which of the following terms refers to a tough membrane that forms on the outer layer of the meninges?
   a. Arachoid meninges
   b. Dura mater
   c. Pia mater
   d. Contra mater

3. The nervous system has how many anatomical divisions?
   a. 2
   b. 1
   c. 3
   d. 4

4. Amyotrophic lateral sclerosis (ALS) is also known as
   a. grand mal seizures.
   b. multiple sclerosis.
   c. Parkinson's disease.
   d. Lou Gehrig's disease.

5. Shingles occurs when _____ is reactivated in the patient's system.
   a. hepatitis A virus
   b. *Streptococcus pneumoniae*
   c. trigeminal neuralgia
   d. herpes varicella-zoster

True/False

T F 1. Infectious conditions of the CNS include encephalitis, meningitis, and brain abscess.

T F 2. Encephalitis, or inflammation of the brain, is usually caused by a virus or may be a sequela of a viral infection.

T F 3. Symptoms of shingles include headache, loss of unilateral nerve and muscle function, speech difficulties and confusion, and possible loss of consciousness.

T F 4. Tumors of the brain arise from abnormal cell development and are benign or malignant.

T F 5. There are 34 pairs of spinal nerves, which originate from the spinal cord.

T F 6. The spinal nerves carry impulses to and from the brain.

T F 7. Taste perception is one of many tests for neurological function.

T F 8. A concussion is more severe than a contusion.

T F 9. Peripheral nervous system disorders include Bell's palsy, trigeminal neuralgia, and shingles.

T F 10. The inferior rectus muscle causes the eye to look up, and the superior rectus muscle causes the eye to look down.

Short Answer

1. An assessment of neurological function involves cranial nerve function. Which areas are tested?

2. What are the three vascular conditions in the brain that cause CVA, or stroke?

Chapter Review (continued)

3. What is the Glasgow Coma Scale?

4. Name three types of epilepsy seizures.

5. Which organs are affected by meningitis?

Research

1. Recent studies suggest that college-bound teens are more likely to contract meningitis while living in dormitories.

Where in your community are vaccinations for meningitis offered?

2. What is the Romberg test, and how would a medical assistant assist the physician in performing this test?

Externship Application Experience

A patient comes to the reception desk with a possible diagnosis of shingles. Children are playing in the same area. What are the implications of allowing this patient to wait in the reception area with children and other adult patients? What is the appropriate action to take?

Resource Guide

American Academy of Neurology
1080 Montreal Ave.
St. Paul, MN 55116
1-800-879-1960
www.aan.com

American Association of Neurosurgery
5550 Meadowbrook Drive
Rolling Meadows, IL 60008
1-888-566-2267
www.neurosurgery.org

American Neurological Association
5841 Cedar Lake Rd., Suite #204
Minneapolis, MN 55416
956-545-6284
www.aneuroa.org

National Multiple Sclerosis Society
733 Third Ave.
New York, NY 10017
1-800-344-4867
www.nationalmssociety.com

National Parkinson Foundation
1501 N.W. 9th Avenue / Bob Hope Road
Miami, FL 33136-1494
1-800-327-4545
www.parkinson.org

National Spinal Cord Injury Association
6701 Democracy Blvd., Suite 300-9
Bethesda, MD 20817
301-588-6959
www.spinalcord.org

National Stroke Association
9707 E. Easter Lane
Englewood, CA 80112
1-800-strokes
www.stroke.org

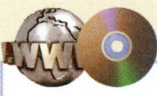

Med**Media**

http://www.MyMAKit.com

More on this chapter, including interactive resources, can be found on the Student CD-ROM accompanying this textbook and on http://www.MyMAKit.com.

CHAPTER 47

Mental Health

Case Study

Michael Yager, CMA (AAMA), is doing a brief rotation in a mental health clinic. He is taking patient information when he meets Yolanda, a high school senior who has brought her 23-year-old brother in for a followup on his recent diagnosis of schizophrenia. While speaking to Yolanda, Michael observes several cuts on her forearms. Yolanda quickly folds her arms when she realizes he has noticed the marks.

Sensing her apprehension, Michael asks Yolanda how her family is coping with the new diagnosis and the changes in her brother. He asks if she has spoken to a counselor or if she would like to. After several minutes of conversation, Yolanda admits that she often cuts herself to deal with the stress of her brother's illness for her and her family. She says the cutting provides relief, and she has sometimes thought that killing herself would be better for her parents because they constantly worry and fight about how to pay for medications, mental health support, and supervision for her brother. Her mother often cries and says she will never be able to retire and travel with her husband because her son will have to live with them forever, "cheating" them out of their golden years, grandchildren, and freedom.

Yolanda tells Michael that she does not wish to speak to anyone about this and makes Michael promise not to tell the physician either. After all, she says, she is not a patient at this clinic, "so it's no one's business."

Objectives

After completing this chapter, you should be able to:

- Define and spell the key terminology in the chapter.
- Define the medical assistant's role in the mental health field.
- Discuss the cognitive functions of the brain.
- Discuss the concept of mental wellness.
- Describe the symptoms and treatment of schizophrenia.
- Describe the symptoms and treatment of various mood disorders.
- Describe the symptoms and treatment of personality disorders.
- Describe the symptoms and treatment of anxiety disorders.
- Describe the forms, symptoms, and treatment of somatoform disorders.
- Explain gender identity disorder.
- Describe mental retardation.
- Describe the forms, symptoms, and treatment of dementia.
- List and describe common mental disorders that originate in childhood.
- Describe disorders related to substance abuse.
- Explain how mental disorders are assessed and diagnosed.
- List the general treatments for mental disorders.

MedMedia

http://www.MyMAKit.com

Additional interactive resources and activities for this chapter can be found on http://www.MyMAKit.com. For a video, audio glossary, tips, legal and ethical scenarios, job scenarios, quizzes, and games related to the content of this chapter, please access the accompanying CD-ROM in this book.

Video
Audio Glossary
Legal and Ethical Scenario: *Mental Health*
On the Job Scenario: *Mental Health*
Multiple Choice Quiz
Games: Crossword, Strikeout, and Spelling Bee
Tips
HIPAA Quiz

✚ MEDICAL ASSISTING STANDARDS

CAAHEP ENTRY-LEVEL STANDARDS	ABHES ENTRY-LEVEL COMPETENCIES
■ Perform within scope of practice (psychomotor) ■ Explore issue of confidentiality as it applies to the medical assistant (cognitive) ■ Apply ethical behaviors, including honesty/integrity in performance of medical assisting practice (affective) ■ Apply local, state and federal health care legislation and regulation appropriate to the medical assisting practice setting (psychomotor) ■ Recognize the importance of local, state and federal legislation and regulations in the practice setting (affective) ■ Describe the normal function of each body system (cognitive) ■ Identify common pathology related to each body system (cognitive) ■ Analyze pathology as it relates to the interaction of body systems (cognitive) ■ Discuss implications for disease and disability when homeostasis is not maintained (cognitive) ■ Describe implications for treatment related to pathology (cognitive) ■ Use language/verbal skills that enable patients' understanding (affective) ■ Apply critical thinking skills in performing patient assessment and care (affective) ■ Document accurately in the patient record (psychomotor) ■ Demonstrate diversity in approaching patients and families (affective) ■ Develop and maintain a current list of community resources related to patients' healthcare needs (psychomotor)	■ Project a positive attitude. ■ Maintain confidentiality at all times. ■ Be a "team player." ■ Be cognizant of ethical boundaries. ■ Exhibit initiative. ■ Adapt to change. ■ Evidence a responsible attitude. ■ Be courteous and diplomatic. ■ Conduct work within scope of education, training, and ability. ■ Interview and take a patient history. ■ Prepare and maintain examination and treatment area. ■ Prepare and administer oral and parenteral medications as directed by the physician. ■ Maintain medication and immunization records.

Introduction

Psychiatry is the branch of medicine that focuses on the diagnosis, treatment, and prevention of mental disorders. **Psychology** deals with normal and abnormal mental processes and behavior. It is the study of the mind, its functional processes, and its relationship to behavior and environmental processes. Patients with mental disorders may be treated by either a **psychiatrist** or a **psychologist,** or by other specialists in the field.

■ The psychiatrist, a medical doctor with special training in the field of psychiatry, diagnoses and treats mental disorders. Treatment may consist of therapy sessions, drug therapy, or electroshock therapy.

■ The psychologist has a doctorate in psychology. Psychologists may specialize in clinical or behavioral psychology, child psychology, development psychology, industrial

Key Terminology

addiction—repetitive and dependent behavior usually involving legal or illegal substance abuse

affect—the observable emotional reaction associated with an experience

antidepressant—medication used to treat depression

antipsychotic—medication used to treat psychotic episodes

cognitive—of or pertaining to the mental processes of judgment, perception, reasoning, and memory

comorbid—denoting coexisting, unrelated medical diseases or conditions

dementia—diminished mental or cognitive functioning with onset after the age of 18 years

dependence—state of addiction to certain drugs; rapid physical withdrawal can cause life-threatening and even fatal reactions

phobia—irrational, obsessive fear of an object, situation, or activity

psychiatrist—medical doctor or physician specializing in the medical treatment of mental illness

psychiatry—branch of medicine that deals with diagnosis, treatment, and prevention of mental disorders

psychologist—specialist in the field of psychology, therapy, and research

psychology—science dealing with normal and abnormal mental processes and behavior

psychosis—abnormal mental coping of the individual who is out of touch with reality

psychotherapeutic—alleviating symptoms of anxiety, depression, and psychosis

psychotherapy—treatment of mental disorders with talk therapy, or counseling

psychotropic—affecting psychic function, behavior, experience, or emotions

tolerance—requiring greater amounts of a substance to achieve the desired effect

Abbreviations

ADHD—attention-deficit hyperactivity disorder

DSM-IV—Diagnostic and Statistical Manual of Mental Disorders

MAO—monoamine oxidase

OCD—obsessive compulsive disorder

ODD—oppositional defiance disorder

PD—personality disorder

PTSD—posttraumatic stress disorder

SAD—seasonal affective disorder

SSRI—selective serotonin reuptake inhibitors

and organizational psychology, educational psychology, social psychology, or forensic psychology. They do not prescribe medications.

- Social workers usually deal with family or behavioral problems.
- Family and marriage counselors are licensed professionals who specialize in couples and family therapy.
- Child therapists specialize in mental health issues concerning children.
- Substance abuse counselors treat individuals with substance abuse history and promote awareness of substance abuse in the general community.
- Correctional rehabilitative counselors usually work within the criminal justice system to counsel prisoners.
- Vocational training counselors assist individuals in finding appropriate vocations and receiving the training to achieve their goals.

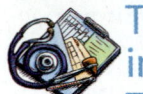

The Medical Assistant's Role in the Mental Health Field

In the field of mental health, many of the opportunities for medical assistants are in the administrative arena, but clinical positions are often available as well (Table 47-1). The psychiatrist may want a patient's weight and certain vital signs obtained. The MA may be assigned to help a patient complete information forms, schedule appointments for diagnostic testing or other services, or obtain precertification. If working with substance abuse counselors, the MA may be responsible for obtaining specimens for screening.

TABLE 47-1 GENERAL GUIDELINES FOR MENTAL HEALTHCARE PROVIDERS

1. Remember that expectations and prejudices complicate communication with the client.
2. You are the *only* person that you can control.
3. Know yourself. This is the most critical aspect of communication with any person.
4. Subtle things about a person's behavior, physical characteristics, and communication style affect our responses to others. Sometimes, we are influenced by things of which we are not aware. What you hear, see, smell, and feel on your first encounter with someone sets up your impression and response to that person.
5. Know which behaviors or traits in others trigger automatic feelings of like and dislike in you.
6. Learn about your biases in communication styles or behavioral patterns. You will probably always have these biases, but you can learn to manage your behavior toward another person's style or behavior.
7. Develop a skill for recognizing your immediate feelings toward others, and develop a set of responses that work in dealing with the situation or person without judgment.
8. Do not judge your clients. You do not have to like your clients, and they do not have to like you. Your goal is to help your clients and to do so fairly. Remember patients' rights.
9. All clients deserve respect and fair treatment.
10. You work in a mental health treatment setting to meet the needs of the client—*not your needs*.
11. Deal with your feelings with someone you trust, *not* with the client. Clients should not help you manage your feelings.
12. Examine your feelings *before* you react.
13. Learn to accept the fact that you do not have to be right; you can "win" even when you appear defeated. Winning an argument with a client is not important, nor is it therapeutic or permissible to argue with clients.
14. You can agree to disagree with others.
15. Remember that the client has to be in agreement with a goal to work on that goal.
16. Feelings are feelings. They are neither right nor wrong, good nor bad. Clients should feel free to tell you their true feelings.
17. People are entitled to feel what they feel. Your job is to help them manage the behavior that results from those feelings.
18. Remember that clients are reacting to illness, hospitalization, loss of control, and fear.
19. Know that people respond to situations with a set of behavioral responses that they have learned throughout life. These may not be healthy responses. The goal is to help the patient to develop healthy coping behaviors.

Source: Miele, Carole G., and England, Teresa, From Nursing Assistant to Clinical Care Associate, *1st Edition © 1999. Reprinted by permission of Pearson Education, Inc. Upper Saddle River, NJ.*

The Anatomy and Physiology of Cognitive Functioning

The brain is a complex organ consisting of many types of neurons and neurotransmitters (Figure 47-1 ◆). Each neuron may be connected by a single synapse, or synaptic gap, to thousands of other synapses for the purpose of communicating the commands of the brain, body, and behavior functions. Neurotransmitters are chemicals that aid in the transmission of electrical impulses from one neuron, or nerve cell, to the next. The neurotransmitter must be received by a receptor on the next neuron in order for a nervous system transmission to cross the synaptic gap. Each neuron may produce a number of neurotransmitters that may be specific or react with many different types of receptors. As the brain processes conscious and unconscious thoughts and memories, the neurons undergo changes that affect the physical structure and chemical substances released by the synaptic gaps. These changes affect the conduction of neuroelectrical impulses and ultimately affect behavior.

The brain maintains the body's homeostasis by reacting to sensory inputs, including emotions and thoughts, with processing and interpretation. Brain impulses signal the autonomic nervous, musculoskeletal, endocrine, and other body systems to respond. As the brain processes different sensory inputs, it prioritizes and places them in different types of memory storage. For example, an image is seen and transmitted from the retina to the thalamus, then to the visual cortex in the occipital lobe of the brain. Simultaneously, the neuron transmissions are analyzed for visual characteristics, such as form and color, as they are analyzed and stored as expressed and implied visual memories, and as memories of the emotional experience. This rapid communication through the neuroelectrical circuitry of the brain is accomplished by excitatory amino acid neurotransmitters such as glutamate and by inhibitory neurotransmitters such as gamma aminobutyric acid and glycine.

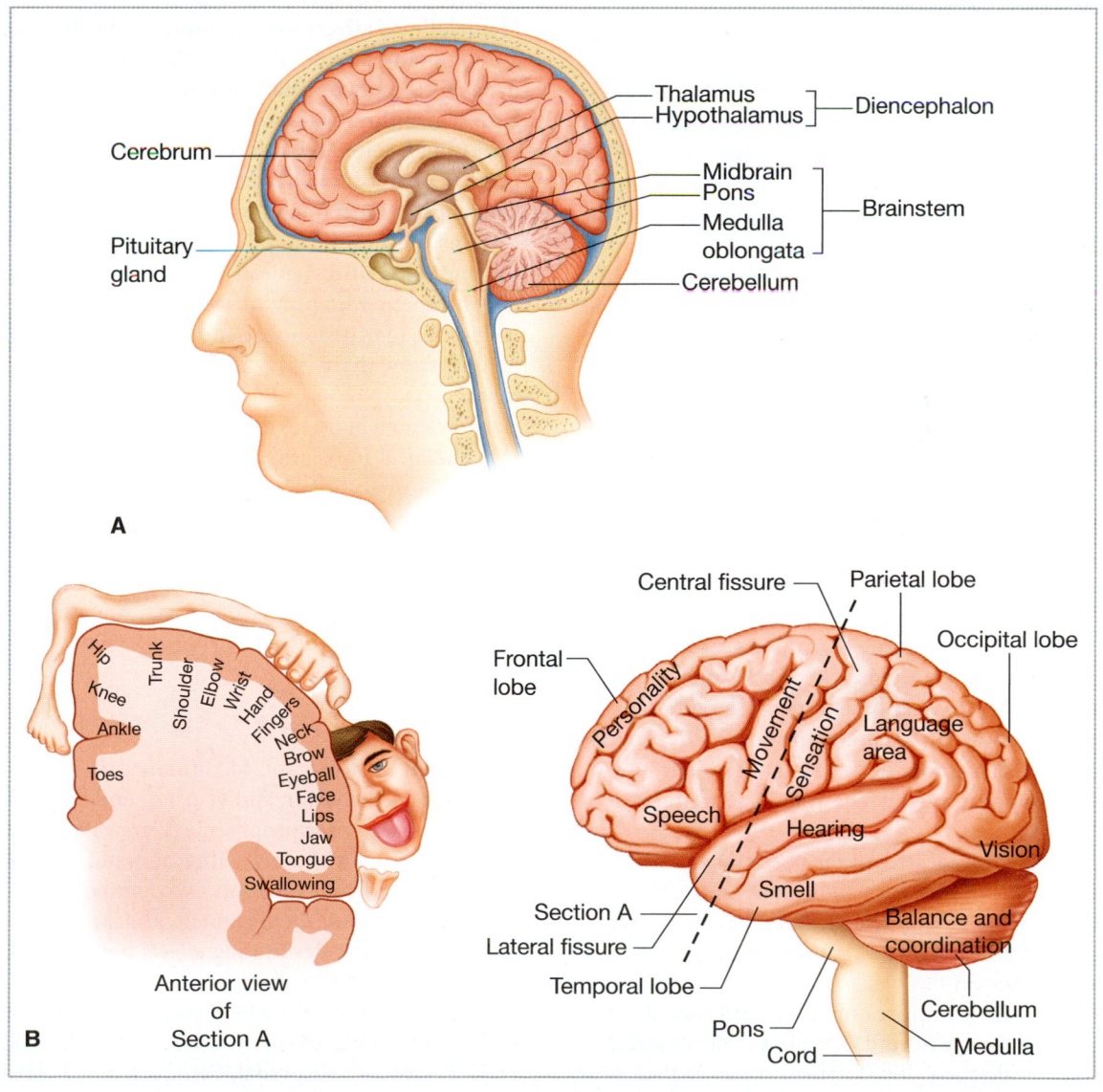

Figure 47-1 ◆ (A) Sagittal section of the brain. (B) Lateral view of the brain.

In addition to excitatory and inhibitory neurotransmitters, there are modulatory neurotransmitters, such as neuropeptides and purines (for example, adenosine), monoamines (norepinephrine, dopamine, serotonin, histamine), and acetylcholine. Neuropeptides and purines aid or inhibit the communication of the neuroelectrical circuitry. Monoamines and acetylcholine function in several ways:

- They determine a person's wakefulness or sleepiness, motivation, and attention span.
- They determine which stimuli are to be stored in memory and the level and type of emotional significance to be attached to each memory.
- They relay emotional feelings throughout the brain that help the patient determine whether to approach, avoid, repeat, fear, cry, or feel neutral in response to events.

Antidepressants, antipsychotics, and other medications utilize the actions of monoamine neurotransmitters to affect emotion and thought processing.

The anatomical regions of the brain are as follows.

- The two cerebral hemispheres contain the frontal, parietal, temporal, and occipital lobes; the basal ganglia; and the cerebral cortical area covering all lobes. The cerebral hemispheres control all the body's voluntary, and some involuntary, activities. Specifically, motion is controlled by the frontal lobes, sensation by the parietal lobes, hearing by the temporal lobes, and vision by the occipital lobes. The basal ganglia are involved in the processing and memory storage of emotions associated with rewarding behaviors such as drinking, eating, and sexual intercourse. The cerebral cortical area is where information from different cortical lobe regions is combined, providing input for logic and planning.
- The middle portion of the brain contains the thalamus, hypothalamus, and hippocampus. The thalamus is a relay station and is also important to perception and pleasure. The hypothalamus, located on the underside of the thalamus, is the master control for the autonomic nervous system. It controls hormone secretion, body temperature, and emotions. The hippocampus acts as a gateway for the passage of new memories into areas of permanent storage in the brain. In addition to converting short-term memory to permanent long-term memory, the hippocampus plays a role in recalling spatial relationships.
- The cerebellum is located on the posterior aspect of the brain. It is responsible for equilibrium and both involuntary and voluntary muscle control. The effects of alcohol on the cerebellum can be seen in the staggering of an intoxicated person.
- The brain stem comprises the pons and medulla and extends into the spinal cord. The pons controls wakefulness, mental alertness, and sleepiness states. As the lowest part of the brainstem, the medulla (medulla oblongata) regulates the heart rate, respirations, blood pressure, and reflexes, including coughing, sneezing, swallowing, and vomiting.

Mental Wellness

Mental wellness is a state of being. It is not necessarily an absence of mental problems but rather a capacity to cope in healthy ways with the pressures of daily living. A positive outlook on life as well as a strong support system, such as family and friends, are helpful. High self-esteem, personal growth, positive relationships with others, and a sense of purpose are also considered elements of mental well-being. Influences on mental health include family life, occupation or working life, and social interactions.

General Mental Disorders

Mental illness affects many families and still carries a stigma among many people. Prior to the advent of antipsychotic drugs of the phenothiazine type in the 1950s, individuals with schizophrenia, for example, were locked away in mental hospitals, often restrained in straitjackets. The new drugs made schizophrenic patients more amenable to treatment and helped return them to society as productive citizens and responsible family members. Antidepressants and other **psychotherapeutic** medications have also improved the outlook for many who previously would have been locked away in mental institutions, abandoned by their families, dismissed from their jobs, and labeled "crazies" or "mental cases."

Research indicates that many mental disorders are caused by a chemical imbalance in the brain. Other causes include heredity and genetic factors, environment, gender, and life experiences. Some mental disorders have no identifiable etiology and no absolute course of treatment. General classifications of mental disorders include schizophrenia, mood disorders, personality disorders, anxiety disorders, somatoform disorders, and gender identity disorder.

Schizophrenia

Disordered or disorganized thinking, inappropriate **affect,** unpredictable behavior, and visual or auditory hallucinations are all symptoms of schizophrenia (Figure 47-2 ◆). The affected person is often out of touch with reality and has difficulty functioning in a normal situation. No definite etiology has been identified; heredity, environment, and stress may be factors. Schizophrenia has devastating effects not only on the patient but on the family as well.

Schizophrenia is treated with antipsychotic medications such as phenothiazines (Thorazine, Compazine, and Mellaril), Haldol, Prolixin, Risperdal, Seroquel, and Zyprexia. Taking medications as prescribed usually controls most symptoms.

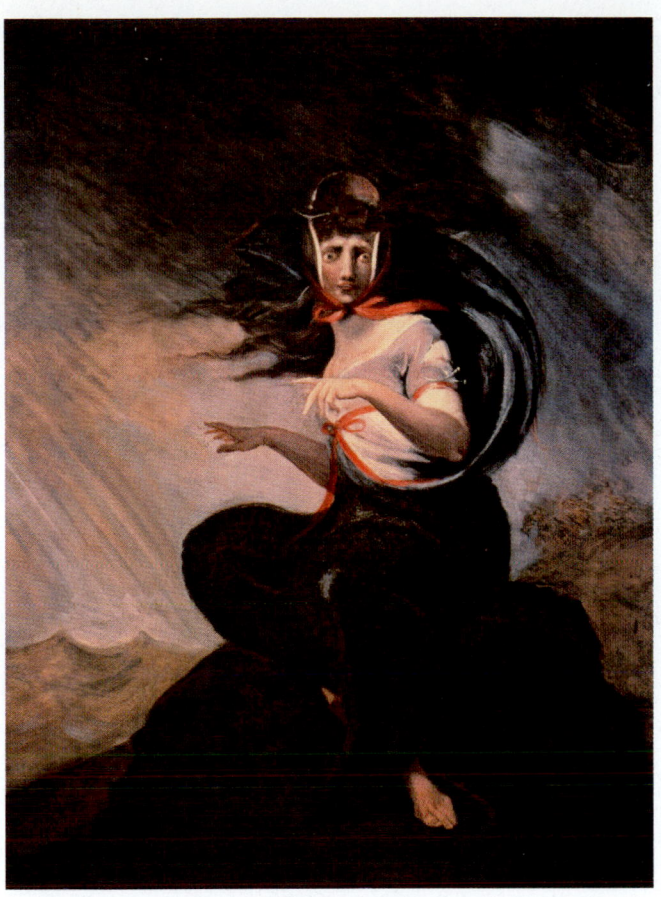

Figure 47-2 ◆ Example of someone suffering from a thought disorder.
Mad Kate, 1806-07 (oil on canvas) by Henry Fuseli (1741–1825) Goethe Museum, Frankfurt/Bridgeman Art Library, London/New York

Family support is also helpful in preventing relapses. See Table 47-2 for intervention strategies for patients who are hallucinating or delusional.

Critical Thinking Question 47-1

What advice and support can Michael offer Yolanda to help her deal with her brother's newly diagnosed condition?

Mood Disorders

Mood disorders involve disturbances in mood level or affect and are the most common mental disorders. Major depressive disorder and bipolar disorder are two mood disorders.

Major Depressive Disorder

Major depressive disorder often is referred to as major, acute, or severe depression. The depressed individual experiences an overwhelming sadness, hopelessness, and despair; has difficulty sleeping and no appetite; feels worthless; and thinks frequently of suicide as an escape from an intolerable situation. A flat affect may be observed.

There is no specific cause for major depressive disorder. However, it is believed that chemical imbalances in the neurotransmitters of the brain, specifically serotonin, may be responsible for the depressive reaction. Devastating life experiences may trigger a strong emotional response. Triggering factors may include unresolved grief, loss of a loved one, loss of a job, loss of a body part or function, and other severe, cruel, and relentless losses. Situational depression often resolves on its own, but

---

TABLE 47-2 INTERVENTION STRATEGIES FOR PATIENTS WHO ARE HALLUCINATING OR DELUSIONAL

1. Communication may be difficult with patients who are experiencing hallucinations because they may talk out loud to themselves, may make gestures or movements that are sudden and startling, or may accuse you or others of saying or doing things that you know are untrue.
2. Never argue or agree with these false perceptions or accusations because when the patient is in a realistic state of thinking, he or she may remember these events. The patient will think you are untrustworthy yourself and will no longer trust you. Even when patients are not in contact with reality, they know that they are experiencing unique perceptions and sensations. Your agreeing that you hear, feel, or see something that is not real will not make this person feel at ease or self-assured.
3. Most hallucinations are frightening or threatening to the person who is having them.
4. The behavior that you see is in response to these threats and fears. Patients need to know that you and the treatment team are working to keep them safe.
5. They need to know that you do not see, hear, or feel what they are experiencing. Simply state, "I know you think you hear your mother's voice, but I don't," or, "I know that you feel bugs crawling on your skin, but I don't see any bugs on you."
6. Initially, you want to investigate the nature of the hallucinations and help the treatment team understand what the patient is experiencing.
7. Once this has been established, do not continue to focus on the false perceptions and sensations.
8. Instead, help the patient to stay focused on reality and eventually divert the thinking to what is real. You may say something like, "I heard what you are experiencing and it must feel terrible, but I am here to help you think about things that we both know are going on around us. Let's talk about _____."
9. Sometimes, patients are plagued by auditory hallucinations, and they are unable to get the voices out of their heads. Try to help the patient focus on your voice. Say something like, "The voices that you are hearing are making you uncomfortable, so try listening to me instead of these voices."
10. It may sound strange, but sometimes you can help distract the patient from the voices by singing with the patient. Let's face it, you can't sing and listen to voices at the same time.
11. Do not allow the patient who is hallucinating to spend too much time alone. This only gives the patient more time to focus on the voices.

continued

TABLE 47-2 INTERVENTION STRATEGIES FOR PATIENTS WHO ARE HALLUCINATING OR DELUSIONAL (CONTINUED)

12. Sometimes, the voices may tell patients that they are evil and must die. Patients who hallucinate hostile voices may make attempts to injure, mutilate, or kill themselves because they are acting on the wishes of the hallucinations.

13. At times, people who respond to hallucinations and delusions are threatening to you and others.

14. You must be aware of the person's personal space and keep a distance that is safe for you and the patient. If you get too close or touch the person, you may be perceived as a threat. The person could strike out or hit you because you have invaded his or her personal space.

15. Patients who have paranoid delusions often feel threatened by others. When this is the case, they may threaten to strike staff or other patients. Pay attention to the body language and the verbal messages of people with delusions.

16. When someone who is extremely suspicious of others says, "Get away from me," it is often quite different in tone and intention than the depressed patient who asks to be left alone.

17. If someone who is hallucinating or has delusional thinking says, "Leave me alone," take it seriously. Do not get in this patient's way. Keep a close watch on the patient, but do not attempt to get too close or to explore for reasons.

18. Patients who have delusions of persecution or have paranoid thinking may think that you and the treatment facility are trying to harm them. They may not eat the food because it could be poisoned. They may refuse medication because they think it is poisoned. They will be argumentative and cannot be persuaded to believe that you want to help them.

19. Do not test the food for this patient. This will only strengthen the belief that even you consider that their delusion is true. Logical thought tells you that if you are willing to eat the food, it must be safe, but this patient's thought process is not logical.

20. Sometimes, you can help this patient to trust the food or medicine by using prepackaged foods and medications.

21. Foods like milk in a carton, canned soda, wrapped sandwiches, and pudding and gelatin in a package are safe to this person. Packaged medications are supplied in unit doses by pharmaceutical companies.

22. Never argue with a delusional thought. Simply state what you believe or know to be true.

23. It is more important to get this patient to say how the delusional thought influences his or her feelings than to argue with the illogical or unreasonable thought process. "So, you think that the food is poisoned. What do you do when you are hungry?" or "You think that the staff wants to kill you. This must be frightening. How can we help you to feel safe?"

24. Always consider your safety and the safety of the patient, other patients, and the staff when a patient is not in contact with reality. The person has a very serious illness that is causing him or her torment and needs your help. You cannot help people if you allow them to hurt you, themselves, or others.

25. Whenever you feel unsafe, other staff and patients probably do too. Let your supervisor know what you feel.

26. Trust your instincts.

Source: Miele, Carole G.; and England, Teresa, From Nursing Assistant to Clinical Care Associate, *1st Edition* © 1999. Reprinted by permission of Pearson Education, Inc. Upper Saddle River, NJ.

care providers must be on the alert for symptoms of potential suicide.

Treatment often includes drug therapy with antidepressant medications: monoamine oxidase (**MAO**) inhibitors, tricyclics, and selective serotonin reuptake inhibitors (**SSRI**). Many of these drugs have serious side effects, and it may take two weeks or more for the condition to improve. Suicidal individuals require constant monitoring and a controlled environment until the crisis stage has been resolved (Table 47-3).

Suicide attempts or expressed suicidal thoughts are cries for help. Table 47-4 lists the typical symptoms of someone contemplating suicide. Occasionally, however, there are no overt

TABLE 47-3 CONSTRUCTIVE APPROACHES TO CARING FOR PATIENTS WHO ARE DEPRESSED

1. Provide interactions and attention that are not associated with compliance or pleasing others' wishes or rules. Often, depressed people do not share their feelings because of the distorted perception that they have nothing to give in return for the "favor" of listening to them.

2. Know that you will identify with the person's depression. When you are emotionally engaged by the client's sadness, you may begin to feel sad yourself. Guard against internalizing the sadness because you will be less therapeutic if you internalize the client's sadness.

3. You will not be helpful if you are also overwhelmed by the person's pain. You may feel sad and empathize with these feelings, especially after the individual has shared his or her emotional pain.

4. Avoid making statements like "I know just how you feel" or "Everything will be all right" or "Just trust in the Lord. He will heal your pain." While these statements express sympathy for the person's sadness, they do not help to make anyone feel

better. They also make the person feel that you view the problem as trivial. They may convey that the problems in this client's life are not important enough to warrant what the person is feeling.

5. You do not know just how the client feels. You are not in the client's life situation.

6. Do not try to minimize the depressed patient's problems, even though the complaints may seem simple to solve. To this person, the problems are very real and may feel insurmountable. When you minimize the problem or the reason for the depression, it does not make the person feel better. It makes the feelings worse. "I must really be inadequate if I can't solve this little problem."

7. Tolerate silences. When you are trying to communicate with people who feel very depressed, there will be many periods of silence. The person may not have enough energy to speak. Thoughts and ideas may come slowly.

8. Your ability to tolerate silences tells the depressed person that you care and that you are willing to accept the person "as is."

TABLE 47-3 CONSTRUCTIVE APPROACHES TO CARING FOR PATIENTS WHO ARE DEPRESSED (CONTINUED)

9. If the client says to you, "Don't bother to talk to me. I don't have anything to say," or asks, "Why bother with me? I'm hopeless," let the person know it's okay not to talk and that you want to sit with him or her quietly for a while. If the client wants to talk, he or she can, and if not, it's okay.

10. Often, people who are depressed feel devalued and have low self-esteem. Sit with the person in silence to demonstrate that this is time well spent. Quiet time assures the client that you are interested and that you care.

11. Tell the client that you will set aside 10 minutes to spend with him or her. "We can sit quietly or have a conversation; I will respect your need for silence." When the 10 minutes are almost up, remind the person that you have just a few minutes left. If nothing is said throughout the entire period of time, simply thank the client for sitting with you. Tell the patient that at a specific hour you will come back and spend another 10 minutes. Be specific about where you will meet.

12. Be sure to return at the stated time. This builds trust. If something prevents you from keeping the appointment, let the patient know you didn't forget your appointment, and explain what kept you away.

13. Do not probe the client for information about the depression. Many questions will make the person feel anxious and unable to answer. This reinforces the client's feelings of inadequacy.

14. When you ask questions the client cannot answer, let the client know it's acceptable not to have an answer: "You can answer that question when you've had more time to think about it."

15. If the client has a tendency to magnify negative aspects of a situation or a task he or she is asked to perform, try to shift the focus to a positive outcome. Shift the focus by emphasizing strategies for solving the problem rather than dwelling on the problem itself. "I know that _____ is a problem—this is one way of resolving this type of problem."

16. Look for and try to help the person find the positive aspects of his or her life. Do not exaggerate strengths. Look for real strengths. "You lost your job, and this was a job you held for _____ years. That is a significant amount of time in one position. You must have been a productive employee for those years."

17. Give genuine praise for efforts made to accomplish activities of daily living (ADLs) or tasks. Do not give false praise. The person will know it is not real.

18. If the patient has not gotten out of bed for several days, offer praise when this behavior occurs. Say something like, "It's good to see you out of bed."

19. When patients cannot accept praise directly, offer it indirectly. Instead of telling the patient, tell another person so that the patient can hear your statement but does not have to directly accept your compliment.

20. When the patient tends to overdramatize everything, use this equation:

$$\text{action} = \text{benefits obtained} \div \text{risks to be taken}$$

In other words, if you ask Mr. Jenkins to get out of bed and he says, "I can't do it," try this: "How badly would you say you feel staying in bed? Rate it on a scale of 0 to 10, with 10 being the worst feeling you have ever experienced." If Mr. Jenkins says any number, there is nothing to lose. If he says 10, say something like, "If staying in bed feels like a 10, try getting out of bed, and we will evaluate how that feels. It can't be worse than a 10."

21. Help the person to realistically look at the action or task you want the person to perform. Evaluate the task in terms of the client's worst fear or what could happen. Help the patient to separate realistic consequences from self-imposed suffering. Present the positive and negative aspects of accomplishing the task. "If you get out of bed and feel worse, you will at least know that you have tried. You may find that it doesn't feel any worse. You will have accomplished something you haven't tried to do in several days, and that's a start. If it feels worse, then we can discuss going back to bed."

22. With depression, the person often avoids activity because he or she feels incapable of completing the task or fears failure. Help the person to look at the extremes on a scale of 0 to 10.

23. Be alert to clues of suicidal ideation, and examine these with the nurse. Suicidal ideation refers to thoughts or ideas of suicide or of killing oneself. An individual may be thinking of suicide as a means of ending his or her emotional pain.

24. Clues may include saying goodbye to significant others, making peace for wrong doings, talking about death as an option, giving away possessions, writing lists of things to do, suddenly appearing happy or "fleeing to health," and asking to be discharged. Fleeing to health refers to a sudden appearance of improvement from the depressed state. The person is said to "flee" to a healthy state when nothing has changed or improved in the person's life or mental condition. It is often used in association with the depressed client who has a sudden change in mood and behavior.

25. People who have made a plan for suicide usually feel a sense of accomplishment, and this may improve their mood and energize their behavior. Be alert to sudden improvements in the mood and energy level of depressed patients. This may be a danger signal. When people are extremely depressed, they usually do not have the organization of thought or the energy level to form a plan for suicide or to act on it.

26. When the energy level and thought organization of the depressed patient improves, he or she is more likely to attempt suicide.

27. If a patient discusses suicide, do not be afraid to ask about these thoughts. Asking about suicide does not give the person the idea to commit the act. Chances are the option of suicide has already been considered.

28. It is more important to find out if the patient is thinking about suicide than to avoid the topic.

29. If a patient expresses suicidal ideas, ask about a plan: "Have you thought of a plan for suicide?" If the person says yes, ask, "What are you considering as a plan?"

30. A patient who has a plan is serious. Even if the person has not thought of a plan but mentions the idea of suicide, *tell your supervisor.*

31. If you ask a question about suicide or a suicidal plan, you *cannot* promise to keep the response a secret, no matter how important you think it is for the patient to share suicidal thoughts. This is worth repeating: You must inform the nurse stat.

32. Whenever any client says, "Promise that you will keep this a secret," you must tell the patient that you *cannot* keep any secrets because the secret could be vital to his or her health and well-being. Say something like this, "I really want you to tell me your thoughts, but I cannot promise that I won't tell anyone involved in your treatment," or "If it is important to

continued

TABLE 47-3 CONSTRUCTIVE APPROACHES TO CARING FOR PATIENTS WHO ARE DEPRESSED (CONTINUED)

your safety or health, I cannot keep the secret; it is up to you to tell me."	must follow your agency's policy and procedures for "suicide watch" or "suicide precautions."
33. If you promise to keep a secret and then find out that the person has ideas of suicide or homicide or that the person has been a victim of abuse or has abused others or that the person has committed a crime, you must tell the person in charge. Now, you are caught in the bind of having to break a promise to a patient. You must tell the patient that someone in authority on the treatment team must know about this "secret." You risk losing the patient's trust when this happens. It is better to tell the patient up front that you cannot promise to keep a secret; this is for the patient's benefit.	37. These special precautions could mean keeping the patient in eyesight at all times, making rounds on the patient every 15 minutes, documenting the patient's whereabouts and condition every 15 minutes on the rounds sheet, or a one-to-one observation.
	38. The treatment team will determine the level of the precautions. If you are assigned, you must adhere closely to these policies.
34. People who express suicidal thoughts are often ambivalent about the wish to die and the wish to live. Ambivalence means having two opposite thoughts and feelings at the same time. It is like sitting on the fence and thinking, "Should I jump, or should I just sit here?"	39. A one-to-one observation means that one staff member is assigned to stay with the patient at all times. This means that you never leave the patient alone, that you stay within an arm's length of the patient, even when he or she is sleeping or in the bathroom or shower. Always follow your agency's procedure, and take this one-on-one observation very seriously.
35. It is important to allow the person time to discuss this ambivalence: "You say you want to die, and you are questioning this; tell me about wanting to live."	40. Safety is the primary issue with all patients and especially patients who are thinking about suicide.
36. Patients who express suicidal thoughts and patients who have made suicide attempts are placed on special precautions. You	41. Every suicide attempt is a cry for help.

Source: Miele, Carole G.; and England, Teresa, From Nursing Assistant to Clinical Care Associate, *1st Edition © 1999. Reprinted by permission of Pearson Education, Inc. Upper Saddle River, NJ.*

symptoms or warning signs. When symptoms *are* present, the individual should not be left alone but should be assisted to a medical or mental health facility until an evaluation, referral, and treatment plan are developed and initiated.

 Critical Thinking Question 47-2

What should Michael tell Yolanda about her self-inflicted injuries and her request that he promise not to tell anyone else? Is he bound by a patient–provider oath?

Postpartum Depression

Postpartum depression is a frequent phenomenon in the first few days or weeks after childbirth. It ranges in severity from crying spells or "new baby blues" through sadness and despair

TABLE 47-4 SYMPTOMS AND WARNING SIGNS OF CONTEMPLATED SUICIDE

- Prolonged depression with episodes of crying, sadness, helplessness, hopelessness, fatigue, weight loss, change in bowel habits toward constipation, and poor concentration
- Episodes of uncharacteristic behavior
- Sudden mood swings, especially to calmness and even happiness
- A vacant stare
- A change in eating and sleeping patterns
- A lack of interest in and withdrawal from social activities
- Reduced interest in sexual activity
- Giving away prized possessions

to **psychosis,** with potentially devastating outcomes. The new mother has feelings of inadequacy and worries about caring for her new infant. She experiences fatigue, loss of appetite, and often a flattened affect and avoids social interaction.

Sudden changes in hormonal balance during and after the birth process along with new infant care responsibilities are thought to trigger the depressive response. Sleep deprivation also plays a role in the condition.

Healthcare providers and family members should be alert for symptoms and should make efforts to assist the new mother. Intervention is important to prevent tragic outcomes, including suicide or infanticide. Most cases resolve quickly when understanding and support are provided, but antidepressant medications may be required.

In Practice

Christine Bass is in the office for her postpartum visit. She delivered a healthy baby girl six weeks ago. As the medical assistant takes her history and prepares her for examination, Christine admits that she has been feeling sad, has lost her appetite, and worries that she many not be a good mother. This patient may be experiencing postpartum depression. What should the medical assistant do? What are some constructive approaches to dealing with this patient?

Seasonal Affective Disorder

Seasonal affective disorder (**SAD**) occurs during the winter months when days are shorter and sunlight is limited. This cyclic form of depression usually has an onset during the autumn months, continues through winter, and eases in the spring. Symptoms include excessive sleepiness and lengthened sleep periods, increased appetite, weight gain, and loss of energy. Phototherapy and exposure to as much natural daylight as possible are used to treat this seasonal depression.

Bipolar Disorder

Bipolar disorder is also referred to as manic-depressive disorder. Intense mood swings are the defining characteristic. During the "manic phase," the individual is highly outgoing, energetic, excited, even euphoric. The need for sleep is minimal, and the thought process is often disturbed and disconnected. The bipolar patient displays bizarre behavior in attitude, dress, and judgment; may spend money to excess; and expresses grandiose thoughts. During the depressive phase, the mood changes to one of sadness and flat affect, with loss of appetite and sleep disturbances. Communication is avoided and activity levels decrease. Suicide is always a concern during the depressive phase.

While this condition may have familial tendencies, alterations in neurotransmitter levels are usually the cause. As with acute depression, various life situations may trigger bipolar episodes. Treatment involves drug therapy to stabilize neurotransmitter levels.

Personality Disorders

Personality disorders (**PDs**) are characterized by behaviors that deviate from accepted and standard patterns of inappropriate behavior. The ten PDs are divided into three classifications, or clusters (Table 47-5).

- Cluster A is also referred to as the Odd Cluster and includes paranoid, schizoid, and schizotypical personalities. Cluster A individuals appear odd and eccentric.
- Cluster B, or the Dramatic Cluster, includes borderline and antisocial personality disorders, narcissistic disorder, and histrionic disorder. Behavior is emotional, dramatic, or erratic.
- Cluster C, the Anxious Cluster, includes avoidant, dependent, and obsessive-compulsive (**OCD**) personality disorders. Individuals appear fearful and anxious.

The etiology of personality disorders is unknown. Although symptoms of PD begin in adolescence, diagnosis should not be confirmed until adulthood. During the assessment process, it is important to distinguish PDs from delusional and psychotic disorders.

Treatment of personality disorders depends on the symptoms. The individual is taught coping mechanisms. Drug therapy for **comorbid** conditions may be helpful.

Anxiety Disorders

Anxiety is a common reaction that most people experience at some point in their lives. When a physical threat is perceived,

TABLE 47-5 CLASSIFICATIONS AND SYMPTOMS OF PERSONALITY DISORDERS

Cluster A	
Paranoid Personality Disorder	Extreme distrust and suspicion of others; belief that others are deliberately trying to exploit, deceive, or harm the individual.
Schizoid Personality Disorder	Flat affect; indifference and detachment; relationships are few and unsatisfying.
Schizotypical Personality Disorder	Similarity to schizoid personality disorder; superstition, paranoia, and anxiety or depression.
Cluster B	
Antisocial Personality Disorder	Total disregard for the rights of others and of the law, failure to conform to social norms, aggression, manipulation, and reckless behavior.
Borderline Personality Disorder	Volatile and unstable relationships characterized by anger, despair, and feelings of rejection and abandonment; poor self-image; impulsive and manipulative behavior.
Histrionic Personality Disorder	Constant need for attention, approval, and reassurance; overly dramatic and theatrical behavior.
Narcissistic Personality Disorder	Pathologic self-love or grandiose self-admiration; exaggerated sense of importance; lack of empathy; tendency to exploit others; rage or humiliation when criticized.
Cluster C	
Avoidant Personality Disorder	Fear of criticism, disapproval or rejection; poor self-image; avoidance of social involvement.
Dependent Personality Disorder	Passivity; reliance on others for decision making; reluctance to disagree with others out of fear of disapproval.
Obsessive-Compulsive Personality Disorder	Preoccupation with orderliness, details and perfection; extreme mental and interpersonal control; tendency to make lists but never complete a task.

anxiety is a natural response. When a reduction in the threat level is not apparent, anxiety can become both a physiologic and psychological condition. Anxiety disorders include generalized anxiety disorder and panic disorder, phobic disorder, obsessive-compulsive disorder, and posttraumatic stress disorder.

Generalized Anxiety Disorder and Panic Disorder

Generalized anxiety disorder, or "free-floating anxiety," is a constant state of anxiety with no apparent cause. Affected individuals worry constantly and find decision making difficult. Physiologic symptoms include difficulty sleeping, hypertension, diarrhea, and tense muscles.

Panic disorder is characterized by a sudden onset of unexplained and severe anxiety that terminates in panic. A person with panic disorder claims to sense impending doom and often expresses the fear that he or she is dying. Physiologic symptoms may consist of trembling, dyspnea, palpitations, chest pain, and dizziness. Panic attacks occur on a regular basis and can become disabling.

Phobic Disorder

Phobic disorder is an unusual fear or anxiety concerning a specific object, situation, or activity that in reality does not present any danger. The fear progresses to the point where it controls the person's life as he or she strives to avoid the feared object or situation altogether. Table 47-6 lists typical **phobias.**

Obsessive-Compulsive Disorder

Unrelenting but unwelcome thoughts and obsessions as well as repeated, compulsive actions are the main feature of obsessive-compulsive disorder. The unsolicited thoughts may be sexual fantasies, or they may revolve around causing harm to others. The person's anxiety is often reinforced by feelings of "going crazy" or "losing my mind." Compulsive, senseless actions or rituals temporarily relieve the anxiety and reduce the stress level. Repeated, excessive hand washing is one example of an OCD symptom.

As with other anxiety disorders, it is not always possible to identify the cause of an OCD. Treatment usually involves drug therapy augmented by **psychotherapy.**

Posttraumatic Stress Disorder

Posttraumatic stress disorder (**PTSD**) is characterized by a delayed response to a traumatic event. The event may be a natural disaster such as an earthquake or hurricane, war, terrorist attack, fire, rape, abuse, car accident, or other kinds of accidents. When personal safety has been compromised in any way, the traumatic shock may precipitate PTSD.

Onset of PTSD may be immediate or delayed. Symptoms include anxiety, denial of the event, fear of being in the proximity of the event, nightmares, flashbacks, reduced appetite, weight loss, and loss of interest in normal activities. Many individuals with PTSD create a safe environment by isolating themselves from society. This condition, which has existed for centuries, was identified and named in the twentieth century when war veterans in great numbers exhibited the symptoms.

Drug therapy is helpful in establishing better sleep patterns. Psychological therapy is directed to helping the patient overcome the traumatic memories and deal with situations and environments that trigger the reaction (Table 47-7). Some cases resolve spontaneously.

Somatoform Disorders

Physical symptoms with no underlying organic etiology are typical of a somatoform disorder. The affected individual has no conscious control over these feelings. Somatization disorder, conversion disorder, hypochondriasis, and factitious disorders are all somatoform disorders.

Somatization Disorder

The condition called somatization disorder is characterized by pain or physical symptoms of illness in more than four body regions or systems and no underlying pathology. These chronic, recurring, multiple complaints have an onset before age 30. Diagnostic tests reveal no cause. Psychotherapy is the usual treatment.

Conversion Disorder

An extremely stressful situation precipitates the onset of conversion disorder, once called hysteria. Physical symptoms—paralysis, tremors, mutism (inability to speak), shortness of breath, difficulty swallowing, nausea, vomiting, temporary blindness, or seizures—create an escape from the situation. The possibility of underlying physical causes must be eliminated. Most of these incidents resolve when the stressful situation has passed. Treatment usually involves psychotherapy.

TABLE 47-6 SOME COMMON PHOBIAS	
Achluophobia	Fear of darkness
Acrophobia	Fear of heights
Agoraphobia	Overwhelming symptoms of anxiety that occur on leaving home; a form of social phobia.
Algophobia	Fear of pain
Arachnophobia	Fear of spiders
Bacteriophobia	Fear of bacteria
Claustrophobia	Fear of closed spaces
Dentophobia	Fear of dentists
Entomophobia	Fear of insects
Felinophobia	Fear of cats
Hematophobia	Fear of blood
Hydrophobia	Fear of water
Iatrophobia	Fear of physicians
Keraunophobia	Fear of thunder and lightning
Melissophobia	Fear of bees
Ophidiophobia	Fear of snakes
Pathophobia	Fear of disease
Pteromerhanophobia	Fear of flying
Pyrophobia	Fear of fire
Thanatophobia	Fear of death
Xenophobia	Fear of strangers
Zoophobia	Fear of animals

TABLE 47-7 THERAPEUTIC APPROACHES TO REDUCE ANXIETY

1. Remember that the person's behavior is aimed at reducing his or her anxiety.
2. The behavior that is displayed is telling others that something needs to be done. The person may be too anxious to make a decision about what to do with this feeling.
3. Unfamiliar and new surroundings and situations can produce anxious behavior. Anxiety increases when the person doesn't know what is expected.
4. Provide concise, clear, and simple directions.
5. Tell the person what is expected and what to expect from a situation or procedure. Tell the individual what is going to happen with each step or what will happen next.
6. Sometimes, what you are asking the person to do is causing anxiety.
7. The person may feel uncertain of what you are asking. Ask the individual what information he or she needs to proceed.
8. When you perceive that a patient is anxious, make a process statement about your perception: "You seem anxious or uncertain about what is happening." A process statement is stating what may be the underlying emotion rather than focusing on the obvious or observed behavior.
9. Allow the individual time to respond. Do not try to rush responses or actions when someone is anxious because this will only increase the anxiety.
10. It may be helpful to give directions about what to do rather than to ask the individual.
11. If you are involved in a discussion with someone who becomes nervous about a topic, it may be helpful to move the discussion off the "hot" topic. You might say, "We don't have to talk about this now. We can talk about this when you feel ready."
12. If there are time constraints, gently let the person know the expected time frame. Sometimes, compulsive actions and rituals cause delay. The client may need to handwash after every step of getting dressed or may need to check the locks and lights numerous times before leaving the room or building.
13. Try not to interrupt a compulsion or ritual because this is what the person feels he or she must do to manage anxiety. When you take away the opportunity to act out the ritual or compulsive behavior, you increase the anxiety.
14. Rituals and compulsions need to be controlled when they are harmful to the patient. If a client handwashes one hundred times a day, the healthy state of the skin might be in jeopardy.
15. Compulsive behavior must be withdrawn gradually. A plan to manage the compulsive behavior is provided by the patient's therapist and doctor.
16. Don't check your watch too often when you are helping an anxious person to communicate feelings or to prepare for an event.
17. Be aware of your frustration with these compulsions and rituals. Do not demonstrate your frustration to the client. This increases the anxiety and the need for the ritual.
18. Get the client started ahead of time so that neither of you becomes frustrated.
19. Do not tell this person about events too far in advance, as this will give him or her more to worry about. Tell the patient in enough time to give direction, to answer questions, and to prepare for the event or procedure.
20. Use a matter-of-fact or businesslike tone of voice when you are assisting someone who is anxious. A cheerful, overly friendly tone or a demanding or bossy attitude can overwhelm the person and will increase anxiety. The individual will wonder what is expected and what must be done in return for your friendliness. If you are demanding, the patient will feel that you cannot manage this display of anxious behavior.
21. It will take time for the anxious person to trust you and to recognize that your only interest is his or her well-being.
22. Your patience, calmness, and assurance of safety will build trust.
23. Do not expect anything in return for your efforts. The person's anxiety will prevent recognition of your efforts to help.

Source: Miele, Carole G.; and England, Teresa, From Nursing Assistant to Clinical Care Associate, 1st Edition © 1999. Reprinted by permission of Pearson Education, Inc. Upper Saddle River, NJ.

Hypochondriasis

Individuals who report pain and symptoms that have no physiologic basis may be diagnosed with hypochondriasis. Although the symptoms are vague, the individuals actually experience them, and negative test results do not allay their fears. They move from physician to physician, looking for one who will verify that a medical condition exists. This abnormal preoccupation with the state of their health can be incapacitating, creating social and occupational dilemmas.

When it has been positively confirmed that there is no underlying pathology, psychotherapy may be helpful. However, it is likely to be rejected by the individual as unnecessary.

Factitious Disorders

Factitious disorders are intentional and fraudulent. Malingering, for example, is the faking or exaggeration of symptoms and complaints for personal and financial gain. Munchausen syndrome is another factitious disorder. Individuals with this syndrome have an extensive knowledge of disease processes and actually injure themselves or ingest or inject a toxic substance to create an illness. Their goal is personal attention from others. Munchausen syndrome by proxy occurs when a child under the care of the individual is administered a toxic substance to create an illness. The caregiver, generally the mother, then seeks medical attention for the child. The resulting personal attention is the caregiver's "reward."

Diagnosis of factitious disorders is difficult as the individual moves from facility to facility seeking care. When this condition is confirmed, psychotherapy may be helpful.

Gender Identity Disorder

Occasionally, an individual experiences gender confusion. A gender identity disorder is characterized by feelings of belonging to the opposite sex, of discomfort or unhappiness in the biological gender role. Girls take on male characteristics, activities, and attire, while boys exhibit a preference for what are considered girls' activities and dress. Low self-esteem and social isolation may accompany these feelings. As the individuals reach maturity, they may take steps to realize their gender preference, including hormonal therapy and sex-change surgery. Psychological counseling helps many patients lead close-to-normal lives in their new gender roles. It also helps when family members recognize the condition as an illness and accept the gender change.

Mental Retardation

Mental retardation occurs as the result of an interruption in the intellectual growth of the child, during prenatal development or the birth process or after birth. Genetic aberrations and inborn errors of metabolism, exposure of the mother and fetus to infection, and any compromise to the oxygen and nutritional supply to the developing brain are possible causes.

Observation of a possible developmental disability is confirmed with standardized testing instruments such as Stanford-Binet, Wechsler Intelligence Scales for Children, and the Kaufman Assessment Battery for Children. The final diagnosis must be made before the age of 18 and must include deficiencies in behavioral areas as well as intellectual function.

Children with mental retardation show signs of lower-than-normal acquisition of intellectual and interpersonal skills. Behavioral performance in the areas of self-care, hygiene, safety, self-direction, and communication is at a lower level than expected for the age group. The children are often not diagnosed until they have problems in school. Many are educable, however, and are encouraged to learn coping and independent living skills. Others who are more severely impaired may require custodial care.

There is no cure or drug therapy for mental retardation, as the compromised brain cells cannot be replaced or repaired. Any concurrent mental disorders should be addressed and treatment options explored and implemented.

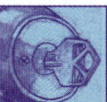

Keys to Success
UNDERSTANDING STANFORD-BINET

The Stanford-Binet scale is a standardized test used to assess the intelligence and **cognitive** abilities of children and young adults. It provides schools and treatment facilities with a beginning point for a child's therapy or education. Results are reported in a numerical format:

110 to 90—average
90 to 70—below average
70 to 50—mild retardation
50 to 35—moderate retardation
35 to 20—severe retardation
below 20—profound retardation

Dementia

Dementia is reduced mental or cognitive functioning that has an onset after the age of 18. Causes of dementia include Alzheimer's disease, vascular compromise, traumatic insult, and the aging process. Vascular disease, trauma, tumors, metabolic conditions, toxins, infections, or organic diseases may be responsible for the interruption of blood flow to the brain. As with mental retardation, symptoms are varied and may have sudden or subtle onset.

Alzheimer's Disease

Alzheimer's disease usually has an insidious inset. In this progressive degenerative disease of the brain, mental and physical functioning is reduced. Early signs include gradual loss of short-term memory, inability to concentrate or to learn new things, and progressively more severe personality changes. Communication becomes difficult, and the individual displays restlessness and disorientation. As the disease progresses, the patient may become hostile and combative. Motor skills also decline and eventually the patient is bedridden.

The onset of Alzheimer's usually occurs after the age of 60, and incidence is greater among the aging. No identifiable cause has yet been found. Diagnosis is difficult. Once symptoms indicate the onset of Alzheimer's, all other organic brain disorders must be ruled out. Recent advances in imaging studies make it possible to visualize an Alzheimer's-affected brain. On autopsy, neurofibrillary tangles and senile plaques and deposits of amyloid material are found in the brain tissue.

There is no cure for Alzheimer's. Treatment is supportive, with drug therapy to enhance memory and reduce anxiety and depression. As symptoms progress, custodial care may be required. Throughout the disease process, therapy is helpful for both the patient and the family to deal with the symptoms and projected outcome of the disorder.

Vascular Dementia

Vascular dementia may be the result of decreased blood flow to the brain. Often atherosclerosis causes narrowed or stenosed arteries and prevents normal oxygenation of cerebral tissue. Typical symptoms of dementia are loss of intellectual faculties, memory lapses, and personality changes. This often progressive condition creates anxiety, depression, and irritability. As the individual ages, the condition usually worsens and the patient loses interest in personal hygiene, appearance, and surrounding activities.

As with Alzheimer's, there is no cure for vascular dementia. Surgical procedures to remove the offending plaque help to prevent further damage from oxygen deprivation by increasing blood flow to the brain tissue and may arrest the progression of the condition. Drug therapy to increase blood flow to the cerebral arteries may be helpful. However, once brain cells have been destroyed, they cannot be replaced. Custodial care may be required. Consistency in care and environment is essential for optimum effect, and counseling is helpful for both the family and the individual.

Dementia due to Head Trauma

Dementia as the result of decreased blood flow to the brain may be caused by a traumatic insult to the skull and brain. The insult may be a closed or open head injury and includes fractures of the skull, hematomas, concussions, and contusions. As in vascular dementia, reduced blood flow leads to decreased oxygenation and nutrition to the brain cells, which die as a result of ischemia.

The symptoms of this type of dementia are similar to those of vascular dementia, except for the insidious onset of the latter. Most cases of severe traumatic insult have an abrupt onset as pressure builds in the cranium or the blood flow is acutely diminished. Treatment is directed to reducing pressure on the brain and in stopping bleeding from the tissue. As with other forms of dementia, once brain cells die from ischemia, there is no way to restore function. Treatment is supportive. Drug therapy relieves concurrent psychological circumstances. Consistency in care and daily routines is essential for optimal outcome. Counseling of the individual and the family are helpful in coping with the situation.

Mental Disorders Occurring During Childhood

Certain childhood disorders are considered mental disorders. These include, but are not limited to:

- Learning disorders, including stuttering, a communication disorder
- Pervasive development disorders, of which the most common is autistic spectrum disorder
- Attention-deficit hyperactivity disorder (**ADHD**), which is not specifically a childhood disorder but has its onset during childhood
- Oppositional defiant disorder (**ODD**), a significant childhood disorder that usually predicts poor outcomes such as dropping out of school, delinquency, and substance abuse

Children with any of these disorders, described in Table 47-8, may be seen by a psychiatrist or psychologist for initial evaluation. Other mental health care providers may eventually be involved in treatment.

TABLE 47-8 MENTAL DISORDERS THAT OCCUR IN CHILDHOOD

Condition	Signs and Symptoms	Cause	Treatment
Learning disorders, including communication disorders	Child learns in nonstandard manner; has normal or superior intelligence but functions at lower level than expected, usually in one area such as reading or math; often has low self-esteem as a result. Stuttering: abnormal speech pattern in which words or sounds are repeated or prolonged.	Often unidentifiable; possibly abnormality in cognitive processing, or problems with vision, hearing, memory, language comprehension, or attention mechanisms. Stuttering: may be familial tendency; occurs mostly in boys; exacerbated by anxiety in parents and others.	Tutoring; drug therapy for hyperactivity; speech therapy for stuttering, or problem may resolve on its own.
Pervasive development disorders	Lack of emotion, nonverbal communication, social interaction, eye contact; poor or absent verbal skills; resistance to physical contact; withdrawal and obsessive behavior before age 3.	Unknown; occurs more often in males.	Behavioral therapy that includes parents and teaches child adaptive responses; community resources for family.
Attention-deficit hyperactivity disorder	Onset before age 7 but can persist into adulthood; persistent inattention, impatience, hyperactivity, impulsivity; difficulty concentrating; fidgeting, excessive talking.	Unknown etiology; tendency to run in families.	Drug therapy, behavior therapy.
Oppositional defiant disorder	Argumentative behavior, defiance of adult supervision or guidance, tendency to blame others.	ADHD, stress related to parents and family, negative parent temperament, negative child temperament, ineffective child management.	Early treatment with drugs (Risperdal and Zyprexia) and psychotherapy; committed parental involvement and stable home environment; generally poor outcome otherwise.

Substance-Related Disorders

Substance abuse occurs among people from every educational, professional, ethnic, racial, and social background. The economic cost to society is immeasurable. **Tolerance, dependence, and addiction** are often the end results of abuse, as well as destruction of the family unit and social relationships. Criminal activity is another possible outcome.

Substance-related disorders involve alcohol, prescription drugs, and other drugs (Table 47-9).

■ Alcohol abuse applies to all forms of alcohol, such as beer, liquor, wine, coolers, and spirits. Some addicts have been known to go so far as to drink aftershave lotion, some cough and cold medications, or vanilla, which contain a tiny amount of alcohol.

■ Prescription drugs are subject to abuse, particularly those with **psychotropic** qualities. Analgesics, sedatives, stimulants, and mood-altering drugs are among the drugs commonly abused. Inhalants and other chemical substances may also be abused.

■ Illegal substances frequently abused include cannabis, hallucinogens, designer drugs, and natural and synthetic opioids. Other, nonillegal substances that are readily available are caffeine and nicotine.

These substances have the capacity to alter behavior, impair judgment, and create medical problems. Social and family relationships suffer and may deteriorate. Operating machinery and motor vehicles while under the influence of mood-altering drugs causes accidents, injuries, and even catastrophic events. When drug use is suspected in any of these events, drug screening may be performed.

TABLE 47-9 SUBSTANCES THAT ARE COMMONLY ABUSED

Classification	Substance	Use	Medical Use	Tolerance	Physical Dependence	Psychological Dependence
Sedatives	Alcohol	Reduce tension	No	Yes	Yes	Yes
	Barbiturates	Relax in social situations, cause relaxation and sleep	Yes	Yes	Yes	Yes
Stimulants	Amphetamines ■ Speed ■ Crank ■ Dexedrine ■ Methamphet-amine	Increase feelings of confidence and alertness, decrease fatigue, stay awake, increase endurance, stimulate sex drive	Yes	Yes	No	Yes
	Cocaine		No	Minimal	No	Yes
	Crack cocaine		Yes	Yes	Yes	Yes
Narcotics	Opium, heroin, morphine, Demerol, Dilaudid, hydrochloride, Percodan, codeine	Reduce physical pain, reduce anxiety and tension, aid sleep	Yes (except heroin)	Yes	Yes	Yes
	Methadone	Treatment for heroin addiction	Yes	Yes	Yes	Yes
Hallucinogens	Marijuana, hashish, peyote, LSD, PCP	Relax; change mood, thoughts, and behavior; "mind expansion," "tripping"	No (THC, the active ingredient in marijuana, is used to reduce nausea associated w/ terminally ill patients)	No	No	Yes
Tranquilizers (antianxiety drugs)	Librium, Valium, Ativan, Serax, Zanax	Reduce anxiety, induce sleep	Yes	Yes	Yes	Yes

Source: Miele, Carole G.,; and England, Teresa, From Nursing Assistant to Clinical Care Associate, *1st Edition © 1999. Reprinted by permission of Pearson Education, Inc. Upper Saddle River, NJ.*

The treatment and outcome of all substance abuse are variable, depending on the substance being abused and the client's cooperation and support systems. Drug therapy and psychotherapy are usually part of the treatment plan. The patient may be placed in a detoxification center or other controlled environment; however, success rates are unpredictable.

Patients going through substance withdrawal and others with psychological problems may experience periods of anger and angry behavior. Healthcare providers must be alert to impending angry behavior and use constructive approaches to help manage that anger and provide safety for themselves, the patient, and any others in the surrounding environment. The MA may find the suggestions in Table 47-10 to be helpful for such situations.

TABLE 47-10 CONSTRUCTIVE APPROACHES TO PATIENTS EXHIBITING ANGRY BEHAVIOR

1. Remember that the person may be reacting to frustration that is beyond his or her impulse control. The anger may be misplaced and may have nothing to do with you.
2. Sometimes, the patient displays this anger because of the belief that you can and will handle it to help him regain control.
3. *Always pay attention to your feelings and intuition when you feel threatened by a hostile or physically threatening person.* If you feel physically threatened, get help before attempting to control the outburst.
4. If you sense that the person is acting out because he or she is threatened by hallucinations or delusional thinking, try to reassure the client that he or she is safe. Assure the client that you do not want to cause him or her harm.
5. Set limits on behavior, not feelings. Let the person know that you recognize the anger or frustration but that you cannot allow this person to hurt others.
6. Be willing to accept the person and the feelings, not the behavior.
7. Do not get drawn into an argument. If you do, the patient has "one up on you." The client has caused you to lose your temper and self-control. Anytime you argue or lose your temper with a patient, the patient wins. You are there to teach appropriate and healthy coping skills. You are perceived in a negative and unprofessional way when you forget this fact. You can expect that patients will not be able to act rationally, but *you* are expected to be rational.
8. Remain in control. Be aware of your body language, voice tone, and volume. The louder you get, the louder the client needs to be to dominate the situation.
9. Try to reduce the possibility of an audience. Try to remove the client to an area where others cannot see his or her loss of control. When the situation is over, the person will be embarrassed. The client may be angry with you because you let other clients see the display of hostility.
10. Do not attempt to do this alone. Have other staff help you to remove the person to a more private area.
11. If the client is physically violent, you or other clients could be injured.
12. When the available staff assemble to manage the violent or potentially violent client, you *must* plan your actions. Determine who will verbally direct the situation. Plan for the real possibility that the client will not cooperate with directions. Determine the number of staff needed, and decide how each staff member will respond to control the client's violent behavior.
13. Remember that other clients will be frightened by the hostile outburst. They want to see that the staff is in control of the person and situation.
14. Try to determine the reason for the outburst. Ask questions in a matter-of-fact but controlled tone of voice.
15. Do not engage the person in explaining this behavior in the heat of the moment.
16. If the patient identifies that you are frightened and uncomfortable, don't say, "I am not afraid," if you are. Simply state that his or her language or behavior is threatening and that you want to help him or her regain control.
17. Examine your attitude. Patients are very perceptive of rejection and hostility. Talk about your feelings with a neutral person to cool down before you face the patient again.
18. Be safe, and believe threats.
19. Get help from other staff. Follow the guidelines and procedures of the facility for controlling physical threats or actual acts of violence.
20. Keep a safe distance from a patient who is verbally threatening. Do not stand too close.
21. Make process statements rather than judgments. Say, "You are angry because you didn't get _____," rather than, "You didn't get _____, so now you are acting out to get _____."
22. First, try to deal with the fact that the person is angry. Then move on to find out why.
23. Sometimes, demanding behavior is in the form of passive, whining behavior that demands your reassurance and support. You may begin to feel that nothing you do for this client is satisfactory.
24. The client may try to control the amount of time that you spend with him or her. This person views the amount of time spent as an indication of personal worth.
25. Let the person know that you are interested and concerned by providing frequent and short interactions.
26. Whining is a style of passively demanding attention. When this is the case, give praise and spend more time with the individual when he or she is not whining. Assess the situation, and find out what the need is. Attend to the need, not the whining behavior.
27. Be kind and courteous, but set limits. Be specific about the amount of time you are prepared to provide.
28. If the person wants something *now* and you cannot do it now or the need is not immediate, tell the person when you will have time to meet the request. Do not say, "I will do this later." Explain when later is: "I will be able to help you with this at 1:00 P.M."
29. Process behavior that doesn't make sense to you with other staff so that, as a team, you will understand the possible underlying reasons for the behavior. *All behavior has a purpose.*

Source: Miele, Carole G., and England, Teresa, From Nursing Assistant to Clinical Care Associate, 1st Edition © 1999. Reprinted by permission of Pearson Education, Inc. Upper Saddle River, NJ.

Assessment and Diagnosis

The diagnosis and treatment of mental disorders consist of an initial mental health intake questionnaire (Table 47-11), a mental status examination (Table 47-12), and a treatment plan (Table 47-13). Drug therapy, psychotherapy, counseling, group therapy, stress reduction therapy, and relaxation techniques are common treatments for some mental disorders. It is important to include the client in goal setting and decision making related to treatment.

The *Diagnostic and Statistical Manual of Mental Disorders IV* (**DSM-IV**) is the reference manual used by mental health providers to diagnose a wide range of mental disorders. The DSM-IV establishes and updates standard criteria for diagnosis.

TABLE 47-11 SUGGESTED TOPICS FOR MENTAL HEALTH INTAKE

1. Reason for visit or counseling
2. History of counseling/therapy
3. Positive outcomes of previous therapy—what helped or didn't help?
4. Medication history
5. Health issues, physical history
6. Any family history of mental illness
7. Family status and history
8. Support systems available
9. School and work history
10. History of substance use or abuse, personally or family
11. Legal issues
12. Military history
13. History of sexual abuse
14. Sexuality history

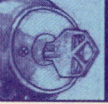

Keys to Success
COMMUNITY SERVICES FOR MENTAL HEALTH CLIENTS

Patients with a history of mental disorders are often unemployed and have no income, no permanent residence, no means of travel, no health insurance, and no way to pay for mental health services and medications. Patients who *do* have insurance may find that coverage is limited. Elderly parents of mentally challenged or disabled children may need assistance in planning for their long-term care. As a medical assistant you should be aware of community and social service agencies to which you can refer these clients.

TABLE 47-12 SUGGESTED MENTAL STATUS EXAMINATION

1. Is the patient oriented to time, person, place, situation?
2. Does the patient exhibit normal or abnormal memory?
3. Does the patient exhibit appropriate insight?
4. Does the patient exhibit appropriate judgment and thinking?
5. Has the patient experienced hallucinations or delusions? ("Do you hear or see things others say are not there?")
6. Has the patient had suicidal thoughts? If so, what does the patient report the thoughts to be?
7. Does the patient report thoughts of homicide?
8. Does the patient express a plan for suicide or homicide?
9. Does the patient have a history of previous suicide attempts?
10. Is there a family history of suicide?

TABLE 47-13 TREATMENT PLAN

■ Develop the treatment plan with input from the client.
■ Determine if therapy will be on an inpatient or outpatient basis, and whether it will be daily, weekly, biweekly, or monthly.
■ Set treatment goals. What does the patient expect to get out of treatment? How will things be different in six months?

Standard Treatments for Mental Disorders

The treatment of mental disorders today is twofold: medication and therapy. Once the patient is assessed and a diagnosis is established, a treatment plan is developed. Many disorders respond to drug therapy alone, and many respond to therapy/counseling. However, many more require the combined actions of drug therapy and counseling or psychotherapy. Some conditions are the result of insult to the brain, especially deprivation of oxygen and nutrition, and the only treatment is supportive care. Disorders caused by chemical imbalance in the brain are treated with drugs, psychotherapy, counseling, group therapy, stress reduction therapy, and relaxation techniques. Those caused by heredity and genetic factors may have no absolute course of treatment. As with other types of disorders and conditions, there may be no identifiable cause and no definitive course of treatment.

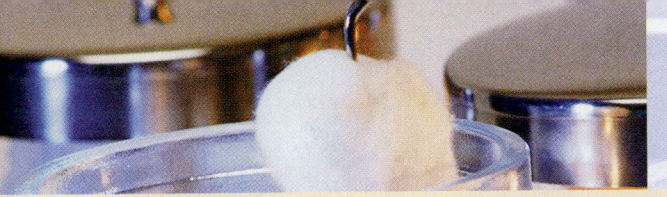

REVIEW

- In the mental health setting, the psychiatrist or psychologist is the primary provider of treatment for mental health disorders. Social workers, family and marriage counselors, child therapists, substance abuse counselors, correctional rehabilitative counselors, and vocational training counselors may also be called on.

- Neurons, or nerve cells, of the brain are connected by synaptic gaps. Each neuron may produce a number of neurotransmitters that may be specific or react with many different types of receptors. As the brain develops and processes thoughts and memories, the neurons undergo changes that affect the physical structure and chemical substances released by the synaptic gaps. These changes ultimately affect behavior.

- Mental wellness is characterized by healthy methods of coping with the pressures of daily living. A positive outlook, strong support systems, strong self-esteem, personal growth, positive relationships, and a purpose in life are all elements of mental well-being.

- General classifications of mental disorders include schizophrenia, mood disorders, personality disorders, anxiety disorders, somatoform disorders, and gender identity disorder. Many mental disorders are caused by a chemical imbalance in the brain and are treated with drugs, psychotherapy, counseling, group therapy, stress reduction therapy, and relaxation techniques. Causes include heredity and genetic factors, environment, gender, and life experiences. Some mental disorders have no identifiable etiology and no absolute course of treatment.

- Symptoms of schizophrenia are disordered or disorganized thinking, inappropriate affect, unpredictable behavior, and visual or auditory hallucinations. Heredity, environment, and stress are possible causes. Schizophrenia is treated with antipsychotic medications.

- Mood disorders involve alterations in mood level. Major depressive disorder is treated with antidepressant medications. Postpartum depression can occur following childbirth. Seasonal affective disorder occurs as daylight hours decrease. Bipolar disorder, or manic-depressive disorder, is characterized by intense mood swings. Alterations in neurotransmitter levels are the usual cause, and drug therapy the usual treatment.

- Personality disorders (PD) are divided into three classifications or clusters. Cluster A includes paranoid, schizoid, and schizotypical personalities. Cluster B includes borderline and antisocial personalities, narcissistic disorder, and histrionic disorder. Cluster C includes avoidant, dependent, and obsessive compulsive personality disorders. The etiology of PDs is unknown. Therapy helps patients develop coping mechanisms. Drugs may be prescribed for comorbid conditions.

- Anxiety is a common reaction to perceived threats but may become a physiologic and psychological condition. Anxiety disorders include generalized anxiety disorder and panic disorder, phobic disorder, obsessive-compulsive disorder, and post-traumatic stress disorder.

- Physical symptoms with no underlying organic etiology are characteristic of a somatoform disorder. Somatization disorder, conversion disorder and hypochondriasis are somatoform disorders. Factitious disorders include malingering, Munchhausen syndrome, and Munchhausen syndrome by proxy. Symptoms are contrived in hopes of personal gain, with no confirmed medical condition.

- The individual with gender identity disorder feels uncomfortable or unhappy in his or her biological role.

- Other mental conditions are caused by lack of oxygen to the brain, genetic aberration, or illness or insult affecting the brain tissue. Mental retardation occurs as the result of an interruption in the child's intellectual growth before, during, or after birth. Dementia is reduced mental or cognitive functioning that has its onset after the age of 18. It may occur as the result of a traumatic insult to the skull and brain that reduces blood flow, oxygenation, and nutrition to the brain.

- Alzheimer's is a progressive degenerative disease of the brain that affects mental and physical functioning. The usual onset is after the age of 60. There is no identifiable cause and no cure.

- Vascular dementia may be the result of decreased blood flow to the brain. Typical symptoms are loss of intellectual faculties, memory lapses, and personality changes. The condition usually worsens with age, and there is no cure.

- Mental disorders that occur in childhood include learning disorders, pervasive development disorder (autistic disorder), attention-deficit hyperactivity disorder, and oppositional defiant disorder. Children with learning disorders tend to function at a lower-than-expected level because of an abnormality in cognitive processing or problems with vision, hearing, memory, language comprehension, and attention.

- Substance-related disorders involve alcohol, prescription drugs, and other drugs. Tolerance, dependence, addiction, and destruction of the family unit and social relationships are often the end results. Drug therapy, psychotherapy, and possible commitment to a detoxification center or other controlled environment are part of the treatment.

- The *Diagnostic and Statistical Manual of Mental Disorders IV* (DSM-IV) is the reference manual used by mental health providers to diagnose mental disorders.

Chapter Review

Multiple Choice

1. The term that means "abnormal mental coping of the individual who is out of touch with reality" is
   a. phobia.
   b. psychotropic.
   c. psychotherapeutic.
   d. psychosis.

2. Which of the following is a medical doctor with special training in the field of psychiatry?
   a. Psychologist
   b. Psychiatrist
   c. Social worker
   d. Counselor

3. In addition to excitatory and inhibitory neurotransmitters, there are modulatory neurotransmitters such as
   a. acetylcholine.
   b. neuropeptides and purines.
   c. monoamines.
   d. all of the above.

4. A patient who reports pain and symptoms with no physiologic basis may be diagnosed with
   a. hypochondriasis.
   b. personality disorder.
   c. malingering.
   d. ADD.

5. The mental disorder characterized by disordered or disorganized thinking, inappropriate affect, unpredictable behavior, and visual or auditory hallucinations is
   a. depression.
   b. bipolar disorder.
   c. schizophrenia.
   d. multiple personality.

True/False

T F 1. A psychologist has a doctorate in psychology.

T F 2. The onset of PTSD is always delayed.

T F 3. A psychologist can prescribe medications for patients.

T F 4. The cerebral hemispheres control all the body's voluntary, and some involuntary, activities.

T F 5. Seasonal affective disorder (SAD) is a cyclic form of depression.

T F 6. Typical symptoms of dementia are loss of intellectual faculties, memory lapses, and personality changes.

T F 7. Neurotransmitters are chemicals that aid in the transmission of electrical impulses from one neuron to the next.

T F 8. Tolerance, dependence, and addiction are often the end results of substance abuse.

T F 9. The cerebellum is located on the posterior aspect of the brain.

Short Answer

1. What is another term for major, acute, or severe depression?

2. List the ten personality disorders.

3. What is the probable cause of vascular dementia?

4. Name two factitious disorders.

5. What is the purpose of the Stanford-Binet Scale?

Research

1. What age groups have the highest level of suicide attempts? Does this information surprise you? Why or why not?

2. In your community, where would family members affected by mental illness (their own or another family member's) find support?

Externship Application Experience

As an extern, you have a brief rotation in a mental health facility. Other students are verbally mocking a male schizophrenic patient who is yelling at a water fountain. The students are openly calling the patient "crazy" and "dummy." What should you do?

Resource Guide

American Psychiatric Association
www.psych.org

American Psychological Association
www.apa.org

National Depressive Manic Depression Association
1-800-826-3632
www.ndmda.org

National Institute of Mental Health
www.nimh.nih.gov

National Alliance for the Mentally Ill
1-800-950-6264
www.nami.org

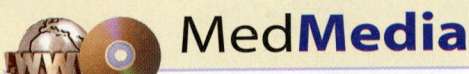

Med**Media**

http://www.MyMAKit.com

More on this chapter, including interactive resources, can be found on the Student CD-ROM accompanying this textbook and on http://www.MyMAKit.com.

CHAPTER 48

Oncology

Case Study

Marilyn has been doing her externship in an oncology office, where she is responsible for taking patient histories and vital signs and assisting the physician. A 45-year-old female patient, Ruth Dillan, asks Marilyn about colorectal cancer. Ruth is concerned because she has experienced a change in her bowel habits and has a strong family history of cancer. Both of her sisters and her mother were diagnosed with cancer in recent years. As worried as she is, however, Ruth has canceled one previous appointment for screening because she is apprehensive about the embarrassment and discomfort of the testing procedures. Ruth asks Marilyn what her chances are of developing cancer. She also asks for specifics about the screening.

Objectives

After completing this chapter, you should be able to:

- Define and spell the key terminology in this chapter.
- Identify the medical assistant's role in the oncology office.
- Describe the different types of malignant neoplasms.
- List and describe routine cancer screening tests.
- Explain tumor markers and how they are used in cancer diagnosis.
- Discuss the staging and grading of malignancies.
- Discuss the role of chemotherapy in cancer treatment.
- Discuss the use of radiation in cancer treatment.
- Discuss the role of surgical intervention in cancer treatment.
- Discuss hormone therapy and immunotherapy as cancer treatments.
- Explain some of the side effects of cancer treatment.
- Describe some recent advances in cancer research.
- Explain hospice care for terminally ill patients.
- Describe the cancer prevention lifestyle.

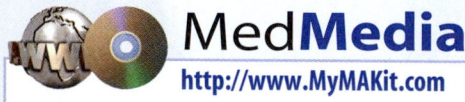

Med**Media**
http://www.MyMAKit.com

Additional interactive resources and activities for this chapter can be found on http://www.MyMAKit.com. For a video, audio glossary, tips, legal and ethical scenarios, job scenarios, quizzes, and games related to the content of this chapter, please access the accompanying CD-ROM in this book.

Video
Audio Glossary
Legal and Ethical Scenario: *Oncology*
On the Job Scenario: *Oncology*
Multiple Choice Quiz
Games: Crossword, Strikeout, and Spelling Bee
Tips
HIPAA Quiz

MEDICAL ASSISTING STANDARDS

CAAHEP ENTRY-LEVEL STANDARDS	ABHES ENTRY-LEVEL COMPETENCIES
■ Perform within scope of practice (psychomotor) ■ Explore issue of confidentiality as it applies to the medical assistant (cognitive) ■ Apply ethical behaviors, including honesty/integrity in performance of medical assisting practice (affective) ■ Apply local, state and federal health care legislation and regulation appropriate to the medical assisting practice setting (psychomotor) ■ Recognize the importance of local, state and federal legislation and regulations in the practice setting (affective) ■ Describe the normal function of each body system (cognitive) ■ Identify common pathology related to each body system (cognitive) ■ Analyze pathology as it relates to the interaction of body systems (cognitive) ■ Discuss implications for disease and disability when homeostasis is not maintained (cognitive) ■ Describe implications for treatment related to pathology (cognitive) ■ Use language/verbal skills that enable patients' understanding (affective) ■ Apply critical thinking skills in performing patient assessment and care (affective) ■ Document accurately in the patient record (psychomotor) ■ Demonstrate diversity in approaching patients and families (affective) ■ Develop and maintain a current list of community resources related to patients' healthcare needs (psychomotor)	■ Project a positive attitude. ■ Maintain confidentiality at all times. ■ Be a "team player." ■ Be cognizant of ethical boundaries. ■ Exhibit initiative. ■ Adapt to change. ■ Evidence a responsible attitude. ■ Be courteous and diplomatic. ■ Conduct work within scope of education, training, and ability. ■ Interview and take a patient history. ■ Prepare patients for and assist physician with routine and specialty examinations and treatments and minor office surgery. ■ Apply principles of aseptic techniques and infection control. ■ Prepare and maintain examination and treatment area. ■ Collect and process specimens. ■ Dispose of biohazardous materials. ■ Practice Standard Precautions. ■ Prepare and administer oral and parenteral medications as directed by the physician. ■ Maintain medication and immunization records.

Key Terminology

benign—noncancerous or noninvasive

cancer—general term for various malignant neoplasms

chemotherapy—treatment of disease and infection with chemical agents; in cancer treatment, use of chemical agents to selectively kill cancer cells

hospice—holistic care of terminally ill patients in a home or homelike setting

malignant—cancerous, invasive, and destructive

metastasis—spread of a disease to adjacent and distal tissues and organs

neoplasm—new growth or tumor

oncology—branch of medicine that deals with the study, diagnosis, and treatment of tumors and cancer

remission—complete or partial disappearance of the clinical characteristics of chronic or malignant disease

tumor—growth characterized by progressive and uncontrolled production of cells

tumor marker—substance produced by tumor cells that can be measured and monitored in blood serum levels to indicate progression of metastases and/or effectiveness of cancer chemotherapy

Introduction

Oncology is the study of **tumors** and **cancer,** which are characterized by uncontrolled cell growth. General types of cancer include carcinomas, sarcomas, lymphomas, leukemias, and melanomas.

Every year 1.3 million Americans are diagnosed with cancer. Twenty-five percent of U.S. deaths (500,000 a year) are caused by cancer. The prevalence of various types of cancer has spurred ongoing research into the nature and causes of this dreaded disease, which in turn has led to important advances in its treatment. Information campaigns have educated the public about lifestyle habits—such as wearing sunscreen and not smoking—that can help reduce the chances of contracting certain types of cancer.

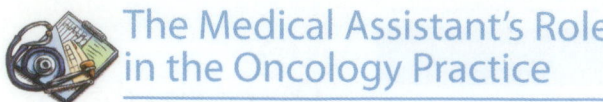

The Medical Assistant's Role in the Oncology Practice

The medical assistant performs several essential functions in an oncology medical practice, which include:

- Obtaining the medical history and vital signs
- Assisting the oncologist as necessary in patient examination and procedures
- Instructing the patient in the removal of clothing before a physical examination and providing a gown and drape
- Providing patients with information on community resources
- Arranging appointments for other tests and procedures
- Collecting specimens, including blood

The Classification and Physiology of Cancers

Cell division and reproduction in the body usually occur at a controlled rate. Cancer, or malignancy, is caused by the rapid and uncontrollable development and reproduction of abnormal cells. These cells take on a different character from the original, normal cell (Figure 48-1 ◆). Abnormal cell growth of this kind is referred to as **malignant** or life-threatening cell growth. As the growth advances, normal cells are deprived of nutrition and crowded out of their normal environment.

The original malignant growth is called the primary site. **Metastasis** creates secondary sites elsewhere in the body. Malignant **neoplasms** are classified according to the type of tissue invaded (Table 48-1).

Benign tumors result from slow growth, and their cellular structure is close to that of adjacent cells. Benign tumor cells are differentiated; that is, they resemble the tissue of origin. These tumors do not necessarily cause symptoms when they are small, but they can cause compression of surrounding tissues and organs as they enlarge. Most benign tumors can be surgically excised, as most are encapsulated and do not invade surrounding tissue. If the entire tumor is removed, it usually does not recur.

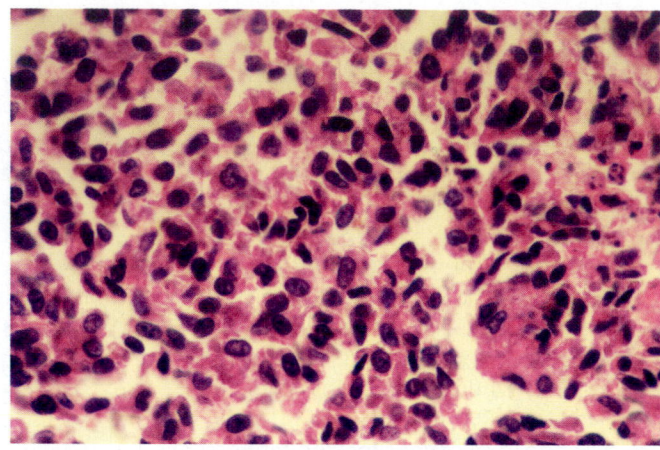

Figure 48-1 ◆ Human cancer cells and tissue.
Source: Phototake NYC

Malignant tumors, also known as cancer, cause symptoms when they invade (often by cell migration through blood and lymph circulation) and destroy local, adjacent, and distal sites of tissue and organs (Table 48-2). When metastasis has occurred, total eradication becomes more difficult, and recurrence is a common problem.

TABLE 48-1 MALIGNANT NEOPLASMS		
Type of Neoplasm	**Tissue of Origin**	**Associated Conditions**
Carcinoma	Epithelial cells	Basal cell carcinoma, squamous cell carcinoma
Glioma	Nervous system, incuding the brain, spinal cord, and nerve tissues	Neurogenic sarcoma, neuroblastoma, glioblastoma, malignant meningioma
Leukemia	Blood precursors (stem cells) in the bone marrow	Acute lymphocytic leukemia, chronic lymphocytic leukemia, acute mylogenous leukemia, chronic mylogenous leukemia
Lymphoma	Lymphoid tissue and lymph vessels	Lymphangiosarcoma, lymphangioendothelioma, malignant lymphoma, lymphosarcoma, reticulum cell sarcoma, Hodgkin's lymphoma, non-Hodgkin's lymphoma
Melanoma	Melanin-producing cells	Malignant melanoma
Sarcoma	Supportive tissue including muscle, cartilage, and bone	Osteogenic sarcoma, angiosarcoma, leiomyosarcoma, rhabdomyosarcoma

TABLE 48-2 DIFFERENCES BETWEEN BENIGN AND MALIGNANT TUMORS

Benign Tumors (Figure 48-2 ◆)	Malignant Tumors (Figure 48-3 ◆)
Tumor cells appear similar to normal cells.	Tumor cells do not resemble normal cells.
Tumor cells are differentiated.	Tumor cells are undifferentiated.
Tumor cells exhibit slow growth.	Tumor cells exhibit rapid growth.
Tumor cells grow adjacent to each other.	Tumor cells infiltrate surrounding tissue.
Tumor expands but does not destroy tissue.	Tumor growth causes ulceration and necrosis of tissue.
Tumor is smooth and movable as a unit.	Tumor is irregularly shaped and more difficult to move.
Tumor recurrence is rare after surgical excision.	Tumor recurrence is common after surgical excision.
Symptoms are related to tumor location, size, and compression on tissue or organs.	Symptoms are related to tumor location, size, and compression, which cause severe pain, cachexia (weight loss), and death.

Cancer has several possible causes:

- Repeated exposure to carcinogens over a long period of time, such as those inhaled during smoking (lung cancer) and certain physical agents such as radiation
- Genetic cellular mutations due to aging
- Immune system diseases such as AIDS, which causes lymphomas
- Hormones, as in breast cancer
- Certain viruses such as human papillomavirus, a possible precursor to cervical cancer

Radiation disrupts DNA and cellular replication. In the form of ultraviolet rays, X-rays, and radioactive materials, it can be carcinogenic. Overexposure to the sun's UV rays raises the

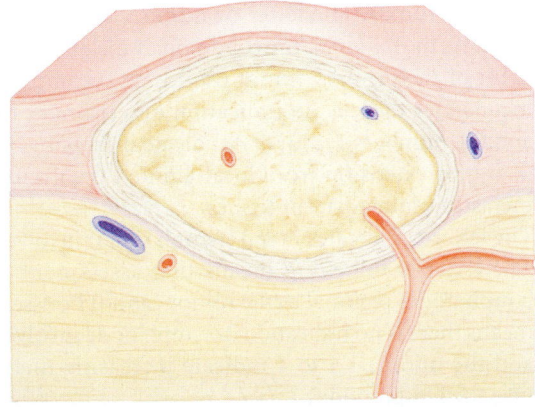

Figure 48-2 ◆ Benign tumor.
Source: Dorling Kindersley Media Library

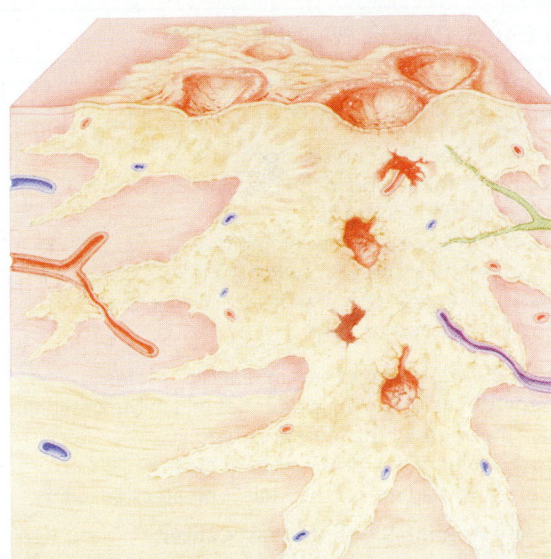

Figure 48-3 ◆ Malignant tumor.
Source: Dorling Kindersley Media Library

risk of basal, squamous, and melanoma skin cancer. Greater amounts of skin pigmentation provide greater protection from the harmful effects of ultraviolet rays; thus, fair-skinned people with higher exposure to the sun are at greater risk of skin cancer.

The incidence of cancer has a tendency to rise with age. Often a silent invader, it may not be diagnosed until it has progressed to an advanced stage. It takes on many forms and has variable outcomes, depending on the tissue or area of the body involved and the degree to which the cancer has metastasized at the time of diagnosis.

Specific types of cancers are discussed in other chapters of this book.

Diagnostic Procedures

In general, the detection, diagnosis, and treatment of cancer in an early stage offer a better prognosis and a greater chance for cure. Public education about the signs and symptoms of cancer is designed to encourage individuals to seek medical evaluation earlier (Table 48-3). Prognosis is usually reported statistically as the percentage of patients with that cancer who are still alive after a certain period of time. The patient may be cured of the disease, in **remission,** or still undergoing treatment.

Cancer detection employs general and specific techniques of physical examination, medical history-taking, and laboratory screening tests. Screening examinations can detect cancers of the breast, rectum, colon, prostate, cervix, testis, tongue, mouth, and skin early, when treatment is more likely to succeed. These cancers account for approximately half of all new cancer cases.

If cancer is suspected, additional diagnostic investigation is achieved with imaging techniques (mammograms,

TABLE 48-3 CANCER WARNING SIGNALS

The American Cancer Society lists the following seven danger signs and symptoms of cancer:

1. Unusual bleeding or discharge
2. A lump or thickening in the breast or elsewhere
3. A sore that does not heal
4. Change in bowel or bladder habits
5. Persistent hoarseness or cough
6. Persistent indigestion or difficulty swallowing
7. Change in a wart or mole

The ABCDs of Abnormalities in Warts or Moles:
Asymmetry: half of the mole does not match the other half
Border: the edges of the mole are irregular
Color: the color of the mole is not uniform
Diameter: the diameter of the mole is greater than 6 mm

The Early Warning Signs of Breast Cancer:
- A lump that can be seen in the breast or felt within the breast
- Changes in the breast's skin color or texture
- A depression or dimpling of the skin of the breast
- Changes in the appearance of the nipple, such as retraction or inversion (pulling in)
- Bloody or spontaneous discharge of any color from the nipple
- Swelling of the breast or of the lymph nodes (in the armpit)

ultrasonograms, MRIs, PET scans) and most decisively by biopsy of the lesion. Blood tests are used to evaluate hormone levels and tumor markers.

Routine Diagnostic Screening

Routine diagnostic screening for cancer includes the following tests:

- Colorectal screening: A fecal screening for occult blood is recommended on a yearly basis. Physicians generally order a flexible sigmoidoscopy or colonoscopy every three years after the age of 50. However, a different recommendation may be made, based on medical history, presenting symptoms, and family history.
- Barium enema or lower gastrointestinal X-ray studies.
- Mammogram screening: Mammograms are generally prescribed yearly after the age of 40, but the patient's medical history, presenting symptoms, and family history may dictate a different recommendation. Medicare, a federally sponsored healthcare plan for senior citizens over 65, chronically disabled patients, and patients with end-stage renal disease, pays for annual mammograms.
- Pap smear and pelvic examination: These are generally ordered annually for sexually active females for life. Medicare covers these procedures only every two years.
- PSA screening and digital rectal examination: These are usually prescribed for males annually after the age of 50. Medicare will only pay annually for PSA screening.

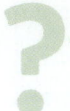

?—Critical Thinking Question 48-1—

Even though Ruth is not yet in the 50-year-old age bracket, should she still be tested for colorectal cancer?

Tumor Markers

Tumor markers, also referred to as *cancer markers,* are proteins, hormones, and other substances produced by tumors and released into the blood. They are used as screening tools to determine the progress of cancer treatment or the recurrence of a tumor. Tumor marker blood studies are usually ordered after a tumor has been diagnosed. Routine use of tumor markers in the diagnostic arena includes PSA screening tests for males and Pap smears for females.

Tumor markers for various forms of cancer include CA19-9, a marker for colorectal, gastric, and pancreatic cancer; CA125, a marker for ovarian cancer as well as for cancer of the uterus, cervix, lung, breast, and digestive tract; and carcinoembryonic antigen, a marker for colorectal cancer, especially when it has metastasized.

These markers are not always an indication of cancer cell or tumor activity. They are only used to monitor tumor growth. Tumor markers may be elevated in benign conditions such as inflammatory bowel disease, pancreatitis, liver disease, endometriosis, pelvic inflammatory disease, menstruation, and inflammation of the pleura.

Staging and Grading Malignant Tumors

Malignancies are staged and graded to determine the prognosis and optimum course of treatment for each patient. Staging identifies the type of cancer and the degree to which it has metastasized. It evaluates the size and extent of the primary tumor, the extent of lymph node involvement, and the extent and number of metastases at distant sites. The most commonly used staging system is the TNM system.

- The letter T indicates the size, depth, and location of the primary tumor. The letter or number following the T indicates the nature of the condition. X means that assessment of the primary tumor cannot be accomplished; 0 means that there is no indication of a primary tumor; and the numbers 1, 2, 3, or 4 indicate increasing degrees of tumor extension from local, limited involvement to metastasis into adjacent tissues.
- The letter N indicates nodal (lymph node) involvement. The letter X following means that assessment of the lymph nodes regional to the tumor cannot be assessed; 0 means there is no indication of lymph node involvement; and the numbers 1 to 4 indicate increasing metastasis into the lymph nodes.
- The letter M indicates distant metastasis. An X following means that no distant metastasis can be assessed; 0 means that no distant metastasis has been found; and 1 means that distant metastasis has been determined.

When the TNM staging has been completed, the tumor is designated stage I, II, III, or IV, indicating the prognosis. For example, T2 N2 M0 Stage II would be a good prognosis, whereas T4 N4 M1 Stage IV would indicate less potential for successful treatment and/or survivability.

Grading refers to the differentiation of the cancer cells. Well-differentiated cancer cells retain some of the features of the cells of origin. This grade of cancer signifies a better prognosis than one in which the cells are poorly differentiated and no longer resemble the cells of origin. The latter grade of cancer is usually in a more advanced stage. Grading involves the microscopic evaluation of biopsy tissue. A laboratory pathologist examines the tissue for growth rate and degree of cellular differentiation.

Cancer Treatment

The outlook for a cancer patient is more positive when the cancer is diagnosed at an early stage and prompt intervention is initiated. The complete eradication of cancer cells from the body is the goal of cancer treatment. At present, treatment consists of three major methods:

- Chemotherapy
- Radiation therapy
- Surgical removal

Hormonal therapy and immunotherapy may also be considered treatment methods.

There is no cure for many metastatic diseases, but the same treatment modalities may be useful in prolonging or improving the quality of the patient's life. Even after the patient has achieved remission, he or she must be followed closely for several years. Micrometastases that are not eradicated with systemic therapy can lead to eventual recurrence of the cancer.

Critical Thinking Question 48-2

Ruth is concerned about being embarrassed and uncomfortable. She has also canceled a previous appointment. How should Marilyn approach this situation?

Chemotherapy

Single or combination **chemotherapy,** in conjunction with other drug therapy, is used effectively to attack the malignancy at different stages of the cancer cell life cycle (Figure 48-4 ◆).

Several types of antineoplastic agents are used in chemotherapy: alkalating agents, antimetabolites, hormones and hormone antagonists, antitumor antibiotics, plant extracts with antineoplastic activity, and miscellaneous anticancer drugs (Table 48-4). Each therapeutic approach is unique, specific to the patient, and may involve one drug, two or more drugs from the same class, or two or more drugs from multiple classes. In the first round of therapy, the maximum tolerable dose is administered to kill as many cancer cells as possible (Figure 48-5 ◆).

Chemotherapeutic treatment is a challenge as the drugs may cause uncomfortable and undesirable side effects. All the body systems can be affected. Recent advances, however, have reduced some of the undesirable effects.

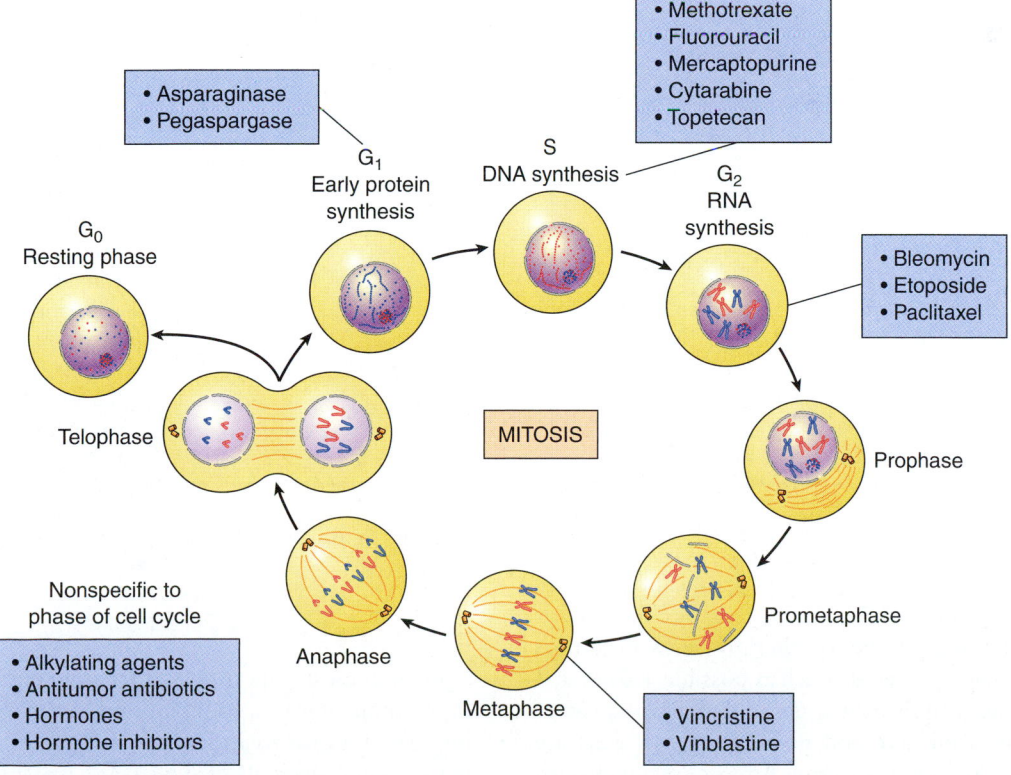

Figure 48-4 ◆ Antineoplastic agents.

TABLE 48-4 ANTINEOPLASTIC DRUGS

Class of Drugs and Common Examples	Mode of Action	Type of Cancer Treated	Side Effects
Alkalating agents: Cytoxan, Leukeran, Alkeran, Emcyt, Zanozar, Myleran, Temodar, Ifex, Mustargen, Platinol, Praplatinoxu	Alter the structure of DNA in cancer cells, preventing them from functioning normally	Hodgkin's disease, non-Hodgkin's lymphoma, leukemias, multiple myeloma, and cancer of the breasts, ovaries, lungs, pancreas, testicles, brain, and bladder	Bone marrow depression with reduction in blood cell formation, RBCs, WBCs, and platelets; effects on epithelial cells lining GI tract, with nausea and vomiting
Antimetabolites: methotrexate, floxuridine, fluorouracil, Cytosar, Gemzar, Leustatin, thiogantine	Similar in structure to essential nutrients and nucleic acids required for cellular growth; block chemical pathways of growth of normal building blocks of the cells, slowing their growth and killing many cancer cells	Leukemia, choriocarcinoma, lymphoma, and cancer of the testicles, breasts, colon, rectum, stomach, pancreas, and lungs; topical (fluorouracil) for basal cell carcinoma	Immunosuppressant action, nausea, vomiting, and anorexia
Hormones and Hormone Antagonists: corticosteroids, estrogen, progestin, and androgens	Usually given as a palliative measure	Glucocorticocoids for leukemias, Hodgkin's, and lymphomas; testosterone for breast cancer; progestin for breast cancer; estrogen for prostate and testicular cancer	
Antitumor Antibiotics: Rubex, Blenoxane, Cosmegan, Cerubidine, Doxil, Ellence, Idamycin, Mutamycin, Valstar	Interact with DNA similarly to alkalating agents	Lymphoma, sarcomas, Kaposi's sarcoma, Wilms' tumor, leukemias, and cancer of the breasts, lungs, testicles, thyroid, bladder, rectum, and ovaries	Similar to those of alkalating agents
Plant Extracts with Antineoplastic Activity: Oncovin, Velban, Navelbine, Taxotere, Taxol, Hycamtin, VePesid, Vumon, Camptosar	Block cell reproduction by impeding cell division	Hodgkin's disease, lymphoma, Wilms' tumor, leukemia, and cancer of the breasts, lungs, ovaries, testicles, colon, and rectum	Lowered resistance to infection, bruising or bleeding, anemia, sore mouth and taste change, diarrhea, malaise and weakness, hair loss, aching joints and muscles, skin changes including rash, numbness or tingling in hands or feet, headaches, allergic reactions, nausea and vomiting
Miscellaneous Anticancer Drugs: tamoxifen	Tamoxifen is an antiestrogenic agent that blocks estrogen receptor in cancer cells	Breast cancer	Nausea and vomiting, hot flashes, vaginal discharge, uterine bleeding, fluid retention and thrombus; may cause increased rate of uterine cancer

Radiation

Radiation X-rays are used to diagnose and treat cancer (Figure 48-6 ◆). Radioactive materials may also be injected or implanted into the body. Radiation therapy destroys tumors while protecting healthy tissue as much as possible. However, it does not always accomplish these goals, usually because of where the tumor is located, and normal, healthy cells are destroyed as well. Also, some cancerous tumors are not affected by safe doses of radiation. Side effects of radiation therapy are hair loss, nausea and vomiting, stomatitis, and internal radiation burns.

Surgery

Surgery alone is only curative for early-stage tumors. Usually, more than one treatment option is employed. Surgery is important for the treatment of solid cancers and is often used in the staging evaluation as well. As a treatment modality, the goal is either cure or palliative symptom control. When

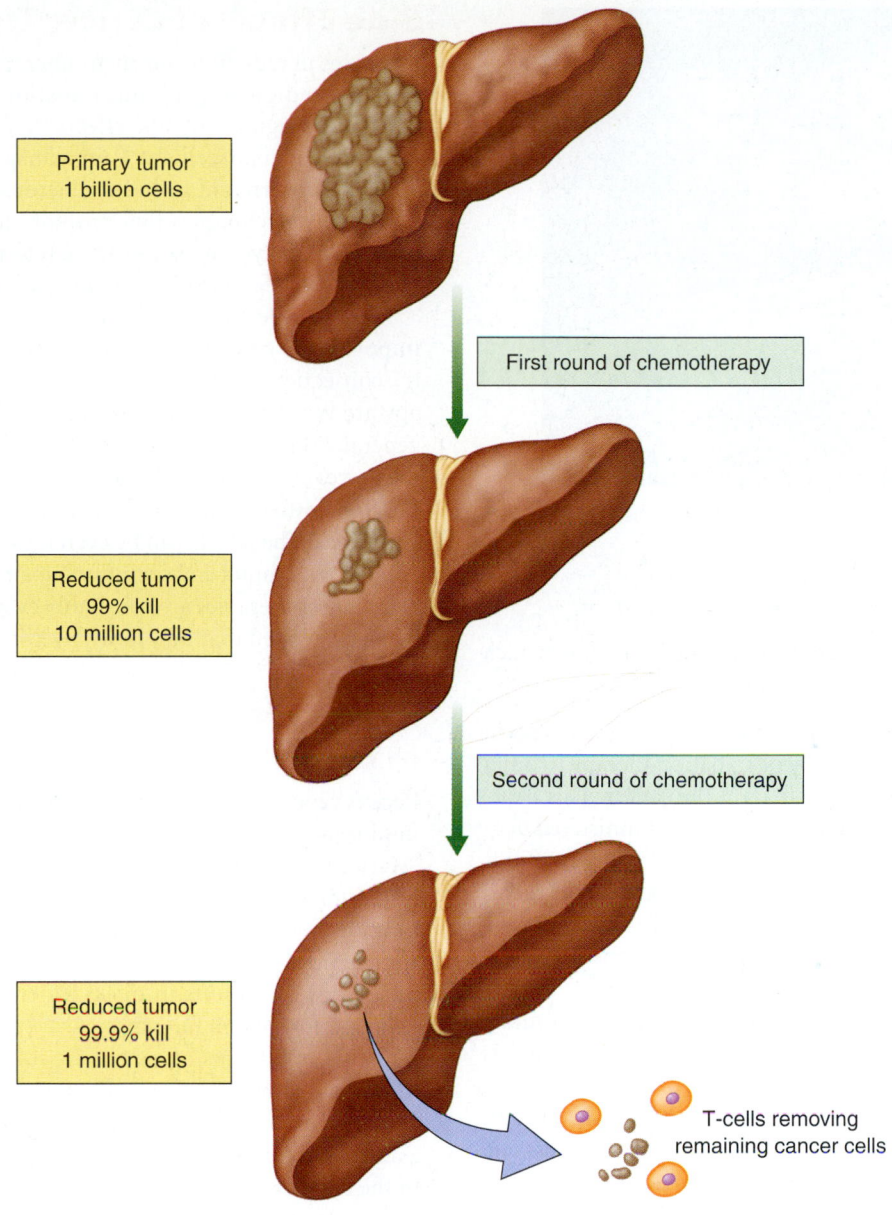

**Primary tumor
1 billion cells**

First round of chemotherapy

**Reduced tumor
99% kill
10 million cells**

Second round of chemotherapy

**Reduced tumor
99.9% kill
1 million cells**

T-cells removing
remaining cancer cells

Figure 48-5 ◆ In the first round of therapy, the maximum tolerable dose is administered to kill as many cancer cells as possible.

surgery is employed as a curative measure, the surgeon tries to achieve negative margins around the tumor, meaning that a certain amount of normal tissue is removed along with the tumor to ensure the entire tumor is removed. If negative margins are not achieved, surgery must be performed again or another type of treatment must be tried. At the time of surgery, the regional lymph nodes may be evaluated in order to determine if the cancer cells have entered the lymphatic system and invaded the nodes. Affected nodes are generally removed. Palliative surgery is performed to relieve troublesome symptoms such as obstruction. Relief can be achieved by tumor resection, bypass, stenting (placing a mesh tube in a vessel to maintain its patency), or laser ablation (removing a growth with laser).

Hormone Therapy and Immunotherapy

The use of hormone therapy and immunotherapy in the treatment of cancer is continually evolving. Hormone therapy can be effective in hormone-dependent cancers such as breast cancer and prostate cancer. It may involve the following:

■ The administration of drugs that suppress hormone synthesis, such as luteinizing hormone-releasing hormone (LHRH) antagonists or aromatase inhibitors, which are used to treat prostate cancer.

■ The administration of drugs that block the action of hormones, such as the estrogen receptor modulator tamoxifen, used to treat breast cancer.

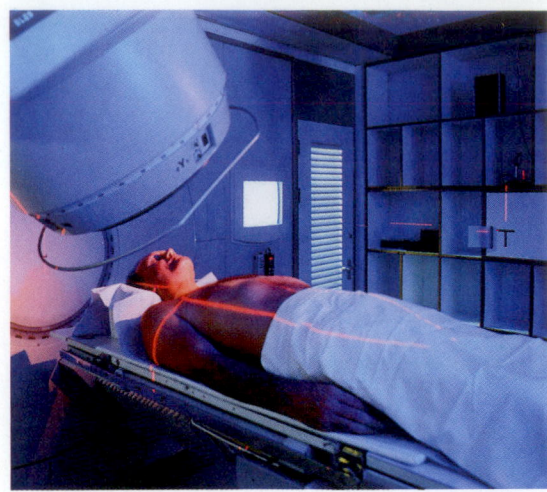

Figure 48-6 ◆ Radiation therapy.
Source: Photolibrary.com

- The surgical removal of hormone-producing glands, such as oophorectomy and orchiectomy.

Immunotherapy, also known as biotherapy, is used in combination with chemotherapy or radiation therapy to build the body's immune system to help fight the cancer. This treatment, still considered experimental, may be administered during the early stages of the disease. Immunotherapy methods include cancer vaccines, monoclonal antibody therapy, and nonspecific, primary, and adjuvant immunotherapy.

Cancer vaccines are similar in application theory to traditional vaccines. Each cancer vaccine contains entire or partial cancer cells or antigens and works to increase the immune response against cancer cells in the body. Cancer vaccinations have not yet been approved for use in the United States.

Monoclonal antibodies are designed to target certain products of cancer cells that are not found in normal cells. The monoclonal antibody is an antibody clone mass-produced in a laboratory setting (as opposed to in the body, in response to antigen presence). When the monoclonal antibody is combined with a B cell that has recognition for a specific antigen, the antibody continues to reproduce and support the immune system. Some monoclonal antibody therapies are still in clinical trial, and others are approved for use in treating specific cancers. Some antibodies currently approved for use are trastuzumab (Herceptin), used for certain breast cancers, and rituximab (Rituxan), used for lymphoma.

Nonspecific immunotherapy can be used as a primary treatment but is often used as adjuvant, or assistive, therapy to other cancer treatments. Cytokines, used in nonspecific immunotherapy, are naturally occurring hormones that regulate the growth and activity of blood and immune system cells. They can also be created in the lab. Cytokines boost the immune system and reduce the side effects of other cancer treatments, including chemotherapy and radiation. They are administered by subcutaneous, intramuscular, or intravenous routes.

Side Effects of Cancer Treatment

Advances in radiation and chemotherapy have diminished the need for radical surgery. But radiation and most anticancer drugs have significant side effects that require constant surveillance and management. Pain management at every stage is a major concern and includes generous use of analgesics and noninvasive techniques that promote relaxation and distraction. Terminally ill persons can be referred to hospice care for compassionate, holistic case management.

One aspect of cancer treatment that is becoming more important as a greater number of patients are being cured is the consequence of therapy. Chemotherapy and radiation therapy are very toxic not only to cancer cells, but to the body in general. Some of the effects of this toxicity are not seen until many years following therapy. Patients are predisposed to develop other malignancies, especially lymphomas and leukemias. The effects can be even more dramatic in children. Growth retardation and cognitive impairment may result. However, cancer therapies are constantly evolving and methods are being developed that may have fewer long-term side effects.

Recent Developments in Cancer Treatment

Recent cancer research has explored the areas of angiogenesis inhibitors and genetic causes. One new approach is based on "starving" a tumor. Experimental studies have shown that inhibiting the growth of new blood vessels that feed the tumor (angiogenesis) causes the tumor to shrink. Since 1994, two angiogenesis inhibitors, angiostatin and endostatin, have produced positive results in mice. Experimental treatments are being performed on humans.

Certain forms of cancer are inherited, such as Wilms' tumor and retinoblastoma; other forms of cancer develop from genetic mutation tendencies that cause common cancers, such as colon cancer and breast cancer, to run in families. Thus, much of the current research is focused on cancer at its genetic roots. Scientists are also investigating genetic switches that cause healthy cells to become disorderly. It has been observed that broken genes can send cells into spirals of cancerous growth. Such genes are proposed targets for therapy.

One recent advance in radiation therapy is particle beam treatment. Higher and more accurately focused doses of neutron energy minimize the side effects of the radiation.

Hospice and Emotional Support

The diagnosis of cancer in any form has a huge impact on the life of the patient and the family. A greatly feared disease, cancer often affects the patient's psychological as well as physical well-being. Many patients elect to fight the disease. Others decide there is no reason to attempt a cure as the cure is often worse than the disease. Religious beliefs, or the absence thereof, may have an impact on the patient's outlook. In all cases the understanding support of family, friends, and health care professionals is essential.

Hospice is the holistic care of terminally ill patients in a home or home-like setting. The philosophy of hospice is to provide quality, palliative care to patients during the final phase of life. Most patients are cancer patients, but hospice care is available to any patient with a terminal condition. Although the emphasis is on the patient, family needs are also addressed. Disease symptoms are managed with nursing-related care, medications, and nutritional support. Pain management integrates emotional, spiritual, and other therapies.

The hospice team is made up of professionals, paraprofessionals, and volunteers who aid the patient and family in holistic terminal care. The team coordinates input from the physician, nurse, chaplain, social worker, home healthcare workers, and volunteers. Team members help patients and their families address physical, social, emotional, and financial needs.

The Cancer Prevention Lifestyle

Some risk factors predisposing a person to cancer can be modified, but others cannot. For example, inherited tendencies cannot be altered. On the other hand, avoiding promiscuous sexual behavior is effective at preventing AIDS and human papillomavirus, the causes of lymphomas and cervical cancer, respectively. Unhealthy lifestyles are likely to increase cancer risk. Healthier lifestyles build the immune system, which fights foreign substances that invade the body, including cancer cells.

Practicing a healthy lifestyle requires education and commitment. The following measures are all part of an effective cancer prevention lifestyle.

- Eliminate tobacco products, both smoking and chewing.
- Avoid secondhand tobacco smoke and other carcinogens.
- Avoid promiscuous sexual behavior and the sharing of contaminated needles.
- Reduce your intake of animal fat. Eat foods high in fiber.
- Eat several servings a day of food from plant sources (vegetables and fruits).
- Limit your intake of alcoholic beverages.
- Exercise regularly and maintain a normal weight.
- Conduct monthly self-examinations (breasts in females, testicles in males) for lumps and abnormal lesions.
- Inspect your skin regularly for changes in pigmentation, lesions, and abnormal growths.
- Apply sunscreen prior to sun exposure. Wear a wide-brimmed hat and long sleeves when you anticipate being out in the sun for extended periods.

In Practice

You are a medical assistant in the Metropolitan Family Practice medical office. Danielle Smith, 50 years old, is in the office today for her annual physical examination. She mentions to the medical assistant that her close friend had recently been diagnosed with cancer and she wants to know how she could prevent developing cancer. What information can you provide for the patient? What resources do you think might be appropriate?

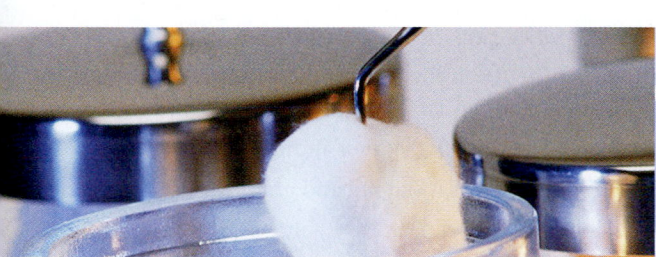

REVIEW

Chapter Summary

- Oncology is the study of malignancies or cancerous growths, including carcinomas, sarcomas, lymphomas, leukemias, and melanomas. Cancer is the rapid and uncontrolled growth and reproduction of abnormal cells. The original malignant growth is the primary site. When a tumor metastasizes, the new sites are known as secondary sites.
- Possible causes of cancer include repeated exposure to carcinogens, genetic cellular mutations due to aging, disease conditions that weaken the immunity system, and certain hormones and viruses. Benign, or nonmalignant, tumors can cause serious symptoms and physiological problems as they grow in size and compress surrounding tissues.

- Detection, diagnosis, and treatment of cancer in earlier stages allow a better prognosis and chance for cure. Screening tests are available for cancers of the breast, rectum, colon, prostate, cervix, testis, tongue, mouth, and skin. Routine diagnostic tests include Pap smears, mammograms, colorectal screening, PSA screening, and others.
- Tumor markers may indicate cancer cell or tumor activity, but are primarily used to monitor tumor growth. Staging identifies the type of cancer and degree of metastasis. Grading determines cellular differentiation and the resulting prognosis.
- The major types of cancer treatment are chemotherapy, radiation therapy, and surgical removal. They may be used alone

Chapter Summary (continued)

or in combination. Combination treatments attack the replication cycle of cancer cells at different times and are often more effective if the patient can tolerate them. Hormonal therapy and immunotherapy are other possible treatments.
■ Both radiation and chemotherapy have serious side effects that must be monitored and managed. As cancer therapies advance, however, some side effects are reduced as well.

■ Hospice programs provide long-term integrated, palliative care to terminally ill patients.
■ Although genetic tendencies toward certain cancers cannot be altered, a cancer prevention lifestyle can help prevent other types of cancer, such as cancer of the lungs, breasts, and skin.

Chapter Review

Multiple Choice

1. The classification *benign* means
   a. cancerous.
   b. noninvasive.
   c. invasive.
   d. destructive.

2. What percentage of U.S. deaths (500,000 a year) are caused by cancer?
   a. 20%
   b. 10%
   c. 15%
   d. 25%

3. Benign tumors result from
   a. slow growth.
   b. rapid growth.
   c. normal growth.
   d. all of the above.

4. Radiation disrupts
   a. cellular replication.
   b. a and c.
   c. DNA.
   d. none of the above.

5. All of the following statements about malignant tumors are true except one. Which one is incorrect?
   a. Tumor cells are undifferentiated.
   b. Tumors are smooth and movable as a unit.
   c. Tumors exhibit rapid growth.
   d. Tumor cells resemble normal cells.

True/False

T F 1. Tumor markers are always an indication of cancer cell or tumor activity.
T F 2. PSA exam and tests are usually prescribed for males annually after the age of 50.
T F 3. Each cancer vaccine contains entire or partial cancer cells or antigens and works to increase the immune response against cancer cells in the body.

T F 4. Oncology is the study of malignancies or cancerous growths, including carcinomas, sarcomas, lymphomas, leukemias, and melanomas.
T F 5. Cancer, or malignancy, is caused by the slow and controllable development and reproduction of abnormal cells.
T F 6. All cancerous tumors are affected by safe doses of radiation.
T F 7. Hormone therapy has not proven to be effective in hormone-dependent cancers such as breast cancer and prostate cancer.
T F 8. Benign tumor recurrence is common after surgical excision.
T F 9. Tumor markers, or cancer markers, are proteins, hormones, and other substances produced by tumors and released into the blood.
T F 10. Mammograms are generally prescribed yearly after the age of 50.

Short Answer

1. What is the term for the holistic care of terminally ill patients in a home or home-like setting?
2. In tumor staging, what does the letter T indicate?
3. What is the difference between staging and grading?
4. List three possible causes of cancer.
5. Name the three major methods of cancer treatment.

Research

1. Is there a support group for breast cancer survivors in your community?
2. In your community, where would a patient find a support group for prostate cancer survivors?

Externship Application Experience

A middle-aged woman visits the medical office. She tearfully states that she has found a lump in her breast. She says, "I'm going to die." What should you do?

Resource Guide

American Cancer Society
1599 Clifton Road NE
Atlanta, GA 30329-4251
404-320-3333 or 800-227-2345
Fax 404-329-7791
www.cancer.org

Cancer Care Incorporated, National Office
275 7th Avenue, 22nd Floor
New York City, NY
212-712-8080 or 800-813-HOPE
Fax 212-712-8495
www.cancercare.org

National Cancer Institute of National Institutes of Health
www.nci.nih.gov/cancerinformation/cancertype/

Cancer Information Service
304-599-1496
800-4-CANCER
Fax 304-599-1552
www.cancer.gov

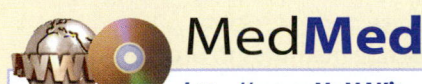

MedMedia

http://www.MyMAKit.com

More on this chapter, including interactive resources, can be found on the Student CD-ROM accompanying this textbook and on http://www.MyMAKit.com.

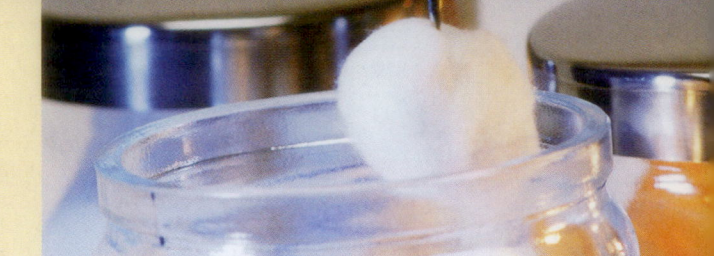

CHAPTER 49

Geriatrics

Case Study

Elora, an RMA (AMT), checks in a patient, Alex Romey, and notices that he is wearing a T-shirt with a slogan that reads: "Do it yourself—I'm retired!" When Elora comments on its humor, Alex explains that this is his last week of work and he plans to wear a different joke shirt each day.

Elora notices that as Alex continues to talk about his past jobs and upcoming retirement, he appears less excited, stops smiling, and starts to look worried. Elora wants to make sure he is prepared for this transition, so she takes a few extra minutes to ask some important questions.

Objectives

After completing this chapter, you should be able to:

- Define and spell the key terminology in this chapter.
- Define the medical assistant's role in a geriatric medical office.
- Discuss the physical changes that take place during aging.
- Explain the psychological aspects of aging.
- Discuss the social components of the aging process.
- Discuss the nutritional needs and problems of the aging person.
- Discuss the economic impact of aging.
- List various cultural views on the place of the elderly in society.
- Describe measures to promote health in geriatric patients.

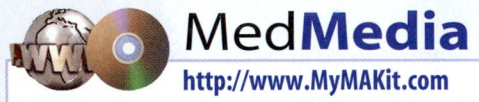

MedMedia

http://www.MyMAKit.com

Additional interactive resources and activities for this chapter can be found on http://www.MyMAKit.com. For a video, audio glossary, tips, legal and ethical scenarios, job scenarios, quizzes, and games related to the content of this chapter, please access the accompanying CD-ROM in this book.

Video
Audio Glossary
Legal and Ethical Scenario: *Geriatrics*
On the Job Scenario: *Geriatrics*
Multiple Choice Quiz
Games: Crossword, Strikeout, and Spelling Bee
Tips
HIPAA Quiz

✚ MEDICAL ASSISTING STANDARDS

CAAHEP ENTRY-LEVEL STANDARDS	ABHES ENTRY-LEVEL COMPETENCIES
▪ Perform within scope of practice (psychomotor) ▪ Explore issue of confidentiality as it applies to the medical assistant (cognitive) ▪ Apply ethical behaviors, including honesty/integrity in performance of medical assisting practice (affective) ▪ Apply local, state and federal health care legislation and regulation appropriate to the medical assisting practice setting (psychomotor) ▪ Recognize the importance of local, state and federal legislation and regulations in the practice setting (affective) ▪ Analyze pathology as it relates to the interaction of body systems (cognitive) ▪ Discuss implications for disease and disability when homeostasis is not maintained (cognitive) ▪ Describe implications for treatment related to pathology (cognitive) ▪ Compare body structure and function of the human body across the life span (cognitive) ▪ Use language/verbal skills that enable patients' understanding (affective) ▪ Apply critical thinking skills in performing patient assessment and care (affective) ▪ Document accurately in the patient record (psychomotor) ▪ Demonstrate diversity in approaching patients and families (affective) ▪ Develop and maintain a current list of community resources related to patients' healthcare needs (psychomotor)	▪ Project a positive attitude. ▪ Maintain confidentiality at all times. ▪ Be a "team player." ▪ Be cognizant of ethical boundaries. ▪ Exhibit initiative. ▪ Adapt to change. ▪ Evidence a responsible attitude. ▪ Be courteous and diplomatic. ▪ Conduct work within scope of education, training, and ability. ▪ Interview and take a patient history. ▪ Prepare patients for and assist physician with routine and specialty examinations and treatments and minor office surgery. ▪ Apply principles of aseptic techniques and infection control. ▪ Prepare and maintain examination and treatment area. ▪ Collect and process specimens. ▪ Dispose of biohazardous materials. ▪ Practice Standard Precautions. ▪ Prepare and administer oral and parenteral medications as directed by the physician. ▪ Maintain medication and immunization records.

✓ COMPETENCY SKILLS PERFORMANCE

1. Role-play sensorimotor changes of the elderly.

Introduction

Life expectancies of different population groups vary, depending on social, economic, environmental, physical, and genetic factors. The average life expectancy in the United States is 76 years. As life expectancy rates continue to rise, it is projected that in the year 2020 16% of the population will be over the age of 65.

Key Terminology

assisted living facility—alternative to long-term care in a nursing home, often the choice for individuals who do not require the 24-hour care provided by skilled nursing facilities

extended care facility—facility that provides 24-hour nursing care; also called nursing home or long-term care facility

geriatrics—science focusing on the aging process; in healthcare, specialty that deals with the disorders of the aging population and their treatment

hemiplegia—paralysis of one side of the body

Medicare—federal health insurance program for those over the age of 65, the disabled, and those with end-stage renal disease

Medigap insurance—insurance for Medicare recipients that covers deductibles and allowable payments not covered by Medicare

orthostatic hypotension—sudden decrease in blood pressure when an individual rises too quickly from a sitting position, usually resulting in light-headedness

paraplegia—paralysis of the lower portion of the body

presbycusis—hearing deficiency normally associated with aging

presbyopia—vision deficiency normally associated with aging

short-term memory—memory of recent events

Abbreviations

CHF—congestive heart failure

LRI—lower respiratory infection

URI—upper respiratory infection

The aging process begins at birth, but becomes more intense during middle age. **Geriatrics** is a medical practice specializing in the treatment and care of older or aging individuals. Some physicians classify themselves as specialists in geriatrics, but most physicians other than pediatricians have geriatric patients in their practice. Patients visiting the medical office may come from independent or **assisted living facilities.** Patients unable to travel may be seen by the physician in a long-term or **extended care facility,** usually on a monthly basis.

The Medical Assistant's Role in the Geriatric Office

As in other specialty medical offices, the medical assistant obtains and charts the patient's history, vital signs, and other pertinent information according to office policy. An important aspect of the MA's role is listening carefully to the patient.

Depending on office policy, the MA may assist aging patients by providing information about community resource agencies that assist the elderly. Local Councils on Aging are a valuable resource that offer social activities and group trips, information sessions, and transportation to grocery stores, shopping centers, and medical care facilities. Many of these agencies also offer financial seminars or services and self-improvement classes.

All patients should be encouraged to document their wishes regarding the extent of medical intervention they desire when they are no longer able to speak for themselves. Advance directives, durable power of attorney, and living wills are discussed in ∞ Chapters 4 and 7. The medical office can be a source of printed information for patients and their families.

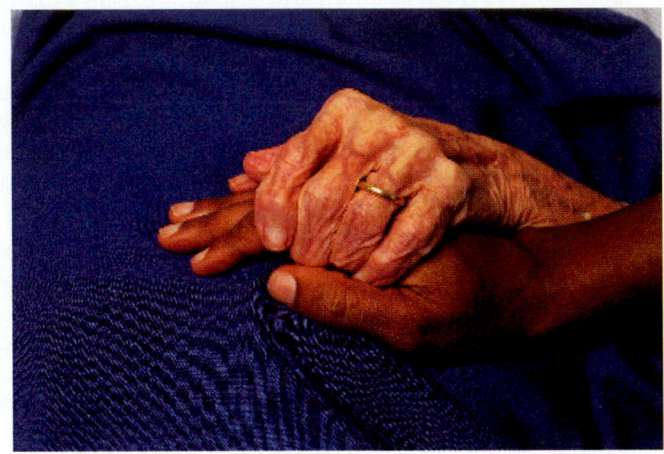

Figure 49-1 ◆ Elderly skin.

The Aging Process

The aging process is an integration of physical, social, and psychological events. Social, economic, and nutritional factors have an effect as well. Some factors—stress, disease, depression—accelerate the process. Others—a healthy diet, exercise, social interaction—can promote a healthier, longer life.

Physical Aspects of Aging

Changes in physical appearance are usually the most obvious changes caused by the aging process. The skin becomes drier, thinner, and less elastic, and it tears easily. Age spots and other changes in pigmentation appear. Wrinkles develop and the skin sags as fat cells and collagen are lost (Figure 49-1 ◆). Dark circles may appear under the eyes, and the eyelids may droop. Hair loss may be total, as in alopecia, or it may involve gradual thinning. In females, supportive tissue is lost in the breasts, which tend to sag as a result. The abdomen thickens in both males and females.

All body systems feel the impact of the aging process.

- The cardiovascular system ages in more than one way. Plaque on vessel walls causes narrowing of the lumen and loss of elasticity. Blood pressure rises, increasing the workload of the heart. The heart itself often enlarges

with the greater workload. It becomes less efficient at pumping blood, circulating nutrients and oxygen, and removing waste from body cells. CHF may result. This sequence moves on to the lungs, which may have experienced some degenerative or disease changes and become less elastic. The exchange of gases through respiration may require greater effort. Higher blood pressure also affects the kidneys or leads to sclerosing in the vessels in the kidneys, resulting in impaired kidney function and related consequences.

- An aging circulatory system contributes to **orthostatic hypotension** when the patient moves too quickly from a resting to an active position.

- Cumulative trauma to all body tissues causes aches and pains, accompanied by reduced range of motion and activity. Muscle tone declines, joints become arthritic and less mobile, and bones are at greater risk for brittleness and breaking due to inactivity. Wear and tear and natural deterioration take their toll on the spinal disks, and the individual stoops and becomes shorter. Hips, knees, ankles and feet are less limber and do not function as well. The fingers become stiff, and the joints are often swollen.

■ The sense of taste, particularly sweet and salty, declines. Vision may be blurred or diminished, and hearing may become impaired. Sensation may also be diminished, which can present certain hazards. For example, an older individual is less able to feel the burning of an overly hot heating pad.

■ As the immune system declines, the body is more susceptible to disease conditions that exacerbate the aging process.

■ As the nervous system ages, the individual finds it harder to control conscious movement. **Short-term memory** may gradually diminish, and custodial care may become necessary.

■ The GI tract has a tendency to slow, resulting in constipation. Spasms of the bladder cause urgency, a prolapsed bladder may lead to infections or incontinence, loss of muscle tone in the sphincter often results in incontinence, and an enlarged prostate may cause urinary retention, frequency, or nocturia.

■ Response time to stimuli is diminished. Tragedies result when elderly drivers fail to respond appropriately in a difficult situation or become confused about the accelerator and brake pedals. Suggesting that the elderly patient stop driving is a task that often falls to the healthcare provider. It is important for the medical assistant to document any discussion with the patient concerning a potentially unsafe situation.

Table 49-1 is a summary of physiological changes in the elderly.

Social and Psychological Aspects of Aging

Social and psychological changes occur as many elderly become more dependent on others for care and financial help. They lose their spouse or companion, other family members, and friends. Retirement often means losing regular social interaction as well as a sense of purpose. Many retired people become

TABLE 49-1 COMMON PHYSIOLOGIC CHANGES IN THE OLDER ADULT

System	Changes	Common Conditions
Cardiac	Decreased cardiac output and efficiency; decreased elasticity of vessel walls, resulting in poor circulation and edema	**CHF,** hypertension, orthostatic hypotension
Endocrine	Increased incidence of metabolic disease, decreased hormonal function, impaired ability to heal	Diabetes type II, thyroid disorders, menopause
Gastrointestinal	Changes in metabolic rate, changes in bowel habits, decreased peristalsis, decreased production of saliva, difficulty chewing and swallowing, loss of teeth, decreased appetite	Cholelithiasis, pernicious anemia, increased drug side effects and adverse interactions with other medications, peptic ulcers, gastroesophageal reflux disease, and colon cancer
Integumentary	Skin: thinning, dryness, decreased elasticity, increased pigmentation (age spots); decreased functioning of sweat and sebaceous glands, adding to dryness; reduced number of fat cells, resulting in often feeling cold (hypothermia); brittle, tough nails; gray or white hair because of loss of pigment; thinning hair or baldness	Seborrheic keratosis, skin tears, photosensitivity, bruising, inability to tolerate temperature extremes, decreased sensitivity to pain, delayed wound healing
Mental Health	Higher incidence of depression due to loneliness, loss of spouse and friends, decreased socialization, loss of sense of usefulness, changes in sleeping patterns	Depression, suicidal thoughts, social isolation
Muscular	Decreased muscle tone and muscle mass, decreased elasticity of ligaments and tendons	Decreasing strength and endurance, related to inactivity, muscle atrophy and fewer muscle cells
Nervous	Diminished sense of touch, pain, temperature, taste, smell, sight (including depth, color, night vision), hearing (delayed auditory response, damage to ossicles, sensoneural damage to auditory nerve); decreased equilibrium and coordination; impaired short-term memory and forgetfulness; slower processing of nervous system impulses; diminished brain size and increased loss of brain cells	Diminished pain perception, touch-related injuries; decreased visual acuity (visual fields, peripheral vision, depth perception, dark adaptation, color discrimination, **presbyopia**), **presbycusis,** (central deafness, conduction deafness), slower musculoskeletal and mental reactions, greater incidence of falls, cerebrovascular accidents (CVA) **paraplegia, hemiplegia,** memory problems, dementia, delirium
Respiratory	Decreased lung capacity, diminished tone in chest wall muscles and diaphragm	Higher risk of contracting **URI** and **LRI,** including pneumonia; advancing stages of emphysema
Skeletal	Softening of the bones, decline in joint flexibility, changes in vertebrae, changes in feet	Osteoporosis, fractures, arthritis, pain on ambulation, shrinking of height
Urinary	Impaired kidney function, diminished bladder tone and sphincter control	Decrease in urinary output, incontinence

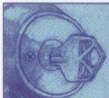

Keys to Success
LISTENING TO THE GERIATRIC PATIENT

Some statements by aging patients demonstrate the complexity and physical effects of aging.

- An 84-year-old female victim of rape tells the emergency department nurse, "If I had my hearing aid in, I would have heard him come in the house. If I had my glasses on, I would have been able to see him. If I had my teeth in, I could have bitten him."

- A 70-year-old male states, "The bones don't work, the ears don't hear, the teeth are falling out, and I can't urinate."

- A 75-year-old female says, "I can't button my clothes, I can't tie my shoes, I can't wear my wedding ring any more because my finger joint is too big, I can't walk in the grocery store without leaning on a grocery cart, I can't open a jar, I can't pick up my granddaughter, and I hurt all the time."

- Two elderly men are discussing how aging is affecting their lives. One comments, "I feel like a baby. I have no teeth, no hair, and I have to wear a diaper or I mess my pants." Listen carefully to what patients report and record it in their charts.

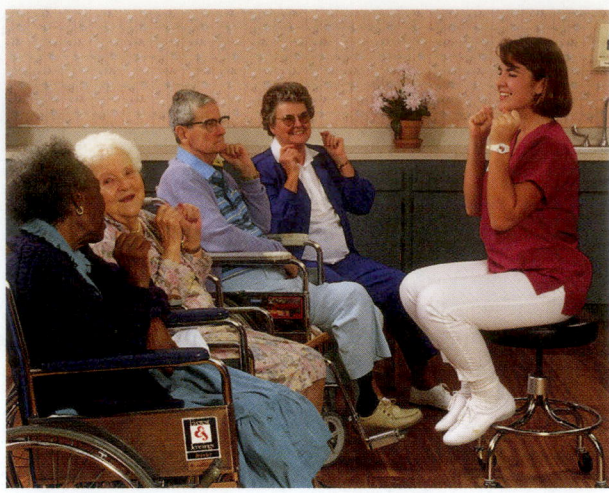

Figure 49-2 ◆ Various groups provide social activities for senior citizens.

Various groups and organizations provide social activities for senior citizens (Figure 49-2 ◆). Local Councils on Aging offer social events and trips. The Red Hat Society is an organization offering activities for women over 50. Other organizations are associated with previous employers or occupations. Many gather for breakfast or lunch, thus providing both social contact and a nutritious meal.

socially isolated and lonely. They must also grapple with a fear of illness and death.

Critical Thinking Question 49-1
What can Elora do to assist the patient during his transition from employment to retirement?

Circulation problems caused by changes in heartbeat or blood supply to the brain may lead to impaired mental functioning. Symptoms of Alzheimer's disease may begin to surface during the aging process. Alzheimer's disease may require long-term or custodial care.

Changes in financial resources and an inability to cope with the physical demands of home upkeep often lead to a change in residence. Familiar surroundings and lifetime attachments are left behind, and the person must learn to cope with the new environment. This major change is often a devastating event for an older person and may lead to depression and occasionally suicide.

An additional impact on social well-being is the often drastic role change that accompanies older age. Self-reliant, independent individuals who have spent most of their lives in a caretaker role suddenly become dependent on their children or others for their care and living arrangements.

Conversations with elderly patients provide clues to their mental status and psychological needs. Elderly persons who have symptoms as the result of a medical condition, a nutritional deficit, or noncompliance with medication administration are sometimes labeled "senile." Patients, especially older patients, should have a complete medical assessment before any psychological diagnosis is made.

Nutritional Aspects of Aging

Nutrition is an important aspect of geriatric care. Many factors contribute to a declining nutritional status:

- Loss of teeth, with a resulting difficulty chewing food
- Poorly fitting dentures
- Decreased secretions and impaired digestive process
- Diminished sensitivity of taste buds
- Solitude during mealtime, eliminating the socialization so helpful in food intake
- Reduced funds for nutritious food
- Inability or diminished desire to prepare meals
- Loss of desire to eat because of depression

Economic Aspects of Aging

The 65th birthday is a dreaded event for many. Our culture has set this age as a rite of passage from activity and regular employment to retirement. Many people look forward to retirement with great anticipation, only to be devastated when the day finally arrives. They feel a loss of identity, self-worth, and financial stability.

Of great concern to the aging population is health insurance. On retirement or at the age of 65, healthcare insurance through an employer is usually no longer available. Ideally, it is replaced by Medicare, the government-sponsored healthcare program. (Refer to ∞ Chapter 17 for a detailed discussion of government insurance.) The **Medicare** system was established

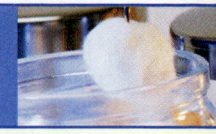

PROCEDURE 49-1 Role-Play Sensorimotor Changes of the Elderly

Theory and Rationale

Americans are living longer and longer. In the year 2000, more than 35 million Americans were older than 65 years. This number is expected to grow to 30% of the total population by the year 2030. As the size of the aging population grows, the need for healthcare will grow as well. There will be a greater need for healthcare professionals who specialize in diseases and disorders of the elderly.

The process of aging has physiological, psychological, and social aspects. The elderly undergo changes in their physical appearance and their ability to cope with their environment. The loss of hearing, taste, smell, and mobility can lead to depression. These changes in sensorimotor abilities impact how the elderly interact with their environment.

Materials

- 2 pairs of laboratory goggles
- yellow tissue paper (such as gift wrap)
- pastel-colored candy
- Vaseline
- earmuffs
- black construction paper
- swimming goggles with one lens blacked out
- heavy dishwashing gloves
- long (50" or more) belt
- walker
- tongue depressors
- ace bandages
- regular print newspaper
- coins (pennies and dimes)
- button-front shirts
- textbook
- tape
- gallon jug of water

Competency

(**Conditions**) With the necessary materials, (**Task**) you will be able to understand the changes that aging patients undergo (**Standards**) within the time determined by the instructor.

1. Vision loss:
   a. Put on the swimming goggles and wait for your partner's directions.
   b. Have your partner stand out of the line of vision and give directions to cross the room and pick up a specific textbook.

2. Vision loss accompanied by hearing loss:
   a. Continue to wear the swimming goggles and put on the earmuffs.
   b. Have your partner stand out of the line of sight and tell you to retrieve a different textbook.

3. Difficulty distinguishing colors:
   a. Remove the goggles and earmuffs. Put on the laboratory goggles, which should be covered with yellow paper to simulate yellowing of the lens.
   b. Have your partner spread the pastel candy on a table and give you directions to pick up specific colors and quantities of each color.

4. Difficulty focusing:
   a. Put on a set of lab goggles that have been smeared with Vaseline.
   b. Without speaking, your partner must get you to walk a specific distance using hand signals.

5. Loss of peripheral vision:
   a. While wearing goggles with black construction paper taped to the sides, have your partner stand out of your line of vision and give you directions to follow.
   b. Have your partner lead you through several turns and doors if possible.

6. Aphasia and partial paralysis:
   a. Bend one arm at the elbow, with your fingertips touching your shoulder. Have another student wrap the ace bandage around your arm, securing it in this position. Bend one leg at the knee with your foot near your buttocks. Have another student secure your leg in place with the belt. Finally, have someone tape your mouth shut.
   b. Your partner should stand several feet away. Communicate to your partner that you need to go to the bathroom.

7. Loss of dexterity:
   a. Put on the dishwashing gloves and try to button a shirt, tie your shoes, and pick up the coins off a flat surface.

8. Problems with mobility:
   a. Use a walker to move across the room.
   b. When you have traveled 2 feet, have your partner hand you a gallon of water to carry.

Patient Education

This exercise will help you better understand the changes that elderly patients are or will be going through.

in 1965 for those over the age of 65, the disabled, and those with end-stage renal disease (ESRD). During their working years, a Medicare tax is deducted from the reported earnings of most individuals, along with the Social Security deduction.

Medicare beneficiaries are encouraged to seek help by calling 1-800-633-4227, the Medicare Helpline, or checking the Medicare website, www.medicare.gov. Medigap insurance is sold by private companies to cover the allowable costs not reimbursed by Medicare. See ∞ Chapter 17 for a more detailed discussion.

Social Security is another federal program for retired Americans. When the Social Security system was implemented in 1935, the age of eligibility for retirement benefits was set at 65 (the earliest qualifying age for Social Security benefits is now 62 years). Social Security was designed as a supplement for retired individuals, those with qualifying disabilities, those unable to work because of a physical disability, and those with end-stage renal disease. Spouses of individuals eligible for Social Security benefits also qualify for benefits when they reach the qualifying age. Those born before January 1, 1938, were eligible for full benefits based on the payments they made throughout their working years. A graduating age schedule applies to those born after January 1, 1938, who also have to work longer to qualify for retirement benefits. Widows and dependent children may be eligible for some benefits as well. It is important to note that eligibility is not automatic; payments must be made into the Social Security program for a minimum of 40 working quarters. Information on Social Security is available online at www.socialsecurity.gov.

Many people retire at 65, others are forced into retirement early, and others continue to work after the age of 65. Some choose to work part-time to supplement their income, while others attempt to live on the fixed income typical of retirement. Many are forced to choose between the essentials of survival (food and shelter) and the medicines they need to stay healthy. Medical care providers should be sensitive to these realities and be alert for signs of financial difficulty, particularly when the patient's health is affected. Many physicians give their Medicare patients pharmaceutical samples when prescribing a new medication. It is an economical way to assess the effect of a drug before prescribing a maintenance regimen. Medical assistants, should also become familiar with services in their community that offer financial and other assistance to the elderly.

Critical Thinking Question 49-2

What can Elora do to make certain the patient has the necessary resources for his retirement and future healthcare coverage?

Cultural Views of Aging

Societal values around the world are reflected in the treatment of the elderly. Table 49-2 lists some of these perspectives on the place of older people in society.

TABLE 49-2 VARIOUS CULTURAL VIEWS OF THE ELDERLY	
Islamic	■ Honor, respect, and stature increase with age. ■ Nursing homes are rare because Muslims care for elderly family members. ■ The eldest son typically cares for the elderly parents.
Chinese	■ Grandparents enjoy a close relationship with their children and grandchildren. ■ The eldest son typically cares for the elderly parents. ■ It is considered shameful not to care for elderly parents.
Indian	■ Elders are respected for their wisdom and often counsel the younger generations. ■ Elders enjoy authority and power and typically control family wealth and arrangement of marriages. ■ Caring for the elderly transmits traditional values and is important to one's status in the afterlife.
Japanese	■ The concept of reciprocity involves being cared for by parents and later caring for the parents. ■ Elders are revered as senior advisors for the family and are given freedom from family duties. ■ The elderly view caring for grandchildren as an honor.
Latino	■ The elderly are considered resources to keep younger generations linked to past traditions. ■ Daughters are expected to care for elderly parents far more than sons are. ■ The elderly do not expect to live with their children, but do expect attention and/or assistance.
Korean	■ Parents are respected and cared for to preserve the family's honor. ■ Health care and financial support are provided by the children.
Native American	■ Elders are respected for their knowledge and wisdom. ■ The elderly pass tradition and cultural values to younger generations. ■ It is a family responsibility to care for the elderly.
Dominant American	■ In an individualistic society, it is embarrassing for the elderly to require assistance. ■ The elderly consider it more desirable to live separately from their children and lead separate lives.
African	■ Elders are respected and honored in families and society and are seen as repositories for wisdom. ■ Large families and lineage groups allow for the elderly family members to be cared for by blood relatives. ■ Elders are elevated to positions of authority in the family and community.

Promoting Health Among the Elderly

Nutrition is a health concern for many elderly. One way to improve the nutritional status of older individuals is to assist them in enrolling in a local "Meals on Wheels" program. This program may differ from community to community, but its basic service is to deliver hot meals and perform regular home visits to provide socialization and check on the status of homebound persons. The local Council on Aging will have information on this program and other food resources.

With the continued increase in the elderly population, many private companies have started to address the concerns unique to aging adults. Living in their home with a caregiver who is scheduled to stop by, help with chores, shopping and companionship are an option. There are also unique living communities that cater specifically to the elderly population. These communities often have a recreational center for group activities, on-site healthcare facility, and aides to help with home maintenance and everyday chores, all while allowing the privacy of living in an individual apartment. There are numerous possibilities available for as much or as little additional help that the elderly patient may need, and the medical assistant should have contact lists available to the patient for researching these possibilities.

Physical activity is another important aspect of the aging process. Many of the elderly become less active and should be encouraged to include some type of moderate exercise, such as walking, in their daily routine as appropriate. Malls and school gyms provide a fairly safe environment for walking. Patients should be cautioned, however, to consult with their physician before beginning an exercise program.

In Practice

The local pharmacist calls the medical office and tells the medical assistant that Mr. Anderson, an elderly patient, is in the pharmacy for a refill on his blood pressure medication. The pharmacist tells the medical assistant that the same prescription was filled just two weeks ago, but the patient states that he is "all out of medicine." What should the medical assistant advise the pharmacist to do?

The elderly are prone to falls. They should be encouraged to eliminate throw rugs in their homes and keep all areas well lit. A grab bar can be of great help moving in and out of the bathtub. Railings or banisters should be installed along steps and stairways. Other safety and assistive devices that can help older individuals maintain their independence (Figure 49-3 ◆) are:

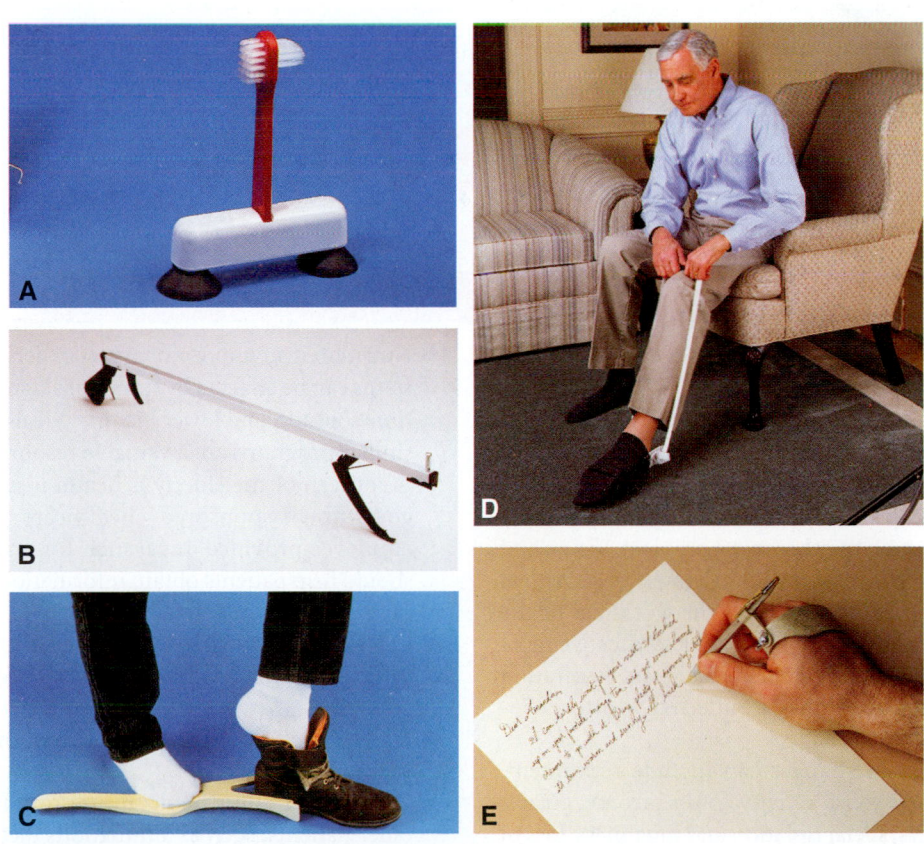

Figure 49-3 ◆ Various assistive devices: (A) a toothbrush; (B) a reaching stick; (C) a shoe holder; (D) a stocking helper; (E) a writing aid.

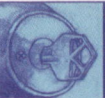

Keys to Success
MYTHS AND MISCONCEPTIONS ABOUT AGING

Certain common beliefs about aging are more accurately seen as myths and misconceptions. Among these are the beliefs that getting older guarantees:

- A decline in activity and enjoyment of life
- Loss of sexuality and capacity for intimacy
- A decline in mental function
- Loss of independence
- Abandonment by family
- Loss of ability to contribute to society
- Mandatory retirement
- Financial insecurity
- Loneliness and depression

    You can better serve older patients by ignoring these stereotypes about growing older.

- Wheelchairs
- Crutches, standard and quad canes
- Walkers

- Handrails and grab bars
- Shower benches and bathtub seats
- Elevated toilet seats and portable commodes
- Extended reachers or grabbers
- Velcro fasteners
- Medication containers with adapted lids
- Large-print and audio books
- Helper dogs
- Adequate lighting with reduced glare
- Grooming, bathing, and dressing devices
- Eating devices

It has been estimated that only 20 to 30% of the elderly are familiar with the Internet. Many have no access to computers. Assisting these individuals to locate facilities that offer help or guidance in this area is a valuable service the MA can offer.

It is important for the MA to become familiar with the normal changes that accompany aging. As part of total patient care, the MA will help older patients identify these changes and how to address or cope with them in order to improve their overall quality of life.

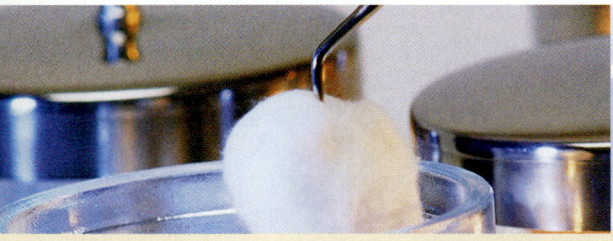

REVIEW

Chapter Summary

- Geriatrics is a medical specialty that focuses on the care and treatment of older or aging patients.
- The aging process becomes more intense during middle age. Physical changes are complex and affect all body systems. The skin becomes thinner and drier, and age spots may appear. The GI tract slows, resulting in constipation. Urinary incontinence or retention may become a problem. Vision and hearing problems are common. Blood vessels become less elastic. High blood pressure increases the workload of the heart, which often enlarges and becomes less effective in its pumping function. The lungs are less elastic and respiration requires greater effort. The bones are affected by osteoporosis and other degenerative changes.
- Social and psychosocial changes can include retirement, decreased physical and social activity, lower income, greater dependence on others, social isolation and loneliness, loss of spouse or companion, and a change in living arrangements.

- Nutrition is an important aspect of geriatric care. Nutritional status can be affected by health problems, loss of teeth, mealtime solitude, and lower income. Meals on Wheels and other similar programs are a valuable resource for the elderly.
- A concern of the elderly is health insurance. Medicare, the government-sponsored healthcare program, replaces employer-provided insurance for many. Medical offices should help patients obtain information regarding insurance programs.
- Medical care providers should be alert for signs of financial difficulty among older patients, especially when health is affected.
- Different cultures have different views on aging and the treatment of elders.
- Promoting healthy habits to improve the quality of life for older patients, such as a nutritious diet and moderate exercise, should be a goal of the medical office.

Chapter Review

Multiple Choice

1. Which of the following means "hearing deficiency normally associated with aging"?
   a. Hemiplegia
   b. Presbyopia
   c. Paraplegia
   d. Presbycusis

2. The average life expectancy in the United States is
   a. 79 years.
   b. 67 years.
   c. 87 years.
   d. 76 years.

3. What percentage of the U.S. population will be over the age of 65 in the year 2020?
   a. 16%
   b. 18%
   c. 20%
   d. 14%

4. An enlarged prostate can cause all of the following except
   a. urinary frequency.
   b. urinary retention.
   c. CHF.
   d. nocturia.

5. The federal healthcare program established in 1965 to serve those over age 65, the disabled, and those with ESRD was
   a. Medicaid.
   b. Medicare.
   c. Social Security.
   d. IRA.

6. As part of their daily routine, the elderly should be encouraged to
   a. avoid exercise.
   b. engage in strenuous exercise.
   c. include moderate exercise.
   d. sleep as much as possible.

7. The U.S. culture has set the age of _____ as a rite of passage from work to retirement.
   a. 65
   b. 70
   c. 55
   d. 60

8. The Social Security system was implemented in
   a. 1935.
   b. 1925.
   c. 1945.
   d. 1955.

True/False

T F 1. Social Security benefits are automatic.

T F 2. The minimum number of working hours for Social Security eligibility is 40 working quarters.

T F 3. Spouses of individuals eligible for Social Security benefits do not qualify at any age.

T F 4. The best way to improve nutritional status of older individuals is to insist that they eat only prepared meals from a restaurant or takeout.

T F 5. It is estimated that only 40% of the elderly are familiar with the Internet.

T F 6. Computers are getting less and less expensive as technology improves, so most elderly people now own one.

T F 7. The aging process becomes more intense during middle age.

T F 8. Aging causes the skin to become thicker and more leathery.

T F 9. *Alopecia* is a condition of total loss of hair.

Short Answer

1. What substance forms on blood vessel walls, causing a loss of elasticity and leading to high blood pressure?

2. Name three gastrointestinal changes that take place in elderly adults.

3. What is the term for the condition that occurs when an elderly patient moves too quickly from a resting to an active position?

4. List three factors that contribute to declining nutritional status among the elderly.

Research

1. Is there a Red Hat Society in your local area?

2. Is there a special society for men of retirement age in your community?

Externship Application Experience

A man brings his elderly mother to the medical office because of a recent history of light-headedness and unsteadiness when standing. He interrupts her as she speaks and insists on answering questions for her. What should you do to obtain the history from the patient herself?

Resource Guide

Administration on Aging
Washington, DC 20201
202-619-0724
www.aoa.gov

American Association of Retired Persons (AARP)
601 E Street NW
Washington, DC 20049
1-800-424-3410
www.aarp.org

American Geriatrics Society
350 Fifth Avenue, Suite 801
New York, NY 10118
212-308-1414
www.americangeriatrics.org

Meals on Wheels Association of America
1414 Prince Street, Suite 302
Alexandria, VA 22314
703-548-5558
www.mowaa.org

National Council on Aging (NCOA)
300 D Street, SW
Suite 801
Washington, DC 20024
202-479-1200
www.ncoa.org

United Seniors Association Inc.
3900 Jamestown Road, #450
Fairfax, VA 22030
1-800-877-2872
www.unitedseniors.org

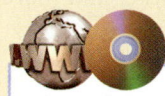

Med**Media**

http://www.MyMAKit.com

More on this chapter, including interactive resources, can be found on the Student CD-ROM accompanying this textbook and on http://www.MyMAKit.com.

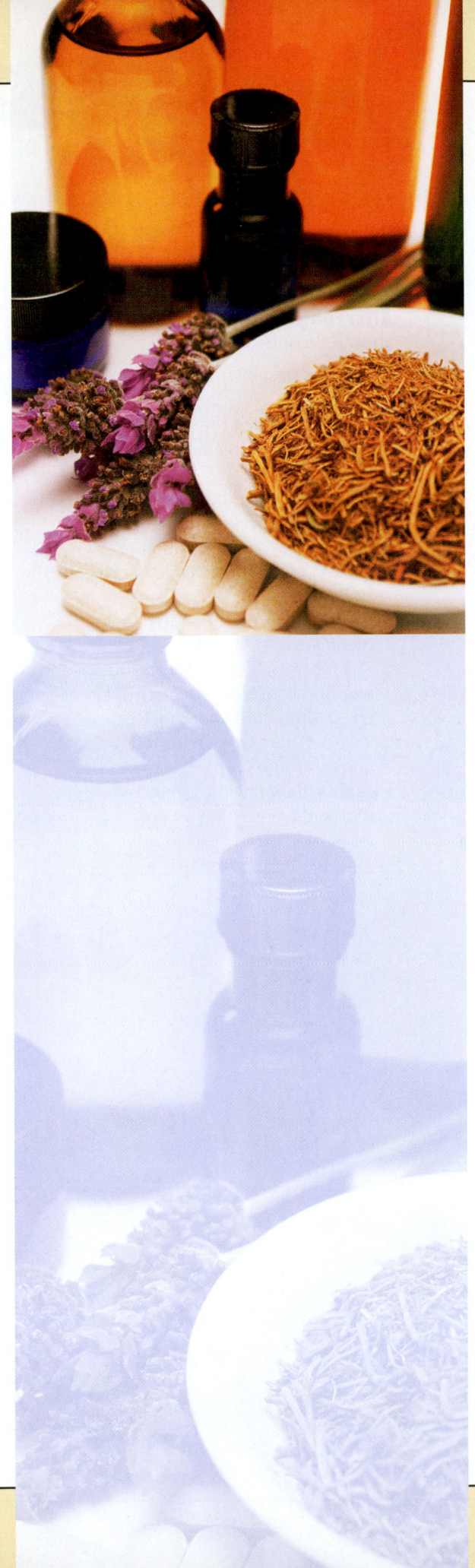

UNIT XI

Nontraditional Medicine

Chapter 50   **Alternative Medicine**

My name is Suzanne Bitters and I am a Registered Medical Assistant. In 1991, having to make a decision to change my direction in life, my cousin handed me a medical assisting textbook telling me, "You are going to love this field." Within a month I was enrolled and starting my new path in life.

I started in the field, getting myself an externship with an internal medicine physician. The doctor was willing to bring me on with no experience. Throughout my time in his practice, I learned professionalism, compassion, as well as the skills necessary to be an accomplished medical assistant. In 1997, I was able to fulfill my promise as I was hired as a medical assisting instructor as well as externship coordinator. Over my nine years teaching, I have in fact helped many students change their lives for the better: Teaching students that they are capable of impacting their patient's lives for the better, and teaching students that this field is never limited except by one's own ambitions.

I retired from teaching and am currently working in a cancer research facility. My position as phlebotomist is again at the forefront, breaking new ground for up-and-coming phlebotomists.

The facility took a chance on me, never having hired a MA/Phlebotomist. They are utilizing all of my skills in ways they did not realize when they hired me. I am on the Emergency Response Team (as well as training the ERT in CPR/FA); I work with the safety committee to make sure all of the labs are OSHA compliant as well as equipped with the most up-to-date safety equipment; I am training the researchers in patient confidentiality/HIPAA compliance; I am able to do vital signs on donors if the research needs it; I write proper protocol to be followed; and I work one-on-one with the researchers in development of their projects, from discussing the techniques needed to take the perfect specimen to which additive in the tubes will provide the right reaction needed to further their cancer research.

Making the decision to become a medical assistant so many years ago was the best decision I ever made. Wanting to be something that my children could be proud of, all of the life issues that came up, all of the hard work and self-doubt that had to be overcome to bring me to this point in my life—I would not change one second of every day.

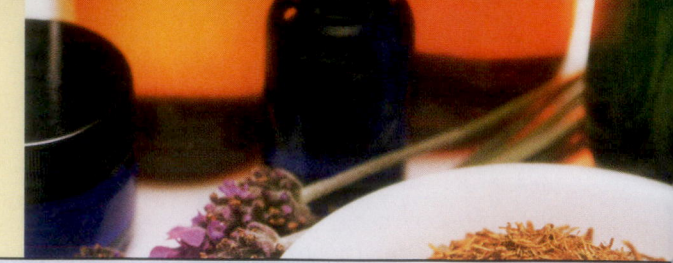

Alternative Medicine

Case Study

Leslie's patient has come in for a followup appointment after completing treatments for a recent motor vehicle accident. During her vitals and assessment, the patient mentions that although she has finished her physical therapy, her neck muscles still get tight and she gets headaches. She also mentions that she would be very interested in an alternative therapy, such as massage, because she is not comfortable with the long-term use of muscle relaxants and other narcotics.

Objectives

After completing this chapter, you should be able to:

- Define and spell the key terminology in the chapter.
- List and describe the five NCCAM classifications of complementary and alternative medicine.
- Describe some types of alternative medicine: Ayurveda, homeopathy, naturopathy, and acupuncture.
- Explain the basic principle of biofeedback.
- Explain how aromatherapy and herbal medicine are used.
- Describe some types of manipulative and body-based therapies: hydrotherapy, acupressure, chiropractic, Craniosacral Therapy, exercise, reflexology, and massage.
- Explain the principle behind energy therapies.

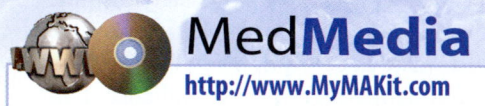

Med**Media**

http://www.MyMAKit.com

Additional interactive resources and activities for this chapter can be found on http://www.MyMAKit.com. For audio glossary, legal and ethical scenarios, job scenarios, quizzes, and games related to the content of this chapter, please access the accompanying CD-ROM in this book.

Audio Glossary
Legal and Ethical Scenario: *Nontraditional Medicine*
On the Job Scenario: *Nontraditional Medicine*
Multiple Choice Quiz
A & P Quiz: The Muscular System; The Skeletal System
Games: Crossword, Strikeout, and Spelling Bee

✚ MEDICAL ASSISTING STANDARDS

CAAHEP ENTRY-LEVEL STANDARDS	ABHES ENTRY-LEVEL COMPETENCIES
▪ Perform within scope of practice (psychomotor) ▪ Explore issue of confidentiality as it applies to the medical assistant (cognitive) ▪ Apply ethical behaviors, including honesty/integrity in performance of medical assisting practice (affective) ▪ Apply local, state and federal health care legislation and regulation appropriate to the medical assisting practice setting (psychomotor) ▪ Recognize the importance of local, state and federal legislation and regulations in the practice setting (affective) ▪ Use language/verbal skills that enable patients' understanding (affective) ▪ Practice Standard Precautions (psychomotor) ▪ Document accurately in the patient record (psychomotor) ▪ Demonstrate diversity in approaching patients and families (affective)	▪ Project a positive attitude. ▪ Maintain confidentiality at all times. ▪ Be a "team player." ▪ Be cognizant of ethical boundaries. ▪ Exhibit initiative. ▪ Adapt to change. ▪ Evidence a responsible attitude. ▪ Be courteous and diplomatic. ▪ Conduct work within scope of education, training, and ability. ▪ Interview and take a patient history. ▪ Apply principles of aseptic techniques and infection control. ▪ Prepare and maintain examination and treatment area. ▪ Dispose of biohazardous materials. ▪ Practice Standard Precautions.

Introduction

Over the last few decades, many alternative forms of medicine have found their way into the U.S. healthcare system. Some have been accepted by the mainstream medical community, but others have been rejected or are regarded with skepticism.

Healthcare consumers are interested in pain relief and, if possible, a cure for their ailments. They are far more educated today about the range of treatments available to them, and many turn to complementary and alternative medicine (**CAM**) when conventional methods fail to meet their needs. They weigh the benefits of conventional medicine, which is sometimes invasive or has undesirable side effects, against the benefits of complementary or alternative methods that are more holistic and usually incorporate natural products and healthy lifestyle habits. Many physicians recommend alternative therapies for their patients to enhance their general health and well-being or to complement conventional treatment.

Alternative medicine has become so popular and in many instances so promising that the government has created the National Center for Complementary and Alternative Medicine (**NCCAM**). Ongoing scientific studies at NCCAM and elsewhere focus on the safety and effectiveness of alternative therapies.

Key Terminology

alternative medicine—systems of medical options varying from traditional medicine, chosen by individuals in place of regularly prescribed modalities and including certain diagnostic procedures and/or accepted and regularly prescribed treatment modalities; examples are aromatherapy, massage therapy, acupuncture, faith healing, and therapeutic touch

complementary medicine—systems of medical options varying from traditional medicine, chosen by individuals along with regularly prescribed modalities; examples include use of herbal remedies such as saw palmetto to promote prostate health

essential oils—oils extracted from flowers and herbs and integrated into an oil base for use in aromatherapy

integrative medicine—systems of medical options that incorporate forms of alternative medicine, complementary medicine, and traditional medicine

Abbreviations

CAM—complementary and alternative medicine

IM—Integrative Medicine

NCCAM—National Center for Complementary and Alternative Medicine

The Medical Assistant's Role in Alternative Medicine

Medical assistants should be aware of the various forms of CAM. When taking a patient history, the MA will need to gather and document information regarding the patient's use of any alternative or complementary medicines or treatments. Harmful interactions may result when conventional and alternative medicine are used simultaneously. The medical assistants will also direct the patient's questions about complementary and alternative therapies to the physician.

Complementary and Alternative Medical Systems

Complementary and alternative therapies are not new concepts; many have been in active use for thousands of years. According to NCCAM, "Complementary and alternative medicine, as defined by NCCAM, is a group of diverse medical and health care systems, practices, and products that are not presently considered to be a part of conventional medicine." **Complementary medicine** works together with conventional medical treatment. An example is massage therapy or relaxation techniques used in combination with pain medication. **Alternative medicine,** such as homeopathy, is practiced in place of conventional medical treatment. **Integrative medicine** incorporates conventional, complementary, and alternative therapies to treat medical conditions. Aromatherapy, reflexology, and music therapy used together in one session are an example of integrative medicine.

NCCAM has classified the various forms of complementary and alternative medicine (CAM) into five categories:

- Alternative medicine: homeopathic and naturopathic medicine, traditional Chinese medicine, Ayurveda
- Mind–body interventions: cognitive behavioral therapy, biofeedback, prayer, meditation, and therapies incorporating art, music, and dance
- Biologically based therapies: aromatherapy, herbal medicine
- Manipulative and body-based methods: acupressure, osteopathic and chiropractic manipulation, hydrotherapy, bodywork, Craniosacral Therapy, exercise, reflexology, various forms of massage
- Energy therapies: biofield therapies, biomagnetic-based therapies

Some of these therapies are described below.

Alternative Medicine

Alternative methods of diagnosis and treatment have been used for centuries. Many of the concepts of ancient as well as nineteenth- and twentieth-century medicine are now recognized as having validity. An example is the use of leeches to eat dead tissue and clean wounds. Nontraditional medical concepts have their origins in cultures all over the world. The Asian medical tradition has contributed several important concepts in alternative medicine, such as acupuncture, acupressure, and the use

of herbs, that are gaining popularity and recognition in the West. This chapter will introduce some of the alternative and complementary practices used today.

Ayurveda

Ayurveda is an ancient healing practice that originated in India. The Sanskrit word *Ayurveda* means "knowledge of life." Ayurvedic practice does not directly treat disease, but focuses on prevention of disease by promoting the return and maintenance of good health. It consists of exercise, nutritional counseling, massage, meditation, and herbal treatments. Ayurveda operates on two principles:

- The mind influences the operation of the body. Negative thoughts can create or aggravate illness. Positive thoughts assist in the return and maintenance of good health.
- Each individual has a specific body type, called *prakriti*, that affects the specific direction of treatment.

According to Ayurvedic principles, the body is made up of *dhatus* (tissues), *malas* (waste products), and *doshas* (energetic forces). The body operates according to the balance of three *doshas*. The *pitta* controls body metabolism, the *kapha* manages the musculoskeletal system, and the *vata* is responsible for cardiovascular, respiratory, digestive, and nervous system functions. The three *doshas,* or *tridoshas,* assist with the creation of all the tissues of the body and remove waste products. They influence all movements, all transformations, all sensory functions, and many of the other activities of the human body and mind. The goal of treatment is to balance the three *doshas*.

The *vata* is the most important of the three *doshas*. *Vata* is the main driver or mover of the body, including the other two *doshas,* the tissues, and the waste products. If the *vata* becomes sufficiently imbalanced, it can throw another *dosha* off balance. If it causes both *pitta* and *kapha* to become imbalanced, this is called a tridoshic imbalance and is the most difficult to overcome.

There are no licensing or accrediting boards for the practice of Ayurveda in the United States. Practitioners with a Bachelor of Ayurveda Medical Studies degree can practice as consultants but not as medical doctors.

Homeopathy

Homeopathic treatment involves the use of natural remedies made from plant, animal, or mineral substances to stimulate the immune system and strengthen the body's healing processes.

Homeopathy is based on the theory that "like cures like"—that large doses of certain substances cause symptoms but smaller, highly diluted doses cure them. Homeopathic remedies are diluted to different strengths, and the practitioner determines which strength to prescribe based on an assessment of the patient. Homeopathy remains a controversial treatment that has not been substantiated by scientific research.

A medical doctor (MD), doctor of osteopathy (DO), or dental surgeon (DDS) can become a Diplomate in Homeopathy (DHt) by passing a written and practical exam. To receive a CCH (Certified in Classical Homeopathy) credential, a candidate must complete 500 hours of training, one to two years experience, and pass a written and practical exam.

Naturopathy

Naturopathy is an eclectic approach that helps the body heal itself by treating psychological, physical, and genetic factors in addition to the disease process. A naturopath may use any of the following approaches: nutritional and lifestyle counseling, acupuncture, exercise, hydrotherapy, osteopathy, homeopathy, herbal medicine, and others.

Naturopaths are licensed primary care practitioners. They determine the cause of the illness, educate the patient about a healthier lifestyle, and select the best treatment. They also refer patients to other healthcare professionals as necessary.

Four years of naturopathic medical school are required to become a Doctor of Naturopathic Medicine (ND). Some states require passing a state or national board examination.

Acupuncture

Acupuncture is an important component of traditional Chinese medicine that has been practiced for over 5,000 years. The insertion of very thin needles into predetermined sites stimulates changes in heart rate, blood pressure, brain activity, blood chemistry, and the immune and endocrine systems (Figure 50-1 ◆).

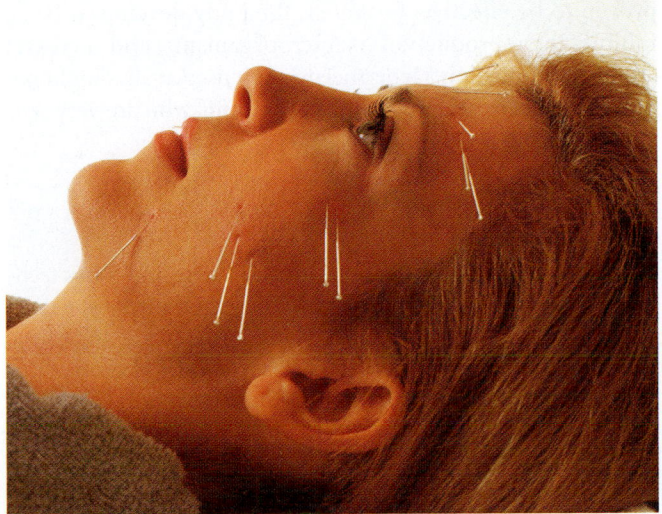

Figure 50-1 ◆ A client receiving acupuncture treatment.
Source: Phototake NYC

Acupuncture helps the body naturally regulate red and white blood cell counts and raise endorphin production. Some health problems or disease processes are treated by as few as one acupuncture treatment; others require many treatments. There is little risk from acupuncture. It is often used in conjunction with conventional medicine for pain management, asthma, drug addiction (illegal, narcotic, alcohol, and nicotine), stroke, and other conditions.

Some private insurance and Medicaid programs reimburse for acupuncture, especially in the treatment of back pain. In most states acupuncturists are licensed separately, but in a few states practitioners of acupuncture must be medical doctors.

Mind–Body Interventions

The focus of mind–body medicine is the ways in which a person's mental, emotional, social, and spiritual health directly affects his or her physiological health. This holistic approach uses techniques that enhance the mind's ability to influence body function and symptoms. For example, positive thinking, along with laughter and personal contact, help to release endorphins, the body's natural antipain mediators.

Biofeedback

Biofeedback is the process of training the client in relaxation, visualization, and meditation techniques. During these activities, body functions such as blood pressure, heart rate, muscle tension, and brain waves are electronically monitored by a biofeedback machine. Audible signals from the machine help the client learn to consciously control his or her body systems and responses. Eventually, the client learns to use the relaxation techniques without biofeedback monitoring. This program has been particularly effective in stress management and has been used to treat migraine headaches, depression, insomnia, and other conditions.

There is no state licensing for biofeedback practitioners. The Biofeedback Certification Institute of America and other groups offer certification.

Integrative Medicine

Integrative Medicine (IM) is used in many U.S. hospitals, universities, and medical schools today. The goal of integrative medicine is to treat the person and not just the disease. With IM, the mind, body, and spirit are treated all at the same time, and conventional and alternative approaches are combined. For example, conventional Western medicine might be used to treat disease along with alternative or complementary treatments, such as yoga, stress reduction techniques, massage, herbal medicine, acupuncture, and biofeedback in an effort to treat the whole person.

Biologically Based Therapies

Natural substances such as herbs, foods, vitamins, and essential oils are the basis for biologically based therapies.

Aromatherapy

Essential oils extracted from flowers and herbs are used in aromatherapy. This branch of herbal healing has been practiced since ancient times, when aromatic plants were burned to drive out evil spirits and purify the air. René Maurice Gattefosse, a French chemist, experimented with essential oils and published his findings in 1928 in a book called *Aromatherapy.*

Aromatherapy affects the autonomic nervous system and stimulates the release of chemicals that are responsible for relaxation and the reduction of pain. Some essential oils have antibacterial or anti-inflammatory properties. Certain oils may be prescribed for complaints such as colds and flu, sinusitis, migraine headaches, insomnia, digestive problems, and muscle aches and pains. Rosemary oil is used for muscle relaxation and pain relief. Jasmine oil helps ease depression, eucalyptus oil and oil of wintergreen relieve congestion, lavender oil relieves anxiety and improves sleep, and peppermint oil relieves nausea and aids in digestion. Lemon, orange, and other citrus oils improve the mood and mental alertness.

Essential oils are extracted in a steam distillation process. They may be added to lotions used in massage treatments. Therapeutic scents can be diffused into the air with spray bottles, diffusers, and baths.

It is important to remember that although aromatherapy is usually considered safe, it is a complementary therapy and should not be used as a substitute for conventional medical care. Essential oils can be quite potent, and some carry potential side effects.

There are no licensing requirements or accrediting boards for the practice of aromatherapy in the United States. Schools usually have their own certification standards.

Herbal Medicine

Throughout history, herbs have been used to treat disease and prevent illness. In the twentieth century the medicinal use of herbs declined as synthetic drugs took their place in conventional medicine. Many people are now turning to natural herbal medicine again.

Herbs are chosen according to their properties and are usually used in combination with other holistic treatments. Some herbs are said to counteract the effects of poor nutrition, stress, and lack of exercise. Others may help repair, strengthen, and rebuild body tissues. Much of the evidence is anecdotal, however. Scientific research has not validated many of the claims of therapeutic benefits to be derived from herbs. Individuals taking herbal supplements should do so with caution. Although side effects are uncommon, they should be discussed with the physician.

There are no herbal medicine licensing or accrediting boards in the United States. In addition, there are no controls or standards for herbal products. The FDA has not given its stamp of approval to any of these products.

Some herbs and their reported benefits are briefly described in Table 50-1. Keep in mind that these benefits have not necessarily been verified.

In Practice

Ms. Smith is in the office complaining of cold symptoms for several days. She states that her mother gave her echinacea and told her that it would help to relieve some of her symptoms. She wants to know if herbs are safe. How should the medical assistant respond to the patient?

Manipulative and Body-Based Methods

Hydrotherapy is a body-based method that uses water to treat disease. Bodywork is a broad term referring to the hands-on manipulation of the musculoskeletal system to promote healing, energy flow, pain reduction, relaxation, and improved health. The following techniques fall into this category: acupressure, Alexander Technique, chiropractic, craniosacral therapy, Feldenkrais Method, foot reflexology, lymphatic massage, Rolfing, shiatsu, sports massage, Swedish massage, Trager approach, and trigger point therapy.

Hydrotherapy

Hydrotherapy, also called water therapy, is available in many forms. It can be offered in a swimming pool, sauna, steam bath, whirlpool, Jacuzzi, or hot tub, or in the form of a hot/cold pack, ice massage, or moist heat pack. Hydrotherapy increases flexibility and strength and accelerates the healing process. It can be used with individuals who cannot withstand the rigors of traditional exercise programs. In conventional medicine, hydrotherapy is usually an addition to physical therapy.

Hydrotherapy by heat stimulates circulation and relaxes the muscles, but prolonged exposure to heat can have the effects of cold therapy. Hydrotherapy by cold reduces swelling and pain, but prolonged application of cold can have the effects of heat therapy. Hydrotherapy-induced hyperthermia has not been proven to be effective. In theory, the body develops a fever, inhibits the reproduction of microorganisms, and increases antibody production. Hyperthermia, if it used at all, should not be induced in the elderly or the very young, who are very sensitive to high temperatures.

Acupressure

Acupressure, or shiatsu, is a traditional Chinese bodywork technique. It is a form of massage and is based on a concept similar to acupuncture. The goal of acupressure is to relieve discomfort by promoting greater balance and circulation of fluids and metabolic energies in the body. Normally, a healing energy or current known as *chi* circulates through body meridians. If it is blocked, disease results. Pressure and massage are applied with the fingers, thumbs, palms, and elbows at appropriate pressure points, often some distance from where the symptom appears. This technique relaxes the involved muscle or tissue, thereby reducing or eliminating pain.

TABLE 50-1 COMMON HERBS USED FOR MEDICINAL PURPOSES

Herb	Reported Properties and Benefits	Herb	Reported Properties and Benefits
Angelica	astringent, diuretic, anti-inflammatory, expectorant, tonic	Licorice	expectorant, antispasmodic, anti-inflammatory, antihepatotoxic, laxative
Bayberry	astringent, antidiarrheal, diaphoretic; stimulates circulatory system, reduces fever, reduces sore throat symptoms (gargle), relieves colitis symptoms	Mustard	irritant, stimulant, diuretic, emetic
Chamomile	anti-inflammatory, antispasmodic, antimicrobial, antianxiety; relieves insomnia, neuralgia, vertigo, motion sickness, stress	Myrrh	antimicrobial, astringent, expectorant; effective in treating mouth infections, pharyngitis, sinusitis, laryngitis, boils, and wound infections
Echinacea	antimicrobial; stimulates immune response to bacterial and viral invasions; increases phagocytosis and white blood cell count	Peppermint	anti-inflammatory, antispasmodic, antiemetic, antimicrobial, analgesic; relieves tension and anxiety
Eucalyptus	antimicrobial, antispermatic, expectorant	Rhubarb root	laxative, astringent
Garlic	antimicrobial, antispasmodic, diaphoretic, hypotensive; improves cardiovascular function and lowers blood cholesterol	Rosemary	antispasmodic, antidepressive, antimicrobial, rubofacient
Ginseng	stimulant, tonic	St. John's wort	anti-inflammatory, astringent; provides pain relief, sedation; relieves anxiety and tension
Gingko	reduces vertigo, headache, tinnitus, anxiety, depression; improves memory, concentration, alertness; dilates blood vessels and increases cardiovascular circulation	Saw palmetto	diuretic, urinary antiseptic; tones and strengthens male reproductive and urinary system; relieves symptoms of hyperplasia of the prostate gland
Goldenseal	antimicrobial, anti-inflammatory, laxative, expectorant, astringent (especially on mucous membranes)	Tea (or ti) tree	antimicrobial on the skin
Horehound	expectorant, antispasmodic; relaxes smooth muscles, especially in bronchi and respiratory tract	Valerian	antispasmodic, hypnotic, sedative, hypotensive
		Vervain	nerve tonic, sedative, antispasmodic, diaphoretic, hypotensive; reduces stress, tension, depression, fever
Lavender	antispasmodic, antidepressive, hypotensive; relieves stress, headaches, depression; promotes sleep	Witch hazel	astringent, anti-inflammatory
		Yarrow	diaphoretic, urinary antiseptic; lowers fever, dilates peripheral vessels and reduces blood pressure; aids in digestive process

Although there are no state licensing requirements for the practice of acupressure, patients should seek a practitioner who has graduated from an accredited school.

Chiropractic

In chiropractic treatment, manipulation and alignment of the spine promote optimum health of the spinal cord and nervous system. Chiropractic treatment corrects misalignments of the spinal column that cause pain, decreased agility, and illness. In addition to vertebral manipulation, massage therapy, heat, cold, and ultrasound may be applied to relieve tension and spasm. Treatment sessions may also include nutrition and exercise counseling.

All states require chiropractors to be licensed. To become a Doctor of Chiropractic (DC), one must graduate from an accredited school and pass national and state board exams.

Craniosacral Therapy

In Craniosacral Therapy, gentle pressure is applied to the areas of the craniosacral system (skull, face, mouth, spine, sacrum, connecting membranes for the cranium and sacrum, and cerebrospinal fluid) to treat tension in these areas and promote CNS health. Following treatment, it is not unusual for the client to experience some worsening of symptoms from pressure

changes that occur during manipulation. Overall, the treatment can lead to a general state of relaxation.

Craniosacral Therapy was developed by John Upledger, an osteopathic physician. No licensing is required to practice Craniosacral Therapy, although the appropriate training and practical and written exams must be completed.

Exercise

All forms of exercise promote health and raise the level of body functioning. The primary focus of exercise can be cardiovascular or endurance training, stretching, or weight training. Cardiovascular training improves the functioning of the cardiovascular and respiratory systems. Activities such as walking, running, dancing, and swimming improve aerobic capacity and physical endurance. Stretching increases joint flexibility. Weight training strengthens bones and muscles. Exercise approaches can include any of the following: hydrotherapy, yoga, qigong, tai chi, chiropractic, polarity therapy, and the Trager approach.

Reflexology

Reflexology restores the body's natural energy flow by stimulating specific reflex points on the foot or hand (Figure 50-2 ◆). Applying pressure to these points can restore function to the areas connected to each point, or zone. Although there are no

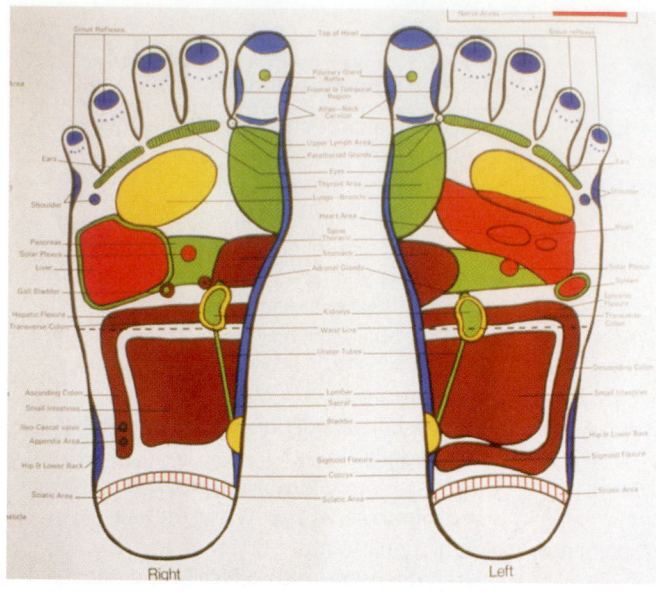

Figure 50-2 ◆ Reflexology points on the sole of the foot.
Source: Photo Researchers, Inc.

state licensing requirements for the practice of reflexology, a certification program followed by a written and practical exam are recommended.

Massage

Massage is the manipulation of muscle and soft tissue to induce relaxation, relieve pain, and promote healing. Done correctly, massage enhances the client's sense of well-being. Types of massage include lymphatic massage, sports massage, and Swedish massage.

Although massage has a number of benefits, there are certain conditions for which it is not appropriate: intoxication, treatment with certain medications, localized tissue inflammation, hematoma, cancer, and others.

Lymphatic Massage

A person with an illness or a sedentary lifestyle may suffer from fatigue and lowered metabolism as a result of the accumulation of waste products in the body. When a healthy flow of lymphatic fluids is restored, waste materials and infectious organisms are more efficiently removed. Lymphatic massage applies pressure and manipulates the muscles to improve the functioning of the lymphatic system. Practitioners massage an area lightly and repeatedly until a small amount of lymphatic fluid surfaces on the skin, then proceed to the next area. Joints are also massaged. A specific order is followed to direct lymphatic flow to the lymph nodes.

Lymphatic massage may not be appropriate if certain conditions exist such as aneurysms, hematomas, tissue damage, or bacterial inflammations.

To perform lymphatic massage, the practitioner must be trained and certified as a Certified Manual Lymph Drainage Therapist (CMLDT). Training in an allied health profession is prerequisite to entering this program.

Sports Massage

Sports massage involves the use of therapeutic massage before, during, and after engagement in sporting activities. Many athletes and sports teams employ a massage therapist or physical therapist who applies massage techniques to loosen up the muscles and relieve fatigue prior to a sporting event. Massage therapy can prepare the athlete for peak performance, reduce muscle tension, promote flexibility, relieve any swelling or edema present, and prevent injuries. During and after the event, the therapist is available to assess any insults to the body and employ massage to promote the healing of strained muscles and keep them in good condition.

Every sporting activity makes different demands on the athlete and uses muscle groups in different ways. The sports massage therapist uses specific techniques to meet different requirements.

Swedish Massage

Swedish massage focuses on general relaxation, stimulating circulation, and enhancing muscle tone. It is effective in reducing muscle tightness. Swedish massage makes use of five main strokes.

- *Effleurage* consists of long, gliding strokes starting at the neck and working down to the base of the spine or from the shoulder down to the fingertips. On the limbs, strokes are directed toward the heart, assisting the blood and lymphatic flow. Effleurage is performed with the whole hand or the thumb pads.
- When performing *petrissage,* the therapist gently lifts muscles up and away from the bones, then follows with a gentle rolling and squeezing action. Kneading and compressing motions, including squeezing, rolling, and pressing, enhance deeper circulation. The goal of petrissage is to increase circulation by clearing toxins from muscle and nerve tissue.
- *Friction,* the most penetrating massage stroke, involves deep circular or transverse movements made with the thumb pads or fingertips. The deep circular movement is performed near joints and other bony areas. Friction breaks down adhesions, or knots, that result when muscle fibers bind together during the healing process, thereby promoting more flexible joints and muscles.
- *Tapotement* is a series of brisk percussive movements. The hands of the therapist alternately strike or tap the muscles, with an invigorating effect. The tapping may be done with the side of the hand, the tips of the fingers, or a closed fist. This technique is used to release tension and muscle spasms.
- In *vibration,* or shaking, the therapist places his or her hands on the limbs or back and performs several seconds of rapid shaking. The goal of this technique is to boost circulation and increase the power of the muscles.

Critical Thinking Question 50-1

What do you think would be the best way for Leslie's patient to find the type of massage that would be most beneficial for her needs?

Energy Therapies

Energy therapies work with the electromagnetic fields that are believed to surround the human body, called biofields. In some energy therapies, such as Reiki, qi gong, and Therapeutic Touch, the biofields are manipulated with the hands. Bioelectromagnetic-based therapies are characterized by more unconventional methods, such as the use of pulsed fields and magnetic fields. It has not been scientifically proven that these so-called biofields exist.

Reiki is a complementary therapy in which a trained practitioner places his or her hands on or above a specific body area and transfers what is called "universal life energy" to the patient. That energy is believed to provide strength, harmony, and balance, which are essential to the treatment of health disturbances. The therapy is derived from ancient Buddhist practice and involves a total of fifteen hand positions covering all body systems.

Therapeutic Touch is a noninvasive, holistic approach to healing that attempts to stimulate the receiver's own powers of recuperation. This modern form of laying on of hands is based on the principle of an energy exchange between people. Therapeutic Touch is believed to reduce or eliminate pain, promote healing, and bring about a relaxation response. Therapeutic Touch is based on the concept that a "human energy field" extends beyond the skin and flows in balanced patterns in health; in illness or injury, it is used up and/or unbalanced. Practitioners of Therapeutic Touch believe they have the ability to restore health by sensing and adjusting these energy fields.

Therapeutic Touch is one of the most visible and popular nontraditional healing techniques practiced by nurses. It is also controversial, and its positive effect may be a result of the positive energy generated by the practitioner.

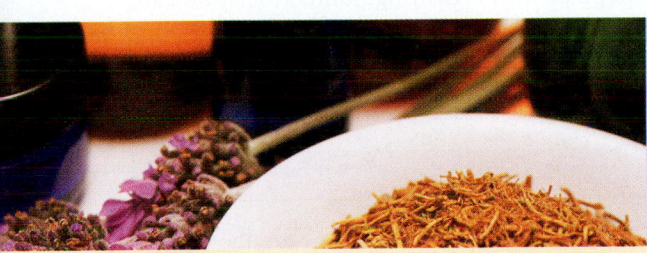

REVIEW

Chapter Summary

- In recent years, alternative, complementary, and integrative therapies have gained popularity and, in some cases, acceptance by the medical community. These forms of medicine have been practiced for many centuries and in many cultures. Medical assistants should be familiar with the various therapies offered in their communities. They should always question patients about any alternative form of treatment they may be receiving. This information should be documented. The MA should be careful not to chastise patients for seeking intervention by any of these methods.

- Alternative treatment modalities such as aromatherapy, massage therapy, acupuncture, faith healing, and therapeutic touch are practiced in place of conventional treatments. Complementary medicine, such as the use of herbal remedies, is used in combination with conventional, regularly prescribed modalities. Integrative medicine brings together conventional, complementary, and alternative therapies to treat medical conditions.

- Ayurveda, homeopathy, naturopathy, and acupuncture are forms of alternative medicine. Ayurveda, an ancient healing practice originating in India, focuses on preventing disease by promoting the return and maintenance of good health. It involves exercise, nutritional counseling, massage, meditation, and herbal treatments. Homeopathy is based on the concept that "like cures like" and uses natural remedies made from plant, animal, or mineral substances to stimulate the body's immune system and healing processes. Naturopathy, an eclectic approach, promotes the concept of the body healing itself and addresses psychological, physical, and genetic factors in addition to the disease process. Acupuncture an important component of traditional Chinese medicine that has been practiced for over 5,000 years. The insertion of very thin needles into predetermined sites stimulates changes in heart rate, blood pressure, brain activity, blood chemistry, and the immune and endocrine systems.

- Other forms of alternative medicine are mind–body interventions, such as biofeedback, and biologically based therapies that feature natural substances such as herbs, foods, vitamins, and essential oils.

- Manipulative and body-based methods include hydrotherapy, acupressure, chiropractic, craniosacral therapy, exercise, reflexology, and different forms of massage.

- Hydrotherapy, or water therapy, is available in many forms, such as sauna, steam bath, hot/cold packs, and ice massage. Hydrotherapy increases flexibility and strength and is useful for individuals who cannot withstand the rigors of traditional exercise programs.

Chapter Summary (continued)

- Acupressure, or shiatsu, is a form of massage based on the concept of healing energy or current (*chi*) circulating through body meridians. If *chi* is blocked, disease results. Pressure and massage are applied at pressure points to dissolve obstructions and reduce or eliminate pain.
- Chiropractic treatment consists of manipulating and aligning the spine to promote optimum health of the spinal cord and nervous system. Craniosacral therapists apply gentle pressure to the craniosacral system to relieve tension in these areas and promote CNS health.
- All forms of exercise promote health and improve body functioning. The primary focus can be cardiovascular or endurance training, stretching, or weight training.
- Reflexology restores the body's natural energy flow by stimulating specific reflex points on the foot or hand.
- Massage, the manipulation of muscle and soft tissue, induces relaxation, relieves pain, and promotes healing. Lymphatic massage is based on the theory that fatigue and lowered metabolism result from the accumulation of waste products in the body. Lymphatic massage improves the functioning of the lymphatic system, thereby removing waste materials and infectious organisms more efficiently. Sports massage involves the application of therapeutic massage before, during, and after engagement in sporting activities. It reduces muscle tension, promotes flexibility, relieves swelling or edema, and prevents injuries. Swedish massage focuses on general relaxation, stimulation of circulation, and enhancing muscle tone. The five main strokes in Swedish massage are effleurage, petrissage, friction, tapotement, and vibration or shaking.
- Energy therapies work with biofields, the electromagnetic fields believed to surround the human body. In some energy therapies, such as Reiki, qi gong, and Therapeutic Touch, the biofields are manipulated with the hands. Other, more unconventional methods rely on the use of pulsed fields and magnetic fields.
- The efficacy of some alternative, complementary, and integrative therapies is not supported by scientific evidence. Most insurance plans do not cover these therapies, but they continue to be popular with a growing number of healthcare consumers.

Chapter Review

Multiple Choice

1. The government branch that controls and evaluates the claims of alternative medicine is
   a. NCCAM.
   b. CAMCC.
   c. NCAM.
   d. CAM.

2. An herb is used as an astringent, diuretic, anti-inflammatory, expectorant, and tonic is
   a. echinacea.
   b. bayberry.
   c. chamomile.
   d. angelica.

3. An herb used for its antimicrobial, antispermatic, and expectorant properties is
   a. chamomile.
   b. bayberry.
   c. eucalyptus.
   d. echinacea.

4. An herb known to lower blood cholesterol is
   a. witch hazel.
   b. lavender.
   c. garlic.
   d. goldenseal.

5. Manipulation and alignment of the spine are the basis of the treatment called
   a. chiropractic.
   b. lymphatic massage.
   c. reflexology.
   d. Swedish massage.

6. A body-based therapy that uses water to treat disease is
   a. acupressure.
   b. hydrotherapy.
   c. chiropractic.
   d. Craniosacral Therapy.

7. A therapy that restores the body's natural energy flow by stimulating specific reflex points on the foot or hand is
   a. chiropractic.
   b. acupressure.
   c. reflexology.
   d. Craniosacral Therapy.

8. The massage stroke that consists of long, gliding strokes is
   a. effleurage.
   b. friction.
   c. petrissage.
   d. tapotement.

9. The massage stroke called *friction* consists of
   a. rapid shaking.
   b. kneading and compression.
   c. tapping or striking.
   d. deep circular movements.

Chapter Review (continued)

10. Massage is not appropriate for conditions such as
    a. fatigue.
    b. localized tissue inflammation.
    c. muscle tightness.
    d. muscle adhesions.

True/False

T F 1. Acupressure, osteopathic, and chiropractic therapies are manipulative and body-based methods.

T F 2. Alternative medicine incorporates conventional, complementary, and alternative therapies to treat medical conditions.

T F 3. According to Ayurvedic principles, the body is made up of dhatus, malas, and doshas.

T F 4. Practitioners with a Bachelor of Ayurveda Medical Studies degree can practice as consultants and medical practitioners.

T F 5. Homeopathic medical treatment uses natural remedies that are all diluted to the same strength.

T F 6. To receive a CCH credential, a candidate must complete 250 hours of training, two to three years experience, and pass written and practical exams.

T F 7. Naturopaths are licensed primary care practitioners.

T F 8. Acupuncture is a traditional Japanese medicine that has been practiced for over 5,000 years.

T F 9. Acupuncture helps the body naturally regulate red and white blood cell counts.

T F 10. Some essential oils possess antibacterial and anti-inflammatory properties.

Short Answer

1. What are essential oils?

2. Which traditional Chinese therapy is used in the treatment of back pain?

3. List the five main strokes used in Swedish massage.

Research

1. Is there a practitioner of hydrotherapy in your community?

2. Is there a practitioner of Ayurveda near you?

Externship Application Experience

A patient comes to you and explains that he has decided not to proceed with the traditional cancer treatments of chemotherapy and medications. A family member has given him a copy of the movie *My Life,* starring Michael Keaton and Nicole Kidman, about a man who attempts to treat his cancer and prepare for death with alternative therapy. How do you respond?

Resource Guide

ACUPRESSURE

American Organization for Bodywork Therapies of Asia (AOBTA)
Laurel Oak Corporate Center, Suite 408
1010 Haddenfield Road
Voorhees, NJ 08043
856-782-1616
www.aobta.org

ACUPUNCTURE/HERBAL MEDICINE

National Acupuncture and Oriental Medical Alliance
14637 Starr Road, SE
Olalla, WA 98359
253-851-6896
www.acuall.org

National Commission for Certification of Acupuncturists (NCCA)
1424 16th Street, NW, Suite 501
Washington D. C. 20036

ALEXANDER TECHNIQUE

North American Society of Teachers of the Alexander Technique (NASTAT)
3010 Hennepin Avenue S., Suite 10
Minneapolis, MN 55408
www.alexandertech.com

AROMATHERAPY

Aromatherapy
836 Hanley Industrial Court
St. Louis, MO 63144

Flower Essence Society
PO BOX 459
Nevada City, CA 95959
800-736-9222
www.flowersociety.org

Nelson Bach USA
Educational Programs
100 Research Drive
Wilmington, MA 01887

Resource Guide (continued)

AYURVEDA

Ayurvedic Institute
11311 Menaul NE, Suite A
Albuquerque, NM 87112

BIOFEEDBACK

Association for Applied Psychophysiology and Biofeedback
10200 W. 44th Avenue, Suite 304
Wheat Ridge, CO 80033

Biofeedback Certification Institute of America
255 W. 98th St
New York, NY 10025
212-222-5665
www.biof.com

CHIROPRACTIC

American Chiropractic Association
1701 Clarendon Boulevard
Arlington, VA 22209
800-986-4636
www.amerchiro.org

CRANIOSACRAL THERAPY

The Upledger Institute, Inc.
11211 Prosperity Farms Road
Palm Beach Gardens, FL 33410-3487
800-233-5880
www.upledger.com

FELDENKRAIS METHOD

Feldenkrais Guild
3611 SW Hood Ave, Suite 100
Portland, OR 97201
800-775-2118

HATHA YOGA

International Association of Yoga Therapists
20 Sunnyside Avenue, Suite A243
Mill Valley, CA 94941

HERBAL MEDICINE

American Holistic Medical Association
6728 Old McLeon Village Drive
McLeon, VA 22101

National Acupuncture and Oriental Medicine Alliance
14637 Starr Road, SE
Olalla, WA 98359

HOLISTIC DENTISTRY

Holistic Dental Association
PO Box 5007
Durango, CO 81301
970-259-1091
www.holisticdental.org

International Academy of Oral Medicine and Toxicology, IAOMT
PO Box 608531
Orlando, FL 32860-8531
407-298-2450
www.iaomt.org

HOMEOPATHY

National Center for Homeopathy
801 N. Fairfax Street, Suite 306
Alexandria, VA 22314

HYDROTHERAPY

Aquatic Exercise Association
PO BOX 1609
Nokomis, FL 34274

HYPNOTHERAPY/HYPNOTISM

American Board of Hypnotherapy
16842 Von Karman Avenue, Suite 475
Irvine, CA 92606

American Society of Clinical Hypnosis
2200 East Devon Avenue, Suite 291
Des Plaines, IL 60018

International Medical and Dental Hypnotherapy Association
4110 Edgeland, Suite 800
Royal Oak, MI 48073-2285

National Guild of Hypnotists
PO Box 308
Merrimack, NH 03054

LYMPHATIC MASSAGE

Dr. Vodder School, North America
PO Box 5701
Victoria, British Columbia
Canada V8R 658

North American Vodder Association of Lymphatic Therapy
356 Waterbury Drive
East Lake, OH 44095

NATUROPATHY

American Association of Naturopathic Physicians
2366 Eastlake Avenue, Suite 322
Seattle, WA 98102

NUTRITIONAL COUNSELING

American Association of Nutritional Consultants
810 South Buffalo Street
Warsaw, IN 46580

American Dietetic Association
216 West Jackson Boulevard, Suite 800
Chicago, IL 60606-6995

Ayurvedic Institute
11311 Menaul NE, Suite A
Albuquerque, NM 87112

National Acupuncture and Oriental Medicine Alliance
14637 Starr Road, SE
Olalla, WA 98359

REFLEXOLOGY

International Institute of Reflexology
5650 First Avenue, North
St. Petersburg, FL 33710

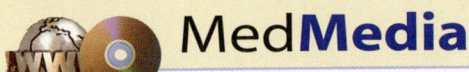

MedMedia

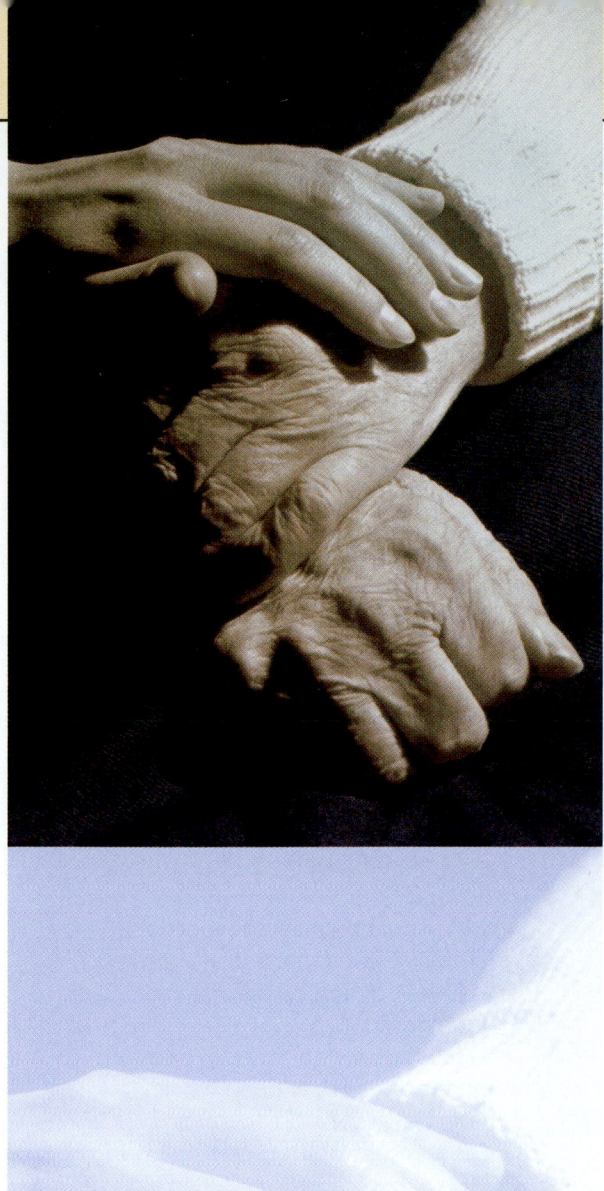

UNIT XII

Career Strategies

Chapter 51   **Competing in the Job Market**

My name is David Jensen. When I decided to become a medical assistant many years ago, I thought that it would be easy to find a job. After I got into the medical assisting program, I found out differently. Being a male, I found it was very difficult to break into the medical assisting field. I talked to many people and ultimately volunteered in a clinic working as an MA. It was a great experience for me, working with patients and doctors who showed me that I was indeed in the field that was right for me.

When I finished the medical assisting program and had volunteered for about six months, I started looking for employment in the area clinics. After applying for several positions through the hospital clinics where I had done my volunteer work, I had an interview. I was called back for a second interview and was hired for an on-call position. I was very happy that I was hired, since that was my goal when doing the volunteer work. It is not always easy to land a job right out of school, but hard work does pay off.

Working as a medical assistant is a very rewarding job. I look forward to going to work each day and planning out how I am going to run the doctors' schedules. I get enjoyment out of talking and listening to my patients and relaying that information to the doctors so they may better assess the plan of treatment. The computer is of great importance in the practice of the clinic and doctors; the MA must have a great knowledge of terminology and computer applications to make the day go smoothly.

The best thing about working as a medical assistant is the respect and the trust that comes with the job. The doctors, managers, and rest of the staff depend on the MA to keep the day flowing smoothly. Oftentimes, these team members come to the MA for answers or solutions to problems in the office. Medical assisting is a fast-paced and rewarding field.

Competing in the Job Market

Case Study

Karim Yousef, a medical assisting graduate seeking employment in health care, lacks personal transportation. Because Karim must rely on public transportation, he has arrived late to a few interviews. As he prepares his cover letter and resume in response to medical assisting job postings, he is trying to determine the most pertinent information to include in these important documents.

Objectives

After completing this chapter, you should be able to:

- Define and spell the key terminology in this chapter.
- Define the medical assistant's role in competing in the job market.
- Discuss the externship experience, including its benefits for the medical assistant, extern site, and medical assisting program.
- Prepare an attractive and effective resume.
- Write an effective cover letter, and discuss the importance of using cover letters.
- Discuss varied places to look for employment as a medical assistant.
- List the dos and don'ts of an effective interview.
- Discuss the importance of body language and proper dress while interviewing.
- Discuss the importance of following up with a medical office after an interview.
- Develop a plan of action for changing jobs.

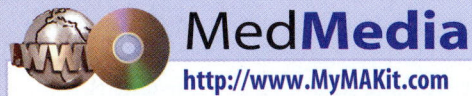

Med**Media**

http://www.MyMAKit.com

Additional interactive resources and activities for this chapter can be found on http://www.MyMAKit.com. For a video, tips, audio glossary, legal and ethical scenarios, on-the-job scenarios, quizzes, and games related to the content of this chapter, please access the accompanying CD-ROM in this book.

Video
Legal and Ethical Scenario: *Competing in the Job Market*
On the Job Scenario: *Competing in the Job Market*
Tips
Multiple Choice Quiz: *Competing in the Job Market*
Audio Glossary
HIPAA Quiz
Games: Spelling Bee, Crossword, and Strikeout

✚ MEDICAL ASSISTING STANDARDS

CAAHEP ENTRY-LEVEL STANDARDS	ABHES ENTRY-LEVEL COMPETENCIES
■ Apply active listening skills (affective) ■ Identify styles and types of verbal communication (cognitive) ■ Identify nonverbal communication (cognitive) ■ Analyze communications in providing appropriate responses/feedback (affective) ■ Demonstrate telephone techniques (psychomotor) ■ Recognize elements of fundamental writing skills (cognitive) ■ Compose professional/business letters (psychomotor)	■ Adapt to change. ■ Project a positive attitude. ■ Use proper telephone technique. ■ Application of electronic technology. ■ Be courteous and diplomatic. ■ Fundamental writing skills.

✓ COMPETENCY SKILLS PERFORMANCE

1. Write an effective resume.
2. Compose a cover letter.
3. Follow up with an employer after an interview.

Key Terminology

advocate—to defend the rights of others

cover letter—document that accompanies a resume to a prospective employer

externship program—final phase of the medical assisting education in an accredited program; consists of hands-on work in a medical office for a specified number of hours

interview—meeting, usually face to face, between an employer and an applicant

mentor—person who supervises an extern in a healthcare facility; also called a preceptor

preceptor—person who supervises an extern in a healthcare facility; also called a mentor

resume—document outlining a job applicant's education and job experience

Introduction

The U.S. Department of Labor predicts that medical assisting will be one of the fastest-growing professions between 2004 and 2014, driven largely by the aging "baby boom" generation. Because older patients tend to seek medical care more often than younger patients, medical offices will be expanding. Medical assisting positions, as a result, will be more and more plentiful and the scope of the position will expand. The scope of practice for any healthcare profession, including medical assisting, consists of the skills and competencies that the professional is licensed, certified, or trained to do. Typically, the scope of practice is defined by the Department of Health within each state. Already, medical assistants are employed in nontraditional organizations, such as insurance companies and inpatient care facilities. The key to finding employment is to make a good impression on potential employers and writer cover letters and resumes that stand out.

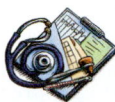

The Medical Assistant's Role in Competing in the Job Market

The employment options available to medical assistants are expanding. Whereas most medical assistants work in ambulatory care settings, there are many other options available to the MA today. When seeking employment, it is important to project a positive, self-confident image to potential employers.

The Externship Experience

Every accredited medical assisting program ends with a 60- to 240-hour **externship program** that allows students to develop hands-on skills in medical offices. Externship students are guests of the sponsoring medical offices. As such, students should behave as they would when hired: as professionals. In successful externships, extern sites, students, and medical assisting programs work together. Some medical assisting students find they are offered employment at their extern site at the end of the externship. The medical assisting student is not paid for the extern work, but earns credit toward graduation from the medical assisting program.

Understanding the Externship Site's Responsibilities

Extern sites are responsible for giving medical assisting students forums in which to exercise their clinical and administrative skills. During externships, medical assistants who work for the extern sites, called **preceptors** or **mentors,** direct externship students and serve as resources when questions or issues arise. Most extern sites are well versed in the responsibilities of externships and take those responsibilities seriously.

HIPAA Compliance

Before launching externships, medical offices should require students to sign a Health Insurance Portability and Accountability Act (HIPAA) agreement that states the students will share no personal patient information with anyone outside the offices.

Outlining the Student's Responsibilities

Externship programs are excellent places for students to showcase their skills to potential employers. To make their externship experiences as robust as possible, students should actively seek involvement in all their sites' clinical and administrative procedures. While most offices allow externship students to participate in all areas of patient care, patients must give their permission (Figure 51-1 ◆).

Whatever duties they undertake, externship students should remain professional, which means arriving on time, being prepared, and dressing in attire that meets extern sites' requirements. Makeup and jewelry should be minimal, hair should be neat and away from the face, and clothing and shoes should be clean and in good repair.

Sometimes, when externships are particularly successful, extern sites offer students permanent positions upon program completion. When employment is not offered but students are interested in working for their extern sites, those students should advise their preceptors of their desire and leave a copy of their resume.

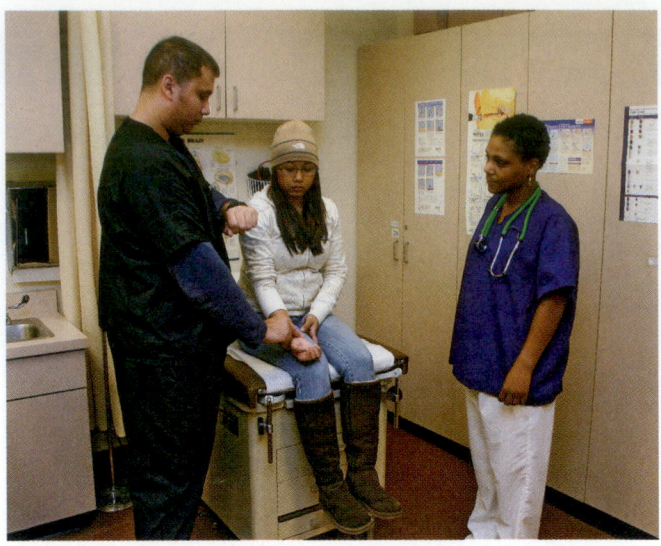

Figure 51-1 ◆ During the externship, the student medical assistant will both observe and participate in caring for patients.

The Responsibilities of the Medical Assisting Program

As externship students' **advocates,** medical assisting program directors are primarily responsible for choosing appropriate extern sites for students. With the help of the mentor, program directors should monitor the extern process closely, making sure students succeed in this important last step in their education. To facilitate the monitoring process and observe students in the clinical environment, many program directors visit students on site. Many programs ask externs to log their learning processes in weekly summaries or to meet periodically with the other externs to share their experiences. Students should bring any concerns to the program director's attention. In turn, directors should address student issues as soon as possible.

Writing an Effective Resume

As a first impression of a job applicant, the **resume** is a critical tool in the job market (Figure 51-2 ◆). Poorly written and prepared resumes suggest that their authors will similarly produce poor quality work in the medical office. As a result, many employers discard resumes with poor grammar, typographical errors, or handwritten corrections. When medical assistants

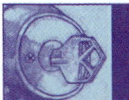

Keys to Success
ASKING QUESTIONS OF THE PHYSICIAN IN FRONT OF THE PATIENT

Medical assisting students should never question the decisions of physicians or other medical assistants in front of patients in the office. Instead, students should pose questions outside patients' hearing range to retain the respect healthcare professionals command.

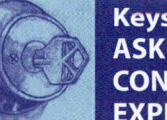

RICHARD CORNELIUS, RMA (AMT)
1234 West Nile Street
Worcester, MA 12345
(808) 555-7890

OBJECTIVE:
To obtain a challenging position in a medical setting that will allow me to gain experience working with a diverse and challenging population of patients.

EDUCATION:
Northridge Community College Medical Assisting Program, Northridge KY (September 1999–June 2001)

EXPERIENCE:

Martinville Pediatrics, Worcester, MA
(March 2005–Present): Clinical medical assistant

Williamsburg Women's Clinic, Northridge, KY
(July 2001–January 2005): Clinical medical assistant

ACTIVITIES:
Member of the PTA since 1997
Member of the AAMA

REFERENCES:
Excellent references are available upon request

Figure 51-2 ◆ Sample resume from a medical assistant.

change phone numbers, for example, they should revise and reprint their resumes, not hand-mark changes. An applicant may be perfect for the job; however; a sub-par resume will sacrifice employment opportunities.

Ideally, resumes are short, preferably one to two pages, as well as impeccably written and presented. Instead of detailing all duties ever performed, resumes should summarize applicants' qualifications and experience and highlight experience most relevant to the open position. Figure 51-3 ◆ provides a framework of some

Keys to Success
ASKING QUESTIONS OR RAISING CONCERNS DURING THE EXTERNSHIP EXPERIENCE

When medical assisting students have questions or concerns during the externship and the mentor cannot address them, those students should raise their issues with the medical assisting program director.

required resume items. In addition to reviewing work history, the resume should stress an applicant's skills and accomplishments. Any perceived shortcomings, such as disabilities or missing skills, should only be raised in the interview. That way, the applicant can point out positive ways in which to address those issues.

 Critical Thinking Question 51-1
Should Karim note his lack of personal transportation on his resume? Why or why not?

Accuracy is also crucial in resume presentation. Applicants should never embellish resume information. Falsifying

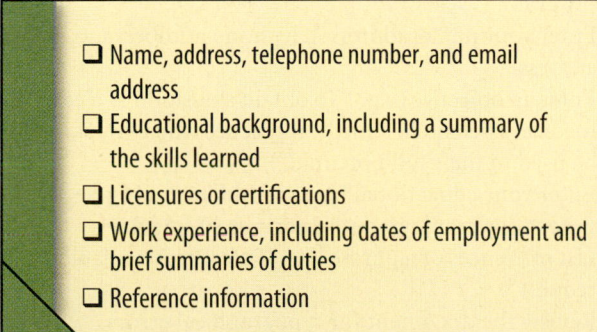

❑ Name, address, telephone number, and email address
❑ Educational background, including a summary of the skills learned
❑ Licensures or certifications
❑ Work experience, including dates of employment and brief summaries of duties
❑ Reference information

Figure 51-3 ◆ Items to include on a resume.

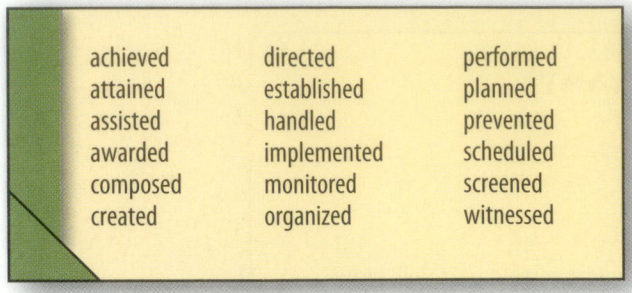

achieved	directed	performed
attained	established	planned
assisted	handled	prevented
awarded	implemented	scheduled
composed	monitored	screened
created	organized	witnessed

Figure 51-4 ◆ Action words.

applications or resumes is grounds for termination in most organizations. Instead of trying to capture employers' attention with erroneous information, applicants should focus on top-notch physical presentation to help get their resumes noticed. In general, however, applicants should defer to good taste and judgment. Resumes printed on lime-green paper may get noticed, but they may also give readers the wrong impression. Action words, in contrast, tend to give the right impression and capture readers' attention in desired ways. Figure 51-4 ◆ lists some action words applicants can use to reflect their skills and experiences properly on resumes.

Keys to Success
FLUENCIES IN LANGUAGES OTHER THAN ENGLISH

Use the resume to list fluencies in languages other than English. Many medical offices, especially those in diverse neighborhoods, seek employees who are fluent in languages other than English.

? —Critical Thinking Question 51-2–
Karim was fired from his last two jobs due to chronic tardiness. Should he mention those terminations on his cover letter? Why or why not?

Preparing a Cover Letter

Often, **cover letters** help job applicants secure opportunities to **interview.** They are, much like resumes, critical job-searching tools. Because cover letters can be critical to job searches, they should accompany all resumes, even those transmitted via e-mail. In addition, like resumes, they should be error-free and professionally presented.

Cover letters are the links between resumes and open jobs. As such, they should address open positions and explain why applicants are the best candidates for those positions. Figure 51-5 ◆ provides an example of a cover letter. Effective cover letters have headings with applicants' full names, addresses, telephone numbers, fax numbers when appropriate, and e-mail addresses. As much as possible, personal e-mail addresses should be professional. Potential employers are more likely to favor patricialocke12@sample.com over crazypatty@sample.com

Identifying Places to Look for Employment

Employment advertisements may appear in a number of venues, including newspapers and employment agencies. Medical assisting programs may also list job postings, and medical offices often advertise open positions on their Websites. To cover all bases, medical assistants should send resumes and cover letters to offices that are not currently hiring. Those resumes may arrive just as open positions become available.

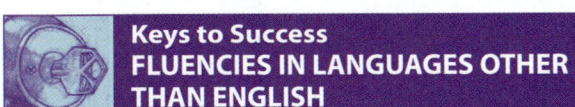

PROCEDURE 51-1 Write an Effective Resume

Theory and Rationale

Every job search starts with a good resume. Many employers see dozens of resumes for one open position in their organizations. To secure interviews, medical assistants need a professional resume with the right information.

Materials

■ computer with word processing software

Competency

(**Conditions**) With the necessary materials, you will be able to (**Task**) compose your resume (**Standards**) correctly within the time allowed by the instructor.

1. Choose a resume template in the word processing program.
2. Enter your name, address, telephone number, and e-mail address.
3. Enter an objective (e.g., "To obtain a position as a certified medical assistant in a medical practice where my skills can be used to their full potential").
4. Enter your educational background, including degrees.
5. Enter your employment history, including dates.
6. List references or a phrase like, "References available upon request."
7. Review the document for typographical errors.
8. Print the resume on quality paper.
9. Review the resume again for typographical errors.

Joan Monson, CMA (AAMA)
2121 1st Avenue South
Seattle, WA 12345
Home Phone: (206) 555-9084
Cell Phone: (206) 555-2434
e-mail: joanmonson@direct.com

Dear Ms. Nielsen:

I enclose my resume in response to your ad for an administrative medical assistant skilled in pediatric medicine.

After working with children extensively for several years, I recently completed my associate degree and obtained a Certificate in Medical Assisting (CMA) distinction. I completed my externship in a pediatric office, because I wish to continue applying my skills with children in the administrative environment.

As followup to this letter, I will call your office next week to determine if my qualifications meet your needs at this time, and to schedule an interview with you. Thank you for your time and consideration. I look forward to meeting you.

Sincerely,

Joan Monson, CMA (AAMA)

Figure 51-5 ◆ Sample cover letter.

 — Critical Thinking Question 51-3—

If Karim lacks personal transportation, how should he seek employment?

Completing Employment Applications

Employment applications are an effective way for employers to capture consistent information from all job applicants (Figure 51-6 ◆). As a result, many employers ask applicants to complete

---

PROCEDURE 51-2 Compose a Cover Letter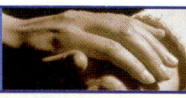

Theory and Rationale

Every resume should include a cover letter. As personalized links between resumes and desired jobs, cover letters allow the medical assistant to tell potential employers why he or she should be chosen for an interview.

Materials

■ computer with word processing software

Competency

(**Conditions**) With the necessary materials, you will be able to (**Task**) compose a cover letter (**Standards**) correctly within the time allowed by the instructor.

1. Using the word processing software, enter the date and name, company, and address of the letter recipient.
2. Compose a letter that addresses the desired job and the reasons the employer should consider you for the position.
3. List any information that directly relates to your ability to perform the desired job.
4. Request an interview.
5. State that you will call the employer to follow up in a few days.

APPLICATION FOR EMPLOYMENT

Mountain View Health Care Center is an equal opportunity employer and upholds the principles of equal opportunity employment. It is the policy of Mountain View Health Care Center to provide employment, compensation and other benefits related to employment based on qualifications and performance, without regard to race, color, religion, national origin, age, sex, veteran status or disability, or any other basis prohibited by federal or state law. As an equal opportunity employer, Mountain View Health Care Center intends to comply fully with all federal and state laws and the information requested on this application will not be used for any purpose prohibited by law. Disabled applicants may request any needed accommodation. This application is intended to allow you, the applicant, to provide Mountain View Health Care Center with the information and data so that your suitability and qualifications can be fairly determined for the position(s) for which you are applying. Please complete this application and answer all questions completely. Please print clearly in ink.

PLEASE PRINT CLEARLY—BE SURE TO SIGN THIS APPLICATION

Date

Name: Last   First   Middle

Social Security No.:   Home Phone:

Address:

   No.   -   Street

City   State   Zip

Have you been previously employed by Mountain View Health Care Center?   ☐ Yes   ☐ No
If "Yes", when?   In what capacity?

How did you learn of the position for which you are applying:
☐ Newspaper/Print Advertisement   ☐ Friend/Relative   ☐ Employment Agency   ☐ Job Service   ☐ Radio/TV Advertisement

EMPLOYMENT DESIRED
Position(s) applied for
Shift Preferences: ☐ First Shift – Days   ☐ Second Shift – Evenings   ☐ Third Shift – Nights
☐ Full-time   ☐ Part-time If "Part time", number of shifts/hours desired:
Date available to start   Salary requested

PERSONAL HISTORY
Are you a United States citizen or do you have an entry permit which allows you to lawfully work in the U.S.?   ☐ Yes   ☐ No
   If applicable, Visa Type: Immigration No.:
Are you at least 18 years old?   ☐ Yes   ☐ No

Are you able to perform all of the duties required by the position for which you are applying, without endangering yourself or compromising the safety, health, or welfare of the Patients or other Staff Persons?   ☐ Yes   ☐ No
   If "No," please explain:

EDUCATION

Name and Location Of School	Graduation Date	Course of Study/ Degree Issued
High School		
College		
Other		

LICENSURE/CERTIFICATION/REGISTRATION

Type of License/Certification	Registration Number

List any special skills or qualifications which you posses and feel are relevant to health care and the position for which you are applying.

Figure 51-6 ◆ Sample employment application.

EMPLOYMENT HISTORY

Please give accurate and complete information. Start with present or most recent employer.

May we contact and communicate with your present employer?   ☐ Yes   ☐ No

Employer   Telephone No.

Address   Employed from   /   to   /

Name of Supervisor   Hourly Pay: Start   Last

Position and Responsibilities

Reason for Leaving

- -

Employer   Telephone No.

Address   Employed from   /   to   /

Name of Supervisor   Hourly Pay: Start   Last

Position and Responsibilities

Reason for Leaving

- -

Employer   Telephone No.

Address   Employed from   /   to   /

Name of Supervisor   Hourly Pay: Start   Last

Position and Responsibilities

Reason for Leaving

- -

MILITARY SERVICE

Branch   From   To

What were your duties?

Did you receive any specialized training?   ☐ Yes   ☐ No
If "Yes", describe:

REFERENCES

Names of friends or relatives, if any, currently employed by Mountain View Health Care Center.

Name   Address   Phone

Name   Address   Phone

Names of co-workers (no relatives) you have worked with and whom we may contact for a reference.

Name   Address   Phone

Name   Address   Phone

Please read the following statements completely and carefully before you initial and sign your name.

The Applicant HEREBY CERTIFIES that the answers given on this Application For Employment, including any statements or answers provided by the Applicant during interview, are true and correct. The Applicant fully authorizes Mountain View Health Care Center to contact any references, past and present employers, persons, schools, law enforcement agencies and any other sources of information which may be relevant to the Applicant and this Application For Employment. It is understood and agreed that any misrepresentation, false statement, or omission by the Applicant will be sufficient reason for rejection of the Application For Employment or for dismissal from employment at any time, without recourse or liability to Mountain View Health Care Center.

I have read, understand and agree to the above statement.   (Please initial here). _____

SIGN HERE _____   DATE _____

Figure 51-6 ◆ (Continued)

employment applications, even when those applicants have submitted resumes.

Before providing any information on job applications, candidates should carefully read all parts of the documents, particularly the instructions. When it comes to entering information, all answers should be well thought out, as well as organized and neatly written in black or blue ink. Every space should contain some type of information. When a section does not apply, applicants should enter "Not applicable" or "N/A." Errors should be neatly crossed through, not scribbled out. Even when applicants have already submitted resumes, they should attach an additional copy to the application they turn in.

The Successful Interview

When resumes succeed in capturing employers' attention, their applicants are generally called for interviews and asked for references. To facilitate the interview process and prepare their references properly, applicants should get their references' permission before using them for job-search purposes. Applicants can use the cover letter to ask prospective employers not to contact their current places of employment.

When potential employers call to schedule interviews, applicants are sometimes unavailable. Therefore, it is crucial for applicants to record professional voicemail messages on appropriate telephones. Cell numbers are generally appropriate contact points for potential employers.

In Practice

Jerome is looking for employment as a medical assistant. He has submitted his resume at several offices and has been waiting for telephone calls requesting interviews. When those calls finally come, the potential employers hear an unprofessional voicemail greeting left by Jerome and his roommate and decide to leave no message. What should Jerome do to increase his chances of gaining employment?

Preparing for the Interview

Before interviewing, medical assistants should research the offices they will be visiting. Knowledge of the facility suggests interest in the practice and may win special attention from the employer. Assume, for example, an office is known for its success with a certain type of therapy. The applicant who asks about that therapy during the interview shows an interest and will likely stand out in the candidate pool. In addition to research, applicants should think of one or two appropriate questions to ask their prospective employers. Figure 51-7 ◆ identifies some questions to avoid, as well as other interview "don'ts." In general, questions about an office's history or industry trends are among the acceptable. Like research, such questions demonstrate applicants' interest. They also prepare applicants should employers ask for questions when the interviews close, and they give employers the chance to talk about themselves.

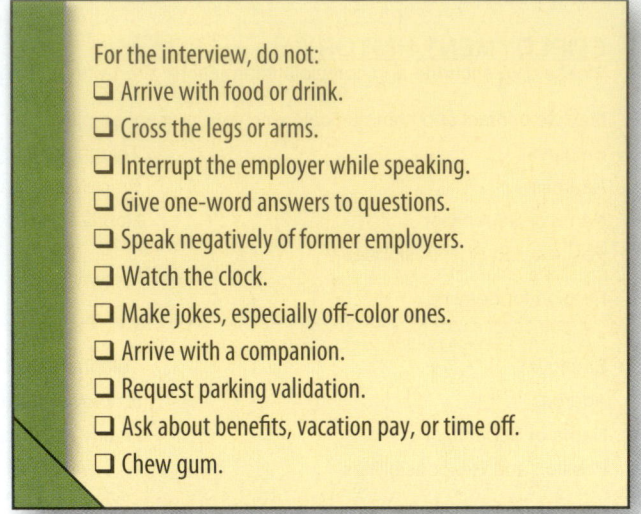

For the interview, do not:
❑ Arrive with food or drink.
❑ Cross the legs or arms.
❑ Interrupt the employer while speaking.
❑ Give one-word answers to questions.
❑ Speak negatively of former employers.
❑ Watch the clock.
❑ Make jokes, especially off-color ones.
❑ Arrive with a companion.
❑ Request parking validation.
❑ Ask about benefits, vacation pay, or time off.
❑ Chew gum.

Figure 51-7 ◆ Interview don'ts.

Dressing for the Interview

When it comes time for the interview itself, several items are vital, including a working black or blue pen, a notepad, at least two copies of the resume, and copies of reference letters, certifications, and awards. Appropriate dress is also a crucial part of the interview. Clothing should be clean and conservative as well as professional. Men should opt for a jacket and tie; women should wear clothing that fits properly and is cut modestly (Figure 51-8 ◆).

Applicants' personal hygiene, like their clothing, must be impeccable. Hands, nails, and teeth should be clean and groomed, and perfumes and colognes should be nearly imperceptible.

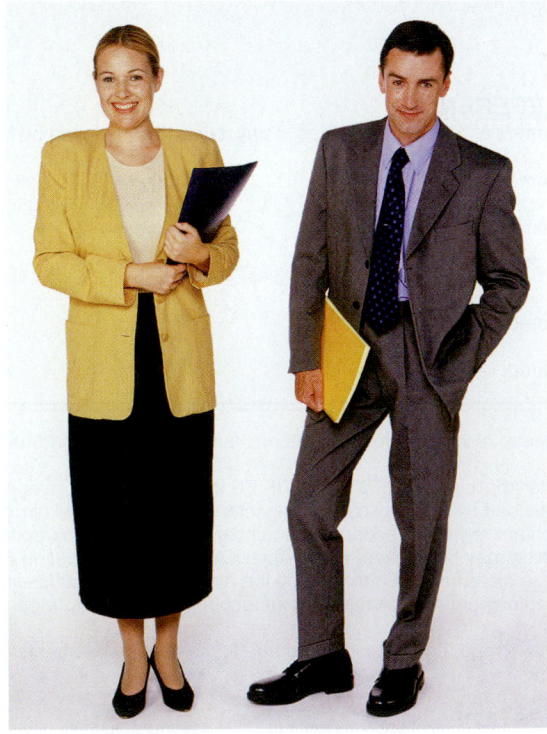

Figure 51-8 ◆ Professional attire is appropriate for the medical office interview.

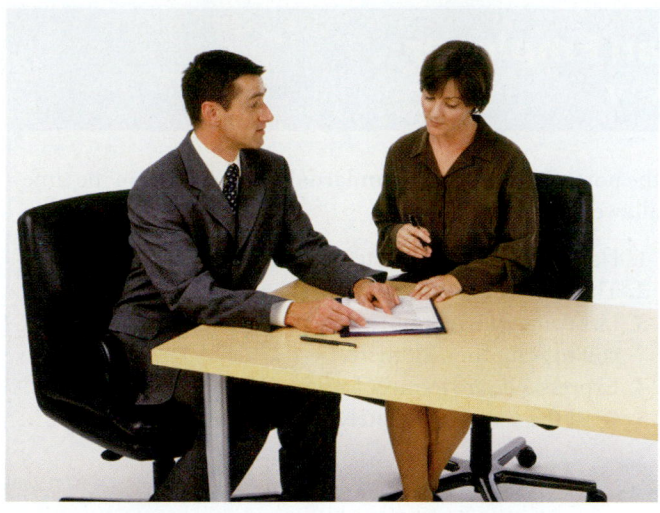

Figure 51-9 ◆ The office manager interviews an applicant.

Smokers should try to erase all evidence of smoke on the clothing and the breath as all applicants should be pleasant and odor free. Men and women both should avoid large jewelry, although earrings, necklaces, and wristwatches are appropriate when tasteful. Tattoos, whenever possible, should be covered; visible piercings other than in the ears are generally undesired and should be removed prior to the interview.

Presenting the Right Image

Upon initial employer meetings, applicants should stand and shake their interviewers' hands. Eye contact should be direct when speaking; avoidance is viewed as deceptive. During the interview, applicants should strive to convey confidence. They should sit straight and speak in a calm, measured tone. Body language communicates a great deal to prospective employers. Even when walking, applicants should maintain proper posture and avoid shuffling. When applicants are prone to nerves, they can take notes on notepads to keep hands busy (Figure 51-9 ◆).

Following Up After the Interview

Interview followup increases the likelihood of hiring. Followup both reminds employers of candidates and allows those candidates to ask questions, extend courtesies, and emphasize their interest in employment. The day after the interview is held, the candidate should send a handwritten thank-you note (Figure 51-10 ◆).

Changing Jobs

Unlike fifty years ago, employees today tend to switch jobs every three to five years. As in all facets of medical assisting, it is important to maintain professional protocol when leaving a job. To leave positions on desired terms, medical assistants should give their employers at least two weeks' notice in writing (four weeks' notice if a supervisory position). During that period, it should be business as usual. Assistants should remain positive and continue performing their duties to the best of their abilities. They should clearly communicate the status of all projects, and they should also clean their workspace and return any office items. Finally, assistants should ask their employers for letters of recommendation (Figure 51-11 ◆).

September 4, 2009

Dear Dr. Bryant:

Thank you for taking the time to interview with me on Monday. I enjoyed hearing about the advances you have made in the area of foot care for diabetic patients. As I stated during our meeting, I am very interested in working in the administrative area of your clinic and feel my qualifications are perfectly suited to what you are looking for in an administrative medical assistant.

If you would like to discuss the position further, I can be reached at (602) 555-0923. I welcome the opportunity to work with you in your clinic and hope that I will hear from you soon.

Sincerely,

Oksana Simonenko, CMA (AAMA)

Figure 51-10 ◆ Sample interview thank-you note.

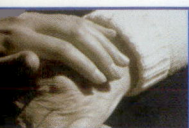

PROCEDURE 51-3 Follow Up with an Employer After an Interview

Theory and Rationale

Many medical offices interview several applicants for a single opening. To stand out in desired ways, medical assistants must find ways to make potential employers remember and want to hire them.

Materials

- note card
- blue or black pen

Competency

(**Conditions**) With the necessary materials, you will be able to (**Task**) follow up after an interview with a thank-you note to the potential employer (**Standards**) correctly within the time allowed by the instructor.

1. Handwrite or type a note to the interviewer.
2. Thank the person for the interview time.
3. List something about the position or office that inspires you to want to work there.
4. Express a desire to meet again.
5. Send the note immediately after the interview.

November 11, 2009

Re: Martin Hawkins, RMA (AMT)

To Whom It May Concern:

I have had the pleasure of working with Martin Hawkins from January 2004 to November 2007 when Martin and his family decided to relocate to Texas.

Martin has demonstrated a tremendous desire to learn, along with a drive to become the best he can be within his chosen profession within the healthcare field. His ability to work both alone and within groups is unsurpassed, and his attention to detail, especially in the area of patient confidentiality, will serve his future employer well.

I would highly recommend Martin Hawkins, RMA, (AMT), for employment in a medical setting. He will make a valued asset to the medical office that recognizes his talents and abilities, and the patients he cares for will be fortunate to have him as their advocate.

Sincerely,

Sharon Tsete, MHA
Clinical Office Manager
Shoreline Family Medicine
(206) 555-9472

Figure 51-11 ◆ Sample recommendation letter.

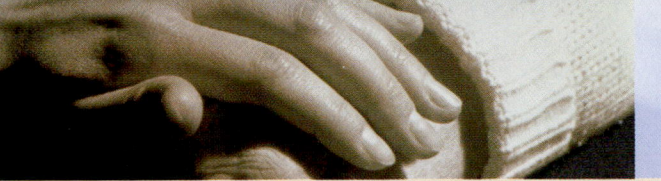

REVIEW

Chapter Summary

- An externship program offers benefits for the medical assistant, the externship site, and the medical assisting program.
- Attractive and effective resumes are critical tools for job seekers, whether those applicants are recently graduated students or established medical assistants.
- When resumes are clear, accurate, and written using action words, they can help medical assisting candidates secure jobs.
- Cover letters, like resumes, support job-searching initiatives by explaining to the potential employer the reasons why the applicant is right for the job.
- Medical assistants can search for job opportunities in varied places, such as newspapers, job fairs, local medical assisting programs, and on the Internet.

- Proper dress and body language are vital while interviewing.
- Interview followup can make the difference between candidates securing the desired position or not. Followup techniques include sending a thank-you note to the potential employer and calling to see if the interviewer has any additional questions of the applicant.
- When medical assistants decide to seek new employment, they should take all steps to leave their employers on good terms. Requesting a recommendation letter upon leaving the office may help secure a future position.

Chapter Review

Multiple Choice

1. During the extern program, the student medical assistant should try to participate in areas devoted to
   a. administration.
   b. clinical procedures.
   c. administration and clinical procedures.
   d. none of the above.

2. Which of the following is an "action" word?
   a. Monitored
   b. Willing
   c. Working
   d. All of the above

3. Which of the following is inappropriate for an interview?
   a. Three-inch pumps
   b. Necktie
   c. Suit jacket
   d. All of the above

4. When job applicants change phone numbers, they should reflect the change on their resumes by
   a. crossing through the old number and handwriting the new one.
   b. whiting out the old number and handwriting the new one.
   c. placing a note over the old number about the change.
   d. retyping the number and reprinting the resume.

True/False

T F 1. The U.S. Department of Labor predicts that medical assisting will be among the fastest growing professions between the years 2004 and 2014.

T F 2. All externship programs require 240 hours for accreditation.

T F 3. Before witnessing patient procedures, student medical assistants should ask for patients' permission.

T F 4. Before starting externship programs, student medical assistants should sign a HIPAA compliance form stating that they will disclose no patient information.

T F 5. Sloppy and poorly written resumes suggest that work in the medical office will be similarly poor.

T F 6. For medical assistants, scrubs are appropriate interview attire.

T F 7. Resumes should reflect competencies such as fluency in sign language.

T F 8. Attractive resumes gain attention through their appearance.

T F 9. To gain attention, resumes should appear on bright paper, like bright pink or red.

T F 10. It is acceptable to leave portions of employment applications blank.

T F 11. Applicants who follow up with the employer after interviews are more likely to be hired.

Short Answer

1. Why is it important to get permission from professional references?
2. What is the purpose of the cover letter?
3. List several places the medical assistant may seek employment.
4. Why is it important to research offices before interviews?
5. Name several items that should not be taken to an interview.

Research

1. Looking at the jobs advertised for medical assistants in your area, what is the starting wage for a new medical assistant?
2. Search online for information on how to compose a professional resume. What information did you find?
3. Ask one of your instructors to review your resume and give you feedback on how you might improve it.

Externship Application Experience

While the medical assisting student is completing an externship in a family practice office, that assistant notices the physician appears to have made an error in a patient's medication. How should the assistant handle this situation?

Resource Guide

Absolutely Health Care (online community for posting resumes)
www.healthjobsusa.com/

Americans with Disabilities Act
www.ada.gov/workta.htm

Monster (Internet site for seeking employment)
www.monster.com

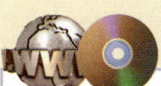

Med**Media**

http://www.MyMAKit.com

More on this chapter, including interactive resources, can be found on the Student CD-ROM accompanying this textbook and on http://www.MyMAKit.com.

Correlation of Text to the General, Clinical, and Administrative Skills of the CMA (AAMA)

General Skills

Communication

Skill	Chapter
Recognize and respect cultural diversity	5, 6, 7, 9, 10, 11, 22
Adapt communications to individual's understanding	3, 5, 6, 7, 8, 9, 10, 11, 22
Employ professional telephone and interpersonal techniques	9, 10
Recognize and respond effectively to verbal, nonverbal, and written communications	5, 6, 7, 8, 9, 10, 11, 22
Utilize and apply medical terminology appropriately	3, 5, 6, 7, 8, 9, 10
Receive, organize, prioritize, store, and maintain transmittable information utilizing electronic technology	8, 9, 11, 12, 13
Serve as communication liaison between the physician and patient	3, 4, 5, 6, 7, 8, 9, 10, 11, 42
Serve as patient advocate professional and health coach in a team approach in healthcare	3, 4, 5, 6, 7, 8, 9, 11, 42

Legal Concepts

Skill	Chapter
Perform within legal (including federal and state statutes, regulations, opinions, and rulings) and ethical boundaries	3, 4, 6, 8, 9, 22
Document patient communication and clinical treatments accurately and appropriately	5, 6, 7, 8, 9, 10, 11, 12, 13
Maintain medical records	12, 13
Follow employer's established policies dealing with the healthcare contract	5, 6, 7, 8, 9, 10, 11, 16
Comply with established risk management and safety procedures	4, 16, 22
Recognize professional credentialing criteria	2, 4, 22
Identify and respond to issues of confidentiality	3, 4 , 5, 6, 7, 8, 9, 10, 11, 12, 13, 14, 22

Instruction

Skill	Chapter
Function as a healthcare advocate to meet individual's needs	5, 6, 7, 8, 9, 10, 11
Educate individuals in office policies and procedures	5, 6, 8, 9, 10, 11, 22
Educate the patient within the scope of practice and as directed by supervising physician in health maintenance, disease prevention, and compliance with patient's treatment plan	5, 6, 7, 42, 43, 44
Identify community resources for health maintenance and disease prevention to meet individual patient needs	5, 6, 7, 10, 11
Maintain current list of community resources, including those for emergency preparedness and other patient care needs	5, 6, 7, 9, 41
Collaborate with local community resources for emergency preparedness	6, 41
Educate patients about their responsibilities relating to third-party reimbursements	17, 20

Operational Functions

Skill	Chapter
Perform inventory of supplies and equipment	15
Perform routine maintenance of administrative and clinical equipment	15
Apply computer and other electronic equipment techniques to support office operations	8, 9, 10, 11,12, 13, 21
Perform methods of quality control	16, 22

Administrative Skills

Administrative Procedures

Skill	Chapter
Schedule, coordinate, and monitor appointments	11
Schedule inpatient/outpatient admissions and procedures	11
Apply third-party and managed care policies, procedures, and guidelines	17
Establish, organize, and maintain patient medical record	12, 13
File medical records appropriately	12, 13
Perform procedural and diagnostic coding for reimbursement	18, 19
Perform billing and collection procedures	17, 18, 19, 20
Perform administrative functions, including bookkeeping and financial procedures	8, 11, 14, 17, 18, 19, 20, 21, 22
Prepare submittal ("clean") insurance forms	17

Clinical Skills

Fundamental Principles

Skill	Chapter
Identify the roles and responsibilities of the medical assistant in the clinical setting	4, 6, 22, 23
Identify the roles and responsibilities of other team members in the medical office	3, 22, 23
Apply principles of aseptic technique and infection control	23, 25, 26, 29
Practice Standard Precautions, including handwashing and disposal of biohazardous materials	23, 25, 26, 29
Perform sterilization techniques	25, 29
Comply with quality assurance practices	4, 25, 26, 29

Diagnostic Procedures

Skill	Chapter
Collect and process specimens	32, 33
Perform CLIA-waived tests	32, 33
Perform electrocardiography and respiratory testing	30, 35, 36
Perform phlebotomy, including venipuncture and capillary puncture	32
Utilize knowledge of principles of radiology	34

Patient Care

Skill	Chapter
Perform initial-response screening following protocols approved by supervising physician	24
Obtain, evaluate, and record patient history employing critical thinking skills	5, 24, 28
Obtain vital signs	24, 28
Prepare and maintain examination and treatment areas	24, 25
Prepare patient for examinations, procedures, and treatments	24, 25, 26
Assist with examinations, procedures, and treatments	24
Maintain examination/treatment rooms, including inventory of supplies and equipment	24
Prepare and administer oral and parenteral (excluding IV) medications and immunizations (as directed by supervising physician and as permitted by state law)	27
Utilize knowledge of principles of IV therapy	27
Maintain medication and immunization records	27
Screen and follow up test results	32
Recognize and respond to emergencies	23, 41

Reprinted with permission of the American Association of Medical Assistants (AAMA).

Registered Medical Assistant (RMA)
Medical Assisting Task List

MEDICAL ASSISTING TASK LIST

The various tasks that medical assistants perform include, but are not necessarily limited to, those on the following list. The tasks presented in this inventory are considered by American Medical Technologists to be representative of the medical assisting job role. This document should be considered dynamic, to reflect the medical assistant's evolving role with respect to contemporary healthcare. Therefore, tasks may be added, removed, or modified on an ongoing basis.

Medical Assistants that meet AMT's qualifications and pass a certification examination are **certified** as a Registered Medical Assistant (RMA).

I. GENERAL MEDICAL ASSISTING KNOWLEDGE

A. Anatomy and Physiology
1. Body systems
2. Disorders and diseases of the body

B. Medical Terminology
1. Word parts
2. Medical terms
3. Common abbreviations and symbols
4. Spelling

C. Medical Law
1. Medical law
2. Licensure, certification, and registration

D. Medical Ethics
1. Principles of medical ethics
2. Ethical conduct
3. Professional development

E. Human Relations
1. Patient relations
2. Interpersonal skills
3. Cultural diversity

F. Patient Education
1. Identify and apply proper communication methods in patient instruction
2. Develop, assemble, and maintain patient resource materials

II. ADMINISTRATIVE MEDICAL ASSISTING

A. Insurance
1. Medical insurance terminology
2. Various insurance plans
3. Claim forms
4. Electronic insurance claims
5. ICD-9/CPT Coding applications
6. HIPAA mandated coding systems
7. Financial applications of medical insurance

B. Financial Bookkeeping
1. Medical finance terminology
2. Patient billing procedures
3. Collection procedures
4. Fundamental medical office accounting procedures
5. Office banking procedures
6. Employee payroll
7. Financial calculations and accounting procedures

C. Medical Secretarial – Receptionist
1. Medical terminology associated with receptionist duties
2. General reception of patients and visitors
3. Appointment scheduling systems
4. Oral and written communications
5. Medical records management
6. Charting guidelines and regulations
7. Protect, store and retain medical records according to HIPAA regulations
8. Release of protected health information adhering to HIPAA regulations
9. Transcription of dictation
10. Supplies and equipment management
11. Medical office computer applications
12. Compliance with OSHA guidelines and regulations of office safety

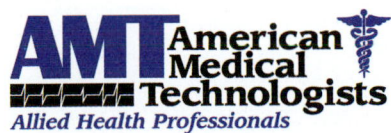

8/05

III.   CLINICAL MEDICAL ASSISTING

A.   Asepsis
1. Medical terminology
2. State/Federal universal blood borne pathogen/body fluid precautions
3. Medical/Surgical asepsis procedure

B.   Sterilization
1. Medical terminology associated with sterilization
2. Sanitization, disinfection, and sterilization procedures
3. Record keeping procedures

C.   Instruments
1. Specialty instruments and parts
2. Usage of common instruments
3. Care and handling of disposable and re-usable instruments.

D.   Vital Signs / Mensurations
1. Blood pressure, pulse, respiration measurements
2. Height, weight, circumference measurements
3. Various temperature measurements
4. Recognize normal and abnormal measurement results

E.   Physical Examinations
1. Patient history information
2. Proper charting procedures
3. Patient positions for examinations
4. Methods of examinations
5. Specialty examinations
6. Visual acuity / Ishihara (color blindness) measurements
7. Allergy testing procedures
8. Normal / abnormal results

F.   Clinical Pharmacology
1. Medical terminology associated with pharmacology
2. Commonly used drugs and their categories
3. Various routes of medication administration
4. Parenteral administration of medications (subcutaneous, intramuscular, intradermal, Z-tract)
5. Classes or drug schedules and legal prescriptions requirements for each
6. Drug Enforcement Agency regulations for ordering, dispensing, storage, and documentation of medication use
7. Drug Reference books (PDR, Pharmacopeia, Facts and Comparisons, Nurses Handbook)

G.   Minor Surgery
1. Surgical supplies and instruments
2. Asepsis in surgical procedures
3. Surgical tray preparation and sterile field respect
4. Prevention of pathogen transmission
5. Patient surgical preparation procedures
6. Assisting physician with minor surgery including setup
7. Dressing and bandaging techniques
8. Suture and staple removal
9. Biohazard waste disposal procedures
10. Instruct patient in pre- and post-surgical care

H.   Therapeutic Modalities
1. Various standard therapeutic modalities
2. Alternative/complementary therapies
3. Instruct patient in assistive devices, body mechanics and home care

I.   Laboratory Procedures
1. Medical laboratory terminology
2. OSHA safety guidelines
3. Quality control and assessment regulations
4. Operate and maintain laboratory equipment
5. CLIA-waived laboratory testing procedures
6. Capillary, dermal, and venipuncture procedures
7. Office specimen collection such as: urine, throat, vaginal, wound cultures – stool, sputum, etc
8. Specimen handling and preparation
9. Laboratory recording according to state and federal guidelines
10. Adhere to the M A Scope of Practice in the laboratory

J.   Electrocardiography
1. Standard, 12 Lead ECG Testing
2. Mounting techniques for permanent record
3. Rhythm strip ECG monitoring on Lead II

K.   First Aid
1. Emergencies and first aid procedures
2. Emergency crash cart supplies
3. Legal responsibilities as a first responder

American Medical Technologists
10700 W. Higgins Road
Rosemont, Illinois 60018
Phone: (847) 823-5169 – Fax: (847) 823-0458
Website: www.amt1.com

How to Become a Successful Student

What Kind of Learner Are You?

In order to become a successful student, it is important to evaluate the type of learner you are. Following are the characteristics of the visual, auditory, and tactile learner.

The visual learner

- Tries to envision the word when spelling it out.
- Dislikes listening for long periods of time.
- Becomes distracted by movement when trying to concentrate.
- May not remember names, but will typically remember faces.
- Prefers face-to-face meetings.
- Prefers to read descriptions when learning new material.
- Likes to look at pictures when learning new material.

The auditory learner

- Tries to sound out a word when spelling it out.
- Enjoys listening rather than talking.
- Becomes distracted by sounds or noises when trying to concentrate.
- Prefers the telephone to face-to-face meetings.
- Prefers verbal instructions.

The tactile learner

- Writes a word out when learning to spell it.
- Uses gestures and expressive movements when talking.
- Becomes distracted by activity when trying to concentrate.
- Prefers to talk while participating in activities.
- Is not necessarily a good reader—prefers stories that are action oriented.
- Tends to figure things out during the process rather than read directions.

Skill Sets

Once you've realized the type of learner you are, take steps to use the skills you have in learning new material.

The visual learner might try

- Looking at pictures or diagrams when learning new material.
- Studying in a quiet room with no distractions.
- Asking for descriptions or asking instructors to explain how a topic might apply in the real world. For example, "Would you demonstrate that skill to the class?"

The auditory learner might try

- Reading aloud or taping his or her voice and playing it back to study new material.
- Taping the instructor's lecture and replaying it later to study.
- Studying in a quiet room with no distractions.
- Working with study groups where students discuss the material they've learned.
- Prefers to hear descriptions when learning new material.

The tactile learner might try

- Writing material down several times in order to memorize it.
- Studying in a quiet area with no distractions.
- Asking the instructor to give examples of how a topic is addressed. For example, "Would you allow the class to role-play that activity so we can see what it feels like?"
- Practicing activities or skills in order to commit them to memory.

Time Management

One of the greatest difficulties for new students is time management and organization of priorities. For those students who have trouble in this area, the following steps may help:

- Set aside blocks of time for studying.
- Take periodic breaks when studying—get up and move around, get a drink, close your eyes for a few moments.
- Prioritize your assignments. Many students find it helpful to write down their assignments and place numbers next to each to indicate the order in which they need to be done.

- Study or read while doing other activities. Students can study or read while exercising, or at the gym.

- Review study material just prior to class on test day.

- Create "to do" lists.

- Use a daily/weekly/monthly calendar. Write down dates of upcoming tests or project due dates then back track to add in dates when certain stages of the project should be completed. For example, if a paper is due four weeks from today, add a note to the calendar for one week from today that the outline should be completed. Two weeks from today that the rough draft should be completed, and so on.

- Look for study partners for each class. Link up with study partners who are "good" students, not those who are not as dedicated as you are to learning the material. Spend time together each week going over the material from the class and studying or preparing for tests or projects.

Students should always be able to consult the course instructor for clarification of subject matter, or for verification of course progress. Students must keep aware of their progress in any given class and take an active part in assuring their own success.

Preparing for the CMA (AAMA) and RMA (AMT) Certification Exams

The AMT Examination

The certification received after passing the AMT examination is Registered Medical Assistant (RMA). This exam consists of 200 to 210 multiple-choice questions. Those questions consist of approximately 43 percent general, 22 percent administrative, and 35 percent clinical topics. The AMT classifies general questions as those pertaining to anatomy and physiology, medical terminology, medical law and ethics, human relations, and patient education. Administrative questions are those pertaining to insurance, financial bookkeeping, and medical reception. Clinical questions are those pertaining to asepsis, sterilization, instruments, vital signs, physical examinations, clinical pharmacology, minor surgery, therapeutic modalities, laboratory procedures, electrocardiography, and first aid. The AMT weighs questions according to the difficulty of the question. The AMT test format consists of either a test booklet with answers written in pencil or on a computer. You have 2 hours to take the computer exam and 3 hours to take the written exam.

Eligibility Requirements

In order to be eligible for the RMA examination, applicants must meet the following requirements:

- Be of good moral character and at least 18 years of age.

- Be a graduate of an accredited high school or acceptable equivalent.

- Meet one of the following criteria:
  - Be a graduate of a medical assisting program that is accredited by the ABHES or the CAAHEP.
  - Be a graduate of a medical assisting program that is accredited by a Regional Accrediting Commission or by a national accrediting organization approved by the U.S. Department of Education. The program must include a minimum of 720 hours of training in medical assisting skills, including a clinical externship.
  - Have been employed in the profession of medical assisting for a minimum of 5 years, with no more than 2 years of that time spent as an instructor in a medical assisting program.

- Applicants who have passed a generalist medical assisting certification examination offered by a medical assisting certification association that is approved by the AMT Board of Directors, and have been working as a medical assistant for 5 years, and who meet the training and experience requirements of the AMT may be considered for the RMA (AMT) certification without further examination.

Application Process

Applications for the RMA examination may be downloaded from the AMT Web site at www.amt1.com/site/epage/15334_315.htm. The application must be filled out and mailed to the AMT at:

American Medical Technologists
10700 West Higgins Road, Suite 150
Rosemont, IL 60018

The application may also be filled out and submitted online at the same Web site. Whether filled out online or downloaded and mailed to the AMT, the applicant must submit all applicable signatures and notarized documents in order to have the application processed. These documents are to be submitted to the AMT along with the payment for the examination. The application fee is currently $90.00.

The AAMA Examination

The certification received after passing the AAMA examination is Certified Medical Assistant (CMA) (AAMA). This exam consists of 300 multiple-choice questions divided into three sections—general, administrative, and clinical. Categories for general questions include anatomy and physiology, medical terminology, medical law and ethics, psychology, and communication. Administrative questions include: data entry, equipment, computer concepts, opening and delivering mail, medical records management, appointment scheduling, finding community resources, managing the physician's professional schedule, office management, office policies and procedures, and medical practice finances. Clinical question areas include principles of asepsis, assisting the physician, preparing patients, maintaining the treatment area, interviewing the patient, collecting and processing specimens, diagnostic testing, preparing and administering medications, handling emergencies, and nutrition. All questions are scored equally.

As of January 5, 2009, the CMA (AAMA) Certification Examination began to be offered via computer-based testing. Candidates are able to select locations and flexible testing times at conveniently located computer-based testing centers throughout the United States.

Eligibility Requirements

In order to be eligible to sit for the AAMA examination, the applicant must have graduated from an accredited medical assisting program. The program must have been accredited by the Commission on Accreditation of Allied Health Education Programs (CAAHEP) or the Accrediting Bureau of Health Educations Schools (ABHES).

Grounds for Denial of Eligibility

The AAMA lists the following reasons for denial of sitting for the examination:

- Obtaining or attempting to obtain certification or re-certification of the CMA (AAMA) credential through fraud or deception.

- Knowingly assisting someone else in obtaining or attempting to obtain certification or recertification of the CMA (AAMA) credential through fraud or deception.

- Making a misstatement of material fact or failure to make a statement of material fact in application for certification or recertification.

- Falsifying information required for admission to the CMA Examination, impersonating another examinee, or falsifying education or credentials.

- Copying answers, permitting another to copy answers, or providing or receiving unauthorized advice about examination content during the CMA Examination.

- Unauthorized possession or distribution of examination materials, including copying and reproducing examination questions and problems.

Generally, individuals who have been found guilty of a felony, or pleaded guilty to a felony, are not eligible to take the CMA exam. The Certifying Board may grant a waiver based upon certain circumstances. In order to apply for this waiver, an applicant must submit the following information to the Certifying Board:

- The age at which the crime was committed.

- The circumstances surrounding the crime.

- The nature of the crime committed.

- The length of time since the conviction.

- The individual's criminal history since the conviction.

- The individual's current employment references.

- The individual's character references.

- Other evidence demonstrating the ability of the individual to perform the professional responsibilities competently and evidence that the individual does not pose a threat to the health or safety of patients.

Application Process

The exam fee for the computer-based test is $125 for CAAHEP and ABHES graduating students, recent CAAHEP and ABHES graduates, and AAMA members. The exam fee is $250 for non-recent CAAHEP and ABHES graduates and non-members. Exam fees are nonrefundable.

After taking the computer-based exam, preliminary pass/fail results will be provided. Official scores will be mailed within five to six weeks directly to candidates.

Recertification

As of 2005, all newly certified and recertifying CMAs (AAMA) will hold their certification through the last day of their birth month in the sixth calendar year following their last certification/recertification. Recertification may be achieved either by sitting for the CMA Examination again or through accumulation of continuing education units (CEUs). If the applicant is recertifying through accumulation of continuing education units, the total points needed is 60. Of that total, 15 points must come from topics in the general category, 15 from the administrative category, and 15 from the clinical category. The remaining 15 points may be accumulated from any of the three categories. In addition, at least 20 of the 60 points must be accumulated from AAMA-approved continuing education units.

When accumulating CEUs, the medical assistant is responsible for keeping documentation of the CEUs earned. This documentation includes the following:

- The date the CEU was obtained.

- The sponsor of the CEU (the group or organization issuing the CEU credits).

- The name of the program attended.

- The amount and type of CEU obtained (general, administrative, clinical).

- The number of CEU credits received from each event.

How to Prepare for the Examination

Just as when studying for any exam, it is important to observe certain techniques in order to achieve the maximum amount from your study time. The following are suggested study tactics:

- Find a quiet place to study.

- Inform those around you that you are not to be disturbed during study time.

- Avoid any possible disruptions, such as having a television or radio on. Turn off the ringer on your telephone.

- Use flashcards to memorize details if this method works for you.

- Use rhymes to memorize details if this method works for you.

- Research medical assisting exam review classes in your area.

- Join or form a study group.

- Purchase a pretest book and use it to take the practice exams. After scoring these practice exams, you will have a better idea of the area(s) you need to focus on for further study.

On the Day of the Exam

- Both of the exams consist of multiple-choice questions. In order to do well on these types of tests, it is important to read the question and each answer thoroughly before making your choice.

- Eliminate the answers you know are wrong. When you have eliminated the wrong answers, consider the answers remaining. Though more than one of them may be correct, remember that one of them is more appropriate than the other.

- Keep an eye on the clock. Considering the number of questions you have to answer, be sure you do not spend more than 45 seconds on any one question. If a question takes longer than that for you to answer, leave it and move on. If you have time after finishing the rest of the questions, come back to consider the ones you skipped.

- Be careful with "all of the above" or "none of the above" answers. If any one of the answers does *not* apply, "all of the above" cannot be the correct choice. Likewise, if even one of the answers *does* apply, "none of the above" cannot be the correct choice.

- Be careful when you see the words, "always," "never," "all," or "none." If you can think of even one exception to the word used, that answer is not correct.

- If you cannot choose between two or more answers, it is in your best interest to guess at the answer. Both the AMT and AAMA take away points for answers left blank.

Translation of English–Spanish Phrases

Would you prefer a morning or an afternoon appointment?
¿Usted prefiere una cita en la manana o' en la tarde?

Are you covered by medical insurance?
¿Tiene aseguranza medica?

Do you need directions to the office?
¿Necesita direccion de nuestra oficina?

Is your visit due to an accident?
¿Es su visita relacionado por un accidente?

What is your home telephone number?
¿Qua les el numero de telefono de su casa?

What is your work telephone number?
¿Qua les el numero de telefono de su trabajo?

Your co-payment for today is $_____.
Su co-pago de este dia es $_____.

Please take a seat, the medical assistant will take you back in just a moment.
Por favor tome asiento, el asistente medico va a tender en un momento.

Can you bring someone with you who speaks English?
¿Puede traer a alguien con usted que pueda abler ingles?

The doctor is running behind schedule, there will be a 20 minute wait.
El doctor esta atrasado, va a ver una espera de viente minutos.

Children may not be left unattended in the reception room.
No dese solos a los ninos en el cuarto de espera.

I need to take a photocopy of your driver's license.
Necesito tomar una fotocopia de su licensia.

Has someone referred you to our office?
¿Quien le recomendo nuestra clinica?

Which doctor did you want to see?
¿Que doctor quiere ver?

Is there a day of the week you would prefer for your appointment?
¿Que dia de la semana prefiere usted su cita?

Please bring your insurance information with you when you come in for your appointment.
Por favor traiga la informacion de su asguranza cuando venga a sue cita.

Please take this slip to the laboratory.
Por favor lleve esta hoja al laboratorio.

This form is our HIPAA privacy agreement.
Este formulario de HIPAA es nuestro aquerdo de privacidad.

I see that you are upset. Let me show you to a private room where we can talk.
Entiendo que esta molesto pasemos a un cuarto privado parea dialogar.

This pamphlet contains written information about your condition.
Este panfieto contiene informacio escrita sobre su condicion.

How long have you had problems with this?
¿Desde cuando tiene este tipo do problemas?

What is your name?
¿Como se llama usted?

Do you speak English?
¿Habla usted ingles?

Can you read English?
¿Sabe usted leer en ingles?

Thank you
Gracias

You are welcome.
De nada

Please
Por favor

It is nice to meet you.
Es un placer conocerle.

Normal Blood Values/Disease Conditions Evaluated for Abnormal Values

Test	Normal Value Range (Conventional)	Normal Value Range (SI units)	Possible Indications
Ammonia (NH_3) - diffusion	20–120 mcg/dl	12–70 mcmol/L	Abnormal levels of Ammonia in the body are used to investigate severe changes in mood and consciousness and to help diagnose the cause of a coma of unknown origin.
Ammonia nitrogen	15–45 µg/dl	11–32 µmol/L	The test for ammonia nitrogen is non-specific and does not indicate a cause. Higher than normal levels simply indicate the body is not effectively metabolizing and eliminating ammonia.
Amylase	35–118 IU/L	0.58–1.97 mckat/L	The normal level of amylase will depend on the method used to collect the data. An increased level may indicate several disorders of the digestive and reproductive systems or cancer of the pancreas. Tubal pregnancies will also cause a rise in the amylase levels. Decreased amylase levels may indicate damage to the pancreas and kidneys.
Anion gap ($Na^+-[Cl^- + HCO_3^-]$) (P)	7–16 mEq/L	7–16 mmol/L	A determination of electrolytes in the blood fluid. Abnormal readings indicate a variety of factors. The test is nonspecific and only tells the physician that there is cause for additional testing. Some factors that cause an abnormal anion gap reading are uncontrolled diabetes, starvation, kidney damage, and ingestion of potentially toxic substances such as antifreeze, excessive amounts of aspirin, or methanol.
Bicarbonate			See *Carbon dioxide content* below
Arterial	21–28 mEq/L	21–28 mmol/L	
Venous	22–29 mEq/L	22–29 mmol/L	
Bilirubin			Increased levels of bilirubin may be an indication of some kind of blockage of the liver or bile duct, hepatitis, trauma to the liver, a drug reaction, or long-term alcohol abuse or some inherited disorders such as Gilbert's,
Conjugated (direct)	0.2 mg/dl	4 mcmol/L	Rotor's, Dubin-Johnson, Crigler-Najjar which will cause an increase in levels. Increased levels of bilirubin in newborns is a critical situation as excessive levels kill developing brain cells and may lead to mental retardation.
Total	0.1–1 mg/dl	2–18 mcmol/L	
Calcitonin	< 100 pg/ml	< 100 ng/L	Increased levels of calcitonin in combination with a thyroid biopsy may be an indication of C-cell hyperplasia.

Test	Normal Value Range (Conventional)	Normal Value Range (SI units)	Possible Indications
Calcium, Total Calcium, Ionized	8.6–10.3 mg/dl 4.4–5.1 mg/dl	2.2–2.74 mmol/L 1–1.3 mmol/L	Increased levels of Calcium in the body indicate an inability to metabolize the intake. This can be due to several factors: hyperthyroidism, sarcoidosis, tuberculosis, excess Vitamin D intake, kidney transplant, and high protein levels (for example, if a tourniquet is used for too long while blood is collected). In this case, free or ionized calcium remains normal.
Carbon dioxide content (plasma)	21–32 mmol/L	21–32 mmol/L	Higher or lower than normal CO_2 levels indicate a problem losing or retaining fluid—disrupting the acid-base balance, which can be an indication of several disorders.
Carcinoembryonic antigen	< 3 ng/ml	< 3 mcg/L	CEA is a protein that is found in embryonic tissues. Increased CEA levels can indicate some non-cancer-related conditions of inflammation of internal organs. Pregnant women who smoke tend to have embryos that have increased levels of CEA. In a normally healthy infant all detectable levels of CEA are gone by birth.
Chloride	95–110 mEq/L	95–110 mmol/L	Increased levels of chloride may indicate dehydration or increased blood sodium. Decreased levels of chloride occurs with prolonged vomiting, chronic diarrhea, emphysema, or other chronic lung disease, and with loss of acid from the body.
Coagulation screen Bleeding time Prothrombin time Partial thromboplastin time (activated) Protein C Protein S	 3–9.5 min 10–13 sec 22–37 sec 0.7–1.4 µ/ml 0.7–1.4 µ/ml	 180–570 sec 10–13 sec 22–37 sec 700–1400 U/ml 700–1400 U/ml	Indicates an inability of the body to develop adequate clotting factors or the inability to produce the correct amount of clotting factors.
Copper, total	70–160 mcg/dl	11–25 mcmol/L	Indication of liver disease.
Corticotropin (ACTH adreno-corticotropic hormone)—0800 hr	< 60 pg/ml	< 13.2 pmol/L	This test is used in conjunction with cortisol to determine if a patient has Cushing's syndrome or Addison's disease.
Coritsol 0800 hr 1800 hr 2000 hr	5–30 mcg/dl 2–15 mcg/dl 50% of 0800 hr	138–810 nmol/L 50–410 nmol/L 50% of 0800 hr	Abnormal levels in coritsol may indicate Cushing's syndrome or Addison's disease.
Creatine kinase Female Male	 20–170 IU/L 30–220 IU/L	 0.33–2.83 mckat/L 0.5–3.67 mckat/L	Creatine kinase is an enzyme found in the heart, brain, skeletal muscle, and other tissues. The body has specific types of CK to indicate which muscles are effected.

Test	Normal Value Range (Conventional)	Normal Value Range (SI units)	Possible Indications
Creatinine kinase isoenzymes, MB fraction	0–12 IU/L	0–0.2 mckat/L	Depending on the ratio, the CK-MB fraction will indicate some form of muscle damage. The specific ratio can indicate if the muscle damage is cardiac or skeletal.
Creatinine	0.5–1.7 mg/dl	44–150 mcmol/L	Increased creatinine levels indicate a disorder with kidney function. Creatinine can also increase temporarily as a result of muscle injury.
			Low levels of creatinine are not common. They may been seen in persons with decreased muscle mass, such as comatose patients. Normal pregnancy will cause the creatinine levels to drop and are not a cause for concern.
Follicle-stimulating hormone (FSH) Female Midcycle Men	2–13 mlU/ml 5–22 mlU/ml 1–8 mlU/ml	2–13 IU/L 5–22 IU/L 1–8 IU/L	Increased levels of FSH and LH (luteinizing hormone) are consistent with primary ovarian failure, which is when ovaries themselves fail. In men this may be an indication of testicular developmental defects or injury.
			Decreased levels of FSH and LH are an indication of secondary ovarian failure, which results in problems with the pituitary or hypothalamic gland. In men this may be an indication of hypothalamic disorders.
Glucose, fasting	65–115 mg/dl	3.6–6.3 mmol/L	Indicates diabetes or pre-diabetes.
Glucose Tolerance Test (Oral), 2 hour	(mg/dl) Normal fasting		Indicates diabetes or pre-diabetes.
Post-drink: Impaired tolerance Indicates diabetes	65–99 < 140 mg/dl 140–199 mg/dl > 200 mg/dl		
Haptoglobin	44–303 mg/dl	0.44–3.03 g/L	If the haptoglobin levels are decreased in combination with several other tests, it may be an indication of hemolytic anemia.
			Haptoglobin will be elevated in many inflammatory diseases, such as ulcerative colitis, acute rheumatic disease, heart attack, and severe infection.
Fibrinogen	200–400 mg/dl	2–4 g/L	Lower than normal fibrinogen levels indicate that the person may not be able to form a stable blood clot after injury. Chronically low levels may indicate an inherited condition such as afibrinogenemia, or to an acquired condition such as liver disease, malnutrition, or some types of cancer. Higher than normal levels of fibrinogen may indicate: acute infections, breast, kidney, or stomach cancer, chronic DIC, inflammatory disorders, myocardial infarction, stroke, or trauma. Fibrinogen concentrations may rise sharply in any condition that causes inflammation or tissue damage.

Test	Normal Value Range (Conventional)	Normal Value Range (SI units)	Possible Indications
Hematocrit (Hct) Female Male Hemoglobin A$_{1C}$	35%–46% 40.0%–50.0% 40.0%–50.0% of total	0.36–0.446 fraction of 1 0.4–0.503 fraction of 1 0.053–0.075	Decreased hematocrit level indicates anemia, such as iron deficiency, but may have other causes such as vitamin or mineral deficiencies, recent bleeding, liver cirrhosis, and malignancies. Abnormally high levels of hematocrit may be an indication of dehydration and can be easily cured by increased fluid intake. *Polycythemia vera*— greater than normal number of red blood cells in a person can also cause a prolonged increase in the hematocrit levels. Higher than normal hematocrit levels are also seen in persons with chronic pulmonary conditions or lung damage. The person's bone marrow will increase production of red blood cells to supply the body with oxygen in response to a lacking pulmonary system.
Hemoglobin (Hb) Female Male	11.6–15.5 g/dl 13.7–16.7 g/dl	121–153 g/L 138–175 g/L	Low levels of Hb are an indication of anemia. Some types of anemia are treated with iron, folic acid, or vitamin B$_{12}$ or B$_6$ supplements. It is normal for women of childbearing age to have temporary decreases during menstrual periods and pregnancy.
Leukocyte count (WBC)	3800–9800/mcl	3.8–9.8 × 10^9/L	Infections usually cause increased WBC counts and may be treated with antibiotics. Leukemias (blood cancer) require chemotherapy and other treatments.
Erythrocyte count (RBC) Female Male	3.8–5.2 × 10^6/mcl 4.3–5.7 × 10^6/mcl	3.8–5.2 × 10^{12}/L 4.3–5.7 × 10^{12}/L	A low ESR can indicate polycythemia, extreme leukocytosis, and some protein abnormalities.
Erythrocyte sedimentation rate (sedrate, ESR) Female Male	30 mm/hr mm/hr	30 mm/hr 20 mm/hr	Elevated ESR level is an indication of inflammation, anemia, infection, pregnancy, and advanced age.
Leukocytes (WBC)	K/uL		Raised levels may indicate infections, inflammation, or cancer. Decreased levels may indicate autoimmune conditions, some severe infections, bone marrow failure, and congenital marrow aplasia. Decreased levels may also occur with certain medications such as methotrexate.
Lymphocytes	of WBC		Chronic high levels may indicate lymphocytic leukemia.
Lipase	7–60 units/L @ 37 C	7–60 units/L @ 37 C	High Lipase levels, with abdominal pain, may indicate acute pancreatitis, slightly raised levels can indicate kidney disease, salivary gland inflammation, or peptic ulcer disease.

Test	Normal Value Range (Conventional)	Normal Value Range (SI units)	Possible Indications
Lipids			A person with high cholesterol has more than twice the risk of coronary heart disease as someone whose cholesterol is below 200 mg/dL.
Total Cholesterol	< 200 mg/dl		
Borderline high	200–239 mg/dl		
High	240–above		
HDL	> 60 mg/dl		Low HDL is considered a major risk factor for heart disease.
High	< 40 mg/dl (men)		
	< 50 mg/dl (women)		
LDL	< 100 mg/dl		If you don't have coronary heart disease or diabetes and have one or no risk factors, your LDL goal is less than 160 mg/dL.
High	> 130 mg/dl		
			If you don't have coronary heart disease or diabetes and have two or more risk factors, your LDL goal is less than 130 mg/dL.
			If you do have coronary heart disease or diabetes, your LDL goal is less than 100 mg/dL.
Triglycerides	> 150 mg/dl		Normal triglyceride levels vary by age and sex. A high triglyceride level combined with low HDL cholesterol or high LDL cholesterol seems to speed up atherosclerosis (the buildup of fatty deposits in artery walls). Atherosclerosis increases the risk for heart attack and stroke. Info on lipids from the American Heart Association.
High	> 200 mg/dl and above		
PSA			PSA is a test indicating the level of protein cells the prostate is producing. The higher the PSA number, the more likely prostate cancer is present. Age, hormonal factors, and medications can alter the test results so a high PSA alone is not a cancer indicator.
0–54 yrs	0.00–2.50 ng/ml		
55–59 yrs	0.00–3.40 ng/ml		
60–64 yrs	0.00–4.10 ng/ml		
65–69 yrs	0.00–5.10 ng/ml		
70 plus yrs	0.00–5.60 ng/ml		
TSH	0.40–5.00 IU/ml		A high TSH result is often due to some type of acute or chronic thyroid dysfunction that causes the thyroid to be underactive. Although rare, a high TSH can be an indication of secondary hyperthyroidism, which is a problem with the pituitary gland.
			A low TSH result can indicate an overactive thyroid gland.
Urea, plasma (BUN)	8.5–25 mg/dl	2.9–8.9 mmol/liter	Increased BUN levels may be due to acute or chronic kidney disease, damage, or failure. Conditions that result in reduced blood flow to the kidneys, such as a recent heart attack, will also result in an increased BUN. Low BUN level are rarely detected because they result from diseases or symptoms, such as dehydration or starvation, that do not warrant a BUN test.
Urinalysis pH	5.0–7.5	5.0–7.5	
Specific Gravity	1.001–1.030	1.001–1.030	Specific gravity is an indication of how well the kidneys are filtering waste products. Reduced specific gravity can indicate diabetes insipidus, certain renal diseases, excess fluid intake, or diabetes mellitus. Raised specific gravity can indicate dehydration, adrenal insufficiency, nephrosis, congestive cardiac failure, or liver disease.

Common Medical Abbreviations

AAO	alert, awake, and oriented		COPD	chronic obstructive pulmonary disease
A&O	alert and oriented		CP	cerebral palsy
ABD	abdomen		CPAP	continuous positive airway pressure
ABG	arterial blood gas		CPR	cardiopulmonary resuscitation
abs	absent		CT	computerized tomography
AC	before eating		CVA	cerebrovascular accident
ACLS	advanced cardiac life support		CXR	chest X-ray
ADH	anti-diuretic hormone		DC	discontinue or discharge
adm	admission		DNR	do not resuscitate
ADR	adverse drug reaction		DOA	dead on arrival
ad lib	as much as needed		DTR	deep tendon reflexes
AFP	alpha-fetoprotein		DVT	deep venous thrombosis
amb	ambulatory		DX	diagnosis
amt	amount		ECG	electrocardiogram
ant	anterior		EMG	electromyogram
ante	before		ENT	ears, nose, and throat
AOB	alcohol on breath		FBS	fasting blood sugar
AP	anteroposterior		FTT	failure to thrive
ASAP	as soon as possible		FU	followup
BCP	birth control pills		Fx	fracture
BE	barium enema		GI	gastrointestinal
bid	twice a day		GSW	gunshot wound
BM	bowel movement		GTT	glucose tolerance test
BMR	basal metabolic rate		HA	Headache
BP	blood pressure		HBP	high blood pressure
BPH	benign prostatic hypertrophy		HCG	human chorionic gonadotropin
BPM	beats per minute		HCT	hematocrit
BS	bowel or breath sounds		HDL	high density lipoprotein
BX	biopsy		HEENT	head, eyes, ears, nose, throat
c	with		Hgb	hemoglobin
CA	cancer		HIV	human immunodeficiency virus
Ca	calcium		HO	history of
CAD	coronary artery disease		H&P	history and physical examination
CAT	computerized axial tomography		HR	heart rate
CBC	complete blood count		HS	at bedtime
CC	chief complaint		HSV	herpes simplex virus
CHF	congestive heart failure		HTN	hypertension
CNS	central nervous system		Hx	history
C/O	complaining of		I&D	incision and drainage

ICU	intensive care unit		**qd**	every day
ID	infectious disease		**qh**	every hour
IG	immunoglobulin		**qid**	four times a day
IM	intramuscular		**qod**	every other day
INF	intravenous nutritional fluid		**R**	right
IV	intravenous		**RA**	rheumatoid arthritis
L	left		**RBC**	red blood cell
LLL	left lower lobe		**R/O**	rule out
LMP	last menstrual period		**ROM**	range of motion
LOC	loss of consciousness or level of consciousness		**ROS**	review of systems
LPN	licensed practical nurse		**RTC**	return to clinic
MAO	monoamine oxidase		**s**	without
MBT	maternal blood type		**SOAP**	subjective, objective, assessment, plan
MI	myocardial infarction or mitral insufficiency		**SOB**	shortness of breath
mL	milliliter		**SQ**	subcutaneous
MMR	measles, mumps, rubella		**STAT**	immediately
MRI	magnetic resonance imaging		**Sx**	symptoms
MRSA	methicillin resistant staph aureus		**T&C**	type and cross
MS	multiple sclerosis		**TB**	tuberculosis
MVA	motor vehicle accident		**tid**	three times a day
NG	nasogastric		**TIG**	tetanus immune globulin
NKA	no known allergies		**TMJ**	temporo mandibular joint
NKDA	no known drug allergies		**TNTC**	too numerous to count
NMR	nuclear magnetic resonance		**TO**	telephone order
NPO	nothing by mouth		**TPN**	total parenteral nutrition
NSAID	nonsteroidal anti-inflammatory drugs		**TSH**	thyroid stimulating hormone
NSR	normal sinus rhythm		**TT**	thrombin time
OB	obstetrics		**Tx**	treatment
OPV	oral polio vaccine		**UA**	urinalysis
OR	operating room		**UAO**	upper airway obstruction
PA	posteroanterior		**UBD**	universal blood donor
PC	after eating		**URI**	upper respiratory infection
PDR	*Physician's Desk Reference*		**US**	ultrasound
PE	physical exam		**UTI**	urinary tract infection
PKU	phenylketonuria		**VO**	verbal order
PMH	previous medical history		**WBC**	white blood cell
PO	by mouth		**WD**	well developed
PR	by rectum		**WF**	white female
PRN	as needed		**WM**	white male
PT	prothrombin time, or physical therapy		**WNL**	within normal limits
Pt	patient		**WO**	written order
PTT	partial thromboplastin time		**yo**	years old
PUD	peptic ulcer disease		**YOB**	year of birth
q	every (e.g., q6h = every 6 hours)		**yr**	year
			ytd	year to date

Medical Terminology Word Parts

Medical terms are like individual jigsaw puzzles. Once you divide the terms into their component parts and learn the meaning of the individual parts, you can use that knowledge to understand many other new terms. Four basic component parts are used to create medical terms:

Root — The basic, or core, part that makes up the essential meaning of the term. The root usually, but not always, denotes a body part. Root words usually come from the Greek or Latin languages. For example, *bronch* is a root that means "the air passages in the lungs" or "bronchial tubes." *Cephal* means "head." An extensive list of root words is given on pages 1153–1156.

Prefix — One or more letters placed before the root to change its meaning. Prefixes usually, but not always, indicate location, time, number, or status. For example, the prefix *bi-* means "two" or "twice." When *bi* is placed before the root *lateral* ("side"), to form *bilateral,* the meaning is "having two sides." An extensive list of prefixes is given on page 1153.

Suffix — One or more letters placed after the root to change its meaning. Suffixes usually, but not always, indicate the procedure, condition, disorder, or disease. For example, the suffix *-itis* means "inflammation," that is, damaged tissue that is red and painful. The medical term *bronchitis* means "inflammation of the bronchial tubes." Another example is the suffix *-ectomy,* which means "removal." Hence, *appendectomy* means "removal of the appendix." An extensive list of suffixes is given on pages 1156–1157.

Combining vowel — A letter used to combine roots with other word parts. The vowel is usually an *o,* but sometimes it is an *a* or *i.* When a combining vowel is added to a root, the result is called a combining form. For example, in the word encephalogram, the root is *cephal* ("head"), the prefix is *en-* ("inside"), and the suffix is *-gram* ("something recorded"). These word parts are joined by the combining vowel *o* to make a word more easy to pronounce. *Cephal/o* is the combining form. An *encephalogram* is an X-ray of the inside of the head.

Analyzing a Medical Term

You can often decipher the meaning of a medical term by breaking it down into its separate parts. Consider the following examples:

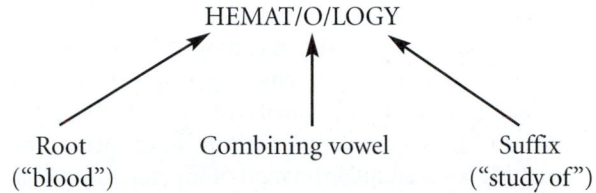

HEMAT/O/LOGY

Root ("blood") Combining vowel Suffix ("study of")

The term *hematology* is divided into three parts. When you analyze a medical term, begin at the end of the word. The ending is called the suffix. Almost all medical terms contain suffixes. The suffix in *hematology* is *-logy,* which means "study of." Now look at the beginning of the word. *Hemat* is the root word, which means "blood." The root word gives the essential meaning of the term.

The third part of this term, which is the letter *o,* has no meaning of its own, but is an important connector between the root (*hemat*) and the suffix (*logy*). It is the combining vowel. The letter *o* is the combining vowel usually found in medical terms.

Putting together the meanings of the suffix and the root, the term *hematology* means "the study of blood."

The combining vowel plus the root is called the combining form. A medical term can have more than one root word; therefore, there can be two combining forms. For example:

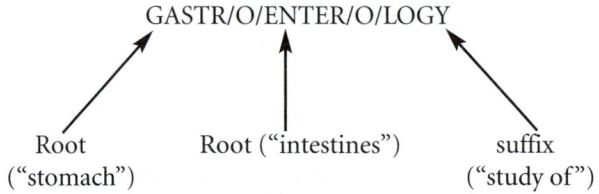

GASTR/O/ENTER/O/LOGY

Root ("stomach") Root ("intestines") suffix ("study of")

The two combining forms are *gastr/o* and *enter/o.* The entire term (reading from the suffix, back to the beginning of the term, and across) means "the study of the stomach and the intestines."

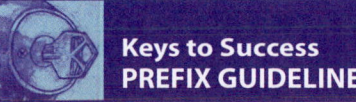

Keys to Success
PREFIX GUIDELINE

A prefix does not require a combining vowel. Do not place a combining vowel between a prefix and a root word.

Rules for Using Combining Vowels

1. A combining vowel is not used when the suffix begins with a vowel (*a-e-i-o-u*). For example, when *neur/o* (nerve) is joined with the suffix *-itis* (inflammation), the combining vowel is not used because *-itis* begins with a vowel. *Neuritis* (new-RYE-tis) is an inflammation of a nerve or nerves.
2. A combining vowel is used when the suffix begins with a consonant. For example, when *neur/o* (nerve) is joined with the suffix *-plasty* (surgical repair), the combining vowel *o* is used because *-plasty* begins with a consonant. *Neuroplasty* (NEW-roh-plas-tee) is the surgical repair of a nerve.
3. A combining vowel is always used when two or more root words are joined. As an example, when *gastr/o* (stomach) is joined with *enter/o* (small intestine), the combining vowel is used with *gastr/o. Gastroenteritis* (gas-troh-en-ter-EYE-tis) is an inflammation of the stomach and small intestine.

Suffixes and Medical Terms Related to Pathology

Pathology is the study of disease and the following suffixes describe specific disease conditions. (A more complete list of suffixes appears on pages 1156–1157.)

Suffix	Meaning
-algia	pain and suffering
-dynia	pain
-ectomy	surgical removal
-graphy	process of recording a picture or record
-gram	record or picture
-necr/osis	death (tissue death)
-scler/osis	abnormal hardening
-sten/osis	abnormal narrowing
-centesis	surgical puncture to remove fluid for diagnostic purposes or to remove excess fluid
-plasty	surgical repair
-scopy	visual examination with an instrument

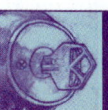
Keys to Success
WORD PART GUIDELINES

1. A single root word with a combining form cannot stand alone. A suffix must be added to complete the term.
2. The rules for the use of combining vowels apply when adding a suffix.
3. When a suffix begins with a consonant, a combining vowel, such as O, is placed before the suffix.

The Double RRs Suffixes

The following suffixes are often referred to as the "double RRs,"

* -rrhage and -rrhagia		Bursting form; an abnormal excessive discharge or bleeding. *Note:* -rrhage and -rhagia refer to the flow of blood.
* -rrhaphy		To suture or stitch.
* -rrhea		Abnormal flow or discharge; refers to the abnormal flow of most bodily fluids. *Note:* Although -rrhea and -rrhage both refer to abnormal flow, they are not used interchangeably.
* -rrhexis		Rupture.

Contrasting and Confusing Prefixes

The following contrasting prefixes can be confusing. Study this list to make sure you know the differences between the contrasting terms. (A more complete list of prefixes appears on page 1153.)

Ab- Means "away from." *Abnormal* means not normal or away from normal.

Ad- Means "toward" or "in the direction." *Addiction* means drawn toward or a strong dependence on a drug or substance.

Dys- Means "bad," "difficult," "painful." *Dysfunctional* means an organ or body that is not working properly.

Eu- Means "good," normal, well, or easy. Euthyroid (you-THIGH-roid) means a normally functioning thyroid gland.

Hyper- Means "excessive" or "increased." *Hypertension* (high-per-TEN-shun) is higher than normal blood pressure.

Hypo- Means "deficient" or "decreased." *Hypotension* (high-poh-TEN-shun) is lower than normal blood pressure.

Inter- Means "between" or "among." *Interstitial* (in-ter-STISH-al) means between, but not within, the parts of a tissue.

Intra- Means "within" "into." *Intramuscular* (in-trah-MUS-kyou-lar) means within the muscle.

Sub- Means "under," "less," or "below." *Subcostal* (sub-KOS-tal) means below a rib or ribs.

Supra- Means "above." *Supracostal* (sue-prah-KOS-tal) means above or outside the ribs.

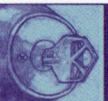

Keys to Success
USING A MEDICAL DICTIONARY

Learning to use a medical dictionary is an important part of mastering the correct use of medical terms. Some dictionaries use categories such as "Diseases and Syndromes" to group disorders with these terms in the titles. For example:

■ Venereal disease would be found under "disease, venereal."

■ Fetal alcohol syndrome would be found under "syndrome, fetal alcohol."

When you come across a term and cannot find it listed by the first word, the next step is to look under the appropriate category.

Singular and Plural Endings

Many medical terms have Greek or Latin origins. As a result of these different origins, the rules for changing a singular word into a plural form are unusual. Additionally, English endings have been adopted for some commonly used terms.

Guidelines to Unusual Plural Forms

	Guideline	Singular	Plural
1.	If the term ends in an *a*, the plural is usually formed by adding an *e*	bursa vertebra	bursae vertebrae
2.	If the term ends in *ex* or *ix*, the plural is usually formed by changing the *ex* or *ix* to *ices*.	appendix index	appendices indices
3.	If the term ends in *is*, the plural is usually formed by changing the *is* to *es*.	diagnosis metastasis	diagnoses metastases
4.	If the term ends in *itis*, the plural is usually formed by changing the *is* to *ides*.	arthritis meningitis	arthritides meningitides
5.	If the term ends in *nx*, the plural is usually formed by changing the *x* to *ges*.	phalanx meninx	phalanges meninges
6.	If the term ends in *on*, the plural is usually formed by changing the *on* to *a*.	criterion ganglion	criteria ganglia
7.	If the term ends in *um*, the plural is usually formed by changing the *um* to *a*.	diverticulum ovum	diverticula ova
8.	If the term ends in *us*, the plural is usually formed by changing the *us* to *i*.	alveolus malleolus	alveoli malleoli

Basic Medical Terms

The following subsections discuss basic medical terms that are used to describe diseases and disease conditions, major body systems, and body direction.

Terms Used to Describe Diseases and Disease Conditions

The basic medical terms used to describe diseases and disease conditions are listed here.

■ A *sign* is evidence of disease, such as fever, that can be observed by the patient and others. A sign is objective because it can be evaluated or measured by others.

■ A *symptom,* such as pain or a headache, can only be experienced or defined by the patient. A symptom is subjective because it can be evaluated or measured only by the patient.

■ A *syndrome* is a set of signs and symptoms that occur together as part of a specific disease process.

■ *Diagnosis* is the identification of disease. To diagnose is the process of reaching a diagnosis.

■ A *differential diagnosis* attempts to determine which of several diseases may be producing the symptoms.

■ A *prognosis* is a forecast or prediction of the probable course and outcome of a disorder.

■ An *acute* disease or symptom has a rapid onset, a severe course, and relatively short duration.

■ A *chronic* symptom or disease has a long duration. Although chronic symptoms or diseases may be controlled, they are rarely cured.

■ A *remission* is the partial or complete disappearance of the symptoms of a disease without having achieved a cure. A remission is usually temporary.

■ Some diseases are named for the condition described. For example, *chronic fatigue syndrome* (CFS) is a persistent overwhelming fatigue that does not resolve with bed rest.

■ An *eponym* is a disease, structure, operation, or procedure that is named for the person who discovered or described it first. For example, Alzheimer's disease is named for Alois Alzheimer, a German neurologist who lived from 1864 to 1915.

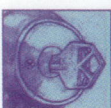

Keys to Success
ACCURACY IN SPELLING

Accuracy in spelling medical terms is extremely important! Changing just one or two letters can completely change the meaning of the word—and this difference could literally be a matter of life or death for the patient.

■ An *acronym* is a word formed from the initial letter or letters of the major parts of a compound term. For example, the acronym AMA stands for American Medical Association.

Terms Used to Describe Major Body Systems

The following is a list of the major body systems and some common related combining forms used with each.

Major Structures and Body System	Related Roots with Combining Forms
Skeletal system	bones (oste/o) joints (arthr/o) cartilage (chondr/o)
Muscular system	muscles(my/o) ligaments (syndesm/o) tendons (ten/o, tend/o, tendin/o)
Cardiovascular system	heart (card/o, cardi/o) arteries (arteri/o) veins (phleb/o, ven/o) blood (hem/o, hemat/o)
Lymphatic and immune systems	lymph, lymph vessels, and lymph nodes (lymph/o), (lymphangi/o) tonsils (tonsill/o) spleen (splen/o) thymus (thym/o)
Respiratory system	nose (nas/o, rhin/o) pharynx (pharyng/o) trachea (trache/o) larynx (laryng/o) lungs (pneum/o, pneumon/o)
Digestive system	mouth (or/o) esophagus (esophag/o) stomach (gastr/o) small intestines (enter/o) large intestines (col/o) liver (hepat/o) pancreas (pancreat/o)
Urinary system	kidneys (nephr/o, ren/o) ureters (ureter/o) urinary bladder (cyst/o, visic/o) urethra (urethr/o)
Integumentary system	glands (aden/o) skin (cutane/o, dermat/o, derm/o) sebaceous glands (seb/o) sweat glands (hidraden/o)
Nervous system	nerves (neur/o) brain (encephal/o) spinal cord (myel/o) eyes (ocul/o, ophthalm/o) ears (acoust/o, ot/o)
Endocrine system	adrenals (adren/o) pancreas (pancreat/o) pituitary (pituit/o) thyroid (thyr/o, thyroid/o) parathyroids (parathyroid/o) thymus (thym/o)
Reproductive system	*Male:* testicles (orch/o, orchid/o) *Female:* ovaries (oophor/o, ovari/o) uterus (hyster/o, metr/o, metri/o, uter/o)

Terms Used to Describe Body Direction

Certain terms are used to describe the location of body parts relative to the trunk or other parts of the anatomy. See Figure H-1 ◆.

Ventral (VEN-tral) refers to the front or belly side of the body or organ (*ventr* means "belly side" of the body and *al* means "pertaining to").

Dorsal (DOR-sal) refers to the back of the body or organ (*dors* means "back of body" and *al* means "pertaining to").

Anterior (an-TEER-ee-or) means situated in the front. It also means on the forward part of an organ (*anter* means "front" or "before" and *ior* means "pertaining to"). For example, the stomach is located anterior to (in front of) the pancreas. *Anterior* is also used in reference to the ventral surface of the body.

Posterior (pos-TEER-ee-or) means situated in the back. It also means on the back portion of an organ (*poster* means "back" or "after" and *ior* means "pertaining to"). For example, the

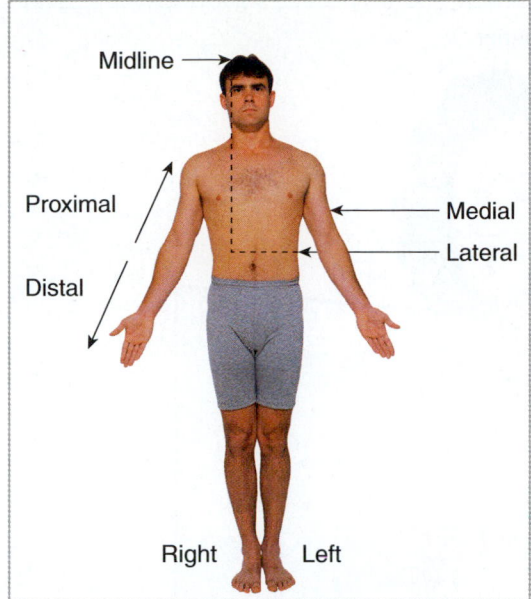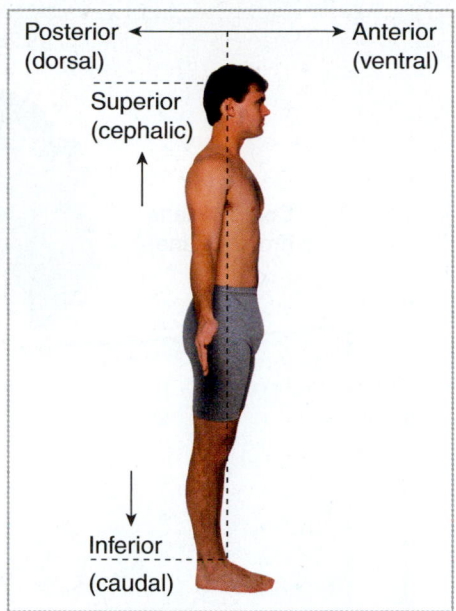

Figure H-1 ◆ Directional anatomical terms.

pancreas is located posterior to (behind) the stomach. Posterior is also used in reference to the dorsal surface of the body.

Superior means uppermost, above, or toward the head. For example, the lungs are superior to (above) the diaphragm.

Inferior means lowermost, below, or toward the feet. For example, the stomach is located inferior to (below) the diaphragm.

Cephalic (seh-FAL-ick) means toward the head (*cephal* means "head" and *ic* means "pertaining to").

Caudal (KAW-dal) means toward the lower part of the body (*caud* means "tail" or "lower part" of the body and *al* means "pertaining to").

Proximal (PROCK-sih-mal) means situated nearest the midline or beginning of a body structure. For example, the proximal end of the humerus (the bone of the upper arm) forms part of the shoulder. Or, it may be easier for you to think of it as "closer to the origin of the body part or the point of attachment of a limb to the body trunk."

Distal (DIS-tal) means situated farthest from the midline or beginning of a body structure. For example, the distal end of the humerus forms part of the elbow.

Medial means the direction toward or nearer the midline. For example, the medial ligament of the knee is near the inner surface of the leg.

Lateral means the direction toward or nearer the side and away from the midline. For example, the lateral ligament of the knee is near the side of the leg.

Bilateral means relating to, or having, two sides.

Planes of the Body

Medical professionals often refer to sections of the body in terms of anatomical planes (flat surfaces). These planes are imaginary lines—vertical or horizontal—drawn through an upright body. The following terms are used to describe a specific body part (see Figure H-2 ◆):

■ Coronal plane (frontal plane): A vertical plane running from side to side; divides the body or any of its parts into anterior and posterior portions.

■ Sagittal plane (median plane): A vertical plane running from front to back; divides the body or any of its parts into right and left sides.

■ Axial plane (transverse plane): A horizontal plane; divides the body or any of its parts into upper and lower parts.

Prefixes, Root Words, and Suffixes

The most common medical prefixes, root words, and suffixes are listed here. Knowing these common prefixes, roots, and suffixes will help you decipher medical terms.

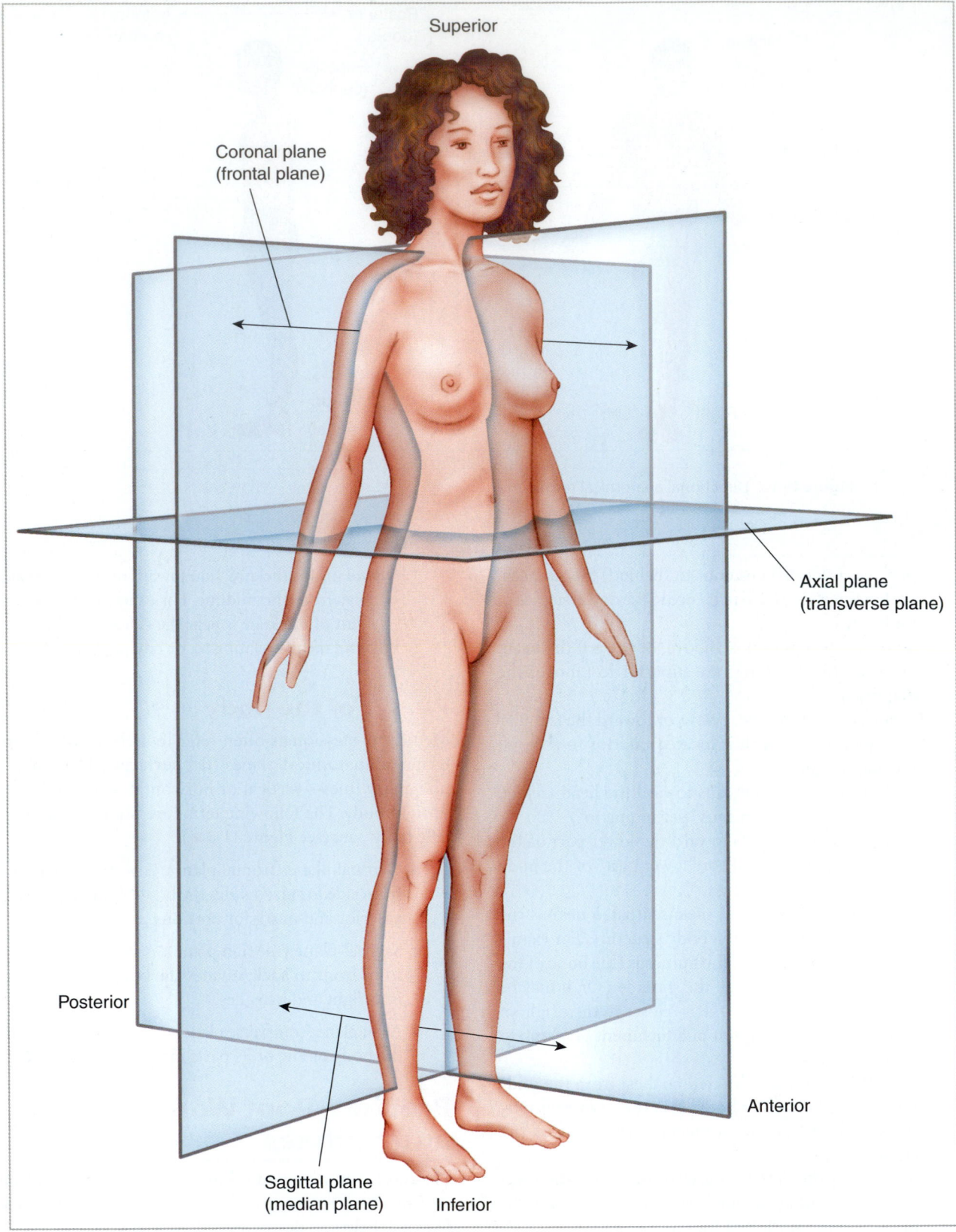

Superior

Coronal plane
(frontal plane)

Axial plane
(transverse plane)

Posterior

Anterior

Sagittal plane
(median plane)

Inferior

Figure H-2 ◆ Anatomical planes.

Prefixes

a	without or absence of	mal	bad
ab	from; away from	meso	middle
ad	to; toward	meta	after; beyond; change
an	without or absence of	micro	small
ante	before	multi	many
anti	against	neo	new
bi	two	nulli	none
bin	two	pan	all; total
brady	slow	para	outside; beyond; around
con	together	per	through
contra	against	peri	surrounding (outer)
de	from; down from; lack of	poly	many; much
dia	through; complete; between; apart	post	after
dis	to undo; free from	pre	before; in front of
dys	difficult; labored; painful; abnormal	pro	before
ec	out	quadri	four
ecto	outside	re	back
endo	within	retro	back; behind
epi	on; upon; over	semi	half
eso	inward	sub	under; below
eu	normal; good	super	over; above
ex	outside; outward	supra	above; beyond; on top
exo	outside; outward	sym	together; joined
extra	outside of; beyond	syn	together; joined
hemi	half	tachy	fast; rapid
hyper	above; excessive	tetra	four
hypo	below; incomplete; deficient	trans	through; across; beyond
in	in; into; not	tri	three
infra	under; below	ultra	beyond; excess
inter	between	uni	one
intra	within		

Root Words

abdomin	abdomen	carcin	cancer
aden	gland	cardi	heart
adren	adrenal gland	caud	tail; toward lower part of the body
adrenal	adrenal gland	cephal	head
aer	air; oxygen; gas	cerebell	cerebellum
alveol	alveolus	cerebr	cerebrum; brain
angi	(blood) vessel; (lymph) vessel	cervic	neck; cervix
ankyl	crooked; stiff; bent	cheil	lip
appendic	appendix	chiro	hand
arteri, arter	artery	cholangi	bile duct
arteriol	arteriole (small artery)	chole	gall; bile
arthr	joint	chondr	cartilage
ather	yellowish; fatty plaque	coccyg	coccyx; tailbone
aur	ear	col	colon; large intestine
aut	self	conjunctiv	conjunctiva
bil	bile	corne	cornea
bio	life	coron	heart; crown of the head
blephar	eyelid	cost	rib
bronch	airway; bronchus	crani	cranium; skull
bronchiol	bronchiole	cutane	skin
burs	bursa	cyan	blue

cyst	bladder; sac	kin	movement
cyt, cyte	cell	kinesi	movement; motion
dacry	tears; tear duct	labi	lips
dactyl	fingers or toes	lacrim	tear duct; tear
dent	tooth	lact	milk
derm	skin	lapar	abdomen
dermat	skin	laryng	larynx
dipl	two; double	later	side
diverticul	diverticulum	lei	smooth
dors	back (of the body)	leuk	white
duoden	duodenum	lingu	tongue
ectop	located away from usual place	lip	fat
edema	swelling	lith	stone; calculus
electr	electricity; electrical activity	lob	lobe
encephal	brain	lymph	lymph
endocrin	endocrine	macr	abnormal largeness
enter	intestines (usually small intestine)	mamm	breast
epiglott	epiglottis	mast	breast
epitheli	epithelium	meat	opening or passageway
erythr	red	melan	black
esophag	esophagus	men	menstruation
esthesi	sensation; feeling; sensitivity	mening	meninges
eti	cause (of disease)	ment	mind
exocrin	secrete out of	mes, meso	middle
faci	face	metr	uterus
fasci	fascia; fibrous band	mon	one
fract	break; broken	morbid	disease; sickness
galact	milk	muc	mucus
gastr	stomach	my, myos	muscle
ger	old age; aged	myc	fungus
geront	old age; aged	myel	bone marrow; spinal cord
gingiv	gums	myelon	bone marrow
glauc	gray	myring	eardrum
gloss	tongue	narc	stupor; numbness
gluc	sweetness; sugar	nas	nose
glyc	sugar; glucose	nat	birth
glycos	sugar; glucose	necr	death (cells; body)
gnos	knowledge; a knowing	nephr	kidney
gonad	gonad; sex glands	neur	nerve
gyn	woman	noct	night
gynec	woman	nyct	night
gyr	turning; folding	nyctal	night
hem	blood	ocul	eye
hemat	blood	onc	tumor
hepat	liver	onych	nail
hidr	sweat	oophor	ovary
hist	tissue	ophthalm	eye
hom	same	or	mouth
home	sameness; unchanging	orth	straight
hydr	water	oste	bone
hyster	uterus	ot	ear
ile	ileum	ox	oxygen
ili	ilium	palpat	touch; feel; stroke
immun	immune	pancreat	pancreas
irid	iris	par, part	bear; give birth to; labor
kerat	horny tissue; hard	parathyroid	parathyroid

path	disease; suffering	spher	round; sphere; ball
pector	chest; muscle	sphygm	pulse
ped	child; foot	spin	spine; backbone to
pelv	pelvis; pelvic bone	spir	breathe
pen	penis	splen	spleen
perine	perineum	spondyl	vertebra; spinal or vertebral column
peritone	peritoneum	staphyl	grapelike clusters
petr	stone; portion of temporal bone	stern	(breastbone)
phac, phak	lens of the eye	steth	chest (muscles)
phag	eat; swallow	stoma	mouth; opening
phalang	finger or toe bone	stomat	mouth; opening
pharyng	pharynx, throat	strab	squint; squint-eyed
phas	speech	synovi	synovia; synovial membrane
phleb	vein	system	system
phot	light	ten, tend	tendon
phren	mind	tendin	tendon
physi	nature	test	testis; testicle
pleur	pleura	therm	heat
pneum	lung; air	thorac	thorax; chest
pneumat	lung; air	thromb	clot
pneumon	lung; air	thym	thymus gland; soul
pod	foot	thyr	thyroid gland
poli	gray matter	thyroid	thyroid gland
polyp	polyp; small growth	tom	cut; section
poster	back (of body)	ton	tension; pressure
prim	first	tone	to stretch
proct	rectum	tonsill	tonsils
pseud	fake; false	top	place; position; location
psych	mind	tox, toxic	poison; poisonous
pulmon	lung	trach, trache	trachea; windpipe
py	pus	trachel	neck; necklike
pyel	renal pelvis	trich	hair
pylor	pylorus	tubercul	little knot; swelling
pyr	fever; heat	tympan	eardrum; middle ear
quadr	four	ulcer	sore; ulcer
rect	rectum	ungu	nail
ren	kidney	ur	urine; urinary tract
retin	retina	ureter	ureter
rhin	nose	urethr	urethra
sacr	sacrum fallopian (uterine)	uria	urination; urine
salping	tube	urin	urine or urinary organs
sanit	soundness; health	uter	uterus
sarc	flesh; connective tissue	uvul	uvula; little grape
scler	sclera; white of eye; hard	vagin	vagina
scoli	crooked; curved	valv	valve
seb	sebum; oil	valvul	valve
seps	infection	vas	vessel; duct
sept	infection; partition; septum	vascul	blood vessel; little vessel
sial	saliva	ven	vein
sinus	inus	versicul	seminal vesicles; blister
somat	body	vertebr	vertebra; backbone
somn	sleep	vesic	urinary bladder
son	sound	vir	poison; virus
sopor	sleep	viril	masculine; manly
sperm	sperm, spermatazoa; seed	vis	seeing; sight
spermat	sperm, spermatazoa; seed		

visc	sticky	ductor	to lead or pull
viscer	viscera; internal organs; sternum	dynia	pain
viscos	sticky	ectasis	stretching out; dilation; expansion
vit	life	ectomy	excision or surgical removal
xanth	yellow	ectopia	displacement
xen	strange; foreign	emesis	vomiting
xer	dry	emia	blood; blood condition
zygot	joined together	gen	producing, forming
		genesis	producing; forming
		genic	producing, forming

Additional Root Words

caus	burning sensation; capable of burning	gnosis	a knowing
cusp	point; cusp	gram	record; X-ray
flexion	bending	graph	instrument used to record
genital	pertaining to birth	graphy	process of recording; X-ray filming
lumb	lumbar; loin region	ictal	seizure; attack
mediastin	mediastinum	ism	state of
tens, tensi	pressure, force, stretching	itis	inflammation
		lepsy	seizure
		logist	specialist

Suffixes

	logy	study of

Suffixes Meaning "Pertaining to"

ac
al, ine
ar, ior
ary, ory
eal, ous
ial
ic
ical, tic

lysis	destruction; reduce; separation
malacia	softening
mania	madness; insane desire
megaly	enlargement
meter	instrument used to measure
metry	measurement
morph	form; shape
oid, ode	resembling
oma	tumor; mass
opia	vision (condition)
opsy	to view
oxia	oxygen
paresis	slight paralysis
pathy	disease
penia	abnormal reduction in number; lack of

Suffixes Meaning "Abnormal Conditions"

ago	abnormal condition, disease
esis	abnormal condition, disease
ia	abnormal condition, disease
iasis	abnormal condition, disease
ion	condition
ism	condition, state of abnormal condition
osis	disease

peps, pepsia	digestion
pexy	surgical fixation; suspension
phagia	eating; swallowing
philia	love
phily	love
phobia	abnormal fear of or adversion to specific objects or things
phonia	sound or voice
phoria	feeling
physis	growth
plasia	formation; development; a growth
plasm	growth; formation; substance
plasty	plastic or surgical repair
plegia	paralysis; stroke
pnea	breathing
porosis	lessening in density; porous condition
praxia	in front of; before
ptosis	drooping; sagging; prolapse
ptysis	spitting

Common Suffixes Used in Medical Terminology

algia	pain, suffering
asthenia	weakness
cele	hernia, protrusion
centesis	surgical puncture to remove fluid
cidal	killing
clasia	break
clasis	break
clast	break
clysis	irrigating; washing
coccus	berry shaped (a form of bacterium)
crine	separate; secrete
crit	to separate
cyte	cell
desis	fusion; to bind; tie together
drome	run; running

rrhage	bursting forth, an abnormal excessive discharge or bleeding	stalsis	contraction; constriction
rrhagia	bursting forth, an abnormal excessive discharge or bleeding	stasis	control; stop; standing still
		stat	to stop
rrhaphy	to suture or stitch	stenosis	narrowing; constriction
rrhea	abnormal flow or discharge	stomy	new artificial opening
rrhexis	rupture	therapy	treatment
schisis	split; fissure	tome	instrument used to cut
sclerosis	hardening	tomy	cutting into; surgical incision
scope	instrument used for visual exam	tripsy	crushing
scopic	visual exam	trophy	nourishment
scopy	visual exam with an instrument	ule	little
sepsis	infection	uria	urine; urination
sis	state of		
spasm	sudden involuntary muscle contraction		

Source: Adapted from Vines, Deborah, Braceland, Ann, Rollins, Elizabeth, and Miller, Susan. *Comprehensive Health Insurance: Billing, Coding, and Reimbursement.* © 2008. Pearson Education. Upper Saddle River, NJ.

Answers to Chapter Case Study Critical Thinking Questions and In-Practice Scenarios

Answers to Case Studies

Chapter 1

CTQ 1-1: Can Janet apply to take the AAMA exam at one of the three times offered this year? Why or why not? If not, explain what steps she might have to take to become eligible.

Answer: Because Janet has never attended an accredited medical assistant school, she would not be eligible to sit for the AAMA exam. She should research her educational options and find a school that is either CAAHEP or ABHES accredited, as required by the AAMA. When she has completed her education, she can submit her transcripts and sit for the exam.

CTQ 1-2: Why has the number of women attending medical school in the United States increased so dramatically since 1970?

Answer: The role of women in healthcare has continued to grow as women have moved into more and more professional positions. The traditional role of women staying home to raise their children has changed on a cultural level, with women moving into fields once dominated by men.

Chapter 2

CTQ 2-1: Referring to the case study at the beginning of this chapter, what evidence supports the argument that medical assistants should have a standardized base of knowledge?

Answer: With dramatic changes in healthcare over the past decade, including shorter hospital stays and managed care, physicians must rely on allied health personnel like medical assistants to help care for patients. With technology advancing and patient safety increasingly a focal point, many physicians today insist on hiring medical assistants who have been formally trained in accredited medical assisting programs.

CTQ 2-2: How do certification discounts on physicians' medical malpractice insurance policies impact job opportunities for medical assistants?

Answer: These discounts encourage physicians to hire certified or registered medical assistants. This places the medical assistant with certification in a better place in the health care market.

CTQ 2-3: How does an externship support the educational goals of an accredited medical-assisting program?

Answer: Externships involve working as a medical assistant under a physician's supervision. Externships can run anywhere from 60 to 240 hours, but many medical-assisting programs require externships of more than 240 hours. While externships are unpaid, students earn credits toward their medical assisting certificates. The externship is an opportunity for the medical assistant to practice his or her newly learned skills in a safe, supervised environment.

Chapter 3

CTQ 3-1: How can Jamie let a potential employer know her level of competence?

Answer: Jamie can clearly outline her skills on her resume as well as mention them in her interview.

CTQ 3-2: How can Jamie let the potential employer know that she will be a responsible employee?

Answer: Jamie can point out areas in former jobs, or during her schooling, where she has shown responsibility.

CTQ 3-3: What are some examples of personal issues that are not mentioned in the above section that should not be brought up while working?

Answer: Examples include relationship issues the medical assistant is experiencing, family problems, financial problems, issues surrounding social activities, or other non-job-related topics.

Chapter 4

CTQ 4-1: How does the case study outlined at the beginning of this chapter illustrate one of the torts in Table 4-2? Please specify the tort.

Answer: The case study illustrates the tort of invasion of privacy. The medical assistant cannot release any information about a patient to another individual without the patient's consent or a court order.

CTQ 4-2: Referring to the case study at the beginning of the chapter, assume that Victoria revealed information about the patient's care to the patient's employer. What is the potential impact on the patient?

Answer: The employer might use the information gained about the patient's care to fire her or to deny her advancement to a better position.

CTQ 4-3: In the case study at the beginning of the chapter, the patient's employer obtained a subpoena for her medical information. How would the medical assistant determine which information to release? What is the proper procedure?

Answer: The medical assistant would want to verify the subpoena has been duly signed. The medical assistant would then seek to determine exactly what information the subpoena covers—the dates of service or condition that are specifically being requested.

CTQ 4-4: Assume that the patient was fired after the medical office gave her employer her private health information without her permission. How should she go about filing a complaint with HIPAA?

Answer: Victoria would need to ask the medical office for a complaint form and file the complaint with the office.

Chapter 5

CTQ 5-1: How can the medical assistant enhance communication with non-native English speakers like Katerina?

Answer: The medical assistant should be careful to use proper English, without using slang terms. The medical assistant might also try writing things down for the patient; often the patient will better understand English she sees written rather than hearing it spoken.

CTQ 5-2: What is the value of written communication for patients like Katerina, who speak English as a second language? What characteristics would make that written communication most effective?

Answer: Often the patient who is not a native English speaker will better understand the written word over the spoken word. A patient may have someone at home who understands English better, and the written communication could be used to help the patient relay to family members the information given by the office. Any written communication should be clear and concise.

CTQ 5-3: How does the reflecting conversation technique help ensure that medical assistants understand the concerns of patients like Katerina? What sort of questions would support this technique?

Answer: Using the reflecting conversation technique, the medical assistant is able to repeat information back to the patient, thereby ensuring that the patient's information was correctly understood. Questions that would support this technique would be, "Mrs. Dow, you said that for 2 weeks you have been having pain in your right shoulder and arm and that the pain has been running down to your right hand. Is that right?"

Chapter 6

CTQ 6-1: In the case study, why do you think the patient looked confused when he noticed that Marina was smoking? Why do you think Marina felt guilty or uneasy about being seen by her patient while smoking? How would you feel if the person teaching you healthy habits and encouraging you did not follow their own advice?

Answer: The patient was mostly confused by Marina's smoking because Marina works in the healthcare field, in naturopathy, and gives patients advice on healthy lifestyle choices. Marina felt guilty about being seen smoking because it is her job to counsel patients against such behavior, and she might have felt like a hypocrite for not following her own advice.

There is a growing trend among employers to refuse to hire smokers or allow smokers to extern at their offices. It is a proven fact that smokers cost more overall than nonsmokers in terms of workdays missed because of smoking-related illness and hospitalizations.

Chapter 7

CTQ 7-1: How should Ori try to educate his mother about the process of organ donation?

Answer: Ori should ask his physician for informational brochures to take home to his mother. She may be more receptive to learning about organ donation in the comfort of her own home and at her own pace.

CTQ 7-2: As you read in the case study, Ori's mother believes that hospitals save money if they let patients die and harvest organs later. Explain why the hospital cannot receive monetary compensation for organs. Also explain the difference between time frames in cold ischemic and warm ischemic donations.

Answer: The hospital does not benefit from "letting a person die" because there is no guarantee that the organs can and will be used in donation. Due to the specific time lines, organs may not all be ideal for donation by the time an emergency situation is managed and the next of kin have been notified. The hospital absorbs the physician's fees and other related costs of organ donation surgery.

According to the Uniform Anatomical Gift Act, the hospital cannot receive compensation for harvested organs. Furthermore, the physician doing the harvesting cannot be the physician who pronounces the patient dead.

CTQ 7-3: Can Ori's mother disregard his signed intent to be an organ donor and refuse to allow the hospital to harvest his organs upon his death?

Answer: Many institutions request permission from family members before procuring any organs. The decision is granted to a family member or guardian in order of priority. Sometimes a family member lower on the priority list may object to the donation. Most institutions abide by the wishes of the family and do not harvest any tissue or organs if all members are not in agreement.

Chapter 8

CTQ 8-1: Referring to the case study at the beginning of this chapter, how can the medical assistant help ensure that the typed letters contain no errors?

Answer: Using spellcheck software and proofreading documents help ensure that a typed letter contains no errors.

CTQ 8-2: What are the possible ramifications to Dr. Jones if the medical assistant does not use accurate grammar, spelling, and punctuation?

Answer: Incorrectly typed letters can result in misunderstanding, misdiagnosis, or even malpractice lawsuits in certain circumstances.

CTQ 8-3: Which courtesy title is appropriate for a letter to a sales representative, and why?

Answer: A letter to a sales representative should use the courtesy title "Mr." or "Ms." These titles are professional and indicate a professional relationship between the sales representative and the medical office.

Chapter 9

CTQ 9-1: If the medical office uses an automated system where callers are greeted by a recording, how can the medical assistant best serve a patient who has a possible emergency?

Answer: The medical assistant must be sure the prerecorded greeting for any automated system includes a message similar to this: "If this is a medical emergency, please hang up and dial 9-1-1 (or other emergency services as appropriate for the area)."

CTQ 9-2: If the medical office mentioned in the case study lacks a triage notebook, how should the medical assistant go about creating one?

Answer: The medical office should hold a staff meeting to discuss the need for the notebook, the conditions that should be listed in the notebook, and the questions to be asked of the patients along with steps for the medical assistant to follow while on each type of telephone call.

Chapter 10

CTQ 10-1: How can the medical assistant demonstrate caring and concern to Marilyn?

Answer: The medical assistant should explain to Marilyn the correlation between filling out the paperwork and receiving appropriate care and diagnosis from the physician. If the patient is unwilling to fill out the paperwork, the medical assistant should take the patient to a private location and ask the questions of the patient, then write down the given answers.

CTQ 10-2: Thinking back to the case study at the beginning of the chapter, how can the medical assistant argue to the physician or office manager that sending new patient history forms before patients' first visits will in fact benefit the office?

Answer: The medical assistant could point out to the physician or office manager that sending the information to the patient will save time for the patient. Also, if the patient is running late when he/she comes in, having the paperwork already filled out will save the office time.

CTQ 10-3: How should the medical assistant respond to Marilyn? What is appropriate for facial expression and tone of voice?

Answer: The medical assistant should explain to Marilyn the importance of having a correct history of the patient. The medical assistant's facial expression and tone of voice should relay concern and compassion rather than impatience.

Chapter 11

CTQ 11-1: If Glenn fails to state his reason for requesting a physician visit, how can the medical assistant determine the time to allot for the appointment?

Answer: Without knowing the reason for the visit, the medical assistant would not know how much time to schedule the patient for. The medical assistant would need to ask Glenn for more information.

CTQ 11-2: How should the medical assistant respond if Glenn refuses to disclose his insurance information?

Answer: In this event, the medical assistant would need to notify the patient of the amount of time he or she was setting aside, clarifying that if the patient's condition or complaint needed more time than that set aside then the patient would need to reschedule for a second visit.

CTQ 11-3: Assume Glenn will be taking the bus to the office. What steps can the medical assistant take to ensure Glenn obtains correct route information?

Answer: The medical assistant should have a list of bus routes available at the front desk in order to give that information to patients.

Chapter 12

CTQ 12-1: Recall the case study at the beginning of this chapter. How would writing "Problem" on the patient's chart work against the physician's office?

Answer: If the patient noticed the word on his chart and asks about it, the medical assistant would be forced to either lie to the patient or to tell the truth—which would likely result in an angry patient.

CTQ 12-2: What are the potential implications of abbreviations for "problem patients"? How does this approach compare to full notes on patient charts, as described in the chapter-opening case study?

Answer: Writing abbreviations on the patient's chart is no better than writing out the entire term. If the patient asks about the abbreviation, the medical assistant would either have to lie to the patient or tell the truth, causing the patient to be either hurt or angry.

CTQ 12-3: Imagine that the medical office has decided to discontinue notes like "Problem" on patient charts. How should the office go about removing such notes from patient files?

Answer: Since using correction fluid or any other method to obliterate portions of the medical record may cause the office to be looked upon with suspicion in the event of a legal case, the only way to remove the notes is to draw a single line through the note as with any other error in the medical chart, and date and sign the correction.

Chapter 13

CTQ 13-1: Recall the case study at the beginning of this chapter. What can you tell Mr. Reardon about the safety of his private patient information as it is contained within the electronic health record? How can you reassure him that his information isn't "out there"?

Answer: The medical assistant should tell Mr. Reardon that his information is well protected as is all information within the medical office computer system. The medical assistant should let Mr. Reardon know that the medical office will not release any information about patients unless the patient directs them to do so, or unless the office receives a court order to release the information.

CTQ 13-2: Recall the case study at the beginning of this chapter. What might you say to Mr. Reardon to convince him the change from paper to electronic medical records is in his best interests?

Answer: The medical assistant should outline the benefits of having medical records electronically instead of on paper. These benefits include the higher level of accuracy in typed entries as opposed to handwritten entries; the ability of more than one staff member to access the patient's file at the same time—which translates into faster insurance processing, and quicker turnaround time for patient inquiries.

CTQ 13-3: Referring to the case study at the beginning of the chapter, what sort of health maintenance reminders do you think a patient such as Mr. Reardon might benefit from receiving?

Answer: A patient such as Mr. Reardon might benefit from receiving reminders about yearly physical exams, regular colonoscopy exams, and yearly flu shots.

CTQ 13-4: Recall the case study at the beginning of this chapter. Do you think you could convince Mr. Reardon that having access to his medical records online might be helpful to him?

Answer: The medical assistant could explain to Mr. Reardon that he might enjoy being able to look at his medical records from home or to be able to allow his family or other physicians to access the medical records. Also, Mr. Reardon might enjoy having the ability to access his medical records while he is traveling away from home, especially in the event of a medical emergency while he is out of town.

Chapter 14

CTQ 14-1: What must the medical assistant know about the medical office's computer needs? How does office need dictate computer choice?

Answer: The medical assistant should know the requirements of any software programs run by the office in addition to the planned budget for the computer system.

CTQ 14-2: What factors would justifiably influence the medical office to fund a flat-screen monitor?

Answer: If the computer monitor was going to be located in a location that is tight on space, a flat-screen monitor might be the appropriate choice.

CTQ 14-3: What type of information can the medical assistant gather to give the physician an accurate idea of printer costs?

Answer: The medical assistant should gather information on the cost of the printer and the cost and availability of the supplies.

Chapter 15

CTQ 15-1: How does rotating the person in charge of inventory each week benefit the medical office's inventory process?

Answer: By rotating the person in charge of the inventory-taking process, the medical office will have a fresh set of eyes looking at the inventory each week. If only one person takes care of inventorying supplies, the office may well run short of items when that one person takes a vacation or is out sick. Also, it is easier for irregularities or thefts to occur if only one person handles the inventory.

Chapter 16

CTQ 16-1: What type of policies and procedures should Monte start identifying for his office?

Answer: Monte should make a list of items that should be included in the book. These might include personnel policies regarding benefits as well as instructions on how certain tasks are handled within the office.

CTQ 16-2: If Monte's office lacks a mission statement, how should he go about explaining its importance to the physician?

Answer: Monte should explain to the physician that a mission statement is helpful in giving all members of the staff a common vision for the clinic.

CTQ 16-3: How should Monte determine which policies should appear in his office's policy manual?

Answer: Monte should make a list of commonly performed tasks in the office, such as an opening and closing routine that should be included in the policy manual.

Chapter 17

CTQ 17-1: How should the medical assistant explain to Martin that his wife will need to add him to her policy if she has not yet done so?

Answer: The medical assistant should explain that it is not typically automatic for a new spouse to be added onto an insurance policy. The medical assistant should encourage Martin to have his wife contact her human resources department to find out the necessary steps to add him to her policy.

CTQ 17-2: Is it advisable to call the insurance carrier of Martin's wife to check on benefits? Why or why not?

Answer: The medical assistant should be able to determine the insurance coverage if he or she calls Martin's wife's insurance carrier.

CTQ 17-3: Assume the medical assistant determined that Martin's wife's insurance plan was not one of the physician's preferred plans. What should the medical assistant say to Martin?

Answer: The medical assistant should explain the non-preferred status of the physician to Martin in addition to explaining how that status affects his coverage in that office.

CTQ 17-4: Using the birthday rule as a guide, what types of questions should the medical assistant ask Martin?

Answer: The medical assistant would need to determine Martin's spouse's date of birth. This information would only be needed if there were children between Martin and his spouse, for whom the medical assistant would need to bill the insurance company.

Chapter 18

CTQ 18-1: Referring to the case study at the beginning of the chapter, what is the potential harm in Mary's guessing at the patient's diagnostic code?

Answer: Mary may be giving the patient a harmful diagnosis, which may cause the patient to lose insurance coverage or be denied insurance one day. Using the wrong diagnosis may also result in the claim being denied, delayed, or underpaid.

CTQ 18-2: When Mary cannot decipher the physician's handwriting, what should she do?

Answer: Mary should go to the physician and ask him or her to translate the notes.

Chapter 19

CTQ 19-1: What should Lydia tell Dr. Anderson about the relationship between appropriate codes and medical chart documentation?

Answer: Lydia should explain to Dr. Anderson that all codes used should be properly reflected in the patient's chart notes. Since insurance companies may request copies of their insured's chart notes at any time, improper coding may result in an audit of the practice.

CTQ 19-2: How would Lydia describe upcoding to Dr. Anderson?

Answer: Upcoding is the act of assigning a higher value code to a procedure with the intent to charge more money than the proper code would earn. Upcoding is illegal and unethical.

Chapter 20

CTQ 20-1: Would Millie be more or less likely to have a balance due if someone in the medical office had discussed a payment plan when services were rendered? Why?

Answer: Millie would be less likely to have a balance due in the office if someone had discussed a payment plan before or at the time services were rendered. If Millie had a financial concern about payment, it could have been raised at that time.

CTQ 20-2: Should medical offices have policies to offer discounts to patients like Millie when those patients agree to pay their full bills via credit card during collection calls? Why?

Answer: Medical offices should have policies in place to offer discounts to patients who pay their bill in full. This practice allows the office to save the future costs of collecting on this account by discounting the bill and having it paid in full now.

CTQ 20-3: Imagine that Millie agrees to pay $100 on her credit card now and $100 per month for the next 4 months. What is the best means the medical assistant has for tracking this agreement?

Answer: The medical assistant should get a written agreement from the patient that outlines the payments agreed to. The medical assistant should then enter this information into a calendar system of some sort in order to follow up on the appropriate days to be certain Millie has sent her payment as agreed.

Chapter 21

CTQ 21-1: What should the medical assistant do with Francie's employee file now that she has provided new information?

Answer: The medical assistant must update Francie's employee file with the new information so that Francie's tax deductions will be correct.

CTQ 21-2: What does the office manager need to do to help Francie ensure that withholding allowances are processed properly?

Answer: Francie must fill out a new W-4 form.

CTQ 21-3: Because the medical assistant, and not an outside agency, handles the medical office's payroll, what can the assistant tell Francie about the time it will take to change her payroll deductions?

Answer: The medical office should have a policy that outlines the length of time it will take for payroll changes to go into effect. Typically, these changes will go into effect no less than 1 week and no more than 2 weeks from the time the employee fills out the change in paperwork.

Chapter 22

CTQ 22-1: As the office manager, how should Juanita address Dr. Whittier's tardiness issue?

Answer: Juanita should speak to Dr. Whittier in a private location and explain how the patients are reacting to the extended wait times.

CTQ 22-2: How could Juanita use a staff meeting to address the issue of Dr. Whittier's tardiness?

Answer: Juanita could bring up the issue at a staff meeting and ask staff members for their input on how to best handle the issue.

CTQ 22-3: Imagine that the chronically late physician, Dr. Whittier, fails to attend the staff meeting at which the issue is addressed. How should Juanita inform him of the staff meeting's discussion?

Answer: Juanita should give Dr. Whittier a copy of the staff meeting minutes, which should outline the discussion and any possible solutions.

CTQ 22-4: How could Juanita communicate to the chronically tardy physician the potential impact of his actions on patient care?

Answer: Juanita could explain to the physician that angry patients will sometimes file malpractice lawsuits. In addition, angry patients may discuss the physician in a negative manner in the community, with their family and friends. This could cause a decrease in the number of patients who see this physician.

Chapter 23

CTQ 23-1: Ian wants to save time and get to the reception area as quickly as possible. But what is the proper procedure for storing personal food items and medications in an office environment?

Answer: It is a violation of OSHA safety standards to store edible items with medications. Ian and all employees should never place personal items in a medication refrigerator. The risk of contaminating both the food and the medications is too great.

CTQ 23-2: Once Ian is on the scene with Cora, who is assessing the patient's vital signs and status, what should he do next?

Answer: Cora is attending to the patient's most immediate needs, so Ian should call 911 or the local area's emergency response number to ensure advanced care will be on the way.

CTQ 23-3: After the situation in the reception area has been taken care of and the patient is no longer in need of medical assistance, how should the incident be recorded, and by whom?

Answer: Cora should document the incident as regulated by office procedures. The documentation should always include the nature of the situation, who was present, who offered aid, and the patient's identity, if known. If the person who received aid was not a patient, Cora should follow office protocol for storing this information. Some offices create a "dummy chart," and others might keep this information in a master file with all incident reports that occur in a certain timeframe.

Chapter 24

CTQ 24-1: What is the proper protocol for Alexis to follow after discovering the soiled chart? Who is responsible for the chart?

Answer: A patient's chart is a legal document in which all treatments and outcomes are recorded. It contains important, irreplaceable information. The situation must be addressed with the office manager or physician, who will know the proper protocol for recreating the documents that were soiled.

CTQ 24-2: Do you think the situation in the case study should be reported to the office manager or physician? Why or why not?

Answer: Alexis needs to take responsibility for her actions. The soiled chart must be recreated in a way that will protect the physician against possible malpractice lawsuits in the future. Recreating the chart may involve contacting the laboratory, hospital, or referring physician and asking for an additional copy of the stained reports. If the reports were created by the physician Alexis works for, he will have to decide the best way to recreate them. If they were computer generated, they may be reprinted. If a transcriptionist typed them, they might have been saved on a disk. Ultimately, everyone in the office is responsible for the patient's chart.

Chapter 25

CTQ 25-1: How do you think Gloria's actions make her patient feel? How much time do you think Gloria really saved by not washing her hands and then not removing the gloves and washing her hands again?

Answer: The patient might feel uncomfortable or rushed, or might even feel like an inconvenience to Gloria. Proper hand washing takes only a few minutes, but it earns the patient's trust and confidence.

CTQ 25-2: In the scenario in the case study, who has been put at risk of possible exposure to strep A by Gloria's actions?

Answer: Gloria's careless actions have put several people at risk: the next person to touch the door handle, the receptionist who took the lab order form, the coworker who may place the pen in his or her mouth, and anyone else who comes in direct contact with surfaces Gloria may have touched with her contaminated gloves.

CTQ 25-3: How would you feel if you were a patient and Gloria enters the exam room and does not wash her hands before examining you?

Answer: This answer will vary from student to student.

Chapter 26

CTQ 26-1: In the case study, is the surgical instrument that Ian placed last, with noticeable moisture on it, considered sterile? Could the moisture possibly indicate that the autoclave is not working properly or that the cycle was not completed properly?

Answer: If the autoclave is run properly, there is no moisture on the instruments at the end of the cycle. Moisture attracts pathogens, so the instrument must be autoclaved again. The autoclave should be checked for mechanical failures or possible operator errors.

CTQ 26-2: Ian left the room to take a phone call after dropping one last instrument on the sterile field. When he reenters the room, is the setup still considered sterile?

Answer: When Ian left the room to answer the phone call without covering the sterile field, he left it open to possible contamination. Ian cannot be certain that the instruments were not touched, so he must start the procedure over with a completely new setup.

Chapter 27

CTQ 27-1: Heidi notes that Claire has been receiving medication refills even though she has missed her follow-up appointments. How would you handle this situation?

Answer: This is generally a simple situation that has been made complex by the patient's pregnancy. First, Heidi should verify who refilled the prescription. Then she should ask if Claire has mentioned taking Zantac to Dr. Wittig, who was not the prescriber. After gathering this information, Heidi can talk to Dr. Wittig about office protocol for allowing continued refills when patients miss follow-up appointments.

CTQ 27-2: Claire has not been seen in Dr. Wittig's office for the past 10 months and is now 7 months pregnant. Dr. Wittig may not be aware that Claire is pregnant and has continued taking Zantac, which may be contraindicated during pregnancy. Now that Heidi is aware of this situation, how should she proceed?

Answer: Heidi should first verify with the patient that she has indeed been taking Zantac twice a day during her pregnancy. She can look up contraindications for Zantac during pregnancy in the *PDR*. Heidi should make sure Dr. Wittig is aware of the patient's continuing use of Zantac.

Chapter 28

CTQ 28-1: Knowing that a normal pulse pressure is between 30 mm Hg and 50 mm Hg, what should Chelsea do next?

Answer: Chelsea should switch arms and take another blood pressure reading. It is possible the patient has an auscultatory gap due to hypertension, or Chelsea may find that she is correct and there is an abnormal blood pressure. Double-checking abnormal findings is always a good idea.

CTQ 28-2: Chelsea heard two distinct blood pressure readings in the same arm. How should she record this in the patient's chart?

Answer: What Chelsea actually heard was an auscultatory gap, common in hypertensive patients. Chelsea should write down exactly what she heard and question her physician/employer about it later. This will be a good learning experience for her.

Chapter 29

CTQ 29-1: Latesha cannot locate the signed informed consent that Gwen "knows" she had the patient sign and promised to bring to Latesha later. How should Latesha handle this situation?

Answer: Even though Gwen is certain that she had the patient sign a consent form, Latesha should verify that it has been done. If the patient is already in the office, there is no harm in having him or her sign a second form. At the very least, Latesha should offer to go back to Gwen's desk to get the form and place it in the patient's chart so that she can be certain that correct protocol has been followed.

CTQ 29-2: Latesha observed Gwen cleaning the room but not sanitizing it or confirming that the counters were disinfected. What should Latesha do?

Answer: The quick cleanup is hazardous to the patient's health and unacceptable practice. Latesha should politely ask Gwen where the disinfectants are kept and should clean and disinfect the room herself so that she knows it has been done properly.

Chapter 30

CTQ 30-1: Jason is scheduling a patient for a laboratory procedure to be done at another location. He has offered the patient several appointment times, but she has rejected each one, saying she has too many other things she needs to do. How should Jason handle this?

Answer: Depending on the kinds of tests that need to be done and the time requirements, Jason should offer the patient specific appointment times. Instead of continuing to list several options, he can ask, "Do mornings or afternoons work better for you?" and follow with "What days of the week are best for you?" This will help save time and avoid frustration.

CTQ 30-2: Jason has called the patient several times this week to make a follow-up appointment to review test results. The physician has specified that she does not want the patient to receive the test results over the phone. But the patient has not returned any of Jason's calls. What can he do?

Answer: Jason should alert the physician and send a certified letter to the patient's home. It is possible that the patient has gone on vacation or is out of town, but a certified letter requesting an appointment for follow-up care protects the physician from a possible lawsuit.

Chapter 31

CTQ 31-1: The sample of *Staphyloccus aureus* taken from the toddler's rash confirms the physician's diagnosis of impetigo. Irene knows what the pathogen will look like and that it will be gram-positive even before she begins the microscopic exam. How does she know this?

Answer: Irene has been working in the microbiology department for several months and remembers that all staph infections stain gram-positive. She knows the pathogen's shape based on its scientific name.

CTQ 31-2: Irene confirms that the patient is positive for an *E. coli* infection in her bladder. What are some possible causes for the bladder infection?

Answer: *E. coli* is the primary cause of UTIs because it is normally found in feces. Patients who do not wipe properly, front to back, are at risk for transferring the pathogen forward to the vaginal opening. Once the pathogen is in the vaginal area, it can spread farther up into the bladder and cause an infection.

Chapter 32

CTQ 32-1: Kathleen is assuming that because the brick-top tube does not contain additives, it will be fine to obtain the prothrombin time sample in. Why is this incorrect?

Answer: Blood-draw tube order is critical to proper testing of blood samples. Mixing up the order of tubes or which tubes samples are drawn in can invalidate results or contaminate other samples. Specifically, prothrombin and other hematology tests must be drawn in light-blue tubes containing EDTA.

Chapter 33

CTQ 33-1: When Gina's patient mentions her urinary frequency and painful urination, what can Gina do to relieve some of her nervousness?

Answer: Gina should inform the patient that there are many treatments that are safe and will give her relief. Gina should also explain the dangers of allowing a possible infection to continue.

CTQ 33-2: Given the patient's complaint, what tests do you think Gina should prepare to perform?

Answer: Gina should always verify what tests the physician would like to have performed on the patient. A urine dip with Chemstrips is standard for all pregnant women, so Gina should continue to perform that test as ordered. She should also keep the unused portion of urine for any additional tests the physician may order.

Chapter 34

CTQ 34-1: Olivia's previous experience with X-rays has made her comfortable with patient preparation, gowning, and draping instructions. The X-ray technician has been ordered to take chest X-rays of a female patient who is believed to have pneumonia. The patient is elderly and has come to the appointment alone. She needs help removing her clothing and getting the drape set up, and is not steady enough on her feet to stand alone in the X-ray room. What instructions or assistance should Olivia give her?

Answer: Prior to beginning the exam, Olivia should make certain that the patient understands why an X-ray is being taken. Then Olivia can explain the X-ray procedure, what clothing needs to be removed, and how the patient will be positioned. Olivia should offer to stay in the room with the patient if she cannot stand unassisted or feels uncomfortable with only the male X-ray technician in the room.

CTQ 34-2: The patient tells Olivia that she is not steady on her feet and would like to have Olivia assist her during the X-ray procedure. What precautions should Olivia take to avoid unnecessary exposure to radiation?

Answer: Olivia should wear a half-apron because only the patient's chest is being X-rayed.

Chapter 35

CTQ 35-1: Knowing that Ray has a history of cardiac surgery and is planning to have dental surgery, what should Rachel's response to his presenting symptoms be?

Answer: With the symptoms that the patient is presenting, in combination with his previous cardiac surgery, endocarditis is a concern. Rachel should chart the patient's complaints and symptoms accurately so that the doctor has all the necessary

information to assess the situation. The patient will probably need to take prophylactic antibiotics before future dental surgeries. Rachel can explain why and how that should be done as the physician directs.

Chapter 36

CTQ 36-1: Keera has been given the directions for obtaining a sputum sample and has observed the technique being performed. Now that it is her turn, what precautions should she take?

Answer: Patients are asked to cough forcefully and bring the sputum up from deep within the lungs. Coughing propels droplets and other infectious material on the person collecting the sample. Keera should wear the correct PPE: gown, gloves, and face mask with eye shield.

CTQ 36-2: Keera has just instructed the patient in the correct way to use a metered dose inhaler (MDI). What other instructions or methods should she mention to the patient?

Answer: Keera should tell the patient that to get the most effective dosage and therefore save money on MDI prescriptions, instructions must be followed very carefully. Keera should also make sure the patient understands the signs and symptoms of oral thrush, which is a common side effect of inhaler misuse.

Chapter 37

CTQ 37-1: The college student who has come in for a Snellen test wears contact lenses. With her left eye, the patient can read to the 20/20 line, making only two errors. With her right eye, she can only read to the 20/40 line and makes three errors. How should Stacy record these results?

Answer: Stacy should record the vision as O.S. 20/20-2 and O.D. 20/50, noting on the chart that the patient wears corrective lens.

CTQ 37-2: The young girl with sand in her eye is frightened about having her eye flushed. She squeezes her eye shut and will not hold still. What are Stacy's options?

Answer: Stacy should explain the procedure in age-appropriate language, assuring the child that the procedure will not hurt and will make her eye feel better. She should also explain that it is very important that she not move while Stacy is cleaning her eye. Stacy can also ask the parent or guardian to assist in holding the child still.

CTQ 37-3: What items should Stacy lay out for the physician so that he can remove the toy from the child's nose?

Answer: The physician will need the proper PPE, such as gloves and a face shield, a light source to get a clear visual of the foreign body, a nasal speculum to gain access, and forceps to grip the object.

Chapter 38

CTQ 38-1: What precautions should Eric take when setting up the patient with AIDS for examination by the physician?

Answer: Regardless of what the chart states, it is important to treat every patient as possibly infected when performing any tasks that put you at risk for infection. The rash is located on the right and left flanks, so Eric should instruct the patient on disrobing from the waist up and provide a drape if he would like to use it.

CTQ 38-2: Before Eric assists the doctor in performing a prick skin test, he must explain the four methods of diagnostic allergy testing. Because the child being tested is a minor, what else does Eric need to do?

Answer: Because the child is a minor, the parent will have to sign a consent form as well as any insurance forms that may or may not cover allergy testing. The methods that may be used to test for a pet allergy are: 1) intradermal, with small amounts of potential antigen under the skin; 2) skin patch, putting a patch soaked with the potential antigen on the skin; and 3) scratch test, placing the potential antigen into a scratch made on the skin. The physician determines the most effective method of testing.

Chapter 39

CTQ 39-1: The mother is very concerned that her children may have lice and is under the impression that they will be labeled "dirty" or that she will be seen as an unfit mother. In addition, she has assumed that all lice are the same and attach to all types of hair. What should Manny tell her about the different kinds of head lice and how they're transmitted?

Answer: Manny can start by explaining that there actually three types of lice, which attach to different areas based on several factors. Head lice are very common and are easily spread among schoolchildren via hats, combs, brushes, and coats. Body lice are a different species and are spread through poor hygiene and close body contact. Pubic lice spread via sexual contact.

CTQ 39-2: The teenage girl with the mole admits to sunbathing regularly in the summer at the lake and describes her mole only as "suspicious." What questions should Manny ask her regarding this condition? What advice should he give?

Answer: Manny should ask the patient to describe what she mean by "suspicious." Using the ABCD rules of mole appearance, he should ask: What color is the mole? Is it evenly colored? What size is the mole? What do the edges look like? Have any of these characteristics changed? If so, when and how? In addition, the patient should be warned about the dangers of long-term sun exposure and educated in the proper use of sun protection.

Chapter 40

CTQ 40-1: Mr. Wiat is apparently unaware of how adult-onset diabetes occurs and what the treatment options are. How should Charles educate him?

Answer: Charles should spend a significant amount of time with this patient. He will need to discuss his lifestyle choices, how they may have contributed to his current condition, and the changes he will need to make. He should ask several open-ended questions to verify that Mr. Wiat understands. To reinforce the information, Charles should also provide reading materials Mr. Wiat can take home and review. Charles should document their conversation in the patient's chart and list the additional resources he has provided Mr. Wiat.

CTQ 40-2: Mr. Wiat seems to be in denial about his condition and how his lifestyle may cause additional health problems and even death. How should Charles proceed in educating him?

Answer: In addition to the discussion about diabetes and the reading materials Charles has provided, Charles may suggest that Mr. Wiat seek additional support in the community through a diabetic counselor who can help him with coping mechanisms, equipment, and further education.

Chapter 41

CTQ 41-1: What questions should Ariko ask Brenna regarding the accident and the child's behavior?

Answer: To provide the physician with an accurate report, Ariko should ask: 1) Is Brenna certain there is no visible injury to the head or extremities, such as bruising, bleeding, or swelling? 2) How is the child reacting? Is she slow, sluggish, or able to talk or walk without assistance? If she has not moved herself, it is important that Brenna not move her to avoid furthering a neck or spinal cord injury. 3) Is the child feeling sleepy? Does she want to take a nap or go to bed? 4) Is there any nausea or vomiting?

CTQ 41-2: After Ariko has collected all the information on the accident as reported by Brenna, how should she advise Brenna?

Answer: Head and neck injuries are a serious matter. Without proper evaluation by a physician, it is impossible to diagnose or rule out a concussion over the phone. A head injury can cause intracranial bleeding, which may take up to 24 hours to produce symptoms. The victim should avoid strenuous activity or taking pain medications that can mask the symptoms and make it more difficult to correctly diagnose. Common symptoms to watch for are nausea, vomiting, sluggishness, confusion, irritability, persistent headache, blurred vision, and seizure activity. Ariko should advise Brenna to watch for those symptoms in her child and relay any other recommendations from the physician. The physician may recommend that the parent take the child to an ER for further evaluation because children cannot adequately describe symptoms that may indicate a serious underlying condition.

Chapter 42

CTQ 42-1: What questions should Reggie ask Serena about her newfound interest in vegetarianism so that he can more accurately assess her nutritional needs?

Answer: Reggie should ask Serena what type of vegetarianism she is interested in. To accurately assess her nutritional needs, he needs to know if she is cutting out meat alone, meat and fish, meat and dairy, or all animal products.

CTQ 42-2: Once Reggie has established what type of vegetarian Serena would like to become, how should he proceed to help her reach her nutritional as well as lifestyle goals?

Answer: Once Serena has established what types of animal products she would like to avoid, Reggie can give her a list of foods to help her maintain adequate protein intake. Depending on her dietary choices, Serena could eat soybeans and other beans, eggs, and dairy products. Reggie should also give Serena brochures and reliable Web site addresses that will help her understand the role of protein in a balanced diet, such as building and repairing tissue.

Chapter 43

CTQ 43-1: Xavier must give information and instructions to the patient, Jorge, who is in pain and will probably not remember most of their conversation in the morning. What is the best approach Xavier can take to make certain Jorge understands his instructions for ankle care, using the brace, and his orthopedic appointment?

Answer: Different people have different styles of learning. Some learn best by hearing, some by seeing, and others by doing. Xavier should carefully explain

each step of self-care, how to use the brace, and why an appointment has been made with another provider. He should ask Jorge if he has any questions. In addition, Xavier should give Jorge written instructions to reinforce his verbal instructions so that Jorge can review them at his leisure when he is feeling better in a few days. Xavier should also instruct Jorge on whom to call should an emergency arise.

CTQ 43-2: What signs and symptoms should Xavier tell Jorge to watch for as his ankle heals? What can Jorge do to relieve some of the pain of his injury?

Answer: Xavier should give Jorge a printed list of signs and symptoms to watch for, as directed by the physician. The list should include measures to relieve discomfort and the signs and symptoms that require immediate medical attention.

Chapter 44

CTQ 44-1: How should Sydney handle the phone call from Mrs. Blakely? How can she reassure her and offer support until Mrs. Blakely can speak to the physician? Should Sydney offer suggestions for nonpharmaceutical therapy?

Answer: Sydney should assure Mrs. Blakely that the latest findings do not mean that everyone who takes hormones will develop cancer. Mrs. Blakely should be offered an appointment to discuss treatment options with the physician, including nonpharmacuetical treatments. Sydney should not offer advice of any kind unless it has been approved by the physician.

Chapter 45

CTQ 45-1: After the physician has diagnosed oral thrush combined with a yeast infection, what should Lucas explain to the mother so that the condition is correctly treated?

Answer: Lucas should explain, without accusation, that the entire course of medication must be taken, even if symptoms subside. If it is not, the child may develop resistance to the medication, which will make further treatment more difficult.

Chapter 46

CTQ 46-1: What the patient thought was an allergic reaction may in fact be a shingles outbreak given her pain level and past history of varicella. What information can Dawn give the patient? How should Dawn handle the information that the patient's boyfriend ruptured some of the blisters?

Answer: Dawn should explain what shingles is and how it is related to varicella. By breaking the skin's integrity and releasing fluid from the blister, Dawn's boyfriend could potentially have infected himself. The boyfriend should be given information on signs and symptoms of infection.

Chapter 47

CTQ 47-1: What advice and support can Charles offer Yolanda to help her deal with her brother's newly diagnosed condition?

Answer: It is clear that Yolanda is in great need of support and professional help. If she does not wish to see a therapist at a mental health clinic, she may feel more comfortable speaking to a school counselor. Regardless of where she receives help, she should be offered the support to protect her mental well-being.

CTQ 47-2: What should Charles tell Yolanda about her self-inflicted injuries and her request that he promise not to tell anyone else? Is he bound by a patient-provider oath?

Answer: Charles should recognize the self-inflicted injuries as a cry for help and alert the physician so that the situation can be properly assessed and it can be determined if Yolanda is a danger to herself. Charles is not bound by a patient-provider oath, as he is not a physician. He should explain that he cannot legally honor Yolanda's request of secrecy and that it is out of concern for her well-being that he must tell the physician. He should assure Yolanda that she will get the help she needs.

Chapter 48

CTQ 48-1: Even though Ruth is not yet in the 50-year-old age bracket, should she still be tested for colorectal cancer?

Answer: It is up to the physician to make the decision to test, but because Ruth has a strong family history of cancer, she is at potentially greater risk. It will be very important for Ruth to monitor her health closely with the help of her physician.

CTQ 48-2: Ruth is concerned about being embarrassed and uncomfortable. She has also canceled a previous appointment. How should Marilyn approach this situation?

Answer: Marilyn should inform Ruth about what the test will entail so she will know what to expect and be less apprehensive. Marilyn should also discuss the missed appointment and find out the reason for it. Ruth may be taking a "head in the sand" approach and is trying to ignore the symptoms so she will not have to face the possibility of a cancer diagnosis.

Chapter 49

CTQ 49-1: What can Elora do to assist the patient during his transition from employment to retirement?

Answer: Elora can politely ask the patient what he plans to do with his free time. Does he have any hobbies? Does he plan to travel? Elora can also give him information on support groups and local community activities designed for individuals of retirement age that he may not be aware of.

CTQ 49-2: What can Elora do to make certain the patient has the necessary resources for his retirement and future healthcare coverage?

Answer: Elora should give the patient some brochures on Social Security and Medicare. Alex may already have them, but making certain is a good idea. He may want to ask about recent changes in Medicare or clear up confusion about his Social Security benefits. The patient should be advised to call the Social Security or Medicare office for additional information.

Chapter 50

CTQ 50-1: What do you think would be the best way for Leslie's patient to find the type of massage that would be most beneficial for her needs?

Answer: There are many different types of massage and many possible settings. Questions the patient should ask herself are: 1) Do I prefer a female or male therapist, or does gender matter? 2) What are my time commitments? Would mornings, afternoons, or evenings work best for me? 3) Do I prefer a softer-touch or a firmer touch? 4) How comfortable am I with being unclothed? (Some therapies can be done on a fully clothed client, and others cannot.) Answering questions like these will help patients tailor the therapy experience to best suit their needs.

Chapter 51

CTQ 55-1: Should Karim note his lack of personal transportation on his resume? Why or why not?

Answer: Karim should not point out his lack of transportation on his resume. This information could be used against Karim and may cost him a chance to interview for the job.

CTQ 55-2: Karim was fired from his last two jobs due to chronic tardiness. Should he mention those terminations on his cover letter? Why or why not?

Answer: Karim should not mention his terminations in his cover letter. If this information comes up in an interview, Karim will have the opportunity to address the topic face to face with the potential employer.

CTQ 55-3: If Karim lacks personal transportation, how should he seek employment?

Answer: Karim should look for employment in a clinic or facility that is within walking distance of his home or is located in a place he can easily access with public transportation.

Answers to In-Practice Scenarios

Chapter 1

Dawn can tell Mrs. Boyan that X-rays were discovered in 1895 by Wilhem Roentgen. This discovery earned Roentgen a Nobel Prize in physics.

Chapter 2

The medical assistant should assure Isaiah that the staff at this facility are professionals who are there to see to the needs of each patient. She should then bring up this conversation in a staff meeting to alert her coworkers and physicians to the conversation so everyone is aware that patients may seek care elsewhere if they do not receive a high level of customer service from everyone in the clinic.

Chapter 3

Sylvia might place her hand on Mr. Paquette's hand or shoulder to show him she feels compassion for his pain. She should allow him to speak or to remain silent, if he prefers. She should offer her condolences and wait until Mr. Paquette is composed before she proceeds with the visit, without hurrying him to do so. Sylvia should also be sure to note the recent loss in Mr. Paquette's chart, as well as share that information with the physician before she enters the room.

Chapter 4

Jan could have refused to add the fraudulent charges to the patient bills. She could have told Dr. Borse that it was illegal and unethical and that she would not participate. Jan likely now knows that the money she made working for Dr. Borse was not worth the shunning she is now experiencing in her community from employers who are reluctant to hire someone who knowingly worked for a physician who committed insurance fraud.

Chapter 5

The medical assistant should remind the coworkers that their conversation can be overheard by patients. This conversation is inappropriate and should not continue in front of the patient.

Chapter 6

Sara should alert the physician to the patient's concerns. If possible, the physician should speak to the patient directly, in order to determine how to work within the patient's financial constraints. The medical assistant may also refer the patient to any local financial assistance programs that may be available.

Chapter 8

Joanne must spell the words correctly. A misspelling can result in incorrect information being sent to the patient, which may result in a misunderstanding that could have a catastrophic consequence.

Chapter 9

The medical assistant should ask Josie if she would like to be moved to a private location to use the telephone. If Josie declines and continues her conversation, the medical assistant should alert the clinical staff to take Josie to a treatment room as soon as possible.

Since Josie is the one talking about her own healthcare issues, there is no violation of HIPAA privacy laws in this scenario. However, it is inappropriate to have a patient discuss these issues, especially in the detail Josie appears to be using, in front of other patients. Some patients may have a queasy stomach, or become frightened by Josie's description of her symptoms.

Chapter 10

Jenny needs to let Marion know that it is not safe to leave a child in the car and that she will not be able to watch her while Marion is in the office. Under no circumstances should Jenny agree to allow Marion to leave the child in the car unattended.

Chapter 11

Dr. Brosnan's office should have clearly documented the missed appointment by Mr. Grissom. The office should also have sent a certified letter to Mr. Grissom alerting him to the importance of the return visit. Documentation that the letter was signed for should have been placed within Mr. Grissom's file. With this information, Mr. Grissom would have a hard time proving that Dr. Brosnan was negligent in not determining whether the vasectomy procedure was a success.

Chapter 12

Dylan should attempt to calm Lynn down and should apologize for the tardiness of the return of her laboratory results. Dylan should offer to transfer Lynn's telephone call to the clinical nurse to hear her results right away, or to the physician, if he or she is available. If Lynn is unwilling to budge from her resolve to change physicians, Dylan should record the following in the patient's chart:

"(Date of the call) Patient called stating she has been waiting for three days for her laboratory results. Patient is unhappy over the unexpected wait time. Offered to transfer patient to the clinical nurse (or physician) and patient declined. Patient states she will be requesting transfer of her medical records to a new physician. Dylan McElvaney, RMA"

Chapter 13

Dr. Jonas could contact the software vendors for all three programs to find out if there is a bridging program he could use that would allow him to translate documents from one system to another. In lieu of that, Dr. Jonas could purchase software that matches one of the two hospitals he rounds within.

Chapter 14

In order to perform this search, Jamie should go to reputable professional medical Web sites online. Dr. Victor is likely subscribed to one or more of these sites and Jamie should visit them all to perform a search for any information pertaining to procedures for scar tissue removal. After locating the information, Jamie should compose a list of the findings and present that list to Dr. Victor, along with information on the Web site where the information was found.

Jamie should begin by visiting only reputable medical information Web sites or search engines. She should be certain to use the key words provided by Dr. Victor and should keep the name of each Web site available to refer to should Dr. Victor have further questions.

Chapter 15

First a policy should be put into place that spells out who will take inventory, how often inventory will be performed, and who is responsible for the ordering of all supplies. The office needs an inventory supply log to track inventory, and a regular system of tracking the supplies being used in the office in order to keep an adequate supply on hand at all times.

Chapter 16

Anka should report the needle stick injury to her supervisor. She should then consult the policy manual to determine the exact steps she should take for documenting her injury, and the need for any testing or vaccinations she may require.

Chapter 17

Since Georgia cannot locate her insurance card while on the phone, the medical assistant should politely let her know that her coverage may vary greatly depending upon the type of health insurance she has. It is important to let her know that with some managed care plans she may not be covered for services in the office; it is impossible to be able to tell her for sure unless it is known which insurance plan she has.

If she still cannot locate the insurance card, confirm her appointment and ask her to call you back if she finds the card prior to her visit. Politely let her know that if she is with a managed care plan that your office is not contracted with, she may be responsible for the entire fee for the visit.

Chapter 18

Anything charted in the medical chart should be charted *only* by the person who performed the service. Since Sharon did not perform or witness the procedure performed on this patient, it would be fraud for her to "jot something" in the medical record in order to make it match what the fee slip says. Instead, Sharon should give the file to the physician and ask him or her to complete the charting for that day.

Chapter 19

Linnea should leave the charts for a coworker to finish, after the coworker has cheked with the physician about the codes. If Linnea is the only coding staff in the office, she should leave the coding on these particular charts until she returns, in order to assure accuracy in the coding. Guessing at the code is never an option, as incorrect coding may lead to improper reimbursement or other delays in payment of the claim.

Chapter 20

Dr. Bowman doesn't understand how fee schedules are made. The medical assistant will need to explain to him how the RBRVS and RVU numbers are assigned by Medicare and how those assigned numbers are standard. He can raise his fees, but until Medicare raises the RSRVS and RVU, he will not receive a higher allowed fee for his services.

Chapter 21

Wendy should recount the funds for the day and if she continues to find them $40 short she should review the receipts written and posted to determine if the error is a posting error. Sometimes asking a coworker to check the work can reveal an error as well.

Chapter 22

Carrie should attempt to move Mrs. Carnes out of the reception area and into a private area as soon as possible. Carrie should remain calm and soothing to Mrs. Carnes and she should let her know that she will take care of the problem as quickly as possible. If the office manager is available, Carrie should take Mrs. Carnes to the office manager's office and should explain the problem to the office manager before leaving Mrs. Carnes there.

Chapter 23

If the spill is minor, Melanie should quickly clean it up before joining the physician. If the spill will take more than a few moments to take care of, Melanie should quickly throw some paper towels over the spill and notify a coworker to the need for clean up before going in with the physician.

Chapter 24

Even though Rocky plans to be in the following morning and believes he can clean the exam rooms before the first patient, it is possible that he may not make it in to work. He may become ill before morning or have some other situation that keeps him from making it to work on time. Most offices have a policy that exam rooms must be cleaned at the end of the day, and Rocky needs to either clean them tonight, or ask a coworker to help out and clean the rooms for him.

Chapter 25

OSHA requires that all health professionals follow "universal blood and body fluid precautions." The medical assistant can reassure the patient that he or she is adhering to standard practice and that wearing gloves is used for the protection of the health professional as well as the patient. This occasion can be used to provide patient education about the importance of standard precautions and infection control.

Chapter 26

Sterilization indicators verify that a dry pack has been placed in the autoclave, that steam has reached the inside of the package, and that sterilization has been achieved. If the strip color has not changed, then the instruments in the dry pack are not sterile and will need to be removed, rewrapped, and sterilized again.

Chapter 27

The three checks are necessary to ensure safe medication administration. The "three checks" require that you (1) check the label when taking the medication from the shelf, (2) check the medication label when preparing it, and (3) check the label when replacing the medication container on the shelf or disposing of the empty container.

Chapter 28

A rectal temperature is considered normal at 99.6 degrees F. Rectal temperatures are usually a degree warmer than oral temperatures because of the internal environment of the rectum. Axillary temperatures are usually a degree lower than oral temperatures as the axilla is more exposed to air. The medical assistant should ask the mother if the child has any other symptoms. If not, then the MA should reassure the mother and provide patient education about normal temperature ranges. The medical assistant should inform the mother that if the child develops an elevated temperature, then the child should be scheduled for an appointment.

Chapter 29

There are three phases in the process of normal healing: the inflammatory, granulation, and contraction phases. The phase described is the granulation phase.

Chapter 30

Quality control is necessary to ensure accuracy of patient test results for blood glucose monitoring. If control results are abnormal, the medical assistant should not use the equipment for the day's testing and should directly report the results to the supervisor. Label the glucometer "Repair" and remove it from the clinical area to prevent use by other staff. An inaccurate glucose reading could directly affect the amount of insulin being administered; accurate readings are essential for the physician to properly diagnose and treat the patient. The glucometer should only be returned to the clinical area after the problem has been corrected. The medical assistant should always follow office policy regarding abnormal quality control findings and discuss the results and next steps with the supervisor and physician.

Chapter 31

The medical assistant should inform the patient that he must be seen by the physician in the office. During the visit, the physician may obtain a throat culture or perform a Rapid Strep test to confirm a diagnosis of "step throat." *Streptococcus pyogenes*, or Group A strep, is the causative agent of the pharyngeal infection.

Chapter 32

LDL cholesterol is considered "bad" cholesterol, and lower blood levels indicate a lower risk of heart disease. HDL cholesterol is "good" cholesterol, and higher levels are beneficial to health. Diet, caloric intake, physical activity, and family heritage all play a factor in the amount of cholesterol formed in the body. Patient education should include verbal and written dietary and physical activity recommendations to help improve the patient's overall cholesterol numbers.

Chapter 33

The testicular self-examination (TSE) is useful in the detection of cancer of the testicles. Testicular cancer is the most common solid tumor found in males age 20 to 34 years. If detected early and treated, testicular cancer is almost 100% curable. If untreated, it may spread to the lymph nodes and lungs. Tumors usually are found on one side, but 2 to 3% are found in both testicles. It is important for men to become familiar with normal size, shape, and weight of each testicle and epididymis. This will help men recognize a change from one self-examination to another, if a change should occur.

Chapter 34

A mammogram is an X-ray of the breast tissue taken to detect possible abnormalities, such as tumors, cysts, and malignant tissue. Baseline mammograms are recommended for women around 35 years of age, and yearly mammograms for women over 40. The medical assistant can describe the technique and the procedure steps and attempt to reassure the patient. A pamphlet or brochure on mammography procedures would be a good resource to share with the patient.

Chapter 35

An electrocardiogram, also called an EKG or ECG, is a simple test that detects and records the electrical activity of the heart. It is used to detect and locate the source of heart problems. Electrical signals in the heart trigger heartbeats. These signals start at the top of the heart in an area called the right atrium. The electrical signals travel from the top of the heart to the bottom. They cause the heart muscle to contract as they travel through the heart. As the heart contracts, it pumps blood out to the rest of the body. An EKG shows how fast the heart is beating. It shows the heart's rhythm (steady or irregular) and where in the body the heartbeat is being recorded. It also records the strength and timing of the electrical signals as they pass through each part of the heart. An EKG is sometimes called a 12-lead EKG (or 12-lead ECG) because the electrical activity of the heart is most often recorded from 12 different places on the body at the same time.

Chapter 36

Reassure the mother that a spirometer is a device that allows the physician to assess Lung Function. Pulmonary Lung Function Tests (PFTs) are performed to diagnose a pulmonary abnormality and/or determine the extent of pulmonary disease. Spirometry is a noninvasive test that measures the exhalation capacity of the lungs and is very helpful in assessing the progression of acute and chronic disorders such as asthma. Refer to Procedure 36-1.

Chapter 37

Cerumen is earwax. Cerumen impaction is a condition in which earwax has become tightly packed in the external ear canal to the point that the canal is blocked. It develops when earwax (cerumen) accumulates in the inner part of the ear canal and blocks the eardrum. It affects between 2 and 6% of the general population in the United States. Cerumen is most likely to become impacted when it is pushed against the eardrum by cotton-tipped applicators, hairpins, or other objects that people put in their ears; and when it is trapped against the eardrum by a hearing aid. Less common causes of cerumen impaction include overproduction of earwax by the glands in the ear canal or an abnormally shaped ear canal. The most important symptom of cerumen impaction is partial loss of hearing. Other symptoms are itching, tinnitus (noise or ringing in the ears), a sensation of fullness in the ear, and pain. The medical assistant can reassure the patient that the condition does not cause permanent hearing loss. The patient can be informed that the most common method of removing impacted cerumen is irrigation. It involves washing out the ear canal with water from a commercial irrigator or a syringe with a catheter attached.

Chapter 38

HIV infection can weaken a person's immune system to the point that it has difficulty fighting off certain infections. These types of infections are known as opportunistic infections because they take the opportunity a weakened immune system gives to cause illness. Some examples of opportunistic infections are *Pneumocystis carinii* pneumonia (PCP) and Kaposi's sarcoma (KS). Opportunistic infections are CDC-defined AIDS indicator illnesses, which mean that an HIV-infected person receives a diagnosis of AIDS after the development of one of them. Refer to Table 38-2 for a list of opportunistic conditions common to AIDS.

Chapter 39

There are many skin disorders that can cause itching. The medical assistant should refer to office policy for placement of patients with potentially contagious disorders. The patient can be placed in a triage area or another designated area. The medical assistant should triage the patient to determine the cause of the pruritic rash and inform the physician of the patient's condition.

Chapter 40

The thyroid gland is located in the neck area on either side of the trachea. Hypothyroidism, the result of underproduction and undersecretion of thyroid hormones, is a common condition. Signs of hypothyroidism include a slowed metabolic rate, low levels of T_3 and T_4, pale, cool skin, slow heart rate, lethargy,

weight gain, intolerance to cold, and possible goiter. The physician may order TSH and T_3 and T_4 levels to determine if this patient has hypothyroidism.

Chapter 41

Place the patient in an exam room and have the patient sit or lie down on the exam table with the feet elevated if possible. Ensure that there is a staff member present with the patient at all times in the event that the patient loses consciousness. The medical assistant should request help, inform the physician of the patient's condition and be prepared to all EMS/911 if needed.

Chapter 42

The medical assistant should inform the physician of the patient's inability to comply with the clear-liquids-only diet. The medical assistant should emphasize the importance of adhering to a clear-liquids-only diet and inform the patient that the colonoscopy exam appointment will have to be rescheduled. All patients scheduled for a colonoscopy exam should be informed that the physician will order a cathartic that must be taken at different intervals during the day before the procedure. The patient will need to increase fluid intake and adhere to a clear-liquids-only diet. He or she will also need to eliminate milk, dairy, and solid foods; red or purple liquids; and fruit juice with pulp.

Chapter 43

A sprain is a partial tear of a ligament and occurs as a result of a traumatic insult to the muscle, tendon, or ligament surrounding a joint. Treatment consists of immobilizing the joint. A strain is the overstretching of a muscle, tendon, or ligament and occurs when a muscle is used or stretched beyond its normal capacity. Treatment includes cool therapy to help to reduce swelling and relieve pain.

Chapter 44

Genital warts are caused by the human papilloma virus (HPV). The medical assistant should inform the patient that genital warts are caused by a virus and cannot be treated by antibiotics (a shot or prescription) and instead must be treated with chemical or surgical removal. Genital warts are contagious and can be transmitted during sexual intercourse; therefore, the patient should be educated on safer sex practices.

Chapter 45

How to Use and Interpret Pediatric Growth Charts

Plot measurements. On the appropriate growth chart, plot the measurements recorded in the data entry table for the current visit.

- ■ Find the child's age on the horizontal axis. When plotting weight-for-length, find the length on the horizontal axis. Use a straight edge or right-angle ruler to draw a vertical line up from that point.

- Find the appropriate measurement (weight, length, stature, head circumference, or BMI) on the vertical axis. Use a straight edge or right-angle ruler to draw a horizontal line across from that point until it intersects the vertical line.

- Make a small dot where the two lines intersect.

Interpret the plotted measurements. The curved lines on the growth chart show selected percentiles that indicate the rank of the child's measurement. For example, when the dot is plotted on the 95th percentile line for BMI-for-Age, it means that only 5 of 100 children (5%) of the same age and gender in the reference population have a higher BMI-for-Age.

According to the data provided, the patient's data plots on the 95th percentile line for Weight-for-Age. Based upon this information, the child appears to be growing appropriately; however, other assessments should be performed to determine the child's overall health status.

Chapter 46

The medical assistant should inform the physician of the patient's status immediately. Stroke is a life-threatening and emergent situation, and the patient's son should be advised to call 911 and seek emergent care.

A *stroke* or cerebrovascular accident (CVA) occurs when the blood supply to a part of the brain is suddenly interrupted by occlusion (an ischemic stroke) or by hemorrhage (a hemorrhagic stroke). A stroke is always serious and can be life threatening. The symptoms that occur following a stroke depend on the area of the brain that has been affected and the extent of the damage. Some of the symptoms that can occur include the following:

- The most common symptom is weakness or paralysis of one side of the body.

- There may be partial or complete loss of voluntary movement and/or feelings in a leg and/or arm.

- A stroke can result in speech problems and weak muscles of the face, which can cause drooling. Numbness or tingling is very common.

- A stroke involving the base of the brain can affect balance, vision, and swallowing functions.

- A stroke can cause difficulty in breathing and even unconsciousness.

Chapter 47

Depression after pregnancy is called postpartum depression or *peripartum depression*. After pregnancy, hormonal changes in a woman's body may trigger symptoms of depression. During pregnancy, the amount of two female hormones, estrogen and progesterone, in a woman's body increases greatly. In the first 24 hours after childbirth, the amount of these hormones rapidly drops back down to their normal nonpregnant levels. Researchers think the fast change in hormone levels may lead to depression, just as smaller changes in hormones can affect a woman's moods before she gets her menstrual period.

Some women don't tell anyone about their symptoms because they feel embarrassed, ashamed, or guilty about feeling depressed when they are supposed to be happy. They worry that they will be viewed as unfit parents. Postpartum or peripartum depression can happen to any woman. The medical assistant can reassure the patient that having postpartum depression does not mean that she is "not a together" mom. Reassure her that she and the baby do not have to suffer. There is help. The medical assistant should document the patient's complaint and symptoms and inform the physician of the patient's status.

Chapter 48

The medical assistant can provide the patient with recommendations for adopting a cancer prevention lifestyle. Some of the recommendations include eliminating tobacco products, reducing the intake of animal fat, exercising regularly, and maintaining a normal weight. For additional information regarding prevention and early detection, patients can visit the American Cancer Society Web site: www.acs.org

Chapter 49

People age 65 and older consume more prescription and over-the-counter (OTC) medicines than any other age group, according to the National Institute on Aging. Older people tend to have more long-term, chronic illnesses such as arthritis, diabetes, high blood pressure and heart disease than do younger people. Because they may have a number of diseases or disabilities at the same time, it is common for older people to take many different drugs. Changes in mental status may result in noncompliance with medication administration. Additionally, the patient may be unclear about the correct dosing for his blood pressure medication and should be advised to return to the medical office for evaluation, appropriate patient education, and a review of medications.

Chapter 50

Throughout history, herbs have been used to treat disease and prevent illness. Many people are now turning to natural herbal medicine. As a matter of fact, more and more patients may present with a history of taking herbs for a variety of different medical conditions. At present, there are no herbal medicine licensing or accrediting boards in the United States, and many herbs have not been approved for use by the FDA.

Chapter 51

Jerome should change his voicemail message to one that is professional, or he should use his mobile telephone number on his resume so that calls will not be received on his home voicemail.

Introduction to Medisoft Advanced (version 12) and Medisoft Simulation

Medisoft Advanced is a medical practice management software program that offers choices of actions through a series of menus. Commands are issued by clicking an option on the menu bar or by clicking a shortcut button on the toolbar. All data, whether a patient's address or a charge for a procedure, is entered into Medisoft through menus on the menu bar or through the buttons on the toolbar. Selecting an option from the menus or toolbar brings up a dialog box. The TAB key is used to move between text boxes within a dialog box.

The menu bar lists the names of the menus in Medisoft: File, Edit, Activities, Lists, Reports, Tools, Window, Services, and Help. Beneath each menu name is a pull-down menu of one or more options.

Menu Bar Titles

The purpose of each menu is briefly described as follows:

File Menu The File menu is used to enter information about the medical office practice when first setting up Medisoft. It is also used to back up data, maintain files, and set up program options.

Edit Menu The Edit menu contains the basic commands needed to move, change, or delete information. These commands are Undo, Cut, Copy, Paste, and Delete.

Activities Menu Most medical office data collected on a day-to-day basis is entered through options on the Activities menu. This menu is used to enter information about patients' office visits, including diagnoses and procedures performed. Transactions, including charges, payments, and adjustments, are also entered via the Activities menu.

Lists Menu Information on new patients, such as name, address, and employer, is entered through the Lists menu. The Lists menu also provides access to lists of codes, insurance carriers, and providers.

Reports Menu The Reports menu is used to print reports about patients' accounts and other reports about the practice.

Tools Menu The calculator is accessed through the Tools menu. Other options on the Tools menu can be used to view the contents of a file as well as a profile of the computer system.

Window Menu Using the Window menu, it is possible to switch back and forth between several open windows.

Services Menu This menu contains links for electronic transmission of insurance claims, electronic prescriptions, and electronic eligibility verification.

Help Menu The Help menu is used to access Medisoft's Help feature.

Basic Medisoft Actions

In this section we discuss some of the basic tasks that all medical office specialists should be able to perform with the Medisoft software.

Saving Data

Information entered into Medisoft is saved by clicking the Save button that appears in most dialog boxes (those in which data is input).

Deleting Data

The majority of Medisoft dialog boxes have buttons for the purpose of deleting data.

Exiting Medisoft

Medisoft is exited by clicking Exit on the File menu or by clicking the Exit button on the toolbar.

Entering Patient Information into Medisoft

Patient information is entered in the Patient/Guarantor dialog box, accessed by clicking Patient/Guarantors and Cases on the **Lists** menu. The Patient List dialog box displays a list of established patients. Information on a new patient is entered by clicking the *New Patient* button at the bottom of the dialog box. The Patient/Guarantor dialog box contains four tabs: the **Name, Address** tab, **Other Information** tab, **Payment Plan** tab, and **Custom** tab (Figure J-1 ◆).

Name, Address Tab

This tab is completed with information provided by a new patient on the practice's patient information form. Most of the information is demographic: name, address, phone numbers, birth date, gender, and Social Security number. Phone numbers must be entered without parentheses or hyphens. The birth date is entered using the eight-digit MMDDCCYY format. The nine-digit Social Security number should be entered *with* hyphens.

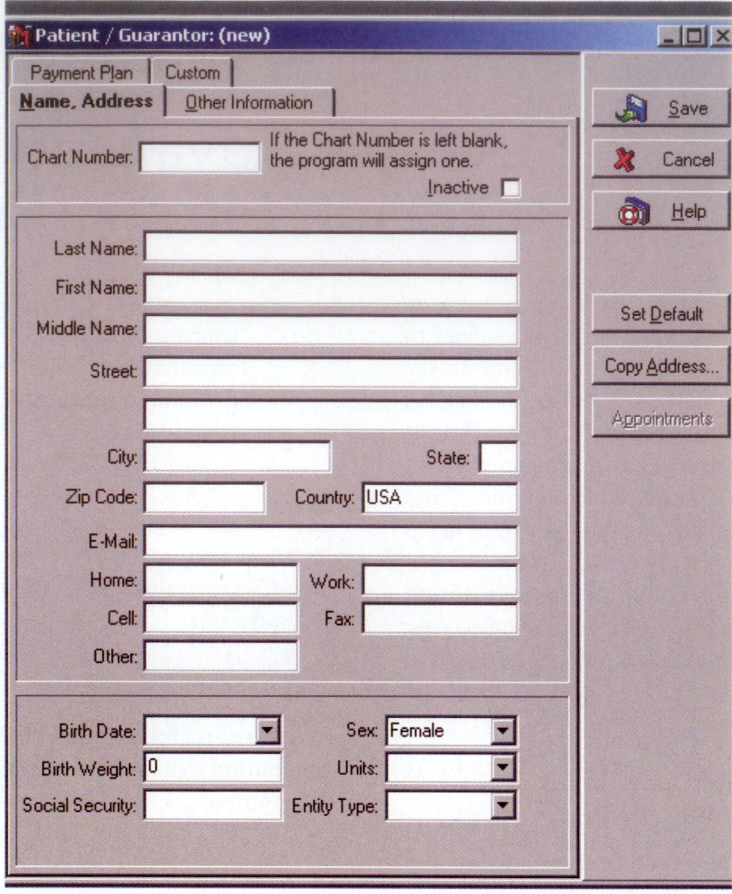

Figure J-1 ◆ The Name, Address tab in the Patient/Guarantor window (dialog box).

Some of the boxes, such as the cell phone number and fax number boxes, are optional.

Chart Number: The chart number is a unique number that identifies each patient. The most common method of assigning a number is to use the first three letters of the last name, the first two letters of the first name, and the digit 0, which represents head of household. If the last name has less than five letters, use more letters of the first name and even of the middle name if necessary. It is not necessary to enter a chart number when entering a new patient. If you choose not to enter one, Medisoft will assign one for you. It is important to note that once the Chart Number is set it cannot be changed. To correct an incorrect chart number, the patient and case information would have to be deleted then re-created with the correct Chart Number.

Other Information Tab

The Other Information tab (Figure J-2 ◆) contains facts about a patient's employment and other miscellaneous information. The major fields in the Other Information tab are:

Type: The Type drop-down list designates whether, for billing purposes, an individual is a patient or a guarantor. A guarantor is someone who is responsible for insurance and payment.

Assigned Provider: The code for the specific doctor who provides care to this patient is selected.

Signature on File: A check mark in the Signature on File check box means that the patient's signature is on file for the purpose of submitting insurance claims.

Signature Date: The date keyed in the Signature Date box is the date the patient signed the release of information form.

Emergency Contact: The name the patient/guarantor has written on the patient information form as an emergency contact is keyed in here, along with any phone numbers provided.

Employer: The name of the patient's employer is selected from the drop-down list of employers stored in the database.

Payment Plan Tab

The Payment Plan tab (Figure J-3 ◆) contains data regarding a patient who has signed a financial agreement to pay the facility the balance on the account over a specific period of time.

Custom Tab

The Custom tab is designed by the particular facility to contain information important to that facility. In the tutorial data

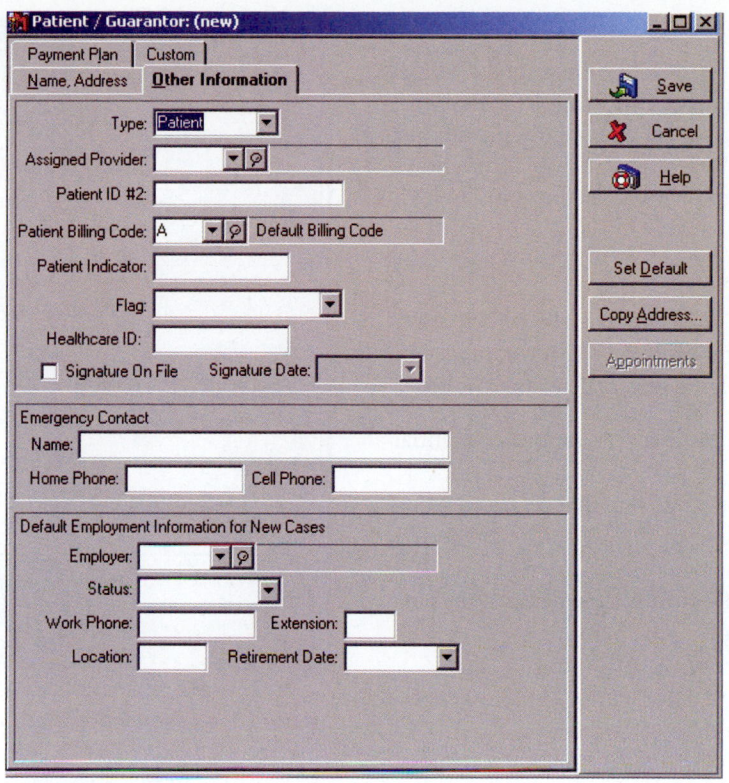

Figure J-2 ◆ The Other Information tab in the Patient/Guarantor window.

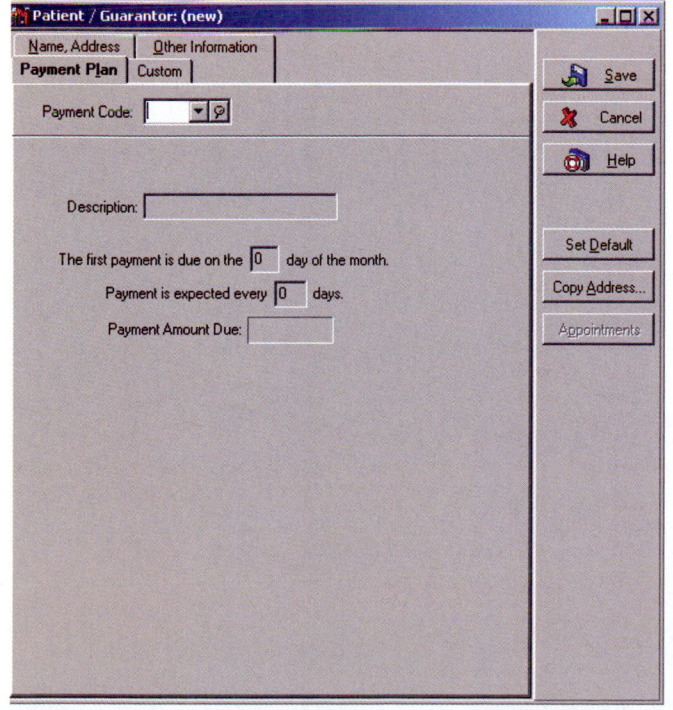

Figure J-3 ◆ The Payment Plan tab in the Patient/Guarantor window.

for Medisoft, the Custom tab contains height, weight, and cigarette smoking data.

Cases

Information about a patient's insurance coverage, billing account, diagnosis, and condition are stored in cases. When a patient comes for treatment, a case is created. Cases are set up to contain the transactions that relate to a particular condition. For example, all treatments and procedures for bronchial asthma would be stored in a case called "Bronchial Asthma." Services performed and charges for those services are entered in the system linked to the bronchial asthma case.

In Medisoft cases are created, edited, and deleted from within the **Patient List** dialog box. When the Case radio button in the Patient List dialog box is clicked, the following buttons appear at the bottom of the Patient List dialog box: Edit Case, New Case, Delete Case, Copy Case, and Close. These buttons perform their respective functions on cases. For example, to create a new case, the New Case button is clicked. Data recorded in the Case dialog box is stored by clicking the Save button on the right side of the Case dialog box.

Entering Case Information

Information on a patient is entered in 11 different tabs within the Case dialog box: Personal, Account, Diagnosis, Policy 1, Policy 2, Policy 3, Condition, Miscellaneous, Medicaid and Tricare, Comment, and EDI. A 12th tab, Custom One, allows the facility to create and design its own Custom tabs as well.

Personal Tab

The Personal tab (Figure J-4 ◆) contains basic information about a patient and his or her employment. The most important boxes that must be completed in the Personal tab are as follows:

Case Number: The case number is a unique sequential number *assigned by Medisoft*.

Description: Information entered in the Description box indicates a patient's complaint, or reason for seeing the physician.

Guarantor: The Guarantor box lists the name of the person responsible for paying the bill.

Account Tab

The Account tab includes information on a patient's assigned provider, referring provider, referral source, as well as other information that may be used in some medical practices but not others (Figure J-5 ◆). The most important boxes that must be completed in the Account tab are as follows:

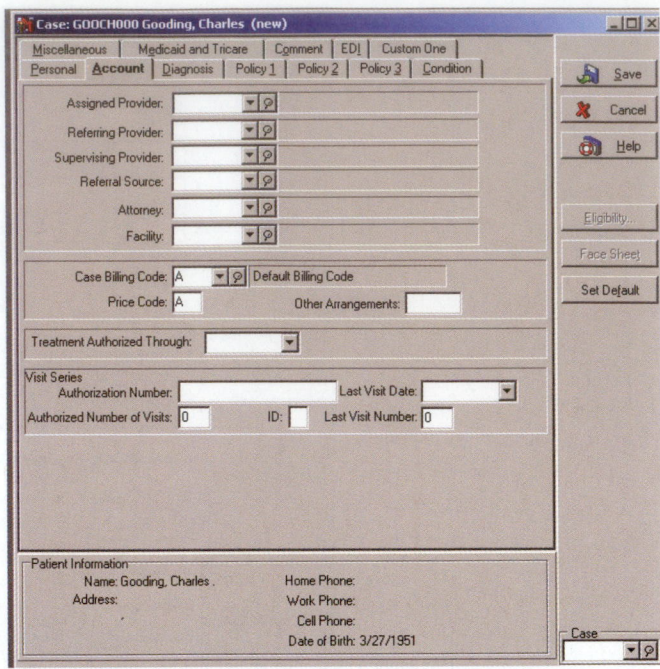

Figure J-5 ◆ Case window, Account tab.

Assigned Provider: The Assigned Provider box is automatically filled in with the code number and name of the assigned provider listed in the Patient/Guarantor dialog box.

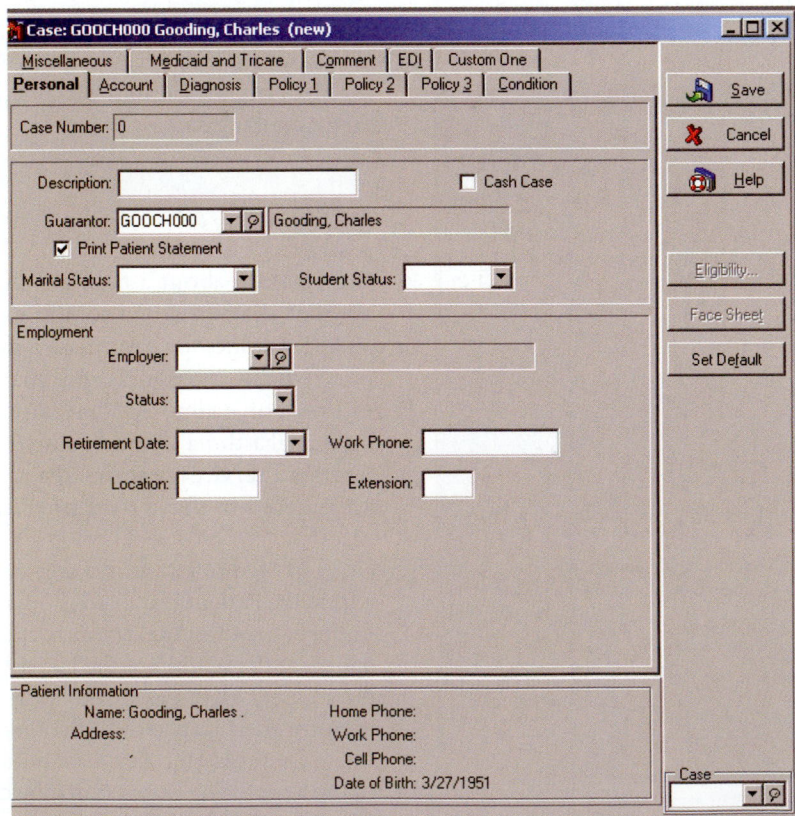

Figure J-4 ◆ Case window, Personal tab.

Referring Provider: If the patient was referred to the facility by another provider, choose the referring provider's name from the drop-down list.

Facility: Choose the correct facility name from the drop-down box for the place the services were rendered.

Authorization Number: For patients whose insurance carrier requires a referral/authorization number for services, the number issued should be entered here along with the number of visits authorized and the referral expiration date.

Diagnosis Tab

The Diagnosis tab contains a patient's diagnosis, information about allergies, and electronic medical claim (EMC) notes (Figure J-6 ♦) . The Allergies and Notes box is the most important box that must be completed in the Diagnosis tab:

Allergies and Notes: If the patient is allergic to anything it should be entered here. This information is taken from the patient information form. Notes regarding payment arrangements, a forgotten copayment, or anything else are entered in this area as well.

You will not complete the Default Diagnosis 1 through 4 boxes. When you are setting up the case, you will not know the patient's diagnosis. After you have posted the charge transaction, the diagnosis code entered into the charge information will be transferred automatically by Medisoft to the Default Diagnosis boxes in this tab.

Policy 1, 2, and 3 Tabs

The Policy tabs are where information about a patient's insurance carrier and coverage is recorded (Figure J-7 ♦). If a patient has more than one insurance policy, the Policy 2 and 3 tabs are used. The following boxes are the most important ones to be completed in the Policy tabs:

Insurance 1: The Insurance 1 box lists the patient's insurance carrier name, which is chosen from the drop-down list.

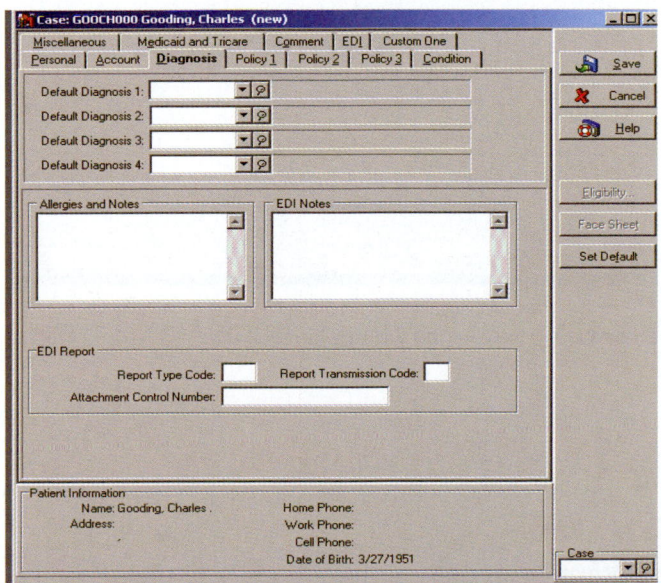

Figure J-6 ♦ Case window, Diagnosis tab.

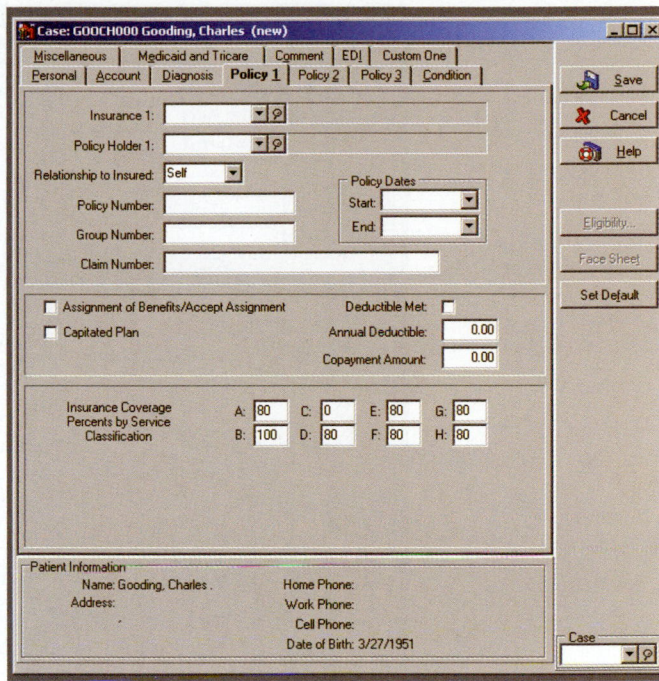

Figure J-7 ♦ Case window, Policy 1 tab.

Policy Holder 1: This box shows the name of the insured person, which is chosen from the drop-down list. (This may or may not be the patient.) The guarantor must be entered in to the Patient List so that he or she can be chosen from the drop-down list here.

Relationship to Insured: This box indicates the patient's relationship to the individual listed in the Policy Holder 1 box.

Policy Number: The patient's insurance policy or ID number is entered in the Policy Number box.

Group Number: If there is a group number for a patient's policy, it is entered in the Group Number box.

Assignment of Benefits/Accept Assignment: Check this box if the patient has assigned insurance benefits to the provider.

Insurance Coverage Percents by Service Classification: The percentage of fees that an insurance carrier covers is entered in the Insurance Coverage Percents … box. The default entry in this box is 80. The default can be changed by highlighting the default entry and keying the correct percentage over the default. Some insurance policies pay different percentages of charges based on the type of service rendered. For example, a carrier may pay 100% for well-man or well-woman exams and 50% for lab charges.

Condition Tab

The Condition tab stores data about a patient's illness, accident, disability, and hospitalization. This information is used by insurance carriers to process claims (Figure J-8 ♦).

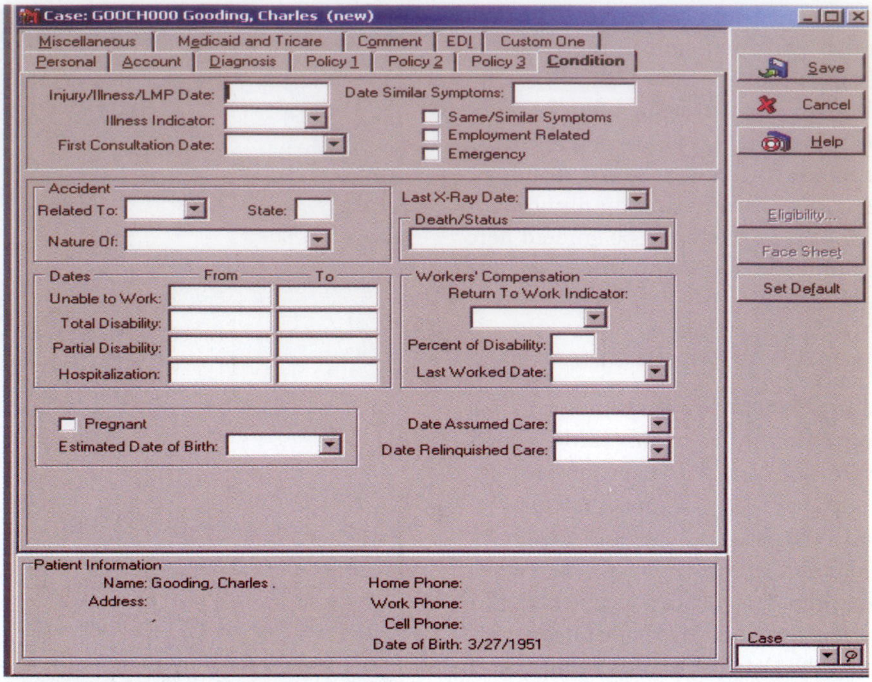

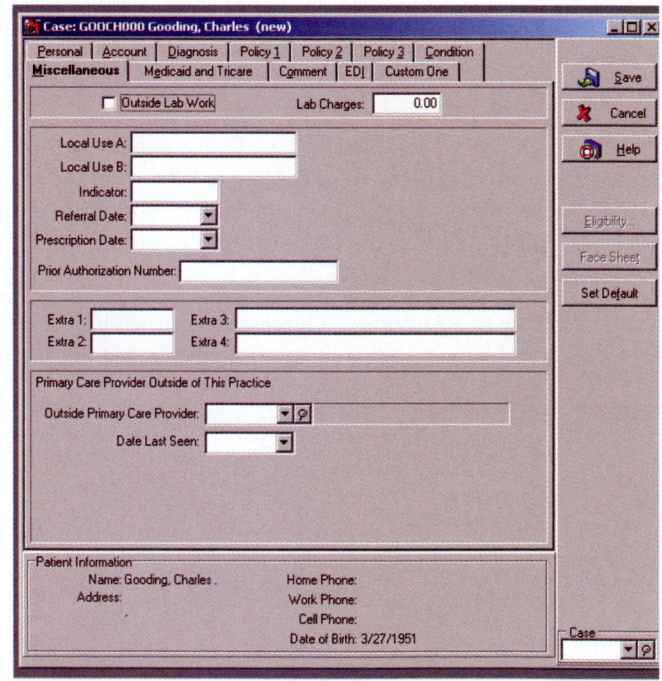

Figure J-8 ◆ Case window, Condition tab.

The top portion of the Condition tab is completed with the date of the illness, injury, or last menstrual period (if the patient is pregnant). Make the appropriate choice from the Illness Indicator drop-down list. If treatment rendered was for an emergency condition, check the box next to Emergency. If the case is for treatment of an accident, select the correct type from the Accident drop-down list. If the "accident" was just a fall at home, it is not considered a true accident. If the Accident box is marked, the insurance carrier may delay processing of the claim to research whether another insurance carrier should be the primary payer. If the case/treatment is workers' compensation related, the boxes for Unable to Work, Total Disability, Partial Disability, and Hospitalization may be completed. The Return To Work Indicator, Percent of Disability, and Last Worked Date all relate to workers' compensation cases.

Miscellaneous Tab

The Miscellaneous tab records a variety of miscellaneous information about the patient and his or her treatment, including outside lab work, prior authorization numbers, and other information (Figure J-9 ◆). For the authorization number to print out on the CMS-1500 form, it must be entered in the Miscellaneous tab.

Medicaid and Tricare Tab

For patients covered by Medicaid or TRICARE, the Medicaid and Tricare tab is used to enter additional information about the government program (Figure J-10 ◆) .

Comment Tab

Any comments or notes pertinent to this patient's case may be entered into the Comment tab (Figure J-11 ◆).

Figure J-9 ◆ Case window, Miscellaneous tab.

EDI Tab

Information necessary for the processing or transmission of electronic data interchange (EDI) data is entered in the EDI tab (Figure J-12 ◆).

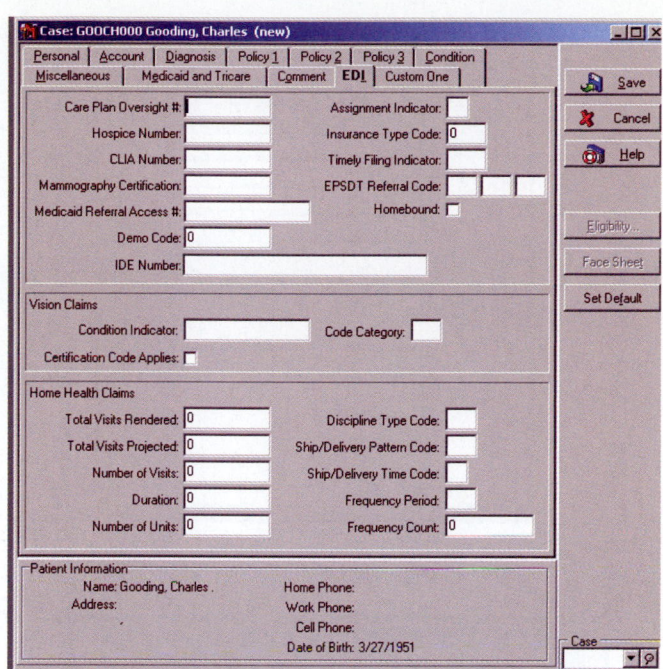

Figure J-10 ◆ Case window, Medicaid and Tricare tab.

Figure J-12 ◆ Case window, EDI tab.

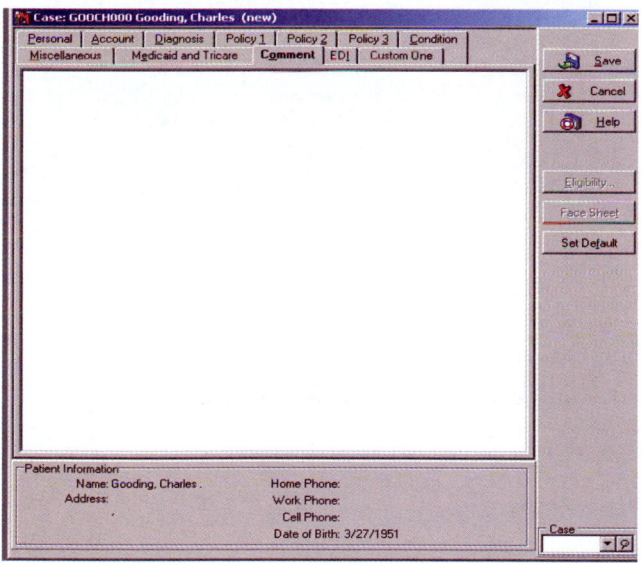

Figure J-11 ◆ Case window, Comment tab.

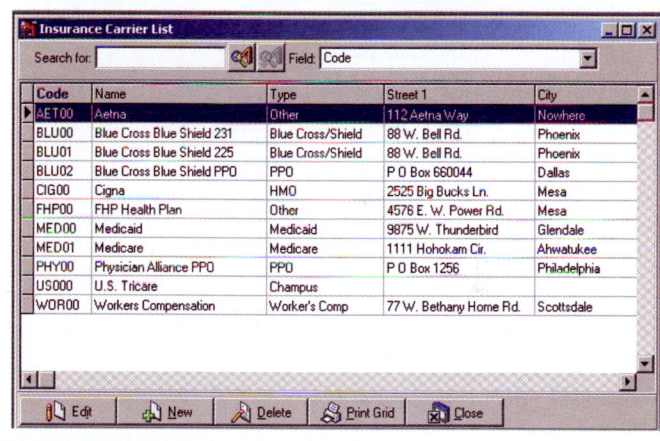

Figure J-13 ◆ Adding an insurance carrier in the Insurance Carrier window.

Adding the Insurance Carriers

If, when you are in the patient's Case window and entering the insurance carrier name, you notice the insurance carrier you are looking for is *not* in the drop-down list, you must go to the **Insurance Carrier List** to add it (Figure J-13 ◆). This can be accessed via a shortcut button or the Lists menu.

Click on the **New** button to add a new carrier name and address.

In the **Address** tab of the new Insurance Carrier window, enter the insurance carrier's name, address, telephone number, fax number, and contact name if you have one (Figure J-14 ◆).

The **Options** tab in the new Insurance Carrier window is vitally important because it is here that you choose the insurance plan type and indicate whether or not "Signature On File" (SOF) should appear on the claim form. SOF indicates that you have the patient's authorization to release this information and that the patient has assigned benefits directly to the provider (Figure J.14). (So the payment for the claim will be sent directly to your provider and not the patient.) "Signature on File" should *always* appear on the claim forms you submit.

The **EDI/Eligibility** tab is used to enter important EDI information for that insurance carrier (Figure J-15 ◆).

The Codes tab is for entering default transactions codes (Figure J-16 ◆).

The Allowed tab may be used to enter the contractual allowed amount per procedure code for that particular insurance carrier (Figure J-17 ◆).

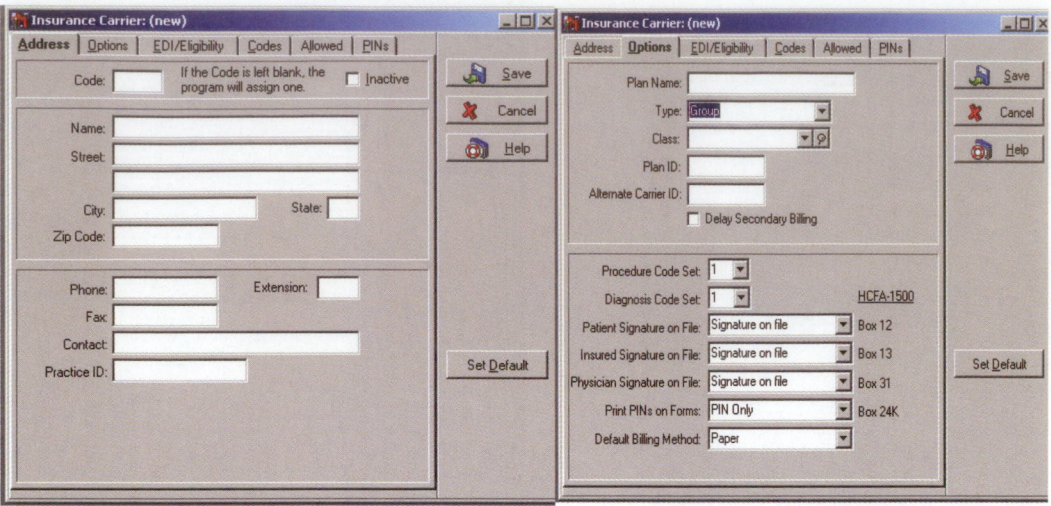

Figure J-14 ◆ New Insurance Carrier window, Address tab (left) and Options tab (right).

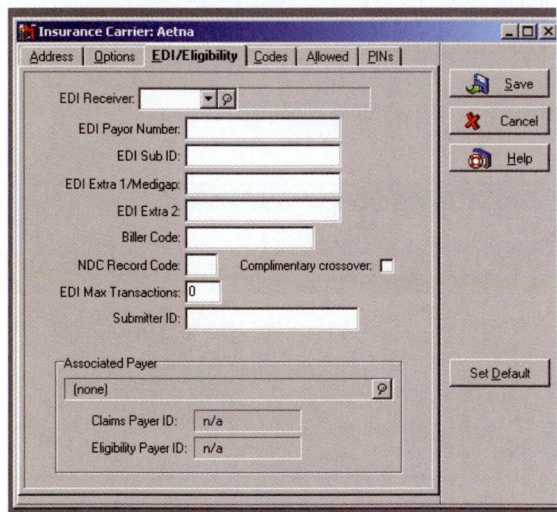

Figure J-15 ◆ Insurance Carrier window, EDI/Eligibility tab.

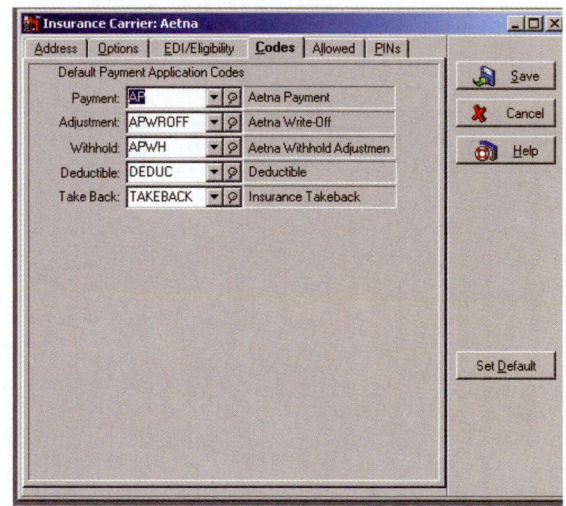

Figure J-16 ◆ Insurance Carrier window, Codes tab.

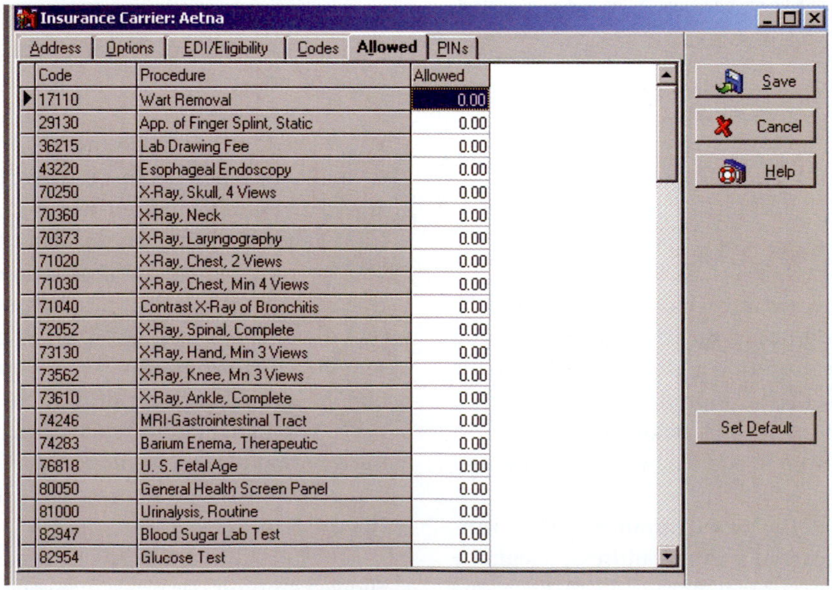

Figure J-17 ◆ Insurance Carrier window, Allowed tab.

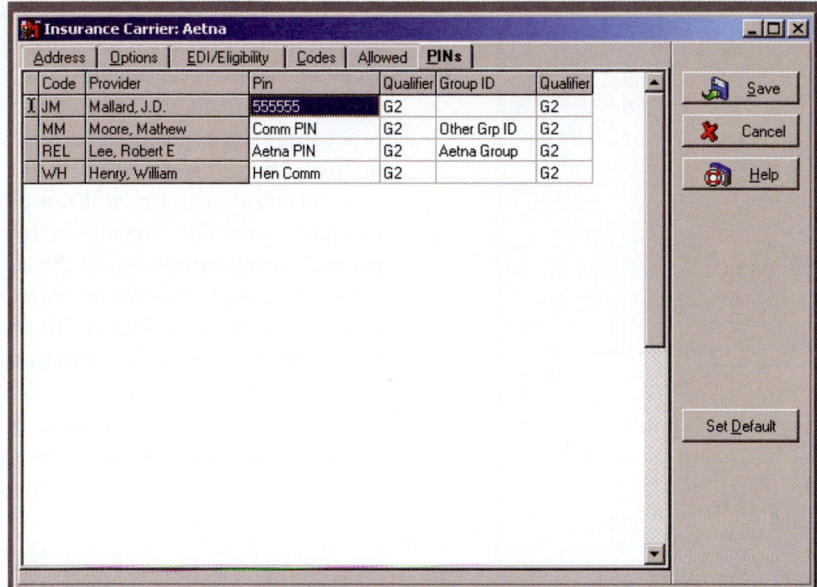

Figure J-18 ◆ Insurance Carrier window, PINs tab.

The **PINs** tab in the Insurance Carrier List is also very important (Figure J-18 ◆). You must first Save your new carrier, then go back in and Edit it to add the provider PINs. PINs are specific to each carrier. Be sure to enter the correct insurance carrier PIN for each participating provider. The appropriate qualifier should also be entered so that it prints on the CMS-1500 claim form.

Entering Employers

When entering patient and case information, it will be necessary to add the patient's or guarantor's employer name/address into Medisoft. This is accomplished in the **Address List,** which is accessed from the taskbar using the Address List shortcut button (Figure J-19 ◆).

The Address List contains not only employer addresses, but also referral sources (other than physicians), facility addresses, and attorney addresses (Figure J-20 ◆).

Click on the **New** button to begin (Figure J-21 ◆). Add the employer name, address and telephone number.

If you are entering an employer (and not a referral source, etc.), in the Type field, be sure Employer is shown (Figure J-22 ◆). Click Save when you have finished entering the information.

You can now select the Employer name from the drop-down list in the Patient List or Case windows.

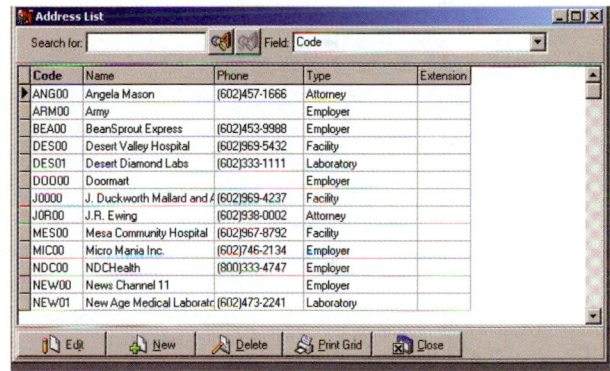

Figure J-20 ◆ Address List window.

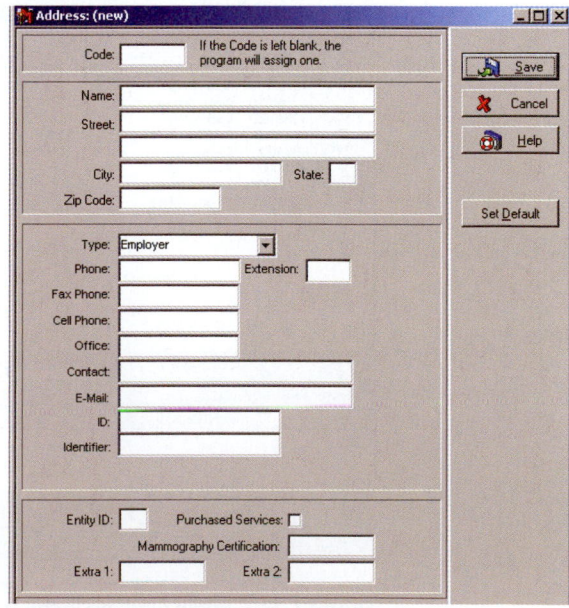

Figure J-21 ◆ New Address window.

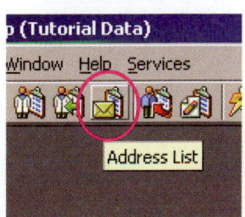

Figure J-19 ◆ Address List shortcut button on the taskbar.

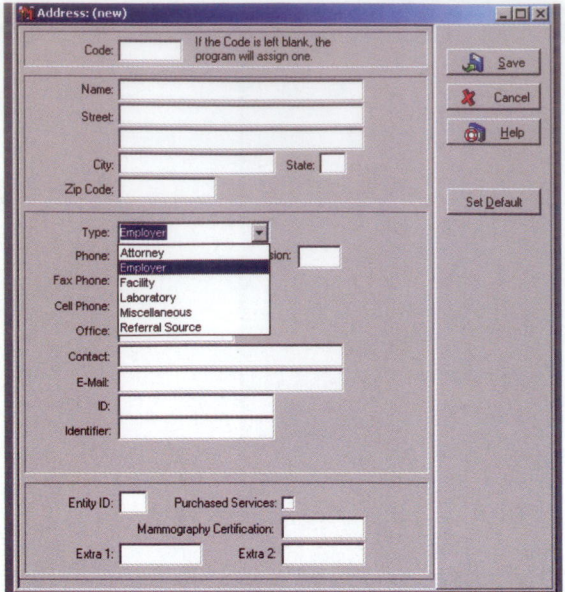

Figure J-22 ◆ In the Type field of the new Address window, be sure to choose "Employer" when entering a new employer.

Reviewing a Completed Superbill

The completed superbill is the primary source of information a medical office specialist needs to record procedure charges. The completed superbill includes the following information: the provider's name, patient's name and chart/account number, date the services were performed, diagnosis, charge amounts, amount of payment received at the time of service, and the next appointment time needed.

After a physician completes a patient exam, he or she will place a check mark (or an X or circle) on the superbill next to the procedures performed. As you may recall, the superbill includes only the most common procedures provided by the medical office. If the physician performs a procedure not listed on the superbill, he or she writes the procedure in the "Other Procedures" area or in a blank space on the form.

Insurance carriers will not pay for treatment without a diagnosis code. The *diagnosis* is the physician's opinion of the patient's condition based on the examination. Therefore, the physician must record this information on the superbill so that it may be included as part of the procedure charge. If a procedure code or diagnosis is not marked on the superbill, you will need to ask the physician to mark it. Never demand that the physician do so and never accuse the physician of forgetting to mark the superbill. Always use respect and tact when addressing members of your medical practice.

Entering a Procedure Charge

After you review a patient's superbill, you are ready to enter the transaction into Medisoft to record the procedure charge and diagnosis code. You will process all transactions (charges, payments, and adjustments) in the **Transaction Entry** window. To access this window, you can use the **Activities** menu and click on Enter Transactions, click the **Transaction Entry** shortcut button or click the **Accounting** menu on the **Medisoft** side bar and choose Enter Transactions.

After you have opened the Transaction Entry window, *the first thing you must do is choose the correct patient's chart number and case number to post a charge to.*

Step 1: Choose a patient chart number and case number (Figure J-23 ◆).

Step 2: After the correct patient and case have been chosen, click on the **New** button in the *middle* of the screen (to access the top of the screen) (Figure J-24 ◆).

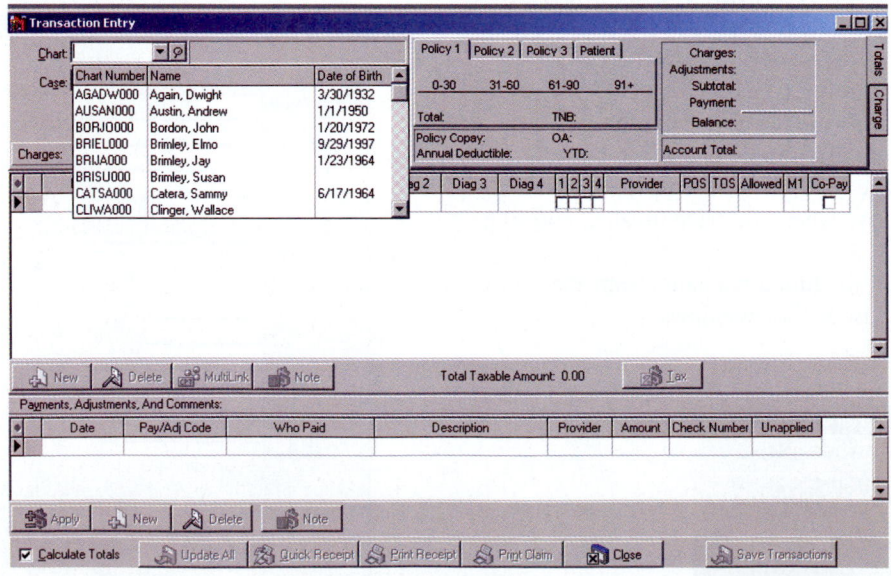

Figure J-23 ◆ Begin working in the Transaction Entry window by choosing a patient chart number and case number.

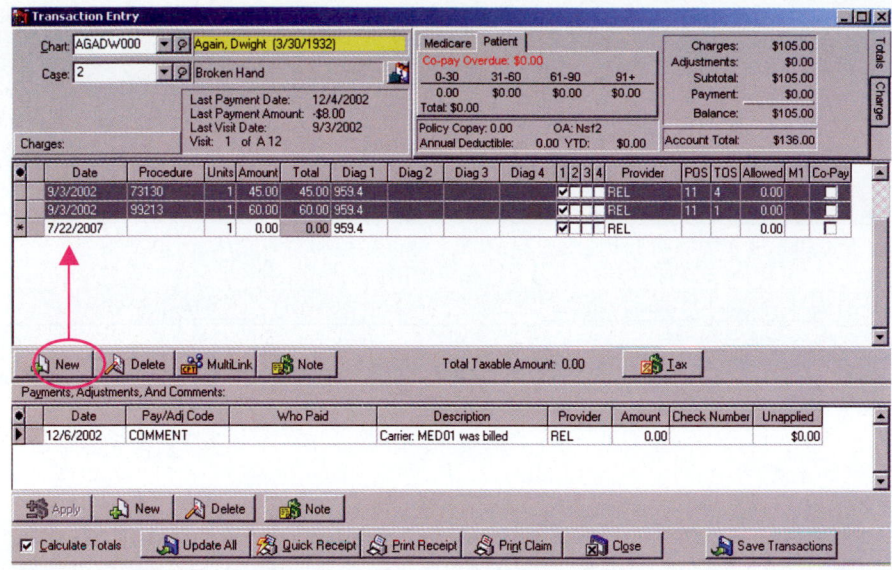

Figure J-24 ◆ After choosing the correct patient and case, choose the New button from the middle of the screen.

Medisoft will add today's date by default to the screen. If the date of service is not today's date, type the correct date in the Date field.

Click your mouse inside the **Procedure** field next to the date. A drop-down menu will be shown. You may either search for the correct procedure code marked on the superbill or type it in.

Once you have entered the CPT® code, press Enter or Tab to be taken to the Units field. Most of the time you will not need to change the default units entry.

Press Tab or Enter to move to the **Amount** field. Medisoft has already entered a dollar amount associated with that CPT code. If this amount is incorrect, key in the correct amount.

Press Tab or Enter again to be taken to the **DIAG1** field. Type in the primary diagnosis code or use the drop-down menu to search for the correct diagnosis. You may enter up to four diagnosis codes per charge transaction.

Tab over to the **Provider** field to make sure the correct provider is being credited with seeing this patient.

The **POS** (place of service) and **TOS** (type of service) fields will automatically be filled in based on the information in the CPT code database.

The **Allowed** amount field is also completed by default per information in the CPT code and insurance database.

The **M1** field is used to enter a two-character CPT modifier if one is marked on the patient superbill.

Complete all of these steps again to enter another procedure charge.

When you have finished entering charges, click on the **Save Transactions** button at the lower right of the screen or the **Update All** button near the lower left side of the window. When the Update All button is used to save transactions, the

Medisoft program checks all fields for missing or invalid information and will display a message if information is needed or invalid.

Posting a Payment

When the patient (or his or her insurance carrier) makes a payment on the patient's account, you must enter this into the accounting software. Payments are posted in the **Transaction Entry** window (Figure J-25 ◆). Remember, you cannot enter a transaction without first choosing a patient chart number and case number. It is important to make sure you have chosen the correct case—especially when posting payments from insurance carriers.

After opening the Transaction Entry window and choosing the appropriate chart and case number, click on the **New** button toward the *bottom* of the window within the Payments, Adjustments, And Comments section.

Medisoft will start a new entry by adding today's date.

Click in the **Pay/Adj Code** field and choose the method of payment (personal check, cash, Aetna payment, etc.).

Tab over to the **Who Paid** field and choose the party that is making the payment.

Enter a description if necessary.

Make sure the correct provider is shown in the **Provider** field.

Enter the amount of the payment in the **Amount** field. Enter a check number if appropriate in the next field.

Next, *you must apply the payment to the correct charge(s)*. To do this, click on the **Apply** button at the bottom left-hand side of the window, to the left of the New button (Figure J-26 ◆).

A new window will open on top of your Transaction Entry window. This is the **Apply Payment to Charges** window. It is here that you can apply the payment to a specific charge or charges. This is called *line item posting*.

CPT is a registered trademark of the American Medical Association.

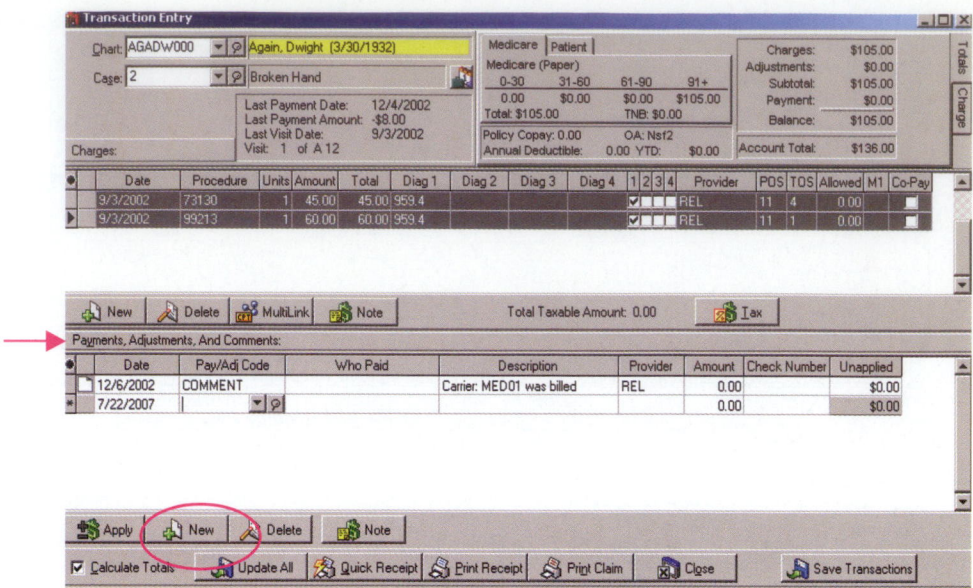

Figure J-25 ◆ Posting payments in the Transaction Entry window.

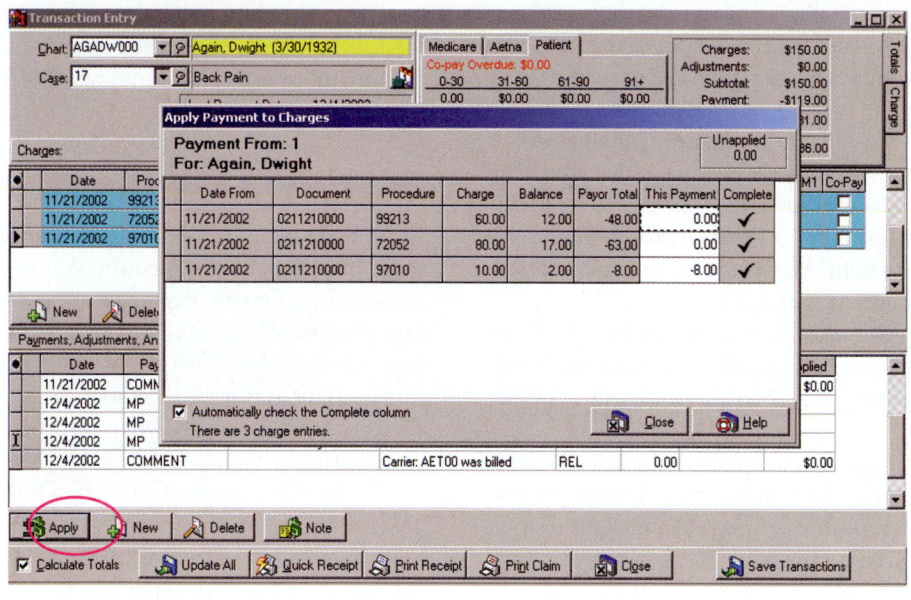

Figure J-26 ◆ Applying a payment to the correct charges.

It is most important to post the payment to the correct date of service and the correct procedure code. One payment can be divided among many charges if it is "broken down" that way on the EOB/ERA or the patient has many separate charges and is paying for all of them.

When you have applied the payment to the correct charge(s), click the **Close** button at the bottom of the Apply Payment to Charges window.

Your **Unapplied** column in the Payment, Adjustment, And Comments section of the Transaction Entry window should read $0.00 if you applied the entire payment. (A patient's account may have an unapplied balance if he or she is prepaying on surgery, for example.) You must now save the payment transaction.

Click on the **Update All** or **Save Transactions** button at the bottom of the window.

Posting an Adjustment

Entering an adjustment into a patient's account is similar to entering a payment and is also performed in the **Transaction Entry** window. To begin, you must first choose the patient chart number and case number.

Click on the **New** button towards the *bottom* of the window.

Medisoft will start a new transaction by entering today's date by default.

In the **Pay/Adj Code** field, select the correct type of adjustment (insurance write-off, charge reversal, courtesy discount, etc.).

Tab over to the **Description** entry field and type a note about why the adjustment is needed.

Tab over to the **Provider** field and choose the correct provider, then tab over to the **Amount** field.

If you are *subtracting* an amount from the patient's account, you will need to enter a *minus (–)* sign before typing the amount. If you are adding an amount to a patient's account, you do not need to enter a plus sign before the amount.

Note: Medisoft will assume all adjustments are positive unless you type in a minus (–) sign before the amount.

When you have entered the amount, click on the **Apply** button at the bottom left of the Transaction Entry window.

When you are applying the adjustment, make sure to choose the correct date(s) of service and CPT code(s). *You must enter a minus sign before the amount in the Apply Adjustment to Charges window.* If you do not, Medisoft will *add* the amount to the patient's account.

When you have entered all of the adjustments, click on the **Close** button to take you back to the Transaction Entry window.

To save all of your hard work, be sure to click on **Update All** or **Save Transactions**.

Using the Enter Deposits and Apply Payments Window

It is easiest to post payments that patients make at the time of service in the Transaction Entry window. However, if you receive a large insurance check that covers claims for many different patients, it is easier to post this in the **Enter Deposits and Apply Payments** window. This window can be accessed by clicking the **Enter Deposits and Apply Payments** shortcut button, opening the **Activities** menu and choosing Apply Deposits/Payments, or by clicking on the **Accounting** shortcut button on the **Medisoft** side bar and choosing Enter Deposits/Payments. A Deposit List window will open (Figure J-27 ◆) that contains the following fields:

Deposit Date: The current date is automatically entered. It can be changed by typing a different date in the field.
Show All Deposits: This check box displays all payments entered regardless of date.
Show Unapplied Only: If this box is checked, only the payments that have not been fully applied to charges are shown.

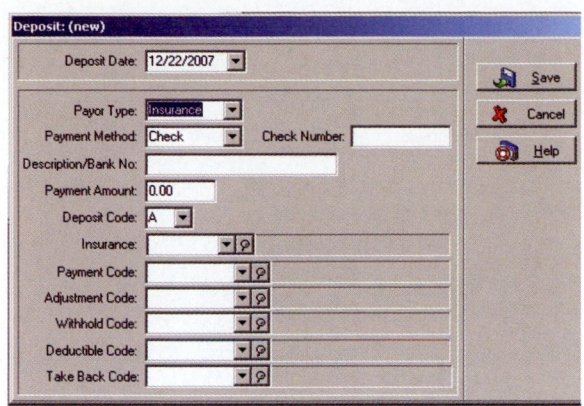

Figure J-28 ◆ New Deposit window.

Sort By: This is a drop-down list that allows you to sort deposits by amount, patient chart number, and payer.
Locate and **Locate Next:** These shortcut buttons allow you to search for a particular deposit.
Detail: This button is used to view a specific deposit in more detail. Highlight the deposit in the window and then click the Detail button.

To enter a new deposit, click on the **New** button at the bottom of the Deposit List window. After the New Deposit window opens (Figure J-28 ◆), you must choose a **Payor Type** (patient, insurance carrier, capitation).

Choose the **Payment Method** (check, cash, credit card, electronic) and Enter or Tab over to the **Check Number** field to enter the check number.

The **Description/Bank No.** field is used to enter an (optional) description of the check.

Enter the dollar amount of the payment in the **Payment Amount** field.

The **Deposit Code** drop-down menu is used by some practices to sort deposits according to practice-defined categories.

Select the insurance carrier making payment from the drop-down menu in the **Insurance** field.

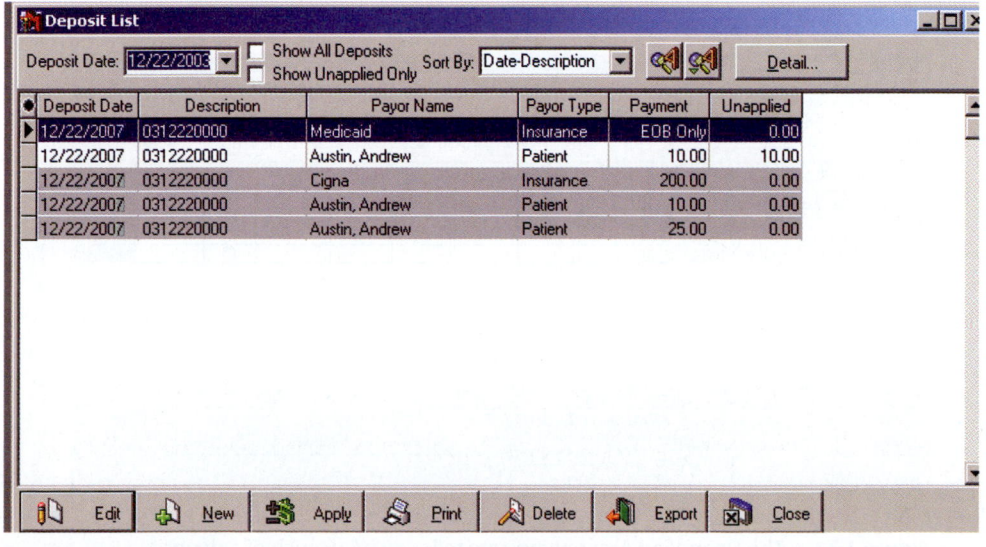

Figure J-27 ◆ Deposit List window (Enter Deposits and Apply Payments).

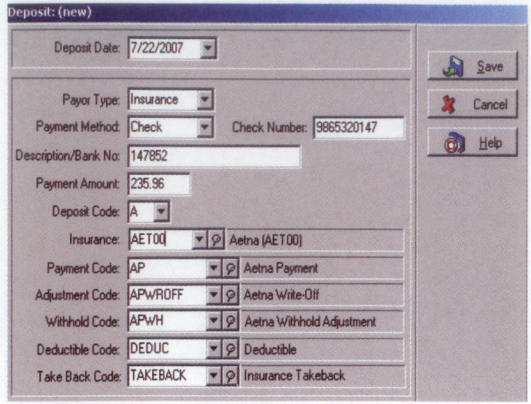

Figure J-29 ◆ The various code fields are filled in automatically when the insurance carrier is selected from the Insurance drop-down box.

After you have selected the carrier, the other **Code** fields are automatically completed (Figure J-29 ◆).

When finished, click **Save.**

After entering the check information, the next step is to apply the payment.

Click the **Apply** button at the bottom of the Deposit List window.

The **Apply Payment/Adjustments to Charges** window (Figure J-30 ◆) is where you will apply payments and adjustments (if needed) to specific patient accounts. You are able to enter payments and adjustments as well as deductibles and withhold information at virtually the same time.

When you have finished entering payment information on one patient, click the **Save Payments/Adjustments** button at the bottom right side of the window.

If you have the **Print Statements Now** box at the bottom of the window checked, after clicking Save, Medisoft will ask what type of statement you would like to print.

If you have another patient to apply payments to, follow the same steps as before.

The **Unapplied Amount** indicator in the top right-hand corner of the window will allow you to keep track of how much you have posted and how much you still have to post (Figure J-31 ◆).

Walkout Receipts

Throughout the simulation at the end of this appendix, you will be responsible for printing a walkout receipt for each

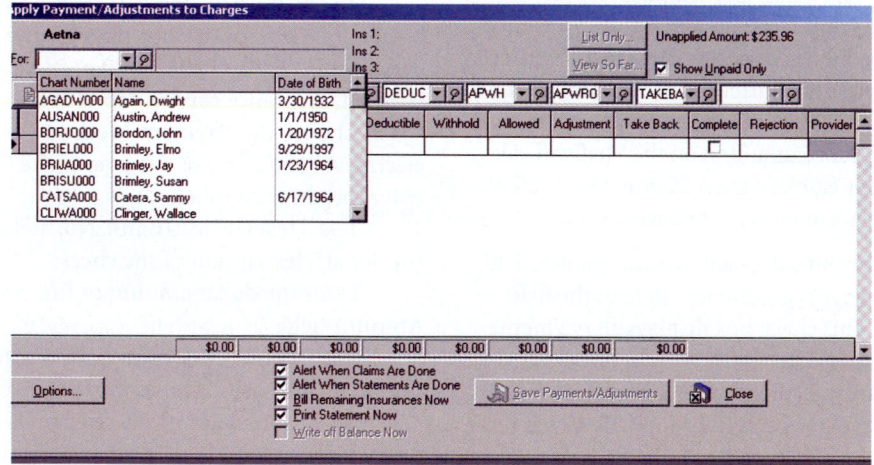

Figure J-30 ◆ The Apply Payments/Adjustments to Charges window.

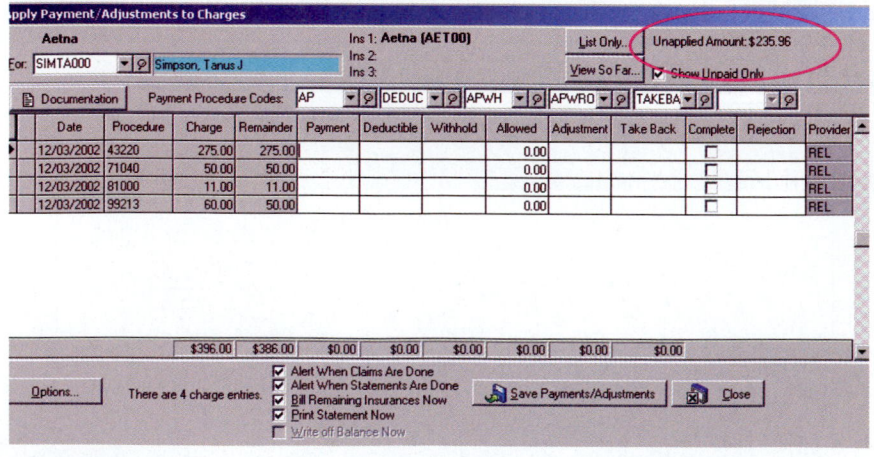

Figure J-31 ◆ The Unapplied Amount indicate tells you how much of a deposit remains to be posted.

| | 9/7/2005 | AP | Aetna -Secondary | Aetna | | REL | -12.00 | | $0.00 |
| | 9/7/2005 | AP | Aetna -Secondary | Aetna | | REL | -17.00 | | $0.00 |

Apply | New | Delete | Note

☑ Calculate Estimates | Update All | **Quick Receipt** | Print Receipt | Print Claim | Close | Save Transactions

Figure J-32 ◆ Quick Receipt button.

patient who has seen the provider. This task is performed in the Transaction Entry window.

After you have posted the patient's charges and/or payments, click the **Quick Receipt** button at the bottom of the window to print a receipt for today's visit only (Figure J-32 ◆). A **Print Report Where?** window will open. After choosing to print to the printer, the receipt will automatically print.

If the patient would like a more comprehensive receipt (one that includes previous visits), click the **Print Receipt** button instead.

When the **Open Report** window opens, choose Walkout Receipt (All Transactions), then click the OK button (Figure J-33 ◆). A **Print Report Where?** window opens after you have clicked OK (Figure J-34 ◆).

After selecting where to print the report, a **Data Selection Questions** window opens. Choose the date ranges for your receipt and click the OK button.

If you choose to preview the report on the screen, you will see a screen similar to that shown in Figure J-35 ◆. To print from the preview screen, click the picture of the printer across the top of the screen. To close the preview screen, click the Close button.

Printing Reports in Medisoft

Let's take a moment to discuss the different reports available in Medisoft.

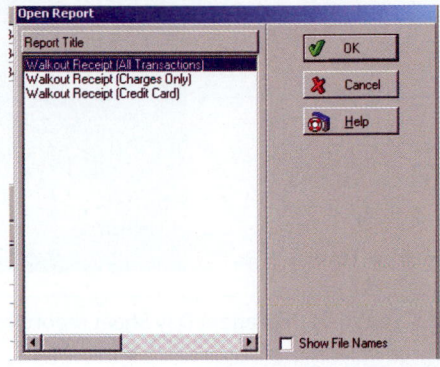

Figure J-33 ◆ Open Report window.

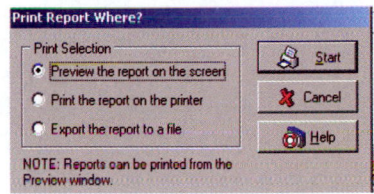

Figure J-34 ◆ Print Report Where? window.

Patient Day Sheet Report

The Patient Day Sheet report can be accessed in either of two ways: by clicking on the **Reports** menu or by clicking the **Daily Reports** menu on the **Medisoft** side bar.

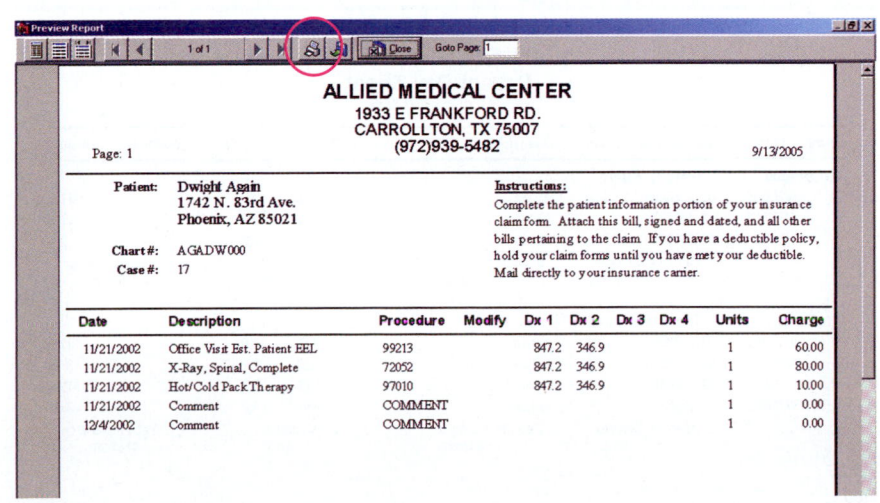

Figure J-35 ◆ Sample walkout receipt.

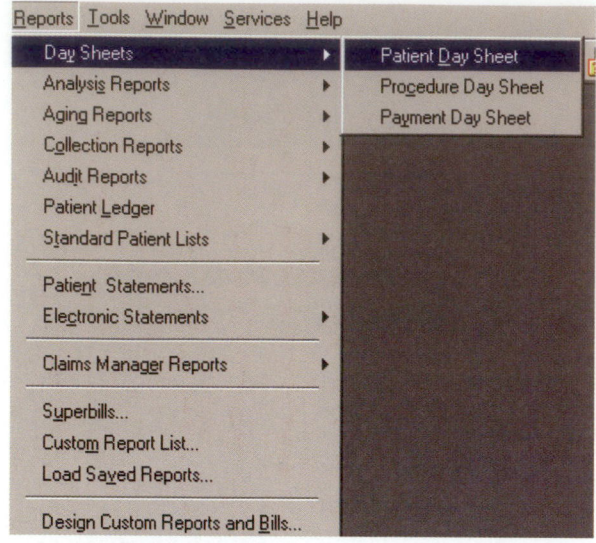

Figure J-36 ◆ Selecting the Patient Day Sheet report from the Reports drop-down menu.

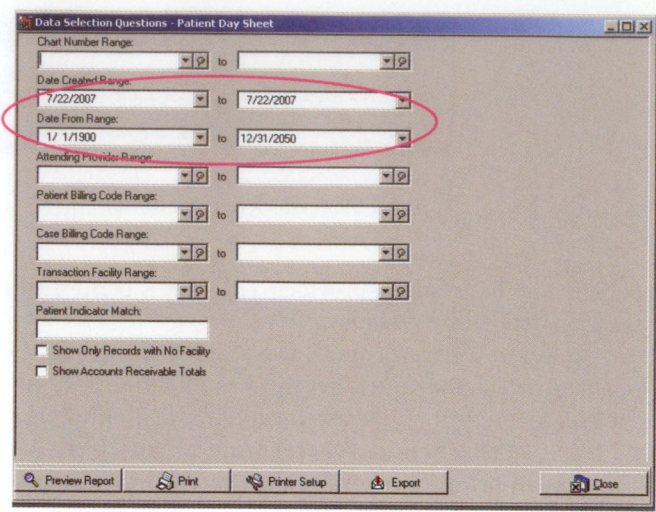

Figure J-37 ◆ Data Selection Questions for Patient Day Sheet Reports.

For the simulation that follows, you will be instructed to stop entering transactions and "batch out." You will need to compile and run the Patient Day Sheet report. This report, as stated earlier in the text, shows all transactions posted in the database for the day. For our purposes, we will use "today's" date.

After clicking on **Patient Day Sheet** in the Reports menu (Figure J-36 ◆), a **Print Report Where?** window will open. After choosing where to print the report (our example printed it to the screen), another window/dialog box will open: **Data Selection Questions: Patient Day Sheet** (Figure J-37 ◆).

Click in the **Date Created Range** field and choose **today's date** for both the From and To boxes, then click the OK button.

Using the arrows at the top of the screen, go to the last page of the report for your totals. Your totals here should match your totals from all the superbills/EOBs you posted throughout the day (Figure J-38 ◆).

Creating and Printing Insurance Claims

During the simulation that follows, you will be responsible for printing paper CMS-1500 claim forms at the end of each day for the patients' accounts you posted charges to. This task is accomplished in the **Claim Management** window.

The Claim Management window can be accessed by clicking the **Claim Management** shortcut button, clicking the **Accounting** button on the **Medisoft** side bar, or by opening the **Activities** menu and clicking Claim Management.

After opening the Claim Management window, the first thing to do is create the insurance claims you want to send. To do this you click the **Create Claims** button at the bottom of the window (Figure J-39 ◆).

The majority of medical practices print claims several times a week. You will notice, again, that you can sort your claim

---

ALLIED MEDICAL CENTER
Patient Day Sheet
9/7/2005 - 9/7/2005

Entry	Date	Document	POS	Description	Provider	Code	Modifier	Amount
AGADW000		**Dwight Again**						
87	9/7/2005	0211210000		Aetna	REL	AP		-12.00
88	9/7/2005	0211210000		Aetna	REL	AP		-17.00
89	9/7/2005	0211210000		Aetna	REL	AP		-2.00
		Patient's Charges $0.00		Patient's Receipts -$31.00		Adjustments $0.00		Patient Balance $105.00
SIMTA000		**Tanus J Simpson**						
90	9/7/2005	0212030000		Aetna	REL	AP		-100.00
91	9/7/2005	0212030000		Aetna	REL	AP		-30.00
92	9/7/2005	0212030000		Aetna	REL	AP		-11.00
93	9/7/2005	0212030000		Aetna	REL	AP		-28.00
		Patient's Charges $0.00		Patient's Receipts -$169.00		Adjustments $0.00		Patient Balance $217.00

Figure J-38 ◆ Sample Patient Day Sheet report.

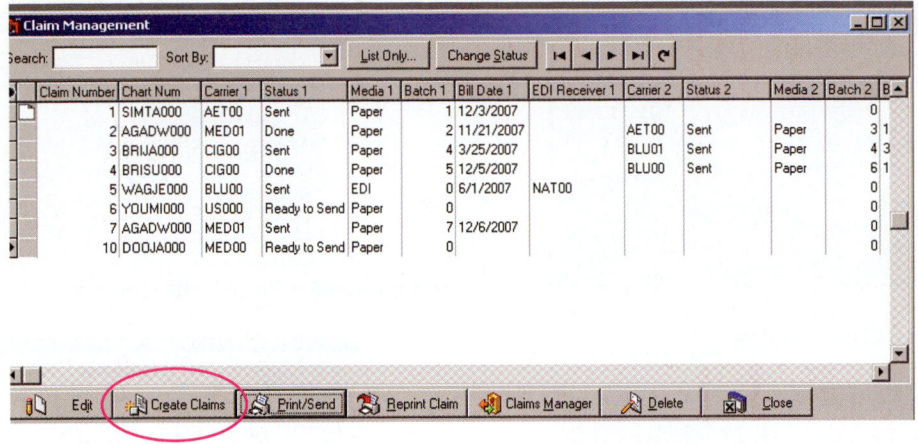

Figure J-39 ◆ To process new insurance claims, click the Create Claims button in the Claim Management window.

report many different ways: by transaction dates, chart numbers, primary insurance carrier—you can even create claims for one particular provider name. For the simulation you will be using today's date in the **Transaction Dates** field (Figure J-40 ◆). After entering the dates, click the **Create** button on the right side of the window.

As you create a claim, the Claim Management window will be automatically updated. It will show the claims you've just created as "Ready to Send" in the Status 1 column of the Claim Management window (Figure J-41 ◆).

The next step is to look over your claims *before* you print them to make sure they are "clean" claims (meaning no information is missing and all information is correct).

To do this, click on the **Print/Send** button at the *bottom* of the Claim Management window (Figure J-42 ◆).

A Print/Send Claims window will open asking you to choose how you wish to send the claims, either on paper or electronically. For our simulation, you will choose the Paper method for claims. Click the OK button on the right side of the window (Figure J-43 ◆).

An Open Report window will open next (Figure J-44 ◆). If you are printing Medicare claims, you will need to choose the CMS-1500 (Primary) Medicare Century report

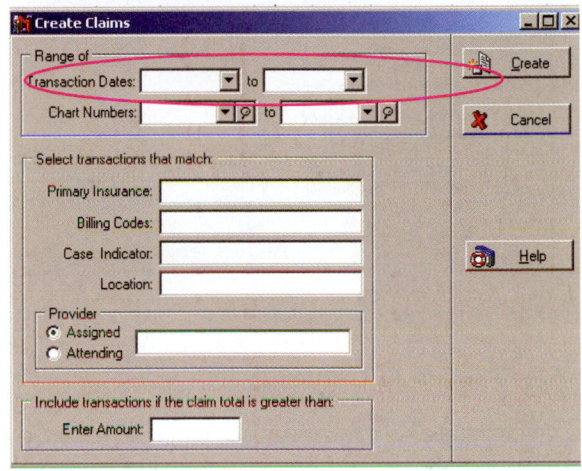

Figure J-40 ◆ The Transaction Dates field in the Create Claims window.

option. If you are printing claims for any other carrier, choose the CMS-1500 (Primary) report option. It is important to choose the correct report type for claims. Medicare prefers a minimum of information on claims, so be sure to choose the correct report/claim format when submitting

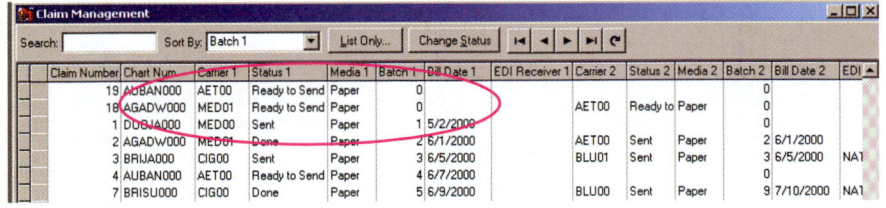

Figure J-41 ◆ The Status 1 column indicates which newly created claims are ready to send to insurance carriers.

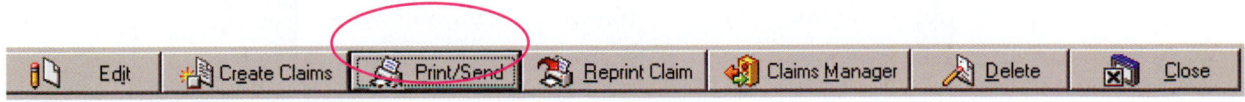

Figure J-42 ◆ Print/Send button at the bottom of the Claim Management window.

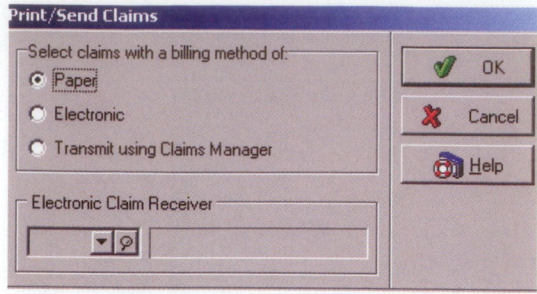

Figure J-43 ◆ Print/Send Claims window.

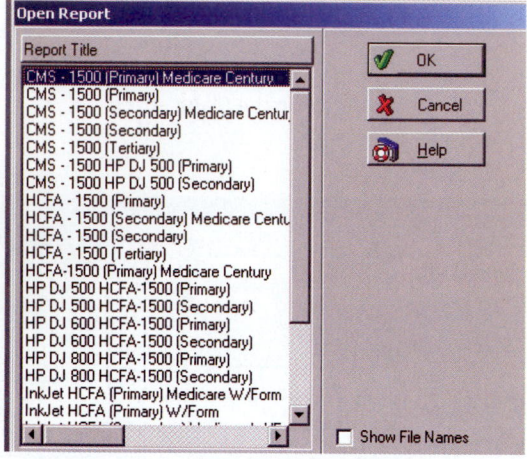

Figure J-44 ◆ Open Report window.

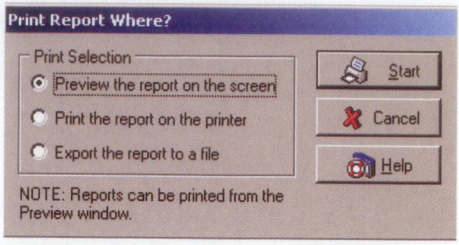

Figure J-45 ◆ Preview the report on the screen.

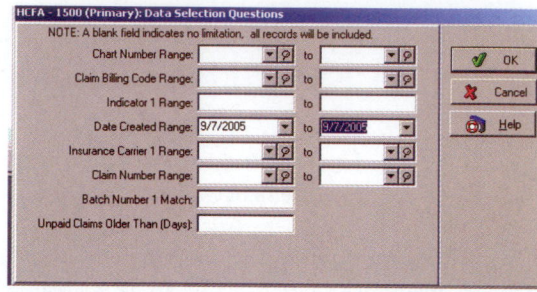

Figure J-46 ◆ Data Selection Questions dialog box.

claims to Medicare. After choosing the report style, click the OK button.

When the **Print Report Where?** window opens, choose to **Preview the report on the screen** and click Start (Figure J-45 ◆). You will look over the claims on the screen to be sure they are clean before printing.

A Data Selection Questions dialog box will open for you to choose which claims you want to preview. Use today's date in the **Date Created Range** fields. You can "filter" those claims you would like to review. Filtering is selecting certain criteria. For

example, you may choose to only review claims for a particular insurance carrier (e.g. Medicaid). In order to do that, you would select the name of the insurance carrier from the drop down menu from the Insurance Carrier 1 Range boxes. This would filter out all the other insurance carrier claims and only show you the claims for the carrier you chose from the drop down menu. You can filter claims by Chart Number Range, Claim Billing Code Range or Claim Number Range. After choosing your filters, click OK (Figure J-46 ◆). If you want to see all claims created, complete only the Date Created Range boxes.

The claims will be shown on the screen in the format you chose. Note that the CMS-1500 locator boxes will not actually show on the screen because they are instead printed on the blank claim form originals that you will insert into your printer when you're ready to print claims. However, you may want to refer to a blank printed claim form while checking your claims on screen to see if any information is missing (Figure J-47 ◆).

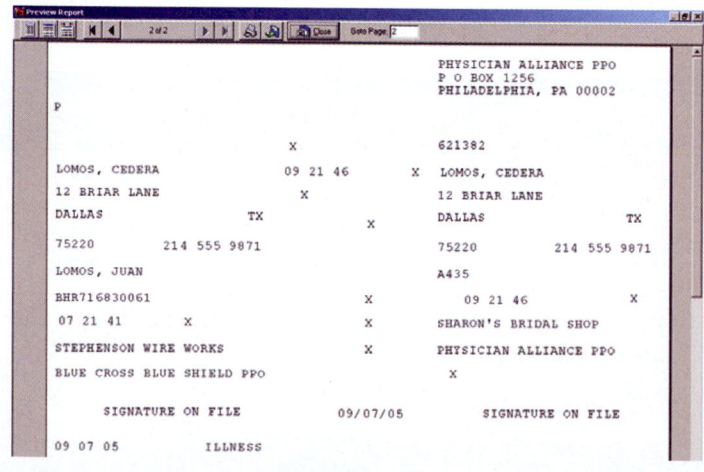

Figure J-47 ◆ Sample CMS-1500 Primary claim printed to screen. Note that the locator boxes do not show on screen.

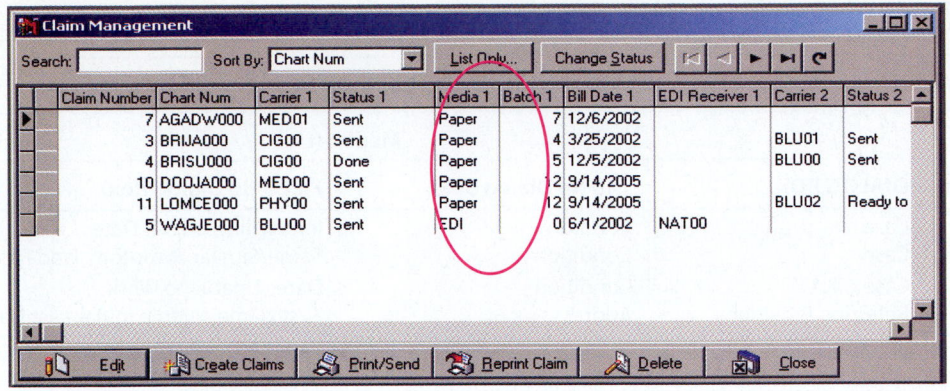

Figure J-48 ◆ Medisoft will update your Claim Management window to indicate that the claims have been sent.

Once you have checked all of your claims and corrected any mistakes if necessary, you are ready to print your claims on CMS-1500 forms that you have loaded into your printer's paper tray.

After you have printed your claims, Medisoft will update your Claim Management window (Status 1 column) to show that the claims have been sent (on paper or electronically) (Figure J-48 ◆).

Table J-1 shows the relationship between the form locators on the CMS-1500 claim form and the dialog boxes in Medisoft. If, when looking over the claim forms before printing, you notice data missing on the claim, consult this table to discern where to enter it in Medisoft.

TABLE J-1	PATIENT/GUARANTOR AND PROVIDER INFORMATION AND THE CMS-1500 FORM		
PATIENT / GUARANTOR INFORMATION AND THE CMS-1500 FORM			
	Medisoft		
CMS Form Locator	**DIALOG BOX**	**TAB (in Dialog Box)**	**FIELD (in Dialog Box)**
1	Insurance Carrier	Options	Type
1a	Case	Policy	Policy Number
2	Patient/Guarantor	Name, Address	Last Name, First Name, Middle Initial
3	Patient/Guarantor	Name, Address	Birth Date, Sex
4	Case	Policy	Policy Holder
5	Patient/Guarantor	Name, Address	Street, City, State, Zip Code, Phones
6	Case	Policy	Relationship to Insured
7	Patient/Guarantor	Name, Address	Street, City, State, ZIP Code, Phones
8	Case	Personal	Marital Status
8	Patient/Guarantor	Other Information	Employment Status
9	Patient/Guarantor	Name, Address	Last Name, First Name, Middle Initial
9a	Case	Policy	Policy Number
9b	Patient/Guarantor	Name, Address	Birth Date, Sex
9c	Patient/Guarantor	Other Information	Employer
9d	Insurance Carrier	Options	Plan Name
10a	Case	Condition	Employment Related
10b	Case	Condition	Accident Related To
10c	Case	Condition	Accident Related To
10d	Case	Miscellaneous	Local Use A, Local Use B
11	Case	Policy	Policy Number
11a	Patient/Guarantor	Name, Address	Birth Date, Sex
11b	Patient/Guarantor	Other Information	Employer
11c	Insurance Carrier	Options	Plan Name
11d	Case	Policy 2	Insurance 2
12	Patient/Guarantor	Other Information	Signature on File
13	Patient/Guarantor	Other Information	Signature on File

continued

TABLE J-1 PATIENT/GUARANTOR AND PROVIDER INFORMATION AND THE CMS-1500 FORM (CONTINUED)

PROVIDER INFORMATION AND THE CMS -1500 FORM

| CMS Form Locator | Medisoft | | |
	DIALOG BOX	TAB (in Dialog Box)	FIELD (in Dialog Box)
14	Case	Condition	Injury/Illness/LMP Date
15	Case	Condition	Same/Similar Symptoms and First Consultation Date
16	Case	Condition	Dates Unable to Work
17	Referring Provider	Address	First Name, Middle Initial, Last Name
17a	Referring Provider	NPI, Qualifiers, PINs, and IDs	Varies with carrier
17b			
18	Case	Condition	Hospitalization
19	Case	Miscellaneous	Local Use A, Local Use B
20	Case	Miscellaneous	Outside Lab Work and Lab Charges
21	Case	Diagnosis	Default Diagnosis 1–4
22	Case	Medicaid	Resubmission Number and Original Reference
23	Case	Miscellaneous	Prior Authorization Number
24A	Transaction Entry	Charge	Dates
24B	Procedure Code	General	Place of Service
24C	Emergency	Condition	Emergency check box
24D	Transaction Entry	Charge	Procedure and Modifiers
24E	Transaction Entry	Charge	Default Diagnosis 1–4
24F	Transaction Entry	Charge	Amount
24G	Transaction Entry	Charge	Units
24H	Case	Medicaid	EPSDT
24I	Provider	PINS	PINs/National Identifier
24J	List/Insurance Carrier List		
25	Provider	PINs and IDs	SSN/Federal Tax ID
26	Patient/Guarantor	Name, Address or Other Information	Chart Number or Patient ID #2
27	Case	Policy	Accept Assignment or Transaction Default
28	Transaction Entry	Charge	Amount
29	Transaction Entry	Payment	Amount
30	Transaction Entry		Case Balance
31	Provider	Address	Signature on File
32	Case	Account	Facility
33	Provider	PINs and IDs	Last Name, Middle Initial, First Name, Street, City, State, Zip Code, Phone

Medisoft Shortcut Buttons

The Shortcut Button toolbar is a quick way to navigate to the most commonly used windows/areas within Medisoft. As a helpful reminder, each button is labeled here with a brief description of what the window is used for.

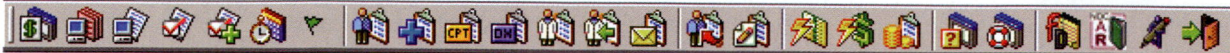

Transaction Entry—Use this window to post charges, payments, and adjustments in patient accounts.

Claim Management—Use this window to create, print, and send insurance claims.

Statement Management—Use this window to print and send statements.

Collection List—Use this window to check on open accounts that require collection follow-up and add tickler notes.

Add Collection List Items—Use this window to add multiple collection items at once to the Collection List based on specific criteria chosen from the screen.

Appointment Book—Use this window to set appointments for the practice's providers.

View Eligibility Verification Results—This feature allows the facility to check a patient's insurance coverage online. It is a fee-based service for which the facility must enroll.

Patient/Case (Guarantor) List—Use this window to add or edit patient, guarantor, or case information.

Insurance Carrier List—Use this window to add or edit insurance carriers in the Medisoft database.

Procedure Code List—Use this window to edit or add procedure, payment, or adjustment codes in the Medisoft database.

Diagnosis Code List—Use this window to add or edit diagnostic codes in the Medisoft database.

Provider List—Use this window to add or edit practice providers in the Medisoft database.

Referring Provider List—Use this window to add or edit names of physicians that refer patients to the practice.

Address List—Use this window to add or edit patient/guarantor, employer, attorney, or facility names to the Medisoft database.

Patient Recall List—Use this window to enter appointment recall information.

Custom Report List—Use this window to view every report choice in Medisoft database.

Quick Ledger—Use this window to quickly view any patient's full financial ledger.

Quick Balance—Use this window to view any patient's financial balance.

Enter Deposits and Apply Payments—Use this window as an alternative way to enter patient/guarantor or insurance payments to patients' accounts.

Show/Hide Hints

Medisoft Help Menu

Edit Patient Notes in Final Draft—If notes were entered anywhere in the system, they may be edited here.

Launch Advanced Reporting—Advanced Reporting provides users with enhanced reporting and data viewing capabilities including ad hoc reporting and a set of standard reports that may be customized by users with the report writer.

Launch Work Administrator—The Work Administrator program lets the staff streamline the work process. Use this feature to organize tasks for users and user groups.

Exit Medisoft Program

Medisoft Menus

Each Medisoft menu is shown here as a navigation reminder. Each menu was explained on page 1177.

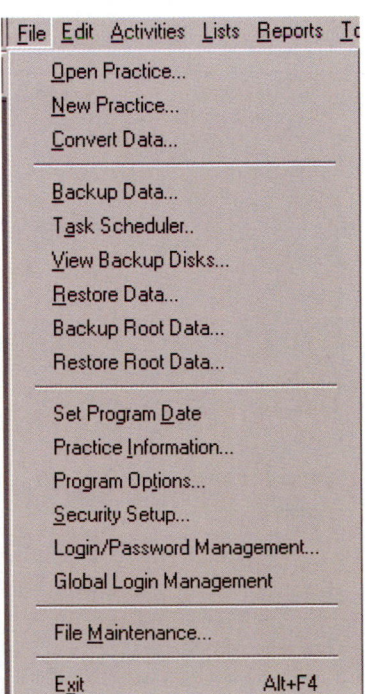

File menu.

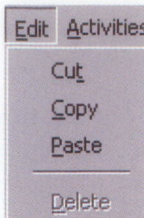

Edit menu.

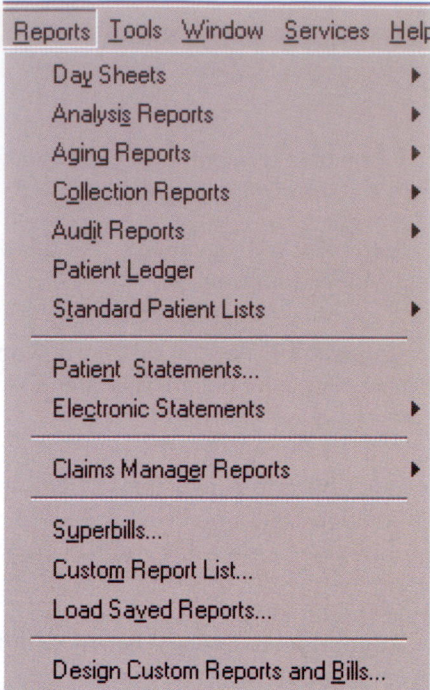

Reports menu.

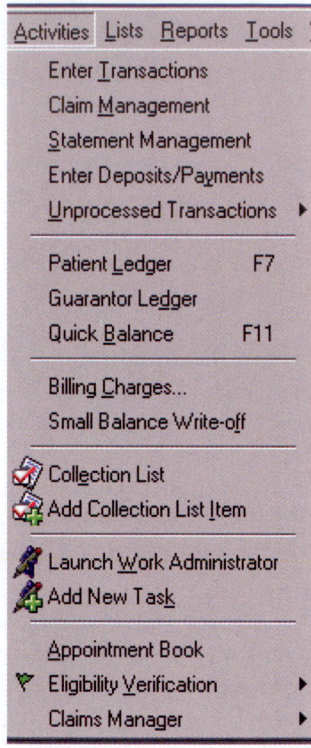

Activities menu.

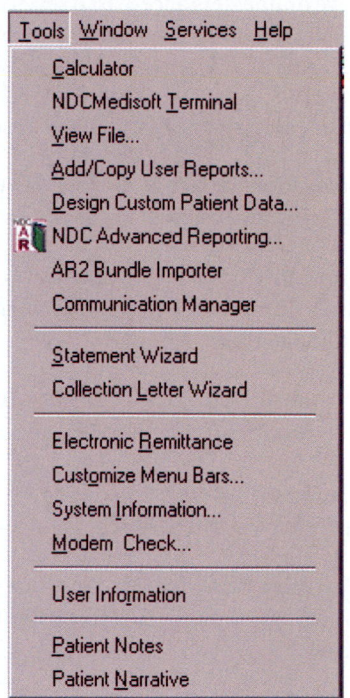

Tools menu.

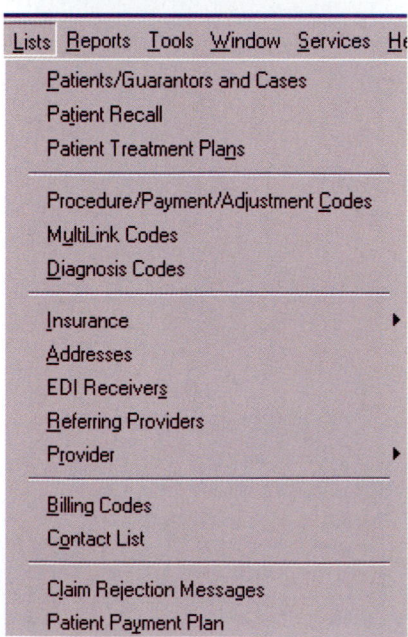

Lists menu.

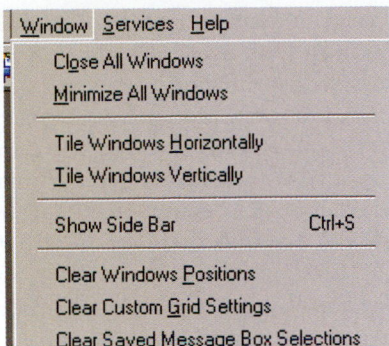

Window menu.

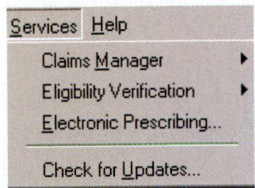

Services menu.

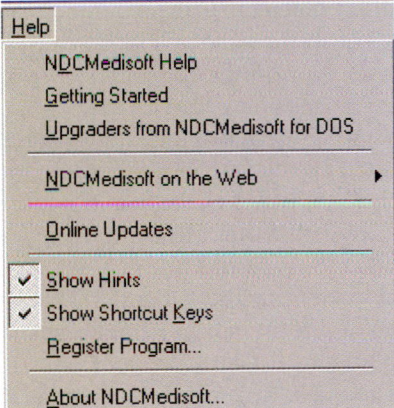

Help menu.

Medisoft Side Bar Shortcut Menus

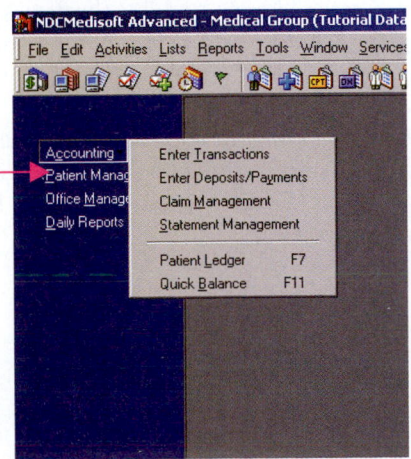

Accounting menu.

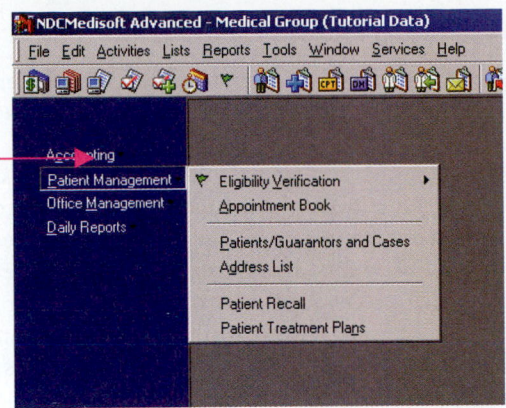

Patient Management menu.

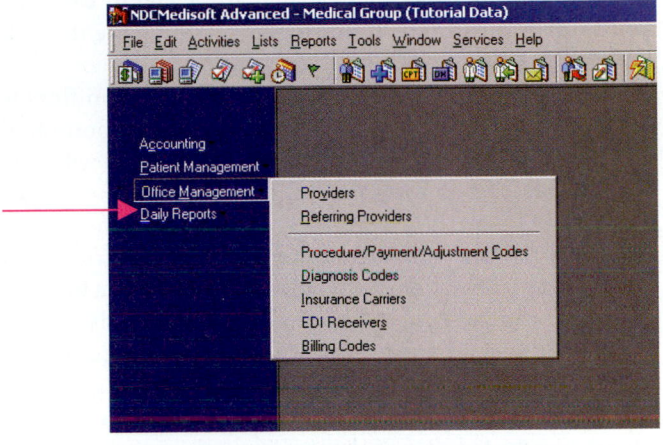

Office Management menu.

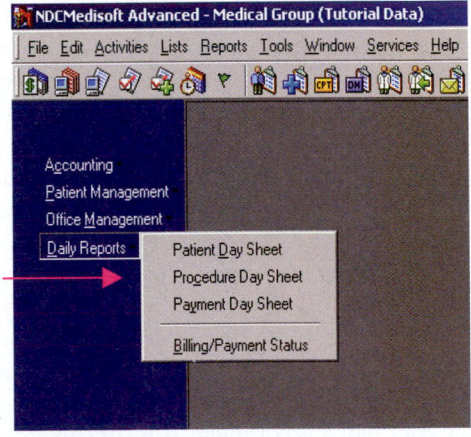

Daily Reports menu.

Simulation Instructions

Please use the patient information forms, encounter forms, and Explanation of Benefits forms located at the end of this appendix to complete this simulation exercise.

For this simulation, you are the medical business office specialist for your medical practice. It is your job to enter all patient demographic information, post charges, payments, and adjustments. **It is necessary to enter the ICD-9 and CPT codes and charges exactly as they appear on the superbills.** This may require you to enter them into the Medisoft database (as a new code) as well as the specific patient's account.

You are responsible for printing a walkout receipt for each patient's account to which you post charges. It is your responsibility to balance your batch at the end of each day and to print insurance claim forms for the patients with insurance.

Some patients may need to come back to the office for follow-up appointments. This will be noted at the bottom of the superbill. If a return appointment is needed, you will need to schedule the appointment for the patient (in Office Hours).

Before class ends each day, you may be instructed to stop posting transactions and "batch out." Access the **Reports** menu and run the **Patient Day Sheet** report for today's date. After printing your report, you will use it to make sure you "balance." To do this, you must separately add up all the charges, payments and adjustments from all the superbills (or EOBs) you posted during the day. Your charges should add up to the amount on the **Total Charges** line on the Patient Day Sheet report. Your payments should equal the negative amount on the **Total Receipts** line of the report, and your adjustments should match the **Total Adjustments** line. If the amounts you totaled from your superbills/EOBs do not match the report totals, you will need to go over the report patient by patient as you look at each patient superbill/EOB to find the discrepancy.

After you have balanced your totals, your instructor may require you to batch your superbills/EOBs and correct Patient Day Sheet report together and turn them in before you leave each day. If this is the case, it means you will have to remove or copy the superbills/EOBs you posted from your textbook. The Patient Day Sheet report is to be placed on top of your superbills/EOBs, followed by your walkout receipts, and stapled together.

Once your batch is complete, it is time to create insurance claims for the patients for whom you entered transaction information. Medisoft allows you to view your insurance claims on screen prior to printing them or sending them electronically. You must look over the claims on the computer screen to make sure there are no errors. If you find any errors, close the claims window and go back to the specific patient's account in the computer and correct it. The claim will automatically be updated with the corrected information. Check your electronic claim batch again to make sure all claims are correct. When you are sure there are no errors, print the claims.

Paper clip your CMS-1500 forms to the bottom of your batch material and turn it in to your instructor.

Tips for Entering Information into Medisoft Advanced

1. First, look over the patient information form. Check the Address List to see if the employer name is already listed in Medisoft. If it is not, add the employer to the Address List.
2. Check the Insurance Carrier List to see if the patient's primary and secondary insurance carrier is already listed in Medisoft. Remember the insurance carrier address must be **exactly the same** as what is written on the patient information form. If the carrier is not listed, add the carrier(s) to the Insurance Carrier List.
3. Check to see if the patient has a Referring Physician (or PCP) listed on the patient information form. If one is listed, check the Referring Provider List to see if the physician is already listed in Medisoft. If the provider is not listed, add the provider.
4. Add the patient to the Patient/Guarantor List if the patient is new. If the patient is not the guarantor, add the guarantor to the Patient/Guarantor List.
5. Make a new Case for the patient. Entering the employer, insurance carrier, and referring provider **prior** to making a patient case allows you to have all the data already entered when you come to the drop down menus (in the case and the patient/guarantor list) for employer, insurance carrier, etc. This saves the hassle of closing the patient case, opening the Address Book (or Insurance Carrier List, etc.), adding the data, saving and closing the window and then opening the patient case again.

Before beginning the simulation, you will need to enter your physician's information into the Medisoft database. Open the **Provider List** (accessed either by shortcut button or Lists menu) and click **New.**

Enter the following information in the *Address* folder in the window:

Your Name

1933 E. Frankford Rd. #110
Carrollton, TX 12345

office telephone: 972-555-5482
home phone: 214-555-8888

cell phone: 469-555-3657
fax: 972-555-5416

Medicare Participating,
Signature on File
Specialty: General Practice

License no.: B1740

In the *Default PINs* folder enter: 75-1234567 for Federal Tax ID Indicator

Medicare PIN: B94765   Medicaid: K89J2   UPIN: B94765

NPI: 1234569860

Be sure to save any data entered. All of the patients you enter during the simulation will be seeing you.

There are two more things to do before you begin. Open the File menu in Medisoft and click on Practice Information. Click in the Practice name box. Enter your name as Your Name Medical Clinic.

Click the Save button on the right side of the window.

Go the Address List and enter a new Facility. The facility will be Your Name Medical Clinic, with the address on Frankford Road that you entered for the Practice Name. Click Save and exit the Address List.

You are ready to begin the simulation.

Allied Medical Center
REGISTRATION FORM
(Please Print)

Today's date:		PCP:

PATIENT INFORMATION

Patient's last name: DUPONT	First: MARGARET	Middle: B	☐ Mr. ☒ Mrs.	☐ Miss ☐ Ms.	Marital status (circle one) Single / (Mar)/ Div / Sep / Wid

Is this your legal name? ☒ Yes ☐ No	If not, what is your legal name?	(Former name):	Birth date: 09/21/1946	Age:	Sex: ☐ M ☒ F

Street address: 12 BRIAR LANE		Social Security no.: 717-87-0054	Home phone no.: (214) 555-9871

P.O. box:	City: DALLAS	State: TX	ZIP Code: 12345

Occupation: MANAGER	Employer: SHARON'S BRIDAL SHOPPE	Employer phone no.: (214) 555-8878

Chose clinic because/Referred to clinic by (please check one box):	☐ Dr.	☒ Insurance Plan	☐ Hospital

☐ Family	☐ Friend	☐ Close to home/work	☐ Yellow Pages	Other

Other family members seen here: LISA DUPONT	**REASON FOR THIS VISIT:** Persistent cough

INSURANCE INFORMATION
(Please give your insurance card to the receptionist.)

Person responsible for bill: SELF	Birth date: / /	Address (if different):	Home phone no.: ( )

Is this person a patient here? ☒ Yes ☐ No

Occupation:	Employer:	Employer address:	Employer phone no.: ( )

Is this patient covered by insurance? ☒ Yes ☐ No

Please indicate primary insurance:	PHYSICIAN ALLIANCE PPO	Claims Mailing Address:	P O BOX 1256	Philadelphia, PA	12345
		PHONE: 800-555-5522			

Subscriber's name: SELF	Subscriber's S.S. no.:	Birth date: / /	☐ M ☐ F	Group no.: A435	Policy no.: 621382	Co-payment: $10.00

Patient's relationship to subscriber:	☒ Self	☐ Spouse	☐ Child	☐ Other

Name of secondary insurance (if applicable): BLUE CROSS BLUE SHIELD TX PPO	Subscriber's name and DOB: FRANK DUPONT 07/21/1941	☒ M ☐ F	Group no.: 126	Policy no.: BHR716830061

Patient's relationship to subscriber:	☐ Self	☒ Spouse	☐ Child	☐ Other Claims Mailing Address: P O BOX 660044 DALLAS 12345

IN CASE OF EMERGENCY

Name of local friend or relative (not living at same address): SHARON THELANER	Relationship to patient: SISTER	Home phone no.: (469) 555-3259	Work phone no.: (817) 555-8114

The above information is true to the best of my knowledge. I authorize my insurance benefits to be paid directly to the physician. I understand that I am financially responsible for any balance. I also authorize ALLIED MEDICAL CENTER or insurance company to release any information required to process my claims.

Maggie Dupont

_____
Patient/Guardian signature   *Date*

ENCOUNTER FORM

Patient Information		Payment Method		Visit Information	
Patient ID number		**Primary**		Visit date	
Patient name	Margaret Dupont	Primary ID number	621382	Visit number	
Address	12 Briar Lane	Primary group number	A435	Rendering physician	
City/State	Dallas, TX 12345	**Secondary**	BCBS TX	Referring physician	
Phone number	214-555-9871	Secondary ID number	BHR716830061	Reason for visit	Cough
Date of birth	09/21/1946	Secondary group no.	126		
Age		Cash/credit card			
		Other billing			

E/M Modifiers	Procedure Modifiers	DIAGNOSIS:
21 — Prolonged E&M Service	22 — Unusual, excessive procedure	
24 — Unrelated E/M service during postop.	50 — Bilateral procedure	ACUTE SINUSITIS 461.9
25 — Significant, separately identifiable E/M	51 — Multiple surgical procedures in same day	
32 — Mandated Service	52 — Reduced/incomplete procedure	
57 — Decision for surgery	55 — Postop. management only	
	59 — Distinct multiple procedures	

CATEGORY	CODE	MOD	FEE	CATEGORY	CODE	MOD	FEE
Office Visit — New Patient				**Wound Care**			
Minimal office visit	99201			Debride partial thickness burn	11040		
20 minutes	99202			Debride full thickness burn	11041		
30 minutes	99203			Debride wound, not a burn	11000		
45 minutes	99204	X	135.00	Unna boot application	29580		
60 minutes	99205			Unna boot removal	29700		
Other				Other			
Office Visit — Established				**Supplies**			
Minimal office visit	99211			Ace bandage, 2"	A6448		
10 minutes	99212			Ace bandage, 3"-4"	A6449		
15 minutes	99213			Ace bandage, 6"	A6450		
25 minutes	99214			Cast, fiberglass	A4590		
40 minutes	99215			Coban wrap	A6454		
Other				Foley catheter	A4338		
General Procedures				Immobilizer	L3670		
Anoscopy	46600			Kerlix roll	A6220		
Audiometry	92551			Oxygen mask/cannula	A4620		
Breast aspiration	19000			Sleeve, elbow	E0191		
Cerumen removal	69210			Sling	A4565		
Circumcision	54150			Splint, ready-made	A4570		
DDST	96110			Splint, wrist	S8451		
Flex sigmoidoscopy	45330			Sterile packing	A6407		
Flex sig. w/ biopsy	45331			Surgical tray	A4550		
Foreign body removal—foot	28190			Other			
Nail removal	11730			**OB Care**			
Nail removal/phenol	11750			Routine OB care	59400		
Trigger point injection	20552			Postpartum care only (separate procedure)	59430		
Tympanometry	92567			Ante partum 4–6 visits	59425		
Visual acuity	99173			Ante partum 7 or more visits	59426		
Other				Other			
Other				Other			

Other Visit Information: _____

Lab Work to Order: _____

Referral to: _____

Provider Signature: _____

Next Appointment: _____ RETURN IN A FEW DAYS IF NOT BETTER _____

Fees:

Total Charges: $135.00

Copay Received: $ 10.00

Other Payment: $_____

Total Due: **$125.00**

Allied Medical Center 1933 E.Frankford Rd. Carrollton, TX 12345 **972-555-5482**

Allied Medical Center
REGISTRATION FORM
(Please Print)

Today's date: _____   PCP: _____

PATIENT INFORMATION

Patient's last name: SMYTH	First: SAMANTHA	Middle: M	☐ Mr. ☐ Mrs.	☐ Miss ☐ Ms.	Marital status (circle one) (Single)/ Mar / Div / Sep / Wid

Is this your legal name? ☐ Yes ☐ No	If not, what is your legal name?	(Former name):	Birth date: 03/17/1968	Age:	Sex: ☐ M ☒ F

Street address: 9401 Winding Valley	Social Security no.: 455-94-8204	Home phone no.: (972) 555-9871

P.O. box:	City: PLANO	State: TX	ZIP Code: 12345

Occupation: FOOD SERVER	Employer: WENDY'S HAMBURGERS	Employer phone no.: (972) 555-8936

Chose clinic because/Referred to clinic by (please check one box):	☐ Dr.	☐ Insurance Plan	☐ Hospital

☐ Family	☐ Friend	☐ Close to home/work	☐ Yellow Pages	Other

Other family members seen here: _____

REASON FOR THIS VISIT: Cholesterol check

INSURANCE INFORMATION

(Please give your insurance card to the receptionist.)

Person responsible for bill: SAMANTHA SMYTH	Birth date: 03/17/1968	Address (if different): Same	Home phone no.: ( )

Is this person a patient here?   ☐ Yes   ☐ No

Occupation:	Employer:	Employer address:	Employer phone no.: ( )

Is this patient covered by insurance?   ☐ Yes   ☐ No

Please indicate primary insurance:	NONE	Claims Mailing Address:	
		PHONE:	

Subscriber's name:	Subscriber's S.S. no.:	Birth date: / /	☐ M ☐ F	Group no.:	Policy no.:	Co-payment: $

Patient's relationship to subscriber:	☐ Self	☐ Spouse	☐ Child	☐ Other

Name of secondary insurance (if applicable):	Subscriber's name and DOB:	☐ M ☐ F	Group no.:	Policy no.:

Patient's relationship to subscriber:	☐ Self	☐ Spouse	☐ Child	☐ Other Claims Mailing Address:

IN CASE OF EMERGENCY

Name of local friend or relative (not living at same address): CARRIE TINKHAM	Relationship to patient: FRIEND	Home phone no.: (972) 555-1502	Work phone no.: (972) 555-0074

The above information is true to the best of my knowledge. I authorize my insurance benefits to be paid directly to the physician. I understand that I am financially responsible for any balance. I also authorize ALLIED MEDICAL CENTER or insurance company to release any information required to process my claims.

Samantha Smyth

_____   _____
Patient/Guardian signature   Date

ENCOUNTER FORM

Patient Information		Payment Method		Visit Information	
Patient ID number		**Primary**		Visit date	
Patient name	Samantha Smyth	Primary ID number		Visit number	
Address	9401 Winding Valley	Primary group number		Rendering physician	
City/State	Plano, TX 12345	**Secondary**		Referring physician	
Phone number	972-555-9871	Secondary ID number		Reason for visit	Cholesterol Check
Date of birth	03/17/1968	Secondary group no.			
Age		Cash/credit card	CHECK		
		Other billing			

E/M Modifiers	Procedure Modifiers	DIAGNOSIS:
21 — Prolonged E&M Service	22 — Unusual, excessive procedure	Hypercholesteremia 272.00
24 — Unrelated E/M service during postop.	50 — Bilateral procedure	
25 — Significant, separately identifiable E/M	51 — Multiple surgical procedures in same day	
32 — Mandated Service	52 — Reduced/incomplete procedure	
57 — Decision for surgery	55 — Postop. management only	
	59 — Distinct multiple procedures	

CATEGORY	CODE	MOD	FEE	CATEGORY	CODE	MOD	FEE
Office Visit — New Patient				**Wound Care**			
Minimal office visit	99201			Debride partial thickness burn	11040		
20 minutes	99202			Debride full thickness burn	11041		
30 minutes	99203			Debride wound, not a burn	11000		
45 minutes	99204			Unna boot application	29580		
60 minutes	99205			Unna boot removal	29700		
Other				Other			
Office Visit — Established				**Supplies**			
Minimal office visit	99211			Ace bandage, 2"	A6448		
10 minutes	99212	X	35.00	Ace bandage, 3"–4"	A6449		
15 minutes	99213			Ace bandage, 6"	A6450		
25 minutes	99214			Cast, fiberglass	A4590		
40 minutes	99215			Coban wrap	A6454		
Other				Foley catheter	A4338		
General Procedures				Immobilizer	L3670		
Anoscopy	46600			Kerlix roll	A6220		
Audiometry	92551			Oxygen mask/cannula	A4620		
Breast aspiration	19000			Sleeve, elbow	E0191		
Cerumen removal	69210			Sling	A4565		
Circumcision	54150			Splint, ready-made	A4570		
DDST	96110			Splint, wrist	S8451		
Flex sigmoidoscopy	45330			Sterile packing	A6407		
Flex sig. w/ biopsy	45331			Surgical tray	A4550		
Foreign body removal—foot	28190			Other			
Nail removal	11730			OB Care			
Nail removal/phenol	11750			Routine OB care	59400		
Trigger point injection	20552			Postpartum care only (separate procedure)	59430		
Tympanometry	92567			Ante partum 4–6 visits	59425		
Visual acuity	99173			Ante partum 7 or more visits	59426		
Other	82465	X	30.00	Other			
Other				Other			

Other Visit Information:_____

Lab Work to Order:_____

Referral to: _____

Provider Signature: _____

Next Appointment:_____ RETURN IN A FEW DAYS IF NOT BETTER _____

Fees:

Total Charges: $65.00

Copay Received: $_____

Other Payment: $65.00 CK #1235

Total Due: $0

Allied Medical Center
REGISTRATION FORM
(Please Print)

Today's date: _____   PCP: _____

PATIENT INFORMATION

Patient's last name: BAILEY	First: EILEEN	Middle: B	❑ Mr. ❑ Mrs.	❑ Miss ❑ Ms.	Marital status (circle one) Single / Mar / Div / Sep / (Wid)

Is this your legal name? ❑ Yes ❑ No	If not, what is your legal name?	(Former name): EILEEN STANFORD	Birth date: 04/26/1961	Age:	Sex: ❑ M ❑ F

Street address: 2531 BENT TREE COURT	Social Security no.: 555-63-2112	Home phone no.: (972) 555-6058

P.O. box:	City: DALLAS	State: TX	ZIP Code: 12345

Occupation: SUPERVISOR	Employer: DISCOUNT COMPUTER WAREHOUSE	Employer phone no.: (972) 555-6577

Chose clinic because/Referred to clinic by (please check one box): ❑ Dr. ❑ Insurance Plan ❑ Hospital

❑ Family ❑ Friend ❑ Close to home/work ❑ Yellow Pages Other

Other family members seen here: _____

REASON FOR THIS VISIT: Yearly Physical

INSURANCE INFORMATION
(Please give your insurance card to the receptionist.)

Person responsible for bill: EILEEN BAILEY	Birth date: / /	Address (if different): Same	Home phone no.: ( )

Is this person a patient here? ❑ Yes ❑ No

Occupation:	Employer:	Employer address:	Employer phone no.: ( )

Is this patient covered by insurance? ❑ Yes ❑ No

Please indicate primary insurance:	PHYSICIAN CHOICE EPO	Claims Mailing Address:	P O BOX 9873	Dover, OH	12345
		PHONE: 800-555-8637			

Subscriber's name: EILEEN BAILEY	Subscriber's S.S. no.: 555-63-2112	Birth date: 04/26/1961	❑ M ❑ F	Group no.: K1047	Policy no.: 13056	Co-payment: $

Patient's relationship to subscriber: ❑ Self ❑ Spouse ❑ Child ❑ Other

Name of secondary insurance (if applicable):	Subscriber's name and DOB:	❑ M ❑ F	Group no.:	Policy no.:

Patient's relationship to subscriber: ❑ Self ❑ Spouse ❑ Child ❑ Other   Claims Mailing Address:

IN CASE OF EMERGENCY

Name of local friend or relative (not living at same address): MALCOLM JOHNSON	Relationship to patient: FRIEND	Home phone no.: (214) 555-5277	Work phone no.: (214) 555-8788

The above information is true to the best of my knowledge. I authorize my insurance benefits to be paid directly to the physician. I understand that I am financially responsible for any balance. I also authorize ALLIED MEDICAL CENTER or insurance company to release any information required to process my claims.

Eileen Bailey

_____   _____
Patient/Guardian signature   Date

ENCOUNTER FORM

Patient Information		Payment Method		Visit Information	
Patient ID number		**Primary**	Physician's Choice EPO	Visit date	
Patient name	Eileen Bailey	Primary ID number	13056	Visit number	
Address	2531 Bent Tree Ct	Primary group number	K1047	Rendering physician	
City/State	Dallas, TX 12345	**Secondary**		Referring physician	
Phone number	972-555-6058	Secondary ID number		Reason for visit	Yearly Physical
Date of birth	04/26/1961	Secondary group no.			
Age		Cash/credit card	CHECK		
		Other billing			

E/M Modifiers	Procedure Modifiers	DIAGNOSIS:
21 — Prolonged E&M Service	22 — Unusual, excessive procedure	Routine Exam V70.0
24 — Unrelated E/M service during postop.	50 — Bilateral procedure	
25 — Significant, separately identifiable E/M	51 — Multiple surgical procedures in same day	
32 — Mandated Service	52 — Reduced/incomplete procedure	
57 — Decision for surgery	55 — Postop. management only	
	59 — Distinct multiple procedures	

CATEGORY	CODE	MOD	FEE	CATEGORY	CODE	MOD	FEE
Office Visit — New Patient				**Wound Care**			
Minimal office visit	99201			Debride partial thickness burn	11040		
20 minutes	99202			Debride full thickness burn	11041		
30 minutes	99203			Debride wound, not a burn	11000		
45 minutes	99204			Unna boot application	29580		
60 minutes	99205	X	160.00	Unna boot removal	29700		
Other				Other			
Office Visit — Established				**Supplies**			
Minimal office visit	99211			Ace bandage, 2"	A6448		
10 minutes	99212			Ace bandage, 3"-4"	A6449		
15 minutes	99213			Ace bandage, 6"	A6450		
25 minutes	99214			Cast, fiberglass	A4590		
40 minutes	99215			Coban wrap	A6454		
Other				Foley catheter	A4338		
General Procedures				Immobilizer	L3670		
Anoscopy	46600			Kerlix roll	A6220		
Audiometry	92551			Oxygen mask/cannula	A4620		
Breast aspiration	19000			Sleeve, elbow	E0191		
Cerumen removal	69210			Sling	A4565		
Circumcision	54150			Splint, ready-made	A4570		
DDST	96110			Splint, wrist	S8451		
Flex sigmoidoscopy	45330			Sterile packing	A6407		
Flex sig. w/ biopsy	45331			Surgical tray	A4550		
Foreign body removal—foot	28190			Other			
Nail removal	11730			OB Care			
Nail removal/phenol	11750			Routine OB care	59400		
Trigger point injection	20552			Postpartum care only (separate procedure)	59430		
Tympanometry	92567			Ante partum 4–6 visits	59425		
Visual acuity	99173			Ante partum 7 or more visits	59426		
Other	82465			Other			
Other				Other			

Other Visit Information:_____
Lab Work to Order:_____
Referral to: _____
Provider Signature: _____
Next Appointment:_____ AS NEEDED _____

Fees:
Total Charges: $160.00
Copay Received: $ 32.00
Other Payment: $_____
Total Due: **$128.00**

Allied Medical Center
REGISTRATION FORM
(Please Print)

Today's date:	PCP:

PATIENT INFORMATION

Patient's last name: CATHER	First: JIM	Middle: S	☐ Mr. ☐ Mrs.	☐ Miss ☐ Ms.	Marital status (circle one) Single / (Mar) / Div / Sep / Wid		
Is this your legal name? ☒ Yes ☐ No	If not, what is your legal name? JAMES CATHER		(Former name):	Birth date: 10/01/1953	Age:	Sex: ☐ M ☐ F	
Street address: 425 LAVENDER STREET			Social Security no.: 188-38-3833		Home phone no.: (972) 555-3394		
P.O. box:	City: GARLAND		State: TX		ZIP Code: 12345		
Occupation: SALESPERSON	Employer: MERRY MILER VANS		Employer phone no.: (972) 555-3337				

Chose clinic because/Referred to clinic by (please check one box):	☒ Dr. LESLIE MCNEICE	☐ Insurance Plan	☐ Hospital
☐ Family ☐ Friend ☐ Close to home/work ☐ Yellow Pages	Other **AUTH # A569874, 30 DAYS, 3 VISITS**		

Other family members seen here:	
	REASON FOR THIS VISIT: Hyperglycemia check up

INSURANCE INFORMATION
(Please give your insurance card to the receptionist.)

Person responsible for bill: JIM CATHER	Birth date: / /	Address (if different): SAME	Home phone no.: ( )
Is this person a patient here? ☐ Yes ☐ No			
Occupation:	Employer:	Employer address:	Employer phone no.: ( )
Is this patient covered by insurance? ☐ Yes ☐ No			

Please indicate primary insurance:	PHYSICIAN ALLIANCE HMO	Claims Mailing Address:	P O BOX 65	TOLEDO, OH	12345
	PHONE: 800-555-9865				

Subscriber's name: SAME AS PATIENT	Subscriber's S.S. no.: 188-38-3833	Birth date: / /	☐ M ☐ F	Group no.: 145	Policy no.: 188383833	Co-payment: $25.00
Patient's relationship to subscriber:	☐ Self	☐ Spouse	☐ Child	☐ Other		

Name of secondary insurance (if applicable):	Subscriber's name and DOB:	☐ M ☐ F	Group no.:	Policy no.:
Patient's relationship to subscriber: ☐ Self ☐ Spouse ☐ Child ☐ Other	Claims Mailing Address:			

IN CASE OF EMERGENCY

Name of local friend or relative (not living at same address): MARILYN CATHER	Relationship to patient: SIBLING	Home phone no.: (214) 555-3329	Work phone no.: (469) 555-8200

The above information is true to the best of my knowledge. I authorize my insurance benefits to be paid directly to the physician. I understand that I am financially responsible for any balance. I also authorize ALLIED MEDICAL CENTER or insurance company to release any information required to process my claims.

Jim Cather

Patient/Guardian signature	*Date*

ENCOUNTER FORM

Patient Information		Payment Method		Visit Information	
Patient ID number		**Primary**	Physician's Alliance HMO	Visit date	
Patient name	Jim Cather	Primary ID number	188383833	Visit number	
Address	425 Lavender St	Primary group number	145	Rendering physician	
City/State	Garland, TX 12345	**Secondary**		Referring physician	Leslie McNeice
Phone number	972-555-3394	Secondary ID number		Reason for visit	Hyperglyc-emia CK
Date of birth	10/01/1953	Secondary group no.			
Age		Cash/credit card			
		Other billing			

E/M Modifiers	Procedure Modifiers	DIAGNOSIS:
21 — Prolonged E&M Service	22 — Unusual, excessive procedure	Hyperglycemia 790.6
24 — Unrelated E/M service during postop.	50 — Bilateral procedure	
25 — Significant, separately identifiable E/M	51 — Multiple surgical procedures in same day	
32 — Mandated Service	52 — Reduced/incomplete procedure	
57 — Decision for surgery	55 — Postop. management only	
	59 — Distinct multiple procedures	

CATEGORY	CODE	MOD	FEE	CATEGORY	CODE	MOD	FEE
Office Visit — New Patient				**Wound Care**			
Minimal office visit	99201			Debride partial thickness burn	11040		
20 minutes	99202			Debride full thickness burn	11041		
30 minutes	99203			Debride wound, not a burn	11000		
45 minutes	99204			Unna boot application	29580		
60 minutes	99205			Unna boot removal	29700		
Other				Other			
Office Visit — Established				**Supplies**			
Minimal office visit	99211			Ace bandage, 2"	A6448		
10 minutes	99212			Ace bandage, 3"-4"	A6449		
15 minutes	99213			Ace bandage, 6"	A6450		
25 minutes	99214	X	65.00	Cast, fiberglass	A4590		
40 minutes	99215			Coban wrap	A6454		
Other				Foley catheter	A4338		
General Procedures				Immobilizer	L3670		
Anoscopy	46600			Kerlix roll	A6220		
Audiometry	92551			Oxygen mask/cannula	A4620		
Breast aspiration	19000			Sleeve, elbow	E0191		
Cerumen removal	69210			Sling	A4565		
Circumcision	54150			Splint, ready-made	A4570		
DDST	96110			Splint, wrist	S8451		
Flex sigmoidoscopy	45330			Sterile packing	A6407		
Flex sig. w/ biopsy	45331			Surgical tray	A4550		
Foreign body removal—foot	28190			Other			
Nail removal	11730			**OB Care**			
Nail removal/phenol	11750			Routine OB care	59400		
Trigger point injection	20552			Postpartum care only (separate procedure)	59430		
Tympanometry	92567			Ante partum 4–6 visits	59425		
Visual acuity	99173			Ante partum 7 or more visits	59426		
Other	93000	X	45.00	Other			
Other	82954	X	12.00	Other			

Other Visit Information: _____

Lab Work to Order: _____

Referral to: _____

Provider Signature: _____

Next Appointment: _____

Fees:

Total Charges: $122.00

Copay Received: $ 25.00

Other Payment: $ _____

Total Due: $ 97.00

Allied Medical Center 1933 E.Frankford Rd. Carrollton, TX 12345 **972-555-5482**

Allied Medical Center
REGISTRATION FORM
(Please Print)

Today's date: _____ PCP: _____

PATIENT INFORMATION

Patient's last name: BAE	First: YONG	Middle: JOON	☒ Mr. ☐ Mrs.	☐ Miss ☐ Ms.	Marital status (circle one) Single / (Mar) / Div / Sep / Wid

Is this your legal name? ☒ Yes ☐ No	If not, what is your legal name?	(Former name):	Birth date: 02/23/1972	Age:	Sex: ☒ M ☐ F

Street address: 4549 EXPLORER DRIVE #110	Social Security no.: 661-39-2520	Home phone no.: (469) 555-0719

P.O. box:	City: FRISCO	State: TX	ZIP Code: 12345

Occupation: SUPERVISOR	Employer: SUGARLAND DAIRY FARM	Employer phone no.: (903) 555-8663

Chose clinic because/Referred to clinic by (please check one box):	☒ Dr. MALCOLM MAZOW	☐ Insurance Plan	☐ Hospital

☐ Family	☐ Friend	☐ Close to home/work	☐ Yellow Pages	Other **REFERRAL # FOR TODAY–1644401**

Other family members seen here:

REASON FOR THIS VISIT: Shoulder Pain

INSURANCE INFORMATION
(Please give your insurance card to the receptionist.)

Person responsible for bill: PATIENT	Birth date: / /	Address (if different): SAME	Home phone no.: ( )

Is this person a patient here? ☒ Yes ☐ No

Occupation:	Employer:	Employer address:	Employer phone no.: ( )

Is this patient covered by insurance? ☒ Yes ☐ No

Please indicate primary insurance:	METLIFE HMO	Claims Mailing Address:	P O BOX 6983	NEWARK, DE	12345

PHONE: 800-555-6897

Subscriber's name: SELF	Subscriber's S.S. no.: 661-39-2520	Birth date: / /	☐ M ☐ F	Group no.: 62440	Policy no.: 661392520-01	Co-payment: $10.00

Patient's relationship to subscriber: ☒ Self ☐ Spouse ☐ Child ☐ Other

Name of secondary insurance (if applicable):	Subscriber's name and DOB:	☐ M ☐ F	Group no.:	Policy no.:

Patient's relationship to subscriber: ☐ Self ☐ Spouse ☐ Child ☐ Other   Claims Mailing Address:

IN CASE OF EMERGENCY

Name of local friend or relative (not living at same address): YUJIN JEONG	Relationship to patient: MOTHER	Home phone no.: (214) 650-9801	Work phone no.: ( )

The above information is true to the best of my knowledge. I authorize my insurance benefits to be paid directly to the physician. I understand that I am financially responsible for any balance. I also authorize ALLIED MEDICAL CENTER or insurance company to release any information required to process my claims.

Yong Joon Bae

Patient/Guardian signature   _Date_

ENCOUNTER FORM

Patient Information		Payment Method		Visit Information	
Patient ID number		**Primary**	MetLife HMO	Visit date	
Patient name	Yong Joon Bae	Primary ID number	661392520-01	Visit number	
Address	4549 Explorer Dr	Primary group number	62440	Rendering physician	
City/State	Frisco, TX 12345	**Secondary**		Referring physician	Malcolm Mazow
Phone number	469-555-0719	Secondary ID number		Reason for visit	Shoulder Pain
Date of birth	02/23/1972	Secondary group no.		Auth # for today: 1644401	
Age		Cash/credit card			
		Other billing			

E/M Modifiers	Procedure Modifiers	DIAGNOSIS:
21 — Prolonged E&M Service	22 — Unusual, excessive procedure	Bursitis, Shoulder 726.10
24 — Unrelated E/M service during postop.	50 — Bilateral procedure	
25 — Significant, separately identifiable E/M	51 — Multiple surgical procedures in same day	
32 — Mandated Service	52 — Reduced/incomplete procedure	
57 — Decision for surgery	55 — Postop. management only	
	59 — Distinct multiple procedures	

CATEGORY	CODE	MOD	FEE	CATEGORY	CODE	MOD	FEE
Office Visit — New Patient				**Wound Care**			
Minimal office visit	99201			Debride partial thickness burn	11040		
20 minutes	99202			Debride full thickness burn	11041		
30 minutes	99203			Debride wound, not a burn	11000		
45 minutes	99204			Unna boot application	29580		
60 minutes	99205			Unna boot removal	29700		
Other				Other			
Office Visit — Established				**Supplies**			
Minimal office visit	99211			Ace bandage, 2"	A6448		
10 minutes	99212			Ace bandage, 3"-4"	A6449		
15 minutes	99213	X	45.00	Ace bandage, 6"	A6450		
25 minutes	99214			Cast, fiberglass	A4590		
40 minutes	99215			Coban wrap	A6454		
Other				Foley catheter	A4338		
General Procedures				Immobilizer	L3670		
Anoscopy	46600			Kerlix roll	A6220		
Audiometry	92551			Oxygen mask/cannula	A4620		
Breast aspiration	19000			Sleeve, elbow	E0191		
Cerumen removal	69210			Sling	A4565		
Circumcision	54150			Splint, ready-made	A4570		
DDST	96110			Splint, wrist	S8451		
Flex sigmoidoscopy	45330			Sterile packing	A6407		
Flex sig. w/ biopsy	45331			Surgical tray	A4550		
Foreign body removal—foot	28190			Other			
Nail removal	11730			OB Care			
Nail removal/phenol	11750			Routine OB care	59400		
Trigger point injection	20552			Postpartum care only (separate procedure)	59430		
Tympanometry	92567			Ante partum 4–6 visits	59425		
Visual acuity	99173			Ante partum 7 or more visits	59426		
Other				Other			
Other				Other			

Other Visit Information:_____

Lab Work to Order:_____

Referral to: _____

Provider Signature: _____

Next Appointment:_____

Fees:

Total Charges: $45.00

Copay Received: $10.00

Other Payment: $_____

Total Due: **$35.00**

Allied Medical Center 1933 E.Frankford Rd. Carrollton, TX 12345 **972-555-5482**

Source: Adapted from Vines, Deborah, Braceland, Ann, Rollins, Elizabeth, and Miller, Susan. *Comprehensive Health Insurance: Billing, Coding, and Reimbursement.* © 2008. Pearson Education. Upper Saddle River, NJ.

abrasion (ah-BRAY-zhun)—open wound in which the outer layer of skin is scraped away, leaving underlying tissue exposed.

absorption (ab-SORP-shun)—passage of digested food products through the wall of the intestine into the bloodstream.

abstract—the process of locating data in multiple source documents and accurately transferring it to a form.

abuse—improper behavior and billing practices that result in financial gain but are not fraudulent.

accept assignment—physician agrees to accept the amount approved by the insurance company as payment in full for a given service.

accommodation (ah-kom-oh-DAY-shun)—the adjustment of the lens of the eye to various distances.

accounts receivable—the amount of money that is owed to the medical practice.

accredited—the process of becoming accredited with an overseeing agency. Accredited programs must provide education along the guidelines of the agency that offers the accreditation. In medical assisting, being accredited allows a program to bestow a certificate in medical assisting to the graduate.

Accrediting Bureau of Health Education School—accrediting agency offering medical assistant education programs the ability to offer a certified medical assisting certificate.

active patient files—normally refers to patient files for patients who currently have appointments to be seen, or who have been in to see the physician recently.

acuity (ah-KYOO-ih-tee)—keenness or sharpness.

acupuncture—a procedure adapted from Chinese medicine in which needles are inserted into various areas of the body for therapeutic purposes.

acute (ah-KYOOT)—sharp, severe, sudden; having a sudden onset and usually of short duration.

acyanotic (A-sigh-ah-NOH-tik)—pertaining to an absence of cyanosis.

ADA form—the standard billing form from the American Dental Association for use in billing for dental services.

add-on code—a CPT code designated by the plus sign (+) that cannot be used alone; must be used together with another CPT code.

addendum—something that has been added on to a patient's medical record after the date of the visit.

addiction (ah-DICK-shun)—repetitive and dependent behavior usually involving legal or illegal substance abuse.

administrative—pertaining to office functions (e.g., computer operation, medical records management, coding and billing).

administrative duties—medical assisting duties such as computer applications, medical records management, coding and billing, and medical law and ethics.

administrative law—laws that are passed by governmental agencies.

advance beneficiary notice—a form patients sign agreeing to pay for covered Medicare services that may be denied due to medical necessity or frequency.

Advance Beneficiary Notice (ABN)—also known as a waiver, this form must be signed by any Medicare recipient prior to a physician performing services that may not be covered by Medicare. If this form is not signed, physicians may not bill the patient for the services.

advance directives—documents outlining a patient's wishes regarding healthcare in the event the patient is unable to speak for themselves.

adverse outcome—a treatment outcome that is different (worse) than what was expected.

adverse reaction—unexpected or dangerous reaction to a drug.

advocate—standing up for the rights of another.

aerobe—organism able to survive and grow only in the presence of oxygen.

affect—emotional expression associated with facial and body behaviors.

afferent nerves (AFF-er-ent)—sensory nerves that carry impulses to the central nervous system.

agenda—a schedule or list of items to be addressed during a meeting.

aging report—a report showing how much money is owed to the medical practice and how long those accounts have been outstanding.

aiquot—representative sample of a well-mixed specimen.

alimentary canal (al-ih-MEN-tar-ree)—tube-like structure of the gastrointestinal system that originates in the mouth and terminates at the anus.

alimentation (al-ih-MEN-tay-shun)—entire process of providing nourishment to the body that includes mastication, swallowing, digestion, and absorption.

allergen (ah-LER-jin)—substance that is not necessarily harmful, such as dust or eggs, but that produces a hypersensitive reaction in some individuals.

allowed amount—the dollar amount for a service that an insurance company considers acceptable and uses to determine benefit payments; also called approved amount.

alphabetic index—alphabetical listing of CPT codes by procedure name, condition, eponym, and acronym.

alternative medicine—systems of medical options varying from traditional medicine, chosen by individuals in place of regularly prescribed modalities and including certain diagnostic procedures and/or accepted and regularly prescribed treatment modalities; examples are aromatherapy, massage therapy, acupuncture, faith healing, and Therapeutic touch.

Ambu bag—bag-valve-mask unit used to provide ventilation to a non-breathing patient or to assist ventilations for a patient whose breathing (respiratory effort) is inadequate to support life.

ambulatory care centers—healthcare clinics where patients are seen for short visits.

American Association of Medical Assistants (AAMA)—national professional association for medical assistants.

American Medical Technologists (AMT)—professional association for individuals who work as medical technologists.

American Red Cross—humanitarian organization that provides emergency assistance, including disaster relief, inside the United States.

Americans with Disabilities Act—federal law that outlines how patients or employees with disabilities must be treated or accommodated.

amino acids (ah-MEE-no)—chief components of protein, synthesized in the body and obtained from the diet.

amniocentesis (am-nee-oh-sen-TEE-sis)—procedure in which a needle is inserted into the amniotic sac to withdraw amniotic fluid for testing; used to identify genetic abnormalities, often neural tube deficits and Down syndrome, in the fetus; also used to determine the sex of the fetus.

amphiarthrosis (am-fee-ARTH-roh-sis)—condition of slight joint movement in all directions.

amplitude (am-plih-tood)—abundance, amount, extent, fullness, or size.

anaerobe—organism that survives and grows in the absence of oxygen.

analgesic (an-al-JEE-zik)—pain reducing.

anaphylaxis(an-ah-fih-LAK-sis)—severe allergic reaction.

anastomosis(ah-nas-toh-MOH-sis)—surgical joining of two tubular structures.

anatomy—the study of the structure and organization of living organisms.

ancillary coverage—insurance coverage for services provided by other than a physician or hospital, such as dental, vision, or chiropractic care.

and—interpreted as *either/and/or* in a diagnostic code description.

anesthesia (an-ess-THEE-zee-ah)—partial or complete loss of sensation.

aneurysm (AN-yoo-rizm)—weakening and dilation of an artery.

angina (AN-jeye-nah)—left-sided chest pain brought on by exertion.

angiography (AN-jee-awg-rah-fee)—radiograph of the vessels usually with contrast medium.

angioplasty (AN-jee-oh-plas-tee)—procedure in which a balloon on the distal aspect of a cardiac catheter is inflated to compress plaque against coronary artery walls, increasing the lumen of the artery.

ankylosis (ang-kih-LOH-sis)—condition of joint immobility.

annotation—the process of reading a document and highlighting pertinent information for someone else.

anorexia (an-oh-REK-see-ah)—diminished desire to eat or diminished appetite.

anterior (an-TEE-ree-or)—toward the front.

antibody (AN-tih-bawd-ee)—substance produced by the body in response to a specific antigen.

anticoagulant (an-tee-koh-AG-yoo-lant)—substance that inhibits blood clot formation.

antidepressant—medication used to treat depression.

antigen (AN-tih-jen)—foreign substance that stimulates the production of antibodies against it when it is introduced into the body.

antipsychotic (an-tee-sy-KAWT-ik)—medication used to treat psychotic episodes.

antipyretic (AN-tih-pi-ret-ik)—fever reducing.

antisepsis—the practice of using antiseptic to prevent growth and reproduction of bacteria and viruses.

antiseptic—substance that prevents growth and reproduction of bacteria and viruses.

antiseptic (an-tih-SEP-tick)—agent that inhibits the growth and reproduction of microorganisms.

anuria (an-YOO-ree-ah)—absence of urine.

anus (AY-nəs)—terminal aspect of the gastrointestinal tract through which dietary waste is expelled.

anxiety—fear of the unknown; a feeling of fear or worry about the future.

apex (AY-pex)—pointed end of the ventricles.

apical (ay-pih-ih-kal)—at the apex of the heart.

apnea (AP-nee-ah)—inability to breathe.

appeal—a process that varies from one insurance plan to the next. The process of asking for a review of a denied service or claim, in an attempt to see the insurance company's denial reversed or overturned.

appendage (A-pen-dij)—anything attached to a larger or major body part.

approved amount—see allowed amount.

approximation—joining together of surgical wound edges.

arrhythmia (ah-RITH-mee-ah)—absence of rhythm.

arteriosclerosis (ar-tee-ree-oh-skleh-ROH-sis)—arterial hardening caused by the buildup of atherosclerotic plaque.

arthritis (ar-THRY-tis)—inflammation of a joint.

arthrography (ar-THRAWG-rah-fee)—radiographic examination of a joint.

articular (ar-TIK yoo-lar)—pertaining to a joint.

artifact—appearance of electrical activity or waveforms from sources outside the heart.

asepsis (**ay-SEP-sis**)—surgical practice that keeps objects and areas sterile or free from microorganisms using sterile technique.

aseptic (ay-SEP-tick)—without germs (literally, without sepsis).

aseptic technique—technique used before and during sterile procedures to prevent microorganism contamination and the possibility of infection; also known as sterile technique.

assault—the threat of touching or doing harm to another without their consent.

assessing—determining what your patient needs to learn and what you will need to have on hand to teach them.

assignment of benefits—request made by a patient to allow the insurance carrier to pay the healthcare professional directly rather than issuing monies to the patient.

assisted living facility—alternative to long-term care in a nursing home, often the choice for individuals who do not require the 24-hour care provided by skilled nursing facilities.

associate degree—degree awarded by community colleges after a course of study of approximately 2 years.

assumption of risk—a defense to medical malpractice; the physician must prove the patient was fully informed as to the risks involved in the procedure.

asthma (AZ-mah)—lung disease characterized by wheezing and shortness of breath; often caused by an allergic response; also known as reversible airways obstruction.

astrology—the practice of studying the planets and stars in an attempt to understand how things work on earth.

asystole (ah-SIS-tole)—absence of cardiac activity; cardiac standstill, without systole.

atherosclerosis (ar-TEER-ee-oh-skleh-ROH-sis)—buildup of plaque in the arteries over a period of years.

atony (ay-TO-nee)—lack of normal tone or strength in a muscle.

atrium (plural: atria) (AY-tree-um)—right or left upper chamber of the heart.

atrophy (AT-roh-fee)—decrease in size of normal muscle mass.

attitude—a state of mind, a way of carrying oneself.

audiologist (AW-dee-AWL-oh-jist)—professional trained to assess hearing levels.

audiometry (AW-dee-AWM-eh-tree)—measuring and testing hearing acuity.

audit—a review process that verifies that every detail of a CPT code is clearly documented in the medical record.

auditors—persons who work for an agency, such as the IRS, who perform the task of reviewing a person's or company's bank or tax records.

augmented lead (AWG-men-TED)—unipolar lead, one positive electrode; has very low voltage and must therefore be augmented by the electrocardiograph to equal the voltage of the other leads.

aura (AW-ruh)—warning of impending seizure.

aural (AW-ral)—pertaining to the ear.

auscultation (AWS-kul-TAY-shun)—listening to various areas of the body.

autoclave (aw-to-CLAVE)—device used to sterilize instruments under steam and pressure.

autoclave load—wrapped or unwrapped instruments, packs, and supplies placed in an autoclave to be sterilized.

autoimmunity—(AW-toh-ih-MYOON-ih-tee)—body's negative reaction to its own cells.

automatic dialer—a telephone feature allowing the user to program commonly called numbers into their system; also called a speed dialer.

automatic routing unit—telephone equipment that allows callers to self-select their call destinations via an automated, electronic prompt system.

automaticity—ability of the heart to initiate and maintain rhythmic activity without the nervous system.

autopsy—examination of a corpse in order to determine the cause of death.

aveolus (plural: alveoli) (al-VEE-oh-lus)—microscopic air sacs that are the primary unit of gas exchange in the lungs.

avulsion (ah-VUL-shun)—open wound in which skin or tissue is torn loose or pulled completely from underlying tissue.

axillary (AK-sil-air-ee)—pertaining to the axilla (armpit); under the arm.

bactericidal (bak-TEER-ih-side-al)—capable of killing or destroying bacteria.

balance billing—billing a patient for the dollar difference between the provider's charge and the insurance approved amount; usually not permitted for participating providers.

bar code scanners—devices used to scan or view a bar code, which then enters the information into a computer.

battery—the act of touching or abusing another person without their consent.

battery backup systems—a battery system that protects the computer in the event of a power surge or power outage.

beneficiary—person who is eligible to receive benefits/services under an insurance policy.

benign (bee-NINE)—noncancerous or noninvasive.

bilateral—refers to something that is occurring on both sides of the body.

bilirubin (BIl-ih-ROO-bin)—substance formed by breakdown of hemoglobin.

binocular (bih-NOK-yoo-lar)—having two eyepieces (on a microscope).

bioethics—issues surrounding life and death situations in healthcare, such as cloning, artificial insemination, or abortion.

biofeedback—using monitoring devices to gain some voluntary control over that function.

birthday rule—a rule used by insurance companies when processing claims for minors who are covered under both parents' insurance plans. The parent with the birthday earlier in the year is the primary carrier, and the parent with the later birthday is the secondary carrier under this rule.

blood pressure—pressure the blood exerts on the vessel walls as a result of the pumping action of the heart.

bloodborne pathogens—pathogens carried in the bloodstream.

body (of letter)—main portion of a business letter.

body language—the way in which our nonverbal actions tell others how we feel.

body mechanics—procedures for standing and efficient body movement, including lifting, pushing, or pulling, that prevent injury and maintain required energy levels for long employment.

body substance isolation (BSI)—procedures, equipment, and supplies used to prevent the transmission of communicable diseases by preventing direct contact with all body substances such as blood, body fluids, drainage from wounds, feces, urine, sputum, and saliva.

bolus (BOH-lus)—mass of masticated food that is swallowed.

bradycardia (BRAD-ee-KAR-dee-ah)—heart rate below 60 beats per minute (BPM).

brochure—a printed document containing information about a topic within the medical office.

bronchiole (BRONG-kee-ole)—airway less than 1 mm in diameter.

bronchitis (brong-KY-tis)—lung disease characterized by large volumes of pulmonary secretions and air trapping; can be chronic or acute in nature.

bronchodilator (BRONG-koh-DY-lay-tor)—medication that dilates the walls of the bronchi.

bronchus (plural: bronchi) (brong-KUSS)—one of two primary airways that branch into the lungs.

buffer time—an appointment scheduling method of leaving certain times of day open to accommodate things like patients who call for same-day appointments or physicians who need to catch up on charting.

bundling—combining multiple services under a single all-inclusive CPT code and one charge.

bursa (plural: bursae) (BER-sah)—a sac filled with synovial fluid that reduces friction and provides ease of movement between tendons and ligaments, ligaments and bone, and other tissues.

bursitis (ber-SIGH-tis)—inflammation of bursa(e).

cadaver—a dead body used for dissection, study, and tissue samples.

caduceus—emblem of the medical profession.

call forwarding—telephone feature allowing the user to forward incoming calls to a different number.

calorie (also called small calorie)—energy released from the metabolism of proteins, fats, and carbohydrates; amount of heat required to raise 1 gram of water 1 degree Celsius.

cancer—general term for various malignant neoplasms.

cannula (KAN-yoo-lah)—tube or sheath.

capitation plans—healthcare plans where the provider is paid a set fee per month per member patient. When the patient comes in for a visit, there may be an additional copayment collected. Other than the possible copayment, no other payment comes from the insurance company or the patient when the patient comes in for care.

carbohydrates—simple and compound sugars that are the primary source of energy for metabolism.

cardiac catheterization (KAR-dee-ak) (KATH-eh-ter-ih-ZAY-shun)—diagnostic procedure in which a catheter is threaded through a major artery back to the heart through the aorta; catheter may be threaded into the left ventricle or into the coronary arteries.

cardiomegaly (KAR-dee-oh-MEG-ah-lee)—enlarged heart.

cardiomyopathy (KAR-dee-oh-my-AWP-ah-thee)—diseases of the myocardium.

carditis (KAR-DI-tis)—inflammation of the heart.

caretaker—person or entity responsible for determining when and if a patient needs specific types of healthcare; also called gatekeeper or primary care provider (PCP).

carrier—person who has the capacity to transmit a disease and is usually unaware of infection.

cartilage (KAR-tih-lij)—smooth, elastic connective tissue that covers the ends of the bones.

carve outs—services that are reimbursed in addition to the base rate for the patient.

cast—a plaster or fiberglass device used to immobilize a body part.

catastrophic—expensive healthcare for large, usually unforeseen events such as accidents, treatment for terminal illnesses, or long-term illness.

categorically needy—Medicaid-eligible patients who qualify for cash assistance as well as medical services.

category—a division of a subsection within the tabular index, consisting of a three-digit code.

category I codes—CPT codes numbered 00100 to 99999 representing widely used services and procedures approved by the FDA.

category II codes—supplemental tracking codes that can be used for performance measurement; four numbers followed by the letter F, such as 1002F.

category III codes—temporary codes for data collection and tracking the use of emerging technology, services, and procedures; four numbers followed by the letter T, such as 0162T.

cauterization (kaw-ter-ih-ZAY-shun)—destruction of tissue with a caustic, electric current, hot iron, or by freezing.

Centers for Disease Control (CDC)—agency of the Public Health Operating Division of the U.S. Department of Health and Human Services that studies and monitors diseases and disease prevention and works to protect public health and safety.

Centers for Medicare and Medicaid Services—federal agency responsible for monitoring laws and regulations surrounding Medicare and Medicaid services.

central processing unit (CPU)—the computer's ability to process information.

centrifuge (SEN-tri-fuj)—instrument that spins substances at high speed to separate them into layers according to density.

cephalgia (SEF-al-AL-jee-ah)—diffuse acute or chronic pain in any part of the head, commonly known as *headache*.

cerebral (sa-REE-bral)—pertaining to the cerebrum, the forepart of the brain.

certificate of coverage—a letter from the insurance company that provides proof of type and timeframe of coverage when a patient terminates a health insurance policy.

certified letter—a letter sent via the postal service sent certified is one that must be signed for by the recipient.

Certified Medical Assistant (CMA)—a graduate of an accredited medical assisting program who has passed the AAMA certification examination.

cerumen (sa-ROO-men)—earwax; waxy substance secreted in external ear canal.

cervix (SER-viks)—entrance to the uterus.

chapter—one of seventeen major sections of ICD-9-CM Volume I tabular list, organized by body system and etiology.

charge slip—also called an encounter form or a routing slip. These forms vary from one office to the next and usually contain the procedural and diagnostic codes commonly used in that clinic. A charge slip is generated on each patient coming in for care each day; these are a record of the charges and diagnoses for that patient for that date of service. Usually completed by the healthcare provider who performed the service.

charitable contributions—donations, including cash, that are given to charitable organizations.

charting—documentation of all the events of a patient's visit.

checklist—a preprinted reminder list of activities or steps to take to perform a task.

chemical name—official pharmaceutical name for a drug based on its chemical composition.

chemical waste—waste drugs, cleaning solutions, and germicides.

chemotherapy (KEE-moh-THAIR-ah-pee)—treatment of disease and infection with chemical agents; in cancer treatment, use of chemical agents to selectively kill cancer cells.

chief complaint—the main reason the patient has come in for care.

chiropractic—healthcare profession that focuses on correcting misalignments of the spine.

chloroform—early method of general anesthesia.

cholecystography (koh-lee-sis-TOG-rah-fee)—radiograph of the gallbladder, using oral contrast; often referred to as gallbladder series.

cholesterol (koh-LES-ter-all)—steroid alcohol formed in the liver and also found in plant and animal fats; may be responsible for fatty deposits of plaque in blood vessels.

chronic (KRAW-nik)—of long duration, often with slow progression.

chyme (KIME)—mixture of partially digested food and enzymes that enters the small intestines.

cilia (SIL-ee-ah)—hairlike processes projecting from the epithelial cells.

circular E—yearly booklet published by the IRS that outlines the proper federal tax deductions to be taken from an individual's wages, depending upon marital status and number of exemptions.

civil law—laws that relate between two or more citizens.

clean claim—insurance claim form (either electronic or on paper) that contains no data errors nor omissions.

clinical duties—medical assisting duties such as drawing blood samples, taking vital signs, and assisting with surgery.

clonic (CLAWN-ik)—alternating muscular contraction and relaxation.

close-ended question—question that can be answered with yes or no.

closed patient files—normally refers to patient files for patients who will not be returning to the clinic.

closed wound—wound that involves trauma to the underlying tissue without a break in the skin or mucous membrane or exposure of the underlying tissue.

closing—ending portion of a business letter.

cluster scheduling—a scheduling method allowing patients with similar appointments to be clustered around the same time of day.

coagulation (koh-ag-YOU-late-shun)—blood clot formation.

cognitive—of or pertaining to the mental processes of judgment, perception, reasoning, and memory.

coinsurance—percentage of the medical charges the patient will be responsible for according to their insurance plan contract.

cold sterilization (ster-ih-lih-ZAY-shun)—sterilization with a chemical sterilant, performed when heat cannot be used.

collagen (KAWL-lah-jen)—fibrous connective tissue.

collection agency—company that will pursue overdue accounts for a fee.

colonoscopy (KOH-lon-AWS-koh-pee)—visual examination of the colon using a colonoscope.

colostomy (koh-LOSS-toh-mee)—surgically created opening connecting the colon to the abdominal surface for fecal evacuation.

colostrum (kuh-LOS-trum)—fluid secreted by the breasts after delivery, before milk production, that contains antibodies and provides the infant with immunological protection.

combination code—a single code that describes two or more conditions that frequently occur together.

commercial insurance—see private insurance.

commercial law—laws that relate to businesses or companies.

Commission of Accreditation of Allied Health Education Programs (CAAHEP)—accrediting agency offering medical assistant education programs the ability to offer a certified medical assisting certificate.

common descriptor—the portion of a standalone code before the semicolon that is shared with the indented codes that follow.

common law—laws that stem from the English legal system.

community college—educational institution that provides 2-year undergraduate education, offering certificates, diplomas, and associate's degrees.

community property laws—laws that cause one spouse to be financially responsible for the debts of the other.

comorbid—denoting co-existing, unrelated medical diseases or conditions.

comparative negligence—defense to medical malpractice where the physician proves the patient was partly responsible for their own injury.

compassion—using empathy to sense others' concerns or feelings.

competence—the ability to perform one's job up to standard.

competency—list of skills that accredited programs must teach students.

complementary and alternative medicine—referred to as CAM, natural remedies and methods that do not use medications or surgeries to care for or cure disease and illness.

complementary medicine—systems of medical options varying from traditional medicine, chosen by individuals along with regularly prescribed modalities; examples include use of herbal remedies such as saw palmetto to promote prostate health.

complete protein (kem-PLEET PRO-teen)—protein containing all the essential amino acids.

compress (kom-PRES)—folded piece of material used to apply dry or moist heat or cold therapeutic applications.

compulsory—required attendance.

computed tomography—CT scan; two-dimensional X-rays.

computer peripherals—devices that connect to the computer to add some function or use.

computer viruses—programs written for the purpose of disrupting a computer's functions.

conduction (kon-DUK-shun)—heat transfer by direct contact through fluids, solids, or other substances.

conduction system (con-DUK-shun)—wiring and paths that initiate and maintain rhythmic contraction of the myocardium.

conductivity (con-duk-TIV-ih-tee)—ability of a cardiac cell to transfer impulses to the next cell, allowing all areas of the heart (myocardium) to depolarize at one time.

conference call—telephone feature allowing three or more persons in different locations to participate in a call.

confidentiality—state of keeping what one person says from being heard by anyone else.

conscience clauses—clauses that allow persons who work in health care to refuse to work in situations with which they have a religious objection.

Consolidated Omnibus Budget Reconciliation Act (COBRA)—Consolidated Omnibus Budget Reconciliation Act. Allows workers to continue their health insurance coverage (at their own expense) after being fired, laid off, or having quit.

constitutional law—laws based on the U.S. Constitution.

consultation—visit between the patient and the healthcare provider where a discussion, but not an examination, takes place.

consumer-directed healthcare—health insurance plans that place the patient in charge of how their healthcare dollars are spent.

contact information—patient's address and phone numbers.

contamination—making a sterile field unclean or having pathogens placed in it.

continuing education—educational program designed to further knowledge in a particular area.

contract—agreement, either verbal or in writing, between two parties.

contract law—laws pertaining to contracts.

contractility—ability of the heart muscle to shorten or reduce in size.

contraindication—condition for which a drug should be administered.

contrecoup (KON-tra-coo)—event on the opposite side, injury in which traumatic impact on the head is strong enough to make the brain strike the opposite side of the cranium and bounce back to strike the impacted side.

contributory factor—three secondary criteria, in addition to the key components, that may influence the selection of an E&M code; include presenting problem, counseling/coordination of care, and physicians' face-to-face time with patients and families.

contributory negligence—defense to medical malpractice where the physician proves that the injury wouldn't have happened if not for the actions of the patient.

controlled substance (or schedule drug)—drug identified by the Federal Controlled Substances Act as having a potential for abuse; requires strict adherence to procedures for storage, prescription, administration, and disposal.

controlled substances—narcotics, stimulants, and certain sedatives.

convection (kon-VEKT-shun)—heat transfer by air.

conventions—ICD-9-CM coding rules, abbreviations, symbols, or formatting intended to ensure consistency in coding.

conversion factor—a constant dollar value multiplied by the relative value unit to determine the price of individual services.

coordination of benefits—the process of determining which insurance policy should be billed first, second, or third when a patient is covered by multiple policies.

coordination of care—a contributory factor in E&M coding that describes physicians' work in arranging care with other providers.

copayment—set dollar fee per visit or service the patient will be responsible for according to their insurance plan contract.

coronary artery bypass (KOR-ah-nair-ee) (AR-toh-ree)—surgery in which the ischemia or obstruction in the coronary arteries is bypassed with a graft of a vessel.

coronary artery disease (KOR-ah-nair-ee) (AR-toh-ree)—condition in which the coronary arteries are narrowed by constriction caused by plaque buildup.

counseling—a contributory factor in E&M coding that describes physicians' discussion with patients and family members regarding diagnosis, treatment options, instructions and followup.

courtesy—polite behavior.

cover letter—letter to accompany the resume when sent to an employer.

covered—services potentially eligible for reimbursement.

CPR mouth barrier—disposable barrier device used to prevent infection.

CPT codes—*Current Procedural Terminology;* a book that is updated every year, contains all nondental procedure codes approved by the Centers for Medicare and Medicaid Services.

CPT-4 book—procedural coding book used in all healthcare settings in the United States.

crash cart—wheeled cart that contains emergency medical equipment.

credibility—quality of believing a person is and does what they say they will do.

crescentic—crescent-shaped; term used to describe abnormalities found on biopsy of the kidney in rapidly progressive glomerulonephritis.

criminal law—laws dealing with crimes.

cross-referencing—method of tracking and finding patient files for those patients who may have more than one last name.

cryosurgery (KRY-oh-SER-jer-ee)—freezing lesions with nitrous oxide.

cryotherapy (KRY-oh-THAIR-ah-pee)—the use of cold applications to prevent or reduce swelling and pain.

cryptorchism (also cryptorchidism) (krip-TOHR-kiz-em)—a condition in which one or both of the testes fail to descend into the scrotal sac during fetal development.

cutting—using a knife or surgical scissors to separate or divide tissues.

cyanosis (sigh-ah-NOH-sis)—bluish tint in skin or mucous membrane, usually appearing in fingernail beds, oral mucous membranes, and circumoral tissue (tissue surrounding the mouth) and indicating excessive deoxygenated hemoglobin or reduced hemoglobin in the blood.

cyanotic (sigh-ah-NOH-tik)—characterized by cyanosis, or a blue tint in the skin, which indicates reduced blood oxygen.

cystitis (sis-TY-tis)—inflammation of the urinary bladder.

damages—the amount of money a patient is awarded for the damages they have sustained.

day sheet—used with a manual pegboard system.

deaf—unable to hear, or having a diminished sense of hearing.

debit—an addition to an account, usually performed in order to remove a credit balance.

debris (de-BREE)—organic or inorganic extraneous material that interferes with the proper functioning or cleaning of supplies or equipment.

decerebrate posture (de-SER-eh-brate)—posture characteristic of brain injury in which the patient is rigid, with head retracted and arms and legs extended.

decibel (DES-ih-bel)—unit for measuring the intensity of sound.

decontamination—use of physical means or chemical agents to remove, inactivate, or destroy pathogens on a surface or object to the point where they are no longer capable of transmitting infectious disease, thereby rendering the surface or object safe for handling, use or disposal.

décor—the way an office is decorated.

decorticate posture (de-KOR-tih-kate)—posture characteristic of brain injury in which the patient is rigid, with clenched fists, flexed arms, and extended legs.

deductible—amount of money the patient must pay to the provider out of pocket for healthcare services before health insurance benefits begin to pay.

deductions—number of withholding allowances an individual wishes to have withheld from their wages.

defamation of character—to say negative things about another person that causes that person some form of harm.

defibrillator—device that delivers an electric shock to a patient.

degenerative (dee-JEN-er-ah-tiv)—impaired in function or condition over time.

delegate—to assign projects to others.

dementia (dee-MEN-she-ah)—diminished mental or cognitive functioning with onset after the age of 18 years.

denied—a claim processed by an insurer and determined not eligible for payment.

dependability—the quality of following through with what is expected of you.

dependence (dee-PEN-dens)—state of addiction to certain drugs; rapid physical withdrawal can cause life-threatening and even fatal reactions.

dependent—a family member or other individual who qualifies for coverage on the insured's policy; also called beneficiary. See also insured; policyholder.

depolarization (dee-POHL-ar-ih-ZAY-shun)—condition in which the cardiac cell environment becomes positive.

dermatitis (DER-mah-TY-tis)—skin inflammation.

dermatologist (DER-mah-TALL-oh-jist)—physician who specializes in the treatment of skin diseases and conditions.

dermatology (DER-mah-TALL-oh-jee)—study and treatment of integumentary system diseases and conditions.

dermatome (DER-mah-tohm)—specific area of skin stimulated by a segment of the spinal cord.

dermatophytoses (DER-mah-to-FI-to-ses)—superficial fungal infections of the skin and its appendages.

dermis (DER-mis)—middle layer of the skin.

diagnosis (DY-ag-NOH-sis)—conclusion made about the patient's condition by interpretation of data.

dialysis (dy-AL-ih-sis)—cleansing of waste products from the blood with a dialysis machine, or dialyzer.

diaphoresis (DY-ah-foh-REE-sis)—profuse sweating.

diaphragm (DY-ah-fram)—primary muscle of breathing; separates chest and abdominal cavities.

diarthrosis (DY-ar-THROH-sis)—condition of bone joints moving freely.

diastole (dy-AS-tole)—period of ventricular relaxation.

diastolic (dy-ah-STOL-ik)—pertaining to relaxation of the heart muscle; lowest reading of the blood pressure.

Dietary Supplement and Education Act—federal act enacted in 1990 directing how nutritional supplements are to be labeled.

dietary supplements—vitamins, herbs, or minerals administered in a variety of ways to alleviate symptoms or to maintain health in a natural, noninvasive manner.

digestion (DY-jest-shun)—physical and chemical conversion of food into substances that can be used by the body.

diluent (dh-LOO-ent)—diluting agent.

direct telephone lines—telephone numbers that reach a person directly, rather than routing the calls through an operator or receptionist.

disability insurance—insurance that covers lost wages and certain other benefits due to a disability that prevents the individual from working.

disability policies—policies that cover an individual's lost income in the event of a temporary or long-term disability.

discovery rule—legal term pertaining to medical malpractice cases; this is the period of time within which a patient has to file a medical malpractice lawsuit from the day the injury was discovered, rather than the date of the injury itself.

discriminating—acting against a person's interest solely because of a perceived difference, such as race, gender, or economic status.

disinfection—method of decontamination that destroys or inhibits pathogenic microorganisms but does not kill spores and some viruses; used sometimes as an alternative to autoclave sterilization.

dissection (dy-SEK-shun)—cutting into smaller parts for study and analysis of each part.

distal (diss-TALL)—away from the center.

distal tubule (DISS-tal)—farthest tubule from the glomerulus.

documenting—process of writing in the patient's chart.

double booking—scheduling more than one patient for the same appointment time.

downcode—to assign a code for a lower level of service than was actually performed; done by some insurance companies to save money; done by some physicians to avoid fraud or abuse charges.

drug—any substance capable of producing a change in function when administered to a living organism; commonly, a term for a substance used to treat or prevent disease; in the medical office, synonymous with the term *medication.*

drug samples—small samples of drugs given to physicians by pharmaceutical companies to be dispensed to patients.

dual fee schedule—a facility or healthcare provider having two fees for the same service.

dumb—unable to speak.

duress—act of coercing someone into an act.

dyscrasia (dis-KRAY-zee-ah)—abnormal blood or bone marrow condition, such as leukemia.

dysfunction (dis-FUNK-shun)—abnormal or impaired function.

dyspepsia (dis-PEP-see-ah)—painful digestion.

dysphagia (dis-FAH-jee-ah)—difficulty swallowing.

dysphasia (dis-FAY-zee-ah)—difficulty speaking.

dyspnea (DISP-nee-ah)—difficulty breathing.

dysrhythmia (dis-RITH-mee-ah)—abnormal, irregular, or disturbed heart rhythm.

e-billing—health insurance claims that are sent electronically.

E-codes—diagnosis codes used to indicate the external cause of an illness or poisoning.

ecchymosis (EK-ih-MOH-seez)—bruise; area of bleeding under the skin.

echocardiogram (EK-oh-KAR-dee-oh-gram)—type of sonogram used to study the internal structures of the heart.

effacement (eh-FAYS-ment)—thinning of the cervix during the labor process.

efferent nerves (EFF-er-ent)—motor nerves that carry impulses from the central nervous system to the peripheral nervous system.

ejection fraction—measurement of the fraction of the total amount (volume) of blood filling the ventricle that is ejected during the ventricular contraction.

elective procedure—procedure that will benefit the patient but does not need to be scheduled immediately.

electrolytes (ee-LEK-troh-lites)—substances present in the bloodstream, cells, and tissues that are involved in homeostatic changes in acid-base balance, movement of tissue fluid, and activities of the cells and cellular walls.

electromyography (ee-LEK-troh-my-AWG-rah-fee)—procedure in which a needle is inserted into muscle tissue to record electrical activity.

electronic mail—e-mail; electronically sending a message from one person to another using computers.

electronic medical records—medical records that are kept electronically, on a computer.

electronic sign-in sheet—device attached to a computer allowing a person to sign their name so it appears in the computer.

electronic signature—electronic version of a person's signature to be used in electronic medical records.

eligibility—the process to determine if a patient is qualified to receive coverage/paid benefits according to the insurance policy guidelines.

elimination (ee-LIM-ih-NAY-shun)—expulsion of waste products from the body.

embolism (EM-boh-lizm)—condition in which an embolus that is moving through the vascular system becomes lodged in a vessel.

embolus (plural: emboli) (EM-boh-lus)—mass of material or tissue in a vessel; may be a blood clot, air, fat, bone fragments, bacterial clumps, amniotic fluid, or other materials.

embryo (EM-bree-oh)—initial physical stage of human development following fertilization of the ovum until the end of the seventh or eighth week.

emergency surgery—any urgent condition perceived by the physician as requiring immediate medical or surgical evaluation or treatment.

emesis (EM-eh-sis)—regurgitation of partially digested food from the stomach; vomit.

empathy—understanding of and sensitivity to the feelings, thoughts, and experiences of others.

emphysema (EM-fih-SEE-mah)—disease of chronic airways obstruction (COLD) in which air is trapped; usually caused by either smoking or heredity.

employee handbook—also called a policy manual; list of policies regarding employment within the office.

emulsification (ee-MUL-sih-fih-KAY-shun)—transformation of ingested particles of fat into small globules with bile.

encounter form—also called a charge slip or a routing slip. These forms vary from one office to the next and usually contain the procedural and diagnostic codes commonly used in that clinic. A charge slip is generated on each patient coming in for care each day; these are a record of the charges and diagnoses for that patient for that date of service. Usually completed by the healthcare provider who performed the service.

end stage renal disease (ESRD)—total or nearly complete failure of the kidneys.

endocarditis (EN-doh-kar-DY-tis)—inflammation of the endocardium.

endocrine glands (EN-doh-krin)—glands that secrete and release hormones directly into the bloodstream; also known as ductless glands.

endometrium (en-doh-MEE-tree-um)—lining of the uterus.

endorphin (en-DOR-fin)—proteins in the brain that have analgesic properties.

endorsement stamp—rubber stamp that contains the banking information for the receiving agency.

endoscope (en-doh-SKOPE)—fiber-optic instrument used to visualize the internal aspect of the GI tract.

endosteum (en-doh-STEE-um)—membrane lining the inner portion and marrow cavity of the bone.

epidemiology (ep-ih-DEE-mee-awl-oh-jee)—branch of science that studies the incidence, spread, and control of disease in a population.

epidermis (EP-ih-DER-mis)—outermost layer of the skin.

epistaxis (ep-ih-STAKS-is)—nosebleed.

epithelial (ep-ih-THEE-lee-al)—pertaining to the epithelium (cells covering the external and internal surfaces of the body).

ergonomic—designed for proper posture of the body while using the equipment.

escort—to accompany someone.

essential oils—oils extracted from flowers and herbs and integrated into an oil base for use in aromatherapy.

established patient—patient who has seen the same provider, or another provider of the same specialty in the same practice, within the past three years.

ether—early method of general anesthesia.

etiology—cause of a disease or illness.

eukaryotes (yoo-CARE-ee-oats)—group of microorganisms, such as fungi and parasites, that have organized nuclear material and organelles to assist in reproduction.

eupnea (YOOP-nee-ah)—normal breathing.

evaluation—process of verifying a patient's progress.

Evaluation and Management (E&M)—CPT codes used for billing physician services to evaluate and manage patient care, such as office visits.

evidence-based medicine—theory of medicine that states health care methods should be scientifically proven to work.

exacerbation (eg-ZAS-er-BAY-shun)—increasing severity and recurrence of symptoms.

examination—a key component E&M coding that describes the complexity of the physical assessment of the patient.

examples—asking the patient to give an example of how they are feeling.

excitability—response of cardiac cell to electrical stimulus.

exclusions—procedures or services that are not covered under a particular insurance plan.

exclusive provider organization—healthcare institutions that combine both providers and facilities, requiring patients to obtain care exclusively at a covered facility with a covered provider.

exocrine glands (EK-soh-krin)—glands that secrete substances through ducts, such as sweat glands.

expert witnesses—witness in a lawsuit who is considered an expert in their given field.

expiration dates—the date something expires; the date it should not be used past.

explanation of benefits—list sent from the insurance company to the healthcare provider (with payment for the services) outlining how the claim for a patient's services was processed. A copy of the EOB is sent to the insured as well.

expressed consent—agreement, either verbally or in writing.

expressed contract—agreement to a contract, either verbally or in writing.

extended care facility—facility that provides 24-hour nursing care; also called nursing home or long-term care facility.

external hard drives—devices that attach to a computer system to allow extra hard drive capacity.

externship program—the final phase of the medical assisting education in an accredited program; consists of hands-on work in a medical office for a specified number of hours.

face-to-face time—a contributory factor in E&M coding that measures the amount of time the provider spent in the presence of the patient and/or family, as opposed to time spent documenting the visit or arranging referrals.

Fair Debt Collection Act—laws outlining how debts may be legally collected.

Fair Labor Standards Act—passed by Congress passed in 1938; addressed several issues relating to workers, including setting a federal minimum wage.

faith healer—practitioners who use prayer, rather than medicine, to heal their patients.

fats—food component that is a source of energy and aids in growth and development by providing fatty acids.

feces (FEE-seez)—waste product of digestion that is expelled through the rectum and anus.

Federal Insurance Contributions Act (FICA)—addresses Social Security withholding taxes.

federal minimum wage—dollar amount, set by Congress, that is the minimum amount an employer may pay an employee per hour in wages.

Federal Unemployment Tax Act (FUTA)—addresses federal unemployment tax withholdings.

fee-for-service—term used to identify the process of insurance companies paying providers a fee for each individual service provided to a covered patient.

fee schedule—the list of approved fees insurance carriers agree to pay to participating providers who agree to contract with the carrier.

feedback—relating to another person what you think you heard them say.

fetus (FEE-tus)—human child in utero from embryonic stage until birth.

fiber—nondigestible substances found in food, such as cellulose and pectin, that provide bulk and roughage for the evacuation of fecal waste.

fibrillation (FIB-rih-LAY-shun)—irregular contractions of the heart; ECG shows waveforms without definite pattern or shape. Atrial fibrillation: atria are quivering and do not have a forceful beat to push blood into ventricles. Ventricular fibrillation: lethal arrhythmia; ventricles are quivering and do not contract with force to push blood into aorta. Rhythm is chaotic, with no recognizable P waves, QRS complexes, or T waves; without immediate intervention and conversion of rhythm, asystole will follow.

financial information—information about a patient consisting of their health insurance identification numbers and policy numbers.

first-listed—the diagnosis that is chiefly responsible for the outpatient services provided; formerly called primary diagnosis.

fistula (FIS-tyoo-lah)—abnormal tube-like structure connecting one body structure to another or to the surface of the body.

fixed appointment scheduling—a scheduling system of giving every patient a specific appointment time.

flank—region in the lateral aspect of the midback, between the ribs and the upper border of the ilium.

flash drives—small, external computer storage devices; also called thumb drives.

flatulence (FLAT-yoo-lents)—excessive gas or air generated in the stomach or intestinal tract.

flex spending account—account set up by employers. Employees are allowed to place pretax earnings into these accounts and then submit receipts to the employer for allowed medical expenses.

flexibility—willingness to change direction or plans when needed or requested.

flexible spending account—also called healthcare reimbursement account.

flow charts—graphs that are used in the patient's medical record to track things such as weight gain or growth of a newborn.

fluoroscopy (floor-AWS-koh-pee)—radiographic study in which structures are visualized in motion.

focus (plural: foci) (FOH-kus)—specific site; the origin of an electrical cardiac impulse.

follicle (FAWL-ih-kl)—small hollow or cavity with secretory functions (e.g., hair follicle, ovarian follicle, gastric follicle, etc.).

fomites (FOH-mites)—nonliving objects that may transmit infectious material.

font—typestyle used within a word processing program.

fontanelle (FAWN-tah-NEL)—"soft spot" on the cranium of a newborn or infant; area of the skull that is not covered by bone at birth but where the cranial bones eventually come together, allowing for the growth of the brain and skull.

forgiven—with regard to collections, to forgive an account is to stop attempting to collect from the debtor.

form locators—the boxes to be completed on the CMS-1500 claim form.

formulary—tiered list of drugs covered by a particular insurance company. Normally, generic or less expensive drugs are covered at a higher rate (with a smaller copay, if any), whereas name brand or more expensive drugs are covered at a lower rate (with a higher copay). Each insurance company constructs their own formulary list. Some insurance plans will *only* cover preferred (lower cost) drugs.

fossil—ancient mineralized remains of plants, animals, or other organisms.

Four Ds of negligence—refers to malpractice; patients must prove duty, dereliction of duty, direct cause, and damages.

fraud—deceitful act made to conceal the truth; in billing, to intentionally bill for services that were never given, including billing for a service that has a higher reimbursement than the service produced.

front desk—place in a medical office where the receptionist welcomes the patients as they enter.

fundal height (FUN-dal)—height of the fundus from the top of the symphysis pubis to the highest point at the top of the uterus; used to estimate the size of the fetus.

garnished—to have monies withheld from a person's wages due to a court order.

gastric (GAS-trik)—pertaining to the stomach.

gastroenterology (gas-troh-en-ter-ALL-oh-jee)—the study of diseases affecting the gastrointestinal tract.

gastroscopy (gas-TRAWS-koh-pee)—visual examination of the stomach using a gastroscope.

gatekeeper—see caretaker.

generic drugs—lower cost, non-name brand prescription drugs that duplicate their brand-name counterparts in active ingredient and effect.

generic message—telephone answering messages that are not specific to any individual office.

generic (nonproprietary) name—pharmaceutical name for a medication, often a shortened chemical name; used by all manufacturers that produce the medication; never capitalized.

geographic adjustment factor (GAF)—a numeric multiplier used by Medicare to adjust fees for the varying costs of practicing medicine in different areas of the country.

Geographical Practice Cost Index (GPCI)—Medicare system of adjusting fees based on the country in which the health care provider practices.

geriatrics (JAIR-ee-AT-riks)—science focusing on the aging process; in healthcare, specialty that deals with the disorders of the aging population and their treatment.

germicide (JER-mih-side)—agent used to kill germs.

glomerulonephritis (gloh-mair-yoo-loh-neh-FRYE-tis)—inflammation and possible infection of the glomerulus.

glomerulus (gloh-MAIR-yoo-lus)—tuft or cluster of capillaries inside the capsule of the nephron.

glucometer (gloo-koh-MEAT-er)—instrument used to measure blood glucose levels.

gluconeogenesis (gloo-kon-ee-oh-JEN-eh-sis)—conversion of noncarbohydrate sources stored in the liver into glucose.

Good Samaritan Act—laws that protect a person when they perform life-saving care to a stranger outside the medical setting.

-gravida (GRAV-ih-dah)—combining form meaning a pregnant female or pregnancy.

gross pay—amount of money a person earns before any taxes or deductions are taken out.

group health insurance—a commercial insurance policy with rates based on a group of people, usually offered by an employer.

guidelines—specific instructions at the beginning of each section of the CPT manual that define terms and describe specific information about how to use codes in that section.

gynecologist (guy-neh-KOL-oh-jist)—physician specializing in the medical care of the female reproductive system, diseases, and disorders.

gynecology (guy-ne-KOL-oh-jee)—branch of medicine pertaining to the female reproductive system, diseases, and disorders.

hands-free telephone device—headsets or headphones that contain both a speaker and a microphone, worn by an individual who is using a telephone and does not wish to hold the receiver.

hardship agreement—agreement a patient signs to indicate an inability to pay full healthcare costs due to financial hardship.

hazard—something that is dangerous, or possibly dangerous.

HCFA 1500 form—former name for the CMS-1500 claim form.

Health Care Financing Administration—former name for the Centers for Medicare and Medicaid Services.

Health Insurance Portability and Accountability Act (HIPAA)—legislation that addresses patient privacy.

health maintenance organization—type of managed care plan that provides health insurance coverage. Healthcare providers contract with HMOs to provide care to covered patients.

health-related calculators—programs that allow the user to determine information about health-related conditions, such as target body weight.

health savings account—tax-free savings accounts used for medical expenses in conjunction with a high-deductible health plan.

Healthcare Common Procedure Coding System (HCPCS)—contains coding for all procedures and services.

healthcare reimbursement account—see flexible spending account.

healthcare savings account—similar to a flex-spending account. Employees are allowed to place pretax earnings into an account set up by their employer. They then submit receipts to the employer for covered medical expenses. This type of account can normally roll over from one year to the next if the employee does not use all of the funds and can often be taken with the employee from one job to another.

hematemesis (hee-mah-TEM-ah-sis)—vomiting of blood, an indication of bleeding in upper GI tract.

hematocrit (hee-MAT-oh-krit)—volume of RBCs in a given volume of blood, expressed as a percent of total blood volume.

hematology (hee-mah-TAWL-oh-jee)—study of blood.

hematopoiesis (hee-mah-toh-poy-EE-sis)—formation of blood cells.

hematopoietic (hee-mah-toh-poy-etic)—pertaining to normal blood cell development in the bone marrow.

hematuria (hee-mah-TYOO-ree-ah)—blood in the urine.

hemiparesis (hem-ee-par-EE-sis)—loss of nerve and muscle function on one side of the body.

hemiplegia (hem-ee-PLEE-jee-ah)—paralysis of one side of the body.

hemoglobin (hee-moh-GLOH-bin)—iron-containing substance found in RBCs whose function is to carry oxygen from the lungs throughout the body.

hemolytic (HEE-moh-LIT-ik)—pertaining to the breakdown of RBCs.

hemoptysis (hee-MAWP-tih-sis)—coughing up blood from the respiratory tract.

hemostasis (hee-moh-STAY-sis)—process by which the body spontaneously stops bleeding and maintains the blood in a fluid state within the vascular compartment.

hemostat (HEE-moh-stat)—instrument used to stop blood flow.

hepatomegaly (HEP-ah-toh-MEG-ah-lee)—enlargement of the liver.

HIPAA compliant—in line with laws regarding patient confidentiality.

Hippocrates—"Father of Medicine"; Greek physician who began moving the practice of medicine to a scientific nature.

Hippocratic oath—oath of ethics thought to be written by Hippocrates. Still recited at medical school graduations.

history—a key component E&M coding that describes the background, onset, and progression of the patient's current condition.

hold feature—telephone feature allowing the user to place callers on hold, allowing the user to take other telephone calls.

holistic—natural, nonmedical treatment.

homeostasis (HOH-mee-oh-STAY-sis)—interaction between body systems that maintains optimum body function.

hormones (HOR-mohnz)—chemical messengers secreted by the endocrine glands.

hospice—facility or service provided for patients who are given a diagnosis of a terminal illness, with 6 months or less to live. Services may be provided in the hospice facility, in the hospital, skilled nursing facility, or the patient's home. Care is normally palliative (comfort-based) in nature.

hospital services—patient care provided by a licensed acute care hospital.

hourly—amount of money to be paid to an employee per hour worked.

Human Genome Project—project designed to map out the human genes.

hydronephrosis (high-droh-neh-FROH-sis)—enlargement of the kidney caused by retention of urine due to an obstruction.

hyperglycemia (hy-per-gly-SEE-mee-ah)—condition in which blood glucose is elevated above normal.

hypertension (hy-per-TEN-shun)—elevated blood pressure.

hyperthermia (hu-per-THERM-ee-a)—condition in which body temperature is much higher than normal for a prolonged period of time.

hypnosis—artificially induced altered state of consciousness, usually accompanied by an increased receptiveness to suggestion.

hypoglycemia (hy-poh-gly-SEE-mee-ah)—condition in which blood glucose is below normal.

hypotension (hy-poh-TEN-shun)—below-normal blood pressure.

hypothalamus (hy-poh-THAL-ah-mus)—very small structure in the midbrain, below the thalamus, that controls many body functions and endocrine processes.

hypothermia (hy-poh-THERM-ee-a)—condition in which body temperature is below normal for a prolonged period of time.

hypoxemia (hy-pawk-SEE-mee-ah)—reduced oxygen content in the blood.

identification numbers—numbers given by the insurance carrier that identify the insured. These numbers have taken the place of using the insured's Social Security number.

ileostomy (ill-ee-OSS-toh-mee)—surgical opening of the ileum onto the surface of the abdomen for the elimination of fecal material.

immunity (im-YOO-nih-tee)—ability to resist disease.

immunocompetence (im-yoo-noh-COM-petence)—body's ability to fight infection; capacity for normal immune response.

immunodeficiency (im-yo-noh-deh-FISH-en-see)—inability of the immune system to function normally to protect the body from infection.

immunohematology (im-yoo-noh-HEE-mah-TAWL-oh-jee)—study of antigens, antibodies, and their interactions.

implementation—putting a plan into place.

implied consent—agreement implied by the patient for examination and treatment when presenting for a routine visit; also, in an emergency, consent that it is assumed the patient would give if the patient could do so.

implied contract—to agree to a contract by one's actions, without speaking or writing.

inactive patient files—normally refers to patient files for patients who have not been in to see the physician for an extended period of time.

incision (in-SIZH-un)—open wound with smooth edges made with a knife or other sharp object.

incomplete protein—protein lacking one or more of the essential amino acids.

incontinence (in-CON-tih-nens)—involuntary leakage of urine or feces.

incubation—period of time between exposure to infection and the appearance of symptoms.

indecipherable—unreadable.

indemnity—see fee-for-service.

indented code—a CPT code whose description is indented three spaces under another (standalone) code and whose definition includes the portion before the semi-colon (;) in the standalone code; done to save space in the CPT manual.

indigestion (in-dy-JES-chun)—inability to digest, often with pain in the gastrointestinal (GI) tract.

individual insurance—a commercial insurance policy with rates based on individual health criteria.

individual practice association—HMOs that are the most decentralized and involve contracting with individual physicians to create a healthcare delivery system.

infection (in-FEK-shun)—invasion of the body by a pathogenic microorganism.

infectious waste—any garbage exposed to bodily fluids or any laboratory cultures or blood products.

informed consent—consent given by a patient after all potential treatments and outcomes have been discussed for a specific medical condition, including risks and possible negative outcomes.

initiative—taking it upon oneself to begin a task, without being asked by someone else to do it.

innervate—stimulate.

inpatient—a person who is admitted to the hospital for a minimum of 24 hours.

inspection (in-SPEK-shun)—visual examination of both the external surface of the body and the interior portions of body cavities.

instructional notes—directions in the tabular index that appear in parentheses before or after a code entry to point the user to alternative codes for closely related procedures or to codes that must or must not be used together.

insured—term used to identify the person who holds or owns an insurance policy. See policy holder.

integrative medicine—systems of medical options that incorporate forms of alternative medicine, complementary medicine, and traditional medicine.

integumentary (in-TEG-you-men-tair-ee)—pertaining to the skin, hair, and nails.

integumentary system (in-TEG-yoo-MEN-tair-ee)—the skin and its supporting structures (nails, hair, and sebaceous and sweat glands).

intentional tort—to purposefully hurt or harm another.

interatrial septum (in-ter-AY-tree-al-SEP-tum)—wall between the right and left atria.

interdisciplinary—multiple healthcare specialties.

interest—to charge a percentage fee each month on overdue account balances.

Internal Revenue Service—federal agency responsible for collecting federal taxes due from individuals and companies.

international law—laws pertaining to two or more countries.

Internet search engines—Web sites that search the Internet for information based on words entered by an individual.

internodal pathway—the three tracts that carry the electrical impulse as it leaves the SA node, transmit the impulse to the AV node, and distribute it throughout the atria; the three divisions are the anterior, middle, and posterior divisions.

interphalangeal (IN-ter-fah-LAN-jee-al)—between the joints of the fingers or toes.

interventriclular septum (in-ter-ven-TRIK-yoo-lar SEP-tum)—wall between the right and left ventricles.

interview—a meeting, usually face-to-face, between an employer and an applicant.

intradermal (IN-trah-DER-mal)—between the layers of the skin.

intraocular (in-trah-AWK-yoo-lar)—within the eye.

intraoperative—pertaining to patient care during surgery.

intrinsic factor—substance secreted by the gastric mucosa that is necessary for the absorption of vitamin B$_{12}$ and the development of RBCs.

invasion of privacy—to give out information about another person without permission.

inventory—supplies that are on hand; counting the supplies that are in the office.

ischemic (is-KEYH-mik)—pertaining to a decreased blood supply to tissue due to impaired circulation to the organ or part.

isoelectric line—flat, horizontal line on an ECG strip representing the beginning and ending point of all waves of the ECG cycle.

jaundice (JAWN-dis)—yellowing of skin and mucous membranes resulting from deposit of bile pigment; usually a symptom of a biliary disease process.

job application—a paper to fill out when applying for a job; contains questions about the applicant.

Joint Commission for the Accreditation of Healthcare Organizations (JCAHO)—this organization is mandatory for hospitals; an accrediting agency that identifies patient care and safety standards.

keratin (KAIR-ah-tin)—tough protein substance found in hair, nails, and horny tissue.

keratinocyte (KAIR-ah-tin-oh-site)—any skin cell that produces keratin, the hard protein material found in the skin, hair, and nails.

key component—three primary determining criteria in selecting an E&M code; include history, examination, and medical decision making.

kidney (KID-nee)—one of two-bean shaped organs located retroperitoneally that filter blood, remove waste products, and manufacture urine.

kilocalorie—1000 calories; amount of heat required to raise 1 kilogram of water 1 degree Celsius.

laceration (LAS-er-aa-shun)—open wound in which the skin and underlying tissue are torn and skin integrity is broken.

laryngeal nerve—nerve that controls the muscles of the larynx in the throat; controls the ability for making vocal sounds.

laryngologist (lar-in-JOL-oh-jist)— physician specializing in disorders and diseases of the throat.

last number redial—telephone feature allowing the user to push one button to dial the last number dialed from that telephone.

late effect—current condition that is the result or byproduct of a previous, resolved condition.

lavage (la-VAZH)—washing out of a cavity.

ledger card—used with manual pegboard systems; each patient has their own ledger card to track services rendered and payments made.

legible—writing that others can read.

lesion (LEE-shun)—tissue abnormality that may be hard or soft, small or large, flat or raised, crusted or filled with fluid or pus, and, when associated with skin, on or within the skin tissue.

letterhead—professional quality stationery containing the name, address, and telephone number of the medical office.

Level I codes—same as CPT.

Level II codes—HCPCS alphanumeric codes created by CMS to bill supplies, drugs, and certain services.

Level III codes—HCPCS alphanumeric codes created by regional Medicare carriers; being phased out under HIPAA.

liability insurance—covers injuries that occur on, in, or because of the insured's property.

licensed—process of registering as a healthcare professional. Those professionals who are bound by law to be licensed in order to practice.

lifetime maximum benefit—amount of money allowed by an insurance carrier for a covered member's covered expenses over the course of the member's lifetime. Often set at $1 million.

ligament (LIG-ah-ment)—a tough, elastic tissue that connects ends of bones.

limiting charge—the maximum amount a Medicare non-PAR provider may bill the patient on an unassigned claim; 115% of the non-PAR fee schedule.

lipids (LIP-ids)—fat-related substances not soluble in water (triglycerides, fats, oils, phospholipids, sterols).

lithotripsy (LITH-oh-trip-see)—breaking up a renal calculus with ultrasound waves aimed at the calculus from outside the body.

litigation—legal action taken against another.

local anesthesia (LOH-kal) (AN-es-thee-zee-ah)—absence of feeling or pain in a localized area of tissue without the loss of consciousness.

logo—artwork used by the medical office in its letterhead or on other printed materials.

Long, Crawford W.—U.S. physician who developed the use of general anesthesia.

long-term care facilities—healthcare facilities designed to care for patients who need care on a long-term basis and may not be able to be cared for in their home.

long-term disability insurance—insurance that covers lost wages and certain other benefits due to a disability that prevents the individual from working, usually for more than one year.

lower gastrointestinal tract (GAS-troh-in-TES-tih-nal) (TRAKT)—small and large intestines.

loyalty—devotion to another; standing by another even in hard times.

M codes—identify neoplasm type and tumor behavior, used by tumor registries.

magnetic resonance imaging—method of using powerful magnets to provide two-dimensional images of the inside of objects.

magnetic therapy—therapy with magnets.

main term—words by which conditions and diseases are alphabetized in ICD-9-CM Volume II; may be name of condition, eponym, acronym, or synonym, but not an anatomical site.

maintained—to keep something in good working order.

malfeasance—performing an incorrect treatment.

malignant (mah-LIG-nant)—cancerous, invasive, and destructive.

malignant hypertension (mah-LIG-nant) (hy-per-TEN-shun)—rapidly developing, severe elevation of blood pressure, often fatal.

malnutrition (MAL-noo-TRISH-un)—condition of excess or deficient nutrient and caloric intake.

malpractice insurance policy—liability insurance that covers injuries patients receive due to acts or omissions by healthcare providers.

malpractice premium—amount of money an insurance carrier charges a healthcare provider in exchange for a malpractice insurance policy.

malware—computer programs written with the purpose of destroying computers or their programs.

mammogram (MAM-moh-gram)—radiograph of breast tissue.

managed care—a system of healthcare delivery focused on reducing costs by transferring risk to the provider; may limit the type and frequency of care members may receive.

manifestation—outward or associated condition resulting from an underlying disease.

massage—using the hands to relax the muscles of the body.

matrix—process of blocking out times in the appointment schedule when the provider is unavailable or out of the office.

Mayo stand—stand that holds a flat metal tray for setting up a sterile field for instruments and supplies; usually has an open side that allows it to be moved over a gurney or table.

Medicaid—a joint federal and state program that helps with medical costs for some people with low incomes and limited resources.

medical asepsis—the practice of reducing the number of pathogens and the transmission of disease; also known as clean technique.

medical decision making (MDM)—a key component E&M coding that describes the complexity establishing a diagnosis and/or selecting a management option.

medical information—information about a patient's medical care and history.

medical management software—software the medical office uses to perform day-to-day functions.

medical necessity—criteria establishing when a service is appropriate.

medical record—legal document consisting of medical information obtained from the patient via consultations, examinations, and tests.

medical research program—program where research is conducted to determine the effectiveness or harm of certain medications or medical treatments.

medical savings account—tax free savings account for small employers and self-employed used for medical expenses in conjunction with a high-deductible health plan.

medically needy—Medicaid-eligible patients who are eligible for medical services, but not cash assistance.

Medicare—federal program covering medical expenses for the elderly, those with end-stage renal disease, and those with a long-term disability. Part A covers hospitalization; Part B covers medical, laboratory, and equipment expenses; and Part D covers prescription drugs.

Medicare managed care plan—managed care plan for Medicare recipients. Less costly than Medicare Part B benefits, and with more restrictions.

Medigap insurance—insurance for Medicare recipients that covers deductibles and allowable payments not covered by Medicare.

meditation—deep concentration on a matter.

megakaryocytes (meg-ah-KAIR-ee-oh-sites)—large bone marrow cells that play an important role in the production of platelets in the bone marrow.

melanin (MEL-ah-nin)—pigment (color) in the skin and hair.

melanocytes (mel-AN-oh-sights)—cells that produce melanin.

melena (me-LEE-nah)—black, tarry stools.

member—the person who owns the insurance policy.

memo—interoffice note.

menarche (men-ARSH)—onset of menses or menstrual cycle during adolescence.

menopause (MEN-oh-pawz)—cessation of menses.

menses (MEN-seez)—cyclic shedding of the uterine lining (endometrium) when fertilization of the ovum does not occur.

mensuration (men-ser-AY-shun)—measurement.

mentor—the preceptor; person who supervises the extern within the healthcare facility during the program.

merit—with regard to malpractice, when a case has substance or is more likely to be found in the patient's favor.

metabolism (meh-TAB-oh-lizm)—process of changing nutrients from food into substances for anabolic or catabolic activity.

metastasis (meh-TASS-tah-sis)—spread of a disease to adjacent and distal tissues and organs.

microbiology—the study of microorganisms.

microorganism—organism that can be viewed under a microscope, but not by the naked eye.

mineral (MIN-er-al)—element essential to every cell, naturally occurring in nature, and used by the body in the processes of blood clotting, muscle contraction, and nervous system impulse conduction.

misfeasance—performing a procedure incorrectly.

mission statement—a written statement that describes the office's reason for existence.

mitral valve prolapse (MY-tral VALV PROH-laps)—valvular disorder in which cusps of mitral valve prolapse into right atrium, failing to close and resulting in back pressure into left atrium.

modified wave scheduling—scheduling system where two or three patients are scheduled at the beginning of each hour, followed by single patient appointments every 10 to 20 minutes for the rest of that hour.

modifier—two-digit alphanumeric codes appended to CPT or Level II codes to further describe circumstances.

modifying term—descriptive words in the alphabetic index that appear indented under the main term to further describe the service or procedure.

monocular—having one eyepiece (on a microscope).

morbidity—the cause of illness or injury.

morphology (mor-FAWL-oh-jee)—the study of shape or form; in microbiology, a method of classifying bacteria according to shape.

mortality—the cause of death.

multidisciplinary—many disciplines; multiple specialties.

multifocal—originating from more than one area or focus.

multiple coding—a diagnosis that requires more than one ICD-9-CM code to completely describe it; often indicated by a second code in slanted brackets.

mycology (my-CALL-oh-jee)—study of fungi, such as yeast and molds.

myelography (MY-eh-LAWG-rah-fee)—radiographs of the spinal cord using a contrast medium.

myocardial infarction (my-oh-CAR-dee-al in-FARC-shun)—death of myocardial tissue due to obstructed blood supply to the tissue.

myocarditis (my-oh-car-DYE-tis)—inflammation of the myocardium.

narrative—type of medical charting where the healthcare provider writes a narrative version of contact with the patient.

nasal septum (NAY-zal SEP-tum)—cartilage wall that divides the nasal cavity.

national commercial insurance carrier—insurance plans available from a variety of companies nationwide. These can be purchased by groups or individuals. Benefits will vary greatly.

national conversion factor—number released by Medicare each year that determines fee schedules for all healthcare services.

national standard—providing a standard that is used throughout the United States.

naturopath—type of therapy that uses natural remedies to treat illness.

negligence—term to describe medical malpractice.

negotiated fee schedule—a common reimbursement method in managed care whereby the MCO develops a list of fees for providers that they agree to accept in the participating provider contract. Fees may be determined based on a percentage of the provider's usual fee or arrived at through negotiation.

neoplasia (NEE-oh-PLAY-zee-ah)—abnormal cell development.

neoplasm—the medical term for an abnormal growth of new tissue; often referred to as a tumor.

neoplasm (NEE-oh-plazm)—new growth or tumor.

nephrologist (neh-FRAWL-oh-jist)—physician specializing in the treatment of kidney diseases and conditions.

nephrology (neh-FRAWL-O-jee)—study of the kidney and the diseases that affect it.

nephrons (NEF-rawnz)—microscopic tubular structures of the kidney.

net pay—amount of an individual's paycheck after all deductions and taxes are taken out.

neuralgia (nyoo-RAL-jee-ah)— sharp, stabbing, or burning pain that occurs along the course of a nerve.

neuritis (nyoo-RY-tis)—inflammation of a nerve or nerves.

neurology (nyoo-RAWL-oh-jee)—study of the nervous system.

neuron (NOOR-on)—nerve cell; basic unit of the nervous system.

neurotransmitter (noo-roh-TRANS-mit-ter)—chemicals that aid in the transmission of electrical impulses from one neuron, or nerve cell, to the next.

new patient—patient who has not seen the same provider, or another provider of the same specialty in the same practice, for more than three years.

new patient checklist—preprinted list of information needed from a new patient when they call to schedule an appointment.

no carbon required (NCR)—paper that, when written on, makes an exact copy beneath it, without the need for carbon paper.

nocturia (nok-TOO-ree-ah)—increased urine output at night.

non-covered—services not eligible for reimbursement under any circumstance.

noncompliance—when a patient refuses to follow the physician's instructions.

noncritical—pertaining to objects that do not touch the patient or touch only intact skin.

nonessential modifiers—words in parentheses after a main term in the ICD-9-CM, clarifying the main term, but need not be present in the medical record.

nonfeasance—delaying treatment or failing to perform a treatment.

noninvasive (non-in-VAY-siv)—pertaining to a procedure or technique that does not require entry into the body by incision or inserting an instrument.

nonparticipating provider—healthcare provider who has not contracted with a particular health insurance carrier.

nonpathogen (non-PATH-oh-jen)—harmless organism that does not cause disease.

nontherapeutic research—research programs that do not create any benefit for the patients in the study; these studies are designed to test if the drug or treatment is harmful to the healthy participant/patient.

nontoxic—not harmful to the body.

normal flora—generally harmless microorganisms common in the human body.

nosocomial infection (NOS-oh-koh-mee-al) (in-FEK-shun)—infection resulting from the hospitalization of a patient.

not elsewhere classified (NES)—diagnosis code that cannot be found elsewhere in the coding book.

not otherwise specified (NOS)—a general code used when details are not available in the medical record.

notice—with regard to legal cases, notice means notice of an impending lawsuit filed.

nuchal rigidity (NOO-kal)—severe and painful rigidity of the neck in which the head is bent forward toward the chest.

nurse practitioner—registered nurse who has completed advanced education and training in the management of common medical illnesses.

obesity (oh-BEE-sih-tee)—excess body weight 20-30 percent above average for gender, age, and height, with abnormal amounts of body fat.

obliterate—to make the original entry completely unreadable.

observation status—a designated type of care in which a patient is hospitalized for monitoring, but not formally admitted.

obstetrician (awb-steh-TRISH-an)—physician specializing in the medical care of women during pregnancy, including prenatal, delivery and postnatal care.

obstetrics (awb-STET-riks)—branch of medicine pertaining to the medical care of women during pregnancy, including prenatal, delivery and postnatal care.

ocular—pertaining to the eye; also, the microscope's eyepiece.

office brochure—pamphlet outlining the staff and services offered within a clinic.

Office of the Insurance Commissioner—each state has its own Insurance Commissioner. This office oversees all aspects of insurance within the state, including health insurance.

office policy—an agreed-upon policy used within the office so all similar situations are handled in the same way.

oliguria (ol-ig-YOO-ree-ah)—diminished urine output, less than 400 ml per day.

omission—something left out.

Omnibus Budget Reconciliation Act—passed by Congress in 1993; created a formula by which all healthcare service fees are calculated.

oncology (ong-KALL-oh-jee)—branch of medicine that deals with the study, diagnosis, and treatment of tumors and cancer.

open-ended question—a question that requires more than a simple yes or no answer.

open hours—scheduling method that allows patients to come in at their leisure, without a set appointment time.

open wound—break in the skin or mucous membrane that exposes underlying tissues.

opening the office—the steps to take to be sure the office is opened properly at the beginning of the day.

ophthalmologist (OFF-thal-MAWL-oh-jist)—physician who specializes in the treatment of eye diseases and disorders.

ophthalmoscope (off-THAL-moh-skohp)—instrument used to examine the eyes.

opportunistic pathogen (AWP-or-too-NIS-tik PATH-oh-jen)—normally nonpathogenic microorganism that causes disease in a host whose immune resistance has been lowered by certain disorders or treatments.

optician (op-TISH-un)—trained professional who grinds lens, inserts the lens into frames, and fits the patient's glasses.

optometrist (op-TAWM-eh-trist)—licensed professional (Doctor of Optometric Medicine) who examines eyes, tests for visual acuity, and prescribes and adapts lens for patients.

oral (AW-ral)—by mouth.

organ—a group of tissues making up a structure that has a particular function in the body.

organelle—a very small organ-functioning unit within a living cell; mitochondria organelles are responsible for the metabolism of lipids and the synthesis (building) of proteins.

organizational chart—breakdown of the chain of command in a business.

orthopedics (or-thoh-PEE-diks)—the study and treatment of diseases and disorders of the musculoskeletal system.

orthopnea (or-THAWP-nee-ah)—ability to breathe only in a standing or upright sitting position.

orthostatic hypotension (or-thoh-STAT-ik hy-poh-TEN-shun)—sudden decrease in blood pressure when an individual rises too quickly from a sitting position, usually resulting in light-headedness.

OSHA—Occupational Safety and Health Administration; a federal agency responsible for oversight of safety in the workplace.

osteoblast (AWS-tee-oh-blast)—a precursor cell in bone formation.

otic (O-tik)—pertaining to the ear.

otolaryngologist (OH-toh-LAIR-in-GAWL-oh-jist)—physician who specializes in the treatment of ear and throat diseases.

otologist (O-tol-O-jist)—physician who specializes in the treatment of ear diseases.

otorhinolaryngologist (OH-toh-RY-noh-LAIR-in-GAWL-oh-jist)—physician who specializes in ear, nose, and throat diseases.

otoscope (OH-toh-skohp)—instrument used to examine the ears.

outliers—exceptional circumstances that cost far more or less than the average.

outpatient—patient who has not been formally admitted to a facility, such as office visits, emergency department, and observation status.

outsourced—sending work outside of the office to a separate company.

overhead—amount of money it costs to sustain a business (rent, salaries, utilities, etc.).

over-the-counter medications—nonprescription medications that can be purchased anywhere without a physician's prescription; examples include antacids, cold remedies, and aspirin.

overtime—wages paid to an individual beyond a regular 40-hour work week; usually paid at 1.5 times the normal hourly wage of that individual.

overweight—general term for early stage of excess body weight above standard for gender, age, and height.

ovum (plural: ova) (OH-vum)—human gamete (egg).

pacemaker—implantable device used to regulate the heartbeat.

packing slip—list of the supplies that were ordered and included in a shipment.

palliative (PAL-ee-ah-tiv)—relieving pain or discomfort.

palpation (pal-PAY-shun)—examination involving touch; examiner uses the hands and fingers to feel both the surface of the body (for abnormalities or irregularities) and various organs (for size, location, and tenderness) and feel generally for masses or lumps and assessing the texture and temperature of the tissue.

palpitations (pal-pih-TAY-shuns)—irregular and often erratic heartbeat felt by the patient.

palsy (PAWL-zee)—tremors; temporary or permanent loss of ability to control or make muscle movement.

para- (PAIR-ah)—combining form signifying the number of deliveries after the 20th week of gestation.

paraplegia (PAIR-ah-PLEE-jee-ah)—loss of sensation and motor activity (paralysis) of the lower trunk and lower extremities.

parasitology (PAIR-ah-si-TAWL-oh-jee)—branch of biology that studies parasites.

parent code—see standalone code.

participating provider—healthcare provider who has contracted with a particular health insurance carrier.

past timely filing limits—the time beyond which an insurance claim will be accepted by an insurance carrier. Usually set at one year from the date of service, though some plans will not accept claims beyond 90 days from the date of service.

pasteurization—method of heating liquids in order to kill bacteria.

patent (PAY-tent)—open.

pathogen (PATH-oh-jen)—disease-causing microorganism.

pathogenicity—ability of an organism to cause disease.

patient billing statements—statements sent to patients, usually monthly, indicating the amount of money they owe to the clinic or provider for healthcare services.

patient information—the information contained within the patient's medical record.

patient status—classification of patients as new or established.

Patient's Bill of Rights—laws pertaining to patients' rights regarding their healthcare.

payer number—unique identifying number assigned to each insurance carrier for the purpose of directing electronic claims.

payroll—process of calculating wages and deductions; calculating the amount to be paid to employees for work performed.

payroll taxes—monies withheld from employees' wages for federal income taxes, Social Security, and Medicare.

pediatrician (pee-dee-ah-TRISH-an)—physician who specializes in treating children from birth to age 20.

pediatrics (pee-dee-AT-riks)—medical specialty that focuses on the care and treatment of children from birth through age 20.

pegboard accounting system—manual system of bookkeeping.

penicillin—antibiotic drug useful in killing some forms of bacteria.

per case—payment method used for hospitals. Under this method, the hospital receives a pre-established amount per patient for the entire stay, based on the patients' diagnosis, regardless of how long they are in or what services are provided.

per diem—payment method whereby the facility is paid a flat amount per day the patient remains, regardless of what services are provided.

percussion (per-KUSH-un)—examination consisting of tapping the fingertips lightly but sharply against the body to assess the size and location of underlying organs.

pericarditis (pair-ee-kar-DY-tis)—inflammation of the pericardium.

perineum (pair-ah-NEE-um)—area between the vaginal orifice and the anus.

periorbital edema—abnormal, excessive fluid surrounding the eye that usually occurs in the morning upon waking.

periosteum (pair-ee-AH-stee-um)—a fibrous membrane covering the outside of bone tissue.

peristalsis (pair-ih-STAL-sis)—rhythmic, involuntary, wave-like motion in the hollow tubes of the body that assists the passage of contents.

personal digital assistants (PDAs)—small, portable devices used to keep and transmit information.

personal information—includes a patient's name, birthdate, gender, marital status, occupation, next of kin, and any other items collected for personal identification. It may also include any comments the medical assistant might write in the patient's file regarding the patient's language or cultural background, or such information that pertains to the patient's healthcare.

personal protective equipment (PPE)—protective clothing and equipment such as gloves, gowns, and masks that are worn to prevent contamination by blood and other body fluids.

personal space—unseen "bubble" around each of us that outlines the perimeter we are not comfortable with others entering.

personnel file—file to be kept on all employees in a company; includes original applications, federal withholding requests, dates and copies of evaluations.

personnel manual—also called an employee handbook, a list of policies relating to employment in an individual office.

petechiae (peh-TEE-kee-eye)—small hemorrhages under the skin.

pH—measurement of hydrogen ion concentration in a substance or solution; a pH of 7.0 is considered neutral, below 7.0 is considered acidic, and above 7.0 is considered alkaline.

phagocytic (FAG-oh-sit-ick)—having the ability to ingest particulate material, such as bacteria.

phagocytosis (FAG-oh-sy-toh-sis)—the engulfing and destruction of microorganisms or foreign matter by phagocytic cells.

pharmaceuticals—drugs, medicines, chemical compounds.

pharmacology—the study of drugs and their effects on the human body.

phlebotomist (fleh-BAWT-oh-mist)—individual trained to draw blood.

phlebotomy (fleh-BAWT-oh-mee)—process of blood collection, sometimes defined as "an incision into a vein".

phobia (FOH-bee-ah)—irrational, obsessive fear of an object, situation, or activity.

photometer (foh-TOHM-eh-ter)—instrument used to measure the intensity of light rays; an electronic component of many instruments.

physical status modifier—two-digit alphanumeric codes (P1 to P6) appended to anesthesia codes that indicate the health status of the patient at the beginning of the procedure.

physician services—patient care provided by a licensed physician.

physician's assistant—nonphysician clinician licensed to practice medicine under a physician's supervision.

Physician's Desk Reference **(PDR)**—published every year, containing up-to-date information on all drugs available for legal sale in the United States.

physiology—study of the mechanical, physical, and biochemical functions of living organisms.

planning—researching the actions or steps needed to implement something.

plasma (PLAZ-mah)—liquid portion of anticoagulated blood.

plasmapheresis (PLAZ-mah-feh-REE-sis)—daily replacement of blood plasma in the body with other fluids or donated plasma for two or more weeks.

point of service—an insurance offering in which a patient has access to multiple plans, such as an HMO, PPO, and indemnity, and may choose to use any of them for any given service.

policy—statement of guidelines, or rules, on a given topic in the office.

policy and procedure manuals—manuals kept in the office, outlining the ways staff should handle/perform certain activities.

policy number—number given by insurance carriers that identify a group of insureds.

policyholder—same as the member or the insured; term used to identify the person who holds or owns an insurance policy.

polyps (POLL-ips)—fingerlike growths on the mucous membranes throughout the body.

polyuria (pol-ee-YOO-ree-ah)—excessive urine production and frequent, urgent, and excessive urinary output.

portal hypertension (POR-tal hy-per-TEN-shun)—condition of increased blood flow pressure through the blood vessels of the liver (portal circulation), often caused by cirrhosis of the liver or compression of the hepatic blood vessels.

portability—being able to take an insurance policy from one employer to another.

postage meter—electronic machine capable of printing postage in the office.

postictal (post-IK-tal)—pertaining to the period immediately following a seizure.

posting—adding charges or payments to a patient's account.

postnatal/postpartum (post-NAY-tal)—after childbirth.

postoperative period—the number of days following a procedure during which follow-up visits are bundled with the primary procedure and are not billed separately.

postoperative (post-op) (post-OP-er-ah-tiv)—pertaining to patient care following surgery.

practitioner—a person who practices in a profession, such as medicine.

pre-existing condition—condition for which a patient received treatment in a certain period prior to beginning coverage with a new insurance plan. Rules vary from one insurance plan to another.

preapprovals—process of calling a patient's insurance carrier prior to a service in order to obtain preapproval or authorization for the service to be performed.

preauthorization—approval for treatment or service obtained from an insurance company before the care is provided.

precedence—to decide a legal case in court, which then relates to all cases that come after it.

preceptor—mentor; person who supervises the extern within the healthcare facility during the program.

precertification—see preauthorization.

precordical lead—ECG lead that views the heart in a horizontal plain.

preferred—services or providers covered at a higher (less cost to the patient) fee.

preferred provider organization (PPO)—organization that contracts with independent providers to perform services for members at discounted rates.

preferred providers—physician who has signed a contract to accept the conditions outlined by a managed care health plan.

premature ventricular contraction (PVC)—a beat that comes early in the cardiac cycle, is not preceded by a P wave, and has a widened and distorted QRS complex; sometimes referred to as premature ventricular complex or premature ventricular beat (PVB).

premium—dollar amount paid to the insurance company to have coverage in force; usually paid monthly; employers may pay part or all of the premium as an employee benefit.

prenatal (pree-NAY-tal)—prior to birth.

preoperative (pre-op) (pree-OP-er-ah-tiv)—pertaining to preparation before surgery.

presbycusis (PREZ-bee-ah-KOO-sis)—hearing deficiency normally associated with aging.

presbyopia (prez-bee-OH-pee-ah)—vision deficiency normally associated with aging.

presenting problem—a contributory factor in E&M coding that consists of a disease, condition, illness, injury, symptom, sign, finding complaint, or other reason for the encounter, as stated by the patient.

primary care provider—term used to define the physician, usually a general or family practice doctor, who oversees all care needed or desired by their patient. The primary care provider is referred to as the PCP and many managed care plans require the PCP be the one to determine when the patient needs care or services, such as a referral to a specialist.

primary diagnosis—see *first-listed*.

primary insurance—insurance plan that pays first for a covered patient's services.

principal diagnosis—the reason determined, after study, to be responsible for an inpatient stay.

private insurance—insurance not provided by the government but by an independent not-for-profit or for-profit company; also called commercial insurance.

problem-oriented medical record charting—type of medical record charting that focuses on the patient's healthcare problems and addresses those problems at each visit.

procedural coding—coding for services and procedures in health care.

procedure—list of steps describing how to perform a given task or project.

procedures—services such as surgery or therapy performed on a patient by a healthcare provider.

proctology (prok-TALL-oh-jee)—medical practice specializing in disorders of the rectum and anus.

prodromal—pertaining to symptoms during the period immediately preceding onset of a disease condition.

professional appointments—appointments the doctor makes with other healthcare providers, associates, or colleagues.

professional courtesy—to give a patient a discount, or free service, due to the fact that he or she is a healthcare professional.

professional distance—keeping a professional relationship with patients.

professionalism—acting in a business-like manner in the workplace.

prognosis (prawg-NOH-sis)—an outcome prediction for the course of a disease and patient recovery (literal meaning: knowledge before).

progress notes—notes in the patient's medical chart outlining progress or complaints.

projectile vomiting—vomiting with uncontrollable force.

prokaryote (pro-CARE-ee-oat)—group of microorganisms, such as bacteria, that lack an organized nucleus and cytoplasmic organelles.

proofreader's marks—list of marks commonly used when proofreading documents.

proofreading—the process of reading and reviewing a document for possible errors.

prostatitis (PRAWS-tah-TY-tis)—inflammation and/or infection of the prostate gland.

prosthesis (plural: prostheses) (praws-THEE-sis)—artificial replacement for a body part.

protein (PROH-teen)—food component composed of amino acids; provides a source of energy and assists in building and renewing body tissues.

proteinuria (PROH-tee-NYOO-ree-ah)—presence of abnormally large amounts of protein in the urine.

proximal tubule (PRAWK-sih-mal TOO-byool)—tubule closest to glomerulus.

psychiatrist (sigh-KY-ah-trist)—medical doctor or physician specializing in the medical treatment of mental illness.

psychiatry (sigh-KY-ah-tree)—branch of medicine that deals with diagnosis, treatment, and prevention of mental disorders.

psychologist (sigh-KALL-oh-jist)—specialist in the field of psychology, therapy, and research.

psychology (sigh-KALL-oh-jee)—science dealing with normal and abnormal mental processes and behavior.

psychosis (sigh-KOH-sis)—abnormal mental coping of the individual who is out of touch with reality.

psychotherapeutic (sigh-koh-THAIR-ah-pew-tik)—alleviating symptoms of anxiety, depression, and psychosis.

psychotherapy (sigh-koh-THAIR-ah-pee)—treatment of mental disorders with talk therapy, or counseling.

psychotropic (sigh-koh-TROW-pik)—affecting psychic function, behavior, experience, or emotions.

public health—the overall health of a community.

public law—laws pertaining to citizens.

pulmonary function testing (PUL-moh-nair-ee)—testing performed to evaluate airflow and lung volume.

purge—to remove closed or inactive patient medical records from the medical office.

purulent (PYOOR-yoo-lent)—containing pus.

pyelonephritis (pye-eh-loh-neh-FRYE-tis)—inflammation and/or of the pelvis of the kidney.

pyogenic (pye-oh-JEN-ik)—pus-forming.

pyuria (py-YOO-ree-ah)—pus in the urine.

quadriplegia (kwod-rih-PLEE-jee-ah)—paralysis of the entire trunk and all four extremities.

qualified—diagnosis statement accompanied by terms such as possible, probable, suspected, rule out (R/O), or working diagnosis indicating the physician has not determined the root cause.

quality improvement programs—programs designed to improve the quality of a service, such as patient care.

quarterly payroll reports—reports of amount of taxes withheld from employees' wages to be filed quarterly (four times per year).

radial (RAY-dee-al)—at the wrist over the radial artery.

radiation (ray-dee-AY-shun)—radiant energy.

radioactive waste—any waste contaminated with radioactive material.

radiocarbon dating—procedure that uses the measure of carbon in a substance to determine its age.

radiograph (rah-dee-O-grahf)—developed X-ray film.

radiography (ray-dee-OG-rah-fee)—study or practice of radiology using x-rays.

radiologist (rah-dee-ALL-oh-jist)—physician who specializes in radiology.

radiology (ray-dee-ALL-oh-jee)—medical specialty that uses radiant energy forms, ultrasound, and magnetic waves to study, diagnose, and treat disease and injury.

radiolucent (ray-dee-oh-LOO-cent)—easily penetrated by x-rays.

radiopaque (ray-dee-oh-PAYK)—capable of obstructing the passage of x-rays.

radium—radioactive chemical element.

range of motion—the full extent of any joint potential for movement, including actions such as flexion, extension, circumduction, adduction, and abduction.

rapport—mutual trust and affection for one another.

reactive (ree-AK-tiv)—able to respond to a stimulus.

reasonable and necessary skill and care—care a reasonable person would render to a patient; the skills a healthcare provider is expected to have.

reception area—waiting area for patients in the medical office.

receptionist—medical staff member who greets patients, answers the telephone, and directs the office flow.

recertification—process of renewing a certificate.

reduction (ree-DUK-shun)—the process of open or closed manipulation that returns bony ends to correct anatomical position before healing.

reference initials—in a professional letter, these are the initials of the author of the letter followed by the initials of the person who typed the letter (AJF/cmm).

referral—one healthcare provider sending a patient to another provider. Usually required for coverage with a specialist in managed care plans.

referred pain—pain that is felt in a different area from the injured or diseased part of the body.

reflecting—repeating to the patient what you believe they are saying to you.

registered medical assistant (RMA)—credential given a medical assistant who has passed the RMA certification examination.

regulatory laws—laws regarding government regulations.

reimbursement—payment sent to the healthcare provider for services rendered.

rejected—a claim that is returned to the provider without processing due to a technical error.

relative value unit (RVU)—unit of measure assigned to medical services based on the resources required to provide it; includes work, practice expense, and liability insurance.

remission (rih-MISH-un)—complete or partial disappearance of the clinical characteristics of chronic or malignant disease.

remotely—to access something, such as a computer system, while away from the office.

renal (REE-nal)—pertaining to the kidney.

renal calculus (plural: calculi) (REE-nal) (KAL-kyoo-lus)—kidney stone.

repolarization (ree-POHL-ar-ih-ZAY-shun)—return of the cardiac cell to the resting state.

res judicata—Latin for the thing has been decided.

resource-based relative value scale—national standard scale developed by the Centers for Medicare and Medicaid Services in order to determine the fee paid for services.

resource-based relative value scale—the methodology Medicare uses to establish physician fees, based on the relative value unit, the geographic adjustment factor, and the conversion factor.

respect—to hold another in a place of high esteem.

respite care—temporary care provided by an outside party to relieve the usual caregiver.

respondeat superior—Latin for let the master answer.

responsibility—taking ownership of ones actions.

resume—professional document outlining the educational and job experience of an applicant for a job.

retirement plan—benefit provided by an employer whereby money (either from the employer only or from both the employer and the employee) can be put aside for the employee's eventual retirement.

rhinologist (ry-NAWL-oh-jist)—physician who specializes in the treatment of nasal passage and sinus diseases.

rhythm—time interval between pulses or breaths.

risk factor—condition or situation that makes a person particularly vulnerable to certain diseases or disorders.

risk management—identifying possible risks that may cause injury to a patient or employee in a healthcare setting.

role delineation chart—list created by the AAMA that identifies all clinical, administrative, and general procedures medical assistants are trained for.

route—to direct telephone calls to a particular extension.

rubber stamp signature—rubber stamp image of a person's signature to be used when obtaining the actual signature is not possible.

salaried—employee who is paid a set amount for a period of time regardless of the hours worked.

salutation—greeting that begins a professional letter (Dear _____).

sanitization (san-ih-ty-ZA-shun)—method of decontamination that reduces the numbers of microorganisms on an object or surface; removes organic material from equipment or instruments and must be performed before disinfection and sterilization.

saturated fats—fats derived from animal sources that are solid at room temperature.

scanners—similar to a copier; capable of taking an exact image of a photo or document and placing it into the computer.

scope of practice—the range of skills a particular healthcare professional is expected to have and operate within.

sebaceous glands (she-BAY-shus) (GLANDS)—small glands in the dermis that secrete sebum, usually through ducts that empty into the hair follicles.

secondary diagnoses—conditions, diseases, or reasons for seeking care in addition to the first-listed diagnosis; they may or may not be related to the first-listed diagnosis.

secondary insurance—insurance plan that pays second for a covered patient's services.

section—one of six major divisions of the CPT manual: evaluation and management; anesthesia; surgery; radiology; pathology and laboratory; medicine.

security envelope—envelope that cannot be seen through.

segregation—keeping two parties apart due to differences, such as race or gender.

self-insurance—type of insurance where, rather than purchasing a commercial insurance policy an employer sets aside a large reserve fund to directly reimburse employees for medical expenses.

semicolon (;)—a punctuation mark in a standalone code; the part of the definition before the semicolon is used by the indented codes that follow.

sentinel event—an event in the healthcare setting where someone was injured, or could have been injured.

sepsis (SEP-sis)—febrile state characterized by pathogens in the bloodstream.

sequela (plural: sequelae) (see-KWELL-ah)—outcome.

sequelae—an abnormal condition resulting from a previous injury, condition, or disease.

serology (seer-HL-oh-gee)—laboratory science in which blood serum is tested for the presence of antibodies.

serum (SEER-um)—liquid portion that remains when the blood has been allowed to clot.

served—with regard to legal cases, being served is to be given notice of an impending lawsuit filed.

service animal—animal that has been trained to assist a person with a handicap.

settled—when an offer of money is extended and accepted in order to drop a legal lawsuit.

sexual harassment—unwanted sexual attention or comments in the workplace.

shaman—religious or spiritual figure.

shingling—process of attaching small pieces of paper to standard-size sheets of paper so the small items are easy to locate in patients' charts.

short-term memory—memory of recent events.

side effect—effect other than the therapeutic effect.

sign—a physical sign of a condition that can observed or measured by a physician.

sign-in sheet—place where patients sign their name upon entry to the office; may be on paper or electronic.

sinoatrial (SA) node (sigh-noh-AY-tree-al)—pacemaker of the heart.

skilled nursing facility—a licensed facility that primarily provides inpatient, skilled nursing care to patients who require medical, nursing, or rehabilitative services but does not provide the level of care or treatment available in a hospital.

slack time—appointment scheduling method of leaving certain times of day open to accommodate things like patients who call for same-day appointments or physicians who need to catch up on charting.

sliding fee scale—a provider's fee schedule that charges varying fees for a service based on a patient's financial ability to pay.

small claims court—the place to file claims against a debtor who owes a small amount of money; the amount of money varies from one state to another.

soak—procedure in which the total body or body part is immersed in water for heat or cold therapeutic applications.

SOAP note charting—type of charting that takes into account the patient's subjective and objective findings, the provider's assessment of the patient's condition, and the prescribed plan of action for treatment.

social information—information about a patient's social habits such as tobacco, drug, or alcohol use.

Social Security Act—passed by Congress in 1935 as a means to provide financial security to workers and their families; provides for a process where money is taken from an employee's wages in order to give it back to them after retirement.

solid waste—paper, cans, cups and other garbage from non-clinical areas.

sonography (soh-NAWG-rah-fee)—use of ultrasound waves to view internal body structures.

speaker telephone—allows the user to place the caller on a speaker, which permits anyone in the room with the user to hear and be heard by the caller.

special instructions—directions within each section describing specific rules and definitions for use of codes within a particular category or subcategory.

specialist—healthcare provider who specializes in a particular area, such as a cardiologist (heart) or dermatologist (skin).

spectrophotometric (SPEK-troh-foh-tom-met-rick)—the measurement or estimate of the amount of color in a solution.

speed dial—telephone feature allowing the user to program commonly called numbers into their system; also called an automatic dialer.

spell check—software that comes with most word processing programs enabling the user to verify the correct spelling of many words.

sphygmomanometer (sfig-moh-mah-NOM-eh-ter)—instrument used to measure blood pressure.

splint—a temporary orthopedic device used to immobilize, restrain, and support any extremity of the body.

spore—capsule formed by some bacteria as a protective shell during their resting state; under favorable conditions the bacteria become active again.

staff model HMO—employs salaried physicians who treat members in facilities owned and operated by the HMO.

standalone code—a CPT code that contains a full description and is not dependent on another code for complete meaning.

standard of care—legal term to describe the type of care a reasonable healthcare provider is expected to provide under the same situation.

Standard Precautions—precautions that replace Body Substance Isolation and Universal Precautions in institutional healthcare settings such as hospitals and nursing homes; the first level of care combines Universal and Body Substance Isolation Precautions, and the second consists of Transmission-based Precautions.

standardized—uniform practice.

staph (STAFF)—*Staphylococcus*.

status epilepticus (STAT-us EP-ih-LEP-tih-kus)—continuous seizure activity.

statute of limitations—time within which a patient has to file a lawsuit after an injury has occurred.

stem cells—cells that are capable of forming into any other cell type.

stenosis (steh-NOH-sis)—narrowing or constriction of a passage.

stent—device implanted in a vessel to maintain its patency (openness).

stereotyping—holding an opinion of another person based solely on something about their group status, such as race, gender, or economic status.

sterilant—chemical sterilizing agent.

sterile—free from all living microorganisms and bacterial spores.

sterile field—microorganism-free environment used during procedures to prevent contamination by pathogens.

sterilization—process of destroying all microbial forms of life, for which the autoclave is most commonly used.

sterilization indicator—different forms of tape or inserts (strips or tubes, for example) that provide verification of an autoclave's effectiveness.

stethoscope(STETH-oh-skohp)—instrument used to listen to sounds within the body.

stop loss—the maximum amount the patient must pay out-of-pocket for copayments and coinsurance.

strep—*Streptococcus*.

subcategory—a division of a category within the tabular index.

subcategory—a four-digit code in ICD-9-CM tabular list.

subclassification—a five-digit code in ICD-9-CM tabular list.

subcutaneous (sub-kyoo-TAY-nee-us)—under the epidermal and dermal layers of the skin.

subcutaneous tissue—deepest layer of the skin.

subject line—in a professional letter, this is the subject of the letter.

sublingually (sub-LING-gwa-lee)—under the tongue.

subpoena—court order demanding someone's appearance in court, or for copies of the medical record to be sent to a third party.

subscriber—same as the member or the insured; a term used to identify the person who holds or owns an insurance policy.

subsection—subdivisions within a CPT section of the tabular index.

subterm—indented two spaces under the boldfaced main term in the ICD-9-CM and further describes the condition, in terms of etiology, co-existing conditions, anatomic site, episode, or similar descriptor.

super bill—also called an encounter form or a routing slip. These forms vary from one office to the next and usually contain the procedural and diagnostic codes commonly used in that clinic. A charge slip is generated on each patient coming in for care each day; these are a record of the charges and diagnoses for that patient for that date of service. Usually completed by the healthcare provider who performed the service.

supporting documentation—Copies sent to an insurance company at its request (and with the patient's permission) in order to determine the medical necessity of a requested procedure. Usually consists of medical chart notes, lab reports, operative reports, or pathology reports.

surgical package—refers to all services that are covered under one surgical code.

suspected condition—condition the physician suspects the patient may have.

sympathy—feeling pity for another person.

symptom (SIMP-tum)—a perceptible change in the body related by the patient.

synarthrosis (sihn-ar-THROS-is)—condition of absent joint movement.

synonyms—words of equivalent meaning.

systole (SIS-tole)—contraction of the myocardium.

systolic (sis-TOL-ik)—pertaining to contraction of the heart; highest reading of the blood pressure.

tabular index—the numerical listing of all CPT codes, accompanied by guidelines and notes.

tabular list—Volume I of ICD-9-CM that lists all diagnostic codes in numerical order.

tachycardia (tak-ee-CAR-dee-ah)—heart rate above 100 beats per minute (BPM).

tachypnea (ta-kip-NEE-ah)—rapid breathing.

take home pay—the amount of an individual's paycheck after all deductions and taxes are taken out.

tax audits—a function of the IRS where an individual or company's records are reviewed to verify that taxes were paid correctly.

technical educational programs—programs designed to teach skills to students without the need for higher education. Also called vocational programs.

temperature—measurement of body heat produced and lost during metabolism, respiration, elimination, and environmental fluctuation.

ten-key calculator—calculator, usually electronic, that has the keys from 1 to 0 laid out similar to a telephone key pad.

tendon (TEN-dun)—tough, elastic tissue that connects muscle to bone.

testis (plural testes, also called testicle) (TES-tis)—oval structure in the scrotal sac that produces sperm.

tetany (TET-ah-nee)—painful, intense, spasmodic muscle contractions.

therapeutic effect—the desired or intended effect.

thermodynamics—the use of cryotherapy or thermotherapy for therapeutic treatment.

thermometer—instrument used to measure body temperature.

thermotherapy (ther-moh-THAIR-ah-pee)—the use of heat application to increase circulation to an area and promote healing.

thesaurus—resource for locating alternate words that have similar meanings.

third party administrator—a company that processes paperwork for claims for a self-insured employer.

thromboembolism (thorm-boh-EM-boh-lizm)—obstruction of a blood vessel by a thrombus.

thrombosis (THROM-boh-sis)—condition of having a blood clot in a blood vessel.

thrombus (plural: thrombi) (THROM-bus)—blood clot in the vessel that can form an obstruction in the vessel.

thumb drives—also called flash drives; small-sized external storage devices.

tickler file—reminder method for keeping track of events needing attention in the future.

time clock—piece of equipment where an employee uses a card to have arrival and departure from work times stamped for the purposes of payroll.

tissue (TISH-yoo)—a group of cells that act together for a particular body function.

tolerance (TAHL-er-ans)—requiring greater amounts of a substance to achieve the desired effect.

tonic (TAWN-ik)—pertaining to muscular tension.

tort law—laws that relate to one party injuring another.

tort of outrage—to intentionally inflict emotional upset on another.

total parenteral nutrition (par-EN-ter-all) (NEW-try-shun)—nutrition ingested by means other than oral intake.

toxic effect—potential harmful or life-threatening effect.

tracing claims—process of calling an insurance company when an insurance claim has not been paid in a timely manner.

trade (brand, proprietary) name—name registered by a manufacturer for use only by that manufacturer; has a registered trademark symbol; first letter is always capitalized.

traditional laws—also known as common law.

training manual—a book that details the type of training needed to use a certain piece of equipment and the date and signature indicating when an individual employee was trained.

transcribe—to listen to a spoken word (usually via tape recording) and type it into a printed document.

transcription machines—machine that allows the user to listen to a tape while typing the words into a printed document.

transdisciplinary duties—general medical assisting duties, such as acting in a professional manner, treating patients with respect, and protecting patient privacy.

Transmission-based Precautions—care based on symptoms of disease and transmission method of the pathogen, such as contact, droplet, air, vector, or common vehicle.

transplant—method of removing an organ from a donor and implanting it into a recipient.

traveler's checks—checks that are more secure for use during travel.

treatment regimen—prescribed or recommended plan of treatment made by the healthcare provider.

triage (TREE-azh)—sorting and setting priorities for treatment for patients who are on the phone or at the reception desk.

triage notebook—notebook kept near the administrative medical assistant responsible for answering incoming telephone calls. The notebook contains questions and steps to follow in the event a caller has a potentially life-threatening condition. The purpose of the notebook is to allow the administrative medical assistant to determine if the patient needs to be seen in the office or referred to emergency medical services.

triaging—process of sorting patients into a priority order based upon their needs.

TRICARE—health insurance administered by the U.S Department of Defense for active duty military personnel, retired service personnel, and their eligible dependents. Formerly known as Civilian Health and Medical Program (CHAMPUS).

triglycerides—chief form of fat found in foods.

trigone (TRY-gohn)—triangular area in floor of urinary bladder where ureters enter and urethra exits.

tumor (TOO-mor)—growth characterized by progressive and uncontrolled production of cells.

tumor marker—substance produced by tumor cells that can be measured and monitored in blood serum levels to indicate progression of metastases and/or effectiveness of cancer chemotherapy.

turbidity (TUR-bid-i-tee)—cloudiness, lack of clarity.

turgor (TER-gor)—normal appearance of the skin and its ability to return to normal after being pinched.

ultramicroscopic—requiring magnification with an electron microscope to be seen.

ultrasonic cleaning—use of ultrasound waves to loosen contaminants.

ultrasound—method of using sound waves to portray 3-D images.

unbundling—billing multiple services with separate CPT codes and separate charges that should be combined under a single CPT code and one charge.

uncertain—see *qualified*.

uncollectible—account that the clinic does not believe will ever be paid.

undue influence—to persuade someone to do something he or she does not want to do.

unemployment insurance—insurance that allows employees to be paid unemployment benefits in the event they should lose their job.

unifocal—originating from same area or focus.

unintentional tort—to harm another person accidentally.

Universal Precautions—the CDC's original guidelines for preventing the transmission of AIDS and other blood-borne diseases.

unsaturated fats—fats derived from plant sources that are liquid at room temperature.

upcode—to code and bill for a higher level of service than was actually provided.

upper gastrointestinal tract (GAS-troh-in-TES-tih-nal)—oral cavity (mouth), esophagus, duodenum, and stomach.

ureter (YOO-ree-ter)—tube leading from the kidney to the urinary bladder.

urethra (yoo-REE-thrah)—tube leading from urinary bladder to outside the body.

urgent care clinics—facilities, such as emergency rooms, that care for patients who have urgent care needs.

urinalysis (YOO-rih-NAL-ih-sis)—visual and chemical examination of the urine.

urinary bladder (YOO-rih-nair-e BLAD-er)—receptacle for urine that has been manufactured by the kidneys.

urinary meatus (YOO-rih-nair-e mee-AY-tus)—external sphincter of the urethra.

urobilinogen—derivative substance formed by conversion of direct bilirubin by bacteria in the intestinal tract.

urologist (yoo-RALL-oh-jist)—physician who specializes in treating urinary system diseases and conditions and conditions involving the male reproductive system.

urology (yoo-RALL-oh-jee)—study of the urinary system in males and females and the diseases that affect it.

user manual—document that describes how something (e.g., equipment) is used.

usual, customary, and reasonable (UCR) fee—a fee determined by third-party payers to reimburse providers based on the provider's normal fee, the range of fees charged by providers of the same specialty in the same geographic area, and other factors to determine appropriate fees in unusual situations.

V-codes—used to classify the reason for the visit, other than the disease or illness.

venipuncture (VEEN-ih-punk-cher)—method of obtaining venous blood for analysis of hematology and chemistry studies.

venous (VEE-nus)—pertaining to blood vessels that carry blood toward the heart.

ventricle (VEN-trik-el)—right or left lower chamber of heart.

verify—take steps to confirm something, such as a patient's healthcare coverage.

virology—specialized branch of microbiology that studies viruses and associated diseases.

viruses—ultramicroscopic, nonliving organisms classified as microorganisms because they contain DNA or RNA and are capable of parasitic metabolism and reproduction.

vitamins—components required for metabolism, growth, and development.

vocational programs—educational programs designed to teach skills to students without the need for higher education. Also called technical educational programs.

W-2 form—federal form that is given to each employee by January 31st for wages paid in the previous year; this form is sent in by each employee with their federal tax return.

W-4 form—federal form filled out by all employees to indicate their marital status and the number of exemptions they wish to claim for the purpose of federal tax withholding.

wages—amount of money paid to an employee for work performed.

waiting period—period of time after a new health insurance plan begins during which certain services are not covered. Varies from one health plan and policy to another.

waiver—see advance beneficiary notice.

warranty—period within which a piece of equipment will be repaired without cost to the buyer.

wave scheduling—scheduling system where patients are scheduled only during the first half of each hour.

with—interpreted as *both, together with* in a diagnostic code description.

withholding allowances—the number of exemptions, such as children, an employee wishes to claim on federal tax forms.

worker compensation—insurance coverage for job-related illness or injury provided by law by employers for employees. Covers medical expenses, lost wages, and job retraining for injuries received by employees while on the job.

write off—to remove a balance from a patient account.

X-ray—form of electromagnetic radiation that travels in waves at the speed of light and can penetrate matter and produce a visible image on film.

yoga—a natural therapy that consists of a series of exercises designed to promote control over the body and mind.

zygote (ZEYE-goat)—the fertilized ovum created by the union of the male and female sex cells (sperm and ovum).

References

Books and Manuals

American Association of Medical Assistants. (2003). *AAMA role delineation study: Occupational analysis of the medical assisting profession.* Chicago, IL: Author.

Badasch, S.A., & Chesebro, D.S. (2004). *Introduction to health occupations: Today's health care worker.* Upper Saddle River, NJ: Pearson Education.

Beaman, N., & McPhillips, L.F. (2007). *Pearson's Comprehensive Medical Assisting.* Upper Saddle River, NJ: Pearson Education.

Beasley, B.M. (2003). *Understanding EKGs: A practical approach* (2nd ed.). Upper Saddle River, NJ: Pearson Education.

Berman, A., Snyder, S., Kozier, B., & Erb, G. (2008). *Fundamentals of nursing: Concepts, process, and practice* (8th ed.). Upper Saddle River, NJ: Pearson Education.

Ellis, K.M. (2007). *EKG plain and simple* (2nd ed.). Upper Saddle River, NJ: Pearson Education.

Fisher, L. E. (1980). *The Hospitals.* New York: Holiday House.

Fremgen, B. (1998). *Essentials of medical assisting: Administrative and clinical competencies.* Upper Saddle River, NJ: Prentice Hall.

Fremgen, B.F., & Frucht, S.S. (2009). *Medical terminology: A living language* (4th ed.). Upper Saddle River, NJ: Pearson Education.

Garza, D., & McBride, K. B. (2005). *Phlebotomy handbook: Blood collection essentials* (7th ed.). Upper Saddle River, NJ: Pearson Education.

Grubbs, P.A., & Blasband, B.A. (2005). *The long term nursing assistant* (3rd ed.). Upper Saddle River, NJ: Pearson Education.

Harris, P. R., & Moran, R. T. (1977). *Managing Cultural Differences.* Houston, TX: Gulf Publishing Co.

Holland, A. (2000). *Voices of Qi: An Introductory Guide to Traditional Chinese Medicine.* Northwest Institute of Acupuncture and Oriental Medicine. New York: North Atlantic Books.

Holland, N., & Adams, M.P. (2007). *Core concepts in pharmacology* (2nd ed.). Upper Saddle River, NJ: Pearson Education.

Ladewig, P.A., London, M.L., & Davidson, M.R. (2006). *Contemporary maternal-newborn nursing care* (6th ed.). Upper Saddle River, NJ: Pearson Education.

Limmer, D., & O'Keefe, M.F. (2007). *Emergency care* (10th ed.). Upper Saddle River, NJ: Pearson Education.

Maciocia, G. (2005). *The Foundations of Chinese Medicine: A Comprehensive Text for Acupuncturists and Herbalists.* London: Churchill Livingstone.

Martini, F.H. (2009). *Fundamentals of anatomy and physiology* (8th ed.). Upper Saddle River, NJ: Benjamin Cummings Publishing Company.

Miele, C., & England, T. (1999). *From nursing care to clinical care associate.* Upper Saddle River, NJ: Brady.

Mulvihill, M.L. et al. (2006). *Human diseases: A systemic approach* (6th ed.). Upper Saddle River, NJ: Pearson Education.

Olds, S.B., London, M.L., Ladewig, P.W., & Davidson, M.R. (2008). *Maternal-newborn nursing and women's health care* (7th ed.). Upper Saddle River, NJ: Pearson Education.

Porter, R. (1999). *The Greatest Benefit to Mankind: A Medical History of Humanity from Antiquity to the Present.* New York: W.W. Norton and Company.

Ramont, R., Niedringhaus, D., & Towle, M. (2006). *Comprehensive nursing care.* Upper Saddle River, NJ: Pearson Education.

Silverthorn, D.U. (2009). *Human physiology: An integrated approach* (4th ed.). Upper Saddle River, NJ: Benjamin Cummings Publishing Company.

Smith, S.F., Duell, D.J., & Martin, B.C. (2008). *Clinical nursing skills: Basic to advanced skills* (7th ed.). Upper Saddle River, NJ: Pearson Education.

Tabloski, P.A. (2006). *Gerontological nursing.* Upper Saddle River, NJ: Pearson Education.

Turley, S.M. (2003). *Understanding pharmacology for health professionals* (3rd ed.). Upper Saddle River, NJ: Pearson Education.

Vallejo-Manzur, F., et al. (2003). "The resuscitation greats. Andreas Vesalius: The concept of an artificial airway." *Resuscitation* 56:3–7. Tamaulipas, Mexico: Autonomous University of Tamaulipas.

Vines, D., Bracleand, A., Rollins, E., & Miller, S. (2008). *Comprehensive health insurance: Billing, coding, and reimbursement.* Upper Saddle River, NJ: Pearson Education.

Wells, S. (2001). *Out of the Dead House: Nineteenth-Century Women Physicians and the Writing of Medicine.* Madison: University of Wisconsin Press.

Wolgin, F. (2005). *Being a nursing assistant* (9th ed.). Upper Saddle River, NJ: Pearson Education.

Zucker, E. (2006). *Being a homemaker home health aide* (6th ed.). Upper Saddle River, NJ: Pearson Education.

Internet-Based References

www.alz.org: Alzheimer's Association

www.alsa.org: The ALS Association

www.amrad.org: Amateur Radio Research and Development Corporation Telecommunications for the Deaf

www.aapc.com: American Academy of Professional Coders

www.aama-ntl.org: American Association of Medical Assistants

www.aamt.org: American Association of Medical Transcription

www.diabetes.org: American Diabetes Association

www.ahima.org: American Health Information Management Association

www.americanheart.org: American Heart Association

www.aha.org: American Hospital Association

www.lungusa.org: American Lung Association

www.amt1.com: American Medical Technologists

www.apdaparkinson.org: American Parkinson Disease Association

www.cdc.gov: Centers for Disease Control and Prevention

www.cms.hhs.gov: Centers for Medicare and Medicaid Services

www.cebm.net: Centre for Evidence-Based Medicine

www.cfhi.org: Child Family Health International

www.epicsystems.com: Epic

www.ftc.gov: Federal Trade Commission

www.hpso.com: Health Care Providers Service Organization

www.hhs.gov/ocr/hipaa: Health Insurance Portability and Accountability Act

www.americanhospice.org: Hospice

www.ornl.gov/sci/techresources/Human_Genome/home.shtml: Human Genome Project

www.ingenix.com: Ingenix

www.iom.edu: The Institute of Medicine

www.jointcommission.org/SentinelEvents: Joint Commission

www.medrecinst.com: Medical Records Institute

http://nccam.nih.gov: National Center for Complementary and Alternative Medicine

www.payroll-taxes.com: Payroll-Taxes.com

www.pbs.org/healthcarecrisis/history.htm: PBS's Health Care Crisis: Health Care Timeline

www.powermed.com: PowerMed

www.citizen.org: Public Citizen

www.shrinershq.org/Hospitals/_Hospitals_for_Children: Shriner's Hospital for Children

www.skillpath.com: SkillPath Seminars

www.sorryworks.net: Sorry Works

www.tricare.org: U.S. Department of Defense Military Health System

www.hhs.gov/ocr/hipaa: U.S. Department of Health and Human Services

www.usdoj.gov: U.S. Department of Justice

www.dol.gov: U.S. Department of Labor

www.bls.gov: U.S. Department of Labor Bureau of Labor Statistics

www.dot.gov: U.S. Department of Transportation (USDOT)

www.nlm.nih.gov/medlineplus: U.S. National Library of Medicine

www.who.org: World Health Organization

Index

Numbers in italics refer to figures; those followed by t refer to tables.

A

AAMA. *See* American Association of Medical Assistants (AAMA)
AAPC. *See* American Academy of Professional Coders (AAPC)
Abbreviations, 127–28
    to avoid, 128t
    in charting, 199
ABCD. *See* Airway, breathing, circulation, defibrillation (ABCD)
Abdomen
    disorders of, 937t
    divisions of, *938*
ABG. *See* Arterial blood gases (ABG)
ABHES. *See* Accrediting Bureau of Health Education Schools (ABHES)
ABN. *See* Advance beneficiary notice (ABN)
Abortus, 984, 994
Above knee amputation (AKA), 950
Abrasion, 571, 588, 868, 891
Absorption, 915
Abstracting, 261, 291
Abuse, 342, 344–45
    reporting by physicians, 51
Accept assignment, 261, 279
Accidental injury files, 177
Accommodation, 541, 565
Accounts payable (AP), 401–405
    checkbook register, 402
    deposit slip preparation, 404–405, 407
    endorsement stamps, 405
    ordering and receiving supplies, 404, 407
    writing checks, 406
Accounts receivable (AR), 371
    managing, 377
    trial balance, 374
Accredited programs, 23
Accrediting Bureau of Health Education Schools (ABHES), 4, 13, 15
Acid-fast bacillus (AFB), 771, 780
Acquired immune deficiency syndrome (AIDS), 41, 56, 431, 464, 621, 825, 1083
    Americans with Disabilities Act and, 60
    caring for patients with, 469
    medical sepsis and, 467–69
    opportunistic conditions common to, 828
    transmission prevention strategies, 828
ACS. *See* American Cancer Society (ACS)
ACTH. *See* Adrenocorticotropic hormone (ACTH)
Actinic keratosis (AK), 836, 845, 848t, *849*
Active listening, 74
Active patient files, 191, 203
Acuity, 794
Acupressure, 1102–1103
Acupuncture, 1101
Acute, 89, 91
Acyanotic, 1011
ADA. *See* American Dental Association (ADA); Americans with Disabilities Act (ADA)
Addiction, 1068
Adding machines, 240
Addition, 1055
Add-on code, 342, 346, 352
ADEA. *See* Age Discrimination in Employment Act (ADEA)
ADH. *See* Antidiuretic hormone (ADH)
ADHD. *See* Attention-deficit hyperactivity disorder (ADHD)

ADHI. *See* Association for Healthcare Documentation Integrity (ADHI)
Administrative competencies, 3, 13, *14*
Administrative law, 40, 42
Administrative procedures, 253, *254*
Administrative skills, 23
Adolescents, disclosing medical information of, 56
Adrenal glands, 858
    disorders, 863
Adrenocorticotropic hormone (ACTH), 856, 858
Advance beneficiary notice (ABN), 261, 263, 280, *281*
Advance medical directives, 40, 60, 108–11, 191, 193
    durable power of attorney for healthcare, 108
    living wills, 108, 110
Adverse effects, 412, 425
    coding, 335–36, 336t
Adverse reactions, 322
Advocate, *34*, 1113, 1114
    medical assistant as, 22
AED. *See* Automatic external defibrillation (AED)
Aerobes, 459, 460
AFB. *See* Acid-fast bacillus (AFB)
Affect, 1037, 1041, 1055, 1058
Afferent nerves, 89, 91
A-fib. *See* Atrial fibrillation (A-fib)
AFP. *See* Alpha-fetoprotein (AFP)
Age
    electrocardiograph and, 749
    immunity and, 832
    influence of, 78
    nutritional status and, 935
Age Discrimination in Employment Act (ADEA), 412, 417
Agendas, 412, 414
Agglutination, 636, 639
Aging process, 1088–92
    cultural views of, 1092, 1092t
    economic aspects of, 1090, 1092
    myths and misconceptions about, 1094
    nutritional aspects of, 1090
    physical aspects of, 1088–89
    social and psychological aspects of, 1089–90
Aging reports, 371, 373
AHA. *See* American Hospital Association (AHA)
AHIMA. *See* American Health Information Management Association (AHIMA)
AIDS. *See* Acquired immune deficiency syndrome (AIDS)
Airway, breathing, circulation, defibrillation (ABCD), 869, 874, 880
AK. *See* Actinic keratosis (AK)
AKA. *See* Above knee amputation (AKA)
ALARA. *See* As low as reasonably achievable (ALARA)
Alcohol, nutrition and, 934–35
Alcohol-based hand rubs, 494
Alimentary canal, 915, 917, 920t
Alimentation, 915, 921
Aliquot, 675, 695
Allergens, 824, 825, 831
Allergic reactions, 831–32
    emergency interventions for, 901–902
    preventing, 716
Allergies, 823–34
    diagnosis and treatment, 832
    food, 935–36, 936t

Allied health associations
    American Academy of Professional Coders (AAPC), 22
    American Health Information Management Association (AHIMA), 22
    American Medical Technologists (AMT), 21
    Association for Healthcare Documentation Integrity (ADHI), 22
    requirements of, 21–22
Allowed amount, 261, 266
    calculating, 268
Alphabetic index, 342
Alpha blockers, 507
Alpha-fetoprotein (AFP), 100, 985
ALS. *See* Amyotrophic lateral sclerosis (ALS)
Alternative medicine, 1098–1109
    acupuncture, 1101
    aromatherapy, 1102
    ayurveda, 1100
    biologically based therapies, 1101–1102
    definition of, 1099
    energy therapies, 1105
    herbal medicine, 1102, 1103t
    homeopathy, 1100–1101
    integrative medicine, 1101
    manipulative and body-based methods, 1102–1104
    mind-body interventions, 1101
    naturopathy, 1101
Alveolus/alveoli, 770, 771
Alzheimer's disease, 1066
Ambu bag, 868, 876
Ambulation, assistive aids for, 969, 972, 974–75, 977–78
Ambulatory care, 62
    Clinical Laboratory Improvement Amendments Act and, 62
    Joint Commission on the Accreditation of Healthcare Organizations and, 62
American Academy of Pediatrics, 1024
American Academy of Professional Coders (AAPC), 22, 323, 338
American Association of Medical Assistants (AAMA), 4, 9
    code of ethics, 9, 62
    definition of medical assistant, 12
    founding of, 20
    history of, *21*
American Cancer Society (ACS), 89, 97, 944, 945t
American Dental Association (ADA), 263
American Health Information Management Association (AHIMA), 22, 57, 323, 338
American Heart Association (AHA), 556, 736, 869, 874, 878, 944
American Hospital Association (AHA), 4, 8, 62
    Patient Bill of Rights, 10
American Medical Association (AMA), 4, 224, 304, 343, 344
    code of ethics by, 8–9
    ethical viewpoints, *64*
    history of, 8–9
    hygiene and, 24
    milestones in, *8*
    recognition of medical assistant profession by, 21
American Medical Technologists (AMT), 4, 13, 21
American Public Health Association (APHA), 323
American Red Cross, 3, 9, 869
American Sign Language (ASL), 68, 71
    alphabet, *73*

American Society of Anesthesiologists (ASA), 343, 359
Americans with Disabilities Act (ADA), 41, 60, 157, 412, 417, 431, 433, 434t
    reception area and, 169
    requirements, 60
    seeing-eye dogs and, 75
    telecommunication relay services and, 154
Amino acids, 915, 927
Amniocentesis, 984, 1003
Amphiarthrosis, 949, 954
Amplitude, 730, 746
Ampules, 524–28, 531–32
    intravenous therapy and, 526, 531–32
    medication withdrawal from, 525–26
Amputations, 891, 962
AMT. *See* American Medical Technologists (AMT)
Amyotrophic lateral sclerosis (ALS), 1038, 1047
Anaerobe, 459
Analgesic, 89, 91
Anaphylactic shock, 886–87, 887, 887t
Anaphylaxis, 868, 874
Anastomosis, 915, 938
Ancillary coverage, 261, 265, 276
And, in coding, 322, *330*
Anerobes, 460
Anesthesia, 3, 6, 571, 578–79
    coding for, 359–60
    local, 572, 579, 579t
Aneurysms, 730, 744
Angina, 730, 735
Angiography, 712, 715–16
Angioplasty, 730, 735
Angry patients, communicating with, 78
Ankylosis, 824, 830t
Annotation, 117, 134, 136
Anorexia, 915, 935
Answering service, 143
Anterior, 730
Anteroposterior view (AV), 712
Anthropometry, 541, 542
Antibody, 824, 825
Anticoagulants, 636, 642
Antidepressant, 1055, 1058
Antidiuretic hormone (ADH), 856, 858
Antigens, 824, 825
Antineoplastic drugs, 1079t–1080t
Antipsychotic, 1055, 1058
Antipyretic, 824, 831
Antisepsis, 3, 7
Antiseptic, 3, 7
Anuria, 675, 680
Anus, 915, 920
Anxiety, 68, 84
    reduction of, 1065t
Anxiety disorders, 1063–64
    generalized anxiety disorder and panic disorder, 1064
    obsessive-compulsive disorder, 1064
    phobic disorder, 1064, 1064t
    posttraumatic stress disorder, 1064
Apex, 730, 744
APHA. *See* American Public Health Association (APHA)
Apical pulse, 541, 550, 552–53
    digitalis patients and, 550
Appeal, 40, 261
Appendages, 836, 837
Approved amount, 261
Approximation, 571, 573
Aromatherapy, 1102
Arrhythmias, 730, 735, 737–38, 737t–738t
    classification of, 738t
    identification of, 756–58, 765
    treatment, 738
Arterial blood gases (ABG), 731, 744, 771, 779, 781–82, 782t
Arteriosclerosis, 730, 735, 742–43
Arthritis, 949, 961
Arthrography, 712, 716
Articular, 949, 954

Artifacts, 730, 747, *749,750*
ASA. *See* American Society of Anesthesiologists (ASA)
Asepsis, 459, 464. *See also* Medical asepsis; Surgical asepsis
    medical *versus* surgical, 479t
    surgical, 477–501
Aseptic, 478, 479
ASL. *See* American Sign Language (ASL)
As low as reasonably achievable (ALARA), 712, 720
Assault, 40, 42, 43t
Assessment, 89
    hearing, 561
    pain, 92–93
    in physical examination, 564–67
    pulmonary, 777, 779–88
Assignment of benefits, 261
Assisted living facility, 1087, 1088
Assistive aids, for ambulation, 969, 972, 974–75, 977–78
    canes, 975, *976*, 977
    crutches, 969, 972–73, 973t, 974–75, 976
    walkers, 975, 977, 978
Associate degree, 3, 13
Association for Healthcare Documentation Integrity (ADHI), 22
Assumption of risk, 40, 48
Asthma, 770, 773, 774t
Asystole, 730, *765*
Atelectasis, 778t
Atherosclerosis, 735, 742–43
Atony, 949, 954
Atrial fibrillation (A-fib), 731, *759*
Atrioventricular node (AV), 731, 735
Atrium, 730, 732
Atrophy, 949, 956
Attention-deficit hyperactivity disorder (ADHD), 1056, 1067
Attitude, 35
Audiologist, 794, 808
Audiometry, 794, 795, 808, 811
Audit, 342, 355
Auditors, 393, 395
Augmented leads, 730, 744, *746*, 752t
Aura, 1037, 1047
Aural temperature, 541, 548–49
Auscultation, 541, 564–65
Authorization, obtaining from insurance companies, 303
Autism, 1025
Autoclave, 478, 479
    indicator tapes, *486*
    load, 478, 484
    loading and operating, 488–89
    requirements for sterilization, 484t
    sterilization, 483–84, 487
Autoimmune diseases, 828, 829t–831t, 831
Autoimmunity, 824
Automatic dialer, 140, 141
Automatic external defibrillation (AED), 869, 876, 879–80
Automaticity, 730, 733
Automatic routing units, 140, 142
Autonomic receptors, 508t
AV. *See* Anteroposterior view (AV); Atrioventricular node (AV)
Avulsion, 571, 588, 868, 891
Awards, medical malpractice, 47
    compensatory, 47
    nominal, 47
    punitive, 47
Axillary, 541, 543, 949
    temperature, 546
Ayurveda, 1100

B

Bacillus Calmette-Guérin (BCG), 771, 786
Bacteria, 619–20
Bactericidal, 459, 463

Bacteroides, 620
Balance billing, 261, 267, 305, *307*
Bandages
    pressure, 890, 895
    tubular, 893–95
Bank accounts, access via Internet, 405–406
Banking procedures
    petty cash, 406, 408
    reconciling statements, 406–408
Bankruptcy, 379
Bar-code scanners, 223, 226
Barium enema, 724
Barium swallow, 724
Barriers, to professionalism, 36
    inappropriate discussions, 36, *37*
    personal business at work, 36
    personal problems, 36
    procrastination of duties, 36
Barton, Clara, 9
Basal cell carcinoma (BCC), 836, 846, *850*, 851t
Basic unit, Time, Modifying circumstances (B*T*M), 343, 359
Basophil, *639*
Battery, 40, 43t
Battery backup systems, 223, 226
BBB. *See* Bundle branch block (BBB)
BCC. *See* Basal cell carcinoma (BCC)
BCG. *See* Bacillus Calmette-Guérin (BCG)
BEA. *See* Below elbow amputation (BEA)
Beats per minute (BPM), 542, 550
Behavior, professional, 34–36
    attitude, 35
    compassion, 34
    competence, 34
    cooperation, 35
    honesty, 34
    loyalty, 35
    prioritizing tasks, 36
    professional demeanor, 35
    respect, 35
    responsibility, 35
Bell's palsy, 1050
Below elbow amputation (BEA), 950
Below knee amputation (BKA), 950
Beneficiary, 261, 266
Benign, 1075, 1076
Benign prostatic hypertrophy (BPH), 676, 704, 707t
Beta blockers, 507
Bilateral procedure, 342, 354
Biliary tract, 922t
Bilirubin, 675, 697
Billing, 370–89
    computerized systems, 373–74
    fee schedules, 374–75
    insurance company overpayment, 387
    manual systems, 373
    overpayment on accounts, 385, 387
    participating provider agreements, 375
    patient identification and, 377
    patient refund, 386
    patient statements, 379
    payment basics, 373
Binocular, 613
Bioethics, 40, 64
Biofeedback, 1101
Biopsy, 571, 572
Bipolar disorder, 1063
Birthday rule, 261, 290
BKA. *See* Below knee amputation (BKA)
Black lung, 773
Blackwell, Elizabeth, contributions of, 10
Blackwell, Emily, contributions of, 10
Bladder calculi, 683t
Bleeding, 887–89
    direct pressure to, 888
    epistaxis, 889
    internal, 888–89
    pressure bandage for, 890
    pressure points, 888, *889*, 890t
    vaginal, 996

Blood
    anatomy and physiology of, 638–42
    capillary puncture collection, 653–56
    cell malformation, 639–40
    cells, 638–39
    cholesterol measurement, 667–68
    collection equipment and procedures, 642–56
    disorders, 1028, 1030t
    evacuation system and, 646–49
    flow through heart, *733*
    glucose, 665, 666–67, 668
    immunohematology and, 640, 642
    order of draw, 642, 644t
    plasma, 638
    platelets, 639
    special-needs testing, 653
    studies, 756, 757t
    tourniquets, 642
    typing and grouping, 669, 669t
    in urinalysis, 697
    vacutainer tubes, additives for, 643t
    venipuncture, 643–46
Blood bank technologist, 27
Bloodborne pathogens, 459, 460, 461t
Blood chemistry testing, 665, 668–69
    automated chemistry analyzers, 665, 668–69
    immunology testing, 669
Blood pressure, 541, 553–57
    average values of, 556t
    classification of, 556t
    diastole, 553
    errors in reading, 557
    Korotkoff sounds, 555–56
    measurement, 557–58
    systole, 553
    therapy, 736
    variations in, 556t
Blood smear, 659–60
    preparation of, 662
    with Wright's stain, 661–62
Blood urea nitrogen (BUN), 597, 602, 680
Blue Cross/Blue Shield plans, 274, *275*
BMI. *See* Body mass index (BMI)
Body, 117, 121
    organization of, *641*
    planes, 723t
Body fluids (humors)
    Hippocrates and, 4
    potentially infectious, 4
Body language, 24, 68, 412, 424
    in different cultures, 24t, 73
    eye contact, 73
    facial expressions, 73
    gestures, 73
    posture, 73–74
    using and reading, 71–74
Body mass index (BMI), 89, 916, 934
Body mechanics, 432, 433, 949, 952, 978, 980
Body movements, 723t
Body Substance Isolation (BSI), 459, 465
Bolus, 915, 918
Bones, 952–54
BPH. *See* Benign prostatic hypertrophy (BPH)
BPM. *See* Beats per minute (BPM)
Braces, 963
Bradycardia, 730
Braille, 71, *73*
Brain
    abscess, 1048–49
    diagram of, *1057*
    tumors, 1049
Breast, 987, *988*
    cancer, 999t
    disorders and conditions, 998–99, 1001
Breast self-exam (BSE), 985, 1000–1001
Brochure, 249, 250, 251
Bronchi, 771
Bronchiectasis, 775t
Bronchioles, 770, 771
Bronchitis, 770, 773, 775t

Bronchodilator, 770
Bronchus, 770
Brown v. Board of Education, 42
BSE. *See* Breast self-exam (BSE)
B*T*M. *See* Basic unit, Time, Modifying
    circumstances (B*T*M)
Buerger's disease, 744
Buffer time, 174, 180
BUN. *See* Blood urea nitrogen (BUN)
Bundle branch block (BBB), 731, 758t
Bundling, 261, 280, 342, 352
Burns, 895–97
    coding, 336–37
    rule of nines and, 336–37, 896, *897*
Bursa, 949, 954
Bursitis, 949, 954
Business associate agreement, HIPAA, 59–60
Business letter
    body, 121
    closing, 122
    components of, 120–24
    composing, 124
    courtesy titles, 122t
    reference initials, 122, *123*
    salutation, 121
    sample, *123*,*125*,*126*,*127*
    state abbreviations, 122t
    style, 124

C

CAAHEP. *See* Committee for Accreditation of Allied
    Health Education Programs (CAAHEP)
CAB. *See* Coronary artery bypass (CAB)
CABG. *See* Coronary artery bypass graft (CABG)
CAD. *See* Coronary artery disease (CAD)
Cadaver, 3, 5, 104, 105
Caduceus symbol, *5*
Calcium (Ca), 951, 954
Call forwarding, 140, 142
Calories, 915, 933
CAM. *See* Complementary and alternative medicine
    (CAM)
Cancer, 1075
    breast, 999t
    cervical, 998
    classification and physiology of, 1076–77
    hospice and emotional support, 1082–83
    prevention lifestyle, 1083
    prostate, 705t
    skin, 846, 848, 851t
    uterine, 998
    warning signals, 1078t
Cancer treatment, 1079–82
    chemotherapy, 1079
    developments in, 1082
    hormone therapy and immunotherapy,
        1081–82
    radiation, 1080, *1082*
    side effects of, 1082
    surgery, 1080–81
Canes, 975, *976*, 977
Cannula, 571, 576
Capillary puncture, 653–56
Capitation plans, 261, 287
Carbohydrates, 915, 922, 929
Carbon dioxide (CO_2), 597, 602
Cardiac arrest, sudden, 735–36
Cardiac catheterization, 730, 745
Cardiology, 729–68
    anatomy and physiology of heart, 732–35
    arrhythmias/dysrhythmias, 756–65
    diagnostic tests, 744–56
    diseases and disorders of heart, 735–44
Cardiomegaly, 730, 737
Cardiomyopathy, 730, 737
Cardiopulmonary resuscitation (CPR), 41, 53, 394,
        395, 869, 874–76, 874t, 878–79
Cardiovascular (CV), 542

Carditis, 824
Caretaker, 261, 272
Carrier, 459, 461
Cartilage, 949, 953
Carve outs, 261, 287
Casts, 949, 963, 964–66
    care of, 964t
    removal of, 966, 967
CAT. *See* Computerized axial tomography (CAT)
Catastrophic, 262, 265, 276
Categorically needy, 262, 283
Category, 322, 329, 342, 349
Category I codes, 342, 345
Category II codes, 342, 345
Category III codes, 342, 345
Catheterization, 689, 690–93
    cardiac, 745
Cauterization, 836
CBC. *See* Complete blood count (CBC)
C1 (cervical vertebra), 951
CCP. *See* Certification Continuation Program
    (CCP)
CCS-P. *See* Certified Coding Specialist-Physician
    based (CCS-P)
CD. *See* Compact disc (CD)
CDHP. *See* Consumer-directed healthcare plans
    (CDHP)
Centers for Disease Control (CDC), 224, 437, 459,
        464, 484, 786
    alcohol-based hand rubs and, 494
    standard precautions, 466
Centers for Medicare and Medicaid Services (CMS),
    41, 62, 263, 278, 324, 343, 372, 375
Central nervous system (CNS), 1038, 1039
Central nervous system (CNS), disorders and
    diseases of, 1045–50
    amyotrophic lateral sclerosis, 1047
    brain abscess, 1048–49
    brain tumors, 1049
    cerebrovascular accident/stroke, 1045–46
    disk disorders, 1050
    encephalitis, 1048
    epilepsy, 1046–47
    headache, 1047–48
    head trauma, 1049–50
    infectious conditions of, 1048–49
    meningitis, 1048
    multiple sclerosis, 1047
    Parkinson's disease, 1047
    spinal cord injuries, 1050
    transient ischemic attack, 1046
Central processing unit (CPU), 224
Centrifuge, 597, 603
Cephalgia, 1037, 1047
Cerebral, 89
Cerebrospinal fluid (CSF), 825, 829t, 1038, 1039
Cerebrovascular accident/stroke (CVA), 869, 903,
        1038, 1045–46
    aspirin and, 903, 1046
    causes of, *1046*
    symptoms, *904*
Certificate of coverage, 262, 268
Certification Continuation Program (CCP), 15
Certification examination
    for Certified Medical Assistant, 15
    for Registered Medical Assistant, 15
Certified Coding Specialist-Physician based
    (CCS-P), 323, 338
Certified laboratory consultant (CLC), 21
Certified letter, 371
Certified medical administrative specialist (CMAS),
    21
Certified Medical Assistant (CMA), 4, 13
    certification examination for, 15
    general, clinical, and administrative skills of, *14*
    licensing and certification for, 27
Certified Medical Transcriptionist (CMT), 22
Certified nursing assistant (CNA), 27
Certified office laboratory technician (COLT), 21
Certified professional coder (CPC), 22, 338

Cerumen, 794, 807
Cervix, 984, 986, 992
Cesarean section (C-section), 985, 992, 1005
CHAMPVA, 262, 263, 265, 285, 291
Chapters, 322, 329
Character
    defamation of, 40, 43t
    of medical assistants, 12
Charge slip, 262, 291
Charitable contributions, 393, 400
Charting, 95, 445
    abbreviations in, 199
    clinical visit, 449–55
    coding and, 337
    errors, 204
    five Cs of, 193
    forms of, 196–98
    medical history, 449–55
    narrative style, 196
    patient communication, 199
    problem-oriented medical record charting,
        197–98
    procedures, 453, 455
    with SOAP, 196–97, 198
    telephone calls, 149
Checklists, 25, 157, 159
Chemical name, 503, 506
Chemotherapy, 1075, 1079
CHF. See Congestive heart failure (CHF)
Chief complaint, 191, 193, 322, 327, 450
Children
    blood disorders, 1028, 1030t
    choking and, 881
    communicating with, 79
    congenital heart conditions, 1028, 1029t
    congenital neurological disorders/neural tube
        defects in, 1025, 1027t–1028t
    consent for, 43
    contagious diseases of, 1025, 1026t–1027t
    CPR for, 874t, 877
    disclosing medical information of, 56
    dosage calculation for, 515
    immunizations for, 1021, 1022,1023,
        1024—1025
    intramuscular injections for, 534–35
    management in reception room, 168–69
    mental disorders in, 1067, 1067t
    monitoring growth development, 1012–17
    physical, developmental, and emotional growth
        of, 1012–17
    poisons and, 906
    positioning and securing for examination,
        1030–31
    stool collection, 625
    urine collection from, 689, 1031–33
    working with, 79
Chinese medicine, early, 4
Chiropractic, 1103
Chlamydia, 707t
Choking, universal sign for, 881
Cholecystography, 712, 716, 725
Cholesterol, 915, 929
    blood, 667–68
Chronic, 89, 91
Chronic obstructive pulmonary disease (COPD),
        771, 773, 884, 886
Chyme, 915, 922
Cilia, 459, 463
Circular E, 393, 400, 402,403
Civilian Health and Medical Program of the
        Veterans Administration (CHAMPVA).
        See CHAMPVA
Civil law, 40, 42
    commercial law, 42
    contract law, 42
Civil Rights Act of 1964, 60
Civil service (CSRS), 263, 286
Claims
    completing computerized, 314
    patient registration, 287, 288, 289

processing, 287–91
    tracing, 307
Classes, accredited, 15t
CLC. See Certified laboratory consultant (CLC)
Clean claim, 262
Clerical supplies, stocking, 244
CLIA. See Clinical Laboratory Improvement
        Amendments (CLIA)
Clinical and Laboratory Standards Institute (CLIS),
        642
Clinical competencies, 3, 13, 14
Clinical dietitian, 27
Clinical Laboratory Improvement Amendments
        (CLIA), 41, 62, 597, 598–600, 637
    ambulatory care and, 62
    certificates, 599
    high-complexity tests, 599
    moderate-complexity tests, 599
    PPMP tests, 598–99
    quality control and assurance, 599–600
    waived tests, 598, 599
Clinical procedures, 252, 253
Clinical skills, 22
Clinical visit, 444–57
    charting medical history and, 449–55
    consent, 448
    documenting, 453–55
    examination and treatment areas, 447
    recurrent, 566
    standard medical office and, 446
    triage, 447–48
Clonic, 1037
Closed patient files, 191, 203
Closed wound, 571, 589
Close-ended questions, 68, 74
Closing, 117, 122
Cluster scheduling, 174, 179
CMA. See Certified Medical Assistant (CMA)
CMAS. See Certified medical administrative
        specialist (CMAS)
CMS. See Centers for Medicare and Medicaid
        Services (CMS)
CMS-1500 claim form, 291, 292,301,302, 308,
        309–13
    instructions for completing, 293t–299t
CMT. See Certified Medical Transcriptionist (CMT)
CNA. See Certified nursing assistant (CNA)
CNS. See Central nervous system (CNS)
CO₂. See Carbon dioxide (CO₂)
Coagulation, 636, 638
Coal Miner's Health and Safety Act, 773
COBRA, 263, 270
Code of ethics
    AAMA, 9, 62
    AMA, 8–9
Cognitive functioning, 1055, 1066
    anatomy and physiology of, 1057–58
Coinsurance, 262, 267, 268
Cold sterilization, 478, 485
Collagen, 836, 837
Collections, 375–77
    bankruptcy and, 379
    bounced checks and, 381–82
    collection agency, 371, 383
    contacting nonpaying patients, 382
    from estates, 384–85
    forgiving deductibles and copayments, 378
    interest, 381
    letters, 382–83
    in managed care, 378–85
    medical assistants and, 372
    nonpayment, 380
    professional courtesy and, 379
    small claims court and, 387
    uncollectible accounts, 383
Colonoscopy, 915, 937, 938–40
Color blindness, 801–2
Colostomy, 915, 916
Colostrum, 984
Colposcopy, 571, 572

COLT. See Certified office laboratory technician
        (COLT)
Combination coding, 322, 332
Commercial insurance, 262
Commercial law, 40, 42
Committee for Accreditation of Allied Health
        Education Programs (CAAHEP), 4,
        13, 15
Common descriptor, 342, 349
Common law, 40, 42
Communication
    with angry or distressed patients, 78
    charting patient, 199
    with coworkers, 81–82
    with culturally diverse patients, 77–78
    with emotionally challenged patients, 79
    factors hindering, 75
    five Cs of, 69
    with geriatric patients, 79
    with grieving patients, 79–80
    with hearing-impaired patients, 76, 77
    interpersonal skills, 67–87
    medical assistant role in, 69
    with mentally ill patients, 78
    nonverbal, 70–74
    with other facilities, 82
    with patients via interpreters, 77–78
    with patients with speech impairments, 76–77
    with physically challenged patients, 75–76
    professional, 80–81, 81
    professionalism and, 12
    with sight-impaired patients, 76, 77
    in special circumstances, 75–80
    verbal, 69–70
    with young patients, 79
Community college, 3, 13
Community hospitals, 8
Community property laws, 371, 387
Community resources, 81
Comorbid, 1055, 1063
Compact disc (CD), 224, 225
Comparative negligence, 40, 48
Compassion, 34
Compensation, 85
Competence, 34
Competencies
    administrative, 3, 13
    clinical, 3, 13
    general, 14
Complementary and alternative medicine (CAM),
        1099, 1100
Complementary medicine, 1099, 1100
Complete blood count (CBC), 597, 602
Complete protein, 915, 927
Compress, 949, 968, 969t, 970–71
Compulsory, 249
Computed tomography (CT), 712, 717, 717t
Computerized axial tomography (CAT), 712, 717
Computerized billing systems, 373–74
Computer peripherals, 223, 226–27
    bar-code readers, 226
    digital cameras, 226
    electronic sign-in sheets, 226–27
    scanners, 226
Computers, in medical office, 222–33
    case study, 222
    ergonomics, 231
    maintaining, 227, 228
    medical assistants and, 224
    peripherals, 226–27
    personal digital assistants and, 231
    personal use in, 231
    privacy, HIPAA and, 59
    security, 228–29
    software, 227–28
    system components, 224–26
Computer viruses, 223, 229
Concussions, 1049–50
Conduction, 541, 542
Conduction system, 730, 733, 734

Conductivity, 730, 733
Conference calls, 140, 141
Confidentiality
    maintaining, 53–57
    patient, 24
    telephone procedures and, 153
Conflicting orders, charting, 205
Congestive heart failure (CHF), 731, 736, 884, 1087
Conscience clauses, 40, 62
Consent, 448
    for cardiac procedures, 756
    for children and mentally incompetent adults, 43
    classification of, 43–44
    expressed, 41, 43
    form, 43, 573
    implied, 41, 43, 44, 573
    informed, 41, 44, 573
    parties who can sign, 43
    signing forms, 44, 47
Consolidated Omnibus Budget Reconciliation Act
        (COBRA). See COBRA
Constipation, 831t
Constitutional law, 40
Consumer-directed healthcare plans (CDHP), 262,
        263, 273–74
Contamination, 459, 465, 481
Contraception, 988–91
Contractility, 731, 733
Contraction, 571
Contract law, 40, 42
Contracts
    expressed, 41, 52, 54
    in healthcare, 52–53
    implied, 41, 52
    terminating, 53
    verbal, 53
Contraindications, 503, 506
Contrast studies, 713, 715, 715t
    abdominal, 724
Contrecoup, 1037, 1050
Contributing factors, 342, 357
Contributory negligence, 40, 48
Controlled substances, 89, 93, 503, 509, 512, 512t
Contusions, 1049–50
Convection, 541, 542
Conventions, 322, 324
    punctuation, 329
Conversion, 85
    factor, 262
Conversion disorder, 1064
Cooperation, 35
Coordination of benefits (COB), 262, 290
Coordination of care, 342, 357
Copayments, 157, 165, 262, 267, 378
COPD. See Chronic obstructive pulmonary disease
        (COPD)
Coronary artery bypass (CAB), 731, 744, 745
Coronary artery bypass graft (CABG), 731, 744
Coronary artery disease (CAD), 731, 735
Counseling, 342, 357
Covered, 262, 280
Cover letter, 1113, 1116, 1117
Coworkers
    communication with, 81–82
    disclosing personal information about, 144
CPC. See Certified Professional Coder (CPC);
        Certified professional coder (CPC)
CPR. See Cardiopulmonary resuscitation (CPR)
CPT. See Current Procedural Terminology (CPT)
CPT-4 manual, 342
    alphabetical index, 346
    appendices, 346
    coding with, 344
    organization of, 345–46
    tabular index in, 345
CPU. See Central processing unit (CPU)
Cranial nerves, 1040t
Craniosacral therapy, 1103
Crash cart, 870–71
Credentials, 412, 418

Credit, 375–77
    medical assistants and, 372
Criminal law, 40, 42
    felonies, 42
    misdemeanors, 42
Cross-referencing, 191, 199
Crutches, 969, 972–73, 973t, 974–75, 976
Cryosurgery, 571, 573, 836, 1005–1006
Cryotherapy, 949, 968
Cryptorchism, 675, 706
Crystals, 699, 700, 701
C&S. See Culture and sensitivity (C&S)
CSA. See Federal Controlled Substances Act (CSA)
C-section. See Cesarean section (C-section)
CSF. See Cerebrospinal fluid (CSF)
CSRS. See Civil service (CSRS)
CT. See Computed tomography (CT)
Culture
    aging and, 1092, 1092t
    body language and, 24t, 73
    breastfeeding and, 996
    communicating with diverse patients, 77–78
    electrocardiograph and, 749
    gynecological examinations and, 1003
    influence of, 78
    patient education and, 95–96
Culture and sensitivity (C&S), 597, 625–26
    pediatric, 1029
    urine, 631
    wound or throat, 628–29
Curie, Marie, 9, 10
Current Procedural Terminology (CPT), 41, 64,
        120, 263, 343, 344, 353–55, 372
Cutting, 571, 575
CV. See Cardiovascular (CV)
CVA. See Cerebrovascular accident/stroke (CVA)
Cyanosis, 868, 884
Cyanotic, 1011
Cystitis, 675, 679
Cystoscopy, 685

D

Damages, 40, 47
Date of birth (DOB), 597, 604
Day sheet, 371
D&C. See Dilatation and curettage (D&C)
DEA. See Drug Enforcement Administration (DEA)
Debridement, 571, 573
Debris, 478, 480
Decerebrate posture, 1037, 1049
Decibels (dB), 794
Decontamination, 431, 436
    laundry, 439
    steps, 485
Decorticate posture, 1037, 1049
Deductible, 262, 265–66
    calculating, 268
    forgiving, 378
Deductions, 393, 395, 400–401
Deep-vein thrombosis (DVT), 731, 742
DEERS. See Defense enrollment eligibility reporting
        system (DEERS)
Defamation of character, 40, 43t
Defense enrollment eligibility reporting system
        (DEERS), 263, 284
Defense mechanisms, 84, 85
    compensation, 85
    conversion, 85
    denial, 85
    displacement, 85
    identification, 85
    overcompensation, 85
    projection, 85
    rationalization, 85
    regression, 85
    repression, 85
    substitution, 85
    suppression, 85

Degenerative, 794, 797
Degenerative joint disease (DJD), 951
Dehydration, consequences of, 932
Delegate, 412, 413
Demeanor, professional, 35
Dementia, 1055, 1066–67
    Alzheimer's disease, 1066
    from head trauma, 1067
    vascular, 1066
Denial, 85
Denied claim, 262, 307, 315
Dental assistant, 27
Dental hygienist, 27
Department of Health and Human Services
        (DHHS), 464, 916, 932
Dependence, 1055, 1068
Dependents, 262, 266
Depolarization, 731, 734
Depression, 1060t–1062t
Dermal temperature, 549
Dermatitis, 836, 839, 839t–840t
Dermatologist, 836
Dermatology, 835–54
    anatomy and physiology of skin, 837–38
    definition of, 836
    diseases and disorders of skin, 839–50
Dermatome, 1037, 1051
Dermatophytoses, 836, 842
Dermis, 459, 463
DGA. See Dietary Guidelines for Americans (DGA)
DHHS. See Department of Health and Human
        Services (DHHS)
DHL, 133
Diabetes mellitus (DM), 323
    coding, 338
    cost of supplies, 863
Diagnostic and Statistical Manual of Mental
        Disorders (DSM-IV), 1056, 1070
Diagnostic coding
    for burns, 336–37
    combination coding, 332
    determining correct, 326–28
    diabetes mellitus, 338
    E codes, 335
    for evaluation and management services,
        355–59
    for fractures, 336
    history of, 323
    hypertension, 332–33
    inpatient services, 338
    late effects, 337
    medical assistants and, 323
    multiple coding, 332
    neoplasms, 333
    obstetrics, 337–38
    perform, 332
    poisonings and adverse effects, 335–36
    professional certification in, 338–39
    secondary diagnoses, 331–32
    signs and symptoms, 332
    for special situations, 331–38
    V codes, 333–35
Diagnostic procedures, 445, 596–611
    cardiac, 744–56, 757t
    Clinical Laboratory Improvement
        Amendments (CLIA) and, 598–600
    hospital laboratory setting, 602–603
    in-house ordering, 605–606
    musculoskeletal, 963
    for obstetrics and gynecology, 1001,
        1003–1004
    for oncology, 1077–79
    ordering, 604–606
    pediatric, 1029–33
    physician office laboratory, 603–604
    precertification, 606
    pulmonary, 777, 779–88
    regulations and laboratory safety, 602
    requisition form for, 607
    scheduling with outside agencies, 606

Diagnostic procedures (continued)
    screening and follow-up of results, 606, 608
    for urinary system, 685–701
Dialysis, 675, 682–83
Diaphoresis, 541
Diaphragm, 770, 771
Diarrhea, 831t
Diarthrosis, 949, 954
Diastole, 541, 553, 731, 735
Dietary Guidelines for Americans (DGA), 916, 932
Dieting
    fad, 934
    information, 96
    special diets, 941t
    therapeutic, 944, 945t
Differential white blood cell count (diff), 597, 603
Differentiated cell count, 659–60
Digestion, 915
Digestive system, *917*
    diseases and conditions of, 926t–927t
Digital rectal examination (DRE), 676, 704
Digital versatile/video disc (DVD), 224, 225
Dilatation and curettage (D&C), 572, 573, 1005
Diluent, 636, 657
Direct telephone lines, 140, 142
Disability
    definition of, 286
    electrocardiograph and, 749
Disability insurance, 262, 286–87
    medical assistants and, 286–87
Discovery rule, 40, 48
Discriminating, 68, 75
Disinfectants, 482t
Disinfection, 478, 479, 481–82
    alcohol, 482
    glutaraldehyde, 482
    hydrogen peroxide, 482
    phenolics, 482
    procedures, 483
    sodium hypochlorite, 482
Displacement, *85*
Dissection, 571, 575
Distal, 571
Distal tubule, 675, 677
Distance
    intimate, *70*
    personal, *70*
    professional, 81
    public, *71*
    social, *70*
Distressed patients, communicating with, 78
DJD. *See* Degenerative joint disease (DJD)
DM. *See* Diabetes mellitus (DM)
DME. *See* Durable medical equipment (DME)
DNR. *See* Do not resuscitate (DNR)
DOB. *See* Date of birth (DOB)
Do not resuscitate (DNR), 41, 60, 104
Dosage calculation, 512–15
    pediatric, 515
Dots per square inch (DPI), 224
Double booking, 174, 179
Downcode, 342, 344
DPI. *See* Dots per square inch (DPI)
Drainage, 571, 588
Draping
    for minor surgery, 576
    for physical examination, 561
DRE. *See* Digital rectal examination (DRE)
Dressings and bandages, 589–90
Drug Enforcement Administration (DEA), 26, 503, 504
Drugs, 503, 504
    absorption, 505, 505t
    antineoplastic, 1079t–1080t
    classification, 507–9, 510t–511t
    controlled substances, 509, 512
    distribution, 506
    effects of, 506
    excretion, 506
    functions of, 506
    metabolism, 506

movement processes, *505*
nomenclature, 506–7
reference sources, 507
samples of, 244
schedule, 509
urine test for, 701
DSM-IV. *See Diagnostic and Statistical Manual of
    Mental Disorders* (DSM-IV)
Dual fee schedule, 371, 372
Duodenum, 920
Durable medical equipment (DME), 26, 263, 343, 364
Durable power of attorney for healthcare, 108, *109*
Duress, 41, 43t
Duties, procrastination of, 36
DVD. *See* Digital versatile/video disc (DVD)
DVT. *See* Deep-vein thrombosis (DVT)
Dyscrasia, 636, 640
Dysfunction, 824
Dyspepsia, 915, 936
Dysphagia, 824, 831t, 915, 936
Dysphasia, 824
Dyspnea, 770, 777
Dysrhythmias, 731, 749, 753
    identification of, 756–58, 765

E

EAP. *See* Employee Assistance Programs (EAP)
Ear
    anatomy and physiology of, 807
    diagnostic procedures, 808
    diagram of, *808*
    diseases and disorders of, 807–808, 809t–810t
    instillation of medication, 813–14
    irrigation, 812–13
    treatments, 808
Ear, nose, and throat (ENT), 771
Ecchymosis, 824, 829t
ECG. *See* Electrocardiogram (ECG/EKG)
Echocardiogram, 712, 719, 755–56
E codes, 322, 335
ED. *See* Emergency department (ED)
EDC. *See* Estimated date of confinement (EDC)
EDD. *See* Expected date of delivery (EDD)
Education
    associate degree, 3, 13
    certification examination, 15
    community college, 3, 13
    latex allergy and, 473
    multiple medical-assisting statuses, 15
    patient, 13, 94–99
    requirements for medical assistants, 13, 15
    technical, 4, 13
    vocational programs, 4, 13
Edwin Smith Papyrus, 4
EEOC. *See* Equal Employment Opportunity
    Commission (EEOC)
E/EX. *See* Examination (E/EX)
EF. *See* Ejection fraction (EF)
Effacement, 984, 992
Efferent nerves, 89, 91
Egyptian medicine, early, 4
EHR. *See* Electronic health records (EHR)
EIN. *See* Employer identification numbers (EIN)
Einthoven, Willem, 6
Einthoven's triangle, 738, *739*
Ejection fraction (EF), 731, 756
EKG. *See* Electrocardiogram (ECG/EKG);
    Electrocardiograph (EKG)
Elderly
    communicating with, 79
    physiologic changes in, 1089t
    promoting health among, 1093–94
    sensorimotor changes of, 1091
Elective procedures, 262, 268
Elective surgery, 571, 573
Electrocardiogram (ECG/EKG), 117, 175, 177, 731,
    744–48, 1038
    artifacts, 747, *749,750*

interpreting waveforms on, 746–47
leads, 745t
performing, 750–52
Electrocardiograph (EKG), 6, 1038
Electrocardiograph technologist, 27
Electrocautery, 571, 573
Electroencephalograph technologist, 27
Electroencephalography (EEG), 1043–45
Electrolytes, 675, 679, 915, 922
Electromyography (EMG), 824, 825, 829t
Electronic health records (EHR), 211, 212
    functions of, *216*
    HIPAA compliance and, 214–15
Electronic mail (e-mail), 117, 134
Electronic media claims (EMC), 263, 300
Electronic medical records (EMR), 191, 196,
    210–21, 211, 213
    access to, 212
    backing up computers and, 215
    benefits of, 216–18
    communication and, 218
    conversion from paper to, 213–14
    correcting, 219
    diagnostic equipment and, 218
    functions of, *216*
    HIPAA compliance and, 214–15
    marketing purposes and, 218
    online, 218
    paper charting *versus,* 212–13
    personal digital assistants with, 216
    saving time with, 217–18
    training for, 213–14
Electronic scheduling, 177–78
Electronic signatures, 191, 196, 211, 216
Electronic sign-in sheets, 223, 226–27
Eligibility, 262, 289
Elimination, 915, 921
ELISA, 468
E-mail. *See* Electronic mail (e-mail)
Embolism, 731, 742
    antiembolism stockings, 743
Embolus, 731, 742
    pulmonary, 778t
Embryo, 984, 992
EMC. *See* Electronic media claims (EMC)
Emergency care, 867–913
    equipment for, 870–71
    intervention, 871–907
    medical office preparedness, 870–71
    resources, 870
Emergency department (ED), 869, 870
Emergency intervention, 871–907
    acute abdominal pain, 904–905
    allergic reactions, 901–902
    assessment, 871, 873
    bleeding, 887–89
    chest pain, 881, 883–84
    CPR, AED, and obstructed airway, 874–81
    diabetic coma or insulin shock, 905
    foreign bodies, 906–907
    head injuries, 904, *905*
    musculoskeletal injuries, 898–901
    neurological, 902–903
    open wounds, 889, 891–92, 895
    OSHA guidelines, 873–74
    oxygen administration, 885–86
    poison control centers, 906
    poisoning and overdose, 905–906
    psychosocial, 907
    respiratory distress, 884–86
    shock and anaphylactic shock, 886–87
    thermal injuries, 895–98, 899t
Emergency Medical System (EMS), 870
Emergency medical technician (EMT), 27
Emergency plans, 434–36
    disasters, 434–35
    fire and electrical safety, 434
    incident reports, 435, 436t
    workplace security, 435
    workplace violence, 435

Emergency preparedness, 908–909
    earthquakes, 908
    environmental exposure plan, 910
    fire, 908
    floods, 909
    hurricanes, 909
    mock-environmental exposures, 909
    terrorism, 909
Emergency surgery, 571, 573
Emesis, 478, 485, 916, 936
EMG. See Electromyography (EMG)
Emotionally challenged patients, communicating
    with, 79
Emotional stages, of life cycle, 83t
Empathetic listening, 74
Empathy, 3, 12
Emphysema, 770, 773, 774t, 779
Employee Assistance Programs (EAP), 412, 423
Employer identification numbers (EIN), 41, 58
Employment applications, 1117, 1118, 1119, 1120
Employment law, 60
EMR. See Electronic medical records (EMR)
EMT. See Emergency medical technician (EMT)
Emulsification, 916, 922
Encephalitis, 1048
Encounter form, 262, 291
Endocarditis, 731, 738–39
Endocrine glands, 856, 857–59, 859t–860t
    adrenal, 858
    parathyroid, 858
    pineal, 859
    pituitary, 857
    thymus, 859
    thyroid, 858
Endocrine system
    anatomy and physiology of, 857–59
    disorders, 859–63, 860t
Endocrinology, 855–66
Endometrium, 984, 986
Endorphins, 89, 91
Endorsement stamps, 393, 405
Endoscopes, 478, 482
Endoscopic retrograde cholangiopancreatography
    (ERCP), 916, 937
Endosteum, 949, 954
End stage renal disease (ESRD), 262, 263, 265, 676,
    682, 1092
Energy therapies, 1105
English as a Second Language, 71
ENT. See Ear, nose, and throat (ENT)
Environmental Protection Agency (EPA), 237, 244,
    602
EOB. See Explanation of benefits (EOB)
Eosinophil, 639
EPA. See Environmental Protection Agency (EPA)
Epidemiology, 3, 6
Epidermis, 459, 462
Epilepsy, 1046–47
Epistaxis, 868, 889
Epithelial, 459, 462
EPO. See Exclusive provider organization (EPO)
Equal Employment Opportunity Commission
    (EEOC), 412, 417
Equipment
    adding machines, 240
    case study, 236
    copy machines, 240
    fax machines, 239–40
    inventory of, 239
    leasing versus buying, 239
    maintenance log for, 238
    malfunction, 240, 446
    replacement or buying of, 239
    training employees, 238
    working with, 238–39
ERCP. See Endoscopic retrograde
    cholangiopancreatography (ERCP)
Ergonomics, 223, 231
Erikson, Erik, 84, 84t
Erythrocytes, 636, 638

Erythrocyte sedimentation rate (ESR), 597, 603,
    662, 664–65
    Westergren method for, 664–65
Esophagus, 919–20
ESR. See Erythrocyte sedimentation rate (ESR)
ESRD. See End stage renal disease (ESRD)
Essential oils, 1099
Established patients, 140, 145, 174, 343, 355, 356
    scheduling appointments, 176–77, 180
Estimated date of confinement (EDC), 985, 991
Estimated time of arrival (ETA), 869, 884
Ether, 3, 6
Ethics, 62–66
    bioethics, 64
    case study, 39
    considerations, 62–63
    medical assistant role in, 42
    model, 63–64
    patient rights and, 10
    physician-patient relationship and, 52
    raising issues in healthcare, 64
Etiology, 322
Eukaryotes, 613, 618
Eupnea, 770, 777
Evaluation, 89, 94
Evaluation and Management (E&M), 343
    coding for, 355–59
Exacerbation, 1037, 1047
Examination and treatment areas, preparing and
    maintaining, 447
Examination (E/EX), 343, 356
Examples, 68, 74
Excitability, 731, 733
Exclusions, 262, 268
Exclusive provider organization (EPO), 262, 263,
    272t, 273
Exercise, 96–97, 1103
Exhalation, 773
Exocrine glands, 856, 858
Expected date of delivery (EDD), 985, 991
Expert witnesses, 48
Expiration, 541, 553
    dates, 237, 244
Explanation of benefits (EOB), 262, 263, 305, 306
Exposure control plan, 437–41
    engineering and work practice controls, 437–38
    hazard communication program, 439–40
    Hepatitis B vaccinations, 439
    housekeeping and laundry decontamination,
        439
    Infection Control Practices, 437
    personal protective equipment, 438
    postexposure evaluation and follow-up, 441
    Standard Precautions, 437
    training and record keeping, 440
Expressed consent, 41, 43
Expressed contracts, 54, 41, 52
Extended care facility, 1087, 1088
Extended life, 103–14
    advance medical directives, 108–11
    case study, 103
    hospice, 111
    organ and tissue donations, 104–107, 107–108
    transplant costs, 107
Externship program, 3, 13, 1113, 1114, 1115
Eye
    anatomy and physiology of, 795–97
    color blindness, 801–802
    diagnostic procedures, 798, 800–802
    diagram of, 796
    disorders and diseases of, 797, 798t–800t
    instillation of medication, 806
    irrigation, 804–805
    movements in head injuries, 1050
    patching, 807
    treatments, 802–803
    visual acuity, 798, 800
Eye, ear, nose, and throat (EENT), 793–822
Eye contact, 73
Eyewash stations, 873

F

Face-to-face time, 343
Facial expressions, 73
Factitious disorders, 1065
Fainting, response to, 888
Fair Debt Collection Act, 371, 383, 384
Fair Labor Standards Act (FLSA), 393, 394
FAS. See Fetal alcohol syndrome (FAS)
Fasting blood sugars (FBS), 637, 648, 856, 862
Fats, 916, 922
    saturated, 916, 928
    unsaturated, 916, 929
Fax machines, in medical office, 239–40, 241
FB. See Foreign body (FB)
FBS. See Fasting blood sugars (FBS)
FDA. See Food and Drug Administration (FDA)
Feces, 916, 922
Federal Controlled Substances Act (CSA), 503, 509,
    520
Federal Emergency Management Agency (FEMA),
    869, 908
Federal employee retirement system (FERS), 263,
    286
Federal Express (FedEx), 133
Federal Insurance Contributions Act (FICA), 393,
    395
Federal Tort Claims Act of 1946, 48
Federal Unemployment Tax Act (FUTA), 393, 395
Feedback, 68, 70
Fee-for-service plans, 262, 271
Fee schedule, 262, 266, 304–305, 371, 374–75
    charge-based fee structure, 304
    resource-based fee structures, 304
    resource-based relative value scale, 304–305
Felonies, 42, 42t
FEMA. See Federal Emergency Management Agency
    (FEMA)
Female reproductive system
    anatomy and physiology of, 985–87
    breast, 987, 988
    diagram of, 986, 987
    menstrual cycle, 987–88
FERS. See Federal employee retirement system
    (FERS)
Fetal alcohol syndrome (FAS), 1011, 1029
Fetal heart tones (FHT), 985, 992
Fetus, 984, 985
FHT. See Fetal heart tones (FHT)
Fiber, 916, 927
Fibrillation, 731
FICA. See Federal Insurance Contributions Act
    (FICA)
File storage systems, 202
Filing systems, 199–202
    alphabetic, 199, 200
    numeric, 200, 202
    shingling items for, 200, 201
    subject, 201
Finances, patient education and, 96
Financial information, 191, 192
Fire and electrical safety, 434
    PASS method of firefighting, 435
First-listed, 322
Fistula, 675
Fixed-appointment scheduling, 174, 179
FL. See Form locators (FL)
Flank, 675
Flash drives, 223, 225
Flatulence, 916, 936
Flexible spending accounts (FSA), 262, 263, 274–75,
    275
Flora, normal, 613, 618–19, 618t
Flow charts, 191, 198
FLSA. See Fair Labor Standards Act (FLSA)
Fluoroscope, 720
Fluoroscopy, 712, 713, 717
Fluorouracil treatment, 852
FNB. See Food and Nutrition Board (FNB)
Focus, 731, 758

Follicles, 459, 463
Follicle-stimulating hormone (FSH), 856, 857
Fomites, 459, 461
Font, 117, 124–25, *127*
Fontanelle, 1011
Food
    allergies, 935–36
    categories and sources, 928t
    intolerances, 935–36, 936t
    labels, 932–33
Food and Drug Administration (FDA), 41, 42, 192, 207, 224, 343, 602
Food and Nutrition Board (FNB), 916, 932
Food Guide Pyramid, 931–33
Foreign body (FB), 794, 797, 799t, 906–907
Form locators (FL), 262, 263, 291
Formulary, 262, 277
Four Ds of negligence, 41, 47
    damages, 47
    dereliction of duty, 47
    direct cause, 47
    duty, 47
Fractures (Fx), 899, 901, 951
    coding, 336
    types of, 961t–962t
Fraud, 41, 43t, 343, 344–45
    insurance, 371, 378
Front desk reception, 157–72
    appropriate patients in, 167
    case study, 157
    check-out, 169
    closing office, 169, 170
    escorting patients, 165
    greeting and registering patients, 163–64
    HIPAA compliance, 159–60
    maintaining, 167–69
    managing difficult patients, 165
    notifying of delays, 165
    opening office, 159, 160
    patient file preparation, 159
    payment collection, 165, 167
    receptionist characteristics, 159
Frostbite, 897–98, 898t
FSA. *See* Flexible spending accounts (FSA)
FSH. *See* Follicle-stimulating hormone (FSH)
Fundal height, 984, 992
Fungi, 620
Fusobacterium, 620
FUTA. *See* Federal Unemployment Tax Act (FUTA)
Fx. *See* Fractures (Fx)

G

GAF. *See* Geographic adjustment factor (GAF)
Gallbladder, *922*
Garnish, 393, 401
Gastric, 916, 922
Gastroenterology, 914–48
Gastrointestinal system (GI), 916
    anatomy and physiology of, 917–22
    diagnosis and treatment for disorders, 936–45
    diseases and disorders of, 922, 923t–927t
    functions of, 921–22
    nutrition and, 927–36
Gastroscopy, 916, 937
Gatekeeper, 26, 262, 272
Gender identity disorder, 1065–66
General competencies, *14*
General hospitals, 8
Generic messages, 140, 143
Generic (nonproprietary) name, 262, 503, 506
Genital herpes, 707t
Geographic adjustment factor (GAF), 262, 263, 304
Geographical practice cost index (GPCI), 371, 375
Geriatric patients. *See* Elderly
Geriatrics, 1086–96
    aging process, 1088–92
    definition of, 1087
Germicides, 478, 481

Gestures, 73
GH. *See* Growth hormone (GH)
GHB A1c. *See* Glycohemoglobin/glycosylated hemoglobin (GHB A1c)
GI. *See* Gastrointestinal system (GI)
Glasgow Coma Scale, 902, 902t, 1043
Global period, 343, 361
Global surgical concept, 343, 361
Glomerulonephritis, 675
Glomerulus, 675, 677
Glucometer, 597, 604, 666–67
    quality control methods and, 600–601
Gluconeogenesis, 856, 861
Glucose, 696
Glycohemoglobin/glycosylated hemoglobin (GHB A1c), 856, 862
Gonorrhea, 707t
Good Samaritan act, 41, 53, 437, 870
Government insurance, 278
Gowning, for physical examination, 561
GPCI. *See* Geographical practice cost index (GPCI)
Gram, Hans C.J., 621
Gram reaction, 619t
Gram stain, 621, 623
Granulation, 572
Gravida (g), 984, 985, 994
Grief, Kübler-Ross's five stages of, *80*
    acceptance, *80*
    anger, *80*
    bargaining, *80*
    denial, *80*
    depression, *80*
Grieving patients, communicating with, 79–80
Gross pay, 393, 395
Group A Streptococcus, 619, 630
    rapid testing for, 630
Group health insurance, 262, 265, 269
Growth hormone (GH), 856, 857, 860
Guidelines, 343, 350
Gynecologist, 984, 985
Gynecology, 984

H

Hair follicle, *838*
Hammurabi Code, 10
Hands-free telephone devices, 140, 141
Hand washing
    antisepsis and, 7
    beginning of, in healthcare, 7
    childbirth fever and, 7
    procedures, 470, *471*
    surgical, 493–94
Hardship agreement, 371, 378, *379*
Hardware, 224–26
    drives, 225
    hard drive, 225
    keyboard, 224
    memory, 225
    monitor, 224
    printer, 225–26
Harvesting, organ and tissue, 105
Harvey, William, 6
Hazards, 157, 167
HBV. *See* Hepatitis B virus (HBV)
HCFA. *See* Health Care Financing Administration (HCFA)
HCPCS. *See* Health Care Common Procedure Coding Systems (HCPCS)
Hct. *See* Hematocrit (Hct)
HDL. *See* High density lipoproteins (HDL)
Headache, 1047–48
Head trauma, 1049–50
    concussions and contusions, 1049–50
    dementia due to, 1067
Healing
    based on supernatural, 4
    early practices, 3–4
    phases of, 589t

Healthcare
    antisepsis use in, 7
    contracts in, 52–53
    employment law and, 60
    hand washing in, 7
    raising ethical issues in, 64
    role of medical assistant in, 3
    team members, 26–28
    women in, 9–10
Health Care Common Procedure Coding Systems (HCPCS), 343, 364, 365t
Healthcare facilities, copy machines in, 240
Health Care Financing Administration (HCFA), 263, 278, 597, 598
Healthcare reimbursement account (HRCA), 262, 263, 274
Health insurance
    benefits, 274
    Blue Cross/Blue Shield plans, 274
    claim forms, 291–304
    consumer-directed healthcare plans, 273–74
    copayments, 267
    coverage types, 276–78
    deductibles, 266–67
    disability, 286–87
    exclusions, 268
    exclusive provider organizations, 273
    fee-for-service plans, 271
    fee schedules and approved amounts, 266
    flexible spending accounts, 274–75
    government, 278
    group, 265
    health maintenance organizations, 272–73
    health savings accounts and, 274
    history of, 265
    individual, 265, 270
    managed care plans, 271
    medical savings accounts, 274
    Medicare coverage, 278–83
    members, 266
    plans, 271–76
    point-of-service options, 273
    pre-existing conditions, 268
    preferred provider organization, 271–72
    premiums, 266
    private, 269–70
    projecting future costs of, 316–17
    reimbursement methods, 287
    stop loss and lifetime maximum, 267–68
    terminology, 265–69
    third-party liability, 275–76
    today, 265
    waiting period, 268
Health insurance coverage, 276–78
    alternative care, 277–78
    ancillary coverage, 276
    catastrophic, 276
    dental, 277
    home health care, 276
    hospital, 276
    major medical, 276
    medical, 276
    outpatient, 276
    prescription drug, 276–77
    specialized policies, 276
    surgical, 276
    vision, 277
Health Insurance Portability and Accountability Act (HIPAA), 4, 24, 41, 56, 57–60, 192, 193, 211, 224, 237, 249, 263, 323, 372, 394, 1113, 1114
    business associate agreement, 59–60
    compliance, 15, 24, 36, 59, 81, 95, 131, 134, 142, 153, 159–60, 178, 204, 226, 268, 285, 300, 405
    computer compliance, *59*
    computer privacy and, 59
    electronic health records and, 214–15
    fax machines and, 240

office policies and procedures and, 251
patient health information and, *229*
penalties for violations, 60
personal employee information and, 396
privacy officer, 59
records violation, 59
sample compliant fax cover sheet, *58*
Title II, 58–59
Health maintenance organizations (HMO), 4, 26, 262, 263, 265, 271, 272–73, 272t
group model, 273
individual practice, 273
network model, 273
staff model, 273
Health-related calculators, 223, 230
Health savings account (HSA), 262, 263, 274
Hearing assessment, 561
Hearing impaired, 68, 71
assisting, 808
communicating with patients, 76, 77
Heart
anatomy and physiology of, 732–35
apex, 744
blood flow through, *733*
cardiac rhythms, 758t, *759–65*
conduction, 733–35
congenital conditions, 1028, 1029t
layers of, *734*
rate, factors affecting, 551t
valves, 733, *740*
Heart, diseases and disorders of, 735–44
angina, 735
arrhythmias, 737–38
cardiomyopathy, *737*
congestive heart failure, 736
coronary artery disease, 735
hypertension/hypertensive heart disease, 736
infective disorders, 738–39
myocardial infarction, 735
pulmonary edema, 736
sudden cardiac arrest, 735–36
valvular disorders, 739–40
vascular disorders, 740, 742–44
Heat exhaustion, 898, 899t
Height, 559–60
Heimlich maneuver, 876, 880–81
Hematemesis, 916, 936
Hematocrit (Hct), 597, 599, 603, 662
Hematology, 635–72
anatomy and physiology of blood, 638–42
basic laboratory testing, 656–65
blood chemistry testing, 665, 668–69
blood collection equipment and procedures, 642–56
definition of, 636, 637
Hematopoiesis, 949, 954
Hematopoietic, 824, 828
Hematuria, 675
Hemiparesis, 1037, 1045
Hemiplegia, 1087
Hemoglobin (Hgb), 597, 599, 603, 637, 638
Hemolytic, 824, 831
Hemopneumothorax, 770, 777
Hemoptysis, 731, 740, 770, 777, 778t
Hemostasis, 636, 639
Hemostat, 572, 574
Hemothorax, 770, 777
Hepatitis B virus (HBV), 431, 436, 464, 465
vaccinations, 439
Hepatomegaly, 916
Hepatotoxicity, 770
Herbal medicine, 1102, 1103t
Hgb. *See* Hemoglobin (Hgb)
Hierarchy of human needs. *See* Maslow's hierarchy of needs
High density lipoproteins (HDL), 916, 929
HIPAA compliant, 157, 164
Hippocrates, 4–5
Hippocratic Oath, 5, 10, *11*
Histoplasmosis, 776t

History (H), 343, 356
HIV. *See* Human immunodeficiency virus (HIV)
HMO. *See* Health maintenance organizations (HMO)
Hold feature, 140, 142–43
Holistic approach, to healthcare, 91
mind-body connection, 91
Holter monitor, 749, 753–54
Homeopathy, 1100–1101
Homeostasis, 459
Honesty, 34
Hormone replacement therapy (HRT), 988
Hormones, 856, 857
therapy, 1081–82
Hospice, 104, 111, 262, 279, 1075, 1082–83
Hospitals
general or community, 8
history of American, 8
laboratory setting, 602–603
organ and tissue donation in, 107–108
research, 8
scheduling services and admissions, 183–84, 185
services, 262, 265
specialty, 8
teaching, 8
HRCA. *See* Healthcare reimbursement account (HRCA)
HSA. *See* Health savings account (HSA)
Human immunodeficiency virus (HIV), 41, 56, 431, 436, 467, 468, 482, 621
Americans with Disabilities Act and, 60
caring for patients with, 469
transmission prevention strategies, 828
Humors (body fluids), 4
Hydronephrosis, 675, 683
Hydrotherapy, 1102
Hygiene, 24
Hyperglycemia, 862t, 868, 905
Hypersensitivity, 831–32
Hypertension, 541, 556, 736, 868, 889
coding, 332–33
malignant, 541, 556
portal, 916
risk factors, 736t
Hypertensive heart disease, 736
Hyperthermia, 868, 895, 898
Hyperventilation, 884, 886
Hypochondriasis, 1065
Hypoglycemia, 862t, 868, 905
Hypotension, 541, 556
orthostatic, 1087, 1088
Hypothalamus, 856, 858
Hypothermia, 868, 895, 898, 899t

I

ICD-9-CM, 120, 263, 300, 605
appendices, 326
contents of, 325t
ICD-10 *versus*, 324t
supplementary code listings, 325–26
volumes of, 324–26
ICD-9-CM coding, 321–40
with book, 324
case study, 321
I&D. *See* Incision and drainage (I&D)
IDDM (type 1). *See* Insulin-dependent diabetes mellitus (IDDM (type I))
Identification, *85*
Ileostomy, 916
Imaging, medical, 711–24
Immune system, 463
anatomy and physiology of, 825–27
Immune system, diseases and disorders of, 827–28, 829t–831t, 831–32
autoimmune diseases, 828, 829t–831t, 831
hypersensitivity and allergic reactions, 831–32
immunodeficiency diseases, 827–28, 827t
Immunity, 459, 463

Immunizations, 1021, *1022, 1023,* 1024–1025
coding for, *363*
documentation of, 1024
Immunocompetence, 770, 786
Immunodeficiency diseases, 824, 827–28, 827t
Immunohematology, 636, 640, 642
Immunology, 823–34
testing, 669
Immunotherapy, 1081–82
Implementing, 89, 94
Implied consent, 41, 43, *44,* 573
Implied contracts, 41, 52
Inactive patient files, 191, 203
Incident reports, 435, 436t
Incision, 572, 868, 891–92
Incision and drainage (I&D), 572, 573
Incomplete protein, 916, 927
Incontinence, 675, 683
Incubation, 459, 461
Indecipherable, 191, 192, 211, 217
Indemnity, 262
Indented code, 343, 349, *350*
India ink, 624
Indigestion, 3
Indirect questions, *75*
Individual health insurance, 262, 265, 270
Individual practice association, 262
Infants
growth measurement, 1018–20
immunizations for, 1021, *1022, 1023,* 1024–1025
routine visits for, 1018–29
Infection, 460
cycle of, 460–62
natural defenses against, 462–63
nosocomial, 465
opportunistic, 469t
of urinary system, 679–80, 679t–680t
Infection control
asepsis and, 464
precautions, 464–65
Infection Control Practices, 437
Infection control procedures, 253–54
personal protective equipment, 465
Infective heart disorders, 738–39
endocarditis, 738–39
myocarditis, 739
pericarditis, 739
rheumatic fever and heart disease, 739
Infertility, 991
Inflammatory, 572
Influenza, 776t
vaccination, 786
Information
financial, 192
misfiled, 203
patient, 192
personal, 192
social, 192
Informed consent, 41, 47, 573
form, *45*
obtaining, 44
preparation of form, 46
Infusion therapy, 529–30
Inhalation, *773*
Inhalers, 786–88
Injections, 522, 523t
gloving for, 524
intramuscular, 534–35
reconstitution of powdered drug for, 529
subcutaneous, 532–33
Z-track, 535–36
Innervate, 1037, 1042
Inpatient admissions, scheduling, 186
Inpatient services, 262, 276, 338, 343, 355
Inspection, 541, 564
Inspiration, 541, 550
Instructional notes, 343, 349, *350*
Instruments, surgical, 574–76
clamping and grasping, 574–75
cutting, 575–76

Instruments, surgical (continued)
dilating, probing, and visualizing, 576
wrapping, 485, 487
Insulin-dependent diabetes mellitus (IDDM (type I)), 856, 861
Insurance billing, 260–320
case study, 260
documenting calls in, 291
electronically, 300, 302, 304
medical assistants and, 264
Office of Insurance Commissioner and, 315
posting payments, 305
processing claims, 287–91
reconciling payments and rejections,307, 314
supporting documentation in, 314–15
verification of benefits, 289–90
Insurance fraud, 371, 378
Insured, 262, 266
Integrative medicine (IM), 1099, 1100, 1101
Integumentary system, 460, 462–63, 836, 837
burns, 895–97
conditions of, 851–52
frostbite, 897–98, 898t
heat exhaustion, 898
hyperthermia, 898
hypothermia, 898
Intentional tort, 41, 42, 43t
Interatrial septum, 731
Internal bleeding, 888–89
Internal Revenue Service (IRS), 41, 263, 394
W-4 form, 397–98
International Classification of Diseases, 9th ed., *Clinical Modification* (ICD-9-CM). *See* ICD-9-CM
International law, 41
Internet
bank accounts via, 405–6
online postage and, 133
patient education and, 98, 99
search engines, 223, 229
web resources, 230
Internodal pathway, 731, 734
Interpersonal communication skills, 67–87
active listening, 74
case study, 67
with coworkers, 81–82
developmental stages of life cycle and, 82–84
interviewing patients, 74–81
nonverbal communication, 70–74
with other facilities, 82
verbal communication, 69–70
Interphalangeal, 824, 830t
Interpreters
communicating via, 76–77
scheduling, 184–85
Interventricular septum, 731, 735
Interviews, 1113, 1116, 1120–21
close-ended questions, 74
dressing for, 1120–21
effective listening skills in, 75
follow up after, 1121, 1122
open-ended questions, 74
of patients, 74–81
preparing for, 1120
presenting image in, 1121
reflecting technique, 74
techniques, 74–75
Intimate distance, *70*
Intradermal testing, 770, 783, 784–86, 786
Intramuscular injections, 534–35
Intraocular, 794
Intraoperative, 572
Intravenous pyelogram (IVP), 685, 712, 725
Intravenous therapy, 522, 526, 531–32
Intrinsic factor, 824, 830t, 916, 922
Invasion of privacy, 41, 43t
Inventory, 237
IRS. *See* Internal Revenue Service (IRS)
Ischemic, 104, 105
Ishihara Color Vision Test, 804

Isoelectric line, 731, 746
IVP. *See* Intravenous pyelogram (IVP)

J

Jaundice, 675, 693, 916, 926
JCAHO. *See* Joint Commission on the Accreditation of Healthcare Organizations (JCAHO)
Job market
changing jobs in, 1121
competing in, 1112–24
cover letter preparation and, 1116, 1117
employment advertisements and, 1116–17
employment applications and, 1117, *1118, 1119,* 1120
externship program, 1114, 1115
interview and, 1120–21
resume writing and, 1114–17
Job opportunities, 13
Joint Commission on the Accreditation of Healthcare Organizations (JCAHO), 41, 62, 224, 425
abbreviations and, 127–28
ambulatory care and, 62
pain assessment and management, 93
prescriptions and, 517
regulations and laboratory safety, 602
Joints, 954–56
synovial movements, *955*
Journal of the American Medical Association (JAMA), 4, *8,* 224

K

Kaposi's sarcoma, 468, *469*
Kaufman Assessment Battery for Children, 1066
Keratin, 836, 837
Keratinocytes, 460, 462
Ketones, 697
Key components, 343, 355
Kidneys, 675, 677
function, 677–79
nephrons, 677–78
Kilocalorie, 916
Kirby-Bauer disc diffusion (KBDD), 626
KOH. *See* Potassium hydroxide (KOH)
Korotkoff sounds, 555–56, 556t
Kübler-Ross, Elizabeth, 80
stages of grief, *80*

L

Labor and delivery (L&D), 985
Laboratory, coding for, 363
Laboratory testing
hematology testing, 657
manual tests, 657, 662, 665
performing basic, 656–57, 662, 665
Laceration, 572, 588, 868, 891–92
Language
sign, 71
symbolic, 71
Large intestine, 916, 920
Laryngologist, 794, 795
Last menstrual period (LMP), 985, 992
Last number redial, 140, 141
Late effects, 322, 337
Latex allergy, 471, 473
Lavage, 1011, 1025
Law
administrative, 40, 42
civil, 40, 42
commercial, 40, 42
common, 40, 42
constitutional, 40
contract, 42
criminal, 40, 42

employment, 60
international, 41
public, 41
public *versus* private, 42
regulatory, 41
sources of, 42
tort, 41, 42
traditional, 41, 42
LC. *See* Limiting charge (LC)
L&D. *See* Labor and delivery (L&D)
LDL. *See* Low-density lipoproteins (LDL)
Leadership styles, 413–14
Learning environment, in patient education, 95
Ledger cards, 371, 373
Left eye (OS), 794, 800
Left lateral view (LL), 712
Left lower leg (LLL), 951
Left lower quadrant (LLQ), 916, 937t
Left upper extremity (LUE), 951
Left upper quadrant (LUQ), 916, 937t
Legionellosis/Legionnaire's disease, 774t
Lesion, 836
Letterhead, 117, 120, *245*
Leukocytes, 636, 638, 697
Level I codes, 343
Level II codes, 343, 346, 364t
Level III HCPCS codes, 343, 364
Level of consciousness (LOC), 869, 902–3
LGI. *See* Lower gastrointestinal tract (LGI)
LH. *See* Luteinizing hormone (LH)
Liability insurance, 262, 265
Licensed practical nurse (LPN), 26
Licensed vocation nurse (LVN), 26
Licenses
for Certified Medical Assistant, 27
for Registered Medical Assistant, 27
revoking, 51
Licensure, 27
Life cycle, developmental stages of, 82–84
defense mechanisms, 84, *85*
emotional, 83t
Maslow's hierarchy of needs, 84
physical, 83t
Life-prolonging declarations, 110, *111*
Lifestyle, 96
Lifetime maximum, 267–68
benefit, 262
Ligaments, 949, 954
Limited-scope radiography, 722
Limiting charge (LC), 262, 263, 279
Lipids, 916, 922
Listening
active, 74
effective skills in interviews, 75
empathetic, 74
Lithotripsy, 675, *684*
Living wills, 108, 110, *110, 111*
LL. *See* Left lateral view (LL)
LLE. *See* Lower left extremity (LLE)
LLL. *See* Left lower leg (LLL)
LLQ. *See* Left lower quadrant (LLQ)
L1 (lumbar vertebra), 951
LMP. *See* Last menstrual period (LMP)
LOC. *See* Level of consciousness (LOC)
Local anesthesia, 572, 579, 579t
Logo, 117
Long-term care, 262, 265
Low-density lipoproteins (LDL), 916, 929
Lower gastrointestinal tract (LGI), 916, 920–21
Lower left extremity (LLE), 951
Lower respiratory infection (LRI), 1087
LP. *See* Lumbar puncture (LP)
LPN. *See* Licensed practical nurse (LPN)
LRI. *See* Lower respiratory infection (LRI)
LS. *See* Lumbosacral (LS)
LUE. *See* Left upper extremity (LUE)
Lumbar puncture (LP), 1038, 1043, 1044
Lumbosacral (LS), 951
LUQ. *See* Left upper quadrant (LUQ)
Luteinizing hormone (LH), 856, 857, 985, 988

M

LVN. *See* Licensed vocation nurse (LVN)
Lymphatic system, *826*
Lymphocyte, *639*

MAC. *See* Medicare administrative contractor (MAC)
Magnetic resonance imaging (MRI), 712, 717–18
Mailing, written communication, 128–29
    annotation, 134, 136
    choosing type of service, 133
    classification of mail, 132–33
    delivery options, 133–34
    managing correspondence, 134
    multiline optical character readers and, 133
    online postage, 133
    opening and sorting, 136
    postage meters, 132
    restricted materials, 133
    USPS-approved abbreviations, 133, *134*
    window envelopes, 128, 135
    zip codes, 133
Mainframe computers, *224*
Maintained, 237
Main term, 322, 343, 346, *348*
Male reproductive system, 701–707
    anatomy and physiology of, 702–703
    diagram of, *702*
    diseases and disorders of, 704–707, 705t–706t
    internal structures, 703
    penis, 702
    scrotum, 702
    sexually transmitted diseases, 706, 707t
    testicular self-examination, 703–704
Malfeasance, 41, 44
Malignant, 1075, 1076
Malignant hypertension, 541, 556
Malnutrition, 916, 935
Malpractice insurance policy, 41, 45
    for medical assistants, 47
    types of, 45–46
Malware, 223, 229
Mammogram, 712, 715, 722
Mammography, 715, 722
Managed care, 262, 271
    collections in, 378–85
    referral, 303
Managed care organization (MCO), 263, 271, 272t
Management
    guidelines for, 93
    of medical records, 190–209
    pain, 93–94
Manifestation, 322, 329
Manipulative and body-based methods, 1102–1104
    acupressure, 1102–1103
    chiropractic, 1103
    craniosacral therapy, 1103
    exercise, 1103
    hydrotherapy, 1102
    massage, 1104
    reflexology, 1103–1104
Mantoux test, 783, 784–86
Manual billing systems, 373
MAO. *See* Monoamine oxidase (MAO)
Maslow's hierarchy of needs, 84
Massage, 1104
    lymphatic, 1104
    sports, 1104
    Swedish, 1104
Material safety data sheet (MSDS), 431, 439
    example of, *440*
    labeling, *438*
Matrix, 174, 177, 178
Mayo stand, 478, 490, 572, 574
MCH. *See* Mean corpuscular hemoglobin (MCH)
MCHC. *See* Mean corpuscular hemoglobin concentration (MCHC)
MCO. *See* Managed care organization (MCO)

M codes, 322
MCV. *See* Mean corpuscular volume (MCV)
MDI. *See* Metered dose inhaler (MDI)
MDM. *See* Medical decision making (MDM)
Mean corpuscular hemoglobin concentration (MCHC), 637, 657
Mean corpuscular hemoglobin (MCH), 637, 657
Mean corpuscular volume (MCV), 637, 657
Measles-mumps-rubella vaccine (MMR), 1011
Medicaid, 262, 265, 283–84
Medical administration, 502–39
Medical asepsis, 458–76
    AIDS and, 467–69
    cycle of infection, 460–62
    definition of, 460
    hepatitis and, 465, 467
    infection control and, 464–65
    latex allergy and, 471, 473
    natural defenses against infection, 462–63
    surgical asepsis *versus*, 479t
Medical assistant
    as advocate, 22, *34*
    body language, reading, *72*
    character of, 12
    computer use and, 224
    definition of term, 12
    educational programs for, 13
    educational requirements for, 13, 15
    job opportunities for, 13
    malpractice insurance for, 47
    with multiple statuses, 15
    physical requirements of, 12
    professionalism and, 33
    qualities of, 23–24, 23t
    responsibilities of, understanding, 22–23
    role of, 20
    scope of practice for, 12
Medical assistant profession, 2–18
    as career, choosing, 22–25
    competencies for, 3
    history of, 20–21
    recognition of, by AMA, 21
    role in healthcare, 3
    standards, 20
    today, 19–31
Medical billing software, 331
Medical decision making (MDM), 343, 356–57
Medical history
    charting, 449–55
    hospitals and, 8
    organizations in, 7–9
Medical imaging, 711–24
    equipment, 719–20
    radiographic records, filing and loading, 725, 726
    radiology, 713–19
    safety precautions and patient protection, 720–22
Medical information, 191
Medical laboratory technician (MLT), 21
Medical laboratory technologist, 27
Medical law, 39–66
    advance directives, 60
    ambulatory care, 62
    Clinical Laboratory Improvement Amendments Act, 62
    conscience clause, 62
    employment law, 60
    Health Insurance Portability and Accountability Act (HIPAA), 57–60
    Joint Commission on the Accreditation of Healthcare Organizations, 62
    medical malpractice, 44–48
    Patients' Bill of Rights, 62
Medically needy, 262, 283
Medical malpractice, 44–48
    assumption of risk as defense, 48
    awards, 47
    contributory and comparative negligence, 48
    defending against claims, 47–48

    immunity from negligence suits, 48
    insurance policy, 45–46
    malfeasance, 44
    misfeasance, 44
    nonfeasance, 45
    payouts, *52*
    preventing claims, 47
    proving, 46–47
    res judicata and *res ipsa locitur,* 48
    respondeat superior, doctrine of, 45
    standard of care and, 48
    statute of limitations, 48
Medical management software, 223, 227
Medical necessity, 262, 280
Medical office
    case study, 411
    clinical visit and, 446
    computers in, 222–33
    creating policies and procedures for, 251–55
    effective time management in, 25
    equipment, 238–39
    fax machines in, 239–40, 241
    logging supplies, 242–44
    managing, 411–27
    preparedness, 870–71
    quality in, 424–25
    reporting office incidents, 425
    risk management in, 424–25
    scheduling issues, 419
    sexual harassment in, 421–22
    staffing, 415–19
    staff meetings in, 414–15
    supply inventory, 242–43
    surgery performed in, 572–73, 573t
    uniformity in, 251
Medical office manager, 413
Medical practice specializations, 28, 28t
Medical records, 191
    abbreviations, in charting, 199
    active, inactive, and closed files, 203
    adding to, 205
    charting, 196–99, 199, 205
    conducting research with, 207
    correcting, 204–5, 206
    electronic, 210–21
    filing documents in, 202
    filing systems for, 199–202
    flow charts in, 198
    information in, 192–93
    management, 190–209
    "owning," 205
    paper records to electronic storage, 203
    preparation and maintenance of, 195–96
    prescription refill requests in, 205–206
    progress notes in, 198
    purpose of, 193
    releasing, 206–207
    retaining, 204
    signing off on, 193, 196
Medical records technician, 27
Medical research programs, 191, 207
Medical savings accounts (MSA), 41, 58, 262, 263, 274
Medical secretary, 27
Medical supplies
    expired, 243
    inventory of, 242–43
    receiving shipment, 244
    storing, 243–44
    tracking with software, 244
Medical technologist (MT), 21
Medical transcription, 241–42
Medical transcriptionist, 27
Medicare, 262, 265, 278–83, 1087, 1090, 1092
    Advantage Plan (Part C), 280
    billing and, 364
    Medigap plans, 281
    other health insurance and, 281
    Part A, 279
    Part B, 279–80

Medicare (continued)
  Part C, 280
  Part D, 280
  providers participating in, 281–83
Medicare administrative contractor (MAC), 263, 278
Medicare secondary payer (MSP), 263, 282
Medication administration
  ampules and vials, 524–28, 531–32
  forms and routes of, 520–36, 522t
  infusion therapy, 529–30
  injection, 522
  intravenous, 522
  oral, 521–22
  parenteral, 521, 522–24
  prescription, 517–19
  safety guidelines for, 516–17, 519
  sublingual, 521
  of Z-track injection, 535–36
Medications
  abbreviations and symbols in dosing, 513t
  administration for children, 1033
  apothecary/metric equivalents, 513t
  avoiding errors, 520
  buying online, 230
  cost of, 536
  dosage calculation, 512–15
  ear, 813–14
  errors, preventing, 96
  eye, 806
  over-the-counter, 26
  rectal suppositories, 940, 943–44
  withdrawal from ampules and vials, 525–28
Medicine
  alternative, 1098–1109
  coding for, 363
  complementary, 1099, 1100
  contributors to, 4–6
  early Chinese, 4
  early Egyptian, 4
  early healing practices, 3–4
  early Native American, 4
  healing based on supernatural, 4
  herbal, 1102
  Hippocrates and, 4–5
  history of, 3–7
  integrative, 1099, 1100, 1101
Medigap insurance, 281, 1087
Megakaryocytes, 824, 829t
Melanin, 836, 837
Melanocytes, 836, 851t
Melanocyte-stimulating hormone (MSH), 856, 858
Melanoma, 851, 851t
Melena, 916, 936
Member, 262, 266
Memo, 117, 128, 130
Men
  catheterization of, 691–93
  reproductive system of, 701–707
Menarche, 984, 986
Meningitis, 1048
Menopause, 984, 986
Menses, 984, 986
Menstrual cycle, 987–88, 989
  disorders, 988, 990t
Mensuration, 541
Mental disorders, 1058–69
  angry behavior and, 1069t
  anxiety disorders, 1063–64
  assessment and diagnosis, 1070
  in childhood, 1067, 1067t
  dementia, 1066–67
  gender identity disorder, 1065–66
  hallucination or delusion, 1059t–1060t
  mental retardation, 1066
  mood disorders, 1059–60, 1062–63
  personality disorders, 1063, 1063t
  schizophrenia, 1058–59
  somatoform disorders, 1064–65
  substance-related disorders, 1068–69, 1068t
  treatments for, 1070

Mental health, 1054–73
  cognitive functioning, 1057–58
  community services and, 1070
  guidelines for providers, 1056t
  mental disorders, 1058–69
  mental status examination, 1070t
  mental wellness, 1058
Mentally ill patients, communicating with, 78
Mentally incompetent adults, consent for, 43
Mental retardation, 1066
Mentor, 1113, 1114
Mercury thermometers, 441
Metabolism, 915, 916
Metastasis, 1075, 1076
Metered dose inhaler (MDI), 771
MI. See Myocardial infarction (MI)
Microbiology, 612–34
  definition of, 613
  normal flora, 615–19
  pathogens, 619–21
  scientific nomenclature and morphology, 615
  specimen collection, storage, and transport, 624–31
Microcomputers, 224
Microhematocrit, 662–64
Microorganisms, 460
  identification of, 626
  transmission of, 462
Microscopes, 603–604
  maintenance, 617
  microbiology and, 612–34
  specimen preparation for examination, 621–24
  structure and parts of, 614–16
  types of, 614, 615t
  using, 616–17
Mind-body connection, 91
Mind-body interventions, 1101
  biofeedback, 1101
Minerals, 916, 927, 929t–931t
Minicomputers, 224
Minor surgery, 570–93
  assisting during, 579–84
  implied and informed consent, 573
  performed in medical office, 572–73, 573t
  preoperative care and patient preparation, 573–79
  recovery/postoperative care, 584, 588–89
  sutures and suture removal, 582–84
Miscommunication, patient, 95
Misdemeanors, 42
Misfeasance, 44
Mission statement, 249, 251
Mitral valve prolapse (MVP), 731
MLOCR. See Multiline optical character readers (MLOCR)
MLT. See Medical laboratory technician (MLT)
MMR. See Measles-mumps-rubella vaccine (MMR)
Modified wave scheduling, 174, 180
Modifiers, 343, 345, 352
  CPT, 353–55
Modifying terms, 343, 346
Monoamine oxidase (MAO), 1056, 1060
Monocular, 613, 614
Monocyte, 639
Mood disorders, 1059–60, 1062–63
  bipolar disorder, 1063
  major depressive disorder, 1059–60, 1061
  postpartum depression, 1062
  seasonal affective disorder, 1062–63
Morbidity, 322
Morphology, 613, 619
Mortality, 322
Mouth, 917–18
  diseases of, 818
  infectious conditions of, 819t
MRI. See Magnetic resonance imaging (MRI)
MS. See Multiple sclerosis (MS)
MSA. See Medical savings accounts (MSA)
MSDS. See Material safety data sheet (MSDS)
MSH. See Melanocyte-stimulating hormone (MSH)

MSP. See Medicare secondary payer (MSP)
MT. See Medical technologist (MT)
MUGA scan, 756
Multifocal rhythms, 731, 737, 764
Multiline optical character readers (MLOCR), 117, 133
Multiple coding, 322, 328, 332
Multiple sclerosis (MS), 825, 829t, 1047
Muscles, 956–58, 956t, 957–58. See also Musculoskeletal system
Musculoskeletal injuries, 898–901
  fractures, 899, 901
  splint application, 900–901
  sprains, strains, and dislocations, 901
Musculoskeletal system
  anatomy and physiology of, 952–58
  appendicular skeleton, 952
  axial skeleton, 952
  bones, 952–54
  diagnostic procedures, 963
  joints, 954–56
  muscles, 956–58, 956t
  neoplasia, 961
  traumatic conditions, 961–62
  treatment of conditions, 963–80
Musculoskeletal system, diseases and disorders of, 958, 958t–960t, 961
  congenital and developmental, 958t–959t
  degenerative and inflammatory, 959t–960t
  infectious, 960t
MVP. See Mitral valve prolapse (MVP)
Myco-bacterium tuberculosis, 462
Mycology, 613, 620
Myelography, 712, 717
Myocardial infarction (MI), 731, 735
Myocarditis, 731, 739
MyPyramid food guide, 98, 931–33

N

Nail bed structure, 838
Narrative, 191, 196
Nasal cannula, 789
Nasal septum, 794
National Center for Complementary and Alternative Medicine (NCCAM), 1099, 1100
National Childhood Vaccine Injury Act, 51
National Commission for Certifying Agencies (NCCA), 4, 13
National conversion factor, 371, 375
National First Aid Society, 9
National Institute on Drug Abuse (NIDA), 89, 98
National Organization for Competency Assurance (NOCA), 13
National provider identifier (NPI), 263, 278
National resources, 80
National standard, 371, 375
Native American medicine, early, 4
Natural defenses against infection, 462–63
  general health and, 463
  immune system, 463
  integumentary system, 462–63
Naturopathy, 1101
Nausea and vomiting (N&V), 825, 916
NCCA. See National Commission for Certifying Agencies (NCCA)
NCCAM. See National Center for Complementary and Alternative Medicine (NCCAM)
NCR. See No carbon required (NCR)
Nebulizers, 786–87, 788–89
Needlestick Safety and Prevention Act, 437
Negligence, 41, 42
  comparative, 40, 48
  contributory, 48, 49
  four Ds of, 41, 47
  immunity from suits, 48
Negotiated fee schedule, 262, 287
Neoplasia, 949, 961

Neoplasms, 322, 1075, 1076, 1076t
  benign, 845, 848t–849t
    coding, 333, *334*
Nephrologist, 675, 676
Nephrology, 675, 676
Nephrons, 675, 677–78
Nerves
  afferent, 89, 91
  cranial, 1040t
  efferent, 89, 91
Nervous system, *92*
  anatomy and physiology of, 1038–41
  central, 1039
  cranial nerves, 1040t
  diagram of, *1039*
  disorders and diseases of, 1045–51
  divisions of, *507*
  functions of, 1041
  neuron, 1040–41
  peripheral, 1039–40
  reactions, 508t
Net pay, 393, 395
Neuralgia, 836, 1037, 1050
Neuritis, 824, 830t
Neurological emergencies, 902–903
  CVA and TIA, 903
  decreased level of consciousness, 902–903
  seizures, 903
Neurology, 1036–53
  assessment of neurological system, 1041–44
  electroencephalography, 1043–44
  examinations, 1042
  Glasgow Coma Scale, 1043
  lumbar punctures, 1043, 1044
Neuromuscular junction, *957*
Neuron, 1037, 1040–41
Neurotransmitters, 1037, 1041
Neutrophil, *638*
New patient checklist, 174, 175
New patients, *174*, 343, 355, *356*
  scheduling appointments, 175–79
NIDA. *See* National Institute on Drug Abuse
    (NIDA)
NIDDM (type II). *See* Non-insulin dependent
    diabetes mellitus (NIDDM (type II))
Nightingale, Florence, 8, 9
Nitrite, 697–98
Nitroglycerin, 883–84
NOCA. *See* National Organization for Competency
    Assurance (NOCA)
No carbon required (NCR), *372, 373*
Nocturia, 675, 680
Nomogram chart, *516*
Non-covered, 262, 280
Noncritical, 478, 482
Nonessential modifiers, 322, 328
Nonfeasance, 41, 45
Non-insulin dependent diabetes mellitus (NIDDM
    (type II)), 856, 861
Noninvasive, 770, 779
Non-participating physician/provider (NPN), 262,
    263, 271
Nonpathogens, 460
Nonsufficient funds (NSF), 372, 381, 385
Nontherapeutic research, 191, 207
Nonverbal communication, 70–74
  body language, 71–74
  personal space, 70–71
  symbolic language, 71
  therapeutic touch, 74
  writing, 71
Normal flora, 613, 618–19, 618t
Normal saline (NS), 869
Normal sinus rhythm (NSR), 731
Nose
  anatomy and physiology of, 814
  diagnosis, 815
  diseases and disorders of, 814–15
  nasopharyngeal specimen, 817
  treatment, 815

No-show appointments, 181, 183
Nosocomial infections, 460, 465
Not otherwise specified (NOS), 322, 329
NP. *See* Nurse practitioner (NP)
NPI. *See* National provider identifier (NPI)
NPN. *See* Non-participating physician/provider
    (NPN)
NS. *See* Normal saline (NS)
NSF. *See* Nonsufficient funds (NSF)
NSR. *See* Normal sinus rhythm (NSR)
Nuchal rigidity, 1037, 1048
Nuclear medicine, 719
Nuclear medicine technologist, 27
Numerical pain level chart, *93*
Nurse, 26
  licensed practical, 26
  licensed vocation, 26
  registered, 26
Nurse practitioner (NP), 21, 26
Nutrition, 927–36
  aging and, 935, 1090
  alcohol and, 934–35
  diseases and disorders involving, 935
  food allergies and intolerance, 935–36
  health and, 933
  patient instruction in, 940
N&V. *See* Nausea and vomiting (N&V)

O

Obesity, 916, 934
OB/GYN. *See* Obstetrics and gynecology
    (OB/GYN)
Obliterate, 191, 205
OBRA. *See* Omnibus Budget Reconciliation Act
    (OBRA)
Observation status, 343, 355
Obsessive compulsive disorder (OCD), 1056, 1063,
    1064
Obstetrician, 984, 985
Obstetrics
  coding, 337–38
  definition of, 984
Obstetrics and gynecology (OB/GYN), 983–1009,
    985
  breastfeeding, 996
  contraception, 988–91
  diagnostic procedures, 1001, 1003–1004
  diseases and disorders, 996, 997t–998t, 998,
    1001
  female reproductive system, 985–87
  infertility and, 991
  menstrual cycle, 987–88, *989*
  pregnancy and birth process, 991–96
  psychological considerations in, 1006
  routine assessment, 1001
  treatment modalities, 1004–1006
Obstructive conditions, of urinary system, 683,
    683t–684t, 685
Occupational Safety and Health Act, 432
Occupational Safety and Health Administration
    (OSHA), 237, 238, 249, 251, 363, 431, 519
  asepsis and infection control, 464
  bloodborne pathogen standards, 436–37
  emergency intervention, 873–74
Occupational therapist (OT), 27
Occupational therapy assistant, 27
OCD. *See* Obsessive compulsive disorder (OCD)
OCR. *See* Optical character recognition (OCR)
Oculars, 613, 614–15
OD. *See* Right eye (OD)
ODD. *See* Oppositional defiant disorder (ODD)
Office brochure, 174, 176
Office fee slip, *166*
Office manager, 27
Office of Insurance Commissioner, 315
Office policies and procedures, 157, 169, 170,
    248–57
  case study, 248

  medical assistants and, 250
  for medical office, 251–55
  patient information pamphlets, 250
  personnel manual, 250
  sample, 255t
Oliguria, 675, 680
Omnibus Budget Reconciliation Act (OBRA),
    371, 374
Oncology, 1074–85
  classification and physiology of cancers,
    1076–77
  definition of, 1075
  diagnostic procedures, 1077–79
Open-ended questions, 68, 74
Open hours, 174, 179
Open wounds, 572, 588, 889, 891–92, 895
  abrasions, 891
  avulsions and amputations, 891
  impaled objects, 892
  lacerations and incisions, 891–92
  puncture, 892
  soft tissue injuries, 892
  traumatic injury, 892, 895
Operative report, *194*, 316
Ophthalmologist, 794, 795
Ophthalmoscope, 445, 446, *801*
Opportunistic pathogens, 613, 619
Oppositional defiant disorder (ODD), 1067
Optical character recognition (OCR), 117,
    291–92, 300
Optician, 794, 795
Optional surgery, 572, 573
Optometrist, 794, 795
Oral administration, 521–22, 530–31
Oral temperature, 541, 543, 544–45
Organ and tissue donation, 104–7, 105t
  donor information, 106
  harvesting, 105
  hospitals and, 107–108
  issues and concerns, 105–107
  Uniform Anatomical Gift Act, 107
  universal donor card, *106*
Organelles, 613, 618
Organizational chart, 249, 251–52, *253*
Organizations
  American Medical Association, 8–9
  American Red Cross, 9
  in medical history, 7–9
Organ Procurement and Transplant Network
    (OPTN), 108
Organs, 104, 105
Organ transplantation, history of, *105*
Orthopedics, 949–82
Orthopnea, 770, 777
Orthostatic hypotension, 1087, 1088
OS. *See* Left eye (OS)
O₂ sat. *See* Oxygen saturation (O₂ sat)
OSHA. *See* Occupational Safety and Health
    Administration (OSHA)
Osteoblasts, 949, 953
OT. *See* Occupational therapist (OT)
Otic, 794
Otolaryngologist, 794, 795
Otologist, 794, 795
Otorhinolaryngologist, 794, 795
Otoscope, 445, 446, *810*
Ototoxicity, 770
Outliers, 263, 287
Outpatient, 263, 276, 343, 355
Outsource, 393, 395
Overcompensation, *85*
Over-the-counter (OTC) medications,
    26, 503
  prescription *versus*, 506
Overtime, 393, 394
Overweight, 916, 934
Ovum, 984, 985
Oxygen saturation (O₂ sat), 771, 779,
    782–83
Oxygen therapy, 789–90

P

PA. *See* Physician's assistant (PA)
PAC. *See* Premature atrial contractions (PAC)
Packing slip, 237, 243
PaCo₂. *See* Partial pressure of carbon dioxide (PaCo₂)
Pain, 91–94
  acute, 91
  assessment, 92–93, *93*
  body response to, 91
  chronic, 91
  management, 93–94
  management, patient teaching, 94
  numerical pain level chart, *93*
  phantom, 92–93
  physical, 91
  psychological, 91–92
  referred, 91
  types of, 91–92
  Wong/Baker FACES rating scale, *93*
  words to describe, 92t
Palliative, 104, 111
Palpation, 541, 564
Palpitations, 731
Palsy, 1037, 1047
Pancreas, disorders of, 861–63
PaO₂. *See* Partial pressure of oxygen (PaO₂)
Paper charting
  conversion from, 213–14
  electronic *versus,* 212–13
  office workflow and, *214*
Paper scheduling, 177–78
Pap Smear (Papanicolaou test), 985, 1001–1003
Para (p), 985, 994
Paraplegia, 1037, 1050, 1087
Parasites, 620–21
Parasitology, 613, 620
Parasympathetic reactions, 1041t
Parathyroid glands, 858
  disorders, 861
Parathyroid hormone (PTH), 856, 858
Parent code, 343, 349
Parenteral administration, *521,* 522–24
Parkinson's disease, 1047
Partial pressure of carbon dioxide (PaCo₂), 771, 781
Partial pressure of oxygen (PaO₂), 771, 781
Partial thromboplastin time (PTT), 597, 603
Participating provider, 263, 267
Pasteurization, 3, 7
Past timely filing limits, 263, 300
Patent, 868, 884
Pathogenicity, 613, 619
Pathogens, 431, 432, *461,* 619–21
  bacteria, 619–20
  bloodborne, 459, 460, 461t
  common, 619t
  fungi, 620
  opportunistic, 613, 619
  parasites, 620–21
  viruses, 621
Pathology, coding for, 363
Patient billing statements, 371, 379, 382
Patient Care Partnership, 41, 62
Patient-centered care
  holistic approach to healthcare, 91
  pain and, 91–94
  wellness, 90
Patient education, 13, 94–99
  culture and, 95–96
  dieting and weight-loss information, 96
  documenting step, 94
  environment for, 95
  evaluation step, 94
  exercise information, 96–97
  finances and, 96
  hepatitis and, 465
  for home tests, 599
  implementing step, 94
  Internet and, 98, 99

latex allergy and, 473
  lifestyle and, 96
  medical assistant role in, 90
  medication errors, preventing, 96–97
  mind and body, 94
  miscommunication, 95
  patient skills and abilities, 95
  planning step, 94
  preventive medicine and, 96
  sample medication teaching tool, *97*
  smoking and substance abuse, 97–98
  stress reduction, 97
  teaching resources, 95
  time needed, determining, 95
Patient files, 159
  active, 203
  closed, 203
  documenting, 290
  inactive, 203
Patient health information (PHI), 224
Patient information, 191, 192
  pamphlets, 250
  sensitive, 197
Patient rights, ethics and, 10
Patients
  calling, 149–52
  chronically late, 180
  confidentiality, 24
  dismissing for nonpayment, 380
  established, 145, 176–77
  with HIV/AIDS, 469
  inappropriate discussions in front of, 36
  interviewing, 74–81
  letters to, 125
  new, 175–79
  in physician-patient relationship, 52
  positioning of, 561–64
  professional communication, maintaining, 80–81
  proper charting and, 95
  refusal of treatment by, 44
  safety, 437
  specimen collection and, 624, 625
  telephone use by, 144
  transportation for, 185
  in wheelchair, assisting, 979
Patients' Bill of Rights, 10, 62, *63*
Patient scheduling, 173–88
  adequate time and, 177
  appointment matrix and, 177, 178
  cluster, 179
  color-coding and, *178*
  correcting, 181
  documenting no-show appointments, 181
  double booking, 179
  efficiency in, 185
  fixed appointment, 179
  follow up for no-show appointments, 181, 183
  hospital services and admissions, 183–84
  inpatient admissions, 186
  interpreters and, 184–85
  managing physician's professional schedule, 183
  medical assistants and, 175
  methods of, 179–83
  modified wave, 180
  new patient appointments, 175–79
  with open hours, 179
  paper and electronic, 177–78
  patient and office needs in, 177
  reminder systems, 180–81
  rescheduling missed, 183
  sample book, *182*
  slack or buffer time in, 180
  specialty referral, 184
  transportation scheduling and, 185
  triage and, 180
  wave, 179–80
Patient status, 343, 355
Payer number, 263, 289

Payment contract, *376*
Payments
  posting, 305
  reconciling, 307, 314
Payroll, 392–410
  calculating, 399–400, 405
  Circular E, 400
  computing deductions, 400
  definition of, 393
  garnishing wages, 401
  history of, 394–95
  medical assistants and, 394
  new employee records, 395, 400
  other deductions, 400–401
  present-day employment issues and, 395
  processing, 394–401
  recording employee work hours, 399
  software to compute, 401
  taxes, 393, 395, *396–97*
  updating employee records, 395–96
PCP. *See* Primary care physician (PCP)
PD. *See* Personality disorders (PD)
PDR. *See* Physician's Desk Reference (PDR)
Peak expiratory flow (PEF), 771
Peak flow testing, 782–83, *784*
Pediatrician, 1011
Pediatrics, 1010–35
  definition of, 1011
  diagnostic procedures, 1029–33
  diseases and conditions in, 1025, 1026t–1028t, 1028–29, 1029t
  immunizations, 1021, *1022, 1023,* 1024–1025
  physical, development, and emotional growth, 1012–17
  routine visits (well-baby checks), 1018–29
PEF. *See* Peak expiratory flow (PEF)
Pegboard accounting systems, 371, 373
Penis, 702
Per case, 263, 287
Percussion, 541, 565
Per diem, 263, 287
Performance evaluations, of medical staff, 420, 421
Pericarditis, 731, 739
Perineum, 985, 986
Periorbital edema, 675
Periosteum, 949, 953
Peripheral nervous system, diseases of, 1050–51
  Bell's palsy, 1050
  shingles (herpes zoster), 1051
  trigeminal neuralgia, 1050–51
Peripheral nervous system (PNS), 1038, 1039–40
Peripherals, 224
Peristalsis, 916, 920
Personal digital assistants (PDA), 216, 223, 224, 231
Personal distance, *70*
Personal information, 191, 192
  disclosing about coworkers, 144
Personal injury protection (PIP), 263, 275
Personality disorders (PD), 1056, 1063, 1063t
Personal protective equipment (PPE), 438, 460, 465, 467, 468, 602
Personal safety measures, 432
  body mechanics, 432, 433
Personal space, 68, 70–71
  therapeutic touch and, 74
  typical measurements in United States, 71
Personal telephone calls, 154
Personnel file, 393, 395
Personnel manual, 249, 250, *252*
PET. *See* Positron emission tomography (PET)
Petechiae, 824, 829t
Petty cash, 406, 408
PFT. *See* Pulmonary function testing (PFT)
pH, 478, 479, 696
Phagocytic, 636, 639
Phagocytosis, 460, 463, *826*
Phantom pain, 92–93
Pharmacist, 26, 27
Pharmacology, 502–39
  abbreviations, 518t

basic, 505–12
definition of, 503
medication measurement and conversion, 512–15
Pharmacy technician, 27
Pharynx, 919
PHI. *See* Patient health information (PHI)
Phlebitis, 740, 742
Phlebotomist, 27, 636, 637
Phlebotomy, 636, 637
Phobias, 1055, 1064, 1064t
Photometer, 597, 604
Physical examination
assessment methods used in, 564–67
assisting physician in, 565–67
draping, 561
gowning, 561
positioning patient, 561–64
preparation for, 561–64
Physically challenged patients, communication with, 75–76
Physical pain, 91
Physical requirements, of medical assistant, 12
Physical stages, of life cycle, 83t
Physical status modifier, 343, 359
Physical therapist (PT), 27, *28*
Physical therapy assistant, 27
Physical therapy (PT), 951
assistive aids for ambulation, 969, 972, 974–75, 977–78
body mechanics and, 978, 980
modalities, 966, 968, 968t, 972, 974–75, 977–78
prostheses and, 977–78
Physical urinalysis
appearance, 693–94
odor, 694
specific gravity, 694–95
Physician assistant (PA), 21
Physician office laboratory (POL), 597, 603–604
Physician-patient relationship, 52
Physicians, 26
assisting in physical examination, 565–67
first woman, 10
managing professional schedule for, 183
in physician-patient relationship, 52
public duties and consequences of, 50–52
reporting abuse, 51–52
reporting vaccine injuries, 51
revoking medical licenses, 52
services of, 263, 265
Physician's assistant (PA), 26
Physician's Desk Reference (PDR), 117, *120*, 503, 507
Piaget, Jean, 83t
Pigmentation disorders, 845, 847t
Pineal gland, 859
PIP. *See* Personal injury protection (PIP)
Pituitary gland, 857
disorders, 860
PJC. *See* Premature junctional contractions (PJC)
Place of service (POS), 343
codes, 358t–359t
Planning, 89, 94
Plant remedies, 3, *5*
Plasma, 636, 638
Plasmapheresis, 676
Platelets, 639, 658–59
Pleuritis, 777t
PMN. *See* Polymorphonuclear WBCs (PMN)
PMS. *See* Premenstrual syndrome (PMS)
Pneumonia, 776t
Pneumonoconiosis, 775t
Pneumothorax, 770, 777
PNS. *See* Peripheral nervous system (PNS)
Point of service (POS), 263, 271, 272t, 273
Poison control centers, 906
Poisoning, coding, 335–36, 336t
POL. *See* Physician office laboratory (POL)
Policy, 249
Policyholder, 263, 266
Politics, office, 37

Polymorphonuclear WBCs (PMN), 637, 638
Polyps, 916, 939
Polyuria, 676
POMR. *See* Problem-oriented medical record (POMR)
Portability, 41, 58
Portal hypertension, 916
POS. *See* Point of service (POS)
Positioning, of patients, 561–64
children, 1030–31
radiographic terms, 723t
for surgery, 576
for X-rays, 722
Positron emission tomography (PET), 712, 719
Postage meters, 117, 132
Posteroanterior view (PV), 712
Postictal, 1037, 1047
Posting, 372, 373, 374
adjustments, 385
collection agency payment, 386
Postnatal/postpartum, 985
Postoperative (post-op) care, 343, 361, 572, 584, 588–89
dressings and bandages, 589
patient teaching and dismissal, 588
wound healing, 588–89
Postpartum depression, 1062
Postpartum (PP), 985
Posttraumatic stress disorder (PTSD), 1056, 1064
Posture, 73–74
Potassium hydroxide (KOH), 614, 621
PP. *See* Postpartum (PP)
PPD. *See* Purified protein derivative (PPD)
PPE. *See* Personal protective equipment (PPE)
PPMP. *See* Provider-performed microscopy procedures (PPMP)
PPO. *See* Preferred provider organization (PPO)
PR. *See* P-R interval (PR)
Practitioner, 3, 6
Preapprovals, 174, 184
Preauthorization, 263, 290
Precedents, 41, 42
Brown v. Board of Education, 42
Roe v. Wade, 42
Preceptor, 1113, 1114
Precertification, 263, 290
Precordial leads, 731, 744
Pre-existing conditions, 263, 268
Preferred provider, 263, 267
Preferred provider organization (PPO), 263, 271–72, 272t
Pregnancy, 991–96
breastfeeding, 996
complications of, 994, 995t–996t
delivery, 992, *993*
obstetrical history, 992, 994
prenatal exam, 994
urine test, 1004
Premature atrial contractions (PAC), *760*
Premature junctional contractions (PJC), *760*
Premature ventricular contraction (PVC), 731, 757
Premenstrual syndrome (PMS), 985, 988
Premium, 263, 266
Prenatal, 985
Prenatal exam, 994
Preoperative (pre-op) care, 572
anesthesia, 578–79
instruments and, 574–76
patient preparation, 573–79
positioning and draping, 576
room preparation, 574
skin preparation, 577–78
Presbycusis, 1087
Presbyopia, 1087
Prescription drug coverage, 276–77
Prescriptions, 517–19
calling in, 149
documenting refill requests, 205–206
pads, safeguarding, 519
pregnancy and, 518
preparation of, 520

Presenting problem, 343, 357
Pressure bandages, 890, 895
Pressure points, 888, *889*, 890t
Preventive care, 263, 265
Preventive medicine, 96
Primary care physician (PCP), 4, 21, 26, 263, 291
Principal diagnosis, 323, 338
P-R interval (PR), 731, 747, *748*
Privacy
computer, 59
invasion of, 41, 43t
Private health insurance, 269–70
coverage sources, 269–70
Private insurance, 263
Private law, public law *versus,* 42
Problem-oriented medical record (POMR), 445, 452
charting, 192, 197–98
Procedural coding, 341–67, 343
for anesthesia, 359–60
definition of, 342
determining correct, 346–52
fraud and abuse, 344–45
history of, 344
medical assistants and, 344
for medicine, 363
for pathology and laboratory, 363
for radiology, 362
reimbursement and, 365
for special situations, 359–64
standardized, 342
for surgery, 360–62
unlisted, 364
Procedures, 249, 343
administrative, 253, *254*
charting, 453, 455
clinical, 252, 253
codes, *326*
diagnostic, 596–611
disinfection, 483
infection control, 253–54
preparing patients for, 185
quality improvement, 254
risk management, 254
for using transfer forceps, 492–93
Procrastination, of duties, 36
Proctology, 916
Prodromal, 460, 676, 1038, 1048
Professional courtesy, 372, 379
Professional distance, 68, 81
Professionalism, 10, 12
barriers to, 36
character and, 12
characteristics of, 34–36
communication and medical terminology, 12
definition of, 33
medical assistant role in, 33
physical requirements, 12
scope of practice for medical assistants, 12
on telephone, 147–48
in workplace, 32–38
Prognosis, 3, 5, 445, 449
Progress notes, 192, 198
Projectile vomiting, 1038, 1049
Projection, *85*
Prokaryotes, 613, 618
Proofreader's marks, 117, 126, *129*
Proofreading, 117, 125–26, 131
Prostate
cancer, 705t
diseases of, 704, 705t
Prostate-specific antigens (PSAS), 89, 90, 704
Prostatitis, 676, 704, 707t
Prosthesis, 949, 962, 977–78
Proteins, 916, 922
complete, 927
incomplete, 927
Proteinuria, 676, 696
Proteus, 620
Prothrombin time (PT), 597, 603

Provider-performed microscopy procedures (PPMP), 597, 599–600
Proximal tubule, 676, 677
PSAS. *See* Prostate-specific antigens (PSAS)
Psychiatrist, 1055
Psychiatry, 1055
Psychological pain, 91–92
Psychologist, 1055
Psychology, 1055
Psychosis, 1055, 1062
Psychosocial emergencies, 907
    alcohol intoxication, 907
    depression, 907
    domestic violence, 907
    psychotic behavior, 907
    rage, 907
    sexual abuse and rape, 907
    suicide, 907
Psychotherapeutic, 1055, 1058
Psychotherapy, 1055, 1064
Psychotropic, 1055, 1068
PT. *See* Physical therapist (PT); Physical therapy (PT); Prothrombin time (PT)
PTH. *See* Parathyroid hormone (PTH)
PTSD. *See* Posttraumatic stress disorder (PTSD)
PTT. *See* Partial thromboplastin time (PTT)
Public distance, *71*
Public law, 41
    private law *versus*, 42
Pulmonary edema, 736, 886
Pulmonary function testing (PFT), 770, 771, 777, 779
Pulmonary system
    anatomy and physiology of, 771–73
    gas exchange mechanics, 773
    lower airways, 771–72
    smoking and, 773
    upper airway, 771
Pulmonary system, diseases and disorders of, 773–77
    chronic obstructive pulmonary disease, 773
    infectious and inflammatory conditions, 776, 776t–777t
    lower respiratory obstructive diseases, 773, 774t–775t, 777
    malignancies, 776–77
    mechanical insults, 777, 778t
Pulmonology, 769–92
    assessment and diagnosis, 777, 779–88
    inhalers and nebulizers, 786–87
    oxygen therapy, 789–90
Pulse, 541, 544, 550
    apical, 552–53
    radial, 551–52
    ranges, 550t
Pulse oximetry, 781–7823
Puncture, 572, 588
Purchase order, preparation of, 243
Purge, 192, 203
Purified protein derivative (PPD), 771, 784–85, 786
Purulent, 794
PV. *See* Posteroanterior view (PV)
PVC. *See* Premature ventricular contraction (PVC)
Pyelonephritis, 676, 679
Pyogenic, 1038, 1048
Pyuria, 676

Q

QNS. *See* Quantity not sufficient (QNS)
QRS interval or waveform, 731, 747, *748*
QS. *See* Quantity sufficient (QS)
Quadriplegia, 1038, 1050
Qualified diagnoses, 323, 327
Qualities, of medical assistants, 23–24, 23t
Quality assurance, 599–600
Quality care, access to, *51*
Quality control, 599–601
Quality improvement procedures, 254

Quantity not sufficient (QNS), 614
Quantity sufficient (QS), 614
Quarterly payroll reports, 393, 395
Questions
    close-ended, 74
    indirect, *75*
    open-ended, 74

R

RA. *See* Rheumatoid arthritis (RA)
Radial pulse, 541, 550, 551–52
Radiation, 712
    exposure time, 721
    shields, 721–22
    sources of, 720t
Radiation therapy, 1080, *1082*
Radiographic records, filing and loading, 725, 726
Radiographs, 712, 713, 715, 722
Radiography, 712, 713
    flat-plate findings, 713t
    limited-scope, 722
Radiologist, 712, 713
Radiology, 712, 713–19
    angiography, 715–16
    arthrography, 716
    cholecystography, 716
    coding for, 362
    computed tomography, 717
    equipment, 719–20
    fluoroscopy, 717
    magnetic resonance imaging, 717–18
    mammography, 715
    nuclear medicine, 719
    radiographs and contrast studies, 713, 715
    sonography, 718–19
    X-rays, 713
Radiolucent, 712, 713
Radiopaque, 712, 713
Random access memory (RAM), 224, 225
Range of motion (ROM), 949, 951, *955*, 956
Rapport, developing, 22
Rationalization, *85*
Raynaud's disease, 744
RBC. *See* Red blood cells (RBC)
RBRVS. *See* Resource-based relative value scale (RBRVS)
RDA. *See* Recommended dietary allowance (RDA)
Reactive, 824, 825
Read-only memory (ROM), 224, 225
Reception area, 157
Receptionist, 157, 159
Recommended dietary allowance (RDA), 916, 932
Records
    disclosing minors' information, 56
    faxing, 57
    guarding superprotected information in, 56
    HIPAA violation, 59
    improper disclosure of, 57
    maintaining confidentiality through, 53–57
    releasing, 53–55, 56
    request for, 57
    subpoenas of, 56
Recovery, 584, 588–89
Rectal suppositories, 940, 943–44
Rectal temperature, obtaining, 547
Red blood cells (RBC), 597, 603, 638
Reduction, 950, 963
Reference initials, 117, 122, *123*
Referrals
    managed care, 303
    preparing, 290–91
Referred pain, 89, 91
Reflecting, 68, 74
Reflexology, 1103–1104
Refractometer, 694–95
Registered Medical Assistant (RMA), 4, 13, 21
    certification examination for, 15
    licensing and certification for, 27

Registered nurse (RN), 21, 26
Registered phlebotomy technician (RPT), 21
Regression, *85*
Regulatory law, 41
Reimbursement, 365
Rejected claim, 263, 307
Rejections, reconciling, 307, 314
Relative value unit (RVU), 263, 304, 343, 344, 372, 375
Remedies, plant, 3, *5*
Remission, 1075, 1077
Renal, 676
Renal calculi/calculus, 676, 683t, 685
Renal diseases, 680–85, 681t–682t
    dialysis and, 682–83
Repeat offender providers, 50
Repolarization, 731, 734
Repression, *85*
Research hospitals, 8
Research nontherapeutic, 207
Res ipsa locitur, 48
Res judicata, 41, 48
Resource-based relative value scale (RBRVS), 263, 304–305, 374
Resources
    community, 81
    national, *80*
    teaching, 95
Respect, 35
Respirations, 550, 553, 554
Respiratory distress, 884–86
    COPD, 886
    hyperventilation, 884, 886
    pulmonary edema, 886
    shortness of breath, 884
Respiratory syncytial virus (RSV), 1011, 1025
Respiratory system, *772*
Respiratory therapist, 27
Respite care, 263, 279
Respondeat superior, 41, 45
Responsibilities, of medical assistant, 22–23, 35
Resume, 1113, 1114–17
Rheumatic fever and heart disease, 739, 830t
Rheumatoid arthritis (RA), 825, 951
Rhinologist, 794, 795
Rhythm, 542, 550, 551t
Right eye (OD), 794, 800
Right lateral view (RL), 712
Right lower extremity (RLE), 951
Right lower leg (RLL), 951
Right lower quadrant (RLQ), 916, 937t
Right upper extremity (RUE), 951
Right upper quadrant (RUQ), 916, 937t
Risk, assumption of, 40, 48
Risk factors, 89, 90t
Risk management procedures, 254
RL. *See* Right lateral view (RL)
RLE. *See* Right lower extremity (RLE)
RLL. *See* Right lower leg (RLL)
RLQ. *See* Right lower quadrant (RLQ)
RMA. *See* Registered Medical Assistant (RMA)
Roentgen, Wilhem, 7
Roe v. Wade, 42
Role Delineation Chart, 4
ROM. *See* Range of motion (ROM); Read-only memory (ROM)
Rotation sites, *523*
Route, 140, 142
RPT. *See* Registered phlebotomy technician (RPT)
RSV. *See* Respiratory syncytial virus (RSV)
RUE. *See* Right upper extremity (RUE)
Rule of nines, in coding burns, 336–37, 896, *897*
RUQ. *See* Right upper quadrant (RUQ)
RVU. *See* Relative value unit (RVU)

S

SA. *See* Sinoatrial node (SA)
SAD. *See* Seasonal affective disorder (SAD)

Safe Medical Devices Act, 602
Safety
    laboratory, 602
    medical imaging and, 720–22
Safety, in medical office, 430–43
    emergency plans, 434–36
    exposure control plan, 437–41
    general office, 432–33
    OSHA bloodborne pathogen standards, 436–37
    personal measures, 432
Salutation, 117, 121
Sanitization, 478, 479–81
    materials for, 480
Saturated fats, 916, 928
Scanners, 223, 226, 237
Scarlet fever, 6
SCC. See Squamous cell carcinoma (SCC)
Scheduling, patient, 173–88
SCHIP. See State Children's Health Insurance
    Program (SCHIP)
Schizophrenia, 1058–59
SCID. See Severe combined immunodeficiency
    disease (SCID)
Scrotum, 702–703, 703
Seasonal affective disorder (SAD), 1056, 1062–63
Sebaceous glands, 836, 837, 839
Secondary diagnoses, 323, 327
    coding, 331–32
Section, 323, 343, 345
Security
    computer, 228–29
    workplace, 435
Security envelopes, 393, 401
Seeing-eye dogs, 75
Segregation, 41, 42
Seizures, 903
    tonic-clonic, 1047
Selective serotonin reuptake inhibitors (SSRI),
    1056, 1060
Self-insurance, 263, 269
Semicolon, 343, 349
Semmelweiss, Ignaz, 7
Sentinel events, 412, 425
Sepsis, 868, 886
Septum, 770, 771
Sequela, 323, 337, 676
Serology, 613, 621
Serum, 636, 638
Service animals, 157, 169
Settled, 41, 46
Severe combined immunodeficiency disease
    (SCID), 825
Sexual harassment, in medical office, 412, 421–22
Sexually transmitted diseases (STD), 41, 56, 998,
    999t
    male, 706, 707t
Shaken baby syndrome, 876
Shingles (herpes zoster), 1051
Shingling, 192, 200, 201
Shock, 886–87
    anaphylactic, 887, 887t
    assisting patients in, 887
    classifications of, 886t
    symptoms of, 887t
    treatment for, 887t
Shortness of breath (SOB), 869, 884, 1025
Short-term memory, 1087, 1089
Side effects, 503, 506
    of cancer treatment, 1082
    of Viagra, 706
Sight-impaired patients, communicating with, 76,
    77
Sigmoidoscopy, 940, 942
Sign-in sheets, 157, 163–64
Sign language, 71
Signs, 323, 327, 445, 450t–451t, 453
    coding, 332
Signs and symptoms (S&S), 916
Sinoatrial node (SA), 731, 734
Skilled nursing facility, 263, 279

Skills
    administrative, 23
    clinical, 22
Skin, 462–63
    anatomy and physiology of, 837–38
    cosmetic treatment, 852
    layers of, 463t
    preparation for surgical procedure, 577–78
    shaving, 578
    structure of, 837, 838
Skin, diseases and disorders of, 839–50
    benign neoplasms, 845, 848t–849t
    cancerous disorders, 846, 848, 851t
    dermatitis, 839, 839t–840t
    fungal conditions, 842, 843t–844t
    infectious skin disorders, 841, 842t–843t
    parasitic conditions, 842, 845, 846t
    pigmentation disorders, 845, 847t
Slack time, 174
SLE. See Systemic lupus erythematosus (SLE)
Sleep apnea, 778t
Sliding fee scale, 263, 265
Small claims court, 387
Small intestine, 916, 920, 921
Smoking
    effects of, 773
    patient education and, 97–98
Snellen charts, 802, 803
Soak, 950, 968, 969t
SOAP note charting, 192, 196–97, 198, 347, 445,
    452–53
SOB. See Shortness of breath (SOB)
Social distance, 70
Social information, 192
Social Security Act, 394
Social Security Disability Insurance (SSDI), 264,
    286
Social security number (SSN), 597, 606
Social worker, 27
Software, 224, 227–28
    medical billing, 331
    packages, 228
    payroll calculation, 401
    tracking supplies with, 244
    training on, 228
Somatoform disorders, 1064–65
    conversion disorder, 1064
    factitious disorders, 1065
    hypochondriasis, 1065
    somatization disorder, 1064
Sonography, 712, 713, 718–19, 718t
Speaker phone, 140, 142
Special instructions, 343, 350, 351
Specialist referral
    appointments, 184
    preparation of, 82
Specializations, medical practice, 28, 28t
Specialty hospitals, 8
Specimen collection, storage, and transport, 624–31
    fecal occult blood testing, 625, 626–28
    stool, 624–28
Specimens
    general handling of, 687
    transporting, 656
    urinalysis and, 685–89
Specimen smear, 621, 622
Spectrophotometric, 636, 657
Speech impaired, 68
Speech impaired patients, communicating with,
    76
Speed dial, 140, 141, 142
Spell-check, 117, 118
Sphygmomanometer, 445, 446, 555
Spinal cord injuries, 1050
Spirometry, 218, 780–81
Splints, 900–901, 950, 963
Spore, 478
Sputum, 780
Squamous cell carcinoma (SCC), 836, 846, 851, 851t
S&S. See Signs and symptoms (S&S)

SSDI. See Social Security Disability Insurance
    (SSDI)
SSI. See Supplemental Security Income (SSI)
SSN. See Social security number (SSN)
SSRI. See Selective serotonin reuptake inhibitors (SSRI)
Staffing, medical office, 415–19
    disciplining and terminating, 420–21, 422
    employment references and, 418, 420
    employment resources, 423
    hiring, 418
    job advertisements, 415, 416
    job descriptions for, 415
    performance evaluations, 420, 421
    providing references, 423–24
    recruiting and interviewing candidates, 416–17
    supervising, 419
    training, 419
Staff meetings, in medical office, 414–15
    agendas, 414
    directing, 415
    minutes, 414–15
Staff model HMO, 263
Standalone code, 343, 349, 350
Standardized, 342, 343
Standard of care, 41, 47, 48, 192, 193
Standard Precautions, 437, 460, 465, 466
Stanford-Binet scale, 1066
Staph, 613, 618, 738, 851
Staphylococcus aureus, 462, 618, 619
State Children's Health Insurance Program
    (SCHIP), 263, 284
Status epilepticus, 868, 902
Statute of limitations, 41, 48, 192, 204
    on healthcare debt, 377t
    in states, 49t–50t
STD. See Sexually transmitted diseases (STD)
Stem cells, 640
Stenosis, 731, 739
Stent, 731, 735
Stereotyping, 68, 75
Sterilant, 478, 492
Sterile, 460, 463, 479
Sterile dressing, 589–90
Sterile field, 479, 489–90
    creation of, 490–92
    guidelines for, 486
Sterile gloving, 497–98
Sterile gowning, 495
    gloves and, 496–97
Sterile scrub, demonstrating, 493–94
Sterile tray preparation, 485, 485t, 487, 580–82
Sterilization, 479, 483–85
    autoclave, 483–84
    cold, 485
    indicators, 479, 485
    methods of, 484–85
Stethoscope, 445, 446
Stomach, 920
Stop loss, 263, 267–68
Strep, 613, 738
Streptococcus pneumoniae, 620, 1048
Stress reduction, patient education and, 97
Stress testing, 755
Stroke. See Cerebrovascular accident/stroke (CVA)
Subcategory, 323, 329, 343, 349
Subclassification, 323, 329
Subcutaneous, 824
Subcutaneous injections, 532–33
Subcutaneous tissue, 460, 463
Subheading, 343, 349
Subjective, objective, assessment, and plan (SOAP).
    See SOAP note charting
Subject line, 117, 121
Sublingually, 542, 544
Sublingual medication administration, 521
Subpoenas, 192, 193
    of medical records, 56
Subscriber, 263, 266
Subsection, 343, 349, 361
Substance abuse, patient education and, 97–98

Substitution, *85*
Subterm, 323
Sudden cardiac arrest, 735–36
Superbill, 263, 291, 372, 373
Supercomputers, *224*
Supernatural, healing based on, 4
Superprotected information, guarding, 56
Supplemental Security Income (SSI), 264, 286
Supply inventory, 242–43
Suppression, *85*
Surge protection, 226
Surgery
    cancer, 1080–81
    coding for, 360–62
    elective, 571, 573
    emergency, 571, 573
    minor, 570–93
    optional, 572, 573
Surgical asepsis, 477–501
    alcohol-based hand rubs, 494
    definition of, 478
    medical asepsis *versus,* 479t
    practice of, 479
    preparation of surgical field, 485–86
    sanitization, disinfection, and sterilization, 479–85
    sterile tray preparation, 485, 485t, 487
    wrapping instruments, 485, 487
Surgical field, preparation of, 485–86
Surgical hand washing, 493–94
Sutures, 582–84
    assisting physician with, 584–86
    removal, 582–84, 586–88
Sydenham's chorea, 6
Symbolic language, 71
    Braille, 71
    sign language, 71
Sympathetic reactions, 1041t
Sympathy, 68, 74
Symptoms, 323, 327, 445, 450, 450t–451t
    abbreviations for, 453t–454t
    coding, 332
Synarthrosis, 950, 954
Syphilis, 707t
Syringes, *524*
Systemic lupus erythematosus (SLE), 825
Systole, 542, 553, 731, 735

T

T₃. *See* Triiodothyronine (T₃)
T₄. *See* Thyroxine (T₄)
Tabular index, 343, 351
Tabular list, 323, 330
Tachycardia, 731
Tachypnea, 770, 777
Talismans, *6*
Tasks, prioritizing, 36
Tax Equity and Fiscal Responsibility Act (TEFRA), 264, 265, 271
TB. *See* Tuberculosis (TB)
TBSA. *See* Total body surface area, of burns (TBSA)
Teaching hospitals, 8
Teaching resources, 95
Team members, 26–28
    nurse, 26
    nurse practitioner, 26
    pharmacist, 26
    physician, 26
    physician's assistant, 26
Technical education programs, 4, 13
Teeth, 918, *919*
TEFRA. *See* Tax Equity and Fiscal Responsibility Act (TEFRA)
Telecommunication relay services, 154
Telephone procedures, 139–56
    answering telephone, 144–49
    appropriate phrases, *148*
    calling in prescriptions, 149
    calling patients, 149–52

    documenting calls, 149
    emergency calls, 146–47
    with emotional patients, 149
    handling difficult callers, 148–49
    with hard-to-understand callers, 148
    improper, *144*
    leaving messages, 151
    long distance or toll-free calls, 151, 153
    messages, 149, *150*, 151
    patient confidentiality and, 153
    patient telephone use, 144
    personal calls, 154
    prioritizing calls, 145, *146*
    professional manner, 147–48
    screening calls, 144
    telecommunications relay services, 154
    telephone system features, 141–44
    triage, 146
    using directory, 152–53
Teletypewriter system (TTY), 140, 154
Temperature, 542–44
    aural, 543, 548–49
    axillary, 546
    conversion, 543t
    dermal, 549
    electronic digital thermometer and, 544–47
    oral, 542–43
    ranges, 543t
    rectal, 547
    thermometers, 544
Temperature, pulse, respirations (TPR), 542
Tendons, 950, 953
Termination, of contracts, 53
Termination-of-care letter, sample, *55*
Testes, 676, 702
Testicles, 702
Tetany, 950, 954
Thallium scan, 756
Therapeutic diets, 944, 945t
Therapeutic effects, 503, 506
Therapeutic touch, 74
Thermodynamics, 950, 952, 968–69
Thermometer, 445, 446
Thermotherapy, 950, 968
Thesaurus, 117
Third-party administrator (TPA), 263, 264, 269
Third-party liability (TPL), 264, 275–76
Throat
    anatomy and physiology of, 815, 818
    culture, 628–29
    diagnosis and treatment, 818
    diseases and disorders of, 816t, 818
    infectious conditions of, 819t
Thromboangiitis obliterans. *See* Buerger's disease
Thrombocytes, 636, 638
Thromboembolism, 731, 742
Thrombophlebitis, 742
Thrombosis, 731
Thrombus, 731, 735
Thumb drives, 223, 225
Thymus gland, 859
Thyroid gland, 858
    disorders, 861
Thyroid-stimulating hormone (TSH), 858
Thyroxine (T₄), 856, 858
TIA. *See* Transient ischemic attack (TIA)
Tickler file, 372, 382
Time clocks, 394, 399
Time management, in medical office, 25
Tinnitus, 794
Tissues, 104, 105
Tolerance, 1055, 1068
Tonic, 1038
Tonic-clonic seizures, 1047
Tonometer, *801*, 802
Tort law, 41, 42
Tort of outrage, 41, 43t
Tort reform, 48, 50
    capping money awarded, 48, 50
    repeat offender providers, 50

Total body surface area, of burns (TBSA), 323, 336
Total parenteral nutrition (TPN), 916, 933
Tourniquets, 642
Toxic effects, 503, 506
TPA. *See* Third-party administrator (TPA)
TPL. *See* Third-party liability (TPL)
TPN. *See* Total parenteral nutrition (TPN)
TPR. *See* Temperature, pulse, respirations (TPR)
Trade (brand, proprietary) name, 503, 506
Traditional law, 41, 42
Transcribe, 237, 241
Transcription machines, 237, 241
Transfer forceps, usage procedure, 492–93
Transient ischemic attack (TIA), 869, 903, 1046
Transmission-based precautions, 460, 465
Transplant costs, 107
Treatment, refusal of, 44
Trepanning, 4
Triage, 140, 146, 445, 447–48
    conducting, 180
    notebook, 140, 146, *147*, 175, 180
TRICARE, 263, 265, 284, 291, 304
Trichomoniasis, 707t
Trigeminal neuralgia, 1050–51
Triglycerides, 916, 928
Trigone, 676, 677
Triiodothyronine (T₃), 856, 858
TSH. *See* Thyroid-stimulating hormone (TSH)
T1 (thoracic vertebra), 951
Tuberculosis (TB), 771, 776t, 777t
Tubular bandages, 893–95
Tumor markers, 1075, 1078
Tumors, 1075
    benign *versus* malignant, 1077t
    staging and grading malignant, 1078–79
Turbidity, 676
Turgor, 542, 565
T wave, *749*
Tympanometer, *814*
Tympanometry, 814

U

UA. *See* Urinalysis (UA)
UCG. *See* Urine chorionic gonadotropin (UCG)
UCR. *See* Usual, customary, and reasonable (UCR) fee
UGI. *See* Upper gastrointestinal tract (UGI)
Ultramicroscopic, 613, 618
Ultrasonic cleaning, 479, 481
Ultrasonography, 969, 971
Ultrasound, 712, 713
Ultrasound technician, 27
Ultraviolet (UV), 836, 837
Unbundling, 263, 280, 343
Uncertain, 323, 327
Uncollectible accounts, 372, 383
Undue influence, 41, 43t
Unemployment insurance, 394, 395
Unifocal rhythms, 731, 737, *763*
Uniform Anatomical Gift Act, 107
Uniforms, 24
Unintentional tort, 41, 42
Unique provider identification number (UPIN), 264, 278
United Network for Organ Sharing (UNOS), 106, 108
United Parcel Service (UPS), 117, 133
United States Postal Service (USPS), 117, 132
Universal Precautions, 460, 464, 469
    and Body Substance Isolation, 437
Universal resource locator (URL), 224
Universal system bus (USB), 225
Unsaturated fats, 916, 929
Upcode, 343, 344
UPIN. *See* Unique provider identification number (UPIN)
Upper gastrointestinal tract (UGI), 916, 917–20
    duodenum, 920
    esophagus, 919–20

mouth, 917–18
pharynx, 919
stomach, 920
teeth, 918, *919*
Upper respiratory infection (URI), 1087
UPS. *See* United Parcel Service (UPS)
Ureters, 676, 677
Urethra, 676, 677
URI. *See* Upper respiratory infection (URI)
Urinalysis (UA), 676, 685–701
catheterization, 689, 690–93
characteristics of, 689t
with chemical test strips, 695–99, 697t
clean-catch specimen collection, 687–88
crystals, 699, *700*, 701
microscopic findings in urine, 700t
physical, 689, 693–94
sediment examination, 698–701
specimen collection, 685–89
24-hour specimen collection, 688–89
Urinary bladder, 676, 677
Urinary meatus, 676, 677
Urinary system
anatomy and physiology of, 677–80
diagnostic procedures for, 685–701
infections of, 679–80, 679t–680t
kidney function, 677–79
neurogenic bladder and incontinence, 683
obstructive conditions, 683, 683t–684t, 685
renal diseases, 680–85
urine formation, 678–79
Urinary tract infections (UTI), 614, 619, 676
Urine chorionic gonadotropin (UCG), 985
Urine collection, pediatric, 1031–33
Urine cultures, 631
Urine pregnancy test, 1004
URL. *See* Universal resource locator (URL)
Urobilinogen, 676, 697
Urologist, 676
Urology, 676
Urticaria, *832*
U.S. Department of Agriculture (USDA), 196, 931
U.S. Pharmacopoeia and National Formulary (USP-NF), 503, 506, 507
USDA. *See* U.S. Department of Agriculture (USDA)
User manual, 237
USP-NF. *See* U.S. Pharmacopoeia and National Formulary (USP-NF)
USPS. *See* United States Postal Service (USPS)
Usual, customary, and reasonable (UCR) fee, 263, 264, 265, 304, 343, 344
UTI. *See* Urinary tract infections (UTI)
UV. *See* Ultraviolet (UV)

V

Vaccination information sheet (VIS), 1011
Vaccinations, 786
Vaccines
reporting injuries, 51
storing, 1025
Vaginal bleeding, 996
Valvular disorders, of heart, 739–40
van Leeuwenhoek, Antoni, 6
Vascular dementia, 1066
Vascular disorders, of heart, 740, 741t–742t, 742–44
aneurysms, 744
arteriosclerosis and atherosclerosis, 742–43

Buerger's disease, 744
embolisms, deep-vein thrombosis and thromboembolism, 742
phlebitis, 740, 742
Raynaud's disease, 744
thrombophlebitis, 742
V codes, 323, 333–35
Venipuncture, 636, 637, 643–46
evacuated tube, 643–44
needle and syringe, 644
performing, 648–50
reactions to, 644
sites, 646
syringe method for, 650–52
winged infusion (butterfly), 644, 645–46
Venous, 868, 887
Ventricle, 731, 732
Ventricular fibrillation (V-fib), 731, 758t, *764*
Ventricular tachycardia (V-tach), 731, 758t, *764*
Verbal contracts, 53
Verified Internet Pharmacy Practice Site (VIPPS), 224, 230
Vertigo, 794
Vesalius, Andreas, 6, *6*
V-fib. *See* Ventricular fibrillation (V-fib)
Viagra, 706
Vials, 524–28, 531–32
Violence, workplace, 435
VIPPS. *See* Verified Internet Pharmacy Practice Site (VIPPS)
Virology, 613
Viruses, 613, 618, 621
Viruses, computer, 229
VIS. *See* Vaccination information sheet (VIS)
Vision screening, pediatric, 1020–21
Visual acuity, 561, 798, 800, 803
Visually impaired, assisting, 808
Vital signs, 540–69
blood pressure, 553–57
definition of, 542
hearing assessment, 561
measurement, 542–61
pediatric, 1020–21
physical examination preparation and, 561–64
pulse, 544, 550
respirations, 550, 553
temperature, 542–44
visual acuity, 561
weight and height, 557, 559–60
Vitamins, 916, 927, 929t–931t
Vocally impaired, 68, 71
Vocational programs, 4, 13
Voicemail, 143–44
Voiding cystogram, 686
V-tach. *See* Ventricular tachycardia (V-tach)

W

Wages, 394, 395
garnished, 401
Waiting period, 263, 268
Waiver, 263, 280
Walkers, 975, 977, 978
Warranty, 237
Wave scheduling, 175, 179–80
WBC. *See* White blood cells (WBC)
Wechsler Intelligence Scales for Children, 1066
Weight, 557, 559–60

Weight-loss information, 96
Wellness, 90, 90t
guidelines, 90t
W-2 form, 394, 401, *404*
W-4 form, 394, 397–98, *398–99*
White blood cells (WBC), 638–39
differential, 657
performing count, 597, 603, 657, 658–59
WHO. *See* World Health Organization (WHO)
With, in coding, 323, *330*
Withholding allowances, 394, 397
Women
catheterization of, 690–91
in healthcare, 9–10
heart attacks in, 883
Wong/Baker FACES rating scale, *93*
Wood, Alexander, 6
Workers' compensation insurance, 263, 265, 285–86
Workplace
inappropriate discussions in, 36, *37*
personal business in, 36
personal problems in, 36
professionalism in, 32–38
World Health Organization (WHO), 4, 10, 237, 244
Wounds
closed, 589
culture of, 628–29
healing, 588–89
open, 588, 889, 891–92, 895
Wright's stain, 661–62
Write off, 372, 383
Writing, as means of communication, 71, 72
Written communication, 116–38
abbreviations in, 127–28
business letter, 120–24
case study, 116
electronic mail, 134
fonts in, 124–25
letters to patients, 125
mailing, 128–29
medical assistants and, 118
medical-term plurals, 120, *121*
memo, 128, *130*
numbers in correspondence, 119–20
for patients and professionals, 118–20
photocopying, 128
proofreading, 125–26, 131
sample level, *119*
sentence structure, 119
spell-check, 118
spelling, grammar, and punctuation use, 118, *121*

X

X-rays, 712, 713, 714–15
assisting with, 722
first image, *8*
medical value of, 7
preparation of room, 722

Z

Z-track injection, 535–36
Zygote, 985

Videos Found on Student CD

Video Title	Use with Chapter #	Affective Skill*
A Medicare Mystery	**17:** Insurance Billing and Authorizations	Cognitive and critical thinking skills
Assisting with the Gynecological Exam	**44:** Obstetrics and Gynecology	• Show awareness of patients' concerns regarding their perceptions related to the procedure being performed.
Collecting Money	**20:** Billing, Collections and Credit	• Demonstrate sensitivity and professionalism in handling accounts receivable activities with clients.
Coping with Sales Calls	**16:** Office Policies and Procedures	• Demonstrate sensitivity appropriate to the message being delivered. • Use appropriate body language and other nonverbal skills in communicating with patients, family, and staff.
Crutch Instruction	**43:** Orthopedics and Physical Therapy	• Use language/verbal skills that enable patients' understanding.
Disposing of Medical Waste in the Medical Office	**23:** The Clinical Environment and Safety	• Recognize the importance of local, state, and federal legislation and regulations in the practice setting
Electrocardiogram and Holter Monitor	**35:** Cardiology and Cardiac Testing	• Explain the rationale for performance of a procedure to the patient.
Exam Room Preparation	**28:** Vital Signs	BASIC KNOWELDGE (Cognitive and psychomotor)
Facing Emergencies	**41:** Emergency Care	• Demonstrate awareness of how an individual's personal appearance affects anticipated responses.
Getting Precertification	**17:** Insurance Billing and Authorizations	• Demonstrate assertive communication with managed care and/or insurance providers. • Communicate in language the patient can understand regarding managed care and insurance plans.
Getting Along with Coworkers	**5:** Interpersonal Communication **12:** Medical Records Management	• Use appropriate body language and other nonverbal skills in communicating with patients, family and staff • Implement time management principles to maintain effective office function
Handwashing & Gloving	**25:** Medical Asepsis **26:** Surgical Asepsis	BASIC KNOWELDGE (Cognitive and psychomotor)
Housekeeping 101	**5:** Interpersonal Communication	• Use appropriate body language and other nonverbal skills in communicating with patients, family and staff • Demonstrate empathy in communicating with patients, family and staff
Injections	**27:** Pharmacology and Medication Administration	• Verify ordered doses/dosages prior to administration • Show awareness of patients' concerns regarding their perceptions related to the procedure being performed

Video Title	Use with Chapter #	Affective Skill*
Insurance Coding	**18:** ICD-9-CM Coding **19:** Procedural Coding	• Work with physician to achieve the maximum reimbursement
Patient Care	**3:** Professionalism in the Workplace	• Demonstrate empathy in communicating with patients, family and staff • Apply active listening skills • Use appropriate body language and other nonverbal skills in communicating with patients, family and staff
Pediatrics	**45:** Pediatrics **37:** EENT	• Demonstrate respect for individual diversity incorporating awareness of one's own biases in areas including gender, race, religion, age and economic status. • Use language/verbal skills that enable patients' understanding • Show awareness of patients' concerns regarding their perceptions related to the procedure being performed.
Pharmacology	**27:** Pharmacology and Medication Administration	• Demonstrate sensitivity to patient rights.
Protecting Patient Privacy	**4:** Medical Law and Ethics	• Demonstrate awareness of the consequences of not working within the legal scope of practice • Recognize the importance of local, state, and federal legislation and regulations in the practice setting
Patient Reception	**9:** Telephone Procedures **10:** Front Desk Reception	• Demonstrate empathy in communicating with patients, family and staff • Demonstrate sensitivity appropriate for the message being delivered • Demonstrate sensitivity to patient rights
Sanitation, Disinfection, Sterilization	**26:** Surgical Asepsis	BASIC KNOWELDGE (Cognitive and psychomotor)
Scheduling Patients	**11:** Patient Scheduling	• Implement time management principles to maintain effective office function
Specimens	**31:** Microscopes and Microbiology	• Display sensitivity to patient rights and feelings in collecting specimens.
Spirometer ing their perceptions	**36:** Pulmonology and Pulmonary Testing	• Show awareness of patients' concerns regard-related to the procedure being performed
Surgical Scrub	**26:** Surgical Asepsis	BASIC KNOWELDGE (Cognitive and psychomotor)
Surgical Field	**26:** Surgical Asepsis	BASIC KNOWELDGE (Cognitive and psychomotor)
Syringe Prep	**27:** Pharmacology and Medication Administration	BASIC KNOWELDGE (Cognitive and psychomotor)
Taking Patient Histories	**24:** The Clinical Visit: Office Preparation and the Patient Encounter	• Demonstrate empathy in communicating with patients, family and staff • Use appropriate body language and other nonverbal skills in communicating with patients, family and staff